Taylor and Kelly's Dermatology for Skin of Color

Taylor and Kelly's Dermatology for Skin of Color

Third Edition

Editors

Susan C. Taylor, MD
Bernett Johnson Endowed Professor of Dermatology
Vice Chair of Community Engagement and Academic Excellence
Department of Dermatology
Perelman School of Medicine
University of Pennsylvania
Philadelphia, Pennsylvania, USA
President, American Academy of Dermatology
Founder, Skin of Color Society
Founding Director, Skin of Color Center

Henry W. Lim, MD
Former Chair, Department of Dermatology
Henry Ford Health
Detroit, Michigan, USA
President, International League of Dermatological Societies
London, United Kingdom

Mc Graw Hill

Taylor and Kelly's Dermatology for Skin of Color, Third Edition

1 2 3 4 5 6 7 8 9 DSS 30 29 28 27 26 25

ISBN 978-1-265-03968-4
MHID 1-265-03968-2

This book was set in Minion Pro by KnowledgeWorks Global Ltd.
The editors were Dimana Tzvetkova and Kim J. Davis.
The production supervisor was Richard Ruzycka.
Project management was provided by Abhishek Singh, KnowledgeWorks Global Ltd.
The designer was Alan Barnett; the cover designer was W2 Design.
This book is printed on acid-free paper.

Library of Congress Cataloging-in-Publication Data

Names: Taylor, Susan C., editor. | Lim, Henry W., 1949- editor.

Title: Taylor and Kelly's dermatology for skin of color / editors, Susan C. Taylor, Henry W. Lim.

Other titles: Dermatology for skin of color

Description: Third edition. | New York : McGraw Hill, [2025] | Includes bibliographical references and index. | Summary: "This book serves as a definitive resource on skin of color dermatology and addresses the challenges associated with skin of color dermatology"—Provided by publisher.

Identifiers: LCCN 2024048637 (print) | LCCN 2024048638 (ebook) | ISBN 9781265039684 (hardcover ; alk. paper) | ISBN 9781265039851 (ebook)

Subjects: MESH: Skin Diseases | Ethnic and Racial Minorities | Skin Pigmentation—physiology

Classification: LCC RL71 (print) | LCC RL71 (ebook) | NLM WR 140 | DDC 616.5—dc23/eng/20241209

LC record available at https://lccn.loc.gov/2024048637

LC ebook record available at https://lccn.loc.gov/2024048638

Dedication

This third edition of *Taylor and Kelly's Dermatology for Skin of Color* is dedicated to the trailblazers and visionaries globally who had the foresight and determination to establish and nurture the subspecialty of dermatology focused on skin of color. Their unwavering commitment to advancing knowledge and understanding in this vital area has paved the way for improved care, research, and education.

To the pioneers who recognized the unique challenges and complexities faced by individuals with diverse skin types: your dedication has not only enriched our field but has also transformed countless lives. Your contributions have inspired a generation of dermatologists worldwide to embrace the importance of inclusivity and representation in dermatology practice, ensuring that all patients receive equitable care tailored to their specific needs.

We honor your relentless pursuit of excellence, your resilience in the face of adversity, and your passion for advocating for those often overlooked. May your legacy continue to inspire future generations of dermatologists, guiding them to push boundaries, challenge norms, and champion diversity within our specialty.

Susan C. Taylor
Henry W. Lim

Contents

Contributors

Tahirah Abdullah, PhD
Associate Professor of Psychology
University of Massachusetts Boston
Core Faculty
Center for Multicultural Training in Psychology
Boston, Massachusetts, USA

Katrina Abuabara, MD, MA, MSCE
Associate Professor
Department of Dermatology
University of California-San Francisco
San Francisco, California, USA
Adjunct Associate Professor
UC Berkeley School of Public Health
Berkeley, California, USA

Susuana T. Adjei, MD
HES/Lake Granbury Medical Center
Department of Dermatology
Dallas, Texas, USA

Antara Afrin, BS
College of Human Medicine
Michigan State University
Grand Rapids, Michigan, USA

Crystal Aguh, MD
Department of Dermatology
Johns Hopkins School of Medicine
Baltimore, Maryland, USA

Tashmeeta Ahad, BM BCh, MA (Cantab), MRCP (UK)(Derm)
Department of Dermatology and Skin Science
University of British Columbia
Vancouver Coastal Health Research Institute
Vancouver, British Columbia, Canada

Maggi Ahmed, MD, PhD
Department of Dermatology
University of Massachusetts Medical School
Worcester, Massachusetts, USA

J. Michael Alberto Bell, MD, MS
Department of Dermatology
Howard University Hospital
Washington, DC, USA

Samantha Jo Albucker, BA
Tulane University School of Medicine
New Orleans, Louisiana, USA

Ama Alexis, MD
Clinical Assistant Professor of Pediatrics
Weill Cornell Medical College
Cornell University
Ithaca, New York, USA

Andrew F. Alexis, MD, MPH
Professor of Clinical Dermatology
Weill Cornell Medical College
Vice-Chair for Diversity and Inclusion
Department of Dermatology
Weill Cornell Medicine
New York, New York, USA

Nora S. Ali, MD, FAAD
Dermatology Consultants
St. Paul, Minnesota, USA

Saira Alvi, BA
University of Missouri-Kansas City School of Medicine
Kansas City, Missouri, USA

Chia-Chun Ang, MBBS, MMed (Int Med), MRCP (UK), FAMS
Department of Dermatology
Singapore General Hospital
Outram Road, Singapore

Alejandra Avila, MD
Dr. Phillip Frost Department of Dermatology and Cutaneous Surgery
University of Miami Miller School of Medicine
Miami, Florida, USA

Hilary E. Baldwin, MD
Medical Director
Acne Treatment and Research Center
Brooklyn, New York, USA
Department of Dermatology
Rutgers Robert Wood Johnson Medical School
New Brunswick, New Jersey, USA

Diane Baras
L'Oreal Recherche
Typology Manager for Instrumental Make Up Evaluation
Chevilly-Larue, France

Naiara S. Barbosa, MD
Department of Dermatology
Mayo Clinic
Jacksonville, Florida, USA

Victoria Barbosa, MD, MPH, MBA
Associate Professor
Director, Hair Loss Program
Director, Diversity, Equity and Inclusion
University of Chicago Section of Dermatology
Chicago, Illinois, USA

Tatiana M. Barrera, BA
School of Medicine
University of California, Riverside
Riverside, California, USA
University of Pennsylvania
Philadelphia, Pennsylvania, USA

Jessica B. Brown-Korsah, MD
Department of Dermatology
Perelman School of Medicine
University of Pennsylvania
Philadelphia, Pennsylvania, USA

Cheryl M. Burgess, MD, FAAD
Center for Dermatology and Dermatologic Surgery
Washington, DC, USA

Daniel Butler, MD
Assistant Dean Student Affairs
Associate Professor
University of Arizona College of Medicine
Tucson, Arizona, USA

Laurence Caisey
L'Oreal Recherche
Worldwide Director for Makeup Evaluation
Chevilly-Larue, France

Valerie D. Callender, MD
Department of Dermatology
Howard University College of Medicine
Washington, DC, USA
Callender Dermatology and Cosmetic Center
Glenn Dale, Maryland, USA

Janeth R. Campbell, BS, MS
Georgetown University School of Medicine
Washington, DC, USA

Hafsa M. Cantwell, MD
Assistant Professor
Department of Dermatology
University of California, Irvine
Irvine, California, USA

Avrom S. Caplan, MD
Ronald O. Perelman Department of Dermatology
NYU School of Medicine
New York, New York, USA

Angad Chadha, MD, FAAD
Assistant Professor
Section of Dermatology
University of Chicago
Chicago, Illinois, USA

Henry Hin-Lee Chan, MD, PhD, FRCP
Department of Medicine
LKS Faculty of Medicine
The University of Hong Kong
Hong Kong SAR, China
Wellman Center for Photomedicine
Massachusetts General Hospital, Harvard Medical School
Boston, Massachusetts, USA

Mandy W. M. Chan, MBBS, MRCP, FAMS
Department of Medicine
LKS Faculty of Medicine
The University of Hong Kong
Hong Kong SAR, China

David J. Chandler, MBChB, DTM&H, MRCP
Dermatology Department
University Hospitals Sussex NHS Foundation Trust
West Sussex, United Kingdom
Department of Global Health and Infection
Brighton and Sussex Medical School
Brighton, United Kingdom

Aileen Y. Chang, MD
Associate Professor
Department of Dermatology
University of California, San Francisco School of Medicine
San Francisco, California, USA

Aheli Chattopadhyay, BS
Fourth Year Medical Student
Dermatology Research Fellow
University of California San Francisco
San Francisco, California, USA

Anna L. Chien, MD
Vice-Chair for Quality, Safety, & Service
Medical Director, JH Dermatology at Howard County
Columbia, Maryland, USA
Associate Professor
Department of Dermatology
Johns Hopkins School of Medicine
Baltimore, Maryland, USA

Maya Childs, BS
Department of Dermatology
Perelman School of Medicine
University of Pennsylvania
Philadelphia, Pennsylvania, USA

Keith A. Choate, MD, PhD
Department of Dermatology
Yale University School of Medicine
New Haven, Connecticut, USA

Kayla St. Claire, MD, MBA
Department of Dermatology
Wayne State University
Detroit, Michigan, USA

Annelise Colvin, MD
Resident
Dermatology Residency Program
University of California, San Francisco
San Francisco, California, USA

Edward W. Cowen, MD, MHSc
Senior Clinician and Head, Dermatology Consultation Service
National Institute of Arthritis and Musculoskeletal and Skin Diseases
National Institutes of Health
Bethesda, Maryland, USA

Sebastian Cruz, MD
Department of Dermatology
University of Southern California
Los Angeles, California, USA

Sindhuja Sominidi Damodaran, MD
Department of Dermatology
Mayo Clinic
Rochester, Minnesota, USA

Jennifer David, DO, MBA
Cone Health MedCenter
Greensboro, North Carolina, USA

DiAnne S. Davis, MD, FAAD
Bare Dermatology
Dallas, Texas, USA

Owen R. Dean, MD
Resident
University of Minnesota Combined Medicine-Dermatology Residency Program
Minneapolis, Minnesota, USA

Mansee Desai, MD
Department of Dermatology
Loma Linda University
Loma Linda, California, USA

Yemisi Dina, MD
Department of Dermatology
Johns Hopkins Medicine
Baltimore, Maryland, USA

Jewell Dinkins, MS
Meharry Medical College
Nashville, Tennessee, USA

Ncoza C. Dlova, MBChB, FCDerm, PhD
Professor and Head
Department of Dermatology
University of KwaZulu Natal
Durban, South Africa

Arturo R. Dominguez, MD
Department of Dermatology
Department of Internal Medicine
UT Southwestern Medical Center
Dallas, Texas, USA

Erica Dommasch, MD
Fenway Institute, Fenway Health
Department of Dermatology
Beth Israel Deaconess Medical Center
Harvard Medical School
Boston, Massachusetts, USA

Grace Y. Duan, BA
Pritzker School of Medicine
University of Chicago
Chicago, Illinois, USA

Kevin Puerta Durango, BS
Department of Dermatology
Perelman School of Medicine, University of Pennsylvania
Philadelphia, Pennsylvania, USA
Geisel School of Medicine at Dartmouth
Hanover, New Hampshire, USA

Alicia Edwards, BS, MS
Howard University College of Medicine
Washington, DC, USA

Nada Elbuluk, MD, MSc
Professor of Clinical Dermatology
Founding Director, Skin of Color and Pigmentary Disorders Program
Founding Director, Dermatology Culture and Engagement Program
Department of Dermatology
University of Southern California Keck School of Medicine
Los Angeles, California, USA

Iain Noel Encarnacion, MS
Eastern Virginia Medical School
Norfolk, Virginia, USA

Valerie Sofia Encarnacion-Cortes
Medical Sciences Campus School of Medicine
University of Puerto Rico
San Juan, Puerto Rico

Maria L. Espinosa, MD
Department of Dermatology
Henry Ford Health
Detroit, Michigan, USA

Jessica C. Evans, MS
Department of Dermatology
UT Southwestern Medical Center
Dallas, Texas, USA

Adaora Ewulu, MD
Department of Dermatology
UC Irvine
Irvine, California, USA

Sabrina Guillen Fabi, MD, FAAD, FAACS
Volunteer Assistant Clinical Professor of Dermatology
University of California, San Diego
San Diego, California, USA

Joseph W. Fakhoury, MD
Department of Dermatology
Henry Ford Health
Detroit, Michigan, USA

Alana Ferreira, BA
Perelman School of Medicine
University of Pennsylvania
Philadelphia, Pennsylvania, USA

Richard H. Flowers, MD
Associate Professor in Dermatology
University of Virginia Health System
Charlottesville, Virginia, USA

Negar Foolad, MD, MAS
Skin of Color Fellow
Duke Department of Dermatology
Duke University Medical Center
Durham, North Carolina, USA

Esther E. Freeman, MD, PhD
Department of Dermatology
Massachusetts General Hospital
Harvard Medical School
Medical Practice Evaluation Center
Mongan Institute, Massachusetts General Hospital
Boston, Massachusetts, USA

Cheri Frey, MD
Assistant Professor
Program Director
Department of Dermatology
Howard University
Washington, DC, USA

Aditi Tushar Gadre, MD
Wake Forest University School of Medicine
Winston-Salem, North Carolina, USA

Ameya Gangal, BS
Department of Dermatology
Emory University School of Medicine
Atlanta, Georgia, USA

Algin Garrett, MD
Forefront Dermatology
Glen Allen, Virginia, USA

Maria Fernanda Reis Gavazzoni Dias MD, MsC, PhD
Professor of Dermatology
Fluminense Federal University
Rio de Janeiro, Brazil
Head of alopecia outpatient clinic at Antonio Pedro University Hospital
Niteroi, Rio de Janeiro, Brazil

Andrea Gelabert-Mora, MD
Department of Dermatology
Broward Health Medical Center
Fort Lauderdale, Florida, USA
San Juan Bautista School of Medicine
Turabo Gardens Caguas, Puerto Rico
Dermatology Research Fellow
University of California San Francisco
San Francisco, California, USA

Donald A. Glass, II, MD, PhD
Associate Professor
Department of Dermatology
University of Texas Southwestern Medical Center
Dallas, Texas, USA

Chee Leok GOH, MBBS, MD, MRCP(UK), FACD(Hon)
Emeritus Consultant Dermatologist, National Skin Centre
Clinical Professor, YLL School of Medicine
National University of Singapore
Adjunct Professor, LKC Medicine
Nanyang Technical University
Singapore, Singapore

Sarah Gonzalez, MD
Wayne State University School of Medicine
Detroit, Michigan, USA

Wilce Gonzalez, BA
Ronald O. Perelman Department of Dermatology
New York University Grossman School of Medicine
New York, New York, USA

Jeromy Gotschall, BA
Perelman School of Medicine
University of Pennsylvania
Philadelphia, Pennsylvania, USA

Pearl E. Grimes, MD
Director, The Vitiligo and Pigmentation Institute of Southern California
Director, The Grimes Center for Medical and Aesthetic Dermatology
Clinical Professor of Dermatology, University of California, Los Angeles
President, Global Vitiligo Foundation
Los Angeles, California, USA

Karina Grullon-Perez, MD
University of Miami at Holy Cross
Oakland Park, Florida, USA

Linna L. Gali, MD, MS, FAAD
Senior Staff Physician
Division of Mohs and Dermatological Surgery
Department of Dermatology
Henry Ford Health
Detroit, Michigan, USA

Aditya K. Gupta, MD, PhD, FAAD
Department of Medicine
University of Toronto
Toronto, Ontario, Canada

Rachel Hammer, MD, MFA
Assistant Professor of Psychiatry and Internal Medicine
Tulane University School of Medicine
New Orleans, Louisiana, USA

Iltefat Hamzavi, MD
Department of Dermatology
Henry Ford Health
Detroit, Michigan, USA

Candrice R. Heath, MD, FAAP, FAAD
Associate Professor
Department of Dermatology
Howard University
Washington, DC, USA

Shanae N. Henry, MS
Howard University College of Medicine
Washington, DC, USA

Drew Hicks, MS, RD
Mayo Clinic Alix School of Medicine
Rochester, Minnesota, USA

Robert Hight, MS
Chicago, Illinois, USA

Andrea Nadine Hinton, MD
Clinical Assistant Professor
Department of Dermatology
Stanford University
Stanford, California, USA

San Honde, DCM, ADDV
Dermatology Officer,
Illovo Sugar Company,
Nkhota Koto, Malawi

Jennifer L. Hsiao, MD
Department of Dermatology
University of Southern California
Los Angeles, California, USA

Kimberly Huerth, MD, MEd
Gateway Aesthetic Institute and Laser Center
Salt Lake City, Utah, USA

Elizabeth Behar Houshmand, MD, FAAD
Houshmand Dermatology and Wellness
Dallas, Texas, USA

Arielle Carolina Mora Hurtado, BS
Medical Student
University of Wisconsin School of Medicine and Public Health
Madison, Wisconsin, USA

Sotonye Imadojemu, MD
Brigham and Women's Hospital
Harvard Medical School
Boston, Massachusetts, USA

Brenda Umenita Imo, MS
Georgetown University School of Medicine
Washington, DC, USA

Camille E. Introcaso, MD
Associate Professor of Medicine, Division of Dermatology
Cooper Medical School of Rowan University
Camden, New Jersey, USA

Jahdonna Isaac, MD
Department of Dermatology
Howard University College of Medicine
Washington, DC, USA

Shanelle Jackson, MD
College of Human Medicine
Michigan State University
Grand Rapids, Michigan, USA

Tiaranesha K. Jackson, MPH
University of Illinois College of Medicine
Peoria, Illinois, USA

Mustufa A. Jafry, MD
Department of Dermatology
Henry Ford Health
Detroit, Michigan, USA

Natalia Jaimes, MD
Dr. Phillip Frost Department of Dermatology and Cutaneous Surgery
Sylvester Comprehensive Cancer Center
University of Miami Miller School of Medicine
Miami, Florida, USA

Tarannum Jaleel, MD, MHSc
Assistant Professor
Duke Department of Dermatology
Director, Hidradenitis Suppurativa Medical and Procedural Clinic
Director, Sponsored Clinical Trials Education
Duke University Medical Center
Durham, North Carolina, USA

Jyothi Jayaraman, DNB
Assistant Professor
Department of Dermatology, Venereology & Leprosy
Father Muller Medical College
Mangalore, India

Mia Jenkins, MS
Georgetown University School of Medicine
Washington, DC, USA

Toni Jenkins, MD, MS
Howard University College of Medicine
Washington, DC, USA

Bwanali Haji Ntaibu Jereni, MBBS, MMED
Dermatologist,
Princess Marina Hospital
University of Botswana
Gaborone, Botswana

Sunil Kalia, MD, MHSc, FRCPC
Department of Dermatology and Skin Science
University of British Columbia
Vancouver Coastal Health Research Institute
Vancouver, British Columbia, Canada

Sewon Kang, MD
Noxell Professor & Chairman
Department of Dermatology
Johns Hopkins School of Medicine
Dermatologist-in-Chief
Johns Hopkins Hospital
Baltimore, Maryland, USA

Sara Saheb Kashaf, PhD
Pritzker School of Medicine
University of Chicago
Chicago, Illinois, USA

Lana Kashlan, MD, FAAD
SkinExperts Polyclinic
Dubai, United Arab Emirates

Shamaila Khan, PhD
Clinical Associate Professor of Psychiatry
Boston University School of Medicine
Program Director
Center for Multicultural Training in Psychology
Boston Medical Center
Boston, Massachusetts, USA

Ellen J. Kim, MD
Professor of Dermatology
Vice Chair of Clinical Operations
Director of Penn Cutaneous Lymphoma and Photopheresis Service
Department of Dermatology
Perelman School of Medicine
University of Pennsylvania
Philadelphia, Pennsylvania, USA

Juliana Kim, MD
UT Southwestern Medical School
Dallas, Texas, USA

Chesahna Kindred, MD, MBA
Medical Director
Kindred Hair & Skin Center
Marriottsville, Maryland
Associate Professor
Department of Dermatology
Howard University
Washington, DC, USA

Robert S. Kirsner, MD, PhD
Chairman and Harvey Blank Professor
Dr. Phillip Frost Department of Dermatology and Cutaneous Surgery
Professor of Public Health Sciences
Director, University of Miami Hospital and Clinics Wound Center
University of Miami Miller School of Medicine
Miami, Florida, USA

Ariel Knowles, MBBS
University of Texas Southwestern Medical Center
Dallas, Texas, USA

Vanesa Kodra, MS-PA
Viva Eve Dermatology
New York, New York, USA

Shannon Kody, MD
Department of Dermatology
Oregon Health & Science University
Portland, Oregon, USA

Lucinda L. Kohn, MD, MHS
Assistant Professor of Dermatology
Section of Pediatric Dermatology
Children's Hospital Colorado
Centers for American Indian and Alaska Native Health
University of Colorado School of Medicine
Aurora, Colorado, USA

Abraham M. Korman, MD
Department of Dermatology
Ohio State University
Columbus, Ohio, USA

Daniela Kroshinsky, MD, MPH
Department of Dermatology
Massachusetts General Hospital
Boston, Massachusetts, USA

Loren Krueger, MD
Department of Dermatology
Emory University School of Medicine
Atlanta, Georgia, USA

Roopal V. Kundu, MD
Professor of Dermatology and Medical Education
Northwestern University Feinberg School of Medicine
Chicago, Illinois, USA

Shawn G. Kwatra, MD
Associate Professor of Dermatology and Oncology
Director, Johns Hopkins Itch Center
Johns Hopkins University School of Medicine
Baltimore, Maryland, USA

Jeffery Kwock, MD
Resident Physician
Duke Department of Dermatology
Duke University Medical Center
Durham, North Carolina, USA

Jorge Larrondo, MD, MSc
Department of Dermatology
Wake Forest Baptist Health
Winston-Salem, North Carolina
Department of Dermatology
Clínica Alemana-Universidad del Desarrollo
Santiago, Chile

Johnathan J. Ledet, MD
Saint Francis Health System
Tulsa, Oklahoma, USA

Becky Li, MD
Department of Dermatology
Howard University
Washington, DC, USA

Viviane Liao, BA
Department of Dermatology
Johns Hopkins University School of Medicine
Baltimore, Maryland, USA

Henry W. Lim, MD
Former Chair, Department of Dermatology
Henry Ford Health
Detroit, Michigan, USA
President, International League of Dermatological Societies
London, United Kingdom

Jordan S. Lim, MB BCh, BAO
Department of Dermatology
Emory University
Atlanta, Georgia, USA
Department of Dermatology
Atlanta Veterans Affairs
Decatur, Georgia, USA

Shari R. Lipner, MD, PhD
Department of Dermatology
Weill Cornell Medicine
New York, New York, USA

Walter Liszewski, MD
Assistant Professor of Dermatology (Medical Dermatology) and
Preventive Medicine (Cancer Epidemiology and Prevention)
Northwestern University Feinberg School of Medicine
Chicago, Illinois, USA

Porcia B. Love, MD, FAAD
Medical Director
River Region Dermatology and Laser
Montgomery, Alabama, USA
Clinical Assistant Professor
UAB School of Medicine
Montgomery Regional Medical Campus
Montgomery, Alabama, USA

Janet E. Lubov, MD, MS
Department of Dermatology
University of Iowa
Iowa City, Iowa, USA

Harvey Lui, MD, FRCPC
Department of Dermatology and Skin Science
University of British Columbia
Vancouver Coastal Health Research Institute
Vancouver, British Columbia, Canada

George Luong, MD
Resident Physician
Department of Internal Medicine
Tulane University
New Orleans, Louisiana, USA

Ramesh Bhat M., MD, DNB, MNAMS
Vice Dean and Professor
Department of Dermatology, Venereology & Leprosy
Father Muller Medical College
Mangalore, India

Lauren M. Madigan, MD
Department of Dermatology
University of Utah
Salt Lake City, Utah, USA

Kathyana Santiago Mangual, BA
David Geffen School of Medicine
University of California Los Angeles
Los Angeles, California, USA

Spero M. Manson, PhD
Distinguished Professor of Public Health and Psychiatry
Director, Centers for American Indian & Alaska Native Health
Colorado Trust Chair in American Indian Health
Colorado School of Public Health at the University of Colorado
Anschutz Medical Campus
Aurora, Colorado, USA

Benjamin Gallo Marin, AB
The Warren Alpert Medical School of Brown University
Providence, Rhode Island, USA

Justin W. Marson, MD
Department of Dermatology
SUNY Downstate Health Sciences University
Brooklyn, New York, USA

Cathy M. Massoud, MD
Assistant Professor of Dermatology and Dermatopathology
Director of the RIH Inpatient
Dermatology Consult Service
Department of Dermatology
The Warren Alpert Medical School of Brown University
Providence, Rhode Island, USA

Melissa M. Mauskar, MD
Department of Dermatology
Department of Obstetrics and Gynecology
UT Southwestern Medical Center
Dallas, Texas, USA

Mayra B. C. Maymone, DDS, MD, DSc
Department of Dermatology
Warren Alpert Medical School of Brown University
Providence, Rhode Island, USA

Tiffany T. Mayo, MD, MS, FAAD
Associate Professor
Department of Dermatology
The University of Alabama at Birmingham
Birmingham, Alabama, USA

Joni Mazza-McCrann, MD, FAAD
Mara Dermatology
Mount Pleasant, South Carolina, USA

John McDowell, DDS, MS
Professor Emeritus of Dentistry
University of Colorado School of Dental Medicine
Aurora, Colorado, USA

Lynn McKinley-Grant, MD, MA, FAAD
Associate Professor of Dermatology
College of Medicine, Howard University
Consultant, Duke Department of Dermatology
Duke University Medical Center
Durham, North Carolina, USA

Shanice McKenzie, MD
Department of Dermatology
University of Southern California
Los Angeles, California, USA

Amy J. McMichael, MD
Department of Dermatology
Wake Forest, University School of Medicine
Winston-Salem, North Carolina, USA

Robert G. Micheletti, MD
Departments of Dermatology and Medicine
Perelman School of Medicine
University of Pennsylvania
Philadelphia, Pennsylvania, USA

Ginat W. Mirowski, DMD, MD
Department of Oral Pathology, Medicine and Radiology
Department of Dermatology
Indiana University School of Medicine
Indianapolis, Indiana, USA

Hope Mitchell, MD, FAAD
Mitchell Dermatology
Perrysburg, Ohio, USA

Richard Mizuguchi, MD
Assistant Clinical Professor
Department of Dermatology
Mount Sinai Medical School
New York, New York, USA

Tasneem F. Mohammad, MD
Department of Dermatology
Henry Ford Health System
Detroit, Michigan, USA
Clinical Assistant Professor
Department of Medicine
Michigan State University
East Lansing, Michigan, USA

Mourad Mokni
Professor of Dermatology
Faculty of Medecine
University al Manar
Department of Dermatology
La Rabta Hospital
Tunis, Tunisia

Rochelle C. Monteiro, MD
Professor
Department of Dermatology, Venereology & Leprosy
Father Muller Medical College
Mangalore, India

Karla L. Valdés Morales, MD
Centro Dermatologico Dr. Ladislao de la Pascua
Mexico City, Mexico

Anisa Mosam, MBCHB, MMed, FC Derm, PhD
Professor
Department of Dermatology
Nelson R Mandela School of Medicine,
University of KwaZulu Natal
Durban, South Africa

Jenny E. Murase, MD
Associate Clinical Professor of Dermatology
University of California, San Francisco (UCSF)
Director of Medical Dermatology Consultative Services and Patch Testing
Palo Alto Foundation Medical Group
Palo Alto, California, USA

Christina M. Murphy, MD
Department of Dermatology
Perelman School of Medicine, University of Pennsylvania
Philadelphia, Pennsylvania, USA

Lina Naga, MD, FAAD
Skin DC
Arlington, Virginia, USA

Kim Nichols, MD, FAAD
Board-Certified Dermatologist and founder of NicholsMD of Greenwich
Greenwich, Connecticut, USA

Rajiv I. Nijhawan, MD
Associate Professor
Department of Dermatology
UT Southwestern Medical Center
Dallas, Texas, USA

Ugonna Nwannunu, BS
Howard University College of Medicine
Washington, DC, USA

Allen S.W. Oak, MD, MTR, FAAD
Department of Dermatology
Perelman School of Medicine
University of Pennsylvania
Philadelphia, Pennsylvania, USA

Ivie Obeime, DO
Department of Dermatology
Wake Forest Baptist Health
Winston-Salem, North Carolina, USA

Charissa N. Obeng-Nyarko, MS
Department of Dermatology
Perelman School of Medicine
University of Pennsylvania
Philadelphia, Pennsylvania
Florida State University College of Medicine
Tallahassee, Florida, USA

Adebola Ogunbiyi, FMCP, FWACP
Professor
Department of Dermatology
University of Ibadan
Oyo State, Nigeria

Temitayo A. Ogunleye, MD
Associate Professor
Department of Dermatology
Perelman School of Medicine
University of Pennsylvania
Philadelphia, Pennsylvania, USA

Ashley E. Ojeaga, MD, MPH, FAAD
Kelsey Seybold Clinic
Houston, Texas, USA

Uche Rowland Ojinmah, MBBS, FMCP
Lecturer, Consultant Dermatologist
College of Medicine, University of Nigeria, Enugu Campus
Department of Dermatology
University of Nigeria Teaching Hospital, Ituku-Ozalla
Enugu, Nigeria

Chidubem A.V. Okeke, MD
Department of Dermatology
Howard University College of Medicine
Washington, DC, USA

Ginette A. Okoye, MD
Department of Dermatology
Howard University College of Medicine
Washington, DC, USA

Christine Olagun-Samuel, BA
MD Candidate
New York University Grossman School of Medicine
New York, New York, USA

Deega Omar, MPH
Department of Dermatology
Perelman School of Medicine
University of Pennsylvania
Philadelphia, Pennsylvania, USA

Oluwakemi Onajin, MD
Section of Dermatology
University of Chicago
Chicago, Illinois, USA

Chinwe Laura Onyekonwu, MBBS, FMCP, MPH
Senior Lecturer/Consultant Physician/Dermatologist
College of Medicine, University of Nigeria, Enugu Campus
Department of Dermatology
University of Nigeria Teaching Hospital, Ituku-Ozalla
Enugu, Nigeria

Ogechukwu Opaigbeogu, MD
Department of Dermatology
Tulane University School of Medicine
New Orleans, Louisiana, USA

Alex G. Ortega-Loayza, MD, MCR
Department of Dermatology
Oregon Health & Science University
Portland, Oregon, USA

Gladys Angela Ozoh, BM, BCH, FWACP
Senior Lecturer, Dermatologist
College of Medicine, University of Nigeria, Enugu Campus
Department of Dermatology
University of Nigeria Teaching Hospital, Ituku-Ozalla
Enugu, Nigeria

Kelly K. Park, MD, MSL
Affiliate Assistant Professor
Stritch School of Medicine
Loyola University of Chicago
Chicago, Illinois, USA
Adjunct Assistant Professor
Department of Medicine
Northeast Ohio Medical University
Rootstown, Ohio, USA
Park Dermatology, PLLC
Lake Forest, Illinois, USA

Jennifer J. Parker, MD, PhD, MPH
Department of Dermatology
Temple University Lewis Katz School of Medicine
Philadelphia, Pennsylvania, USA

Helena Pasieka, MD, MS
Departments of Dermatology & Medicine
Uniformed Services University
Bethesda, Maryland, USA
Georgetown University School of Medicine
Department of Dermatology
MedStar Washington Hospital Center/Georgetown University
The Burn Center
MedStar Washington Hospital Center
Washington, DC, USA

Lauren Payne, MD, MS, FAAD
Clinical Assistant Professor
George Washington University School of Medicine
Howard University Hospital
Flourish Dermatology and Aesthetics
New Orleans, Louisiana, USA

Klint Peebles, MD
Department of Dermatology
Kaiser Permanente Mid-Atlantic Permanente Medical Group
Rockville, Maryland, USA

Miriam Keltz Pomeranz, MD
Ronald O. Perelman Department of Dermatology
NYU Grossman School of Medicine
New York, New York, USA

Sneha Poondru, BA
Northwestern University Feinberg School of Medicine
Chicago, Illinois, USA

Alba Posligua-Alban, MD
Department of Dermatology
University of New Mexico Hospital
Albuquerque, New Mexico, USA

Domenica Del Pozo, MD, MPH
Lewis Katz School of Medicine
Temple University
Philadelphia, Pennsylvania, USA

Kyla N. Price, MD
Department of Dermatology
Keck School of Medicine
University of Southern California
Los Angeles, California, USA

Ellen N. Pritchett, MD, MPH
Associate Professor
Department of Dermatology
Howard University College of Medicine
Washington, DC, USA

Sara D. Ragi, MS
The Warren Alpert Medical School of Brown University
Providence, Rhode Island, USA

Shobita Rajagopalan, MD, MS, MPH
Senior Physician Internal Medicine/Infectious Disease
Associate Medical Director/STD Clinical Chief
Division of HIV and STD Programs
Los Angeles County Department of Public Health
Manhattan Beach, California, USA

Jasmine Rana, MD, MMSc
Clinical Assistant Professor
Department of Dermatology
Stanford University
Redwood City, California, USA

Supriya Rastogi, MD
Schweiger Dermatology Group
New York, New York, USA

Nithya Ravindran, DO
Assistant Clinical Professor of Psychiatry
Charles R. Drew University School of Medicine
Los Angeles, California, USA

Camille Robinson, MD
Duke University School of Medicine
Durham, North Carolina, USA

Ciara G. Robinson, MD
Department of Dermatology
Henry Ford Health
Detroit, Michigan, USA

Larimar Rodriguez, MD
Department of Dermatology
University of New Mexico School of Medicine
Albuquerque, New Mexico, USA

Ellen K. Roh, MD
Assistant Professor in Dermatology
Massachusetts General Hospital
Harvard Medical School
Boston, Massachusetts, USA

Misha Rosenbach, MD
Endowed Chair
Professor of Dermatology & Rheumatology
Vice Chair of Education
Perelman School of Medicine
University of Pennsylvania
Philadelphia, Pennsylvania, USA

Arturo P. Saavedra, MD, PhD, MBA
Endowed Professor in Dermatology
Chair of Dermatology
University of Virginia Health System
Charlottesville, Virginia, USA

Regina Casz Schechtman, MD, PhD
Department of Dermatology, State Universitário of Rio de Janeiro, UERJ
Rio de Janeiro, Brazil
Institute of Dermatology
Pontifical Catholic University of Rio de Janeiro
PUC Rio
Rio de Janeiro, Brazil

John T. Seykora, MD, PhD
Department of Dermatology
Perelman School of Medicine
University of Pennsylvania
Philadelphia, Pennsylvania, USA

Dwana R. Shabazz, MD, MPH
Renascance Dermatology, PC
Fairfax, Virginia, USA

Hadir Shakshouk, MBBS
Department of Dermatology
Oregon Health & Science University
Portland, Oregon
Department of Dermatology, Venerology and Andrology
Alexandria University
Alexandria, Egypt

Norhan Shamloul, MD
Department of Dermatology
Penn State Hershey Medical Center
Hershey, Pennsylvania, USA

Divya Sharma, MD
Resident Physician
Department of Medicine
Riverside Methodist Hospital
Columbus, Ohio, USA

William D. Shipman, III, MD, PhD, FAAD
Skin & Beauty Center
Pasadena, California
Department of Dermatology
University of Southern California
Los Angeles, California, USA

Nanette Silverberg, MD
Clinical Professor of Dermatology and Pediatrics
Icahn School of Medicine at Mount Sinai Chief,
Pediatric Dermatology
Mount Sinai Health Systems
New York, New York, USA

Meena Singh, MD
KMC Hair Center
Mission, Kansas, USA

Ashley Slack, MD
Howard University College of Medicine
Washington, DC, USA

Stephanie Smith, DNP, FNP-BC
Lead Nurse Practitioner
NicholsMD of Greenwich
Greenwich, Connecticut, USA

Olayemi Sokumbi, MD
Departments of Dermatology and Laboratory Medicine and Pathology
Mayo Clinic
Jacksonville, Florida, USA

Jaime Soto, MD
Professor Emeritus of Dermatology
HMC – UNG – Bogotá Colombia
Chair FUNDERMA, Fundación Nacional de Dermatología
Santa Cruz de la Sierra, Bolivia

Yacine Sow, MD
Department of Dermatology
University of California San Francisco
San Francisco, California, USA

Courtney Squirewell, BS
Howard University College of Medicine
Washington, DC, USA

Nivedita Sriram, BS
University of Texas Southwestern Medical Center
Dallas, Texas, USA

Benjamin Eduardo Swaby, MD, MS
Georgetown University School of Medicine
Washington, DC, USA

Nicole Syder, MD
Keck School of Medicine of University of Southern California
Los Angeles, California, USA

Sumayah Taliaferro, MD
Atlanta Dermatology & Aesthetics, PC
Atlanta, Georgia, USA

Alice Tan, BS
Department of Dermatology
Massachusetts General Hospital
Boston, Massachusetts, USA

Nicholas Tan, BS
Fenway Institute, Fenway Health
Boston, Massachusetts, USA
Department of Dermatology
Beth Israel Deaconess Medical Center
Boston, Massachusetts, USA
Case Western Reserve University School of Medicine
Cleveland, Ohio, USA

Marta Taye, BA
Department of Dermatology
Emory University School of Medicine
Atlanta, Georgia, USA

Susan C. Taylor, MD
Bernett Johnson Endowed Professor in Dermatology
Vice Chair for Community Engagement and Academic Excellence
Department of Dermatology
Perelman School of Medicine
University of Pennsylvania
Philadelphia, Pennsylvania, USA

Cristina Thomas, MD
Department of Dermatology
Department of Internal Medicine
UT Southwestern Medical Center
Dallas, Texas, USA

Gail Todd, BSc (Agric), MBChB. FFDerm (SA), PhD
Emeritus Professor
Department of Medicine
University of Cape Town
Cape Town, South Africa

Christina Topham, MD
Department of Dermatology
University of Utah
Salt Lake City, Utah, USA

Antonella Tosti, MD
Dr. Phillip Frost Department of Dermatology and Cutaneous Surgery
University of Miami
Miami, Florida, USA

Patricia Treadwell, MD
Professor Emeritus of Dermatology and Pediatrics
Department of Dermatology
Indiana University School of Medicine
Indianapolis, Indiana, USA

Stephen K. Tyring, MD, PhD
University of Texas Health Science Center
Department of Dermatology &
Center for Clinical Studies
Houston, Texas, USA

Neelam A. Vashi, MD
Department of Dermatology
Boston University School of Medicine
Boston, Massachusetts, USA

Rebecca Vasquez, MD
Department of Dermatology
University of Texas Southwestern Medical Center
Dallas, Texas, USA

Benjamin G. Vazquez, MD, FAAD
Assistant Professor of Dermatology
Oregon Health & Sciences University
Portland, Oregon, USA

Natalie M. Villa, MD
Assistant Professor
Department of Dermatology
Dartmouth Hitchcock Medical Center
Lebanon, New Hampshire, USA

Christopher Wachuku, MS
Rutgers, Robert Wood Johnson Medical School
New Brunswick, New Jersey, USA

Chloe Walker, MD, MHS
Clinical Research Fellow
River Region Dermatology and Laser
Montgomery, Alabama, USA

Carl Washington, MD
Dermatology Associates of Georgia
Atlanta, Georgia, USA
Adjunct Associate Professor
Department of Dermatology
Emory University School of Medicine
Atlanta, Georgia, USA

Jeffrey M. Weinberg, MD
Department of Dermatology
Mount Sinai Beth Israel
Clinical Professor of Dermatology
Mount Sinai School of Medicine
New York, New York, USA

Sydney A. Weir, MSPH, MD
Marnix E. Heersink School of Medicine
University of Alabama
Birmingham, Alabama, USA

Victoria P. Werth, MD
Department of Dermatology
Hospital of the University of Pennsylvania and Corporal Michael J. Creszenz VAMC
Philadelphia, Pennsylvania, USA

Jessica R. Williams, MS
Department of Dermatology
Howard University College of Medicine
Washington, DC, USA

Mikayla Woodard, BS
Morehouse School of Medicine
Atlanta, Georgia, USA

Amy Woods, MD
Program Director/Clinical Assistant Professor
Child and Adolescent Psychiatry Fellowship
Charles R. Drew University School of Medicine
Los Angeles, California, USA

Kaelynn Workman, BS
Case Western Reserve University School of Medicine
Cleveland, Ohio, USA

Scott Worswick, MD
Clinical professor of dermatology
Department of Dermatology
University of Southern California
Los Angeles, California, USA

Joyce Xia, BS
Department of Dermatology
Massachusetts General Hospital
Boston, Massachusetts, USA

Marita Yaghi, MD
Dermatology Resident Physician
Department of Dermatology
Larkin Community Hospital
South Miami, Florida, USA

Angeline Anning Yong, MBBS, MPH
Dermatologist and Dermatologic Surgeon
Angeline Yong Dermatology
Gleneagles Medical Centre
Singapore, Singapore

John Montgomery Yost, MD, MPH
Clinical Associate Professor
Director, Nail Disorders Clinic
Department of Dermatology
Standford University
Stanford, California, USA

Kelly Z. Young, MD, PhD
Department of Dermatology
University of Michigan
Ann Arbor, Michigan, USA

John G. Zampella, MD
Assistant Professor of Dermatology
Ronald O. Perelman Department of Dermatology
Preston Robert Tisch Center for Men's Health
New York University Grossman School of Medicine
New York, New York, USA

Megan Zhao, MD
Perelman School of Medicine
University of Pennsylvania
Philadelphia, Pennsylvania, USA

Preface

The Eurocentric focus of clinical dermatology, research, images, and literature has, until recently, largely neglected skin of color dermatology. This oversight has resulted in a significant lack of reliable information regarding the pathology, physiology, diagnosis, and treatment of cutaneous diseases in darker skin types. However, by the late twentieth century, a renewed interest in ethnic skin began to emerge, reflecting the changing demographics of patient populations worldwide. The term "skin of color" was coined to be inclusive of a wide variety of racial and ethnic groups including Asian, Black, Hispanic, and Native populations. Foundational publications have established the groundwork for understanding ethnic and dark skin types, while organizations such as the Skin of Color Society, the Dermatology section of the National Medical Association, and the American Academy of Dermatology have been instrumental in advancing knowledge in this area.

The first edition of *Dermatology for Skin of Color*, published in 2009 and edited by A. Paul Kelly and Susan C. Taylor, served as a comprehensive textbook and photographic atlas authored by a diverse group of nationally and internationally recognized experts. It became the definitive resource on skin of color dermatology, aimed at educating and serving the global medical community. As our world grows increasingly multiracial, multicultural, and multiethnic, dermatologists face the ongoing challenge of recognizing differences in disease presentations between darker and lighter skin, distinguishing normal from pathological conditions, identifying treatments that are both effective and carry minimal side effects, and interacting with patients in a culturally competent manner.

The third edition of *Dermatology for Skin of Color* further expands our knowledge of the field and is a comprehensive up-to-date resource. We anticipate that this textbook will continue be an invaluable resource for dermatologists, medical students, residents, fellows, physician extenders, and the broader medical community in addressing the challenges associated with skin of color dermatology.

Susan C. Taylor
Henry W. Lim

Acknowledgments

We are honored to present the third edition of *Dermatology for Skin of Color*, featuring 105 chapters that provide a comprehensive overview of all aspects of skin of color dermatology. This edition addresses cultural and basic science considerations, skin, hair, and nail disorders, cosmetic and procedural dermatology, unique population factors, and global dermatology. This achievement is made possible by the dedication of our outstanding authors and stellar section editors: Victoria Barbosa, Valerie Callender, Cheryl Burgess, Nada Elbuluk, and Rebecca Vasquez. This project would not have been possible without the invaluable support of our exceptional colleagues at McGraw Hill.

Finally, I wish to express my deepest gratitude to my wonderful family: my husband, Kemel Winston Dawkins; my daughters, Morgan Elizabeth and Madison Lauren; my sister, Flora Taylor; my nephew, Noah Toney; and my nieces, Simone and Nicole Toney—with whom all things are possible.

"It always seems impossible until it is done." Nelson Mandela

Susan C. Taylor

It is a privilege and a pleasure to join Susan Taylor again in editing the third edition of *Dermatology for Skin of Color*. My current position as the President of International League of Dermatological Societies gives me a unique insight on the importance of skin of color dermatology that is being emphasized and appreciated by global dermatology community. This textbook has now become a standard textbook on this topic.

The excellent contribution of the international experts as authors and the efforts of our superb section editors, Victoria Barbosa, Valerie Callender, Cheryl Burgess, Nada Elbuluk, and Rebecca Vasquez, have made editing this textbook a joy. The team from McGraw Hill has been most helpful in bringing this book to fruition.

My deep gratitude goes to my wife Mamie Wong Lim, MD, who is a loving wife and mother to our children, Christopher and Kevin, and grandmother to Julian, Madelaine, Dylan, and Collin. Her patience and support have made this and many other projects possible.

Henry W. Lim

Foreword

Currently, individuals with skin of color constitute the majority of the global population. The term "skin of color" encompasses people with generally darker skin pigmentation, including Africans, African Americans, Asians, Latinos, Middle Eastern, Pacific Islanders, and indigenous people as compared to Caucasians. By the year 2050, the U.S. Census Bureau has projected that individuals with skin of color will constitute 50% or more of the U.S. population. Hence, there is a critical and profound need in dermatology and medicine for a textbook that provides an in-depth discussion of the biology and unique presentations, manifestations, and nuanced treatments for skin diseases in darker skin types. A comprehensive understanding of skin diseases in individuals with skin of color is no doubt essential for any level of equity in healthcare.

The third edition of *Taylor and Kelly's Dermatology for Skin of Color*, edited by my internationally recognized, esteemed, and revered colleagues Drs. Susan Taylor and Henry Lim is, no doubt, unparalleled in its depth of data and presentation for skin diseases in patients with skin of color. This textbook has been recognized by the Association of Academic Publishers for excellence in both clinical medicine and biology and life sciences.

The highly distinguished section editors include Drs. Victoria Barbosa, Cheryl Burgess, Valerie Callender, Nada Elbuluk, and Rebecca Vasquez. The third edition, with 105 updated and detailed chapters, addresses epidemiology, cultural considerations, structure, function, and biology, a broad spectrum of cutaneous, hair, scalp and nail disorders, pigmentary diseases, infections, mucosal conditions, cosmetic and procedural dermatology, and much more. It also addresses healthcare disparities, cultural competence, and the ongoing need for inclusivity in healthcare and delivery.

We are truly indebted to Drs. Taylor and Lim and the Section Editors for this foundational, comprehensive, and inclusive work. This magnificent treatise addresses the diverse spectrum and treatment of skin diseases in skin of color around the globe. It is an essential textbook for medical students, residents, clinicians, scientists, and researchers in dermatology and in the house of medicine.

To paraphrase Dr. Vivek Murthy, we must ensure that every person in society has access to high-quality healthcare, regardless of who they are or where they come from.

Pearl E. Grimes, MD
Director, The Vitiligo & Pigmentation Institute of Southern California
Clinical Professor of Dermatology
University of California, Los Angeles

SECTION 1

Definitions, Epidemiology, and Cultural Considerations

CHAPTER 1 Defining Skin of Color

Tatiana M. Barrera
Yacine Sow
Susan C. Taylor

KEY POINTS

- *Skin of color* (SOC) is an umbrella term for people of diverse racial and ethnic backgrounds whose skin color is not "white."
- SOC is a term that seeks to provide a voice for underserved, underrepresented, and understudied populations.
- Modern research led to the vitamin D-folate hypothesis and supports an evolutionary process behind skin color in response to ultraviolet radiation.
- Biological differences in SOC patients and social determinants of health may impact the development, prevention, management, and treatment of dermatologic conditions in this patient population.
- A strong understanding of the unique biological, clinical, and psychosocial components of dermatologic care for SOC patients is needed to provide excellent patient care.

INTRODUCTION

The term *skin of color* (SOC) encompasses people of diverse racial and ethnic backgrounds whose skin color is not "white" and may include those who identify as Hispanic/Latine, Black/African, Asian/Pacific Islander, Middle Eastern, American Indian/Native American/Native Alaskan, Indigenous Australian, and biracial/multiracial.[1] People with SOC often share genetic polymorphisms and unique biological skin, hair, and nail properties. Moreover, their shared experiences with identity formation and social determinants of health influence the prevalence and manifestation of dermatologic conditions among SOC populations and individuals. Of note, SOC does not seek to define any race, ethnicity, or culture. Rather, it serves as an umbrella term to provide an opportunity for increased research, improved quality of care, and boosted morale in historically marginalized populations in dermatology.

DEMOGRAPHICS AND SKIN OF COLOR POPULATIONS

According to the U.S. Census Bureau, the fastest-growing racial/ethnic group consists of people who identify as mixed race, followed by Asians and Hispanic/Latine, both of which are estimated to double within the next four decades.[2] While the non-Hispanic White population is projected to remain the single largest race group until 2060 [**Figure 1-1**], people of color will make up the majority of the U.S. population beginning in 2045.[2]

Census data on race are based on self-identification, and categories generally reflect a social definition of race.[3] While SOC can encompass people of various race categories, race is not a surrogate for biological/genetic inheritance or inherent risk factors. Ethnicity incorporates social, religious, dietary, linguistic, and other variables to identify individuals and populations. However, both race and ethnicity may be too broad. For example, people racially categorized as Asian/Pacific Islanders (Indian, Bangladeshi, Pakistani, Chinese, or Pacific Islanders) share some—but not all—cultural, religious, and ethnic values.

Race and ethnic categories are historical, evolving over time to include, exclude, or rename different people groups based on sociopolitical and economic factors. In the early 20th century, the already prevalent "one drop rule" was codified into law in the United States, whereby a person with even the smallest trace of ancestral "black blood" was categorized as Black and ergo a slave. The iniquitous racial and ethnic hierarchical classification of human groups has led to many abuses in politics, medicine, and beyond—traumatic experiences shared among people with SOC for centuries. However, despite the controversy surrounding racial and ethnic categories, they may serve a purpose in epidemiologic studies for understanding shared behaviors, beliefs, and practices within ethnoracial communities.

Moreover, race and ethnicity may function as a source of social identity for human groups, as well as highlight the impact of social determinants of health, racial, and ethnic discrimination, and the need for diversity, equity, and inclusion efforts in medicine and dermatology.

Still, neither race nor ethnicity determines the skin color of individuals or populations. Even the seemingly benign term "ethnic skin" used in medical literature to describe SOC is problematic and not an appropriate substitute considering the great variety of skin colors that can be seen in a single ethnicity. For instance, the ethnicity Hispanic/Latine includes individuals with vastly different skin colors and hair textures who identify as Afro-Latine (race: Black), Mestizo (race: Mixed [White and Indigenous]), Asian Hispanic (race: Asian), and Indigenous (race: American Indian). Among Africans, for example, the skin of Nilo-Saharan pastoralists is one of the most darkly pigmented on Earth. Yet south of them, the Khoisan hunter-gatherers have relatively light skin.[4,5] These phenotypic variations may be explained by the origin, evolutionary adaptation, and genetics of skin color.

SKIN PIGMENTATION

It is postulated that early modern humans (*Homo sapiens*) originated from eastern and southern Africa approximately 300 to 350 thousand years ago and had eumelanin-rich, dark skin to protect their naked and mostly hairless bodies from the harmful effects of ultraviolet radiation (UVR).[6] Around 80 to 100 thousand years ago, humans emigrated from Africa to neighboring regions where they encountered diverse environmental and geographic conditions. This led to their genetic adaptation under natural selection, resulting in variable phenotypes including height, immunity, hemoglobin levels, and skin color.[5] The most widely accepted evolutionary theory explaining human origins and skin pigmentation is the vitamin D-folate hypothesis [**Table 1-1**].[6,7]

As early humans migrated to regions with less and more variable UVR, the selective pressure to maintain adequate levels of photosensitive vitamin D and folate led to their decreased need for UVR photoprotection. Over time, this resulted in the depigmentation and lighter skin of humans residing in the northern and southern hemispheres.[6] Studies testing the vitamin D-folate hypothesis demonstrate support for an evolutionary multiplex of exposomal (ie, nongenetic) and genetic factors that contributed to the adaptive phototype of human skin in response to varying UVR regions.[7]

One of the most variable phenotypes in humans is constitutive skin color (ie, the color of skin that results from genetically determined

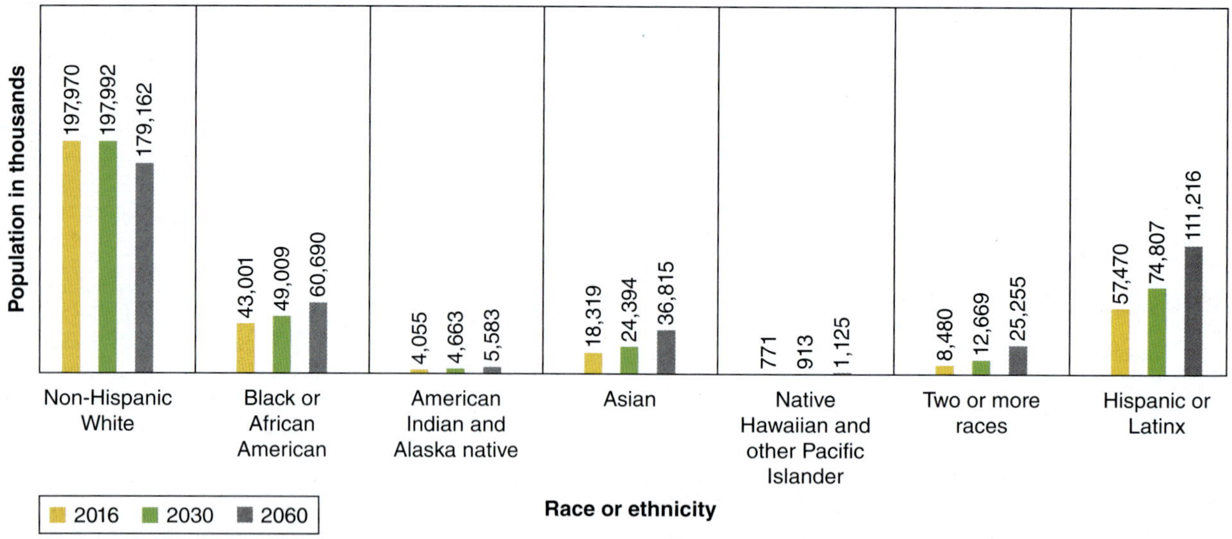

FIGURE 1-1. The changing racial and ethnic demographics in the United States from 2016 to 2060. This figure shows how the racial and ethnic demographics in the United States are changing, with Hispanic/Latinx and Asian populations expected to double by 2060. (Adapted from Vespa J, Medina L, Armstrong DM. Demographic turning points for the United States: population estimates and projections for 2020 to 2060. U.S. Census Bureau. 2020:25-114. https://www.census.gov/content/dam/Census/library/publications/2020/demo/p25-1144.pdf.)

quantities and qualities of synthesized melanin). Constitutive skin color strongly correlates with latitude and UVR intensity.[6] Among the over 150 genes identified in the natural selection for pigmentation and protection from UVR are the genes *p53*, *MC1R*, *SLC45A2* and *SLC24A5*, *KITLG*, *TYRP1*, *MFSD12*, and *MITF*. (See Chapter 15.[8,9])

Some genes tied to skin pigmentation and color have been found in greater proportion among SOC populations with shared ancestry but from differing geographic regions—a phenomenon that may be explained by the migrations of early humans.[6,8-10] The Arabian Peninsula, for example, was once a crossroad between Europe, Africa, and Asia. It is perhaps no surprise that modern-day Iranians share skin pigmentation genes in common with European, African, and South Asian neighboring populations.[11] The dark pigmentation observed in populations of African, South Asian, and Austro-Melanesian descent is associated with variations in multiple genes, including *HERC2*, *OCA2*, *MFSD12*, and *DDB1*. Gene variants may also explain the great range of skin colors observed within those populations. For example, studies identified that allelic variations in one of the introns of HERC2 (a protein that influences the expression of the melanosome-regulating gene *OCA2*) contribute to skin color differences observed among the darker Ethiopian Nilo-Saharans and the lighter Botswanan KheoSans.[4]

During the 19th century, people from northern and northwestern European regions traveled and migrated to regions with greater sun exposure. They settled in modern-day southern Europe and Africa, the Americas, and Australia.[6] Their admixing with established indigenous peoples ensued, as did the transatlantic slave trade. This increased exposure to UVR, and reincorporation of genes favoring the selection of darker skin colors led to the repigmenting of people with lighter skin.[6]

TABLE 1-1 The vitamin D-folate hypothesis (BH4 – Tetrahydrobiopterin)

Three core tenants	Role in human biology	Selective pressures
1. An inadequate **folate** status negatively impacts reproductive success	Folate is essential for: • Biosynthesis of DNA • DNA repair • DNA methylation • Production and regeneration of BH4	• Females: neural tube defects during pregnancy • Males: decreased sperm count and reduced motility • Low folate ⟶ less BH4 ⟶ decreased melanin biosynthesis and further loss of folate with exposure to ultraviolet radiation (UVR) ⟶ greater DNA damage • Dark skin exposed to low UVR experiences minimal folate loss; light skin exposed to low UVR experiences less severe folate loss[a] • Result: higher folate levels in response to a lower folate requirement to maintain melanin biosynthesis[a]
2. An inadequate **vitamin D** level in pregnant individuals may affect fertility	Vitamin D is essential for: • Absorption and retention of calcium and phosphorus • Bone growth, mineralization, and remodeling • Modulation of cell growth, neuroimmune function, and glucose metabolism	• Fetal skeletal development requires adequate calcium status ⟶ pregnant individuals experience a 4-5× increase in vitamin D levels • Pelvic bone structure: inadequate vitamin D in early life ⟶ increased risk of pelvis malformation ⟶ prevents vaginal childbirth • Result: to compensate for impaired vitamin D synthesis in dark skin, vitamin D-dependent genes interact with pigmentation single nucleotide polymorphisms[a]
3. Skin pigmentation is a phenotypic adaptation resulting from the natural selective pressures of environment **(diet and UVR)** and a complexity of genes	• Diet: consumption of essential vitamins • UVR and vitamin synthesis/degradation: • Vitamin D: photosynthesized by ultraviolet (UV) B (<310 nm with peak sensitivity at 285-295 nm) • Folate: photodegraded by UVA and UVB	• Initial selective pressure: UVR-induced photodegradation of folate in skin vasculature ⟶ darker skin phenotypes advantageous at tropical latitudes • Later selective pressures: humans emigrated from Africa ⟶ less pigmentation needed for vitamin D photosynthesis in the skin

[a]Extension of the original Vitamin D-folate hypothesis.[7]

Source: From Lucock MD, Jones PR, Veysey M, et al. Biophysical evidence to support and extend the vitamin D-folate hypothesis as a paradigm for the evolution of human skin pigmentation. *Am J Hum Biol.* 2022;34(4):e23667.

Other factors such as wars, famine, immigration, modern travel, and infectious disease have moved people to regions near and far, resulting in admixed populations with shared ancestry.[6,12] Thus, a multitude of shared gene polymorphisms influence the wide-ranging phenotypic skin tones observed in people with SOC. For instance, a large, population-based genome-wide association study identified one specific polymorphism of *MFSD12* that had previously only been found among East Asians and Native Americans as the gene most associated with the skin color of highly admixed Latin Americans.[9]

The study of selective pressures and human adaptations has contributed to the advancement of medicine, helping us gain insight into the genetic factors that influence a population's risk and disease prevalence. We now better understand how local adaptations in humans have influenced the association between obesity and diabetes or between sickle cell trait and protection against malarial infection.[5] Dermatologic conditions are no exception. The unique and shared genetic adaptations among people with SOC contribute to their differences and similarities in the biological and structural features of skin, hair, and nails (see 2nd edition Chapters 11, 14, 15).

PREDISPOSITION FOR PIGMENTARY DISORDERS IN SKIN OF COLOR

All human skin, regardless of color, shares foundational biological structures and functions. However, there are key differences that impact dermatologic disease prevention, prevalence, management, and treatment in SOC populations.

The vast array of human skin colors and tones [**Figure 1-2**] results from different combinations of light absorption and reflection from key chromophores: melanin, carotenoids, hemoglobin, oxyhemoglobin, and opsin.[13] Skin pigmentation depends on the synthesis and deposition of the pigment melanin in the epidermis by melanocytes. Darker skin is linked to higher melanin content and eumelanin levels and greater size of melanosomes.[9] The size, distribution, and stages of melanosomes vary across people groups of different ethnoracial descent and skin color. (See Chapter 15.[14])

To maintain cutaneous homeostasis, the regulation of melanogenesis depends on the interactions and crosstalk among melanocytes and other cutaneous cell types (eg, keratinocytes and dermal fibroblasts).[15] Furthermore, signaling pathways, such as paracrine regulation via local pro-opiomelanocortin (POMC) production, contribute to pigmentation in response to UVR.[9,10] These processes not only result in the increased cutaneous melanin pigment observed in people with SOC but also augment the predisposition for pigmentary disorders in this population.

Both intra- and extracutaneous factors have been linked to pigmentary disorders and their prevalence among patients with SOC. For example, dermal fibroblasts are known to secrete messenger molecules responsible for regulating skin pigmentation and are thought to play a key role in the development of pigmentary disorders.[15] In addition, recent studies suggest that high-energy visible (HEV) light (380-500 nm) may contribute to pigmentary disorders.[13] When HEV light interacts with the OPSN3 protein-coupled receptor, a calcium-dependent cascade is activated that ultimately increases the expression and sustained activity of tyrosinase and pigment-specific genes, thereby increasing melanogenesis.[13,16] Moreover, in darker skin types, pigmentation induced by HEV light is more intense and sustained compared to that by UVA-1.[13] Thus, HEV light photoprotection may prevent and treat HEV-light-induced hyperpigmentation, a common dermatologic concern in SOC patients.[13]

SKIN OF COLOR CLASSIFICATIONS

Scientific classifications of humans have historically been based on skin color. The earliest of these classifications was the formal taxonomy of humans by Carl Linnaeus in the 1700s, dividing early humans into four groups based on geography and skin color: *Homo Europaeus albescens*, *Homo Americanus rubescens*, *Homo Asiaticus fuscus*, and *Homo Africanus niger*.[12] During the early 20th century, verbal descriptions of skin color (eg, black, brown, red, yellow, white) were replaced by classification systems that matched a person's skin to standardized, colored glass tiles or strips of paper.[17] Since then, many classification systems have been created to categorize skin types and tones, each with its strengths and weaknesses. Among the most widely used skin classification systems is the Fitzpatrick skin phototype classification system (FST).

In 1975, Dr. Thomas Fitzpatrick developed a scale, based on skin propensity to tan or burn, that could help clinicians identify the appropriate dose of UVR for psoriasis treatment. The original scale consisted of four categories (skin types I-IV) representing "white skin" only, with brown and black skin categories later included as skin types V and VI, respectively [**Table 1-2**].[18] As practical and simple as the FST is, it has inherent clinical and ethnoracial limitations.

Several weaknesses exist in the application of FST to describe an individual's photosensitivity, particularly for those with darker skin types. FST types V and VI are inaccurately labeled as having little to no propensity to burn on sun exposure, but individuals with darker skin indeed do report sunburning.[19] In addition, people tend to underestimate their ultraviolet (UV) skin sensitivity and experience recall errors.[10] Because counseling on photoprotection is often guided by FST, its use as a standard assessment tool may promote health disparities, and incorrect sun reactivity classification by the clinician may lead to a patient receiving incomplete or inaccurate information.

Furthermore, the FST does not include other descriptors of skin attributes that are of particular concern to patients with SOC, such as those

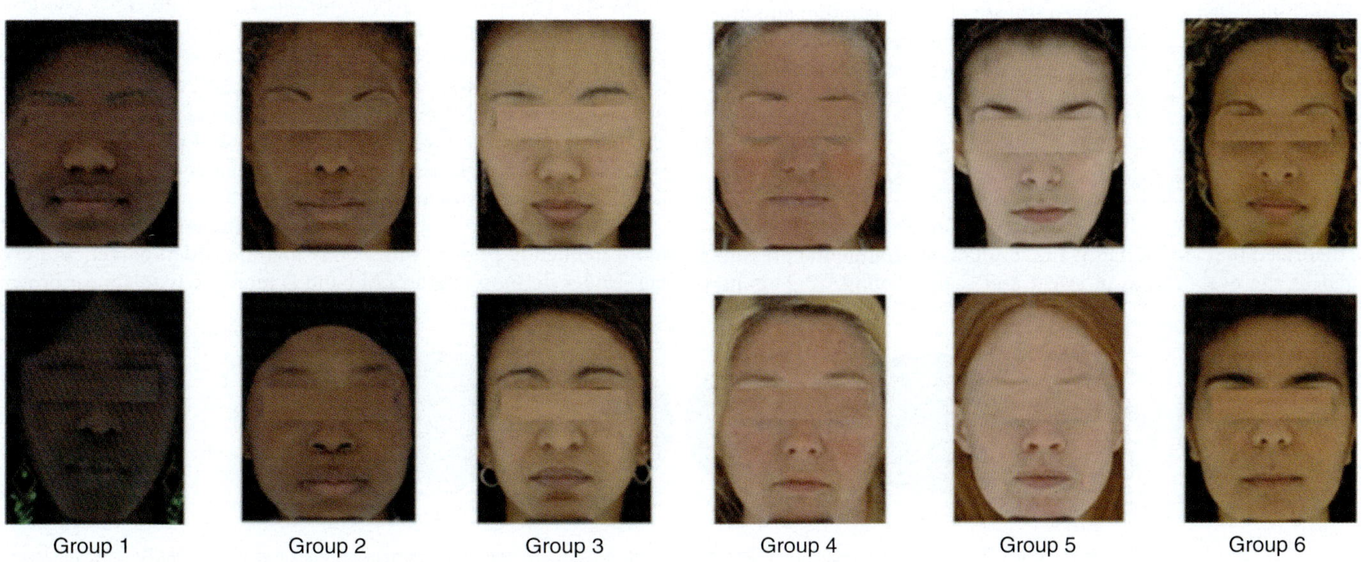

FIGURE 1-2. The six groups of skin tones. A reflection of the diversity in skin color.

TABLE 1-2 Classification of Fitzpatrick's skin phototypes (FST)

SPT	Basic skin color	Response to sun exposure
I	Pale white	Burn easily, do not tan
II	White	Burn easily, tan with difficulty
III	White	May burn initially but tan easily
IV	Light brown/olive	Hardly burn, tan easily
V	Brown	Usually do not burn, tan easily
VI	Black	Do not burn, become darker

Source: Reproduced with permission from Wolff K, Johnson RA, Saavedra AP, Roh EK. *Fitzpatrick's Color Atlas and Synopsis of Clinical Dermatology*. 8th ed. New York: McGraw Hill; 2017.

related to the skin's moisture, aging, and propensity to scar or pigment (eg, postinflammatory hyperpigmentation). Thus, other skin type classification systems have been developed that consider additional skin attributes.

Dr. Fitzpatrick recognized that race and ethnicity were sociocultural and political constructs, without a scientific basis.[18] Nevertheless, the addition of FST types V and VI established a precedent for people of similar ethnoracial groups to be grouped into a single FST category. One study found that approximately one in three physicians report using FST to describe a patient's race/ethnicity.[20] FST, however, cannot serve as a proxy for race. The entire range of self-reported FST types (I-VI) has been observed in people with SOC.[21] Furthermore, data reporting race do not consistently correlate with objective measures of pigmentation or with self-reported FST of all skin colors.[10,21] The lack of consistency is complicated by the subjective nature of the FST questionnaire. A person's desired skin color or experiences of colorism may influence their answer choices.[22] Their inability to distinguish their constitutive versus facultative skin color may also lead to self-reported FST inconsistencies.

Questions designed to determine FST may not be fully applicable to all races and ethnicities. Data show that culturally adapted FSTs that include considerations of skin colors and tones, beliefs, practices, and language differences are a better fit.[20,21,23] Terms such as "sunburn" and "tan" are not universal. Neither is the concept of tanning. Based on the subjects' responses, a study of an Indian population replaced questions on tanning habits after finding them to be irrelevant in a culture that favors light skin. Instead, they expanded hair and eye colors.[20] Another study analyzing the validity of the FST scale among Mestizo Ecuadorians (>90% FST III and IV) determined that questions on freckles (a consequence of sun exposure) decreased the questionnaire's internal consistency and construct validity.[23] This suggests that alternative descriptors to burning and tanning (eg, skin itching, tenderness, or darkening) may be a better fit for FST questionnaires given to individuals with SOC.[20]

Nevertheless, FST continues to be the standard of skin type classifications in clinical dermatology, given its ease of administration and practicality. However, for research purposes and to prevent conflating UV phototyping with skin color, more objective measurements of pigmentation, such as spectrometry and colorimetry, are preferred.[10,18]

HAIR IN SKIN OF COLOR POPULATIONS

Like skin, human hair evolved in response to environmental pressures. It is theorized that curled hair is the result of environmental pressures related to the evaporation of sweat and scalp cooling.[24,25] This may explain why despite great geographic distances, the hair of populations in high-temperature regions share similar measurable degrees of curl [**Figure 1-3**].[24] For example, the tightly coiled hair observed in Melanesians of the Solomon Islands is very similar to that of many African populations.

Genes also play a major role in the pleomorphic nature of hair. Hair types, shapes, and colors can vary greatly in admixed populations, yet be similar among people of shared descent. The CANDELA cohort found that some of the same single nucleotide polymorphisms (SNPs) that influence the skin color of Latin Americans also contribute to hair color. Other SNPs, such as those in trichohyalin and EDAR (a cell surface receptor of tumor necrosis factor expressed in skin and hair follicles), are strongly associated with hair fiber thickness and hair shapes.[24] These SNPs may code for the differing hair shapes commonly observed across East Asian, Native American, and Latin American populations—all of which share genetic ancestry.[24] Furthermore, across different SOC populations, a single SNP can influence more than one anatomic hair region. A pilot study of a male, Pakistani Punjabi population identified that *beard* thickness in this population was associated with intron variants of a locus that had previously been linked to *eyebrow* thickness in Latin Americans.[26] As the admixing of people increases, so will the genetic diversity of hair. These genetic differences are an important factor to consider when addressing prevention strategies, clinical trials, and treatment regimens in SOC populations.

As with evolutionary and genetic factors, the biological structure and function of the hair phenotypes observed in people with SOC are also similar. All hair colors are observed in the hair of SOC populations. Hair colors ranging from blond to brown and black all contain small amounts of pheomelanin, but the degree of pigmentation depends on the eumelanin content (higher in black hair; lower in blond hair).[9,24,25] Compared to hair shafts of lighter-haired individuals, the shafts of dark hair are densely occupied by melanosomes.[25] Hair with any degree of curl results from a curved, asymmetric follicle.[24] Of note, dark or curly hair phenotypes are not unique to SOC populations; they may be observed in those who identify as White or who have fairer skin. However, there are hair pathologies that disproportionately affect patients with SOC with these hair phenotypes (eg, pseudofolliculitis barbae and traction alopecia in tightly coiled hair).[27] Having a firm grasp of the genetic and biological differences will provide the foundation of knowledge to then further appreciate the social determinants of health that drive these disparities.

NAILS IN SKIN OF COLOR POPULATIONS

The melanocytes in the distal matrix of nails are more active in darker skin than in white skin, contributing to increased melanin deposition in the nail plate and the greater prevalence of pigmented nail lesions in SOC populations.[28,29] Hence, longitudinal melanonychia (LM), also known as melanonychia striata, is rare in white skin but is more prevalent in older adults with dark skin.[28,29] Clinically, the appearance of LM does not differ much from subungual melanoma. However, the lack of clinical and dermoscopic knowledge of how LM presents differently in SOC compared to light skin has led to more patients with SOC undergoing nail matrix biopsies for benign lesions.[29]

It is important to consider that patients with darker skin who have LM more frequently present with bands that are wider, darker, and evolving. Under dermoscopy, an LM band is more likely to appear brown in

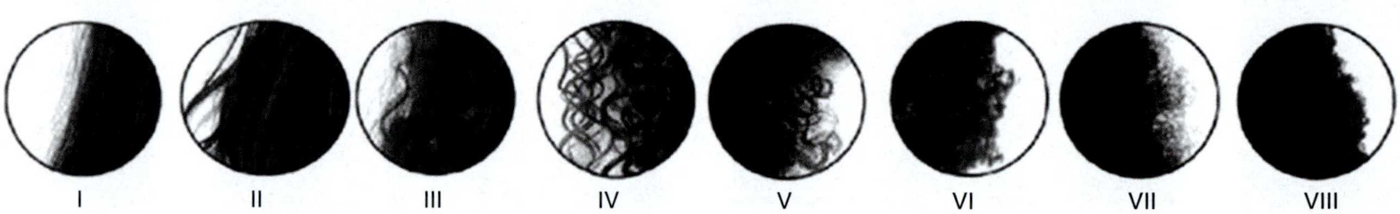

FIGURE 1-3. Hair types in people with skin of color. The eight types of human hair in terms of degree and type of curl, as described by Loussouam et al. (Reproduced with permission from Loussouarn G, Garcel AL, Lozano I, et al. Worldwide diversity of hair curliness: a new method of assessment. *Int J Dermatol.* 2007;46(suppl 1):2-6.)

the nails of patients with SOC, versus the gray hue that is observed in their White counterparts.[29] Thus, differentiating a common LM from a nail apparatus melanoma in dermoscopy may impact outcomes in SOC patients.[28,29] (See Chapter 25.)

THE PSYCHOSOCIAL COMPONENT OF SKIN OF COLOR

SELF-IDENTITY IN SKIN OF COLOR INDIVIDUALS AND COMMUNITIES

Over time, skin color has gone from an indicator of geographic origin and environment to one of cultural and behavioral differences.[12] Skin color and hair type are some of the major attributes that define a person's individual and group identity.[12,30] As a visually dominant species, humans readily notice interindividual differences in skin color and use it as a characteristic for identifying distinct individual and group differences.[30] A study of over 900 diverse college students found that participants perceived their typicality/atypicality within their ethnic group based on factors such as their skin color, hair, and facial features.[31] Though in and of itself "color" is value neutral, skin colors carry profound cognitive associations that affect how people with SOC identify themselves and how they are identified by others.[12]

Hair can also serve as a public marker of identity and core values; thus, clinicians should practice cultural humility when providing hair information and scalp examinations to patients with SOC. For example, in Black communities, a child's hair may be viewed as an outward representation of their parents' parenting skills.[32] We must also be aware that patients with tightly coiled hair may present with natural and protective hairstyles that make partitioning hair or examining the scalp more challenging.[33]

Furthermore, the psychological and psychosocial ramifications of skin and hair play a critical role in SOC patients with dermatologic conditions. An individual with SOC whose perception of skin tone is shaped by community views that favor lighter skin may be more inclined to use skin-lightening products, resulting in deleterious health consequences. Likewise, a patient for whom hair holds spiritual value may experience spiritual distress or mental health challenges when faced with alopecia.[30] Practicing cultural sensitivity and humility in dermatology promotes equitable care, respects a patient's identity, facilitates diagnosis and management, and improves patient outcomes (see Chapter 3).

SOCIAL DETERMINANTS OF HEALTH

The dermatologic inequities experienced among communities of color may be explained by social determinants of health (SDOHs): the conditions in which people are born, grow, live, learn, work, play, and age. Environmental and occupational exposures play a critical role in the differences in disease manifestation and anatomic variation of dermatologic conditions. For example, higher risks of keratinocyte cancers are seen among outdoor workers, and 40% of U.S. outdoor workers identify as having SOC.[34,35] Other SDOHs commonly shared among people with SOC are barriers to financial stability and access to dermatologic care. The 2020 U.S. Census estimates that Black, Asian, and Hispanic (any race) SOC populations are among the most underinsured (eg, Medicaid, Medicare, Veterans Affairs) and uninsured populations.[36] Data demonstrate that underinsured or uninsured patients are less likely to visit an outpatient dermatologist for their condition and are more likely to experience longer treatment wait times, fewer treatment options, and worse dermatologic outcomes.[37,38] All populations may be exposed to financial barriers to medical care access, but in the United States, those who identify as American Indian, Black or African American, or Hispanic/Latine are among the lowest income earners.[35] In addition to finances affecting the insurance types and dermatology services affordable or accessible to many SOC populations, they also affect their access to prescription and over-the-counter skin care products.

The Centers for Disease Control and Prevention describes racism as one of the major negative influences on the SDOHs experienced by communities of color, driving health inequities and increasing the risk of poor health outcomes among people with SOC.[39] Racism contributes to *colorism*, that is, the overt and subconscious prejudice or discrimination against individuals with a darker skin tone among members of the same ethnic or racial group.[6,12] The racism and colorism experienced among SOC populations have profound health consequences—from the systemic and dermatologic adverse effects associated with mercury-containing skin bleaching creams to the need for legislation to protect patients with natural hair from workplace discrimination.[30,40]

THE IMPACT OF SKIN OF COLOR ON DERMATOLOGY AND MEDICINE

SOC is not limited to the skin tones, hair types, races, or ethnicities of individuals. Rather, it is an umbrella term that seeks to provide a voice for these underserved, underrepresented, and understudied populations. Dermatologic conditions in SOC patients may have unique clinical presentations compared to those observed in non-Hispanic White patients. The dermatologic concerns and needs of SOC patients, which are shaped in part by history, identity, and SDOHs, may also differ from those of White patients. A strong understanding of the unique biological, clinical, and psychosocial components of SOC is needed to provide excellent dermatologic care. Our goal is that the materials presented in this textbook will enrich your knowledge and appreciation of the importance of SOC in dermatology. In so doing, we will help improve diagnosis and treatment, strengthen patient-physician relationships, bolster physician-physician relationships, and support holistic and culturally mindful care for people with SOC.

REFERENCES

1. Brown-Korsah JB, McKenzie S, Omar D, Syder NC, Elbuluk N, Taylor SC. Variations in genetics, biology, and phenotype of cutaneous disorders in skin of color. Part I: genetic, biological, and structural differences in skin of color. *J Am Acad Dermatol.* 2022;87(6):1239-1258.
2. Vespa J, Medina L, Armstrong DM. Demographic turning points for the United States: population estimates and projections for 2020 to 2060. U.S. Census Bureau. 2020:25–114. https://www.census.gov/content/dam/Census/library/publications/2020/demo/p25-1144.pdf.
3. U.S. Census Bureau. About the topic of race. https://www.census.gov/topics/population/race/about.html. Accessed August 15, 2022.
4. Feng Y, McQuillan MA, Tishkoff SA. Evolutionary genetics of skin pigmentation in African populations. *Hum Mol Genet.* 2021;30(R1):R88-R97.
5. Fan S, Hansen MEB, Lo Y, Tishkoff SA. Going global by adapting local: a review of recent human adaptation. *Science.* 2016;354(6308):54-59.
6. Jablonski NG. The evolution of human skin pigmentation involved the interactions of genetic, environmental, and cultural variables. *Pigment Cell Melanoma Res.* 2021;34(4):707-729.
7. Lucock MD, Jones PR, Veysey M, et al. Biophysical evidence to support and extend the vitamin D-folate hypothesis as a paradigm for the evolution of human skin pigmentation. *Am J Hum Biol Off J Hum Biol Counc.* 2022;34(4):e23667.
8. Naik PP, Farrukh SN. Influence of ethnicities and skin color variations in different populations: a review. *Skin Pharmacol Physiol.* 2022;35(2):65-76.
9. Pavan WJ, Sturm RA. The genetics of human skin and hair pigmentation. *Annu Rev Genomics Hum Genet.* 2019;20:41-72.
10. Del Bino S, Duval C, Bernerd F. Clinical and biological characterization of skin pigmentation diversity and its consequences on UV impact. *Int J Mol Sci.* 2018;19(9):2668.
11. Fernandes V, Brucato N, Ferreira JC, et al. Genome-wide characterization of Arabian Peninsula populations: shedding light on the history of a fundamental bridge between continents. *Mol Biol Evol.* 2019;36(3):575-586.
12. Jablonski NG. Skin color and race. *Am J Phys Anthropol.* 2021;175(2):437-447.
13. Austin E, Geisler AN, Nguyen J, et al. Visible light. Part I: properties and cutaneous effects of visible light. *J Am Acad Dermatol.* 2021;84(5):1219-1231.
14. Jothishankar B, Stein SL. Impact of skin color and ethnicity. *Clin Dermatol.* 2019;37(5):418-429.
15. Kapoor R, Dhatwalia SK, Kumar R, Rani S, Parsad D. Emerging role of dermal compartment in skin pigmentation: comprehensive review. *J Eur Acad Dermatol Venereol.* 2020;34(12):2757-2765.

16. Setty SR. Opsin3: a link to visible light-induced skin pigmentation. *J Invest Dermatol.* 2018;138(1):13-15.
17. Swiatoniowski AK, Quillen EE, Shriver MD, Jablonski NG. Technical note: comparing von Luschan skin color tiles and modern spectrophotometry for measuring human skin pigmentation. *Am J Phys Anthropol.* 2013;151(2):325-330.
18. Fitzpatrick TB. The validity and practicality of sun-reactive skin types I through VI. *Arch Dermatol.* 1988;124(6):869-871.
19. Bello O, Sudhoff H, Goon P. Sunburn prevalence is underestimated in UK-based people of African ancestry. *Clin Cosmet Investig Dermatol.* 2021;14:1791-1797.
20. Ware OR, Dawson JE, Shinohara MM, Taylor SC. Racial limitations of Fitzpatrick skin type. *Cutis.* 2020;105(2):77-80.
21. Sommers MS, Fargo JD, Regueira Y, et al. Are the Fitzpatrick skin phototypes valid for cancer risk assessment in a racially and ethnically diverse sample of women? *Ethn Dis.* 2019;29(3):505-512.
22. Sacksner JP, Kaundinya T, Daftary K, Jackson KL, Kundu RV. Skin tone preferences and their influence on skin care behaviors. *Arch Dermatol Res.* 2022;314(10):961-966.
23. Fors M, González P, Viada C, Falcon K, Palacios S. Validity of the Fitzpatrick skin phototype classification in Ecuador. *Adv Skin Wound Care.* 2020;33(12):1-5.
24. Westgate GE, Ginger RS, Green MR. The biology and genetics of curly hair. *Exp Dermatol.* 2017;26(6):483-490.
25. Koch SL, Shriver MD, Jablonski NG. Variation in human hair ultrastructure among three biogeographic populations. *J Struct Biol.* 2019;205(1):60-66.
26. Jawad M, Adnan A, Rehman RA, et al. Evaluation of facial hair-associated SNPs: a pilot study on male Pakistani Punjabi population. *Forensic Sci Med Pathol.* 2023;19(3):293-302.
27. Sharma D, Dalia Y, Patel TS. Ethnic equity implications in the management of pseudofolliculitis barbae. *J Am Board Fam Med.* 2022;35(1):173-174.
28. Leung AKC, Lam JM, Leong KF, Sergi CM. Melanonychia striata: clarifying behind the Black curtain. A review on clinical evaluation and management of the 21st century. *Int J Dermatol.* 2019;58(11):1239-1245.
29. Lee DK, Chang MJ, Desai AD, Lipner SR. Clinical and dermoscopic findings of benign longitudinal melanonychia due to melanocytic activation differ by skin type and predict likelihood of nail matrix biopsy. *J Am Acad Dermatol.* 2022;87(4):792-799.
30. Gupta MA, Gupta AK. The color of skin: psychiatric ramifications. *Clin Dermatol.* 2019;37(5):437-446.
31. Mitchell LL, Kathawalla UK, Ajayi AA, et al. Ethnic-racial typicality and its relation to ethnic identity and psychological functioning. *Cultur Divers Ethnic Minor Psychol.* 2018;24(3):400-413.
32. Jones NL, Heath CR. Hair at the intersection of dermatology and anthropology: a conversation on race and relationships. *Pediatr Dermatol.* 2021;38(S2):158-160.
33. Grayson C, Heath C. An approach to examining tightly coiled hair among patients with hair loss in race-discordant patient-physician interactions. *JAMA Dermatol.* 2021;157(5):505-506.
34. Loney T, Paulo MS, Modenese A, et al. Global evidence on occupational sun exposure and keratinocyte cancers: a systematic review. *Br J Dermatol.* 2021;184(2):208-218.
35. U.S. Bureau of Labor Statistics. Labor force characteristics by race and ethnicity, 2020: BLS Reports. https://www.bls.gov/opub/reports/race-and-ethnicity/2020/home.htm. Accessed August 17, 2022.
36. Keisler-Starkey K, Bunch LN. Health Insurance coverage in the united states: 2020. U.S. Census Bureau. 2021:60-274. https://www.census.gov/content/dam/Census/library/publications/2021/demo/p60-274.pdf.
37. Tripathi R, Knusel KD, Ezaldein HH, Scott JF, Bordeaux JS. Association of demographic and socioeconomic characteristics with differences in use of outpatient dermatology services in the United States. *JAMA Dermatol.* 2018;154(11):1286-1291.
38. Creadore A, Desai S, Li SJ, et al. Insurance acceptance, appointment wait time, and dermatologist access across practice types in the US. *JAMA Dermatol.* 2021;157(2):181-188.
39. Centers for Disease Control and Prevention. Racism and health. https://www.cdc.gov/healthequity/racism-disparities/index.html. Accessed September 12, 2022.
40. Watson Coleman B. Text - H.R.2116 - 117th Congress (2021-2022): Creating a Respectful and Open World for Natural Hair Act of 2022. http://www.congress.gov/. Accessed September 12, 2022.

CHAPTER 2

Epidemiology of Cutaneous Diseases

Andrea Gelabert-Mora
Aheli Chattopadhyay
Katrina Abuabara

KEY POINTS

- *Incidence, prevalence, morbidity, mortality,* and *burden of disease* are epidemiologic concepts that describe patterns of disease and are important to objectively quantify disease trends and public health measures.
- Both observational and experimental study designs contribute to evidence-based medicine, and the best study design depends on the nature of the clinical question.
- Cutaneous diseases affect over two billion people worldwide, approximately one in four individuals.
- The Global Burden of Disease Study standardized the assessment of disease morbidity across settings and measures disease burden in disability-adjusted life years, which combines years of life lost and years with disability.
- There are temporal and geographic differences in the global burden of cutaneous disease; high socioeconomic index countries are burdened by inflammatory skin disease, whereas low socioeconomic index countries are burdened by infectious skin diseases.
- Spectrometers and colorimeters measure skin color but are not widely available; simple, validated measures for skin color are needed to better understand the epidemiology of disease among patients with skin of color (SOC).
- Patients with SOC are more likely to suffer from eczematous, adnexal, or follicular skin diseases and less likely to receive systemic treatments, regardless of insurance status. Cutaneous malignancies, although less prevalent in patients with SOC, are often found at later stages, leading to worse outcomes and higher morbidity and mortality.
- Dermatologist availability and insurance type limit access to dermatologic care, especially among lower socioeconomic groups and racial/ethnic minoritized individuals in the United States.

MEASURES OF DISEASE

Disease frequency is often described using the concepts of incidence and prevalence. *Incidence* is defined as the number of new cases in a population over a defined period. *Prevalence* is the total number of existing cases in a population, either at one point in time (point prevalence) or over a specified time interval (period prevalence).[1] *Mortality* refers to the number of deaths attributable to a disease.

The cumulative impact of a disease with respect to its prevalence, morbidity, mortality, and the economic cost to society is measured by the *burden of disease.*[2] One of the most commonly used measures of disease burden is the disability-adjusted life year (DALY). DALYs measure the gap between the current state of the population and an ideal scenario in which everyone reaches the average life expectancy in perfect health, assuming that the greater the time lived with an illness, the greater the burden of disease.

EPIDEMIOLOGIC STUDY DESIGNS

OBSERVATIONAL STUDIES

Epidemiologic study designs can be broadly divided into two main categories: observational studies and experimental studies [**Figure 2-1**]. *Observational studies* examine associations between exposures and

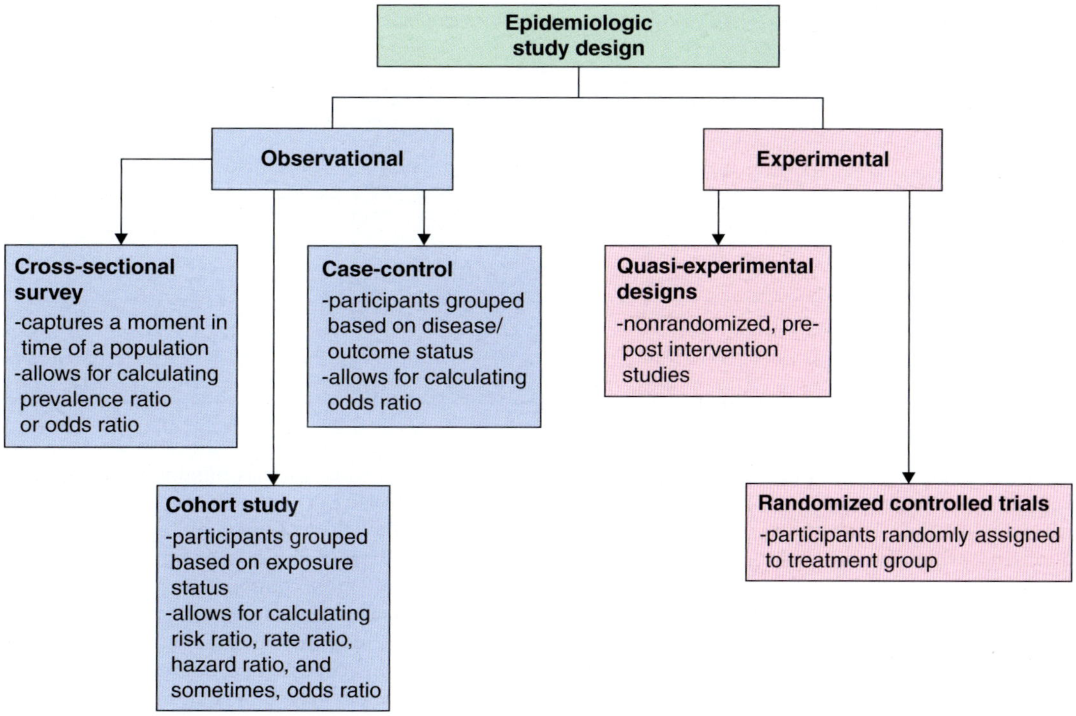

FIGURE 2-1. Epidemiologic study designs are divided into two main categories: observational and experimental studies.

outcomes without experimental intervention. Within the category of observational studies are *cohort studies* that identify subjects based on an exposure and examine whether the outcome of interest develops; *case-control studies* that identify subjects based on the outcome of interest and compare prior exposures; and *cross-sectional studies* that record exposures and outcomes of a population for a moment in time, often with the use of a survey.[1] These studies use measures of relative risk such as odds ratios, risk ratios, rate ratios, prevalence ratios, and hazard ratios to compare outcomes and exposures. *Case reports* and *case series* describe a single case or group of cases, respectively, and do not typically include a comparison group.

EXPERIMENTAL STUDIES

Experimental studies involve an intervention, be it behavioral or biomedical. *Randomized controlled trials* randomly assign individuals to treatment and/or control groups, and the process of randomization can result in unbiased assessments of treatment efficacy if randomization is successful and minimizes potential confounding. Additional techniques to strengthen the validity of results include blinding, which refers to withholding information on what treatment is given to each group to reduce bias in perceptions of treatment efficacy and outcome assessment, and a crossover design, in which individuals receive both the treatment and the control over differing time frames in random order, which allows for comparison of treatment groups within individuals and reduces potential confounding. Systematic reviews and meta-analyses use clearly defined criteria to extract results from the literature and statistically combine findings of multiple studies. *Quasi-experimental* designs aim to infer causality by leveraging situations that have near-random variation in treatment assignment rather than experimentally randomizing participants to treatment groups.[3]

HIERARCHY OF EVIDENCE

Epidemiologic study types are sometimes arranged in an "evidence hierarchy," with randomized controlled trials (RCTs), or meta-analyses of RCTs, constituting the highest level of evidence and case series and case reports contributing the lowest level of evidence. Although RCTs may be the gold standard when evaluating the efficacy of a treatment, they are costly and often have limited generalizability because they aim to answer a very specific question in a selected population.[4] Moreover, many important clinical questions cannot be answered through an interventional trial. For example, patients cannot be randomized to have disease; therefore, questions about the natural history of disease and comorbidities can only be addressed by observational study designs. In addition, case studies and case series can be useful for rare diseases and for generating hypotheses about novel treatment approaches. Therefore, when evaluating the strength of evidence, rather than relying on an evidence hierarchy, one should consider whether the study design is appropriate for the question and generalizable to the population of interest and whether multiple studies have found consistent results.

GLOBAL BURDEN OF CUTANEOUS DISEASE

AN INTRODUCTION TO GLOBAL BURDEN OF DISEASE

The Global Burden of Disease (GBD) study aims to standardize the quantification of disease impact to improve health systems and eliminate disparities globally. Hosted by the Institute of Health Metrics Evaluation at the University of Washington and funded by the Bill and Melinda Gates Foundation, it is a living database that relies on data collected and analyzed by a consortium of more than 7000 researchers in 195 countries and, as such, allows for comparisons of disease impact over time, across age groups, and across populations.

Disease burden is measured by DALYs, which represent the sum of years of life lost (YLL) to a disease and the years living with disability (YLD). One DALY is equivalent to 1 year of healthy life lost, and it is a useful metric for comparison because it represents both the prevalence of a given disease and the relative harm it causes in terms of both the impact on quality of life and life expectancy. The GBD categorizes cutaneous diseases based on International Classification of Diseases, Tenth Revision (ICD-10) codes and uses a sophisticated statistical modeling tool to estimate DALYs, including for areas with sparse or unreliable data.

Cutaneous diseases are grouped into 12 subcategories by the GBD, and melanoma and keratinocyte cancers are categorized separately under the category of neoplasms. The 12 cutaneous disease subcategories reported in the 2019 GBD are as follows: dermatitis, bacterial skin diseases, viral

TABLE 2-1 Overall ranking of deaths, years lost to disease (YLD), and disability-adjusted life years (DALYs) attributable to cutaneous diseases and cutaneous malignancies in 1990, 2010, and 2019 for both sexes, globally

Disease category	Year	Deaths	YLD	DALYs
Cutaneous diseases	1990	20th	7th	20th
	2010	20th	6th	21st
	2019	20th	7th	21st
Melanoma skin cancer	1990	96th	141st	143rd
	2010	92nd	134th	133rd
	2019	89th	133rd	129th
Nonmelanoma skin cancer	1990	106th	140th	155th
	2010	94th	141st	148th
	2019	92nd	137th	140th

skin diseases, fungal skin diseases, pruritus (itching without explained cause), urticaria, scabies, acne vulgaris, psoriasis, decubitus ulcer, alopecia areata, and other skin diseases. The category "other skin diseases" includes skin conditions that are less frequent or lack data availability but may have high individual burden, such as bullous diseases, connective tissue diseases, and severe cutaneous drug reactions.[5]

BURDEN OF CUTANEOUS DISEASES

The collective burden of skin diseases can be summarized with multiple metrics. In 2019, cutaneous diseases affected two billion people worldwide, approximately one in four individuals.[6] In the United States, over 92 million individuals suffered from cutaneous diseases in 2019, and an additional three million suffered from cutaneous malignancies.[6] Cutaneous diseases collectively contribute a large burden—over 42 million DALYs annually[6]—and this has been fairly consistent over time [**Table 2-1**]. From 1990 to 2019, cutaneous diseases as a group ranked 11th among all noncommunicable diseases in terms of the disease burden, between sense organ diseases such as blindness and hearing loss (10th largest contributor to DALYs) and substance use (12th largest contributor to DALYs).[6] Although cutaneous diseases affect individuals of all ages, the burden is largest among children and teens. In contrast, cutaneous malignancies are more common among older adults [**Figure 2-2**]. There are also regional and socioeconomic differences: regions with higher socioeconomic index have a higher burden from inflammatory skin diseases whereas infectious skin conditions, account for the most burden in low-middle sociodemographic index countries.[7,8]

Overall mortality from cutaneous diseases contributed to 1.3 per 100,000 deaths worldwide in 2019 and has remained fairly constant since 1990 [Table 2-1].[6] Mortality from skin cancers, which are counted separately from cutaneous diseases, contributed another 100,000 deaths in 2019: approximately 62,000 from malignant skin melanoma and 56,000 from nonmelanoma skin cancers.[6] In the United States, Black/African American patients over 65 years had increased rates of mortality from nonneoplastic skin diseases compared to Whites.[9]

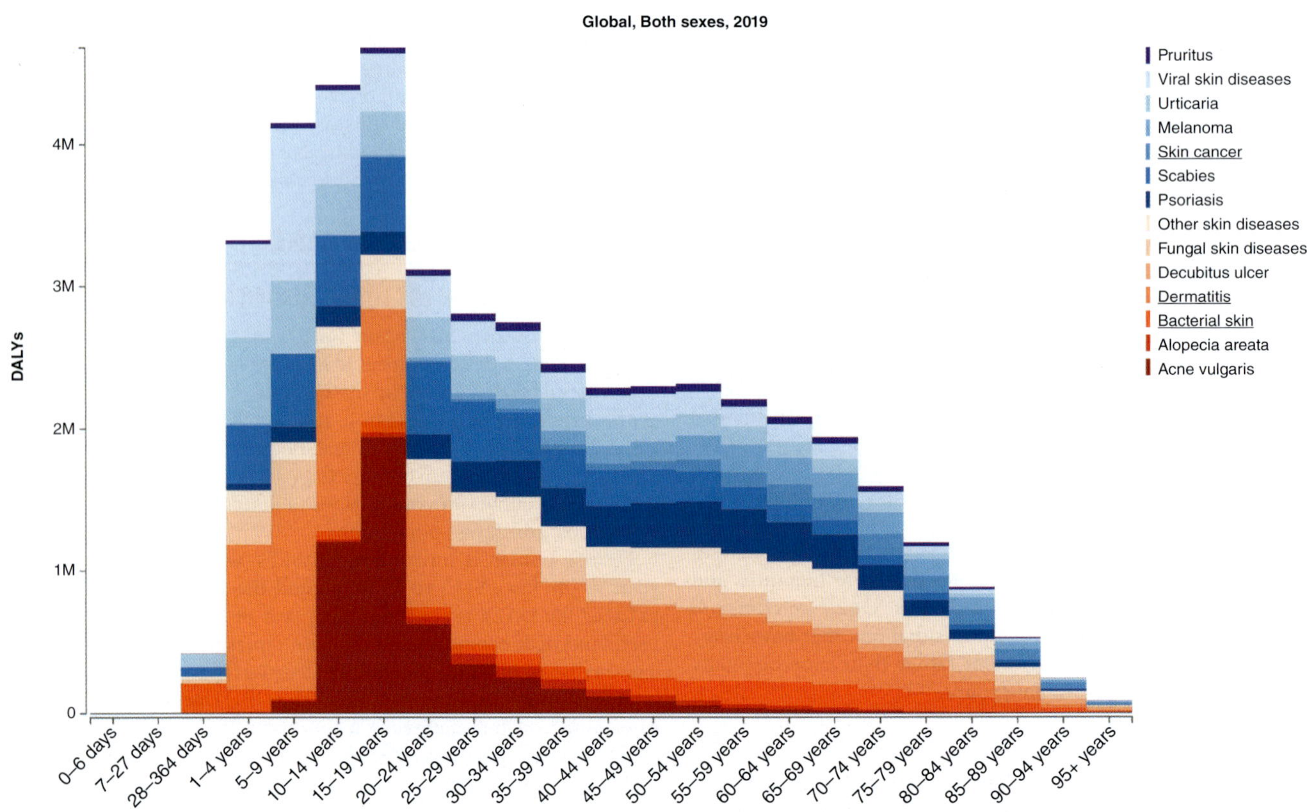

FIGURE 2-2. Global disability-adjusted life years (DALYs) attributed to cutaneous diseases, malignant skin melanoma, and nonmelanoma skin cancer by group ages in 2019. A bimodal curve for most cutaneous diseases can be observed, with a peak in early childhood and a second peak in adulthood. (Source: Institute for Health Metrics and Evaluation. Used with permission. All rights reserved.)

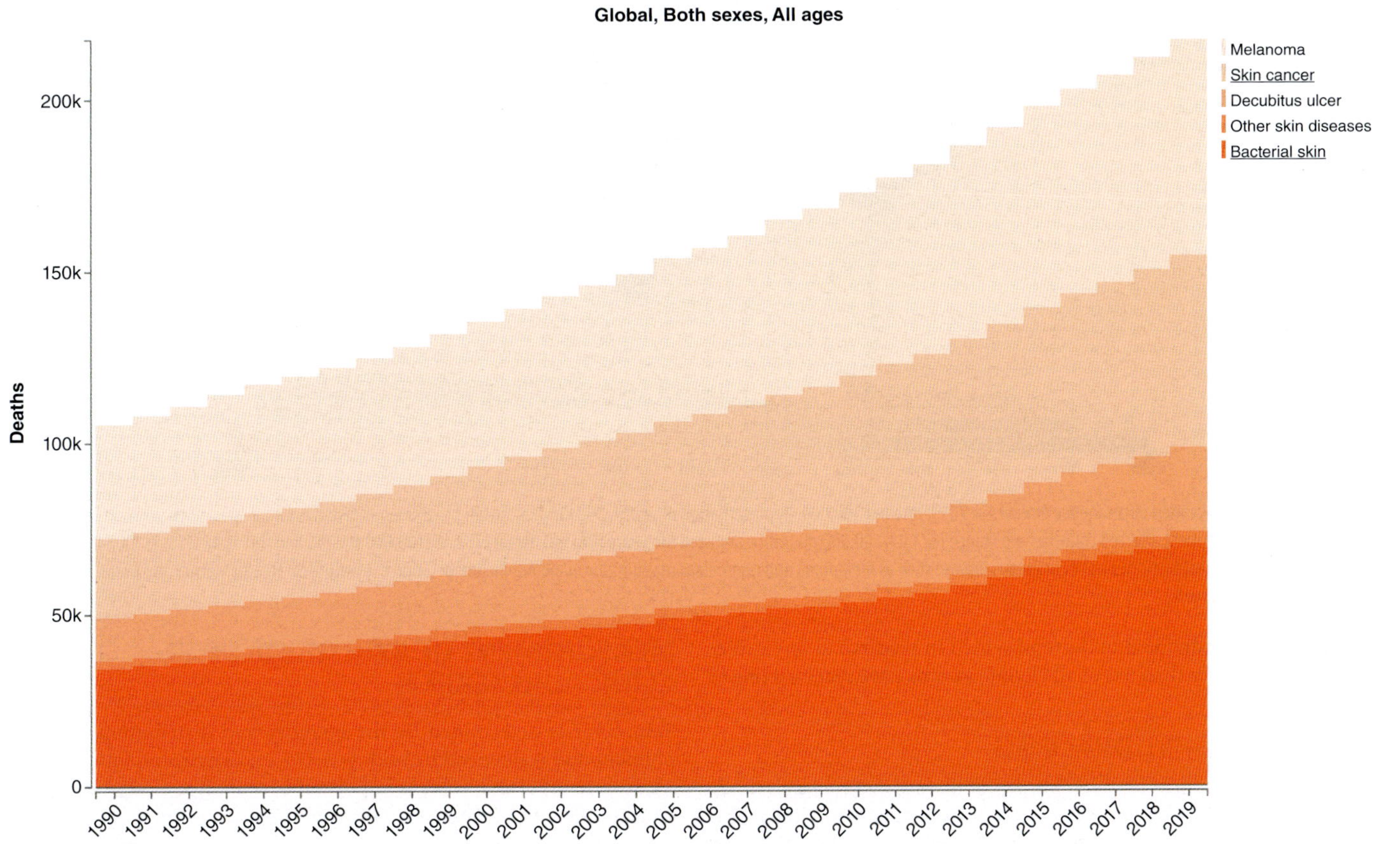

FIGURE 2-3. Global mortality attributed to cutaneous disease from 1990 to 2019 for both sexes and all ages. Values were reported for bacterial skin diseases, decubitus ulcer, and other skin diseases. For completeness and comparison, malignant skin melanoma and nonmelanoma skin cancer values were plotted. There has been a consistent rise in mortality attributed to bacterial skin diseases. The Global Burden of Disease (GBD) only reported mortality values for the plotted diseases. (Source: Institute for Health Metrics and Evaluation. Used with permission. All rights reserved.)

BURDEN BY SUBCATEGORY OF CUTANEOUS DISEASE

Globally, dermatitis, acne vulgaris, scabies, and viral skin diseases are the most burdensome categories of cutaneous diseases.[6] Among these, dermatitis is the largest contributor: it contributes 10 million DALYs worldwide. In 2017, dermatitis ranked as the 59th leading cause of global burden. For comparison, this was just below the burden from measles and above cirrhosis and other chronic liver diseases.[10] There is a bimodal age distribution with a peak in early infancy and second peak in late adulthood, and the burden appears to be increasing over time in both children and older adults.[11] Acne vulgaris is the second most burdensome cutaneous disease. It primarily affects men and women ages 10 to 24 years; although in adults, acne mostly impacts women older than 30.[12] The burden of acne vulgaris is highest in higher income regions such as North America and Western Europe.[12]

Melanoma and nonmelanoma skin cancers are ranked 25th and 28th, respectively, out of 33 measured neoplasms in the 2019 GBD study.[13] Burden from malignant skin melanoma in Europe has increased slightly by 1%, and in Asia, Africa, and North and South America, melanoma rates have increased over 2% since 1990.[6] Overall, both categories of cutaneous malignancy have increased in rank for DALYs and death counts globally since 1990 [**Figure 2-3**]. Melanoma rose to 129th in all causes of global DALYs in 2019, compared to 143rd in 1990, Similarly, nonmelanoma skin cancer rose to 140th in all causes of global DALYs, compared to 155th in 1990 [Table 2-1].[6]

BURDEN BY REGION

Because of their population size, China and India have the largest absolute numbers of people with cutaneous diseases. However, Europe and the Americas have the highest population-adjusted rates of cutaneous disease (608/100,000 DALYs and 599/100,000 DALYs, respectively). The most affected countries are France (871/100,000 DALYs), Israel (782/100,000 DALYs), and Denmark (772/100,000)[6] [**Figure 2-4**]. Europe had a high burden of cutaneous inflammatory disease, with dermatitis and psoriasis as its leading causes. In the United States, dermatitis, and psoriasis were also leading causes, in addition to viral skin diseases the leading cause of disability due to a skin condition.[6] In Africa and Asia, acne vulgaris and dermatitis, respectively, were most burdensome [**Figure 2-5**].[6]

EQUITY IN CLINICAL RESEARCH

REPRESENTATION IN FUNDING AND PUBLICATIONS

Studies have found that research funding and the number of research publications do not always match the burden of dermatologic diseases. For example, the share of National Institutes of Health (NIH) funding for melanoma research is four times more than the relative burden, whereas dermatitis, acne, and fungal skin diseases are relatively underfunded. In contrast, funding for nonmelanoma skin cancers, viral skin diseases, and psoriasis is roughly equivalent to their relative burden.[14] Similarly, the number of melanoma publications in the top dermatology journals far exceeds the relative burden; for psoriasis, it is about equal; and the share of the literature focused on most other cutaneous conditions is much smaller than their relative contribution to disease burden globally.[15]

There are also disparities in representation among researchers in dermatology. From 2007 to 2018, academic dermatology appointments in the United Staes rose by 53%, but White dermatologists made up 68% of these appointments. White dermatologists additionally composed the majority of academic chair and full professor positions (79% of each).[16] To allow for a more diverse workforce that may help to reduce disparities in research focus, in 1989, the NIH introduced diversity supplements, which award additional funding to existing grants, whereby a principal investigator can provide research opportunities, training, and

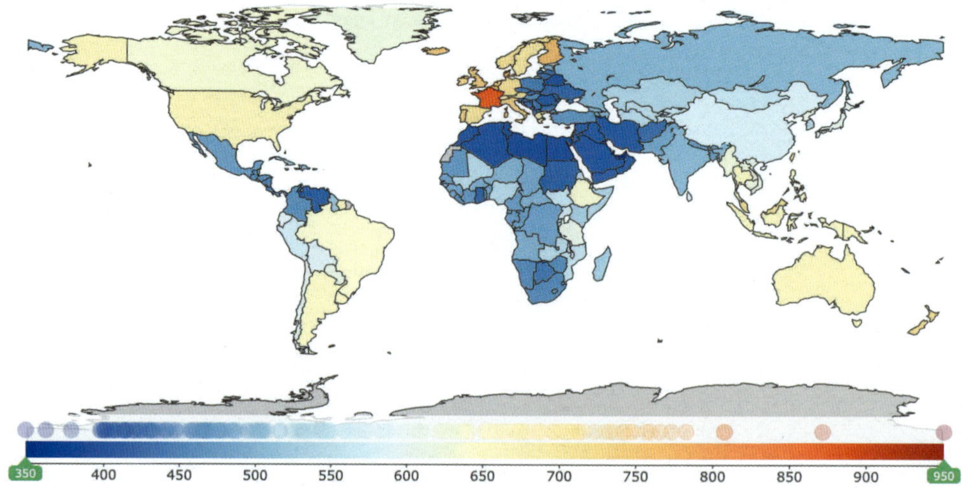

FIGURE 2-4. Global burden of cutaneous diseases in 2019, rate per 100,000. Representation of worldwide burden caused by cutaneous diseases for all ages, both sexes, in 2019. Values are adjusted per 100,000. The most affected countries are France (871.44/100,000 disability-adjusted life years [DALYs]), Israel (782.55/100,000 DALYs), and Denmark (772.9/100,000). A limitation of this illustration is that neoplastic causes of cutaneous disease such as melanoma and nonmelanoma skin cancer are not included. (Source: Institute for Health Metrics and Evaluation. Used with permission. All rights reserved.)

mentorship to an individual underrepresented in research at any career stage. However, fewer than 5% of all eligible awards have received one of these supplements.[17]

REPRESENTATION IN CLINICAL TRIALS

In addition to imbalances between burden of disease and research funding, there may be unequal representation of participants in clinical trials. A recent review found that although the percentage of participants in dermatology clinical trials who are not White increased from 19% to 27% from 2005 to 2019, the proportion of participants who identify as African American, Pacific Islander, American Indian, or Hispanic/Latine has remained low.[18] Psoriasis trials are the least diverse, whereas eczema trials were the most diverse; only 12% of psoriasis trials versus 71% of eczema trials reported at least 20% of participants who were not White.[19] There may be multiple reasons for differential participation in trials, including differences in the distribution of disease, lack of trust in health systems, and lack of time or financial flexibility to participate.[20]

MEASUREMENT OF SKIN OF COLOR IN CLINICAL RESEARCH

Skin color is determined by the quantity and distribution of melanin pigment and influenced by both genetics and environmental exposures. Measurement of skin color is important because it can contribute to both clinical care and research; for example, changes in skin color can be indicators of dermatologic disease severity or response to treatment.[21]

HISTORY OF THE FITZPATRICK SCALE

The Fitzpatrick scale is the most widely cited measure related to skin pigmentation; however, it was originally developed to measure the skin's ability to darken after phototherapy. While it may be useful for assessing response to light treatments including lasers, it has been shown to be a poor indicator of skin color and is not recommended for this purpose, especially among patients of African and Asian descent.[22]

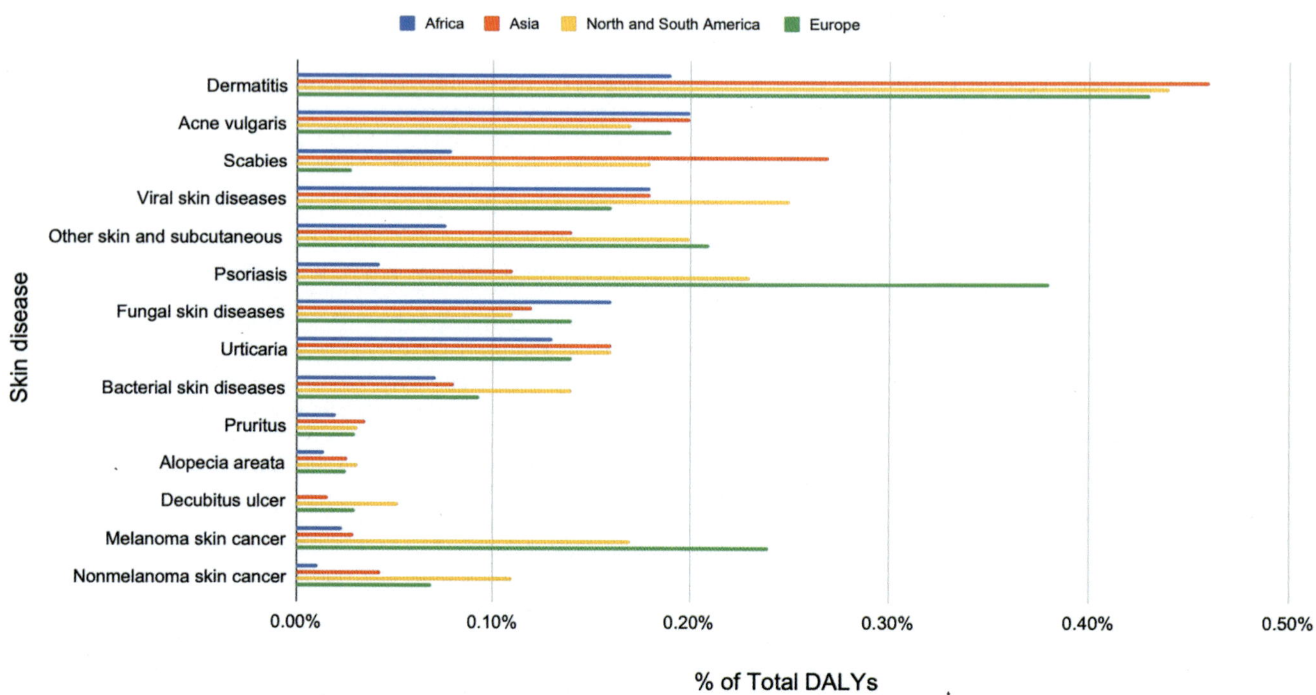

FIGURE 2-5. Comparison of total disability-adjusted life years (DALYs) per region evaluated by 15 of the highest prevalent skin diseases. The four regions evaluated were Africa, Asia, North and South America, and Europe.[6] (Source: Institute for Health Metrics and Evaluation. Used with permission. All rights reserved.)

SKIN COLOR MEASUREMENT BY COLORIMETRY

Colorimeters and spectrophotometers can be used to obtain noninvasive, reproducible, and more objective measures of skin color. Colorimetry can provide a quantitative measurement of skin color that incorporates erythema, level of pigmentation, total melanin content, and tanning ability. Spectrophotometers are colorimetric devices that measure the spectral composition of light in skin, thus conferring a measure of absolute color. Colorimetry and spectrophotometry are not only standardized techniques for skin color measurement but also useful tools for assessing healing, bruises, and efficacy of treatment in patients with darker skin and melasma or atopic dermatitis.[21] Unfortunately, the drawbacks of these measures are that they are not widely available in clinical practice and require frequent calibration.

EPIDEMIOLOGY OF CUTANEOUS DISEASES IN SKIN OF COLOR

Despite longstanding awareness of the importance of differences in the epidemiology of cutaneous diseases in skin of color (SOC), comprehensive data are still lacking.[23] While further research is needed to gain a better understanding of the disparities experienced by patients with SOC, some studies suggest differences in epidemiologic trends in these populations. A retrospective cohort study conducted in the outpatient Henry Ford Health System in United States sought to identify the most common dermatologic diagnoses among over 60,000 new patients between 2013 and 2016 by race/ethnic category. They found that Black/African Americans exhibited a higher prevalence of eczema or dermatitis, adnexal disease (acne, hidradenitis suppurativa, rosacea, and hyperhidrosis), and follicular disorders (alopecia areata, androgenic alopecia, cicatricial alopecia, and hirsutism).[24] In contrast, Blacks and Hispanics had lower rates of skin cancer. Similarly, other studies have found that although White patients have the highest overall skin cancer rates, patients with SOC are more likely to be diagnosed at later stages and have worse outcomes.[25,26]

Patients with SOC may present with morphology that is less commonly taught and therefore less likely to be recognized by providers. For example, patients with SOC and atopic dermatitis tend have more truncal and extensor involvement, along with distinct lesions of papular or perifollicular morphology,[27] as compared to the classically described presentation involving flexural lesions more commonly highlighted in textbooks. Recognition of erythema is another example that is important for the diagnosis of multiple dermatologic conditions such as psoriasis, cutaneous T-cell lymphoma, hidradenitis suppurativa, and melanoma. Among Black, Asian, and Hispanic/Latine patients, erythema may appear more violaceous or hyperpigmented and can be overlooked during clinical examination, leading to delays in diagnosis among patients with SOC.[28] Multiple studies have shown that photographs of patients with darker skin tones are less common in dermatology textbooks[29] and the medical literature,[30] which can lead to underrecognition and misdiagnosis of dermatologic conditions among patients with SOC.[31-33]

Treatment patterns have also been reported to vary in patients with SOC for common cutaneous conditions. For example, multiple studies have found that patients who identify as Black or Hispanic/Latine or had Medicaid (as compared to White patients or those with private insurance) were less likely to receive acne prescriptions.[34,35] Another study found that patients with SOC were less likely to receive isotretinoin, regardless of insurance status.[36] There have been similar findings for other common conditions. For example, a large, cross-sectional U.S. study found that patients with SOC were also less likely to receive new systemic treatments such as biologics for psoriasis and atopic dermatitis than White patients.[28]

ACCESS TO DERMATOLOGIC CARE

BARRIERS TO ACCESS

The availability of dermatologists and socioeconomic factors create challenges for patients of color to access dermatologic care. On average, there are 3.4 dermatologists per 100,000 people in the United States, which is slightly less than the number needed to adequately care for the population.[37] This average obscures geographic disparities: dermatologists in the United States are primarily concentrated in costal urban areas and near academic centers and are less likely to practice in areas that have lower socioeconomic status, lower education levels, and a higher proportion of minoritized people. For example, it was found that 75% to 100% of counties with Black/African American, Hispanic/Latine American, and Native American majorities have no dermatologists.[38] These disparities are reflected in the number of dermatologist visits: in the United States, White individuals are twice as likely as Hispanic/Latine and Black individuals to have seen a dermatologist.[39] Insurance status also impacts dermatologist accessibility: compared to patients with private insurance, those with Medicaid are less likely to be able to schedule an appointment[39] and often have to wait longer for their appointments,[40] including for surgical treatment of melanoma.[41] Additional factors including clinician bias, language barriers, and distrust of the medical profession may also impact rates of care. Access to dermatologists is critical, as dermatology visits can reduce adverse events, hospitalization, and, in cases such as melanoma, even death.

WORKPLACE DIVERSITY IN DERMATOLOGY

The American Association of Medical Colleges (AAMC) identifies racial and ethnic groups that are underrepresented in medicine (URM) relative to their numbers in the general population, which most commonly include Black, Hispanic/Latine, and Native American individuals. There are about one-third as many URM dermatologists as in the general population, and dermatology ranks below nearly every other medical specialty in terms of diversity.[42] This is important because race-concordant visits are associated with increased patient satisfaction and patient perception that their physician is engaged[43] but remain a challenge to implement due to the lack of workplace diversity in dermatology.

There has been a push for dermatology residency programs to address the lack of diversity by holistic review of prospective candidates and recruitment and retention of diverse mentors. Multiple dermatologic organizations are working together advance inclusivity in dermatology through programming, education, and advocacy.

CONCLUSION

Epidemiology is the study of diseases in a population in relation to the characteristics of individuals and their environment. It is used to understand the pathogenesis of diseases, improve diagnostic accuracy, help reduce risk factors, and identify the best therapeutic approaches. Epidemiologic studies can be experimental or observational in nature and can determine incidence, prevalence, morbidity, and burden of disease, which are valuable measures of disease frequency that can inform research and clinical practice. From 1990 to 2019, the global burden of cutaneous diseases has remained constant, although regional and socioeconomic differences exist. Dermatitis, acne vulgaris, and scabies contribute the largest nonfatal burden globally, whereas melanoma and nonmelanoma skin cancer are the leading causes of mortality.

Data on the epidemiology on SOC are limited by the lack of standardized, widely available measurement tools. Skin color measurement has clinical and investigative relevance, as it may serve as an indicator of disease severity or treatment progression. To this end, objective measures such as colorimetry provide a more useful measure of skin color than the previously developed Fitzpatrick scale but are not widely available in general clinical practice. Moreover, racial and ethnic minoritized individuals are underrepresented in clinical trials and are less likely to access dermatologic care due to a variety of issues including insurance barriers and a lack of dermatologists in areas with a higher proportion of historically marginalized individuals. Efforts to diversify the dermatology workforce and research could help to mitigate healthcare disparities.

REFERENCES

1. Gordis L. *Epidemiology*. 5th ed. Philadelphia, PA: Elsevier/Saunders; 2014.
2. Hessel F. Burden of disease. In: Kirch W, ed. *Encyclopedia of Public Health*. Dordrecht, the Netherlands: Springer Netherlands; 2008:94-96.
3. Glanville J, Eyers J, Jones AM, et al. Quasi-experimental study designs series—paper 8: identifying quasi-experimental studies to inform systematic reviews. *J Clin Epidemiol*. 2017;89:67-76.
4. Naik HB, Abuabara K. Systematic reviews of case reports and case series: from anecdote to evidence. *Br J Dermatol*. 2018;178(2):317-318.
5. Hollestein LM, Nijsten T. An insight into the global burden of skin diseases. *J Invest Dermatol*. 2014;134(6):1499-1501.
6. The Institute for Health Metrics and Evaluation. GBD compare data visualization. In: University of Washington, ed. Bill & Melinda Gates Foundation, trans. Seattle, WA: IHME; 2020.
7. Urban K, Chu S, Giesey RL, et al. Burden of skin disease and associated socioeconomic status in Asia: a cross-sectional analysis from the Global Burden of Disease Study 1990-2017. *JAAD Int*. 2021;2:40-50.
8. Xue Y, Zhou J, Xu BN, et al. Global burden of bacterial skin diseases: a systematic analysis combined with sociodemographic index, 1990-2019. *Front Med (Lausanne)*. 2022;9:861115.
9. Lott JP, Gross CP. Mortality from nonneoplastic skin disease in the United States. *J Am Acad Dermatol*. 2014;70(1):47-54.e41.
10. Laughter MR, Maymone MBC, Mashayekhi S, et al. The global burden of atopic dermatitis: lessons from the Global Burden of Disease Study 1990-2017. *Br J Dermatol*. 2021;184(2):304-309.
11. Chan LN, Magyari A, Ye M, et al. The epidemiology of atopic dermatitis in older adults: a population-based study in the United Kingdom. *PLoS One*. 2021;16(10):e0258219.
12. Layton AM, Thiboutot D, Tan J. Reviewing the global burden of acne: how could we improve care to reduce the burden? *Br J Dermatol*. 2021;184(2):219-225.
13. Institute for Health Metrics and Evaluation. GBD results. https://www.healthdata.org/data-tools-practices/interactive-visuals/gbd-results/. Accessed August 2, 2024.
14. Hagstrom EL, Patel S, Karimkhani C, et al. Comparing cutaneous research funded by the US National Institutes of Health (NIH) with the US skin disease burden. *J Am Acad Dermatol*. 2015;73(3):383-391.e381.
15. Pulsipher KJ, Szeto MD, Rundle CW, Presley CL, Laughter MR, Dellavalle RP. Global burden of skin disease representation in the literature: bibliometric analysis. *JMIR Dermatol*. 2021;4(2):e29282.
16. Lu JD, Tiwana S, Das P, Siddiqi J, Khosa F. Gender and racial underrepresentation in academic dermatology positions in the United States: a retrospective, cross-sectional study from 2007 to 2018. *J Am Acad Dermatol*. 2020;83(5):1513-1516.
17. Hill KA, Desai MM, Chaudhry SI, Nguyen M, Boatright D. NIH diversity supplement awards by year and administering institute. *JAMA*. 2021;326(23):2427-2429.
18. Ferguson JE, Vetos D, Ho BV, et al. Trends in diversity of participants in dermatology clinical trials over time: a systematic review. *J Am Acad Dermatol*. 2022;86(6):1403-1405.
19. Chen V, Akhtar S, Zheng C, Kumaresan V, Nouri K. Assessment of changes in diversity in dermatology clinical trials between 2010-2015 and 2015-2020: a systematic review. *JAMA Dermatol*. 2022;158(3):288-292.
20. George S, Duran N, Norris K. A systematic review of barriers and facilitators to minority research participation among African Americans, Latinos, Asian Americans, and Pacific Islanders. *Am J Public Health*. 2014;104(2):e16-31.
21. Ly BCK, Dyer EB, Feig JL, Chien AL, Del Bino S. Research techniques made simple: cutaneous colorimetry: a reliable technique for objective skin color measurement. *J Invest Dermatol*. 2020;140(1):3-12.e11.
22. Reddy KK, Lenzy YM, Brown KL, Gilchrest BA. Chapter 9. Racial considerations: skin of color. In: Goldsmith LA, Katz SI, Gilchrest BA, Paller AS, Leffell DJ, Wolff K, eds. *Fitzpatrick's Dermatology in General Medicine*. 8th ed. New York, NY: The McGraw Hill Companies; 2012.
23. Taylor SC. Epidemiology of skin diseases in people of color. *Cutis*. 2003;71(4):271-275.
24. Gaulding JV, Gutierrez D, Bhatia BK, et al. Epidemiology of skin diseases in a diverse patient population. *J Drugs Dermatol*. 2018;17(10):1032-1036.
25. Shao K, Hooper J, Feng H. Racial and ethnic health disparities in dermatology in the United States. Part 2: disease-specific epidemiology, characteristics, management, and outcomes. *J Am Acad Dermatol*. 2022;87(4):733-744.
26. Qian Y, Johannet P, Sawyers A, Yu J, Osman I, Zhong J. The ongoing racial disparities in melanoma: an analysis of the Surveillance, Epidemiology, and End Results database (1975-2016). *J Am Acad Dermatol*. 2021;84(6):1585-1593.
27. Vachiramon V, Tey HL, Thompson AE, Yosipovitch G. Atopic dermatitis in African American children: addressing unmet needs of a common disease. *Pediatr Dermatol*. 2012;29(4):395-402.
28. Bell MA, Whang KA, Thomas J, Aguh C, Kwatra SG. Racial and ethnic disparities in access to emerging and frontline therapies in common dermatological conditions: a cross-sectional study. *J Natl Med Assoc*. 2020;112(6):650-653.
29. Adelekun A, Onyekaba G, Lipoff JB. Skin color in dermatology textbooks: an updated evaluation and analysis. *J Am Acad Dermatol*. 2021;84(1):194-196.
30. Lester JC, Jia JL, Zhang L, Okoye GA, Linos E. Absence of images of skin of colour in publications of COVID-19 skin manifestations. *Br J Dermatol*. 2020;183(3):593-595.
31. Kaufman BP, Guttman-Yassky E, Alexis AF. Atopic dermatitis in diverse racial and ethnic groups—variations in epidemiology, genetics, clinical presentation and treatment. *Exp Dermatol*. 2018;27(4):340-357.
32. Tadesse GA, Cintas C, Varshney KR, et al. Skin Tone Analysis for Representation in Educational Materials (STAR-ED) using machine learning. *NPJ Dig Med*. 2023;6(1):151.
33. Martin GC, Kirgis J, Sid E, Sabin JA. Equitable imagery in the preclinical medical school curriculum: findings from one medical school. *Acad Med*. 2016;91(7):1002-1006.
34. Patel VM, Schwartz RA. Disparities in access to a dermatologist for acne care in the United States. *Int J Dermatol*. 2017;56(6):e131-e133.
35. Barbieri JS, Shin DB, Wang S, Margolis DJ, Takeshita J. Association of race/ethnicity and sex with differences in health care use and treatment for acne. *JAMA Dermatol*. 2020;156(3):312-319.
36. Fleischer AB, Simpson JK, McMichael A, Feldman SR. Are there racial and sex differences in the use of oral isotretinoin for acne management in the United States? *J Am Acad Dermatol*. 2003;49(4):662-666.
37. Glazer AM, Farberg AS, Winkelmann RR, Rigel DS. Analysis of trends in geographic distribution and density of US dermatologists. *JAMA Dermatol*. 2017;153(4):322-325.
38. Vaidya T, Zubritsky L, Alikhan A, Housholder A. Socioeconomic and geographic barriers to dermatology care in urban and rural US populations. *J Am Acad Dermatol*. 2018;78(2):406-408.
39. Tripathi R, Knusel KD, Ezaldein HH, Scott JF, Bordeaux JS. Association of demographic and socioeconomic characteristics with differences in use of outpatient dermatology services in the United States. *JAMA Dermatol*. 2018;154(11):1286-1291.
40. Creadore A, Desai S, Li SJ, et al. Insurance acceptance, appointment wait time, and dermatologist access across practice types in the US. *JAMA Dermatol*. 2021;157(2):181-188.
41. Adamson AS, Zhou L, Baggett CD, Thomas NE, Meyer AM. Association of delays in surgery for melanoma with insurance type. *JAMA Dermatol*. 2017;153(11):1106-1113.
42. Xierali IM, Castillo-Page L, Zhang K, Gampfer KR, Nivet MA. AM last page: the urgency of physician workforce diversity. *Acad Med*. 2014;89(8):1192.
43. Cooper LA, Roter DL, Johnson RL, Ford DE, Steinwachs DM, Powe NR. Patient-centered communication, ratings of care, and concordance of patient and physician race. *Ann Intern Med*. 2003;139(11):907-915.

CHAPTER 3

Culturally Informed Dermatological Care

Shamaila Khan
Tahirah Abdullah

KEY POINTS

- Disparities in dermatologic diseases can be partially accounted for by the quality of the patient-physician interaction and necessitate that clinicians be more culturally informed or aware.
- Cultural competence is the ability to engage knowledgeably with people across cultures.

- Cultural humility involves understanding that a clinician will never be fully competent about the evolving and dynamic nature of a patient's experiences.
- Cultural competence must be embedded in a framework of cultural humility to be effective.
- A crucial way to build cultural competence and cultural humility into a healthcare system is with representation.

INTRODUCTION

Patient populations around the world are becoming increasingly diverse, introducing a variety of health behaviors that are influenced by a patient's cultural background and identities. Clinicians and healthcare organizations have a growing responsibility to improve inclusive efforts to better serve patients, and studies have suggested culturally attuned care improves patient adherence, satisfaction, and, ultimately, health outcome.[1] Yet, almost half (47%) of dermatologists and dermatology residents surveyed reported that they had not received adequate training to prepare them to work with communities of color, in particular Black patients' dermatological concerns.[2] In addition, another study revealed that only about half of dermatology chief residents (52.4%) reported that their residency programs include skin of color explicitly as part of the training curriculum.[3]

In U.S. society, there is often an implicit and unconscious perception of lighter skin tones as the norm or standard. This perception can contribute to the disproportionately fewer depictions of skin of color in dermatology textbooks and dermatologists receiving less training with persons of color.[4] As a result, dermatologists may be more prone to diagnostic challenges when treating patients with skin of color and may inadvertently communicate exclusionary messages, whether through biases or misunderstandings. Thus, there is a clear need for dermatologists to receive training with a specific focus on the unique presentations and needs of patients with skin of color.

As such, this chapter will briefly explore the historical context of colorism, which continues to shape the experiences of patients, dermatologists, and their interactions. It will also examine multicultural frameworks such as cultural competence and cultural humility, highlighting their relevance and value in guiding clinical care within healthcare systems influenced by social challenges that affect access and outcomes.

COLORISM

Colorism is of great importance when considering the understandings and meanings one may internalize and ascribe to their skin color. Colorism is defined as discrimination, preferential treatment, and privileging due to skin complexion, such that lighter complexions are preferred and privileged over darker complexions.[5] In the United States, the history of colorism is rooted in slavery, wherein ascribed inferiority as a result of darker skin color was used as a justification for enslaving Africans. Further, enslaved people were stratified by skin color and those with darker skin were required to do manual, outdoor labor, while those with lighter skin were required to do domestic tasks.[6] Despite the legal abolition of slavery in the United States in 1865, colorism remains ever-present in U.S. society. While perceptions of "light" and "dark" skin are subjective, several studies suggest that people of color with lighter complexions have more favorable outcomes than those with darker complexions, including higher financial earning, higher educational attainment, and shorter prison sentences.[6-9]

Colorism is also deeply intertwined with ideals of beauty that have been shaped by history and the global promotion of Eurocentric beauty standards. These ideals have influenced skin-lightening practices worldwide. The global market for skin-lightening products—many of which suppress melanin production—continues to thrive, particularly in Africa, Asia, Latin America, and the Caribbean. Despite known health risks, these products remain in demand. In recent years, however, there has been a growing movement to challenge these beauty standards and celebrate the beauty of darker skin tones. Notably, countries such as South Africa, Ghana, Rwanda, and India have taken legislative steps to ban or regulate harmful skin-lightening products.[10-12]

In dermatology, awareness of colorism is essential—especially as more patients with richly pigmented skin seek care for pigmentation concerns, such as hyperpigmentation and hypopigmentation. Dermatologists must consider how societal attitudes toward skin color may influence patients' cosmetic concerns and treatment choices. The use of skin-lightening agents on healthy skin also raises important ethical questions about the role of dermatologists in reinforcing or challenging colorist beauty ideals.

Pause for self-reflection: What messages have you heard explicitly or implicitly about skin color? What has reinforced those messages? What can you do to counteract those messages?

CULTURAL COMPETENCE AND HUMILITY

Lack of cultural competence and humility in the training curricula can prevent dermatologists from effectively treating patients with darker skin and may perpetuate patients' historically rooted fears of being exploited. Given that 50% of the United States is estimated to be populated by people of color by 2050,[13] it is even more pertinent to consider the upstream determinants of care of cultural competence and humility [**Figure 3-1**]. A commitment to other-oriented awareness has been made apparent in healthcare overall,[14] and this necessitates that providers be equipped to recognize and treat illnesses in patients of every skin tone.

CULTURE AND WHY WE NEED THIS IN HEALTHCARE

Culture is the conceptual system developed by a community or society to structure individuals and how they view the world. It involves a particular set of beliefs, norms, and values that influence ideas about relationships, how people live their lives, and the way people organize their world.[15] Culture is not an apparent entity to which people belong or do not belong. People belong to multiple cultural groups and manage multiple cultural expectations on an ongoing basis. These expectations, or cultural norms, are the explicit or implicit and unspoken rules or standards. The word "culture" is sometimes applied to groups formed on the basis of age, race, gender, socioeconomic status, disability, sexual orientation, faith/religion, language, or other social identities [refer to Figure 3-1]. Clinicians ought to understand that each patient embraces their culture(s) in a unique way and that there is considerable diversity within and across races, ethnicities, and culture heritages and that there are subcultures that exist within larger culture.

Disparities in dermatologic diseases, as discussed in Chapter 11, can be partially accounted for by the quality of the patient-physician interaction and necessitate that clinicians be more culturally attuned or aware. Culturally responsive skills can improve patient engagement in healthcare services, therapeutic relationships between patients and clinicians, and treatment retention and outcomes. Cultural competence and humility are essential ingredients in decreasing overall disparities in healthcare. In addition to the other-oriented awareness, it is critical that clinician's self-awareness also be necessitated and considered, when working with patients. As per Khan,[16] to address this other-oriented and self-oriented awareness, the notions of cultural competence and cultural humility in tandem are necessary for effective treatment, as further explicated below.

CULTURAL COMPETENCE

Cultural competence is loosely defined as the ability to engage knowledgeably with people across cultures. It's a product of the 1960s and 1970s, grounded in the sociopolitical climate of the civil rights movements. It has also been referred to as "a set of behaviors, attitudes, and policies that ... enable a system, agency, or group of professionals to work effectively in cross cultural situations" (p. 13).[17] The term hence became ubiquitous in healthcare, with an assumption that the more knowledge we have about another culture, the greater the competence in practice. However, cultural competence has been critiqued for several reasons. First, it suggests that

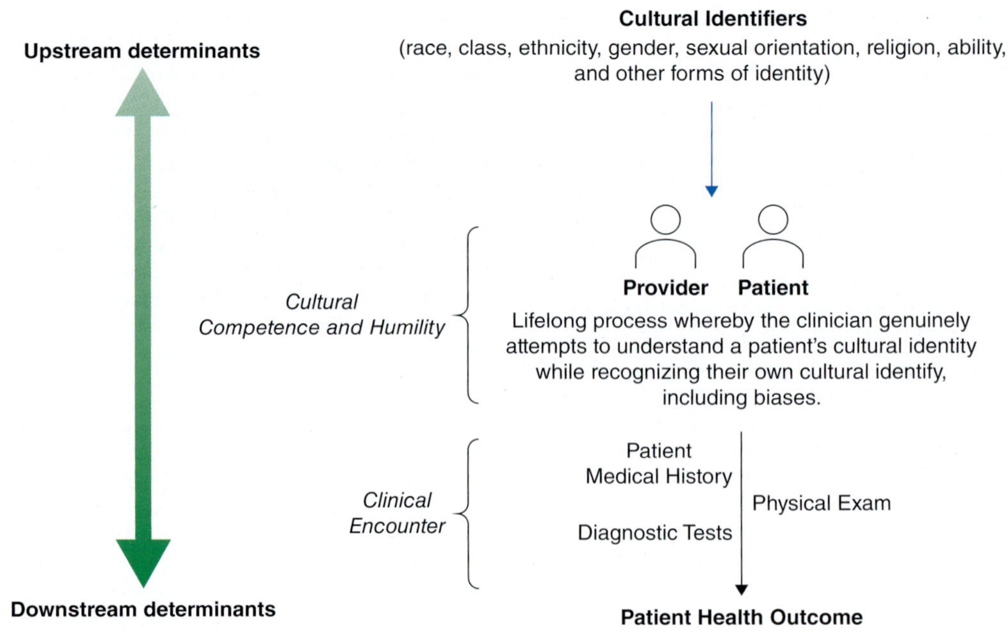

FIGURE 3-1. Cultural competence and cultural humility.

there is categorical knowledge a person could attain about a group of people, and this oversimplification leads to stereotyping and bias. Cultural competence also does not fully address the complex social and historical factors that influence patient experiences, and thus provides a superficial, identity-only means of increasing knowledge and awareness. Further, the language of "competence" suggests that there is an endpoint to becoming fully culturally knowledgeable and aware. The reality is that this would be impossible given the sheer amount of variation in culture and identity, the individual differences in the ways culture and identity are expressed, the ever-changing nature of culture and identity itself, the language used to describe it, and how it is constructed in a given society at a given time.

These critiques contributed to the shift from cultural competence frameworks to those of cultural humility and sensitivity. The term "cultural humility" was introduced in 1998 as a dynamic and lifelong process focusing on self-reflection and personal critique, acknowledging one's own biases. It recognizes the shifting nature of intersecting identities and encourages ongoing curiosity rather than an endpoint. Cultural humility involves understanding the complexity of identities—that even in sameness there is difference—and that a clinician will never be fully competent about the evolving and dynamic nature of a patient's experiences.

HOW TO DEVELOP CULTURAL HUMILITY

At its base, cultural humility means opening a conversation in a way that genuinely attempts to understand a person's identities related to race and ethnicity, gender, sexual orientation, socioeconomic status, education, social needs, and others. An awareness of the self is central to the notion of cultural humility—who a person is informs how they see another.

Culturally attuned clinicians are aware of their own cultural backgrounds and values, their privileged and marginalized identities, and they acknowledge their own assumptions and biases about other individuals and cultures. Moreover, they aim to understand how their assumptions and biases impact their capacity to provide culturally responsive services to patients from similar or diverse cultural backgrounds. Clinicians ought to begin the process of becoming culturally attuned by identifying and exploring their own cultural history and worldview along with understanding how this informs their clinical worldview, shaping their perceptions of the treatment process. Hence, understanding ourselves as clinicians and how our culture and values impact the clinical process is a key component of being a culturally aware and attuned clinician. As such, the writers of this chapter identify as: (1) A Pakistani American, Muslim, cisgender, heterosexual, married, immigrant, nondisabled woman, who has lived in three different continents. (2) A Black, African American, Muslim, cisgender, heterosexual, married, nondisabled woman who was born and raised in the U.S. South.

We have dug deep and explored aspects of our identities and the associated marginalized and privileged parts, and the ways in which these may possibly play out in our clinical work with patients. Despite this, there is an awareness that we may still have blind spots that may lead to biases. How the individual clinician and patient see and understand health and illness is very much tied to their respective cultural beliefs and views. As culture impacts the way in which an individual beholds the world, it also naturally impacts the way that the individual sees health and illness. A clinician who is aware, attuned, and can appreciate the role of culture as it may impact the patient's receptivity to treatments, is much better positioned to form a strong working alliance with the patient, and in the long run, gain the patient's cooperation in their own treatment. It is pertinent for clinicians to recognize that all cultures have systems of health beliefs that explain what causes illness, how it can be managed, or treated, and who ought to be involved in the process.

With this awareness, a clinician can ask questions about how they receive the patient: Who is this person? What knowledge and awareness do I have about their culture? What thoughts and feelings emerge from me about them?

Pause for self-reflection: Which parts of my identity am I aware of? Which are most salient? Which parts of my identity are privileged and/or marginalized? How does my sense of identity shift based on context and settings? What are the parts onto which people project? And which parts are received well, by whom? What might be my own blind spots and biases?

CULTURAL COMPETENCE AND CULTURAL HUMILITY TOGETHER

Despite the aforementioned valid critiques of cultural competence, some aspects drawn from the movement provide important guidance. For instance, a "culturally competent" clinician needs to have knowledge and awareness of:

- health-related beliefs, practices, and cultural values of diverse populations;
- illness and diagnostic incidence and prevalence among culturally/ethnically diverse populations;
- treatment efficacy data (if any) of culturally and ethnically diverse populations.

Still, cultural competence must be embedded in a framework of cultural humility to be effective. A clinician operating with cultural humility must listen with interest and curiosity, have an awareness of their own possible biases and attempt a nonjudgmental stance about what they hear, and recognize their inherent status of privilege as a provider and be willing to be taught by their patients. Utilizing one of these frameworks without the other misses the mark, and effective interventions would uphold both. However, intertwining cultural humility and competence into healthcare, ideally, would go beyond individual clinicians and their patients.

RELATIONSHIP BETWEEN CULTURAL HUMILITY AND STRUCTURAL HUMLITY

Racism, sexism, ableism—all of these 'isms and others—are embedded in the world at large and trickle down to national levels, state levels, institutions, and systems of care and how policies and procedures are established. It is imperative that healthcare clinicians are aware of and troubled by these inequities.

Cultural humility as already noted facilitates respect and appreciation for diversity that is active, multifaceted, and shifting. Embracing this approach on a systemic level is equally critical in evaluating and resolving systemic practices that may contribute to health disparities at large. For this reason, clinical training is in need of a shift from a sole focus on the individual encounter to include the organization, the institutions and policies, as well as of neighborhoods and cities, for clinicians to more effectively impact health disparites.[18]

The variables of race, class, gender, ethnicity, religion, ability, and their intersections are shaped both by the interactions of two persons in a room and by the larger structural contexts in which their interactions take place. According to Yan Li et al, these include, and are not limited to, "the historical evolution of healthcare for people with skin of color, systemic discriminatory practices, the current landscape of financial payers and care reimbursement (private vs public insurances), healthcare organizational infrastructure (for-profit vs public/municipal facilities, etc), the settings in which care is delivered (medical facilities, schools, correctional facilities, home based), and the demographics of the workforce providing care" (p. 252).[19] Structural humility therefore challenges health professionals to work "outside of the four walls of the clinic" in order to collaborate and seek the expertise of others (including patients, community-based organizations or other non-health sector agencies, ie, like housing agencies or schools) when responding to aspects of the infrastructure that perpetuate disparities.[20] Structural humility builds upon the existing social determinants of health (see Chapter 11), cultural competency, and cultural humility. It conveys that to reduce disparities in health, we must also address the systems and structures outside the control of the individual patient [**Figure 3-2**].

BUILDING CULTURAL COMPETENCE AND HUMILITY IN HEALTHCARE INSTITUTIONS

A crucial way to build cultural competence and humility into a healthcare system is with representation. A diverse workforce is essential, but it doesn't stop there. It includes revising our curriculums, trainings, policies, and procedures to reflect a broader range of experiences; it includes having a diverse student body, faculty, and administrators; and it includes not just recruitment but retention of students/faculty from underrepresented and communities made vulnerable. To truly be multiculturally attuned clinicians who uphold values of cultural humility and cultural competence, promote health equity, and work to improve access to care necessitates that clinicians understand how these 'isms are operational within the systems in which they provide services. For this, cultural competence and humility/sensitivity trainings are essential on an individual as well as on a systemic and structural level. One challenge is that healthcare executives, clinicians, and others working in the system aren't having honest, authentic conversations about systemic or individual biases because it makes them uncomfortable. Everyone has biases. Avoiding or concealing them only escalates the problem. Instead, healthcare institutions and providers need to raise them to the surface and become more comfortable with having uncomfortable conversations to effect change.

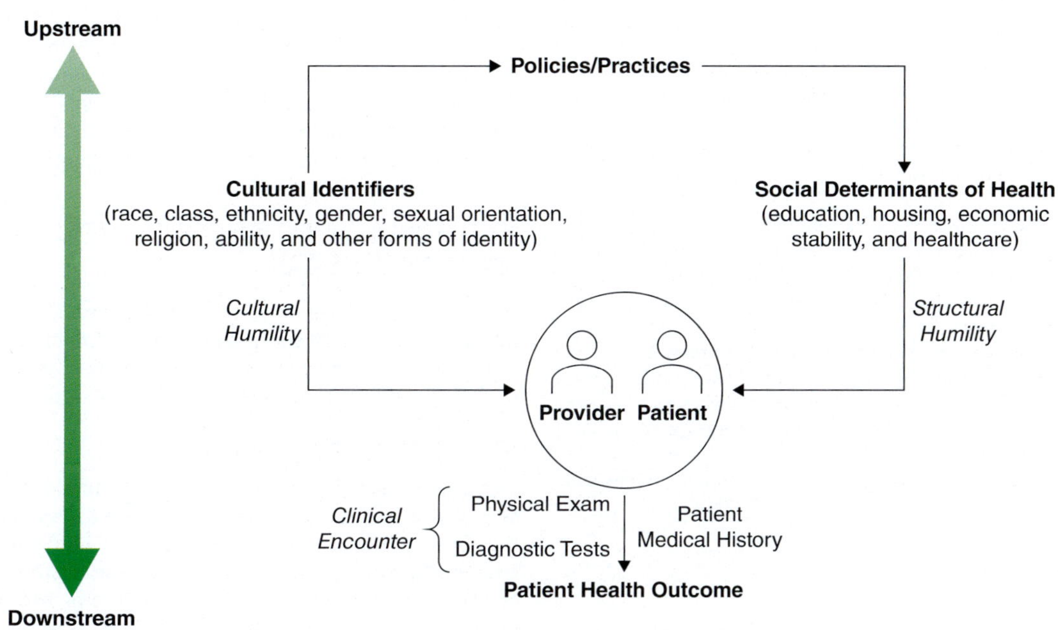

FIGURE 3-2. Determinants of equitable patient care.

It's imperative to reckon with the complexity of these cultural terms and not shift to either-or binaries amid already problematic and polarized us-them dichotomies at the core of these challenges.

REFERENCES

1. McKesey J, Berger TG, Lim HW, McMichael AJ, Torres A, Pandya AG. Cultural competence for the 21st century dermatologist practicing in the United States. *J Am Acad Dermatol.* 2017;77(6):1159-1169.
2. Buster KJ, Stevens EI, Elmets CA. Dermatologic health disparities. *Dermatol Clin.* 2012;30(1):53-59.
3. Nijhawan RI, Jacob SE, Woolery-Lloyd H. Skin of color education in dermatology residency programs: does residency training reflect the changing demographics of the United States? *J Am Acad Dermatol.* 2008;59(4):615-618.
4. Paradies Y, Ben J, Denson N, et al. Racism as a determinant of health: a systematic review and meta-analysis. *PloS One.* 2015;10(9):e0138511.
5. Dixon AR, Telles EE. Skin color and colorism: global research, concepts, and measurement. *Annu Rev Sociol.* 2017;43(1):405-424.
6. Ryabov I, Goza, FW. Phenotyping and adolescence-to-adulthood transitions among Latinos. *Race Soc Probl.* 2014;6:342-355.
7. Hunter M. The persistent problem of colorism: skin tone, status, and inequality. *Sociol Compass.* 2007;1(1):237-254.
8. Ryabov I. Colorism and educational outcomes of Asian Americans: evidence from the National Longitudinal Study of Adolescent Health. *Soc Psychol Educ.* 2016;19:303-324.
9. Viglione J, Hannon L, DeFina, R. The impact of light skin on prison time for Black female offenders. *Soc Sci J.* 2011;48(1):250-258.
10. Garcia SE. Rwanda cracks down on skin bleaching agents by seizing cosmetics. The New York Times. https://www.nytimes.com/2019/01/09/world/africa/skin-bleaching-banned-rwanda.html. Accessed September 24, 2023.
11. Pandey G. Fair and Lovely: can renaming a fairness cream stop colourism? BBC News. https://www.bbc.com/news/world-asia-india-53182169. Accessed January 3, 2024.
12. Pollock S, Taylor S, Oyerinde O, et al. The dark side of skin lightening: an international collaboration and review of a public health issue affecting dermatology. *Int J Women's Dermatol.* 2021;7(2):158-164.
13. U.S. Census Bureau. U.S. Census Bureau projections show a slower growing, older, more diverse nation a half century from now. http://www.census.gov/newsroom/releases/archives/population/cb12-243.html. Accessed August 29, 2022.
14. Williams DR, Rucker TD. Understanding and addressing racial disparities in health care. *Health Care Financ Rev.* 2000;21(4):75-90.
15. U.S. Department of Health and Human Services. Mental Health: Culture, Race, and Ethnicity. A Supplement to Mental Health: A Report of the Surgeon General. HHS Publication No. (SMA) 01-3613. Rockville, MD: U.S. Department of Health and Human Services, Substance Abuse and Mental Health Services Administration, Center for Mental Health Services; 2001.
16. Khan S. Cultural humility vs. cultural competence—and why providers need both. Health City Newsletter. https://www.bmc.org/healthcity/policy-and-industry/cultural-humility-vs-cultural-competence-providers-need-both?utm_campaign=healthcity&utm_medium=morning-buzz&utm_source=morning-buzz&utm_content=Cultural-Humility. Accessed January 3, 2024.
17. Cross, TL, Bazron, BJ., Dennis, KW, Isaacs MR. *Towards a Culturally Competent System of Care: A Monograph on Effective Services for Minority Children Who Are Severely Emotionally Disturbed*, Vol. 1. Washington, DC: Georgetown University Child Development Center; 1989.
18. Metzl JM, Hansen H. Structural competency: theorizing a new medical engagement with stigma and inequality. *Soc Sci Med.* 2014;103:126-133.
19. Yan Li AS, Lang Q, Cho J, Nguyen VS, Nandakumar S. Cultural and structural humility and addressing systems of care disparities in mental health services for Black, Indigenous, and People of Color Youth. *Child Adolescent Psychiatry Clin N Am.* 2022;31(2):251-259.
20. Amarasekera U. Helen Hansen: developing structural humility in medicine. *Lancet.* 2022;399(10340):2007.

CHAPTER 4

Historical and Sociocultural Influences on Healthcare Practices: An Overview

Karla L. Valdés Morales
Valerie Sofia Encarnacion-Cortes
Aileen Y. Chang
Rebecca Vasquez

KEY POINTS

- The modern-day healthcare system is heavily influenced by historical events and paradigms that have shaped the health and perception of ethnoracial communities.
- Learning about the culture of different ethnic groups (along with the difficulties they may face) can challenge existing perceptions and improve patient-physician communication along with health outcomes.
- The social ecological model represents a framework for understanding how exposures across different levels (individual, interpersonal, community, societal) and other domains may contribute to disease distribution among ethnoracial groups.
- With intentional effort, dermatologists can make meaningful adjustments within education, the community, the workforce, health policy, and research to advance health equity.

INTRODUCTION

Numerous studies have shown that communities of color, especially minoritized ethnoracial groups, experience burdens of disease and health risk at disproportionate rates. While the sources of these disparities are complex, they can be traced to historical and sociocultural influences on health and healthcare practices.[1] Improving the overall health of communities of color relies not only on understanding their cultural perspectives on health, communication preferences, and traditional practices but also on the role of social determinants of health that drive disparities in health outcomes. This chapter (and subsequent chapters in this section) will explore the impact of historical and sociocultural influences among communities of color that contribute to health. The final section of this chapter will conclude with a discussion on the social ecological model, which presents a framework for understanding how exposures across different levels (including the individual, group/community, and the physical, social, and political environments) may contribute to disease distribution among ethnoracial groups.[2] The goal is to consider this approach while working toward elucidating and eliminating the drivers of illness among communities in order to promote health equity.

HISTORICAL INFLUENCES ON HEALTH AND HEALTHCARE

Before we can engage in meaningful dialogue about health and dermatologic care across diverse populations, it's important to understand the historical roots of how race has been socially constructed and applied in ways that continue to shape healthcare systems today.[3,4]

HISTORY OF RACE IN AMERICA

The modern concept of race in America developed alongside the rise of global economic systems such as colonialism and slavery. During the Enlightenment era, figures like Carl Linnaeus introduced early attempts to classify human populations into distinct categories.[5] These classifications—though now understood to be pseudoscientific—were used by early American settlers to support social and legal distinctions among groups, particularly between those of European descent and Indigenous peoples or individuals of African ancestry. Over time, these racial categories became embedded into law and policy, contributing to a societal structure in which access to opportunity and resources—including healthcare—was unevenly distributed. While civil rights legislation in the 1960s prohibited discrimination, implementation and enforcement have varied, and disparities continue to affect historically marginalized populations.[3,4]

As dermatologists, recognizing how these systemic factors have contributed to present-day differences in access, diagnosis, and outcomes is essential. A deeper understanding of these social determinants can help us provide more equitable, informed, and patient-centered care.

BIAS AND DISCRIMINATION

Clinicians are not exempt from holding biases, even towards racial and ethnic minoritized communities. Preconceived ideas among healthcare providers about behavior and attitudes from different racialized or ethnic groups may impact medical treatments and recommendations. Examples include undertreatment of pain in Black/African Americans related to false beliefs about biological differences between Black people's skin compared to their non-Hispanic White counterparts, underdiagnosis of diabetes among Asian Americans due to the model minority myth (stereotype that misleadingly portrays Asian Americans, as a collective group, as having achieved better social and health outcomes than other minoritized groups), and delayed recognition of anorexia nervosa in Black and Latine/Hispanic adolescents due to stereotypical association with upper middle class, White adolescents (see Chapter on Psychiatric Aspects of Skin of Color).[6-8] Some degree of bias has also been reported in the practice of dermatology, where according to a survey of 80 dermatologists, significantly more testing (including human immunodeficiency virus (HIV) and rapid plasma regain (RPR) testing) was recommended for patients with psoriasis who had medium to dark skin tones versus light skin tones.[9] This pattern may reflect longstanding trends in medical education materials, where images of sexually transmitted infections are disproportionately shown in patients with skin of color.[10]

How a clinician's attitude, expectations, and behavior in relation to a patient's racial and ethnic origin, along with a patient's own perceptions of a clinician of a particular cultural background, can affect and compromise the care delivering and care receiving process.[1] As a result, over the years, there has been an emphasis on developing an awareness of biases in the professional setting in order to mitigate disparities and promote health equity (see Chapter 3).

CULTURAL INFLUENCES ON HEALTH AND HEALTHCARE

How patients understand skin health, how they take care of their skin health, and how they make decisions related to their skin health are highly influenced by cultural perspectives, family traditions, social structure, and their worldview.[11,12] When caring for communities of color, improving misconceptions regarding skin conditions (especially skin cancer), together with satisfying expectations regarding delivery of care, are a just few important components to consider. For instance, in a study to learn about melanoma knowledge and perception among participants of skin of color (including an equal number of Black/African American, Latine/Hispanic, and Asian individuals for a total of 120 participants), many were not aware they could get melanoma on acral sites, let alone skin cancer, and requested more culturally relevant content from both providers and public materials (ie, images of acral melanoma in a person of color).[13-15] With respect to expectations regarding delivery of care, in a study surveying Black women being treated for hair loss, patients had a negative perception of the care they received from previous providers who did not offer to touch their hair, were unaware of their traditional hair routines, and lack shared life experiences.[16] Further studies to enhance strategies that improve delivery of culturally sensitive care in dermatology are needed.

Mistrust of clinicians based on historic factors such as persecution, segregation, and medical experimentation, as well as current issues of racism and discrimination, also play a role with respect to how different ethnoracial groups perceive their health and when they decide to seek care or medical evaluations.[1] These attitudes, although not generalizable to all members of a group, may pose health risks for communities of color. In caring for diverse populations, providers should employ cultural humility to address their patients, avoid cultural stereotyping, and consider both historic and sociocultural factors that influence health and healthcare practices.

CROSS-CULTURAL COMMUNICATION

Communication styles differ greatly among different cultural identities, and include both direct (verbal) and indirect (nonverbal) forms of communication. Although direct forms of communication may be preferred among individuals living in Western Europe and the United States, many individuals living outside of these regions rely heavily on indirect forms of communication, in which meanings are conveyed but not explicit, using body language, tone of voice, or other cues.[17] In addition, healthcare providers belong to professional cultures with their own medical terms or language. These terms are not familiar to patients or the larger community and hinder understanding of both written and spoken health messages that can be even further hindered when other cultural differences exist. The LEARN (Listen, Explain, Acknowledge, Recommend, Negotiate) model is a tool that was developed to help improve cross-cultural communication across different cultural identities [see **Table 4-1**].[17,18] In addition, a diverse medical workforce with fluency in non-English languages and mixed cultural backgrounds could improve cross-cultural communication that can enhance patient-provider communication and improve patient health outcomes.

TRADITIONAL MEDICINE AND RELIGION/SPIRITUALITY

Culturally based health practices have been in use since ancient times and continue to be an important means by which health is both maintained and sought.[19] Traditional medicine, as defined by the World Health Organization, is the collective knowledge, skills, and practices based on the theories, beliefs, and experiences indigenous to different cultures used in the maintenance of health, including prevention, diagnosis, improvement, or treatment of physical and mental illness.[20] Some traditional medicine systems are supported by huge volumes of literature and practical skills; others have been passed down from generation to generation through verbal teaching. In some parts of the world, much of the population continues to rely on their own traditional medicine to

TABLE 4-1 The LEARN model for cross-cultural communication[17,18]

	Definition	Other considerations
Learn	Assess patient's understanding of their skin condition	– Establish what is important to the patient – Observe body language and nonverbal cues
Explain	Convey your own perceptions of the skin condition	– Use translator when possible if language/communication challenges exist – Confirm understanding
Acknowledge	Be respectful when discussing differences between views	– Acknowledge differences in culture[a] – Show empathy
Recommend	Develop and propose a treatment plan for the patient	– Identify possible barriers to plan[b]
Negotiate	Reach an agreement on the treatment plan in collaboration with the patient	– Ensure plan is sensitive to patient's context (ie, incorporate culturally relevant approach) – When in doubt, ask the patient (or family) about their comfort with a particular plan. – Provide opportunity for follow up

[a]Learn about the patient's culture through library research, just as you might research an unfamiliar medical issue. Do so with the understanding that each patient may or may not fit the generalities provided in the literature.

[b]Take a careful history, which should include the patient's social situation and history of alternative therapies, and how healthcare decisions are made in the family. Take care to assess stressors the patient may be experiencing at home or at work.

meet their primary healthcare needs.[20] In the United States, about half of Americans report having tried some form of alternative medicine, such as herbal products, acupuncture, or other remedy, at some point during their lifetime.[21] In the Southwest, the influences of American Indian and Latine/Hispanic cultures are prominent, with traditional healing practices being widespread in both populations. Other widely used traditional medicine systems include those of China, India, and Africa (see Chapters 5-9).[20] The widespread use of traditional medicine necessitates that cultural humility also includes the ability to recognize other personal and professional cultural biases that may inadvertently marginalize patients who want to use traditional medicine.

No less important, religion and spirituality also play a dominant role in the health of many patients—from explaining the cause of a disease to providing a coping mechanism in the face of illness.[22] Because many patients turn to their religious beliefs when difficult healthcare decisions are made, it is vital for healthcare professionals to recognize and accommodate a patient's religious and spiritual needs. Health professionals should provide an opportunity for patients to discuss their religious and spiritual beliefs and tailor their evaluation and treatment to meet their specific needs, where possible.

ACCULTURATION

While acculturation—or the adoption and incorporation of attitudes, beliefs, behaviors, and norms from different cultures or from a new country—may have positive effects with regard to newcomers to the United States, including better socioeconomic profiles and increased occupational opportunities, the opposite is true for health outcomes.[23] Extended time in the United States may expose newcomers or immigrants to harmful sources of psychosocial stress (including racial and anti-immigrant discrimination) and enable adoption of unhealthy behaviors that can contribute to worse health outcomes.[23] For instance, among Latine/Hispanic individuals, acculturation has been linked with skin cancer-related behaviors such that Latine/Hispanic who become more acculturated to U.S. norms may develop less concern about the risk of skin cancer and engage in less sun-safe behavior.[24,25]

PRACTICING CULTURAL HUMILITY

In reality, not everyone with a shared culture will have the same expectation or attitudes about various aspects of their skin health. Understanding the complexities of identities—that even in sameness there is difference—is part of the practice of cultural humility (see Chapter 3 to learn more about cultural humilty). As a result, despite accumulating knowledge on the cultures, perspectives, and religions for different ethnoracial groups, the data do not replace a thorough discussion with patients to understand their individual and possibly culturally diverse beliefs and practices.

UNDERSTANDING DISEASE DISTRIBUTION USING A SOCIAL ECOLOGICAL MODEL

The overall health of individuals, and the populations of which they are part of, is perpetually influenced by and cannot be separated from the lived realities and context of their daily lives. Accordingly, the social ecological model understands health to be affected by the interaction between the individual, the group/community, and the physical, social, and political environments. Multiple frameworks or diagrammatic representations of the social ecological model currently exist.[26-29] "Ecosocial theory," one such framework, helps to conceptualize societal distributions of disease in relation to power, levels, life course, historical generation, biology, and ecosystems [see **Figure 4-1**].[2,30,31]

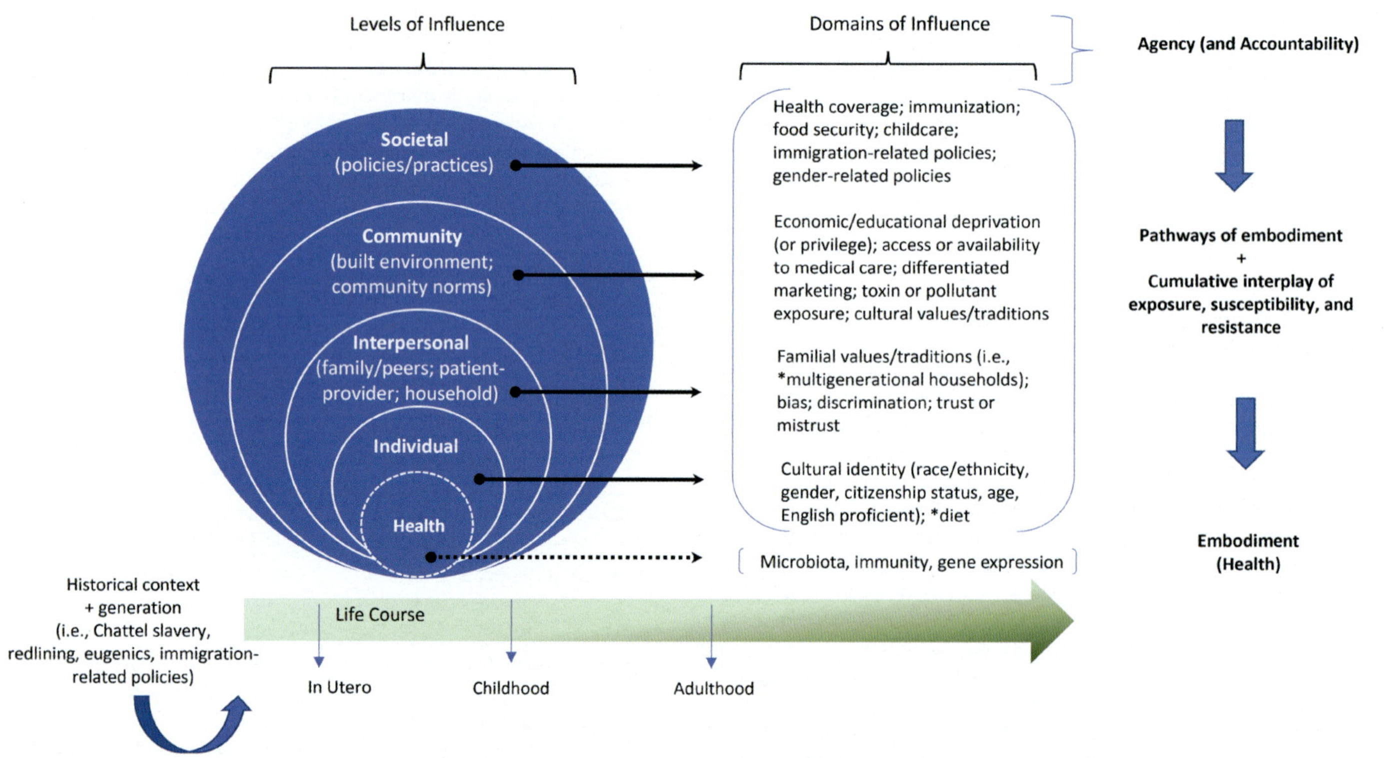

FIGURE 4-1. This figure illustrates how individuals, and the populations of which they are part of, are perpetually influenced by interpersonal relationships, their community, and societal institutions. Key constructs of the ecosocial theory (embodiment; pathways of embodiment; cumulative interplay of exposure, susceptibility, and resistance; accountability and agency) serve to elucidate how disease distributes among different groups/populations, via specified pathways operating at diverse levels/domains and throughout the life course, in historical context. For further explanation of these key constructs, please review Table 4-2. (Adapted from National Institute on Minority Health and Health Disparities Research Framework. 2018. https://www.nimhd.nih.gov/docs/research_framework/research-framework-slide.pdf. Accessed May 26, 2023; Models and Frameworks for the Practice of Community Engagement. 2015. https://www.atsdr.cdc.gov/communityengagement/pce_models.html. Accessed May 26, 2023; Braveman P, Egerter S. *Overcoming obstacles to health: report from the Robert Wood Johnson Foundation Commission to Build a Healthier America*. Princeton, NJ: Robert Wood Johnson Foundation; 2008; Krieger N. Methods for the scientific study of discrimination and health: an ecosocial approach. *Am J Public Health*. 2012;102(5):936-944.) Domains of influence include biological, behavioral, physical/built environment, sociocultural environment, and/or healthcare system.[26] *Multigenerational living and diet may be dually influenced by cultural norms and/or socioeconomic factors.

TABLE 4-2 Key constructs of the ecosocial theory

Key constructs	Explanation
Embodiment	Active process that refers to how an individual literally incorporates, biologically, the material and social world in which they live (from utero to death)
Pathways of Embodiment	Describes the different ways in which both historical and societal arrangements lead to adverse exposures (ie, exposure to toxins or other hazardous conditions) that facilitate embodiment
Cumulative interplay of exposure, susceptibility, and resistance across the life course	Describes how disease occurs in the individual (whether through gene expression, microbiota, or immunity) from embodied exposures over the life course
Accountability and agency	Elucidates policies, laws, or research that may explain disease distribution

Source: Adapted from Krieger N. Methods for the scientific study of discrimination and health: an ecosocial approach. *Am J Public Health.* 2012;102(5):936-944.

Proposed in the mid-1990s, a core foundational construct of the ecosocial theory is "embodiment" or the process by which the outside physical and social world becomes embedded in one's biology (see **Table 4-2** for key constructs of the ecosocial theory).[31] That is, how one's social, physical, and political environment "get under the skin" to contribute to health, thus producing population rates and distributions of health. Embodiment requires explicit consideration of the processes or pathways, simultaneously shaped by historical events, that lead to exposure(s) and facilitate embodiment that has the potential to impact generations. Moreover, the cumulative interplay of exposure with susceptibility and resistance across one's life course may influence biology by interacting with the host's microbiota, immunity, and/or genetics. We therefore live embodied: "genes" do not interact with exogenous (ie, outside the body) environments—only organisms do, with consequences for gene regulation and expression.[31] Finally, the ecosocial theory extends beyond conscious choices or psychosocial "risk factors" and emphasizes accountability to explain disease distribution.[32] It illuminates the impact of ideas, policies, laws, as well as research that can shape inequities in health.[30,31]

In dermatology, disparities in prevalence, incidence, or outcomes may reflect embodied expressions of social injustices or inequities. To illustrate, consider recent evidence implying that air pollutants (including environmental tobacco smoke, volatile organic compounds, and particular matter among others) act as an important risk factor for the development or aggravation of atopic dermatitis (AD).[33] A possible pathway of embodiment includes exposure to air pollutants over one's life course that could facilitate epigenetic changes and damage to the stratum corneum (even while in utero) through the generation of reactive oxygen species.[33,34] Black/African American, Latine/Hispanic, and American Indian communities are more frequently exposed to environmental hazards, pollutants, toxins, and other effects of poor housing, all of which are associated with AD.[35] Additionally, historical events (like redlining) have resulted in census tracts that have higher levels of hazardous air pollutants related to policies dictating highway placement and toxic waste sites targeting these redlined areas that are disproportionately inhabited by communities of color.[35] False beliefs about visible skin disease (like AD), and discrimination against patients from others can lead to social exclusion or isolation among individuals living with AD.[36]

Ultimately, it will take responding to the needs of patients beyond a biomedical model and incorporating social factors of health through advocacy across multiple levels (including patient, community, and system-level activities) so that every individual has a fair and just opportunity to be as healthy as possible.

ADVANCING HEALTH EQUITY

Although advancing health equity may seem like an enormous task, with intentional and empathetic actions, dermatologists can make meaningful adjustments that can directly impact patients' lives [**Figure 4-2**].

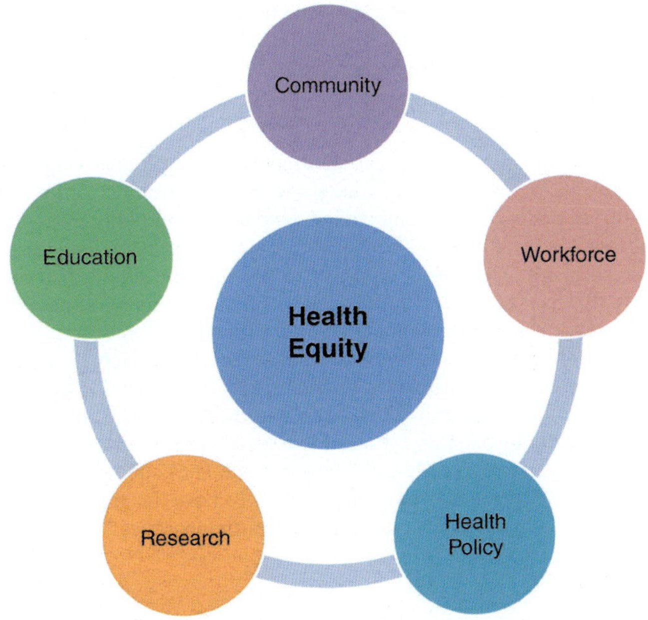

FIGURE 4-2. Advancing health equity through education, community, workforce, health policy, and research.

EDUCATION

Beyond improving recognition or diagnosis of dermatologic conditions across different skin tones, understanding the role of the social determinants of health in influencing individuals' context, choices, and behaviors is a prerequisite to advancing health equity. Yet, residency training programs are still behind on its incorporation into formal curricula.[37] In addition to didactics and activities on how to address bias and communicate effectively across diverse cultural backgrounds, competencies that increase awareness and responsiveness to the social determinants of health (SDOH), as part of Accreditation Council for Graduate Medical Education (ACGME) requirements, could help augment any existing efforts to advance health equity.

COMMUNITY

Healthcare providers can also take action to address the structural/social determinants of health in their local community through practicing awareness, adjustment, assistance, alignment, and advocacy (as outlined by the National Academies of Science, Engineering, and Medicine). Alignment and advocacy are generally considered community-focused activities. An **alignment** activity might include accepting Medicaid insurance and offering timely appointments to beneficiaries to mitigate the lack of access or inaccessibility to timely dermatologic care impacting the community.[38] **Advocacy** could include supporting health policies that expand access to care (ie, universal health coverage or affordable copayments; also see Health Policy section).[38]

While awareness, adjustment, and assistance are patient-focused, they indirectly contribute to the overall health of the local community as they work to neutralize identifiable social risks for individuals who make up the community. For example, in addition to pursuing strategies to **assist** patients with lack of reliable transportation (ie, transport voucher programs), providers can **adjust** their clinic care by offering telehealth services to offset this identifiable social risk, thereby benefitting not only the individual but potentially others in the community.

WORKFORCE

Training alongside people with diverse backgrounds can increase familiarity with different cultures and challenge assumptions, improving effective patient-physician communication and health outcomes. Data also suggest that providers who identify as part of racial and ethnic minoritized groups are more likely to ask about social determinants of health.[39] Beyond trainings to understand the historical and sociocultural factors affecting local communities, we must also recruit and retain more dermatologist from diverse backgrounds.

HEALTH POLICY

Both dermatologists and health organizations can work to leverage their political, social, and economic capital within a community to encourage healthcare or social care organizations to partner and pool resources to empower communities. Within healthcare, actionable items may include advocating for Medicaid expansion to low-income adults (in states where this has yet to happen); inclusion of biologic therapies that effectively treat chronic inflammatory skin conditions on medication formularies; prior authorization processes that are less time/energy intensive; and increased reimbursement for patients with more social risks and/or advocating for reimbursement models that do not penalize health systems that care for patients with multiple social risks. Outside of healthcare, actions related to early child development, fair employment/decent work, and the living environment are likely to have the greatest impact on the social determinants of health and health inequities.[40]

RESEARCH

In addition to recruitment of diverse patient populations in ongoing dermatologic clinical trials, research that goes beyond a biomedical model and addresses the multifactorial nature of the social-ecological influences in health is necessary to eliminate health disparities, hence generating a body of health equity research that can be used to support health policy and ongoing education. Embedded in this research should include studies measuring the impact of stereotype threat, microaggression, and bias (both from a patient and provider perspective) that also contribute to overall health outcomes.

CONCLUSION

Long-standing health inequities remain a challenge in the United States, especially for communities of color.[1] Numerous studies affirm that health outcomes and disparities result not strictly or even primarily from individual behaviors or genetics but from policies, structures, and systems that circumscribe individuals' choices, access, and knowledge.[41] While opportunities to advance health equity through clinical care continue to be important, so is learning about the cultural perspectives of different ethnic groups, along with the challenges they face, which contribute to uncertain health outcomes.

Application of the social ecological model in research could provide a framework to better assess gaps, progress, and opportunities in health equity that spans different levels of influence (individual, interpersonal, community, societal) and domains across place and time. In closing, by becoming familiar with the needs of patients beyond a biomedical model, dermatologists can begin to eliminate health inequities.

REFERENCES

1. Smedley BD, Stith AY, Nelson AR, eds. *Unequal Treatment: Confronting Racial and Ethnic Disparities in Health Care.* Washington, DC: National Academies Press; 2003.
2. Krieger N. *Ecosocial Theory, Embodied Truths, and The People's Health.* Oxford, England: Oxford Unversity Press; 2021.
3. Pritchett EN, Vasquez R. History of race in America. *Dermatol Clin.* 2023;41(2):335-343.
4. Bailey ZD, Krieger N, Agenor M, Graves J, Linos N, Bassett MT. Structural racism and health inequities in the USA: evidence and interventions. *Lancet.* 2017;389(10077):1453-1463.
5. Kelly A, Taylor SC, Lim HW, Serrano A, eds. *Taylor and Kelly's Dermatology for Skin of Color.* 2nd ed. New York, NY: McGraw Hill; 2016. https://accessmedicine.mhmedical.com/content.aspx?bookid=2585&sectionid=211761881. Accessed May 16, 2023.
6. Hoffman KM, Trawalter S, Axt JR, Oliver MN. Racial bias in pain assessment and treatment recommendations, and false beliefs about biological differences between blacks and whites. *Proc Natl Acad Sci USA.* 2016;113(16):4296-4301.
7. Tung EL, Baig AA, Huang ES, Laiteerapong N, Chua KP. Racial and ethnic disparities in diabetes screening between Asian Americans and other adults: BRFSS 2012-2014. *J Gen Intern Med.* 2017;32(4):423-429.
8. Silber TJ. Anorexia nervosa in blacks and hispanics. *Int J Eat Disord.* 1986;5(1): 121-128.
9. Schoenberg E, Wang JV, Duffy R, Keller M. Uncovering unconscious bias and health disparities in the practice of dermatology. *Skinmed.* 2019;17(6): 367-368.
10. Lester JC, Taylor SC, Chren MM. Under-representation of skin of colour in dermatology images: not just an educational issue. *Br J Dermatol.* 2019;180(6): 1521-1522.
11. Agency for Healthcare and Research Quality. https://www.ahrq.gov/health-literacy/improve/precautions/tool10.html. Accessed May 26, 2023.
12. Moy JA, McKinley-Grant L, Sanchez MR. Cultural aspects in the treatment of patients with skin disease. *Dermatol Clin.* 2003;21(4):733-742.
13. Robinson JK, Joshi KM, Ortiz S, Kundu RV. Melanoma knowledge, perception, and awareness in ethnic minorities in Chicago: recommendations regarding education. *Psychooncology.* 2011;20(3):313-320.
14. Robinson JK, Nodal M, Chavez L, Ali Y, Mallett K, Turrisi R. Enhancing the relevance of skin self-examination for Latinos. *JAMA Dermatol.* 2017;153(7):717-718.
15. Buchanan Lunsford N, Berktold J, Holman DM, Stein K, Prempeh A, Yerkes A. Skin cancer knowledge, awareness, beliefs and preventive behaviors among Black and Hispanic men and women. *Prev Med Rep.* 2018;12:203-209.
16. Gorbatenko-Roth K, Prose N, Kundu RV, Patterson S. Assessment of Black patients' perception of their dermatology care. *JAMA Dermatol.* 2019;155(10):1129-1134.
17. Ladha T, Zubairi M, Hunter A, Audcent T, Johnstone J. Cross-cultural communication: tools for working with families and children. *Paediatr Child Health.* 2018;23(1):66-69.
18. Lee S, Martinez G, Ma GX, et al. Barriers to health care access in 13 Asian American communities. *Am J Health Behav.* 2010;34(1):21-30.
19. Kesler DO, Hopkins LO, Torres E, Prasad A. Assimilating traditional healing into preventive medicine residency curriculum. *Am J Prev Med.* 2015;49(5 Suppl 3):S263-269.
20. Che CT, George V, Ijinu TP, Pushpangadan P, Andrae-Marobela K. Chapter 2 - Traditional Medicine. In: Badal S, Delgoda R, eds. *Pharmacognosy*. Boston, MA: Academic Press; 2017:15-30.
21. Americans' health care behaviors and use of conventional and alternative medicine 2017:104. https://www.pewresearch.org/internet/wp-content/uploads/sites/9/2017/02/PS_2017.02.02_Vaccines_FINAL.pdf. Accessed March 16, 2023.
22. Swihart DL, Yarrarapu SNS, Martin RL. Cultural Religious Competence In Clinical Practice. In: *StatPearls.* Treasure Island, FL: StatPearls Publishing; 2023.
23. Lee S, O'Neill AH, Ihara ES, Chae DH. Change in self-reported health status among immigrants in the United States: associations with measures of acculturation. *PLoS One.* 2013;8(10):e76494.
24. Perez MI. Skin cancer in Hispanics in the United States. *J Drugs Dermatol.* 2019;18(3):s117-120.
25. Viola AS, Stapleton JL, Coups EJ. Associations between linguistic acculturation and skin cancer knowledge and beliefs among U.S. Hispanic adults. *Prev Med Rep.* 2019;15:100943.
26. Woolf SH, Aron L, eds. *U.S. Health in International Perspective: Shorter Lives, Poorer Health.* Washington, DC: National Academies Press; 2013.
27. National Institute on Minority Health and Health Disparities Research Framework. 2018. https://www.nimhd.nih.gov/docs/research_framework/research-framework-slide.pdf. Accessed May 26, 2023.
28. Models and Frameworks for the Practice of Community Engagement. 2015. https://www.atsdr.cdc.gov/communityengagement/pce_models.html. Accessed May 26, 2023.
29. Braveman P, Egerter S. *Overcoming obstacles to health: report from the Robert Wood Johnson Foundation Commission to build a healthier America.* Princeton, NJ: Robert Wood Johnson Foundation; 2008.
30. Krieger N. Methods for the scientific study of discrimination and health: an ecosocial approach. *Am J Public Health.* 2012;102(5):936-944.
31. Krieger N. Embodiment: a conceptual glossary for epidemiology. *J Epidemiol Community Health.* 2005;59(5):350-355.
32. Krieger N. Theories for social epidemiology in the 21st century: an ecosocial perspective. *Int J Epidemiol.* 2001;30(4):668-677.
33. Ahn K. The role of air pollutants in atopic dermatitis. *J Allergy Clin Immunol.* 2014;134(5):993-999; discussion 1000.
34. Martinez A, de la Rosa R, Mujahid M, Thakur N. Structural racism and its pathways to asthma and atopic dermatitis. *J Allergy Clin Immunol.* 2021;148(5):1112-1120.

35. Bowers S, Chang AY. The social determinants of health and their Impact on dermatologic health, Part 1: the social determinants of health and their dermatologic implications. *Dermatol Clin*. 2023;41(2):309-316.
36. Germain N, Augustin M, Francois C, et al. Stigma in visible skin diseases - a literature review and development of a conceptual model. *J Eur Acad Dermatol Venereol*. 2021;35(7):1493-1504.
37. Gard LA, Cooper AJ, Youmans Q, et al. Identifying and addressing social determinants of health in outpatient practice: results of a program-wide survey of internal and family medicine residents. *BMC Med Educ*. 2020;20(1):18.
38. Williams J, Amerson EH, Chang AY. How dermatologists can address the structural and social determinants of health-from awareness to action. *JAMA Dermatol*. 2022;158(4):351-352.
39. Palacio A, Seo D, Medina H, Singh V, Suarez M, Tamariz L. Provider perspectives on the collection of social determinants of health. *Popul Health Manag*. 2018;21(6):501-508.
40. Saunders M BB, McHale P, Hamelmann C. *Key policies for addressing the social determinants of health and health inequities*. Copenhagen: WHO Regional Office for Europe; 2017 (Health Evidence Network (HEN) synthesis report 52).
41. Golden TL, Wendel ML. Public health's next step in advancing equity: re-evaluating epistemological assumptions to move social determinants from theory to practice. *Front Public Health*. 2020;8:131.

CHAPTER 5

Historical and Sociocultural Influences on Black American Healthcare Practices

Ameya Gangal
Marta Taye
Loren Krueger

KEY POINTS

- The Black population of the United States (U.S.) has important historical and sociological influences stemming from migration, race-relations, and healthcare disparities that shape skin and haircare.
- Black skin, and skin of color more broadly, remains underrepresented in dermatologic research and educational resources, which may contribute to diagnostic bias and poorer health outcomes when compared to White counterparts.
- Dermatologists should be aware of the historical and sociocultural influences that shape Black American skin and haircare practices and should be prepared to deliver informed, culturally sensitive care.

INTRODUCTION

The Black population of the United States is composed of a diverse group of multinational identities with nuanced sociocultural roots. Black Americans are a heterogeneous ethnic group that include but are not limited to descendants of enslaved Black Africans, Black African immigrants, and Black Caribbean immigrants. The U.S. Black population has steadily grown to almost 47 million individuals in 2019.[1] The Black immigrant population is also projected to grow by 90% between 2020 and 2060. Roughly 80% of Black Americans are a third-generation immigrant group or higher.[2] Immigrants from African and Caribbean countries carry with them cultural norms related to music, food, health, and skin and hair practices that both evolve and remain constant. While much of Black American culture is rooted in Afro-Caribbean practices, this diverse group demonstrates its own unique behaviors related to skin and hair care.

The physician's office is a microcosm of the diversity we observe in these demographic shifts. Understanding the disease processes and health risks of individuals of all skin tones and ethnic groups is vital for successful patient interactions and effective care. To establish meaningful patient-physician relationships, it is important to understand the belief systems and cultural context of the individual patient to recognize patient concerns, communicate effectively, and to make treatment recommendations that will encourage adherence.

DEMOGRAPHICS

In 2022, the world population reached over 7.9 billion people, of which 1.14 billion reside in sub-Saharan Africa and hundreds of millions of individuals of African ancestry live outside of the continent.[3] In total, roughly 16.1% of the world's population can trace their ancestry to sub-Saharan Africa. This number is steadily growing as sub-Saharan African nations account for 8 of the 10 fastest growing international migrant populations since 2010.[4] The statistics regarding populations of African descent are more nuanced than the numbers may suggest. For example, there are several countries in the northern part of the African continent (the Western Sahara, Morocco, Algeria, Tunisia, Libya, Egypt, Sudan, and South Sudan) who may identify with and are heavily influenced, religiously and culturally, by the Middle East, Asia, and Europe. Recent estimates of the African diaspora distribution includes 28 million people of African descent in the Caribbean, 101 million in Central and South America, 49 million in North America, and 14 million in Europe.[5]

In the United States, the population of Black Americans is growing at a rapid pace. In 2020, data from the U.S. Census showed that 46.9 million people identified as Black or African American, encompassing 14.2% of the American population.[6] This represents an 11.7% increase compared to the 2010 census.[6] The Pew Research Center reports the U.S. Black African immigrant population grew 246% between 2000 and 2019 and is expected to reach 9.5 million by 2060. Despite the rapidly rising Black African immigrant population, the Caribbean remains the most common region of birth for U.S. Black immigrants with Jamaica and Haiti being the top nations of birth.[2] It is important to note that "Black immigrants" encompasses single-race Black, multiracial Black, and Black Hispanic people.[2] A rising number of Black Americans have foreign-born connections, with nearly one in five Black people in the United States identifying as immigrants or children of Black immigrants.[2] In general, Black Americans, Africans, and Afro-Caribbeans recognize their common ancestry, with an understanding that they represent distinct ethnic groups. Traditional cultural practices of immigrant populations are maintained but intertwined with and influenced by American life [**Table 5-1**].

The aforementioned statistics on Black Americans included both "Black or African American alone" as well as "... in combination," however, it is important to note these groups are diverse and evolving. The "Black or African American alone" population represented 12.4% of the

TABLE 5-1 Top birthplaces for Black immigrants in the United States in 2000 and 2019

	2000	2019
Jamaica	530,000	760,000
Haiti	410,000	700,000
Nigeria	130,000	390,000
Ethiopia	70,000	260,000
Dominican Republic	80,000	210,000
Ghana	70,000	190,000
Trinidad and Tobago	160,000	170,000
Kenya	30,000	130,000
Guyana	110,000	120,000
Somalia	40,000	110,000

Source: Reproduced with permission from Pew Research Center 2022 analysis of U.S. Census Bureau's 2006-2019 American Community Surveys (ACS).

total population, a 5.6% increase since 2010.[6] Of note, the population of "Black or African American in combination" individuals grew 88.7% since 2010, outpacing the 75% increase since 2000 and highlighting the rapid increase in the country's multiracial population.[6] The increasing identification of a "in combination" group may also suggest multiracial populations may not have been well-captured in prior surveys. Thus, while demographic shift contributes to a greater representation of multiracial groups, improvement in survey design with two separate questions for race and ethnicity allows individuals greater freedom to self-identify and present a more accurate reflection of the nation's demographics. The growing number of multiracial and multiethnic groups has significant implications for healthcare practitioners and the delivery of healthcare services from research and clinical trials to diagnostics and treatments.

Finally, it is important to stress that many people with African ancestry are of mixed race and that racial and ethnic heritage are not always apparent based on the appearance of the individual. The use of racial categories in medicine is often criticized as it rarely correlates to disease and reinforces social divisions, contributing to discrimination.[7] Ethnicity is a fluid, multidimensional concept encompassing cultural, behavioral, and environmental factors that can be attributable to disease but is difficult to measure. There is a great deal of diversity within and among Black American populations. The practice of routinely collecting patient demographic information and allowing patients to self-identify is imperative to the delivery of quality healthcare.

BLACK AMERICANS AND THE HEALTHCARE SYSTEM

Racism, segregation, and injustice are at the core of historical events surrounding the interactions between Black Americans and the healthcare system. Exploitative research practices, perhaps most widely acknowledged through the Tuskegee Study of Untreated Syphilis in the Negro Male, fundamentally undermined Black Americans' trust in the U.S. healthcare system. Other notable historical examples include the lack of consent for Henrietta Lacks' immortal cell line, known as HeLa, which continue to serve as underpinnings for discoveries in cancer research and immunology.[8]

These transgressions and injustice within our healthcare systems continue to have lasting effects. Differences in health outcomes between Black and White Americans are well-documented, particularly in obstetrics, chronic health conditions, cancer, and as recent as the COVID-19 pandemic. For example, infants born to Black mothers are over twice as likely to die during the first year of life when compared to infants born to White mothers.[9] Despite a lower overall incidence, Black women have a twofold higher mortality for endometrial cancer and a 41% higher risk for breast cancer when compared to White women.[10] Black patients with COVID-19 were also significantly more likely to suffer an ischemic stroke when compared to non-Black patients with COVID-19.[11] Mistrust, rooted in disparities in health outcomes, persist as half of Black adults stated that they were not confident that the development of a COVID-19 vaccine was taking the needs of Black people into account.[12] These examples underscore how Black racial identity, and its associated sociocultural implications in the form of systemic racism, inequity in employment, and housing, may impact health outcomes and contribute to mistrust. Despite growing calls for increased diversity of representation among physicians and focused cultural competencies among learners, healthcare providers must also continue to shed light on these disparities through rigorous, inclusive research and targeted clinical interventions.

DISPARITIES IN HEALTHCARE STATUS AND HEALTH SERVICES UTILIZATION FOR PATIENTS WITH SKIN OF COLOR

Despite this growing body of literature, there remains relatively sparse data to describe health disparities for skin and hair conditions. Studies on melanoma have found that 26% of Black American patients present with regional or distant metastases compared to 12% in individuals with lighter skin.[13] Black Americans also present with more advanced nonmelanoma skin cancers, such as squamous cell carcinoma, when compared to White counterparts.[14] Furthermore, Krueger et al found that resident and attending dermatologists were more likely to biopsy nonmalignant conditions and less likely to biopsy malignant conditions in darker skin when compared to lighter skin counterparts.[15] This study suggested a diagnostic bias exists for clinical decision-making in darker skin types when compared to lighter skin types. Additionally, Adamson et al observed that *New England Journal of Medicine* respondents to an image challenge misdiagnosed skin conditions in darker skin types when compared to lighter skin types.[16] Taken together, these data suggest underlying diagnostic biases of providers could contribute to health disparities.

Dermatologic concerns among African American patients also differ from other racial and ethnic groups. In a nationally representative sample, the top five diagnoses among Black Americans were acne, unspecified dermatitis or eczema, seborrheic dermatitis, atopic dermatitis, and dyschromia that differed when compared to White patients who were commonly diagnosed with actinic keratosis, acne, benign neoplasm of skin, unspecific dermatitis or eczema, and nonmelanoma skin cancer [**Figure 5-1**].[17]

In addition to awareness of common conditions, dermatologists should also focus on representation and culturally sensitive care for Black American patients. For example, a mixed-methods focus group-guided study found that Black patients benefitted from specific cultural and medical knowledge regarding hair and skin among providers.[18] However, medical schools, textbooks, and image search engines largely lack representation and educational resources focused on skin of color or Black American skin and hair practices. For example, most textbooks have less than 1% representation of dermatologic conditions in Fitzpatrick V or VI skin types yet darker skin types appear to be overrepresented when compared to lighter skin types for sexually transmitted infections.[19] It is critical to continue to identify and address these biases to better train future healthcare professionals to approach dermatologic conditions with the appropriate clinical and sociological context.

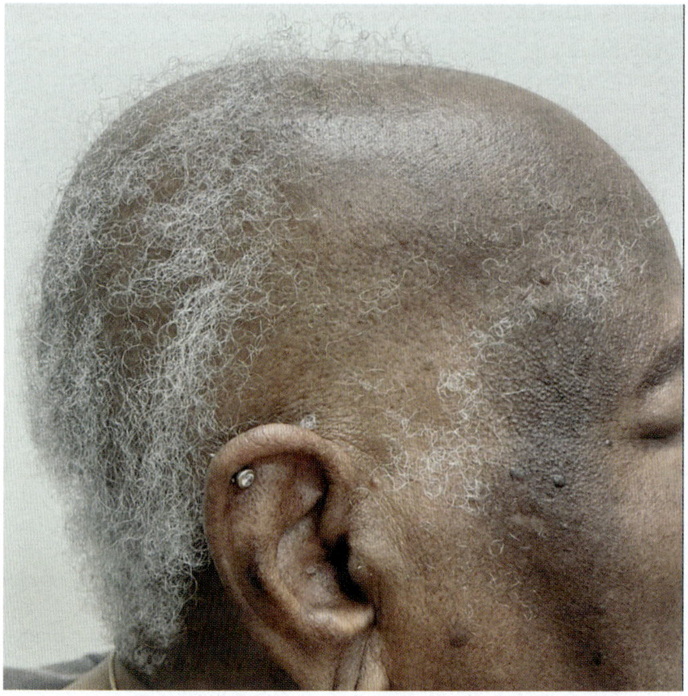

FIGURE 5-1. Dyschromia is a common diagnosis in Black American patients. The patient shown here has brown patches on her bilateral cheeks consistent with maturational hyperpigmentation.

BLACK AMERICAN HAIR AND RACE RELATIONS

Hair has served as a profound marker of identity among Black American communities, particularly Black American women. Evidence of hair as indicator for marital status, age, and societal rank dates to 15th century African traditions. Following enslavement, hair practices often reflected occupation; field slaves often hid their hair while house slaves wore wigs.[20] A major cultural shift took place when Madame C.J. Walker, the first female self-made millionaire in the United States, patented the "hot comb" or "pressing comb." In addition to this mechanical straightening method, chemical straighteners or the "relaxer" was introduced. These forms of hair straightening were used among Black American women throughout the early-mid-20th century to assimilate and convey social standing.[21]

In the mid-20th century, hair also came to be viewed as a symbol of resistance and independence. Distinctive hairstyling, including afros and dreadlocks, challenged the longstanding traditional beauty standards that were reflective of White Americans.[20] Movement away from chemically straightened hair to afros in the 1950s was a sign of pride. Black American men also used longer hair styles, which contrasted against preferences for short hair among White Americans. Relaxers remained widespread throughout the late 20th century, but braids, twists, and extensions remained in fashion. As of the 21st century, a movement toward natural hair styling, which rejects chemical and mechanical modifications—grew in popularity among Black Americans. In 2011, approximately one-third of Black women avoided the use of chemical relaxers or straightening products, an increase from 26% in 2010.[22]

Hair continues to hold significance in U.S. race relations. Today, hairstyles are less explicitly indicative of political or social associations, but these historical underpinnings are critical to understanding the nuance and identity inherent to Black American hair practices.

HAIR STYLING PRACTICES AMONG BLACK AMERICANS

Hairstyling practices such as straightening and the use of heated tools remain prevalent. Straightening can be accomplished with chemicals or through heat-mediated rearrangement of hydrogen and disulfide bonds.[23] Heating tools, including blow dryers, curling irons, flat irons, and hot combs may be used at home. Professional styling can also be used to access tools that heat the hair to over 450°F.

Health consequences related to the use of high heat include scalp and neck burns [**Figure 5-2**]. Excessive heat can also lead to trichorrhexis nodosa, an acquired deformity of the hair shaft that leads to hair breakage over time [**Figure 5-3**]. Areas of hair shaft deformity appear as glistening nodes that can be seen microscopically as pockets of gas that form due to rapid water vaporization. These structurally compromised areas lead to breakage of the hair shaft over time.

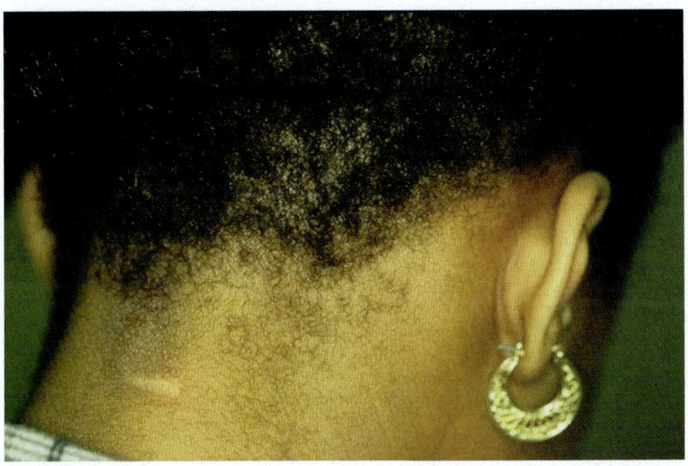

FIGURE 5-2. Chemical burn on a patient's neck resulting from the use of a heated styling appliance.

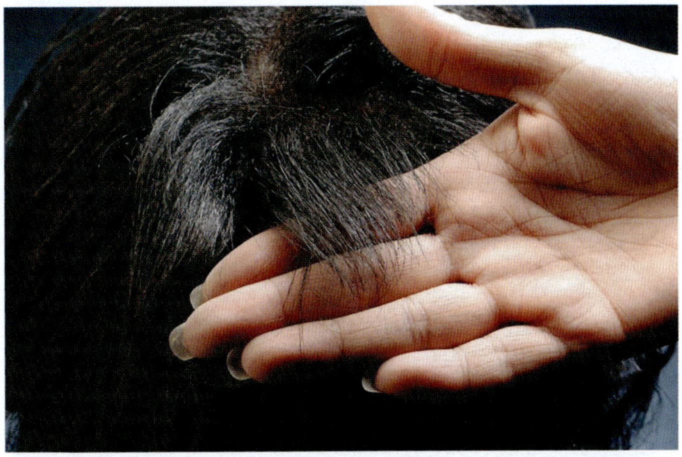

FIGURE 5-3. Hair breakage due to the use of styling tools heated to high temperatures.

A more permanent form of straightening can be achieved with the use of relaxers, during which a strong alkali can permanently rearrange disulfide bonds in the hair. These strong alkalis, such as sodium hydroxide and calcium hydroxide, may also lead to irritant contact dermatitis and chemical burns on the scalp. Even one application of relaxers may also lower the tensile strength of the hair.

Recently, the use of hair straightening products has been linked with higher uterine cancer risk. In a survey study including greater than 33,000 women in the United States, women who reported frequent use of hair straightening products (defined as more than four times in the previous year) were more likely to go on to develop uterine cancer. Major limitations of this study include the lack of diversity among research participants (with <8% of women identifying as Black or African American), the wide assortment of hair straightening practices used (ie, straighteners, relaxers, or pressing products), and the positive family history of breast cancer among participants in the study limiting the generalizability of these results. Further research is necessary to authenticate these findings. Until then, it may be reasonable for patients to extend the duration between hair relaxers application to at least every 12 weeks, during which the product should only be applied to new hair growth to reduce scalp irritation.

Black American hair styling borrows many traditions, such as braids and twists, directly from African culture. Patients choose to wear hair in different styles for many reasons—some may choose to make a statement on fashion or politics while others may opt for comfort or a natural look. Providers should be aware of hair styling as a fundamental component of identity and simultaneously treat and counsel on the complications of hairstyling practices [**Figure 5-4**].

Black American hair structure and practices differ in meaningful ways from White counterparts. Black American hair has an elliptically shaped hair shaft as opposed to the circular shape of White hair. Black American hair shafts may also display notable retrocurvature, which may stem from underlying bilateral asymmetry in structure of keratin fibers.[24] Black American hair may also be more prone to developing knots and splits along the hair shaft.[24] Given the unique hair shaft characteristics of Black American hair, a major misconception among industry leaders, patients, and providers alike is that products, stylings, and beauty perceptions may be one-size-fits-all for both Black and White hair.

Braids and twists, which can be left in place for 6 to 8 weeks or longer, are at times worn by Black Americans. During this period, the hair is relatively protected from "weathering" of heat, chemicals, and mechanical forces, such as combing. However, some patients perceive hair loss during braid removal, which may be a normal finding. Patients should be reassured of the natural course of hair loss, in which individuals can lose approximately 100 strands per day. When hair is worn in braids, these hairs remain trapped in the styling. Hairstyles that place significant tension on the hair, such as tight braids and hair extensions, can

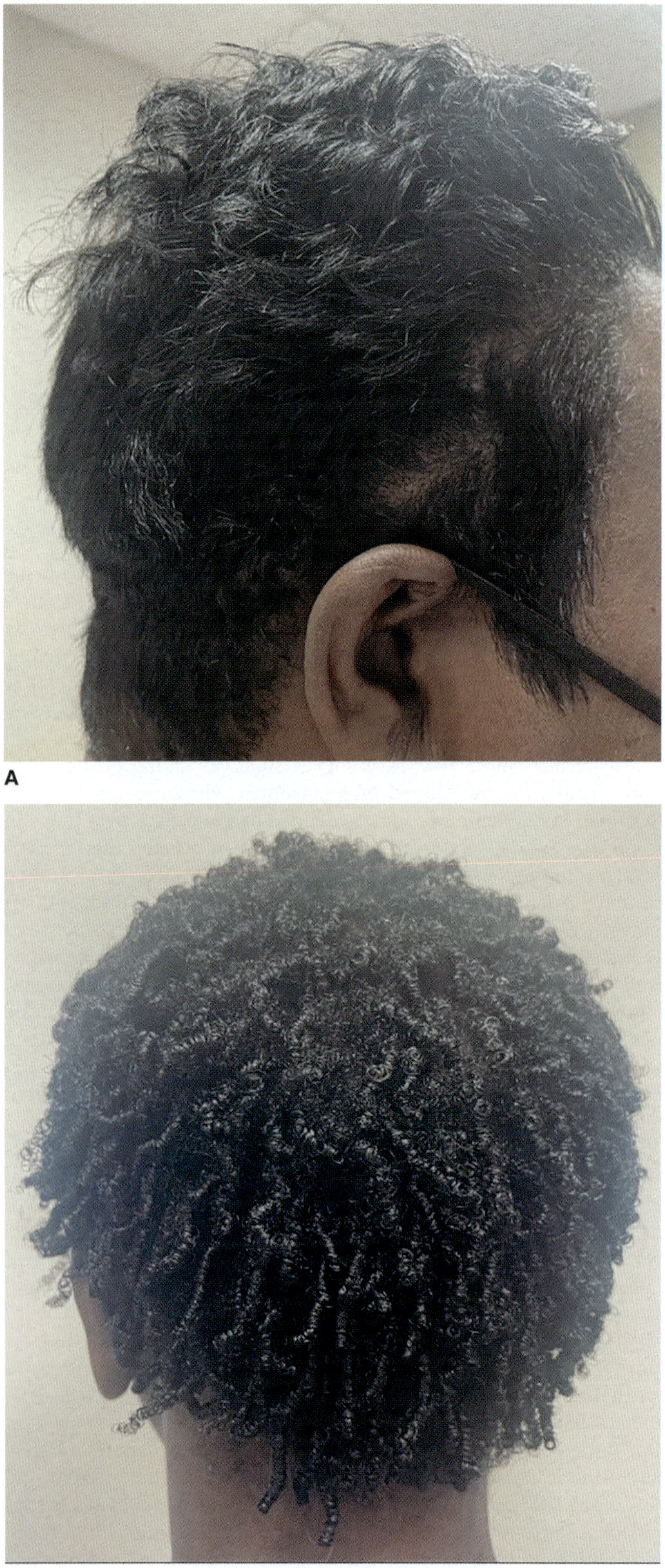

A

B

FIGURE 5-4. Hair styling with chemical relaxers and heat styling **(A)** and natural hair styling **(B)**.

lead to increased hair loss and precipitate traction alopecia. Any sign of erythema, pustules, or scaling on the frontal hairline should prompt removal of the hairstyle in favor of a low-tension option.

Dryness associated with hair washing is another misconception among Black Americans. Sebum travels less easily down the shaft of Black American hair when compared to straighter hair types and therefore requires less frequent washing. Excessive hair washing, particularly with harsher shampoos, may damage hair shafts. Styling techniques using excessive heat, such as blow dryers, cap dryers, curling irons, and flat irons, may similarly cause hair breakage. To counteract the damage related to heat and mechanical forces, patients should be counseled on gentle combing, optimal hair washing frequency, and the use of deep or leave-in conditioners.

Finally, Black Americans may hold misconceptions regarding dry scalp and associated treatments. One common practice to treat dry scalp or hair among Black Americans is greasing—during which an oily product is applied to the scalp. While these products may moisturize the hair shaft, they provide little benefit to the scalp itself. In addition, some products used in greasing may contain mineral oils or petroleum, which contribute to pomade acne or worsen seborrheic dermatitis. Dry scalp among some patients may also be due to seborrheic dermatitis, a condition common among Black Americans. These patients may benefit from prescription medication and targeted over-the-counter products. While greasing remains prevalent, a shift toward "natural" hair among Black Americans has led to the use of natural oils, such as olive, coconut, and argan oils.

In a survey of Detroit-based Black American women, only a third stated they felt their provider understood Black American hair.[25] Dermatologists should be knowledgeable of the diversity of cultural hair practices among Black Americans and be prepared to address potential misconceptions.

MISCONCEPTIONS ABOUT SKIN

No study has comprehensively assessed the prevalence of skin lightening practices among Americans. Current prevalence estimates of skin-lightening cream and bleach use likely underestimate use of skin lightening creams and bleaches due to stigma surrounding the practice. In parts of Africa and the Caribbean, consumers may apply skin lightening creams, including hydroquinone, steroids, and/or bleach, under occlusive dressings and clothing. This application method may further increase the likelihood of adverse effects.

Beyond the problematic nature of skin lightening in the face of beauty standards rooted in colorism, treatment options for skin lightening may hold unforeseen consequences. Hydroquinone can paradoxically lead to bluish-gray hyperpigmentation of the skin, known as exogenous ochronosis. Skin lightening may also be pursued with the use of topical steroids, which can lead to steroid-induced acne and uneven skin hypopigmentation. Bleaching creams may also contain mercury, a harmful compound to developing fetuses. Thorough history-taking regarding skin care practices may aid in mitigating adverse effects of skin lightening practices.

Erroneous beliefs regarding sun exposure and perception of skin cancer risk are central to misconceptions of skin care among Black Americans. Darker pigmentation offers relative protection against sun damage but does not eliminate the possibility of sunburn or photoaging. For example, roughly 1 in 10 Black Americans experience sunburn every year.[26] Dyschromia, including melasma and postinflammatory hyperpigmentation, requires strict adherence to sun protection. However, Black Americans report lower sunscreen use when compared to White Americans across multiple studies.[26-28] Sunscreen use is particularly low in African countries, and prevalence of sunscreen use increases with increasing income and with higher educational levels.[26,28] Tinted sunscreens, specifically those containing iron (ferrous, ferric) oxides, are needed to block visible light, which has been shown to worsen hyperpigmentation in darker skin types.[29] These factors suggest that misconceptions about photodamage in Black Americans may be driven by lack of information regarding sun protection in the prevention of hyperpigmentation.

In addition to misconceptions regarding risk of sun damage, Black Americans report low self-perceived risk of skin cancer.[30] This is concerning given patients of darker skin color and Hispanics are more likely to present with advanced melanoma and experience poorer outcomes when compared to White counterparts. While other melanoma and nonmelanoma skin cancers occur at lower frequencies among Black American populations when compared to White, early education on skin cancer risk and variability in presentation is critical.

CONCLUSION

Black American hair and skin practices stem from a rich cultural and sociopolitical history. Physicians should respect the cultural background of patients, listen to concerns, elicit goals of care, and be prepared to address misconceptions specific to dermatologic care in Black American populations.

REFERENCES

1. Bureau USC. U.S. Census Bureau QuickFacts: United States. https://www.census.gov/quickfacts/fact/table/US/PST045221. Published 2022. Accessed December 13, 2022.
2. C. T. Key findings about Black immigrants in the U.S. Pew Research Center. https://www.pewresearch.org/fact-tank/2022/01/27/key-findings-about-black-immigrants-in-the-u-s/. Published 2022.
3. Bureau USC. U.S. and World Population Clock. https://www.census.gov/popclock/. Published 2022.
4. Connor P. International migration from sub-Saharan African has grown dramatically since 2010. Pew Research Center. https://www.pewresearch.org/fact-tank/2018/02/28/international-migration-from-sub-saharan-africa-has-grown-dramatically-since-2010/. Published 2018.
5. Introduction to the African Diaspora across the world. Institute for Cultural Diplomacy. https://www.culturaldiplomacy.org/index.php?en_programs_diaspora.
6. Race and Ethnicity in the United States: 2010 Census and 2020 Census. United States Census Bureau. https://www.census.gov/library/visualizations/interactive/race-and-ethnicity-in-the-united-state-2010-and-2020-census.html. Published 2021.
7. Agyemang C, Bhopal R, Bruijnzeels M. Negro, Black, Black African, African Caribbean, African American or what? Labelling African origin populations in the health arena in the 21st century. *J Epidemiol Community Health*. 2005;59(12):1014-1018.
8. Henrietta Lacks: science must right a historical wrong. *Nature*. 2020; 585(7823):7.
9. Ely DM, Driscoll AK. Infant mortality in the United States, 2019: data from the period linked birth/infant death file. *Natl Vital Stat Rep*. 2021;70(14):1-18.
10. Giaquinto AN, Miller KD, Tossas KY, Winn RA, Jemal A, Siegel RL. Cancer statistics for African American/Black people 2022. *CA Cancer J Clin*. 2022; 72(3):202-229.
11. Lekoubou A, Pelton M, Ba DM, Ssentongo P. Racial disparities in ischemic stroke among patients with COVID-19 in the United States. *J Stroke Cerebrovasc Dis*. 2021;30(8):105877.
12. Rusoja EA, Thomas BA. The COVID-19 pandemic, Black mistrust, and a path forward. *EClinicalMedicine*. 2021;35:100868.
13. Hu S, Parmet Y, Allen G, et al. Disparity in melanoma: a trend analysis of melanoma incidence and stage at diagnosis among whites, Hispanics, and blacks in Florida. *Arch Dermatol*. 2009;145(12):1369-1374.
14. Gloster HM, Jr., Neal K. Skin cancer in skin of color. *J Am Acad Dermatol*. 2006;55(5):741-760; quiz 761-744.
15. Krueger L, Hijab E, Latkowski JA, Elbuluk N. Clinical decision-making bias in darker skin types: a prospective survey study identifying diagnostic bias in decision to biopsy. *Int J Dermatol*. 2023;62(4):e252-e253.
16. Diao JA, Adamson AS. Representation and misdiagnosis of dark skin in a large-scale visual diagnostic challenge. *J Am Acad Dermatol*. 2022;86(4):950-951.
17. Davis SA, Narahari S, Feldman SR, Huang W, Pichardo-Geisinger RO, McMichael AJ. Top dermatologic conditions in patients of color: an analysis of nationally representative data. *J Drugs Dermatol*. 2012;11(4):466-473.
18. Gorbatenko-Roth K, Prose N, Kundu RV, Patterson S. Assessment of Black patients' perception of their dermatology care. *JAMA Dermatol*. 2019;155(10):1129-1134.
19. Adelekun A, Onyekaba G, Lipoff JB. Skin color in dermatology textbooks: an updated evaluation and analysis. *J Am Acad Dermatol*. 2021;84(1):194-196.
20. C. T. Black Women and Identity: What's hair got to do with it? https://quod.lib.umich.edu/cgi/t/text/text-idx?cc=mfsfront;c=mfs;c=mfsfront;idno=ark5583.0022.105;g=mfsg;rgn=main;view=text;xc=1. Published 2009.
21. Nwadei T, Krueger LD. The importance of hair in Black-White race relations: a historical review and recommendations for US dermatologists. *JAMA Dermatol*. 2022;158(7):723-724.
22. Versey HS. Centering perspectives on Black women, hair politics, and physical activity. *Am J Public Health*. 2014;104(5):810-815.
23. Wang H, Parry DA, Jones LN, Idler WW, Marekov LN, Steinert PM. In vitro assembly and structure of trichocyte keratin intermediate filaments: a novel role for stabilization by disulfide bonding. *J Cell Biol*. 2000;151(7):1459-1468.
24. Quaresma MV, Martinez Velasco MA, Tosti A. Hair breakage in patients of African descent: role of dermoscopy. *Skin Appendage Disord*. 2015;1(2):99-104.
25. Gathers RC, Mahan MG. African American women, hair care, and health barriers. *J Clin Aesthet Dermatol*. 2014;7(9):26-29.
26. Buchanan Lunsford N, Berktold J, Holman DM, Stein K, Prempeh A, Yerkes A. Skin cancer knowledge, awareness, beliefs and preventive behaviors among black and hispanic men and women. *Prev Med Rep*. 2018;12:203-209.
27. Pichon LC, Corral I, Landrine H, Mayer JA, Norman GJ. Sun-protection behaviors among African Americans. *Am J Prev Med*. 2010;38(3):288-295.
28. Calderon TA, Bleakley A, Jordan AB, Lazovich D, Glanz K. Correlates of sun protection behaviors in racially and ethnically diverse U.S. adults. *Prev Med Rep*. 2019;13:346-353.
29. Dumbuya H, Grimes PE, Lynch S, et al. Impact of iron-oxide containing formulations against visible light-induced skin pigmentation in skin of color individuals. *J Drugs Dermatol*. 2020;19(7):712-717.
30. Goldenberg A, Vujic I, Sanlorenzo M, Ortiz-Urda S. Melanoma risk perception and prevention behavior among African-Americans: the minority melanoma paradox. *Clin Cosmet Investig Dermatol*. 2015;8:423-429.

CHAPTER 6

Historical and Sociocultural Influences on Asian American Healthcare Practices

Richard Mizuguchi
Juliana Kim

KEY POINTS

- Asian Americans represent the fastest-growing racial and ethnic group in the United States.
- Asian American are an economically diverse group with wide differences in socioeconomic status partly related to historical immigration policies.
- Asian Americans underutilize dermatology services compared to other racialized groups.
- Alternative or traditional medicine remains a commonly sought out alternative for many Asian Americans.
- Traditional Chinese medicine (TCM) involves topical/oral supplements, dietary therapy, massage, and acupuncture.
- Traditional Asian practices of cupping, coining, and moxibustion can cause bruises and lesions that are sometimes mistaken for physical abuse; however, these are distinguishable by their regular circular appearance.
- Dermatologists who are unfamiliar with TCM may possess some miscomprehension about these health beliefs or practices. It is worthwhile for dermatologists to gain some familiarity with these therapies, as some have shown efficacy in double-blind studies.

INTRODUCTION

The Asian population is the fastest-growing ethnicity and race in the United States. Asians comprise 7% of the population and their number is projected to quadruple by 2060, surpassing 46 million.[1] Because Asians represent a substantial segment of the population, dermatologists should become familiar with historical and sociocultural factors that may inform healthcare practices as well as having a basic knowledge of some of the traditional health practices of Asians.

TABLE 6-1 Asian subgroups based on geography

"East Asian"	China, Japan, North Korea, or South Korea
"Southeast Asian"	Cambodia, Indonesia, Laos, Malaysia, the Philippines, Singapore, Thailand, Vietnam, or Burma
"South Asian"	India, Pakistan, Sri Lanka, Bangladesh, Bhutan, or Nepal
Pacific Islanders	
"Micronesian"	The Commonwealth of the Northern Mariana Islands, Republic of the Marshall Islands, Guam, Republic of Palau, or Federated States of Micronesia
"Polynesian"	New Zealand, Tonga, Tahiti, Hawaii, Samoa, and American Samoa
"Melanesian"	Fiji or Papua New Guinea

The Asian population is a highly heterogeneous group that includes East Asians, Southeast Asians, South Asians, and Pacific Islanders. Pacific Islanders are further subdivided into Micronesians, Polynesians, and Melanesians [**Table 6-1**]. It is important to recognize that each group has unique challenges with access to or utilization of healthcare services. Hesitancy of people in this population to pursue mainstream medicine stems from multiple reasons, including availability or accessibility, communication barriers, cultural attitudes surrounding healthcare, preference for alternative/traditional medicine, and/or social determinants of health (also see Chapter 11) that have long impacted Asian Americans, particularly those with liminal (or "in-between") legal status and with family histories influenced by displacement, colonization, and imperialism.

This chapter will review the historical or sociocultural factors that influence healthcare practices among Asian Americans. The use of traditional Chinese medicine (TCM) will also be discussed. This chapter will primarily focus on East Asian, Southeast Asian, and Pacific Islanders.

SOCIOECOMONIC DISPARITIES AMONG ASIAN AMERICANS

Asian Americans are the highest-earning racial and ethnic group in the United States. However, this status is not shared by all Asians. Between 1970 and 2016, the gap in the standard of living between Asians near the top and the bottom of the income ladder nearly doubled. In the process, Asian Americans have displaced Black Americans as the most economically diverse group with wide differences in socioeconomic status.[2] As such, broad generalizations inherent in the Asian American categorization can obscure the economic reality for many within this large community.

INCOME INEQUALITY AND IMMIGRATION

The pattern of income inequality (a measure of the economic gap between the highest and lowest income groups) across groups can be traced back to differences in immigration and factors related to immigration.[3] Similar to the Latine/Hispanic population (see Chapter 7, Historical and Sociocultural Influences on Latine/Hispanic American Healthcare), Asian Americans have been shaped by immigration policies that have historically favored certain pathways to entry. One of the most influential policies in shaping the distribution of income among immigrants entering the United States occurred during the civil rights movement. The Immigration and Naturalization Act of 1965 (also known as the Hart-Celler Act) overhauled the 1920s immigration quota system based on national-origin and eased immigration access for highly skilled immigrants as well as for people already living in the United States.[4] An inadvertent consequence has been ongoing ethnic differences in wealth and poverty rates with some Asian ethnic groups entering the United States bringing capital investment or by filling highly skilled occupations. In comparison, political refugees from Southeast Asia, who may have immigrated to escape war or political persecution, may have come with fewer economic resources. In addition, family reunification facilitated migration of individuals from similar socioeconomic backgrounds, reinforcing class differences and reproducing the same patterns of distribution of wealth among Asian Americans as in other ethnic groups immigrating to the United States.[5]

Income inequality is important because it has the potential to perpetuate inequities in the social determinant of health (ie, housing, education, employment, health, etc) that impact health and well-being (see Chapter 11).[2] In fact, a recent nationwide analysis found that disparities in self-rated health among Asians living in the United States was partially mediated by socioeconomic status (ie, education level and household income), with South Asians reporting better self-rated health compared to other Asian ethnic groups probably due to higher socioeconomic status.[6] Future policies aimed at mitigating the income inequality among Asian Americans might consider factors related to immigration, including the number of years in the United States, and English language proficiency.[5]

UTILIZATION OF SPECIALTY SERVICES AMONG ASIAN AMERICANS

Compared to White and Black patients, access to specialty providers in healthcare by Asian Americans is limited. In 2016, Asian Americans comprised 4.32% of visits to outpatient specialists, while accounting for 5.97% of the population. Asians comprised 3.13% of visits to dermatologists that same year, while White patients comprised 90.27% and Blacks patients 6.26%, according to the National Ambulatory Medical Care Survey (NAMCS) data [**Figure 6-1**].[7] Several factors may account for underutilization of healthcare services by the Asian American population, including financial constraints (influencing health coverage), communication barriers, and cultural attitudes toward health.

FINANCIAL CONSTRAINTS

The implementation of the Affordable Care Act (ACA) significantly decreased the uninsured rate among the Asian population from 14.7% in 2013 to 6.8% in 2019.[8] However, a study based on the survey responses of 349 Asian Americans in northern California suggested that having health insurance of any type did not change the likelihood that an Asian patient ever saw a dermatologist. After creating a multivariate model accounting for several demographic variables (education level, generation in the United States, etc), insurance status was not predictive of whether a patient visited a dermatologist ($p = 0.22$), while income level trended toward significance ($p = 0.07$). The odds ratio (OR) that an insured patient would see a dermatologist compared to a patient without insurance was not significant (OR = 0.55 [0.22-1.41]). However, those with annual income between 50k and 75k were significantly more likely to see a dermatologist than those with income under 25k (OR = 3.19 [1.24-8.23]).[9] This finding suggests that financial constraints may still be a factor, even after insurance coverage. Another study of patients seeking care for acne demonstrated that Medicaid insurance and self-reported Asian race were the top two factors that decreased the odds of seeing a dermatologist over a nondermatologist physician.[10] In general, socioeconomic status has a large impact on the health of patients, and Asian patients are no exception. Low-income jobs with minimal to no health benefits and long working hours may disproportionately affect already impoverished Asian immigrants and could contribute to barriers seeking medical treatment, including specialty services.[11] Involving social workers in making patients aware of available social services may be helpful.

BARRIERS IN COMMUNICATION

Patients may be reluctant to seek specialty care due to communication barriers with the provider. About 34% of the Asian population have limited English proficiency, which is associated with fewer regular check-ups and unmet healthcare needs. Language barriers are a unique challenge for the Asian population because it encompasses over 100 native languages and dialects. While the Latine/Hispanic population has a similar proficiency rate, there is better access to translation services, as most speak Spanish.[12] Physicians may also misunderstand Asian communication styles. A recent report suggested Asian patients with psoriasis receive significantly less face-to-face time with dermatologists.[13]

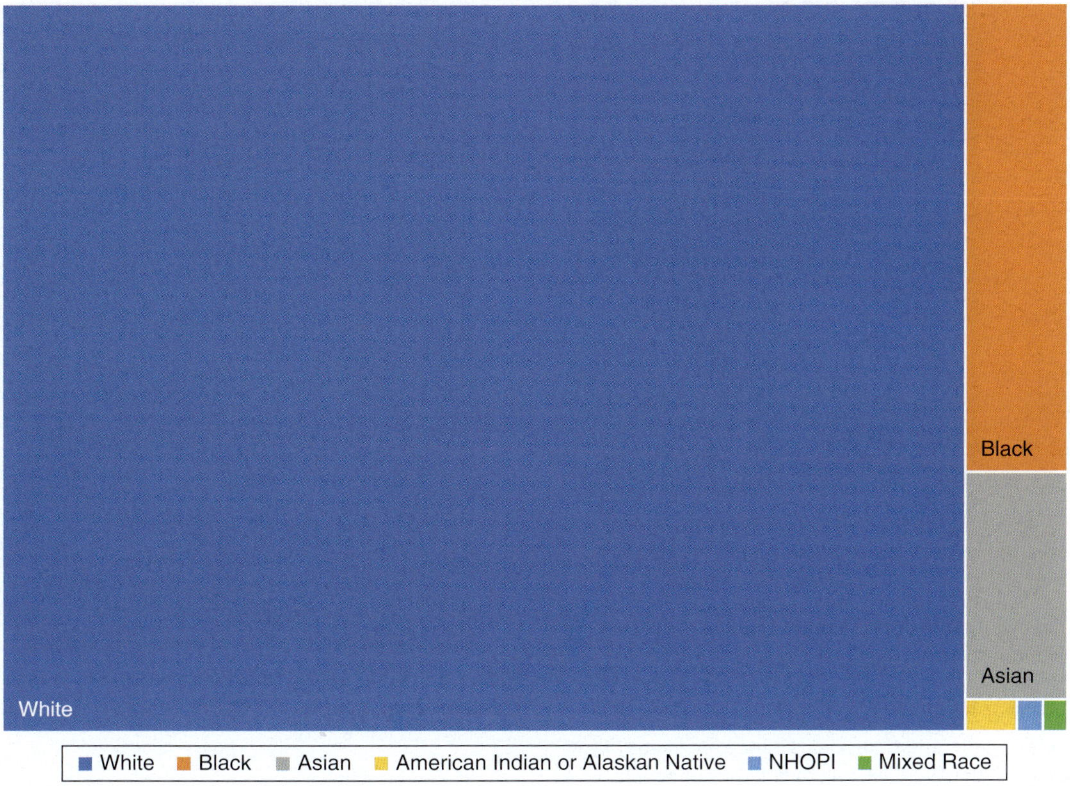

FIGURE 6-1. Proportion of dermatology visits by race. In 2016, Asian-American patients comprised 3.13% of visits to dermatologists, while White patients comprised 90.27% and Black patients 6.26%. NHOPI = Native Hawaiian and Other Pacific Islander.

Asian cultures are highly context-dependent and rely on nonverbal cues. For example, patients may use silence or a flat affect to express the presence of illness. Patients might also nod or smile as a sign of respect rather than agreement with what is being said. A prominent value in many cultures is deference to authority, which includes respecting professionals, like physicians, with higher education. Asians may avoid making direct requests and think it rude to voice disagreement or question the physician. As such, physicians can compensate by asking more questions and eliciting the patient's views on the treatment plan.[14]

CULTURAL ATTITUDES ON HEALTH AND HEALTHCARE

Finally, hesitancy to seek care from any provider in general (including specialist care) may stem from cultural attitudes on health and healthcare. According to a qualitative study exploring barriers to healthcare access in 13 Asian communities, participants reported that going to the physician on a regular basis for routine checkups is not a regular practice in their countries of origin.[15] For example, if a person feels well, there is no need to see a doctor. This cultural practice may prevail even after immigration to the United States and can influence younger generations who live in multigenerational households. Many Asian communities use traditional medicine to manage a diversity of illnesses. Participants in the same qualitative study reported that the use of traditional medicine was ingrained in their culture and, as a result, preferred over Westernized medicine.[15] Some Asian patients resort to Western medicine only if traditional healing fails; others use both traditional and Western medicine. Physicians should therefore become familiar with traditional therapies and inquire about them while taking a history.

DERMATOLOGY AND ASIAN AMERICANS

As the Asian population in the United States quickly rises, it will be crucial to improve access and use of specialty care, especially in dermatology, to help mitigate racial and ethnic health disparities that impact the Asian community. Asian Americans are more likely to present with thicker and distant melanoma compared to their Latine/Hispanic and White counterparts, with lower 5-year survival rates when compared to White Americans alone.[9] Among patients with psoriasis, studies report Asian American patients present with larger body surface area involvement at the time of diagnosis when compared to White patients.[16] With respect to atopic dermatitis, patients identified as Asian or Black were more likely to be admitted for mental health disorders.[17] Asian females report a greater negative impact on self-perception and social functioning from their acne compared to other racial groups.[18]

Physicians can work to optimize care for the Asian population by engaging in conversations regarding the importance of early treatment and preventative health, addressing communication barriers within the community (ie, using a translator or via increased representation of underrepresented groups in medicine from Asian countries, including but not limited to individuals from Laos, Cambodia and Indonesia[19]), and both acknowledging and respecting differences in cultural attitudes about health.

ALTERNATIVE/TRADITIONAL MEDICINE

Alternative or traditional medicine remains a commonly sought out alternative for many Asian Americans, especially among groups that may be more vulnerable to poor healthcare access due to high poverty rates, language barriers, insufficient health literacy, and recent immigration status. Cultural perception of illness, which focuses on holistic healing, may also motivate Asian Americans to use traditional medicine.[20] Finally, Asian immigrants, like many other immigrants and refugees who settled in the United States, tend to visit physicians within their local communities. Therefore, many cultural practices may go unnoticed by healthcare providers outside of the Asian community.[21] However, sometimes an emergency or change in location requires patients to seek treatment from dermatologists outside of their habitual communities. Therefore, the dermatologist

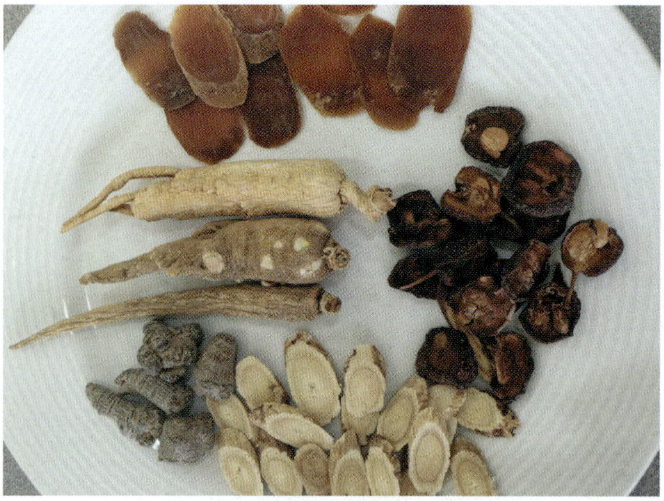

FIGURE 6-2. Chinese herbs. (Image courtesy of Dr. Jianting Tong.)

should become familiar with traditional treatments among the Asian community and potential adverse effects.

TRADITIONAL CHINESE MEDICINE

As an alternative method of therapy, traditional Chinese medicine (TCM) is practiced throughout China and East Asia by millions of people. Until the middle of the 19th century, alternative medicine provided by botanical healers, midwives, chiropractors, homeopaths, and an assortment of other lay healers was the fundamental method used by humans to treat diseases and to preserve their health.[22] The current prevalence of TCM suggests that patients are looking for more therapeutic options than are widely available in conventional healthcare settings[22] and are searching for a more holistic approach to healthcare. Typically, TCM involves medical practices that use herbs, cannabis, dietary therapy, massage, and acupuncture [**Figures 6-2** and **6-3**]. The use of medicinal herbs that are chosen and combined specifically for each individual patient is stressed. Shen Nung's herbal book, dated 2700 BC, is considered the oldest Chinese medical book and contains details of the medicinal uses of over 300 plants [**Figure 6-4**].[23]

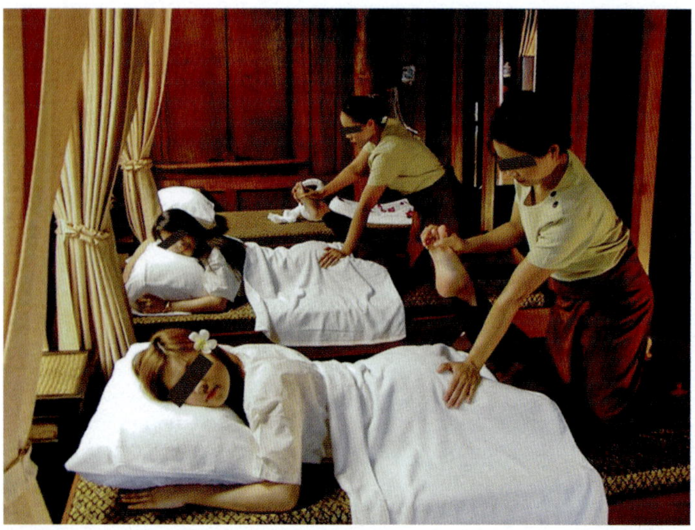

FIGURE 6-3. Thai massage is a system of massage and assisted stretching developed in Thailand and influenced by the traditional medicine systems of India, China, and Southeast Asia. (Used with permission from Marisol LLC, Muscat, Sultanate of Oman.)

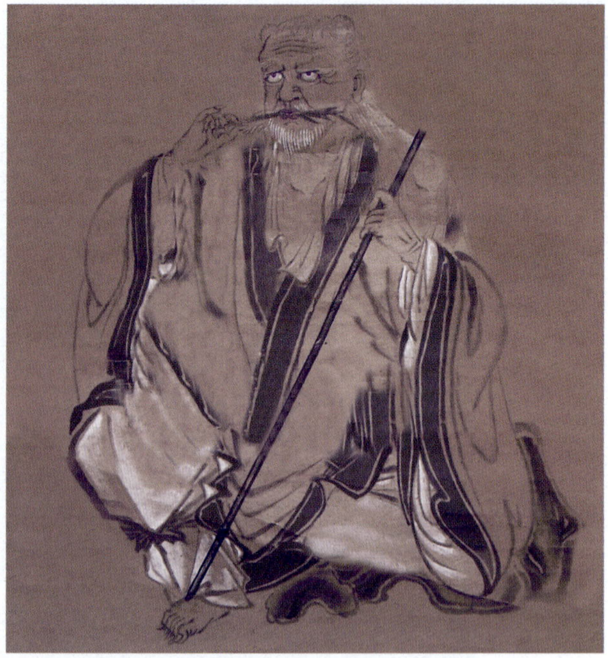

FIGURE 6-4. Shen Nung's herbal book, dated 2700 BC, is considered the oldest Chinese medical book and contains details of more than 300 plants. (Used with permission from Marisol LLC, Muscat, Sultanate of Oman.)

Among the Asian population, TCM is a very popular method of treating systemic and dermatologic diseases. The use of alternative medicine in Western countries ranges between 35% and 69%.[24,25] This popularity, which extends beyond the Asian population, is partly based on the misconception that alternative therapies are always safe and cost less than Western medicine. Additionally, patients who are increasingly frustrated by modern medicine also tend to seek alternative medical therapy. Americans spend over 30 billion a year on alternative therapy, according to the National Institutes of Health (NIH).[26] Due to the increasing popularity of TCM, it is important to address the safety of some of the more common treatments and practices.

Topical/Oral Traditional Medicine Many dermatologists remain unaware of the existence of placebo-controlled studies involving traditional medicine. Sheehan et al,[27] working in conjunction with the Chinese herbalist Luo in London, England, conducted one of the first placebo-controlled, double-blind studies involving atopic dermatitis. Therapeutic agents—including *Potentilla chinensis*, *Tribulus terrestris*, *Rehmannia glutinosa*, *Lophatherum gracile*, *Clematis armandii*, *Ledebouriella seseloides*, *Dictamnus dasycarpus*, *Paeonia lactiflora*, *Schizonepeta tenuifolia*, and *Glycyrrhiza glabra*—were compared with placebo herbs that had had no known efficacy for the treatment of atopic dermatitis. The results revealed that erythema decreased by 91.4% with the active herbs compared with only 10.6% with the placebo herbs. The safety of these agents was demonstrated, and liver function tests, renal function tests, and complete blood cell counts remained stable during the study period.[27]

Herbal Treatments Herbal treatments are becoming increasingly popular and are often used for dermatologic conditions. For instance, furocoumarins, a class of organic chemical compounds produced by various plants, are found in many Chinese herbal medicines that are used in the treatment of psoriasis. Despite the common misconception that herbal remedies have no adverse effects due to their "natural" composition, possible adverse effects such as hepatotoxicity have occurred. The most common adverse reactions with topical herbal treatments are contact dermatitis and irritant dermatitis. Essential oils used topically for aromatherapy and in herbal creams have been responsible for

TABLE 6-2 Rare side effects of traditional Chinese medicine other than allergic reactions or contact dermatitis

Ingredient	Adverse reactions
Arnica extracts, paprika	Sweet's syndrome[a,b]
Arsenic	Arsenic dermatoses[c-e]
Garlic	Urticaria, angioedema[f]
Kakkon-to	Fixed drug eruption[g]
Kombucha tea	Pellagra[h]
Mercury	Mercury poisoning[i]
Piperaceae	Contact leukomelanosis[j]

[a]Greer JM, Rosen T, Tschen JA. Sweet's syndrome with an exogenous cause. *Cutis*. 1993;51:112-114.

[b]Delmonte S, Brusati C, Parodi A, et al. Leukemia-related Sweet's syndrome elicited by pathergy to arnica. *Dermatology*. 1998;197:195-196.

[c]Kew J, Morris C, Aihie A, et al. Arsenic and mercury intoxication due to Indian ethnic remedies. *BMJ*. 1993;306:506-507.

[d]Wong SS, Tan KC, Goh CL. Cutaneous manifestations of chronic arsenicism: review of seventeen cases. *J Am Acad Dermatol*. 1998;38:179-185.

[e]Tay CH. Cutaneous manifestations of arsenic poisoning due to certain Chinese herbal medicine. *Australas J Dermatol*. 1974;15:121-131.

[f]Asero R, Mistrello G, Roncarolo D, et al. A case of garlic allergy. *J Allergy Clin Immunol*. 1998;101:427-428.

[g]Fujimoto N, Tajima S. Extensive fixed drug eruption due to the Japanese herbal drug "kakkon-to." *Br J Dermatol*. 2003;149:1303-1305.

[h]Wood B, Rademaker M, Oakley A, et al. Pellagra in a woman using alternative remedies. *Australas J Dermatol*. 1998;39:42-44.

[i]Ernst E, de Smet PAGM. Risks associated with complementary therapies. In: Dukes MNG, ed. *Meyler's Side Effects of Drugs*. 13th ed. Amsterdam, the Netherlands: Elsevier Science; 1996:1427.

[j]Liao YL, Chiang YC, Tsai TF, et al. Contact leukomelanosis induced by the leaves of Piper Betle L. (Pieperaceae): a clinical and histopathologic survey. *J Am Acad Dermatol*. 1999;40:583-589.

photosensitization.[28] Bergamot has been implicated in some cases because it contains 5-methoxypsoralen, and St. John's Wort, a best-selling herbal antidepressant, has photosensitivity as an adverse effect as well.[29] This may be significant in patients who require phototherapy for dermatologic conditions. The contamination of oral herbal preparations has also been reported, resulting in cases of arsenic and mercury poisoning.[30] Therefore, it is prudent to gain a detailed history of TCM use for patients presenting with either arsenical dermatoses or symptoms of mercury poisoning, because this may determine the cause of the poisoning. Other rare adverse effects are listed in **Table 6-2**.

Oils and Ointments The use of traditional medicated oils and ointments is increasing in the United States. It is important to note that certain brand names do not indicate the actual ingredients contained within the treatments. For instance, the popular brands Tiger Balm and 3-Snake Oil do not actually contain any material from these two animals [**Figure 6-5**]. Topical TCM treatments may also be adulterated with allergens, like balsam of Peru, which is a natural resinous balsam from the trunk of a Central American tree. Allergens such as tea tree oil and ylang-ylang, which are also commonly found in TCM, are now part of the North American standard patch tray.

One of the frequent arguments of using topical TCM by patients is the supposed absence of topical corticosteroids. However, many of the most common and prevalent adulterants in herbal creams are indeed corticosteroids.[31-35] More alarmingly, oral formulations have also been found to contain corticosteroids.[36-38] In a large-scale study from Taiwan, 2609 samples of traditional Chinese remedies were analyzed, and 24% were found to contain corticosteroids, some with significant amounts of clobetasol propionate.[38] In a study from London, 8 of 11 creams analyzed contained dexamethasone at concentrations inappropriate for use on the face or by children.[39] Other investigators reported the presence of triamcinolone acetonide in a phytocosmetic cream marketed in Europe as a skin care cosmetic product.[40] Unfortunately, both adults and infants may use products such as these for long periods of time, unaware of the potential adverse effects.

Acupuncture Acupuncture, used in a number of dermatologic conditions, such as atopic dermatitis, urticaria, and psoriasis,[41] is an ancient system of healing developed over thousands of years as part of traditional medicine in China, Japan, and other Eastern countries. The earliest recorded use of acupuncture date back over 4700 years ago, and it was described by Huang Ti Nei Ching Wen in The Yellow Emperor's Classic of Internal Medicine, which is considered the authoritative text of Ancient Chinese medicine.[42] In the United States, data from the National Health Interview Survey showed a 50% increase in the number of acupuncture users from 2002 and 2012. In 2012, 6.4% of U.S. adults reported they had used acupuncture, and 1.7% reported they had used it in the past 12 months.[43]

The practice of acupuncture is thought to have begun with the discovery that the stimulation of specific areas on the skin affects the functioning of certain organs of the body. Acupuncture uses fine needles to stimulate the body's own healing process through lines of energy in the body or the vital energy—otherwise known as Qi. The Qi is thought to flow through channels known as meridians (meaning the elements of wood, water, metal, fire, and earth). When the free flow of this energy is obstructed, a symptom appears. The aim of acupuncture is to remove these obstructions, thus allowing the energy to flow freely and the symptom to disappear. This is done by the insertion of fine needles into acupuncture meridian points just beneath the skin [**Figures 6-6** and **6-7**]. Magnets are also used on acupuncture meridian points and are most commonly secured with tape or a bandage, as shown in **Figure 6-8**.

Moxibustion, Cupping, and Coining

Moxibustion Moxibustion is a procedure practiced most commonly in Southeast Asia and almost exclusively by the Mien.[44] Moxibustion is a word derived from the words moxa and combustion. Moxa is a herb derived from the plant mugwort, or *Artemisia vulgaris*. It is believed that this herb, when burned on acupuncture points, can restore the flow of Qi. The procedure consists of heat application with use of the herb moxa on acupuncture points. Similar to acupuncture, moxibustion can be used either directly or indirectly to treat a variety of ailments, such as anemia, chronic stasis, acute lymphangitis, and immune suppression.[45] In the direct method, moxa is simply placed on the skin and lighted with an incense stick. The burning moxa is then pinched out or taken away by the therapist before it burns down completely to the skin. In the indirect method, the burning moxa is placed at the head of an inserted acupuncture needle.[46] Patients often report a rush of warmth throughout their body during the treatment. A great deal of training is required for a therapist to master moxibustion techniques. The lesions may mimic physical abuse, similar to cupping and coining,[47] because permanent burn scars can occur from an improper technique.[48] Physicians unfamiliar with these practices may suspect abuse, especially if the patient presenting is a woman or a child. Misdiagnosis could lead to grave consequences; for example, in one case, a false accusation of child abuse resulted in the suicide of a Vietnamese father.[49]

Cupping In cupping, a bottle is placed over a candle and coin with the bottle lip in direct contact with the skin [**Figure 6-9**]. As the candle consumes the oxygen, a vacuum is produced. This vacuum is intended to draw out the "fire wind" (pain). With this procedure, blood is drawn to the surface of the skin by the suction of the glass vessel on the skin. The cups are placed on areas in need of treatment, such as the chest, back, buttocks, chin, and dorsum of the foot. The cups are left on these specific areas of the skin until they adhere to the skin due to the negative pressure. They are then removed, leaving raised red patches that represent superficial skin inflammation. This is thought to reduce inflammation in adjacent organs deeper under the skin. Both pain and infection are thought to be alleviated through the effect of counterirritation.

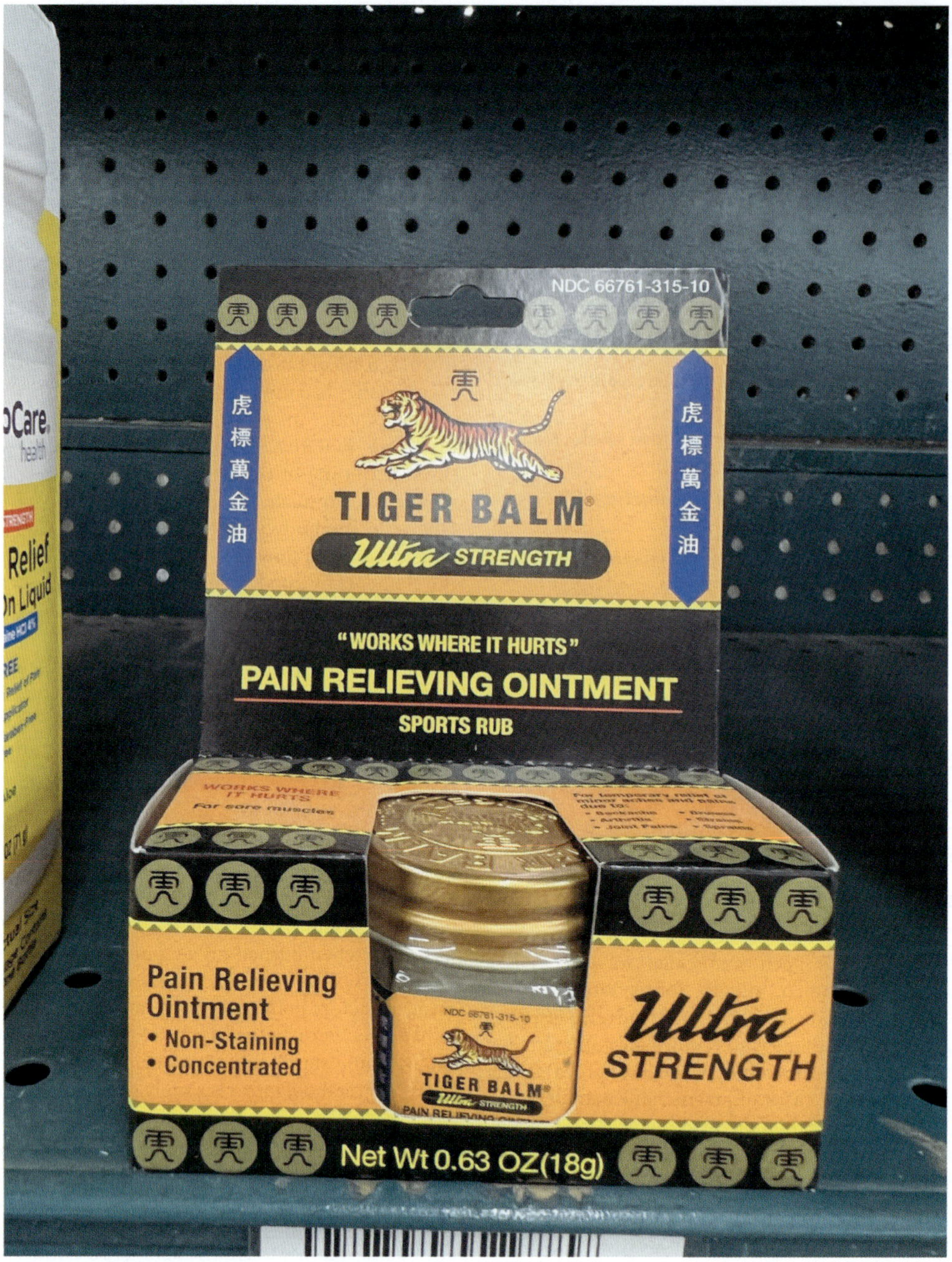

FIGURE 6-5. Tiger Balm is used to treat minor muscle/joint aches or pain.

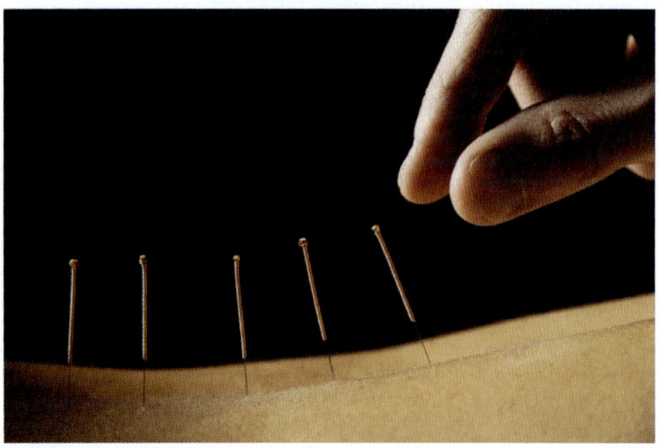

FIGURE 6-6. Acupuncture is an ancient system of healing developed over thousands of years as a part of the traditional medicine.

Coining Coining is a Chinese and Vietnamese practice used commonly to treat a variety of illnesses, including febrile illnesses, headaches, myalgia, and malaise. This remedy is also known as *cao gio* (scaping for wind) in Vietnam. Coining is the process of applying hot mentholated oil or Tiger Balm to the chest and back. The edge of a coin is rubbed over the spine and ribs, producing linear petechiae and ecchymoses [**Figure 6-10**].[50] When found in Vietnamese children, lesions produced by coining have sometimes been misdiagnosed as child abuse, and legal actions have been brought against the parents.[50]

The most common complications of coining have been minor burns. Because many fear criticism from their physicians for practicing coining, the true incidence of the custom is probably much higher in the United States than appreciated. In a survey of a clinic in Washington, DC, coining was the most used among Cambodian (70%), Chinese (35%), and Laotian (10%) patients.[44] Another Asian healing practice, pinching, uses the same principle as coining. In this case, pressure is

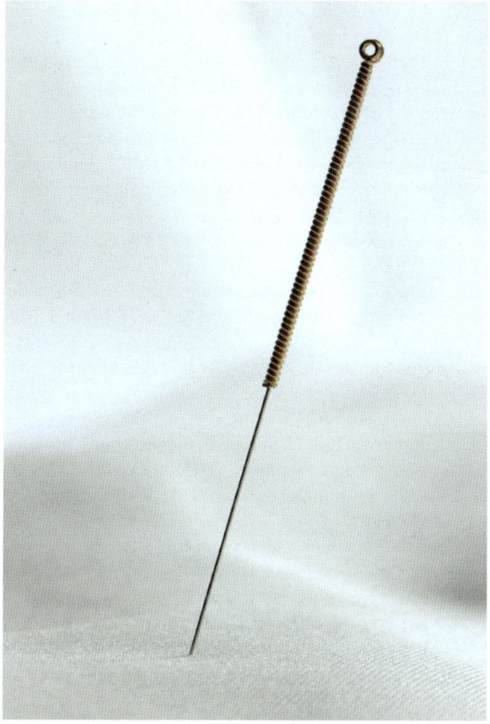

FIGURE 6-7. Needles are commonly used for acupuncture. (Used with permission from Marisol LLC, Muscat, Sultanate of Oman.)

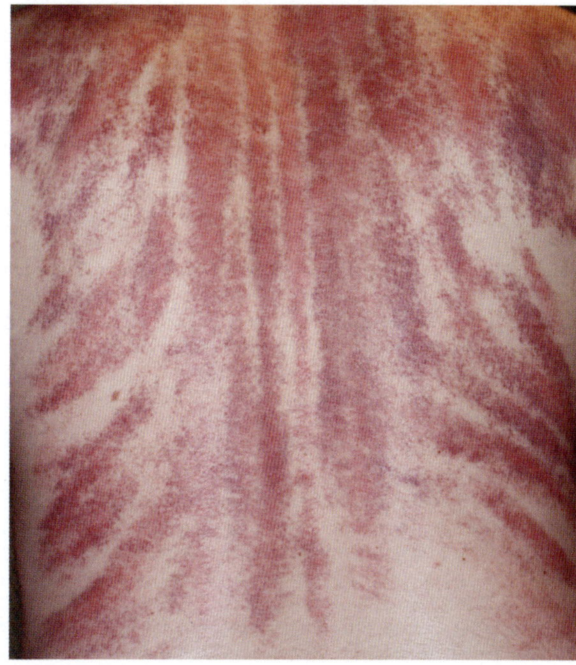

FIGURE 6-10. Coining is a Vietnamese practice used commonly to treat a variety of illnesses, including febrile illnesses, headaches, myalgia, and malaise. (Used with permission from Marisol LLC, Muscat, Sultanate of Oman.)

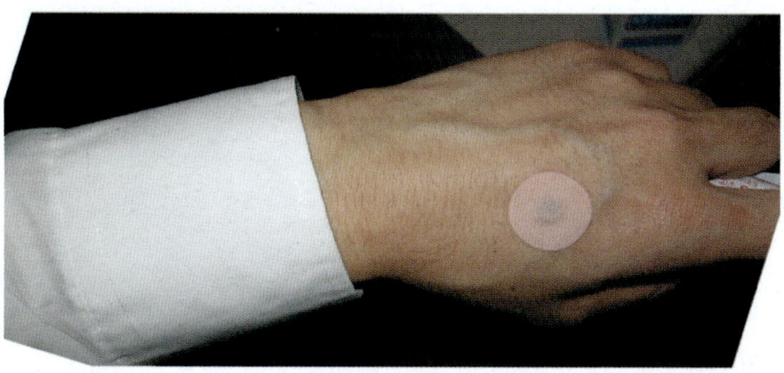

FIGURE 6-8. Magnets are also used on acupuncture meridian points and are most commonly secured with a tape or a bandage.

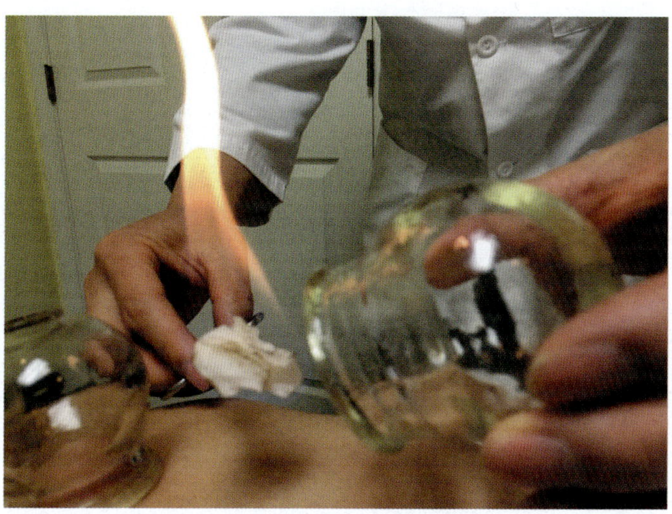

FIGURE 6-9. Cupping therapy. (Image courtesy of Dr. Jianting Tong.)

applied by pinching the skin between the thumb and index finger in order to produce a contusion.

CONCLUSION

With more than 25 different nations represented in the Asian population, it is important to recognize that patients who identify as part of the Asian community may vary widely in terms of their socioeconomic status, language, and health beliefs or practices. An increased awareness of these differences across subgroups within the Asian community is essential to provide competent care. Providers must also become familiar with the role of traditional medicine prevalent in the Asian American community. Finally, research involving Asian Americans may benefit from focusing on smaller-sized ethnic subgroup populations to better anticipate particular needs within the community.

REFERENCES

1. Ruiz AB, Ruiz NG. Key facts about Asian Americans, a diverse and growing population. 2021. https://www.pewresearch.org/fact-tank/2021/04/29/key-facts-about-asian-americans/. Accessed December 12, 2022.
2. Kochhar R, Cilluffo A. Income inequality in the U.S. is rising most rapidly among Asians. 2018. https://www.pewresearch.org/social-trends/2018/07/12/income-inequality-in-the-u-s-is-rising-most-rapidly-among-asians/#:~:text=The%2090%2F10%20ratio%20among,significant%20shift%20from%20the%20past. Accessed December 12, 2022.
3. Yi SS, Ali SH, Chin M, Russo RG, Doan LN, Rummo P. Contrasting the experiences for high- and low-income Asian Americans during COVID-19. *Prev Med Rep*. 2021;24:101519.
4. Banerjee A. Understanding economic disparities within the AAPI community. 2022. https://www.epi.org/blog/understanding-economic-disparities-within-the-aapi-community/. Accessed December 12, 2022.
5. Patraporn V, Ong P, Pech C. Wealth inequality among Asian Americans: the continuing significance of ethnicity and immigration. 2021;31. https://aapr.hkspublications.org/2021/04/16/wealth-inequality-among-asian-americans-the-

continuing-significance-of-ethnicity-and-immigration/. Accessed December 12, 2022.
6. Ahmmad Z, Wen M, Li K. Self-rated health disparities among Asian Americans: mediating roles of education level and household income. *J Immigr Minor Health*. 2021;23(3):583-590.
7. National Center for Health Statistics. Ambulatory health care data. Centers for Disease Control and Prevention; 2016.
8. Chu R, Sommers B. Health insurance coverage changes since implementation of the Affordable Care Act: Asian Americans and Pacific Islanders (Issue Brief No. HP-2021-11). Washington, DC: Office of the Assistant Secretary for Planning and Evaluation, US Department of Health and Human Services, May 24, 2021.
9. Lingala B, Li S, Wysong A, Truong AK, Kim D, Chang AL. Low rate of dermatology outpatient visits in Asian-Americans: an initial survey study for associated patient-related factors. *BMC Dermatol*. 2014;14:13.
10. Patel VM, Schwartz RA. Disparities in access to a dermatologist for acne care in the United States. *Int J Dermatol*. 2017;56(6):e131-e133.
11. Jin XW, Slomka J, Blixen CE. Cultural and clinical issues in the care of Asian patients. *Cleve Clin J Med*. 2002;69(1):50, 53-54, 56-58 passim.
12. Jang Y, Kim MT. Limited English proficiency and health service use in Asian Americans. *J Immigr Minor Health*. 2019;21(2):264-270.
13. Wu KK, Armstrong AW. Differences in face-to-face time spent with a dermatologist among patients with psoriasis based on race and ethnicity. *JAMA Dermatol*. 2022;158(10):1210-1212.
14. Howard University College of Medicine. *BESAFE-Asian Pacific Islander Model Book*. Washington, DC: National Minority AIDS Education and Training Center; 2009.
15. Lee S, Martinez G, Ma GX, et al. Barriers to health care access in 13 Asian American communities. *Am J Health Behav*. 2010;34(1):21-30.
16. Abrouk M, Lee K, Brodsky M, et al. Ethnicity affects the presenting severity of psoriasis. *J Am Acad Dermatol*. 2017;77(1):180-182.
17. Hsu DY, Smith B, Silverberg JI. Atopic dermatitis and hospitalization for mental health disorders in the United States. *Dermatitis*. 2019;30(1):54-61.
18. Gorelick J, Daniels SR, Kawata AK, et al. Acne-related quality of life among female adults of different races/ethnicities. *J Dermatol Nurses Assoc*. 2015;7(3):154-162.
19. Figure 3. Percentage of Asian (alone) applicants to U.S. medical schools by Asian subgroups, academic year 2018-2019. https://www.aamc.org/data-reports/workforce/interactive-data/figure-3-percentage-asian-alone-applicants-us-medical-schools-asian-subgroups-academic-year-2018. Accessed December 27, 2022.
20. Felicilda-Reynaldo RFD, Choi SY, Driscoll SD, Albright CL. A national survey of complementary and alternative medicine use for treatment among Asian-Americans. *J Immigr Minor Health*. 2020;22(4):762-770.
21. Ries AL, Picchi MA, Nguyen LH, Moser RJ, Molgaard CA, Wasserman SI. Asthma in a Vietnamese refugee population. *Am J Respir Crit Care Med*. 1997;155(6):1895-1901.
22. White House Commission on Complementary and Alternative Medicine Policy. Chapter 2: overview of CAM in the United States: recent history, current status, and prospects for the future. https://govinfo.library.unt.edu/whccamp/pdfs/fr2002_chapter_2.pdf. Accessed December 12, 2022.
23. U.S. National Library of Medicine. Classics of traditional Chinese medicine. https://www.nlm.nih.gov/exhibition/chinesemedicine/emperors.html. Accessed December 12, 2022.
24. Ernst E, Pittler MH, Stevinson C. Complementary/alternative medicine in dermatology: evidence-assessed efficacy of two diseases and two treatments. *Am J Clin Dermatol*. 2002;3(5):341-348.
25. Smith N, Shin DB, Brauer JA, Mao J, Gelfand JM. Use of complementary and alternative medicine among adults with skin disease: results from a national survey. *J Am Acad Dermatol*. 2009;60(3):419-425.
26. Nahin RL, Barnes PM, Stussman BJ. Expenditures on complementary health approaches: United States, 2012. *Natl Health Stat Rep*. 2016;(95):1-11.
27. Sheehan MP, Rustin MH, Atherton DJ, et al. Efficacy of traditional Chinese herbal therapy in adult atopic dermatitis. *Lancet*. 1992;340(8810):13-17.
28. Cocks H, Wilson D. Dangers of the intake of psoralens and subsequent UV exposure producing significant burns. *Burns*. 1998;24(1):82.
29. Stevinson C, Ernst E. Safety of hypericum in patients with depression. *CNS Drugs*. 1999;11:125-132.
30. Sakharkar P. Lead Poisoning due to herbal medications. *Indian J Clin Biochem*. 2017;32(4):500-501.
31. Ahmed S, Riaz M. Quantitation of cortico-steroids as common adulterants in local drugs by HPLC. *Chromatographia*. 1991;31:67-70.
32. Wood B, Wishart J. Potent topical steroid in a Chinese herbal cream. *N Z Med J*. 1997;110(1055):420-421.
33. Ernst E. Adverse effects of herbal drugs in dermatology. *Br J Dermatol*. 2000;143(5):923-929.
34. O'Driscoll J, Burden AD, Kingston TP. Potent topical steroid obtained from a Chinese herbalist. *Br J Dermatol*. 1992;127(5):543-544.
35. Hughes JR, Higgins EM, Pembroke AC. Oral dexamethasone masquerading as a Chinese herbal remedy. *Br J Dermatol*. 1994;130(2):261.
36. Vander Stricht BI, Parvais OE, Vanhaelen-Fastre RJ, Vanhaelen MH, Quertinier D. Safer use of traditional remedies. Remedies may contain cocktail of active drugs. *BMJ*. 1994;308(6937):1162.
37. Joseph AM, Biggs T, Garr M, Singh J, Lederle FA. Stealth steroids. *N Engl J Med*. 1991;324(1):62.
38. Huang WF, Wen KC, Hsiao ML. Adulteration by synthetic therapeutic substances of traditional Chinese medicines in Taiwan. *J Clin Pharmacol*. 1997;37(4):344-350.
39. Keane FM, Munn SE, du Vivier AW, Taylor NF, Higgins EM. Analysis of Chinese herbal creams prescribed for dermatological conditions. *BMJ*. 1999;318(7183):563-564.
40. Bircher AJ, Niederer M, Hohl C, Surber C. Stealth triamcinolone acetonide in a phytocosmetic cream. *Br J Dermatol*. 2002;146(3):531-532.
41. Chen CJ, Yu HS. Acupuncture treatment of urticaria. *Arch Dermatol*. 1998;134(11):1397-1399.
42. Veith I. *The Yellow Emperor's Classic of Internal Medicine*. Vol 18. Berkeley, CA: University of California Press; 1984.
43. Acupuncture: what you need to know. https://www.nccih.nih.gov/health/acupuncture-what-you-need-to-know. Accessed December 12, 2022.
44. Buchwald D, Panwala S, Hooton TM. Use of traditional health practices by Southeast Asian refugees in a primary care clinic. *West J Med*. 1992;156(5):507-511.
45. Zhou W. Acute lymphangitis treated by moxibustion with garlic in 118 cases. *J Tradit Chin Med*. 2003;23(3):198.
46. Wilcox L. *Moxibustion: The Power of Mugwort Fire*. Boulder, CA: Blue Poppy Press; 2008.
47. Look KM, Look RM. Skin scraping, cupping, and moxibustion that may mimic physical abuse. *J Forensic Sci*. 1997;42(1):103-105.
48. Conde-Salazar L, Gonzalez MA, Guimarens D, Fuente C. Burns due to moxibustion. *Contact Dermatitis*. 1991;25(5):332-333.
49. Nong The A. "Pseudo-battered child" syndrome. *JAMA*. 1976;236(20):2288.
50. Yeatman GW, Dang VV. Cao Gio (coin rubbing). Vietnamese attitudes toward health care. *JAMA*. 1980;244(24):2748-2749.

CHAPTER 7

Historical and Sociocultural Influences on Latine/Hispanic American Healthcare

Larimar Rodriguez
Alba Posligua-Alban
Benjamin Vazquez
Naiara S. Barbosa

KEY POINTS

- Medical professionals should recognize and understand the historical and sociocultural factors influencing the health and healthcare access of the Latine/Hispanic populations in the United States.
- Immigration policies, unfamiliarity and mistrust of the healthcare system, and cultural or traditional practices are factors that impact how dermatologic care is sought and delivered to Latine/Hispanic individuals.
- Traditional medicine continues to be used by Latine/Hispanic communities to treat dermatologic conditions; therefore, providers should be aware of and inquire about these practices.

- Increased access to care, inclusive research, and higher recruitment of diverse dermatology workforce are crucial to decrease the dermatologic disparities affecting the Latine/Hispanic populations in the United States.

INTRODUCTION

The United States is a multicultural and ethnically diverse country, shaped by centuries of immigration and cultural exchange. Since its colonization in the 17th century, people from around the world have contributed to the nation's evolving identity. Latine or Hispanic individuals accounted for just over half (51.1%) of the U.S. population growth between 2010 and 2020 and currently represent over 18% of the population—a figure projected to rise to more than 26% by 2050.[1,2] As this population continues to grow, it is increasingly important for healthcare providers to understand the unique strengths, needs, and experiences of the communities they serve.

Latine/Hispanic communities in the U.S. have long faced barriers to opportunity, including disparities in employment, housing, and education. Within the healthcare system, they have also encountered challenges such as bias, stereotyping, and communication gaps.[3,4] Language barriers, in particular, can limit access to care, affect comprehension of medical information, and hinder the development of trusting provider-patient relationships. Strengthening cultural humility and communication in clinical practice can help improve care and build stronger connections with Latine/Hispanic patients.

In this chapter, we will explore both historical and sociocultural factors that influence health in this community, examine dermatologic disparities that exist in the Latine/Hispanic populations, and highlight traditional health practices used for dermatologic conditions.

DEFINITIONS

Historically, *ethnicity* has been used to refer to a person's cultural identity (ie, language, customs, and religion) and *race* to classify groups based on ancestral origin and physical characteristics. Conversations on defining *race* and *ethnicity* and the most appropriate way to incorporate these terms in the medical literature are ongoing, but inclusion of these terms (along with an understanding how these terms emerged in America—see Chapter 1) are necessary to mitigate racial and ethnic disparities across medicine.[5]

The terms *Latino* and Hispanic categorize a heterogeneous population and are used synonymously by the U.S. government to classify individuals of various regions of origin, place of birth, and racial identification.[1] Although the two terms are often used interchangeably, they differ in meaning. *Latino* describes persons whose origin or ancestries are from countries of Latin America.[6] It has also been used when referring to persons from Europe and America where languages derived from Latin are spoken.[6] *Hispanic,* a term that was implemented in the U.S. Census in the 1970s, describes individuals whose origin or ancestries comes from Hispania, regions now occupied by Portugal and Spain, or Spanish-speaking persons with culture or ancestry related to Spain.[6] Critics of the organizing term "Hispanic" have noted that it may oversimplify the wide range of backgrounds and experiences within the communities it is meant to represent. In particular, some argue that the term does not adequately reflect the diverse cultural, historical, and social contexts—especially the differing experiences of those with ancestry rooted in colonizing nations versus those from formerly colonized regions.[7] For example, a White person of Spanish descent who has immigrated to the United States from Spain may experience life differently compared to a Brown-skinned immigrant from Mexico. Following these debates, the term "Latino/a" arose to name those descendants from Latin American populations. More recently, the term has undergone various alterations to eliminate the masculine/feminine binary that is present in the Spanish language to acknowledge all gender expressions. In 2000, "Latin@" gained traction as it could describe both men and women, followed by "Latinx," which is the gender-neutral, widely used term today.[7] "Latine" has since been introduced as a newer term that is synonymous with Latinx but can be pronounced and conjugated in Spanish.

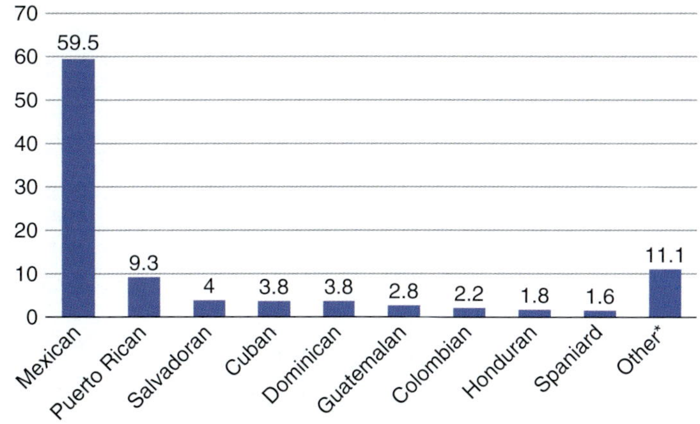

FIGURE 7-1. Percentage of Latine/Hispanic origin groups in the United States, 2021.*Other includes Latine/Hispanic origin groups in the United States with percentages less than 1.5%, including Nicaraguan, Argentinean, Panamanian, Costa Rican, Chilean, Bolivian, Uruguayan, Paraguayan, other South American, and other Central American. (Adapted from https://www.pewresearch.org/fact-tank/2022/09/23/key-facts-about-u-s-latinos-for-national-hispanic-heritage-month/.)

This chapter will focus on persons residing in the United States, most of whom are from Latin American countries [**Figure 7-1**], therefore the terms *Latine* and *Hispanic* will be used interchangeably.

HISTORICAL AND SOCIOCULTURAL FACTORS INFLUENCING HEALTH

There are various historical and sociocultural factors that influence the Latine/Hispanic community in their medical decision-making and access to healthcare in the United States. It is important to consider how immigration policies, unfamiliarity and mistrust of the healthcare system, and cultural or traditional practices impact how dermatologic care is sought out and delivered in this country. Below, we will discuss each of these factors, many of which intersect, and their relevance to working with Latine/Hispanic patients.

IMMIGRATION POLICIES AND BARRIERS TO ESSENTIAL RESOURCES/SERVICES

Immigration policies and practices can directly and indirectly influence the health of Latine/Hispanic immigrants by affecting the availability of material resources (such as food, wages, working conditions and housing), access to institutions essential to health (including education and healthcare) and the way in which Latine immigrants are perceived or discriminated against by others, and their personal perceptions of belonging in a community [**Figure 7-2**].[8] Moreover, these barriers can spill over and affect all Latine/Hispanic individuals. For instance, Latine citizens and noncitizens who live in states with a high number of immigration-related laws have decreased odds of reporting optimal health as compared to Latine respondents in states with fewer immigration-related laws. Regarding families in which members have different immigration statuses, a study in 2017 found undocumented parents were less likely to report optimal health for their child who was a citizen as compared to parents who were either a Legal Permanent Resident or U.S. Citizen.[9] About nine million Americans live in mixed-status families and nearly 10% of babies born each year have one undocumented parent.[10] Of the 62.5 million Latine/Hispanic individuals residing in the United States, it is estimated that just under 13% are undocumented, and Latine communities obtain less insurance than all other ethnoracial groups.[11-13] Furthermore, medical services are provided in large part through employer-based health insurance,

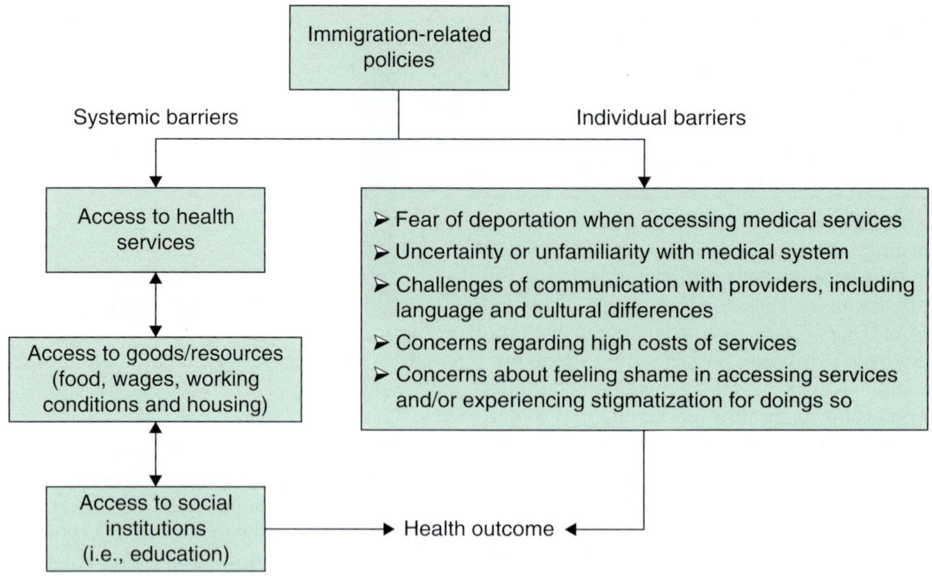

FIGURE 7-2. Pathways through which immigration-related policies relevant to immigrants may influence Latine health. (Adapted from Philbin MM, Flake M, Hatzenbuehler ML, Hirsch JS. State-level immigration and immigrant-focused policies as drivers of Latino health disparities in the United States. *Soc Sci Med.* 2018;199:29-38, Figure 3.)

Medicare, or Medicaid, and any individual that is not covered under one of these will have a challenging time accessing and paying for healthcare services.[11] In 1996, the Illegal Immigration Reform and Immigration Responsibility Act (IIRIRA) and Personal Responsibility and Work Opportunity Reconciliation Act (PRWORA) were implemented, and to this day serve as a major exclusion to the Affordable Care Act (ACA) for immigrants. Only U.S. citizens and long-term immigrants with legal permanent residency or asylum qualify for ACA, meaning that legal permanent residents with less than 5 years residing in the United States, unauthorized immigrants, and student or work visa holders are excluded from the Medicaid expansion, including purchasing their own coverage.[11] It is important to note that in the instances where patients may be eligible for insurance resources, either through an employer or another institution, fear about sharing their information due to their immigration status or the status of immediate family members could still stand in the way of them seeking coverage. As a result, many Latine people who legally qualify for insurance coverage or health services do not enroll.[8]

There are limited health resources available to low-income and undocumented immigrants. Emergency Medicaid is a policy that offers reimbursement to hospitals providing emergency services to individuals who would otherwise qualify for Medicaid if it were not for their immigration status.[14] Healthcare offices should keep a list of institutions and academic hospitals that offer free clinics and low-cost to free medication programs specific to their region.

UNFAMILIARITY AND MISTRUST OF THE HEALTHCARE SYSTEM

Several studies have reported mistrust among Latine/Hispanic communities toward the American healthcare system that can be attributed to personal experiences of discrimination and the larger history of unjust medical treatment and unethical research of Black, Latine/Hispanic, and Indigenous communities by the United States.[15,16] It is also important for healthcare providers to consider that the American healthcare system is vastly different and unfamiliar to those of Latin America on several fronts. Physician assistants and nurse practitioners are not part of the healthcare in Latin America, which can lead to confusion if not properly explained, and cost of medical services tend to be significantly higher in the United States, which can contribute to mistrust in our system.[17] It is imperative that culturally sensitive educational efforts are undertaken by medical providers in the clinical and research settings to gain patient trust and ultimately improve health outcomes. Consenting for medical treatments and procedures should be carefully explained with the help of a certified medical interpreter and, when available, forms and instructions should be offered in Spanish, so that patients can fully understand them.

CULTURAL INSIGHTS AND TRADITIONAL PRACTICES

Latine communities have one of the highest proportions of multigenerational households (>10%) among all ethnoracial groups.[18] Cultural norms encouraging multigenerational living and socioeconomic conditions may contribute to this high percentage. Latine women, who may ascribe to values of "marianismo" (characterized as submissiveness, selflessness, and family- or home-centered), are typically responsible for maintaining the health and well-being of families. Conversely, Latine men may be reluctant to consult physicians for health problems until a visit to an emergency room is needed.

Whether due to affordability, familiarity, reduced linguistic barriers or dissatisfaction with perceived results of modern medical therapy, traditional medicine is often sought after.[19] First-generation Latine/Hispanic individuals or new immigrants are more likely to hold onto these traditional beliefs and practices out of long held respect,[20,21] which are easily passed on in a multigenerational home.

Latine communities also value the importance of communication (including verbal and nonverbal) in interpersonal relationships.[22] Inability to effectively communicate with healthcare professionals, whether due to linguistic barriers or less patient-centered care by the provider, could result in feelings of mistrust, lack of confidence, fear, and therefore worse patient outcomes. Efforts aimed at recruiting healthcare professionals representative of the U.S. population could contribute to improved trust, confidence, and better patient outcomes in this community.[23]

DERMATOLOGY AND LATINE/HISPANIC

LATINE/HISPANIC DERMATOLOGIC DISPARITIES

Significant dermatologic disparities affecting Latine/Hispanic populations exist with one of the most widely acknowledged being morbidity and mortality in cutaneous melanoma. While melanoma is more common in White individuals, Latine/Hispanic patients are more likely to present at a later stage of diagnosis, with increased tumor thickness and poorer survival [**Figure 7-3**].[24] Lately, more efforts have been dedicated to understand such health disparities, especially when there have been advancements in treatment options and universal improvement

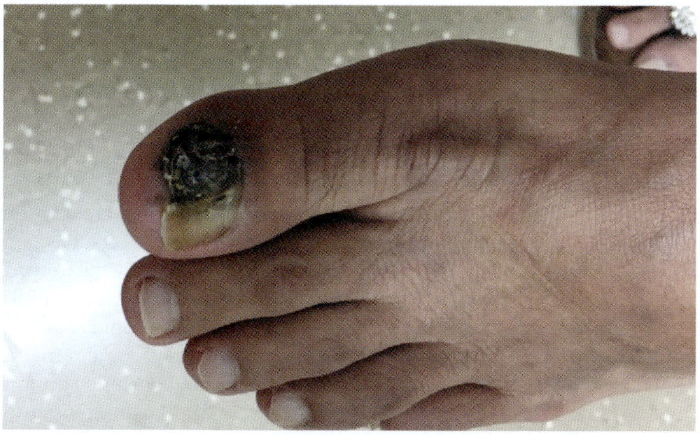

FIGURE 7-3. Acral lentiginous melanoma of the left great toe (with Breslow depth of at least 2.2 mm) on a 54-year Latine woman.

of melanoma outcomes. Many Latine/Hispanic individuals wrongly believe they cannot develop skin cancer due to their darker skin tones and lack of family history, and, therefore, do not use sun protection regularly.[25] During clinical encounters, medical providers should take the time to educate their Latine/Hispanic patients about skin cancer risk and protective measures. Health disparities have also been associated with atopic dermatitis and psoriasis. Among Latine/Hispanic children, risk of persistent atopic dermatitis is higher compared to their non-Hispanic White counterparts.[26] Among Latine/Hispanic adults, hospitalization for psoriasis is more probable compared to non-Hispanic White adults.[23] Keloidal scarring is a complication more frequently seen among communities of color afflicted with hidradenitis suppurativa, including Latine/Hispanic patients. While these studies aim to account for socioeconomic factors, there is likely residual confounders regarding socio-demographic factors impacting historically marginalized populations in the United States, including the Latine/Hispanic community.

ROLE OF TRADITIONAL MEDICINE

Traditional medicines are skills and practices derived from the knowledge, beliefs, and experiences native to different cultures, which are used to better the overall health of those communities.[27] Traditional health beliefs or practices are not monistic and emanate from cultural, familial, religious, and scientific sources.[28] More importantly, many traditional practices have been passed down for hundreds of generations prior to colonization. For many in the Latine community, traditional medicine is inextricably linked to spirituality and religion [**Figure 7-4**]. In Mexico and Central America, for instance, traditional medicine is particularly important for helping mothers through pregnancy and during the birthing process as well as helping the dying to depart this life in peace and move on to the spirit world(s). U.S. providers should also be aware that Latine immigrants may not speak Spanish or Portuguese but may speak a language native to a region and spoken by Indigenous peoples.

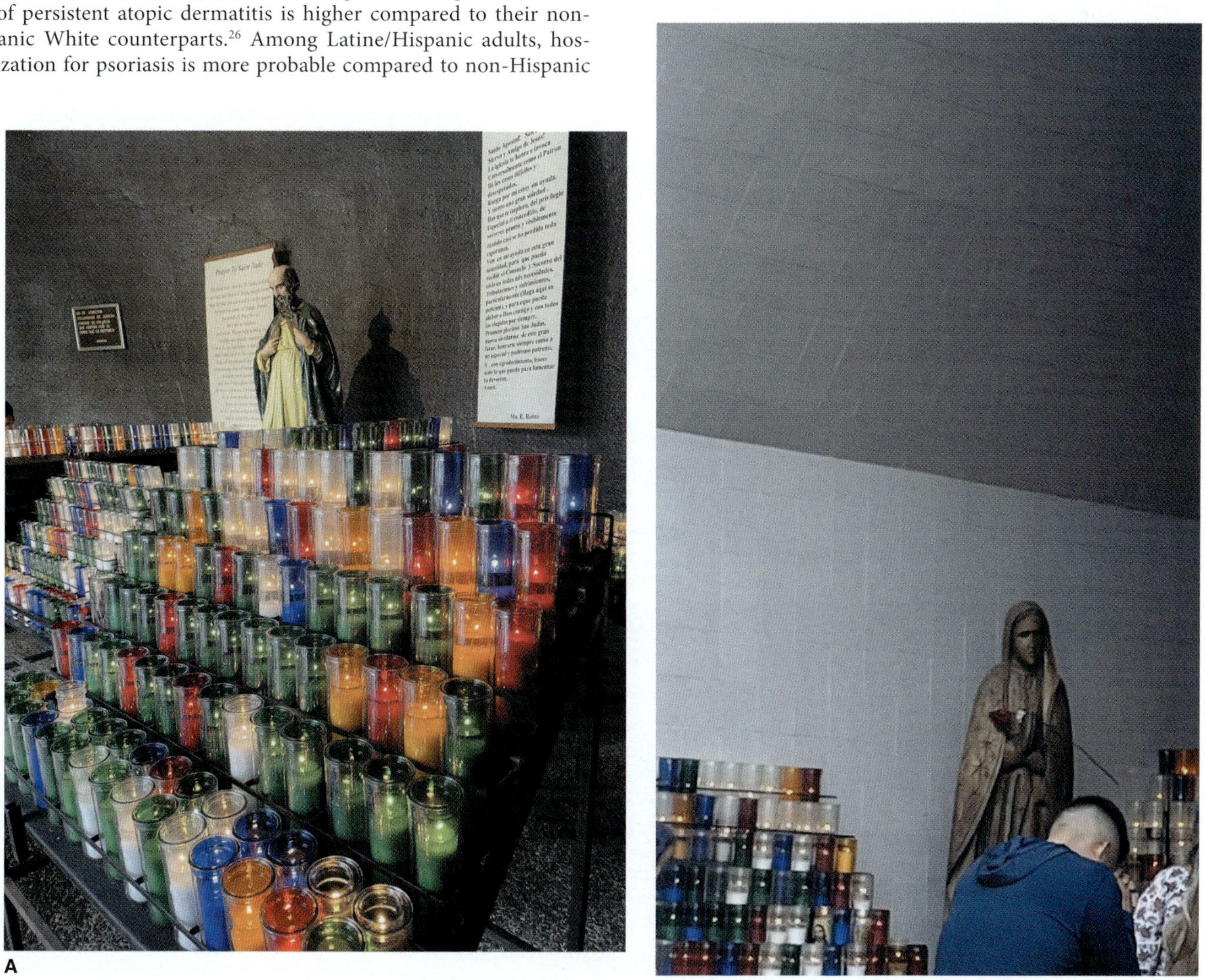

A

B

FIGURE 7-4. Prayer to the Saints **(A)** or the Virgen of Guadalupe **(B)**. For many in the Latine/Hispanic community, religious beliefs or practices are an important mechanism used to gain some emotional stability when facing difficult situations such as poor health.

TABLE 7-1 Types of Latine/Hispanic medicine practitioners

Traditional healer	Description
Santería	Traditional healers thought to hold supernatural forces and can be used to mobilize these beneficial supernatural forces, which can decrease uncertainty and/or stress.
Curandero/a	Professional healer or *sanador* who treats physical illnesses, helps deliver babies, and treats victims to curses with their strong belief in God, herbs, prayer, and other remedies.
Sabador(a)	Deals with the musculoskeletal system treating sprains, bruises, and other pains.
Yebero/a	Herbalist that specializes in herbal remedies.
Huesero/a	Bone specialist that can set bones.

The above descriptions are informed by a combination of the study team's expertise in addition to Fowler et al[28] and Cruz et al.[19]

Traditional healing incorporates culturally known herbs, prayer, and other remedies that may be obtained through a healer [**Table 7-1**].[28] It also acknowledges illnesses that may not be well known among healthcare providers, including but not limited to *mal de aire* (bad or malevolent wind), *susto* and *espanto* (sudden fright), and *mal de ojo* (evil eye).[28] These illnesses are deeply rooted in Latine/Hispanic culture and can carry psychological or religious overtones. When Latine/Hispanic patients are treated by providers unfamiliar with these cultural-specific illnesses, the true nature of their complaint could be lost or mislabeled as fabrications or malingering.

TREATMENTS FOR DERMATOLOGIC CONDITIONS

Natural remedies are used among Latine/Hispanic individuals not only for ailments of the skin but also joint aches, abdominal pain, headaches, among others common ailments.[29] Botanical remedies, and herbs specifically, are the most common traditional-healing products used [**Figure 7-5**].[30] These treatments are typically purchased from local herbal shops (*botánicas* or *hierberías*) commonly found in Latine/Hispanic neighborhoods and involve applying the plants or plant products externally to the skin, even for internal ailments [**Figure 7-6**]. The botanical products can be boiled resulting in solution being used for compresses or are mixed with a variety of oils to be formulated into creams, pastes, or poultices.[31] Other preparations include syrups, salves, capsules, and tablets containing the powdered form of the herb [**Figure 7-7**]. No regulation of herbal products currently exists in the United States, except for dietary supplements, meaning there no standardization of purity, active ingredients, or concentrations of herbal remedies. Vitamins and minerals are widely used as dietary supplements in the Latine/Hispanic community for disease treatment and prevention, with one-a-day multivitamin/multimineral supplements being the most common.[20] **Table 7-2** describes remedies commonly used by many Latine/Hispanic groups for dermatologic conditions and the current scientific evidence that exists supporting effectiveness of such remedies.

CONCLUSION

Despite established prevention measures and ever-improving treatment options, disease-specific dermatologic disparities exist within the Latine/Hispanic community. Historical, structural, and cultural factors affecting this community may contribute to these disparities by influencing access to care or through feelings of uncertainty/mistrust in the U.S. healthcare system. Traditional medicine is often sought after and emanates from cultural, familial, religious, and scientific sources.[32] Beyond training culturally sensitive dermatologists to help ameliorate health disparities in this community, it is imperative that we recruit and retain more dermatologists who identify as Latine/Hispanic and incorporate trainings to understand the history, culture, and social determinants of health affecting the communities we are treating.

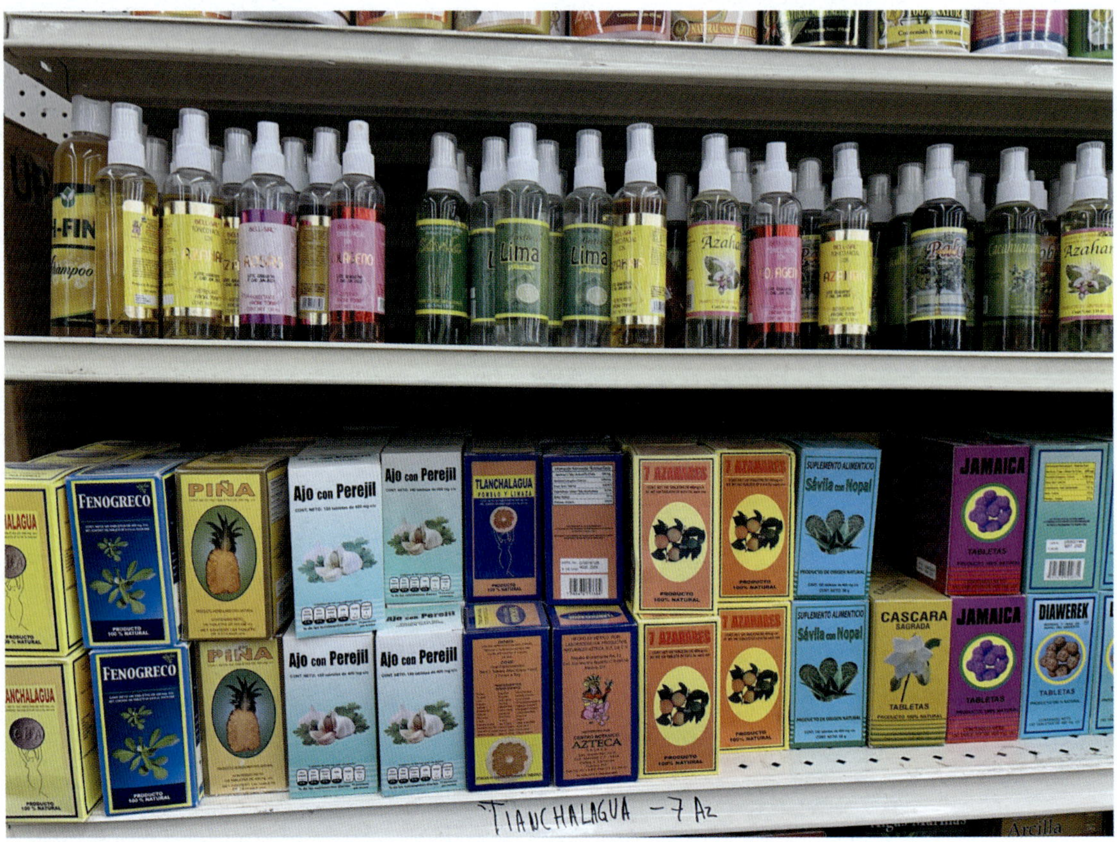

FIGURE 7-5. Botanical remedies used as traditional-healing products.

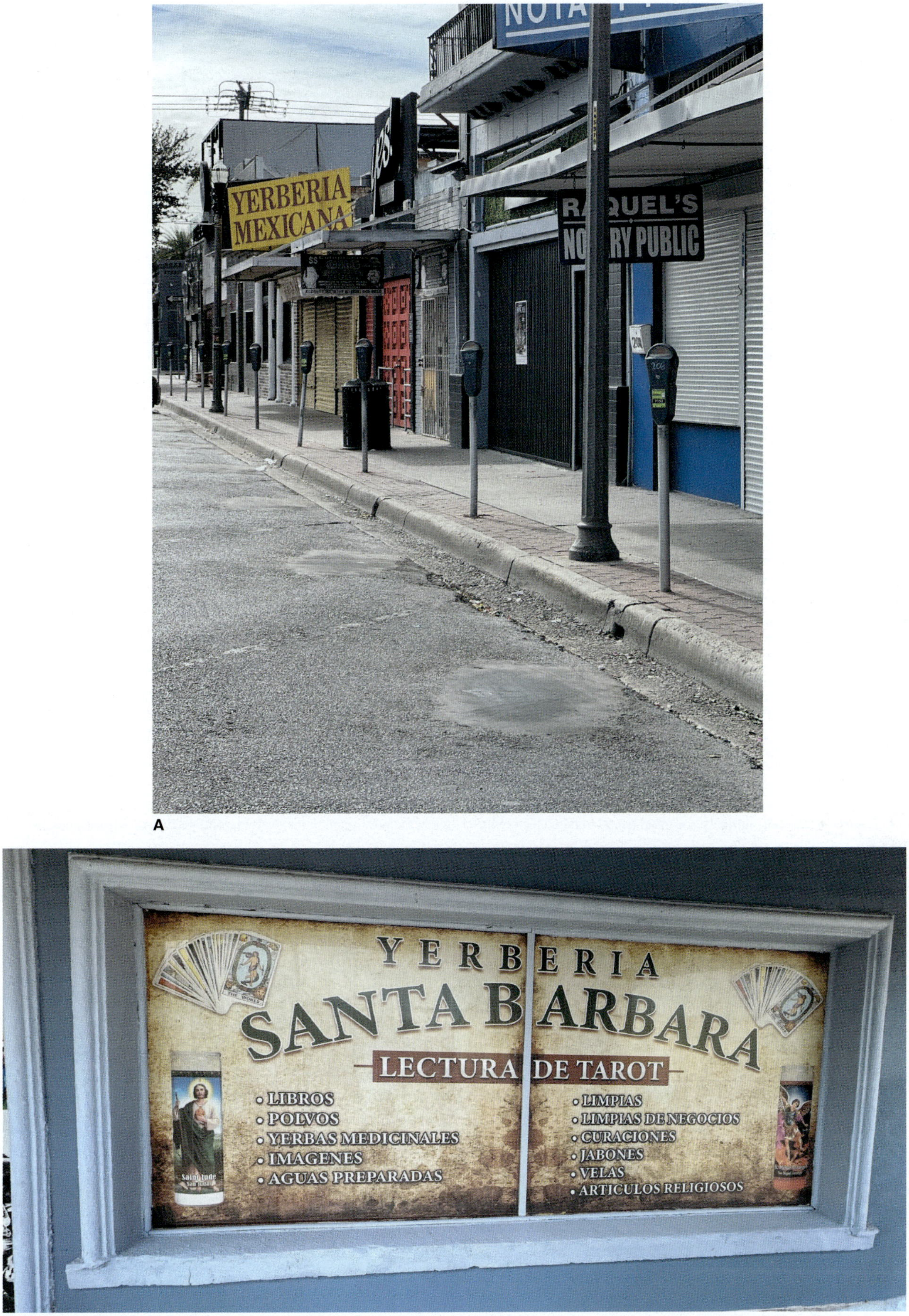
YERBERIA
MEXICANA
A
YERBERIA
SANTA BARBARA
LECTURA DE TAROT
• LIBROS
• POLVOS
• YERBAS MEDICINALES
• IMAGENES
• AGUAS PREPARADAS
• LIMPIAS
• LIMPIAS DE NEGOCIOS
• CURACIONES
• JABONES
• VELAS
• ARTICULOS RELIGIOSOS
B

FIGURE 7-6. **(A)** Local herbal shop found in Latine/Hispanic neighborhood. **(B)** The storefront of a local natural remedies shop, or botánica, in a Latine/Hispanic neighborhood. The items available for sale include medicinal herbs and religious items.

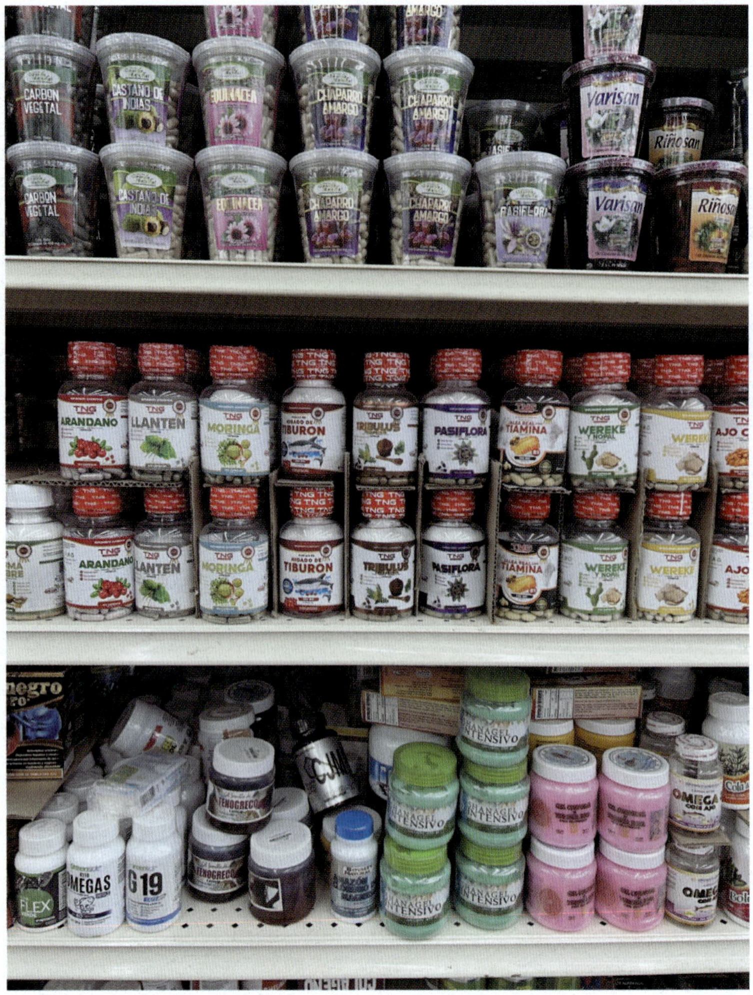

FIGURE 7-7. Capsules and tablets containing the powdered form of select herbs.

TABLE 7-2 Botanicals, minerals, nutrients, and other typical traditional ingredients used by Latine/Hispanic individuals for common dermatologic conditions

	Traditional ingredients used medicinally		
Dermatologic condition	**Ingredient name**	**Spanish name**	**Contraindications**
Acne			
	Aloe vera	*Zábila*	• None with topical use
	Apple cider vinegar	*Vinagre de sidra de manzana*	• Moderate interaction with digoxin, insulin, and potassium-sparing diuretics • Phytophotodermatitis with sun exposure
	Basil	*Albahaca*	• Moderate interaction with anticoagulants
	Garlic	*Ajo*	• Major interaction with isoniazid and NNRTIs • Moderate interaction with oral contraceptive pills, cyclosporine, medications changed by the cytochrome P450 system, and anticoagulants
	Lemon juice	*Jugo de limón*	• Large amounts should not be ingested by those with renal disease • Phytophotodermatitis with sun exposure
	Orange skin	*Piel de naranja*	• Phytophotodermatitis with sun exposure
	Tea tree oil	*Esencias del árbol del té*	• Should not be ingested
Alopecia			
	Aloe vera	*Zábila*	• None with topical use
	Lavender oil	*Aceite esencial de lavanda*	• None
	Onion	*Cebolla*	• Moderate interaction with aspirin, lithium, antidiabetic agents, and anticoagulants
	Rosemary	*Romero*	• Possible exacerbation of seizure disorders
	Thyme	*Tomillo*	• May affect thyroid activity
	Castor oil	*Aceite de castor*	• None with topical use

(*Continued*)

TABLE 7-2 Botanicals, minerals, nutrients, and other typical traditional ingredients used by Latine/Hispanic individuals for common dermatologic conditions (*Continued*)

Traditional ingredients used medicinally			
Dermatologic condition	**Ingredient name**	**Spanish name**	**Contraindications**
Arthropod bite and burn			
	Aloe vera	*Zábila*	• None with topical use
	Honey	*Miel*	• None
	Lemon juice	*Jugo de limón*	• Large amounts should not be ingested by those with renal disease • Phytophotodermatitis with sun exposure
	Milk	*Leche*	• None
	Olive oil	*Aceite de oliva*	• None topically
	Sage	*Salvia*	• None
	Tea tree oil	*Esencias del árbol del té*	• Should not be ingested
	Yogurt	*Yogur*	• Moderate interaction with tetracyclines, ciprofloxacin, and immunosuppressants
Atopic dermatitis and pruritis			
	Aloe vera	*Zábila*	• None with topical use
	Apple cider vinegar	*Vinagre de sidra de manzana*	• Moderate interaction with digoxin, insulin, and potassium-sparing diuretics • Phytophotodermatitis with sun exposure
	Arnica	*Árnica*	• Moderate interaction with anticoagulants (aspirin, clopidogrel, ibuprofen, dalteparin, enoxaparin, heparin, and warfarin)
	Burdock	*Bardana*	• Moderate interaction with anticoagulants
	Chamomile	*Manzanilla*	• Moderate interaction with oral contraceptive pills, estrogen, benzodiazepine, CNS depressants, tamoxifen, and warfarin • Minor interaction with medications changed by cytochrome P450 system • Should not be used in patients with conditions worsened by exposure to estrogen (eg, breast cancer, uterine cancer, ovarian cancer, endometriosis, and fibroids)
	Cornstarch	*Maicena*	• None
	Lavender oil	*Aceite esencial de lavanda*	• None
	Oatmeal	*Avena*	• Should not be used on large open wounds
	Olive oil	*Aceite de oliva*	• None topically
	Witch hazel	*Agua de hamamelis*	• None
Bacterial infection			
	Tea tree oil	*Esencias del árbol del té*	• Should not be ingested
Fungal infection			
	Lavender oil	*Aceite esencial de lavanda*	• None
	Vinegar	*Vinagre*	• Moderate interaction with digoxin, insulin, and diuretics
	Yogurt	*Yogur*	• Moderate interaction with tetracyclines, ciprofloxacin, and immunosuppressants
	Garlic	*Ajo*	(Listed above)
	Burdock	*Bardana*	• Moderate interaction with anticoagulants
	Tea tree oil	*Esencias del árbol del té*	• Should not be ingested
	Thyme	*Tomillo*	• May affect thyroid activity
Psoriasis			
	Garlic	*Ajo*	(Listed above)
	Aloe vera	*Zábila*	• None with topical use
	Oatmeal	*Avena*	• Should not be used on large open wounds
	Olive oil	*Aceite de oliva*	• None topically
	Fish oil	*Aceite de pescado*	• Moderate interaction with oral contraceptive pills, antihypertensives, and tetrahydrolipstatin (orlistat) • Minor interaction with anticoagulants
	Arnica	*Árnica*	(Listed above)
	Burdock	*Bardana*	• Moderate interaction with anticoagulants
	Zinc	*Zinc*	• Moderate interaction with quinolones, tetracycline, cisplatin, and penicillamine • Minor interaction with amiloride
Scar			
	Aloe vera	*Zábila*	• None with topical use
	Garlic	*Ajo*	(Listed above)
	Honey	*Miel*	• None
	Lemon juice	*Jugo de limón*	• Large amounts should not be ingested by those with renal disease • Phytophotodermatitis with sun exposure

(*Continued*)

TABLE 7-2 Botanicals, minerals, nutrients, and other typical traditional ingredients used by Latine/Hispanic individuals for common dermatologic conditions (*Continued*)

	Traditional ingredients used medicinally		
Dermatologic condition	**Ingredient name**	**Spanish name**	**Contraindications**
	Milk	*Leche*	• None
	Orange skin	*Piel de naranja*	• Phytophotodermatitis with sun exposure
	Persimmons	*Nísperos*	• Moderate interaction with antihypertensives
	Rose hips	*Rosa de Castilla*	• Moderate interaction with vitamin C
Verruca			
	Garlic	*Ajo*	(Listed above)
	Onion	*Cebolla*	• Moderate interaction with aspirin, lithium, antidiabetic agents, and anticoagulants
	Aloe vera	*Zábila*	• None with topical use
	Lemon juice	*Jugo de limón*	• Large amounts should not be ingested by those with renal disease • Phytophotodermatitis with sun exposure
	Castor oil	*Aceite de castor*	• None with topical use

Abbreviations: CNS, central nervous system; NNRTI, nonnucleoside reverse transcriptase inhibitor.

Source: Data from Howell et al[30] and Dole et al.[29]

REFERENCES

1. Bureau UC. 2020 Census Illuminates Racial and Ethnic Composition of the Country. Census.gov. https://www.census.gov/library/stories/2021/08/improved-race-ethnicity-measures-reveal-united-states-population-much-more-multiracial.html. Accessed July 12, 2022.
2. Vespa J, Medina L, Armstrong DM. Population Estimates and Projections. Current Population Reports. P25-1144. Issued March 2018.
3. Institute of Medicine (US) Committee on Understanding and Eliminating Racial and Ethnic Disparities in Health Care. *Unequal Treatment: Confronting Racial and Ethnic Disparities in Health Care*. Washington, DC: National Academies Press; 2003.
4. Boonyasai R, Azam I, Hahn C, et al. 2021 National Healthcare Quality and Disparities Report. https://www.ahrq.gov/sites/default/files/wysiwyg/research/findings/nhqrdr/2021qdr.pdf. Accessed January 7, 2025.
5. Flanagin A, Frey T, Christiansen SL, AMA Manual of Style Committee. Updated guidance on the reporting of race and ethnicity in medical and science journals. *JAMA*. 2021;326(7):621-627.
6. RAE. Diccionario de la lengua española (2001). Diccionario esencial de la lengua española. https://www.rae.es/drae2001/. Accessed July 23, 2022.
7. Smith K. Latinx vs. Hispanic: a history of terms. https://facingtoday.facinghistory.org/latinx-vs.-hispanic-a-history-of-terms. Accessed September 24, 2022.
8. Perreira KM, Pedroza JM. Policies of exclusion: implications for the health of immigrants and their children. *Annu Rev Public Health*. 2019;40:147-166.
9. Hill J, Rodriguez DX, McDaniel PN. Immigration status as a health care barrier in the USA during COVID-19. *J Migr Health*. 2021;4:100036.
10. Philbin MM, Flake M, Hatzenbuehler ML, Hirsch JS. State-level immigration and immigrant-focused policies as drivers of Latino health disparities in the United States. *Soc Sci Med 1982*. 2018;199:29-38.
11. Terriquez V, Joseph TD. Ethnoracial inequality and insurance coverage among Latino young adults. *Soc Sci Med 1982*. 2016;168:150-158.
12. Baker B. Estimates of the unauthorized immigrant population residing in the United States: January 2015-January 2018. https://www.dhs.gov/sites/default/files/publications/immigration-statistics/Pop_Estimate/UnauthImmigrant/unauthorized_immigrant_population_estimates_2015_-_2018.pdf. Accessed January 7, 2024.
13. Krogstad JM, Passel JS, Noe-Bustamante L. Key facts about U.S. Latinos for National Hispanic Heritage Month. Washington. DC: Pew Research Center. https://www.pewresearch.org/fact-tank/2022/09/23/key-facts-about-u-s-latinos-for-national-hispanic-heritage-month/. Accessed November 23, 2022.
14. Khullar D, Chokshi DA. Immigrant health, value-based care, and emergency Medicaid reform. *JAMA*. 2019;321(10):928-929.
15. Oakley LP, López-Cevallos DF, Harvey SM. The association of cultural and structural factors with perceived medical mistrust among young adult Latinos in rural Oregon. *Behav Med*. 2019;45(2):118-127.
16. Funk C, Lopez MH. 3. Hispanic Americans' trust in medical scientists and views about the potential for researcher misconduct. Washington, DC: Pew Research Center Science & Society. https://www.pewresearch.org/science/2022/06/14/hispanic-americans-trust-in-medical-scientists-and-views-about-the-potential-for-researcher-misconduct/. Accessed September 26, 2022.
17. Radcliffe S. Healthcare: Mexico vs. the United States. Healthline. https://www.healthline.com/health-news/mexico-healthcare-system. Accessed October 3, 2022.
18. Lofquist, D. A. (2012). Multigenerational households: 2009-2011 (ACSBR/11-03). U.S. Census Bureau. Retrieved from https://www.census.gov/library/publications/2012/acs/acsbr11-03.html . Accessed January 7, 2024.
19. Cruz ML, Christie S, Allen E, Meza E, Nápoles AM, Mehta KM. Traditional healers as health care providers for the Latine community in the United States, a systematic review. *Health Equity*. 2022;6(1):412-426.
20. Green RR, Santoro N, Allshouse AA, Neal-Perry G, Derby C. Prevalence of complementary and alternative medicine and herbal remedy use in Hispanic and Non-Hispanic White women: results from the study of women's health across the nation. *J Altern Complement Med N Y N*. 2017;23(10):805-811.
21. Ortiz BI, Shields KM, Clauson KA, Clay PG. Complementary and alternative medicine use among Hispanics in the United States. *Ann Pharmacother*. 2007;41(6):994-1004.
22. Centers for Disease Control and Prevention (U.S.), Office for the Associate Director of Communication, Division of Communication Services. Cultural insights; communicating with Hispanics/Latinos. https://stacks.cdc.gov/view/cdc/13183. Accessed November 23, 2022.
23. Bray JK, Cline A, McMichael AJ, Feldman SR. Differences in healthcare barriers based on racial and/or ethnic background for patients with psoriasis. *J Dermatol Treat*. 2021;32(6):590-594.
24. Sanchez DP, Maymone MBC, McLean EO, et al. Racial and ethnic disparities in melanoma awareness: a cross-sectional survey. *J Am Acad Dermatol*. 2020;83(4):1098-1103.
25. Buchanan Lunsford N, Berktold J, Holman DM, Stein K, Prempeh A, Yerkes A. Skin cancer knowledge, awareness, beliefs and preventive behaviors among Black and Hispanic men and women. *Prev Med Rep*. 2018;12:203-209.
26. Kim Y, Blomberg M, Rifas-Shiman SL, et al. Racial/ethnic differences in incidence and persistence of childhood atopic dermatitis. *J Invest Dermatol*. 2019;139(4):827-834.
27. World Health Organization. Traditional, complementary and integrative medicine. World Health Organization. https://www.who.int/health-topics/traditional-complementary-and-integrative-medicine. Accessed July 24, 2022.
28. Fowler AL, Mann ME, Martinez FJ, Yeh HW, Cowden JD. Cultural health beliefs and practices among Hispanic parents. *Clin Pediatr (Phila)*. 2022;61(1):56-65.
29. Dole EJ, Rhyne RL, Zeilmann CA, Skipper BJ, McCabe ML, Low Dog T. The influence of ethnicity on use of herbal remedies in elderly Hispanics and non-Hispanic whites. *J Am Pharm Assoc Wash DC 1996*. 2000;40(3):359-365.
30. Howell L, Kochhar K, Saywell R, et al. Use of herbal remedies by Hispanic patients: do they inform their physician? *J Am Board Fam Med JABFM*. 2006;19(6):566-578.
31. Trotter RT. Curanderismo: a picture of Mexican-American folk healing. *J Altern Complement Med N Y N*. 2001;7(2):129-131.
32. Feldmann JM, Wiemann CM, Sever L, Hergenroeder AC. Folk and traditional medicine use by a subset of Hispanic adolescents. *Int J Adolesc Med Health*. 2008;20(1):41-51.

CHAPTER 8

Impact of Historical and Sociocultural Influences on American Indian Healthcare Practices

Lucinda L. Kohn
Spero M. Manson
Camille E. Introcaso

KEY POINTS

- American Indians and Alaska Natives (AI/AN) are racially minoritized people who are members of sovereign Tribal Nations, and who have a specific, defined relationship with the United States federal and state governments.
- AI/AN have experienced overwhelming historical trauma and loss due to European colonization, westward expansion of U.S. settlers, and centuries of racist, negligent, and patronizing U.S. policies concerning Tribal Nations.
- Based on centuries of treaties, the U.S. Constitution, and other legislation, the U.S. government is required to provide healthcare for members of federally recognized Tribes; however, the healthcare system for AI/AN is severely underfunded and short-staffed. Access to specialty care, including dermatology, is particularly limited.
- AI/AN experience overwhelmingly adverse social determinants of health in almost all contexts, resulting in dramatic disparities in health outcomes, yet many AI/AN populations demonstrate tremendous resiliency in their ability to create supportive social communities.
- Dermatologists can help address the health disparities faced by AI/AN by recognizing and educating themselves about the historical and cultural context of AI/AN communities and by respectfully and humbly engaging with Tribes and individuals to form sustainable relationships to provide direct care, training, and research support.

INTRODUCTION AND LAND STATEMENT

We acknowledge this chapter was written on the traditional territories and ancestral homelands of the Cheyenne, Arapaho, Ute, and Lenni-Lenape nations. As authors who are American Indian (SMM) and allies of American Indians and Alaska Natives (LLK and CEI), we humbly acknowledge that our chapter does not capture all aspects of caring for diverse groups of Native peoples.

DEFINITIONS

AI and AN are racially minoritized populations who are identified by a specific political relationship with the United States. Two fundamental principles define this unique population: Tribal sovereignty and the federal trust relationship between the United States and Tribal governments. Tribal Nations are sovereign governments, meaning they are independent nations with control over their own territory and constituents. Tribes' authority to self-govern arises from the U.S. Constitution, government-to-government treaties, executive orders, Supreme Court decisions and case law, and U.S. legislation. The federal trust responsibility compels the federal government to protect Tribal self-governance, lands, assets, resources, and to provide Tribal members with healthcare and basic needs.[1]

An individual must be a member of a federally recognized Tribe to experience the benefits of the trust responsibility, including access to healthcare. Yet, not all individuals who identify as AI/AN are eligible for the benefits of the federal trust responsibility. Some AI/AN belong to Tribes that are not recognized by the federal government. Individuals may also have Tribal heritage and celebrate Tribal culture but might not meet Tribally defined criteria for membership.

HISTORICAL PERSPECTIVE

AI/AN people in the United States are not a monolithic culture but share a collective past and elements of current cultural identity that include overwhelming historical trauma and loss. The following summary of the U.S. government and Tribal history is intended to convey the weight that every AI/AN carries today. Although these concepts may be difficult for the uninitiated reader to grasp, they are central to AI/AN identity. Even AI/AN children have an awareness of sovereignty and the loss of culture, life, and land that occurred from the establishment and growth of the United States.

RELOCATION

Prior to European colonization, North America was home to thousands of Tribes. Since the arrival of European settlers and the colonization they imposed on the continent, AI/AN have suffered waves of involuntary and violent relocation. Prior to and during the 1700s, European settlers occupied Native lands through violence and without permission. In the 1800s, the federal government forced Tribes to relinquish large tracts of land in the east, south, and Great Plains regions, and move to barren reservations in the West.[2] The Indian Removal Act of 1830 led to the infamous Trail of Tears that forced more than 100,000 AI from their homes and resulted in more than 15,000 deaths.[1,3] In the late 1800s, the Dawes Act converted hundreds of thousands of acres of Tribal lands to small parcels for individual ownership, which enabled and encouraged settlers to push into AI/AN territories despite treaties that guaranteed Native peoples rights to the land on which they lived. Nearly two-thirds of reservation land were forcibly wrested from Tribes and transferred to non-Native occupants.[2] Current reservations [**Figure 8-1**] represent a fraction of the United States in areas typically distant from Tribes' traditional homelands, and often resource-poor, that plays a major role in the adverse social determinants of health experienced by AI/AN.[4]

CULTURAL ASSIMILATION

In the late 1800s to early 1900s, the United States pushed to assimilate AI/AN into mainstream American life. The federal government funded and operated boarding schools located far from reservations with the expressed goal of cultural eradication. Children were forcibly removed from their families and forbidden to participate in their traditional cultures, including speaking Native languages, wearing Native dress or hairstyles, and practicing Native religion. Schools prioritized teaching manual labor, which limited AI/AN education and employment opportunities. Children endured emotional, sexual, and physical abuse and neglect; indeed, many died. The United States has only recently begun to recognize the death toll from these boarding schools. In 2022, a federal document reported that thousands of AI/AN children were buried in unmarked graves on school grounds. The trauma to AI/AN culture and identity caused by boarding schools continues to have repercussions among Native people today.[5]

The 1940s to the 1960s comprised the Termination Era, which was a dark time in U.S. and Native history. During Termination, Congress unilaterally dissolved treaties with more than 100 previously recognized Tribes, resulting in the end of promised federal protection, support, and healthcare for more than 11,000 people and the loss of more than 1.3 million acres of reservation land. The Indian Relocation Act of 1956 lured most of these people into urban environments in further efforts to assimilate AI/AN into U.S. culture. Many Tribes have not been able to reestablish federal recognition because the federal government destroyed records of their treaties and existence.[6] In the late 1960s, the U.S. policies toward Tribes began to change, and now the United States has largely recognized Tribal sovereignty and has increasingly allowed Tribes to self-govern.[2] This chapter discusses the current era in more detail below.

The history of AI/AN and the United States is fraught with injustices and colors how AI/AN currently interact with state and federal governments, including our healthcare systems. AI/AN often approach

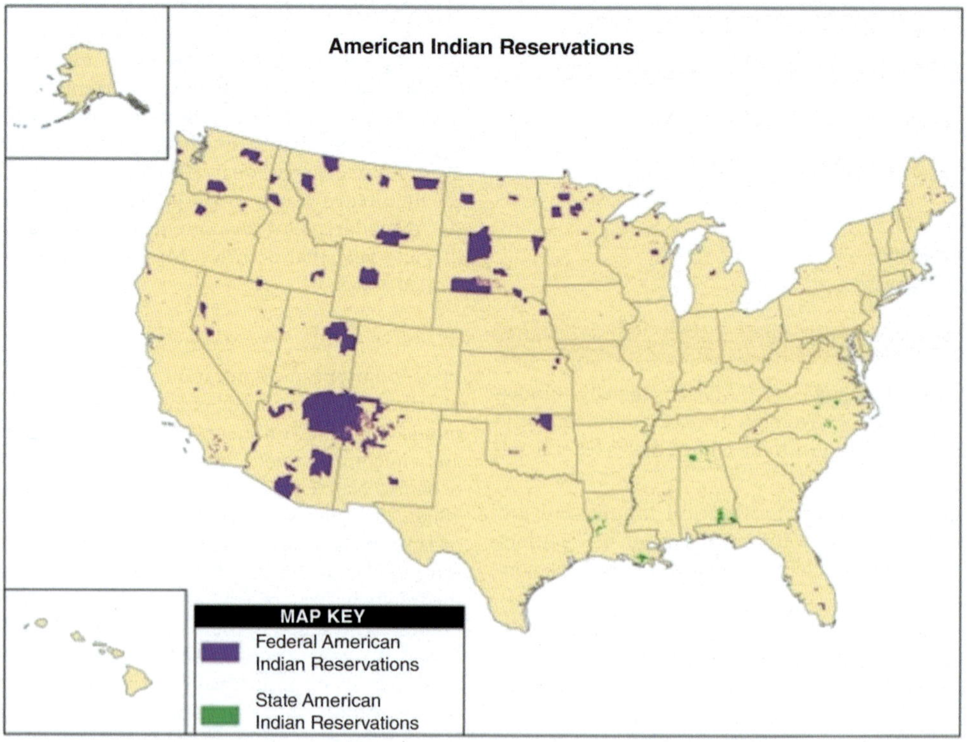

FIGURE 8-1. Map of federal- and state-recognized American Indian reservations.

government institutions, and people who work for those institutions, with mistrust. When healthcare providers interact with AI/AN communities, it is critical to understand the weight of history and lasting impact of intergenerational trauma as we seek to establish respectful, safe, and effective physician-patient and physician or researcher-Tribal relationships.

CURRENT ERA

POPULATION

As of 2020, there are 574 federally recognized sovereign Tribal Nations and 334 federally and state recognized AI/AN reservations located across 35 states.[7] The size of Tribal Nations ranges widely, from the Navajo Nation with approximately 400,000 enrolled members and a reservation located in parts of Arizona, New Mexico, and Utah, to a few California rancherias that consist of only one or two families. Economic conditions vary significantly; poverty is extensive.[2]

Of the 331.5 million people who were counted in the 2020 U.S. Census, 9.7 million people (2.9% of the U.S. population) identified as AI/AN alone or in combination with another race.[8] It must be noted that due to rurality and mistrust of government programs, AI/AN have historically been undercounted in the U.S. Census; this is true of the 2020 U.S. Census as well.[9] Not all AI/AN live on reservations or in the rural communities that border reservations. Due to economic and educational opportunities that are not present on reservations and relocation during the Termination Era, many AI/AN are in metropolitan areas. In 2020, more than 7 out of every 10 AI/AN live in or near cities.[10]

HEALTHCARE

Treaties between Tribal Nations and the United States in the 1700s and 1800s promised physicians, medical supplies, and hospitals in exchange for land. Despite these treaties, healthcare services for AI/AN have lacked funding and providers both historically and today. In 1880, only four hospitals and 77 physicians served AI. In the 1900s, federal efforts to support AI/AN healthcare delivery increased after surveys revealed that more AI were dying than being born. In 1922, Congress passed the Snyder Act, which authorized the Bureau of Indian Affairs to direct healthcare programs for AI. In 1968, the Indian Health Service (IHS) was created out of the U.S. Public Health Service to provide healthcare for AI/AN living on reservations. In 1976, Congress passed the Indian Health Care Improvement Act, which improved funding for IHS programs, and created the Urban Indian Health Program. In 1992, the Indian Self-Determination and Education Assistance Act (Public Law 93-638) provided Tribes the option to administer their own healthcare systems and schools. While these programs face challenges of limited funding, the results of Tribal control have been positive.[2] With Tribal control, healthcare improves, and more healthcare facilities, community programs, and preventative programs are added. Today, many Tribes prefer to run their own programs, including healthcare and governmental units.

Currently, the IHS is a separate agency within the Department of Health and Human Services and is responsible for providing federal health services to AI/AN. There are 170 IHS and Tribally managed healthcare service units; nearly 80% are Tribally operated [**Table 8-1**]. As of 2019, there are 776 physicians, 104 physician assistants, and 798 dentists who are employed by the IHS.[11]

Yet, the healthcare provided by the IHS is not comprehensive. The IHS offers limited specialty care, including dermatology. Currently, the IHS employs three dermatologists, most likely in a part-time capacity. Many of the systemic failures in IHS are related to funding. Unlike Medicaid

TABLE 8-1 Types of IHS and Tribal healthcare facilities (July 2020)[11]

Type of facility	IHS	Tribal
Hospital	24	22
Health center	51	279
Health station	24	79
Alaska village clinic	0	59
School health center	12	6
Youth regional treatment centers	6	6

and Medicare, the IHS is not an entitlement program and its funding does not keep pace with inflation. In 2019, the IHS spent $4078 per capita and Urban Indian Health Organizations spent $672 per capita, compared to the general population with a median of $8436 by Medicaid and $11,142 by Medicare.[11-13] IHS focuses its efforts on primary and emergency services, limited specialty care, and narrow prescription drug coverage. In addition to funding shortfalls, the IHS faces a 25% clinician vacancy rate, which includes core clinicians such as primary care clinicians, midwives, dentists, and pharmacists.[14] Geographic isolation and low salaries have made it difficult for IHS facilities to attract qualified staff and AI/AN are significantly underrepresented in health professions. State expansion of Medicaid through the Affordable Care Act of 2010 improves access to healthcare for AI/AN who are residents in states that have adopted Medicaid expansion.[15]

SOCIAL DETERMINANTS OF HEALTH

The conditions in which we live, work, learn, and play comprise the social determinants of our health. Natural and built environments, food cultures, community support systems, and access to education, employment, and healthcare all significantly factor into a person's health.[16] AI/AN face centuries of federal, state, and local government policies that have created barriers to healthcare, education, and economic opportunities; degraded natural and built living environments; and sought to destroy cultural communities. AI/AN experience overwhelmingly adverse social determinants of health in almost all contexts, and yet many AI/AN populations demonstrate tremendous resiliency in their ability to create supportive social communities.

NEGATIVE SOCIAL DETERMINANTS OF HEALTH

By almost every measure of health status, from infant mortality, to rates of infections such as HIV, viral hepatitis, and tuberculosis, to mortality from colon, breast, and other cancers, to overall life expectancy, AI/AN have worse outcomes compared to the U.S. population at large.[17,18] Differences in genetics or physiology do not account for these poor outcomes; these disparities are best explained by the social determinants of health faced by AI/AN, namely disparities in economic stability, education, neighborhood and built environment (access to clean water, housing, nutritious foods, and transportation), and healthcare access and quality. AI/AN experience the highest rates of poverty of any racial group, with 24% of AI/AN living in poverty in 2020 compared to 12.8% of the overall population.[19] AI/AN are also less likely to achieve a high school or bachelor's degree compared to the overall U.S. population.[20] In 2017, 13% of AI/AN living on reservations lacked access to safe water or adequate sanitation facilities, compared to only 0.6% of non-AI/AN Americans.[21] Twenty-five percent of AI/AN experience food insecurity, which is more than twice the rate of the overall population.[22] American Indians and Alaska Natives face tremendous obstacles when attempting to access the healthcare system due to inadequate facilities and limited numbers of providers.[23]

American Indian and Alaska Native health has also been affected by government policies on food and environmental issues. Treaties have required federal government programs to provide supplemental food for AI/AN for generations. Unfortunately, commodity food is typically low in nutritional value and high in sugar and fat.[4] Combined with the loss of access to traditional food culture due to forced relocation and assimilation, these programs contributed to high rates of obesity, cardiovascular disease, and diabetes among AI/AN.[3] Government policies concerning mining and land allocation have led AI/AN living on reservations to be exposed to heavy metals, particularly uranium, at significantly higher rates than other communities.[24] Environmental health injustices faced by AI/AN, including lack of access to safe water and exposure to air pollution, have been worsened by climate change, which brings extreme weather, natural disasters, and vector-borne disease.[3] Current federal policies allowing energy companies to build pipelines on AI/AN land increase the risk of environmental hazards for those communities.

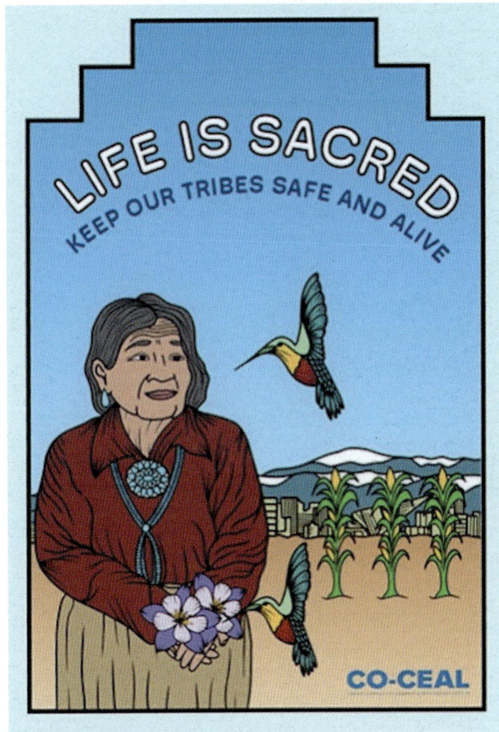
LIFE IS SACRED
KEEP OUR TRIBES SAFE AND ALIVE
CO-CEAL

FIGURE 8-2. COVID vaccination poster. (Designed by Marcus Trujillo (Pueblo of Laguna) of Haatzee Designs. Used with permission of The Denver American Indian/Alaska Native Colorado COVID-19 Community Engagement Alliance workgroup (AI/AN CO-CEAL) workgroup.)

POSITIVE SOCIAL DETERMINANTS OF HEALTH

Despite centuries of persecution, attempts at cultural eradication, and blatant racism, AI/AN maintain strong, supportive communities positively affecting AI/AN health. The fact that AI/AN populations achieved both the highest first-dose and full vaccination rates against the SARS CoV-2 virus of any racialized or ethnic group in the United States provides a recent measurable example of this strong and supportive community. From the early days of the COVID pandemic, Tribal governments adopted safety measures including stay-at-home orders and mask mandates in efforts to protect vulnerable community members. When COVID vaccines became available in 2021, AI/AN communities moved quickly to immunize their members. Tribal leaders employed culturally tailored messages focused on the need for all members to take measures to care for elders, and the community responded [**Figure 8-2**].[25] These efforts were the result of the work and attitudes of local AI/AN champions, but this success was also driven by two key factors: (1) the U.S. government fulfilled its treaty obligations to pay for healthcare and provided vaccinations, and (2) Tribal governments were allowed the autonomy to develop the programs themselves. Although AI/AN communities are working to improve their living, working, and learning conditions, achieving parity in social determinants of health for AI/AN will require U.S. recognition of Tribal sovereignty and fulfillment of treaty rights to allow for Tribal self-determination and appropriate expenditures on healthcare, education, and economic development.

DERMATOLOGY AND AMERICAN INDIANS AND ALASKA NATIVES

CUTANEOUS DISEASE IN AI/AN

The current literature on cutaneous diseases and treatments in AI/AN is sparse and includes research done on AI/AN populations without their expressed consent. We summarize relevant observations here as a background to dermatologic issues facing AI/AN.

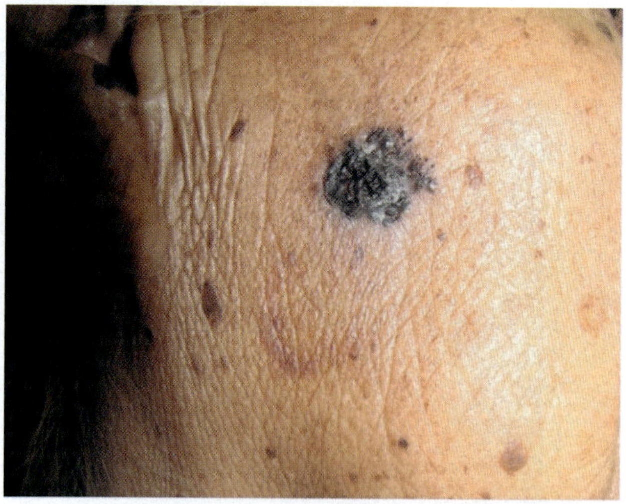

FIGURE 8-3. Pigmented basal cell carcinoma on the right cheek of a *Diné* (Navajo) woman.

Photosensitive disorders are reported at rates higher in AI/AN compared to other populations. Actinic prurigo, an immunologically mediated, scarring condition characterized by pruritic papules on sun exposed skin and mucous membranes, is more common in AI/AN.[26] Some studies report a prevalence of actinic prurigo of more than 1% in some Tribes; an association with HLA-DR4 in these groups and others has been reported. There appears to be a distinct subset of actinic prurigo in AN, specifically the Inuit people, who experience a later onset of lesions, more ocular involvement and less favorable prognosis.[26,27]

Cutaneous malignancies, particularly melanoma, have been reported to have a lower incidence in the AI/AN population compared to the White population. However, AI/AN patients present with thicker primary melanomas, have a higher rate of metastasis at time of presentation, and a decreased overall 5-year survival compared to non-Hispanic White patients.[26] Although acral lentiginous melanoma occurs more often in AI/AN than in White patients, superficial spreading melanoma is the most common subtype of melanoma reported in AI/AN, and the trunk is the most commonly reported site.[26] As in other populations with highly pigmented skin, pigmented basal cell carcinoma is the most common subtype of basal cell carcinoma seen in AI/AN [**Figure 8-3**].

A number of other conditions, specifically hypertrophic scarring, acanthosis nigricans, and systemic lupus erythematosus, have been reported to occur in AI/AN at higher rates than the general population. In addition to these disorders, AI/AN may also experience higher morbidity from chronic inflammatory skin diseases such as acne, hidradenitis suppurative, psoriasis, and atopic dermatitis, in part due to the poor social determinants of health highlighted above, including poor access to dermatology care, dry climates, and lack of access to nutritious foods and environments that foster physical activity. Future collaborations between dermatologists, researchers, and AI/AN communities will hopefully further describe important dermatologic issues facing these communities and promote improvements in care.

TRADITIONAL MEDICINE AND DERMATOLOGY

Traditional medicine has been practiced by AI/AN throughout history. Like many aspects of AI/AN cultures, during the 1800s and early 1900s, traditional medicine on reservations was criminalized; traditional healers and their patients were punished by fines and imprisonment.[28] Despite efforts to eradicate traditional medicine, contemporary studies indicate the majority of many AI/AN communities engage with traditional medicine in some way. Although beliefs and conventions around medicine and healing vary widely, common themes and practices are evident. Traditional medicine and healing are therapeutic processes using sacred, cultural knowledge and practices passed from one traditional healer to another.[29] These processes identify and treat imbalances that cause physical, mental, and spiritual distress in patients. Ceremonies involving prayer, the use of herbal remedies, and the central importance of the relationship between patient and traditional healer are three common institutions found among diverse AI/AN.[30] Traditional healers are identified by the community served; the spiritual and cultural knowledge they possess is considered sacred and private.[31] Understanding the role of traditional medicine in our patients' lives is critical for dermatologists trained in the evidence-based, biomedical model of healthcare. However, some patients might fear their doctor's judgement and be reluctant to volunteer this information. Directly and humbly asking patients how they engage with traditional medicine starts this important conversation. Indeed, the cultural case formulation developed as part of American Psychiatric Association's Diagnostic and Statistical Manual offers a concrete example of how such aspects of the lived experience may be solicited and inform the process of care.[32] The challenges for dermatologists can arise if traditional medicine conflicts with Western medicine; however, dermatologists can and should choose to respect their patient's autonomy if the patient prioritizes spiritual needs over science-based values. When a dermatologist recognizes and openly engages with an AI/AN patient's traditional medicine practices, they have the opportunity to educate themselves, maximize benefit, minimize harm if necessary, and strengthen their relationship with the patient.[30]

COLLABORATING WITH TRIBES ON RESEARCH AND HEALTHCARE PROGRAMS

A long history of harmful government programs have led Tribes to distrust healthcare and research programs. Today's healthcare providers must approach their service to AI/AN with humility, compassion, and a willingness to listen and learn. Additionally, healthcare providers have a responsibility to be discerning of the healthcare system in which they practice. Dermatologists might be tempted to offer free healthcare services for a limited time to AI/AN communities in desperate need of dermatology care, but these so-called voluntourism efforts have been criticized by the global health community to be unsustainable, impede local economic development, and offer poor quality of healthcare to patients. Instead, practicing dermatologists should endeavor to serve the AI/AN communities by training more AI/AN dermatologists, and providing sustainable, ethical, and culturally concordant dermatology care to AI/AN communities and patients. A potential solution is to build sustainable partnerships between dermatologists at universities and Tribes or Urban Indian Health Organizations so that dermatology care is delivered to AI/AN and AI/AN students have opportunity for mentorship and experience in dermatology. These collaborations should fully credit Tribal partners and ensure their active voice in programmatic design and implementation. Standards for these clinics should be high. Trainees should not practice beyond their level of training; medical licensure regulations (including Tribal regulations where they exist) must be followed; clinicians should learn, practice, and teach culturally concordant care and maintain the same standards of healthcare as expected on campus; universities need to support faculty members' outreach, program administrative time, and underwrite student expenses like housing and transportation.

Today's researchers must take steps to collaborate with the Tribe communities they work with at all stages of investigation, from development to dissemination of results. This approach requires an investment of time and personnel to build relationships and trust with Tribes and their memberships, which operate with scarce resources and a lasting distrust of outside researchers. Some Tribes have established IRBs and community review boards to have a voice in the inception, design, and final products to ensure the culturally appropriate interpretation of research data and security of research findings.

CONCLUSION

Health inequities exist for AI/AN; they are pronounced for dermatologic care. To bridge this gap, reform is warranted at all levels. Our immediate goals should be to train more dermatologists who identify as AI/AN, build collaborative dermatology programs with Tribes and Urban Indian Health Organizations, and understand the barriers to care arising from the social determinants of health and historical trauma that AI/AN face when we care for them as our patients.

REFERENCES

1. *Tribal Nations and the United States: An Introduction*. Washington, DC: National Congress of American Indians; 2020. https://www.ncai.org/about-tribes.
2. Newton NJ, Anderson R, Goldberg C, LaVelle J, Royster JV, Singer JW. *Cohen's Handbook of Federal Indian Law*. New York, NY: LexisNexis; 2019.
3. Burns J, Angelino AC, Lewis K, et al. Land rights and health outcomes in American Indian/Alaska Native children. *Pediatrics*. 2021;148(5).
4. Warne D, Wescott S. Social determinants of American Indian nutritional health. *Curr Dev Nutr*. 2019;3(Suppl 2):12-18.
5. Federal Indian Boarding School Initiative Investigative Report (May 2022).
6. Myers MD. Federal recognition of Indian Tribes in the United States. *Stan L & Pol'y Rev*. 2001;12:271.
7. Indian entities recognized by and eligible to receive services from the United States Bureau of Indian Affairs (01/28/2022).
8. 2020 Census: Native population increased by 86.5 percent. *Indian Country Today*. https://indiancountrytoday.com/news/2020-census-native-population-increased-by-86-5-percent. Accessed August 4, 2022.
9. National Congress of American Indians. American Indians and Alaska Natives living on reservations have the highest 2020 Census undercount. https://www.ncai.org/news/articles/2022/03/10/american-indians-and-alaska-natives-living-on-reservations-have-the-highest-2020-census-undercount. Accessed August 4, 2022.
10. Urban Indian America: the status of American Indian and Alaska Native children and families today (2008).
11. IHS Profile. https://www.ihs.gov/newsroom/factsheets/ihsprofile/. Accessed January 8, 2025.
12. Medicaid per capita expenditures. https://www.medicaid.gov/state-overviews/scorecard/how-much-states-spend-per-medicaid-enrollee/index.html. Accessed August 4, 2022.
13. Biniek JF, Cubanski J, Neumann T. Traditional Medicare spending fell almost 6% in 2020 as service use declined early in the COVID-19 pandemic. https://www.kff.org/medicare/issue-brief/traditional-medicare-spending-fell-almost-6-in-2020-as-service-use-declined-early-in-the-covid-19-pandemic/. U.S. Gen. Accounting Office: GAO-18-580: Indian Health Service Agency Faces Ongoing Challenges Filling Provider Vacancies. (2018) Accessed August 4, 2022.
14. INDIAN HEALTH SERVICE agency faces ongoing challenges filling provider vacancies (2018).
15. Walker M. For Tribal members in Oklahoma, Medicaid expansion improves access to specialty care. https://www.nytimes.com/2021/09/04/us/politics/oklahoma-medicaid-indian-health-service.html#:~:text=%E2%80%9CThis%20Medicaid%20expansion%20helps%20our,who%20have%20signed%20up%20statewide. Accessed August 4, 2022.
16. World Health Organization. Social determinants of health. https://www.who.int/health-topics/social-determinants-of-health#tab=tab_1. Accessed June 16, 2022.
17. Arias E, Xu J, Curtin S, Bastian B, Tejada-Vera B. Mortality profile of the non-Hispanic American Indian or Alaska Native population, 2019. *Natl Vital Stat Rep*. 2021;70(12):1-27.
18. Centers for Disease Control and Prevention. Health disparities in HIV, viral Hepatitis, STDs, and TB. https://www.cdc.gov/nchhstp/healthdisparities/americanindians.html. Accessed June 26, 2022.
19. US Census Bureau. Selected characteristics of people in poverty in the last 12 months (S1702). https://data.census.gov/cedsci/table?q=poverty&g=0100000US&tid=ACSST5Y2020.S1703. Accessed June 26, 2022.
20. US Department of Health and Human Services. Profile: American Indian/Alaska Native. https://minorityhealth.hhs.gov/omh/browse.aspx?lvl=3&lvlid=62. Accessed June 26, 2022.
21. US Water Alliance. An equitable water future: a national briefing paper. http://uswateralliance.org/sites/uswateralliance.org/files/publications/uswa_waterequity_FINAL.pdf. Accessed July 2, 2022.
22. Jernigan VBB, Huyser KR, Valdes J, Simonds VW. Food insecurity among American Indians and Alaska Natives: a national profile using the current population survey-food security supplement. *J Hunger Environ Nutr*. 2017;12(1):1-10.
23. Kohn LL, Introcaso CE. A cultural context for providing dermatologic care to American Indian and Alaskan Native communities through telehealth. *JAMA Dermatol*. 2019;155(8):884-886..
24. Redvers N, Chischilly AM, Warne D, Pino M, Lyon-Colbert A. Uranium exposure in American Indian communities: health, policy, and the way forward. *Environ Health Perspect*. 2021;129(3):35002.
25. Foxworth R, Redvers N, Moreno MA, Lopez-Carmen VA, Sanchez GR, Shultz JM. Covid-19 Vaccination in American Indians and Alaska Natives - lessons from effective community responses. *N Engl J Med*. 2021;385(26):2403-2406.
26. Kryatova MS, Okoye GA. Dermatology in the north American Indian/Alaska native population. *Int J Dermatol*. 2016;55(2):125-134.
27. Lain ES. Skin diseases among full-blood Indians of Oklahoma. *J Am Med Assoc*. 1913;61(3):168-171.
28. Cloatre E. Traditional medicines, law and the (dis)ordering of temporalities. In: Beynon-Jones Siân M, Grabham E, eds. *Law and Time*. Abington, UK: Routledge; 2019:128-144.
29. Esposito ML, Kahn-John M. How should allopathic physicians respond to Native American patients hesitant about allopathic medicine? *AMA J Ethics*. 2020;22(10):837-844.
30. Esposito ML, Kahn-John M. How should allopathic physicians respond to Native American patients hesitant about allopathic medicine? *AMA J Ethics*. 2020;22(10):E837-844.
31. Tribal Health Research Office. NIH 2019 Traditional Medicine Summit: maintaining and protecting culture through healing. https://dpcpsi.nih.gov/thro/tms. Accessed July 8, 2022.
32. Lewis-Fernández R, Aggarwal NK, Bäärnhielm S, et al. Culture and psychiatric evaluation: operationalizing cultural formulation for DSM-5. *Psychiatry*. Summer 2014;77(2):130-154.

CHAPTER 9

Historical and Sociocultural Influences on Middle Eastern and North African (MENA) Healthcare Practices

Kathyana Santiago Mangual
Elizabeth Behar Houshmand
Nora S. Ali
Lana Kashlan
Lina Naga

KEY POINTS

- The Middle Eastern and North African (MENA) population in the United States is a diverse group, accounting for roughly 3% of the country's immigrant population.
- MENA Americans often face discrimination, language barriers, and cultural stigma that can influence health and healthcare practices.
- The medical beliefs and practices of people from these countries are the result of their rich history, tribal traditions, and the involvement and importance of religion in all aspects of life.
- Traditional religious beliefs and practices play a significant role in the healthcare and treatment choices of MENA communities, especially among first-generation or elderly individuals.
- Understanding and respecting the perspectives, beliefs, and social factors influencing this population can positively impact dermatologic health outcomes and treatment.

INTRODUCTION

The Middle Eastern and North African (MENA) population in the United States comprise a fast-growing and diverse group [**Table 9-1**]. Between 2000 and 2019, the immigrant population from the MENA region doubled from 596,000 to 1.2 million, accounting for roughly 3% of the country's immigrant population. Nearly 68% of MENA immigrants are from the Middle East and the rest are from Northern Africa. Overall, Iraq and Egypt are the top countries of origin for MENA immigrants, followed by Lebanon, Syria, and Jordan.[1,2]

Within the United States, greater than 50% of MENA individuals reside in five states: California (18%), Michigan (10%), New York (9%), Texas (8%), and New Jersey (6%), with approximately one-third living in either California or Michigan. Currently, the U.S. Census classifies MENA people as racially White, although people can identify themselves as MENA in subsequent open-ended items.[3] However, MENA people have a range of different skin colors,[4] and research has shown that MENA Americans and non-MENA White individuals predominantly perceive MENA people as non-White.[5] This places MENA Americans in a unique position—one in which they are largely understudied with regard to research and health disparities but highly visible and often stigmatized in the public.[6]

Factors such as discrimination, language barriers, and cultural stigma contribute to growing health disparities in these populations. Understanding the unique perspectives, beliefs, and social factors influencing this population is an essential component of providing culturally attuned dermatologic care. In this chapter, we will discuss historical and sociocultural factors influencing health and healthcare in MENA communities living in the United States, including traditional religious beliefs and practices that are more likely to be encountered among first-generation or the elderly individuals.

TABLE 9-1 Middle East/North African (MENA) countries[a]

Arab countries[b]	Non-Arab MENA countries	Transnational communities
• Algeria	• Iran	• Assyrians/Chaldeans
• Bahrain	• Israel	• Kurds
• Comoros	• Turkey	• Berber/Amazigh
• Djibouti		
• Egypt		
• Iraq		
• Jordan		
• Kuwait		
• Lebanon		
• Libya		
• Mauritania		
• Morocco		
• Oman		
• Palestine		
• Qatar		
• Saudi Arabia		
• Somalia		
• Sudan		
• Syria		
• Tunisia		
• United Arab Emirates		
• Yemen		

[a]According to the United Census Bureau (https://www2.census.gov/about/partners/cac/nac/meetings/2022-05/discussant-mena-reporting-category.pdf).

[b]Arab countries consists of 22 countries in the Middle East and North Africa where Arabic is the principal (although not the only) language spoken.

HISTORY

Immigrants from MENA countries have been coming to the United States since the 1800s, and immigration has occurred in three major waves. The first, between the late 1800s and early 1900s, brought over 250,000 people from what was then Greater Syria and other regions; these arrivals were mostly Christian laborers, farmers, and merchants seeking economic opportunity. The second wave came after World War II and the 1948 Arab-Israeli War, which displaced tens of thousands of Palestinians who immigrated to the United States. After 1965, when discriminatory immigration laws were reformed, there was a third wave of MENA immigrants, numbering about 250,000. The second and third waves were about 60% Muslim,[7,8] many of whom were educated professionals who were escaping war and political instability in their countries.[1,7-9]

In the early 20th century, identification as racially White was a necessary and conscious effort pursued by prior generations of MENA immigrants to qualify for naturalization and signal their entry into the American mainstream. In 1977, the U.S. Office of Management and Budget's (OMB) original Directive 15 defined White as those with origins in "Europe, the Middle East and North Africa," a definition that essentially remains today. Thus, individuals identifying with the MENA region are routinely categorized as "White" in social science and health research, while the lived experience of MENA groups includes being perceived and treated as non-White, which has implications for health and healthcare.[2]

DISCRIMINATION

MENA Americans have faced substantial xenophobia and discrimination since they first started to immigrate to this country in the 1800s and continue to face a growing risk of hate crimes following the events of September 11, 2001. Progressively greater negative rhetoric and adverse public policies have increased the vulnerability of this ethnic group in the United States. For example, perceived discrimination among MENA Americans after September 11th was found to heighten psychological distress, reduce levels of happiness, contribute to more adverse birth outcomes, and enhance feelings of isolation and stigmatization in this group.[10-14] Discrimination has an impact on health by depriving individuals of access to resources, dignity, and a high quality of life.[3] The literature on the impact of discrimination on Arab American health is a subset of a larger and robust literature on the detrimental role of racism and discrimination on the health of minoritized populations in the United States.[10,15]

HEALTH DISPARITIES

Health Patterns Prior work suggests that MENA Americans have both health and social patterns that are different from the outcomes of others identifying as White non-Hispanic, the group they are asked to identify with on standard surveys.[16] Relative to White non-Hispanic groups, Arab Americans have a higher prevalence of metabolic disorders and cardiovascular disease.[10,16]

Unfortunately, there is a paucity of knowledge related to dermatologic conditions impacting MENA Americans. According to one study including responses from Arab Americans (n = 401) living in Southeast Michigan, the most common self-reported skin conditions (based on diagnoses given previously by a physician) were acne (38%), eczema/dermatitis (26%), warts (20%), fungal skin infections (20%), and melasma (15%).[4] Acne and eczema are also among the most prevalent dermatologic conditions among other communities of color, including Black/African Americans and Hispanic Americans.[17] Another study of Middle Eastern populations in California compared rates of malignancy, including melanoma skin cancer, between Middle Eastern and White non-Hispanic individuals, revealing that California residents of Middle Eastern descent have relatively lower rates of melanoma.[18] This lower incidence may be secondary to a combination of heightened resistance resulting from individuals who may have darker skin pigmentation and limited exposure to sunlight.[18] Of note, it has also been shown that

Middle Eastern women living in California have an incidence of melanoma five times greater than women in their countries of origin.[18] This discrepancy may be due to assimilation into American culture and habits, but it could also be related to differences in data collection methods, such as national cancer registries.[18]

Social Patterns Social risk factors in MENA communities are influenced by socioeconomic status, culture, immigration status, and discrimination. In a recent cross-sectional study including 412 adults living in Southeast Michigan who identified as MENA, prevalent social risks included transportation barriers to healthcare (33%), food insecurity (33%), and financial strain (25%).[3] More social risk factors were evident among those identifying as female ($p<0.01$), with education of some college or less ($p<0.001$), with lower income ($p<0.001$), Arab versus Chaldean descent ($p<0.02$), non-U.S. born ($p<0.05$), in the United States for fewer years ($p<0.003$), originating from Egypt, Syria, Yemen versus other countries ($p<0.001$), and who speak Arabic at home ($p<0.01$). More unmet needs were also evident among those who reported being treated unfairly ($p=0.03$), worried about deportation ($p<0.002$), and those who reported worse health ($p<0.01$).[3] In addition, data using National Health Interview Surveys (n = 1013) from 2011 to 2018 reveal MENA immigrants who do not identify as White and who are not U.S. citizens are less likely to access and utilize healthcare compared to those who identify as White and are U.S. citizens.[2] These findings have implications for developing innovative social needs screening that can best serve MENA sub-populations in the United States.

CULTURAL INSIGHTS

MENA Americans are a diverse group with a tremendous amount of within-group variability (eg, based on socioeconomic status, level of acculturation, education level, religion, country of origin, etc). With these variations in mind, there are some common cultural characteristics that are shared by many MENA groups.

LANGUAGE

The MENA region is linguistically diverse with more than 60 languages being spoken throughout. The four most spoken languages in the region are Arabic (the most widely spoken language in many of the MENA countries); Persian or Farsi (spoken in Iran and by significant Persian-speaking populations in Afghanistan); Hebrew (primarily spoken in Israel); and Turkish (spoken in Turkey as well as in Cyprus).[19] When talking to recent MENA immigrants, the provider should assess language comprehension. If needed, a medical interpreter proficient in both languages (ie, the healthcare provider's and patient's language), as well as one who understands the cultural issues (such as family structures/roles), should be chosen. The U.S. Department of Health and Human Services Office of Minority Health does not allow the use of minor children for interpretation during a medical encounter. In general, it is important to avoid the use of children or other family members as interpreters to avoid inaccurate and biased interpretation that may ultimately lead to an incorrect diagnosis or lack of patient adherence to treatment.[20]

GENDER ROLES AND FAMILY

Traditionally and historically, MENA families have a patrilineal structure, where the male or paternal figure is expected to provide, protect, and make decisions for his family. This is not necessarily true for MENA families living in the United States, particularly for those families who have lived outside of their countries of origin for many years. For some female patients of MENA descent, when a male husband is present, he may answer medical questions directed at the female patient and may also sign any consent forms on her behalf.[21] The woman may avoid eye contact with a male healthcare provider or may not answer his questions directly. This dynamic, like in all cultures, depends on a particular family's structure, religion, and traditions.

While the healthcare delivery system in the United States is oriented toward patient autonomy, decisions regarding healthcare are often made by the family group and are not the responsibility of the individual alone. Arab American mothers have been described as being "the backbone of their families."[22] They are highly respected and are seen as sacred in the family unit for guiding their offspring through their educational and career paths.[22,23] However, family obligations are often given priority and the extended family is often consulted in all important decisions. The cultural values of the individual, family, and relatives may affect the delivery of medical care. However, it should be established with the patient if they want others to be part of the decision-making process or not.[8,24,25]

RELIGION

While MENA groups are portrayed as uniformly Muslim, most MENA groups in the United States come from diverse religious traditions, including Christianity, Judaism, Bahá'í, Druze, and Yazidism, and others adopt no religious tradition. In recent years, the percentage of MENA Americans who are Muslim has increased because most new MENA immigrants tend to be Muslim.[7,8] For American Muslim populations, some traditional beliefs or practices can potentially impact health and healthcare. Practices will vary based on culture, as many American Muslims also come from non-Arab or non-MENA backgrounds [**Table 9-2**].

Prophetic Medicine Prophetic medicine refers to the actions and words of the Muslim prophet, Muhammad. Prophetic medicine treats illness, addresses hygiene, and encourages preventative health. Muslims are encouraged by their religion to seek medical advice whenever they are ill, and they believe that every disease has a cause and a cure. Many Muslims may use prophetic medicine as part of their system of healthcare, alongside seeking modern medical treatment. Physicians and medicine are well-respected in Islam.[26]

Prayer Muslim men and women are obliged to recite prayers five times each day, at home or in a mosque, at various times between dawn and nightfall. Prayer nodules [**Figure 9-1**] are well-known, asymptomatic, chronic skin changes that consist mainly of thickening, lichenification, and hyperpigmentation on the bony prominences, such as the forehead,

TABLE 9-2 Muslim, Middle Eastern and North African (MENA), and South Asian communities in the United States

	Muslim	MENA	South Asian[c]
Refers to country of origin?	No: Refers to religion	Yes: See Table 9-1	Yes: India, Pakistan, Bangladesh, Sri Lanka, Nepal, Bhutan, and Maldives
Race/ethnicity in the United States	Ethnically diverse[a]	White	Asian
Religion	Follower of Islam	Islam; Christianity; Judaism; Bahá'í, Druze; Yazidism; others adopt no religious tradition	Sikh; Hindu; Islam; other religious traditions
Top 10 countries with the largest population of Muslims[b]	Indonesia, Pakistan, India, Bangladesh, Nigeria, Egypt, Iran, Turkey, Algeria, Sudan		

[a]According to a 2019 study, American Muslims are 28% Black or African American, 23% Asian/Chinese/Japanese, 19% White, 14% Arab, 8% Hispanic, 2% Native American/American Indian/Alaska Native, and 5% other.

American Muslim Poll 2019. *Institute for Social Policy and Understanding*. Retrieved August 6, 2023. https://www.ispu.org/research-on-racism-and-the-experiences-and-responses-of-american-muslims/.

[b]Top 10 Countries with the largest number of Muslims: https://worldpopulationreview.com/country-rankings/muslim-population-by-country.

[c]Afghanistan is sometimes positioned within the South Asian region.

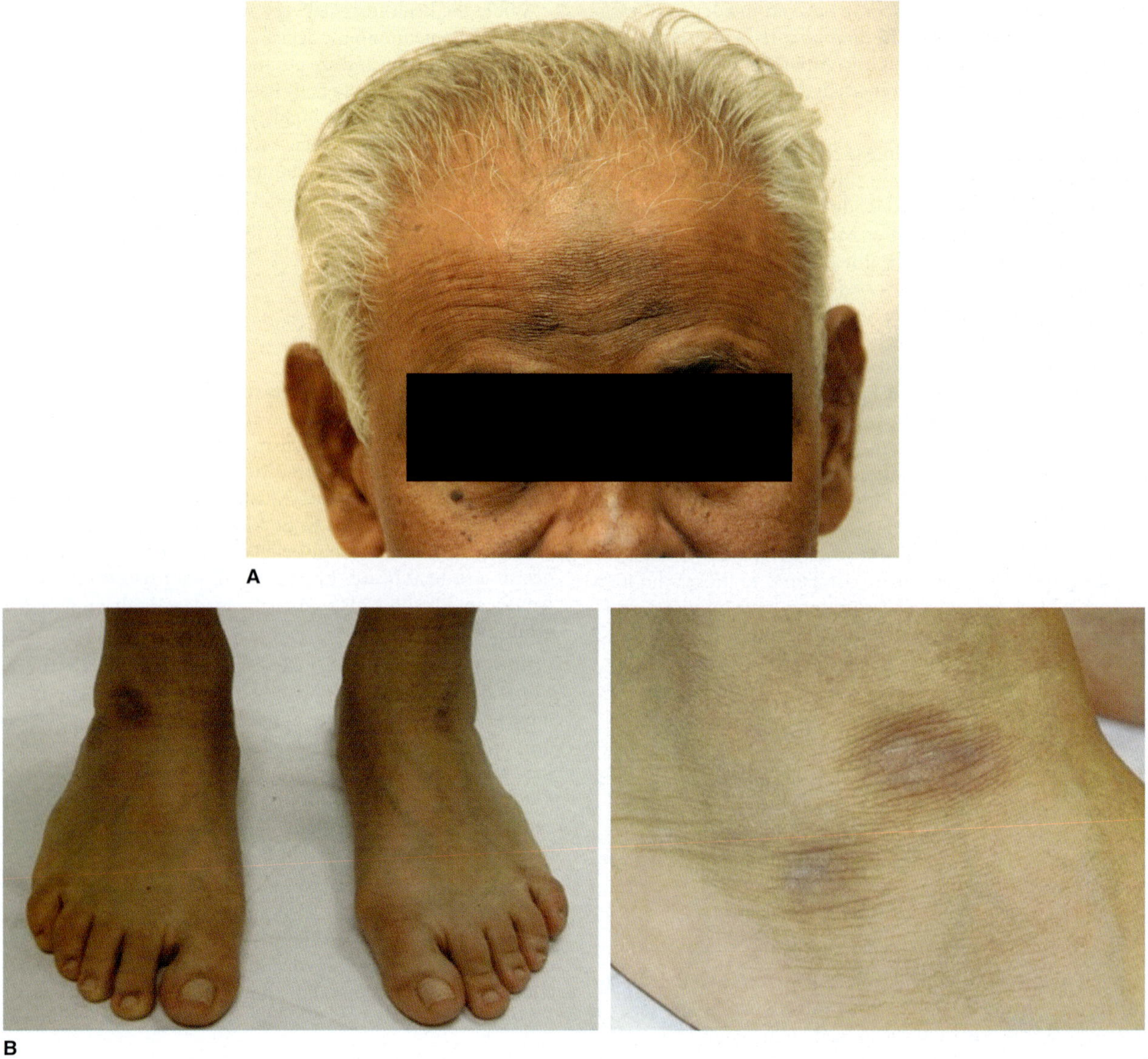

FIGURE 9-1. **(A)** A prayer nodule on the forehead of a man that is acquired after repeated *sajdah*, which is the practice of bending down to touch the head to the floor during prayer. (Used with permission from Nivu Hussain.) **(B)** Left: hyperpigmented and hyperkeratotic plaques over the lateral malleoli of a 41-year old patient. Right: detail of the prayer marks of the right foot. (Reproduced with permission from Fosse N, Rast AC, Kammermann A, et al. Pitfall prayer marks: recognition and appropriate treatment: a case report and review of literature. *Dermatol Ther.* 2020;33(1):e13176, Figure 2.)

the dorsum of the feet, the knees, and the ankles. They develop over a long period of time because of the repeated, extended pressure against hard, rough floors during prayer.[27,28]

Before prayer, Muslims must engage in a cleansing process called ablution or Wudu. The steps of ablution include washing the face, hands, arms, legs, and feet, using running water. The increased prevalence of tinea pedis has been reported in Muslim communities due to the prolonged wetness of the feet caused by frequent ablution.[29] Moreover, the common tradition of sitting cross-legged may, over time, induce a macerated pressure reaction hyperkeratosis in the toe webs of individuals, where the webs become colonized by environmental microorganisms.

Prohibitions in Food and Medications Approved foods in Islam are known as halal [**Figure 9-2**]. Forbidden products, on the other hand, are known as haram. Generally, haram products include alcohol, pork or pork by-products, and illicit substances that cloud one's judgment. The Jewish dietary kosher meat is roughly equivalent to halal meat for Muslims. Most Muslims stringently avoid such products, regardless of their level of religious devotion. Patients may refuse to take medications that contain alcohol or porcine products. This may pose an ethical issue if the patients are not informed of the contents of such medications. This has been a concern in some capsules of isotretinoin that contain porcine gelatin. However, Islamic law will allow the use of such medications only if the patient's condition is critical and there is no other alternative medicine.[30]

Fasting During Ramadan Ramadan, the ninth month of the lunar calendar, is one of the most sacred times for Muslims. As part of their religious practices, Muslims are supposed to refrain from eating or drinking from dawn until dusk. This fasting includes any oral medications or injections. If possible, healthcare providers should discuss safe methods to adapt the medication schedules, or medication doses, of their patients. For example, medications to be taken once or twice per day are preferable because they will not interfere with fasting. It is important to know that acutely or chronically ill patients, people who are traveling, and women who are menstruating, pregnant, or breastfeeding are exempt from fasting. Nevertheless, if a patient chooses to fast under such circumstances, the healthcare provider should discuss with the patient the potential

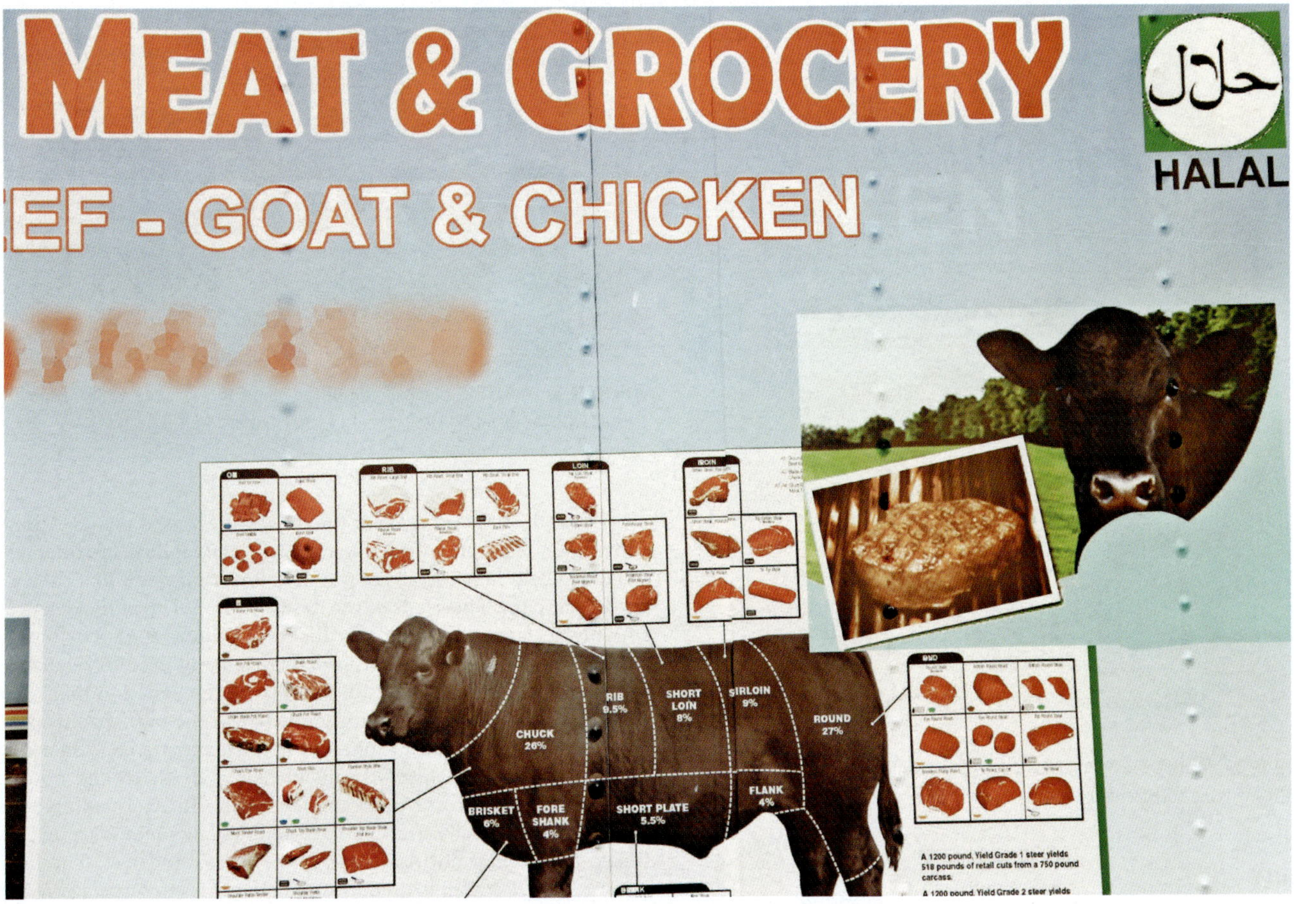

FIGURE 9-2. Halal foods are allowed under Islamic dietary guidelines.

health risks of doing so as medical exemptions are acknowledged in Islam. In a life-threatening situation, the healthcare provider should seek a family member or a leader from the Muslim community to help convey to the patient that complying with treatment does not breach Islamic teachings.[31]

Ruqyah (Spiritual Healing) Many Muslims believe that reading verses from the Quran or reading statements of the Prophet will give the power to heal body, mind, and soul. This is called Ruqyah. Many Muslims use this type of spiritual healing as part of their treatment plan. It is very common to see patients or family members uttering religious words during difficult times, such as in the case of severe illness or before a surgery.[32]

Dress Code In terms of dress code, the Islamic requirement for women is to observe the hijab, that is, dress to cover all parts of the body except the face and hands. Women may wear a head covering (or veil) and a long overgarment called an abaya. Some women will choose to cover their face with the niqab or burqa. Traditionally, women wear this clothing at all times while in public places or around strangers, removing it only when absolutely necessary, such as during a medical examination. In such situations, Muslim patients—both men and women—should be allowed to wear long gowns (preferably floor length with long sleeves) that can be securely tied in the back or should be offered a robe or sheet to preserve their modesty. Alternatively, a patient may choose to wear a shawl or coat over their gown in order to cover up. Still, the practice of hijab will vary greatly among Muslims in the West, from no observance at all to full hijab for some. The use of the hijab can lead to certain dermatoses, including traction alopecia due to tight hair pulling, telogen effluvium related to vitamin D deficiency in the setting of decreased exposure to the sun, allergic contact dermatitis due to pins used to wear the hijab, and seborrheic dermatitis and acne related to occlusion and increased perspiration.[33]

While examining a patient who practices hijab, it is advisable to uncover only one part of the body at a time, recovering the other parts of the body as necessary because patients may feel very uncomfortable exposing large areas of their body. In some cases, female patients may only show one part of the body even if the lesion or condition is widespread. Full body exposure is unacceptable, and any suggestion to expose the whole body will be taken with suspicion. The recognition of these sensitivities by the healthcare provider or technician will help the patient relax.[34]

Touching and Shaking Hands Some Muslim and MENA patients may avoid excessive touching between members of the opposite gender; this includes forms of touching such as shaking hands, hugging, or patting on the shoulder.[34] However, touching and holding hands while walking in the street may be acceptable between members of the same gender and with certain close family members. Because of this, the practitioner may extend their hand as a courtesy, remaining aware that a refusal from the other party to do the same should not be considered insulting.

TRADITIONAL MEDICINE

USE OF TRADITIONAL PLANT AND FOOD PRODUCTS

The use of plants in traditional therapy is common in MENA countries. Many plants and foods traditionally used as home remedies in MENA countries are based on the recommendations of the Prophet Muhammad. Some products are used widely based on these recommendations.[35]

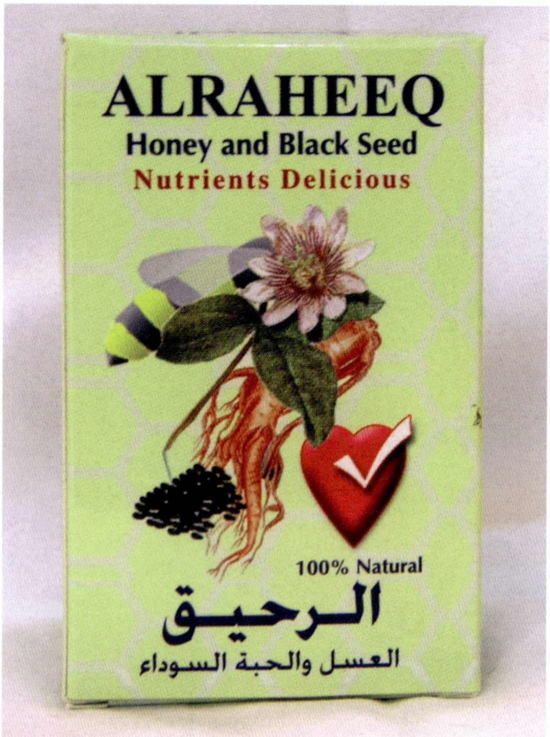

FIGURE 9-3. The use of honey and black seed (Nigella sativa) products is widely used as preventative medicine. (Used with permission from Nivu Hussain.)

HONEY

Honey is widely used as a natural remedy for various ailments, including coughs, to treat burns, heal stomach ulcers, and relieve allergies among MENA communities. The use of honey and black seed (Nigella sativa) products are particularly widespread in the Arab communities as preventative medicines and treatments for a variety of gastrointestinal and dermatologic ailments [**Figure 9-3**].[36,37]

SENNA

Another common plant product used traditionally is senna, which is a shrub that grows to about 1 m in height and is found in hot and humid climates. It is used to relieve constipation, relax the muscles, and improve hair; it is also used as an aid against lice, headaches, rashes, and epilepsy.[38] Senna is also used as a hair conditioner to make the hair thick and glossy and to nourish and strengthen the scalp.

SIWAK

Siwak (also known as miswak) is a twig used as a natural toothbrush, toothpaste, and dental floss. It comes from the Arak tree (*Salvadora persica*), and the twigs are usually a hand span in length and of medium thickness. Siwak contains tannin, which helps to strengthen the gums. It is believed to help remove bad smell from the mouth.[39] Modern medicine has confirmed its benefits in improving dental plaque score and gingival health when it is used as an adjunct to modern teeth brushing [**Figure 9-4**].[40] In addition, the use of siwak was reported to promote gingival health in patients with orthodontic appliances.[41]

HERBS AND SEEDS

Specialized Etara shops are common and sell different mixtures and compounds of herbs [**Figure 9-5**] to cure many diseases. The composition of these products is not standardized and is based on the individual experience and preference of the herbalist.

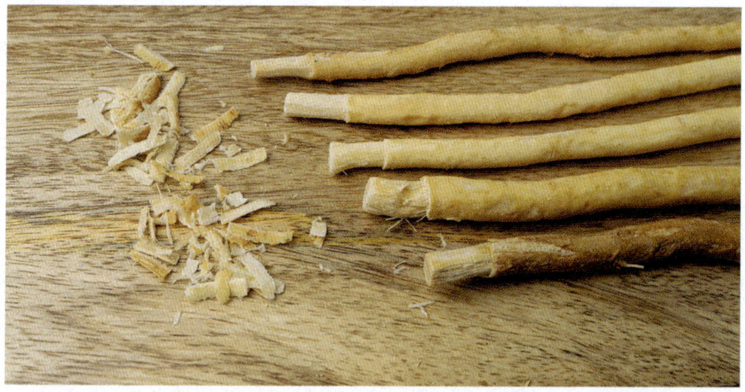

FIGURE 9-4. The trimmed end of the siwak stick is often used for tooth cleaning. (Used with the permission from Ermak Oksana/Shutterstock.)

The following are some of the most widely used plants. The seeds of the senna plant previously mentioned, *Senna italica*, are often used as a laxative, and many Arabs of the Bedouin tribe claim that they will heal stomach pain. The seeds of the desert squash, *Citrullus colocynthis*, are highly acclaimed as a cure for diabetes [**Figure 9-6**]. The bitter sap of the milkweed, *Calotropis procera*, is dried and used to fill aching, hollow teeth; the woody parts of this plant are burned to make charcoal, which was an ingredient for gunpowder in the past. Poultices made of the leaves are applied to joints to heal rheumatism. *Salsola imbricata* and several of the *Suaeda* genus of plants are dried and powdered to be used in snuff form to clear the sinuses. In Arab culture, the best-known cosmetically used plant is henna (*Lawsonia inermis*), which is used to dye hair and to decorate the hands and feet. The poisonous plant *Rhazya stricta* is used in small quantities to settle gastrointestinal problems. An important plant for combating fevers is *Teucrium stocksianum*, a very fragrant herb that is similar to sage. The seeds of the Arab gum tree (*Acacia nilotica*) are grounded to a powder to dry out second-degree burns.[42]

THERAPEUTIC PROCEDURES

HIJAMA (WET CUPPING OR BLOODLETTING CUPPING)

Hijama is a therapeutic procedure where blood is drawn from a small skin incision by a vacuum created with the aid of suction cups [**Figure 9-7**].[43] Hijama can be performed almost anywhere on the body, but it is often done at the site of an ache or pain to ease or alleviate it. Islamic teaching considers cupping to be both a cure and a blessing. Early Muslims used hijama to treat numerous afflictions, including headaches, stomach

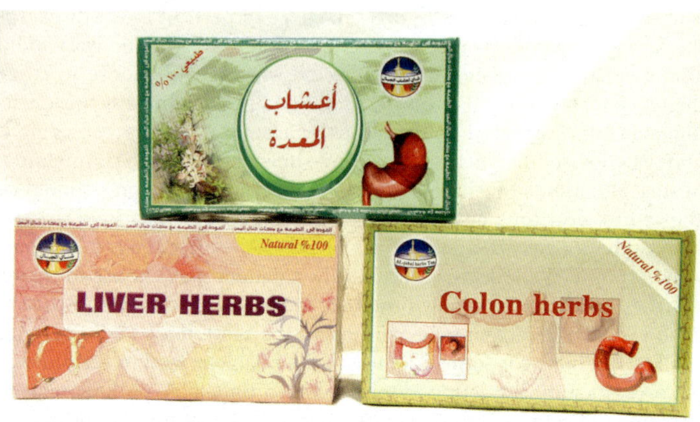

FIGURE 9-5. Different herbal mixtures that are used for treating liver and colon. (Used with permission from Nivu Hussain.)

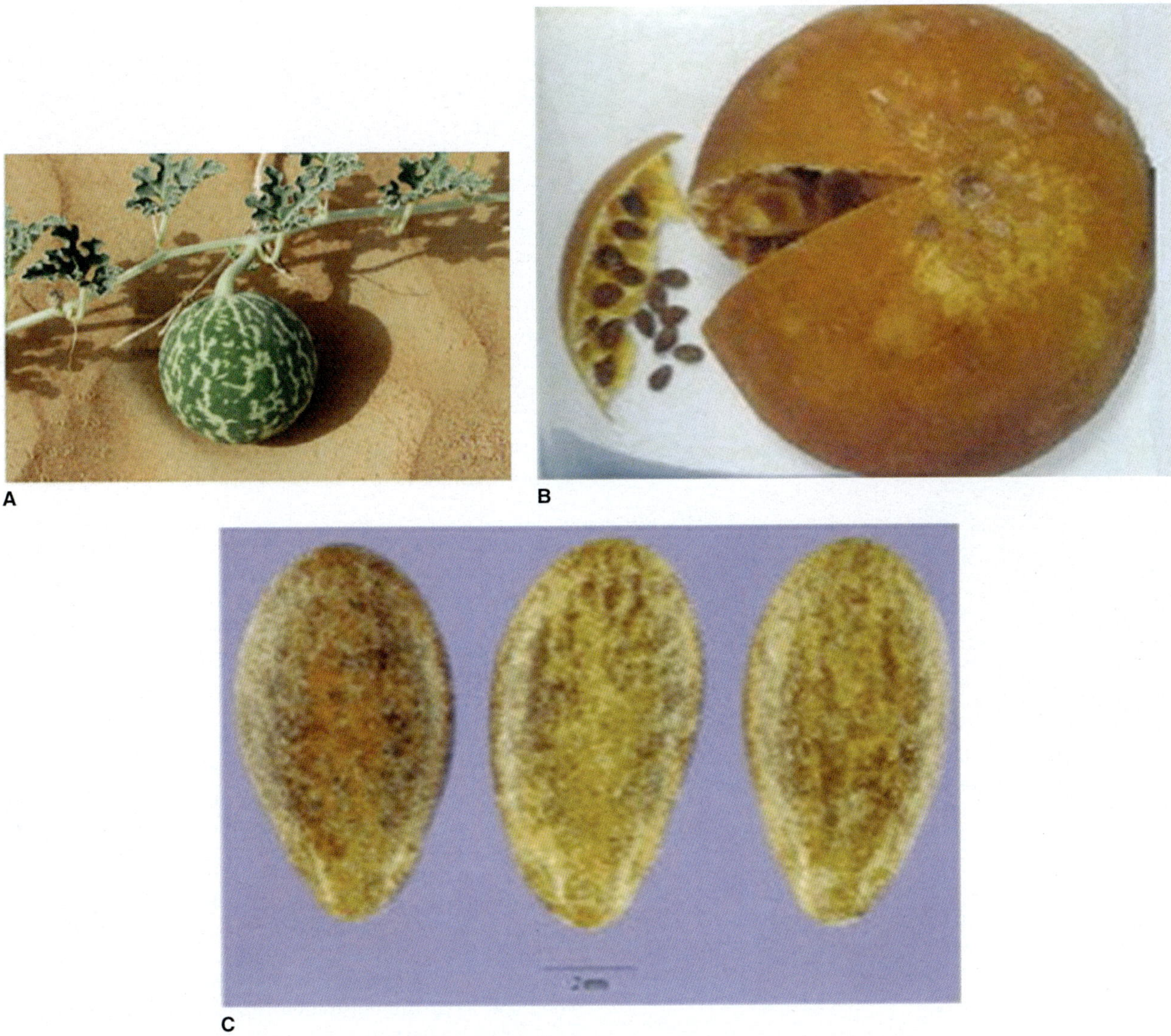

FIGURE 9-6. **(A)** The seeds of the desert squash, *Citrullus colocynthis*, are widely used in different parts of the world for the treatment of diabetes, constipation, leprosy, joint pain, and mastitis, among other conditions. (Reproduced with permission from CiteLi QY, Munawar M, Saeed M, Shen JQ, Khan MS, Noreen S, Alagawany M, Naveed M, Madni A, Li CX. Citrullus colocynthis (L.) Schrad (Bitter Apple Fruit): Promising Traditional Uses, Pharmacological Effects, Aspects, and Potential Applications. Front Pharmacol. 2022 Jan 25;12:791049. Figure 1F.) **(B)** (Reproduced with permission from Hussain AI, Rathore HA, Sattar MZ, Chatha SA, Sarker SD, Gilani AH. Citrullus colocynthis (L.) Schrad (bitter apple fruit): a review of its phytochemistry, pharmacology, traditional uses and nutritional potential. *J Ethnopharmacol.* 2014;155(1):54-66, Figure 1.) **(C)** Reproduced with permission from Photo: Carole Ritchie at USDA PLANTS Database.

problems, poisoning, magic spells, bruising, pain, skin sores, and more. This procedure continues to be practiced by Muslims today, and it is very popular in the Gulf Cooperation Council (GCC) area. Some practitioners claim that dry cupping therapy is beneficial in treating pain, muscular and joint problems, circulatory problems, colds, indigestion, arthritis, congestion in the throat and lungs, headaches, fever, and more. The mechanism of hijama is not exactly known. However, there is a marked difference in the composition of blood drawn through the technique of cupping compared with blood drawn intravenously (eg, via a phlebotomy or venesection), suggesting that hijama may produce its beneficial effect through a mechanism different than that of drawing blood intravenously.[44] Recent studies have suggested a beneficial effect of wet cupping in the treatment of several diseases, such as rheumatoid arthritis,[45] herpes zoster,[46] and low back pain.[47]

KAIY (CAUTERY)

Kaiy, the Arabic term for cautery, is one of the most ancient forms of therapy that is still in use currently. In the Persian Gulf, kaiy involves the use of metal sticks or iron nails that are heated over hot charcoal until they glow red and are then placed on a specified area of the skin for a few seconds.

The choice of location for the application of the metal depends on the patient's individual complaints.[48] This practice was often used in the past to manage internal pain, clean wounds, and treat psychiatric conditions. Although kaiy is rarely seen now, cautery scars can nevertheless still be seen on the skin of elderly people who have come from or been raised in Bedouin areas. The Bedouin are a distinct desert dwelling Arabian ethnic group within the GCC countries.

ORIGINS OF ILLNESSES

HASSAD (ENVY)

One popular belief among the cultures of Persian Gulf countries is hassad (envy or "the Evil eye"). In Islam, hassad occurs when a person envies others for something good that they possess; this envy is accompanied by a wish to inflict misfortune on them or for them to be deprived of their good fortune. Muslims believe that a look or a comment by the envious person may initiate an adverse event, such as an ailment, mental illness, or a failure in relationships or in business. It is not uncommon that, once they have established trust in their healthcare provider, some patients may consider hassad to be the

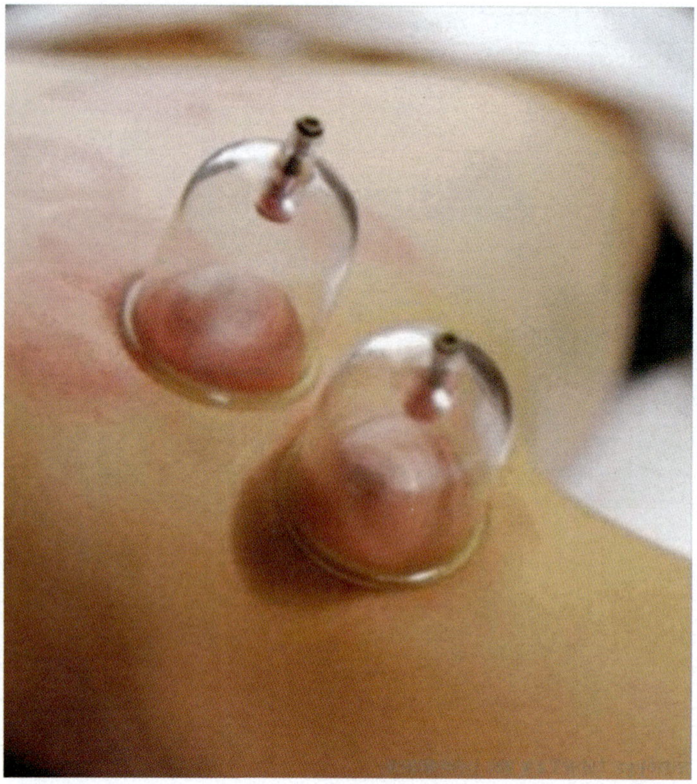

FIGURE 9-7. Circular marks on the back of an individual after *hijama* (bloodletting cupping). (Reproduced with permission from Nisar MK. Cupping (hijama) treatment: benign or sinister? *J Patient Saf.* 2018;14(1):e1-e2, Figure 1.)

cause of their suffering. Dismissing this notion may offend the patient, potentially breaking trust and creating a barrier in the patient-provider relationship. The physician should remain respectful of the patient's beliefs. It is believed that the reversal of hassad is possible by reading special verses of the Quran.[49]

WILL OF GOD

In general, the Islamic view tends to stress the will of God as the origin of all actions, fates, and events. Accordingly, illnesses are often regarded as divine punishment for having committed a sin or as a gift from God to purify the soul. Those who exert patience and accept their illnesses are believed to be praised and rewarded by God. Many Muslims also believe that the cure for their suffering can only be received from God and that any treatment given by a healthcare provider is merely the execution of God's will. Muslims are required to seek medical treatment, while also praying, reading verses of the Quran, and reciting invocations.[26]

JINN AND EVIL FORCES

Although uncommon, some patients believe in the role of unseen forces, mostly jinn or evil spirits, in causing diseases, especially in cases of mental illness and for diseases of unknown cause. Some believe that wearing amulets containing verses from the Quran can protect the individual from the harm of jinn.[49]

BEAUTY STANDARDS AND PRACTICES

SKIN LIGHTENING

Standards of beauty have changed over time, based on the changing cultural values in MENA countries. Despite the influence of the media, which perpetuates a supposedly "global" standard of ideal beauty, there is a distinction in the perception of beauty that is evident in different

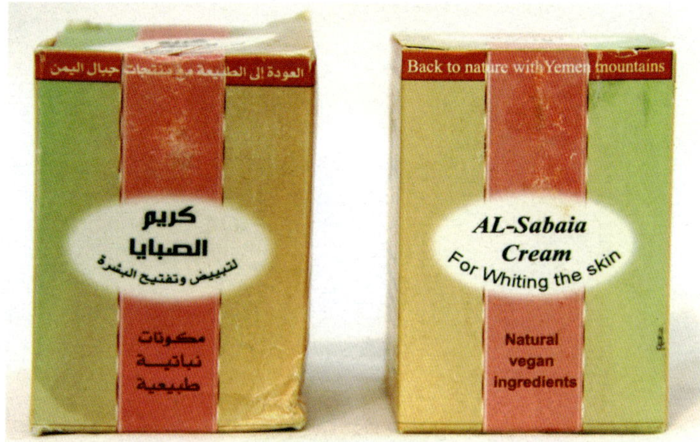

FIGURE 9-8. Skin-lightening creams are often used by many women in attempts to lighten their skin tone. (Used with permission from Nivu Hussain.)

parts of the world. Nevertheless, a lighter complexion is often preferred among many women within the MENA population,[50] especially among individuals with darker skin. This has resulted in a dramatic increase in the use of skin lightening products, even when the safety of such products has not been established, in an attempt to lighten the skin tone [**Figure 9-8**].

HENNA

Henna (*L. inermis*) is a plant that is widely used in MENA countries to dye the hair and temporarily tattoo the skin. The name is often misused for other skin and hair dyes, such as black henna or neutral henna, that do not actually contain henna plant products. Black henna may be derived from the indigo plant (*Indigofera tinctoria*) or *S. italica* and may contain unlisted dyes and chemicals such as p-phenylenediamine (PPD), which can quickly stain the skin black. However, PPD can also cause severe allergic reactions such as blistering, intense itching, permanent scarring, and permanent chemical sensitivities [**Figure 9-9**].[51,52] The U.S. Food and Drug Administration (FDA) specifically forbids PPD to be used for such a purpose.

In several parts of the world, henna is traditionally used in various festivals and celebrations. Decorative henna has been used for over 5000 years and has become a symbol of good luck, health, and sensuality [**Figure 9-10**]. Henna decorating is considered an art form and is practiced widely in many MENA countries. The most popular traditional use of henna is in wedding celebrations and during bridal preparations.[53] For dyeing or tattooing the skin, a paste of henna (either prepared from a dried powder or from the freshly ground leaves) is applied to the skin and left for a period of time ranging from a few hours to overnight. Henna stains can last from a few days to a month depending on the quality of the paste, the individual skin type, and the duration of time that the paste has been left in contact with the skin.[52] Various shades of colors can be procured by mixing henna with the leaves and fruit of other plants, such as indigo, tea, coffee, cloves, and lemon. In addition to its decorative use, henna is also applied to the palms and soles during hot weather because it acts as a cooling agent. As a temporary tattoo, henna is acceptable from the religious point of view; this is in contrast to any permanent tattoos, which are strongly forbidden in some sects of Islam. Many Muslims who have had a permanent tattoo at some point in their life often later seek tattoo removal by laser or surgery.

CONCLUSION

There exists a paucity of knowledge related to medical and health conditions, including dermatologic, impacting MENA Americans. Future research should take the initiative to include data on the MENA population to remedy health disparities that exist in this diverse population.

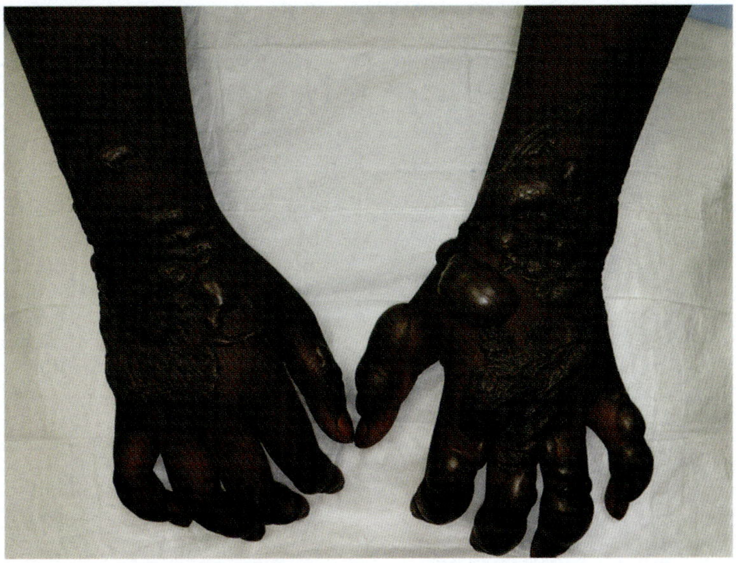

FIGURE 9-9. Allergic contact dermatitis from a henna tattoo. (Reproduced with permission from Allergic Contact Dermatitis to a Henna Tattoo, Perez, Victoria A. et al. Journal of Emergency Medicine, Volume 59, Issue 4, e137-e138. Figure 1.)

In addition, the deeply rooted cultures, beliefs, and practices of people from MENA countries appear to affect many aspects of healthcare practices. Awareness by healthcare providers of the different cultures and beliefs of people from these regions of the world will help to ensure proper care and management of health concerns, including skin conditions.

Acknowledgments

We would like to acknowledge Dr. Ashraf M. Reda and Dr. Faiza Mohamed Al Ali for their work on the previous edition of this chapter, along with Dr. Stephanie Javadi and Dr. Persiana Saffari for their insight and contributions to the current chapter.

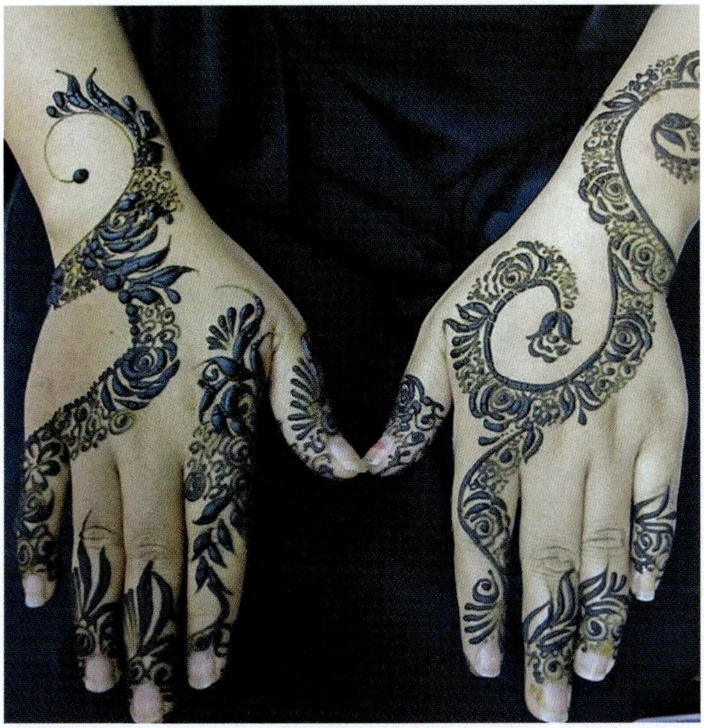

FIGURE 9-10. Decorative henna has been used for over 5000 years and has become a symbol of good luck, health, and sensuality.

REFERENCES

1. Harjanto L, Batalova J. Middle Eastern and North African immigrants in the United States. Migration Policy Institute. https://www.migrationpolicy.org/article/middle-eastern-and-north-african-immigrants-united-states#:~:text=Between%202000%20and%202019%2C%20the,44.9%20million%20as%20of%202019.&text=Sources%3A%20Data%20from%20U.S.%20Census,ACS)%2C%20and%20Campbell%20J. Accessed June 25, 2023,
2. Samari G, Sharif MZ, Alcala HE. Racial and citizenship disparities in health care among Middle Eastern Americans. *Med Care*. 2020;58(11):974-980.
3. Patel MR, Green M, Tariq M, et al. A snapshot of social risk factors and associations with health outcomes in a community sample of Middle Eastern and North African (MENA) people in the U.S. *J Immigr Minor Health*. 2022;24(2):376-384.
4. El-Essawi D, Musial JL, Hammad A, Lim HW. A survey of skin disease and skin-related issues in Arab Americans. *J Am Acad Dermatol*. 2007;56(6):933-938.
5. Maghbouleh N, Schachter A, Flores RD. Middle Eastern and North African Americans may not be perceived, nor perceive themselves, to be White. *Proc Natl Acad Sci USA*. 2022;119(7):e2117940119.
6. Sarsour NY, Hammoud MM. Integration of Arab and Muslim health education into a medical school curriculum. *MedEdPORTAL*. 2021;17(11188):1-9.
7. Minority Rights Group International. Arab and other Middle Eastern Americans. https://minorityrights.org/minorities/arab-and-other-middle-eastern-americans/. Accessed June 25, 2023.
8. Awad GH. The impact of acculturation and religious identification on perceived discrimination for Arab/Middle Eastern Americans. *Cultur Divers Ethnic Minor Psychol*. 2010;16(1):59-67.
9. Foad HS. Waves of immigration from the Middle East to the United States. *Soc Sci Res Netw*. 2013;1(1):1-20.
10. Abuelezam NN. Health equity during COVID-19: the case of Arab Americans. *Am J Prev Med*. 2020;59(3):455-457.
11. Amer MM, Hovey JD. Anxiety and depression in a post-September 11 sample of Arabs in the USA. *Soc Psychiatry Psychiatr Epidemiol*. 2012;47(3):409-418.
12. Padela AI, Heisler M. The association of perceived abuse and discrimination after September 11, 2001, with psychological distress, level of happiness, and health status among Arab Americans. *Am J Public Health*. 2010;100(2):284-291.
13. Lauderdale DS. Birth outcomes for Arabic-named women in California before and after September 11. *Demography*. 2006;43(1):185-201.
14. Abu-Ras W, Abu-Bader SH. The impact of the September 11, 2001, attacks on the well-being of Arab Americans in New York City. *J Muslim Ment Health*. 2008;3(2):217-239.
15. Bailey ZD, Krieger N, Agenor M, Graves J, Linos N, Bassett MT. Structural racism and health inequities in the USA: evidence and interventions. *Lancet*. 2017;389(10077):1453-1463.

16. Awad GH, Abuelezam NN, Ajrouch KJ, Stiffler MJ. Lack of Arab or Middle Eastern and North African health data undermines assessment of health disparities. *Am J Public Health.* 2022;112(2):209-212.
17. Davis SA, Narahari S, Feldman SR, Huang W, Pichardo-Geisinger RO, McMichael AJ. Top dermatologic conditions in patients of color: an analysis of nationally representative data. *J Drugs Dermatol.* 2012;11(4):466-473.
18. Nasseri K, Mills PK, Allan M. Cancer incidence in the Middle Eastern population of California, 1988-2004. *Asian Pac J Cancer Prev.* 2007;8(3):405-411.
19. Northwestern University Weinberg College of Arts and Sciences. Mena languages. https://mena-languages.northwestern.edu/undergraduate/mena-languages/index.html. Accessed June 25, 2023.
20. Giordano S. Overview of the advantages and disadvantages of professional and child interpreters for limited English proficiency patients in general health care situations. *J Radiol Nurs.* 2007;26(4):126-131.
21. Alkhaibari RA, Smith-Merry J, Forsyth R, Raymundo GM. Patient-centered care in the Middle East and North African region: a systematic literature review. *BMC Health Serv Res.* 2023;23:135.
22. Salari S. Invisible in aging research: Arab Americans, Middle Eastern immigrants, and Muslims in the United States. *Gerontologist.* 2002;42(5):580-588.
23. Elmaghraby R, Daas M, Elnajjar A, Elkady R. Cultural considerations in working with Arab American Youth. *Child Adolesc Psychiatr Clin N Am.* 2022;31(4):719-732.
24. Attum B, Hafiz S, Malik A, Shamoon Z. Cultural competence in the care of Muslim patients and their families. *StatPearls.* 2023.
25. Hakim-Larson J, Kamoo R, Nassar-McMillan SC, Porcerelli JH. Counseling Arab and Chaldean American families. *J Ment Health Couns.* 2007;29(4):301-321.
26. Rassool GH. The crescent and Islam: healing, nursing and the spiritual dimension. Some considerations towards an understanding of the Islamic perspectives on caring. *J Adv Nurs.* 2008;32(6):1476-1484.
27. English JS, Fenton DA, Wilkinson JD. Prayer nodules. *Clin Exp Dermatol.* 984;9(1):97-98.
28. Monk BE. Prayer nodules. *Clin Exp Dermatol.* 1982;7(2):225-226.
29. Raboobee N, Aboobaker J, Peer AK. Tinea pedis et unguium in the Muslim community of Durban, South Africa. *Int J Dermatol.* 2002;37(10):759-765.
30. Ogden J. Religious constraints on prescribing medication. *Prescriber.* 2016;27(12):4-54.
31. Abolaban H, Al-Moujahed A. Muslim patients in Ramadan: a review for primary care physicians. *Avicenna J Med.* 2017;7(3):81-87.
32. Çaksen H. Ruqyah and its use among patients with cancer. *J Child Sci.* 2023;13(01):e20-e27.
33. Rehman R, Haque M, Ceresnie M, Hamzavi IH, Fahs F, Mohammad TF. Dermatological considerations and culturally sensitive recommendations for women who wear the hijab. *Br J Dermatol.* 2022;187(6):1003-1004.
34. Padela AI, Rodriguez del Pozo P. Muslim patients and cross-gender interactions in medicine: an Islamic bioethical perspective. *J Med Ethics.* 2011; 37(1):40-44.
35. Ali SA, Parveen N, Ali AS. Links between the Prophet Muhammad (PBUH) recommended foods and disease management: a review in the light of modern superfoods. *Int J Health Sci (Qassim).* 2018;12(2):61-69.
36. Bener A, Janahi I. Association between childhood atopic disease and parental atopic disease in a population with high consanguinity. *Coll Antropol.* 2005;29(2):677-682.
37. Alireza MA. Honey: Food And Medicine. https://www.arabnews.com/node/324985. Accessed June 18, 2023.
38. Al-Jawzīyah IQ. *Medicine of the Prophet.* Johnstone P. Islamic Texts Society; 1998.
39. Haque MM, Alsareii SA. A review of the therapeutic effects of using miswak (Salvadora Persica) on oral health. *Saudi Med J.* 2015;36(5):530-543.
40. Patel PV, Shruthi S, Kumar S. Clinical effect of miswak as an adjunct to tooth brushing on gingivitis. *J Indian Soc Periodontol.* 2012;16(1):84-88.
41. Al-Teen RM, Said KN, Abu Alhaija ES. Siwak as a oral hygiene aid in patients with fixed orthodontic appliances. *Int J Dent Hyg.* 2006;4(4):189-197.
42. Saad B, Said O. *Greco-Arab and Islamic Herbal Medicine: Traditional System, Ethics, Safety, Efficacy, and Regulatory Issues.* Hoboken, NJ: John Wiley & Sons; 2011.
43. Hajar Albinali H. Chairman's reflections: blood-letting. Special section. *Heart Views.* 2004;5(2):74-85.
44. Bilal M, Khan RA, Ahmed A, Afroz S. Partial evaluation of technique used in cupping therapy. *Journal of Basic and Applied Sciences.* 2011;7(1):65-68.
45. Ahmed SM, Madbouly NH, Maklad SS, Abu-Shady EA. Immunomodulatory effects of blood letting cupping therapy in patients with rheumatoid arthritis. *Egypt J Immunol.* 2005;12(2):39-51.
46. Cao H, Zhu C, Liu J. Wet cupping therapy for treatment of herpes zoster: a systematic review of randomized controlled trials. *Altern Ther Health Med.* 2010;16(6):48-54.
47. Farhadi K, Schwebel DC, Saeb M, Choubsaz M, Mohammadi R, Ahmadi A. The effectiveness of wet-cupping for nonspecific low back pain in Iran: a randomized controlled trial. *Complement Ther Med.* 2009;17(1):9-15.
48. Hajar Albinali H. Special section: Arab Gulf traditional medicine cautery. *Heart Views.* 2003;5:178-183.
49. Thomas J, Al-Qarni N, Furber SW. Conceptualising mental health in the United Arab Emirates: the perspective of traditional healers. *Ment Health Relig Cult.* 2015;18(2):134-145.
50. Pollock S, Taylor S, Oyerinde O, et al. The dark side of skin lightening: an international collaboration and review of a public health issue affecting dermatology. *Int J Womens Dermatol.* 2021;7(2):158-164.
51. Singh M, Singh YV, Jindal SK, Narain P, eds. Traditional methods of cultivation and processing of henna. *Henna, Cultivation, Improvement and Trade.* Jodhpur: Central Arid Zone Research Institute; 2005: 21-24.
52. Hema R, Kumaravel S, Gomathi S, Sivasubramaniam C. Gas chromatography – mass spectroscopic analysis of Lawsonia inermis leaves. *New York Sci J.* 2010;3(11):141-143.
53. Werbner P. Ritual, embodiment and creativity in the Muslim diaspora: transnational migrations and symbolic returns. In: Leaman O, ed. *Routledge Handbook of Islamic Ritual and Practice.* 1st ed. London: Routledge; 2022:11.

CHAPTER 10

Psychiatric Aspects of Skin of Color

Nithya Ravindran
Amy Woods
Rachel Hammer

KEY POINTS

- Dermatologists may be the first encounter for a patient who presents with a medical complaint secondary to a primary psychiatric disorder.
- Patients who suffer from psychiatric disorders experience stigma and significant psychosocial burdens that can worsen both their psychiatric and dermatological condition, especially in people with skin of color.
- When discussing psychiatric disorders in patients with skin of color, the impact of racism must be considered along with the impact of diagnoses on a patient's quality of life and psychosocial circumstance.
- Universally, treating patients with an authentic, nonjudgmental, present, and compassionate approach can lead to better engagement and outcomes.
- An integrated and holistic approach is necessary to alleviate disparities in healthcare, including psychiatric health disparities among historically marginalized communities.

INTRODUCTION

Just as the epidermis, melanocytes, and the nervous system all form from common embryologic origins in the ectoderm,[1] skin, skin color, and mental health also have an interconnected relationship. When discussing psychiatric aspects of skin of color, race and racism cannot be ignored. Race categorizes individuals according to genetic ancestry, physical appearance (including variations in skin color), and historical context.[2] And although race does not have a biological basis, it is a proxy for many other factors, all of which directly and indirectly impact health and wellness.

This chapter will start with a discussion on the impact of social constructs on mental health, including disparities found among Black, Latine/Hispanic, and Indigenous (First) people of color (or historically marginalized communities) in the United States. Following this discussion, common primary psychiatric disorders and their associated dermatological findings (such as those in obsessive-compulsive disorders, body dysmorphic disorder, and psychotic disorders) will be reviewed, followed by general medical conditions with cutaneous and psychiatric findings, and finally other topics at the intersection of psychiatry and dermatology [**Figure 10-1**]. Many patients with comorbid psychiatric and dermatological illnesses require management by an interdisciplinary team of specialists, primary care physicians, and mental health providers. We conclude this chapter with an entreaty to consider the value of interdisciplinary care clinics in psycho-dermatology, a clinical domain well-situated within the model of collaborative care, as a way to improve patient care and outcomes at this intersection of medicine and psychiatry.

SOCIOLOGICAL ASPECTS OF SKIN COLOR

IMPACT OF SOCIAL CONSTRUCTS ON MENTAL HEALTH

Skin color is a result of a complex interplay of genetics, biology, and environment; similarly, race is a complex social construct inclusive of an individuals' biological and environmental differences as well as social experiences such as historical context, policies, and structures (also see Chapter 1).[3,4] A person's skin color is often the first and most prominent indicator of one's race. In medicine, race-based differences have long been erroneously attributed to biology. However, since race does not have any relevant biological correlate and is itself a proxy for various genetic, ancestral, historical, and social aspects of a person's life, race-based differences in health is often a clearer reflection of the social system of racism impacting health.[2,5]

Dr. Camara Jones defines racism as the "system of structuring opportunity and assigning value based on the social interpretation of how one looks that unfairly disadvantages some individuals and communities, unfairly advantages other individuals and communities, and saps the strength of the whole society through the waste of human resources."[6]

The health impacts of racism are well documented. A recent review sampling studies done in the United States reported an experience of racism was associated with poorer general and mental health.[7] The association

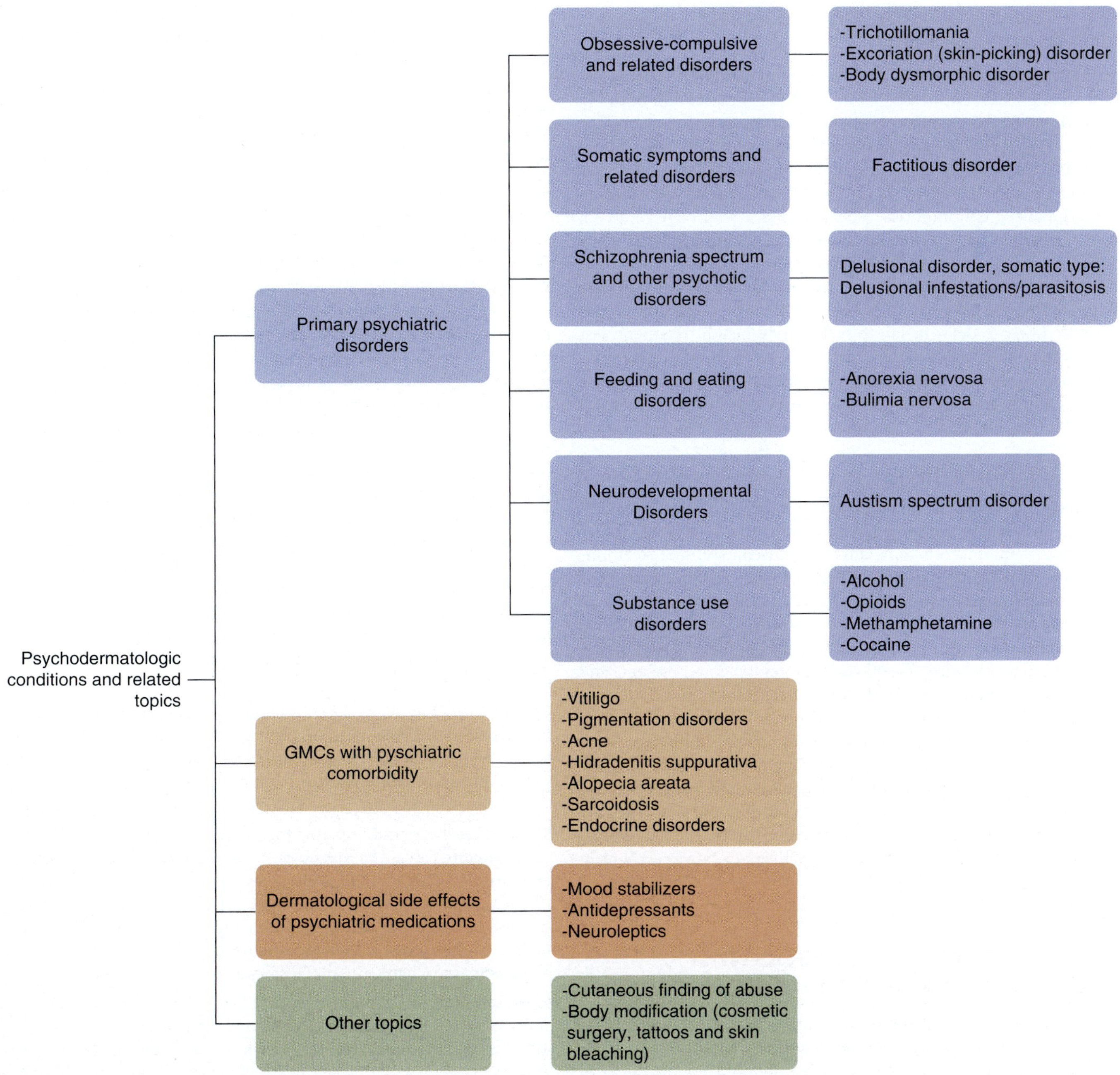

FIGURE 10-1. Psychodermatologic conditions and related topics. GMCs, general medical conditions. (Modified from Bolognia J, Schaffer J, Duncan K, Ko C. *Dermatology Essentials*. 2nd ed. Amsterdam, the Netherlands: Elsevier; 2022.)

was strongest between racism and poorer mental health, especially suicidal ideation, depression, and post-traumatic stress disorder (PTSD), leading the authors to conclude that racism may impact the hypothalamic-pituitary-adrenal (HPA) axis like chronic stress does. This has later general medical consequences such as cardiovascular disease, obesity, and endocrine dysfunction, among others. Racism has also been shown to dysregulate certain neural regions and pathways in the prefrontal cortex, anterior cingulate cortex, amygdala, and thalamus—areas that are implicated in the pathophysiology of anxiety, depression, attention/concentration difficulties, and psychosis. Decades of empirical evidence correlates race-based traumatic stress (RBTS) to emotional dysregulation and psychological distress. In children, racism-related stress (RST) and trauma has a deleterious effect on emotional development and regulation, with greater exposure to RST associated with decreased well-being, increased maladjustment, and increased emotional dysregulation (reactivity, loss of control, rumination, aggression, and anger).[8] It is clear from a neuroscientific, clinical, and sociological review that racism-based stress is harmful to mental health and physical health.

PSYCHIATRIC HEALTH DISPARITIES IN HISTORICALLY MARGINALIZED COMMUNITIES

The cumulative impact of the above is evident in psychiatric health disparities among Black, Latine/Hispanic, and Indigenous communities in the United States. For example, Native Americans were found to be at heightened risk for PTSD and alcohol dependence, Black and Latine/Hispanic patients are diagnosed with schizophrenia at higher rates than mood disorders compared to their White counterparts, and children from marginalized communities, especially Black youth aged 5 to 12, have much higher rates of suicide than White children of the same age.[9,10] Further, individuals from historically marginalized communities in the United States have less access to mental health services, are less likely to receive needed care, more likely to receive poor quality treatment, more likely to delay or fail to seek mental health treatment, less likely to receive the best available treatments for depression and anxiety, and more likely to terminate treatment prematurely. Addressing the problem requires a multi-layered approach at institutional, interpersonal, and internal levels.[10]

APPROACH WITH PATIENTS

In psychiatry, the therapeutic alliance a doctor has with a patient is tantamount to care. It has been shown to affect outcomes such as adherence and response to pharmacotherapy, and often is used to promote relationship insights in patients. External limitations (such as time limits and other clinical/administrative demands) and internal constraints (such as compassion, fatigue, and preoccupation with clinical assessment) can make connecting with patients difficult for all physicians. Universally, treating patients with an authentic, nonjudgmental, present, and compassionate approach can lead to better engagement and outcomes, even within a 15-minute follow-up visit. Especially due to the historical stigma surrounding both psychiatric and dermatological illnesses, having an understanding about the impact of diagnoses on a patient's quality of life and psychosocial circumstance and creating a space to have discussions about this can lead to improved rapport and outcomes. As discussed throughout this chapter, a compassionate and nonjudgmental approach to patients is as important in the delivery of care as arriving at the correct diagnosis and treatment.

PRIMARY PSYCHIATRIC DISORDERS WITH DERMATOLOGICAL MANIFESTATIONS

Often, dermatologists or primary care physicians may be the first encounter for a patient who presents with a medical complaint secondary to a primary psychiatric disorder. It is important for providers to be familiar with the clinical presentation, diagnosis, and management of psychiatric conditions, including obsessive-compulsive disorders, psychotic disorders, somatic disorders, autism spectrum disorder, and eating disorders so that proper care is provided for these patients.

TABLE 10-1 DSM 5-TR Criteria trichotillomania

Recurrent pulling out of one's hair, resulting in hair loss.
Repeated attempts to decrease or stop hair pulling.
The hair pulling causes clinically significant distress or impairment in social, occupational, or other important areas of functioning.
The hair pulling or hair loss is not attributable to another medical condition (eg, a dermatological condition).
The hair pulling is not better explained by the symptoms of another mental disorder (eg, attempts to improve a perceived defect or flaw in appearance in body dysmorphic disorder).

OBSESSIVE-COMPULSIVE AND RELATED DISORDERS

Trichotillomania, excoriation disorder, and body dysmorphic disorders are three disorders within the obsessive-compulsive and related disorders that have cutaneous manifestations. Both trichotillomania and excoriation disorder involve recurrent body-focused repetitive behaviors. Body dysmorphic disorder is the perceived physical deficit or flaw.

Trichotillomania Trichotillomania is a primary psychiatric condition characterized by hair loss due to recurrent pulling out of one's hair. See **Table 10-1** for diagnostic criteria.

Epidemiology The prevalence of trichotillomania among adults and adolescents in the United States is between 1% and 2%. In self-identified samples, the prevalence between women and men is 10:1; however, the ratio is closer to 2:1 in community samples. In children there is a 1:1 ratio. Onset typically coincides with puberty.[11]

Clinical Features Patients will typically present to a dermatologist before seeing a psychiatrist or psychologist with the chief complaint of hair loss.[12] Patients can either engage in conscious or unconscious hair pulling.[12,13] People who engage in unconscious hair pulling will not recall pulling their hair out. They may remember playing or twisting their hair. In conscious hair pulling, the behavior may be associated with rituals such as looking for a particular kind of hair to pull (eg, texture) or removal by a particular manner (eg, at the root). Patients may visually inspect the hair or manipulate it in their mouth.[11] Conscious hair pulling is usually triggered by strong emotions (eg, anger, anxiety, boredom) or stressors (eg, school or family).[11,13] Patients may feel a sense of relief from their emotional state shortly after engaging in hair pulling.[11] Children often engage in this behavior privately, so caregivers may only report that hair is falling out.[12] The most common sites for hair pulling include scalp (crown, parietal area) [**Figure 10-2**], eyebrows, eyelashes, or even the pubic region.[11,12] The affected area may have hairs of various lengths, and the borders of the area may also be irregular and geometric.[13]

Differential Diagnosis The differential diagnosis for trichotillomania includes alopecia areata, tinea capitis, traction alopecia, telogen effluvium, other psychiatric conditions (eg, obsessive-compulsive disorder, stereotypic movement disorder, psychotic disorder).[11,12]

Diagnosis For patients aged 10 to 17, using The National Institute of Mental Health Trichotillomania Symptoms Severity Scale (NIMH-TTS) questionnaire can aid in diagnosis.[12] For adults, the Massachusetts General Hospital Hair-pulling Scale assesses the severity of symptoms.[14] If the diagnosis is not clear from physical exam and history, dermoscopy can also be used. Typical dermoscopic presentations of trichotillomania include broken hairs, frayed ends, flame hairs, coiled hairs, and irregular black dots (see Chapter 25 on Dermoscopy in Skin of Color).[12]

Management It is important to establish rapport with the patient and caregivers and provide psychoeducation to combat stigma as the initial steps in management. First-line treatment is Habit Reversal Training (HRT), a skill-based psychotherapy focusing on reversing the unwanted behavior. Support groups can be helpful for patients as well as caregivers.[12]

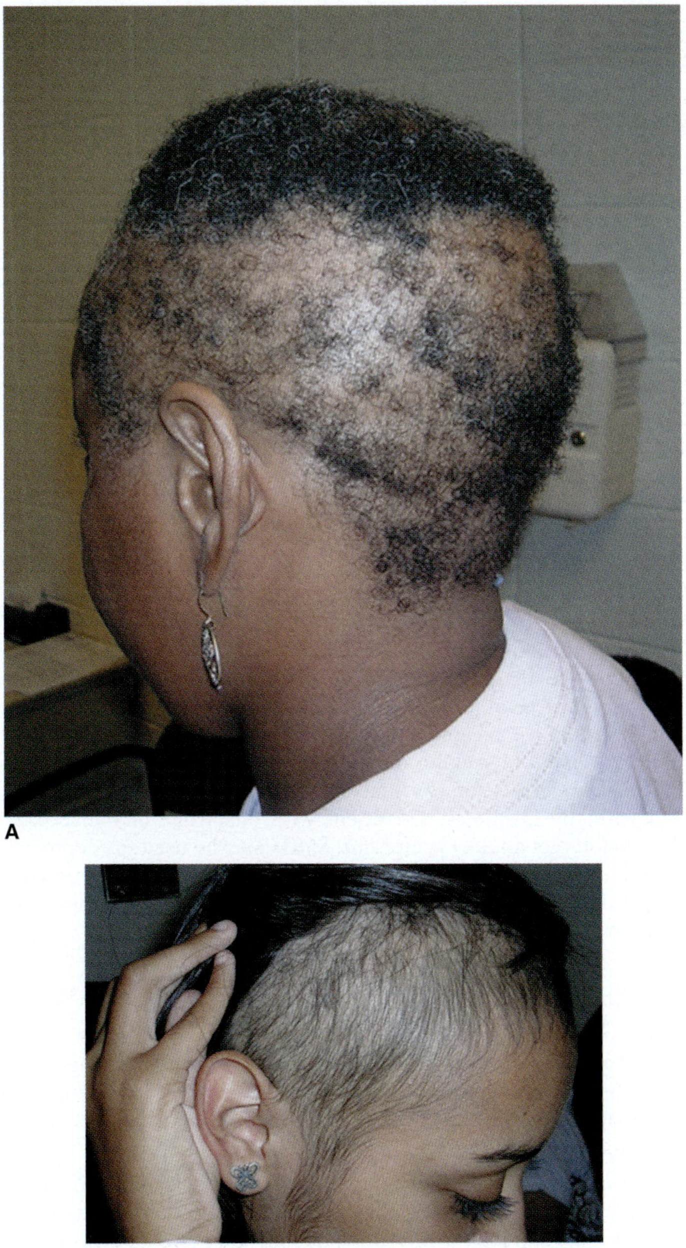

A

B

FIGURE 10-2. Trichotillomania. **(A)** Chronic hair loss in a woman with trichotillomania. **(B)** Trichotillomania in a college student who is currently taking four Advanced Placement courses simultaneously. (From Usatine RP, Smith MA, Mayeaux EJ Jr, Chumley HS. *The Color Atlas and Synopsis of Family Medicine*. 3rd ed. New York, NY: McGraw Hill; 2019, Figures 196-4 and 196-5. Part A: Reproduced with permission from E.J. Mayeaux, Jr., MD. Part B: Reproduced with permission from Richard P. Usatine, MD.)

Currently, there are no FDA-approved medications for the treatment of trichotillomania. Treatment with *N*-acetylcysteine 1200 to 2400 mg/day has demonstrated significant improvement in adults with trichotillomania but did not show such effect in pediatric patients. Other medications that have been used to treat trichotillomania include selective serotonin reuptake inhibitors (SSRIs), clomipramine, and antipsychotics.[12,15]

There has been little research on variations in the symptomology of trichotillomania in the Black community, especially in Black women. For many Black women, racial discrimination regarding their natural hair can influence their self-esteem, self-worth, and perception of attractiveness.[16] Race/ethnicity may influence how patients with trichotillomania cope with the diagnosis and seek help.[15] Further, inadequate access to care may prevent persons of marginalized communities from receiving medical and mental healthcare.[14]

TABLE 10-2 DSM 5-TR criteria excoriation (skin-picking) disorder

Recurrent skin picking resulting in skin lesions.
Repeated attempts to decrease or stop skin picking.
The skin picking causes clinically significant distress or impairment in social, occupational, or other important areas of functioning.
The skin picking is not attributable to the physiological effects of a substance (eg, cocaine) or another medical condition (eg, scabies)
The skin picking is not better explained by symptoms of another mental disorder (eg, delusions or tactile hallucinations in psychotic disorder, attempts to improve a perceived defect or flaw in appearance in body dysmorphic disorder, stereotypies in stereotypic movement disorder, or inattention to harm oneself in nonsuicidal self-injury).

Excoriation (Skin-Picking) Disorder Excoriation disorder results from recurrent skin picking that results in lesions of the skin. **Table 10-2** outlines the diagnostic criteria.

Epidemiology The U.S. prevalence is 2.1% with higher rates seen in woman than men.[11] Onset is most common in childhood or adolescence; however, it can occur in adulthood as well.[15]

Clinical Features Most often, the disorder begins following a primary dermatological condition (eg, acne) that initiates the site for skin picking, most commonly on the face [**Figure 10-3**]. Any area of the body could be a site, limited by accessibility (eg, arms, back, shoulders, legs). The scars are often angulated around the borders.[11,15]

Differential Diagnosis The differential diagnosis for excoriation disorder includes delusions (eg, parasitosis), tactile hallucinations (eg, formication), obsessive-compulsive disorder, stereotypic movement disorder resulting in self-injurious behavior, dermatitis artefacta (also known as factitious dermatitis), substance use-related (eg, cocaine), and scabies.[11]

Management There are no FDA-approved medications for excoriation disorder. In a randomized control trial, *N*-acetylcysteine 1200 to 3000 mg/day was shown to significantly reduce symptoms. Habit Reversal Training (HRT) has shown some benefit in reducing symptoms. SSRIs have shown mixed results in reducing symptoms. It is important to manage any

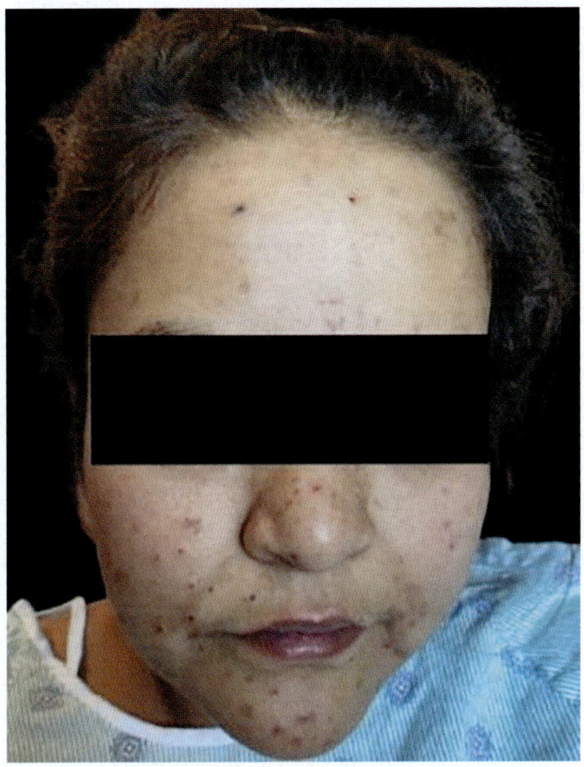

FIGURE 10-3. Acne excoriée (skin picking) disorder.

TABLE 10-3 DSM 5-TR criteria body dysmorphic disorder

Preoccupation with one or more perceived defects or flaws in physical appearance that are not observable or appear slight to others.
At some point during the course of the disorder, the individual has performed repetitive behaviors (eg, mirror checking, excessive grooming, skin picking, reassurance seeking) or mental acts (eg, comparing their appearance with that of others) in response to the appearance concerns.
The preoccupation causes clinically significant distress or impairment in social, occupational, or other important areas of functioning.
The appearance preoccupation is not better explained by concerns with body fat or weight in an individual whose symptoms meet diagnostic criteria for an eating disorder.

secondary complications such as infection, bleeding, and inflammation.[15] Historically marginalized communities of color are less likely to receive treatment. The exact cause for this is unclear but could be related to lack of access, mistrust, stigma, or bias within healthcare delivery.[14]

Body Dysmorphic Disorder Body dysmorphic disorder (BDD) is the perceived physical deficit or flaw that is not observable by others. Diagnostic criteria is shown in **Table 10-3**.

Epidemiology The prevalence among U.S. adults is 2.4%.[11] Among cosmetic dermatology patients, the prevalence of body dysmorphic disorder is 14%.[15] The age of onset is usually during adolescence; however, the diagnosis can be delayed between development of symptoms and when the patient seeks medical treatment.[11,17]

Clinical Features Concern for acne or dyschromia on the face is common with BDD patients. Patients with BDD often seek treatment from dermatologists for cosmetic procedures to treat their perceived problem area.[15] BDD patients who receive cosmetic treatments are often unsatisfied with results or believe symptoms have worsened. This can result in multiple unnecessary procedures or treatments. The Body Dysmorphic Disorder Questionnaire can be used to aid in the diagnosis of BDD by dermatologists.[17]

Differential Diagnosis The differential diagnosis for BDD includes obsessive-compulsive disorder, social anxiety, major depressive disorder, psychotic disorders, and eating disorders.[11,15]

Management Patients with BDD often lack insight into their disorder and thus may not appreciate the need or value of seeing a psychiatrist for treatment. It is important to build rapport with the patient in an empathetic and nonjudgmental manner. Cognitive Behavioral Therapy is first-line treatment. Patients may also benefit from the use of SSRIs; however, they may require higher doses of medication (eg, fluoxetine ≥ 60 mg/day) and response can take 6 to 9 weeks.[15]

SOMATIC SYMPTOMS AND RELATED DISORDERS

Factitious Disorder Factitious disorder (FD) results when a person falsifies illness in themselves or another person without any obvious external reward. **Table 10-4** lists the diagnostic criteria for both FDs imposed on self and FD imposed on another.

Epidemiology FD has a prevalence of 0.3% among dermatology patients. More commonly seen in women than men with 8:1 ratio. FD commonly develops in adolescence.[18]

Clinical Features Dermatitis artefacta is a dermatologic FD. Patients present with excoriation, blisters, ulcers, erythema, edema, panniculitis, localized crusting, eczematous lesions, nodules, ecchymoses, and purpura. Most common sites are the face, lower extremities, upper extremities, and hands. The presenting history provided by the patient is often vague and inconsistent with the presentation of known dermatoses.[15,18] In the case of FD imposed on another person, the victim is often a child or an elderly person.[19]

Differential Diagnosis FD is a diagnosis of exclusion. Collateral information from previous providers or family can be helpful in aiding in the diagnosis as well as minimizing invasive procedures. The differential

TABLE 10-4 DSM 5-TR criteria factitious disorder imposed on self and factitious disorder imposed on another

Factitious disorder imposed on self	Factitious disorder imposed on another
Falsification of physical or psychological signs or symptoms, or induction of injury or disease, associated with identified deception.	Falsification of physical or psychological signs or symptoms, or induction of injury or disease, in another, associated with identified deception.
The individual presents themselves to others as ill, impaired, or injured.	The individual presents another individual (victim) to others as ill, impaired, or injured.
The deceptive behavior is evident even in the absence of obvious external rewards.	The deceptive behavior is evident even in the absence of obvious external rewards.
The behavior is not better explained by another mental disorder, such as delusional disorder or another psychotic disorder.	The behavior is not better explained by another mental disorder, such as delusional disorder or another psychotic disorder.

Note: The diagnosis is given to the perpetrator not the victim.

diagnosis includes excoriation disorders, obsessive-compulsive disorder, primary skin disease (eg, pyoderma gangrenosum and panniculitis), or malingering.[15]

Management Treatment starts with managing any acute dermatologic conditions produced by the disorder. Direct confrontation regarding the diagnosis is not recommended until a supportive environment free of judgment has been established. This can ensure that the patient is receptive to recommendations for treatment, particularly related to seeking mental health treatment. Often, patients will reject referrals for psychiatric treatment due to stigma associated with the diagnosis. Treatment with buspirone or benzodiazepines can target anxiety symptoms; SSRIs may be used for depressive symptoms or compulsive behaviors. Low doses of second-generation antipsychotics can also be beneficial. Adjunctive psychotherapy is recommended.[15]

SCHIZOPHRENIA SPECTRUM AND OTHER PSYCHOTIC DISORDERS

Delusional Disorder, Somatic type: Delusional Infestations or Parasitosis Delusions are fixed false beliefs. The somatic subtype of delusional disorder results when patients have a fixed belief that they have an infestation or parasite. **Table 10-5** lists the full diagnostic criteria of this disorder.

Epidemiology The onset of delusional disorder typically occurs in late adulthood (age > 50); however, it can also develop in adolescence or in young adults, although earlier presentations are more likely to be secondary to substance abuse.[20]

Clinical Features Patients present with cutaneous dysesthesias such as formication (the feeling of bugs crawling on the skin), itching, tingling, or a biting sensation on their skin, scalp, or in body orifices.[20] Morgellons disease is a variant of delusional infestation where patients believe there are fibers embedded in and protruding from their skin. The most

TABLE 10-5 DSM 5-TR Criteria delusional disorder, somatic type: delusional infestations or parasitosis

The presence of one (or more) delusions with a duration of 1 month or longer.
Criterion A for schizophrenia has never been met. Note: Hallucinations, if present, are not prominent and are related to the delusional theme (eg, the sensation of being infested with insects associated with delusions of infestation).
Apart from the impact of the delusion(s) or its ramifications, functioning is not markedly impaired, and behavior is not obviously bizarre or odd.
If manic or major depressive episodes have occurred, these have been brief relative to the duration of the delusional periods.
The disturbance is not attributable to the physiological effects of a substance or another medical condition and is not better explained by another mental disorder, such as body dysmorphic disorder or obsessive-compulsive disorder.

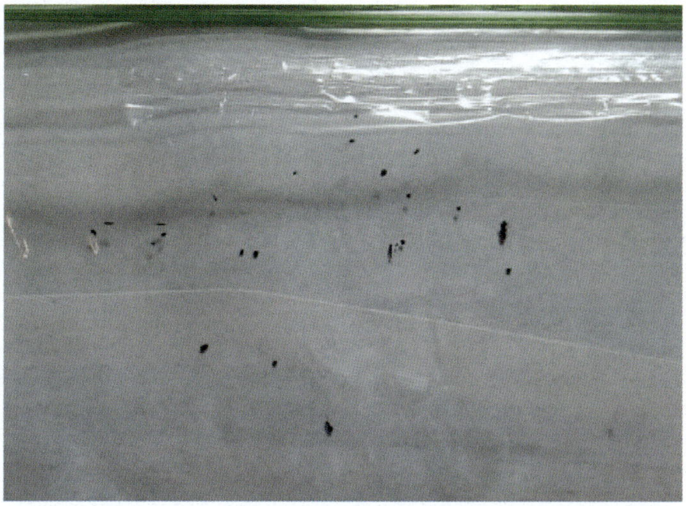

FIGURE 10-4. Specimen sign in patient with delusional infestations. Clothing lint and other debris contained in plastic bag. (Courtesy of Dr. Rebecca Vasquez.)

common symptom is pruritus. Patients often use sharp objects, harsh chemicals, or fingernails to scratch and relieve the sensation, which may result in cutaneous damage or lesions.[15,20] Patients may bring in a "specimen" as proof of infestation and may feel disappointed or dismissed to learn of negative results [**Figure 10-4**]. It is common for patients to share their delusion with someone close to them, referred to as "folie a deux."[20]

Differential Diagnosis The differential includes schizophrenia and other psychotic disorders, neurocognitive disorders, hypothyroidism, anemia, vitamin B_{12} deficiency, hepatitis, severe renal disease, diabetes, HIV, syphilis, and substance abuse.[20]

Management Treatment should involve Cognitive Behavioral Therapy, second-generation antipsychotics, treatment for primary medical conditions, as well as treatment for dermatologic complications of the disorder (eg, ulcers, infections). In severe cases, patients may be at elevated risk for suicide and should be monitored closely and hospitalized if indicated.[20]

FEEDING AND EATING DISORDERS

Anorexia Nervosa and Bulimia Nervosa Anorexia nervosa is characterized by intentional restriction of food intake leading to significantly low body weight and fear of gaining weight. It has a mortality rate of 6.6%, the highest among all psychiatric disorders.[21] Bulimia nervosa is characterized by binge-eating episodes with a lack of control during those episodes. Patients will also engage in compensatory behavior to avoid weight gain such as purging, excessive exercise, laxative or diuretic use. Both bulimia nervosa and anorexia nervosa have cutaneous complications resulting from starvation, hormonal changes, and overuse of diuretics/laxatives [see **Table 10-6**].[21]

It is important to rule out other medical issues that can mimic eating disorders such as hyperthyroidism, inflammatory bowel disease, immunodeficiency, malabsorption, chronic infections, Addison's disease, malignancy, and diabetes. Usually, people with a primary medical condition resulting in weight loss will express concern over the lost weight, so patients who lack concern should raise suspicion for eating disorders.[21]

There is clinical bias regarding eating disorders. The stereotype of an eating disorder patient being White, affluent, and female has led to an underdiagnosis of eating disorders in men and in people from communities of color that have been marginalized. Considering again that eating disorders have the highest mortality rate of all psychiatric disorders, clinical bias can have grave consequences. In addition, patients with eating disorders who are of average weight or even overweight may experience delayed diagnosis.[22] It is important to screen patients of all genders, all body types, and all ethnic and racial groups for eating disorders. Screening tools such as the SCOFF [see **Table 10-7**] and Eating Attitudes Test (EAT-26) questionnaires are easily administered in the primary care and dermatology settings.[23]

Family-based therapy and treatment of comorbid psychiatric conditions is standard of care. In some cases, inpatient treatment for medical or psychiatric reasons may be warranted, in particular with patients at risk for refeeding syndrome.

TABLE 10-6 Cutaneous manifestations of eating disorders[21]

Xerosis	Paronychia	Scurvy
Lanugo-like body hair	Generalized pruritus	Acrodermatitis enteropathica
Telogen effluvium	Acquired striae distensae	Russell sign (knuckle calluses)
Carotenoderma	Slower wound healing	Petechiae
Acne	Prurigo pigmentosa	Livedo reticularis
Hyperpigmentation	Edema	Interdigital intertrigo
Seborrheic dermatitis	Linear erythema craquelé	Acral coldness
Acrocyanosis	Perniosis	Pellagra

Source: Strumia R. Dermatologic signs in patients with eating disorders. Am J Clin Dermatol. 2005;6(3): 165-173.

TABLE 10-7 The SCOFF questionnaire[23]

SCOFF questionnaire for quick screening of eating disorders in the primary care setting	
S	Do you make yourself **S**ick because you feel uncomfortably full?
C	Do you worry you have lost **C**ontrol over how much you eat?
O	Have you recently lost more than **O**ne stone (approx. 12 lbs) in a 3 month period?
F	Do you believe yourself to be **F**at when others say you are too thin?
F	Would you say that **F**ood dominates your life?

[a]One point for every "yes"; a score of ≥2 indicates a likely case of anorexia nervosa or bulimia.

Source: Reproduced with Permission from Hill LS, Reid F, Morgan JF, Lacey JH. SCOFF, the development of an eating disorder screening questionnaire. Int J Eat Disord. 2010;43(4):344-51.

NEURODEVELOPMENTAL DISORDERS

Autism Spectrum Disorder Autism spectrum disorder (ASD) is a neurodevelopmental disorder that is characterized by impairments in social communication and restricted, repetitive behaviors. It is also associated with several genetic disorders with dermatologic manifestations, as well as nutritional and hormonal disorders [see **Table 10-8**].

Often pediatric and adult patients with ASD have a difficult time finding providers who are comfortable meeting the needs of this population. For example, patients with ASD commonly have tactile sensory sensitivities that can make relatively benign dermatologic conditions and treatment intolerable for some patients. Patients with tactile hypersensitivity may have difficulty tolerating topical treatments or irritation from dermatologic disorders, which can increase their maladaptive behaviors.[24] **Table 10-9** provides practical tips for providers to improve the clinical encounter when working with people with ASD.

TABLE 10-8 Genetic disorders with skin manifestations and ASD

Angelman syndrome
Prader-Willi syndrome
Tuberous sclerosis
Neurofibromatosis type 1
Hypomelanosis of Ito
Velocardialfacial syndrome
Cornelia de Lange syndrome
PTEN hamartoma tumor syndrome
Turner syndrome
Klinfelter syndrome

TABLE 10-9 Tips to improve clinical encounters with patients with Autism spectrum disorder (ASD)[24]

Identify sensitivities before a visit (ie, loud noises, smells) and minimize them if possible
Avoid unnecessary touching, give warning, and narrate what you are doing during physical exam
Limit the number of people the person must interact with
Reduce the number of questions asked
Schedule the patient in the morning to minimize wait time and crowds in waiting room
Use social stories to communicate procedures to patients
Have a clear understanding of how the patient communicates and how to best communicate with them. Do not assume their communication abilities
Use clear and concrete language
Work with families/caregivers to develop treatment plans that meet the unique needs of the patient
Allow patients to take breaks during exam or interview
Provide pain management before procedures
Minimize unnecessary testing or frequency of testing

Source: Accordino RE, Lucarelli J, Yan AC. Cutaneous Disease in Autism Spectrum Disorder: A Review. Pediatr Dermatol. 2015;32(4):455-460.

SUBSTANCE USE DISORDERS

Substance use disorders (SUDs) are a complex group of psychiatric conditions comprising interactions of genetic, neurobiological, psychological, and environmental factors.[25] These group of psychiatric disorders and the individuals who experience them have been highly stigmatized due to misconceptions about SUDs. Current evidence points to a disruption in the brain's reward pathways causing chronic, debilitating, relapsing, and remitting illness. SUD is the individual's persistent use of a substance despite consequences resulting from its use. The main symptom clusters are summarized in **Table 10-10**.

Epidemiology Within the past three decades, the worldwide prevalence of alcohol, opioid, cocaine, and amphetamine use disorders have all increased. Alcohol use disorder is the most prevalent of all SUDs worldwide.[25] Among U.S. adults, the 12-month prevalence of high-risk drinking is 17.4% for Native Americans, 15.1% for Black Americans, 13.5% for Latine/Hispanic, 12.3% for non-Latine/Hispanic Whites, and 7.2% for Asians and Pacific Islanders.[11] The COVID-19 pandemic has only exacerbated this, with most Americans reporting that they use alcohol and drugs at about the same rate or more since the pandemic began.[26]

TABLE 10-10 DSM 5 Symptom categories of substance use disorders

Grouping	Symptoms
IMPAIRED CONTROL OF SUBSTANCE USE	• Substance is taken in larger amounts or over a longer period than was originally intended • Persistent desire to cut down or regulate substance use with multiple unsuccessful attempts • Great deal of time obtaining, using, or recovering from a substance • Intense desire for the substance, more likely occurring in environments where previously obtained/used
SOCIAL IMPAIRMENT	• Failure to fulfill major obligations at work, school, or home • Continued use despite persistent or recurrent social/interpersonal problems caused/worsened by substance • Important social, occupational, or recreational activities given up or reduced because of substance use
RISKY USE	• Recurrent substance use in physically hazardous situations • Persistent/recurrent physical or psychological problems caused/worsened by substance
TOLERANCE	• Markedly increased dose of the substance needed to achieve desired effect
WITHDRAWAL	• Physiological/psychologic syndrome occurs when blood/tissue concentrations of substance decline after sustained, prolonged, heavy use

Worldwide, the prevalence of opioid use disorder is over 26 million people and has increased by 47.3% in the past two decades. In 2017, the United States Department of Health and Human Services declared a public health emergency due to the increase in opioid overdose deaths.[25] The steep increase in opioid use and correlative overdose deaths has been attributed to opioid overprescription, fueled by the manufacturers of Oxycontin.[27] The resultant public health crisis called for evidence-based interventions, such as "buy back" programs, Prescription Drug Monitoring Programs for physicians, harm reduction methods (such as supervised injection sites, wider public awareness of and availability of overdose reversal medication, naloxone), and decreased criminal sentencing for nonviolent drug offenses. Historically, similar substance use epidemics, such as the cocaine epidemic of the 1980s and the heroin epidemic of 1970s that have plagued communities of color, have led to harsher penalties and criminalization rather than public health interventions. Many scholars have criticized disparities in the public health response to these epidemics and have implicated systemic and interpersonal racism as the cause.[27] Likewise, prevalence of cocaine use disorder affects 5.8 million people worldwide and has increased by close to 40% in the past two decades.[25]

Clinical Features The following section summarizes the psychiatric and cutaneous findings common with chronic use alcohol, opioids, amphetamines, and cocaine. The cutaneous findings associated with each SUD is also listed in **Table 10-11**.

Alcohol Use Disorder (AUD) Many cutaneous manifestations of chronic alcohol use are due to vascular changes such as vasodilation, hepatic or biliary dysfunction, and accidental injuries.[28] The most representative lesion of AUD is spider telangiectasia or spider nevi, characterized by a pinpoint macule surrounded by radiating arterioles. These can occur on the face, upper chest/clavicular area, arms, hands, abdomen, and legs. Chronic alcohol is also a risk factor for many cancers including non-melanoma skin cancer and squamous cell carcinoma of the oral cavity.[28]

AUD is often comorbid with bipolar disorder, schizophrenia, antisocial personality disorder, depression, and most anxiety disorders. Use of alcohol is a strong risk factor for suicide, and there is an association among alcohol use, possession of firearms, and suicide by firearms.[11] Awareness and identification of cutaneous markers can prompt early detection and intervention.

Opioid Use Disorder Opioids include substances such as natural opioids (morphine and codeine), semi-synthetic opioids (oxycodone, hydrocodone, hydromorphone, and oxymorphone), synthetic opioid (methadone, tramadol, and fentanyl), and heroin, an opioid synthesized from morphine. Opioids are used for their analgesic and psychoactive properties and have a high potential for dependence and abuse due to the euphoric "high," especially experienced with more immediate routes of administration (intranasally or intravenously [IV]).

Heroin is the most widely used opioid worldwide, and it can be administered intranasally or intravenously (IV). Distribution of injection sites appears to follow a temporal pattern during the individual's substance use with the cubital fossa of the nondominant arm being the first location to administer, then upper arms, then hands, followed by neck, foot, and leg, and lastly groin, toes, or fingers.[29] Due to stigma and to avoid discovery, many individuals may choose injection locations that are hidden by clothing or use deliberate subcutaneous injection (skin popping) to hide track marks. Cutaneous manifestations of opioid use are listed in Table 10-11, and most are consequences of aseptic administration or venous thrombosis, including necrotizing cellulitis/fasciitis [**Figure 10-5**]. Nonpitting edema of the back of the hands, also called "puffy hand syndrome," has been described in individuals who use heroin and is thought to be caused by quinine, an adulterant in heroin.[29,30]

Methamphetamine Use Disorder Methamphetamine ("meth") is a synthetic compound that is generally inhaled, smoked, or injected IV producing a euphoric feeling and enhanced performance. At high doses, amphetamines can cause hallucinations, delirium, aggression, anxiety, and cardiovascular arrest. Many of the cutaneous findings of meth use are resultant from inhalation or smoking of the substance.[31]

TABLE 10-11 Common dermatological findings of substance use disorders

Alcohol	• Pinpoint/spider telangiectasias • Ecchymoses • Palmar erythema • Caput medusae • Facial erythema and flushing • Jaundice • Pruritis (due to elevated bile acids) • Nail changes ("Terry's nails" blanching of nail bed, with distal 2 mm is pink and multiple transverse white bands parallel to the lunula, red lunula) • Hyperpigmentation (either diffusely or in blotchy circumscribed areas with freckling, areolar pigmentation, and perioral/periorbital pigmentation)
Opioid	• Pruritis (especially of face and genitals), • Ulcers • Necrotizing cellulitis/fasciitis • Pemphigus vegetans • Toxic epidermal necrolysis • Necrolytic migratory erythema • Acanthosis nigricans • Venous thrombosis, subsequent scarring and hyperpigmentation of veins used for intravenous (IV) injection ("track marks") • Nonpitting edema of back of hands ("puffy hand syndrome") • Abscesses • Cutaneous findings of endocarditis (Janeway lesions and Osler's nodes)
Meth-amphetamine	• Intense pruritis • Body odor • Weight loss • Premature aging • Hyperhidrosis • Formication of the face • Acne excoriѐe • Lichenoid drug eruptions • Poor dentition
Cocaine	• Halitosis • Frequent lip smacking • Cuts and burns on the lips • Madarosis (loss of lateral eyebrow) • Palmar and digital hyperkeratosis • Midline destructive lesions of nasal septum • Nasal verrucae ("snorter's warts") due to human papillomavirus (HPV) • Vasculitis • Urticarial vasculitis, eosinophilic granulomatosis with polyangiitis (EGPA), necrotizing granulomatous vasculitis, palpable purpura, and Buerger disease • Pyoderma gangrenosum • Scleroderma • Cocaine-induced formication or tactile hallucination of insects crawling on skin • Levamisole induced necrotic vasculitis (characteristically over external ears, cheeks, nose, and breasts)

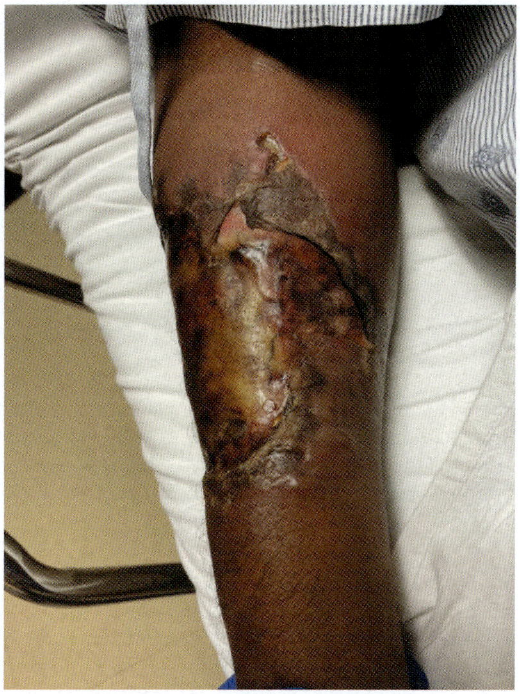

FIGURE 10-5. Necrotizing cellulitis/fasciitis after injection of heroin in the arm. (Courtesy of Dr. Rebecca Vasquez.)

These include intense pruritus, formication of the face, acne excoriѐe, and lichenoid drug eruptions. Poor dentition is also common and likely due to a combination of xerostomia, bruxism, and poor dental hygiene resulting in dental caries and enamel erosions in people who use meth.[31]

Cocaine Use Disorder Cocaine is a sympathomimetic that produces intense feelings of euphoria, confidence, and wakefulness. Cocaine can be administered via inhalation of fine powder ("snorting"), by subcutaneous injection or IV, or by smoking crack cocaine through a heated glass pipe ("freebasing").[30]

Chronic use of cocaine in powder or crack formulations has significant systemic effects including cerebrovascular and cardiovascular disease. Cutaneous findings that dermatologists may notice are listed in Table 10-11 and include consequences of heat exposure from smoke accessories, hot fume exposure, or nasal lesions due to inhalation of cocaine. Nasal verrucae ("snorters' warts") caused by human papillomavirus infection are thought to be transmitted via the inhalation vehicle (ie, rolled dollar bills) used to snort cocaine. Vascular inflammatory syndromes such as urticarial vasculitis, eosinophilic granulomatosis with polyangiitis (EGPA), necrotizing granulomatous vasculitis, palpable purpura, and Buerger disease have been described,[30] as well as reports of pyoderma gangrenosum [**Figure 10-6**]. Cocaine use can unmask or cause scleroderma. Chronic users of cocaine and other stimulants can experience formication, a tactile hallucination of insects crawling on skin. Care must be taken to distinguish delusional parasitosis from substance-induced formication.

Levamisole, an antiparasitic medication, has been identified as a dangerous adulterant in up to 70% of seized cocaine in the United States, as reported by the Drug Enforcement Agency.[30] Levamisole is thought to be added to cocaine to potentiate its effects but can have devastating consequences such as agranulocytosis, a distinctive necrotizing vasculitis of retiform purpuric lesions affecting the external ears and cheeks, and high titers of perinuclear antineutrophil antibodies or anti-myeloperoxidase antibodies.[31]

Management Treatment of SUDs demands a multidisciplinary approach. Chronic management includes treatment and prevention of systemic consequences and comorbidities, pharmacotherapy to curb cravings and manage withdrawal symptoms, and psychotherapy to

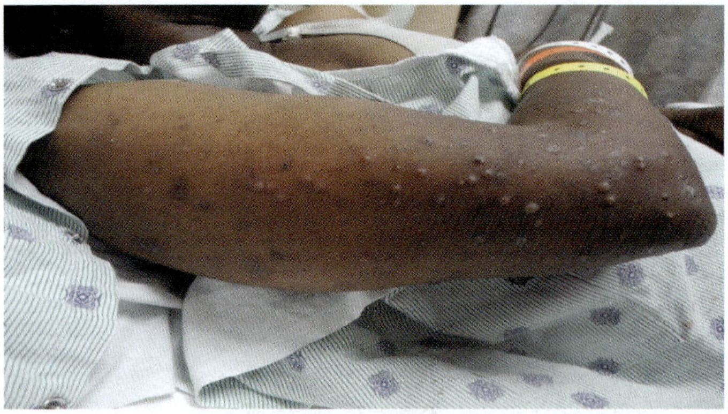

FIGURE 10-6. Pyoderma gangrenosum associated with levamisole-adulterated cocaine. (Reproduced with permission from Jeong HS, Layher H, Cao L, Vandergriff T, Dominguez AR. Pyoderma gangrenosum (PG) associated with levamisole-adulterated cocaine: clinical, serologic, and histopathologic findings in a cohort of patients. *J Am Acad Dermatol.* 2016;74(5):892-898, Figure 1A.)

enhance motivation for cessation/abstinence, promote support systems, and prevent relapse. Medication-assisted treatment (MAT) options for opioid use disorder include synthetic opioid methadone and opioid partial agonist buprenorphine/naloxone. Group support and therapy (such as Alcoholics Anonymous or Narcotics Anonymous) assists many in relapse prevention and maintenance of sobriety.[18]

Care must be taken to refer any individual with a SUD to the appropriate level of care and maintain a nonjudgmental approach to relapse and recovery. Since SUDs are highly stigmatized, gaining trust and establishing rapport are crucial for engaging patients in treatment.

GENERAL MEDICAL CONDITIONS WITH CUTANEOUS FINDINGS AND PSYCHIATRIC COMORBIDITY

Many common chronic dermatologic conditions affecting appearance and self-image, such as psoriasis, eczema, hyperhidrosis, hidradenitis suppurativa, and herpes simplex, are associated with higher rates of depression and anxiety symptoms. Thus, screening for mental health morbidity and referral to mental health care and increased psychosocial support is recommended. We consider here several specific conditions that have uniquely severe psychiatric comorbidity and have relevance to skin of color.

VITILIGO

Vitiligo is an autoimmune condition that attacks melanocytes and results in marked loss of skin pigmentation, more easily noticeable in individuals with darker skin (see Chapters 56 to 59 on disorders of pigmentation). Individuals with this disorder can experience shame and higher rates of depression and anxiety related to the seemingly uncontrollable and unpredictable course of the disease.[32] People with vitiligo, especially children, may socially isolate because of "anticipated rejection." The extent of psychosocial comorbidities supports screening for early diagnosis and a multidisciplinary approach to treatment strategies.

PIGMENTATION DISORDERS

There are numerous inherited disorders affecting skin pigmentation: oculocutaneous albinism, ocular albinism, and piebaldism, among others (also see Chapter 103). Oculocutaneous albinism has an autosomal recessive inheritance pattern resulting in disrupted biosynthesis of melanin with great phenotypic variety. Similar to vitiligo, individuals with albinism may experience discrimination or stigma in their families and in greater society. This is particularly severe in Africa, and in some regions represents a public health emergency.[33,34] In Tanzania, for example, where the prevalence of albinism is highest in the African continent, People with Albinism (PWA) are being murdered and mutilated for use of their bones and hair in religious ceremonies. Children with albinism may be abandoned by their families. Many international advocacy organizations are working to protect PWA in Africa, they include: Under the Same Sun, the National Albinism Alliance, Standing Voice and Salif Keita Foundation, along with the United Nations Human Rights Commission.

ACNE VULGARIS

Acne vulgaris is an inflammatory disease of the skin on the face and trunk, most common in teenagers, with prevalence estimated at 9% of the population worldwide and 85% of people ages 12 to 24.[35] Acne can cause permanent scarring and dyschromia, with the latter more likely to develop among patients with darker skin types. Acne can negatively affect self-esteem and self-image,[36] and is associated with increased rates of anxiety, depression, and suicidal ideation. A recent meta-analysis suggests isotretinoin, once thought to potentially cause or worsen depressive symptoms, is likely not causative, but correlative, and treatment should be considered safe in patients with depression and acne.[37]

HIDRADENITIS SUPPURATIVA

Hidradenitis suppurativa (HS) is a chronic inflammatory disorder of the hair follicles characterized by debilitating, recurrent nodules, abscesses, and sinus tracts primarily affecting the intertriginous areas of the body. Prevalence of the disease varies from 0.05% to 4% in the general population, with data demonstrating increased prevalence, and possibly increased disease burden, in historically marginalized communities of color.[38] Psychiatric comorbidities associated with HS include depression and anxiety, as well as substance-related disorders, alcohol abuse, and suicide. Screening for these comorbidities, psychiatric referral and adequately managing pain could help improve the well-being of HS patients.[39]

ALOPECIA AREATA

Alopecia areata is an autoimmune disease that causes nonscarring hair loss on the scalp and at other body sites. Recent studies suggest alopecia areata is more common in individuals racialized as Black compared to their White counterparts.[40] In alopecia areata, the onset and progression of inflammation at the hair follicles is unpredictable. While 80% of people affected recover hair growth after a year, the uncertainty and distress associated with temporary disfigurement and hair loss is associated with adjustment disorders. It is estimated that overall psychiatric comorbidity with alopecia areata is common; up to 40% suffer major depression, and up to 60% suffer anxiety disorders, including an increased risk for obsessive-compulsive disorder.[41] It is not known if increased stress can cause alopecia areata; epidemiological reviews demonstrate that half of people with alopecia areata have psychiatric disorders prior to onset of hair loss, and half develop afterward.

SARCOIDOSIS

Sarcoidosis is a multisystem disease of granulomatous inflammation that disproportionately affects Black people as compared with other racialized groups, and Black women more than men (see Chapter 35 on sarcoidosis).[42] Cutaneous manifestations of the disease are usually papules, nodules or plaques on the face, extremities, and trunk.[43] Erythema nodosum is the most common presentation of disease on the skin in sarcoidosis, in the form of tender nodules on the lower legs. Sarcoidosis is often complicated by chronic fatigue (CF) symptoms and depression, with prevalence of CF in 70% of patients with sarcoidosis.[44]

ENDOCRINE DISORDERS

Multiple disorders of hormone balance result in neurocutaneous findings that may be clues to the diagnosis. Disruptions of the HPA axis are often associated with psychiatric symptoms. In brief, we summarize in **Table 10-12** several classic presentations of rashes associated with neuroendocrine disruption and psychiatric sequelae.[45]

TABLE 10-12 Common dermatological findings associated with endocrine disorders

		Dermopathy	Associated psychiatric comorbidity
Thyroid diseases	Graves disease- hyperthyroidism	Pretibial myxedema Flushing Palmar erythema Hyperhidrosis Diffuse scalp hair thinning Onycholysis Thyroid acropachy Generalized pruritus Chronic urticaria	Anxiety Mania w or w/o Psychosis
	Hypothyroidism	Asteatotic eczema Cold, mottled skin Carotenemia Myxedema Macroglossia Loss of lateral third of eyebrows Coarse brittle hair	Depression Cognitive impairment Coma (when severe)
Pituitary disorders	Acromegaly	Gingival hyperplasia Coarse facial features Cutis verticis gyrata Hyperpigmentation Acanthosis nigricans Hyperhidrosis Hypertrichosis Nail changes	Depression, anxiety, and psychosis
Pancreatic disorders	Diabetes mellitus	Necrobiosis lipoidica diabeticorum (NLD) Diabetic dermopathy Diabetic bullae Scleredema Acanthosis nigricans (IMAGE) Carotenemia Lipodystrophy Eruptive xanthomas Cutaneous infections (bacterial, candidal, dermatophytes)	Major depression
Adrenal disorders	Cushing syndrome	Moon facies Dorsocervical fat pad Supraclavicular fat pad Easy bruising Delayed wound healing Skin atrophy Striae distensae Hyperpigmentation Acanthosis nigricans Steroid acne	Mania w or w/o psychosis Depression Cognitive impairment
	Addisons disease-adrenal insufficiency	Diffuse cutaneous hyperpigmentation Hair hyperpigmentation Mucosal hyperpigmentation Loss of axillary and pubic hair Longitudinal hyperpigmented nail bands Vitiligo	Major depression Cognitive impairment
Reproductive hormone disorders	Polycystic Ovarian Syndrome	Hirsutism Acne vulgaris Androgenetic alopecia Acanthosis nigricans	Major depression Generalized anxiety Social phobia Obsessive-compulsive disorder Eating disorder Bipolar disorder Psychotic disorders
	Menopause	Xerosis Advanced collagen loss/aging Vulvovaginal atrophy/dryness	Major depression
Other	Carcinoid syndrome	Flushing Venous telangectasia Persistent brawny edema of face	Mania w or w/o psychosis Cognitive impairment

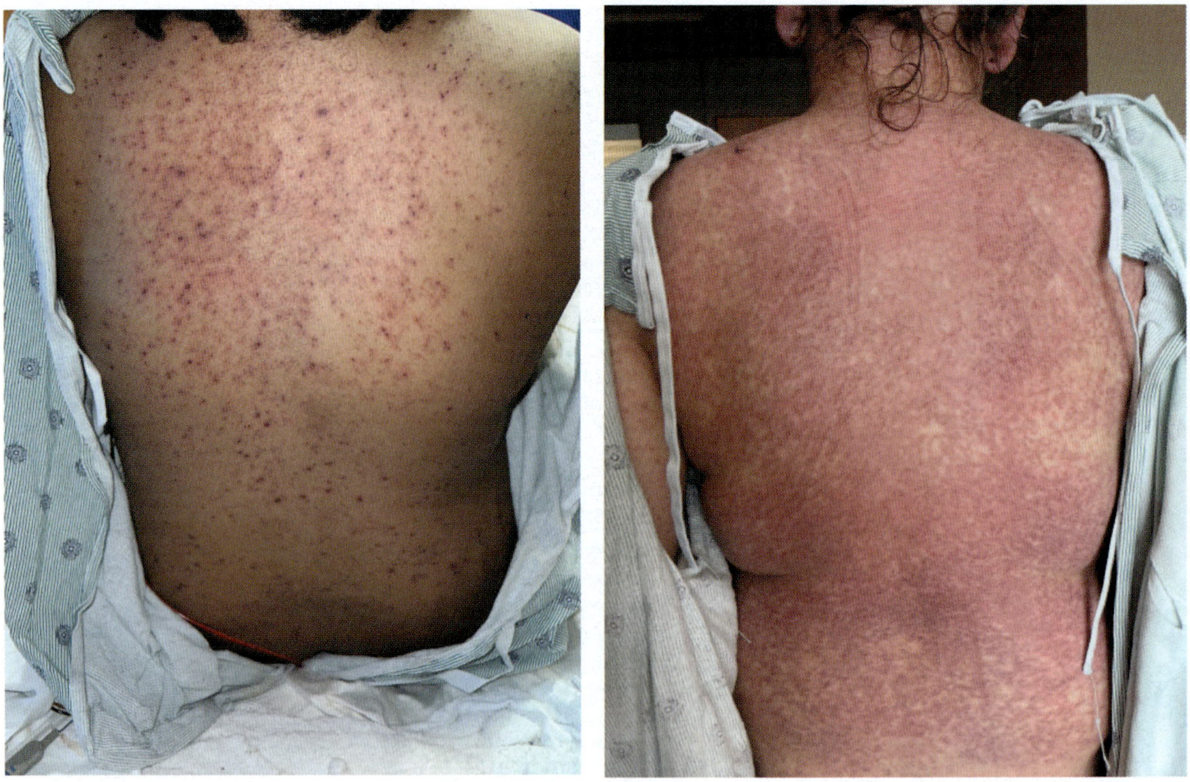

A B

FIGURE 10-7. Neuroleptic associated with SJS. **(A)** Black/African American women with a history of posttraumatic stress disorder and bipolar disorder admitted for Stevens-Johnson syndrome after treatment with lamotrigine. **(B)** Latina/Hispanic women with past medical history of depression admitted for Stevens-Johnson syndrome/toxic epidermal necrolysis due to lamotrigine. (Courtesy of Dr. Cristina Thomas.)

DERMATOLOGIC SIDE EFFECTS OF PSYCHOTROPIC MEDICATIONS

Drug reactions occur more frequently at the skin than at any other site in the body, and this remains true for psychotropic medication (also refer to Chapter 81). The incidence of clinically relevant cutaneous drug reactions attributable to psychiatric medications is 0.1%,[46] with mood stabilizers accounting for 39% of these reactions, 29% to antidepressants and 19% to neuroleptics. People of color appear to be at highest risk of developing cutaneous drug reactions, possibly due to differences in HLA subtypes, but robust studies examining this trend are lacking.[47] Possible psychiatric sequelae include PTSD, depression, or anxiety, especially after more severe adverse reactions.

MOOD STABILIZERS

Most cutaneous drug reactions caused by psychotropic medications are due to lamotrigine.[47] Lamotrigine is an antiepileptic and mood stabilizer used in bipolar disorder. Every patient initiated on lamotrigine must be educated on the risk of developing epidermal necrolysis, also known as Stevens-Johnsons syndrome (SJS) or toxic epidermal necrolysis (TENS). The incidence is low, estimated as 0.8% to 0.33% from reports issued by FDA clinical trials, and the risk of SJS/TENS may be mitigated when dosing guidelines are followed. Patients prescribed lamotrigine should be informed to stop taking the medication and seek emergency attention if confluent, purpuric lesions appear on the face, neck, soles, and palms or in mucosal surfaces [**Figure 10-7**].[48] The average time from drug initiation to onset of rash is 16 days, with less than 2% of cases occurring more than 1 month after starting lamotrigine. The rash may be associated with fever, malaise, pharyngitis, anorexia, or lymphadenopathy. With these accompanying symptoms, drug-induced hypersensitivity syndrome (DIHS) should be considered in the differential. The risk of SJS/TENS increases significantly when valproic acid and/or carbamazepine are co-administered with lamotrigine.[48]

Lithium remains a mainstay for treatment of bipolar disorder. It may cause or worsen acne and psoriasis.[49] The overall incidence of cutaneous reactions with lithium is low, 0.01%, and in addition to acneiform eruptions, hidradenitis suppurativa, folliculitis, alopecia or hair texture changes, and maculopapular eruptions may occur.[47]

Other antiepileptic mood stabilizers used for bipolar disorder include valproic acid and carbamazepine, both of which are associated with more benign cutaneous reactions. Approximately, 13% to 24% of patients prescribed valproic acid report alopecia. Less commonly, changes in hair/nail pigmentation or urticarial rashes is noticed.[47] Carbamazepine is more likely to cause exanthematous eruptions; typically, these start on the face as diffuse, pruritic macules approximately 10 days after drug initiation and spread to the trunk. The course of these drug-induced exanthems is usually benign and resolves with stopping the drug. Carbamazepine is also associated with SJS/TENS; specific cross-reactivity has been noted with co-administration of phenytoin and should be avoided.[50] Oxcarbazepine may be a safer alternative to carbamazepine and less likely to cause drug eruptions.

ANTIDEPRESSANTS

Antidepressants are some of the most prescribed medications, and the incidence of cutaneous drug reactions is quite low, estimated around 0.054%.[46] The most common adverse reactions are exanthematous eruptions and urticaria with or without angioedema. Bupropion and the tricyclic antidepressants are most likely to cause a rash (3.7-4%), and the least likely are fluoxetine, paroxetine, sertraline, and venlafaxine (0.01%).[47] Bruising can occur in patients on selective serotonin reuptake inhibitors (SSRIs) due the inhibition of SSRIs on platelet aggregation. Patients starting SSRIs may also notice increased photosensitivity on face, neck, and other sun-exposed areas of skin. Hair loss and changes in nail growth has been observed, as has hirsutism and hyperhidrosis in those on paroxetine and fluoxetine.[51] Serotonin-norepinephrine reuptake inhibitors (SNRIs) should be considered as alternatives for patients who experience cutaneous side effects to SSRIs as the cutaneous side effects are exceedingly rare for SNRIs. Mirtazapine causes acne in 1% of patients, and exfoliative dermatitis and alopecia rarely.

ANTIPSYCHOTICS

The most common cutaneous drug reactions attributed to antipsychotics are photosensitivity and pigmentation changes. Chlorpromazine has been noted to cause hyperpigmentation starting as browning of skin color that transforms over time into blue-gray skin color changes in 0.1% to 0.2% of patients and increased photosensitivity in 25% of patients. Alternative antipsychotics such as loxapine should be considered in patients experiencing pigmentation changes. These changes may not be well-appreciated in people with darker skin color and are not considered toxic or harmful or associated with increased risk of cutaneous malignancy. Pigmentation of the cornea and eyelids may also occur and may be irreversible.[52]

OTHER TOPICS

ABUSE

Although neglect remains the most common form of abuse in children and elders, both neglect and physical abuse can have lasting effects on an individual's psychological and physical health. In the United States, the annual incidence of child physical abuse is approximately 126,000 to 225,000 children. Worldwide, 13% of the 1.2 million deaths of children younger than 15 years is thought to be due to child abuse/neglect.[53] Among adults, nearly 4 million people (over 90% of them female) are victims of domestic violence and 2 million adults over age 65 are victims of elder abuse.[53]

Common cutaneous identifiers of physical abuse include head injuries (black eyes, especially bilaterally and including trauma to nose or superior orbital ridge). Defensive injuries such as bruising, purpura, sprains, dislocations, and fractures to the wrist or forearms, palms, and soles can be indicative of domestic abuse. Also raising suspicion are repeated injuries, in varying stages of healing, and similar distribution. Cutaneous morphology more unique to elder abuse include bed sores (decubitus ulcers) and strangely patterned alopecia. Inquiry is warranted if history is not consistent with the extent of injury.

In children, consequences of accidental injury must be differentiated from abuse. Accidental injury is more likely to occur in the distal arms and legs, knees, elbows, and forehead. Bruises on the trunk, buttocks, neck folds, palms/soles, thighs, genitalia, ear lobes, neck, and cheeks are uncommon and should therefore raise suspicion of abuse. Other physical findings suspicious of child abuse include subconjunctival hemorrhage beyond 1 and 2 weeks of life and petechiae in the periorbital region (often accompanied by retinal hemorrhage). Suspicion of sexual trauma should be raised in children with physical findings of chafing, abrasions, or bruising of inner thighs and genitalia, scarring, tears, or distortion of the hymen, scarring of the fossa navicularis or urethra, injury to or scarring of the posterior fourchette, scarring or tears of the labia minora, and enlargement of the hymeneal opening. Genital warts onset after age 5 is also suspicious of sexual trauma in children. Burns, in small circular patterns, may indicate inflicted burn by cigarette or another hot object. Bilateral, stocking and glove burns result when children's feet or hands are forcibly held under hot water not allowing them to withdraw.[53]

In cases of suspected child abuse, care must be taken to interview the child and family from a trauma-informed and nonjudgmental approach. Consequences of abuse in children include PTSD, attention-deficit and hyperactivity disorder, depression/anxiety, and development of oppositional deviant disorder/conduct symptoms and personality disorders in adulthood. Adults who experience trauma and physical abuse have risk factors for PTSD, but also chronic pain, mood disorders, and heart disease. Treatment often includes pharmacotherapy (SSRIs, alpha-agonists, or stimulants) and psychotherapy (in the form of trauma-focused CBT or play therapy). Documentation should include specific and detailed history, physical description of injuries and distribution as well as consented photographs due to likelihood of the medical record being included in forensic investigation.

BODY MODIFICATION

Cosmetic Surgery According to the American Society of Plastic Surgeons, in the year 2020 cosmetic surgical procedures use increased by a total of 22%. Trends indicate that for certain procedures, the numbers have skyrocketed, such as cheek implant (malar augmentation), which increased by 938% between 2000 and 2020; dermabrasion increased by 231% in the same period; lower body lift, which increased by 3974%; and upper arm lift, which increased by 4174% in the past 20 years.[54] The top five cosmetic surgical procedures in 2020 include nose reshaping, eyelid surgery, facelift, and liposuction. Also growing during this period was the growing use of social media, especially among adolescents and young adults.

There is emerging evidence that use of social media and photo editing applications may be associated with increased acceptance and consideration of cosmetic surgery, especially in those who spent significant amount of time on social media, followed many accounts, and were less satisfied with their appearance.[55,56]

Tattoos Although tattoos have been part of many indigenous cultures for centuries, in the Western world within the past two decades, there has been a clear shift in social acceptance of tattoos. They are no longer associated with subcultures such as prisoners, gangs, military, or those considered socially marginalized. In fact, as many as 3 out of 10 Americans aged 18 to 24 and 4 out of 10 Americans aged 26 to 40 has a tattoo.[57] Tattoos can be categorized as cosmetic, traumatic, or decorative. Tattoos are also increasingly seen as artful self-expression and the motivations to get one include family, life journey, emotional healing, commemoration of others/loss, willpower, and connection to heritage.[58] In this context, tattoos may also function to provide a sense of empowerment and healing.[58]

As prevalence of tattoos increase, so does the demand for their removal. Fortunately, technology such as pico-lasers have emerged as effective tools for removal of unwanted tattoos.[59]

Skin Bleaching As discussed in the introduction and Chapter 3, skin bleaching is prevalent in many communities of color, especially in countries with a history of colonialism. The consequence of these practices not only include psychological distress and harm to people of all skin colors but also local irritation or allergic reaction, carcinogenicity, permanent depigmentation, kidney and liver malfunction, blood poisoning, convulsion, and even coma.[60] Intervention should include addressing personal and interpersonal bias of lighter skin color, addressing messaging underlying marketing of lighter skin and skin-lightening products, increased public health messaging regarding the harm of skin bleaching, and stricter pharmaceutical regulation of lightening agents.[60]

PSYCHOCUTANEOUS CLINICS

Psychiatrists and primary care clinicians have appreciated that to fully address the disparities in healthcare, an integrated and holistic approach is necessary. Recently, clinics that integrate psychiatry and dermatology to better address psychocutaneous concerns have been established.[61] The top five most common referral reasons to these clinics include: excoriation (skin picking) disorder, itch, delusional disorder, trichotillomania, and psoriasis. The final psychiatric diagnoses for those who were referred to and eventually seen were excoriation (skin picking) disorder, depression, anxiety disorder, tobacco use disorder, and OCD (obsessive-compulsive disorder).

Among the patients who were seen in the clinic, around half of them needed long-term treatment and half only needed a one-time consultation with treatment recommendations. Treatments offered included topical or systemic dermatological medications, psychiatric medications (antidepressants, antianxiety, and neuroleptics), and therapy (CBT, behavioral modification, mindfulness, and other relaxation techniques, and/or family therapy).[62]

This collaboration among dermatologists, psychiatrists, and therapists has been shown to not only improve treatment outcomes but also improve patients' satisfaction with healthcare services, quality of life, and more effective healthcare expenditure.

CONCLUSION

It is clear from the above review that at the intersection of dermatology and psychiatry, illnesses and disorders require compassionate, nuanced, and personal care. Patients who suffer from these illnesses experience stigma and significant psychosocial burdens that can worsen both their dermatological and psychiatric conditions, especially true in people with skin of color. Addressing structural and interpersonal racism in medicine, which impacts not only risk factors for illness but also access to adequate, compassionate care, is essential to alleviate these health disparities.

REFERENCES

1. Garza L. Developmental biology of the skin. In: Kang S, Amagai M, Bruckner AL, et al, eds. *Fitzpatrick's Dermatology*. 9th ed. New York, NY: McGraw Hill Education; 2019. accessmedicine.mhmedical.com/content.aspx?aid=1161320534. Accessed August 23, 2022.
2. Deyrup A, Graves JL. Racial biology and medical misconceptions. *N Engl J Med*. 2022;386(6):501-503.
3. Kelly A, Jamoussi M. Skin of color: a historical perspective. In: Kelly A, Taylor SC, Lim HW, Serrano A, eds. *Taylor and Kelly's Dermatology for Skin of Color*. 2nd ed. McGraw Hill; 2016.
4. Amutah C, Greenidge K, Mante A et al. Misrepresenting race — the role of medical schools in propagating physician bias. *N Engl J Med*. 2021;384(9):872-878.
5. Eneanya ND, Boulware LE, Tsai J, et al. Health inequities and the inappropriate use of race in nephrology. *Nat Rev Nephrol*. 2022;18(2):84-94.
6. Jones CP. Toward the science and practice of anti-racism: launching a national campaign against racism. *Ethn Dis*. 2018;28(Suppl 1):231-234.
7. Paradies Y, Ben J, Denson N, et al. Racism as a determinant of health: a systematic review and meta-analysis. *PLoS One*. 2015;10(9):e0138511.
8. Roach EL, Haft SL, Huang J, Zhou Q. Systematic review: the association between race-related stress and trauma and emotion dysregulation in youth of color. *J Am Acad Child Adolesc Psychiatry*. 2023;62(2):190-207.
9. McGuire TG, Miranda J. New evidence regarding racial and ethnic disparities in mental health: Policy implications. *Health Affairs*. 2008;27(2):393-403.
10. Alvarez K, Polanco-Roman L, Samuel Breslow A, Molock S. Structural racism and suicide prevention for ethnoracially minoritized youth: a conceptual framework and illustration across systems. *Am J Psychiatry*. 2022;179(6):422-433.
11. *Diagnostic and Statistical Manual of Mental Disorders, Text Revision*. 5th ed. Washington, DC: American Psychiatric Association Publishing; 2022.
12. Henkel ED, Jaquez SD, Diaz LZ. Pediatric trichotillomania: review of management. *Pediatr Dermatol*. 2019;36(6):803-807.
13. Mosca M, Martin K, Hadeler E, Hong J, Brownstone N, Koo J. Review of the diagnosis and management of pediatric psychodermatologic conditions: part I. *Pediatr Dermatol*. 2022;39(1):17-21.
14. Grant JE, Valle S, Aslan IH, Chamberlain SR. Clinical presentation of body-focused repetitive behaviors in minority ethnic groups. *Compr Psychiatry*. 2021;111:152272.
15. Kuhn H, Mennella C, Magid M, Stamu-O'Brien C, Kroumpouzos G. Psychocutaneous disease: Clinical perspectives. *J Am Acad Dermatol*. 2017;76(5):779-791.
16. Neal-Barnett A, Statom D, Stadulis R. Trichotillomania symptoms in African American women: are they related to anxiety and culture? *CNS Neurosci Ther*. 2011;17(4):207-213.
17. Herbst I, Jemec GBE. Body dysmorphic disorder in dermatology: a systematic review. *Psychiatr Q*. 2020;91(4):1003-1010.
18. Boland RJ, Verduin ML, Ruiz P, Shah A, Sadock BJ, Teton Data Systems. *Kaplan & Sadock's Synopsis of Psychiatry*. 12th ed. Philadelphia: Wolters Kluwer; 2022.
19. Boyd AS, Ritchie C, Likhari S. Munchausen syndrome and Munchausen syndrome by proxy in dermatology. *J Am Acad Dermatol*. 2014;71(2):376-381.
20. Torales J, García O, Barrios I, et al. Delusional infestation: clinical presentations, diagnosis, and management. *J Cosmet Dermatol*. 2020;19(12):3183-3188.
21. Strumia R. Dermatologic signs in patients with eating disorders. *Am J Clin Dermatol*. 2005;6(3):165-173.
22. Sim L. Our eating disorders blind spot: sex and ethnic/racial disparities in help-seeking for eating disorders. *Mayo Clin Proc*. 2019;94(8):1398-1400.
23. Hill LS, Reid F, Morgan JF, Lacey JH. SCOFF, the development of an eating disorder screening questionnaire. *Int J Eat Disord*. 2010;43(4):344-351.
24. Accordino RE, Lucarelli J, Yan AC. Cutaneous disease in autism spectrum disorder: a review. *Pediatr Dermatol*. 2015;32(4):455-460.
25. Degenhardt L, Charlson F, Ferrari A, et al. The global burden of disease attributable to alcohol and drug use in 195 countries and territories, 1990–2016: a systematic analysis for the Global Burden of Disease Study 2016. *Lancet Psychiatry*. 2018;5(12):987-1012.
26. Center for Behavioral Health Statistics and Quality. (2021). *2020 National Survey on Drug Use and Health (NSDUH): Methodological Summary and Definitions*. Rockville, MD: Substance Abuse and Mental Health Services Administration. https://www.samhsa.gov/data/.
27. Hansen H, Netherland J. Is the prescription opioid epidemic a white problem? *Am J Public Health*. 2016;106(12):2127-2129.
28. Smith KE, Fenske NA. Cutaneous manifestations of alcohol abuse. *J Am Acad Dermatol*. 2000;43(1):1-18.
29. Del Giudice P. Cutaneous complications of intravenous drug abuse. *Br J Dermatol*. 2004;150(1):1-10.
30. Hennings C, Miller J. Illicit drugs: What dermatologists need to know. *J Am Acad Dermatol*. 2012;69(1):135-142.
31. Frank N, Hennings C, Miller JL. Drug abuse. In: Kang S, Amagai M, Bruckner AL, Enk AH, Margolis DJ, McMichael AJ, Orringer JS, eds. *Fitzpatrick's Dermatology*. 9th ed. McGraw Hill; 2019.
32. Ezzedine K, Eleftheriadou V, Jones H, et al. Psychosocial effects of vitiligo: a systematic literature review. *Am J Clin Dermatol*. 2021;22(6):757-774.
33. Brilliant M. Albinism in Africa: a medical and social emergency. *Int Health*. 2015;7(4):223-225.
34. Imafidon E. Dealing with the other between the ethical and the moral: albinism on the African continent. *Theor Med Bioeth*. 2017;38(2):163-177.
35. Eichenfield DZ, Sprague J, Eichenfield LF. Management of acne vulgaris: a review. *JAMA*. 2021;326(20):2055-2067.
36. Dunn LK, O'Neill JL, Feldman SR. Acne in adolescents: quality of life, self-esteem, mood, and psychological disorders. *Dermatol Online J*. 2011;17(1):1.
37. Huang Y, Cheng Y. Isotretinoin treatment for acne and risk of depression: a systematic review and meta-analysis. *J Am Acad Dermatol*. 2016;76(6):1068-1076.e9.
38. Kilgour JM, Li S, Sarin KY. Hidradenitis suppurativa in patients of color is associated with increased disease severity and healthcare utilization: a retrospective analysis of 2 U.S. cohorts [published correction appears in JAAD Int. 2021;3:88]. *JAAD Int*. 2021;3:42-52.
39. Phan K, Huo YR, Smith SD. Hidradenitis suppurativa and psychiatric comorbidities, suicides and substance abuse: systematic review and meta-analysis. *Ann Transl Med*. 2020;8(13):821.
40. Lee H, Jung SJ, Patel AB, Thompson JM, Qureshi A, Cho E. Racial characteristics of alopecia areata in the United States. *J Am Acad Dermatol*. 2020;83(4):1064-1070.
41. Villasante Fricke AC, Miteva M. Epidemiology and burden of alopecia areata: a systematic review. *Clin Cosmet Investig Dermatol*. 2015;8:397-403.
42. Hena KM. Sarcoidosis epidemiology: race matters. *Front Immunol*. 2020;11:537382.
43. Valeyre D, Prasse A, Nunes H, Uzunhan Y, Brillet P, Müller-Quernheim J. Sarcoidosis. *Lancet*. 2014;383(9923):1155-1167.
44. Drent M, Lower EE, De Vries J. Sarcoidosis-associated fatigue. *Eur Respir J*. 2012;40(1):255-263.
45. Lause M, Kamboj A, Fernandez Faith E. Dermatologic manifestations of endocrine disorders. *Transl Pediatr*. 2017;6(4):300-312.
46. Lange-Asschenfeldt C, Grohmann R, Lange-Asschenfeldt B, Engel R, Rüther E, Cordes J. Cutaneous adverse reactions to psychotropic drugs. *J Clin Psychiatry*. 2009;70(9):1258-1265.
47. Mitkov MV, Trowbridge RM, Lockshin BN, Caplan JP. Dermatologic side effects of psychotropic medications. *Psychosomatics*. 2014;55(1):1-20.
48. Huang, CW, Tsai JJ, Lai ML. Lamotrigine-related skin rashes in adults. *Kaohsiung J Med Sci*. 2002;18(11):566-572.
49. Garnis-Jones S. Dermatologic side effects of psychopharmacologic agents. *Dermatol Clin*. 1996;14(3):503-508.
50. Sierra NM, García B, Marco J, Plaza S, Hidalgo F, Bermejo T. Cross hypersensitivity syndrome between phenytoin and carbamazepine. *Pharm World Sci*. 2005;27(3):170-174.
51. Warnock JK, Morris DW. Adverse cutaneous reactions to antidepressants. *Am J Clin Dermatol*. 2002;3(5):329-339.

52. Huff LS, Prado R, Pederson JF, Dunnick CA, Lucas LM. Chlorpromazine-induced skin pigmentation with corneal and lens opacities. *Cutis.* 2014;93(5):247-250.
53. M. MacArthur K, Grossberg A. Physical abuse. In: Kang S, Amagai M, Bruckner AL, et al. eds. *Fitzpatrick's Dermatology*. 9th ed. McGraw Hill; 2019.
54. ASPS National Clearinghouse of Plastic Surgery Procedural Statistics. 2020 plastic surgery statistics report. plasticsurgery.org. https://www.plasticsurgery.org/documents/News/Statistics/2020/plastic-surgery-statistics-full-report-2020.pdf. Published 2022. Accessed August 12, 2022.
55. Chen J, Ishii M, Bater K, et al. Association between the use of social media and photograph editing applications, self-esteem, and cosmetic surgery acceptance. *JAMA Facial Plast Surg.* 2019;21(5):361-367.
56. Walker CE, Krumhuber EG, Dayan S, Furnham A. Effects of social media use on desire for cosmetic surgery among young women. *Curr Psychol.* 2019;40(7):3355-3364.
57. Roggenkamp H, Nicholls A, Pierre JM. Tattoos as a window to the psyche: How talking about skin art can inform psychiatric practice. *World J Psychiatry.* 2017;7(3):148-158.
58. Alter-Muri S. The body as canvas: motivations, meanings, and therapeutic implications of tattoos. *Art Ther.* 2019;37(3):139-146.
59. Hsu VM, Aldahan AS, Mlacker S, Shah VV, Nouri K. The picosecond laser for tattoo removal. *Lasers Med Sci.* 2016;31(8):1733-1737.
60. Van Hout MC, Wazaify M. Parallel discourses: leveraging the black lives matter movement to fight colorism and skin bleaching practices. *Public Health.* 2021;192:1-2.
61. Mostaghimi L. Psychocutaneous medicine clinic: Wisconsin experience. *J Acad Consult Liaison Psychiatry.* 2021;62(5):522-527.
62. Patel A, Jafferany M. Multidisciplinary and holistic models of care for patients with dermatologic disease and psychosocial comorbidity: a systematic review. *JAMA Dermatol.* 2020;156(6):686-694.

CHAPTER 11 Social Determinants of Health and Health Disparities

Jennifer J. Parker
Chidubem A.V. Okeke
Jessica R. Williams
Ellen N. Pritchett

KEY POINTS

- Social determinants of health (SDOH) are the nonmedical conditions (including housing, education, employment, income, quality health services, etc) that contribute to an individual's lived experience and overall health.
- For many communities of color, disparities across the SDOH can be traced back to complex social and historical factors.
- SDOH are important contributors of racialized health disparities in the United States, including dermatologic disparities in skin cancer and inflammatory skin conditions.
- To realize health equity, where every person can attain their full potential health, efforts to address the SDOH are essential.

INTRODUCTION

Social determinants of health (SDOH) are the conditions in which people are born, live, work, socialize, worship, and age that have a major impact on a person's health, well-being, and quality of life. Complex interactions and feedback loops exist among the social determinants. For instance, low income may reduce or restrict access to care, which may lead to poor health and loss of employment, thereby further decreasing income.[1] SDOH explain many of the observed disparities in health, healthcare access and quality, and premature death particularly among historically marginalized groups.[2] These disparities are widespread throughout medicine and in the field dermatology.

As the United States becomes more diverse and pluralistic, it is increasingly important to understand how SDOH contribute to health disparities—especially those affecting historically marginalized communities of color (as defined in Chapter 1). Moreover, many of these same groups have multiple social identities (eg, race, ethnicity, gender, socioeceomic, sexual orientation, etc). These intersecting identities should be taken into account when considering the SDOH that a patient may face. This chapter will explore SDOH and review their impact on differing outcomes in dermatologic disease among diverse communities.

TABLE 11-1 Key terminology and definitions

Term	Definition
Social determinants of health	According to the U.S. Department of Health and Human Services and the World Health Organization, SDOH are conditions in the environments where people live, learn, work, play and age that influence a wide range of health and quality-of life-risks and outcomes.
Structural determinants of health	The social, economic, and political mechanisms that generate social class inequalities in society.
Historically marginalized racial and ethnic groups	Blacks/African Americans, American Indians and Alaska Natives, Latine/Hispanics, Native Hawaiians, and other Pacific Islanders.
Structural racism	A system in which public policies, institutional practices, cultural representations, and other norms work in various, often reinforcing ways to perpetuate racial group inequity.

TERMINOLOGY

The terminology around health equity is evolving over time [**Table 11-1**]. According to the latest guidance from the American Medical Association, it is recommended that the term "White" be used as an equity-focused alternative to the word Caucasian.[3,4] The term "Black/African American (AA)" will be used herein to refer to African Americans and persons of African descent. The term Latine/Hispanic "L/H" will be used to describe the ethnic identity of people with Latin American or Spanish ancestry. It is important to note that L/H patients may prefer to identify using other terms including national origin. "American Indian or Alaska Native (AI/AN)" will be used throughout this chapter to refer to Native peoples and Indigenous (First) peoples.

SOCIAL DETERMINANTS OF HEALTH

SDOH are the nonmedical conditions that contribute to an individual's lived experience and overall health. These factors include housing, transportation, education, language proficiency, employment or income, access to nutritious food and opportunities for physical activity, access to quality healthcare, and experiences of social inclusion and nondiscrimination (including citizenship status). In the United States, differences in the SDOH can have a greater impact on certain communities [**Table 11-2**].

HOUSING, TRANSPORTATION, EDUCATION, AND FOOD SECURITY

Compared to White individuals, members of racially and ethnically diverse communities tend to have lower rates of home ownership [Table 11-2]. They are also more likely to live in multi-family housing and report not having access to a household vehicle. Additionally, individuals who identify as Black or African American, Latine/Hispanic, and American

TABLE 11-2 Social determinants of health among ethnoracial groups

Social determinants of health	White	Asian	Black/AA	Latine/Hispanic	AI/AN
Home ownership percentage rate[1]	77	69*	48*	55*	63*
Percent of individuals (ages 25 and older) who completed some post-secondary education (ie, some college or Bachelor's degree or higher)[1,a]	68	74	58	45	52
Percent of adults (18 years and older) with food insecurity[2]	4	4	12*	8*	N/A
Percent of individuals living in crowded housing[1]	3	12*	8*	18*	16*
Percent of individuals living in a household without vehicle access[1]	4	9*	12*	7*	8*
Percent of nonelderly population (0-64 years of age) who is a noncitizen[1]	1	26*	4*	19*	0.6*
Percent of individuals living in a household where no one ages 14 or older speaks English well[1]	1	16*	1*	13*	2*
Percent of children (17 years and younger) who have experienced two or more adverse childhood experiences by race/ethnicity as reported by parents[3]	15	6*	24*	19*	N/A
Percent of adults (18 years and older) reporting four or more adverse childhood experiences in selected states[4]	19	11*	22*	22*	31*

Abbreviations: AA, African American; AI/AN, American Indian or Alaskan Native; KFF, Kaiser Family Foundation.

*Indicates statistically significant difference from White population at the $p < 0.05$ level.

[1]Source: KFF analysis of 2021 American Community Survey, 1-Year Estimates.

[2]Source: KFF analysis of 2021 National Health Interview Survey.

[3]Source: 2020-2021 National Survey of Children's Health data query.

[4]Source: KFF Analysis of 2021 Behavioral Risk Factor Surveillance System.

[a]Statistical analysis not reported for percent of individuals who completed some post-secondary education.

[b]Note: Adverse childhood experiences (ACEs) are potentially traumatic events, such as experiencing violence, abuse, neglect; witnessing violence; or growing up in a household with substance use problems or mental health problems.

Indian or Alaska Native generally have lower levels of educational attainment and experience higher rates of food insecurity when compared to their White and Asian counterparts [Table 11-2].[5]

CITIZENSHIP AND LANGUAGE PROFICIENCY

Among the nonelderly (ages 64 years or younger), L/H and Asian people have the highest percentage of noncitizens (19% and 26%, respectively) [Table 11-2]. Noncitizen immigrants are less likely to be insured due to limited access to both private and public health coverage.[6-8] Nonelderly L/H and Asian people are also more likely to live in a household where those 14 years or older have limited English proficiency. Compared to people who only speak English, individuals with limited English proficiency have fewer physician visits, lower rates of cancer screenings, and are less likely to have a regular healthcare provider.[6]

BUILT ENVIRONMENT AND SAFETY

Communities of color (both children and adults) are more likely to report adverse childhood experiences (ACEs) defined as traumatic events such as experiencing violence, abuse, or neglect; witnessing violence; or growing up in a household with substance use problems or mental health problems.[9] According to published data, the more ACEs an individual encounters, the higher at risk they are for negative health and well-being.[5]

HEALTH COVERAGE AND ACCESS TO DERMATOLOGY

Disparities in health coverage persist for some communities of color despite gains in health coverage across racial and ethnic groups with the Affordable Care Act (ACA). In 2019, nonelderly AI/AN and L/H individuals had the highest uninsured rates at 22% and 20%, respectively.[10] Nonelderly White and Asian people had the lowest uninsured rates at 8% and 7%, respectively. Between 1991 and 2016, annual visits to dermatologist increased by 68% by White patients.[11] Another study in 2018 revealed White patients were twice as likely to visit an outpatient dermatologist compared to Black/AA and L/H patients.[12]

In the last few decades, research has revealed consistent associations between health and the SDOH across time, geography, and a variety of health outcomes.[13] At least 80% of health outcomes are determined by modifiable social, economic, and physical environmental factors outside of the clinical setting.[13] For certain communities, especially those from historically underserved groups, disparities across the SDOH can be traced to past practices, systems, or policies (structural discrimination, including structural racism) that have impacted access to housing, education, health services, income or good-paying jobs, and exposure to environmental pollutants and chronic stressors [**Figure 11-1**].[14]

DEFINING HEALTH DISPARITIES

Health disparities can be described as "potentially avoidable differences in health—or in the major socially determined influences on health—between groups of people who have different relative positions in social hierarchies according to wealth, power, or prestige." Because these differences adversely affect the health or health risks of groups already at a disadvantage by virtue of their underlying social positions, they are particularly unfair.[15,16] In the United States, these differences among population groups in the attainment of full potential health are reflected in disparities in length of life; quality of life; rates of disease; disability and death; severity of disease; and access to treatment across medicine, including dermatology.

In contrast to racial disparities, racial differences have little to do with being unfair. Nonetheless, racial differences are considerably more difficult to discuss because of the social construct that defines race and the lack of a precise definition of a health disparity in the medical literature. Within this context, racial differences require focused study to understand their causes, impact, and mitigation.[17,18]

DISEASE-SPECIFIC HEALTH DISPARITIES

MELANOMA

Melanoma, the third most common skin cancer seen across all racialized groups, has an incidence of 26 per 100,000 individuals in non-Hispanic White patients, versus 7.4 in AI/AN, 4.6 in L/H, 1.3 in Asians, and 1.0 in non-Hispanic Blacks/AA.[19,20] While the incidence is lower in skin of color, these patients typically present with a more advanced stage of

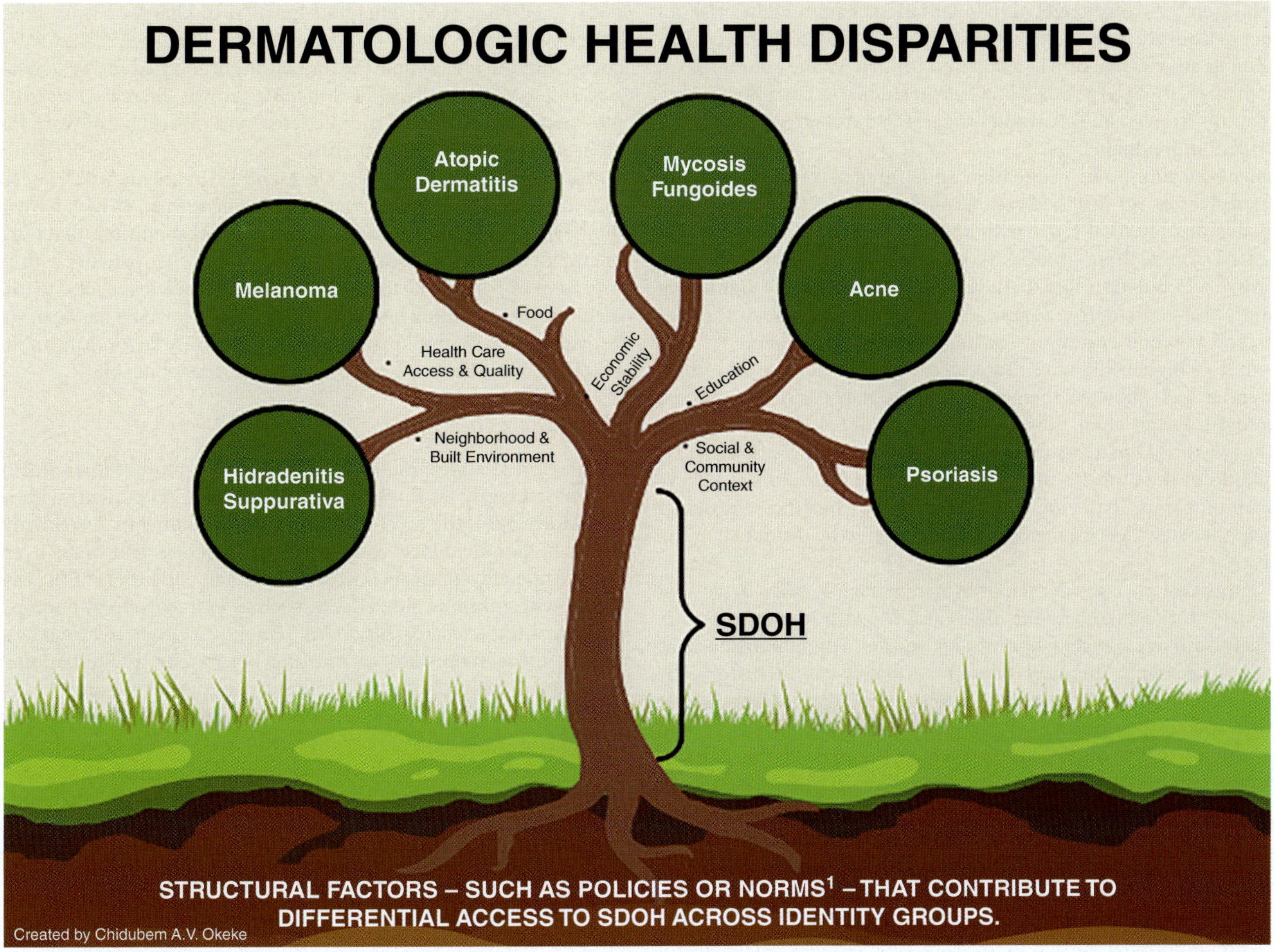

[1]Examples include discriminatory housing policies, unequal school funding, limited access to care in low-income areas, and clinical trial designs that do not reflect diverse patient populations.

FIGURE 11-1. Dermatologic health disparities tree diagram that shows the relationship between structural factors, social determinants of health, and disease disparities.

cancer and have a poorer prognosis compared to White patients.[21] For example, AI/AN persons were more likely to present with stage IV melanoma compared with White patients and have a greater risk of disease-specific mortality, even though the incidence of melanoma is lower.[21,22]

Disparities in melanoma survival rates among racial and ethnic groups also exist, with worse 5-year survival rates in Black/AA individuals (58.5%) compared to White individuals (84.4%). Additionally, differences in clinical presentation of melanoma between racial and ethnic groups (eg, acral involvement in patients with skin of color versus trunk and lower extremity involvement in White patients) may contribute to delayed detection, and, thereby, disparities in survival rates.

Socioeconomic status (SES) is an important social determinant of access to routine cancer screening, incidence, and mortality rates of melanoma.[23] Lower SES correlates with more advanced stages of melanoma seen on initial presentation as well as increased mortality rates.[23] In a study of L/H and Non-Hispanic White California residents, the incidence of melanoma was higher in Non-Hispanic Whites, but melanoma thickness was larger at the time of diagnosis in L/H.[24] Of the two groups, most Non-Hispanic White individuals had a higher SES compared to the L/H group. Individuals from the lower SES had more nodular melanoma while those from the higher SES had more superficial spreading melanoma.[24]

Additionally, outcomes and treatment options may also vary based on insurance type and race. Patients with Medicare health maintenance organizations received a melanoma diagnosis at an earlier disease stage than patients with Medicare fee-for-service.[25] Patients with Medicare were less likely to be treated with chemotherapy compared with patients who had private insurances.[23] Patients with stage IA and IB/II melanoma who were also insured under Medicaid or Medicare were less likely to receive a sentinel lymph node biopsy.[26] More recently, data queried from the National Cancer Database to study receipt of immunotherapy in patients with newly diagnosed metastatic melanoma found that Black patients, recipients of Medicaid, and low-income patients were significantly less likely to receive immunotherapy.[27]

Multiple studies demonstrate that L/H and Black/AA individuals tend to have less information and understanding of melanoma.[23] Patients without a history of melanoma were surveyed on their self-perception of the likelihood that they could get skin cancer. Those who were older, Black/AA, and/or with a lower educational attainment did not think they were at risk.[28] Individuals who are educated about malignant melanoma and who are knowledgeable about potential interventions are more likely to perform self-skin examinations.[29]

ATOPIC DERMATITIS

Atopic dermatitis (AD), also known as eczema, affects 7% to 14% of adults and approximately 20% of children worldwide of all ethnicities.[30] The prevalence is notably higher among historically marginalized racial and ethnic communities, particularly Black/AA, compared to White patients.[31,32] Research suggest that non-Hispanic Black/AA children have an earlier onset, higher prevalence, risk and severity of AD compared to

White children.[33,34] Additionally, L/H populations have a higher risk for persistent and severe disease.[34] Similarly, AI/AN populations have a disproportionate prevalence of AD compared to their White counterparts. Despite the paucity of large-scale population studies to corroborate this, extrapolations from small U.S. studies suggest that AD affects 8% to 11% of the AI/AN individuals.[35]

Income, education, and occupation show graded associations with AD severity across all levels of socioeconomic status (SES). Research findings demonstrate that those with lower SES have a decreased prevalence of AD.[36] Yet, these groups are more likely to experience severe symptoms.[29,37] Population-based studies show a statistically significant association between children (ages 1-17) from households with higher incomes and parental education level and eczema prevalence.[38-40] Possibly, people of higher SES have more access to medical care and information about AD, allowing them to recognize flares and present to a dermatologist earlier than those lower on the SES ladder.[34] Interestingly, a survey of AD patients reported that those with increased disease severity did not see a healthcare provider because they did not believe their symptoms were "bad enough," did not think a healthcare provider could help them, or their care was either not covered by insurance or too expensive.[41]

It is important to consider environmental factors that drive disease severity in those with lower SES. Families with low incomes are more likely to live in rented homes and reside in neighborhoods of low-quality housing.[42] This may disproportionately expose historically marginalized communities to multiple triggers that exacerbate atopic dermatitis and lead to poorer outcomes.[36] A study by Silverberg and Simpson found that local exposures such as the presence of garbage on the streets and dilapidated housing were associated with increased eczema severity.[40] Additionally, a study of 201 pediatric AD patients (age 0-18) showed that elements such as air pollution and residential segregation were associated with increased AD severity in Black/AA children.[37]

AD has a chronic disease course and it is associated with an increased financial and emotional burden in lower-income families.[43] The cost of an emergency department visit for AD is two to three times more expensive than that for an outpatient visit.[41] Studies show that Black/AA, L/H, and lower SES patients with more severe eczema are more likely to visit the emergency department or urgent care and receive prescriptions than White patients with atopic dermatitis.[32,44-46]

This trend can be further explained by the disparities in insurance coverage. Adults with severe AD are more likely to be uninsured and denied converge for cost of AD medications.[45] An analysis of U.S. healthcare claims databases between 2011 and 2016 detected discrepancies in the management of AD between commercially insured and Medicaid-insured patients.[47] Furthermore, Medicaid formularies exclude many medications recommended by guidelines.[48] Results showed that ED and urgent care center utilization was higher in Medicaid-insured AD patients than commercially insured AD patients (10.8% vs 3.2%, respectively), and Medicaid-insured patients were less likely receive specialist care.

HIDRADENITIS SUPPURATIVA

The overall prevalence of hidradenitis suppurativa (HS) is 0.1% in the United States.[49] It disproportionately affects females, young adults (30-39 years), and Black/AA patients.[50] The prevalence of HS in Black/AA patients is three times higher than White patients (0.3% vs 0.1%, respectively).[50,51] The prevalence of HS in Asians, Pacific Islanders, Native Americans, L/H Americans, and Native Hawaiians is lower at 0.04%.[50]

Disease severity, as indicated by higher Hurley stages, is worse in Black/AA and L/H patients.[49,52] Black/AA and L/H patients also have greater levels of healthcare utilization, including outpatient and emergency department visits and inpatient hospitalizations for HS flares, when compared to White patients.[49,53]

Overall HS is more common in individuals of low SES.[54] Low SES, derived from mean household income and real estate value on a neighborhood level, was associated with axillary involvement and high body mass.[55] Another study analyzed hospital discharges across the United States from 1999 to 2014 and found that Black/AA patients from zip codes with the lowest quartile for income accounted for 41% of hospitalizations.[56] Additionally, slower income growth, increased risk of unemployment, higher annual indirect cost, and more days of work loss have all been reported for HS patients.[57]

Adverse SDOH among Black/AA and L/H patients with HS can result in or confound poor patient outcomes. Patient with HS may have low SES due to more debilitating disease and comorbid conditions that lead to loss of employment and educational opportunities,[52] or patients with low SES may have worse HS due to health care barriers, such as access to expensive medications, including biologics. Additionally, low SES has been shown to be associated with smoking and obesity, which are factors known to trigger HS. Thus, low SES may be a risk factor for developing HS.[55]

MYCOSIS FUNGOIDES

In the United States, multiple retrospective cohort studies and population-based registries show that Black/AA and L/H patients with mycosis fungoides (MF), the most common type of cutaneous T cell lymphoma, have a higher incidence, younger age at diagnosis, and worse overall and disease-specific survival compared to White patients.[58,59] Effective treatments with minimal side effects, such as extracorporeal photopheresis, are less often used for Black/AA patients[60]. Other treatments such as topical nitrogen mustard, carmustine, bexarotene, and radiation therapy may cause long-term postinflammatory dyspigmentation.[20]

The role of SDOH in MF patients has not been well described. For example, one study of a large, racially and socioeconomically diverse cohort of 440 patients with MF found that Medicaid insurance was a significant independent predictor of disease progression and shorter progression-free survival.[61] Conversely, a retrospective study of 157 patients with MF/Sezary syndrome found that demographic and socioeconomic factors were not associated with MF prognosis.[62]

PSORIASIS

Psoriasis mostly occurs in individuals of European ancestry followed by Black/AA and L/H individuals. Although there are similarities in psoriasis between different racial and ethnic groups, there are significant differences in the presentation (see Chapter 26) and quality of life impact.[63] For example, lower scores on the Dermatology Life Quality Index (DLQI) is consistently observed in Black/AA and L/H individuals compared to White individuals even when accounting for body surface area involved and severity of disease.[63] In addition, other social factors like lower educational attainment have been associated with severity of psoriasis.[64] In addition, lower SES status along with lower educational attainment led to seeing fewer physicians and decreased systemic treatment.

ACNE

Acne is most common in adolescents affecting approximately 85% of teenagers.[65] Furthermore, acne is one of the top five dermatologic diagnoses for all major U.S. racial and ethnic groups. However, visits by Black/AA and L/H patients to dermatologists for acne were less as compared to Asians and Pacific Islanders and White patents.[66] In one study by Barbieri et al,[67] almost 30,000 patients were examined for associations between patient demographic and socioeconomic characteristics with healthcare utilization and acne treatment during 1 year of follow-up. The findings revealed that although non-Hispanic Black/AA patients were more likely to be seen by a dermatologist (OR = 1.20, 95% CI, 1.09-1.31) than non-Hispanic White patients, they received fewer prescriptions for acne medications (IRR = 0.89, 95% CI, 0.84-0.95).[67] In addition, Black/AA patients were more likely to receive topical retinoids and topical antibiotics compared to oral antibiotics, spironolactone, and isotretinoin. A similar phenomenon is noted in the pediatric dermatology population.[68] Furthermore, a cross-sectional study of AI/AN revealed an elevated rate of acne scarring when compared with a large cohort of racially and ethnically diverse patients, which could reflect a lack of access to early care.[69]

UNDERREPRESENTATION IN RESEARCH

More research is needed to measure the impact that SDOH have on differences in outcomes across racial and ethnic groups. It is worth noting that historically marginalized groups are often underrepresented during clinical trials and studies.[49,70] The continued lack of representation may result in the development of interventions and therapeutics that do not consider the sociodemographic influences of disease and therefore are not efficacious in all patient groups.

FUTURE DIRECTIONS

Despite decades of efforts to address health disparities, evidence of racial and ethnic health disparities are routinely documented in the U.S. Examples of these disparities in dermatology are highlighted above. In order to realize health equity, "where every person has the opportunity to attain their full potential health," efforts to address the SDOH are essential.[71] Immediate interventions to address the SDOH have been explored within other fields of medicine and may prove to be beneficial for the specialty of dermatology.[15] For example, Promotores de Salud (or community health workers), led by the Health and Human Services (HHS) Office of Minority Health, promote their increased engagement in health education, outreach, and access to healthcare for racially and ethnically diverse populations and their communities. The model demonstrated improvement in healthcare access and outcomes and enhancement in quality of life for people living in poor, underserved, and minoritized communities.[72]

This research should also account for historical and structural factors that have shaped economic and social policies in the U.S. and may continue to influence the lived experiences of many historically marginalized communities. Per the National Academies of Science, Engineering, and Medicine, healthcare providers can address SDOH through five approaches—awareness, adjustment, assistance, alignment, and advocacy.[73] Using this framework, collaboration among researchers, leaders in the community, healthcare providers, and educators could create opportunities to enhance strategic thinking to mitigate inequities in the SDOH based on evidence.[15,74]

Finally, diversifying, developing, and retaining a culturally attuned workforce and ensuring linguistic competence could help further mitigate health disparities driven by inequities in the SDOH.

REFERENCES

1. Catalyst N. Social determinants of health (SDOH). *NEJM Catalyst Innovations in Care Delivery*; 2017.
2. Sauaia A, Dellavalle RP. Health care inequities: an introduction for dermatology providers. *Dermatol Clin*. 2009;27(2):103-107.
3. Colleges AMAaAoAM. Advancing health equity: guide on language, narrative and Concepts; 2021.
4. Flanagin A, Frey T, Christiansen SL, AMA Manual of Style Committee. Updated guidance on the reporting of race and ethnicity in medical and science journals. *JAMA*. 2021;326(7):621-627.
5. Hill L, Artiga S, Halder S. Key facts on health and health care by race and ethnicity: social determinants of health. Kaiser Family Foundation. Social Determinants of Health Web site. https://www.kff.org/report-section/key-facts-on-health-and-health-care-by-race-and-ethnicity-social-determinants-of-health/. Published 2022. Accessed March 7, 2023.
6. Foiles Sifuentes AM, Robledo Cornejo M, Li NC, Castaneda-Avila MA, Tjia J, Lapane KL. The role of limited english proficiency and access to health insurance and health care in the affordable care act era. *Health Equity*. 2020;4(1):509-517.
7. Kaiser Family Foundation. Health coverage and care of immigrants. Racial Equity and Health Policy Website. https://www.kff.org/racial-equity-and-health-policy/fact-sheet/health-coverage-and-care-of-immigrants/#:~:text=Although%20noncitizen%20immigrants%20are%20as,both%20public%20and%20private%20coverage. Published 2020. Accessed Janurary 14, 2023.
8. Ku L. Why immigrants lack adequate access to health care and health insurance. Migration Information Source Website. https://www.migrationpolicy.org/article/why-immigrants-lack-adequate-access-health-care-and-health-insurance. Published 2006. Accessed December 30, 2022.
9. Planalp C, Stewart A. The Kids Aren't Alright: Adverse Childhood Experiences and Implications for Health Equity. Robert Wood Johnson Foundation; 2023. Accessed May 11, 2023. https://shadac-pdf-files.s3.us-east-2.amazonaws.com/s3fs-public/publications/ACES_Health%20Equity%20Brief.pdf
10. Hill L, Artiga S, Halder S. Key facts on health and health care by race and ethnicity: health coverage and access to and use of care. https://www.kff.org/report-section/key-facts-on-health-and-health-care-by-race-and-ethnicity-health-coverage-and-access-to-and-use-of-care/. Published 2022. Accessed March 7, 2023.
11. Conway J, Roy B, Barazani L, Wu A, Cline A, Moy J. High demand: identification of dermatology visit trends from 1991-2016 National Ambulatory Medical Care Surveys. *SKIN J Cutaneous Med*. 2020;4(6):552-555.
12. Tripathi R, Knusel KD, Ezaldein HH, Scott JF, Bordeaux JS. Association of demographic and socioeconomic characteristics with differences in use of outpatient dermatology services in the United States. *JAMA Dermatol*. 2018;154(11):1286-1291.
13. Hood CM, Gennuso KP, Swain GR, Catlin BB. County health rankings: relationships between determinant factors and health outcomes. *Am J Prev Med*. 2016;50(2):129-135.
14. Vela MB, Erondu AI, Smith NA, Peek ME, Woodruff JN, Chin MH. Eliminating explicit and implicit biases in health care: evidence and research needs. *Annu Rev Public Health*. 2022;43:477-501.
15. Cooper LA, Purnell TS, Showell NN, et al. Progress on major public health challenges: the importance of equity. *Public Health Rep*. 2018; 133(1_suppl):15S-19S.
16. Braveman P. Health disparities and health equity: concepts and measurement. *Annu Rev Public Health*. 2006;27:167-194.
17. Taylor AL. Racial differences and racial disparities: the distinction matters. *Circulation*. 2015;131(10):848-850.
18. Hebert PL, Sisk JE, Howell EA. When does a difference become a disparity? Conceptualizing racial and ethnic disparities in health. *Health Aff (Millwood)*. 2008;27(2):374-382.
19. Siegel RL, Miller KD, Fuchs HE, Jemal A. Cancer statistics, 2021. *CA Cancer J Clin*. 2021;71(1):7-33.
20. Shao K, Hooper J, Feng H. Racial and ethnic health disparities in dermatology in the United States. Part 2: Disease-specific epidemiology, characteristics, management, and outcomes. *J Am Acad Dermatol*. 2022;87(4):733-744.
21. Cormier JN, Xing Y, Ding M, et al. Ethnic differences among patients with cutaneous melanoma. *Arch Intern Med*. 2006;166(17):1907-1914.
22. Kryatova MS, Okoye GA. Dermatology in the North American Indian/Alaska Native population. *Int J Dermatol*. 2016;55(2):125-134.
23. Harvey VM, Patel H, Sandhu S, Wallington SF, Hinds G. Social determinants of racial and ethnic disparities in cutaneous melanoma outcomes. *Cancer Control*. 2014;21(4):343-349.
24. Pollitt RA, Clarke CA, Swetter SM, Peng DH, Zadnick J, Cockburn M. The expanding melanoma burden in California hispanics: Importance of socioeconomic distribution, histologic subtype, and anatomic location. *Cancer*. 2011;117(1):152-161.
25. Kirsner RS, Wilkinson JD, Ma F, Pacheco H, Federman DG. The association of Medicare health care delivery systems with stage at diagnosis and survival for patients with melanoma. *Arch Dermatol*. 2005;141(6):753-757.
26. Bilimoria KY, Balch CM, Wayne JD, et al. Health care system and socioeconomic factors associated with variance in use of sentinel lymph node biopsy for melanoma in the United States. *J Clin Oncol*. 2009;27(11):1857-1863.
27. Haque W, Verma V, Butler EB, Teh BS. Racial and socioeconomic disparities in the delivery of immunotherapy for metastatic melanoma in the United States. *J Immunother*. 2019;42(6):228-235.
28. Buster KJ, You Z, Fouad M, Elmets C. Skin cancer risk perceptions: a comparison across ethnicity, age, education, gender, and income. *J Am Acad Dermatol*. 2012;66(5):771-779.
29. Uphoff E, Cabieses B, Pinart M, Valdes M, Anto JM, Wright J. A systematic review of socioeconomic position in relation to asthma and allergic diseases. *Eur Respir J*. 2015;46(2):364-374.
30. Bylund S, Kobyletzki LB, Svalstedt M, Svensson A. Prevalence and incidence of atopic dermatitis: a systematic review. *Acta Derm Venereol*. 2020;100(12):adv00160.
31. Brunner PM, Guttman-Yassky E. Racial differences in atopic dermatitis. *Ann Allergy Asthma Immunol*. 2019;122(5):449-455.
32. Kaufman BP, Guttman-Yassky E, Alexis AF. Atopic dermatitis in diverse racial and ethnic groups-variations in epidemiology, genetics, clinical presentation and treatment. *Exp Dermatol*. 2018;27(4):340-357.

33. Steinberg AD, Klinman DM. Pathogenesis of systemic lupus erythematosus. *Rheum Dis Clin North Am*. 1988;14(1):25-41.
34. Wegienka G, Havstad S, Joseph CL, et al. Racial disparities in allergic outcomes in African Americans emerge as early as age 2 years. *Clin Exp Allergy*. 2012;42(6):909-917.
35. Martinez A, de la Rosa R, Mujahid M, Thakur N. Structural racism and its pathways to asthma and atopic dermatitis. *J Allergy Clin Immunol*. 2021;148(5):1112-1120.
36. Chung J, Simpson EL. The socioeconomics of atopic dermatitis. *Ann Allergy Asthma Immunol*. 2019;122(4):360-366.
37. Tackett KJ, Jenkins F, Morrell DS, McShane DB, Burkhart CN. Structural racism and its influence on the severity of atopic dermatitis in African American children. *Pediatr Dermatol*. 2020;37(1):142-146.
38. Fu T, Keiser E, Linos E, et al. Eczema and sensitization to common allergens in the United States: a multiethnic, population-based study. *Pediatr Dermatol*. 2014;31(1):21-26.
39. Hammer-Helmich L, Linneberg A, Thomsen SF, Glumer C. Association between parental socioeconomic position and prevalence of asthma, atopic eczema and hay fever in children. *Scand J Public Health*. 2014;42(2):120-127.
40. Silverberg JI, Simpson EL. Associations of childhood eczema severity: a US population-based study. *Dermatitis*. 2014;25(3):107-114.
41. Baker LC, Baker LS. Excess cost of emergency department visits for nonurgent care. *Health Aff (Millwood)*. 1994;13(5):162-171.
42. Pacheco CM, Ciaccio CE, Nazir N, et al. Homes of low-income minority families with asthmatic children have increased condition issues. *Allergy Asthma Proc*. 2014;35(6):467-474.
43. Filanovsky MG, Pootongkam S, Tamburro JE, Smith MC, Ganocy SJ, Nedorost ST. The financial and emotional impact of atopic dermatitis on children and their families. *J Pediatr*. 2016;169:284-290.e5.
44. Fischer AH, Shin DB, Margolis DJ, Takeshita J. Racial and ethnic differences in health care utilization for childhood eczema: an analysis of the 2001-2013 medical expenditure panel surveys. *J Am Acad Dermatol*. 2017;77(6):1060-1067.
45. Silverberg JI, Gelfand JM, Margolis DJ, et al. Atopic dermatitis in US adults: from population to health care utilization. *J Allergy Clin Immunol Pract*. 2019;7(5):1524-1532.e2.
46. Chovatiya R, Begolka WS, Thibau IJ, Silverberg JI. Financial burden and impact of atopic dermatitis out-of-pocket healthcare expenses among black individuals in the United States. *Arch Dermatol Res*. 2022;314(8):739-747.
47. Siegfried EC, Paller AS, Mina-Osorio P, et al. Effects of variations in access to care for children with atopic dermatitis. *BMC Dermatol*. 2020;20(1):24.
48. Kamara M, Kuo AM, Stein SL, et al. Disparities in availability of skin therapies found in public assistance formularies. *J Am Acad Dermatol*. 2022;87(2):411-417.
49. Kilgour JM, Li S, Sarin KY. Hidradenitis suppurativa in patients of color is associated with increased disease severity and healthcare utilization: a retrospective analysis of 2 U.S. cohorts. *JAAD Int*. 2021;3:42-52.
50. Garg A, Kirby JS, Lavian J, Lin G, Strunk A. Sex- and age-adjusted population analysis of prevalence estimates for hidradenitis suppurativa in the United States. *JAMA Dermatol*. 2017;153(8):760-764.
51. Vlassova N, Kuhn D, Okoye GA. Hidradenitis suppurativa disproportionately affects African Americans: a single-center retrospective analysis. *Acta Derm Venereol*. 2015;95(8):990-991.
52. Soliman YS, Hoffman LK, Guzman AK, Patel ZS, Lowes MA, Cohen SR. African American patients with hidradenitis suppurativa have significant health care disparities: a retrospective study. *J Cutan Med Surg*. 2019;23(3):334-336.
53. Udechukwu NS, Fleischer AB, Jr. Higher risk of care for hidradenitis suppurativa in African American and non-Hispanic patients in the United States. *J Natl Med Assoc*. 2017;109(1):44-48.
54. Wertenteil S, Strunk A, Garg A. Association of low socioeconomic status with hidradenitis suppurativa in the United States. *JAMA Dermatol*. 2018;154(9):1086-1088.
55. Deckers IE, Janse IC, van der Zee HH, et al. Hidradenitis suppurativa (HS) is associated with low socioeconomic status (SES): a cross-sectional reference study. *J Am Acad Dermatol*. 2016;75(4):755-759.e1.
56. Anzaldi L, Perkins JA, Byrd AS, Kharrazi H, Okoye GA. Characterizing inpatient hospitalizations for hidradenitis suppurativa in the United States. *J Am Acad Dermatol*. 2020;82(2):510-513.
57. Tzellos T, Yang H, Mu F, Calimlim B, Signorovitch J. Impact of hidradenitis suppurativa on work loss, indirect costs and income. *Br J Dermatol*. 2019;181(1):147-154.
58. Sun G, Berthelot C, Li Y, et al. Poor prognosis in non-Caucasian patients with early-onset mycosis fungoides. *J Am Acad Dermatol*. 2009;60(2):231-235.
59. Hinds GA, Heald P. Cutaneous T-cell lymphoma in skin of color. *J Am Acad Dermatol*. 2009;60(3):359-375; quiz 376-358.
60. Buechler CR, Sagher E, Tisack A, et al. Contribution of socioeconomic risk factors within a diverse mycosis fungoides cohort from Detroit, Michigan. *J Am Acad Dermatol*. 2022;87(4):897-900.
61. Agi C, Kuhn D, Chung J, Zampella J, Hinds G. (2014). Racial differences in the use of extracorporeal photopheresis for mycosis fungoides. Journal of Dermatological Treatment, 26(3), 266–268. https://doi.org/10.3109/09546634.2014.946381.
62. Geller S, Lebowitz E, Pulitzer MP, et al. Outcomes and prognostic factors in African American and black patients with mycosis fungoides/Sezary syndrome: retrospective analysis of 157 patients from a referral cancer center. *J Am Acad Dermatol*. 2020;83(2):430-439.
63. Kaufman BP, Alexis AF. Psoriasis in skin of color: insights into the epidemiology, clinical presentation, genetics, quality-of-life impact, and treatment of psoriasis in non-white racial/ethnic groups. *Am J Clin Dermatol*. 2018;19(3):405-423.
64. Mahe E, Beauchet A, Reguiai Z, et al. Socioeconomic inequalities and severity of plaque psoriasis at a first consultation in dermatology centers. *Acta Derm Venereol*. 2017;97(5):632-638.
65. Knutsen-Larson S, Dawson AL, Dunnick CA, Dellavalle RP. Acne vulgaris: pathogenesis, treatment, and needs assessment. *Dermatol Clin*. 2012;30(1):99-106, viii-ix.
66. Narahari S, Gustafson CJ, Feldman SR. What's new in antibiotics in the management of acne? *G Ital Dermatol Venereol*. 2012;147(3):227-238.
67. Barbieri JS, Shin DB, Wang S, Margolis DJ, Takeshita J. Association of race/ethnicity and sex with differences in health care use and treatment for acne. *JAMA Dermatol*. 2020;156(3):312-319.
68. Kuo A, Silverberg N, Fernandez Faith E, Morgan R, Todd P. A systematic scoping review of racial, ethnic, and socioeconomic health disparities in pediatric dermatology. *Pediatr Dermatol*. 2021;38 Suppl 2:6-12.
69. Zullo SW, Maarouf M, Shi VY. Acne disparities in Native Americans. *J Am Acad Dermatol*. 2021;85(2):499-501.
70. Okeke CAV, Perry JD, Simmonds FC, et al. Clinical trials and skin of color: the example of hidradenitis suppurativa. *Dermatology*. 2022;238(1):180-184.
71. Jackson CS, Gracia JN. Addressing health and health-care disparities: the role of a diverse workforce and the social determinants of health. *Public Health Rep*. 2014;129 Suppl 2:57-61.
72. Community Health Worker National Workforce Study. In: Protection. USDoHaHSHRaSABoH; 2007.
73. Committee on Educating Health Professionals to Address the Social Determinants of Health; Board on Global Health; Institute of Medicine; National Academies of Sciences, Engineering, and Medicine. A Framework for Educating Health Professionals to Address the Social Determinants of Health. Washington (DC): National Academies Press (US); 2016 Oct 14. Available from: https://www.ncbi.nlm.nih.gov/books/NBK395983/ doi: 10.17226/21923.
74. Braveman P, Gottlieb L. The social determinants of health: it's time to consider the causes of the causes. *Public Health Rep*. 2014;129 Suppl 2(Suppl 2):19-31.

CHAPTER 12

Advancing Exellence in Dermatology

Tiaranesha K. Jackson
Tatiana M. Barrera
Susan C. Taylor

KEY POINTS

- An underpinning of excellence in dermatology is clinicians, researchers, resident physicians, and departmental and organizational leadership who provide diverse thoughts, experiences, and approaches to enrich healthcare.
- Knowledge gaps regarding skin of color dermatology may negatively impact patient care and perpetuate health disparities among populations made vulnerable.

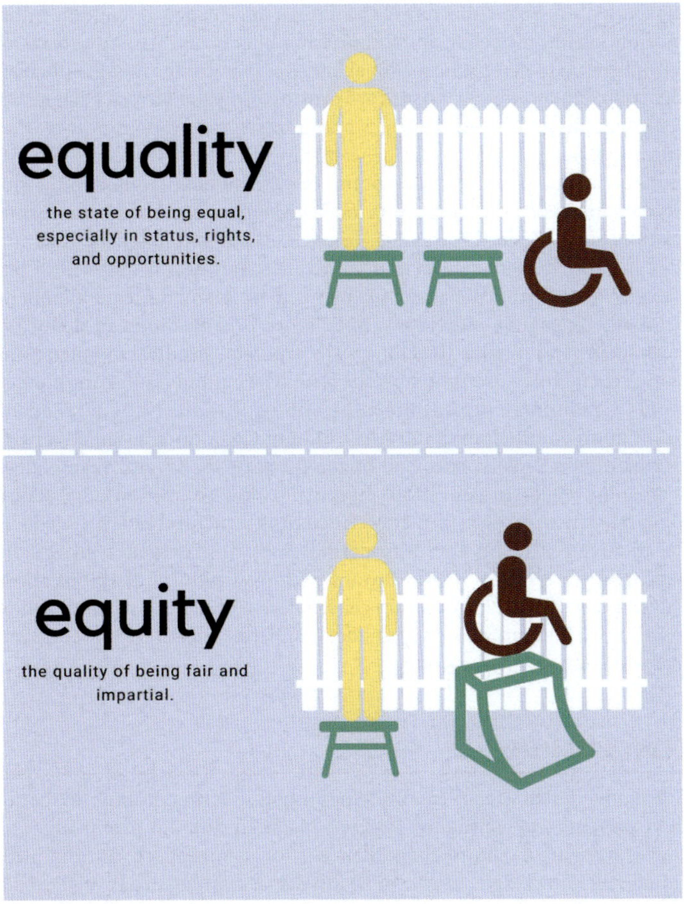
equality
the state of being equal, especially in status, rights, and opportunities.
equity
the quality of being fair and impartial.

FIGURE 12-1. The definition of equality versus equity.[2]

INTRODUCTION

Excellence in patient care, education, and research in dermatology depends on creating a professional environment where people with varied backgrounds, perspectives, and experiences are welcomed, supported, and able to contribute fully. Achieving health equity means recognizing that different patients may require different resources or approaches to achieve similar health outcomes [**Figure 12-1**]. To provide high-quality care, the dermatology workforce must be prepared to address the needs of all patients.[1] Without this readiness, patients—particularly those with skin of color—are at risk for delayed diagnoses, limited access to treatment, and poorer outcomes. These persistent gaps have motivated the inclusion of this chapter. Dermatology remains one of the least racially and ethnically representative specialties.[3] This imbalance is seen across all areas of the field, including clinicians, trainees, department leadership, and researchers. Therefore, in this chapter we will review research on representation and inclusion in dermatology, explore reasons for gaps in knowledge related to skin of color, and offer strategies for integrating this understanding into clinical care, education, and training—ultimately to ensure better outcomes for all patients.

REPRESENTATION OF SKIN OF COLOR (SOC) IN DERMATOLOGY AND MEDICINE

Diagnosis of disease in SOC begins with learning nuances in darker skin tones. Dermatology is unique in that the study of skin, hair, and nails is visual and has been historically depicted on white skin.[4] Moreover, many key features of skin disease are influenced by skin tone. Limited representation of disease on darker skin in dermatologic educational materials disadvantages students beginning in medical school and persists through residency training and beyond. For example, a subacute, shawl sign eruption of dermatomyositis presenting with hyperpigmentation often suggests postinflammatory disease in lighter skin but may indicate active disease in darker skin. The similar presentation (hyperpigmentation) but different recommendations for treatment (active vs maintenance) of this rash are clinically important yet difficult to recognize without appropriate SOC training. Nevertheless, in a study published in 2021, among textbooks commonly used by dermatology residents, such as Rook's Textbook of Dermatology or Fitzpatrick's Dermatology, only 4.5% to 19.9% of dermatologic images illustrate dark skin, while the overwhelming majority of images show pathology on lighter skin tones.[4] Online resources such as DermNet NZ and VisualDx demonstrated a larger range for inclusion of dark skin at 2.8% and 28.5%, respectively. A similar underrepresentation of SOC images has been noted in medical student resources.[5] Urgent inclusion and visual representation of diverse skin and hair types in curricula, textbooks, and educational resources is vital, as lack of representation may influence dermatologist's ability to recognize pathologies in skin of color. Ultimately, diagnosis and grading of severity is delayed, inaccurate, or completely missing, which impacts treatment selection and outcomes of dermatologic disease in SOC populations.

In addition to all dermatologists achieving excellence in the identification, diagnosis, and treatment of disease in SOC patients, there is need for equity and inclusion of clinicians underrepresented in medicine (URiMs), defined as racialized or ethnic populations who have lower numbers in the medical profession relative to their numbers in the general population. However, URiMs make up only 8.1% of all U.S. dermatologists.[3] Race concordant patient-dermatologist interactions are preferred and helpful to establish rapport with patients of color.[6] SOC patients report higher levels of trust, satisfaction, and adherence when paired with physicians of the same ethnoracial background.[7] A diverse workforce also expands cultural competency and humility.[7] Yet, dermatology has been slow to respond to changing demographics, and the dermatologic workforce does not reflect the diversity seen in the general population.

Even though the number of students entering medical school who are URiM has increased, a sizeable gap remains. Latine/Hispanics, Blacks, and American Indians/Alaska Natives make up 18.9%, 13.6%, and 1.3% of the U.S. population, respectively.[8] In 2022, only 7% of U.S. medical school matriculants were Latine/Hispanic, 9.4% Black, and 0.2% American Indian or Alaska Native,[9] none of which reflect the growing diversity of the country. When medical institutions fail to promote inclusivity in medical schools and the dermatologic workforce, they may jeopardize quality of care.

People of color are underrepresented in dermatologic clinical trials, and the dearth of involvement contributes to inadequate care for SOC populations. Among U.S. randomized control trials investigating common dermatologic disorders, racial/ethnic diversity remains unchanged from the years 2010-2015 to 2015-2020.[10] Inequitable representation of current population demographics persists even in dermatologic trials for conditions that are more common in people of color, such as atopic dermatitis.[11] There is also limited research on dermatologic conditions that disproportionately affect or present differently in SOC patients. Research focused on SOC is particularly lacking in darker skin types,[11] and few, if any, randomized controlled trials investigate central centrifugal cicatricial alopecia, hidradenitis suppurativa, and keloids, conditions that primarily affect SOC populations. Dermatologists should take caution when extrapolating information from clinical trials that do not adequately represent SOC. Many challenging factors may explain the decreased participation of SOC populations in clinical trials, such as limited access to healthcare and historical mistreatment in research; though daunting, low representation of these groups is a great disparity consistently identified in the literature, and we must address it. Whatever the reason, low participation in clinical research trials limits treatment for SOC and indicates the serious need for inclusivity in medical research.

GAP OF KNOWLEDGE REGARDING SOC

Insufficient knowledge to adequately treat patients with SOC is prevalent and linked to inadequate medical training. A recent survey of 125 dermatology residents representing 46 programs across the United States found that resident confidence in treating patients with SOC was significantly lower compared to treating patients with white skin, regardless of graduation year.[12] This confidence disparity was present across all categories, such as detecting suspicious lesions and making treatment recommendations. However, resident physicians in programs with SOC curricula reported significantly higher confidence compared to those who did not receive formal SOC education. This reveals another concern: not all U.S. dermatology residencies incorporate SOC curriculum. A 2008 study revealed that only 52% of dermatology residency programs had lectures or didactics focused on diseases in patients with SOC, and even fewer programs (33%) surveyed had a dedicated SOC rotation.[13] In 2022, the needle had moved marginally, with 63.2% of residency programs reporting SOC-related didactics, 44% a rotation where residents primarily saw patients with SOC, and 11.2% a dedicated SOC rotation.[14]

The low confidence for diagnosing and treating dermatologic conditions in SOC extends to other regions of the world too. A national Australian survey of dermatologists demonstrated a need and desire for more training in medical, cosmetic, and procedural aspects of SOC dermatology.[15] Likewise, recent data from members of the Irish Association of Dermatology showed only 23.2% received training in SOC dermatology, and the majority lacked confidence in diagnosing and managing skin conditions in patients with SOC.[16] Even more, research shows the discrepancy in diagnosing skin conditions in SOC begins in medical school,[17] which suggests diversity in educational content should start earlier in a clinician's education and training process.

HOW CAN THE FIELD OF DERMATOLOGY FOSTER A CULTURE OF EXCELLENCE?

Recent efforts have focused on increasing representation of racial and ethnic diversity among medical students and dermatologic trainees who are considered URiM, but individuals that have disabilities, are first generation in the United States, are first in their immediate family to attend college, or who identify as LGBTQIA must also be adequately represented. As aforementioned, the racial/ethnic makeup of dermatology is still not representative of the U.S. population; thus, academic institutions should sustain their recruitment focus. Underrepresentation must be addressed at the medical school level since the demographics of resident physicians reflect such trends. Similar efforts are needed in other elements of the dermatologic workforce—academic faculty, researchers, departmental leadership—to further promote ethnoracial and broader equity in medicine. However, focusing solely on increased representation without providing equitable support to maintain such diversity is detrimental to trainees and patients; for instance, it may even create more disparities such as increased dismissal of URiMs from residency programs.

Increasing representation of SOC in dermatologic training is another critical strategy to advance a culture of excellence in dermatology, and major goal of this textbook. Currently, there is a concerted effort to include more diverse images in educational materials. To address gaps in SOC, in 2022, the American Academy of Dermatology (AAD) released a SOC Curriculum. Several medical schools and dermatology residency programs have joined the effort, creating and implementing their own SOC curriculum. Ideally, trainings for practicing clinicians and students incorporate SOC rather than offer supplemental or optional SOC materials. However, SOC images alone are insufficient in training a clinically competent and culturally mindful dermatologist. One study recently found that equal representation of Fitzpatrick skin type images in a supplemental curriculum did not improve diagnostic accuracy in SOC,[18] hence the need for integration and equity, not equality. This underscores the importance of expanding dermatologic training to include equitable representation of SOC in clinical research, clinical exposure to SOC, curricula on social determinants of health, and diverse academic faculty/staff dedicated to mentoring and training clinicians.

The ability of the clinician to demonstrate cultural competence and practice cultural humility also plays an important role in fostering a culture of excellence in dermatology. Cultural competence indicates the ability to engage with people from different cultures and recognize cultural influence on healthcare behaviors. Cultural humility is an ongoing process of self-reflection to determine personal biases and how one's thoughts/behaviors contribute to the quality of care provided to patients (see Chapter 3). Several evidenced-based strategies and frameworks propose how we can better integrate social care into healthcare delivery.[19] By using patient-centered language and avoiding outmoded terminology rooted in racism, we can improve communication and strengthen the physician-patient relationship.[20] Medical teams that bridge cultural and linguistic gaps not only improve patient satisfaction, adherence, and health outcomes[21] but also provide an educational and inclusive environment for team members.

Finally, engaging individuals and larger organizations in advocacy work inside and outside the clinic walls is pivotal. Medical organizations play a crucial role in setting the stage for advocacy and mobilizing change agents.[22] Prominent organizations, beginning with the National Medical Association and including the AAD, Skin of Color Society and Women's Dermatologic Society, have had ongoing efforts for several years. However, some major organizations have been slow to acknowledge that a focus on structural discrimination (including structural racism) is essential to advance health equity in dermatology.[23] As evidence grows, the path forward requires action toward ending structural discrimination. Our hope is that the information shared here will serve as a call to action for all health organizations, providers, and researchers to develop and utilize a comprehensive strategy.

CONCLUSION

Advancing Exellence in Dermatology equips dermatologists to better serve patients and colleagues. Progress has been slow but promising. The key to fostering a culture of excellence is for us to, collectively and individually, acknowledge our role in health disparities that negatively impact patients of color and take subsequent action to end these disparities.

REFERENCES

1. Lester JC, Taylor SC, Chren MM. Under-representation of skin of colour in dermatology images: not just an educational issue. *Br J Dermatol.* 2019;180(6):1521-1522.
2. Dictionary.com. Equity definition & meaning. https://www.dictionary.com/browse/equity. Accessed September 12, 2022.
3. Lopez S, Lourido JO, Lim HW, Ferguson NN, Pandya AG, Vasquez R. The call to action to increase racial and ethnic diversity in dermatology: a retrospective, cross-sectional study to monitor progress. *J Am Acad Dermatol.* 2022;86(3):e121-e123.
4. Alvarado SM, Feng H. Representation of dark skin images of common dermatologic conditions in educational resources: a cross-sectional analysis. *J Am Acad Dermatol.* 2021;84(5):1427-1431.
5. Jones VA, Clark KA, Shobajo MT, Cordova A, Tsoukas MM. Skin of color representation in medical education: an analysis of popular preparatory materials used for United States Medical Licensing Examinations. *J Am Acad Dermatol.* 2021;85(3):773-775.
6. Gorbatenko-Roth K, Prose N, Kundu RV, Patterson S. Assessment of Black patients' perception of their dermatology care. *JAMA Dermatol.* 2019;155(10):1129-1134.
7. Gronbeck C, Feng PW, Feng H. Assessment of dermatologist-patient race and ethnicity concordance in the Medicare population. *J Am Acad Dermatol.* 2022;86(3):651-653.
8. U.S. Census Bureau. QuickFacts: United States. https://www.census.gov/quickfacts/fact/table/US/PST045221. Accessed August 5, 2022.
9. AAMC. 2021 FACTS: applicants and matriculants data. https://www.aamc.org/data-reports/students-residents/interactive-data/2021-facts-applicants-and-matriculants-data. Accessed August 4, 2022.
10. Chen V, Akhtar S, Zheng C, Kumaresan V, Nouri K. Assessment of changes in diversity in dermatology clinical trials between 2010-2015 and 2015-2020: a systematic review. *JAMA Dermatol.* 2022;158(3):288-292.
11. Montgomery SNB, Elbuluk N. A quantitative analysis of research publications focused on the top chief complaints in patients with skin of color. *J Am Acad Dermatol.* 2021;85(1):241-242.

12. Gupta R, Ibraheim MK, Dao H, Patel AB, Koshelev M. Assessing dermatology resident confidence in caring for patients with skin of color. *Clin Dermatol.* 2021;39(5):873-878.
13. Nijhawan RI, Jacob SE, Woolery-Lloyd H. Skin of color education in dermatology residency programs: does residency training reflect the changing demographics of the United States? *J Am Acad Dermatol.* 2008;59(4):615-618.
14. Ibraheim MK, Gupta R, Dao H, Patel A, Koshelev M. Evaluating skin of color education in dermatology residency programs: data from a national survey. *Clin Dermatol.* 2022;40(2):228-233.
15. Rodrigues MA, Ross AL, Gilmore S, Daniel BS. Australian dermatologists' perspective on skin of colour: results of a national survey. *Australas J Dermatol.* 2018;59(1):e23-e30.
16. O'Connor C, Gallagher C, Bourke J, Murphy M. Confidence of Irish dermatologists in caring for patients with skin of colour. *Clin Exp Dermatol.* 2022;47(1):169-171.
17. Fenton A, Elliott E, Shahbandi A, et al. Medical students' ability to diagnose common dermatologic conditions in skin of color. *J Am Acad Dermatol.* 2020;83(3):957-958.
18. Mullen BL, Gorman BG, Soares AA, et al. Equal representation of low and high Fitzpatrick skin type images in a supplemental curriculum does not improve overall high Fitzpatrick diagnostic accuracy. A prospective study. *Int J Dermatol.* 2023;62:e210-e212. doi:10.1111/ijd.16211
19. National Academies of Sciences, Engineering, and Medicine; Health and Medicine Division; Board on Health Care Services; Committee on Integrating Social Needs Care into the Delivery of Health Care to Improve the Nation's Health. Integrating social care into the delivery of health care: moving upstream to improve the nation's health. http://www.ncbi.nlm.nih.gov/books/NBK552597/. Accessed August 10, 2022.
20. Barton M, Boos MD. Towards a more inclusive environment in the dermatology clinic: an introduction to using thoughtful language in the practice of dermatology. *Dermatol Clin.* 2022;40(1):103-108.
21. McKesey J, Berger TG, Lim HW, McMichael AJ, Torres A, Pandya AG. Cultural competence for the 21st century dermatologist practicing in the United States. *J Am Acad Dermatol.* 2017;77(6):1159-1169.
22. Desai SR, Khanna R, Glass D, et al. Embracing diversity in dermatology: Creation of a culture of equity and inclusion in dermatology. *Int J Womens Dermatol.* 2021;7(4):378-382.
23. Bailey ZD, Feldman JM, Bassett MT. How structural racism works — racist policies as a root cause of U.S. racial health inequities. *N Engl J Med.* 2021;384(8):768-773.

SECTION 2

International Dermatology for Skin of Color

CHAPTER 13

Global Perspectives and Insights on Dermatology for Skin of Color

Harvey Lui
Tashmeeta Ahad
Sunil Kalia

KEY POINTS

- Cultural customs in different parts of the world lead to a spectrum of unique cutaneous manifestations and effects that may be unfamiliar to healthcare professionals.
- Healthcare systems around the world are heterogeneous with disparate capacities and approaches for skin of color patients.
- Photoprotection is universally beneficial, but the specific goals and methods must be matched according to skin phenotype in addition to individual cultural customs and preferences.
- Dermatologic care for Indigenous persons is fragmentary and insufficiently studied.
- International organizations for dermatology serve to harmonize global standards of care and promote competency with "Dermodiversity" in all its forms.

UNDERSTANDING GLOBAL INFLUENCES AND EFFECTS

HISTORICAL PERSPECTIVES AND CONSEQUENCES

The ethnocultural diversity of various global regions has been historically shaped by human migrations involving conquest and colonialism. The effects have been enduring, deeply entrenched, and more often than not nonbeneficent. Since the end of World War II, colonial territories and their sociopolitical structures have been incrementally dismantled; subsequent civil rights movements around the world led to further improvements in civil freedoms and equity. For dermatology, more recent seminal events including the murder of George Floyd in 2020 catalyzed a fundamental shift in attitudes and actions toward more meaningful inclusiveness, especially for patients and health practitioners from disadvantaged groups.

Ethnocultural diversity varies widely among different countries and continents [**Figure 13-1**].[1] East Asian and European countries are relatively homogeneous in ethnocultural terms. Africa is considered the most ethnically diverse of all continents because of its multiplicity of distinct cultural and linguistic groups. On a global level, dermatology practitioners encounter varying degrees of patient diversity according to their country or region of practice. Ongoing globalization trends will progressively heighten ethnocultural diversity throughout the world, including in North America where the prevailing majority population has arisen from successive waves of immigration over the last half millennium.

Specific ethnic groupings are only vaguely correlated with human skin color, whereas anthropologic studies demonstrate a relatively strong relationship between skin color and geographic latitude for indigenous populations.[2] The biologic basis for variations in skin color is primarily accounted for by long-term evolutionary pressures in response to geographic variations in solar radiation flux on the skin. Effective, compassionate, and ethical clinical practice mandates an appreciation of the complex, nuanced, and evolving interplay between biologically determined skin color and disparate psychosocial and socioeconomic interactions.

THE GLOBAL RELEVANCE AND EFFECTS OF SKIN COLOR

The visual appearance of the skin is one of the physical traits through which individuals are identified and find expression. The color of a person's skin is readily apparent and can be objectively quantified in terms of various optical parameters.[3] Skin color truly occurs on a continuum and therefore attempts to categorize individuals based solely on color will be fraught and misleading.

Skin color can almost reflexively trigger assumptions and inferences about a person that are arbitrary and inaccurate at best, and injurious at worst. Societal perceptions about the significance of a person's skin color are both pervasive and consequential. Having darker colored skin essentially imposes socioeconomic and ethnocultural disadvantages that influence many aspects of life, including the restoration and maintenance of health.

This chapter explores global aspects and insights within dermatology that affect persons who broadly and phenotypically manifest skin that is visibly darker than individuals with light-colored "white" skin. Specific diseases that disproportionately or differentially affect skin of color are covered extensively in other chapters; this chapter focuses on global influences and origins as a framework for recognizing and appreciating worldwide "Dermodiversity."

CULTURAL AND RELIGIOUS INTERSECTIONS WITH DERMATOLOGY

Understanding diverse cultural and religious practices is foundational for healthcare providers, as it can impact health behaviors in multiple ways. First, interactions between healthcare providers and patients' varying cultural and religious attitudes may influence dermatological care, patient satisfaction, and adherence to treatment. Second, lack of awareness of certain cultural practices may lead to misdiagnoses or incorrect diagnoses. Third, cultural and therapeutic practices may cause or exacerbate dermatoses, for example, contact dermatitis and atopic eczema. Familiarity with specific cultural practices [**Table 13-1**] around the world will better enable an enlightened approach to caring for skin patients of color.

CULTURAL AND RELIGIOUS COMPETENCY AND SENSITIVITY

Cultural competency involves recognizing the social and cultural factors that may influence healthcare. This requires healthcare providers to understand and respect patients' diverse religious beliefs, cultural practices, attitudes, and varying health preferences. Studies have demonstrated that enhanced cultural competency among physicians leads to improved patient satisfaction, adherence, and treatment outcomes.[4,5] There are only a handful of qualitative studies that delve into the attitudes of diverse religious and ethnic groups. Even so, it is crucial to acknowledge the heterogeneity within these groups as attitudes can vary significantly within them. Individual patient preferences should always be obtained to avoid reinforcing preconceived notions or stereotypes.

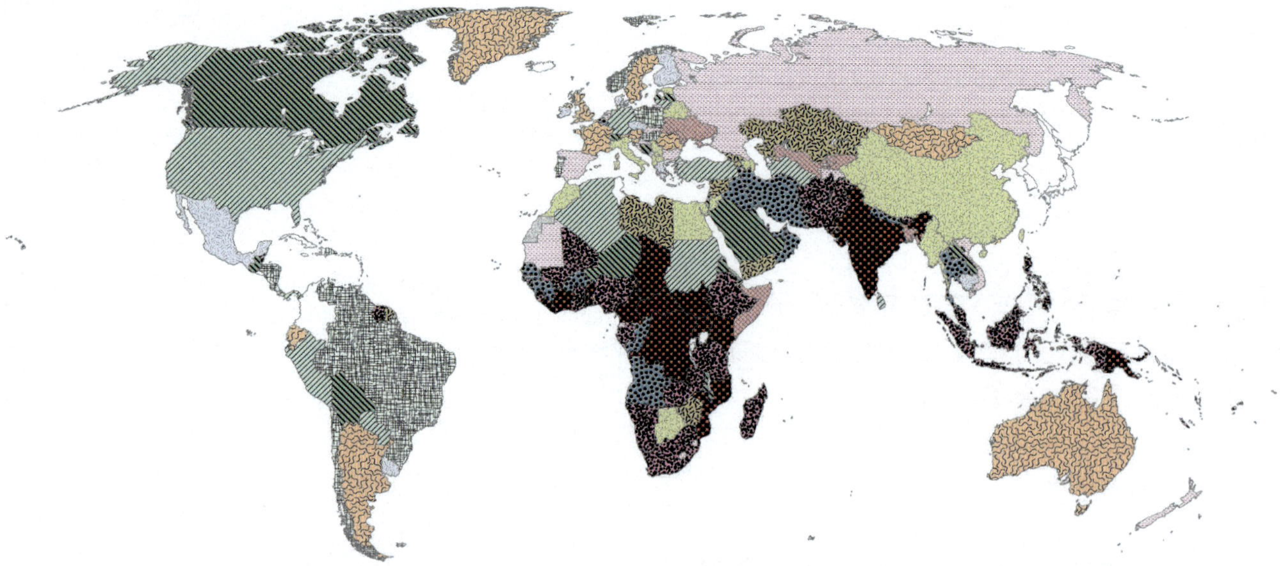

FIGURE 13-1. Global ethnolingual diversity by country; color shading intensity is linearly proportional to diversity index. Adapted from https://commons.wikimedia.org/wiki/File:Ethnologue_18_linguistic_diversity_index_BlankMap-World6.svg based on data from Fennig et al.[1]

In a qualitative study surveying Muslim patients in the United States, attitudes varied, although certain themes were prevalent.[6] Modesty was a prominent priority among Muslim women; patients felt more comfortable with clinicians of the same gender, particularly for examinations involving private body sites. Approaches including performing physical examinations in phases, providing blankets for modesty, asking women whether they are comfortable with removing hijabs/veils before examining, and asking patients' preferences before bringing additional male trainees into the clinic room can help improve culturally competent care.[7]

Islam promotes the observance of a halal diet, which involves consuming bovine and poultry meat prepared in accordance with Islamic principles and abstaining from porcine and alcohol-containing products. Fasting during the month of Ramadan is one of the "Five Pillars" of Islam and is widely observed by Muslims. Certain Muslim patients may avoid medications that do not align with a halal diet, such as isotretinoin, which may contain porcine gelatin. Patients may also prefer to adjust oral medication schedules around fasting periods during the month of Ramadan.[6] However, most Muslim patients will prioritize medical needs despite these customs. This prioritization is driven by the understanding that maintaining one's health and well-being is a fundamental aspect of Islamic teachings and "necessity makes the forbidden permissible."[8]

Family dynamics may mean that members may want to shield older patients from negative prognoses and may be observed in cultures such as some Latin families.[9]

Highly negative cultural biases and misapprehensions toward noticeable skin diseases can also exist within certain ethnocultural settings. For example, vitiligo leads to profound social isolation of not only the patient but also their entire family due to misguided stigmatization over contagiousness. These attitudes are particularly common in South Asia and the Middle East. For persons with albinism, societal attitudes and behavior can even be life-threatening. In certain parts of Africa, these patients are murdered because of the odious superstition that possessing the body parts of someone with albinism will bestow wealth and power.[10] Although this example is extreme, negative attitudes about having skin disease are harmful and dangerous in many ways.

BEAUTY AND ESTHETICS AROUND THE WORLD

Perceptions of beauty vary among diverse cultures and ethnic groups and can evolve when these groups intersect. For example, among East Asians, the "double eyelid" operation that results in a more "Western" appearance has gained in popularity, not only in North America but also in Asian countries.[11] In South Asian, African, and Middle Eastern regions, lighter or fairer skin has traditionally been considered more desirable, giving rise to the use of skin lightening products including medically-unsupervised chronic used of topical corticosteroids leading to significant side effects. However, there are ongoing efforts to challenge and redirect these societal preferences and pressures.

These physical beauty standards may in part stem from vestigial colonial influences in these regions, which may have historically led to beauty or attractiveness being equated to looking more "Caucasian."[12] Pop culture also heavily influences cosmetic preferences, especially among youth, and evolves with time and trends. Direct motivations for esthetic enhancement may relate to perceived higher social standing, success in professional and personal life, marriage prospects, increased self-esteem, and family and peer influences.[13]

GLOBAL HEALTH SYSTEMS AND PHILOSOPHIES FOR TREATING SKIN DISEASE

Dermatology as a medical discipline is fundamentally a Western-based approach to skin disease that relies on formalized, rational scientific principles to guide clinical practice. Globally, there are many other medical practice systems, beliefs, and philosophies that are offered or promoted to those afflicted with skin disease [**Table 13-2**]. Health systems around the world vary, both in terms of the specific care techniques employed as well as how they can be accessed. Patients with skin of color may experience limited or restricted access to standard dermatologic care for a multitude of reasons (eg, affordability, insufficient practitioners, location), and/or seek care from so-called alternative practitioners because of personal beliefs or preferences. They may also pursue more than one healing approach simultaneously. Black patients have shown higher levels of satisfaction when reviewed by race-concordant or skin of color dermatologists, emphasizing the need for greater diversity among the dermatology workforce.[14]

Varying regulatory standards and marketing priorities for pharmaceutical products around the world contribute to global disparities in the availability of up-to-date drugs and devices. In addition, inadequate enforcement of pharmaceutical and device regulations in some countries can expose patients to harm as in the case of the unregulated widespread availability of potent topical corticosteroids in India.[15]

TABLE 13-1 Global range and origins of selected ethnocultural-specific dermatologic practices and manifestations

Predominant ethnocultural group or geographic origin[a]	Practice or custom	Purpose	Dermatologic manifestations or conditions	Specific features	Cross reference
COSMETIC OR ETHNO-SPECIFIC ALTERATIONS TO THE SKIN					
Africa, South Asia, Middle East	Skin lightening and bleaching	• Achieve lighter skin color	• Exogeneous ochronosis • Squamous cell carcinoma • Skin atrophy • Striae • Chemical burns • Contact dermatitis	Face or diffuse applications over the body	Ch. 59
Africa	Hot combing	• Hair straightening	• Chemical burns • Hair breakage • Contact dermatitis • Scarring and nonscarring alopecia	Scalp	Ch. 5, 42
Africa, South Asia, Middle East	Threading	• Hair removal	• Irritant contact dermatitis • Pseudofolliculitis barbae • Folliculitis • Acne • Flat warts	Face, especially eyebrows	Ch. 45
Africa	Scarification	• Decorative, medicinal purposes, or tribal affiliation	• Scarring • Cutaneous infections	Uses sharp tools or burning with hot metal that may induce keloid formation	
Africa	Ritual tattooing	• Decorative	• Contact dermatitis • Keloids • Foreign body reaction	Various sites (eg, gingival tattooing in Ethiopian women)	
Worldwide	Male circumcision	• Faith affirmation (especially Judaism and Islam) • Preventative health	• Decreased risk of sexually transmitted infections and genital carcinoma • Treatment or prevention of penile dermatoses	Variably practiced around the world	
East Asia	Double eyelid surgery	• Achieve a more Western appearance	• Scarring risk		
RITUALS, CUSTOMS, AND DECORATIVE ADORNMENTS THAT MAY AFFECT THE SKIN					
Muslim	Prayer	• Faith expression	• Localized lichenification, nodules, and hyperpigmentation	Prostration, bowing, and sitting lead to localized lesions over the central forehead, malleolus, left dorsal foot	Ch. 9
Muslim	Prayer	• Ablution: preprayer purification	• Ritual washing may cause xerosis or exacerbate eczema	Face, arms, feet	
Muslim	Hijab	• Conceal hair for modesty • Faith affirmation	• Traction alopecia • Seborrheic dermatitis • Contact dermatitis	Hijabs can be removed during medical evaluation with patient consent	Ch. 9
Sikh	Turban	• Protects the hair and keeps it clean • Faith affirmation	• Traction alopecia • Seborrheic dermatitis • Contact dermatitis	Male Sikhs do not cut their hair	
South Asia/ Middle East	Temporary henna dye tattoos	• Decorative	• Irritant or allergic contact dermatitis especially to para-phenylenediamine • Contact urticaria, erythema multiforme, hypertrichosis, and skin necrosis are less common complications	Hands, feet, or forearms	Ch. 9
South Asia	Bindi application	• Decorative dot worn on forehead	• Contact dermatitis from dot sticker	Forehead	
Hindu	Kumkum application (synonymous with sindoor)	• Application of red powder to symbolize marital status in women	• Irritant or allergic contact dermatitis	Frontal hairline part and forehead	
East Asia	Cupping or coining	• Extraction or release of toxins or stagnant blood by applying suction or abrading the skin	• Well-demarcated circular or linear purpuric or hyperpigmented patches	Back, extremities	Ch. 6

[a]Although prevalent worldwide to varying degrees, these practices are categorized according to their predominant group or geographic origin.

Source: Adapted in part from Vashi et al[16] and Budair.[17]

TABLE 13-2 Selected global healthcare approaches and systems with reference to skin of color

Approach or method	Source or origin	Underlying philosophy and principles	Skin of color aspects
Dermatology (as a medical specialty)	Western societies	• Scientific methodology and evidence • Formalized training standards for practitioners • Legal regulation	• Incomplete or insufficient access by patients of color (multifactorial) • Limited access to novel therapies and/or inadequate enforcement of regulations may selectively disadvantage or harm persons of color
Complementary or alternative medicine[a]	Worldwide	• Healing does not require biologic plausibility, testability, or repeatability • Emphasizes holistic integration with lifestyle alterations	• For those unable to access conventional medicine or who feel that Western approaches are culturally insensitive
Traditional folk medicine	Indigenous societies	• Treatments based on historical tradition and experience • Strong reliance on spirituality • Extensive use of botanical products	• Used predominantly by Indigenous patients of color
Traditional Chinese medicine	China	• Achieving balance and bodily harmony using herbal medicine, acupuncture, exercise, massage, and dietary practices • Greater emphasis on organ function rather than anatomy • All therapies are nonstandardized	• High familiarity and use among East Asian patients • Nonstandard products may contain undisclosed adulterants that may be toxic or allergenic
Ayurvedic medicine	India	• Disease is due to imbalances in bodily forces known as vaata (air), pitta (bile/fire), and kapha (phlegm) • Practice dictated by ancient texts	• High familiarity and use among South Asians • Medicinal products may contain toxic or allergenic substances

[a]Complimentary or alternative medicine can also be considered a broad category that encompasses all forms of non-Western-based medicine including those listed in the remainder of this table.

PHOTOPROTECTION AROUND THE WORLD

Photoprotection as an intentional health prevention strategy was initially driven by the need to decrease sunburns in those with light skin. Topical sunscreens became the key technologic solution to this goal and were subsequently demonstrated to also mitigate the risks of skin cancer and photoaging, albeit based on clinical evidence derived solely from White populations. Since skin color is inherently an evolutionary consequence of terrestrial solar flux, it stands to reason that photoprotection needs will vary significantly on a global basis due to skin color diversity. Beyond sunburns and carcinogenesis, sun-induced pigmentation is an important consideration for photoprotection that is of much greater relevance for persons with darker skin. In current practice, photoprotection is usually approached monolithically with minimal consideration of global and individual differences in skin photoreactivity. Attitudes toward sun exposure and cultural norms for clothing and exposing bare skin in public are yet additional dimensions that shape sun protection practices around the world. Climate change and pollution must also be accounted for if human skin is to be protected on a global scale. The concept of "personalized photoprotection" addresses the varying needs to the diverse global population.[18]

GLOBAL ATTITUDES TOWARD SUN EXPOSURE

Behavioral attitudes toward sun exposure appear to be influenced by the physiologic effects of UV radiation on facultative pigmentation (ie, tanning) and what those sun-induced changes are perceived to confer on individuals. Globally, these attitudes and preferences can be almost antithetical. For example, recreational tanning in Western society remains popular among younger people, who consider the acquisition of a tan to confer attractiveness and health, whereas in Asia and even Africa, lighter skin is desired for a range of different sociologic reasons.

The preference for lighter skin may be the primary reason for photoprotection and reflects the higher adherence in Asian countries like Japan. A study evaluating 2338 Japanese people suggested that up to 83% of individuals used some form of photoprotection.[18] It is also customary for Asians to use parasols outdoors as part of their routine sun protection regimen. In contrast, in a study evaluating Asian Americans, over two-thirds of individuals reported never or rarely wearing sunscreen or seeking shade. This highlights the cultural rather than ethnic variation in photoprotection adherence.[19]

Intentional photoprotection is least practiced by Africans and South Asians with black or dark brown skin color, which may be due to their perception of having a lower risk for skin cancer, the mistaken belief that dark skin does not tan or sunburn, or the lack of economic ability to purchase photoprotective clothing or sunscreens. Tanning occurs even in heavily melanized individuals, but the sun-induced change in skin color appears to be much less apparent than for tans in medium-complected skin. Lived experiences and self-acknowledgement of society's negative biases against dark skin color are likely a strong deterrent for these individuals to look even darker. Persons with skin of color may lack the socioeconomic means for pursuing recreational activities involving the sun. Finally, there is the possibility that sun exposure is biologically and physically more uncomfortable for people with darker skin.[20]

PHOTOPROTECTION GOALS VARY ACCORDING TO SKIN COLOR

Skin cancer occurs much more frequently in fair skin because its lower constitutive melanin content allows more ultraviolet radiation to be absorbed by the epidermis. In contrast, in individuals with darker skin, skin cancer is far less often related to ultraviolet radiation exposure and more likely related to other carcinogenic factors (eg, genetics, human papillomavirus, chronic inflammation, or immunosuppression). Thus, the goals for photoprotection in skin of color individuals are to minimize hyperpigmentation, sunburn, and photoaging more so than to prevent skin cancer.[21] In Asia and Africa, photoprotection is especially important for ameliorating skin conditions such as postinflammatory pigmentation, melasma, photosensitive eruptions, and vitiligo.

GLOBAL VARIATION IN PHOTOPROTECTION STRATEGIES BY GEOGRAPHY AND ETHNICITY

Generally speaking, photoprotection is usually practiced by avoiding sun exposure during peak hours (10 to 2 o'clock), seeking shade, wearing protective clothing, donning sunglasses, and applying sunscreen. It can be difficult to seek shade in regions without natural foliage or in jurisdictions where limited financial resources preclude the construction of shade structures. With global warming, this is of particular concern in regions becoming more arid such as the Sahara Desert and the Amazon rainforest. Further effort is needed to restore natural foliage in these areas or access funding to implement shade structures for both photoprotection and curbing heat stress.

Differences in sun protective clothing practice and sunscreen recommendations vary globally, based on ethnic background or skin color tones. In North America, the clothing recommended is usually wide-brimmed hats and long-sleeved shirts. However, head coverings can vary among different ethnic groups. Conventional western styled hats may not be appropriate for groups such as Jews and Sikhs who tend to wear kippahs and turbans or chunni, respectively. American Indians are known to wear warbonnets. Even within an ethnic group or religion, such as with Muslim women, head coverings may vary in form, that is, hijab, niqab, dupatta, chador, or burqa. Although the primary purpose of these coverings is not for photoprotection, their routine use can be photoprotective to varying degrees. Rather than using garments, members of the Himba tribe in Africa are known to cover their hair and whole body with mud to protect their skin from the sun, along with clothes mostly made of goat skin. Ovahimba women cover their bodies, hair, and personal attire with *otjise,* a red ochre-powder mixed with clarified butter. *Otjise* has been shown to yield an SPF of up to 15, with potentially higher effective levels of photoprotection, since the material is usually applied at a thickness greater than the standard used during standardized SPF testing (ie, 2 mg/cm^2).[22] Overall, Western culture tends to use slogans such as "slip, slap, slop" to encourage use of specific protective clothing, garments, and sunscreen, but there is limited understanding of the relative effectiveness of different head coverings or other specific forms of skin protection.

BARRIERS TO SUNSCREEN USE BY PERSONS OF COLOR

Advances have been made to make sunscreens more cosmetically acceptable in darker skin individuals, although barriers still exist. Common reasons for darker skin individuals to use sunscreen are to prevent tanning, minimize exacerbation of pigmentary conditions, and mitigate photoaging. Prevention of these conditions requires attenuation of ultraviolet A (UVA) and visible light in addition to UVB. U.S. Food and Drug Administration regulations have limited the availability of UV filters in UVA I and visible regions, leaving only mineral filters and tinted sunscreens as viable options for protecting against these longer wavelengths of light. Mineral filters add to the barrier of using sunscreens in dark skin because they impart a semi-opaque and noticeable white cast when applied to the skin. Tinting with iron oxides helps with better skin color matching; however, staining of clothing and imprecise skin tone matching may still render these formulations unacceptable to darker skin of color users. Using sunscreens in global climate zones that are humid as well as sunny can be challenging due to the effects of perspiration on sunscreen adherence to the skin. The cost of sunscreens is a further barrier to sunscreen use that disproportionately affects people of lower socioeconomic means or those who live in low-income countries, especially within Africa.

FUTURE PHOTOPROTECTION TRENDS

Global warming with hotter ambient temperatures necessitates collaboration by the photoprotection community with other public health concerns such as heat stroke, heat exhaustion, and cardiovascular diseases. These health issues are of greater significance in countries situated in the tropics and subtropical regions where the prevailing population has darker skin; Africa is expected to be the continent most affected by global warming,[23] and warrants special consideration for photoprotection recommendations. Methods such as wearing protective clothing or even using sunscreens may exacerbate heat stress, and thus sun avoidance or developing shade structures may be more appropriate strategies. Furthermore, as governmental and other agencies increase infrastructural support and funding for shade structures to reduce heat stress, lower the carbon cost of air conditioning, and prevent heat-related illness, there will be a concomitant photoprotection effect that should be highlighted and promoted to decision-makers.

INDIGENOUS CARE IN DERMATOLOGY

One key consequence of human migration is the coexistence of peoples who originally inhabited a given land over thousands of years and individuals who migrated by volition or coercion to that same land where they ultimately settled. Indigenous peoples in their own native lands have undergone forced assimilation and adoption of European culture as a result of colonialism, which also involved the slave trade. According to the United Nations, there are 476 million indigenous people worldwide accounting for 6.2% of the global population.[24] In the United States, the U.S. Census Bureau specifically recognizes persons who are descended from the original peoples of continental America as American Indians and Alaska Natives; for Hawaii, the equivalent individuals are Native Hawaiians. Various terms used for and by people who have historical continual links with a given land prior to colonialism include indigenous, aboriginal, native, and First nations. Using the term "American Indian," as is done by the U.S. Census bureau, is considered by some to be problematic and inaccurate because indigenous persons in the United States bear no relationship with people from the Indian subcontinent.

Indigenous peoples around the world are highly diverse, but they almost universally share lived experiences of discrimination, oppression, and subjugation in all aspects of their lives including healthcare and its social determinants. Collectively the net effect has been referred to as cultural genocide. These experiences date back to colonial times, with forced tuberculosis treatments involving relocation of Indigenous people away from their native land and families, or the continued coercion of Indigenous women into tubal ligation. These negative encounters and with continued cultural clashes have led to mistrust of the healthcare system by Indigenous people. With increasing recognition of the mistrust of the healthcare system by the Indigenous community, barriers to accessing the healthcare system, and discovery of the undisclosed burials of indigenous children in government-sponsored Indian Residential Schools,[25] there has been an acceleration of the need to equalize and prioritize healthcare access among indigenous people. The United Nations has formulated the Declaration on the Rights of Indigenous Peoples[26] to delineate and define their specific rights; while nonlegally binding, the declaration provides a moral and specific framework for working respectfully with these peoples in a spirit of mutual reconciliation.

In addition to the multiplicity of healthcare challenges faced by indigenous persons of color, the scope and epidemiology of their dermatologic issues remain inadequately studied and addressed. Specific examples of conditions that may have genetic, environmental, and cultural underpinnings for indigenous patients include actinic prurigo, atopic dermatitis, pyodermas, and focal epithelial hyperplasia (Heck disease). Actinic prurigo occurs throughout North and South America indigenous populations and has been correlated with certain HLA subtypes that may be common to these people.[27] It is analogous to but clinically distinct from polymorphous light eruption. In Canada, atopic dermatitis with secondary infection has been cited as an example of a condition that is not only highly prevalent among indigenous children but also inadequately treated by existing healthcare systems and professionals.[28] Similarly, in Australia cutaneous infections and infestations (ie, impetigo and scabies) in Aboriginal children are among the highest in the world.[29] Heck's disease, focal epithelial hyperplasia is distinctly found among indigenous children in the Americas and is related to a predisposition to HPV 13/32 mucosal infections.[30] These specific examples are well documented in the literature, but systematic approaches to understanding the scope of dermatologic burdens in indigenous persons appear to be nonexistent to date in countries and regions with high proportions of settler classes. In addition, better representation of indigenous people in clinical trials is required, especially for skin conditions disproportionately affecting Indigenous peoples.[31]

GLOBAL DERMATOLOGY ORGANIZATIONS

In addition to traditional academic institutions that focus on scholarly aspects of the specialty via formal education and research, professional dermatology organizations serve to promote the clinical, continuing educational, and political needs of practicing dermatologists. Two longstanding organizations are dedicated to global dermatologic activities: the International League of Dermatological Societies (ILDS) and the International Society for Dermatology (ISD); these have been in existence since 1935 and 1959, respectively. Both organizations host major quadrennial international congresses (eg, World Congress of Dermatology, International Congress of Dermatology) with the first one dating back to 1889 in Paris. These congresses bring together dermatologists internationally with programs that specifically and intentionally recruit participants from around the world.

The World Health Organization, which is part of the United Nations, addresses dermatological issues that have global impact through official relations with the ILDS. These initiatives aim not only at harmonizing dermatologic care via standardizing terminology through the ICD-11 (International Classification of Diseases, 11th revision)[32] but also at highlighting certain diseases from underserviced populations and/or with broad global impact. On May 24, 2025, World Health Assembly of WHO approved a resolution recognizing "Skin Diseases as a Global Public Health Priority," further highlighting the recognition of the importance of skin diseases and their burdens globally.[33] Persons with skin of color are often disproportionately affected by neglected tropical diseases, access to essential medicines, and poor awareness of the specific manifestations and impacts of diseases occurring in darker skin. The ILDS, through its International Foundation for Dermatology, also builds capacity for dermatology in sub-Saharan Africa via an advanced and formalized dermatology training center (Regional Dermatology Training Center) in Tanzania that specifically addresses localized diseases and populations in a culturally relevant environment. The *International Journal of Dermatology* (of the ISD) and more recently the *JAAD International* journal (a companion publication to the *Journal of the American Academy of Dermatology*) have been an important instrument for highlighting dermatologic manifestations on a global level, especially from countries that are otherwise underrepresented in other peer-reviewed publications.

CONCLUSION

Globalism is neither inherently good nor bad, but it is consequential and directly impacts patients afflicted by skin disease. It can be exploitive and discriminatory as evidenced by myriad historical events and precedents that have culminated in systematized healthcare disparities. Alternatively, understanding and promoting global aspects of dermatology can be an opportunity for unifying and enlightening both practitioners and patients through the collective sharing of experiences and expertise from around the world as a manifestation of dermodiversity.

REFERENCES

1. Fennig CD, Simons GF, Lewis MP. Ethnologue 18ed. SIL International; 2015.
2. Jablonski NG. The evolution of human skin and skin color. *Annu Rev Anthropol.* 2004;33(1):585-623.
3. Ly BCK, Dyer EB, Feig JL, Chien AL, Del Bino S. Research techniques made simple: cutaneous colorimetry: a reliable technique for objective skin color measurement. *J Invest Dermatol.* 2020;140(1):3-12.e1.
4. McKesey J, Berger TG, Lim HW, McMichael AJ, Torres A, Pandya AG. Cultural competence for the 21st century dermatologist practicing in the United States. *J Am Acad Dermatol.* 2017;77(6):1159-1169.
5. Taylor SC, Heath C. Cultural competence and unique concerns in patients with ethnic skin. *J Drugs Dermatol JDD.* 2012;11(4):460-465.
6. El-Banna G, Rezaei SJ, Chang M, Merrell SB, Bailey EE, Kibbi N. Perceptions of US-Based Muslim Patients of Their Dermatology Care. *JAMA Dermatol.* 2024;160(1):45-53.
7. Rehman R, Chabaan A, Hamzavi I, Fahs F, Mohammad TF. The etiquette of hijab: recommendations to improve care in dermatology clinics. *Br J Dermatol.* 2022;186(1):176-177.
8. The Qur'an 2:173 (Translation by A. Bewley, The Noble Qur'an : A New Rendering of its Meaning in English. London, UK: Ta-Ha Publishers, 2016.
9. Alexis AF, Barbosa VH, eds. *Skin of Color: A Practical Guide to Dermatologic Diagnosis and Treatment.* Springer; 2013.
10. Brilliant MH. Albinism in Africa: a medical and social emergency. *Int Health.* 2015;7(4):223-225.
11. Nguyen MQ, Hsu PW, Dinh TA. Asian blepharoplasty. *Semin Plast Surg.* 2009;23(3):185-197.
12. Fakhro A, Yim HW, Kim YK, Nguyen AH. The evolution of looks and expectations of Asian eyelid and eye appearance. *Semin Plast Surg.* 2015;29(3): 135-144.
13. Dimitrov D, Kroumpouzos G. Beauty perception: a historical and contemporary review. *Clin Dermatol.* 2023;41(1):33-40.
14. Gorbatenko-Roth K, Prose N, Kundu RV, Patterson S. Assessment of black patients' perception of their dermatology care. *JAMA Dermatol.* 2019;155(10):1129-1134.
15. Kumar S, Goyal A, Gupta YK. Abuse of topical corticosteroids in India: Concerns and the way forward. *J Pharmacol Pharmacother.* 2016;7(1):1-5.
16. Vashi NA, Patzelt N, Wirya S, Maymone MBC, Kundu RV. Dermatoses caused by cultural practices: cosmetic cultural practices. *J Am Acad Dermatol.* 2018;79(1):19-30.
17. Budair FM. Dermatoses due to Arabic cultural and traditional practices. *Indian J Dermatol Venereol Leprol.* 2019;85(5):448-454.
18. de Troya-Martín M, Rodríguez-Martínez A, Rivas-Ruiz F, Subert A, Arellano-Mendoza MI, Calzavara-Pinton P, de Gálvez MV, Gilaberte Y, Goh CL, Lim HW, Schalka S, Wolf P, González S. Personalized Photoprotection: Expert Consensus and Recommendations From a Delphi Study Among Dermatologists. *Photodermatol Photoimmunol Photomed.* 2025 Jan;41(1):e70001. doi: 10.1111/phpp.70001. PMID:39868505;PMCID:PMC11771696.
19. Ng W, Ikeda S. Use of sun-protective items by Japanese pedestrians: a cross-sectional observational study. *Arch Dermatol.* 2011;147(10):1167-1170.
20. Ono K, Viet CT, Ye Y, et al. Cutaneous pigmentation modulates skin sensitivity via tyrosinase-dependent dopaminergic signalling. *Sci Rep.* 2017;7(1):9181.
21. Passeron T, Lim HW, Goh CL, et al. Photoprotection according to skin phototype and dermatoses: practical recommendations from an expert panel. *J Eur Acad Dermatol Venereol.* 2021;35(7):1460-1469.
22. Rifkin RF, d'Errico F, Dayet-Boulliot L, Summers B. Assessing the photoprotective effects of red ochre on human skin by in vitro laboratory experiments. *South Afr J Sci.* 2015;111(3/4):1-8.
23. Tzachor A, Richards CE, Gudoshava M, et al. How to reduce Africa's undue exposure to climate risks. *Nature.* 2023;620(7974):488-491.
24. United Nations. Indigenous peoples. United Nations. https://www.un.org/en/fight-racism/vulnerable-groups/indigenous-peoples. Accessed December 21, 2023.
25. Austen I. 'Horrible history': mass grave of indigenous children reported in Canada. The New York Times. https://www.nytimes.com/2021/05/28/world/canada/kamloops-mass-grave-residential-schools.html. Published May 28, 2021. Accessed December 21, 2023.
26. UN General Assembly. United Nations declaration on the rights of indigenous peoples: resolution adopted by the General Assembly. https://www.refworld.org/legal/resolution/unga/2007/en/49353. Accessed May 20, 2025.
27. Valbuena MC, Muvdi S, Lim HW. Actinic prurigo. *Dermatol Clin.* 2014;32(3):335-344, viii.
28. Asiniwasis RN, Heck E, Amir Ali A, Ogunyemi B, Hardin J. Atopic dermatitis and skin infections are a poorly documented crisis in Canada's Indigenous pediatric population: it's time to start the conversation. *Pediatr Dermatol.* 2021;38 Suppl 2:188-189.
29. Bowen AC, Mahé A, Hay RJ, et al. The global epidemiology of impetigo: a systematic review of the population prevalence of impetigo and pyoderma. *PloS One.* 2015;10(8):e0136789.
30. Sethi S, Ali A, Ju X, Antonsson A, Logan R, Jamieson L. An update on Heck's disease-a systematic review. *J Public Health Oxf Engl.* 2022;44(2):269-285.
31. Elhage KG, Davis MS, Hakimi M, et al. Ethnoracial representation in hidradenitis suppurativa clinical trials. *Arch Dermatol Res.* 2023;315(6):1793-1796.
32. White JML, Lui H, Chute CG, Jakob R, Chalmers RJG. The WHO ICD-11 classification of dermatological diseases: a new comprehensive online skin disease taxonomy designed by and for dermatologists. *Br J Dermatol.* 2022;186(1):178-179.
33. World Health Organization. (2025). Skin diseases as a global public health priority. Seventy-eighth World Health Assembly, Agenda item 13.4, WHA78.15, 27 May 2025. Available at: https://apps.who.int/gb/ebwha/pdf_files/WHA78/A78_R15-en.pdf (accessed August 22, 2025)

SECTION 3

Structure, Function, and Biology

CHAPTER 14

Biology of Keratinocytes

Yacine Sow
Christopher Wachuku
Susan C. Taylor

KEY POINTS

- Keratinocytes play an essential role in the skin's function of structure, protection, and immunomodulation.
- Keratinocytes contribute to stratum corneum structure, lipids, and melanin dispersion with differences demonstrated in populations with skin of color.
- Differences of keratinocyte interactions with melanocytes and fibroblasts may account for increased prevalence of keloids and variety of pigmentary disorders among individuals with skin of color.

Keratinocytes are derived from the ectoderm and can be distinguished from melanocytes and Langerhans cells by their larger size, ample cytoplasm, and intercellular bridges [**Figure 14-1**].[1] They are the most abundant cell within the epidermis—making up greater than 90% of the population of cells.[1] Hemidesmosomes anchor keratinocytes to the basement membrane, while desmosomes anchor keratinocytes to each other. Present in all four layers of the epidermis, keratinocytes proliferate and differentiate in response to inflammation, injury, or neoplasia, thus playing an essential role in protection, structure, and immunomodulation. This functional epidermal barrier protects internal organs against environmental damage by ultraviolet (UV) radiation, heat, water loss, and microbial organisms.

KERATINOCYTE DIFFERENTIATION

Keratinocytes proliferate in the basal layer of the epidermis and then undergo gradual differentiation. During this process, the cell morphology changes and keratinocytes begin to produce keratin, cytokines, growth factors, and interleukin factors.[2] The differentiation process is critical for epidermal stratification and the formation of the stratum corneum. Differentiation involves a series of complex processes that yield gradual changes in keratinocyte characteristics and function. Keratinocytes withdraw from the cell cycle, initiate expression of differentiation markers, and move suprabasally as they become components of the stratum spinosum, stratum granulosum, and eventually corneocytes in the stratum corneum [**Figure 14-2**].[2,3] Cell cycle withdraw describes the end of replication that occurs during the terminal differentiation of keratinocytes, while in the basal layer of the epidermis.[3]

Keratinocytes in the stratum basale are arranged in a single layer along the basement membrane.[1,2] They contain dark-staining round to oval nuclei, and the cytoplasm is more basophilic compared to the adjacent keratinocytes in the stratum spinosum. Keratinocytes in the stratum basale are connected to other nearby keratinocytes by intercellular bridges formed by desmosomes and to the basement membrane by hemidesmosomes.[1] In the stratum spinosum, keratinocytes adhere to other keratinocytes via desmosomes. Compared to the stratum spinosum, keratinocytes in the stratum granulosum are flatter, more irregular in shape and have deeply basophilic keratohyalin granules. Keratinocytes in this layer release Odland bodies, lamellar granules, and keratinosomes, which all create a water permeability barrier and facilitate cell adhesion in the stratum corneum.[1] As keratinocytes differentiate, mature, and migrate upward to the stratum corneum, the nucleus and other organelles dissolve.[2] In the stratum corneum, keratinocytes are completely keratinized and have no nuclei.[1,2] Desmosomes also begin to disappear and become nonfunctional in this layer. Enzymes in the upper stratum corneum break down the components of lamellar granules that function in facilitating cell adhesion, resulting in the desquamation of the uppermost cells.[1] Corneocytes are keratinocytes that have fully differentiated and lost their nucleus and cytoplasmic organelles. Corneocytes will eventually desquamate and shed off as new ones come in.[1,2] In humans, it is estimated that keratinocytes turn over from stem cells to desquamation every 40 to 65 days.[2]

Filaggrin is an intermediate filament-associated protein that aids in keratinocyte differentiation. One study found that cell lines expressing filaggrin exhibited increased sensitivity to apoptotic stimuli. Yet, filaggrin expression alone was insufficient to induce apoptosis in keratinocytes.[4] Thus, filaggrin primes cells for apoptosis due to its keratin binding ability. Because filaggrin is expressed where keratinocytes are in transition between nucleated granular and anucleate cornified layers, it is thought that filaggrin aids in the terminal differentiation process.[4]

Studies have investigated the differences of thickness, density, and compactness of the stratum corneum in patients with skin of color and White individuals. Among White and Black individuals, thickness of the stratum corneum is thought to be similar.[5] Yet, a comparative study

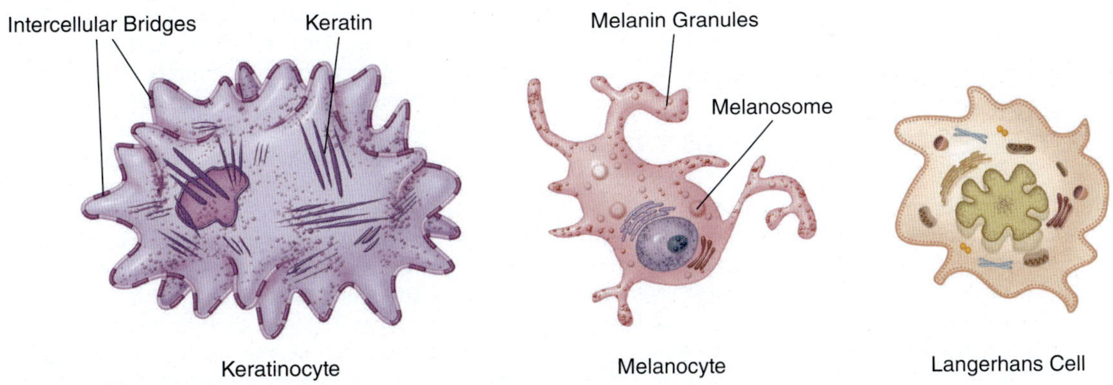

FIGURE 14-1. Three types of cells in the epidermis. Keratinocytes can be distinguished from melanocytes and Langerhans cells in the epidermis by their larger size, intercellular bridges, and ample cytoplasm. (Illustration provided by Kenya Thrasher.)

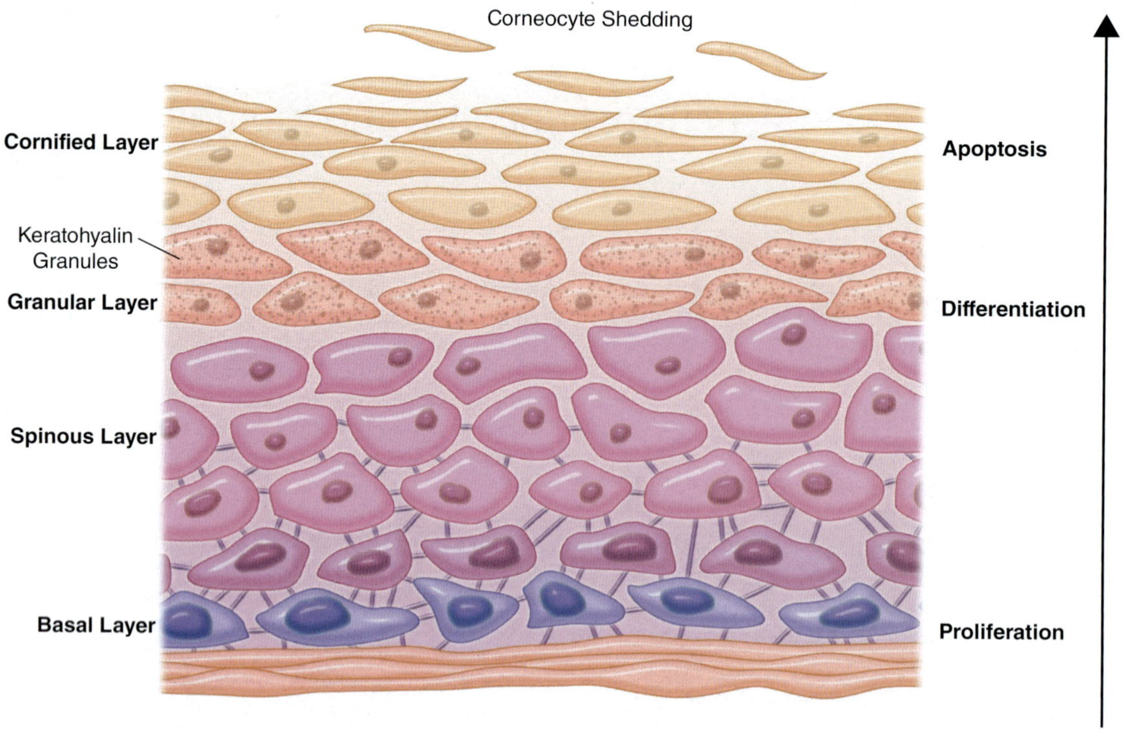

FIGURE 14-2. Keratinocyte differentiation process. Stratified epidermis consists of multiple layers of epidermal keratinocytes characterized by increasing advancement of cell differentiation. Cells undergo extensive nuclear, organelle, and molecular alterations as they gradually move to the upper layers. (Illustration provided by Kenya Thrasher.)

investigating the number of tape strips required to completely remove the stratum corneum (a measure of the number of layers of the stratum corneum) demonstrated a greater variability in tape strippings in Black subjects compared to White subjects. Black participants required a higher number of tapes strippings than White participants.[5] Light microscopy findings also demonstrated a greater average number of stratum corneum layers in the skin of Black individuals compared with the skin of their White counterparts.[5] This led to the conclusion that since thickness was equal in both groups, the stratum corneum in the skin of Black individuals is more cohesive and compact.[5] This observation was confirmed when comparing individuals with skin phototypes V and VI with those of phototypes II and III.[6] Subjects with darker skin phototypes required more tape strippings to disrupt the epidermal barrier.[6] Yet, they found no statistically significant differences in the number of strippings between White and Asian subjects.[6] Although these data led investigators to conclude that more cornified compact cell layers in individuals with darker skin could display more efficient epidermal barrier function and faster recovery from barrier damage, it must be taken into consideration that they rely on only two studies published over a quarter century ago.[6] Hence, more robust contemporary studies must be performed to validate these data to determine if structural epidermal differences indeed exist related to skin phototype and/or race.

KERATINOCYTE STRUCTURAL PROTEINS & FUNCTIONAL INTERACTIONS

KERATIN

Keratin is a key protein that makes up the structural components of hair, nails, and skin. Keratinocytes express a specific set of type I and type II keratins that serve as major contributors to their mechanical properties.[7] Keratins are the major components of the epithelial cytoskeleton and play a vital role in mechanical integrity at the cellular and tissue level.[1,7] Keratins account for up to 80% of the protein in differentiated keratinocytes and are arranged in tonofilaments that provide internal cellular structure.[1,7] Keratin filaments are believed to strengthen epithelial cells against various types of mechanical stress (eg, indentation, strain, and local deformation).[7] One study examined the structure and function of keratinocytes that lacked keratins to investigate this hypothesis. The study found a substantial softening of keratin deficient keratinocytes.[7] On reexpression of the basal epidermal keratin pair, the mechanical properties were restored, indicating that expression of a single keratin pair is sufficient for almost complete reconstitution of their mechanical properties.[7] Removing keratin pairs also demonstrated that elasticity, effective spring constant, and cell viscosity are significantly affected by keratins, leading to softened, less viscous cells in their absence.[7] Another study demonstrated the importance of an intact keratin network for mechanical integrity and barrier function.[8] In keratin deficient cells, there was an increased wound area and an inefficient overall wound closure. The loss of the keratin network led to impaired, fragmented cell-cell junctions and triggered a profound change in the overall cellular cytoskeletal architecture.[8] Keratin filaments thus impact cytoarchitecture and grant epithelial cells their mechanical resilience and ability to withstand various forms of stress.[9]

LIPIDS

Lipids are synthesized in the keratinocytes during epidermal differentiation and then extruded into the extracellular domains, forming lipid-enriched extracellular layers. Epidermal lipids play roles in cell structure, growth and differentiation, cohesion, and desquamation, and in the formation and function of a permeability barrier. Lipids present in the epidermis include phospholipids, ceramides, cholesterol, cholesterol esters, cholesterol sulfate, triglycerides, and fatty acids [**Figure 14-3**].[10,11] The phospholipids are major structural components of keratinocytes' plasma membrane and membranous organelles.[11] Vesicles release lipids that spread out over the cell surface and waterproof the epidermal layer.[10,11] This epidermal water barrier prevents water loss and dehydration. Lipids in the stratum corneum are composed primarily of ceramides, cholesterol, cholesterol esters, and fatty acids, which prevent desiccation and limit the penetration of various noxious environmental agents.[10]

Investigators have reported that the composition of epidermal lipids vary between racial groups, with the lowest ceramide level found in individuals of African descent,[12] followed by Whites. Asians had the highest ceramide level.[13] Ceramide levels are inversely correlated with transepidermal water loss.[12,13] This suggests that darker skin has poor water

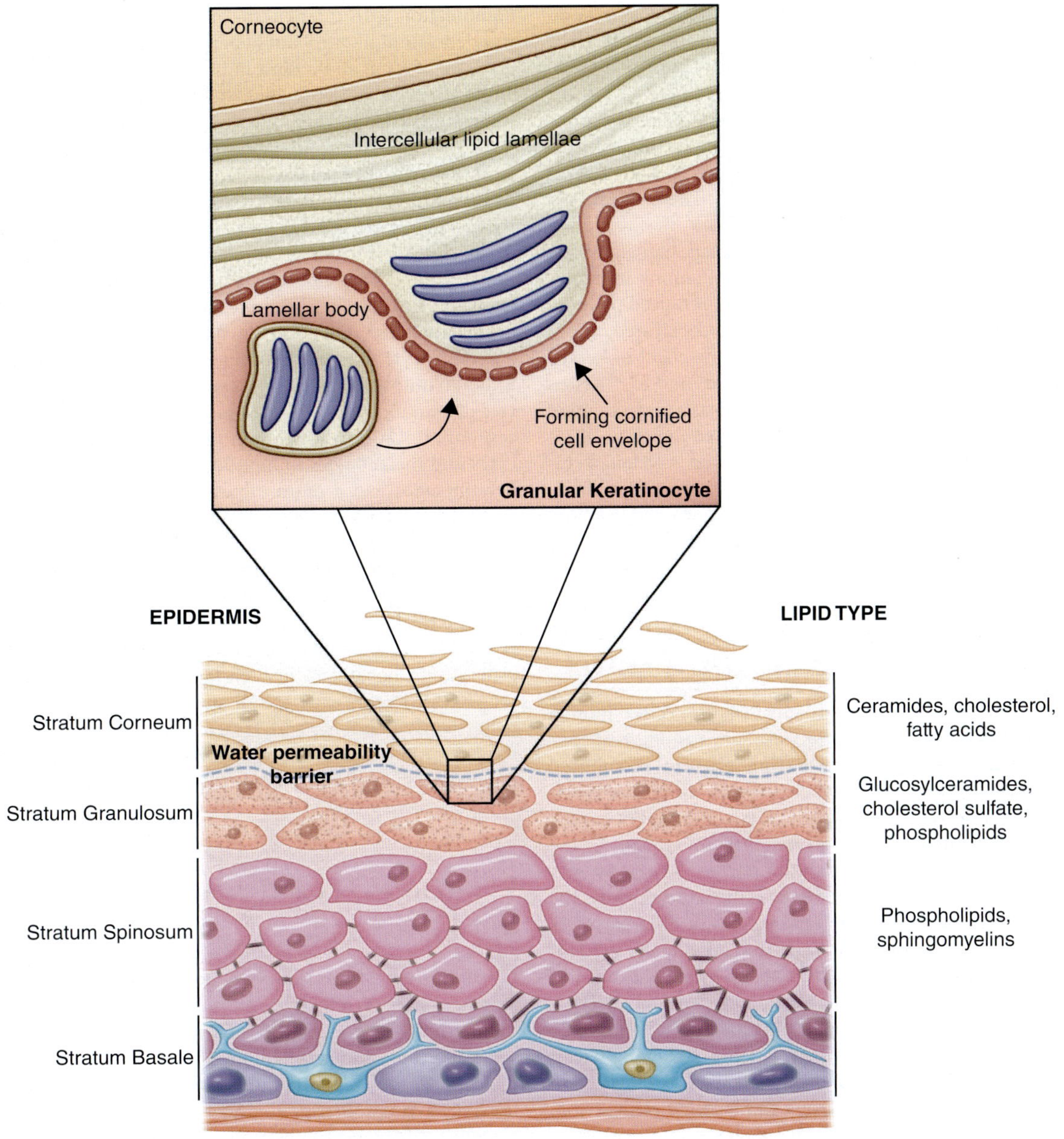

FIGURE 14-3. Main lipid components of the epidermis. Main lipid components in various layers of the epidermis. Lamellar bodies are secreted from keratinocytes, resulting in the formation of the water permeability barrier. (Illustration provided by Kenya Thrasher. Adapted from Vietri Rudan M, Watt FM. Mammalian epidermis: a compendium of lipid functionality. *Front Physiol.* 2022;12:804-824.)

retention capacity and the highest evaporative water loss.[6] Ceramide levels and cohesion in the uppermost stratum corneum layers were similar in the skin of White and East Asian individuals.[13] Xerosis and scaliness among individuals of African descent may be attributed to low ceramide levels, larger corneocyte size, and greater corneocyte density, suggesting a slower desquamation rate.[12] Qualitative and quantitative changes in these lipids, specifically reduced ceramide levels, have resulted in impaired barrier function and water retention capacity and have been shown to be a characteristic of dry skin, especially in patients with atopic dermatitis.[14] The level of ceramides appears to influence cellular cohesion and thus may influence the amount of scaliness.

ANTIMICROBIAL PEPTIDES

Cathelicidin is an antimicrobial peptide produced constitutively by neutrophils and is inducible in keratinocytes in response to infection.[15] Keratinocyte cathelicidin contributes to the innate immune defense of skin against bacterial pathogens.[15] A study aimed to evaluate the potential contribution of keratinocyte cathelicidin to keratinocyte antimicrobial activity demonstrated that cathelicidin-deficient mice were more susceptible to group A streptococcus infection compared to mice with intact cathelicidin.[15] Keratinocytes isolated in culture and found to inhibit the growth of *Staphylococcus aureus* were partially dependent on their ability to synthesize and activate cathelicidin. Cathelicidin predominantly resides in granules of the superficial epidermis and partially localizes in lamellar bodies. Lamellar bodies may act as storage sites for cathelicidin, which offers a potential mechanism for extracellular secretion upon injury or during keratinocyte differentiation and stratum corneum formation.[16] The clinical consequence of defective antimicrobial peptide production by keratinocytes is evident in patients with atopic dermatitis.[15,16] Patients with atopic dermatitis are relatively deficient in cathelicidin, which may explain the increased susceptibility to bacterial and viral infection of involved skin.[15]

FIBROBLASTS

In healthy skin, keratinocytes maintain skin homeostasis through active crosstalk with fibroblasts.[17] Fibroblasts allow deposition and resorption of the extracellular matrix (ECM), which is continually renewed under homeostatic conditions.[17] Enhanced ECM deposition is an essential part of the reparative process in damaged tissues. The traumatic loss of keratinocytes and the subsequent reepithelialization process are spatially and chronologically timed to regulate fibroblast activation and ECM deposition.[17] Keratinocyte survival was reported to be increased in the presence of fibroblasts secondary to reduced apoptosis, reduced expression of Bcl2, and enhanced expression of p53.[17] Keratinocyte proliferation, adhesion, cadherin expression, and keratinocyte differentiation were also enhanced in the presence of fibroblasts.[17] These effects are mainly mediated by keratinocyte growth factor (KGF).

The crosstalk between keratinocytes and fibroblasts has also been studied in keloids, a condition that is more prevalent among individuals with skin of color. Keloid cells were obtained from removed patients' tissue, keratinocytes and fibroblasts were isolated and cultured, and a transwell co-culture system was used to investigate the effect of keratinocytes on collagen production using a "scar-in-a-jar" model.[18] When keloid keratinocytes were added to normal skin fibroblasts, expression of collagen was significantly upregulated; but when added to keloid fibroblasts, collagen I production was significantly reduced.[18] Keloid keratinocytes appear to decrease collagen production by keloid fibroblasts, suggesting that both keratinocytes and fibroblasts are disrupted in keloid pathogenesis. More specifically, the synthesis of type I collagen (COL1A) in fibroblasts is at least partly regulated by soluble factors released by keratinocytes, and these pathways are altered in keloid disease.[18]

KERATINOCYTE DIFFERENCES IN SKIN OF COLOR

Skin color is one of the most visually distinctive features of the human race. To assess the mechanisms of skin color variation, Yoshida et al constructed human skin substitutes (HSS) by grafting mixtures of cultured keratinocytes and melanocytes from a combination of donor skin types, together with light skin-derived fibroblasts.[19] HHS composed of keratinocytes acquired from dark skin had a greater melanin content in the epidermis and a significantly increased maturation stage of melanosomes compared to keratinocytes acquired from light skin.[19] Additionally, the patterns of melanosome distribution in keratinocytes of different races varied. Melanosomes are predominantly dispersed individually in keratinocytes derived from dark skin while distributed in membrane clusters in those acquired from light skin.[19,20] The size and shape of melanosomes also vary in skin of differing colors. Individuals with lighter skin typically show small, spherical melanosomes, whereas individuals with darker skin have larger elliptical melanosomes dispersed singly, and those with golden-brown skin typically have a combination of the two.[21] Genetic expression of melanogenic cytokines and melanin synthesis-related proteins (ie, microphthalmia-associated transcription factor, tyrosinase, pmel-17, endothelin-1, proopiomelanocortin, stem cell factor) were higher in the darker skin-derived keratinocytes.[19] It was previously demonstrated that the amount of tyrosinase does not differ between Black and White individuals; however, this same study suggests that the genetic expression for tyrosinase was elevated in human skin substitutes composed of keratinocytes derived from darker skin compared to those derived from lighter skin.[19] Ultimately, this in vivo xenograft system demonstrated that keratinocytes play a significant role in skin color determination by producing cytokines involved in melanogenesis and regulating the melanosome pattern of distribution in the epidermis.[19]

Studies investigating physiological factors that regulate skin pigmentation found one receptor expressed on keratinocytes that seems to be closely involved with melanosome transfer: a seven transmembrane G-protein coupled receptor protease (proteinase) activated receptor-2 (PAR-2) that regulates phagocytosis in keratinocytes.[22] PAR-2's role in melanosome transfer explains why individuals with darker skin exhibit a higher expression of PAR-2 compared to those with lighter skin.[22] Additionally, the transcription factor Foxn1/Whn/Hfh11 expressed in keratinocytes is identified as a regulator of keratinocyte growth and differentiation and of melanocyte recruitment and induction of pigmentation in the skin via basic fibroblast growth factor (bFGF) production.[23] Increasing evidence has demonstrated the role of keratinocytes in skin pigmentation via the keratinocyte growth factor (KGF) alone or in combination with interleukin-1α.[24,25] This growth factor induces melanin deposition in vitro and hyperpigmented lesions in vivo. A moderate increase of KGF and a high induction of its receptor has been demonstrated in solar lentigo lesions, suggesting its involvement in the onset of hyperpigmented spots.[24]

Human epidermal melanocytes play a role in protecting the skin from the effects of solar UV radiation and other environmental toxins or inflammatory agents. An elaborate network of paracrine factors synthesized by epidermal keratinocytes and dermal fibroblasts regulate the survival of melanocytes.[26] While melanocytes protect epidermal keratinocytes and dermal fibroblasts from the damaging effects of solar radiation, keratinocytes and dermal fibroblasts regulate the stress response of melanocytes.[26] For instance, basic fibroblast growth factor (bFGF) is a keratinocyte-derived paracrine factor that stimulates melanocytes to undergo mitosis by activating a specific tyrosinase kinase receptor.[27] The role of keratinocytes is further supported by a study that investigated the response to UVB irradiation in melanocytes co-cultured with keratinocytes and melanocytes in monoculture.[28] Melanocytes co-cultured with keratinocytes had a more robust increase in pigmentation, suggesting that the tanning response to UVB is modulated by keratinocyte-derived paracrine factors. Disruption of the paracrine network results in pigmentary disorders due to abnormal regulation of melanin synthesis and compromise of melanocyte survival or genomic stability.[25,26] Dysregulation of paracrine factors such as alpha- melanocyte stimulating hormone (α-MSH), Dickkopf-related protein 1 (DKK1), endothelin-1 (End-1), eicosanoids, hepatocyte growth factor (HGF), keratinocyte growth factor (KGF), nitric oxide (NO), stem cell factor (SCF), tumor necrosis factor-alpha (TNF-α), and secreted frizzled-related protein 2 (sFRPs) has been implicated in multiple pigmentary disorders including hyperpigmentation, melasma, post-inflammatory hyperpigmentation, solar lentigines, and vitiligo.[23-27]

KERATINOCYTE PATHOLOGY

ACNE

Desquamation of keratinocytes, increase in circulating androgens, and follicular hyperkeratosis create an environment within the pilosebaceous unit that is favorable for *Cutibacterium acnes* colonization.[29] *C. acnes* secretes various inflammatory molecules and chemotactic factors that initiate the local inflammatory response and possibly induce keratinocyte hyperproliferation.[29] Several early reports provide histological evidence for hyperproliferation of keratinocytes in acne lesions, demonstrating a higher expression of Ki67 (a proliferation marker protein) and certain keratins. One study looked at the expression of keratinocyte proliferation, mitosis, and apoptosis markers among individuals with acne vulgaris.[30] Cell proliferation rate, measured by the expression of Ki67 and phosphor-histone H3, was identical between the acne and control groups.[30] Interestingly, their findings demonstrated the absence of increased keratinocyte proliferation in acne vulgaris.[30] Therefore, alternative mechanisms may be responsible for infundibular hyperkeratinization in acne pathogenesis.[30]

Traditionally, acne was treated as a homogenous disease across all skin types. Yet, Perkins et al revealed that acne has a difference in presentation and sequelae among various racial and ethnic groups.[31] Investigators found that Black women had larger, more visible pores,[31] which supports another study's findings that individuals of African descent have greater gland pore size and sebaceous glands.[32] Some factors that play a role in acne pathogenesis and clinical presentation exhibit racial differences. For instance, there is a positive correlation between sebum secretion and acne severity;[31] investigators reported 60% to 70% greater lipid content in the hair follicles of Blacks compared to White individuals.[32] Even though Hispanics have a similar acne prevalence to African Americans, there have been no pathogenetic or histological studies on the quality of acne seen in this ethnicity. East Indian women in the Perkins et al study were less likely to have acne, which is consistent with another recent study from India demonstrating a low prevalence of

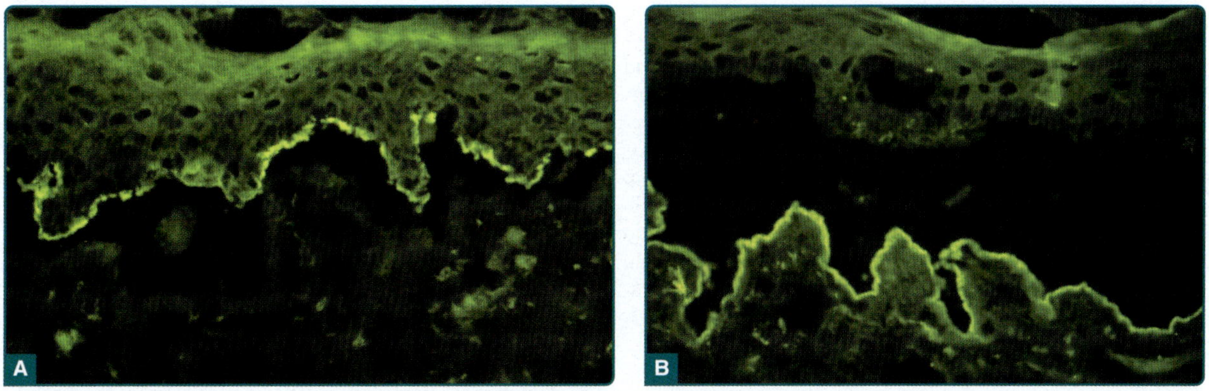

FIGURE 14-4. Bullous pemphigoid. **(A)** Indirect immunofluorescence demonstrating IgG antibodies from bullous pemphigoid serum binding to the epidermal side (roof) of the artificial blister (BP180 and BP230 of hemidesmosomes). **(B)** IgG antibodies from epidermolysis bullosa acquisita (EBA) serum binds to the floor of the split (collagen VII of anchoring fibers). (Reproduced with permission from Kang S, Amagai M, Bruckner AL, et al, eds. *Fitzpatrick's Dermatology.* 9th ed. New York, NY: McGraw Hill; 2019, Figure 54-6.)

acne vulgaris.[31] Acne sequelae, such as dyspigmentation and scarring, are more prevalent among African American individuals compared to any other groups. A survey of African American women with acne vulgaris revealed that postinflammatory hyperpigmentation was a more common complaint than acne itself when seeking dermatologic care.[33] Previously, it was remarked that papulopustular acne was far more common among White patients compared to African American patients. Yet, another study found that African American patients had marked histological inflammation in comedonal acne lesions, despite no signs of inflammation on clinical exam.[34] Specifically, histological findings showed extensive inflammation surrounding papules and pustules and away from the lesion, foreign body granulomas with giant cells, and epidermal melanin granules and melanophages extending into the dermis in areas of hyperpigmentation.[34] It is hypothesized that a heightened inflammatory response may explain why mild to moderate acne in individuals of African descent results in scarring and hyperpigmentation.[34]

AUTOIMMUNE BLISTERING DISORDERS

Pemphigus vulgaris and bullous pemphigoid are autoantibody-mediated blistering skin diseases. In pemphigus vulgaris, keratinocytes in the epidermis and mucous membranes lose cell-cell adhesion, while in bullous pemphigoid, the basal keratinocytes lose adhesion to the basement membrane. Bullous pemphigoid autoantibodies target hemidesmosome proteins within the dermal-epidermal junction, designated BP180 and BP230 [**Figure 14-4**].[35,36] Pemphigus vulgaris is caused by autoantibodies that target keratinocyte proteins, desmoglein 1 (Dsg 1), and desmoglein 3 (Dsg 3).[36] Desmogleins are transmembrane glycoproteins that are an integral part of desmosomes required for cell-to-cell adhesion. The binding of circulating immunoglobulin G (IgG) autoantibodies to intercellular adhesion molecules (ie, desmogleins) leads to the loss of keratinocyte-to-keratinocyte adhesion resulting in acantholysis.[36] Acantholysis clinically presents as bullae that are prone to rupture.

The causative factors of pemphigus vulgaris (PV) is unknown, but patients at risk have a genetic predisposition.[36] The occurrence of PV may be related to ethnicity and geographic location. Ashkenazi Jews have an increased incidence of PV,[36] while individuals living in India, Southeast Europe, and the Middle East are at greatest risk.[36] In Tunisia, PV is more common in women compared to men by a ratio of 4:1, whereas the global prevalence of PV is equal among men and women.[36] A case series of patients with skin of color with blistering skin disorders presented with more dramatic, long-lasting pigmentary sequelae, which may reflect the deeper level of blistering [**Figure 14-5**].[37] The typical therapeutic regimen for blistering disorders includes topical steroids. Potent corticosteroids can induce hypopigmentation, a side effect that is more apparent in darker skin phototypes.[37]

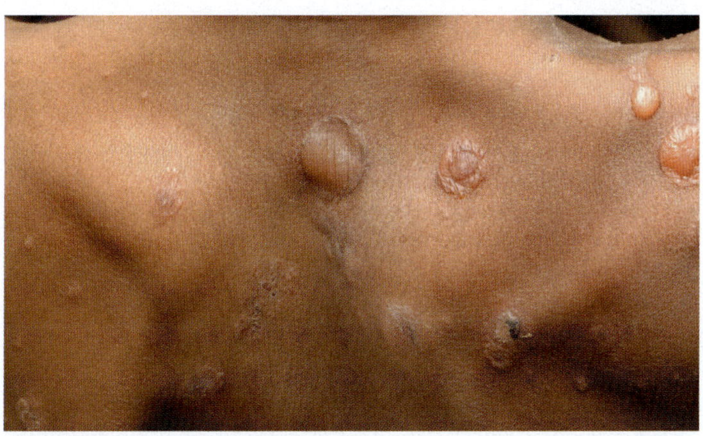

FIGURE 14-5. Pemphigus vulgaris lesions. (Source: Used with the permission from SCIENCE PHOTO LIBRARY/Science Source)

TABLE 14-1 Possible clinical implications in patients with skin of color based on epidermal differences [12,38,39]

Skin of color	Properties	Possible clinical implications
African descent	More compact cell layers	Superior barrier function, decreased penetration, more resistance to irritants, and faster barrier recovery
	Reduced ceramides	Increased transepidermal water loss and weaker epidermal barrier function.
	High maturation index[a]	Superior barrier function, improved recovery from stressors
	Less keratinocyte differentiation[b]	Increased scaliness
	Increased desquamation	Increased dry skin/ashiness
Asian descent	Less compact cell layers	Slower barrier recovery, weak barrier function
	Increased ceramides	Less dryness
	Low maturation index (East Asian)[a]	Weak barrier function, increased skin sensitivity
	High degree of differentiation[b]	Less scaliness

[a]Maturation index is a measure of the amount of cross-linking in the cornified envelope.

[b]Differentiation is a measure of the amount of proteolytic activity required for corneodesmosome degradation.

CONCLUSION

In summary, keratinocytes serve an important role in the structure and function of the epidermis. Keratinocytes form a barrier against environmental damage through production and interactions with structural proteins, enzymes, lipids, and antimicrobial peptides. The keratinocyte differentiation process develops the layers of the epidermis: stratum spinosum, stratum granulosum, and eventually corneocytes in the stratum corneum. Within the epidermis, keratinocytes interact with other cell types contributing to immunomodulation, wound healing, and pigmentation. Racial and skin phototype differences in the structure, function, and interactions of the keratinocytes have been documented. These differences, detailed in **Table 14-1**, have implications for clinical disease and treatment of skin of color.

REFERENCES

1. McManus LM, Mitchell RN. Skin: basic structure and function. In: *Pathobiology of Human Disease: A Dynamic Encyclopedia of Disease Mechanisms*. 2014.
2. Halprin KM. Epidermal "turnover time"–a re-examination. *Br J Dermatol.* 1972;86(1):14-19.
3. Albers KM, Greif F, Setzer RW, Taichman LB. Cell-cycle withdrawal in cultured keratinocytes. *Differ Res Biol Divers.* 1987;34(3):236-240.
4. Kuechle MK, Presland RB, Lewis SP, Fleckman P, Dale BA. Inducible expression of filaggrin increases keratinocyte susceptibility to apoptotic cell death. *Cell Death Differ.* 2000;7(6):566-573.
5. Weigand DA, Haygood C, Gaylor JR. Cell layers and density of Negro and Caucasian stratum corneum. *J Invest Dermatol.* 1974;62(6):563-568.
6. Reed JT, Ghadially R, Elias PM. Skin type, but neither race nor gender, influence epidermal permeability barrier function. *Arch Dermatol.* 1995;131(10):1134-1138.
7. Ramms L, Fabris G, Windoffer R, et al. Keratins as the main component for the mechanical integrity of keratinocytes. *Proc Natl Acad Sci USA.* 2013;110(46):18513-18518.
8. Karsch S, Büchau F, Magin TM, Janshoff A. An intact keratin network is crucial for mechanical integrity and barrier function in keratinocyte cell sheets. *Cell Mol Life Sci CMLS.* 2020;77(21):4397-4411.
9. Wang F, Zieman A, Coulombe PA. Skin Keratins. *Methods Enzymol.* 2016;568:303-350.
10. Wertz PW. Lipids and barrier function of the skin. *Acta Derm Venereol Suppl (Stockh).* 2000;208:7-11.
11. Vietri Rudan M, Watt FM. Mammalian epidermis: a compendium of lipid functionality. *Front Physiol.* 2021;12:804824.
12. Muizzuddin N, Hellemans L, Van Overloop L, Corstjens H, Declercq L, Maes D. Structural and functional differences in barrier properties of African American, Caucasian and East Asian skin. *J Dermatol Sci.* 2010;59(2):123-128.
13. Jungersted JM, Høgh JK, Hellgren LI, Jemec GBE, Agner T. Ethnicity and stratum corneum ceramides. *Br J Dermatol.* 2010;163(6):1169-1173.
14. Imokawa G, Abe A, Jin K, Higaki Y, Kawashima M, Hidano A. Decreased level of ceramides in stratum corneum of atopic dermatitis: an etiologic factor in atopic dry skin? *J Invest Dermatol.* 1991;96(4):523-526.
15. Braff MH, Zaiou M, Fierer J, Nizet V, Gallo RL. Keratinocyte production of cathelicidin provides direct activity against bacterial skin pathogens. *Infect Immun.* 2005;73(10):6771-6781.
16. Braff MH, Di Nardo A, Gallo RL. Keratinocytes store the antimicrobial peptide cathelicidin in lamellar bodies. *J Invest Dermatol.* 2005;124(2):394-400.
17. Russo B, Brembilla NC, Chizzolini C. Interplay between keratinocytes and fibroblasts: a systematic review providing a new angle for understanding skin fibrotic disorders. *Front Immunol.* 2020;11:648.
18. Alghamdi MA, Al-Eitan LN, Stevenson A, et al. Secreted factors from keloid keratinocytes modulate collagen deposition by fibroblasts from normal and fibrotic tissue: a pilot study. *Biomedicines.* 2020;8(7):E200.
19. Yoshida Y, Hachiya A, Sriwiriyanont P, et al. Functional analysis of keratinocytes in skin color using a human skin substitute model composed of cells derived from different skin pigmentation types. *FASEB J Off Publ Fed Am Soc Exp Biol.* 2007;21(11):2829-2839.
20. Thong HY, Jee SH, Sun CC, Boissy RE. The patterns of melanosome distribution in keratinocytes of human skin as one determining factor of skin colour. *Br J Dermatol.* 2003;149(3):498-505.
21. Reddy KK, Lenzy YM, Brown KL, Gilchrest BA. Racial considerations: skin of color. In: Goldsmith LA, Katz SI, Gilchrest BA, Paller AS, Leffell DJ, Wolff K, eds. *Fitzpatrick's Dermatology in General Medicine.* 8th ed. The McGraw Hill Companies ; 2012.
22. Babiarz-Magee L, Chen N, Seiberg M, Lin CB. The expression and activation of protease-activated receptor-2 correlate with skin color. *Pigment Cell Res.* 2004;17(3):241-251.
23. Yamaguchi Y, Hearing VJ. Physiological factors that regulate skin pigmentation. *BioFactors Oxf Engl.* 2009;35(2):193-199.
24. Cardinali G, Kovacs D, Picardo M. Mechanisms underlying post-inflammatory hyperpigmentation: lessons from solar lentigo. *Ann Dermatol Venereol.* 2012;139 Suppl 4:S148-S152.
25. Duval C, Chagnoleau C, Pouradier F, Sextius P, Condom E, Bernerd F. Human skin model containing melanocytes: essential role of keratinocyte growth factor for constitutive pigmentation-functional response to α-melanocyte stimulating hormone and forskolin. *Tissue Eng Part C Methods.* 2012;18(12):947-957.
26. Upadhyay PR, Ho T, Abdel-Malek ZA. Participation of keratinocyte- and fibroblast-derived factors in melanocyte homeostasis, the response to UV, and pigmentary disorders. *Pigment Cell Melanoma Res.* 2021;34(4):762-776.
27. Fajuyigbe D, Lwin SM, Diffey BL, et al. Melanin distribution in human epidermis affords localized protection against DNA photodamage and concurs with skin cancer incidence difference in extreme phototypes. *FASEB J Off Publ Fed Am Soc Exp Biol.* 2018;32(7):3700-3706.
28. Duval C, Régnier M, Schmidt R. Distinct melanogenic response of human melanocytes in mono-culture, in co-culture with keratinocytes and in reconstructed epidermis, to UV exposure. *Pigment Cell Res.* 2001;14(5):348-355.
29. Webster GF. The pathophysiology of acne. *Cutis.* 2005;76(2 Suppl):4-7.
30. Persson G, Johansson-Jänkänpää E, Ganceviciene R, et al. No evidence for follicular keratinocyte hyperproliferation in acne lesions as compared to autologous healthy hair follicles. *Exp Dermatol.* 2018;27(6):668-671.
31. Perkins AC, Cheng CE, Hillebrand GG, Miyamoto K, Kimball AB. Comparison of the epidemiology of acne vulgaris among Caucasian, Asian, Continental Indian and African American women. *J Eur Acad Dermatol Venereol JEADV.* 2011;25(9):1054-1060.
32. Rawlings AV. Ethnic skin types: are there differences in skin structure and function? *Int J Cosmet Sci.* 2006;28(2):79-93.
33. Taylor SC, Cook-Bolden F, Rahman Z, Strachan D. Acne vulgaris in skin of color. *J Am Acad Dermatol.* 2002;46(2 Suppl Understanding):S98-S106.
34. Halder RM, Holmes YC, Bridgeman-Shah S, Kligman A. A clinicohistopathological study of acne vulgaris in black females. Published online 1996.
35. Kasperkiewicz M, Ellebrecht CT, Takahashi H, et al. Pemphigus. *Nat Rev Dis Primer.* 2017;3:17026.
36. Ingold CJ, Khan MA. *Pemphigus Vulgaris.* In: *StatPearls.* StatPearls Publishing ; 2022. Accessed August 12, 2022. http://www.ncbi.nlm.nih.gov/books/NBK560860/.
37. Tamazian S, Simpson CL. Autoimmune bullous disease in skin of color: a case series. *JAAD Case Rep.* 2020;6(11):1173-1178.

CHAPTER 15

Biology of Melanocytes

Christopher Wachuku
Tiaranesha Jackson
Susan C. Taylor

KEY POINTS

- Melanocytes are complex cells responsible for producing melanin within specialized organelles called melanosomes.
- There are differences in size, distribution, and grouping of melanosomes and melanin that contribute to variations in skin color.
- Multiple other factors such as hormones, genetics, and environment can affect skin pigmentation.

MELANOCYTE BASICS

Melanocytes are complex cells that reside within the basal layer of the epidermis. Their primary function is the production of pheomelanin and eumelanin. Embryologically, melanocytes derive from neural crest

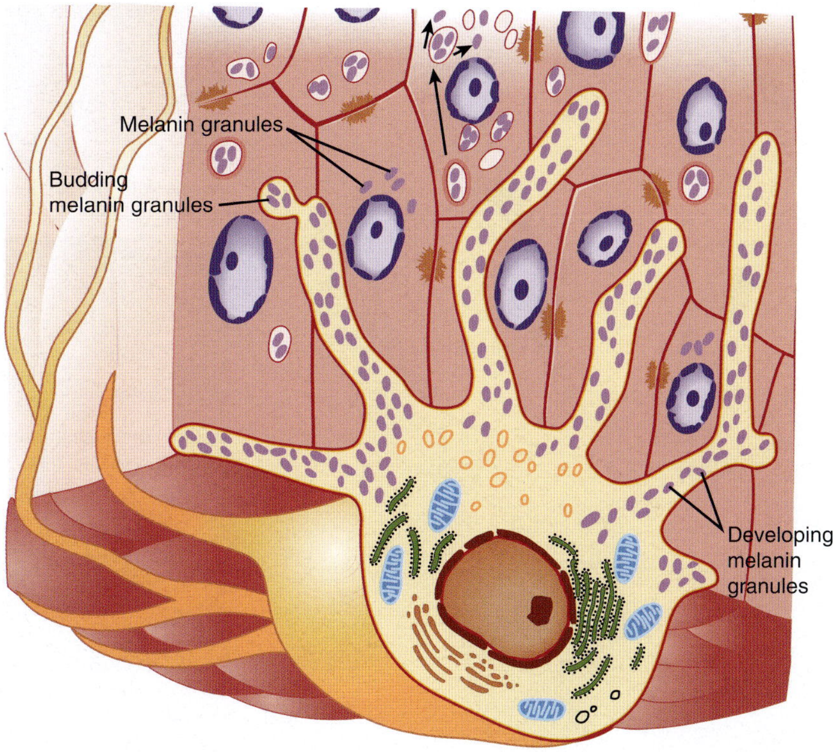

FIGURE 15-1. The melanocyte. The melanocyte resides in the stratum basale of the epidermis. Melanocytes produce melanosomes containing melanin granules that are distributed to surrounding keratinocytes through dendritic processes. (Reproduced with permission from Junqueira LC et al. *Basic Histology.* 10th ed. New York, McGraw-Hill; 2003.)

cells and arise from the neural tube.[1] Transient neural trunk cells migrate along the dorsolateral pathway, located in between the embryo somites and ectoderm, then differentiate into melanoblasts, and later into melanocytes.[2] Subsequently, the newly developed melanoblasts translocate to various structures including the stratum basal of the epidermis, hair matrix, outer root sheath of the hair follicles, various mucous membrane epithelia, leptomeninges, cochlea of the inner ear, and the uveal tract of the eye [**Figure 15-1**].

MELANOSOMES

STRUCTURE AND FUNCTION

Melanocyte contains melanosomes, the specialized organelle responsible for the storage and synthesis of melanin. The "epidermal melanin unit" is composed of one melanocyte connected by dendrites to approximately 36 keratinocytes.[3,4] It is the distribution of melanin to the surrounding keratinocytes that provides both the pigmentation of the skin as well as protection from the effects of UV radiation.

The melanosome is a lysosome-related organelle that undergoes four stages of development. Prior to the first stage, nascent melanosomes are assembled by the Golgi apparatus where they receive the necessary enzymes, including tyrosinase, the rate-limiting enzyme for melanogenesis, and other structural proteins for melanogenesis to occur.[5] Stage I melanosomes are nonpigmented, irregular fibrous structures with features of late endosomal multivesicular bodies.[6] During stage II, these fibers develop into elongated parallel arrays that can be seen on electronic microscopy.[6] Stage III marks the beginning of melanin deposition resulting in darkening and thickening of the fibers.[6] Stage IV melanosomes are mature and fully melanized [**Figure 15-2**].[6]

MELANOSOME TRANSFER

Melanosomes are transferred to surrounding keratinocytes through dendrites.[5,7] Before transfer to the keratinocytes, melanocytes initially transfer melanosomes from the site of formation in the center of the cell (the perinuclear area) to the tips of the dendrites.[7] Transportation of these organelles occurs along microtubules and is facilitated by Rab27a and motor proteins, such as kinesins.[8,9] Afterward, the melanosomes, via intercellular cell-to-cell transfer, are transferred to the keratinocytes.

There are four proposed models for the intercellular transfer of melanosomes into human keratinocytes that include the cytophagocytosis model, membrane fusion model, shedding-phagocytosis model, and the exocytosis-endocytosis model.[7,10] The cytophagocytosis model purports that keratinocytes phagocytize the melanosomes contained in the dendrites of the melanocyte.[7] In the membrane fusion model, a temporary conduit, formed by membranes of the melanocyte and keratinocyte, connects the cytoplasms of both cells allowing melanosome transfer.[7] In the shedding-phagocytosis model, the melanocyte sheds the melanosome, which the keratinocyte incorporates through phagocytosis.[7] Finally, in the exocytosis-endocytosis model, the content of the melanosomes is released by the melanocyte into the extracellular space through exocytosis with the subsequent incorporation of the released melanin into the keratinocyte via phagocytosis.[7] Various studies support each of the aforementioned theories; however, further investigation is required to elucidate the exact mechanism of melanosome-to-keratinocyte transfer [**Figure 15-3**].

MELANOSOME VARIATIONS

Variations in melanosome density, size, and distribution have implications regarding skin color [**Figure 15-4**]. The number of melanocytes across human skin colors are constant.[11] In individuals with light skin, early stage I and II melanosomes predominate. They are small, grouped together, and degraded faster in the stratum spinosum. However, in darker skin, stage III and late stage IV melanosomes predominate and they are larger, individually distributed, slowly degraded, and remain for longer periods within the stratum corneum. African Americans of lighter skin color have been found to have a combination of single, large, and sometimes aggregated melanosomes.[12] One study found a statistically significant increase in the size of an average melanosome in darkly pigmented skin compared to lightly pigmented skin.[13] The distribution of melanosomes in the epidermis varies by race with melanosomes limited to the stratum basale and absent in the layers of the upper epidermis

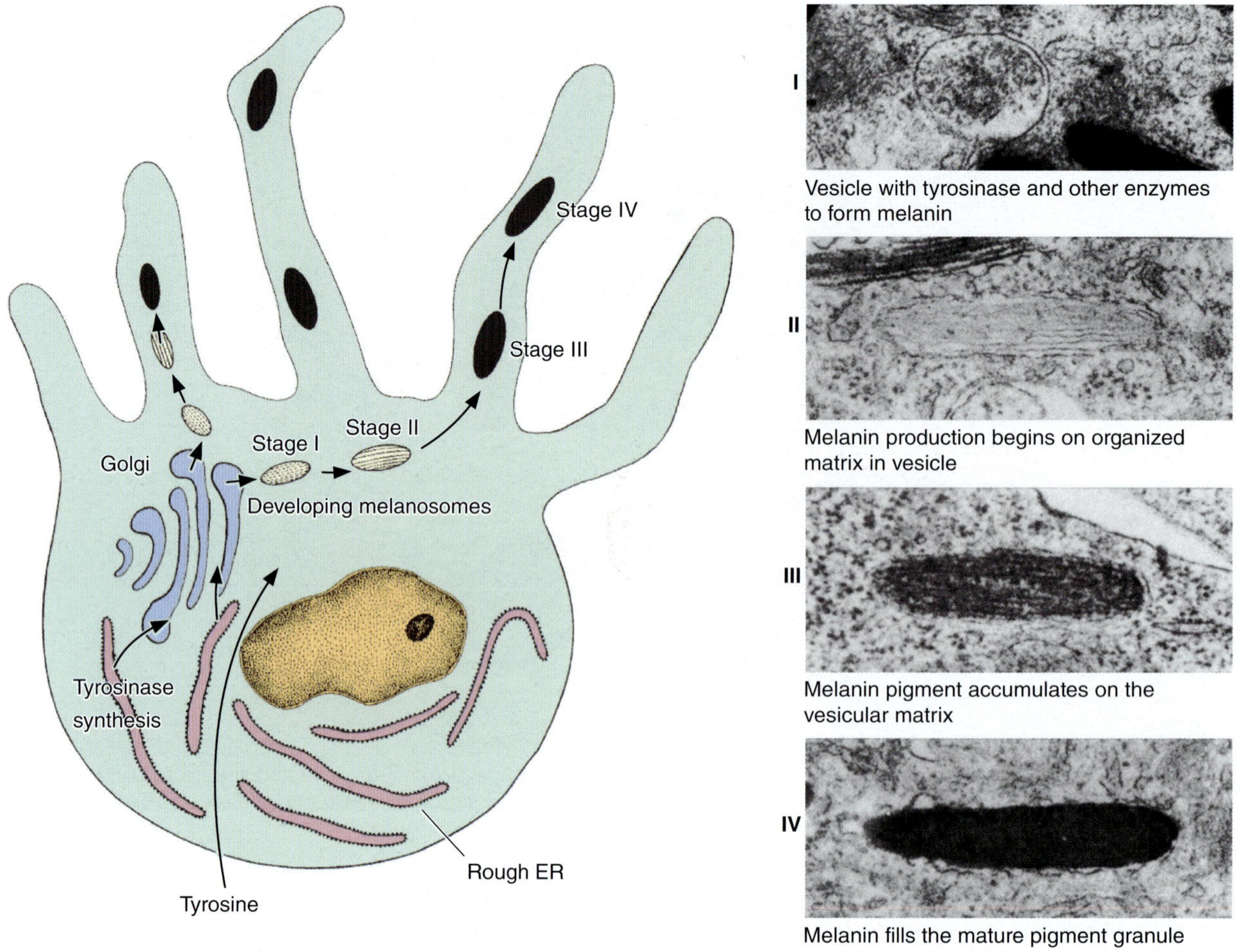

FIGURE 15-2. Melanosome stages I to IV. The four stages of melanosome maturation illustrated and described via electron microscopy. (Reproduced with permission from Mescher AL. *Junqueria's Basic Histology Text and Atlas*. 16th ed. New York, NY: McGraw Hill; 2021, Figure 18-7.)

in white individuals, as compared to melanosomes distributed throughout all epidermal layers in those of African descent.[14]

In addition, sun exposure may impact the distribution and groupings of melanosomes. It was shown that regardless of ethnicity, chronically photo-exposed skin showed a small, however consistent, increase in melanosome size.[13] In sun-exposed, deeply-tanned white skin, the distribution of melanosomes was found to be similar to that of those individuals with darker skin colors.[14,15] A study of tanned individuals of Thai descent supported this through the findings of dense clusters of melanosomes in the basal layer, dispersal of melanosomes throughout the epidermal layers, and increased pigmentation within the stratum corneum.[16] This supports the notion that prolonged sun exposure may result in melanosome organization similar to individuals of darker skin tones [**Table 15-1**].

MELANIN

The mechanism of melanin synthesis involves the tyrosinase-catalyzed conversion of tyrosine to dihydroxyphenylalanine (L-DOPA) to L-dopaquinone, both of which are rate-limiting steps.[6,20,21] The availability of cysteine during melanogenesis determines the subsequent synthesis of pheomelanin or eumelanin.[21,22] Cysteine is a required substrate for the synthesis of pheomelanin [**Figure 15-5**].[23] In general, pheomelanin-rich melanosomes are circular in shape, while eumelanin-rich melanosomes are oblong.[24] Eumelanin is brown-black in color, more abundant in darkly pigmented skin, and provides superior photoprotection through reduced transmission of light as compared to red-yellow pheomelanin, which is not photostable.[22,25] In addition to this, pheomelanin synthesis has been linked to increased reactive oxidant species (ROS). The synthesis of pheomelanin utilizes antioxidants, such as glutathione, to deliver cysteine. This leads to decreased glutathione stores, and as a result, less protection against ROS and DNA damage, leading to tumorigenesis.[26] Individuals with red hair have been associated with mutations in the melanocortin 1 receptor (*MC1R*) gene, leading to decreased eumelanin production and higher quantities of the less photoprotective pheomelanin.[24,27] Eumelanin aids in scattering and absorbing 50% to 75% of ultraviolet (UV) radiation, along with protecting against UV radiation-generated free radicals.[24] One study assessed the quality and composition of melanin in various skin colors (excluding Fitzpatrick type I skin). The investigators determined that in some light-skinned individuals, there is an increased rate of eumelanin turnover in keratinocytes due to increased degradation by lysosomal enzymes, hence photoprotection in these individuals is diminished.[24]

The quantity, density, and distribution of melanosomes and melanin impacting skin color also play a role in photoprotection and skin cancer occurrence. Melanin provides an endogenous form of protection from UV radiation.[28–31] It has been postulated that individuals with white skin are approximately 70 times more likely to develop skin cancer on sun-exposed areas.[32] This is supported by the epidemiological findings of skin cancers typically occurring in acral, nonphotoexposed areas within individuals of color.[32,33] One study assessing the differences between Black and White skin concluded that in Black skin melanin provides a sun protection factor (SPF) of 13.4 as compared to 3.4 in White skin.[30] Within individuals of color, the increased number of nonclustered, stage IV melanosomes are capable of absorbing more UV radiation than the small, clustered melanosomes within lighter skin-toned individuals.[30] The reduced proportion of melanosomes in the upper epidermal layers in individuals with lighter skin results in decreased photoprotection, thus increasing the likelihood

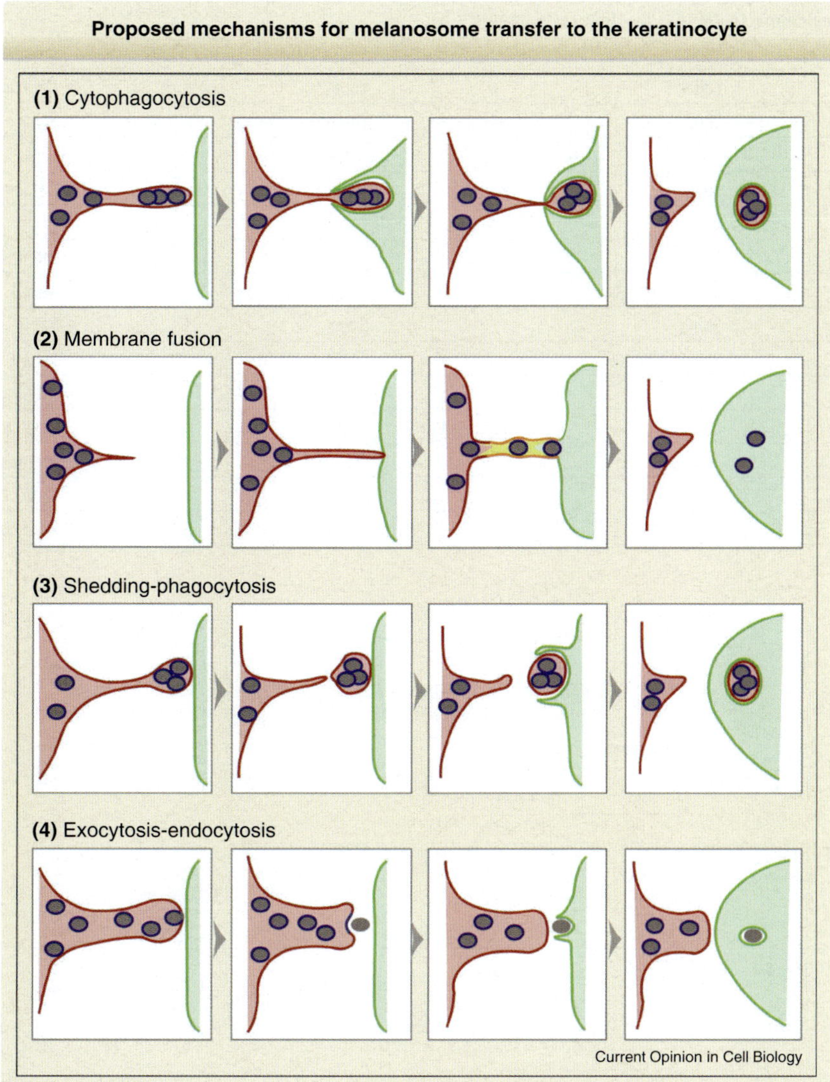

FIGURE 15-3. The currently proposed mechanism(s) of melanosomes transfer to surrounding keratinocytes. (Reproduced with permission from Wu X, Hammer JA. Melanosome transfer: it is best to give and receive. *Curr Opin Cell Biol.* 2014;29:1-7.)

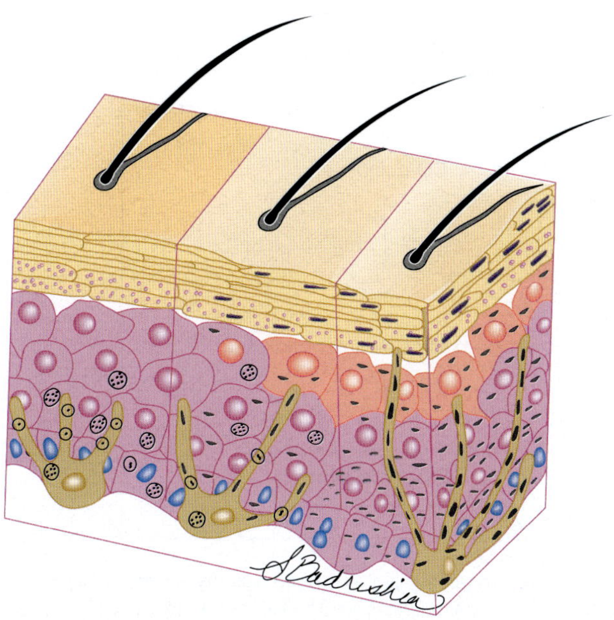

FIGURE 15-4. Schematic representation illustrating the differences in melanosome organization in dark skin (right), tan skin (middle), and light skin (left).

of UV-induced DNA damage and carcinogenesis.[33] The melanosome and melanin content throughout the layers of the epidermis play a significant role in protection against UV-induced DNA damage and skin cancer.[31]

PIGMENTARY INFLUENCES

HORMONES

Hormonal, environmental, and genetic factors contribute to the melanization of human skin. Alpha-melanocyte stimulation hormone (α-MSH) and adrenocorticotrophic hormone (ACTH) impact melanogenesis.[34] These peptide hormones interact with the melanocortin 1 receptor (MC1R) on the surface of melanocytes to stimulate melanin production.[34] These interactions lead to activation of the cAMP/PKA signaling pathway that allow for changes in gene expression and protein phosphorylation through the use of transcription factor gene product microphthalmia-associated transcription factor (MITF).[20] MITF transcriptionally activates genes that catalyze the conversion of tyrosine into melanin.

Despite epidermal melanocytes lacking estrogen or progesterone receptors, it has been postulated that sex hormones may play a role in cutaneous pigmentation.[35] Clinical findings, such as the increased

TABLE 15-1 Comparison of the epidermal contents across three racial groups[17–19]

Characteristic	White descent	African descent	Asian descent
Stratum corneum thickness	Equal	Equal	Data not available
Stratum corneocyte size	Equal	Equal	Equal
Stratum corneum layers	Less	More	Less
Stratum corneum lipids	Low	High	Data not available
Ceramide concentration	High	Low	High
Melanin	Low	High	Intermediate
Melanosomes	Small, aggregated	Large, dispersed	Mixed
Melanocyte number	Same	Same	Same
Melanosome distribution	Stratum basale	Entire epidermis	Mixed
Vitamin D production	High	Low	Intermediate
Minimal erythema dose	Low	High	Intermediate
Photodamage	High	Minimal	Intermediate
Glutathione (reduced state)	High	Low	Data not available
Glutathione reductase	High	Low	Data not available

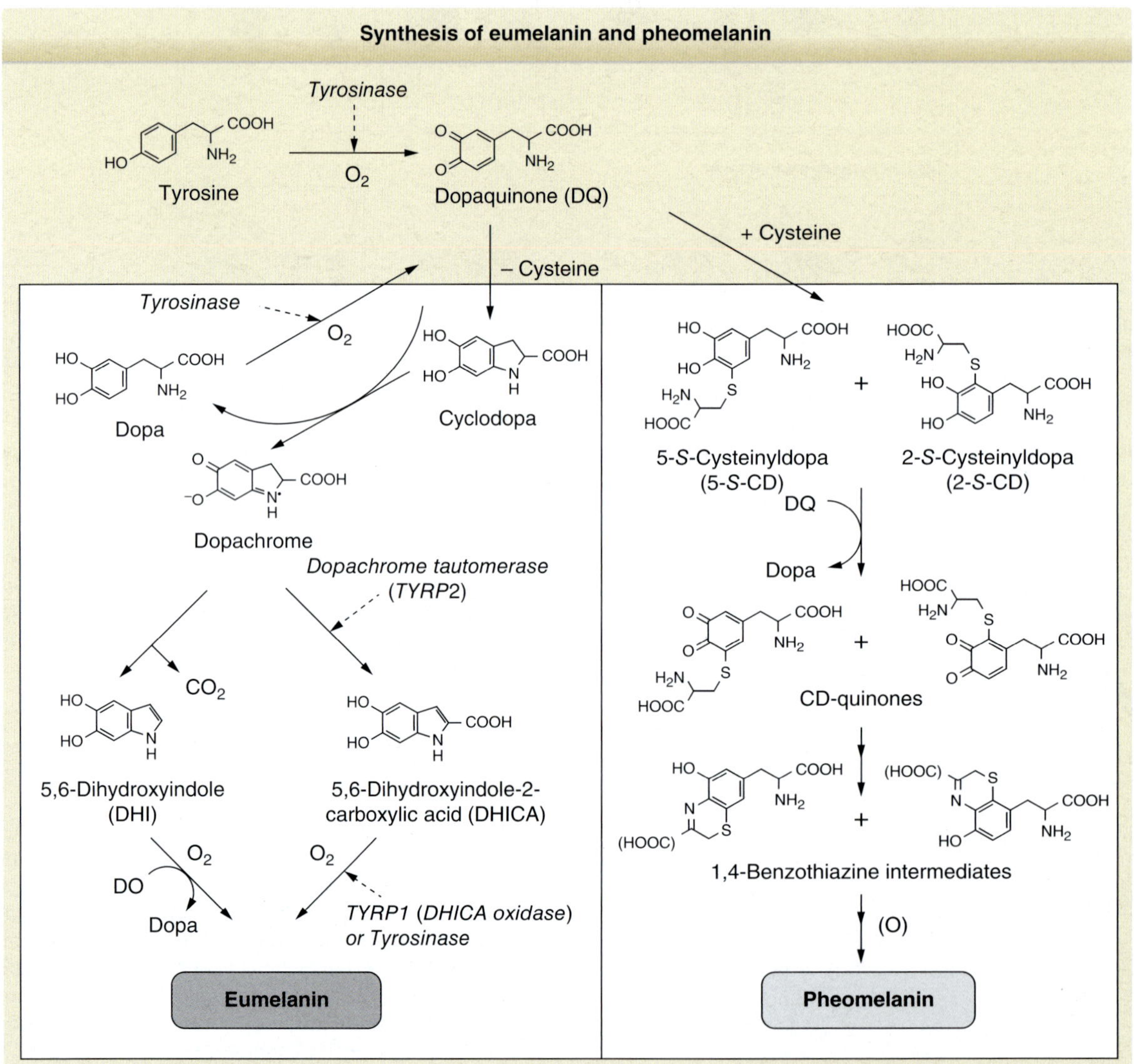

FIGURE 15-5. Diagram of eumelanin and pheomelanin synthesis from tyrosine. The initial rate-limiting step of melanin synthesis involves the conversion of tyrosine into dopaquinone (DQ). DQ, through a series of the illustrated steps, is converted into eumelanin and pheomelanin. (Reproduced with permission from Ito S, Wakamatsu K. Chemistry of mixed melanogenesis-pivotal roles of dopaquinone. *Photochem Photobiol*. 2007; 84(3):582-92.)

occurrence of melasma with the use of oral contraceptives or pregnancy, have been observed suggesting that α-MSH-independent pigmentation mechanisms may exist.[36] One study investigated the possible association of estrogen on melanocytes through an organotypic skin model created utilizing human primary epidermal keratinocytes and melanocytes within native human stroma.[35] It was noted that treatment of primary human melanocytes with 17B-estradiol caused a dose-dependent increase of melanin while treatment with progesterone resulted in a dose-dependent decrease in melanin production.[35] These findings were attributed to the possible mechanism of estrogen, progesterone, and α-MSH converging on the G protein-coupled receptor (GPCR) pathway activating adenylate cyclase.[35] Consecutively, this results in increased cAMP levels leading to downstream transcriptional gene activations inducing gene expression necessary for melanin synthesis.[35] Further robust studies are needed to continue investigating the involvement of sex hormones with melanin and skin pigmentation.

ENVIRONMENT

Variations in environment play a large role in skin pigmentation. Human populations at lower latitudes, compared to higher latitudes, are known to have darker skin pigmentation.[37] This has been attributed to the need to accumulate more vitamin D in regions with less UV radiation further from the equator where UV radiation is, in comparison, less abundant.[37] In addition, it has been postulated that deeply pigmented skin is an adaptation to protect against UV-induced photolysis of essential nutrients, particularly folate.[37] This suggests that the multitude of skin pigmentations could be an adaptation of different levels of UV radiation.[37] Darker pigmentation, in this regard, would be an evolutionary means to alleviate the pathogenic effects of UV radiation such as skin cancer or nutrient photolysis.[37]

Dermal fibroblasts have also been recently identified to have a role in skin pigmentation. Dermal fibroblasts are primarily responsible for the synthesis and maintenance of the collagen and noncollagen extracellular matrix that provides the structural foundation for the skin and tissues throughout the body.[38] Fibroblasts have been found to secrete various cytokines, proteins, and growth factors that bind to melanocyte receptors and activate intracellular signaling cascades.[38] One study used a reconstructed epidermis model that was cultured with UVA-exposed fibroblasts to demonstrate that these fibroblasts resulted in an increased number of melanocytes and dermal-epidermal junctional remodeling.[39] Another study also demonstrated in vitro that photo-exposed fibroblasts resulted in increased pigmentation through the increase in epidermal melanin content and melanogenic gene expression.[40]

GENETICS

Recent genome wide association studies have made progress in investigating the genetic differences of skin pigmentation. Traditionally, most of the knowledge considering the genetics of human pigmentation has come from studying predominately European populations. However, recently these studies have expanded into various populations around the globe. Over 150 genes, including the TYR gene responsible for tyrosinase, have been implicated in the skin color differences within humans.[41,42] The *MC1R* gene has been shown to be a gene responsible for red hair color.[24,34,43] Additional genes associated with human pigmentation include but are not limited to *BNC2, DCT, IRF4, KIT, KITLG, MITF, POMC, SLC24A4*, and *TPCN2*.[43] However, pigmentation is not only attributed to those genes but also variations within the genes resulting in numerous alleles that contribute to our phenotypical appearance. For instance, the *M1CR* gene is highly polymorphic and has been associated with at least 200 different variants.[44] Recent studies within Africans have identified numerous alleles in genes that result in the lightening and darkening of the skin.[41,45] One large study of Africans recently identified a large amount of single nucleotide polymorphisms in *SLC24A5*, a gene that was previously linked with pigmentation in Europeans.[45] The consistent migration of humans throughout the globe have contributed to the various polymorphisms that have resulted in the wide-ranging phenotypes we see in human pigmentation. The *SLC24A5* gene has now been found to be responsible for 25% to 38% of the variation in skin color among Europeans and Africans.[46,47] Another genome wide association study of over 6000 individuals of Latin American descent found that gene variants of *TYR, TYRP1, OCA2/HERC2, SLC45A2, SLC24A5*, and *IRF4* were responsible for the phenotypical variation of hair, skin, and eye pigment observed.[48] These genetic differences are continuing to be studied, yet show a breadth of potential information to be discovered.

Disruption of the factors that mediate and influence melanogenesis result in a variety of pigmentation disorders including but not limited to postinflammatory hyperpigmentation, melasma, vitiligo, and albinism. Numerous other disorders of dyspigmentation will be discussed in later chapters.

SUMMARY

Melanocytes are multi-faceted cells that reside in the basal layer of the epidermis. Through melanosomes, they are responsible for synthesizing the melanin that provides us with multiple functions including skin color and endogenous protection against UV radiation. People of various backgrounds have differences in the size, distribution, and organization of melanosomes and melanin that contribute to individual appearances and protection against the sun. The pigmentation of human skin is influenced by various factors that include hormones, genetics, and environment. The disruption of melanocyte activity and melanogenesis can lead to a variety of pigmentary disorders that can occur across different populations.

REFERENCES

1. Mort RL, Jackson IJ, Patton EE. The melanocyte lineage in development and disease. *Development.* 2015;142(7):1387-1387.
2. Larue L, Kumasaka M, Goding CR. β-catenin in the melanocyte lineage. *Pigment Cell Res.* 2003;16(3):312-317.
3. Jimbow K, Quevedo WC, Fitzpatrick TB, Szabo G. Some aspects of melanin biology: 1950–1975. *J Invest Dermatol.* 1976;67(1):72-89.
4. Nordlund JJ. The melanocyte and the epidermal melanin unit: an expanded concept. *Dermatol Clin.* 2007;25(3):271-281, vii.
5. Costin GE, Hearing VJ. Human skin pigmentation: melanocytes modulate skin color in response to stress. *FASEB J.* 2007;21(4):976-994.
6. Marks MS, Seabra MC. The melanosome: membrane dynamics in black and white. *Nat Rev Mol Cell Biol.* 2001;2(10):738-748.
7. Wu X, Hammer JA. Melanosome transfer: it is best to give and receive. *Curr Opin Cell Biol.* 2014;29:1-7.
8. Kuroda TS, Fukuda M. Rab27A-binding protein Slp2-a is required for peripheral melanosome distribution and elongated cell shape in melanocytes. *Nat Cell Biol.* 2004;6(12):1195-1203.
9. Wu X, Bowers B, Rao K, Wei Q, Hammer JA. Visualization of melanosome dynamics within wild-type and dilute melanocytes suggests a paradigm for myosin V function in vivo. *J Cell Biol.* 1998;143(7):1899-1918.
10. Van Den Bossche K, Naeyaert JM, Lambert J. The quest for the mechanism of melanin transfer: revelations of the pigmentation synapse. *Traffic.* 2006;7(7):769-778.
12. Masson P. Pigment cells in man. *Ann N Y Acad Sci.* 1948;4:15-51.
13. Alaluf S, Atkins D, Barrett K, Blount M, Carter N, Heath A. Ethnic variation in melanin content and composition in photoexposed and photoprotected human skin. *Pigment Cell Res.* 2002;15(2):112-118.
14. Montagna W, Carlisle K. The architecture of black and white facial skin. *J Am Acad Dermatol.* 1991;24(6):929-937.
15. Herzberg AJ, Dinehart SM. Chronologic aging in black skin. *Am J Dermatopathol.* 1989;11(4):319-328.
16. Kotrajaras R, Kligman AM. The effect of topical tretinoin on photodamaged facial skin: the Thai experience. *Br J Dermatol.* 1993;129(3):302-309.
17. Muizzuddin N, Hellemans L, Van Overloop L, Corstjens H, Declercq L, Maes D. Structural and functional differences in barrier properties of African American, Caucasian and East Asian skin. *J Dermatol Sci.* 2010;59(2):123-128.
18. Taylor SC. Skin of color: biology, structure, function, and implications for dermatologic disease. *J Am Acad Dermatol.* 2002;46(2):S41-S62.

19. Whitmore SE, Sago NJG. Caliper-measured skin thickness is similar in white and black women. *J Am Acad Dermatol.* 2000;42(1):76-79.
20. Buscà R, Ballotti R. Cyclic AMP a key messenger in the regulation of skin pigmentation. *Pigment Cell Res.* 2000;13(2):60-69.
21. D'Alba L, Shawkey MD. Melanosomes: biogenesis, properties, and evolution of an ancient organelle. *Physiol Rev.* 2019;99(1):1-19.
22. Hunt G, Kyne S, Ito S, Wakamatsu K, Todd C, Thody AJ. Eumelanin and phaeomelanin contents of human epidermis and cultured melanocytes. *Pigment Cell Res.* 1995;8(4):202-208.
23. Prota G. Recent advances in the chemistry of melanogenesis in mammals. *J Invest Dermatol.* 1980;75(1):122-127.
24. Nasti TH, Timares L. MC1R, eumelanin and pheomelanin: their role in determining the susceptibility to skin cancer. *Photochem Photobiol.* 2015;91(1):188-200.
25. D'Mello S, Finlay G, Baguley B, Askarian-Amiri M. Signaling pathways in melanogenesis. *Int J Mol Sci.* 2016;17(7):1144.
26. Morgan AM, Lo J, Fisher DE. How does pheomelanin synthesis contribute to melanomagenesis? *BioEssays News Rev Mol Cell Dev Biol.* 2013;35(8):672-676.
27. Wolf Horrell EM, Boulanger MC, D'Orazio JA. Melanocortin 1 receptor: structure, function, and regulation. *Front Genet.* 2016;7:95.
28. Olson RL, Gaylor J, Everett MA. Skin color, melanin, and erythema. *Arch Dermatol.* 1973;108(4):541-544.
29. Mitchell RE. The skin of the Australian Aborigine; a light and electronmicroscopical study. *Australas J Dermatol.* 1968;9(4):314-328.
30. Kaidbey KH, Agin PP, Sayre RM, Kligman AM. Photoprotection by melanin–a comparison of black and Caucasian skin. *J Am Acad Dermatol.* 1979;1(3):249-260.
31. Fajuyigbe D, Lwin SM, Diffey BL, et al. Melanin distribution in human epidermis affords localized protection against DNA photodamage and concurs with skin cancer incidence difference in extreme phototypes. *FASEB J.* 2018;32(7):3700-3706.
32. Halder RM, Bang KM. Skin cancer in blacks in the United States. *Dermatol Clin.* 1988;6(3):397-405.
33. Brenner M, Hearing VJ. The protective role of melanin against UV damage in human skin. *Photochem Photobiol.* 2008;84(3):539-549.
34. Sturm RA, Teasdale RD, Box NF. Human pigmentation genes: identification, structure and consequences of polymorphic variation. *Gene.* 2001;277(1-2):49-62.
35. Natale CA, Duperret EK, Zhang J, et al. Sex steroids regulate skin pigmentation through nonclassical membrane-bound receptors. *eLife.* 2016;5:e15104.
36. Sheth VM, Pandya AG. Melasma: a comprehensive update: part I. *J Am Acad Dermatol.* 2011;65(4):689-697.
37. Jablonski NG, Chaplin G. The evolution of human skin coloration. *J Hum Evol.* 2000;39(1):57-106.
38. Wang Y, Viennet C, Robin S, Berthon JY, He L, Humbert P. Precise role of dermal fibroblasts on melanocyte pigmentation. *J Dermatol Sci.* 2017;88(2):159-166.
39. Salducci M, André N, Guéré C, et al. Factors secreted by irradiated aged fibroblasts induce solar lentigo in pigmented reconstructed epidermis. *Pigment Cell Melanoma Res.* 2014;27(3):502-504.
40. Duval C, Cohen C, Chagnoleau C, Flouret V, Bourreau E, Bernerd F. Key regulatory role of dermal fibroblasts in pigmentation as demonstrated using a reconstructed skin model: impact of photo-aging. *PLoS One.* 2014;9(12):e114182.
41. Martin AR, Lin M, Granka JM, et al. An unexpectedly complex architecture for skin pigmentation in Africans. *Cell.* 2017;171(6):1340-1353.e14.
42. Naik PP, Farrukh SN. Influence of ethnicities and skin color variations in different populations: a review. *Skin Pharmacol Physiol.* 2022;35(2):65-76.
43. Pavan WJ, Sturm RA. The genetics of human skin and hair pigmentation. *Annu Rev Genomics Hum Genet.* 2019;20(1):41-72.
44. Tagliabue E, Gandini S, García-Borrón JC, et al. Association of melanocortin-1 receptor variants with pigmentary traits in humans: a pooled analysis from the M-skip project. *J Invest Dermatol.* 2016;136(9):1914-1917.
45. Crawford NG, Kelly DE, Hansen MEB, et al. Loci associated with skin pigmentation identified in African populations. *Science.* 2017;358(6365):eaan8433.
46. Juzeniene A, Setlow R, Porojnicu A, Steindal AH, Moan J. Development of different human skin colors: a review highlighting photobiological and photobiophysical aspects. *J Photochem Photobiol B.* 2009;96(2):93-100.
47. Feng Y, McQuillan MA, Tishkoff SA. Evolutionary genetics of skin pigmentation in African populations. *Hum Mol Genet.* 2021;30(R1):R88-R97.
48. Adhikari K, Mendoza-Revilla J, Sohail A, et al. A GWAS in Latin Americans highlights the convergent evolution of lighter skin pigmentation in Eurasia. *Nat Commun.* 2019;10:358.

CHAPTER 16

Dermis

Yacine Sow
Susan C. Taylor

KEY POINTS

- Although few definitive conclusions can be made with sparse research, biological differences of the dermis among individuals with different skin types do exist.
- Dermal differences include varied structural organization and concentration of dermal components.
- Racial differences in dermis structure, cellularity, glands, and hair follicles have been observed.

The dermis is a layer of the skin that lies between the epidermis and subcutaneous tissue. It is a highly vascular structure divided into two layers: a superficial papillary region and a deeper, thicker region known as the reticular dermis. The structure of the dermis provides strength and flexibility, while its vasculature helps maintains the epidermis by transporting nutrients. Depending on the body site, thickness of the dermis ranges from 0.5 to 5 mm, as a thin dermis is found on the eyelid, and a thick dermis is present on the back.[1] The dermis is composed of interstitial (collagen and elastic fibers, ground substance) and cellular (fibroblasts, macrophages, mast cells, plasma cells, lymphocytes, dermal dendritic cells, and histiocytes) components that contribute to structural and immunomodulatory functions of the skin. Glands (sweat glands, sebaceous glands, apocrine glands, and apoeccrine glands), hair follicles, and lymphatic vessels are also present in the dermis. Dermis mechanoreceptors and thermoreceptors play a role in tactile and thermoregulatory feedback, respectively.[2,3]

DERMAL STRUCTURE AND FUNCTION IN SKIN OF COLOR

The dermis is a fibrous structure composed of collagen, elastic tissue, and reticular fibers.[4] There are scant data examining potential racial and ethnic differences in dermal structure and cell types. Data that have been published are over a quarter century old and must be repeated to be able to draw definitive conclusions regarding differences, if indeed they exist. Data that are commonly cited are based on work published in 1991 by Montagna et al who obtained punch biopsy specimens from the malar eminences of Black and White women and compared morphology.[5] Black subjects had thick, compact dermis yielding a clear distinction between the papillary and reticular layers.[5,6] This structural distinction was less evident in the skin of White individuals.[6] Notably, another study utilizing a skinfold caliper measuring device on a small number of subjects found no difference in overall dermis thickness between Black and White females.[7] In the dermis of Black individuals, collagenous fiber bundles are arranged orthogonally and run mostly parallel to the skin's surface as compared to a horizontal laminar organization in the skin of Whites.[6] Additionally, the collagenous fiber bundles in the reticular dermis of Black participants are smaller than those in White participants.[6] Interestingly, all Black subjects had collagenous fiber fragments in the dermal interstices but were sparse in the dermis of White subjects.[6] These fiber fragments were thought to be proteoglycans. The racial differences in collagen-proteoglycan interactions may account for the firmness (turgor) in the skin of Black individuals.[6] Investigators also found that dermal elastic fibers were more abundant in the skin of White individuals, even among the younger subjects in their 20s. Even the skin of older Black subjects had fewer elastic fibers than that of older White individuals. Elastotic fibers (degenerated elastic fibers) in sun-exposed areas are one of the key indices of dermal photodamage. The reduction in extracellular proteoglycans and resorption of elastotic material can decrease dermal volume, resulting in rhytids.[6] Since these events occur primarily in the sun-exposed skin of White individuals, the presence of collagenous fiber fragments in the dermal interstices may explain why the sun-exposed skin in Black individuals is less prone to dermal photodamage and wrinkles. Dermal vasculature also has some racial variations. In Black individuals, the dermis of appears to have more superficial blood vessels compared to their White counterparts.[8] Additionally, the dermis contains larger, more dilated lymph vessels, especially on the face.[8]

Racial differences in dermal cell types have also been noted. Montagna et al also found that fibroblasts in Black female facial skin were more abundant than in White female facial skin.[5] Yet, White individuals showed greater interindividual variability in fibroblast quantity. Black subjects had more defined, larger fibroblasts and macrophages than White subjects.[5] Specifically, the fibroblasts in Black skin were hypertrophied and contained extensive rough endoplasmic reticulum, Golgi bodies, and vesicles.[5] Fibroblast hyperactivity in the skin of Black individuals is thought to be due to the interaction between other cell types (ie, mast cells, cytokines, and other fibroblasts). This could account for the predisposition of keloids among individuals of African descent. Although investigators reported no significant differences in the number or size of mast cells between the two racial groups, macrophages in the papillary dermis were larger and more numerous among Black individuals.[5]

While the number and size of mast cells are constant between Black and White individuals, there is a difference in the size of mast cell granules. Sueki et al did find a statistically significant difference in mast cell granule size between the skin of Black and White particpants.[9] Biopsies of normal buttock skin were obtained from four Black males and three White males. A quantitative assessment of mast cell granules and electron micrographs found that mast cells in the skin of Black participants contained larger granules than those in the skin of White participants.[9] Additionally, mast cells in Black individuals contained larger granules, a larger percentage of parallel-linear striations, and a smaller percentage of curved lamellae.[9] While the clinical significance of parallel-linear striations and curved lamellae variation is unknown, racial variation in mast cell granule size may reflect the difference in their rates of degranulation and regranulation.[9] The role of mast cells in aberrant fibrosis in diseases such as hypertrophic scars,[10] keloids,[11] scleroderma,[12,13] and chronic graft-versus-host disease have been documented.[14] Mast cell granules contain mediators such as histamine, fibroblast growth factor, and tryptase that also contribute to clinical disease pathogenesis. Specifically, tryptase has been described to stimulate the proliferation of fibroblasts. In keloid biopsies, tryptase-positive mast cells are interspersed among collagen bundles throughout the dermis.[15] Although the density of tryptase-positive mast cells in keloid was not significantly different from that in normal skin, the much thicker dermis of a keloid suggests greater total mast cell number under a given epidermal area.[9,11,15] Sueki et al found that the density of tryptase-labeled gold particles was significantly higher in the skin of Black participants, which may explain why patients of African descent have a higher predisposition to keloids.[9]

The dermis has 1.5-4 $\times$ 10^6 sweat glands subdivided into eccrine and apocrine glands.[1] Sweat glands consist of a coiled acinar secretory structure in the dermis and a straight duct that connects this acinar structure to the surface of the epidermis.[16] Although eccrine glands are sweat glands present throughout the body; they are most numerous on the soles of the feet. Derived from the embryonic ectoderm, eccrine glands are simple, tubular, and coiled and help to maintain homeostasis primarily by stabilizing temperature.[17] As the body's internal temperature increases, sweat glands release water to the skin's surface.[18] It then quickly evaporates, subsequently cooling the skin and blood beneath as a means of thermoregulation. Eccrine sweat glands can produce at least 500 to 750 mL in a day while also participating in ion and nitrogenous waste excretion.[18]

Apocrine sweat glands are large, branched, and predominantly localized to the axillary and perineal regions. Given that apocrine sweat glands start to function at puberty under the stimulation of sex hormones, they are also referred to as odoriferous sweat glands and known for producing malodorous perspiration.[18] The viscous, protein-rich product expelled from the gland may develop an odor after exposure to bacteria. Both types of sweat glands play a regenerative role in skin damage. In second-degree cutaneous burns that extend into the reticular dermis, skin regeneration occurs via skin appendages such as hair follicles, sebaceous glands, and sweat glands. Epithelial cells surrounding these appendages produce more cells that progress to form a new epithelium, a process that takes approximately 1 to 3 weeks.[1,18]

Another type of gland in the mid-dermis is the sebaceous gland, which almost always develops alongside a hair follicle with an outlet emptying into the follicular canal. The association between a sebaceous gland and the hair follicle is known as the pilosebaceous unit.[19] The embryonic development of the sebaceous gland lies in the process of ingrowth of ectodermal cells into the mesoderm.[19] Sebaceous glands are found all over the human body except on the palms and soles. Sebaceous glands are more frequently on the face and scalp.[19] The number of sebaceous glands remains constant throughout life, whereas their size increases with age.[19] Sebaceous glands are unique because their primary cellular unit, the sebocyte, engages in lipid synthesis and metabolism, a function usually reserved for adipocytes.[19] Additionally, products of the sebaceous gland are synthesized via holocrine secretion, a process characterized by purposeful self-destruction of the sebocyte.[19]

Sebaceous glands produce squalene and fatty acids critical for maintaining skin homeostasis, lubrication, and defense against environmental and infectious injury.[19,20] The gland's main product, sebum, helps to seal moisture and prevent skin desiccation.[19] Sebum also contains antimicrobial substances, free fatty acids, and matrix metalloproteinases that help protect the skin from external insults.[19] Sebaceous glands are important sites of androgen processing and modulation. Androgens regulate sebaceous gland function through binding to nuclear androgen receptors.[21] These receptors stimulate cell proliferation and lipogenesis in the sebaceous gland. The role of androgens is evident in acne vulgaris, the most common pathology relating to sebaceous glands. High levels of androgen production stimulate sebaceous glands to increase sebum production and produce sebum plugs, resulting in open and closed comedones.[18,21]

ECCRINE GLANDS

Documented racial differences in the quantity, structure, and function of eccrine sweat glands are limited. Given the established premise that race evolved due to environmental selection, it is plausible that differences in sweat glands between races exist due to adaptation to hot, humid climates versus colder climates. The theory of environmental adaptation is appreciated among the Ainu, a Japanese ethnic group representing a mixture of races. Ainu people born in Japan who migrated to the tropics had the same number of sweat glands as Ainu born in Japan who continued to live in Japan.[22] However, Ainu born in the tropics had more sweat glands than the other groups.[22] Considerably, most literature suggests no significant differences in eccrine glands between races. A 1965 study measured active eccrine sweat gland activity among 30 African American and 29 White males to determine whether sweat gland activity was a possible factor in racial differences in skin conductance.[23] There was no significant difference in the number of active sweat glands between races, but the intragroup relationship between sweat gland count and skin conductance was significantly higher among African American males.[23,24]

When evaluating the functional activity of eccrine sweat glands, Robinson et al reported higher rates of sweating by White Americans compared with Black Americans when engaging in physical labor.[25] McCance et al also measured sweat production on the forearm of subjects from Uganda and compared it to age- and gender-matched European and continental Indian subjects. Similarly, they found that White Europeans had a higher sweating rate than Black and Indian subjects.[26] Interestingly, measurement of pilocarpine-stimulated sodium concentration in sweat revealed that the Black Africans had significantly lower sodium concentration in their sweat compared with White Europeans and Asian Indians.[26] This suggests more efficient electrolyte conservation observed among individuals of African ancestry.[27] Evaluating the quantity of sweat production did not produce consistent results across all investigations. Herrmann et al found no significant difference between 4 Black and 16 White male Americans in the onset and quantity of sweat produced.[28]

A considerable limitation of this study was its small sample size. Kawahata and Adams studied racial differences in sweat gland functional activity and distribution. They found a greater density and number of active sweat glands in White males compared to Black males.[29] White women exceeded any other group in these measurements, regardless of race or sex.[29]

Another method used to compare eccrine sweat glands is through skin resistance measurements. Electrophysiologic studies can evaluate these differences considering that skin resistance correlates with greater eccrine gland activity. Each study found a higher skin resistance in Black subjects compared to White subjects, implying that Black subjects have greater eccrine gland activity.[24,30–32] When assessing Hispanic subjects of Mexican and Spanish origin, average skin resistance was between that of White and Black subjects. Since Spanish subjects are considered White, while Mexicans represent racial admixture, pigmentation may play a role in skin resistance. Ultimately, these studies demonstrated a higher skin resistance among dark-skinned individuals compared to light-skinned individuals.

Notably, most studies evaluating the racial differences in eccrine sweat glands were conducted from 1930 to 1960, and all have contradictory findings and relatively small sample sizes. Additionally, acclimatization needs to be taken into consideration when measuring sweat gland functionality, as this will influence the onset and type of sweating process. Thus, it is probable that individuals in the tropics have a greater density of actively sweating glands rather than real differences in gland numbers. These less-than-optimal investigative conditions cannot clearly determine whether observed racial differences are due to ancestry or genetics, environmental adaptations, or both.

APOCRINE GLANDS

Literature regarding racial differences in apocrine gland function and number is limited. In 1926, Homm completed a histologic analysis of samples taken from four apocrine-bearing areas of the body and observed that apocrine glands occurred three times as often in Black subjects compared to White subjects.[30] Interestingly, none of the specimens were obtained from the axillae, which is the area of the body with the greatest number of apocrine glands. Hurley and Shelley also investigated apocrine gland structure and function among Black and White subjects. They reported larger apocrine glands and greater number of secretions in Black subjects than in White subjects.[33] The researchers engaged in subjective measurements of appraisal and determined that secretions from Black subjects were more turbid.[33] The lack of investigator-blinded, objective assessment of apocrine gland function and size makes it difficult to draw any clinically or statistically significant conclusions.

The secretion of apocrine glands contains proteins and fatty acids that interact with bacterial enzymes on the skin surface to produce odoriferous molecules, commonly known as "body odor." Studies have suggested that human axillary odor is influenced by genetic factors, specifically the *ABCC11* gene, which encodes an ATP-driven efflux transporter localized in human apocrine sweat glands.[34] The ABCC11 protein is known to transport a variety of small molecules that play a role in the generation of axillary malodor and earwax (cerumen) phenotype. A single nucleotide polymorphism substitutes glycine for arginine, producing the G180R variant of ABCC11. This genetic polymorphism results in a dry, white earwax phenotype that is highly prevalent (80-95%) among Chinese, Korean, and Japanese populations.[34] G180R homozygous individuals produce significantly less characteristic axillary odor. Notably, this G180R variant is rare among individuals of European and African descent. Based on the ethnic variations of *ABCC11*, it is hypothesized that axillary odorants produced by East Asians would differ from those obtained from European and African descent. Prokop-Prigge et al enrolled 30 healthy adult males (10 African American, 10 White, and 10 East Asian) subjects and analyzed their *ABC11* genotype and quantified substances of axillary sweat using liquid chromatography mass spectrometry.[35] Results found that characteristic axillary odorants quantitatively varied with respect to ethnicity. This study's findings aligned with the prediction that East Asian donors exhibited lower levels of axillary odorants.[34,35] Despite exhibiting the same *ABCC11* genotype, there were still marked differences in the levels of characteristic axillary odors between African American and White donors. A major contributor to axillary odor, *E*-3M2H (*E*-3-methyl-2-hexenoic acid), was significantly higher in African Americans compared to Whites.[35] There were also significant differences in the number of individuals who produced detectable levels of 3H3M (3-hydroxy-3-methylhexanoic acid), with African Americans having the highest levels, followed by Whites and then East Asian participants.[35] Further expanding on the ethnic differences in body odor, Jacoby et al decided to investigate the levels of *apoD* in axillary skin extracts. *ApoD* serves as a carrier protein of the major axillary odorants, *E*-3M2H (*E*-3-methyl-2-hexenoic acid).[36] Their results demonstrated that Chinese individuals had diminished and nondetectable *ApoD* levels, while Europeans and African subjects had detectable levels of *apoD* in axillary skin extracts.[36]

SEBACEOUS GLANDS

Similar to eccrine glands, racial differences in sebaceous gland size and activity are limited, contradictory, and have small sample sizes. Kligman and Shelley compared surface sebum levels during a 4-hour period in five Black and five White subjects. Results demonstrated that Black individuals had higher surface sebum levels compared to White subjects.[20] Histological evidence from forehead biopsy specimens from two Black subjects revealed larger sebaceous glands in comparison to two White subjects.[20] Approximately 30 years later, Pochi and Strauss also measured sebum production on the foreheads of 30 Black males.[37] Compared to 373 White male subjects, they found a trend toward increased mean sebum production among African American males.[37] However, when they compared 37 Black females to 209 White females, they found a trend toward decreased mean sebum production.[37] When controlling for race, only 4 of the 67 Black subjects had sebum production values that exceeded the range of two standard deviations from the mean of White patients.[37] Another study by Abedeen et al used a sebutape and a sebumeter to measure the rate of sebum production in three different racial groups.[38] They found no statistical difference in sebum excretion rate between African Americans, Northern Asian, and White subjects.[38]

Sebum is an etiologic factor in the development of acne vulgaris. Understanding the racial and ethnic differences in sebum production may predict trends in acne prevalence among patients with skin of color. A study of acne vulgaris demonstrated differences in acne presentation among Asian, White, Continental Indian, and African American women.[39] African American women were found to have larger, more visible pores than other groups, which supports previous studies that showed that Black subjects had greater gland pore size and sebaceous glands.[39,40] There was also a positive correlation between sebum secretion and acne severity, which supports other studies that report 60% to 70% greater lipid content in the hair follicles of Black individuals compared to White subjects.[41] Consistent with these reports, Hillebrand et al found that African Americans showed significantly more sebum excretion compared to East Asians, whereas Hispanics had the lowest.[42]

Sebum is a semisolid mixture of squalene, cholesterol, cholesterol esters, wax esters, and triglycerides. Race may contribute to differences in sebum composition. One study investigating the effect of race on sebum composition found that Japanese subjects have a greater predominance of straight-chain fatty acids in their sebum and a greater quantity of C16 iso-branched chain fatty acids.[43] Additionally, Japanese men appeared to have a greater sebaceous gland activity (measured as the ratio of wax esters to cholesterol esters) compared to Whites.[43] Another study sought to identify lipid components of sebum that could correlate with ethnic skin hydration and barrier. Investigators found significant differences in six fatty acids in the wax ester fraction among African American women.[44] Sapienic acid (16:1, n10), the most prevalent fatty acid in sebum, is significantly higher in African American subjects and correlated with higher sebum output.[44] Considering that sapienic acid is the most abundant fatty acid in sebum, it is usual that levels are higher among subjects with higher sebum output. African American women also had higher amounts of oleic acid (18:1, n9) and myristic acid

(14:0).[44] It is well understood that *C. acnes* colonizes the pilosebaceous unit and contributes to a higher lipid outlet. African Americans have a higher amount of specific fatty acids in wax esters, demonstrating that bacterial fatty acids may be incorporated into sebaceous wax synthesis.[44] Different ethnoracial groups may have variations in skin microflora.[44]

HAIR FOLLICLES IN SKIN OF COLOR

Hair is a keratinous filament primarily made of dead, keratinized cells that grows out of the epidermis. Strands of hair originate in an epidermal penetration of the dermis called the hair follicle. Hair follicles that produce terminal hairs extend into the deep dermis and sometimes even the subcutis.[45] Terminal hair is thick, coarse hair that grows on the scalp, eyelashes, and eyebrows. The terminal hair variant may also grow on the face, armpits, pubic area, chest, and belly under the influence of androgenic hormones during puberty.

Hair has been deemed a more distinctive phenotypical characteristic than skin color. Just as hair color and structure are different among racial groups, hair follicle density and morphology may also vary. According to prior reports, Whites had significantly more hair follicles in the forehead region than Asians and Africans.[46,47] White participants also had a statistically significant increased percentage of hair follicle orifices on the forehead surface.[46] Two studies confirmed that Whites had increased follicular infundibulum than Africans and Asians on the scalp.[47,48] Considerably, the infundibulum of Whites patients is filled with sebum and desquamated cells.[48]

Additionally, hair follicles have different cross-sectional shapes. A round follicle is likely to produce a straight strand of hair, a flattened or oval-shaped follicle is likely to produce wavy to curly hair, and a very flat, oval, elliptical follicle is likely to produce tight curls or kinky hair.[49] The hair of Asian individuals is likely to have round to slight oval-shaped follicles, Whites are likely to have oval-shaped follicles, and individuals of African descent are likely to have elliptical hair follicles that sit at an oblique angle, with the concavity toward the epidermis.[49] Ethnoracial differences in hair follicle shape explains why individuals of African descent and Hispanic origin are genetically predisposed to pseudofolliculitis barbae. Pseudofolliculitis barbae is a chronic inflammatory condition with a multifactorial etiology, as the shape of the hair follicle, hair cuticle, and direction of hair growth all play a role in the inflammatory response.[50] When shaving, the hair develops a tip that grows out of the follicle, curves downward, and re-enters the epidermis (extrafollicular penetration) or the dermis (transfollicular penetration).[50] The ensuing inflammatory response is seen clinically by the presence of perifollicular papules and pustules.

In summary, differences in dermal structure, function, activity, cell type, glands, and hair follicles have been observed among different racial groups. These differences can have therapeutic implications. **Tables 16-1** and **16-2** summarize these findings and their implications for clinical disease.

TABLE 16-1 Comparison of dermal structure between individuals of European and African descent[5,6,9]

Characteristic	European descent	African descent
Dermis	Thin and less compact	Thick and compact
Papillary and reticular layer	Less distinct	More distinct
Collagen fiber bundles	Large	Small, close stacking; proteoglycans between collagen fibrils
Fiber fragments	Sparse	Prominent and numerous
Mast cell granules	Smaller	Larger
Melanophages	Few	Numerous and larger
Lymphatic vessels	Moderate, dilated	Dilated empty channels
Fibroblasts	Few	Numerous large, binucleated and multinucleated
Elastic fibers	Several, elastosis Normal arrangement in papillary dermis Surround secretory eccrine glands	Few, elastosis uncommon Abnormal arrangement in papillary dermis Surround secretory eccrine glands
Superficial blood vessel	Sparse to moderate	Numerous, mostly dilated

TABLE 16-2 Therapeutic implications of structural/functional characteristics in individuals with skin of color[6]

Structural/functional differences	Clinical implications
Epidermis	
Increased melanin content	Lower rates of skin cancer
Increased melanosome dispersion	Pigmentation disorders due to both biologic predispositions and cultural practices
Dermis	
Multinucleated and larger fibroblasts	Greater incidence of keloids
Thick and compact dermis	Less rhytids of the skin

REFERENCES

1. Lai-Cheong JE, McGrath JA. Structure and function of skin, hair and nails. *Medicine*. 2013;41(6):317-320.
2. Iheanacho F, Vellipuram AR. *Physiology, Mechanoreceptors*. In: *StatPearls*. StatPearls Publishing; 2022. Accessed September 3, 2022. http://www.ncbi.nlm.nih.gov/books/NBK541068/.
3. Jänig W. Peripheral thermoreceptors in innocuous temperature detection. *Handb Clin Neurol*. 2018;156:47-56.
4. Brown TM, Krishnamurthy K. *Histology, Dermis*. In: *StatPearls*. StatPearls Publishing; 2022. Accessed September 3, 2022. http://www.ncbi.nlm.nih.gov/books/NBK535346/.
5. Montagna W, Carlisle K. The architecture of black and white facial skin. *J Am Acad Dermatol*. 1991;24(6 Pt 1):929-937.
6. Montagna W, Prota G, Kenney JA, eds. *Black Skin: Structure and Function*. Academic Press; 1993.
7. Whitmore SE, Sago NJ. Caliper-measured skin thickness is similar in white and black women. *J Am Acad Dermatol*. 2000;42(1 Pt 1):76-79.
8. Basset A, Liautaud B, Ndiaye B. *Dermatology of Black Skin*. Oxford University Press; 1986.
9. Sueki H, Whitaker-Menezes D, Kligman AM. Structural diversity of mast cell granules in black and white skin. *Br J Dermatol*. 2001;144(1):85-93.
10. Kischer CW, Bunce H, Shetlah MR. Mast cell analyses in hypertrophic scars, hypertrophic scars treated with pressure and mature scars. *J Invest Dermatol*. 1978;70(6):355-357.
11. Craig SS, DeBlois G, Schwartz LB. Mast cells in human keloid, small intestine, and lung by an immunoperoxidase technique using a murine monoclonal antibody against tryptase. *Am J Pathol*. 1986;124(3):427-435.
12. Nishioka K, Kobayashi Y, Katayama I, Takijiri C. Mast cell numbers in diffuse scleroderma. *Arch Dermatol*. 1987;123(2):205-208.
13. Akimoto S, Ishikawa O, Igarashi Y, Kurosawa M, Miyachi Y. Dermal mast cells in scleroderma: their skin density, tryptase/chymase phenotypes and degranulation. *Br J Dermatol*. 1998;138(3):399-406.
14. Choi KL, Giorno R, Claman HN. Cutaneous mast cell depletion and recovery in murine graft-vs-host disease. *J Immunol*. 1987;138(12):4093-4101.
15. Huang C, Murphy GF, Akaishi S, Ogawa R. Keloids and hypertrophic scars: update and future directions. *Plast Reconstr Surg Glob Open*. 2013;1(4):e25.
16. Kobielak K, Kandyba E, Leung Y. *Skin and Skin Appendage Regeneration*. In: *Translational Regenerative Medicine*. Elsevier; 2015:269-292.
17. Cui CY, Schlessinger D. Eccrine sweat gland development and sweat secretion. *Exp Dermatol*. 2015;24(9):644-650.
18. Hodge BD, Sanvictores T, Brodell RT. *Anatomy, Skin Sweat Glands*.
19. Hoover E, Aslam S, Krishnamurthy K. *Physiology, Sebaceous Glands*. In: *StatPearls*. StatPearls Publishing; 2022. Accessed September 3, 2022. http://www.ncbi.nlm.nih.gov/books/NBK499819/.
20. Kligman AM, Shelley WB. An investigation of the biology of the human sebaceous gland. *J Invest Dermatol*. 1958;30(3):99-125.
21. Makrantonaki E, Ganceviciene R, Zouboulis C. An update on the role of the sebaceous gland in the pathogenesis of acne. *Dermatoendocrinology*. 2011;3(1):41-49.

22. Kawahata A, Sakamoto H. Some observations on sweating of the Aino. *Jpn J Physiol.* 1951;2(2):166-169.
23. Johnson LC, Landon MM. Eccrine sweat gland activity and racial differences in resting skin conductance. *Psychophysiology.* 1965;1(4):322-329.
24. Johnson LC, Corah NL. Racial differences in skin resistance. *Science.* 1963;139(3556):766-767.
25. Wilson JW, Dill DB, Nielsen M, Robinson S. Adaptations of white men and Negroes to prolonged work in humid heat. *Am J Trop Med Hyg.* 1941;s1-21(2):261-287.
26. McCance RA. The effect of salt deficiency in man on the volume of the extracellular fluids, and on the composition of sweat, saliva, gastric juice and cerebrospinal fluid. *J Physiol.* 1938;92(2):208-218.
27. Calhoun DA, Oparil S. Racial differences in the pathogenesis of hypertension. *Am J Med Sci.* 1995;310 Suppl 1:S86-S90.
28. Herrmann F, Prose PH, Sulzberger MB, Mandol L, Medoff G. Studies on sweating. IV. A new quantitative method of assaying sweat-delivery to circumscribed areas of the skin surface. *J Invest Dermatol.* 1951;17(4):241-249.
29. Kawahata A, Adams T. Racial variations in sweat gland distribution. *Exp Biol Med.* 1961;106(4):862-865.
30. Homma H. On apocrine sweat glands in White and Negro men and women. *Bull Johns Hopskins Hosp.* 1926;38(5):365-371.
31. Janes CL, Worland J, Stern JA. Skin potential and vasomotor responsiveness of black and white children. *Psychophysiology.* 1976;13(6):523-527.
32. Juniper K, Dykman RA. Skin resistance, sweat-gland counts, salivary flow, and gastric secretion: age, race, and sex differences, and intercorrelations. *Psychophysiology.* 1967;4(2):216-222.
33. Shelley WB, Hurley HJ. The physiology of the human axillary apocrine sweat gland. *J Invest Dermatol.* 1953;20(4):285-297.
34. Martin A, Saathoff M, Kuhn F, Max H, Terstegen L, Natsch A. A functional ABCC11 allele is essential in the biochemical formation of human axillary odor. *J Invest Dermatol.* 2010;130(2):529-540.
35. Prokop-Prigge KA, Mansfield CJ, Parker MR, et al. Ethnic/Racial and genetic influences on cerumen odorant profiles. *J Chem Ecol.* 2015;41(1):67-74.
36. Jacoby RB, Brahms JC, Ansari SA, Mattai J. Detection and quantification of apocrine secreted odor-binding protein on intact human axillary skin. *Int J Cosmet Sci.* 2004;26(1):37-46.
37. Pochi PE, Strauss JS. Sebaceous gland activity in black skin. *Dermatol Clin.* 1988;6(3):349-351.
38. Abedeen S, Gonzalez M, Judodihardjo H, Gaskell S, Dykes P. Racial variation in sebum excretion rate. *Program and abstracts of the 58th Annual Meeting of the American Academy of Dermatology.*
39. Perkins AC, Cheng CE, Hillebrand GG, Miyamoto K, Kimball AB. Comparison of the epidemiology of acne vulgaris among Caucasian, Asian, Continental Indian and African American women. *J Eur Acad Dermatol Venereol.* 2011;25(9):1054-1060.
40. Rawlings AV. Ethnic skin types: are there differences in skin structure and function? *Int J Cosmet Sci.* 2006;28(2):79-93.
41. Goulden V, Stables GI, Cunliffe WJ. Prevalence of facial acne in adults. *J Am Acad Dermatol.* 1999;41(4):577-580.
42. Hillebrand G. The age-dependent changes in skin condition in African Americans, Caucasians, East Asians, Indian Asians and Latinos. *IFSCC Mag.* 2001;4:259-266.
43. Yamamoto A, Serizawa S, Ito M, Sato Y. Effect of aging on sebaceous gland activity and on the fatty acid composition of wax esters. *J Invest Dermatol.* 1987;89(5):507-512.
44. Pappas A, Fantasia J, Chen T. Age and ethnic variations in sebaceous lipids. *Dermatoendocrinol.* 2013;5(2):319-324.
45. Martel JL, Miao JH, *Badri T. Anatomy, Hair Follicle.* In: *StatPearls*. StatPearls Publishing; 2023. Accessed December 24, 2023. http://www.ncbi.nlm.nih.gov/books/NBK470321/.
46. Mangelsdorf S, Otberg N, Maibach HI, Sinkgraven R, Sterry W, Lademann J. Ethnic variation in vellus hair follicle size and distribution. *Skin Pharmacol Physiol.* 2006;19(3):159-167.
47. Luther N, Darvin ME, Sterry W, Lademann J, Patzelt A. Ethnic differences in skin physiology, hair follicle morphology and follicular penetration. *Skin Pharmacol Physiol.* 2012;25(4):182-191.
48. Teichmann A, Jacobi U, Ossadnik M, et al. Differential stripping: determination of the amount of topically applied substances penetrated into the hair follicles. *J Invest Dermatol.* 2005;125(2):264-269.
49. Cloete E, Khumalo NP, Ngoepe MN. The what, why and how of curly hair: a review. *Proc Math Phys Eng Sci.* 2019;475(2231):20190516.
50. Perry PK, Cook-Bolden FE, Rahman Z, Jones E, Taylor SC. Defining pseudofolliculitis barbae in 2001: a review of the literature and current trends. *J Am Acad Dermatol.* 2002;46(2):S113-S119.

CHAPTER 17

Biology of Hair

Allen S.W. Oak
Deega Omar
John T. Seykora

KEY POINTS

- Hair follicles serve a vital role in regulating skin homeostasis and represent a rich reservoir of stem cells that contribute to the hair cycle and wound healing.
- Embryonic hair development and the postembryogenic hair cycle are highly regulated with multiple pathways that continuously relay the signal between the epidermis and the dermis.
- All hair follicles share similar microanatomic features. The keratin filament structure and the amino acid content of hair are consistent across all ethnic groups.
- The architectural and physical properties (eg, tensile strength) of hair differ significantly in individuals of different ethnic backgrounds. The lipid content of hair and the hair density also demonstrate significant ethnic variability.

INTRODUCTION

The hair and its associated adnexal structures aid in thermoregulation, and the scalp hairs also provide photoprotection. Furthermore, hair serves an important role in how a person is perceived in various social contexts, and hair abnormalities (eg, hirsutism and alopecia) cause significant psychosocial stress. Physiologically, the hair follicle serves as a rich reservoir of stem cells that play a crucial role during the hair cycle and wound healing.

ANATOMY OF THE HAIR FOLLICLE [FIGURE 17-1]

In humans, there are three types of hair: lanugo, vellus, and terminal. Lanugo hair, which is long, fine and unpigmented, is the first type of hair to arise in humans and is typically not seen outside the perinatal period. While the presence of lanugo hair in a newborn is considered a normal physical exam finding, most lanugo hairs are shed into the amniotic fluid prior to birth. After the shedding of lanugo hairs, hair follicles continue to cycle. These hair follicles generate vellus (<30 μm in diameter) or terminal (>60 μm in diameter) hairs seen in adults. A sudden appearance of lanugo hairs in an adult may represent a sign of internal malignancy.[1]

All hair follicles share similar microanatomic features. Starting from the level of the interfollicular epidermis, the hair follicle contains (vertical section, listed superior to inferior) an infundibulum, an isthmus, a suprabulbar area, and a bulb [Figure 17-1]. The sebaceous gland is at the level of the junctional zone, which serves as the demarcating region between the infundibulum and the isthmus. The hair bulb resides at the base of the follicle and encompasses the matrix and the dermal papilla (DP), a cluster of specialized mesenchymal cells. The secondary hair germ (SHG, also called secondary germ), which anatomically separates the bulge from the underlying DP, forms at the end of catagen and persists through telogen.

Housed in the bulb, the transit-amplifying cells of the hair matrix give rise to progeny cells that migrate upward toward the skin surface. These matrix-derived cells undergo epidermal keratinization (ie, differentiation pattern of epidermal keratinocytes as they migrate upward and progress in a stepwise manner through the following layers: the basal layer, spinous layer, granular layer, and the stratum corneum). The hair shaft is a rigid structure consisting of terminally differentiated keratinocytes formed in this manner. Most of the hair shaft is visibly exposed to the skin surface, where the shaft emerges from the follicular ostium.

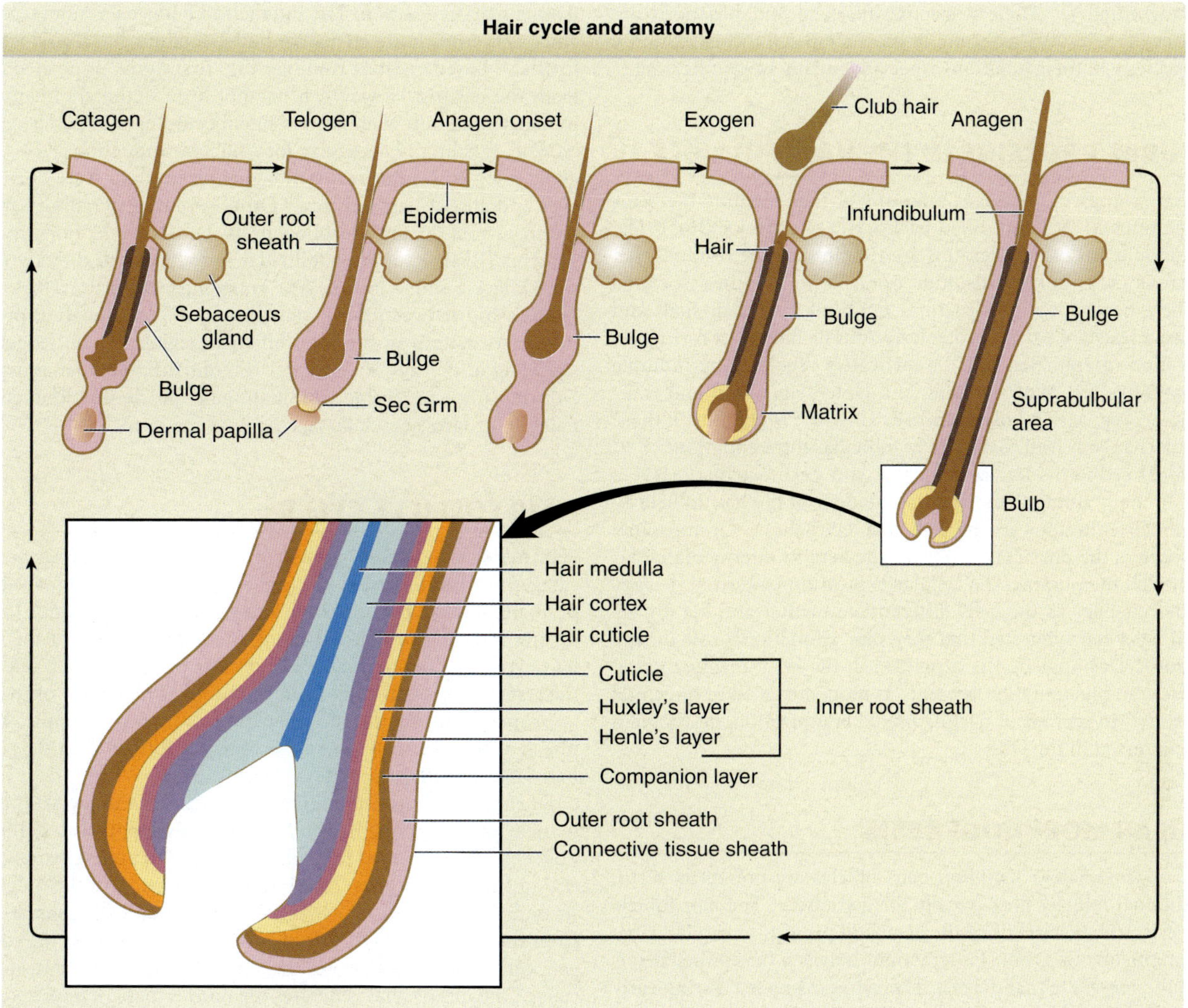

FIGURE 17-1. Hair follicle cycling and hair anatomy. Sec Grm, secondary germ. (Reproduced with permission from Kang S, et al. *Fitzpatrick's Dermatology*. 9th ed. New York, NY: McGraw Hill; 2019, Figure 7-2.)

The hair shaft consists of the following cylindrical layers: the centermost medulla, the outermost cuticle, and the cortex in the middle. The cuticle layer covers and protects the hair shaft from weathering. Cuticular damage causes the hair shaft to fracture, split, and break. The hair shaft cortex serves as the site of keratinization. The cortex, which contains melanin, is an intricate network of hair-specific type I and type II keratin intermediate filaments.[13] Its structural integrity contributes to the mechanical strength of the hair shaft. The medulla, centrally located within the cortex, is often absent in vellus hair.[2] The structure of the hair shaft influences its interactive properties with light (ie, absorption, reflection, and refraction).[3]

The hair shaft is surrounded by the inner root sheath (IRS) and the outer root sheath (ORS).[13] The IRS, which contains trichohyalin granules, consists of at least three concentric layers (listed innermost to outermost): the IRS cuticle (interlocks with the hair shaft cuticle), Huxley's layer, Henle's layer. Henle's layer is surrounded by the companion layer, which is intimately associated with the ORS. The companion layer and the ORS keratinocytes both express CK75.[4] Recent single-cell RNA-sequencing data also raise the possibility that the companion layer may be a component of the ORS.[5] The ORS, which surrounds the IRS, is continuous with the epidermis at the level of the infundibulum.

The rigid IRS guides the differentiating matrix cells as they migrate upward from the bulb. Multiple signaling pathways (eg, epidermal growth factor receptor signaling, BMP signaling, and Notch signaling) are involved in IRS differentiation.[6–8] GATA-3, a transcription factor known for its role in T-cell lineage determination, was also identified to play a crucial role in the lineage determination of IRS cells.[9]

The hair bulb, particularly the degree of its axial asymmetry, demonstrates significant ethnic variance and its asymmetric architecture is associated with increased hair shaft curvature.[10] The DP plays a critical role in guiding the behavior of the matrix, and the number of DP cells is positively correlated with the size of the hair follicle.[11] The matrix generates the hair shaft and all epithelial compartments of the hair follicle except the ORS, which likely is derived from multiple stem cell populations (eg, nestin-positive cells in the bulge).[12,13] The differentiation pattern of ORS cells is distinct from that of matrix-derived cells. Unlike matrix-derived keratinocytes that undergo epidermal keratinization, the ORS keratinocytes only begin to keratinize at the level of the isthmus. The ORS keratinocytes undergo trichilemmal keratinization (ie, abrupt keratinization without forming a granular layer), which is also observed in pilar cysts. During anagen, melanocyte stem cells in the bulge generate melanocytes in the upper portion of the matrix.[14–16] These highly melanogenic cells are responsible for follicular melanogenesis during anagen. The melanized secretory granules are transferred to precortical keratinocytes that form the hair shaft. Within the hair shaft, melanin is predominantly found in the cortex.

The hair follicle houses stem cells that play a vital role during the hair cycle and wound healing. Hair follicle stem cells were first identified in the bulge,[17] the region of the ORS that also serves as the insertion site of the arrector pili muscle. The bulge contains epithelial and melanocytic stem cells that become the transit-amplifying cells of the hair matrix. These cells divide prolifically and reform the lower portion of the hair follicle during anagen.[1,5] Multiple hair follicle stem populations (eg, Lrig1+ cells in the infundibulum and Lgr6+ stem cells in the isthmus) have been identified.[18,19] Their respective markers and functions are reviewed elsewhere.[20,21] At least some of these stem cell niches exhibit a degree of plasticity in their function, especially during wound healing.[22]

STRUCTURAL PROTEINS IN THE HAIR FOLLICLE

The hair shaft expresses abundant amounts of hair keratins (keratins 31-37 and keratins 81-86, also called trichocytic or hard keratins). The head and tail domains of hair keratins are rich in cysteine residues that form numerous cross-linking disulfide bonds with keratin-associated proteins. These bonds provide structural rigidity for the hair shaft and grant increased resistance from proteolysis.[23,24] The hair shaft formation (ie, cornification of epithelial cells) is intricately regulated by multiple signaling pathways (eg, Wnt signaling and Notch signaling) and transcription factors (eg, Msx2, Foxn1, and Hoxc13).[25-27] Mutations in these regulatory mechanisms lead to defects in follicular differentiation.[25,28]

Desmosomal cadherins (ie, desmogleins and desmocollins) serve a critical role in maintaining the structural integrity of the hair follicle by forming cell-cell adhesions in the follicular epithelium. Desmosomal cadherins serve as the physical anchor for the keratin intermediate filaments on the cell membrane. The cellular expression pattern of desmoglein isotypes changes as the cells differentiate further and keratinize. Therefore, it has been suggested that they play a functional role during differentiation.[29] Desmoglein 4 is expressed in the keratinizing zone of the hair cortex, and its mutation presents as monilethrix-like congenital hypotrichosis.[30,31] In regions of trichilemmal keratinization, desmoglein 3 is highly expressed in the ORS.[29]

FOLLICULAR MORPHOGENESIS

In humans, approximately 5 million hair follicles are present at birth, and no additional follicles are typically formed after.[32] The hair follicle morphogenesis, which starts from the head and progresses caudally in a wavelike fashion, involves robust interactions between the epithelial epidermis and the mesenchymal dermis. The genes expressed during early embryogenesis establish the precise spacing, distribution, and future phenotype of hair follicles.[33]

Based on murine studies, Paus and colleagues previously defined and characterized eight distinct stages of hair follicle morphogenesis.[34] This widely used classification system, which is also used to describe follicular morphogenesis in humans, defines the morphologic traits and the immunohistochemical staining pattern of each stage between stage 0 (pregerm) and stage 8 (hair follicle at maximal length with a visible hair shaft emerging from the follicular ostium). Stage 1 is defined by the focal thickening of the epidermis (ie, a placode) that becomes visible around E13.5 in mice and between 10 and 11 weeks of gestation on the human scalp.[35] A collection of Wnt-responsive dermal fibroblasts (ie, a dermal condensate) forms below the placode shortly after. The dermal condensate becomes the DP seen in adult hair follicles. The establishment of a reciprocal signaling loop between the placode and the dermal condensate, as well as the intricate sequence of events that drive morphogenesis, are reviewed elsewhere.[36,37] Of note, an alternative classification system with 10 stages of hair follicle morphogenesis was proposed by Saxena et al in 2019.[38] This alternative classification system defines stage 0 as the unspecified epidermis before the pregerm stage and further splits the pregerm stage into two distinct stages (stage 1: pre-placode, and stage 2: pre-placode/pre-dermal condensate).

Many current concepts regarding follicular development were built based on findings from a groundbreaking series of studies that examined the epithelial-mesenchymal interactions using embryonic cells from two different species (ie, heterotransplant studies) or those from different body regions from the same species (eg, hair-bearing region and a hair-free region).[39] These studies revealed that while the dermis generates the signal needed to initiate development (ie, the "first signal"), the epidermis dictates the hair follicle morphology. For instance, a mouse dermis from a hair-bearing region induced placode formation in the epidermis from a hair-free region. The interaction between a mouse dermis and a chick epidermis initiated feather bud formation, but it could not progress further.[39] Based on these findings, the "first signal" is posited to originate from the dermis. However, it has not been definitely identified, and it remains uncertain whether this signal is uniform or patterned.

Wnt signaling is necessary for follicular induction. K14-*Dkk1* transgenic mice with impaired Wnt signaling in utero were born with open eyes and absent hair follicles.[40] Other essential signaling pathways play a crucial role during morphogenesis. For example, bone morphogenic proteins (BMPs) suppress follicular induction and directly inhibit Wnt signaling via induction of Wnt antagonist Dkk1.[41,42] This antagonistic relationship between BMP signaling and Wnt signaling prevents hair follicle formation in the interfollicular region. Sonic hedgehog (SHH) signaling also plays an essential role during follicular morphogenesis. *Shh* null mice were able to initiate hair follicle development, but they failed to progress beyond stage 2.[43]

HAIR FOLLICLE CYCLE

Hair follicles cycle continuously through three stages: anagen (growth), catagen (involution), and telogen (rest). In a regulated manner, the nonpermanent lower portion (bulb and the suprabulbar region) is destroyed during the catagen phase. During the anagen phase of the subsequent hair cycle, this nonpermanent or cycling portion is then reformed from the reservoir of stem cells from the bulge. The length of the hair cycle is proportional to the length of the hair. For example, the anagen phase of human scalp hair (2-8 years) is longer than that of eyebrow hair (2-3 months).

During the catagen phase, the follicular keratinocytes in the nonpermanent portion of the hair follicle undergo apoptosis.[44] Follicular melanogenesis also ceases as follicular melanocytes undergo apoptosis. At the end of the catagen phase, the lowermost portion of the bulge forms the secondary hair germ. The SHG, which anatomically separates the bulge from the underlying DP,[45] persists through telogen. At the onset of anagen, cells from the bulge and the SHG give rise to the transit-amplifying cells of the matrix that generates the nonpermanent lower portion of the follicle. The SHG, which is more closely located to the dermal papilla, proliferates first at the onset of anagen.[46] Its increased proximity to the dermal papilla, which triggers proliferation, is believed to contribute to this sequence of events. Following depilation-induced injury, the SHG cells are capable of regenerating the bulge.[45] The onset of catagen is regulated by FGF5 and EGFR signaling.[47-49] As such, deficiency in FGF5 or transforming growth factor alpha (EGFR ligand) prolongs the anagen phase.

It is not certain how the matrix can sustain its high proliferation rate for such a prolonged duration. It has been hypothesized that the bulge continuously replenishes the matrix in a manner similar to that seen in the corneal limbus (ie, the conveyor belt model).[50,51]

During the telogen or resting stage, the hair shaft matures into a club hair and is encased by the permanent portion of the hair follicle. The telogen stage typically lasts 2 to 3 months and is accompanied by hair shedding (also called the exogen phase). About 5% to 15% of scalp hair follicles are in the telogen phase at any time, and approximately 50 to 150 scalp hairs are shed daily.

MODULATORS OF HAIR CYCLE AND GROWTH

Androgenetic alopecia (AGA), also called pattern alopecia, is associated with shortening the anagen phase with progressive miniaturization of hair follicles.[52] In AGA, the reservoir of bulge-derived progenitor cells diminishes while the stem cell population in the bulge is maintained.[53] Follicular sensitivity to androgens (eg, testosterone and dihydrotestosterone) are implicated in the pathogenesis of AGA, and those with androgen deficiency do not develop AGA.[54] While the mechanism for androgen dependency for AGA has not been established, the current therapeutic strategy for the medical management of AGA involves the

TABLE 17-1 Summary of characteristics of hair of various racial groups

Race	Morphology	Lipid content	Tensile strength	Hair density	Growth rate
European	Straight, wavy, or curly; ovoid or round cross-section	Low	High	226 ± 73 hairs/cm^2	367 ± 56 μm/day
African	Helical, coiled, or spiraled; flattened cross-section	Low, but high squalene content	Low	161 ± 50 hairs/cm^2	280 ± 50 μm/day
Asian	Straight; round cross-section	High	High	175 ± 54 hairs/cm^2	411 ± 43 μm/day

pharmacologic blockade of androgens and their target receptors. In men, 5α-reductase inhibitors (eg, finasteride and dutasteride) are used to suppress dihydrotestosterone synthesis.[55,56] In women, spironolactone is used for its antiandrogenic effect.

Minoxidil, which prolongs the anagen phase through an unknown mechanism, is also used topically to treat AGA.[57] The off-label use of oral minoxidil at a low dose (2.5-5 mg) may also be efficacious in AGA management.[58] Metabolites of arachidonic acid have been implicated in hair cycle regulation. The peak in prostaglandin D2 level triggers the onset of catagen, and prostaglandin Fα induces anagen onset.[59,60] Bimatoprost, a PGF2α analog, is FDA-approved to treat hypotrichosis of the eyelashes.

ETHNIC VARIATIONS IN HAIR

Ethnic differences have been identified in the structural and functional components of hair follicles. The Asian hair is typically straight and round in cross-section[61] [**Table 17-1**]. The African hair is helical, coiled, or spiraled and is flattened in cross-section. The European hair is straight, wavy, or curly and is ovoid or round in cross-section.[62] The hair shaft in those of African descent shows the greatest percentage of section variability, with regular constrictions in its cross-section along the entire shaft. To examine the ethnic differences in hair shaft morphology, a comprehensive analysis was carried out using hair samples from seven ethnic populations in Asia, Africa, Europe, North America, Papua New Guinea, and the Solomon Islands.[63] The hair diameter, medullation (ie, presence or absence of a medulla), and crimp (ie, the number of times the direction of curvature changes for a given length) had significant F-ratios of 19.6, 25.4, and 47.1, respectively. The most striking parameter was the average curvature (ie, the inverse of the average radius of curvature), which had an F-ratio of 364.8.

The physical properties of the hair shaft also differ based on ethnic background. Using 3-mm-long hair samples from people of African, Asian, and Caucasian descent, Franbourg and colleagues[61] investigated the degree of radial swelling of hair in water and its response to mechanical stress. In a study performed by Franbourg and colleagues,[61] African hair had the lowest radial swelling rate, with similar swelling rates in Asian and Caucasian hairs. Ethnic differences in the hair tensile strength were also examined. In dry conditions (45% relative humidity), African hair displayed lower breaking stress than Asian and Caucasian hairs. Increased microscopic signs of structural damage (eg, breaks, knots and longitudinal splits) were also identified in African hair compared to those from other ethnic groups.[64] Knots were identified almost exclusively in African hair (10-16% vs. 0.15% in Caucasian and Asian hair).

Despite significant ethnic differences in hair morphology and properties, the biochemical composition of the hair shaft is almost identical across all ethnic groups. Amino acid composition analysis from hair shafts from those of African, Asian, and Caucasian descent identified no significant differences.[65,66] Furthermore, an X-ray analysis of the keratin structure did not reveal any intrinsic differences between hair samples from African, Asian, and Caucasian individuals.[61] The distribution of cystine-rich residues was also highly similar in these ethnic groups.[67]

Ethnic difference in integral hair lipids (eg, fatty acids, cholesterol sulfate, ceramides, and cholesterol) of the cuticle was examined. These hydrophobic lipids are believed to maintain hair integrity by moisturizing the cuticle.[68] Asian hair had higher levels of integral hair lipids than African and Caucasian hair. The African hair had the lowest lipid content overall, but its level of squalene was elevated. After UV exposure, the lipid content of all hair samples diminished. However, the Asian hair samples with the highest lipid content showed fewer signs of structural damage (eg, focal lift of the cuticle edge). On the other hand, the African hair samples showed more signs of UV-induced damage.

The hair density also demonstrates ethnic variability. A retrospective analysis of healthy scalp hair density revealed that African Americans have a significantly lower mean density of hair follicles than Caucasians (22.4 vs 35.5 per transverse section of a 4-mm punch biopsy, respectively).[69] Similar findings were reported in a study by Loussouarn and colleagues. In this study, greater hair density was observed in Caucasians than those in Asians and Africans (mean ± standard deviation [SD]: 226 ± 73, 175 ± 54, and 161 ± 50 hairs/cm^2, respectively).[70] Africans also tended to have higher telogen counts than Asians and Caucasians (mean ± SD: 14% ± 9%, 12% ± 7%, and 12% ± 8%, respectively). Furthermore, African hair demonstrated the lowest rate of growth (280 ± 50 μm/day) compared to those of Caucasian hair (367 ± 56 μm/day) or Asian hair (411 ± 43 μm/day).[70] This difference in the rate of growth was also observed in vitro.[10]

Despite profound ethnic differences in the tensile strength of hair and its susceptibility to stress-induced damage, there are only minute ethnic differences in its chemical composition. Significant differences in the hair shaft's architectural qualities (ie, curliness) and lipid composition represent likely etiologies for these observed ethnic variations.

REFERENCES

1. Slee PHTJ, van der Waal RIF, Schagen van Leeuwen JH, et al. Paraneoplastic hypertrichosis lanuginosa acquisita: uncommon or overlooked? *Br J Dermatol.* 2007;157(6):1087-1092.
2. Shimomura Y, Christiano AM. Biology and genetics of hair. *Annu Rev Genomics Hum Genet.* 2010;11:109-132.
3. Schlake T. Determination of hair structure and shape. *Semin Cell Dev Biol.* 2007;18(2):267-273.
4. Sperling LC, Hussey S, Sorrells T, Wang J-a, Darling T. Cytokeratin 75 expression in central, centrifugal, cicatricial alopecia–new observations in normal and diseased hair follicles. *J Cutan Pathol.* 2010;37(2):243-248.
5. Joost S, Annusver K, Jacob T, et al. The molecular anatomy of mouse skin during hair growth and rest. *Cell Stem Cell.* 2020;26(3):441-457.e7.
6. Luetteke NC, Phillips HK, Qiu TH, et al. The mouse waved-2 phenotype results from a point mutation in the EGF receptor tyrosine kinase. *Genes Dev.* 1994;8(4):399-413.
7. Genander M, Cook PJ, Ramsköld D, et al. BMP signaling and its pSMAD1/5 target genes differentially regulate hair follicle stem cell lineages. *Cell Stem Cell.* 2014;15(5):619-633.
8. Pan Y, Lin MH, Tian X, et al. γ-Secretase functions through notch signaling to maintain skin appendages but is not required for their patterning or initial morphogenesis. *Dev Cell.* 2004;7(5):731-743.
9. Kaufman CK, Zhou P, Pasolli HA, et al. GATA-3: an unexpected regulator of cell lineage determination in skin. *Genes Dev.* 2003;17(17):2108-2122.
10. Thibaut S, Gaillard O, Bouhanna P, Cannell DW, Bernard BA. Human hair shape is programmed from the bulb. *Br J Dermatol.* 2005;152(4):632-638.
11. Chi W, Wu E, Morgan BA. Dermal papilla cell number specifies hair size, shape and cycling and its reduction causes follicular decline. *Development.* 2013;140(8):1676-1683.
12. Legué E, Nicolas JF. Hair follicle renewal: organization of stem cells in the matrix and the role of stereotyped lineages and behaviors. *Development.* 2005;132(18):4143-4154.
13. Li L, Mignone J, Yang M, et al. Nestin expression in hair follicle sheath progenitor cells. *Proc Natl Acad Sci USA.* 2003;100(17):9958-9961.

14. Slominski A, Wortsman J, Plonka PM, Schallreuter KU, Paus R, Tobin DJ. Hair follicle pigmentation. *J Invest Dermatol.* 2005;124(1):13-21.
15. Zocco M, Blanpain C. Identifying the niche controlling melanocyte differentiation. *Genes Dev.* 2017;31(8):721-723.
16. Botchkareva NV, Khlgatian M, Longley BJ, Botchkarev VA, Gilchrest BA. SCF/c-kit signaling is required for cyclic regeneration of the hair pigmentation unit. *FASEB J.* 2001;15(3):645-658. doi:10.1096/fj.00-0368com
17. Cotsarelis G, Sun TT, Lavker RM. Label-retaining cells reside in the bulge area of pilosebaceous unit: implications for follicular stem cells, hair cycle, and skin carcinogenesis. *Cell.* 1990;61(7):1329-1337.
18. Snippert HJ, Haegebarth A, Kasper M, et al. Lgr6 marks stem cells in the hair follicle that generate all cell lineages of the skin. *Science.* 2010;327(5971):1385-1389.
19. Füllgrabe A, Joost S, Are A, et al. Dynamics of Lgr6 + progenitor cells in the hair follicle, sebaceous gland, and interfollicular epidermis. *Stem Cell Rep.* 2015;5(5):843-855.
20. Daszczuk P, Mazurek P, Pieczonka TD, Olczak A, Boryń ŁM, Kobielak K. An intrinsic oscillation of gene networks inside hair follicle stem cells: an additional layer that can modulate hair stem cell activities. *Front Cell Dev Biol.* 2020;8:595178.
21. Oak ASW, Cotsarelis G. Wound-induced hair neogenesis: a portal to the development of new therapies for hair loss and wound regeneration. *Cold Spring Harb Perspect Biol.* 2023;15(2):a041239.
22. Rompolas P, Mesa KR, Greco V. Spatial organization within a niche as a determinant of stem-cell fate. *Nature.* 2013;502(7472):513-518.
23. Powell BC, Rogers GE. The role of keratin proteins and their genes in the growth, structure and properties of hair. *EXS.* 1997;78:59-148.
24. Bragulla HH, Homberger DG. Structure and functions of keratin proteins in simple, stratified, keratinized and cornified epithelia. *J Anat.* 2009;214(4):516-559.
25. Jave-Suarez LF, Winter H, Langbein L, Rogers MA, Schweizer J. HOXC13 is involved in the regulation of human hair keratin gene expression. *J Biol Chem.* 2002;277(5):3718-3726.
26. Schneider MR, Schmidt-Ullrich R, Paus R. The hair follicle as a dynamic miniorgan. *Curr Biol.* 2009;19(3):R132-R142.
27. Lee J, Tumbar T. Hairy tale of signaling in hair follicle development and cycling. *Semin Cell Dev Biol.* 2012;23(8):906-916.
28. Guo L, Degenstein L, Fuchs E. Keratinocyte growth factor is required for hair development but not for wound healing. *Genes Dev.* 1996;10(2):165-175.
29. Wu H, Stanley JR, Cotsarelis G. Desmoglein isotype expression in the hair follicle and its cysts correlates with type of keratinization and degree of differentiation. *J Invest Dermatol.* 2003;120(6):1052-1057.
30. Shimomura Y, Sakamoto F, Kariya N, Matsunaga K, Ito M. Mutations in the desmoglein 4 gene are associated with monilethrix-like congenital hypotrichosis. *J Invest Dermatol.* 2006;126(6):1281-1285.
31. Bazzi H, Getz A, Mahoney MG, et al. Desmoglein 4 is expressed in highly differentiated keratinocytes and trichocytes in human epidermis and hair follicle. *Differentiation.* 2006;74(2-3):129-140.
32. Paus R, Cotsarelis G. The biology of hair follicles. *N Engl J Med.* 1999;341(7):491-497.
33. Stark J, Andl T, Millar SE. Hairy math: insights into hair-follicle spacing and orientation. *Cell.* 2007;128:17-20.
34. van der Veen C, Handjiski B, Paus R, et al. A comprehensive guide for the recognition and classification of distinct stages of hair follicle morphogenesis. *J Invest Dermatol.* 1999;113(4):523-532.
35. Gay DL, Yang CC, Plikus MV, et al. CD133 expression correlates with membrane beta-catenin and E-cadherin loss from human hair follicle placodes during morphogenesis. *J Invest Dermatol.* 2015;135(1):45-55.
36. Chen D, Jarrell A, Guo C, Lang R, Atit R. Dermal β-catenin activity in response to epidermal Wnt ligands is required for fibroblast proliferation and hair follicle initiation. *Development.* 2012;139(8):1522-1533.
37. Holbrook KA, Minami SI. Hair follicle embryogenesis in the human. Characterization of events in vivo and in vitro. *Ann N Y Acad Sci.* 1991;642:167-196.
38. Saxena N, Mok KW, Rendl M. An updated classification of hair follicle morphogenesis. *Exp Dermatol.* 2019;28(4):332-344.
39. Hardy MH. The secret life of the hair follicle. *Trends Genet.* 1992;8(2):55-61.
40. Andl T, Reddy ST, Gaddapara T, Millar SE. WNT signals are required for the initiation of hair follicle development. *Dev Cell.* 2002;2(5):643-653.
41. Mukhopadhyay M, Shtrom S, Rodriguez-Esteban C, et al. Dickkopf1 is required for embryonic head induction and limb morphogenesis in the mouse. *Dev Cell.* 2001;1(3):423-434.
42. Botchkarev VA, Botchkareva NV, Roth W, et al. Noggin is a mesenchymally derived stimulator of hair-follicle induction. *Nat Cell Biol.* 1999;1(3):158-164.
43. St-Jacques B, Dassule HR, Karavanova I, et al. Sonic hedgehog signaling is essential for hair development. *Curr Biol.* 1998;8(19):1058-1069.
44. Lindner G, Botchkarev VA, Botchkareva NV, Ling G, van der Veen C, Paus R. Analysis of apoptosis during hair follicle regression (catagen). *Am J Pathol.* 1997;151(6):1601-1617.
45. Ito M, Cotsarelis G, Kizawa K, Hamada K. Hair follicle stem cells in the lower bulge form the secondary germ, a biochemically distinct but functionally equivalent progenitor cell population, at the termination of catagen. *Differentiation.* 2004;72(9-10):548-557.
46. Greco V, Chen T, Rendl M, et al. A two-step mechanism for stem cell activation during hair regeneration. *Cell Stem Cell.* 2009;4(2):155-169.
47. Luetteke NC, Qiu TH, Peiffer RL, Oliver P, Smithies O, Lee DC. TGF alpha deficiency results in hair follicle and eye abnormalities in targeted and waved-1 mice. *Cell.* 1993;73(2):263-278.
48. Hollis DE, Chapman RE. Apoptosis in wool follicles during mouse epidermal growth factor (mEGF)-induced catagen regression. *J Invest Dermatol.* 1987;88(4):455-458.
49. Hébert JM, Rosenquist T, Götz J, Martin GR. FGF5 as a regulator of the hair growth cycle: evidence from targeted and spontaneous mutations. *Cell.* 1994;78(6):1017-1025.
50. Reynolds AJ, Jahoda CA. Hair follicle stem cells: characteristics and possible significance. *Skin Pharmacol.* 1994;7(1-2):16-19.
51. Waters JM, Richardson GD, Jahoda CAB. Hair follicle stem cells. *Semin Cell Dev Biol.* 2007;18(2):245-254.
52. Ellis JA, Sinclair R, Harrap SB. Androgenetic alopecia: pathogenesis and potential for therapy. *Expert Rev Mol Med.* 2002;4(22):1-11.
53. Garza LA, Yang CC, Zhao T, et al. Bald scalp in men with androgenetic alopecia retains hair follicle stem cells but lacks CD200-rich and CD34-positive hair follicle progenitor cells. *J Clin Invest.* 2011;121(2):613-622.
54. Hamilton JB. Male hormone stimulation is prerequisite and an incitant in common baldness. *Am J Anat.* 1942;71(3):451-480.
55. Chen W, Zouboulis CC, Orfanos CE. The 5 alpha-reductase system and its inhibitors. Recent development and its perspective in treating androgen-dependent skin disorders. *Dermatology.* 1996;193(3):177-184.
56. Sato T, Sonoda T, Itami S, Takayasu S. Predominance of type I 5alpha-reductase in apocrine sweat glands of patients with excessive or abnormal odour derived from apocrine sweat (osmidrosis). *Br J Dermatol.* 1998;139(5):806-810.
57. Messenger AG, Rundegren J. Minoxidil: mechanisms of action on hair growth. *Br J Dermatol.* 2004;150(2):186-194.
58. Randolph M, Tosti A. Oral minoxidil treatment for hair loss: a review of efficacy and safety. *J Am Acad Dermatol.* 2021;84(3):737-746.
59. Sasaki S, Hozumi Y, Kondo S. Influence of prostaglandin F2alpha and its analogues on hair regrowth and follicular melanogenesis in a murine model. *Exp Dermatol.* 2005;14(5):323-328.
60. Garza LA, Liu Y, Yang Z, et al. Prostaglandin D2 inhibits hair growth and is elevated in bald scalp of men with androgenetic alopecia. *Sci Transl Med.* 2012;4(126):126ra34.
61. Franbourg A, Hallegot P, Baltenneck F, Toutain C, Leroy F. Current research on ethnic hair. *J Am Acad Dermatol.* 2003;48(6 Suppl):S115-S119.
62. Lindelöf B, Forslind B, Hedblad MA, Kaveus U. Human hair form. Morphology revealed by light and scanning electron microscopy and computer aided three-dimensional reconstruction. *Arch Dermatol.* 1988;124(9):1359-1363.
63. Hrdy D. Quantitative hair form variation in seven populations. *Am J Phys Anthropol.* 1973;39(1):7-17.
64. Khumalo NP, Doe PT, Dawber RP, Ferguson DJ. What is normal black African hair? A light and scanning electron-microscopic study. *J Am Acad Dermatol.* 2000;43(5 Pt 1):814-820.
65. Gold RJ, Scriver CG. The amino acid composition of hair from different racial origins. *Clin Chim Acta.* 1971;33(2):465-466.
66. Hrdy D, Baden HP. Biochemical variation of hair keratins in man and non-human primates. *Am J Phys Anthropol.* 1973;39(1):19-24.
67. Khumalo NP, Dawber RPR, Ferguson DJP. Apparent fragility of African hair is unrelated to the cystine-rich protein distribution: a cytochemical electron microscopic study. *Exp Dermatol.* 2005;14(4):311-314.
68. Ji JH, Park TS, Lee HJ, et al. The ethnic differences of the damage of hair and integral hair lipid after ultra violet radiation. *Ann Dermatol.* 2013;25(1):54-60.
69. Sperling LC. Hair density in African Americans. *Arch Dermatol.* 1999;135(6):656-658.
70. Loussouarn G, El Rawadi C, Genain G. Diversity of hair growth profiles. *Int J Dermatol.* 2005;44 Suppl 1:6-9.

CHAPTER 18

Biology of Nails

Andrea Nadine Hinton
Jasmine Rana
John Montgomery Yost

KEY POINTS

- The nail unit is a complex appendage comprised of four major components: the proximal and lateral nail folds, the nail matrix, the nail bed, and the nail plate.
- Given the position of the nail unit directly overlying the periosteum of the distal phalanx, the nail may manifest pathologic changes in numerous inflammatory, neoplastic, drug-induced, and endocrinologic conditions in the nail unit and underlying bone.
- The nail matrix is an immune-privileged site that serves as the origin of nail plate development as well as the locus of nearly all the melanocytes present in the nail unit.
- In skin of color, nail matrix melanocytes are similar in number to those of other patients, but they contain mature and active melanosomes that are more likely to produce nail plate pigmentation.
- Longitudinal melanonychia can be a benign manifestation of melanosome activity in patients of color; its presence in multiple nails reduces, but does not eliminate, the probability of melanoma.
- Although melanoma of the nail unit is uncommon, it tends to arise in acral locations, including nails, disproportionately in skin of color.
- Over 90% of melanonychias arise from the distal rather than the proximal nail matrix.

INTRODUCTION

The nail is a highly keratinized unit that, like its evolutionary predecessors—including the hoof and claw—serves as a mechanism of protecting the digits from trauma and other iatrogenic insults. In mammals, the nail has evolved to serve additional critical functions, including increasing tactile sensation, aiding digital and pedal biomechanics, and augmenting dexterity.[1,2] Nail changes can be seen in numerous disease processes; thus, significant efforts have been made to understand the structure and function of the nail unit in order to further characterize the pathophysiology of numerous disorders.

ANATOMY AND EMBRYOLOGY OF THE NAIL

A framework for understanding the biology and anatomy of the nail is key to evaluating relevant pathology. The nail unit is a complex appendage composed of four main components:

1. The proximal and lateral nail folds;
2. The nail matrix;
3. The nail bed; and
4. The nail plate.

Together, these overly the distal phalanx [**Figure 18-1**]. Because the nail unit lies immediately above the periosteum of the distal phalanx, disorders of the bone and nail are closely intertwined. The shape of the distal phalangeal bone also determines the shape and transverse curvature of the nail.

The digits, nails, and nail folds are formed early in embryonic development [**Figure 18-2**]. The development and structure of the nail unit has been compared to that of the follicular hair unit and is also intimately tied to the development of the associated digit and limb.[1,2] The nail arises from the same primitive epidermis that gives rise to hair, sweat glands, and stratum corneum. A seminal paper previously hypothesized that the primary nail field, which is the earliest precursor to the nail and composed of thickened epidermis delineated by proximal, lateral, and distal grooves, arose at the ninth week of gestation.[3] However, recent research has indicated that this critical unit arises as early as the seventh week of gestation.[4] This is followed by development of the distal ridge and nail plate by roughly the 12th week of gestation; the nail plate extends to cover the majority of the nail bed between 17 and 20 weeks of gestation. The development of the toenails lags behind that of the fingernails by 2 to 9 weeks, depending on stage of development.[4] Defects early in development of the nail, which may range from abnormalities of the Wnt/β-catenin pathway to those of the curvature of the nail, can result in congenital disorders. These occasionally have particular significance in skin of color; for instance, congenital curved nail of the fourth toe has been reported to occur nearly exclusively in East Asian populations.[5]

NAIL FOLDS

There are three main nail folds within the nail unit: the proximal nail fold and the two lateral nail folds. The epithelium of the proximal nail fold is identical to the surrounding skin but lack pilosebaceous units. The dorsal aspect is continuous with the skin of the dorsal digit, while the ventral aspect covers the germinative matrix and covers approximately one-fourth of the nail plate. Histologically, the border between the proximal nail fold and the nail matrix is demarcated by disappearance of the granular layer in the latter.

The proximal nail fold is also continuous with the eponychium, commonly referred to as the cuticle, which comprises cornified epithelium and prevents separation of the nail plate from the nail fold. Distally, the hyponychium, defined as the cutaneous margin underlying the free edge of the nail, serves a similar function to seal the nail plate to the digit and serve as a barrier to the subungual space [Figure 18-1].[2,6] Any iatrogenic (eg, nail plate avulsion) or pathologic (eg, lichen planus, scleroderma) disruption of the eponychium and hyponychium can result in dorsal and ventral pterygium, respectively, in which the surrounding epithelium adheres to the nail bed and compromises nail plate growth.

NAIL MATRIX

The nail matrix is a critical component of the nail unit. It is positioned underneath the proximal nail fold, cuticle, and nail plate, overlays the distal phalanx, and is proximal to the nail bed [Figure 18-1]. The convex margin of the matrix is called the lunula, which may be visualized as a half-moon shape through the proximal aspect of several nail plates, most commonly the thumbs and great toes.

Histologically, nail matrix keratinocytes divide in the basal cell layer and keratinize in the absence of a granular layer. The site of keratinization of nail matrix onychocytes can be clearly distinguished in histologic

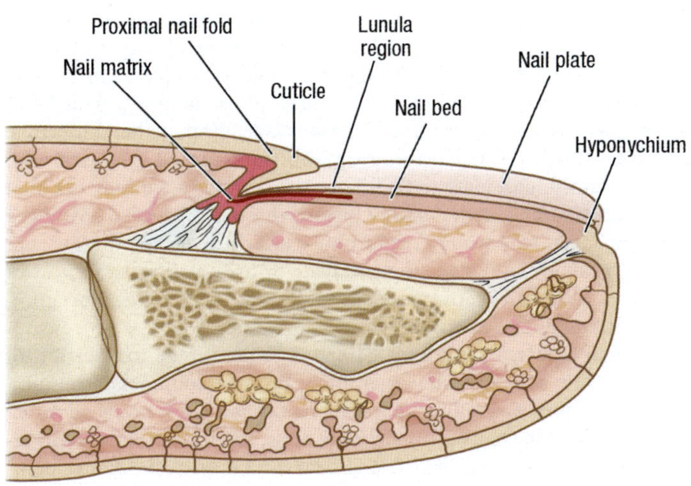

FIGURE 18-1. Nail anatomy.

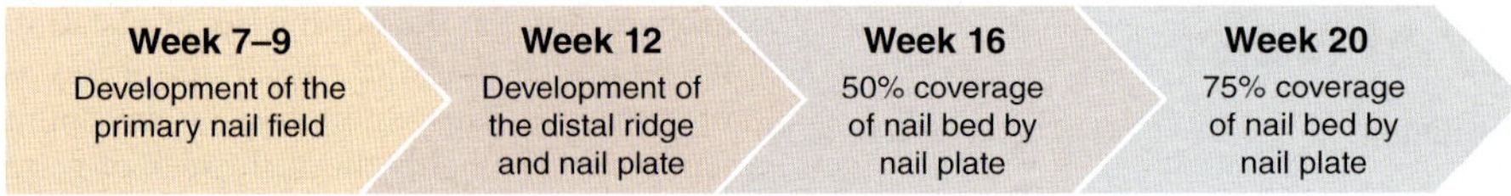

FIGURE 18-2. Fingernail embryology, by week of gestation.

sections as superficial compartments of eosinophilic cells with condensed nuclei. These cells demonstrate fragmentation of their nuclei and condensation of their cytoplasm as they progress to mature onychocytes.[7] Many nail pathologies are the result of abnormal keratinization of the nail unit, including nail psoriasis, chronic onycholysis, and squamous cell carcinoma.

In culture, nail matrix keratinocytes are larger and have a greater proliferation rate than epidermal keratinocytes. At the ultrastructural level, nail matrix cells contain a higher euchromatin-to-heterochromatin ratio and a lower nucleus-to-cytoplasm ratio than epidermal keratinocytes.[8] Both soft keratins (typically found in the epithelium) and hard keratins (similar to keratins found in hair) are produced by nail matrix keratinocytes. In humans, the proximal nail matrix is composed of soft keratins K10, K14, K16, K17, K1, K5, and K6, while the distal matrix contains soft keratins K10, K14, K20, K1, and K5 and the hard keratin Ha1.[9]

The nail matrix has been well established as the source for most of the nail plate development. The maturation and differentiation of nail matrix keratinocytes occurs distally along a beveled axis, such that the proximal nail matrix produces the dorsal nail plate, and the distal nail matrix produces the ventral nail plate. When cultured in serum-containing medium, nail matrix cells produce an outgrowth of epithelium and a spontaneous migration phenomenon associated with a tendency to stratify in a semilunar area that resembles the architecture of the nail matrix.[9]

In recent studies, the nail matrix has been felt to serve as a niche for nail stem cells, analogous to the bulge of the pilosebaceous unit.[2] A growing body of evidence suggests that the proximal nail matrix in particular serves as a site of immune privilege,[2] with immunohistochemical stains of the apparatus in one study showing marked downregulation of MHC class II and CD209 expression by Langerhans cells, as well as decreased activity of innate immune cells.[10] This may explain, in part, the relative rarity of nail unit involvement in diseases such as pemphigus vulgaris due to decreased antigen presentation; of note, this finding varies between ethnic groups, with populations from India, Iraq, and the United States noted to have more frequent involvement of pemphigus vulgaris than ethnic Polish people, perhaps due to difference in MHC class II expression.[11]

NAIL BED

The nail bed is a few cell layers thick and, like the nail matrix, lacks a granular layer. It contains a rich network of nerve endings and longitudinally oriented vessels. Though previous research suggested that the nail bed lacks melanocytes, recent studies suggest a paucity of these cells, which are confined to the basal layer of the epidermis, in the nail bed. Epithelial rete ridges in the nail bed interlock with grooves on the nail plate to facilitate a firm attachment between nail plate and nail bed. After nail avulsion, the nail bed may develop a granular layer, which may compromise attachment. For this reason, efforts are made to replace the nail plate or use a nail prosthesis after biopsies of the nail matrix and bed to decrease the risk of pterygium and promote normal regrowth.

The nail bed was previously estimated to contribute to one-fifth of nail thickness and mass; however, more recent immunohistochemical studies examining keratinocyte proliferation via Ki-67 reveal minimal contribution of the nail bed to nail plate mass, and instead support development of the nail plate via the nail matrix.[12] Of interest, splinter hemorrhages have been reported in a higher frequency in skin of color for unknown reasons and appear as longitudinal streaks due to disruption of the vasculature in the nail bed that then assumes the shape of grooves and ridges between the nail plate and bed.[13]

NAIL PLATE

The nail plate represents the colloquial "nail" as understood by most observers. The nail plate is a hard, semi-transparent sheet made of onychocytes, or compact keratinized epithelial cells. The nail plate covers both the nail bed and nail matrix. It is curved along both the longitudinal and transverse axes, as guided by the proximal and lateral nail folds. This allows it to be embedded into the nail folds at each margin, providing strong attachment. Acquired ingrown nails from ill-fitting footwear can compromise this attachment laterally, resulting in associated inflammation, pain, and infection. Of note, the curvature of the toenail is greater than that of the fingernail. The transverse curvature of the nail is influenced by age, handedness, and gender.[14]

The nail plate is generally organized into three layers—dorsal, intermediate, and ventral—in accordance with the orientation of underlying filaments. The dorsal surface of the nail plate is smooth, though it may develop a variable number of longitudinal ridges with age.[15] In contrast, the ventral surface has prominent longitudinal ridging, which increases the total surface area upon which the nail plate is able to attach to the nail bed as described above. The distal aspect of the nail tends to be thicker than its proximal aspect.

In general, there are a number of factors that influence thickness of the nail plate, including mechanical forces and repetitive trauma, vascular supply, underlying chronic disease, and infection.[15,16] As previously noted, the origin of the nail plate is felt to be primarily driven by the nail matrix, but remains under debate, with recent research suggesting that multiple components, including the nail matrix, the ventral aspect of the proximal nail fold, and the nail bed contribute to its production to varying degrees.[2]

The dorsal plate has a relatively high calcium, phospholipid, and sulfhydryl group content, with a paucity of acid phosphatase activity, all of which contribute to its tensile strength and hard texture. The phospholipid content may provide some water resistance; however, overall nails are quite permeable and vulnerable to the effects of repeat water insults.[17]

In contrast, the intermediate nail plate has higher acid phosphatase activity than its dorsal counterpart, likely corresponding to the number of retained nuclear remnants. The intermediate plate cells are eosinophilic and move both upward and forward with nail growth. The nail plate has been found to have a superficial dry compartment and a deep humid one.

NEUROVASCULAR SUPPLY

The nail unit has an abundant blood supply provided by two dorsolateral and two ventrolateral digital arteries. The palmar digital arteries provide the main blood supply to the fingers, while the nail fold is supplied by a superficial arcade. The distal and subungual arcades, arising from an anastomosis of the palmar arch and the dorsal nail fold, supply the subungual region. Substantial anastomotic connection is provided through glomus bodies, which contain nerve endings and arteriovenous anastomoses that regulate capillary circulation in response to temperature. The glomus bodies are found predominately in the dermis, with a density varying from 90 to 500 per mm^2 and typical length of 300 μm.[18] They are particularly important in maintaining blood supply to the periphery in cold weather, and abnormalities are implicated in numerous pathologic processes, most notably connective tissue disease and glomus cell tumors that are located commonly in the nail unit. Paired digital nerves give rise to the cutaneous sensory nerves, which have a parallel course to the digital vessels. There is a very high density of nerve endings in the nail folds and nail bed; thus, good anesthesia is paramount to successful biopsies of the nail unit.

CHEMICAL AND PHYSICAL PROPERTIES

The onychocytes of the nail are composed primarily of keratins, which are low-sulfur filamentous proteins with a horizontal parallel orientation. Because of this orientation, the nail is more susceptible to transverse splitting. The keratins are embedded in nonkeratin proteins, which are rich in sulfur, glycine, and tyrosine. The hardness of the nail plate is largely due to the hard, hair-like keratins, which comprise 80% to 90% of the nail keratins. The soft, skin-like keratins comprise the remaining 10% to 20%.[19]

The normal water content of the nail ranges from 7% to 18%, lower than the 15% to 25% in the epidermis. Most of the water is localized to the intermediate nail plate, which has been found to be 1000 times more permeable to water than the skin.[20,21] The porosity of the nail causes the nail to be both readily hydrated and readily dehydrated. The nail also contains trace organic elements, including iron, zinc, and calcium, which do not contribute to the hardness of the nail. The total fat content of the nail plate varies from 0.1% to 5%, in comparison with the stratum corneum, which has 10% fat content.[18] The primary lipid in the nail is cholesterol.

The physical properties of the nail plate are hardness, strength, and flexibility. The presence of hard keratins and cysteine-rich high-sulfur proteins determines the hardness of the nail. The strength is attributed to the curved axis in the longitudinal and transverse orientations and the firm adhesion of the onychocytes, while nail hydration and membrane phospholipids contribute to flexibility.[22] The compact ultrastructure of the nail plate also limits its permeability to topical therapeutics like antifungals, which has inspired research into drug enhancers to alter keratin and lipid conformations such as urea, salicylic acid, and dimethylsulfoxide (DMSO).

The ultrastructure of the nail plate varies in each of its three layers.[19] The dorsal nail plate contains flat onychocytes with a shorter diameter perpendicular to the nail plate surface. Intermediate plate cell adhesion is provided by desmosomes and interdigitations of the cell membranes. The ventral nail plate is very thin and composed of soft keratins, which may make it more susceptible to pathologic processes. The ventral nail plate provides firm attachment to the underlying nail bed.

In clinical practice, the brittle nail, which is caused by disruption of corneocytes as well as altered lipid and keratin content in the nail plates, is a frequent chief complaint of patients presenting with nail disorders. While nearly any nutritional deficiency can result in brittle nails or other nail dystrophies, supplements such as calcium, biotin, collagen, and vitamin E have limited data to suggest efficacy in treating nail disease.[23]

NAIL GROWTH

Fingernails grow at 2 to 3 mm/month versus 1 mm/month for toenails, which in a healthy individual leads to a complete replacement of the fingernails in approximately 4 to 6 months and of toenails in 12 to 18 months.[20] Because of this slow rate of growth, diseases of the nail matrix require significant time to both become apparent and resolve. The rate of nail growth is typically greatest during the second and third decades. After age 50, the rate of nail growth decreases sharply.[21] Many conditions have been associated with either increased or decreased rate of growth [**Table 18-1**].[24]

TABLE 18-1 Conditions affecting rate of nail growth

Decreased growth rate	Increased growth rate
Inflammatory/Infectious	*Inflammatory/Infectious*
Lichen planus	Psoriasis
Measles	Pityriasis rubra pilaris
Mumps	Epidermolytic hyperkeratosis
Onychomycosis	
Systemic diseases of manifestations	*Systemic diseases or manifestations*
Atherosclerosis	Hyperthyroidism
Tobacco use disorder	Arteriovenous shunting
Peripheral vascular disease	Digital clubbing
Malnutrition	Hyperpituitarism
Exogenous sources	*Exogenous sources*
Medications	Medications
Prolonged cold exposure	Onychophagia
Other	*Other*
Yellow nail syndrome	Pregnancy

MELANOCYTES

In the nail, melanocytes are less dense and more frequently dormant than in the rest of the skin epidermis. Because the nail matrix is covered by the nail plate and the nail fold at the proximal areas, these melanocytes are presumed not to be stimulated by ultraviolet radiation. It has been postulated that this is the reason the population of DOPA (dihydroxyphenylalanine)-positive (ie, pigment-producing) melanocytes is fewer in the nail matrix than in the epidermis.[25]

Classically, increased melanocyte *activity* can reflect benign changes of the nail (ie, melanocytic activation), whereas increased melanocyte *proliferation* or *hyperplasia* can result in either banal (ie, nevus or lentigo) or pathologic (ie, melanoma) entities. Given this, defining the density of melanocytes in the nail unit has become a particular area of research interest. It has been demonstrated that melanocytes are present in multiple components of the nail unit, including the nail matrix and, in much lower numbers, the nail bed.[26] The relative absence of melanocytes in the nail bed may account for the similarity in appearance of healthy nail plates across skin types [**Figure 18-3A** and **B**].

Most longitudinal melanonychia arises from the distal nail matrix, which reflects the fact that melanocytes populate the distal matrix most densely, where they are present in both the basal and suprabasal layer. Historical studies have estimated a density of 208 to 576 melanocytes/mm^2 by DOPA-stain[27]; more recent studies have estimated a density of about 6.86 melanocytes per 1 mm length of the nail matrix (or, 47.04 melanocytes/mm^2).[26] In contrast, melanocytes in the nail bed are confined to the basal layer, with markedly lower detection rates by staining with HMB-45, at just 0.43 melanocytes/mm (0.185 melanocytes/mm^2). Ongoing research has been limited by specificity in melanocytic marker staining, yielding widely variable results even within individual studies. For instance, a recent study of a Colombian population suggested that staining by H&E underestimates the number of melanocytes, with a nearly tripled population of 12.4 melanocytes/linear mm found in via staining with anti-MITF versus 4.6/linear mm with H&E, 9.8/linear mm with HMB-45.[28]

Longitudinal melanonychia refers to band-like pigmentation of the nail from the proximal nail fold to the distal end of the nail plate. It may be caused by, more commonly, melanocyte *activation*, as detailed below, or by melanocyte *proliferation*. Melanocyte activation can be triggered by numerous causes, including infection, inflammation, trauma, and medications, most commonly chemotherapeutic agents, antihypertensives, antibiotics, and/or antiretrovirals. However, longitudinal melanonychia may also be a benign phenomenon, particularly in patients of color, and especially in those of African or Asian descent [**Figure 18-4**]. Studies have reported that, for instance, in Black Americans, incidence of longitudinal melanonychia was 96% by age 50, in Japanese patient populations, between 11% and 23% (without age specifications), in patients of Chinese descent evaluated in Canada, incidence of 1.7% over age 50, and in a study of over 600 White patients, was entirely absent.[29]

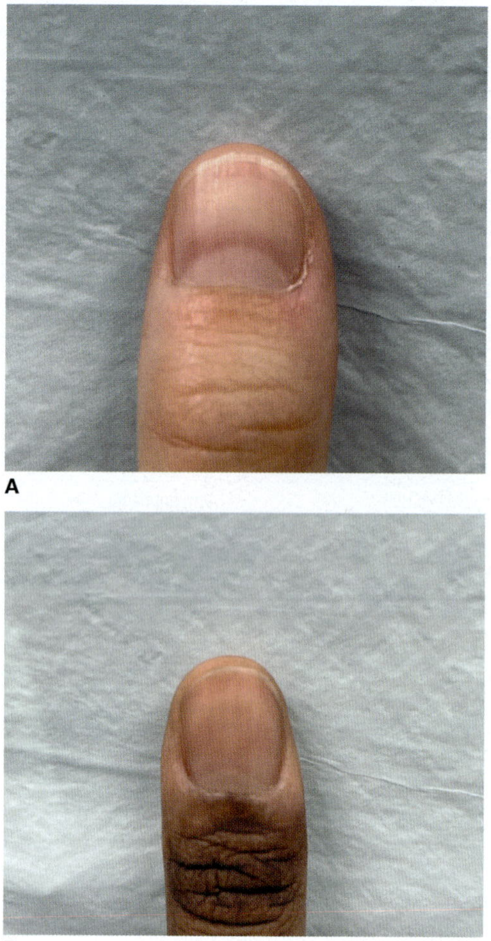

A

B

FIGURE 18-3. **(A)** and **(B)** Normal nail across phototypes.

Visible longitudinal melanonychia in the nail plate is ultimately due to presence of melanosomes (intracellular organelles that contain pigment) transferred from activated melanocytes, often in the matrix, to growing distal onychocytes distally. Although this has not been studied well across multiple skin tones, classic teaching is the number of melanocytes is the same across skin types, but the composition and the ultra-structure of melanosomes varies, which may account for the increased frequency of physiologic longitudinal melanonychia in skin of color and cuticular hyperpigmentation.[30]

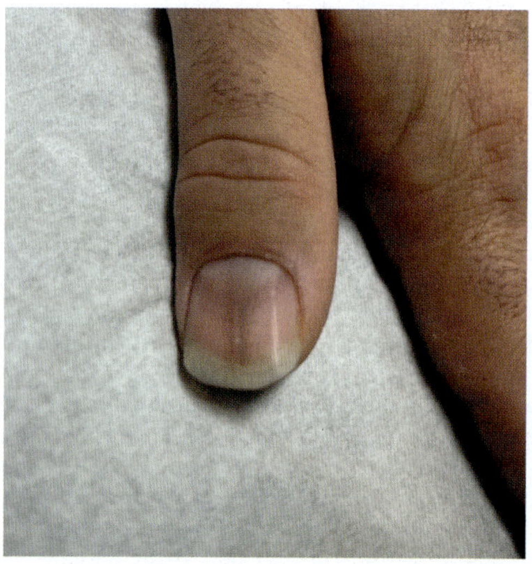

FIGURE 18-4. Longitudinal melanonychia.

REFERENCES

1. Sellheyer K, Nelson P. The concept of the onychodermis (specialized nail mesenchyme): an embryological assessment and a comparative analysis with the hair follicle. *J Cutan Pathol.* 2013;40:463-471.
2. Saito M, Ohyama M, Amagai M. Exploring the biology of the nail: an intriguing but less-investigated skin appendage. *J Dermatol Sci.* 2015;79(3):187-193.
3. Zaias N. Embryology of human nail. *Arch Dermatol.* 1963;87:37-53.
4. Munteanu O, Filipoiu FM, Cirstoiu MM, Băloiu AI, Petrescu IA, Bohiltea RE. A comprehensive study regarding the intrauterine development of nails. *Organogenesis.* 2021;17(1-2):14-19.
5. Hirata Y, Shiiya C, Miyamoto J, Saito M. Congenital curved nail of the fourth toe: report of three cases and review of the literature. *J Dermatol.* 2022;49(9):925-927.
6. Martin B. Nail histopathology. *Actas Dermosifiliogr.* 2013;104(7):564-578.
7. Haneke E. Anatomy of the nail unit and the nail biopsy. *Semin Cutan Med Surg.* 2015;34(2):95-100.
8. Picardo M, Tosti A, Marchese C, et al. Characterization of cultured nail matrix cells. *J Am Acad Dermatol.* 1994;30:434-440.
9. de Berker D, Wojnarowsha F, Sviland L, et al. Keratin expression in the normal nail unit: markers of regional differentiation. *Br J Dermatol.* 2000;142:89-96.
10. Ito T, Ito N, Saathoff M, et al. Immunology of the human nail apparatus: the nail matrix is a site of relative immune privilege. *J Invest Dermatol.* 2005;125:1139-1148.
11. Pietkiewicz P, Bowszyc-Dmochowska M, Gornowicz-Porowska J, Dmochowski M. Involvement of nail apparatus in pemphigus vulgaris in ethnic poles is infrequent. *Front Med (Lausanne).* 2018;5:227.
12. de Berker D, Angus B. Proliferative compartments in the normal nail unit. *Br J Dermatol* 1996;135:555-559.
13. Haber R, Khoury R, Kechichian E, Tomb R. Splinter hemorrhages of the nails: a systematic review of clinical features and associated conditions. *Int J Dermatol.* 2016;55(12):1304-1310.
14. Murdan S. Transverse fingernail curvature in adults: a quantitative evaluation and the influence of gender, age, and hand size and dominance. *Int J Cosmet Sci.* 2011;33(6):509-513.
15. de Berker DA, André J, Baran R. Nail biology and nail science. *Int J Cosmet Sci.* 2007;29(4):241-275.
16. de Berker D, Mawhinney B, Sviland L. Quantification of regional matrix nail production. *Br J Dermatol.* 1996;134:1083-1086.
17. Lee DY, Park JH, Shin HT, Jang KT, Shim JS. Immunohistochemical study of epithelial markers in longitudinal and transverse sections of the human nail unit. *Clin Exp Dermatol.* 2012;37:688-689.
18. Dawber RPR, de Berker DA, Baran R. Science of the nail apparatus. In: Baran R, Dawber RPR, deBerker DAR, eds. *Diseases of the Nails and Their Management.* Oxford, England: Blackwell Science; 2001:1-47.
19. Lynch MH, O'Guin W, Hardy C, et al. Acidic and basic hair/nail ("hard") keratins: their colocalization in the upper cortical and cuticle cells of the human hair follicle and their relationship to "soft" keratins. *J Cell Biol.* 1986;103:2593-2606.
20. Jemec GBE, Serup J. Ultrasound structure of the human nail plate. *Arch Dermatol.* 1989;125:643-646.
21. Spruit D. Measurement of water vapor loss through human nail in vivo. *J Invest Dermatol.* 1971;56:359-361.
22. Finlay AY, Frost P, Keith AD. Assessment of factors influencing flexibility of human fingernail. *Br J Dermatol.* 1980;10:357-365.
23. Muddasani S, Lin G, Hooper J, Sloan SB. Nutrition and nail disease. *Clin Dermatol.* 2021;39(5):819-828.
24. Zaiac MN, Walker A. Nail abnormalities associated with systemic pathologies. *Clin Dermatol.* 2013;31:627-649.
25. Higashi N. Melanocytes of nail matrix and nail pigmentation. *Arch Dermatol.* 1968;97:570-574.
26. Perrin C, Michiels JF, Boyer J, Ambrosetti D. Melanocytes pattern in the normal nail, with special reference to nail bed melanocytes. *Am J Dermatopathol.* 2018;40(3):180-184.
27. Higashi N, Saito T. Horizontal distribution of the dopa-positive melanocytes in the nail matrix. *J Invest Dermatol.* 1969;53:163-165.
28. Rodríguez G, Vargas EJ, Abaúnza MC, Díaz Quijano DM, Melo-Uribe M. Immunohistochemical identification of nail matrix melanocytes. *J Eur Acad Dermatol Venereol.* 2018;32(9):1602-1607.
29. Leung AKC, Lam JM, Leong KF, Sergi CM. Melanonychia striata: clarifying behind the Black Curtain. A review on clinical evaluation and management of the 21st century. *Int J Dermatol.* 2019;58(11):1239-1245.
30. Hashimoto K. Ultrastructure of the human toenail: I. Proximal nail matrix. *J Invest Dermatol.* 1971;56:235-246.

CHAPTER 19

Biology of Wounds and Wound Care

Marita Yaghi
Robert S. Kirsner

KEY POINTS

- Chronic wounds are a rising concern across all racial and ethnic groups, with disproportionate complications often observed in patients with skin of color (SOC).
- The core biology of wound healing is consistent across skin tones, but the clinical manifestations and sequelae, such as keloids and hypertrophic scars, are more prevalent in dark pigmented skin.
- Post-inflammatory hyperpigmentation (PIH) is a common and often distressing outcome of wound healing in patients with darker skin types.
- Traditional visual cues of inflammation (e.g., erythema) may be muted or altered in SOC, making wound assessment more challenging.
- Culturally competent care and skin tone-sensitive diagnostic approaches are essential for equitable and effective wound management.

INTRODUCTION

Beyond pigmentation, the integumentary system has relatively few differences across racial groups. As such, the underlying biology remains the same but directed knowledge and skills are required for the proper assessment of patients with diverse skin color.[1]

Diversity in skin color often translates into disparities in patients with wounds. For instance, detecting erythema might pose a challenge in darker-pigmented skin when it might be visually obvious in lighter-pigmented skin. Similarly, skin necrosis at the wound edge might go undiagnosed in patients with darker-pigmented skin. The failure to timely detect signs of infection or inflammation may lead to life-threatening infections, ultimately translating into worse patient outcomes. For example, significant delays in pressure ulcer healing affect patients with darker-pigmented skin; these outcomes were notably worse than what was expected based on clinical assessment.[2] Additionally, diabetic foot ulcers result in more amputations in patients with darker-pigmented skin as compared to their light-pigmented skin counterparts.[3]

Wounds compromise the integrity of the integumentary system. As such, they disturb the protective barrier against the environment that the skin offers to the inner body, making it vulnerable to foreign allergens and pathogens. Extensive wounds may additionally jeopardize other important functions of the skin, including fluid homeostasis, thermoregulation, immune surveillance, sensory detection, and healing. This may result in significant morbidity and mortality. It is estimated that 8.2 million Medicare beneficiaries suffered from a wound or related infection in 2014 alone, with cost projections reaching $96.8 billion dollars.[4] Furthermore, chronic wounds occur mostly in the elderly population, suggesting an increasing prevalence as the U.S. population becomes increasingly older.[4,5]

This chapter summarizes the basic biology of wound healing, and guides wound assessment and treatment, highlighting special considerations for patients with skin of color.

WOUND TYPES AND EPIDEMIOLOGY

A wound is defined as a break in the skin. Hence, dermatologists routinely create wounds in their day-to-day practice performing diagnostic biopsies, therapeutic surgery, and aesthetic procedures. Numerous other extrinsic factors lead to the development of wounds, such as trauma with sharp or pointed objects, chemical or thermal burns, or friction. Poor nutrition, some medications, such as high doses of glucocorticoids, or radiation therapy may alter the skin structure and predispose it to wound formation. Patients may also create wounds themselves, either factitiously or as a result of drug abuse, but also inadvertently in the setting of severe pruritus, for example.

Some skin diseases, such as epidermolysis bullosa or autoimmune blistering diseases (eg, pemphigus, bullous pemphigoid), lead to wounds. More commonly, vascular insufficiency leads to ulceration that often becomes chronic. In the United States, chronic wounds affect approximately 6.5 million patients.[6] Lower extremity ulcers have a prevalence of 1% to 2% in the general population,[7] with venous insufficiency accounting for 80% as leg ulcers.[8] They represent a significant financial burden on the U.S. healthcare system with direct annual costs reaching as high as $14.9 billion.[9] Diabetes mellitus is another important intrinsic factor, which leads to the development of foot ulcers secondary to peripheral neuropathy with or without peripheral vascular disease. The 5-year mortality of new-onset diabetic foot ulcers has been reported to reach 55% and increase to 74% if patients undergo lower extremity amputations, showing rates higher than those seen with several malignancies such as prostate, breast, or colon cancer.[10]

THE BIOLOGY OF WOUND HEALING

The phenomenon of *repair* largely governs wound healing in children and adults. In contrast, fetuses in the first two trimesters experience *regeneration* following injury.[11] Fibrosis, scarring, and possible loss of adnexal structure depending on wound depth, which occur with wound *repair*, fundamentally separate both phenomena, resulting in loss of normal skin morphology and function. Fetal skin, on the other hand, heals without visible scars.[12]

Wound healing is a complex and dynamic process, which involves the interplay of hematopoietic cells and soluble mediators recruited to the damaged site with local parenchymal cells and the extracellular matrix (ECM). These elements will take part in a series of cellular and molecular events that can be temporally categorized into three major phases: inflammation, proliferation, and remodeling. These will be described in the rest of this chapter.

Cutaneous wound depth determines the healing ability of the skin and quality of repair. Wounds limited to the epidermis are called erosions and heal rapidly through epidermal regeneration with no scar formation. Wounds that extend into the dermis heal slower and potentially with scar, depending on the extent and depth of dermal injury. When adnexal structures remain preserved in dermis, this is called a *partial-thickness* wound, and epithelial cells from those adnexal structures serve as a reservoir,[13] allowing reepithelialization from both the wound edges and from the adnexa in with wound. In contrast, *full-thickness* wounds are characterized by complete dermal loss along with adnexa eliminating the adnexal reservoir of epithelial cells. Consequently, reepithelization only occurs from the wound edges and additional wound contracture occurs as does the potential for worse scarring.

Contraction is hypothesized to be mediated by both mechanical and biological factors, the latter involving the differentiation of particular fibroblasts into myofibroblasts.[14] As the wound contracts, its area decreases via centripetal movement of preexisting tissue as opposed to the formation of new tissue. This can result in cosmetically disfiguring and functional problematic contractures.[15]

Tissue repair mechanisms that govern regeneration in human embryos (as opposed to repair) remain largely unelucidated. Further insight into these mechanisms could potentially lead to therapeutics that not only support wound repair but also restore the skin's original morphology and adnexal structures.

HEMOSTASIS AND INFLAMMATION

Tissue injury causes blood vessel disturbance and consequent leakage of blood constituents and release of vasoactive factors into the injury site. Rapid local vasoconstriction preventing exsanguination is the first response

TABLE 19-1 Chemical mediators released by platelets that play a role in wound healing

Chemical mediator	Action
Platelet factor 4 (PF-4)	Neutrophil and macrophage recruitment Monocyte differentiation Reactive oxygen species (ROS) formation
Platelet-derived growth factor (PDGF)	Neutrophil and macrophage recruitment Fibroblast recruitment and proliferation Angiogenesis Granulation tissue formation
Vascular endothelial growth factor (VEGF)	Angiogenesis Macrophage recruitment
Hepatocyte growth factor (HGF)	Keratinocyte proliferation
Fibroblast growth factor (FGF)	Fibroblast and keratinocyte proliferation Matrix deposition Angiogenesis
Transforming growth factor-β1 (TGF-β1)	Keratinocyte proliferation Epidermis remodeling and regeneration

to injury and step toward the reestablishment of *hemostasis*.[16] Platelets are then activated upon contact with the exposed sub-endothelial collagen of damaged blood vessels, which leads to their aggregation and initiation of the clotting cascade. This results in the formation of a fibrin-rich blood clot that plugs severed vessels, shields against bacterial invasion, and releases key mediators, such as growth factors and proinflammatory cytokines, that act as chemotactic agents targeting blood leukocytes and fibroblasts and guiding their behavior during early wound repair [**Table 19-1**].[17–21] This process lasts from minutes to hours after skin damage.

Injured necrotic and apoptotic cells release damage-associated molecular patterns (DAMPs), initiating *inflammation*,[22] which typically may last up to 3 days. DAMPs, such as High-Mobility Group Box-1 (HMGB-1), S100 proteins, and heat shock proteins, activate Toll-like receptor-3 (TLR-3), TLR-4, and TLR-9 upregulated on the surface of keratinocytes in acute wounds.[23–26] This leads to additional inflammatory cytokine production and release,[27] further augmented by the effects of intracellular Ca^{2+} at the wound edges and the release of hydrogen peroxide, a reactive oxygen species (ROS), by the wounded cells.[22] Neutrophils and macrophages are then recruited in large numbers at the site of injury. Neutrophils will first cleanse the area from foreign particles, including bacteria, and cellular debris. Upon completion of particle clearance, generation of granulocyte chemotactic factors ceases, and the remaining neutrophils recede. Monocyte accumulation, separately driven by selective monocyte chemotactic agents, follows and further contributes to the wound debridement process. They differentiate into tissue macrophages upon adherence to the ECM, which produce and secrete cytokines and growth factors: interleukin-1 (IL-1), platelet-derived growth factor-BB (PDGF-BB), transforming growth factor alpha (TGF-α), transforming growth factor beta (TGF-β), and fibroblast growth factor (FGF).[28] The latter are crucial for the initiation of the next phase of skin repair.

While neutrophils and macrophages play a critical role in combatting infection and aiding in growth factor generation and release, excessive inflammation may be harmful.[29] For example, if microorganisms or indigestible particles are lodged in the wound site, neutrophils will be prompted to release substantial amounts of digesting enzymes and toxic oxygen side-products, causing further damage to the injured tissue. This is further supported by in vivo experiments demonstrating faster wound healing in the presence of fewer inflammatory cells, particularly in situations where the wound remains sterile.[30]

PROLIFERATION

The *proliferation* phase overlaps with the end of the inflammation phase. It aims at creating new tissue to fill the wound space internally and closes the cutaneous defect superficially, effectively restoring the skin's function as a protective barrier from the outside environment.

Reepithelialization Reepithelialization of the wound is one of the main features of the proliferation phase and begins within hours following injury, overlapping with the inflammatory phase. Epithelial cells will move from the surrounding epidermis to cover the denuded surface, working at rapidly reestablishing an epidermal surface. This process of keratinocyte migration and proliferation originating at the wound edges is driven by epidermal-mesenchymal interaction[31] and characterized by marked phenotypic and functional alterations. The resultant prevention of further water loss and wound protection from colonization by outside pathogens substantially decreases patient morbidity and mortality, particularly in those with a large cutaneous defect. To initiate migration, keratinocytes retract their intracellular filaments and dissolve their intercellular junctional adhesion molecules (desmosomes).[32] These migrating cells also undergo dissolution of their hemidesmosomal links to the underlying basement membrane and form peripheral actin filaments to facilitate their movement. Already present collagen-binding receptors will be replaced by other integrins with enhanced adherence to the provisional wound matrix. Additionally, front-to-rear polarity replaces top-to-bottom polarity, allowing for lateral movement.[33] All these phenotypic alterations offer migrating keratinocytes plasticity and flexibility, while maintaining a functioning intracellular scaffold, essential for their lateral migration over the wound site.[34] These alterations also phenotypically distinguish the migrating keratinocytes from the terminally differentiated keratinocytes and basal cells of the normal stratified epidermis. If a large surface of epidermis is lost and if dermal structures remain, keratinocytes will also migrate from hair follicles and other adnexal structures.

Wound keratinocytes express cell surface receptors for various integrins and α2β1 collagen receptors on their basal surface.[35] The latter are normally found on the lateral sides of basal keratinocytes but redistribute upon contact with dermal collagen fibers. These receptors allow wound keratinocytes to migrate over a provisional matrix of fibronectin, tenascin, vitronectin and type I collagen.[36] If a wound eschar is present, it will block the lateral migration of keratinocytes. Instead, wound keratinocytes will need to dissect through the wound to reach the underlying viable dermal tissue, separating the fibrin/fibronectin-rich eschar from the underlying dermis in the process.[37] The absence of αvβ3 integrin receptor for fibrin/fibronectin on the surface of keratinocytes prevents their interaction with these eschar matrix proteins.[37] Consequently, the migrating wound cells will avoid moving along the eschar surface. In lieu, these epidermal cells will produce collagenase, specifically matrix metalloproteinase-1 (MMP-1), plasminogen activator, and stromelysin proteases to degrade attachments to underlying basement membrane as well as the surrounding ECM and reach the underlying collagen-rich dermis.[38] Intriguingly, the amount of MMP-1 produced by wound keratinocytes greatly increases upon their contact with dermal collagen, generating a positive feedback loop that promotes further provisional fibrin-rich wound bed degradation.[39] This was observed in superficial skin ulcers and burn wounds, where high levels of MMP-1 mRNA were expressed in areas in direct contact with dermal collagen.[40] Migrating keratinocytes will then continue to travel along the type I collagen containing wound edge via their α2β1 collagen receptors. Their migration upon reaching the fibronectin-rich newly formed granulation tissue of the wound will continue, mediated by the fibronectin receptor α5β1 taking over the regulation of cellular traction forces.[41]

Once migrations occurs, keratinocytes will proliferate at the wound edges.[42] The release of autocrine or paracrine growth factors by recruited macrophages, dermal fibroblasts, and neighboring keratinocytes may also play a role in epidermal cell proliferation [**Table 19-2**],[43–46] further augmented by some growth factors from the circulation acting as a hormone, such as insulin-like growth factor (IGF). Animal models have been useful in identifying the role of growth factors in stimulating re-epithelialization,[47] particularly those investigating knock-out mice models.[48]

As epithelialization progresses, keratinocyte basement membrane proteins reappear in a very ordered sequence from the margin of the wound inward in a zipper-like fashion.[47] Migration also terminates when keratinocytes from opposing edges meet.[16] The epidermal cells then revert to their normal phenotype, attaching to the reestablished underlying basement membrane through hemidesmosomes junctional proteins,

TABLE 19-2 Growth factors involved in keratinocyte proliferation

Growth factor	Source
Transforming growth factor-α (TGF-α)	Keratinocytes
Transforming growth factor-β (TGF- β)	Keratinocytes
Keratinocyte growth factor (KGF)	Fibroblasts, macrophages
Insulin-like growth factor 1 (IGF-1)	Fibroblasts
Hepatocyte growth factor (HGF)	Fibroblasts, macrophages
Heparin-binding epidermal growth factor (HB-EGF)	Fibroblasts, macrophages
Vascular endothelial growth factor (VEGF)	Keratinocytes, macrophages

α6β4 integrin, and 180-kDa bullous pemphigoid antigen[49] and to the underlying neodermis through type VII collagen fibrils.[50] Finally, keratinocytes will undergo terminal differentiation.[51]

Not all epidermal keratinocytes participate in the reepithelialization process. Only interfollicular stem cells, transient amplifying cells, and early differentiated cells have the ability to form a differentiated epidermis and primarily contribute to wound healing.[52,53] These cells commit early on to the differentiation process and undergo specific changes that mark late terminal differentiation.[54] Furthermore, only specific stem cell compartments in the hair follicle contribute to wound healing through keratinocyte differentiation. Stem cells in the lower bulge area and in the isthmus above the bulge area greatly contribute to the keratinocyte pool,[55] while keratin-15 (Krt-15) and Krt-19 positive bulge-region stem cells only play a minor role.[56,57] These findings highlight the complexity underlying wound reepithelization and help shed light on the capability of repair as influenced by the depth of injury.

Granulation Tissue Formation Fibroblasts are the main cell types that replace the temporary fibrin/fibronectin-rich matrix with longer-lasting *granulation tissue*. The latter derives its name from the granular appearance of the newly formed tissue when it is examined, which can be attributed to the presence of innumerable micro-capillaries forming within this neostroma. This process occurs approximately 4 days following injury and consists of two overlapping phenomena: *fibroplasia* and *neovascularization*.

Macrophages, platelets, fibroblasts, and endothelial cells work interdependently within the wound space to facilitate tissue repair. As mentioned in the section on *inflammation*, the arrival of peripheral blood platelets and monocytes, which differentiate into macrophages, to the site of injury is essential to establish conditions for continued synthesis and release of growth factors. These supplement the pool of cytokines released by the injured and activated parenchymal cells themselves, resulting in ECM construction by fibroblasts, necessary to support cell ingrowth, as well as new blood vessel formation, necessary for cellular oxygenation and metabolism. For example, migrating wound epidermal cells produce vascular endothelial growth factor (VEGF), TGF-β, and PDGF-BB, to which endothelial cells and fibroblasts respond, respectively. The provisional ECM also promotes granulation tissue formation by positive feedback regulation of integrin ECM receptor expression.[58] Once fibroblasts and endothelial cells express the appropriate integrin receptors, they invade the fibrin/fibronectin-rich wound space.

Fibroplasia Fibroplasia is defined as the formation of granulation tissue by fibroblasts. Paracrine and autocrine interactions of fibroblasts with provisional matrix molecules and growth factors, specifically PDGF and TGF-β,[58] drive their proliferation, appropriate integrin receptor upregulation, and migration into the wound space. This process relies on both paracrine and autocrine signaling, as macrophages, platelets,[12,47] and fibroblasts themselves[59] are major sources synthesizing and secreting these growth factors. Multiple intricate cooperative biologic phenomena occur within fibroblasts as they respond to these growth factors, including the release and activation of additional cytokines and modulation of cell-surface cytokine receptors.

The interaction of PDGF-BB, FGF-2, and TGF-β with fibronectin and thrombin in the provisional matrix drives the proliferation of fibroblasts[58,60] and the expression of proteoglycans[61] and α5β1 and αvβ3 integrin receptors on their surface,[62] allowing for fibroblast migration along the provisional ECM fibrils into the wound space. In vitro investigations have demonstrated enhanced DNA synthesis and mitosis of dermal fibroblasts following treatment with exogenous FGF-2 and PDGF, via activation of the mitogen-activated protein kinase/extracellular-signal-regulated kinase (MEK/ERK) and phosphatidylinositol 3-kinase (P13K)/Akt signaling pathways.[63] A similar effect was observed in cultured human fibroblasts treated with TGF-β1.[64] Furthermore, the addition of recombinant FGF-2 to cutaneous wounds in knock-out animal models with delayed repair responses restored the repair process, effectively recruiting fibroblasts to the wound site and increasing granulation tissue formation.[65–68]

Structural molecules of the provisional matrix also drive fibroplasia. Hyaluronic acid promotes both fibroblast proliferation and motility, through the CD44 cellular glycoprotein,[69] while fibronectin acts as a conduit for cell migration through interaction with cellular β1, β3, and β5 integrin receptors.[62] The binding of fibroblasts to fibronectin stimulates the production of collagen and proteoglycans. In addition to changing the mechanical environment, these molecules interact with one another, as proteoglycans may facilitate collagen fibrillogenesis.[70] The presence of fibronectin within the ECM appears to be a critical rate-limiting step in fibroblast activation, and thus the formation of granulation tissue.[71] Given the role of fibroblasts in ECM remodeling, this highlights the dynamic reciprocity governing the fibroblasts and provisional matrix interaction.[72]

Active proteolytic degradation of the cross-linked fibrin clot is required to cleave a path for fibroblast migration. It is driven by a variety of fibroblast-derived enzymes in conjunction with serum-derived plasmin, including plasminogen activator, interstitial collagenase-1, and -3 (MMP-1 and MMP-13, respectively), the 72-kDa gelatinase A (MMP-2), and stromelysin (MMP-3). For instance, the plasminogen activator protease clears fibrin from the wound,[73] while MMP-13 cleaves native helical collagens throughout repair.[74] High levels of MMP-1 have been found within fibroblasts at the interface of granulation tissue with the provisional matrix in burn wounds,[42] and many stromal cells stain for MMP-1 and MMP-13 in chronic ulcers.[75] Metalloproteinase secretion and activity are highly regulated for optimal fibroplasia, a task mainly accomplished by cytokines: PDGF stimulates the synthesis and release of these proteinases, while TGF-β downregulates their activity. Downregulation of MMP-1 seems to be important for normal tissue remodeling as high levels of MMP-1 have been found in chronic nonhealing wounds.[76] MMP-8, if increasingly expressed, causes breakdown of type I collagen detrimentally impacting wound repair.[77] In contrast, double knock-out of MMP-13 and plasminogen activator resulted in more delayed healing as compared to single knock-out of plasminogen activator alone.[78] Thus, proper regulation of the overlapping activity of the various MMP proteases is necessary for proper tissue repair in cutaneous wounds.

Once fibroblast have migrated into the wound site, they begin the process of protein synthesis and granulation tissue formation. α3β1 and α5β1 integrin receptors to fibronectin from the provisional matrix become downregulated on the surface of the fibroblasts, effectively replaced by α2β1 collagen receptors.[58,79] Thus, a phenotypic switch from migratory to profibrotic occurs within fibroblasts, allowing for collagen synthesis. PDGF stimulates heightened upregulation of α2β1 collagen receptors, but not α3β1 and α5β1 fibronectin receptors,[58] while TGF-β induces high levels of collagen synthesis.[80] As both these cytokines are sourced from the provisional extracellular matrix, this further supports the hypothesis of dynamic reciprocity between fibroblasts and the provisional matrix governing fibroplasia.[72] This results in the gradual supersession of the fibronectin-rich provisional matrix by a collagenous matrix.[79] IL-4 can induce a modest increase in type I and III collagen production by fibroblasts[81]; thus, mast cells present in the healing wound milieu might also contribute to the collagen production. Collagen deposition halts once abundant collagen matrix is synthesized by fibroblasts, through a direct suppression of fibroblast function,[82,83] despite the presence of TGF-β.[82] This might be spurred by γ-interferon as demonstrated in both in vitro and in vivo models.[84]

On day 10 of the wound healing process, fibroblasts develop pyknotic nuclei, a marker of apoptosis.[85] This suggests that programmed cell death apoptosis is the mechanism responsible for the transition from a fibroblast-rich granulation tissue to a relatively acellular scar.[86] Although signals for wound fibroblast apoptosis have not been elucidated, fibroplasia in wound repair is clearly tightly regulated, whereas in fibrotic diseases, such as keloids, morphea, and scleroderma, these processes become dysregulated. Evidence suggests that fibroblast apoptotic signals in hypertrophic scars and keloids are disrupted.[87]

Neovascularization As fibroplasia occurs, new blood vessels are formed to meet the metabolic demands of the highly proliferative healing tissue. This is referred to *angiogenesis*. Hypoxia and COX-2 trigger angiogenesis,[88] which is then driven by many soluble factors within the wound bed.[89] Various cell types play a role in the process, such as endothelial cells in the vicinity of the wound edge but also activated macrophages, fibroblasts, and keratinocytes.[90] Increasing evidence suggest that the provisional ECM also plays a role in regulating angiogenesis.[89]

In healthy tissues, mature blood vessels are maintained in a quiescent state and surrounded by a collagen type IV and laminin coat.[91] Upon injury, proangiogenic factors come into contact with endothelial cells, which start to proliferate and migrate forming vascular sprouts.[92] Upon contact with neighboring sprouts, these structures will fuse, reestablishing blood flow; nonperfused sprouts will regress by apoptosis.[92]

Many soluble factors promote angiogenesis in wound repair [**Table 19-3**][12,47,93] and take part the various steps of the process. Upon injury, FGF is release from damaged cells and surrounding ECM.[94] Recruited platelets release multiple growth factors, such as PDGF, VEGF, TGF-α, TGF-β, FGF, and angiopoietin.[95–98] Additionally exposure to thrombin upon eschar formation triggers endothelial cells upregulation of VEGF cell-surface receptors and release of gelatinase A (MMP-2),[99] which promotes the local dissolution of the basement membrane surrounding mature blood vessels. These factors work together in complex coordinated pathways to drive angiogenesis. For instance, TNF-α induces PF-4 that stimulates angiogenesis through NO,[100] whereas low oxygen tension stabilizes hypoxia inducible factor-1α (HIF-1α), which induces increased expression of VEGF.[101] Recruited inflammatory cells within the wound bed further amplify angiogenesis. Macrophages and monocytes release PDGF, VEGF, Ang-1, TGF-α, FGF, IL-8, and TNF-α along with proteases to degrade the dense fibrin network of the provisional matrix to drive endothelial migration.[102] Macrophage dysfunction and failure to release VEGF-A has been shown to cause reduced capillary formation in knock-out mice models.[103] Altogether, these factors stimulate endothelial proliferation, migration, and vascular tube formation.

Proteolytic enzymes, such as MMP-2 and FGF-2, dissolve the basement membrane of mature blood vessels surrounding the wound, allowing the proliferating endothelial cells to sprout through and migrate into the wound bed. FGF-2 stimulates endothelial cells to release plasminogen activator and procollagenase. Plasminogen activator converts plasminogen and procollagenase to plasmin and active collagenase, respectively, and these two proteases digest the basement membrane surrounding the endothelial cells. Additionally, FGF2, along with other chemoattractant factors, triggers the movement of endothelial cells into the provisional matrix. This migration is allowed by the upregulation of the cell-surface αvβ3, αvβ5, and αvβ1 integrins, which have the ability to recognize provisional ECM proteins, notably fibrin and fibronectin.[28,104–106]

As they move into the wound matrix, endothelial cells proliferate and form vascular sprouts. Upon meeting with neighboring neovessels, vascular sprouts connect and attach through a process known as anastomosis, essentially forming continuous tubular structures that further connect forming vascular loops. These differentiate into mature afferent and efferent limbs. Mitogens, such as FGF and VEGF, stimulate endotheliocyte proliferation and allow for a continual supply of cells needed for capillary extension[107] while TGF-β is hypothesized to support cellular phenotypic switches allowing for capillary tube formation. Fibronectin within the ECM also triggers phenotypic alterations such as endothelial cells pseudopodia extension.[108] Macrophages support the process by guiding vessel tips together.[109] The ECM releases its reservoir of metalloproteinases, dissolving the matrix surrounding the sprouting vessels and clearing a path for further progression.[108] Maturation and stabilization of the newly formed capillaries is governed by angiopoietin.[110] Binding of angiopoietin to its receptor Tie-2 on activated endothelial cells triggers the production of PDGF and recruitment of pericytes and smooth muscle cells, which form a stabilizing mural structure around the immature blood vessels.[111–114] As blood vessels mature, blood flow begins providing the necessary oxygenation and nutrients for continuous fibroplasia.

With terminal stages of healing, angiogenesis is suppressed, and capillaries undergo regression as characterized by mitochondrial swelling, apoptosis, and necrosis of the endothelial cells at the distal tips of the capillaries. Platelets adhere to degenerating endothelial cells and macrophages phagocytose superfluous vessels.[115,116] Numerous ECM molecules,[117] including thrombospondin,[118] also play a regulatory role in endothelial cell apoptosis. Further angiogenesis is also suppressed by blood vessels mural pericytes and components,[93] notably the collagen XVIII breakdown byproduct endostatin.[119]

REMODELING

Once reepithelialization of the wound surface is complete, the wound is usually considered healed clinically. However, wounds continue to undergo tissue maturation or *remodeling* for up to a year, mainly comprising neovasculature regression, ECM deposition, reconstitution of granulation tissue to form scar tissue[22] and wound contraction. Scar formation is the ultimate outcome of skin wound repair in humans in the postembryonic period. Cutaneous scars lack epidermal appendages and harbor a distinct collagen pattern from that of unwounded skin. Fibroblasts are the major cell type responsible for the remodeling process.

Toward the end of fibroplasia, fibroblasts undergo a phenotypic switch characterized by the deposition of large actin microfilaments along the cytoplasmic face of their plasma membrane and the establishment of cell-cell and cell-matrix linkages.[79,120] These changes are prompted by both mechanical tension and the action of PDGF[121] and initiate the differentiation of fibroblasts into stress fiber-expressing protomyofibroblasts, which in turn become myofibroblasts. The presence of TGF-β in the wound milieu[79,120] triggers myofibroblasts to express alpha-smooth muscle actin (α-SMA) specifically.[122]

Myofibroblasts synthesize a multitude of MMP and their inhibitors (TIMP), targeting specific components of the ECM for degradation.[123,124] Keratinocytes and recruited macrophages also secrete proteases that take part in collagen remodeling. Put simply, proteolytic MMPs degrade the ECM collagen III, making way for concurrent collagen I deposition. Three MMPs have been identified to have the ability to cleave native collagen: MMP-1 or classic interstitial collagenase, which cleaves types I, II, III, XIII, and X collagens; neutrophil collagenase (MMP-8), which cleaves types I, II, and III collagen; and a novel collagenase that is prominent in chronic wounds (MMP-13).[75] Although MMP-8 is hypothesized to be the predominant collagenase in healing wounds, it remains currently unclear as to the specific role of each collagenase in ECM

TABLE 19-3 Angiogenesis stimulators and inhibitors in wound healing

Angiogenic stimulators	Angiogenic inhibitors
FGF-1	Thrombospondin-1
FGF-2	Tissue inhibitors of matrix metalloproteinases
TGF-α	Interferon-α (INF-α)
TGF-β	INF-β
PGE2	INF-γ
TNF-α	Endostatin
VEGF	Angiostatin
EGF	
Angiogenin	
Angiotropin	
Angiopoietin-1	
IL-8	
Lactic acid	
Nitric oxide (NO)	

remodeling.[123] For example, in knock-out mice models, a deficiency of MMP-13 alone did not impair the remodeling process.[125] In contrast, a double knock-out of MMP-13 and the plasminogen activating system created an additional delay of healing compared with knock-out of only the plasminogen activating system.[78]

Modulatory factors involved in the expression of MMPs and TIMPs include cytokines such as TGF-β, PDGF, IL-1, and the ECM. For instance, increased TGF-β secretion has translated into increased TIMP-1, type I and type III procollagen formation in diabetic skin animal models.[126] Type I collagen from the ECM induces the expression of α2β1 collagen receptors on fibroblasts as well as their expression of MMP-1.[58,127] Overall, these regulatory interactions are of utmost importance as imbalances of MMP and their inhibitors expression lead to aberrant ECM remodeling and possibly chronic wounds.[128,129]

Myofibroblast appearance corresponds to the initiation of connective tissue compaction and wound contraction. This process occurs toward the end of fibroplasia, prompting granulation tissue synthesis by fibroblasts to slow down significantly.[122] Myofibroblasts possess α5β1 integrin receptors to the ECM fibronectin and α1β1 and α2β1 receptors to collagen[121] and link to each other through direct adherens desmosome junctions.[79] Collagen bundles, in turn, join end-to-end with preexisting collagen bundles within the dermis at the wound edge through covalent crosslinks.[130] These cell-cell, cell-matrix, and matrix-matrix links provide a network across the wound that allows for the coordinated transmission of the traction forces initiated by myofibroblasts on their pericellular matrix, effectively leading to wound contraction. The ability to generate strong contractile forces and focal adhesions has been attributed specifically to α-SMA filaments in myofibroblasts.[131]

As the healing process concludes, fibroblasts and myofibroblasts undergo apoptosis.[131] Aberrant programmed cell death causing continued ECM secretion and excessive wound contraction has been implicated in the pathogenesis of abnormal scar formation, clinically manifesting as hypertrophic scars or keloids.[85,132] Additionally, following wound repair, the skin fails to resume its initial composition and strength. The collagen composition of intact skin in adults is approximately 80% type I collagen and only 10% type III collagen.[133] In wounded skin, granulation tissue shows approximately 30% type III collagen with only 10% type I collagen. As healing evolves, the ratio of type III to type I collagen increases drastically, as does the tensile strength of the scar.[134] Additionally, collagen fibers in intact skin are also oriented is a basket weave fashion, in contrast with the parallel deposition observed in the dermis of healed wounds. The results is a lower breaking strength, only up to 80% of prewounding strength postinjury.[133,135]

CHRONIC WOUNDS

Delays in the natural wound healing process can lead to chronic wounds and generally occur in the context of a wide range of underlying pathologies. Chronic wounds are associated with heightened patient morbidity and represent a major socioeconomic burden both to patients and the healthcare system.[136] Therefore, an effective therapeutic approach focusing on both the core underlying disease and localized wound care is essential. Both systemic factors and elements from the local microenvironment can result in the development of chronic wounds. Venous insufficiency, advanced age, atherosclerosis, and diabetes mellitus are some of the most common systemic factors influencing wound repair. Less common factors are vasculitis, hypercoagulability, malnutrition, and medications causing an immunosuppressive state. Local microenvironment disturbances include inadequate blood supply, the presence of necrotic tissue, increased proteolytic activity, mechanical irritation, pressure, bacterial components, local toxins, and growth factor deficiency. Smoking has also been linked to delayed wound healing.

Careful wound examination and directed investigations of possible underlying pathologies are essential to identify the disease entity causing delayed wound healing. In the case of a longstanding or recalcitrant wound, laboratory work-up [**Table 19-4**] including a blood count, a complete metabolic panel, vitamin levels, and a microbiology swab (if an infection is suspected) might be warranted, along with vascular studies in the case of lower extremity wounds. Histologic examination, preferably of the wound border and including normal skin, might also be necessary to rule out unusual diagnoses, such as squamous cell carcinoma or atypical mycobacterial infections.

TABLE 19-4 Laboratory tests for chronic wounds

Hematology	Complete blood count with differential
	Blood smear
	Sedimentation rate
	Glucose 6 phosphate dehydrogenase
	Protein C, Protein S
	Fibrinogen and D-Dimers
	Prothrombin time/partial thromboplastin time
	Cryoglobulins/cryofibrinogens
	Antiphospholipid antibodies
	Serum protein electrophoresis
	Antithrombin 3
Chemistry	Complete metabolic panel
	Glucose levels
	Liver function tests
	Lipids
	Glycosylated hemoglobin HbA_{1c}
	Amylase, lipase
	Iron, Ferritin
	Parathyroid hormone
Nutritional assessment	Albumin
	Prealbumin
	Transferrin
	Vitamins
	Minerals
Microbiology	Bacterial culture
	Fungal culture, including mycobacterial culture
Histopathology	Wound edge biopsy
Vascular studies	Ankle-brachial index
	Lower extremity arterial duplex ultrasonography
	Lower extremity venous duplex ultrasonography with reflux

Erythema surrounding a wound might be a sign of concurrent wound infection or cellulitis as the underlying cause of delayed wound healing. While redness is easy to identify in lighter skin tones, it may be harder to identify in patients with darker-pigmented skin. Thus, careful comparison of the area surrounding a wound to the rest of the patient's skin tone might lead to improved clinical assessment in patients with darker skin. In addition, the prevalence of pathologies underlying delayed wound healing differ across racial and ethnic backgrounds. For instance, higher rates of undernutrition were noted in African American elderly with chronic wounds as compared to their Hispanic and non-Hispanic Whites counterparts.[137] One study has found that 85% of patients with delayed wound healing at suture removal had a history of use of skin-lightening products.[138] Physician awareness of these differences and disparities is essential to guide appropriate management of chronic wounds among racial and ethnic groups.

SCARRING

Excessive fibrosis and scarring lie on the opposite end of the spectrum of dysfunctional wound healing as compared to chronic wounds and represent an additional significant healthcare challenge. Clinically, excessive scarring manifests with the presence of hypertrophic scars or keloids. Hypertrophic scars are raised, highly vascularized scars confined to the original wound boundaries. They harbor abundant inflammatory cells and fibroblasts depositing excessive and disorganized ECM and might regress over time.[22] In contrast, keloids grow beyond the original parameters of the wound and rarely decrease in size. The pathology of keloids is characterized by hyalinized collagen, nonflattened epidermis, nonfibrotic papillary dermis, and a tongue-like advancing edge of hyalinized collagen under normal epidermis.[139] In addition to the clinical presentation, the composition in α-smooth muscle actin distinguishes hypertrophic scars (70% expression) from keloids (45%). Although the exact pathogenesis behind excessive scarring has not been identified, soluble mediators within the wound environment, exterior mechanical forces, and genetic predisposition are thought to be implicated.

As outlined in the section on *wound remodeling*, "stop signals" triggered by closure of the dermal defect and completion of reepithelization lead fibroblasts and myofibroblasts to undergo apoptosis. Absence or dysfunction of these signals, halting apoptosis, may lead to continued remodeling and consequent excessive scarring.[132,140] Fibroblasts within hypertrophic scars exhibit resistance to apoptosis and overexpress tissue transglutaminase, which stabilizes the newly formed granulation tissue and makes it resistant to enzymatic breakdown.[87] In addition, excessive periostin expression, an ECM protein induced by TGF-β in human dermal fibroblasts, has been uncovered in hypertrophic scars and keloids.[141,142] Higher levels of hypoxia inducible factor (HIF)-1α have also been found in keloids and are thought to mediate pro-fibrotic state in dermal fibroblasts via the TGF-β1/SMAD3 pathway.[143]

Mechanical strain during wound healing is also hypothesized to be implicated in hypertrophic scar formation,[144] but the literature remains divided. It has been proposed that keratinocytes secrete growth factors that act on fibroblasts, playing a role into excessive scar formation. This process is thought to be mediated by the integrin-focal adhesion kinase (FAK) pathway.[22] Mechanical forces during wound healing lead to excessive activation of FAK in fibroblasts and downstream phosphatidylinositol 3-kinase (PI3K)/Akt and mitogen-activated protein kinases (MAPK) activation, leading to hypertrophic scar formation.[22] Decreased FAK signaling in nonhealing wounds and increased FAK degradation in diabetic foot ulcer wounds leading to abnormal skin architecture support this theory.[22]

While excessive scarring occurs among people throughout the world, certain demographics display a greater incidence than others. The prevalence of hypertrophic scars ranges from 5% to 37% in lighter-skinned individuals and are slightly more common in those with darker-pigmented skin [**Figure 19-1**].[145] Although the literature remains divided, there does not appear to be a genetic cause for the occurrence of hypertrophic scars.[146]

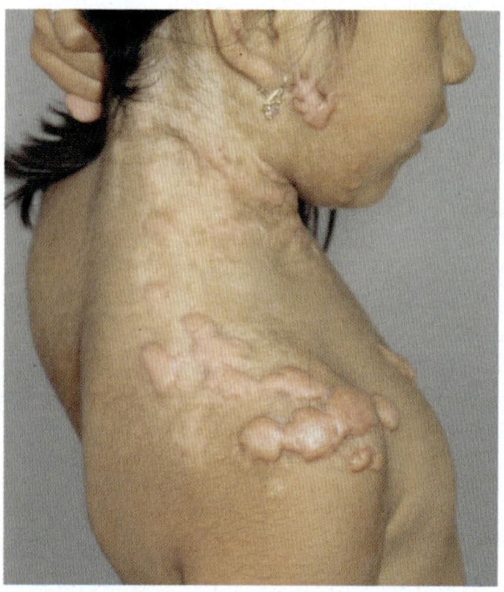

FIGURE 19-1. Scarification from a thermal burn on the posterior neck and upper back of a young Hispanic girl showing both keloids and hypertrophic scars.

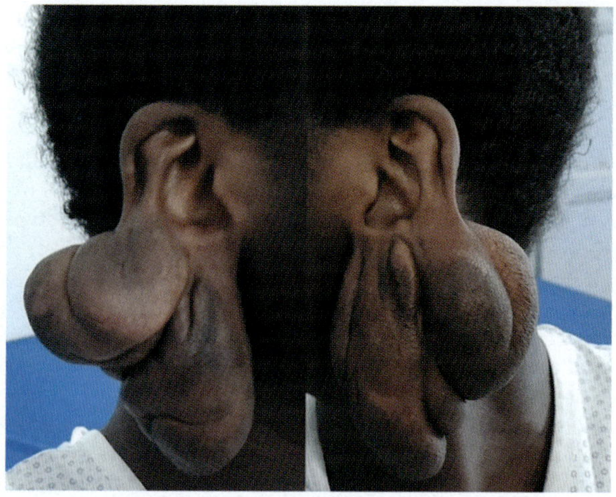

FIGURE 19-2. Earlobe keloids in an African American following piercing placement causing severe disfigurement and altered function. (Reproduced with permission from Montero JA et al. Extensive keloid and hypertrophic mixed scarring pattern in ear lobes of a 14-year-old African female: a case report. *Fetal Pediatr Pathol.* 2023;42(2):270-274.)

Keloids, on the other hand, occur almost exclusively in daker-skinned individuals, affecting 15% to 20% of the concerned population[147] and by a ratio ranging from 5:1 to 16:1 as compared to lighter-skinned individuals.[148] As such, genetics play a significant role in keloid susceptibility. However, despite numerous attempts to investigate the genetics governing keloid formation, no single genetic cause has been ascertained so far. A number of chromosomal linkage intervals have been identified in some families,[149–151] such as the 10q23.31 in the Han Chinese population.[150,151] The latter region codes for transcription factors Suppressor of Mothers against Decapentaplegic (SMAD) 2, 7, and 4 that play a role in the regulation of TGF-β.[152] However, the various studies failed to replicate findings and no putative gene was identified. The involvement of various Human leukocyte antigen (HLA) class immunogenetics has also been identified across ethnic groups, but again, no single genotype was uncovered.[153–160] HLA alleles are, however, a promising genetic marker and further support immune system dysregulation as the driver of keloid formation.

The presence of hypertrophic scars and keloids is associated with pruritus, pain, disfigurement, and consequent psychological distress to the patient [**Figure 19-2**].[161] A cross-sectional study looking at the burden of keloid disease in patients with no other skin conditions found significant emotional and mental quality of life impairment, specifically in patients with painful or itchy keloids.[162] It is estimated that keloids cost the healthcare system $281 million a year due to loss of productivity.[163] Despite the higher prevalence of keloids in patients with darker-pigmented skin, a recent meta-analysis found no studies on the intersectional interaction between keloids and race and ethnicity within marginalized identities keloid psychosocial and economic burden.[164]

WOUND ASSESSMENT

GENERAL ASSESSMENT

Thorough history-taking and physical examination are essential for the proper assessment of wounds. A full medical history needs to include wound onset, clinical course, and associated symptoms as well as the patient's past medical history, current medications, personal habits including smoking or the use of alcohol, and nutritional habits. Following history-taking, a visual evaluation should include wound anatomical location, size, and morphology (depth, shape, border, base, and color). Leg ulcers secondary to venous insufficiency characteristically present as shallow defects with irregular sloped borders and moderate to heavy exudate, whereas those of arterial origin show a punched out round form and are classically dry. Pyoderma gangrenosum presents with purple rolled borders and a granular erythematous ulcer bed [**Figure 19-3**].

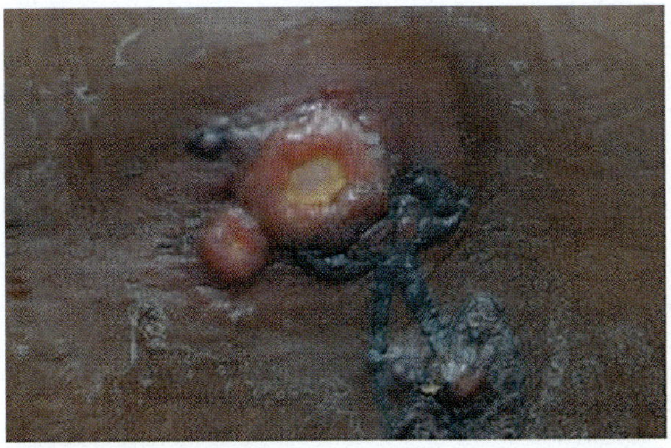

FIGURE 19-3. Pyoderma gangrenosum showing central ulceration and rolled borders in an African American following tattoo placement. (Reproduced with permission from Jacobson S et al. Pyoderma gangrenosum following tattoo placement in a patient with acute myelogenous leukemia. *J Dermatolog Treat.* 2008;19(1):58-60.)

Of equal importance is the examination of the skin surrounding the wound or *periwound* area. Characteristics of the surrounding skin or, including discoloration, temperature, fibrosis, necrosis, edema or signs of dermatitis need to be documented, as they would point to comorbid ongoing conditions potentially affecting the wound and provide valuable information for proper wound care. Tense warm tissue could indicate cellulitis, whereas erythema around the wound could indicate maceration and the need for more absorbent wound dressings.

A full skin exam should be performed to look for lesions, bruising, absence of hair, shiny skin, callus formation, and hypertrophic and keloid scars. Additionally, an evaluation of peripheral pulses, capillary refill time, deep tendon reflexes and the presence of peripheral neuropathy need to be conducted, particularly in leg ulcers. Of equal importance is the documentation of wound progress, either in writing or pictures, as it remains the only way to objectively assess treatment response.[165]

CONSIDERATIONS IN PATIENTS WITH DARKER-PIGMENTED SKIN

No specific guidelines address the assessment of wounds in darker-pigmented skin. This translates into diagnostic delays, missed diagnoses, and consequent disparities in the treatment and healing of wounds in patients with darker-pigmented skin.[2,166]

Erythema is defined as the red appearance of skin caused by the dilation of capillaries near the surface and increased blood flow. It occurs with many skin conditions, namely trauma, inflammation, infection, or rash. Although clearly visible on light skin tones, erythema may not be as obvious in darker skin tones. Recognizing the presence of erythema during the assessment of a wound is, however, crucial for proper disease characterization. For instance, moisture-associated skin damage (MASD) is an umbrella term for irritant-contact dermatitis that incorporates periwound maceration among others. Periwound "redness" remains a cardinal indication of maceration, but consideration needs to be made on how this may present across various skin tones [**Figure 19-4**]. Hence, it is important to remember that paler, darker, or purple discoloration are more likely to be seen in darker skin tones as compared to actual red discoloration in lighter patients.[167] A violaceous gray appearance may also indicate inflammation in dark-pigmented skin [**Figure 19-5**].

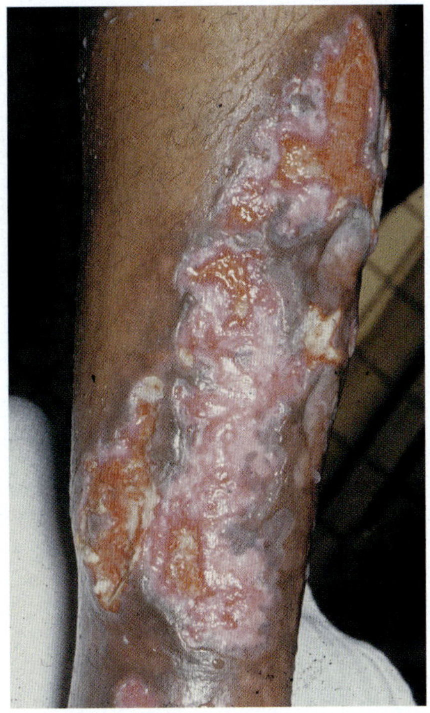

FIGURE 19-5. Venous leg ulcer with gray wound edges indicating inflammation.

Recognizing hemosiderin staining, a sign pointing to a venous etiology in the case of lower extremity ulcers, and differentiating it from erythema are additional challenges in darker-pigmented skin.[168] Relying on additional visual evaluation helps in conducting a proper assessment: while hemosiderin staining usually occurs in close vicinity to the wound edges, injury-related color changes usually extend out a considerable distance and are accompanied by the other signs of inflammation such as warmth, swelling, or induration.

Alternatively, if present alongside a chronic nonhealing wound, pallor might be a sign of insufficient blood flow. In darker-pigmented skin, pallor might present as ashen or gray. In contrast, the skin will present with a yellowish hue in brown-toned skin. On the other hand, it remains important to not miss the presence of eschars or necrosis in darker skin [**Figure 19-6**].

It remains important to remember that dyspigmentation around the wound edges is not necessarily a sign of ongoing inflammation in patients with darker-pigmented skin. Non-Caucasian skin is more susceptible to

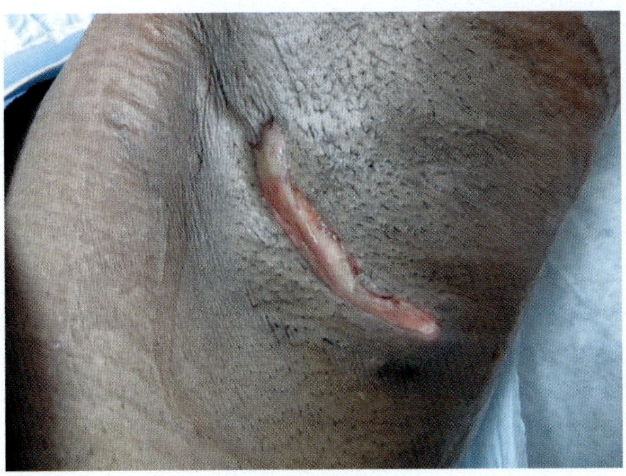

FIGURE 19-4. Maceration and periwound inflammation in a hidradenitis suppurativa deroofing surgical wound presenting as gray discoloration in a darker-pigmented woman.

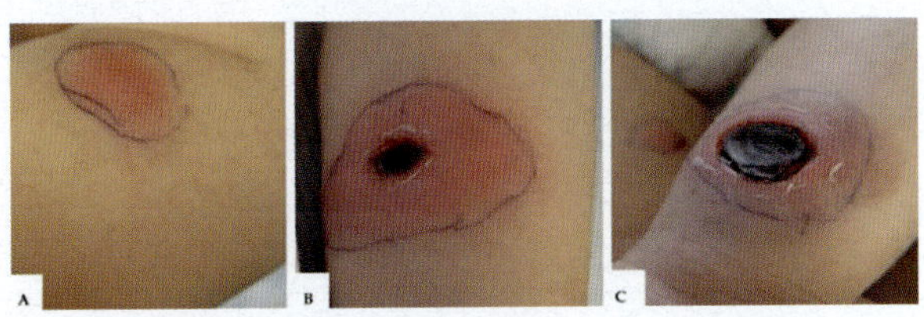

FIGURE 19-6. Wound necrosis caused by ecthyma gangrenosum. (Reproduced with the permission from Martínez-Longoria, C. A., Rosales-Solis, G. M., Ocampo-Garza, J., Guerrero-González, G. A., & Ocampo-Candiani, J. (2017). Ecthyma gangrenosum: a report of eight cases. Anais Brasileiros de Dermatologia, 92(5), 698–700. Figure 2.)

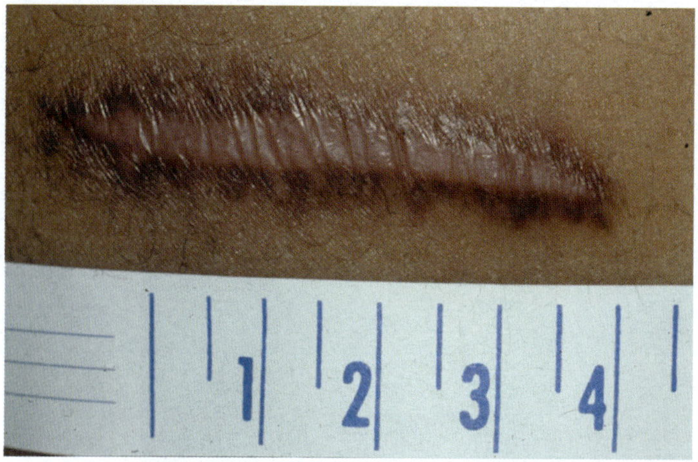

FIGURE 19-7. Four weeks after an incision, a slight hypertrophic scar has developed on the medium-color pigmented skin. The borders of the incision are hyperpigmented, and the center of the incision is hypopigmented.

the development of postinflammatory hyperpigmentation and postinflammatory hypopigmentation than Caucasian skin.[169]

ASSESSING SCARRING

When visually evaluating scars, it is important to note the anatomical site, orientation, length, color, contracture, and healing status (fresh, healing, healed, mature). If present, sinuses, fistulas, granulation tissue, or discharge should prompt into an investigation for possible site infection. The feel and mobility of the scar should also be further assessed, looking at the presence of tenderness, scar tissue thickness, pliability, and mobility, as well as the mobility of the surrounding skin. In addition, patient-reported symptoms of pain or itch need to be assessed.[170] Patients might also present with pathological scarring, namely hypertrophic scars or keloids. As mentioned in the section on *scarring*, these are secondary to aberrances in the remodeling phase of wound healing.

Hypertrophic scars present with an elevation of the plane of the scar, which is thickened and inflammatory but remain confined to the wound boundaries.[171] They usually occur directly after initial repair, tend to follow the line of the incision, and are more common in young patients [**Figure 19-7**]. Additionally, they typically regress over time, resolving 12 to 18 months after they form.[148,171] Interestingly, hypertrophic scars tend to occur very often in healing burn wounds but may also occur in wounds secondary to surgical procedures, trauma, and radiation therapy.

Unlike hypertrophic scars, keloid scars extend beyond the initial margins of the wounds, affecting healthy skin around the scar. They present with a wide range of pigmentation from red to dark brown [**Figure 19-8**]. They also tend to grow larger over time[148] and are associated with pruritus or pain in 40% of cases.[172] While keloids can develop everywhere on the body, wounds occurring on the ear lobe, chest, deltoid region, or in the pubic area are more likely to heal with keloid formation.[173,174] Individuals with darker-pigmented skin have a notable predisposition for keloids,[173] but the underlying mechanisms remain unelucidated. Given the symptoms and psychosocial burden associated with the presence of keloids and hypertrophic scars, it is important to inquire about patient comfort during the assessment of these pathological scars, as further management pertaining to the scar and related symptoms may be needed despite wound closure.

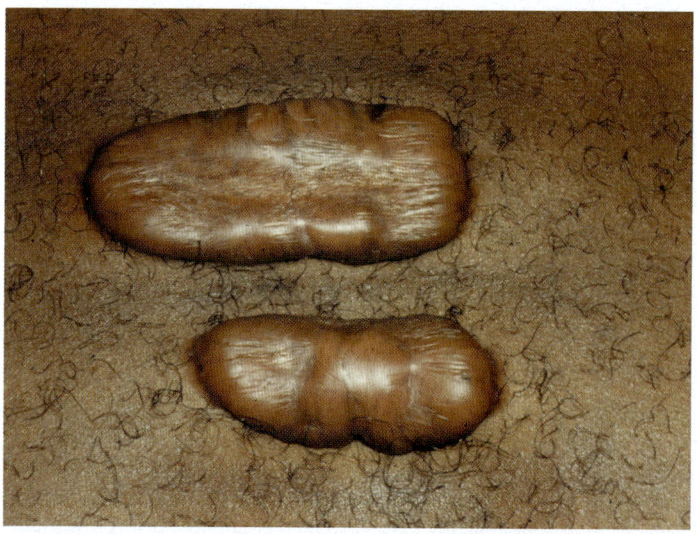

FIGURE 19-8. Horizontal keloids on the chest of a darker-pigmented man.

Pigmentation is an additional consideration in the examination of scars. Disruption of the normal melanogenesis within wounds may result in dyspigmentation affecting the scar, making it more noticeable.[175] This tends to occur more frequently in patient with darker-pigmented skin. In light-skinned individuals, the *neo*-epithelium is more likely to be pearly or silvery and shiny, whereas in patients with darker skin, the color of the newly formed epithelium is more likely to be distinct from the surrounding undamaged epithelium, presenting with hyperpigmented scars. Scar dyspigmentation may have a significant psychological impact.[176] It is therefore important to inquire about patient comfort when they present with abnormally pigmented scar, even in the absence of hypertrophic scars or keloids.

WOUND CARE

A wide range of treatment options are available for acute and chronic wounds, providing therapeutic flexibility to meet the various facades of care. The following section covers several commonly used therapies. Examples of additional adjunctive modalities and their indications be found in **Table 19-5**.

DEBRIDEMENT

Debridement is the removal of devitalized or contaminated tissue or foreign material from the wound or the periwound area. As such, adequate debridement is crucial to reduce bacterial bioburden, remove necrotic tissue, have responsive keratinocytes at the wound edge, and provide a perfused wound bed.[177] There are five types of debridement: surgical, mechanical, autolytic, enzymatic, and biologic.

Surgical debridement, using sharp instruments, remains the fastest method to remove unhealthy tissue. Despite being highly effective when performed by a trained practitioner, it is associated with risks of pain or bleeding. Adequate anesthesia can be achieved by direct infiltration of

TABLE 19-5 Adjunctive wound treatment modalities and their indications

Adjunctive wound treatment	Indication
Compression bandages (Unna boot, four-layer compression system)	Venous leg ulcers
Contact casts	Diabetic foot ulcers
Cyclosporine	Pyoderma gangrenous, vasculitis-related ulcers
Granulocyte colony-stimulating factor	Diabetic foot ulcers
Horse chestnut extract	Venous leg ulcers, lymphedema
Hyperoxygenated fatty acid cream (Mepentol)	Pressure ulcers
Miltefosine	Malignant, fungating ulcers
Mycophenolate mofetil	Pyoderma gangrenosum
Infliximab	Pyoderma gangrenous, vasculitis-related ulcers
Pentoxifylline	Venous leg ulcers
Topical lidocaine/prilocaine	Pain reduction in venous leg ulcers, arterial ulcers, digital ulcers in the setting of sclerosis
Topical metronidazole	Odor control in chronic wounds
Topical tacrolimus	Pyoderma gangrenosum

anesthetic agents locally in most cases.[178] In patients with neuropathy, such as those with diabetic foot ulcers, the use of local anesthesia might not be necessary. An example of *mechanical* debridement is the use of wet-to-dry dressing. However, this type of debridement will remove both necrotic and viable tissue and seems be associated with a higher incidence of infection.[178]

Autolytic debridement relies on the action of enzymatic agents secreted by the wound itself. This is facilitated by the use of occlusive dressings that provide a moist environment, effectively promoting the lytic activity of proteases in wound exudate and liquefaction of necrotic tissue. *Enzymatic* debridement involves the use of topical enzymatic agents to debride the wound. Most debriding agents contain papain, which can solubilize fibrin, denatured collagen and skin, or collagenase, best used to digest collagen and elastin. Currently, only the collagenase Santyl (Smith & Nephew, Inc., Watford, England), derived from *Clostridium histolyticum*, is approved for use by the FDA.[179] These agents should only be applied to the necrotic portion of the wound and not the surrounding normal skin or tissue.[178]

Biologic debridement employs maggots and has been historically used to debride chronic wounds. Maggots use collagenases and trypsin-like enzymes to digest necrotic tissue, secrete antibacterial compounds, such as phenylacetic acid and phenylacetaldehyde, and ingest bacteria, notably MRSA.[180] Maggots raised in a sterile environment are available for medical use but patient's acceptance and comfort remains a major challenge.

DRESSINGS

In addition to their role as a protective barrier between an open wound and the outside world, dressings can be utilized to speed up healing by maintaining a moist environment.

An ideal wound dressing will be free of toxic components, prevents bacterial infection, and provides thermal insulation while allowing oxygen permeability. It will also provide an optimum amount of adhesive material that would avoid injury upon removal and maintain moisture while absorbing excess exudate. It would minimize patient pain during application and removal.[181]

Dressings have various absorptive capacities; therefore, wound depth and amount of exudate should be assessed before prescribing a specific dressing [**Table 19-6**].[182,183] In addition, it is important to assess for the presence of bacterial or microbial colonization in the wound environment as the consequent need for antiseptic-impregnated dressings [**Table 19-7**]. Finally, although wound characteristics often primarily determine the choice of dressing, it remains important to keep in mind cost, access, and patient preference.

GROWTH FACTORS

Growth factors are critical to the wound healing process as they encourage keratinocyte and fibroblast proliferation and augment angiogenesis. Wound exudate normally contains an array of growth factors; the use of occlusive dressings to maintain the wound fluid within the wound bed is therefore crucial to augment healing. The efficacy of topical application of numerous human recombinant growth factors continues to be extensively investigated. Currently, only Becaplermin (Smith & Nephew, Inc., Watford, England), a gel formulation of recombinant human platelet-derived growth factor (PDGF) is approved for the treatment of chronic ulcers by the FDA, specifically nonhealing diabetic foot ulcers.[184]

TOPICAL TIMOLOL

In vivo and in vitro investigations have demonstrated the role of the β2-adrenergic receptor at preventing keratinocyte migration when

TABLE 19-6 Dressing categories, absorptive capacity, indications, and features

Absorptive capacity	Dressing type	Indications	Advantages	Disadvantages
Least absorptive Most absorptive	Film	• Minor burns • Abrasions or lacerations • Lightly exudating wounds • Sutured incision sites after surgery • Donor sites following skin harvesting	• Reducing skin tension on flexor surfaces • Permeable to water vapor	• Nonabsorbent • May adhere to wound bed upon drying
	Hydrogel	• Sutured incision sites after surgery • Minor burns • Dermabrasion • Laser resurfacing	• Fills in wound space • Permeable to water vapor • Nonadherent • Facilitate autolytic debridement • Atraumatic removal • Safe in infected wounds	• May encourage hypertrophic granulation • May cause maceration of periwound skin • May increase the risk for anaerobic infection • Nonadherent
	Hydrocolloid	• Light to moderate exudating wounds • Partial or full thickness wounds • Chronic ulcers with slough or necrotic tissue	• Nonadherent to moist wound base • Maintains moisture by gelling on contact with exudate • Soothing and cooling effect, reducing postoperative pain • Designed to be worn for 1-7 days	• Limit gas exchange between wound bed and environment • May injure fragile skin on removal
	Foam	• Minimally to heavily exudating partial and full thickness wounds • Wounds or fragile skin over bony prominences or friction areas	• Conforms to wound shape • Thermally insulates • Comfortable • Wear time of 1-7 days depending on amount of exudate	• May macerate periwound skin if saturated • Not effective on wounds with dry eschar • May dry the wound bed too much if wound is inappropriately exudative
	Alginates	• Moderately to heavily exudating wounds • Full-thickness burns • Surgical wounds	• Spontaneous sucking ability • Nonadherent • Soluble with saline application for low-trauma dressing change	• May cause mild burning on application • Unpleasant smell
	Gelling fiber	• Moderately to heavily exudating wounds	• Remove harmful bacteria from wound • Respond to wound fluid levels by forming cohesive gel • Available in various sizes • Retain and control exudate level	• May cause irritation • May cause periwound maceration • May cause hypergranulation

TABLE 19-7 Common antiseptics used in select dressings and their coverage

Agent	Coverage spectrum
Chlorhexidine and derivatives	Broad spectrum antibacterial
Hypertonic saline	Broad-spectrum antibacterial
Silver	Broad-spectrum antibacterial, MRSA, VRE
Methylene blue and gentian violet	Broad-spectrum antibacterial, MRSA, VRE, anti-candidal
Povidone-iodine	Broad-spectrum antimicrobial (bacteria, fungi, and viruses)
Honey	Broad-spectrum antimicrobial (bacteria, fungi, and viruses)

activated within the wound environment. Subsequent studies examined the impact of β2-adrenergic receptor blockade with timolol and found accelerated skin reepithelialization in healing recalcitrant wounds of varying etiologies. Specifically, topical timolol (Bausch And Lomb, Inc., Vaughan, ON, Canada) augmented the healing of venous leg ulcers, pyoderma gangrenosum, radiation dermatitis-related, and malignancy-related wounds.[185] The advantage topical timolol offers is its low-cost and ease of availability, making it an ideal agent to supplement the healing of treatment-resistant wounds.

CELL AND TISSUE-BASED THERAPIES

Skin substitutes are a heterogenous group of biosynthetic materials that cover wounds temporarily or permanently and aim to replicate the properties of normal skin.[186,187] Engineered dressings drive autologous regenerative healing by promoting epithelialization from the edge of the ulcer toward the center through the release of cytokines by the donor cells.[188] They also help decrease wound contracture and improve function. There are three types of skin substitutes: epidermal grafts, dermal replacements, and composite grafts. Another classification of tissue-engineered dressings relies on graft cell source: autologous, allogeneic, or xenogeneic.

These cellular substitutes have shown promising results in a variety of chronic wounds, including ulcers, burns, and postsurgical lesions.

There are two types of dermal skin substitutes: xenogeneic and allogeneic. Major components are collagen, glycosaminoglycans, and fibroblasts. Xenogeneic grafts are acellular substitutes composed of porcine (Oasis® Wound Matrix, EZ Derm™, Biobrane®) or bovine (Integra™) collagen. In addition to providing immediate closure, these products protect from potential human pathogens due to their animal origin and allow for the formation of cosmetically better scars.[189] They also carry the advantage of not requiring dressing changes, as they adhere to the wound bed after placement.[189] Allogeneic dermal grafts are cellular substitutes that use cadaveric dermis (AlloDerm®, Graftjacket®) or neonatal foreskin fibroblasts (Dermagraft®). Although they provide numerous advantages such as improved healing time and quality similar to those of xenogeneic grafts, they do carry a risk of graft rejection due to T-cell recognition of donor T-cells.[190]

Bilayered cellular skin substitutes composed of both epidermal and dermal layers. Current products (Apligraf®) use human keratinocytes to compose the epidermal layer and bovine collagen with human fibroblasts to form the dermal layer. These grafts have the ability to produce their own matrix proteins and growth factors and have been successful in the treatment of challenging wounds such as epidermolysis bullosa, pyoderma gangrenosum, burns, and surgical excisions. When used in chronic venous ulcers, Apligraf® has also led to shorter healing periods as compared to compression alone, especially in the case of larger defects.[191] A major disadvantage of these products remains the associated cost and short shelf-life.

WOUND CARE DEVICES

Negative pressure wound therapy (NPWT) is an airtight sealed vacuum-assisted closure system that delivers sub-atmospheric "negative" pressure to the wound bed. It removes interstitial fluid, stimulates angiogenesis, and enhances both blood and lymphatic circulations.[192] There is evidence to support the use of NPWT for acute postsurgical wounds and debrided diabetic foot ulcers.[193]

Hyperbaric oxygen therapy (HBOT) administers patients with oxygen at pressures greater than 1 atmosphere during 45 to 120 minutes long sessions in pressure chambers. It is thought to oxygenate hypoxic tissue, augment fibroblast replication and collagen synthesis, and upregulate growth factors but data remains inconclusive.[194]

COMPLEMENTARY AND ALTERNATIVE MEDICINE

The use of Complementary and Alternative Medicine (CAM) is widespread in the American population, with the National Health Interview Survey 2012-2015 reporting a prevalence of 34% nationwide.[195] People of Hispanic ethnicity use herbal self-care remedies as part of their cultural heritage more commonly than other ethnic groups,[196] although one study has found similar rates of CAM use in Hispanics and Asians.[197] In comparison, people of African American descent are less likely to use home remedies as whole, but the use of CAM remains more common in those who are older, female, college-educated, or insured.[198] Nevertheless, knowledge of CAM treatments with supportive evidence of efficacy is crucial for optimal care delivery.

Aloe vera (*Aloe barbadensis*) is commonly used in many cultures for ulcers or chronic wounds, including thermal burn wounds. Some studies show evidence that aloe vera promotes wound healing in various animal models, possibly through anti-inflammatory effects mediated by a reduction in levels of thromboxane A2 (TXA2), thromboxane B2 (TXB2), and prostaglandin 26 (PG26).[199] This was further supported by clinical studies supporting it as an effective intervention in first- to second-degree burns[200] and chronic ulcers[201] as well as for the prevention of pressure ulcers.[202]

Chamomile (*Matricaria recutita*; *Chamaemelum nobile*) has been shown to work in synergy with antibiotics to control antibiotic-resistant bacteria when applied as ointment to chronic wounds.[203] As an oil, it is also believed to accelerate wound healing and decrease wound contraction through improving the deposition of transforming growth factor-β1 (TGF-β1) and collagen and reducing the ratio of IL-1 and MMP-9 to tissue inhibitor MMP-1.[204]

Honey is commonly applied to wounds to enhance healing. It harbors antimicrobial properties driven by its high sugar content, which generates an osmotic effect leading to bacterial dehydration and low pH (mean of 4.4).[205] In addition, honey immunomodulatory effects lead to the acceleration of wound re-epithelialization and closure, through cytokine and ROS modulation, collagen matrix production enhancement, and augmentation of the migration, proliferation, and chemotaxis of human keratinocytes, fibroblasts, and endothelial cells.[206]

Marigold (*Calendula officinalis*) is a flower native to northern Mediterranean countries and has been proven to hasten to inflammation phase of wound repair in acute wounds through increasing the levels of granulation tissue. In contrast, its efficacy in treating chronic wounds, particularly venous leg ulcers, remains largely controversial.[207]

Tea tree oil, extracted from the leaves of *Melaleuca alternifolia*, is believed to accelerate wound healing.[208] Additionally, it has shown multiple antiseptic properties thought to be mediated by bacterial membrane disruption[209] and promising efficacy in treating *Methicillin-Resistant Staphylococcus aureus* (MRSA) cutaneous infections.[210] It is widely used by patients with hidradenitis suppurativa, a condition more prevalent in patient with darker-pigmented skin, as it reduces swelling and wound severity.[211,212]

MANAGEMENT OF ABERRANT SCARRING

The standard of care for excessive scarring is serial intralesional triamcinolone acetonide injections. Corticosteroids are thought to enable collagenase to be active, enabling collagen.[148] This therapy has been shown to reduce scar volume and height, improve scar pliability, and diminish associated scar pain and itching as well as prevent recurrence.[213,214] Patients usually require multiple injections at 4- to 6-week intervals. Response rates vary with 50% to 100% likelihood of regression within 1 year of treatment and 5-year recurrence rates ranging between 33% and 55%.[213]

Surgical excision or *keloidectomy* is another treatment method. However, it involves the creation of a new wound, which might outcome in a similar or more severe keloid. The surgical technique employed plays a crucial role in the risk of recurrence. Although a wide variety of methods can be employed, including linear closure and flap coverage, excision with grafting, W-plasty and Z-plasty, it is important to establish tension-free wound closure to decrease the risk of recurrence.[215-217] The use of dermal substitutes and epidermal skin grafting following keloid excision has shown promising results.[218] Recurrence rates are usually high with surgery monotherapy.[219] Therefore, it is usually used in combination with other agents.[219]

A few agents have been investigated in combination with intralesional corticosteroids or surgery for the treatment of keloids, and research is still ongoing.[219] In a recent case report, serial combination injections with hyaluronic acid have been shown to fully treat keloids previously refractory to treatment with steroids alone.[220] Mixed data were shown investigating combination therapy with botulinum toxin[221] and verapamil.[222] Interestingly, collagenase injections showed mixed results[223] despite the proposed mechanism of action of collagenase in the setting of keloid treatment with steroids. In situ radiation therapy following excision is an effective adjuvant intervention shown to prevent the regrowth of keloids postsurgically.[224,225] Challenges remain the lack of consensus on an optimal regimen[226,227] and associated side effects such as pigmentary changes, hypertrophic scar formation, telangiectasias, or redness.[228] Steroid injections with bleomycin led to softening and flattening of lesions. However, in patients with Fitzpatrick III to V skin phototype, resultant hyperpigmentation was seen in 71.4% of participants.[229] Therefore, despite its efficacy, bleomycin should be used in caution in patients with darker-pigmented skin, due to the risk of hyperpigmentation. Dyspigmentation was also seen with the use of cryotherapy in surgically treated keloids, specifically in Fitzpatrick IV-IV skin phototypes [**Figure 19-9**].[230] Despite its efficacy at flattening keloids,[231] the risk of hypopigmentation remains an important consideration when treating patients with darker skin.

In patients with a higher susceptibility for aberrant scarring, it remains best to take preventive measures. For instance, surgical incisions along Langer lines (in natural creases) and the use of fine suture material might help avoid excessive scar formation.[148] Additionally, the use of sun protection with early scars on sun-exposed areas might prevent the development of dyspigmentation, especially in darker-pigmented patients.

FUTURE DIRECTIONS

Regenerating the skin and restoring its structural and functional properties within the wounded tissue is the ultimate goal of wound care. Repair following injury leads to abnormal skin formation, and resultant high risk of wound recurrence along a myriad of symptoms such as loss of integral skin function, associated pain, and psychosocial impairment. Despite recent advances, current available therapeutic modalities fail to mimic embryonic wound regeneration, but some promising emerging modalities are currently under investigation, some of which we highlight.

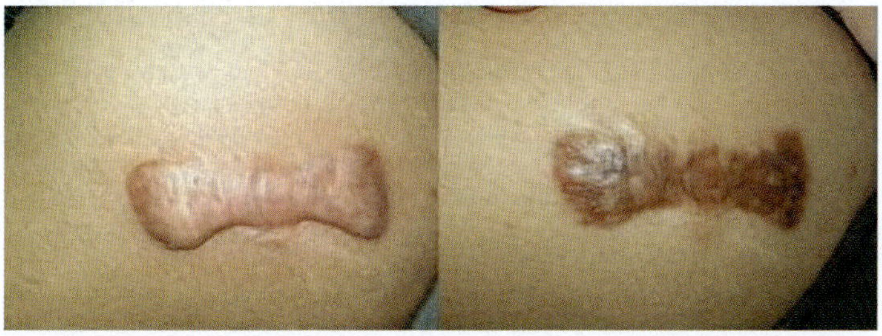

FIGURE 19-9. Keloid pre- and posttreatment with Bleomycin injections in a patient with darker-pigmented skin, showing keloid flattening and hyperpigmentation. (Reproduced with permission from Payapvipapong K et al. The treatment of keloids and hypertrophic scars with intralesional bleomycin in skin of color. *J Cosmet Dermatol.* 2015;14(1):83-90.)

The use of stem cells is a recent approach in wound care. In vitro studies have stimulated induced pluripotent stems cells to differentiate into skin-like cell lines forming multi-differentiated kertatinocytes, hair follicles, sebaceous glands, and fibroblasts. These have translated into facilitated wound healing in animal models by promoting collagen synthesis and angiogenesis.[232] Similarly, mesenchymal stem cells have shown promising results in burn wounds, through decreased levels of anti-angiogenic TNF-α and IFN-γ and increased levels of pro-angiogenic VEGF.[233,234] Adipose-derived stem cells have been shown to increase collagen production by fibroblasts and trigger neovascularization through their ability to differentiate endothelial cells and release VEGF.[235,236] Altogether, such advancements demonstrate that stems cells are extremely promising tools for skin regeneration as part of wound healing.

Resolving the additional burden of scarring on wound care and patient functionality is another aspect being investigated. Recent advances have highlighted the role of *Engrailed-1* expression by fibroblasts in inducing scarring, following the enzyme's activation by mechanical tension within the wound environment. Mechanotransduction signaling blocking has successfully promoted wound healing, with recovery of skin appendages, ultrastructure, and mechanical strength.[237] Translational implications of these discoveries that have demonstrated fully regenerative skin healing are of primordial importance, specifically for patients with darker-pigmented skin who disproportionately suffer from excessive scarring and keloid formation.

Accelerating wound repair is another active area of investigation. For instance, bacteriophages-based therapies are being used to target bacterial biofilms and multidrug-resistant organisms that colonize wounds and delay their healing. These emerging therapies have led to the resolution of wound infections previously resistant to antibiotics and translated into decreased inflammation, improved granulation, and enhanced wound healing.[238]

CONCLUSION

As the leading specialists of the integumentary system, dermatologists should place a greater emphasis on wounds and their care. Specifically, attention should be focused on darker-pigmented patients, mainly aiming at optimizing diagnosis in a timely manner and treatment modality choice. Awareness of the diversity that affects wounds and their healing moves therapeutic efforts away from algorithmic-based care to more personalized care, ultimately resulting in better patient outcome. Education and training outreach efforts ought to be implemented, supplementing subsequent research efforts in wound healing that include patients with darker-pigmented skin.

REFERENCES

1. Bennett MA. Report of the task force on the implications for darkly pigmented intact skin in the prediction and prevention of pressure ulcers. *Adv Skin Wound Care.* 1995;8(6):34-35.
2. Bliss DZ, Gurvich O, Savik K, et al. Racial and ethnic disparities in the healing of pressure ulcers present at nursing home admission. *Arch Gerontol Geriatr.* 2017;72:187-194.
3. Tan T-W, Armstrong DG, Concha-Moore KC, et al. Association between race/ethnicity and the risk of amputation of lower extremities among medicare beneficiaries with diabetic foot ulcers and diabetic foot infections. *BMJ Open Diabetes Res Care.* 2020;8(1):e001328.
4. Nussbaum SR, Carter MJ, Fife CE, et al. An economic evaluation of the impact, cost, and medicare policy implications of chronic nonhealing wounds. *Value Health.* 2018;21(1):27-32.
5. Sen CK. *Human Wounds and Its Burden: An Updated Compendium of Estimates.* Mary Ann Liebert, Inc.; 2019.
6. Sen CK, Gordillo GM, Roy S, et al. Human skin wounds: a major and snowballing threat to public health and the economy. *Wound Repair Regen.* 2009;17(6):763-771.

7. Singer AJ, Tassiopoulos A, Kirsner RS. Evaluation and management of lower-extremity ulcers. *New Engl J Med*. 2017;377(16):1559-1567.
8. Vivas A, Lev-Tov H, Kirsner RS. Venous leg ulcers (Japanese Version). *Ann Intern Med*. 2016;165(3):JITC17-JITC32.
9. Kirsner RS, Margolis D, Masturzo A, Bakewell K. A real-world experience with the bioactive human split thickness skin allograft for venous leg ulcers. *Wound Repair Regen*. 2020;28(4):547-552.
10. Robbins JM, Strauss G, Aron D, Long J, Kuba J, Kaplan Y. Mortality rates and diabetic foot ulcers: is it time to communicate mortality risk to patients with diabetic foot ulceration? *J Am Podiatr Med Assoc*. 2008;98(6):489-493.
11. Degen KE, Gourdie RG. Embryonic wound healing: a primer for engineering novel therapies for tissue repair. *Birth Defects Res C Embryo Today*. 2012; 96(3):258-270.
12. Gurtner GC, Werner S, Barrandon Y, Longaker MT. Wound repair and regeneration. *Nature*. 2008;453(7193):314-321.
13. Morgun EI, Vorotelyak EA. Epidermal stem cells in hair follicle cycling and skin regeneration: a view from the perspective of inflammation. *Front Cell Dev Biol*. 2020;8:581697.
14. Driskell RR, Lichtenberger BM, Hoste E, et al. Distinct fibroblast lineages determine dermal architecture in skin development and repair. *Nature*. 2013;504(7479):277-281.
15. Shin D, Minn KW. The effect of myofibroblast on contracture of hypertrophic scar. *Plast Reconstr Surg*. 2004;113(2):633-640.
16. Wilkinson HN, Hardman MJ. Wound healing: cellular mechanisms and pathological outcomes. *Open Biol*. 2020;10(9):200223.
17. Ren Q, Chan K-w, Huang H, et al. Platelet-derived alpha-granules are associated with inflammation in patients with NK/T-cell lymphoma-associated hemophagocytic syndrome. *Cytokine*. 2020;126:154878.
18. Komi DEA, Khomtchouk K, Santa Maria PL. A review of the contribution of mast cells in wound healing: involved molecular and cellular mechanisms. *Clin Rev Allergy Immunol*. 2020;58(3):298-312.
19. Chicharro-Alcántara D, Rubio-Zaragoza M, Damiá-Giménez E, et al. Platelet rich plasma: new insights for cutaneous wound healing management. *J Funct Biomater*. 2018;9(1):10.
20. Chong DL, Trinder S, Labelle M, et al. Platelet-derived transforming growth factor-β1 promotes keratinocyte proliferation in cutaneous wound healing. *J Tissue Eng Regen Med*. 2020;14(4):645-649.
21. Wu L-W, Chen W-L, Huang S-M, Chan JY-H. Platelet-derived growth factor-AA is a substantial factor in the ability of adipose-derived stem cells and endothelial progenitor cells to enhance wound healing. *FASEB J*. 2019;33(2):2388-2395.
22. Rodrigues M, Kosaric N, Bonham CA, Gurtner GC. Wound healing: a cellular perspective. *Physiol Rev*. 2019;99(1):665-706.
23. Wilgus TA. Alerting the body to tissue injury: the role of alarmins and DAMPs in cutaneous wound healing. *Curr Pathobiol Rep*. 2018;6(1):55-60.
24. Land WG. Use of DAMPs and SAMPs as therapeutic targets or therapeutics: a note of caution. *Mol Diagn Ther*. 2020;24(3):251-262.
25. Chen L, DiPietro LA. Toll-like receptor function in acute wounds. *Adv Wound Care*. 2017;6(10):344-355.
26. Rani M, Nicholson SE, Zhang Q, Schwacha MG. Damage-associated molecular patterns (DAMPs) released after burn are associated with inflammation and monocyte activation. *Burns*. 2017;43(2):297-303.
27. Chen L, Guo S, Ranzer MJ, DiPietro LA. Toll-like receptor 4 has an essential role in early skin wound healing. *J Invest Dermatol*. 2013;133(1):258-267.
28. Clark R, Tonnesen MG, Gailit J, Cheresh DA. Transient functional expression of alphaVbeta 3 on vascular cells during wound repair. *Am J Pathol*. 1996;148(5):1407.
29. Martin P, Leibovich SJ. Inflammatory cells during wound repair: the good, the bad and the ugly. *Trends Cell Biol*. 2005;15(11):599-607.
30. Ashcroft GS, Yang X, Glick AB, et al. Mice lacking Smad3 show accelerated wound healing and an impaired local inflammatory response. *Nat Cell Biol*. 1999;1(5):260-266.
31. Werner S, Krieg T, Smola H. Keratinocyte–fibroblast interactions in wound healing. *J Invest Dermatol*. 2007;127(5):998-1008.
32. Clark R. Wound repair. Overview and general considerations. *The molecular and cellular biology of wound repair*. 1994.
33. Wager L, Leavesley D. MicroRNA regulation of epithelial-to-mesenchymal transition during re-epithelialisation: assessing an open wound. *Wound Pract Res*. 2015;23(3):132-142.
34. Coulombe PA. Wound epithelialization: accelerationg the pace of discovery. *J Invest Dermatol*. 2003;121(2):219-230.
35. Huttenlocher A, Horwitz AR. Integrins in cell migration. *Cold Spring Harb Perspect Biol*. 2011;3(9):a005074.
36. Yamada KM, Clark RA. Provisional matrix. *The Molecular and Cellular Biology of Wound Repair*. Springer; 1988:51-93.
37. Kubo M, Van De Water L, Plantefaber LC, et al. Fibrinogen and fibrin are anti-adhesive for keratinocytes: a mechanism for fibrin eschar slough during wound repair. *J Invest Dermatol*. 2001;117(6):1369-1381.
38. Rousselle P, Braye F, Dayan G. Re-epithelialization of adult skin wounds: cellular mechanisms and therapeutic strategies. *Adv Drug Delivery Rev*. 2019;146:344-365.
39. Petersen MJ, Woodley DT, Stricklin GP, O'Keefe EJ. Enhanced synthesis of collagenase by human keratinocytes cultured on type I or type IV collagen. *J Invest Dermatol*. 1990;94(3):341-346.
40. Stricklin GP, Nanney LB. Immunolocalization of collagenase and TIMP in healing human burn wounds. *J Invest Dermatol*. 1994;103(4):488-492.
41. Di Russo J, Young JL, Wegner JW, Steins T, Kessler H, Spatz JP. Integrin α5β1 nano-presentation regulates collective keratinocyte migration independent of substrate rigidity. *Elife*. 2021;10:e69861.
42. Dejana E. Endothelial adherens junctions: implications in the control of vascular permeability and angiogenesis. *J Clin Invest*. 1996;98(9):1949-1953.
43. Werner S. Keratinocyte growth factor: a unique player in epithelial repair processes. *Cytokine Growth Factor Rev*. 1998;9(2):153-165.
44. Conway K, Price P, Harding KG, Jiang WG. The molecular and clinical impact of hepatocyte growth factor, its receptor, activators, and inhibitors in wound healing. *Wound Repair Regen*. 2006;14(1):2-10.
45. Werner S, Smola H. Paracrine regulation of keratinocyte proliferation and differentiation. *Trends Cell Biol*. 2001;11(4):143-146.
46. Hakvoort T, Altun V, Van Zuijlen P, De Boer W, van Schadewij W, van der Kwast T. Transforming growth factor-beta1,-beta2,-beta3, basic fibroblast growth factor and vascular endothelial growth factor expression in keratinocytes of burn scars. *Eur Cytokine Netw*. 2000;11(2):233-239.
47. Singer AJ, Clark RA. Cutaneous wound healing. *New Engl J Med*. 1999;341(10): 738-746.
48. Grose R, Werner S. Wound-healing studies in transgenic and knockout mice. *Mol Biotechnol*. 2004;28(2):147-166.
49. Litjens SH, de Pereda JM, Sonnenberg A. Current insights into the formation and breakdown of hemidesmosomes. *Trends Cell Biol*. 2006;16(7):376-383.
50. El Ghalbzouri A, Hensbergen P, Gibbs S, Kempenaar J, Schors Rvd, Ponec M. Fibroblasts facilitate re-epithelialization in wounded human skin equivalents. *Lab Invest*. 2004;84(1):102-112.
51. Baum CL, Arpey CJ. Normal cutaneous wound healing: clinical correlation with cellular and molecular events. *Dermatol Surg*. 2005;31(6):674-686.
52. Li A, Pouliot N, Redvers R, Kaur P. Extensive tissue-regenerative capacity of neonatal human keratinocyte stem cells and their progeny. *J Clin Invest*. 2004;113(3):390-400.
53. Arwert EN, Hoste E, Watt FM. Epithelial stem cells, wound healing and cancer. *Nat Rev Cancer*. 2012;12(3):170-180.
54. Morasso MI, Tomic-Canic M. Epidermal stem cells: the cradle of epidermal determination, differentiation and wound healing. *Biol Cell*. 2005;97(3): 173-183.
55. Mascré G, Dekoninck S, Drogat B, et al. Distinct contribution of stem and progenitor cells to epidermal maintenance. *Nature*. 2012;489(7415):257-262.
56. Garcin CL, Ansell DM, Headon DJ, Paus R, Hardman MJ. Hair follicle bulge stem cells appear dispensable for the acute phase of wound re-epithelialization. *Stem cells*. 2016;34(5):1377-1385.
57. Driskell I, Oeztuerk-Winder F, Humphreys P, Frye M. Genetically induced cell death in bulge stem cells reveals their redundancy for hair and epidermal regeneration. *Stem cells*. 2015;33(3):988-998.
58. Xu J, Clark R. Extracellular matrix alters PDGF regulation of fibroblast integrins. *The J Cell Biol*. 1996;132(1):239-249.
59. Pardoux C, Derynck R. JNK regulates expression and autocrine signaling of TGF-β1. *Mol Cell*. 2004;15(2):170-171.
60. Gray AJ, Bishop JE, Reeves JT, Laurent GJ. A alpha and B beta chains of fibrinogen stimulate proliferation of human fibroblasts. *J Cell Sci*. 1993;104(2): 409-413.
61. Clark RA, Lin F, Greiling D, An J, Couchman JR. Fibroblast invasive migration into fibronectin/fibrin gels requires a previously uncharacterized dermatan sulfate-CD44 proteoglycan. *J Invest Dermatol*. 2004;122(2):266-277.
62. Greiling D, Clark R. Fibronectin provides a conduit for fibroblast transmigration from collagenous stroma into fibrin clot provisional matrix. *J Cell Sci*. 1997;110(7):861-870.
63. Chrissouli S, Pratsinis H, Velissariou V, Anastasiou A, Kletsas D. Human amniotic fluid stimulates the proliferation of human fetal and adult skin fibroblasts: the roles of bFGF and PDGF and of the ERK and Akt signaling pathways. *Wound Repair Regen*. 2010;18(6):643-654.
64. Giannouli CC, Kletsas D. TGF-β regulates differentially the proliferation of fetal and adult human skin fibroblasts via the activation of PKA and the autocrine action of FGF-2. *Cell Signal*. 2006;18(9):1417-1429.

65. Hebda PA, Klingbeil CK, Abraham JA, Fiddes JC. Basic fibroblast growth factor stimulation of epidermal wound healing in pigs. *J Invest Dermatol.* 1990;95(6):626-631.
66. Akasaka Y, Ono I, Yamashita T, Jimbow K, Ishii T. Basic fibroblast growth factor promotes apoptosis and suppresses granulation tissue formation in acute incisional wounds. *J Pathol.* 2004;203(2):710-720.
67. Ortega S, Ittmann M, Tsang SH, Ehrlich M, Basilico C. Neuronal defects and delayed wound healing in mice lacking fibroblast growth factor 2. *Proc Natl Acad Sci.* 1998;95(10):5672-5677.
68. McGee GS, Davidson JM, Buckley A, et al. Recombinant basic fibroblast growth factor accelerates wound healing. *J Surg Res.* 1988;45(1):145-153.
69. Kawano Y, Patrulea V, Sublet E, et al. Wound healing promotion by hyaluronic acid: effect of molecular weight on gene expression and in vivo wound closure. *Pharmaceuticals.* 2021;14(4):301.
70. Clark RA. Biology of dermal wound repair. *Dermatol Clin.* 1993;11(4):647-666.
71. McClain SA, Simon M, Jones E, et al. Mesenchymal cell activation is the rate-limiting step of granulation tissue induction. *Am J Pathol.* 1996;149(4):1257.
72. Schultz GS, Davidson JM, Kirsner RS, Bornstein P, Herman IM. Dynamic reciprocity in the wound microenvironment. *Wound Repair Regen.* 2011;19(2): 134-148.
73. Bugge TH, Kombrinck KW, Flick MJ, Daugherty CC, Danton MJS, Degen JL. Loss of fibrinogen rescues mice from the pleiotropic effects of plasminogen deficiency. *Cell.* 1996;87(4):709-719.
74. Toriseva M, Laato M, Carpén O, et al. MMP-13 regulates growth of wound granulation tissue and modulates gene expression signatures involved in inflammation, proteolysis, and cell viability. 2012.
75. Vaalamo M, Mattila L, Johansson N, et al. Distinct populations of stromal cells express collagenase-3 (MMP-13) and collagenase-1 (MMP-1) in chronic ulcers but not in normally healing wounds. *J Invest Dermatol.* 1997;109(1):96-101.
76. Sudbeck BD, Pilcher BK, Welgus HG, Parks WC. Induction and repression of collagenase-1 by keratinocytes is controlled by distinct components of different extracellular matrix compartments. *J Biol Chem.* 1997;272(35): 22103-22110.
77. Danielsen PL, Holst AV, Maltesen HR, et al. Matrix metalloproteinase-8 overexpression prevents proper tissue repair. *Surgery.* 2011;150(5):897-906.
78. Juncker-Jensen A, Lund LR. Phenotypic overlap between MMP-13 and the plasminogen activation system during wound healing in mice. *PLoS ONE.* 2011;6(2):e16954.
79. Welch MP, Odland GF, Clark R. Temporal relationships of F-actin bundle formation, collagen and fibronectin matrix assembly, and fibronectin receptor expression to wound contraction. *The J Cell Biol.* 1990;110(1):133-145.
80. Roberts AB, Sporn MB, Assoian RK, et al. Transforming growth factor type beta: rapid induction of fibrosis and angiogenesis in vivo and stimulation of collagen formation in vitro. *Proc Natl Acad Sci.* 1986;83(12):4167-4171.
81. Postlethwaite A, Holness M, Katai H, Raghow R. Human fibroblasts synthesize elevated levels of extracellular matrix proteins in response to interleukin 4. *J Clin Invest.* 1992;90(4):1479-1485.
82. Clark R, Nielsen LD, Welch MP, McPherson JM. Collagen matrices attenuate the collagen-synthetic response of cultured fibroblasts to TGF-beta. *J Cell Sci.* 1995;108(3):1251-1261.
83. Grinnell F. Fibroblasts, myofibroblasts, and wound contraction. *J Cell Biol.* 1994;124(4):401-404.
84. Granstein R, Murphy G, Margolis R, Byrne M, Amento E. Gamma-interferon inhibits collagen synthesis in vivo in the mouse. *J Clin Invest.* 1987;79(4):1254-1258.
85. Desmouliere A, Redard M, Darby I, Gabbiani G. Apoptosis mediates the decrease in cellularity during the transition between granulation tissue and scar. *Am J Pathol.* 1995;146(1):56.
86. Desmoulière A, Badid C, Bochaton-Piallat M-L, Gabbiani G. Apoptosis during wound healing, fibrocontractive diseases and vascular wall injury. *Int J Biochem Cell Biol.* 1997;29(1):19-30.
87. Linge C, Richardson J, Vigor C, Clayton E, Hardas B, Rolfe KJ. Hypertrophic scar cells fail to undergo a form of apoptosis specific to contractile collagen—the role of tissue transglutaminase. *J Invest Dermatol.* 2005;125(1):72-82.
88. Huang S-P, Wu M-S, Shun C-T, et al. Cyclooxygenase-2 increases hypoxia-inducible factor-1 and vascular endothelial growth factor to promote angiogenesis in gastric carcinoma. *J Biomed Sci.* 2005;12(1):229-241.
89. Tonnesen MG, Feng X, Clark RA. Angiogenesis in wound healing. Elsevier; 2000.
90. Cao Y. Tumor angiogenesis and molecular targets for therapy. *Front Biosci.* 2009;14(10):3962-3973.
91. Carmeliet P. Angiogenesis in health and disease. *Nat Med.* 2003;9(6):653-660.
92. Carmeliet P, Jain RK. Molecular mechanisms and clinical applications of angiogenesis. *Nature.* 2011;473(7347):298-307.
93. Honnegowda TM, Kumar P, Udupa EGP, Kumar S, Kumar U, Rao P. Role of angiogenesis and angiogenic factors in acute and chronic wound healing. *Plast Aesthet Res.* 2015;2:243-249.
94. Tsopanoglou NE, Maragoudakis ME. On the mechanism of thrombin-induced angiogenesis: potentiation of vascular endothelial growth factor activity on endothelial cells by up-regulation of its receptors. *J Biol Chem.* 1999;274(34):23969-23976.
95. Hellberg C, Östman A, Heldin C-H. PDGF and vessel maturation. *Angiogenesis Inhibition.* 2010:103-114.
96. Pintucci G, Froum S, Pinnell J, Mignatti P, Rafii S, Green D. Trophic effects of platelets on cultured endothelial cells are mediated by platelet-associated fibroblast growth factor-2 (FGF-2) and vascular endothelial growth factor (VEGF). *Thromb Haemost.* 2002;88(11):834-842.
97. Li J-J, Huang Y-Q, Basch R, Karpatkin S. Thrombin induces the release of angiopoietin-1 from platelets. *Thromb Haemost.* 2001;85(02):204-206.
98. Nath SG, Raveendran R. An insight into the possibilities of fibroblast growth factor in periodontal regeneration. *J Indian Soc Periodontol.* 2014;18(3):289.
99. Nguyen M, Arkell J, Jackson CJ. Human endothelial gelatinases and angiogenesis. *The Int J Biochem Cell Biol.* 2001;33(10):960-970.
100. Montrucchio G, Lupia E, De Martino A, et al. Nitric oxide mediates angiogenesis induced in vivo by platelet-activating factor and tumor necrosis factor-alpha. *Am J Pathol.* 1997;151(2):557.
101. Andrikopoulou E, Zhang X, Sebastian R, et al. Current insights into the role of HIF-1 in cutaneous wound healing. *Curr Mol Med.* 2011;11(3):218-235.
102. Du Cheyne C, Tay H, De Spiegelaere W. The complex TIE between macrophages and angiogenesis. *Anat Histol Embryol.* 2020;49(5):585-596.
103. Willenborg S, Lucas T, Van Loo G, et al. CCR2 recruits an inflammatory macrophage subpopulation critical for angiogenesis in tissue repair. *Blood.* 2012;120(3):613-625.
104. Brooks PC, Clark RA, Cheresh DA. Requirement of vascular integrin αvβ3 for angiogenesis. *Science.* 1994;264(5158):569-571.
105. Leavesley D, Schwartz M, Rosenfeld M, Cheresh D. Integrin beta 1-and beta 3-mediated endothelial cell migration is triggered through distinct signaling mechanisms. *J Cell Biol.* 1993;121(1):163-170.
106. Weis SM, Cheresh DA. αV integrins in angiogenesis and cancer. *Cold Spring Harb Perspect Med.* 2011;1(1):a006478.
107. Cai J, Ahmad S, Jiang WG, et al. Activation of vascular endothelial growth factor receptor-1 sustains angiogenesis and Bcl-2 expression via the phosphatidylinositol 3-kinase pathway in endothelial cells. *Diabetes.* 2003;52(12): 2959-2968.
108. Kalebic T, Garbisa S, Glaser B, Liotta L. Basement membrane collagen: degradation by migrating endothelial cells. *Science.* 1983;221(4607):281-283.
109. Fantin A, Vieira JM, Gestri G, et al. Tissue macrophages act as cellular chaperones for vascular anastomosis downstream of VEGF-mediated endothelial tip cell induction. *Blood.* 2010;116(5):829-840.
110. Singh H, Tahir TA, Alawo DO, Issa E, Brindle NP. Molecular control of angiopoietin signalling. *Biochem Soc trans.* 2011;39(6):1592-1596.
111. Inoki I, Shiomi T, Hashimoto G, et al. Connective tissue growth factor binds vascular endothelial growth factor (VEGF) and inhibits VEGF-induced angiogenesis. *FASEB J.* 2002;16(2):1-27.
112. Ma J, Wang Q, Fei T, Han J-DJ, Chen Y-G. MCP-1 mediates TGF-β–induced angiogenesis by stimulating vascular smooth muscle cell migration. *Blood.* 2007;109(3):987-994.
113. Korff T, Kimmina S, Martiny-Baron G, Augustin HG. Blood vessel maturation in a 3-dimensional spheroidal coculture model: direct contact with smooth muscle cells regulates endothelial cell quiescence and abrogates VEGF responsiveness. *FASEB J.* 2001;15(2):447-457.
114. Onimaru M, Yonemitsu Y, Fujii T, et al. VEGF-C regulates lymphangiogenesis and capillary stability by regulation of PDGF-B. *Am J Physiol Heart Circ Physiol.* 2009;297(5):H1685-H1696.
115. Stefater III JA, Lewkowich I, Rao S, et al. Regulation of angiogenesis by a non-canonical Wnt–Flt1 pathway in myeloid cells. *Nature.* 2011;474(7352):511-515.
116. Gurevich DB, Severn CE, Twomey C, et al. Live imaging of wound angiogenesis reveals macrophage orchestrated vessel sprouting and regression. *EMBO J.* 2018;37(13):e97786.
117. Cheresh D, Stupack D. Regulation of angiogenesis: apoptotic cues from the ECM. *Oncogene.* 2008;27(48):6285-6298.
118. Koch AE, Polverini PJ, Kunkel SL, et al. Interleukin-8 as a macrophage-derived mediator of angiogenesis. *Science.* 1992;258(5089):1798-1801.
119. Lange-Asschenfeldt B, Velasco P, Streit M, et al. The angiogenesis inhibitor vasostatin does not impair wound healing at tumor-inhibiting doses. *J Invest Dermatol.* 2001;117(5):1036-1041.
120. Hinz B, Pittet P, Smith-Clerc J, Chaponnier C, Meister J-J. Myofibroblast development is characterized by specific cell-cell adherens junctions. *Mol Biol Cell.* 2004;15(9):4310-4320.

121. Tomasek JJ, Gabbiani G, Hinz B, Chaponnier C, Brown RA. Myofibroblasts and mechano-regulation of connective tissue remodelling. *Nat Rev Mol Cell Biol.* 2002;3(5):349-363.
122. Darby IA, Laverdet B, Bonté F, Desmoulière A. Fibroblasts and myofibroblasts in wound healing. *Clin Cosmet Investig Dermatol.* 2014;7:301.
123. Caley MP, Martins VLC, O'Toole EA. Metalloproteinases and wound healing. *Adv Wound Care (New Rochelle).* 2015;4(4). doi:10.1089/wound.2014.0581
124. Visse R, Nagase H. Matrix metalloproteinases and tissue inhibitors of metalloproteinases: structure, function, and biochemistry. *Circ Res.* 2003;92(8): 827-839.
125. Hartenstein B, Dittrich BT, Stickens D, et al. Epidermal development and wound healing in matrix metalloproteinase 13-deficient mice. *J Invest Dermatol.* 2006;126(2):486-496.
126. Ren M, Hao S, Yang C, et al. Angiotensin II regulates collagen metabolism through modulating tissue inhibitor of metalloproteinase-1 in diabetic skin tissues. *Diab Vasc Dis Res.* 2013;10(5):426-435.
127. Langholz O, Röckel D, Mauch C, et al. Collagen and collagenase gene expression in three-dimensional collagen lattices are differentially regulated by alpha 1 beta 1 and alpha 2 beta 1 integrins. *J Cell Biol.* 1995;131(6):1903-1915.
128. Gill SE, Pape MC, Khokha R, Watson AJ, Leco KJ. A null mutation for tissue inhibitor of metalloproteinases-3 (Timp-3) impairs murine bronchiole branching morphogenesis. *Dev Biol.* 2003;261(2):313-323.
129. Telgenhoff D, Shroot B. Cellular senescence mechanisms in chronic wound healing. *Cell Death Differ.* 2005;12(7):695-698.
130. Birk DE, Zycband EI, Winkelmann DA, Trelstad RL. Collagen fibrillogenesis in situ: fibril segments are intermediates in matrix assembly. *Proc Natl Acad Sci.* 1989;86(12):4549-4553.
131. Schultz GS, Wysocki A. Interactions between extracellular matrix and growth factors in wound healing. *Wound Repair Regen.* 2009;17(2):153-162.
132. Wassermann R, Polo M, Smith P, Wang X, Ko F, Robson M. Differential production of apoptosis-modulating proteins in patients with hypertrophic burn scar. *J Surg Res.* 1998;75(1):74-80.
133. Witte MB, Barbul A. General principles of wound healing. *Surg Clin North Am.* 1997;77(3):509-528.
134. Diegelmann RF, Evans MC. Wound healing: an overview of acute, fibrotic and delayed healing. *Front biosci.* 2004;9(1):283-289.
135. Young A, McNaught C-E. The physiology of wound healing. *Surgery (Oxford).* 2011;29(10):475-479.
136. Järbrink K, Ni G, Sönnergren H, et al. The humanistic and economic burden of chronic wounds: a protocol for a systematic review. *Syst Rev.* 2017;6(1):1-7.
137. Molnar JA, Underdown MJ, Clark WA. Nutrition and chronic wounds. *Adv Wound Care.* 2014;3(11):663-681.
138. Kibadi K. Time to removal of sutures from the palmar surface of the hand in dark-skinned patients: results in a prospective cohort of 146 hands. *Hand Surg Rehabil.* 2022;41(1):142-148.
139. Lee JY-Y, Yang C-C, Chao S-C, Wong T-W. Histopathological differential diagnosis of keloid and hypertrophic scar. *Am J Dermatopathol.* 2004;26(5):379-384.
140. Armour A, Scott PG, Tredget EE. Cellular and molecular pathology of HTS: basis for treatment. *Wound Repair Regen.* 2007;15:S6-S17.
141. Crawford J, Nygard K, Gan BS, O'Gorman DB. Periostin induces fibroblast proliferation and myofibroblast persistence in hypertrophic scarring. *Exp Dermatol.* 2015;24(2):120-126.
142. Zhang Z, Nie F, Kang C, et al. Increased periostin expression affects the proliferation, collagen synthesis, migration and invasion of keloid fibroblasts under hypoxic conditions. *International J Mol Med.* 2014;34(1):253-261.
143. Zhao B, Guan H, Liu J-Q, et al. Hypoxia drives the transition of human dermal fibroblasts to a myofibroblast-like phenotype via the TGF-β1/Smad3 pathway Corrigendum in/10.3892/ijmm. 2019.4403. *Int J Mol Med.* 2017;39(1):153-159.
144. Wong VW, Paterno J, Sorkin M, et al. Mechanical force prolongs acute inflammation via T-cell-dependent pathways during scar formation. *FASEB J.* 2011;25(12):4498-4510.
145. Li-Tsang CW, Lau JC, Chan CC. Prevalence of hypertrophic scar formation and its characteristics among the Chinese population. *Burns.* 2005; 31(5):610-616.
146. Brown J, Bayat A. Genetic susceptibility to raised dermal scarring. *Br J Dermatol.* 2009;161(1):8-18.
147. Tuan T-L, Nichter LS. The molecular basis of keloid and hypertrophic scar formation. *Mol Med today.* 1998;4(1):19-24.
148. Kelly AP. Update on the management of keloids. WB Saunders; 2009.
149. Marneros AG, Norris JE, Watanabe S, Reichenberger E, Olsen BR. Genome scans provide evidence for keloid susceptibility loci on chromosomes 2q23 and 7p11. *J Invest Dermatol.* 2004;122(5):1126-1132.
150. Yan X, Gao J, Chen Y, Song M, Liu X. Preliminary linkage analysis and mapping of keloid susceptibility locus in a Chinese pedigree. *Zhonghua Zheng Xing Wai Ke Za Zhi.* 2007;23(1):32-35.
151. Chen Y, Gao J-H, Yan X, Song M, Liu X-J. Location of predisposing gene for one Han Chinese keloid pedigree. *Zhonghua Zheng Xing Wai Ke Za Zhi.* 2007;23(2):137-140.
152. Halim AS, Emami A, Salahshourifar I, Kannan TP. Keloid scarring: understanding the genetic basis, advances, and prospects. *Arch Plast Surg.* 2012;39(03): 184-189.
153. Lu W-S, Cai L-Q, Wang Z-X, et al. Association of HLA class I alleles with keloids in Chinese Han individuals. *Hum Immunol.* 2010;71(4):418-422.
154. Niessen FB, Spauwen PH, Schalkwijk J, Kon M. On the nature of hypertrophic scars and keloids: a review. *Plast Reconstr Surg.* 1999;104(5):1435-1458.
155. Shih B, Bayat A. Genetics of keloid scarring. *Arch Dermatol Res.* 2010;302: 319-339.
156. Zhang G, Jiang J, Luo S, Tang S, Liang J, Yao P. Analyses of CDC2L1 gene mutations in keloid tissue. *Clin Exp Dermatol.* 2012;37(3):277-283.
157. Brown J, Ollier W, Thomson W, Bayat A. Positive association of HLA-DRB1* 15 with keloid disease in Caucasians. *Int J Immunogenet.* 2008;35(4-5):303-307.
158. Laurentaci G, Dioguardi D. HLA antigens in keloids and hypertrophic scars. *Arch Dermatol.* 1977;113(12):1726-1726.
159. McCarty SM, Syed F, Bayat A. Influence of the human leukocyte antigen complex on the development of cutaneous fibrosis: an immunogenetic perspective. *Acta Derm Venereol.* 2010;90(6):563-574.
160. Choo SY. The HLA system: genetics, immunology, clinical testing, and clinical implications. *Yonsei Med J.* 2007;48(1):11-23.
161. Robles DT, Berg D. Abnormal wound healing: keloids. *Clin Dermatol.* 2007;25(1):26-32.
162. Bijlard E, Kouwenberg C, Timman R, Hovius S, van Busschbach J, Mureau M. Burden of keloid disease: a cross-sectional health-related quality of life assessment. *Acta Derm Venereol.* 2017;97(2):225-229.
163. Bickers DR, Lim HW, Margolis D, et al. The burden of skin diseases: 2004: a joint project of the American Academy of Dermatology Association and the Society for Investigative Dermatology. *J Am Acad Dermatol.* 2006;55(3):490-500.
164. Tsuruo S. Quality of life in patients with keloids in the context of marginalized identities: pilot study and literature review.
165. Baranoski S, Ayello EA. *Wound Care Essentials: Practice Principles.* Lippincott Williams & Wilkins; 2008.
166. Bates-Jensen BM, Anber K, Chen MM, et al. Natural history of pressure injury among ethnically/racially diverse nursing home residents: the pressure ulcer detection study. *J Gerontol Nurs.* 2021;47(3):37-46.
167. Beeckman D, Smet S, Van den Bussche K. Incontinence-associated dermatitis: why do we need a core outcome set for clinical research? *Wounds Int.* 2018;9(2):21-25.
168. Sussman C, Bates-Jensen BM. *Wound Care: A Collaborative Practice Manual.* Lippincott Williams & Wilkins; 2007.
169. Halder RM, Nootheti PK. Ethnic skin disorders overview. *J Am Acad Dermatol.* 2003;48(6):S143-S148.
170. O'connor E, Sheena Y, Giele H. Examination of scars. In: Gogalniceanu P, Pegrum J, Lynn W, eds. *Physical Examination for Surgeons: An Aid to the MRCS OSCE.* Cambridge University Press; 2015:359-361.
171. Kinani ME, Duteille F. Scar epidemiology and consequences. *Textbook on Scar Management.* Springer; 2020:45-49.
172. Rockwell WB, Cohen IK, Ehrlich HP. Keloids and hypertrophic scars: a comprehensive review. *Plast Reconstr Surg.* 1989;84(5):827-837.
173. Philandrianos C, Kerfant N, Jaloux Jr C, Martinet L, Bertrand B, Casanova D. Keloid scars (part I): clinical presentation, epidemiology, histology and pathogenesis. 2015;61:128-135.
174. Crockett DJ. Regional keloid susceptibility. *Br J Plast Surg.* 1964;17:245-253.
175. Tyack ZF, Pegg S, Ziviani J. Postburn dyspigmentation: its assessment, management, and relationship to scarring—a review of the literature. *J Burn Care Rehabil.* 1997;18(5):435-440.
176. Chadwick S, Heath R, Shah M. Abnormal pigmentation within cutaneous scars: a complication of wound healing. *Indian J Plast Surg.* 2012;45(02): 403-411.
177. Kirsner RS, Bohn G, Driver VR, et al. Human acellular dermal wound matrix: evidence and experience. *Int Wound J.* 2015;12(6):646-654.
178. Steed DL. Debridement. *Am J Surg.* 2004;187(5):S71-S74.
179. Files R, Files AM, Recalls FS. Label: COLLAGENASE SANTYL ointment.
180. Parnés A, Lagan K. Larval therapy in wound management: a review. *Int J Clin Pract.* 2007;61(3):488-493.
181. Tavakoli S, Klar AS. Advanced hydrogels as wound dressings. *Biomolecules.* 2020;10(8):1169.

182. Sussman G. Technology update: understanding film dressings. *Wounds Int.* 2010;1(4):23-25.
183. Source W. Types of Wound Dressings: Features, Indications and Contraindications. 2018. https://www.biosanas.com.br/uploads/outros/artigos_cientificos/39/fbd0ab65f32286644ee7c39a3d8557d2.pdf.
184. Wieman TJ, Smiell JM, Su Y. Efficacy and safely of a topical gel formulation of recombinant human platelet-derived growth factor-BB (becaplermin) in patients with chronic neuropathic diabetic ulcers: a phase III randomized placebo-controlled double-blind study. *Diabetes Care.* 1998;21(5):822-827.
185. Cahn BA, Kaur R, Hirt PA, et al. Use of topical timolol maleate as re-epithelialization agent for treatment of recalcitrant wounds of varying etiologies. *J Drugs Dermatol.* 2020;19(12):1252-1256.
186. Figus A, Leon-Villapalos J, Philp B, Dziewulski P. Severe multiple extensive postburn contractures: a simultaneous approach with total scar tissue excision and resurfacing with dermal regeneration template. *J Burn Care Res.* 2007;28(6):913-917.
187. Buchanan PJ, Kung TA, Cederna PS. Evidence-based medicine: wound closure. *Plast Reconstr Surg.* 2016;138(3S):257S-270S.
188. Kirsner R, Falanga V, Kerdel F, Katz M, Eaglstein W. Skin grafts as pharmacological agents: pre-wounding of the donor site. *Br J Dermatol.* 1996;135(2): 292-296.
189. Vyas KS, Vasconez HC. Wound healing: biologics, skin substitutes, biomembranes and scaffolds. MDPI; 2014.
190. Benichou G, Yamada Y, Yun S-H, Lin C, Fray M, Tocco G. Immune recognition and rejection of allogeneic skin grafts. *Immunotherapy.* 2011;3(6):757-770.
191. Falanga V, Margolis D, Alvarez O, et al. Rapid healing of venous ulcers and lack of clinical rejection with an allogeneic cultured human skin equivalent. *Arch Dermatol.* 1998;134(3):293-300.
192. Mendez-Eastman S. Guidelines for using negative pressure wound therapy. *Adv Skin Wound Care.* 2001;14(6):314-323.
193. Mervis JS, Phillips TJ. Pressure ulcers: prevention and management. *J Am Acad Dermatol.* 2019;81(4):893-902.
194. Thackham JA, McElwain DS, Long RJ. The use of hyperbaric oxygen therapy to treat chronic wounds: a review. *Wound Repair Regen.* 2008;16(3):321-330.
195. Clarke TC, Black LI, Stussman BJ, Barnes PM, Nahin RL. Trends in the use of complementary health approaches among adults: United States, 2002–2012. *Natl Health Stat Rep.* 2015;(79):1.
196. Green RR, Santoro N, Allshouse AA, Neal-Perry G, Derby C. Prevalence of complementary and alternative medicine and herbal remedy use in hispanic and non-hispanic white women: results from the study of women's health across the nation. *J Altern Complement Med.* 2017;23(10):805-811.
197. Gardiner P, Whelan J, White LF, Filippelli AC, Bharmal N, Kaptchuk TJ. A systematic review of the prevalence of herb usage among racial/ethnic minorities in the United States. *J Immigr Minor Health.* 2013;15(4):817-828.
198. Brown C, Barner J, Bohman T, Richards K. A multivariate test of an expanded Andersen Health Care utilization model for complementary and alternative medicine (CAM) use in African Americans. *J Altern Complement Med.* 2009;15(8):911-919.
199. Bedi MK, Shenefelt PD. Herbal therapy in dermatology. *Arch Dermatol.* 2002;138(2):232-242.
200. Maenthaisong R, Chaiyakunapruk N, Niruntraporn S, Kongkaew C. The efficacy of aloe vera used for burn wound healing: a systematic review. *Burns.* 2007;33(6):713-718.
201. Avijgan M, Kamran A, Abedini A. Effectiveness of Aloe vera gel in chronic ulcers in comparison with conventional treatments. *Iran J Med Sci.* 2016; 41(3 Suppl):S30.
202. Hekmatpou D, Mehrabi F, Rahzani K, Aminiyan A. The effect of Aloe Vera gel on prevention of pressure ulcers in patients hospitalized in the orthopedic wards: a randomized triple-blind clinical trial. *BMC Complement Altern Med.* 2018;18(1):1-11.
203. Kazemian H, Ghafourian S, Sadeghifard N, et al. In vivo antibacterial and wound healing activities of Roman chamomile (Chamaemelum nobile). *Infect Disord Drug Targets.* 2018;18(1):41-45.
204. Gad HA, Abd El-Rahman FA, Hamdy GM. Chamomile oil loaded solid lipid nanoparticles: a naturally formulated remedy to enhance the wound healing. *J Drug Delivery Sci Technol.* 2019;50:329-338.
205. Saikaly SK, Khachemoune A. Honey and wound healing: an update. *Am J Clin Dermatol.* 2017;18(2):237-251.
206. Majtan J. Honey: an immunomodulator in wound healing. *Wound Repair Regen.* 2014;22(2):187-192.
207. Givol O, Kornhaber R, Visentin D, Cleary M, Haik J, Harats M. A systematic review of Calendula officinalis extract for wound healing. *Wound Repair Regen.* 2019;27(5):548-561.
208. Pazyar N, Yaghoobi R, Bagherani N, Kazerouni A. A review of applications of tea tree oil in dermatology. *Int J Dermatol.* 2013;52(7):784-790.
209. Carson CF, Hammer KA, Riley TV. Melaleuca alternifolia (tea tree) oil: a review of antimicrobial and other medicinal properties. *Clin Microbiol Rev.* 2006;19(1):50-62.
210. Halcón L, Milkus K. *Staphylococcus aureus* and wounds: a review of tea tree oil as a promising antimicrobial. *Am J Infect Control.* 2004;32(7):402-408.
211. Slade D, Powell B, Mortimer P. Hidradenitis suppurativa: pathogenesis and management. *Br J Plast Surg.* 2003;56(5):451-461.
212. Katyayan A. HIDRADENITIS SUPPURATIVA. 2021.
213. Coppola MM, Salzillo R, Segreto F, Persichetti P. Triamcinolone acetonide intralesional injection for the treatment of keloid scars: patient selection and perspectives. *Clin Cosmet Investig Dermatol.* 2018;11:387.
214. Arno AI, Gauglitz GG, Barret JP, Jeschke MG. Up-to-date approach to manage keloids and hypertrophic scars: a useful guide. *Burns.* 2014;40(7):1255-1266.
215. Reish RG, Eriksson E. Scar treatments: preclinical and clinical studies. *J Am Coll Surg.* 2008;206(4):719-730.
216. Son D, Harijan A. Overview of surgical scar prevention and management. *J Korean Med Sci.* 2014;29(6):751-757.
217. Ogawa R, Akaishi S, Huang C, et al. Clinical applications of basic research that shows reducing skin tension could prevent and treat abnormal scarring: the importance of fascial/subcutaneous tensile reduction sutures and flap surgery for keloid and hypertrophic scar reconstruction. *J Nippon Med Sch.* 2011;78(2):68-76.
218. Nguyen KT, Shikowitz L, Kasabian AK, Bastidas N. A novel approach to keloid reconstruction with bilaminar dermal substitute and epidermal skin grafting. *Plast Reconstr Surg.* 2016;138(1):235-239.
219. Ojeh N, Bharatha A, Gaur U, Forde AL. Keloids: current and emerging therapies. *Scars Burn Heal.* 2020;6:2059513120940499.
220. Di Stadio A. Ear keloid treated with infiltrated non-cross-linked hyaluronic acid and cortisone therapy. *In Vivo.* 2016;30(5):695-699.
221. Gauglitz G, Bureik D, Dombrowski Y, Pavicic T, Ruzicka T, Schauber J. Botulinum toxin A for the treatment of keloids. *Skin Pharmacol Physiol.* 2012;25(6):313-318.
222. Abedini R, Sasani P, Mahmoudi HR, Nasimi M, Teymourpour A, Shadlou Z. Comparison of intralesional verapamil versus intralesional corticosteroids in treatment of keloids and hypertrophic scars: a randomized controlled trial. *Burns.* 2018;44(6):1482-1488.
223. Kang N, Sivakumar B, Sanders R, Nduka C, Gault D. Intra-lesional injections of collagenase are ineffective in the treatment of keloid and hypertrophic scars. *J Plast Reconstr Aesthet Surg.* 2006;59(7):693-699.
224. Del Toro D, Dedhia R, Tollefson TT. Advances in scar management: prevention and management of hypertrophic scars and keloids. *Curr Opin Otolaryngol Head Neck Surg.* 2016;24(4):322-329.
225. Siotos C, Uzosike AC, Hong H, et al. Keloid excision and adjuvant treatments: a network meta-analysis. *Ann Plast Surg.* 2019;83(2):154-162.
226. Gold MH, Berman B, Clementoni MT, Gauglitz GG, Nahai F, Murcia C. Updated international clinical recommendations on scar management: part 1—evaluating the evidence. *Dermatol Surg.* 2014;40(8):817-824.
227. Gold MH, McGuire M, Mustoe TA, et al. Updated international clinical recommendations on scar management: part 2—algorithms for scar prevention and treatment. *Dermatol Surg.* 2014;40(8):825-831.
228. Liu EK, Cohen RF, Chiu ES. Radiation therapy modalities for keloid management: a critical review. *J Plast Reconstr Aesthet Surg.* 2022;75(8):2455-2465.
229. Payapvipapong K, Niumpradit N, Piriyanand C, Buranaphalin S, Nakakes A. The treatment of keloids and hypertrophic scars with intralesional bleomycin in skin of color. *J Cosmet Dermatol.* 2015;14(1):83-90.
230. van Leeuwen MC, Bulstra AEJ, Ket JC, Ritt MJ, van Leeuwen PA, Niessen FB. Intralesional cryotherapy for the treatment of keloid scars: evaluating effectiveness. *Plast Reconstr Surg Glob Open.* 2015;3(6).
231. Litrowski N, Boullie M, Dehesdin D, De Barros A, Joly P. Treatment of earlobe keloids by surgical excision and cryosurgery. *J Eur Acad Dermatol Venereol.* 2014;28(10):1324-1331.
232. Zhang J, Guan J, Niu X, et al. Exosomes released from human induced pluripotent stem cells-derived MSCs facilitate cutaneous wound healing by promoting collagen synthesis and angiogenesis. *J Transl Med.* 2015;13(1):1-14.
233. Aggarwal S, Pittenger MF. Human mesenchymal stem cells modulate allogeneic immune cell responses. *Blood.* 2005;105(4):1815-1822.
234. Liu L, Yu Y, Hou Y, et al. Human umbilical cord mesenchymal stem cells transplantation promotes cutaneous wound healing of severe burned rats. *PloS ONE.* 2014;9(2):e88348.
235. Kim W-S, Park B-S, Sung J-H, et al. Wound healing effect of adipose-derived stem cells: a critical role of secretory factors on human dermal fibroblasts. *J Dermatol Sci.* 2007;48(1):15-24.

236. Ebrahimian T, Pouzoulet F, Squiban C, et al. Cell therapy based on adipose tissue-derived stromal cells promotes physiological and pathological wound healing. *Arterioscler Thromb Vasc Biol.* 2009;29(4):503-510.
237. Mascharak S, desJardins-Park HE, Davitt MF, et al. Preventing *Engrailed*-1 activation in fibroblasts yields wound regeneration without scarring. *Science.* 2021;372(6540):eaba2374.
238. Pinto AM, Cerqueira MA, Bañobre-Lópes M, Pastrana LM, Sillankorva S. Bacteriophages for chronic wound treatment: from traditional to novel delivery systems. *Viruses.* 2020;12(2):235.

CHAPTER 20

Biology of the Oral Mucosa

Antara Afrin
Mayra B. C. Maymone
Ginat W. Mirowski

KEY POINTS

- Both skin and the oral mucosa are derived from the ectoderm.
- The oral mucosa comprises stratified squamous epithelium, lamina propria or connective tissue, and variably present submucosa.
- The oral mucosa can be classified into masticatory (keratinized epithelium), lining (nonkeratinized epithelium), and specialized mucosa.
- Physiologic oral melanin pigmentation is a normal variation in pigmentation that can affect any mucosal site yet is more common in the gingiva of patients with skin of color.
- Compared to the skin, unique differences in the oral mucosa are the presence of salivary glands, teeth for mastication, the oral microbiome comprising pathogenic and nonpathogenic microorganisms, and the specialized sensory epithelium of the tongue.
- Wound healing in oral mucosa undergoes the same phases of wound healing as the skin. However, this process is often faster and is less susceptible to scarring due to the moist environment, hemostatic properties of saliva, presence of anti-inflammatory cytokines, and abundant vascularity.
- Intrinsic aging of the oral mucosa and salivary glands is noted by decrease in saliva leading to xerostomia.

INTRODUCTION

The functions of oral mucosa are to protect the oral cavity against mechanical trauma, serve as a barrier to environmental, chemical, and biologic stressors, as well as to provide sensory perception and salivary secretion.[1] The unique differences between skin and oral mucosa are the presence of salivary glands that helps create a moist environment that facilitates swallowing, speaking, and digestion, the presence of teeth for mastication, and the presence of oral microbiome, comprising both nonpathogenic and pathogenic microorganisms that maintains homeostasis preventing diseases.[2]

This chapter aims to describe the normal structure and histology of oral mucosa, highlighting specific finding in skin of color individuals. We hope to provide a basic understanding of normal oral mucosa prior to discussing the oral diseases, reactive processes, and infections of oral mucosa discussed in Section 9, Chapter 61.

CLINICAL ANATOMY OF ORAL CAVITY

The oral cavity, also referred to as the buccal cavity, is divided into the lips, the oral vestibule, and oral cavity proper. The lip marks the transition from the skin to the oral cavity. The junction where the outer part of the lip meets skin is referred to as the vermillion border [**Figures 20-1** to **20-3**].[3] Labial and buccal mucosa form the linings of the lips and cheeks, respectively.[4] The vestibule is the region between the lips and the boney arches of the teeth [see **Figure 20-4**]. The oral cavity proper is the area between the dental arches. Within the mandibular arch is the anterior two-thirds of the tongue. The maxillary arch includes the hard palate, the bony roof of the oral cavity proper, which separates the oral cavity from the nasal cavity. The soft palate is continuous with the hard palate [**Figure 20-5**].[5] In the midline at the end of the soft palate, the uvula can be found [**Figure 20-6**].[6] The dental arches are covered by the gingiva, a masticatory mucosa, that overlay the bone. The alveolar bone is protected by the periodontal tissue from mechanical trauma, bacterial invasion, and propioseption.[3]

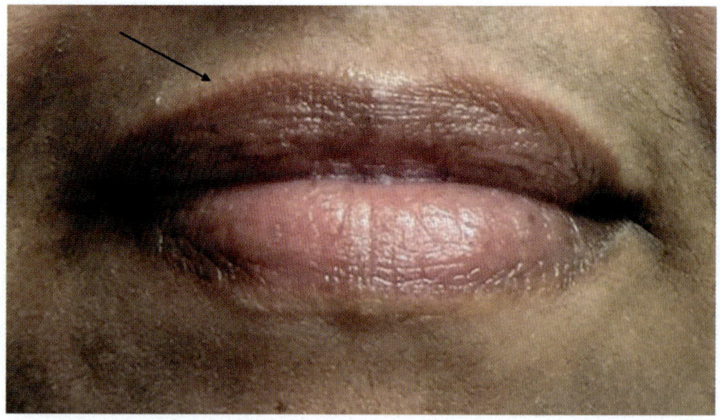

FIGURE 20-1. Vermillion border (marked with black arrow) is the transition between the vermillion of the oral mucosa and skin. (Image courtesy of Neelam Vashi, MD, Department of Dermatology, Boston University, Boston, MA.)

The oral mucosa can be classified into masticatory, lining, and specialized. Masticatory mucosa consists of the hard palate and the attached gingiva [Figures 20-4 and 20-5]. Lining mucosa includes the vestibule buccal and labial mucosa, soft palate, lips, and floor of mouth. The tongue is considered specialized sensory epithelium responsible for the taste.[3] More details of these classifications will be discussed in the sections to follow.

HISTOLOGIC STRUCTURE OF ORAL MUCOSA

Histologically, the oral mucosa comprises three layers: oral epithelium, lamina propria, and submucosa. The vermillion border provides the transition from skin to oral epithelium that serves as lining of the oral

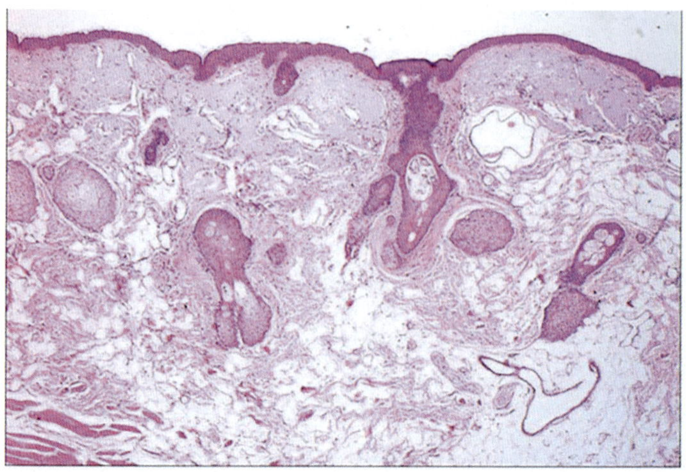

FIGURE 20-2. Histology of cutaneous lip with solar elastosis and villous hair follicles. (Image courtesy of Dr. Ginat Mirowski.)

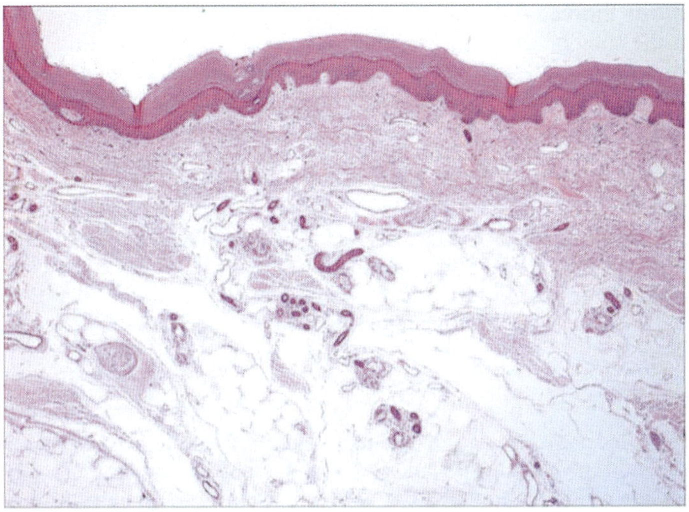

FIGURE 20-3. Histology of vermillion of lip with prominent stratum corneum. (Image courtesy of Dr. Ginat Mirowski.)

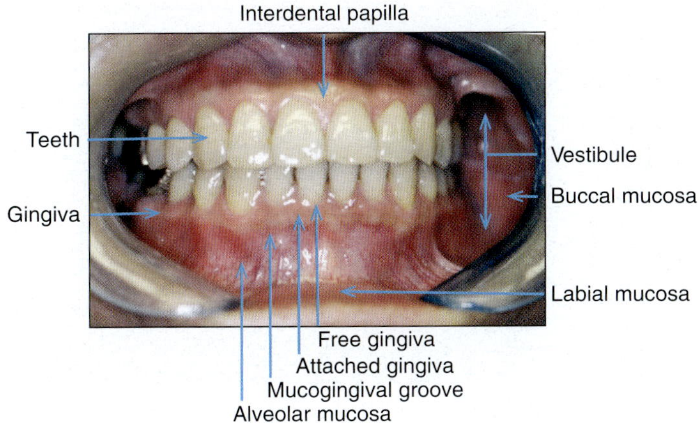

FIGURE 20-4. Oral anatomy.

cavity. The oral epithelium consists of stratified epithelium. Below this layer is the lamina propria, which is composed of loose connective tissue. The deepest layer, the submucosa, is absent at the attached gingiva and hard palate. The salivary and sebaceous glands may be located within the submucosa but originate from the junction of the epithelium and submucosa. The type of mucosa, masticatory, lining, or specialized, is influenced by anatomic location and function. Akin to skin, keratinocytes, melanocytes, Langerhans cells, and Merkel cells are also found in the oral mucosa.[3]

ORAL EPITHELIUM

Anatomic location and function influence modifications in the oral epithelium, such as the degree of keratinization.[3] Keratinized epithelium can be parakeratinized, having a nuclei in the stratum corneum, or orthokeratinized, in which the nuclei are absent. This type of epithelium functions to support mechanical forces and is found in masticatory mucosa. Nonkeratinized epithelium is epithelium that lacks a granular layer. Additionally, the spinous layer of nonkeratinized epithelium is thinner compared to keratinized epithelium. Nonkeratinized epithelium, found in lining or movable mucosa, allows for flexibility needed for speech and swallowing food. Specialized mucosa, found on the dorsum of the tongue, can be either keratinized or nonkeratinized. Melanocytes are found in the basal layer of the oral epithelium. Like the skin,

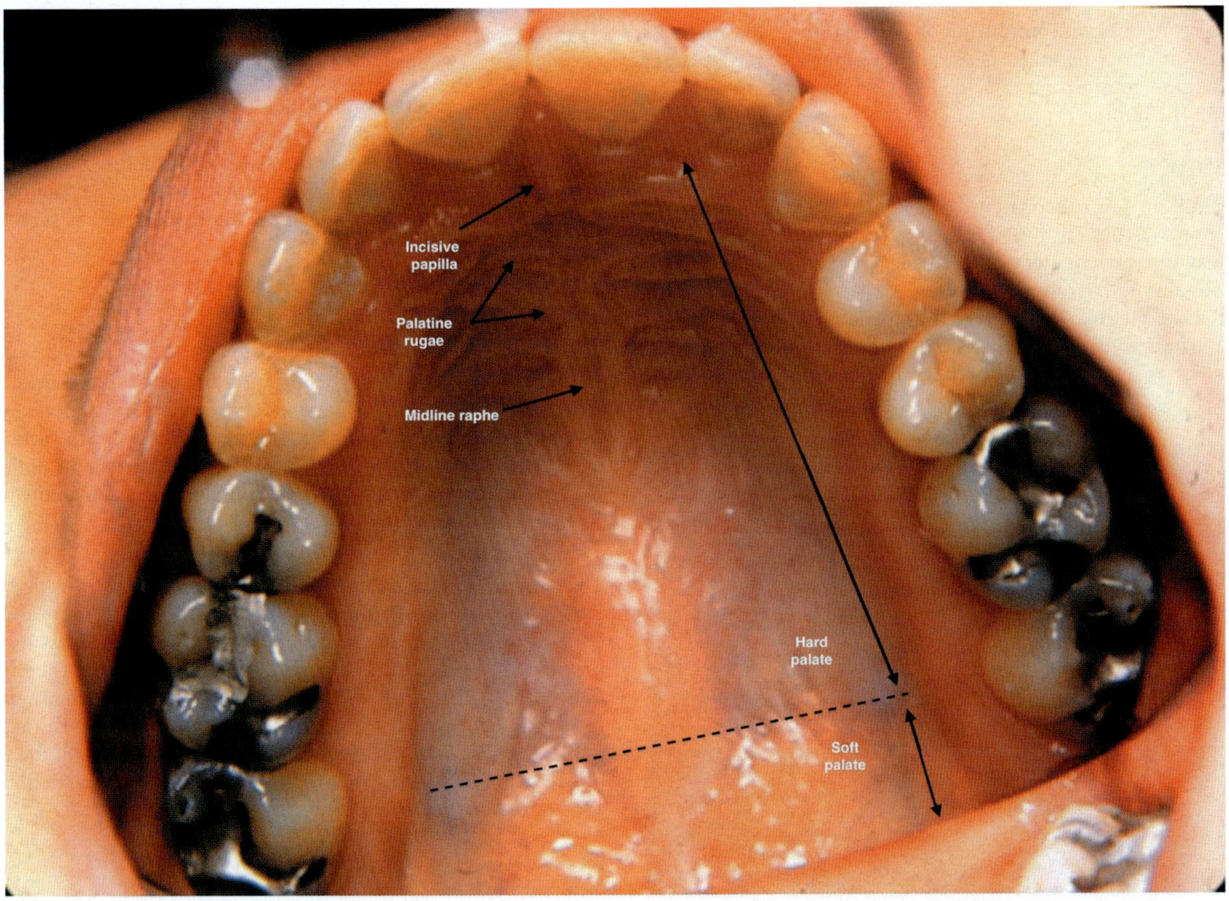

FIGURE 20-5. Hard palate and attached gingiva. (Image courtesy of Dr. Ginat Mirowski.)

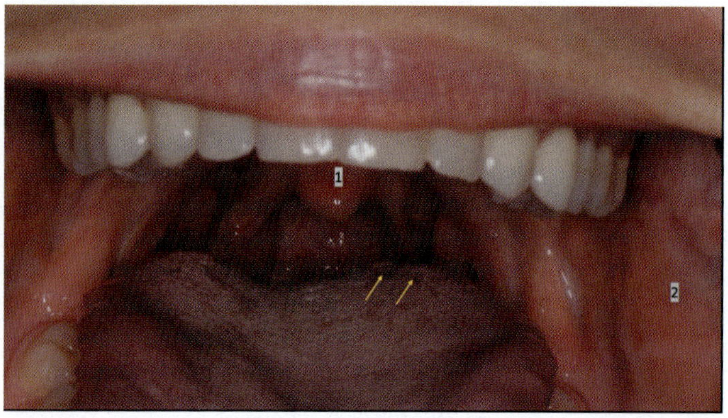

FIGURE 20-6. Posterior oral cavity. (1) Uvula and (2) Buccal mucosa. Circumvallate papillae (arrows).

the density of melanocytes in oral mucosa is consistent in all racialized groups. Increased melanocyte activity and decreased degradation of melanosomes are responsible for the changes in physiologic pigmentation observed in skin of color [**Figure 20-7**].[7-9]

LAMINA PROPRIA

The lamina propria of the mucosa is similar to the dermis of the skin in that they both are dense connective tissue layers. The lamina propria of the mucosa consist of two sublayers: papillary and deeper reticular.[10] The blood vessels present in the lamina propria allow for an inflow of nutrients.[11] Masticatory mucosa generally contains less blood vessels compared to lining mucosa.[12] Fibroblasts are the main cells in the lamina propria. While fibroblasts in the skin originate from mesoderm, the fibroblasts of the lamina propria are derived from the embryonic neural crest. Furthermore, the gene expression of fibroblasts can differ based on the location in the oral cavity depending on type of mucosa present, lining or masticatory.[11] Plasma cells, lymphocytes, neutrophils, mast cells, and monocytes/macrophages, which contribute to antimicrobial benefits of the oral mucosa, are also found in the lamina propria.[9]

SUBMUCOSA

Like the hypodermis or subcutaneous layer of the skin, the submucosa of the oral mucosa contains blood vessels and nerves. The submucosa of the oral cavity also contains minor salivary glands. This layer of the oral mucosa is absent from some areas of the oral cavity, such as the hard palate or attached gingiva. In these regions, the lamina propria attaches directly to the underlying bone.[1]

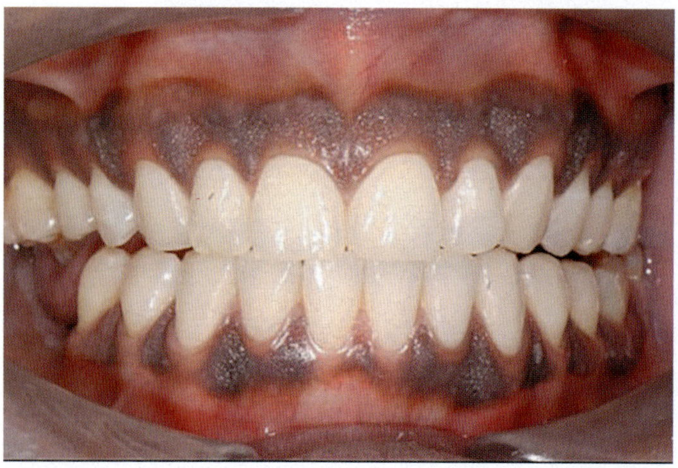

FIGURE 20-7. Physiologic gingival pigmentation. (Image courtesy of Dr. John McDowell.)

Minor Salivary Glands The minor salivary glands can be found in the submucosa. Since the hard palate and gingiva lack this layer, minor salivary glands are not found in these areas. There are up to 1000 minor salivary glands, with each gland having one duct. Von Ebner glands are a type of minor salivary glands that can be found on the dorsum of the tongue. While most minor salivary glands secrete mucous fluid, Von Ebner glands secrete serous fluid and serve a function for taste.

Damage to salivary glands, diseases, and medications that directly or indirectly affects saliva production may lead to altered salivary flow impairing antimicrobial defense, affecting taste, digestion, and mastication. Treatment for xerostomia depends on the causal factor.[13,14]

MAJOR SALIVARY GLANDS

The three paired major salivary glands are the parotid, the submandibular, and the sublingual glands. The major salivary glands are located outside of the oral mucosa but deliver saliva into the mouth through ducts. These major salivary glands are responsible for more than 90% of the salivary secretion. The difference in fluid secretion by each paired glands allow for them to be targeted preferentially by different conditions and drugs.[7,13]

Parotid Glands The parotid glands are largest and are located anterior and inferior to the ears bilaterally. The parotid gland is divided by the facial nerve and posterior facial vein into superficial lobe and deep lobe. The most inferior portion of the superficial lobe is known as the parotid tail and curves around the ramus and under the angle of the mandible. The parotid gland saliva is composed of serous fluid. Stensen's duct is the major excretory duct for the parotid gland and opens into the oral cavity at the level of the buccal mucosa of the maxillary second molar.[7,13]

Submandibular Glands The submandibular glands are located below the floor of the mouth. The main excretory duct of the submandibular glands is Wharton's duct. The submandibular gland consists of the mix of both serous and mucous secretions.[7,13]

Sublingual Glands The sublingual glands are located beneath the tongue and secretes mucous fluid. The ducts of Rivinus allow the sublingual gland to drain into the floor of the mouth. The Bartholin's duct of the sublingual gland joins the Wharton's duct of the submandibular glands to drain both sides of the lateral frenulum. The sublingual glands contain both serous and mucinous acini; however, it secretes mostly mucous secretions.[7,13]

REGIONAL DIFFERENCES IN STRUCTURE

Along with the type of epithelium present, other differences in the oral mucosa are noted in different anatomic regions of the oral cavity. These differences allow for the specific functions that occur in each region. An understanding of the differences will assist clinicians in understanding the appearance, variations, and pathologies that occur in the oral cavity.

VERMILLION LIP AND VERMILLION BORDER

The vermillion zone of the lip consists of keratinized epithelium. However, as the vermillion zone transitions into the oral cavity, the epithelium becomes nonkeratinized. The connective tissue, or lamina propria, of the vermillion lip is highly vascularized.[3] The lip color is due to the presence of melanocytes and variable melanin and, therefore, may have a wide range of colors that changes with race and ethnicities. Additionally, the color of the vermillion lip and the vermillion border can be the same coloration of perioral skin particularly in persons of color.[15]

MAXILLA AND MANDIBLE

The maxilla and mandible bones comprise the upper and lower jaw, respectively. The maxilla separates the oral cavity from the nasal cavity.

The mandible, the largest bone in the human skull, is located inferior to the maxilla. Both the maxilla and mandible are formed from the first pharyngeal arch.[5,16,17] The maxilla and mandible form the alveolar process that are the sockets of the teeth.[18]

GINGIVA

The gingiva plays a role in protecting underlying periodontal tissue against microbial and traumatic aggressions. The gingiva is divided into the free marginal gingiva and attached gingiva [Figure 20-4]. Masticatory keratinized epithelium externally covers the gingiva up the gingival margin and the tip of the interdental papillae. Like the hard palate, the lamina propria of the gingiva attaches directly to the periosteum of the bone. Collagen fibers and ground substance make up 95% of the gingival connective tissue, allowing for structural integrity of this tissue. The marginal end of the gingiva folds over the tooth surface. It attaches to the tooth below the gingival border. On the internal part of the marginal gingiva, there is a smooth collar of junctional epithelium. The junctional epithelium is attached to the enamel. The space found between the tooth and the gingiva is referred to as the gingival sulcus, which is lined by sulcular epithelium that extends up to the free gingival margin. The junctional and sulcular epithelium both are nonkeratinized. The attached gingiva extends from the free gingival groove to the beginning of the alveolar crest. It is continuous with the alveolar mucosa. The mucogingival junction, found along the vestibular and lingual aspects of the alveolar ridge, demarcates the gingiva from the floor of mouth. The gingiva is normally light pink and tightly bound, whereas the alveolar mucosa found on the floor of the mouth is dark red and movable. The amount of melanin produced by melanocytes may cause physiologic variations to this.[12,19]

HARD AND SOFT PALATES

The mucosa of the hard palate is keratinized, which allow it to play a role in both protection and mastication. The lamina propria of the hard palate is directly attached to the periosteum of bone.[3] The hard palate is embryologically formed by fusion of three bones: incisive, palatine, and maxillary [Figure 20-5].[5] The incisive papilla, also called the palatine papilla, is an oval-shaped mucosal prominence. The incisive papilla is found on the distal midline of the hard palate, just posterior to the central incisors [**Figure 20-8**]. The line extending from the incisive papilla is known as the midline raphe. Lateral to the midline raphe, multiple corrugated ridges called the palatal rugae can be found [Figure 20-5]. Tori or boney exostoses can be found present on the center of the hard palate. These are structures of benign excessive bone growth that progress over time in a slow fashion.[6]

In contrast to the hard palate, the soft palate is covered in nonkeratinized mucosa.[7,8] It is embryologically derived from the first three pharyngeal arches. The soft palate appears reddish-pink in coloration and has a homogeneous spongy consistency. In older patients, it may appear yellow due to increased adipose tissue. At the tip of the soft palate, the uvula can be found.[6]

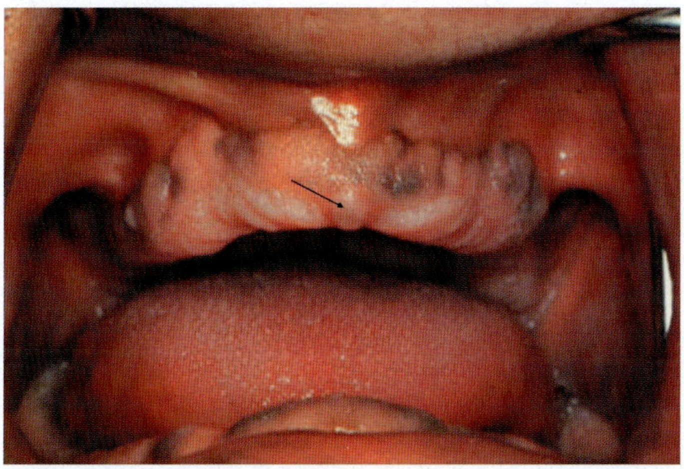

FIGURE 20-8. Edentulous maxilla with incisive papilla in a patient with longstanding edentulous state. Note physiologic pigmentation and stippled attached gingiva. (Image courtesy of Dr. Ginat Mirowski.)

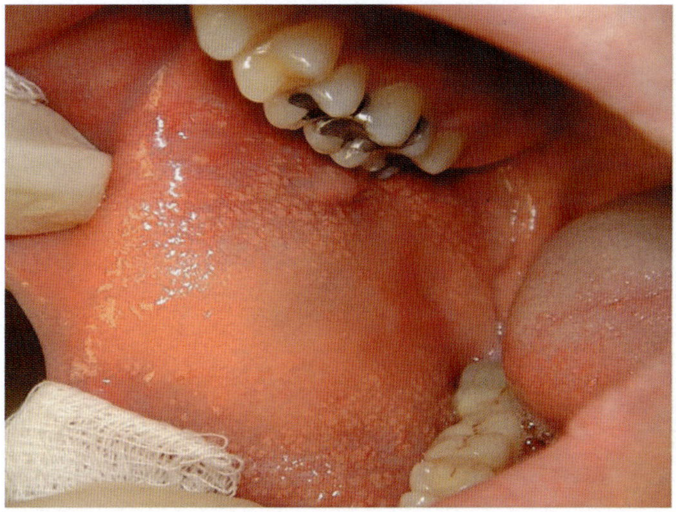

FIGURE 20-9. Fordyce spots (small yellow papules on buccal mucosa). (Image courtesy of Dr. Ginat Mirowski.)

Cleft palate, or a cleft in the hard and/or soft palates, occurs when the palatal shelves of the maxillary processes fail to fuse.[5] This can extend anteriorly through the dental arch and involve the lips as well.[20]

BUCCAL AND LABIAL MUCOSA

Nonkeratinized lining epithelium lines both the buccal and labial mucosa.[3] Fordyce granules, or ectopic benign sebaceous glands, are more prevalent in the lamina propria of the labial mucosa than of the buccal mucosa [**Figure 20-9**]. Similarly, while minor salivary glands can be found in the submucosa of both regions, these are also more prevalent in the labial mucosa. Linea alba buccalis is a variable whitish horizontal line that reflects the occlusal plane and can be found in the buccal mucosa.[9]

Thought to be a variation of normal buccal mucosa, leukoedema is characterized by whitish-gray appearance of buccal and labial mucosa that subsides when stretched. It is more common in individuals of African descent, likely due the darker oral mucosa making the white leukoedema changes more noticeable.[21]

FLOOR OF MOUTH

The mucosa of the floor of the mouth is very thin and classified as lining mucosa.[8,9] Given the increased permeability of nonkeratinized epithelium, this makes the floor of the mouth a great location for drug delivery. This increased permeability also presents with a challenge as it increases risk of carcinogens penetrating through.[22] The floor of the mouth also contains the Rivinus, Bartholin, and Wharton ducts.[23]

TONGUE

The tongue's specialized epithelium comprises both keratinized and nonkeratinized epithelium.[3] The ventral or undersurface and sulci of the tongue are nonkeratinized, whereas the dorsum is keratinized.[7,8] The anterior two-thirds of the tongue is derived from ectoderm and the posterior one-third is of endoderm origin. The junction of these two areas is demarcated by the sulcus terminalis. The dorsal aspect of the tongue is mostly covered by filiform (small, <1 mm, elongated and keratinized) papillae giving the hairy or velvety surface appearance. The overgrowth of the filiform papillae is a benign finding known as hairy tongue. Hairy tongue of variable colors such as black hairy tongue is due to acquired pigmentation. The pigmentation may be the result of bacterial overgrowth or exogenous pigment deposition,

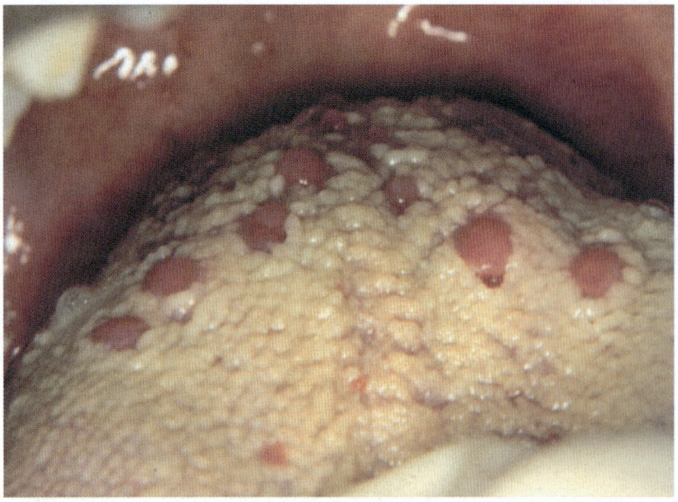

FIGURE 20-10. Dorsal tongue. Circumvallate papillae (red papules) arranged in a "V" distribution with foramen cecum visible at base of the inverted "V." (Image courtesy of Dr. Ginat Mirowski.)

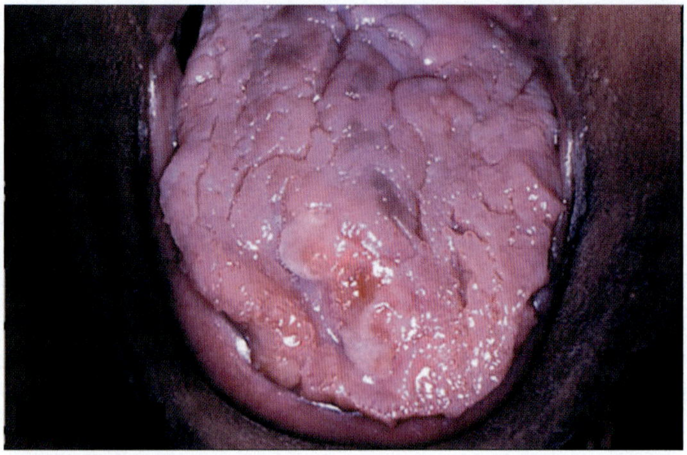

FIGURE 20-11. Fissured tongue. (Image courtesy of Dr. John McDowell.)

such as caffeine, liquorish, or bile (described in detail in Chapter 61). On the other hand, loss of filiform papillae due to inflammation is known as geographic tongue or benign migratory glossitis. Another normal benign variant known as fissured, plicated, or scrotal tongue, is characterized by asymptomatic fissures on dorsal tongue and common with increase in age. At the junction between the anterior two-thirds of the dorsal tongue and the posterior one-third of the tongue, arranged in an inverted V shaped distribution, are the circumvallate papillae [**Figure 20-10**]. Scattered over the anterior tongue surface, the fungiform papillae are small, red, or brown, dome-shaped structures. Deposition of melanin at the tips of the fungiform papillae is often noted in skin of color individuals. This is a form of physiologic pigmentation. Foliate papillae are located on latero-posterior aspects of the tongue. These appear as vertical folds. All the papillae on the tongue except the filiform papillae are responsible for taste.[7]

Foramen Cecum The foramen cecum is located at the junction of the anterior two-thirds of the tongue that meets the posterior one-third. The foramen cecum is the site where the thyroid tissue begins to form.[17]

Varicosities Varicosities are benign vascular dilatations and may consist of veins, arteries, or lymphatic vessels. In the oral cavity, oral varix typically refers to venous varicosities as they are the most common. Hypertrophy of the structures result in an increase of the diameter. Adults are more likely to present with oral varix, which present as irregular, blue/purple lesions typically on the ventral aspect of the tongue, buccal mucosa, and lips. These lesions may often be referred to as "caviar tongue."[24]

PHARYNX

The posterior of the oral cavity is formed by the pharynx [Figure 20-6]. The lingual and palatine tonsils are posterior aspects of the circumvallate papillae. Along with the tongue, taste buds are also found in the pharynx.[25] The oropharyngeal arch and the palatoglossal arch are soft tissue pillars that are found anterior and posterior to the tonsils.

MUCOSAL TURNOVER AND CHEMOTHERAPY

The oral mucosal epithelium has a higher turnover rate estimated on average of 2 to 6 days, which is important in the defense against adhesion of microorganisms.[26] The fast proliferative property of the oral mucosa makes it particularly vulnerable to chemotherapy medications, leading to erosions and ulcerations often seen in areas of frequent trauma such as the soft palate, tongue, and buccal mucosa resulting in severe discomfort to patients. In addition, chemotherapy drugs and radiation may damage the fibroblast and blood vessels causing fibrosis and decrease blood flow affecting healing and increasing the risk of oral infections.[27,28]

ORAL MUCOSAL AND WOUND HEALING

The wound healing process in the oral mucosa undergoes the same phases of wound healing as the skin. However, wound healing often occurs faster in the oral mucosa and is less susceptible to scarring.[11] This is attributed to the moist environment, hemostatic properties of saliva, presence of anti-inflammatory cytokines, and abundant vascularity. Interestingly the presence of a balanced oral microbiome leads to higher expression of antimicrobial peptides enhancing barrier function. Moreover, the oral epithelium has more cell layers and higher basal cell proliferation rate promoting faster reepithelization. The oral epithelium is influenced by external factors including smoking and affected by diseases like pemphigus vulgaris, paraneoplastic pemphigus, Stevens-Johnson syndrome, and drug-induced hypersensitivity syndrome that alter the oral mucosal environment and increase the susceptibility to opportunistic infections such as candidiasis and herpes simplex.[1]

AGING OF ORAL MUCOSA AND SALIVARY PRODUCTION

The oral cavity is protected from photodamage and photoaging; however, intrinsic changes in its structures are noticeable with aging.[29] Over time, there is a flattening of the epithelium, possible reduction of oral mucosa permeability, reduction of skin vasculature, and perfusion. These changes could contribute to a more pale vermillion lip observed with aging.[30] Salivary glands also undergo age-related degeneration of the acini, characterized by atrophy of the acini and ductal dilatation. Moreover, the salivary composition changes with aging demonstrated by a decrease in mucin, antioxidants enzymes, and reduction of receptors reducing saliva stimulation and secretion that may increase susceptibility to oral mucosa inflammation with age.[31] Common conditions affecting the elderly are likely related to intrinsic aging and include decrease in saliva leading to xerostomia, lingual varicosities, fissured tongue [**Figure 20-11**], and frictional keratosis.

SUMMARY

In summary, the oral mucosal acts as a physical, biological, and immune barrier to the oral cavity. Understanding of normal oral mucosa anatomy, physiologic variations in individuals with skin of color, and the unique environment to which the oral cavity is exposed is essential to comprehend oral diseases presentation and management. Additionally, awareness of the changes seen with oral mucosa aging may help minimize the oral discomfort that can be associated this inevitable process.

ACKNOWLEDGMENTS

We would like to acknowledge and thank Dr. Lin and Dr. Bibb for their excellent work writing the previous chapter on the biology of oral mucosa.

REFERENCES

1. Brizuela M, Winters R. *Histology, Oral Mucosa*. In: *StatPearls*. StatPearls Publishing; 2022.
2. Şenel S. An overview of physical, microbiological and immune barriers of oral mucosa. *Int J Mol Sci*. 2021;22(15):7821.
3. Dawson DV, Drake DR, Hill JR, Brogden KA, Fischer CL, Wertz PW. Organization, barrier function and antimicrobial lipids of the oral mucosa. *Int J Cosmet Sci*. 2013;35(3):220-223.
4. Turabelidze A, Guo S, Chung AY, et al. Intrinsic differences between oral and skin keratinocytes. *PLOS ONE*. 2014;9(9):e101480.
5. Helwany M, Rathee M. *Anatomy, Head and Neck, Palate*. In: *StatPearls*. StatPearls Publishing; 2022.
6. Madani M, Berardi T, Stoopler ET. Anatomic and examination considerations of the oral cavity. *Med Clin North Am*. 2014;98(6):1225-1238.
7. Qin R, Steel A, Fazel N. Oral mucosa biology and salivary biomarkers. *Clin Dermatol*. 2017;35(5):477-483.
8. Groeger S, Meyle J. Oral mucosal epithelial cells. *Front Immunol*. 2019;10. https://www.frontiersin.org/articles/10.3389/fimmu.2019.00208.
9. Otsuka-Tanaka Y, Oommen S, Kawasaki M, et al. Oral lining mucosa development depends on mesenchymal microRNAs. *J Dent Res*. 2013;92(3):229-234.
10. Janssen R, Moisik SR, Dediu D. Modelling human hard palate shape with Bézier curves. *PLoS One*. 2018;13(2):e0191557.
11. Waasdorp M, Krom BP, Bikker FJ, van Zuijlen PPM, Niessen FB, Gibbs S. The bigger picture: why oral mucosa heals better than skin. *Biomolecules*. 2021;11(8):1165.
12. Yaprak E, Kasap M, Akpınar G, et al. The prominent proteins expressed in healthy gingiva: a pilot exploratory tissue proteomics study. *Odontology*. 2018;106(1):19-28.
13. Ghannam MG, Singh P. *Anatomy, Head and Neck, Salivary Glands*. In: *StatPearls*. StatPearls Publishing ; 2022.
14. Porcheri C, Mitsiadis TA. physiology, pathology and regeneration of salivary glands. *Cells*. 2019;8(9):E976.
15. Feller L, Masilana A, Khammissa RA, Altini M, Jadwat Y, Lemmer J. Melanin: the biophysiology of oral melanocytes and physiological oral pigmentation. *Head Face Med*. 2014;10(1):8.
16. Soriano RM, M Das J. *Anatomy, Head and Neck, Maxilla*. In: *StatPearls*. StatPearls Publishing ; 2022.
17. Breeland G, Aktar A, Patel BC. *Anatomy, Head and Neck, Mandible*. In: *StatPearls*. StatPearls Publishing ; 2022.
18. Walker WB. *The Oral Cavity and Associated Structures*. In: Walker HK, Hall WD, Hurst JW, eds. *Clinical Methods: The History, Physical, and Laboratory Examinations*. 3rd ed. Butterworths ; 1990.
19. Schroeder HE, Listgarten MA. The gingival tissues: the architecture of periodontal protection. *Periodontol 2000*. 1997;13(1):91-120.
20. Groeger S, Meyle J. Oral Mucosal Epithelial Cells. *Front Immunol*. 2019;10:208.
21. Huang BW, Lin C wei, Lee YP, Chiang CP. Differential diagnosis between leukoedema and white spongy nevus. *J Dent Sci*. 2020;15(4):554-555.
22. Wertz PW. Roles of lipids in the permeability barriers of skin and oral mucosa. *Int J Mol Sci*. 2021;22(10):5229.
23. Chen C-j, Guo P, Chen X-y. Recurrent sublingual ranula or saliva leakage from the submandibular gland? Anatomical consideration of the ductal system of the sublingual gland. *J Oral Maxillofac Surg Off J Am Assoc Oral Maxillofac Surg*. 2015;73(4):675.e1-7.
24. Lazos JP, Piemonte ED, Panico RL. Oral varix: a review. *Gerodontology*. 2015;32(2):82-89.
25. Qin R, Steel A, Fazel N. Oral mucosa biology and salivary biomarkers. *Clin Dermatol*. 2017;35(5):477-483.
26. Harris D, Robinson JR. Drug delivery via the mucous membranes of the oral cavity. *J Pharm Sci*. 1992;81(1):1-10.
27. Naidu MUR, Ramana GV, Rani PU, Mohan IK, Suman A, Roy P. Chemotherapy-induced and/or radiation therapy-induced oral mucositis–complicating the treatment of cancer. *Neoplasia N Y N*. 2004;6(5):423-431.
28. Schrementi ME, Ferreira AM, Zender C, DiPietro LA. Site-specific production of TGF-beta in oral mucosal and cutaneous wounds. *Wound Repair Regen Off Publ Wound Heal Soc Eur Tissue Repair Soc*. 2008;16(1):80-86.
29. Radwan-Oczko M, Bandosz K, Rojek Z, Owczarek-Drabińska JE. Clinical study of oral mucosal lesions in the elderly-prevalence and distribution. *Int J Environ Res Public Health*. 2022;19(5):2853.
30. Gomi T, Imamura T. Age-related changes in the vasculature of the dermis of the upper lip vermilion. *Aging*. 2019;11(11):3551-3560.
31. Toan NK, Ahn SG. Aging-related metabolic dysfunction in the salivary gland: a review of the literature. *Int J Mol Sci*. 2021;22(11):5835.

CHAPTER 21

Photobiology: Acute and Chronic Effects

Maria L. Espinosa
Ciara G. Robinson
Henry W. Lim

KEY POINTS

- Erythema is induced primarily by UVB spectrum (290-320 nm) of sunlight, with UVA2 (320-340 nm) as a minor contributor.
- Immediate pigment darkening (IPD), persistent pigment darkening (PPD), and delayed tanning (DT) are primarily the effect of UVA (320-400 nm) and visible light (VL; 400-700 nm).
- VL induces intense and long-lasting pigmentation in dark-skinned individuals. This effect is enhanced in the presence of UVA1 (340-400 nm).
- Photoprotection against the effect of VL is an active area of investigation and development.

INTRODUCTION

Sunlight reaching the surface of the earth is composed of ultraviolet (UV) radiation, visible light (VL), and infrared radiation (IR). While it has several beneficial effects, such as UVB radiation being essential for the synthesis of Vitamin D and for treatment of inflammatory conditions such as psoriasis, sunlight can also have harmful effects on the skin. These effects vary depending on skin type given that melanin can be protective against some, but not all, of the harmful effects emitted by sunlight. In this chapter, we will review the effects of acute and chronic exposure of solar radiation on the skin and importance of photoprotection, highlighting differences in light versus dark skin types. While UV and visible light can induce photodermatoses, these are covered in Chapter 91.

COMPONENTS OF SUNLIGHT

Ultraviolet (UV) radiation makes up 2% of the sunlight that reaches earth's surface. UV is further divided into UVA (320-400 nm), UVB (290-320 nm), and UVC (200-290 nm) based on the biological activity of wavelengths; UVA is further subdivided into UVA2 (320-340 nm) and UVA1 (340-400 nm)[1] [**Figure 21-1**]. UVA comprises 95% of UV radiation that reaches the earth's surface with UVB making up the remaining. UVC is completely absorbed in the hemisphere, therefore does not reach the surface of the earth and does not cause biological effects in the skin. Visible light (VL) includes wavelengths 400 to 700 nm and comprises 47% of the sunlight that reaches earth's surface.[1] VL is the sunlight that can be perceived by the human eye; it ranges from blue (shortest wavelength) to red (longest wavelength). Infrared radiation makes up most of the sunlight that reaches earth's surface at 51% and consists of wavelengths 760 nm to 1 mm. When solar rays penetrate the skin, they

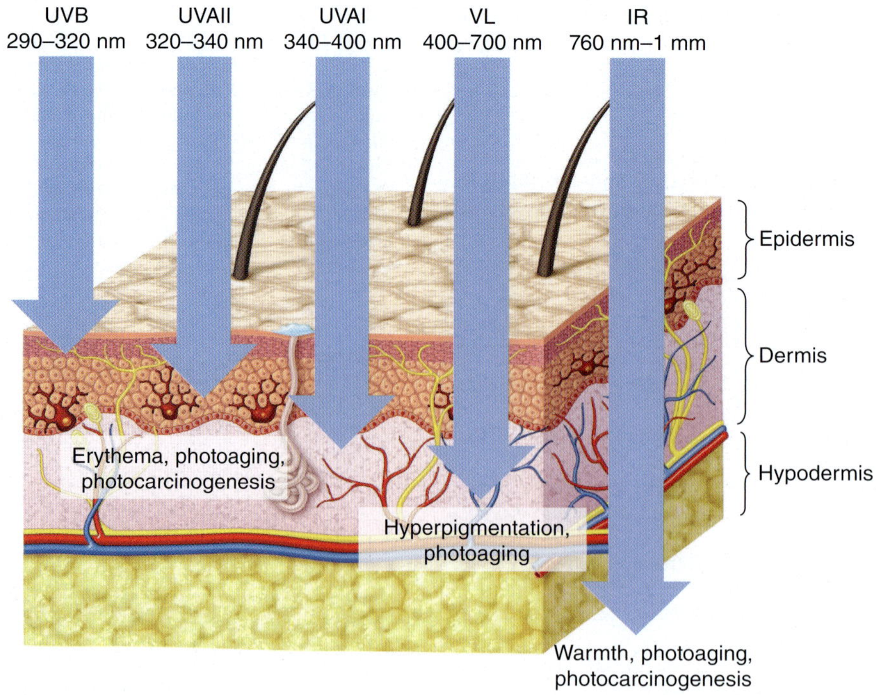

FIGURE 21-1. Components of sunlight and corresponding effects on the skin. (Figure adapted from Taylor SC et al. Misconceptions of photoprotection in skin of color. *J Am Acad Dermatol*. 2022;86(3s):S9-s17.)

are absorbed by molecules such as nucleic acids, proteins, and melanin that act as endogenous chromophores and convert the solar radiation energy to energy that may drive cellular processes, be released as heat, or cause fluorescence that is releasing the absorbed energy as a longer wavelength.[2] Each chromophore has specific wavelength range that it absorbs, known as its absorption spectrum.

SKIN PHOTOTYPE

Melanocytes are neural crest-derived cells located along the basal layer of the epidermis that contain melanosomes which produce two types of melanin: brown-black eumelanin and yellow-red pheomelanin. Melanin is transferred from melanocytes to neighboring keratinocytes for transport to the surface of the epidermis. Eumelanin and pheomelanin are the key players in the determination of skin color; while all humans have the same density of melanocytes, the quantity and quality of melanin production by melanocytes determines a person's skin color.[2] Individuals with dark skin have a higher quantity of melanin along the upper layers of the epidermis and a higher eumelanin/pheomelanin ratio than individuals with light skin. Specifically, studies have shown that ethnic groups with darker skin (African and Indian) have nearly twice as much melanin compared with those with lighter skin (European, Chinese, and Mexican)[3]. See **Chapters 14-16,** which cover the biology of keratinocytes, melanocytes, and the dermis, for more information regarding biological differences in structure and function. A commonly used classification of skin phototypes is the Fitzpatrick skin type (FST) scale that categorizes individuals on the propensity of skin to burn and tan, with FST I to III commonly being grouped as non-skin of color and FST IV to VI being skin of color (SOC), the latter group having higher melanin concentration; however, it should be noted that overlaps do occur [**Table 21-1**].

MOLECULAR MECHANISMS OF SOLAR RADIATION ON THE SKIN

ULTRAVIOLET RADIATION

The effects of ultraviolet radiation on the skin have been widely known. In the acute setting, UV radiation leads to erythema, pigment changes, epidermal hyperplasia, and vitamin D synthesis. Chronic exposure to UV radiation leads to photoaging and photocarcinogenesis.

Acute Effects of UV Radiation **Erythema**, or sunburn, is the result of exposure to any portion of the solar radiation spectrum that results in redness of the skin, tenderness, warmth, or swelling. It is predominantly the effects of UVB, and to a lesser extent, UVA2. UVB is 1000 times more efficient in inducing erythema than UVA radiation due to the fact that shorter wavelength UVB is primarily absorbed in the epidermis, while the longer wavelength UVA, in the dermis.[4] Within the epidermis, there are several chromophores with absorption spectra lying in the UV range with nuclear DNA being the most studied chromophore for UVB.[4] Nuclear DNA absorbs the energy emitted from UVB leading to the formation of pyrimidine

TABLE 21-1 Fitzpatrick skin types

Fitzpatrick skin type	Skin color	Ability to tan	Propensity to sunburn	Eumelanin to pheomelanin ratio
I	White	None	Always	
II	White	With difficulty	High	
III	Beige	Medium tan	Moderate	
IV	Brown	Dark tan	Low	
V	Dark brown	Tans very easily	Very low	
VI	Black	Tans very easily	Exceedingly low	

dimers, resulting in DNA damage. In turn, this leads to the release of cytokines and inflammatory markers including histamine, prostaglandins, and other cytokines, resulting in vasodilation and inflammation that manifests as erythema.[4] In lighter skin types, it is easily recognized by the color changes; however, in darker skin types it is more often associated with warmth, tenderness, and burning of the skin.[4] Duration of erythema varies by skin type; for individuals with non-SOC, it may last for 1 to 2 weeks, whereas for SOC individuals it resolves within 3 days after exposure.[5] UVA exposure results in alterations in DNA induced by reactive oxygen species (ROS). The oxidized DNA base, 8-oxoG, is highly mutagenic and thus is suspected to play a role in the carcinogenic nature of UVA radiation.[6]

Solar radiation also leads to pigmentation changes that may be divided into three separate stages—**immediate pigment darkening (IPD)**, **persistent pigment darkening (PPD)**, and **delayed tanning (DT)**. These changes are most prominent in those with SOC. While all wavelengths except for IR, cause IPD, it is predominantly the effect of UVA and visible light.[4] IPD is a gray color that occurs within a few minutes of sun exposure and lasts for 10 to 20 min. IPD is followed by PPD, which is the brown pigmentation that persists about 2 hours after sun exposure; PPD lasts for 24 hours. Both IPD and PPD are due to the oxidation of preexisting melanin and other melanin precursors. About 3 to 5 days after sufficient sun exposure, delayed tanning arises. In contrast to IPD and PPD, DT is the result of new melanogenesis. Melanin limits the penetration of UV radiation by acting as a neutral density filter along the basal layer of the epidermis. UV radiation leads to the increase in size and activity of melanocytes by activating tyrosine kinase, a key protein in the melanin biosynthetic pathway. This increased amount of melanin leads to delayed tanning within 24 to 72 hours of exposure to UVA and UVB radiation that provides some protection against photocarcinogenesis.[7]

UVB and UVA have also been showed to cause **epidermal hyperplasia** or thickening of the stratum corneum. This epidermal cell proliferation is photoprotective against solar radiation. Studies have shown that UVB causes an initial decrease in epidermal cell proliferation due to DNA damage followed by a rebound increase in epidermal cell proliferation after DNA repair.[8] Literature on the effect of epidermal hyperplasia induced by UVA varies, but it has been shown to also induce hyperplasia when studied in patients with light skin types.[9]

Another effect of UVB radiation is synthesis of vitamin D. Exposure to sunlight, more specifically UVB at action spectrum 290 to 315 nm, results in 7-dehydrocholesterol absorbing UVB photons, which creates previtamin D_3 via splitting of the B ring; previtamin D_3 is rapidly converted to vitamin D_3.[10] Since melanin absorbs UV radiation, individuals with dark skin types make less vitamin D through this pathway when compared to a light-skinned individual.

Chronic Effects of UV Radiation The two primary chronic effects of UV radiation are photoaging and photocarcinogenesis. Multiple UV exposures leads to sustained increase in the expression of collagenase, a 92-kd gelatinase, and stromelysin. These matrix metalloproteinases degrade endogenous collagen, thereby causing photoaging.[11] In Caucasian skin, wrinkles generally appear 10 to 20 years earlier than in Asian skin, while Asian and dark-skinned individuals are more prone to actinic lentigines and hyperpigmentation.[12] An ex vivo study found that when exposed to equivalent doses of UVR, DNA damage was observed throughout the epidermis and the papillary dermis in light to tan skin types, whereas in dark skin types the damage was limited to the suprabasal portion of the epidermis.[13] In vitro studies examining the extent of DNA damage resulting from UVR reveal an inverse relationship between melanin concentration and depth of photodamage, showing the protective effect of melanin in photoaging of individuals with SOC.[14] There are also differences in the extent of facial wrinkling across ethnic groups with Caucasians having the most severity, followed by Hispanics, African Americans, and East Asians[15] [**Figures 21-2** to **21-4**].

UVB is directly absorbed by DNA and results in the formation of dipyrimidine products including cyclobutene pyrimidine dimers (CPD), pyrimidine (6-4) pyrimidone photoproducts, and Dewar valence isomer. CPD is the most abundantly produced and result in mutations and

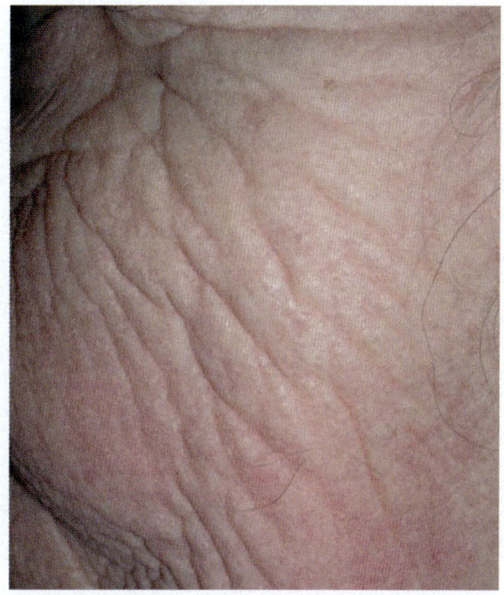

FIGURE 21-2. Photoaging in a 75-year-old White woman. Note deep and coarse wrinkling.

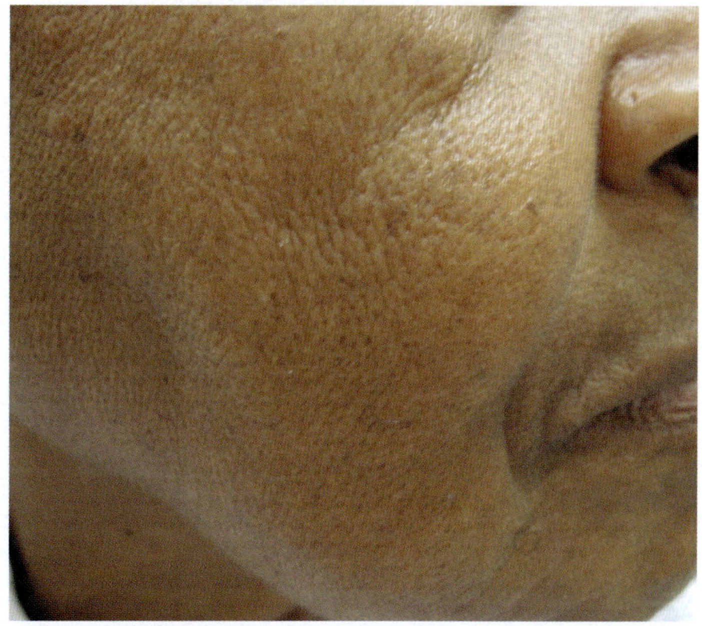

FIGURE 21-3. Photoaging in a 79-year-old Black woman. Note subtle coarse wrinkling.

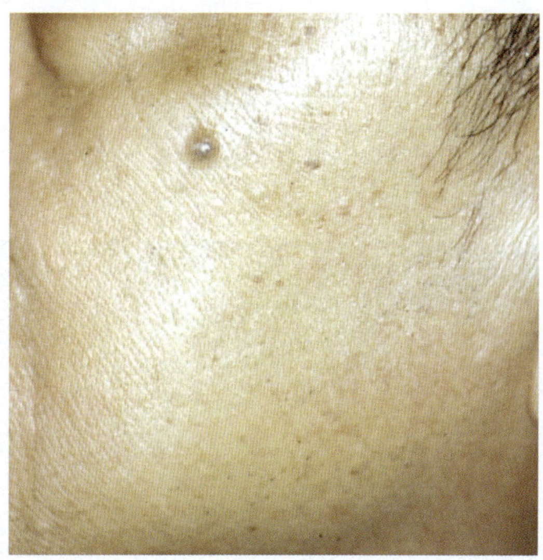

FIGURE 21-4. Photoaging in a 70-year-old East Asian man. Note fine wrinkling on periorbital area and a few small seborrheic keratoses.

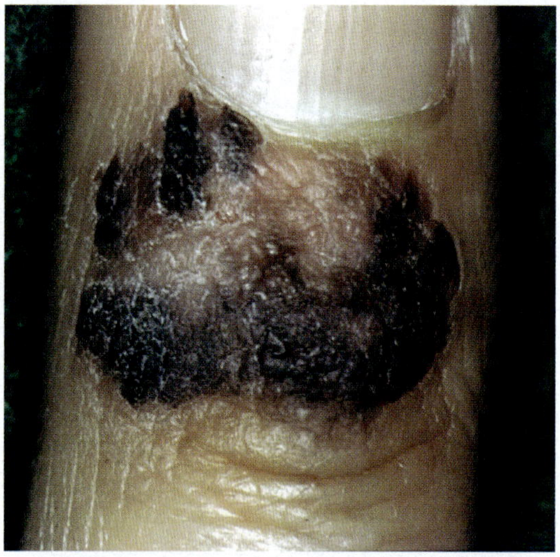

FIGURE 21-5. Pigmented squamous cell carcinoma in situ in an African American man.

cell death if not repaired correctly, therefore contributing to photocarcinogenesis.[16,17] ROS generated by UVA react with guanine to produce 7,8-dihydro-8-oxo-guanosine (8-oxoG), and 8-oxo-7,8-dihydro-2′-deoxyguanosine (8-oxo-dG), both of which are mutagenic. There are two main mechanisms to repair DNA from photodamage. In nucleotide excision repair, endonucleases remove a DNA oligomer containing approximately 30 nucleotides with CPD. A polymerase then synthesizes an intact complementary DNA chain, and a ligase connects the two free DNA chains together. Base excision repair occurs when a damaged base is removed by 8-oxoguuanine glycosylase followed by an apurinic/apyrimidinic endonuclease removing nucleotides near the damaged site that are then resynthesized.[18] DNA repair is more efficient in dark skin than in light skin.[19] It should be noted that the action spectra in inducing DNA damage in mammalian cells by UVB and UVA are not mutually exclusive.[20] Although UVA predominately induces DNA damage through generation of ROS, in vivo, UVA has been shown to also induce pyrimidine dimer formation in human skin.[21] UVB is also known to induce oxidative damage on the DNA.

UV exposure has been associated with the development of actinic keratoses, squamous cell carcinomas (SCCs) [**Figures 21-5** and **21-6**], basal cell carcinomas (BCCs) [**Figure 21-7**], and possibly melanomas. Because melanin acts as a natural UV filter, SOC has the dual benefit of decreased actinic DNA damage as well as reduced UV-induced immunosuppression, together greatly contributing to the decreased rates of skin cancer in SOC. It is uncertain if UV radiation is associated with melanoma incidence in SOC; in a systematic review including 13 studies, only 2 showed weak associations of melanoma in dark skin types, suggesting that UV radiation may not play a large role in the development of melanoma in patients with SOC.[22] For more in-depth discussion of SCC, BCC, and melanoma in SOC, please refer to **Chapters 52** to **54**.

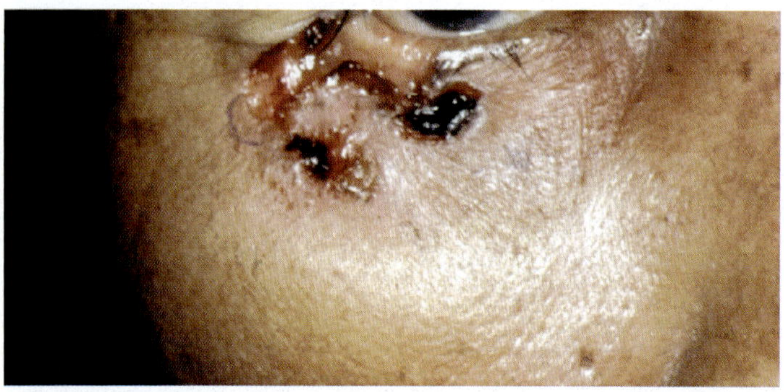

FIGURE 21-6. Pigmented squamous cell carcinoma in a Chinese woman.

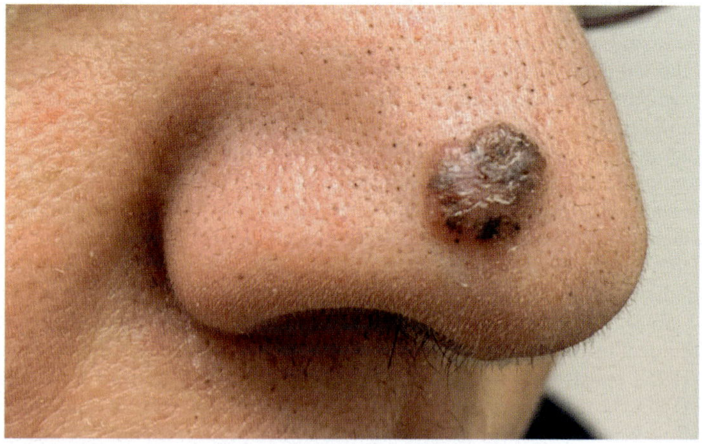

FIGURE 21-7. Pigmented basal cell carcinoma in Arab American woman.

VISIBLE LIGHT

Recently, great strides have been made in the understanding of the effects of visible light on the skin. Acute effects include erythema in light-skinned individuals, and intense and persistent pigmentation in dark-skinned persons, which clinically could contribute to melasma and postinflammatory pigmentation (PIH) seen commonly in dark-skinned individuals. Chronic exposure to visible light can has been shown to contribute to photoaging.[23]

Acute Effects of VL Radiation Pigmentation changes from VL are due to the activation of tyrosine activity, especially in individuals with SOC.[24] Opsin 3 is a key sensor protein present in melanocytes that induces phosphorylation of microphthalmia-associated transcription factor. This phosphorylation increases tyrosinase and dopachrome tautomerase, which form protein complexes most found in the melanocytes of those with darker skin. These complexes prompt sustained tyrosinase activity, explaining the hyperpigmentation seen in darker skin following exposure to blue light.[25] Increased epidermal melanin has been found to be associated with decreased penetration of VL, indicating a protective effect in patients with SOC.[26]

In addition to the independent effects of UVR and VL, there are synergistic effects between VL and UVA1 on erythema and pigmentation compared to those induced by pure VL. A recent research study irradiated patients with skin phototypes IV to VI with visible light in the presence and absence of UVA1. The results demonstrated that combination of VL and UVA1 resulted in more intense pigmentation. A similar study investigated the effects of VL with UVA1 on subjects with skin phototypes I to III. In this study, irradiation resulted in immediate erythema. These studies emphasize contribution of VL and UVA1 to pigmentary conditions (melasma, PIH) in those with dark skin.[27,28]

Chronic Effects of VL Radiation While the long-term cutaneous effects of exposure to visible light are still being studied, we know that it can cause photoaging and could be the action spectrum of some photodermatoses, including chronic actinic dermatitis, cutaneous porphyrias, and solar urticaria. Shorter wavelengths of visible light including blue light (400-500 nm) induce photoaging via increase in ROS formation and altering the extracellular matrix, as well as contribute greatly to pigmentary changes.[23] Longer wavelengths within the visible light spectrum including yellow and red light, 560 to 590 and 620 to 750 nm, respectively, have shown to be photoprotective by reducing inflammation, and promoting wound healing and antioxidation.[23]

INFRARED RADIATION

Acute Effects of IR While further research is warranted on the cutaneous effects of IR, previous studies have demonstrated that exposure is perceived as warmth on the skin. Acute exposure leads to erythema that typically lasts less than 1 hour, heat-related pain due to over-warming of skin, and loss of effective blood circulation. It is thought that the erythema is secondary to vasodilation.[29]

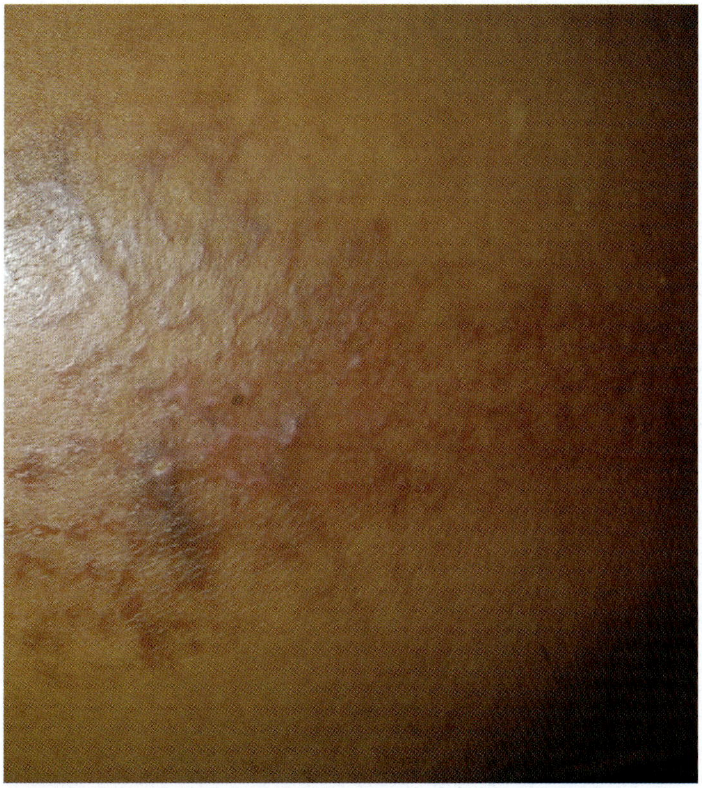

FIGURE 21-8. Erythema ab igne on the thigh as a result of application of heating pad for 3 weeks.

Chronic Effects of IR Long-term exposure to IR radiation on the skin may disrupt the electron flow in the mitochondrial electron transport chain, leading to insufficient in energy production in dermal fibroblasts that ultimately alters the structure and function of the skin. Moreover, IR promotes formation of blood vessels and increases the number of mast cells, which are both associated with photoaging.[29] Other chronic effects include squamous cell carcinoma and *erythema ab igne* [**Figure 21-8**]. These are seen with repeated, frequent exposure to IR. It is important to note that these can result even when an individual does not experience heat on the skin.

SUMMARY OF KEY DIFFERENCES OF THE EFFECTS OF SUNLIGHT ON DIFFERENT SKIN TYPES

As discussed above, sunlight has a multitude of effects on the skin that can vary by skin color based on the protective nature of melanin in darker skin types. This is summarized in **Table 21-2**. Erythema, photoaging, and photocarcinogenesis are more pronounced in light-skinned individuals.

TABLE 21-2 Effects of sunlight on healthy skin of individuals with different skin phototypes

Chronicity	Effects of UV	Effects of VL	Effects of IR
Acute	-Erythema (longer lasting in FST I-III, shorter in FST IV-VI) -immediate pigment darkening (IPD), persistent pigment darkening (PPD), and delayed tanning (DT), most prominent in SOC -Epidermal hyperplasia -Dark-skinned individuals incur less DNA damage due to more efficient DNA repair.	-Immediate erythema in light-skinned subjects -Intense and persistent hyperpigmentation in FST IV-VI	-Warmth
Chronic	-Photoaging and photocarcinogenesis (greater in FST I-III)	-Photoaging	-Photoaging -Photocarcinogenesis

Abbreviations: FST, Fitzpatrick skin type; IR, infrared radiation; UV, ultraviolet radiation; VL, visible light.

TABLE 21-3 Photoprotection for individuals with different skin types

	Light skinned	Dark skinned
SPF	50+	30+
UVA protection	Presence	High
Visible light protection	Presence	High

PHOTOPROTECTION

The effects of sun exposure differ by skin phototype, therefore photoprotection recommendations can be individually tailored, that is, personalized photoprotection [**Table 21-3**]. UVB exposure leads to DNA damage in the upper layers of the epidermis in dark skin but in light skin, damage is also seen in the lower layers of the epidermis where stem cells are present, increasing the risk of developing skin cancers. UVA1 affects all skin types and leads to photodamage by penetrating deeper into the skin than UVB. While higher quantities of melanin provide some intrinsic protection against UVB, the same is not true for visible light and UVA, both of which can result in hyperpigmentation in dark-skin individuals. Tinted sunscreens containing iron oxides, some with pigmentary titanium dioxide, provide a physical barrier between visible light and the skin, making their use of utmost importance in dark-skinned individuals.[30] Other measures include new filters, sunscreens with antioxidants as ingredients, and oral agents such as Polypodium leucotomos. See Chapter 94 for more information regarding photoprotection.

CONCLUSION

This chapter summarizes the acute and chronic cutaneous effects of sun exposure in general and its unique impact on individuals with SOC. Solar radiation leads to erythema, epidermal cell hyperplasia, tanning in the acute setting while prolonged exposure leads to photoaging and photocarcinogenesis. Due to the protective effect of melanin, individuals with SOC are less likely to develop UV-associated skin cancers and photoaging compared with light-skinned individuals but are more prone to the effects of visible light-induced hyperpigmentation. Knowledge of these differences is important for providing patient-centered care and sun protective recommendations for the public.

REFERENCES

1. Diffey BL, Kochevar IE. Basic principles of photobiology. *Photodermatology*. Informa Healthcare USA; 2007.
2. Austin E, Geisler AN, Nguyen J, et al. Visible light. Part I: properties and cutaneous effects of visible light. *J Am Acad Dermatol*. 2021;84(5):1219-1231.
3. Alaluf S, Heath A, Carter N, et al. Variation in melanin content and composition in type V and VI photoexposed and photoprotected human skin: the dominant role of DHI. *Pigment Cell Res*. 2001;14(5):337-347.
4. Hönigsmann H. Erythema and pigmentation. *Photodermatol Photoimmunol Photomed*. 2002;18(2):75-81.
5. Kollias N, Baqer A, Sadiq I. Minimum erythema dose determination in individuals of skin type V and VI with diffuse reflectance spectroscopy. *Photodermatol Photoimmunol Photomed*. 1994;10(6):249-254.
6. Schuch AP, Moreno NC, Schuch NJ, Menck CFM, Garcia CCM. Sunlight damage to cellular DNA: focus on oxidatively generated lesions. *Free Radic Biol Med*. 2017;107:110-124.
7. Bolognia JL, Schaffer JV, Cerroni L, eds. *Dermatology*. vol I. Elsevier; 2018.
8. Epstein JH, Fukuyama K, Fye K. Effects of ultraviolet radiation on the mitotic cycle and DNA, RNA and protein synthesis in mammalian epidermis in vivo. *Photochem Photobiol*. 1970;12(1):57-65.

9. Pearse AD, Gaskell SA, Marks R. Epidermal changes in human skin following irradiation with either UVB or UVA. *J Invest Dermatol.* 1987;88(1):83-87.
10. Holick MF. Vitamin D: a millenium perspective. *J Cell Biochem.* 2003;88(2):296-307.
11. Fisher GJ, Wang ZQ, Datta SC, Varani J, Kang S, Voorhees JJ. Pathophysiology of premature skin aging induced by ultraviolet light. *N Engl J Med.* 1997;337(20):1419-1428.
12. Passeron T, Lim HW, Goh CL, et al. Photoprotection according to skin phototype and dermatoses: practical recommendations from an expert panel. *J Eur Acad Dermatol Venereol.* 2021;35(7):1460-1469.
13. Del Bino S, Sok J, Bessac E, Bernerd F. Relationship between skin response to ultraviolet exposure and skin color type. *Pigment Cell Res.* 2006;19(6):606-614.
14. Yamaguchi Y, Takahashi K, Zmudzka BZ, et al. Human skin responses to UV radiation: pigment in the upper epidermis protects against DNA damage in the lower epidermis and facilitates apoptosis. *FASEB J.* 2006;20(9):1486-1488.
15. Rawlings AV. Ethnic skin types: are there differences in skin structure and function? *Int J Cosmet Sci.* 2006;28(2):79-93.
16. Cadet J, Douki T, Ravanat JL. Oxidatively generated damage to cellular DNA by UVB and UVA radiation. *Photochem Photobiol.* 2015;91(1):140-155.
17. Seité S, Fourtanier A, Moyal D, Young AR. Photodamage to human skin by suberythemal exposure to solar ultraviolet radiation can be attenuated by sunscreens: a review. *Br J Dermatol.* 2010;163(5):903-914.
18. Vechtomova YL, Telegina TA, Buglak AA, Kritsky MS. UV radiation in DNA damage and repair involving DNA-photolyases and cryptochromes. *Biomedicines.* 2021;9(11).
19. Miyamura Y, Coelho SG, Wolber R, et al. Regulation of human skin pigmentation and responses to ultraviolet radiation. *Pigment Cell Res.* 2007;20(1):2-13.
20. Kielbassa C, Roza L, Epe B. Wavelength dependence of oxidative DNA damage induced by UV and visible light. *Carcinogenesis.* 1997;18(4):811-816.
21. Young AR, Potten CS, Nikaido O, et al. Human melanocytes and keratinocytes exposed to UVB or UVA in vivo show comparable levels of thymine dimers. *J Invest Dermatol.* 1998;111(6):936-940.
22. Lopes F, Sleiman MG, Sebastian K, Bogucka R, Jacobs EA, Adamson AS. UV exposure and the risk of cutaneous melanoma in skin of color: a systematic review. *JAMA Dermatol.* 2021;157(2):213-219.
23. Pourang A, Tisack A, Ezekwe N, et al. Effects of visible light on mechanisms of skin photoaging. *Photodermatol Photoimmunol Photomed.* 2022;38(3):191-196.
24. Lim HW, Kohli I, Ruvolo E, Kolbe L, Hamzavi IH. Impact of visible light on skin health: the role of antioxidants and free radical quenchers in skin protection. *J Am Acad Dermatol.* 2022;86(3s):S27-S37.
25. Regazzetti C, Sormani L, Debayle D, et al. Melanocytes sense blue light and regulate pigmentation through opsin-3. *J Invest Dermatol.* 2018;138(1):171-178.
26. Anderson RR, Parrish JA. The optics of human skin. *J Invest Dermatol.* 1981;77(1):13-19.
27. Kohli I, Braunberger TL, Nahhas AF, et al. Long-wavelength ultraviolet A1 and visible light photoprotection: a multimodality assessment of dose and response. *Photochem Photobiol.* 2020;96(1):208-214.
28. Kohli I, Chaowattanapanit S, Mohammad TF, et al. Synergistic effects of long-wavelength ultraviolet A1 and visible light on pigmentation and erythema. *Br J Dermatol.* 2018;178(5):1173-1180.
29. Sklar LR, Almutawa F, Lim HW, Hamzavi I. Effects of ultraviolet radiation, visible light, and infrared radiation on erythema and pigmentation: a review. *Photochem Photobiol Sci.* 2013;12(1):54-64.
30. Taylor SC, Alexis AF, Armstrong AW, Chiesa Fuxench ZC, Lim HW. Misconceptions of photoprotection in skin of color. *J Am Acad Dermatol.* 2022;86(3s):S9-S17.

CHAPTER 22

Genetics of Skin Diseases

William D. Shipman
Keith A. Choate

KEY POINTS

- Differences in disease incidence and prevalence in different racial and ethnic populations provide evidence for a genetic contribution to disease. Furthermore, familial disease clustering and more frequent concordance of disease in monozygotic (MZ) than dizygotic twins supports a genetic component.
- Less than 100% concordance in MZ twins as well as evidence for epigenetic modifications in disease support an environmental contribution.
- Genome-wide linkage and association studies provide evidence for involvement of genes at specific chromosomal regions.
- Systemic lupus erythematosus (SLE), vitiligo, systemic sclerosis (SSc), sarcoidosis, and keloids are genetically complex, with multiple genetic loci and environmental triggers conferring risk for these diseases and their severity.
- In addition to shared genetic susceptibilities, some gene differences are observed mainly within a single disorder, within a single racial group, or within a group of patients with similar clinical symptoms.
- Problems in replicating genetic findings and in elucidating the genetic contribution to the pathogenesis of complex diseases are currently being addressed by analyzing results from different racial group separately; admixture mapping to identify association of specific disease-related variation with ancestry; association studies using panels of single-nucleotide polymorphisms (SNPs) from different racial populations; using subsets of patients with similar clinical symptoms; and using ordered subset analysis to obtain evidence for gene interaction (epistasis) between different genetic loci.

BASIC PRINCIPLES OF GENETICS OF SKIN DISEASE [TABLES 22-1 AND 22-2]

GENETICS AND SKIN OF COLOR

It is well known that genetics plays an important role in many skin diseases. Recent research also shows that genetics may play a unique role in dermatologic conditions in skin of color (based on prevalence, incidence, and presentation of certain conditions in certain ethnic and racial populations). In this chapter, we discuss genetics in dermatology and how it specifically relates to dermatology of skin of color and also provide updates on particular conditions that affect individuals with skin of color.

Genome-wide association studies (GWAS) are employed to identify genomic variants associated with a risk for a disease or a specific trait. Utilizing high-density single-nucleotide polymorphism data in typically large cohorts, GWAS identifies genomic variants that occur more frequently in individuals with a particular disease than in a matched control population. Identifying variants in particular diseases not only provides novel information about potential pathophysiology, epidemiology, and risk, but also has the potential to inform development of new therapeutics.

GWAS and associated studies revolutionized our understanding of many common dermatologic conditions such as psoriasis, atopic dermatitis, and cutaneous and systemic lupus erythematosus. However, there is a lack of diversity in many GWAS studies and as of 2019, 78% of participants in GWAS studies all together have been of

TABLE 22-1 Common genetics terms

Term	Definition
Chromosome	bundles of tightly coiled DNA and proteins found within the nucleus of cells
Gene	the basic unit of inheritance, a portion of DNA that encodes a protein
Allele	one of two or more alternative forms of a particular gene or DNA sequence at a given locus
Karyotype	the number and visual appearance of the complete set of chromosomes in an individual
Locus	the physical location of a gene or a particular sequence of DNA on a chromosome
Single nucleotide polymorphism (SNP)	a single nucleotide alteration in a DNA sequence that is present in at least 1% of the population
Mutation	a change in the DNA sequence that usually results in a disease phenotype
Genotype	the combination of alleles an individual possesses for a specific locus or gene
Phenotype	physical manifestations of a particular genotype
Mosaicism	the presence of two or more genetically distinct sets of cells in one individual
Penetrance	the proportion of individuals in a population who carry a specific gene or gene mutation and express the related trait
Autosomal recessive	a pattern of inheritance where the offspring inherits one mutated copy of a specific gene from each parent and the parents are usually not affected and are known as carriers
Autosomal dominant	a pattern of inheritance where the offspring inherits the genetic trait or condition if only one copy of a mutated gene is inherited, and parents are typically affected
X-linked recessive	a pattern of inheritance where the offspring inherits the genetic trait or condition through mutations on the X chromosome. In males who have a single X chromosome, a mutation will cause the condition, in females who have two X chromosomes, a mutation is needed on both chromosomes to cause the condition. The other is usually considered a "carrier"
X-linked dominant	a pattern of inheritance where the offspring inherits the genetic trait or condition through mutations on a single X chromosome. A mutation is only needed on a single X chromosome in females to cause the trait or condition. Parents are typically affected
Monogenic	disorders or traits caused by variations in a single gene
Polygenic	disorders or traits caused by variations in multiple genes
Admixture	when previously divergent or isolated populations exchange genetic material
Monozygotic/ dizygotic twin concordance	concordance indicates the presence of the same trait in both members of a pair of twins. A higher concordance rate in monozygotic twins than in dizygotic twins is typically accepted as evidence of a genetic component

European descent,[1] raising the possibility that there is considerable missing genetic information from populations at risk for disease. Here we discuss genomic complexity of diseases that are prevalent in individuals with skin of color to highlight important areas to further explore.

TABLE 22-2 Common genetics methodologies

Method	Description
Genome linkage studies	the entire DNA is searched systematically for locations on the chromosome that are inherited in the same pattern as a specific trait
Genome positional cloning	used to detect chromosomal location of disease genes based on the observation that genes that reside physically close together on a chromosome remain linked during meiosis
Genome-wide association studies (GWAS)	observational study of a genome-wide set of genetic variants in different individuals to identify variants associated with risk of disease or a particular trait
Whole exome sequencing	genetic sequencing of all exons, the protein-coding regions, within a genome
Whole genome sequencing	genetic sequencing of nearly all nucleotides of an individual's complete DNA sequence, including noncoding regions
RNA sequencing	uses high-throughput sequencing to detect, quantify, and examine the sequence of messenger RNA in biological samples

GENETICS OF DERMATOLOGIC CONDITIONS IN SKIN OF COLOR

SYSTEMIC LUPUS ERYTHEMATOSUS

Systemic lupus erythematosus (SLE) is a multisystem autoimmune disorder characterized by deposition of autoantibodies that can subsequently lead to tissue injury in the skin, kidneys, joints, lungs, brain, heart, and other organs. The pathogenesis of SLE is complex and includes genetic, environmental, and hormonal influences. Increased prevalence in particular populations and a familial association supports a genetic component. The overall prevalence of SLE is 1 in 2000, but African Americans, Asians, and Hispanics have an increased incidence, estimated to be 1 in 1000 in African American women versus 1 in 4000 in Caucasian American women. In addition, 90% of SLE cases occur in women, possibly suggesting a hormonal influence.[2-4] Phenotypic differences have also been reported in different racial groups, in particular African Americans and Hispanics who have been reported to have more active aggressive disease that can also occur at a younger age.[5] Genetic admixture, which occurs when two or more previously isolated populations intermix,[6] has also been observed in SLE with the observation that Hispanic SLE individuals of Mexican and Central American ancestry have more severe disease than mainland Puerto Rican individuals, although mainland Puerto Rican individuals have more cutaneous manifestations.[7]

Twin and familial studies in SLE have also highlighted a genetic component. The monozygotic to dizygotic twin concordance ratio is high and estimated to be 10, with a monozygotic twin concordance rate between 24% and 58% and a dizygotic twin concordance rate between 2% and 5%, which is similar to nontwin siblings.[8,9] Discordance in monozygotic twins may be explained by epigenetic factors, such as the finding that immune-related genes were less methylated in the lupus-affected twin.[10] Even within the general population, there is a 20- to 40-fold higher SLE risk for a sibling of an individual with SLE compared to an unrelated person underscoring a familial component.[11]

Previously, candidate gene association and genome-wide linkage analysis has been used to identify susceptibility genes and loci of interest for SLE, and in more recent years GWAS and targeted genome scans[12-27] have further elucidated numerous chromosomal regions with linkages to SLE. Throughout the years, several dozens of new SLE loci have been discovered[28,29] and the combination of larger studies and implementation of novel genetic approaches will continue to allow new susceptibility genes and loci to be discovered.

The most common loci associated with SLE include HLA, complement, and Fc-γ low-affinity receptor gene families. In fact, *HLA-DRB1,*

HLA-DQA1, HLA-DQA2, HLA-DQB2, and *HLA-DR3* located at 6p21.32-33, human low-affinity receptors *FcGR2A* and *FcGR3A* at 1q23, and deficiency of complement components C4 and C2 at 6p21, C1q at 1p36, and C1r/s at 12p13 are associated with increased risk of disease.[23,30-34] Individuals with C1q deficiency are at risk of developing SLE at a young age, developing a severe photosensitive rash, and developing rheumatic disease. A proportion of individuals with deficient C4 and C2 also have a stronger risk of developing rheumatic disease.

Variation in gene copy number has been shown to be a heritable source of susceptibility to rheumatic disease. For instance, a low *FcGR3B* copy number has been associated with an increased risk of autoimmune glomerulonephritis in a subset of SLE individuals[35] and C4 copy number is a risk factor for SLE when low and a protective factor when high in European Americans.[36]

In addition to HLA, complement, and Fc-γ low-affinity receptors, numerous other genes and loci have been associated with SLE including genes responsible for T-cell signaling (*PTPN22* 1p13; *STAT4* 2q32.3; *TNFSF4* 1q25.1), B-cell signaling (*IL-10* 1q31-32; *BANK1* 4q24; *BLK* 8p23.1; *RASGRP3* 2p22.3), toll-like receptor (TLR) and interferon (IFN) signaling (*IRF5* 7q32.1; *IRF7* 11p15.5; *IRF8* 16q24.1; *TYK2* 19p13.2; *STAT4* 2q32.3), inflammation activation of interleukin-1β (*NLRP1* 17p3), cell cycle/apoptosis/cell metabolism (*TNFAIP3* 6q23.3; *RASGRP3* 2p22.3; *UBE2LR* 22q), and transcriptional regulation (*JAZF1* 7p15.2-p15.1; *UHRF1BP1* 6p21.31)[28,29,37]

Certain SLE genes and loci have been associated with certain racial and ethnic groups. For instance, the programmed cell death-1 (*PD-1*) alle (2q37 linkage) is associated with individuals of European, Mexican, Spanish descent but not in African Americans.[38,39] SLE individuals stratified for discoid lupus manifestations showed a linkage at 11p13 in African Americans.[40] Other SLE susceptibility linkages associated with racial and ethnic groups include 12q24 in mainly Hispanic and European individuals[19]; *ETS1* (11q24.3) and *WDFY4* (10q11.23) in Chinese individuals[41]; *SLEH1* (11q14), *SLEN2* (2q34-35), and *SLEN3* (11p15.5) in African Americans,[42-45] and *SLEN1* (10q22.3) in Caucasians.[44,45] There are numerous SLE associated loci found across racial and ethnic groups, and larger studies involving racial and ethnic groups are needed to further elucidate heterogeneity in these and other novel loci in examination of diverse population.

The functional effects of SLE susceptibility loci have been studied, providing novel avenues for therapeutic approaches. For instance, several different functional variants of IFN regulatory genes[46,47] have highlighted the role of IFN signaling in SLE contributing to the development of novel therapies for SLE targeting the type I interferon pathway.[47,48]

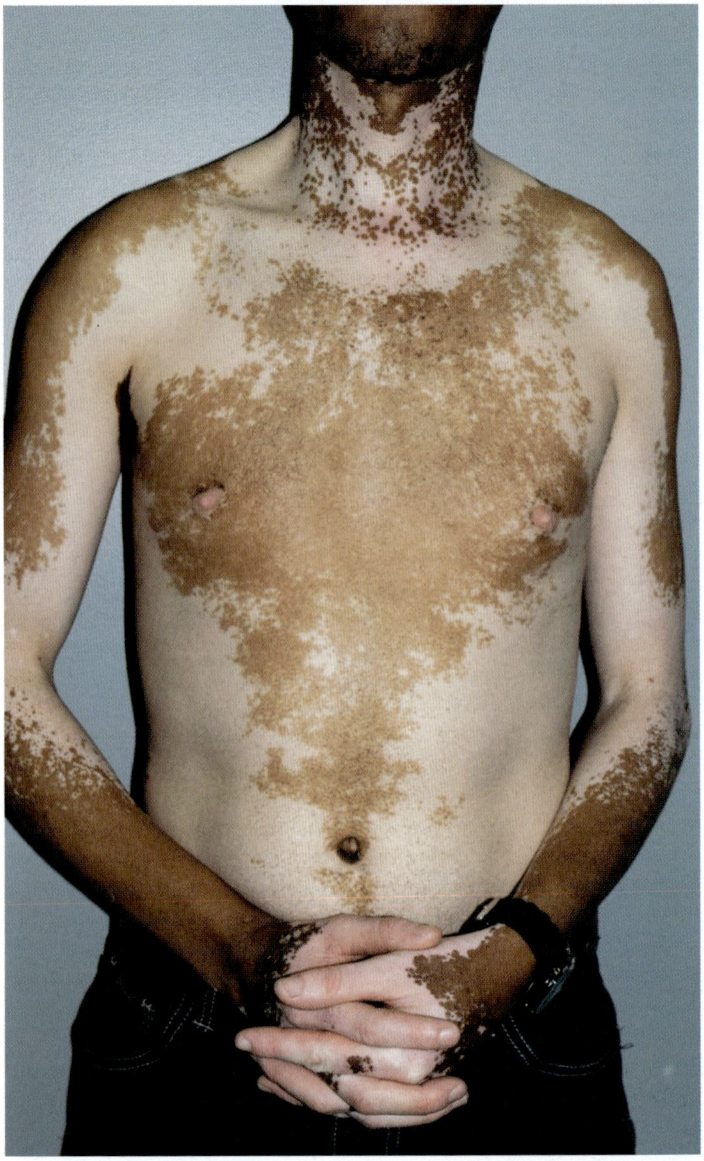

FIGURE 22-1. Vitiligo. Extensive depigmented macules and confluent patches on the neck, hands, arms, and trunk of a skin of color individual with vitiligo. (Photo courtesy of Ncoza Dlova, MBChB, FCDerm, PhD.)

VITILIGO

Vitiligo is an acquired dermatologic disorder characterized by well-circumscribed depigmented macules and patches on the skin due to the dysfunction of melanocytes [**Figure 22-1**]. The pathogenesis is due to a complex interplay of genetic susceptibility, immune dysfunction, and environmental triggers. Worldwide, vitiligo prevalence is estimated to be between 0.2% and 2%.[49] Although most cases of vitiligo, up to 91%, are sporadic, the frequency of developing vitiligo is elevated in close relatives in those affected, estimated to be about 7% in first-degree relatives.[50] Further heritability studies have shown that vitiligo heritability is relatively high and that about 80% of vitiligo risk is genetically based, while the other 20% is due to environmental factors.[51]

The prevalence of vitiligo has also been examined in various racial and ethnic populations. In the Chinese Han population, which represents greater than 90% of the Chinese population, the prevalence of vitiligo was estimated to be 0.19% and evaluation of affected individuals showed that the age of onset was younger when compared to individuals from the United States.[52,53] For individuals in the French West Indies, where 96% of the population is Black Caribbean, the overall prevalence was estimated to be 0.34%, prevalence among relatives was 7%, and the age of onset was later compared to other populations.[54] In the United States, overall prevalence was estimated to be between 0.76% and 1.11%.[55] These studies highlight that there may be differences in the prevalence and age of onset in vitiligo across various racial and geographic populations.

Initially candidate gene studies were utilized to identify two immune-related candidate genes *CTLA4*[56,57] and *PTPN22*,[58] which were later confirmed by GWAS studies. Later additional susceptibility genes such as *FOXD3, NLRP1, PDGFRA, HLA*, and *XBP1* were identified. GWAS studies in vitiligo have revealed numerous loci that contribute to vitiligo risk, some which are shared across populations and some that are specific to certain populations.[51] The majority of these loci encodes genes that are involved in immunoregulation, apoptosis, and melanocyte biology, and the proteins that these genes encode have been shown to form a functional network that suggests melanocyte damage, antigen processing and presentation, immune cell activation, and melanocyte targeting and apoptosis.[51,59]

Epidemiologic studies have shown that vitiligo is associated with other autoimmune diseases such as rheumatoid arthritis, type 1 diabetes, autoimmune thyroid disease, SLE, and Addison's disease. Genetic studies have shown that there are indeed shared genes and loci in vitiligo and other autoimmune diseases such as HLA, *PTPN22, CTLA4, IFIH1, SH2B3, ARID5B, BACH2, IL2RA, IKZF4, UBASH3, C1QTNF6*, among others. In fact, at least 19 of the 47 non-MHC loci associated with vitiligo

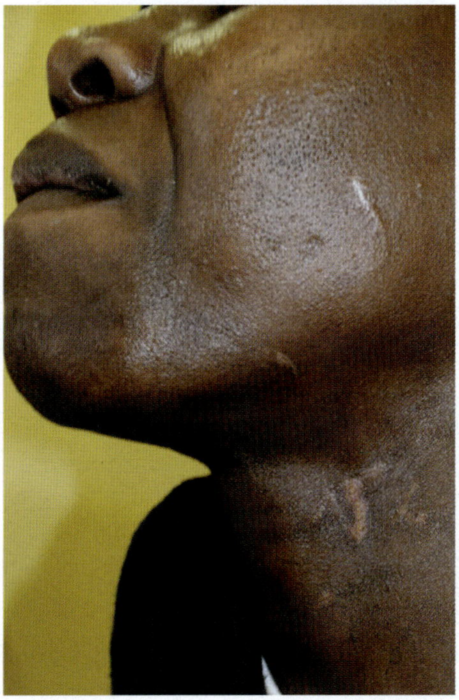

FIGURE 22-2. Scleroderma. Shiny bound-down plaques with pink scarring in the centers on the neck and face of a skin of color individual with scleroderma. (Photo courtesy of Ncoza Dlova, MBChB, FCDerm, PhD.)

in European populations have also been associated with at least one of the above mentioned autoimmune diseases.[51]

SYSTEMIC SCLEROSIS

Systemic sclerosis (SSc) is a chronic autoimmune disease that affects both the skin [**Figure 22-2**] and systemic organs with fibrosis and vascular abnormalities. The clinical phenotype of SSc can range from limited focal cutaneous involvement, as found in localized scleroderma or morphea, to extensive fibrosis of the skin and systemic organs. Although incompletely understood, there is evidence to support a role for genetics in SSc pathogenesis in addition to environmental triggers. This includes a variation in SSc prevalence and incidence among ethnic and racial groups. In the United States, the prevalence of SSc is higher in African Americans compared to Caucasians,[60] while lower prevalence rates have been reported in Japanese individuals.[61] An extremely high prevalence has been reported for Oklahoma Choctaw Native Americans and this was found to be associated with a specific haplotype on chromosome 15q and is thought to be due to the founder effect from generations prior.[62,63] SSc also occurs more frequently in families and a positive family history is the strongest risk factor for the disease.[64,65]

Clinical phenotypes of SSc are also varied among racial and ethnic groups. African Americans and Hispanics in the United States were more likely to have diffuse skin involvement, skin pigmentary changes, digital ulcers, and pulmonary hypertension (African Americans) when compared to Whites who were more likely to have more facial telangiectasias and hypothyroidism.[60,66] Systemically there is also a higher prevalence of SSc renal crisis among African Americans.[67] The variation in racial and ethnic SSc clinical phenotypes may in part be explained by autoantibody production that is also influenced by hereditary factors and varies in different racial groups.[68] Specifically, anticentromere antibodies, which are strongly associated with limited cutaneous SSc and a higher risk for calcinosis and ischemic digital loss with a lower frequency of interstitial pulmonary fibrosis, occur most frequently in Caucasians and occur with less frequency in Hispanic, African American, and Thai individuals. Anti-topoisomerase I autoantibodies occur at higher frequency in Mexican American, African American, Native American, Thai, and Japanese individuals.[68] Chinese individuals also seem to have higher frequencies of anti-topoisomerase I and anti-U1-ribonucleoprotein (U1RNP), which corresponds to a higher risk of more diffuse forms of SSc.[68,69] Anti-nucleolar antibodies such as anti-fibrillarin/anti-U3-RNP is found with higher frequency in SSc individuals of African descent than in Caucasians and is associated with diffuse skin involvement, gastrointestinal dysmotility, myositis, pulmonary hypertension, cardiac involvement, renal disease, younger age or onset, more severe vascular disease, digital ulcers, and less severe lung involvement.[68,70,71] Further characterization of genetic basis and functional significance of differences in autoantibody production among different racial and ethnic groups may help further elucidate disease pathogenesis of SSc.

Several candidate gene mutations and polymorphisms have been identified in SSc including genes encoding class II HLA (6p21), TNF-α (12p13), IL-4 receptor alpha (16p12.1-p11.2), IL-8 receptor 2 (2q35), topoisomerase I (20q12), transforming growth factor beta (19q13.1), and connective tissue growth factor (6q23-27).[37,72] Recent GWAS has also shown risk conferred by variants in *STAT4, IRF5, PTPN22, BANK1, BLK, CD247, TNFSF4.*[37] A role for epigenetics has been implicated in SSc including DNA and histone modification as well as long noncoding RNAs (lncRNAs) and microRNAs (miRNAs).[73] Although there are no reported differences in disease concordance between monozygotic and dizygotic twins, concordance for serum autoantibodies was significantly higher in monozygotic twins.[72,74]

SARCOIDOSIS

Sarcoidosis is a noninfectious granulomatous disorder [**Figure 22-3**] that can occur in individuals of all ages, races, and sexes but in the United States, there is an increased incidence in African Americans (ranging from 35 to 64 per 100,000). In particular, African American women have the highest incidence (107 per 100,000) and have a lifetime risk of 2.7% of developing sarcoidosis, compared to Caucasians in the United States having an incidence ranging from 10 to 14 per 100,000,[75] although wide variations are reported.[76] In addition, sarcoidosis in African Americans tends to be more chronic and severe with a higher mortality rate than other populations.[77]

The pathogenesis of sarcoidosis has several components and is characterized by hyperactivity of the cell-mediated immune system. It is thought that individuals with a genetic susceptibility are exposed to a triggering antigen that leads to activation of macrophages and T-cells and subsequently leading to granuloma formation. Given the variation in disease prevalence and incidence among racial and ethnic groups, familial associations[78] and genetic studies[79,80] highlight a genetic role in the pathogenesis of sarcoidosis. Furthermore twin studies demonstrate a concordance of 14.8% in monozygotic twins compared to 1.2% in dizygotic twins,[81] suggesting a genetic component but also the likely contribution of environmental factors.

Through genome linkage studies and GWAS numerous candidate genes for sarcoidosis have been identified and include loci that involved in immune regulation, antigen presentation, HLA genes, immunoregulatory cytokines, growth factors, and angiotensin-converting enzyme.[79,80] The distribution of HLA class III alleles was observed to be significantly different between African Americans and Caucasians and HLA *DRB1*1501* allele was found to increase risk in Caucasians but be protective in African Americans.[82]

Recent GWAS studies have identified both alleles in sarcoidosis that are both shared and specific to certain racial and ethnic groups. For instance, the susceptibility locus *ANXA11* (10q22.3-q23.1) was initially observed in Caucasian populations.[83] ANXA11 is a member of the annexin family and has been reported to give rise to autoantibodies in several autoimmune disorders.[84] Further GWAS studies found a major susceptibility locus, *ANXA11* (rs1049550), in both African Americans and European Americans but additional SNPs were more significant in African American populations with persistent fibrotic lung disease.[85] Another locus at the minor A allele of SNP rs61860052, within the first intron of *ANXA11*, was found to have a protective effect on sarcoidosis in African Americans.[85]

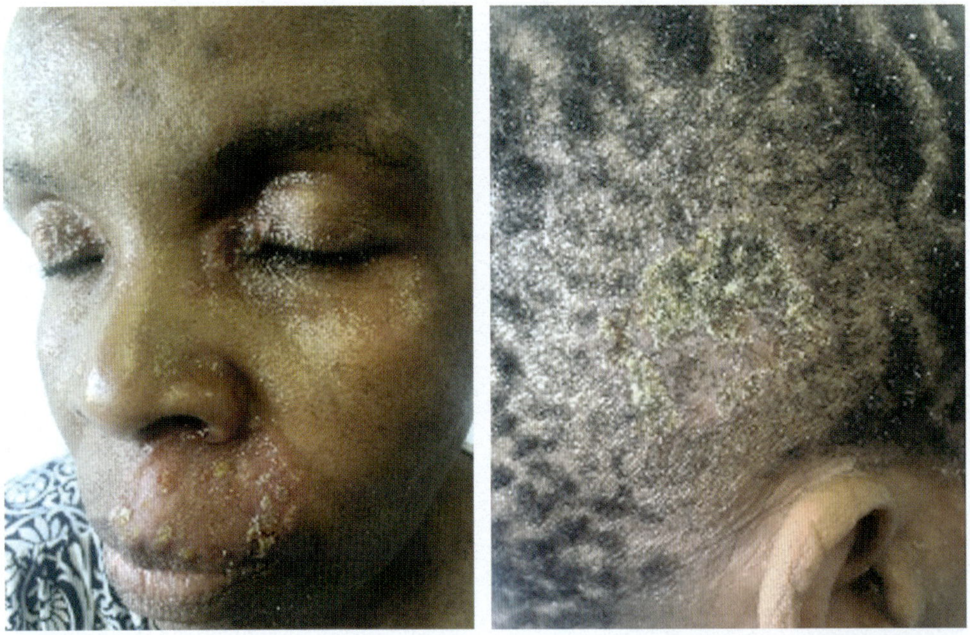

FIGURE 22-3. Sarcoidosis. Multiple smooth pink-brown papules and plaques with overlying crust around the mouth, nose, medial canthus, and eyelids along with a smooth pink-brown plaque with overlying crust and associated hair loss in the scalp of an individual with sarcoidosis. (Photos courtesy of Ncoza Dlova, MBChB, FCDerm, PhD.)

Using GWAS and other shared associations have been found between African and European origin Americans including several class II HLA genes (*DRA*, *DRB5*, and *DRB1*), and *BTNL2*.[86] Specific to African American populations, *Notch4* was found to be a susceptibility gene for sarcoidosis (odds ratio 1.3-1.5).[86]

RNA sequencing and gene-set enrichment analysis of cutaneous sarcoidosis skin has shown activation of interferon-gamma, tumor necrosis factor alpha (TNF-α), IL-6, STAT1, STAT3, and mammalian target of rapamycin complex 1 (mTORC1) signaling and treatment with the JAK-STAT inhibitor tofacitinib resulted in the downregulation of these pathways in a case report.[87] Further work is warranted to identify additional susceptibility loci and to elucidate their role in the pathogenesis of sarcoidosis in various populations.

KELOIDS

Keloids are benign fibrous dermal nodules that typically form at sites of injury and extend beyond the wound itself. Keloids are characterized by delayed onset and are usually symptomatic. The genetic predisposition of keloids is found predominantly in individuals with skin of color, with an estimated prevalence of 4.5% to 16% in Black and Hispanic populations and less than 1% in Caucasians.[88] A study conducted on Japanese populations indicated that those with a family history of keloids were more susceptible to developing keloids[89] and another study in Black African individuals observed that individuals with a family history of keloids were four times more likely to develop keloids.[90] Studies examining multiple pedigrees in multiple racial and ethnic groups observed an inheritance pattern consistent with an autosomal dominant trait with incomplete penetrance and variable expression[91]; however, there are prior studies that report some incidences of autosomal recessive inheritance.[88] The occurrence of keloids at distinct frequencies in different racial and ethnic populations and the observation of inheritance among families highlights a role of heritability in the development of keloids.

Numerous studies have explored the genetic basis of keloids and have identified susceptibility SNPs and genes. In a Japanese population, four SNPs (rs873549, rs1511412, rs94018, and rs8032158) in three chromosomal regions (1q41, 3q22.3-23, and 15q21.3) were associated with the development of keloids.[92] Later, a study on a Chinese Han population identified another two SNPs (rs1442440 at loci 1q41 and rs2271289 at loci 15q21.3) that were associated with the development of keloids.[93] Through whole-genome sequencing, three more SNPs were identified (rs181924090 at loci 11p15.5, *SIRT3*; rs151091483 at loci 17p13.1, *MYH8*; and rs183178644 at loci 6p25, HUS1B) and the genes involved are thought to contribute to keloid proliferation, apoptosis, and collagen generation.[88,94] Further studies observed *LEPR* SNPs (rs1137101, rs1938496, rs7555955) that were not only associated with keloid development but also severity and family history.[95]

Numerous susceptibility genes have been identified in keloid formation including genes related to TGF-beta/SMAD signaling, *NEDD4*, HLA-related genes, and other genes related to fibroblasts function (such as *ASAH1*, *TRAF4*, *HOXA5*, and *ADAM33*).[88] There have also been some genetic mutations associated with keloid formation including mutations of *CXCR1*, *CDC2L1*, *WNT10A*, *p53*.[88]

Although keloids are closely linked to hereditary association and the above-mentioned susceptibility SNPs and genes, epigenetics has been shown to play a role in keloid formation. DNA methylation is the most prominent form of epigenetic alteration found in keloids. The DNA methyltransferase inhibitor 5-aza-2-deoxycytidine appeared to at reverse epigenetic alterations, suggesting that this may be a potential novel therapy.[96] In addition, the use of miRNAs is being explored as another potential treatment. miRNA expression has been shown to be dysregulated in keloid fibroblasts[88,97] and treatment of fibrotic fibroblasts with TNF-α has been shown to reduce fibrosis by modulation of miRNAs.[98] Long noncoding RNA has also been implicated in keloid development and progression of keloids via various signaling pathways [**Table 22-3**].[88]

CENTRAL CENTRIFUGAL CICATRICIAL ALOPECIA

Central centrifugal cicatricial alopecia (CCCA) is a chronic progressive condition resulting in scarring alopecia primarily centered on the crown or vertex and as the disease progresses the alopecia expands in a relatively symmetric fashion [**Figure 22-4**]. Although epidemiologic data for CCCA is limited, it is thought to primarily occur in African American women but can also occur in men.[107-109] Although the prevalence is relatively unknown, small studies have suggested that the prevalence ranges from 2.7% to 15.4% in studies including African American and Black African women.[110-112]

TABLE 22-3 Susceptibility genes, SNPs and mutations associated with keloids

Chrom.	Gene	Method	SNP	Gene function	Race/ Ethnicity	Ref
1q41	–	GWAS	rs873549 rs1442440	–	Japanese Chinese Han	92,93
3q22.3-23	*FOXL2*	GWAS	rs1511412 rs940187	encodes a transcription factor essential for ovary differentiation and maintenance, regulation of CYP19 expression, and eyelid/eyebrow development	Japanese	92
15q21.3	*NEDD4*	GWAS	rs8032158 rs2271289	encodes a ubiquitin ligase enzyme that targets proteins for ubiquitination and degradation	Japanese Chinese Han	92,93
11p15.5	*SIRT3*	GWAS	rs181924090	encodes histone deacetylase found exclusively in mitochondria where it can eliminate reactive oxygen species and inhibit apoptosis	Chinese Han	94
17p13.1	*MYH8*	GWAS	rs151091483	encodes member of the conventional myosin heavy chains and functions in skeletal muscle contraction	Chinese Han	94
6p25	*HUS1B*	GWAS	rs183178644	encodes component of cell cycle checkpoint protein complex involved in cell cycle arrest.	Chinese Han	94
–	*LEPR*	MLDR	rs1137101 rs1938496 rs7555955	encodes leptin receptor protein involved in fat metabolism	Chinese Han	95
7p11	*EGFR*	GWAS	–	encodes epidermal growth factor receptor, a transmembrane glycoprotein receptor involved in cell proliferation and survival	African American	99
2q23	*TNFAIP6*	GWAS	–	–	Japanese	99
15q21.3	*NEDD4*	GWAS	rs8032158	encodes a ubiquitin ligase enzyme that targets proteins for ubiquitination and degradation	Egyptian	100
15q21.2-22.3	*MYO1E*	AM	rs747722 rs28394564	encodes myosin protein involved in intracellular movement and membrane trafficking	African American	101
15q21.2-22.3	*NEDD4*	AM	rs138585173	encodes a ubiquitin ligase enzyme that targets proteins for ubiquitination and degradation	African American	101
11q13.5	*MYO7A*	GWAS	rs35641839	encodes myosin protein involved in intracellular movement and membrane trafficking	African American	101
–	*HLA-DQA1*	PCR-SSP	–	encodes membrane protein involved in critical roles in immune processes by presenting peptides derived from extracellular proteins	Chinese Han	102
–	*HLA-DQB1*	PCR-SSP	–		Chinese Han	102
–	*HLA-DRB1*	PCR-SSOP	–		Caucasian	103,104
8p23.3-p21.3	*ASAH1*	GWAS	–	encodes member of the acid ceramidase family of proteins and is involved in catalyzing degradation of ceramide into sphingosine and free fatty acid	Nigerian Yoruba	105
20p13	*ADAM33*	PCR-RFLP	rs612709	encodes membrane protein implicated in cell-cell and cell-matrix interactions	Chinese Han	106

Abbreviations: AM, admixture mapping; MLDR, multiple ligase detection reaction; PCR-RFLP: PCR-restriction fragment length polymorphisms; SSOP, sequence-specific oligonucleotide probes.

Source: Modified with permission from Liu S, et al. Keloid: Genetic susceptibility and contributions of genetics and epigenetics to its pathogenesis. *Exp Dermatol.* 2022;31(11):1665-1675.

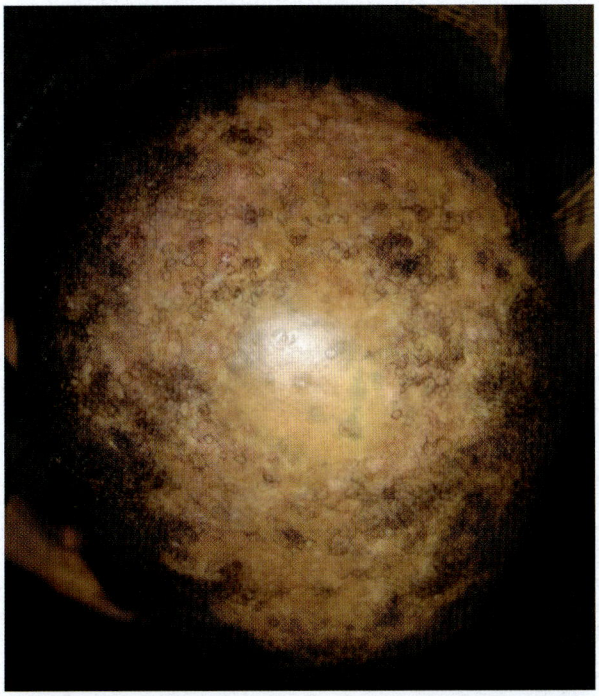

FIGURE 22-4. Central centrifugal cicatricial alopecia (CCCA). A large patch of scarring alopecia with irregular borders, some retained follicles, and areas of erythema on the vertex and frontal scalp of a skin of color individual with CCCA. (Photo courtesy of Ncoza Dlova, MBChB, FCDerm, PhD.)

Initially CCCA was thought to be due to the use of hot combs and was even initially referred to as "hot comb alopecia." However, recent advances have shown that the pathogenesis is likely due to a genetic predisposition, chronic inflammation, and hair care practices that may aggravate or cause progression of disease.[107] A genetic predisposition for CCCA has been proposed due to studies showing family history being a strong risk factor[107] underscoring possible genetic contributions to the disease.

Recent studies have found that women with CCCA have a five times increased odds of having uterine leiomyomas, a known fibroproliferative disease.[113] Using DNA microarray studies of scalp biopsies from individuals with CCCA, upregulation of fibroproliferative genes such as platelet derived growth factor (*PDGF*), collagen I (*COLI*), collagen III (*COLIII*), matrix metalloproteinase 1 (*MMP1*), matrix metalloproteinase 2 (*MMP 2*), matrix metalloproteinase 7 (*MMP7*), and matrix metalloproteinase 9 (*MMP9*).[114] In addition, DNA microarray showed that clinically extensive, severe CCCA was characterized by increased expression of the fibroproliferative genes matrix metalloproteinase 9 (*MMP9*), secreted frizzled-related protein gene (*SFRP4*), and macrophage scavenger receptor 1 gene (*MSR1*) when compared to focal and limited disease.

Using whole exome sequencing and RNA sequencing, mutations in *PADI3*, which encodes peptidyl arginine deiminase, type III (PADI3) was found in 24% of subjects studied with CCCA. PADI3 is an enzyme that post-translationally modifies other proteins that are essential for hair-shaft formation,[115] and loss of function *PADI3* mutations may contribute to the disease pathogenesis in CCCA. Further larger cohort and genomic studies are needed to further elucidate genetic components of CCCA pathophysiology.

CONCLUSION

Genetics play an important role in dermatologic conditions and particularly in skin of color. SLE, vitiligo, SSc, sarcoidosis, keloids, and CCCA—commonly observed diseases in individuals with skin of color—are genetically complex, with multiple genetic loci and environmental triggers conferring risk for the disease and its severity. Identifying genetic susceptibility and genes for specific disorders in skin of color populations is an ongoing and dynamic process that continues to evolve with new genetic advances. The identification of relevant loci in specific groups will allow the enrichment of studies for relevant genes for dermatologic conditions. There is a compelling need to have representative populations in dermatologic genomic studies including in both cases and controls to identify risk alleles specific to different racial and ethnic groups. Inclusion of diverse populations in genomic studies may reveal novel molecular determinants of dermatologic disease, highlight new areas for genetics research in skin of color, and lead to the development of novel therapeutics.

REFERENCES

1. Del Cid S. Lack of diversity in genomics research. *Osmosis Magazine.* 2019(1).
2. Hochberg M. The epidemiology of systemic lupus erythematosus. In: Wallace D, Hahn B, Quismorio F, eds. *Dubois' Lupus Erythematosus.* Baltimore, MD: Williams & Wilkins; 1997:49-65.
3. Rus V. Systemic lupus erythematosus. In: Silman A, ed. *Epidemiology of Rheumatic Diseases.* Oxford, United Kingdom: Oxford University Press; 2001:123-140.
4. Whitacre CC, Reingold SC, O'Looney PA, Task Force on Gender MSaA. A gender gap in autoimmunity. *Science.* 1999;283(5406).
5. Uribe AG, McGwin G, Jr., Reveille JD, Alarcon GS. What have we learned from a 10-year experience with the LUMINA (Lupus in Minorities; Nature vs. nurture) cohort? Where are we heading? *Autoimmun Rev.* 2004;3(4):321-329.
6. Shriner D. Overview of admixture mapping. *Curr Protoc Hum Genet.* 2013;Chapter 1:Unit 1 23.
7. Vila LM, Alarcon GS, McGwin G, Jr., et al. Early clinical manifestations, disease activity and damage of systemic lupus erythematosus among two distinct US Hispanic subpopulations. *Rheumatology (Oxford).* 2004;43(3):358-363.
8. Block SR, Winfield JB, Lockshin MD. Studies of twins with systemic lupus erythematosus: a review of the literature and presentation of 12 additional sets. *Am J Med.* 1975;59.
9. Deapen D, Escalante A, Weinrib L, et al. A revised estimate of twin concordance in systemic lupus erythematosus. *Arthritis Rheum.* 1992;35(3):311-318.
10. Javierre BM, Hernando H, Ballestar E. Environmental triggers and epigenetic deregulation in autoimmune disease. *Discovery Med.* 2011;12(67):535-545.
11. Wandstrat A, Wakeland E. The genetics of complex autoimmune diseases: non-MHC susceptibility genes. *Nat Immunol.* 2001;2:802-809.
12. Cantor RM, Yuan J, Napier S, et al. Systemic lupus erythematosus genome scan: support for linkage at 1q23, 2q33, 16q12-13, and 17q21-23 and novel evidence at 3p24, 10q23-24, 13q32, and 18q22-23. *Arthritis Rheum.* 2004;50(10):3203-3210.
13. Gaffney PM, Kearns GM, Shark KB, et al. A genome-wide search for susceptibility genes in human systemic lupus erythematosus sib-pair families. *Proc Natl Acad Sci.* 1998;95:14875-14879.
14. Moser KL, Neas BR, Salmon JE, et al. Genome scan of human systemic lupus erythematosus: evidence for linkage on chromosome 1q in African American pedigrees. *Proc Natl Acad Sci.* 1998;95:14869-14874.
15. Gaffney PM, Ortmann WA, Selby SA, et al. Genome screening in human systemic lupus erythematosus: results from a second Minnesota cohort and combined analyses of 187 sib-pair families. *Am J Hum Genet.* 2000;66(2):547-556.
16. Gray-McGuire C, Moser KL, Gaffney PM, et al. Genome scan of human systemic lupus erythematosus by regression modeling: evidence of linkage and epistasis at 4p16-15.2. *Am J Hum Genet.* 2000;67(6):1460-1469.
17. Lindqvist AK, Steinsson K, Johanneson B, et al. A susceptibility locus for human systemic lupus erythematosus (hSLE1) on chromosome 2q. *J Autoimmun.* 2000;14(2):169-178.
18. Shai R, Quismorio F, Li L, et al. Genome-wide screen for systemic lupus erythematosus susceptibility genes in multiplex famiiles. *Hum Mol Genet.* 1999;8(4):639-644.
19. Nath SK, Quintero-Del-Rio AI, Kilpatrick J, Feo L, Ballesteros M, Harley JB. Linkage at 12q24 with systemic lupus erythematosus (SLE) is established and confirmed in Hispanic and European American families. *Am J Hum Genet.* 2004;74(1):73-82.
20. Koskenmies S, Lahermo P, Julkunen H, Ollikainen V, Kere J, Widen E. Linkage mapping of systemiic lupus erythematosus (SLE) in Finnish families multiply affected by SLE. *J Med Genet.* 2004;41.
21. Tsao BP, Cantor RM, Grossman JM, et al. PARP alleles within the linked chromosomal region are associated with systemic lupus erythematosus. *J Clin Invest.* 1999;103(8):1135-1140.
22. Tsao BP, Cantor RM, Kalunian KC, et al. Evidence for linkage of a candidate chromosome 1 region to human systemic lupus erythematosus. *J Clin Invest.* 1997;99(4):725-731.
23. Moser KL, Gray-McGuire C, Kelly J, et al. Confirmation of genetic linkage between human systemic lupus erythematosus and chromosome 1q41. *Arthritis Rheum.* 1999;42(9):1902-1907.
24. Criswell LA, Moser KL, Gaffney PM, et al. PARP alleles and SLE: failure to confirm association with disease susceptibility. *J Clin Invest.* 2000;105(11):1501-1502.
25. Graham RR, Langefeld CD, Gaffney PM, et al. Genetic linkage and transmission disequilibrium of marker haplotypes at chromosome 1q41 in human systemic lupus erythematosus. *Arthritis Res.* 2001;3(5):299-305.
26. Magnusson V, Lindqvist AK, Castillejo-Lopez C, et al. Fine mapping of the SLEB2 locus involved in susceptibility to systemic lupus erythematosus. *Genomics.* 2000;70(3):307-314.
27. Johanneson B, Lima G, von Salome J, et al. A major susceptibility locus for systemic lupus erythemathosus maps to chromosome 1q31. *Am J Hum Genet.* 2002;71(5):1060-1071.
28. Ha E, Bae SC, Kim K. Recent advances in understanding the genetic basis of systemic lupus erythematosus. *Semin Immunopathol.* 2022;44(1):29-46.
29. Owen KA, Grammer AC, Lipsky PE. Deconvoluting the heterogeneity of SLE: The contribution of ancestry. *J Allergy Clin Immunol.* 2022;149(1):12-23.
30. Graham RR, Ortmann WA, Langefeld CD, et al. Visualizing human leukocyte antigen class II risk haplotypes in human systemic lupus erythematosus. *Am J Hum Genet.* 2002;71(3):543-553.
31. Magnusson V, Johanneson B, Lima G, et al. Both risk alleles for FcgammaRIIA and FcgammaRIIIA are susceptibility factors for SLE: a unifying hypothesis. *Genes Immun.* 2004;5(2):130-137.
32. Ghebrehiwet B, Peerschke EIB. Role of C1q and C1q receptors in the pathogenesis of systemic lupus erythematosus. *Curr Dir Autoimmun.* 2004;7:87-97.
33. Manderson AP, Botto M, Walport MJ. The role of complement in the development of systemic lupus erythematosus. *Annu Rev Immunol.* 2004;22:431-456.
34. Slingsby JH, Norsworthy P, Pearce G, et al. Homozygous hereditary C1q deficiency and systemic lupus erythematosus. A new family and the molecular basis of C1q deficiency in three families. *Arthritis Rheum.* 1996;39(4):663-670.
35. Fanciulli M, Norsworthy PJ, Petretto E, et al. FCGR3B copy number variation is associated with susceptibility to systemic, but not organ-specific, autoimmunity. *Nat Genet.* 2007;39(6):721-723.
36. Yang Y, Chung EK, Wu YL, et al. Gene copy-number variation and associated polymorphisms of complement component C4 in human systemic lupus erythematosus (SLE): low copy number is a risk factor for and high copy number is a protective factor against SLE susceptibility in European Americans. *Am J Hum Genet.* 2007;80(6):1037-1054.
37. Ortiz-Fernandez L, Martin J, Alarcon-Riquelme ME. A summary on the genetics of systemic lupus erythematosus, rheumatoid arthritis, systemic sclerosis, and Sjogren's syndrome. *Clin Rev Allergy Immunol.* 2023;64(3): 392-411.
38. Prokunina L, Castillejo-Lopez C, Oberg F, et al. A regulatory polymorphism in PDCD1 is associated with susceptibility to systemic lupus erythematosus in humans. *Nat Genet.* 2002;32(4):666-669.
39. Ferreiros-Vidal I, Gomez-Reino JJ, Barros F, et al. Association of PDCD1 with susceptibility to systemic lupus erythematosus: evidence of population-specific effects. *Arthritis Rheum.* 2004;50(8):2590-2597.
40. Nath SK, Namjou B, Kilpatrick J, et al. A candidate region on 11p13 for systemic lupus erythematosus: a linkage identified in African-American families. *J Investig Dermatol Symp Proc.* 2004;9(1):64-67.
41. Yuan YJ, Luo XB, Shen N. Current advances in lupus genetic and genomic studies in Asia. *Lupus.* 2010;19:1374-1383.
42. Kelly JA, Thompson K, Kilpatrick J, et al. Evidence for a susceptibility gene (SLEH1) on chromosome 11q14 for systemic lupus erythematosus (SLE) families with hemolytic anemia. *Proc Natl Acad Sci U S A.* 2002;99(18):11766-11771.
43. Sawalha AH, Namjou B, Nath SK, et al. Genetic linkage of systemic lupus erythematosus with chromosome 11q14 (SLEH1) in African-American families stratified by a nucleolar antinuclear antibody pattern. *Genes Immun.* 2002;3 Suppl 1:S31-S34.
44. Quintero-del-Rio AI, Kelly JA, Garriott CP, et al. SLEN2 (2q34-35) and SLEN1 (10q22.3) replication in systemic lupus erythematosus stratified by nephritis. *Am J Hum Genet.* 2004;75(2):346-348.
45. Quintero-Del-Rio AI, Kelly JA, Kilpatrick J, James JA, Harley JB. The genetics of systemic lupus erythematosus stratified by renal disease: linkage at

10q22.3 (SLEN1), 2q34-35 (SLEN2), and 11p15.6 (SLEN3). *Genes Immun.* 2002;3 Suppl 1:S57-S62.
46. Bronson PG, Chaivorapol C, Ortmann W, Behrens TW, Graham RR. The genetics of type I interferon in systemic lupus erythematosus. *Curr Opin Immunol.* 2012;24(5):530-537.
47. Psarras A, Wittmann M, Vital EM. Emerging concepts of type I interferons in SLE pathogenesis and therapy. *Nat Rev Rheumatol.* 2022;18(10):575-590.
48. Crow MK. Advances in lupus therapeutics: achieving sustained control of the type I interferon pathway. *Curr Opin Pharmacol.* 2022;67:102291.
49. Zhang Y, Cai Y, Shi M, et al. The prevalence of vitiligo: a meta-analysis. *PLoS ONE.* 2016;11(9):e0163806.
50. Alkhateeb A, Fain PR, Thody A, Bennett DC, Spritz RA. Epidemiology of vitiligo and associated autoimmune diseases in Caucasian probands and their families. *Pigment Cell Res.* 2003;16(3):208-214.
51. Spritz RA, Santorico SA. The genetic basis of vitiligo. *J Invest Dermatol.* 2021;141(2):265-273.
52. Zhang XJ, Liu JB, Gui JP, et al. Characteristics of genetic epidemiology and genetic models for vitiligo. *J Am Acad Dermatol.* 2004;51(3):383-390.
53. Laberge G, Mailloux CM, Gowan K, et al. Early disease onset and increased risk of other autoimmune diseases in familial generalized vitiligo. *Pigment Cell Res.* 2005;18(4):300-305.
54. Boisseau-Garsaud AM, Garsaud P, Cales-Quist D, Helenon R, Queneherve C, Claire RC. Epidemiology of vitiligo in the French West Indies (Isle of Martinique). *Int J Dermatol.* 2000;39(1):18-20.
55. Gandhi K, Ezzedine K, Anastassopoulos KP, et al. Prevalence of vitiligo among adults in the United States. *JAMA Dermatol.* 2022;158(1):43-50.
56. Blomhoff A, Kemp EH, Gawkrodger DJ, et al. CTLA4 polymorphisms are associated with vitiligo, in patients with concomitant autoimmune diseases. *Pigment Cell Res.* 2005;18(1):55-58.
57. Kemp EH, Ajjan RA, Waterman EA, et al. Analysis of a microsatellite polymorphism of the cytotoxic T-lymphocyte antigen-4 gene in patients with vitiligo. *Br J Dermatol.* 1999;140(1):73-78.
58. Canton I, Akhtar S, Gavalas NG, et al. A single-nucleotide polymorphism in the gene encoding lymphoid protein tyrosine phosphatase (PTPN22) confers susceptibility to generalised vitiligo. *Genes Immun.* 2005;6(7):584-587.
59. Spritz RA, Andersen GH. Genetics of vitiligo. *Dermatol Clin.* 2017;35(2):245-255.
60. Mayes MD, Lacey JV, Jr., Beebe-Dimmer J, et al. Prevalence, incidence, survival, and disease characteristics of systemic sclerosis in a large US population. *Arthritis Rheum.* 2003;48(8):2246-2255.
61. Tamaki T, Mori S, Takehara K. Epidemiological study of patients with systemic sclerosis in Tokyo. *Arch Dermatol Res.* 1991;283(6):366-371.
62. Arnett FC, Howard RF, Tan F, et al. Increased prevalence of systemic sclerosis in a Native American tribe in Oklahoma. Association with an Amerindian HLA haplotype. *Arthritis Rheum.* 1996;39(8):1362-1370.
63. Moore DF, Steen VD. Racial disparities in systemic sclerosis. *Rheum Dis Clin North Am.* 2020;46(4):705-712.
64. Arnett FC, Cho M, Chatterjee S, Aguilar MB, Reveille JD, Mayes MD. Familial occurrence frequencies and relative risks for systemic sclerosis (scleroderma) in three United States cohorts. *Arthritis Rheum.* 2001;44(6):1359-1362.
65. Broen JC, Coenen MJ, Radstake TR. Genetics of systemic sclerosis: an update. *Curr Rheumatol Rep.* 2012;14(1):11-21.
66. Reveille JD, Fischbach M, McNearney T, et al. Systemic sclerosis in 3 US ethnic groups: a comparison of clinical, sociodemographic, serologic, and immunogenetic determinants. *Semin Arthritis Rheum.* 2001;30(5):332-346.
67. Prisant L, Loebl D, Mulloy L. Scleroderma renal crisis. *J Clin Hypertensioni.* 2003;5(2).
68. Cepeda E, Reveille JD. Autoantibodies in systemic sclerosis and fibrosing syndromes: clinical indications and relevance. *Curr Opin Rheumatology.* 2004;16(6):723-732.
69. Wang J, Assassi S, Guo G, et al. Clinical and serological features of systemic sclerosis in a Chinese cohort. *Clin Rheumatol.* 2013;32(5):617-621.
70. Tormey V, Bunn C, Denton C, Black C. Anti-fibrillarin antibodies in systemic sclerosis. *Rheumatology.* 2001;40:1157-1162.
71. Sharif R, Fritzler MJ, Mayes MD, et al. Anti-fibrillarin antibody in African American patients with systemic sclerosis: immunogenetics, clinical features, and survival analysis. *J Rheumatol.* 2011;38(8):1622-1630.
72. Johnson R, Tew M, Arnett FC. The genetics of systemic sclerosis. *Curr Rheumatol Rep.* 2002;4:99-107.
73. Gibson F, Hanly A, Grbic N, et al. Epigenetic dysregulation in autoimmune and inflammatory skin diseases. *Clin Rev Allergy Immunol.* 2022;63(3):447-471.
74. Feghali-Bostwick C, Medsger TA, Jr., Wright TM. Analysis of systemic sclerosis in twins reveals low concordance for disease and high concordance for the presence of antinuclear antibodies. *Arthritis Rheum.* 2003;48(7):1956-1963.
75. Rybicki BA, Major M, Popovich J, Maliarik MJ, Iannuzzi MC. Racial differences in sarcoidosis incidence: a 5-year study in a health maintenence organization. *Am J Epidemiol.* 1997;145(3):234-241.
76. Brito-Zeron P, Kostov B, Superville D, Baughman RP, Ramos-Casals M, Autoimmune Big Data Study Group. Geoepidemiological big data approach to sarcoidosis: geographical and ethnic determinants. *Clin Expe Dermatol.* 2019;37:1052-1064.
77. Mirsaeidi M, Machado RF, Schraufnagel D, Sweiss NJ, Baughman RP. Racial difference in sarcoidosis mortality in the United States. *Chest.* 2015;147(2): 438-449.
78. Rybicki BA, Iannuzzi MC, Frederick MM, et al. Familial aggregation of sarcoidosis. A case-control etiologic study of sarcoidosis (ACCESS). *Am J Respir Crit Care Med.* 2001;164(11):2085-2091.
79. Iannuzzi MC, Rybicki BA. Genetics of sarcoidosis: candidate genes and genome scans. *Proc Am Thorac Soc.* 2007;4(1):108-116.
80. Calender A, Weichhart T, Valeyre D, Pacheco Y. Current insights in genetics of sarcoidosis: functional and clinical impacts. *J Clin Med.* 2020;9(8).
81. Sverrild A, Backer V, Kyvik KO, et al. Heredity in sarcoidosis: a registry-based twin study. *Thorax.* 2008;63(10):894-896.
82. Rossman MD, Thompson B, Frederick M, et al. HLA-DRB1*1101: a significant risk factor for sarcoidosis in blacks and whites. *Am J Hum Genet.* 2003;73(4):720-735.
83. Hofmann S, Franke A, Fischer A, et al. Genome-wide association study identifies ANXA11 as a new susceptibility locus for sarcoidosis. *Nat Genet.* 2008;40(9):1103-1106.
84. Jorgensen CS, Levantino G, Houen G, et al. Determination of autoantibodies to annexin XI in systemic autoimmune diseases. *Lupus.* 2000;9(7):515-520.
85. Levin AM, Iannuzzi MC, Montgomery CG, et al. Association of ANXA11 genetic variation with sarcoidosis in African Americans and European Americans. *Genes Immun.* 2013;14(1).
86. Adrianto I, Lin CP, Hale JJ, et al. Genome-wide association study of African and European Americans implicates multiple shared and ethnic specific loci in sarcoidosis susceptibility. *PLoS ONE.* 2012;7(8):e43907.
87. Damsky W, Thakral D, Emeagwali N, Galan A, King B. Tofacitinib treatment and molecular analysis of cutaneous sarcoidosis. *N Engl J Med.* 2018;379(26): 2540-2546.
88. Liu S, Yang H, Song J, Zhang Y, Abualhssain ATH, Yang B. Keloid: genetic susceptibility and contributions of genetics and epigenetics to its pathogenesis. *Exp Dermatol.* 2022;31(11):1665-1675.
89. Hirata M, Kamatani Y, Nagai A, et al. Cross-sectional analysis of BioBank Japan clinical data: a large cohort of 200,000 patients with 47 common diseases. *J Epidemiol.* 2017;27(3S):S9-S21.
90. Kouotou EA, Nansseu JR, Omona Guissana E, et al. Epidemiology and clinical features of keloids in Black Africans: a nested case-control study from Yaounde, Cameroon. *Int J Dermatol.* 2019;58(10):1135-1140.
91. Marneros AG, Norris JE, Olsen BR, Reichenberger E. Clinical genetics of familial keloids. *Arch Dermatol.* 2001;137(11):1429-1434.
92. Nakashima M, Chung S, Takahashi A, et al. A genome-wide association study identifies four susceptibility loci for keloid in the Japanese population. *Nat Genet.* 2010;42(9):768-771.
93. Zhu F, Wu B, Li P, et al. Association study confirmed susceptibility loci with keloid in the Chinese Han population. *PLoS ONE.* 2013;8(5):e62377.
94. Teng G, Liu C, Chen M, Ma K, Liang L, Yan T. Differential susceptible loci expression in keloid and hypertrophic scars in the Chinese Han population. *Ann Plast Surg.* 2015;74(1):26-29.
95. Liu J, Cai L, Zhang Z, Ma Y, Wang Y. Association of leptin receptor gene polymorphisms with keloids in the Chinese Han population. *Med Sci Monit.* 2021;27:e928503.
96. Naik PP. Novel targets and therapies for keloid. *Clin Exp Dermatol.* 2022;47(3):507-515.
97. Li C, Bai Y, Liu H, et al. Comparative study of microRNA profiling in keloid fibroblast and annotation of differential expressed microRNAs. *Acta Biochim Biophys Sin (Shanghai).* 2013;45(8):692-699.
98. Zhou R, Wang C, Lv D, Sun Y, Liang Y. TNF-alpha inhibits fibrosis and migration of fibroblasts in hypertrophic scar by miR-141-3p. *Acta Biochim Biophys Sin (Shanghai).* 2021;53(8):1106-1108.
99. Marneros AG, Norris JE, Watanabe S, Reichenberger E, Olsen BR. Genome scans provide evidence for keloid susceptibility loci on chromosomes 2q23 and 7p11. *J Invest Dermatol.* 2004;122(5):1126-1132.
100. Farag AGA, Khaled HN, Hammam MA, et al. Neuronal precursor cell expressed developmentally down regulated 4 (NEDD4) gene polymorphism contributes to keloid development in Egyptian population. *Clin Cosmet Investig Dermatol.* 2020;13:649-656.
101. Velez Edwards DR, Tsosie KS, Williams SM, Edwards TL, Russell SB. Admixture mapping identifies a locus at 15q21.2-22.3 associated with keloid formation in African Americans. *Hum Genet.* 2014;133(12):1513-1523.

102. Lu WS, Wang JF, Yang S, et al. Association of HLA-DQA1 and DQB1 alleles with keloids in Chinese Hans. *J Dermatol Sci.* 2008;52(2):108-117.
103. Brown JJ, Ollier WE, Thomson W, Bayat A. Positive association of HLA-DRB1*15 with keloid disease in Caucasians. *Int J Immunogenet.* 2008;35(4-5):303-307.
104. Shih B, Bayat A. Comparative genomic hybridisation analysis of keloid tissue in Caucasians suggests possible involvement of HLA-DRB5 in disease pathogenesis. *Arch Dermatol Res.* 2012;304(3):241-249.
105. Santos-Cortez RLP, Hu Y, Sun F, et al. Identification of ASAH1 as a susceptibility gene for familial keloids. *Eur J Hum Genet.* 2017;25(10):1155-1161.
106. Han J, Han J, Yu D, Xiao J, Shang Y, Hao L. Association of ADAM33 gene polymorphisms with keloid scars in a northeastern Chinese population. *Cell Physiol Biochem.* 2014;34(3):981-987.
107. Ogunleye TA, McMichael A, Olsen EA. Central centrifugal cicatricial alopecia: what has been achieved, current clues for future research. *Dermatol Clin.* 2014;32(2):173-181.
108. Sperling LC, Skelton HG, Smith KJ, Sau P, Friedman K. Follicular degeneration syndrome in men. *Arch Dermatol.* 1994;130:763-769.
109. Dlova NC, Salkey KS, Callender VD, McMichael AJ. Central centrifugal cicatricial alopecia: new insights and a call for action. *J Investig Dermatol Symp Proc.* 2017;18(2):S54-S56.
110. Olsen EA, Callender V, McMichael A, et al. Central hair loss in African American women: incidence and potential risk factors. *J Am Acad Dermatol.* 2011;64(2):245-252.
111. Khumalo NP. Prevalence of central centrifugal cicatricial alopecia. *Arch Dermatol.* 2011;147(12):1453-1454.
112. Nnoruka EN. Hair loss: is there a relationship with hair care practices in Nigeria? *Int J Dermatol.* 2005;44 Suppl 1:13-17.
113. Dina Y, Okoye GA, Aguh C. Association of uterine leiomyomas with central centrifugal cicatricial alopecia. *JAMA Dermatol.* 2018;154(2):213-214.
114. Aguh C, Dina Y, Talbot CC Jr, Garza L. Fibroproliferative genes are preferentially expressed in central centrifugal cicatricial alopecia. *J Am Acad Dermatol.* 2018;79(5):904-912.e1.
115. Malki L, Sarig O, Romano MT, et al. Variant PADI3 in central centrifugal cicatricial alopecia. *N Engl J Med.* 2019;380(9):833-841.

CHAPTER 23

Histology

Kayla St. Claire
Oluwakemi Onajin

KEY POINTS

- Skin is the human body's largest organ and composed of the epidermis, dermis, and hypodermis (subcutaneous fat).
- Variations in skin of color are based on the number and size of melanosomes present in both keratinocytes and melanocytes; melanocytes in individuals of African descent are larger, more dendritic, highly enzymatically reactive and melanosomes are individually distributed.
- Characteristics of hair in individuals of African descent that make it susceptible to dryness and breakage include elliptical shape, smaller diameter, frequent narrow twists, thinner cuticle layer, and slower sebum travel.
- There is an increased prevalence of scarring alopecia among Black women due to suggested lower blood flow to scalp, fewer elastic fibers anchoring hair follicles, and earlier disintegration of the inner root sheath.
- Dyspigmentation from postinflammatory hyperpigmentation disproportionately affects skin of color with greater frequency and severity.

SKIN STRUCTURE AND FUNCTION

The integumentary system is composed of skin and its appendages (sweat glands, sebaceous glands, nails, hair follicles, and mammary glands) that derive from the epidermis. The skin is the largest organ of the body and serves as a protective barrier against pathogens, ultraviolet (UV) radiation, mechanical, and chemical injury. Other functions of the skin include body temperature regulation, vitamin D synthesis, fluid homeostasis, and detection of stimuli. Histologically, the skin is composed of three layers in the following order from superficial (external) to deep (internal): epidermis, dermis, and hypodermis (subcutaneous fat) [**Figure 23-1A** and **B**].

In this chapter, a general overview of skin histology will be given, followed by a section on unique aspects seen in skin of color.

EPIDERMIS

The epidermis, derived from the ectoderm, is composed of four to five layers of stratified squamous epithelial cells, also known as keratinocytes. From deep to superficial, the primary layers are the stratum basale, spinosum, granulosum, and corneum [**Figure 23-2**]. The transit time from the basal layer to the stratum corneum, and from the stratum corneum to desquamation is about 14 days at minimum, respectively. Thus, epidermal regeneration occurs as fast as every 28 days. The epidermis lacks a blood supply and obtains its nutrition from the underlying dermis.

Stratum Basale (Stratum Germinativum) The cells of the basal layer are mitotically active and give rise to other keratinocytes. Histologically,

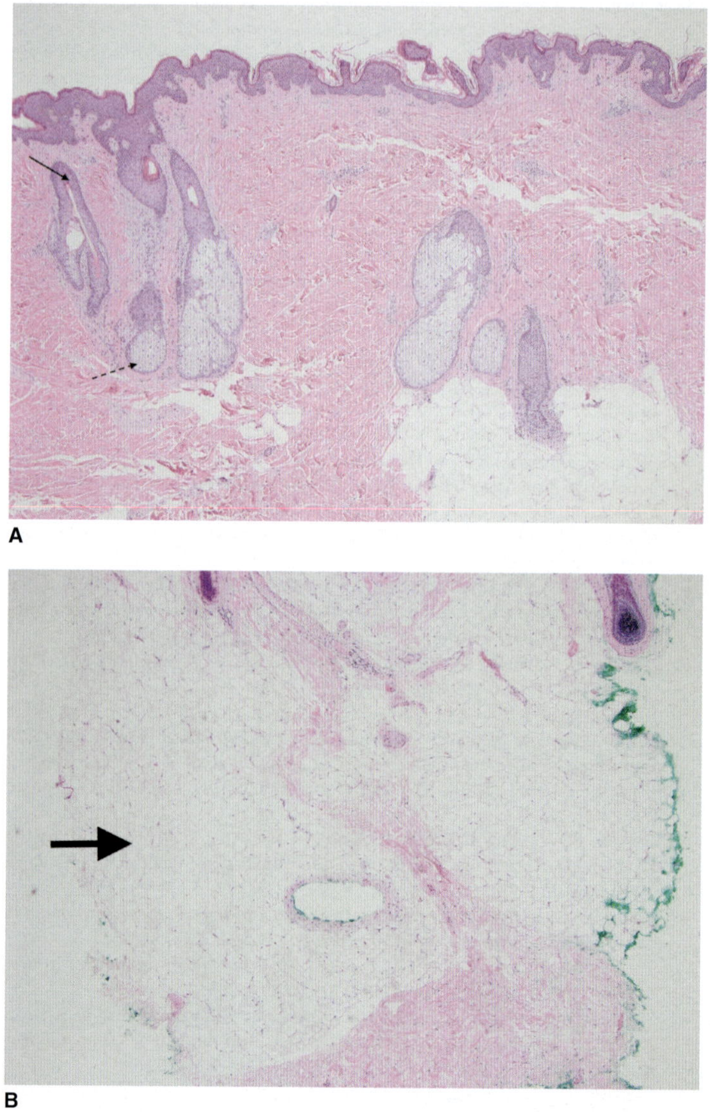

FIGURE 23-1. (A) Normal skin. The skin is composed of the epidermis, dermis, and hypodermis. Skin appendages including sebaceous glands (broken arrow), hair follicles (black arrow) and sweat ducts are present within the dermis. **(B)** Hypodermis: the subcutaneous fat is divided into lobules by vascular fibrous septa. Adipocytes (black arrow) contain a large single globule of lipid that compresses the cytoplasm and nucleus

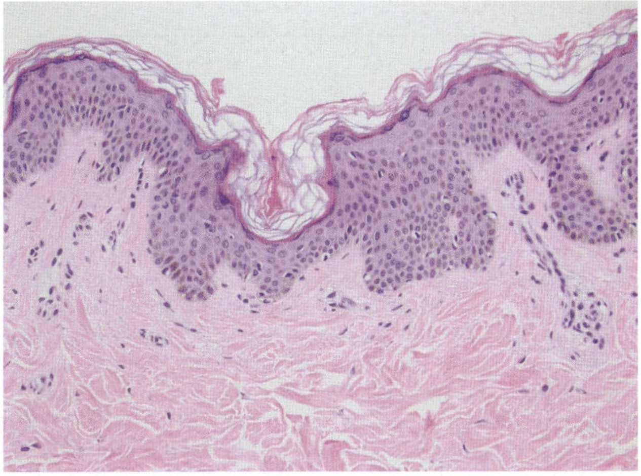

FIGURE 23-2. From deep to superficial, the primary layers of the epidermis are the stratum basale, spinosum, granulosum, and corneum. Keratinocytes constitute the major cell population of the epidermis.

basal cells are columnar or cuboidal, with a round or oval nucleus, coarse chromatin, an indistinct nucleolus, and basophilic cytoplasm.[1] Basal cells present as a single layer above the basement membrane. They are connected to neighboring keratinocytes via desmosomes and to the basement membrane via hemidesmosomes. Melanin is present in the cytoplasm of basal cells as a result of pigment transfer from neighboring melanocytes [**Figure 23-3**].[1]

Stratum Spinosum The spinous or prickle cell layer is named after its characteristic short projections extending from cell to cell that are known as desmosomes. This layer is located superficial to the basal layer and is composed of about 5 to 10 layers of keratinocytes. These keratinocytes are larger than the basal layer with a polyhedral shape, round nucleus, and basophilic cytoplasm.[1]

Stratum Granulosum The granular cell layer contains flattened keratinocytes with cytoplasmic basophilic keratohyalin granules.[2] The thickness of the granular layer is generally proportional to the thickness of the stratum corneum and is typically about one to three layers of keratinocytes.[2]

Stratum Lucidum Considered a subdivision of the stratum corneum, the stratum lucidum presents as a homogenous eosinophilic zone composed of about four to six rows of flattened keratinocytes.[1] It is present in the palms and soles and absent in thin skin.

Stratum Corneum The cornified layer contains about 15 to 20 rows of eosinophilic anucleate keratinocytes that lack cytoplasmic organelles.[3] These cells eventually exfoliate from the surface of the epidermis.

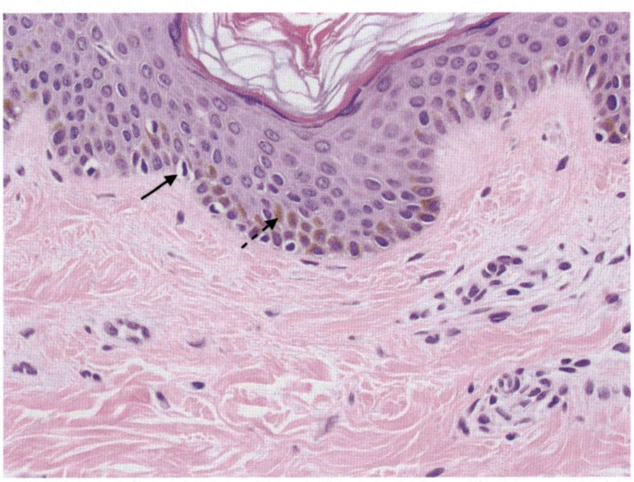

FIGURE 23-3. Skin of color. Melanocytes reside in the basal epidermis. They have elongated or ovoid nuclei surrounded by a clear space (black arrow). Melanin is present in the cytoplasm of basal cells as a result of pigment transfer from neighboring melanocytes (broken arrow).

EPIDERMAL CELLS

Keratinocytes Keratinocytes constitute the major cell population of the epidermis, accounting for approximately 80% of all cells.[4] They are stratified into the above layers. Compared to melanocytes and Langerhans cells, keratinocytes have intercellular bridges and are larger with abundant stainable cytoplasm.[2]

Melanocytes Derived from the neural crest, melanocytes are dendritic cells located in the basal layer of the epidermis, hair bulb, and outer root sheath of hair follicles.[2] They are composed of elongated or ovoid nuclei surrounded by a clear space. The number of melanocytes in relation to basal keratinocytes is typically around 1 to 10 cells, although this varies with body region and increases with exposure to UV radiation.[2] The tyrosine kinase receptor KIT influences melanocyte migration, proliferation, differentiation, and survival. [2] The synthesis of melanin occurs in melanosomes that are lysosome-type organelles. Melanin is produced from its precursor, tyrosine, through a multistep enzymatic process involving tyrosinase, which is a copper-dependent enzyme. At the tips of melanocytic dendrites, the melanosomes containing melanin are phagocytosed and transferred to neighboring basal keratinocytes and hair cortex cells. The epidermal melanin unit is the term used to describe the association of a melanocyte with about 30 to 40 surrounding keratinocytes to which it transfers melanosomes.[5] The major role of melanin is to protect against deleterious effects of nonionizing ultraviolet irradiation.

Langerhans Cells Langerhans cells originate from progenitor cells in the bone marrow similar to other macrophages and monocytes. They are the main antigen-presenting cells of the skin and are primarily present in the stratum spinosum.[1] Once antigens are detected and processed, Langerhans cells migrate to the lymph nodes to active T-cells. These dendritic histiocytes have characteristic reniform (kidney shaped) nuclei and tennis racket-shaped Birbeck granules on electron microscopy.

Merkel Cells Merkel cells are slow-adapting mechanoreceptors that mediate tactile sensation and are scarcely present in the basal layer of the epidermis. They are most heavily concentrated in skin with high hair density and in glabrous epithelium of the digits, lips, oral cavity, and outer root sheath of the hair follicle.[2] It has been postulated that they either originate from differentiated stem cells in the epidermis or are neural crest derived.[2]

DERMAL-EPIDERMAL JUNCTION

The dermal-epidermal junction (DEJ) contains the basement membrane zone, which is a semipermeable barrier that serves to adhere basal keratinocytes to the underlying dermis. It is composed of the lamina lucida, lamina densa, and sublamina densa regions. Additional components include hemidesmosomes, keratin filaments, anchoring filaments, anchoring fibrils (collagen VII), and collagen types I, III, and IV. Defects in any of these constituents can lead to various disease states. Histologically, the DEJ is characterized by an undulating appearance, with epidermal projections (rete ridges) alternating with upwardly protruding dermal papillae [**Figure 23-4**].

DERMIS

Derived from the mesoderm, the dermis is a supportive connective tissue composed of an extracellular matrix that includes collagen, elastic fibers, and ground substance.[2] The dermis consists of two zones, the papillary and reticular dermis. The papillary zone is most superficial, located beneath the epidermis and between the rete ridges. It is thin and has a loose meshwork of predominantly type III collagen admixed with type I collagen and delicate elastic fibers.[1] The reticular zone is thicker with bundles of predominantly type I collagen and broader elastic fibers. The cellular component of the dermis mainly contains fibroblasts, myofibroblasts, macrophages, dermal dendritic cells, and mast cells. Epidermal appendages with their connective tissue sheath, arrector pili

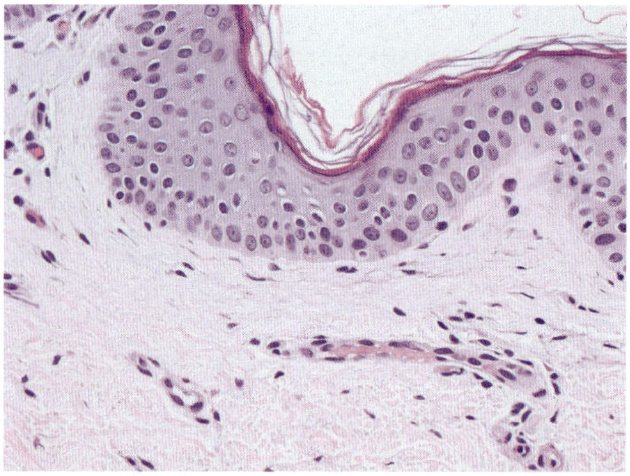

FIGURE 23-4. The derma-epidermal junction is characterized by an undulating appearance, with epidermal projections (rete ridges) alternating with upwardly protruding dermal papillae. The dermis consists of two zones, the thinner, superficial papillary dermis and the thicker reticular dermis composed of bundles of collagen and elastic fibers.

muscles, blood vessels, and nerves are also present within the dermis [Figure 23-1A and 23-4].[2]

DERMAL CELLS

Fibroblasts Fibroblasts are the main dermal cell responsible for synthesis of collagen, elastic tissue, proteoglycan/glycosamingoglycans, and basement membrane.[6] They appear as inconspicuous bipolar spindle cells with elongated ovoid nuclei.[2] Fibroblasts also play a role in proliferation and migration in response to chemotactic, mitogenic, and modulatory cytokines, specifically transforming growth factor beta (TGF-β), keratinocyte growth factor (KGF), granulocyte-macrophage colony-stimulating factor (GM-CSF), interleukin (IL)-6, and fibroblast growth factor (FGF)-10.[6] Fibroblasts produce vascular endothelial growth factor (VEGF) that is important in wound healing, neovascularization, and lymphangiogenesis.[6] Myofibroblasts, a specialized form of fibroblast, are important for wound contraction and reside in granulation tissue.

Mast Cells Mast cells are bone marrow-derived and appear as oval to spindle-shaped cells with a centrally located round to oval nucleus.[2] They are present in the papillary dermis most concentrated around post-capillary venules. Mast cells play an important role in immediate (type 1) hypersensitivity reactions such as anaphylaxis, urticaria, and angioedema. Degranulation of mast cells occurs after many triggers, some of which include cross-linking of IgE on the cell surface, neuropeptides (substance P), and drugs (opiates, aspirin). Mast cells contain mediators that are preformed (histamine, tryptase) and newly formed (prostaglandins, leukotrienes) that upon release exert functions such as vasodilation and smooth muscle contraction.

HYPODERMIS

Also called the subcutaneous fat, the hypodermis plays a role in thermal regulation, insulation, mechanical cushioning, energy storage, and endocrine function. Fat is divided into lobules by vascular fibrous septa. Fat cells, known as adipocytes, contain a large single globule of lipid that compresses the cytoplasm and nucleus [Figure 23-1B]. The cytoplasm contains numerous mitochondria. Adipocytes have important roles in osteogenesis and angiogenesis.[6] Fat comprises both white and brown adipose tissue. Deposits of brown adipose tissue are more common in infants and children and mainly present in the interscapular region, back, thorax, and mediastinum.[6] Brown adipose tissue has different mitochondrial properties and increased heat production.[6]

SKIN APPENDAGES

ECCRINE GLANDS

The secretory eccrine gland is the primary gland responsible for thermoregulatory sweating in humans and waste excretion.[6] Eccrine glands are most concentrated on the palms, soles, forehead, and axillae. Histologically, the eccrine gland is divided into four subunits: a highly vascularized coiled secretory gland, a coiled dermal duct, a straight dermal duct, and a coiled intraepidermal duct (the acrosyringium).[6] The secretory coil is present in the lower dermis and has an outer discontinuous layer of contractile myoepithelial cells that are stimulated by acetylcholine and an inner layer of clear and dark secretory cells.[6] The convoluted and straight dermal ducts are narrow tubes with a slit-like lumina lined by double layers of basophilic cuboidal cells.[1] The intraepidermal portion has a helical course in the epidermis and opens directly onto the surface of the skin. It consists of a single layer of luminal cells and two or three rows of concentrically oriented outer cells.[1] The initial fluid released from secretory cells is isotonic but becomes hypotonic as it reaches the skin surface.

APOCRINE GLANDS

Apocrine glands have low secretory output and their function in humans is unknown. In other mammals, they are responsible for scent production and sexual attraction. These glands are primarily in the anogenital, axillary, periumbilical, breast, vermilion lip, eyelid, and external ear regions.[6] At puberty, apocrine glands become larger, functionally active, and are stimulated by circulating catecholamines. Apocrine glands have a coiled secretory portion and an excretory (ductal) component. The secretory portion is in the lower reticular dermis or subcutaneous fat and is composed of an outer discontinuous layer of myoepithelial cells and an inner layer of cuboidal to columnar eosinophilic cells.[6] The ductal component has a double layer of cuboidal cells and links the gland with the pilosebaceous follicle above the sebaceous duct.[1] Secretory products are released through decapitation secretion. Apocrine secretion is odorless, but unpleasant odor can occur due to breakdown products by cutaneous bacterial flora.[6]

SEBACEOUS GLANDS

These secretory exocrine glands are prominent on the scalp, face, and upper trunk and absent on palms and soles. They are associated with hair follicles and empty into the inferior portion of the infundibulum. Sebaceous glands typically have several lipid-containing lobules leading into a common excretory duct composed of stratified squamous epithelium [Figure 23-1A].[2] They enlarge at puberty due to increased androgen output and are stimulated by various endocrine factors. Secretory products are released via disintegration of cells, known as holocrine secretion. Secretions are mainly composed of triglycerides followed by wax esters and squalene, respectively.[6]

HAIR FOLLICLE

The pilar unit is composed of a hair follicle, sebaceous gland, and arrector pili muscle [**Figure 23-5**]. The hair follicle is divided into three segments: the infundibulum (which extends from the epidermal opening to the sebaceous duct opening), the isthmus (which extends from the sebaceous duct entrance to the insertion of the arrector pili muscle), and the inferior segment (which extends from the arrector pili insertion to the base of the follicle).[1] The inferior segment or hair bulb is composed of five major components: dermal hair papilla, hair matrix, hair shaft (from inward to outward consisting of medulla, cortex, and hair cuticle), inner root sheath (from inward to outward consisting of inner root sheath cuticle, Huxley layer, Henle layer), and the outer root sheath.[2] The hair bulb contains the pluripotent cells of the hair matrix that give rise to the hair and inner root sheath.[2] Melanocytes are mainly present in the upper half of the bulb.[1] The color of hair depends on the amount and distribution of melanin in the hair shaft. The hair shaft is predominantly composed of keratin. The bulge region at the site of the arrector pili muscle insertion contains stem cells that participate in regeneration of the hair follicle during cycling.[2] The hair cycle consists of three phases: anagen, the

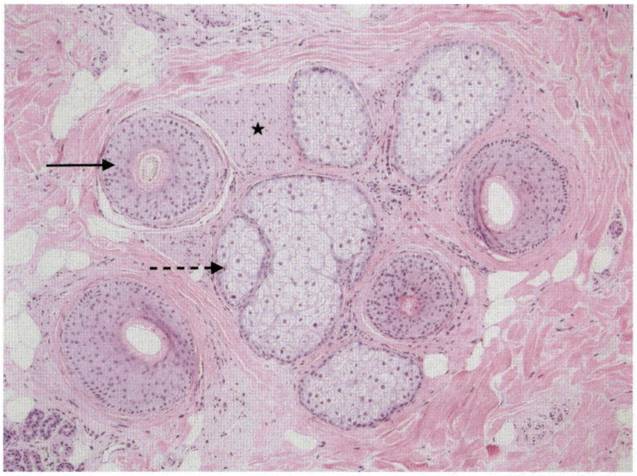

FIGURE 23-5. A cross-section of the hair shaft from a person of African descent has an elliptical shape. The pilar unit is composed of a hair follicle (black arrow), sebaceous gland (broken arrow), and arrector pili muscle (black star).

active growth phase; catagen, the involuting phase; and telogen, the resting phase. After completion of the cycle, a new anagen phase begins with formation of new hair matrix. The duration of normal hair cycle varies based on body location. For the scalp, anagen lasts about 3 years, catagen 3 weeks, and telogen 3 months. In a healthy scalp, about 84% of hairs are in anagen, 2% in catagen, and 14% in telogen.[2] On average, scalp hair grows 1 cm a month and about 100 hairs are lost per day.[7] Curliness of hair is determined by disulfide bonding via cysteine residues.

NAIL UNIT

A region of specialized keratinization, the nail unit has six main components: nail matrix (gives rise to nail plate), nail plate, cuticular system (contains dorsal component, or cuticle, and distal component, or hyponychium), nail bed (includes dermis, underlying bone, and soft tissue underneath nail plate), anchoring system of ligaments between bone and matrix proximally and between grooves distally, and nail folds (proximal, lateral, and distal).[2] The proximal matrix forms the dorsal nail plate and the distal matrix forms the ventral nail plate. Nail thickness is predominantly determined by the matrix.[2] Melanocytes reside in the distal nail matrix. The nail plate is composed of dense, interdigitating corneocytes lacking nuclei or organelles.[2] Fingernails grow about 2 to 3 mm per month, while toenails grow about 1 mm per month.[7]

SKIN OF COLOR PHYSIOLOGY

SKIN PIGMENTATION

The ratio of melanocytes to basal keratinocytes in normal skin is constant (1:10) in all races. Variations in skin of color are based on the number and size of melanosomes present in both keratinocytes and melanocytes. The two forms of melanin pigment are eumelanin and pheomelanin. Eumelanin is a brown or black pigment made from elliptical melanosomes and is found in darker skin types. Pheomelanin is a yellow-red pigment made by round melanosomes and predominates in lighter skin types. In skin of individuals of African descent, melanocytes are larger, more dendritic, and highly enzymatically reactive [Figure 23-3].[2] Additionally, transferred melanosomes within keratinocytes are more individually distributed, whereas in white skin are packaged in membrane-enclosed aggregates.[2]

HAIR

In individuals of African descent, a cross-section of the hair shaft demonstrates an elliptical shape and, while smaller, its diameter varies throughout the hair shaft [Figure 23-5].[8] In addition, the hair shaft is characterized by frequent narrow twists along its longitudinal axis. This, combined with its thinner cuticle layer, makes it more susceptible to knotting and breakage.[8] There are no differences in cysteine content of keratin proteins between different racial groups.[8] There are also no differences in the hair growth cycle; however, studies have shown that hair grows slower on average in Black females compared to those identified as White or Asian.[8] In hair of African descent and other curly hair types, it is harder for sebum to travel from the scalp along the hair shaft, leading to drier hair.[8] There are conflicting studies on differences in sebaceous gland size and activity among different racial groups.[8]

REGIONAL HISTOLOGIC VARIATIONS AND RELEVANCE IN SKIN OF COLOR

SCALP

Histologically, a biopsy from a healthy scalp shows many terminal hairs with their bulbs deeply anchored in the subcutaneous tissue. Sebaceous and eccrine glands are prominent, whereas apocrine glands are scarce and nonfunctional. Bald areas can mimic biopsies from the skin of the face, showing prominence of sebaceous glands and vellus hairs.[9]

Central Centrifugal Cicatricial Alopecia and Traction Alopecia In comparison to other races, there is an increasing prevalence of scarring alopecia in Black women given suggested lower blood flow to scalp, fewer elastic fibers anchoring hair follicles, and earlier disintegration of the inner root sheath.[8] Central centrifugal cicatricial alopecia (CCCA) is the most common cause of scarring alopecia among women of African descent. CCCA begins at the vertex and spreads in a centrifugal pattern leading to permanent hair loss [**Figure 23-6A**]. Horizontal sections are useful to identify early features of CCCA. The most common pathologic findings for CCCA are decreased number of terminal follicles, premature desquamation of the inner root sheath, loss of sebaceous glands, compound follicular structures with perifollicular fibrosis and/or inflammation, and naked hair shafts [**Figure 23-6B**].[10] The prevalence of traction alopecia is highest among women of African descent; it occurs from tension of repeated traumatic hairstyles such as tight braids, weaves, or ponytails. It presents with hair thinning along the frontotemporal hairline. In the early nonscarring phase, there is an increased number of terminal catagen and/or telogen hairs, with normal size and number of follicles, and no significant inflammation.[11] In the end scarring stage, terminal hairs are markedly reduced, some follicles are replaced with connective tissue, sebaceous glands persist in follicular units with loss of their hair-producing epithelium, and there is no significant perifollicular inflammation.[11]

FACIAL SKIN

Generally facial skin has an abundance of pilosebaceous units. Apocrine glands are few. The female face and nonbearded male face show vellus hairs. The bearded male face shows terminal hairs. The forehead is particularly rich in sebaceous glands. The nose has the highest density of sebaceous glands.[9] Eyelid skin is the thinnest and contains cutaneous and conjunctival portions. For eyelid skin, the epidermis is flat, dermis is thin, and hypodermis is usually not present, with bundles of the orbicularis oculi muscle seen in the reticular dermis.[9] The hypodermis is thinner on the forehead and nose but is thicker on the cheek. Skeletal muscle is more superficial on the face; these muscle fibers may be seen particularly in the dermis of the lips and periorbital areas.[2]

Postinflammatory Hyperpigmentation Postinflammatory hyperpigmentation (PIH) is an acquired hypermelanosis that occurs in response to cutaneous inflammation or injury and disproportionately affects skin of color patients with greater frequency and severity. On the face, it commonly occurs with acne, pseudofolliculitis barbae, atopic dermatitis, and impetigo. There are two histopathological patterns of PIH: epidermal and dermal. With epidermal PIH, there is increased production and transfer of melanin to surrounding keratinocytes, which clinically appears tan to dark brown.[12] Dermal PIH results from inflammation that damages basal keratinocytes, releasing

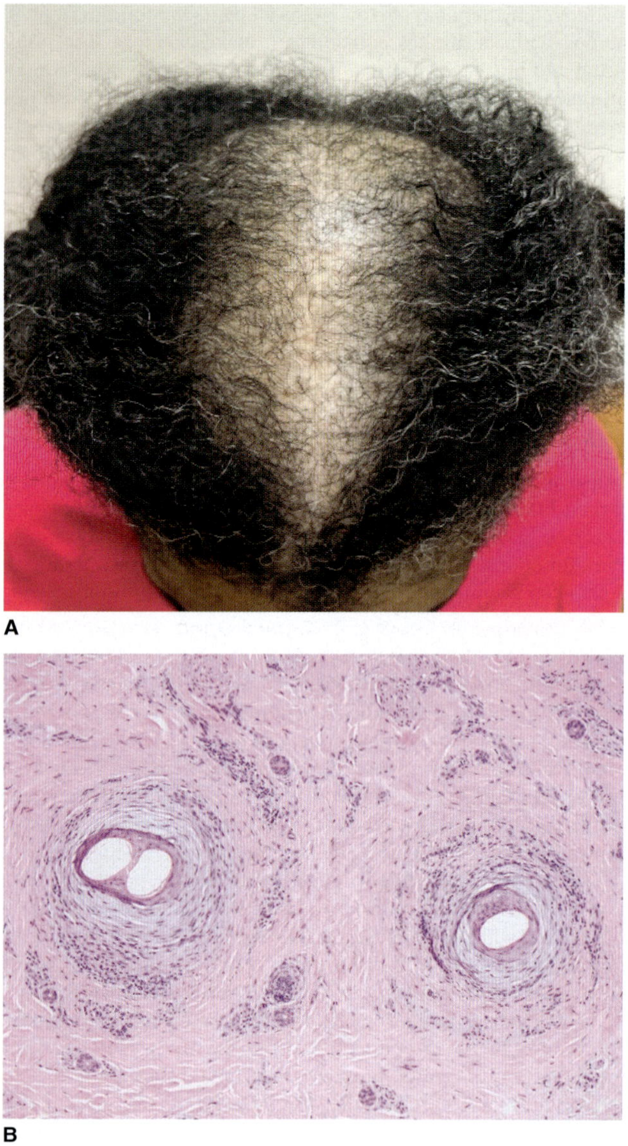

FIGURE 23-6. **(A)** Central centrifugal cicatricial alopecia (CCCA): CCCA begins at the vertex and spreads in a centrifugal pattern leading to permanent hair loss. **(B)** Central centrifugal cicatricial alopecia (CCCA): a cross-section of the scalp shows decreased number of terminal follicles, premature desquamation of the inner root sheath, loss of sebaceous glands, polytrichia with perifollicular fibrosis and inflammation.

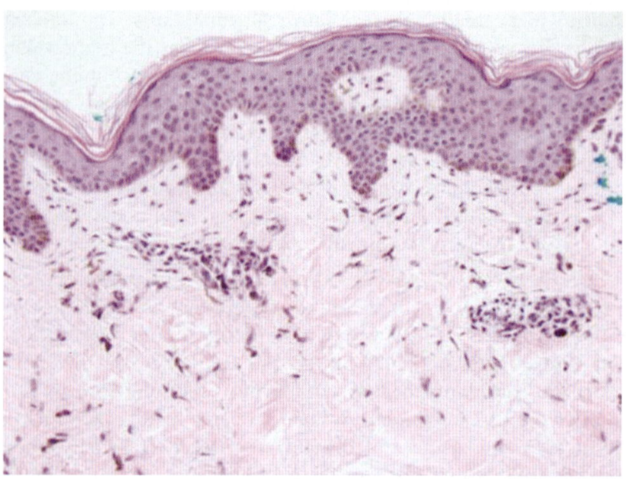

FIGURE 23-7. Postinflammatory hyperpigmentation: there is perivascular lymphocytic inflammation with deposition of melanin pigment and melanophages in the superficial dermis.

large amounts of melanin into the upper dermis that is phagocytosed by macrophages (melanophages) [**Figure 23-7**]; this clinically demonstrates a blue-gray appearance.[12] Lichen planus pigmentosus (LPP), a variant of lichen planus, predominantly observed in dark-skinned patients, commonly presents as acquired dark brown to gray-blue macules that coalesce with ill-defined borders. It affects sun-exposed areas, but mainly localizes to the temporal and preauricular face and neck [**Figure 23-8A**].[13] Histologically, LPP displays vacuolar degeneration of the basal layer and a band-like lichenoid or perivascular lymphocytic infiltrate in the papillary dermis with pigment incontinence and melanophages [**Figure 23-8B**].[13]

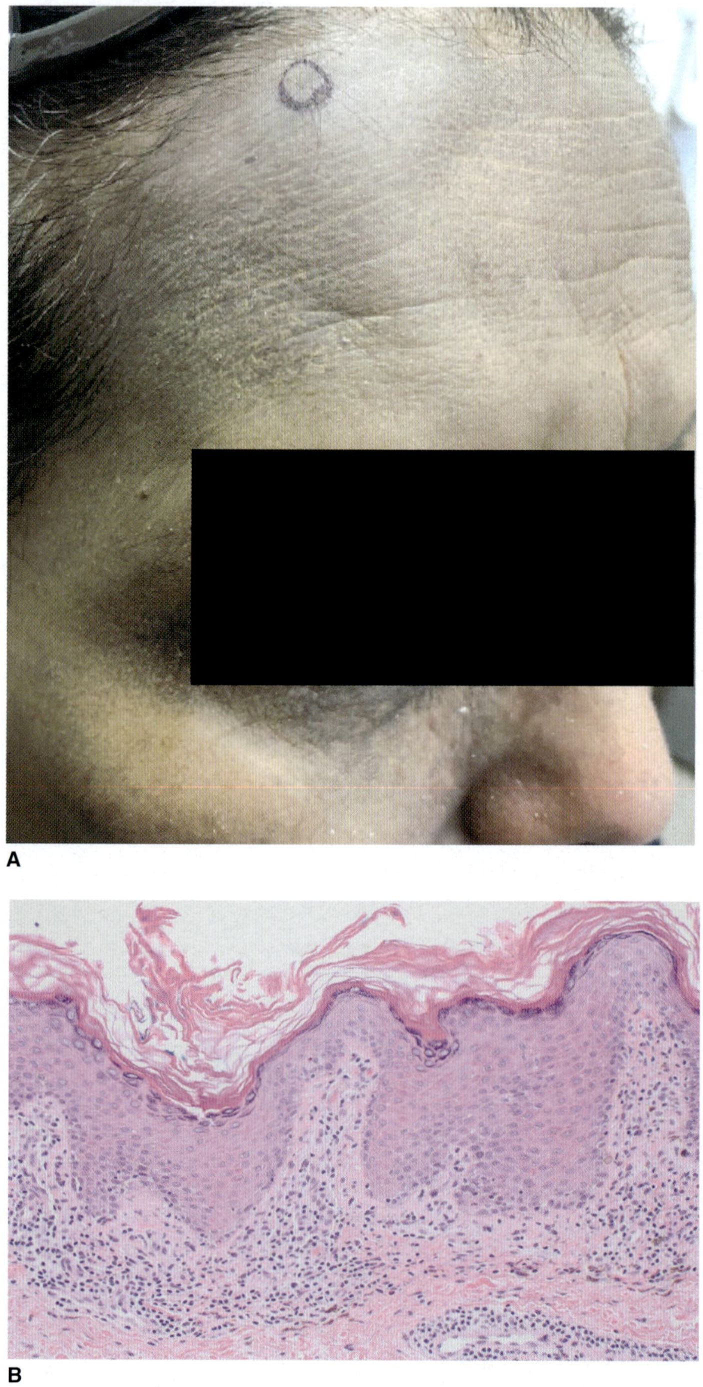

FIGURE 23-8. **(A)** Lichen planus pigmentosus (LPP): dark brown to gray-blue macules localized to temporal face. **(B)** Lichen planus pigmentosus (LPP): there is vacuolar degeneration of the basal layer and band-like lichenoid infiltrate in the papillary dermis with pigment incontinence and melanophages. (Courtesy of Dr. Travis Vandergriff.)

ACRAL SKIN

Skin from the palms and soles is notable for its thick, compact stratum corneum, presence of stratum lucidum, prominent granular layer, and distinguished rete ridges.[9] These areas have abundant eccrine glands and lack pilosebaceous units. Glomus cells (specialized smooth muscle cells derived from Sucquet-Hoyer canals) are present in the dermis and they are responsible for shunting blood from arterioles to venules, bypassing capillaries. Meissner corpuscles are located in the dermal papillae and are mechanoreceptors responsible for light touch. Subcutaneous tissue of digits are rich in Pacinian corpuscles that are sensory receptors that detect deep pressure and vibration.

Acral Lentiginous Melanoma Acral lentiginous melanoma (ALM) is the most common type of melanoma in Black, Asian/Pacific Islander, and Latine/Hispanic populations. Early ALM presents as an asymmetric brown macule or patch with irregular borders and variegated pigmentation [**Figure 23-9A**].[14] Diagnosing early ALM may be challenging given its location (frequently at the sole), subtle histopathologic features, dermatoglyphic pattern of furrows and ridges, and inadequate specimen size, sectioning, or sampling of the pigmented lesion. The following architectural and cytologic features may aid in diagnosis of ALM: (a) melanocytic nuclei are hyperchromatic and larger than keratinocytes, (b) melanocytes have angulated and vertically arranged nuclei with thick, elongated, uneven dendrites, (c) melanocytes' thick, elongated

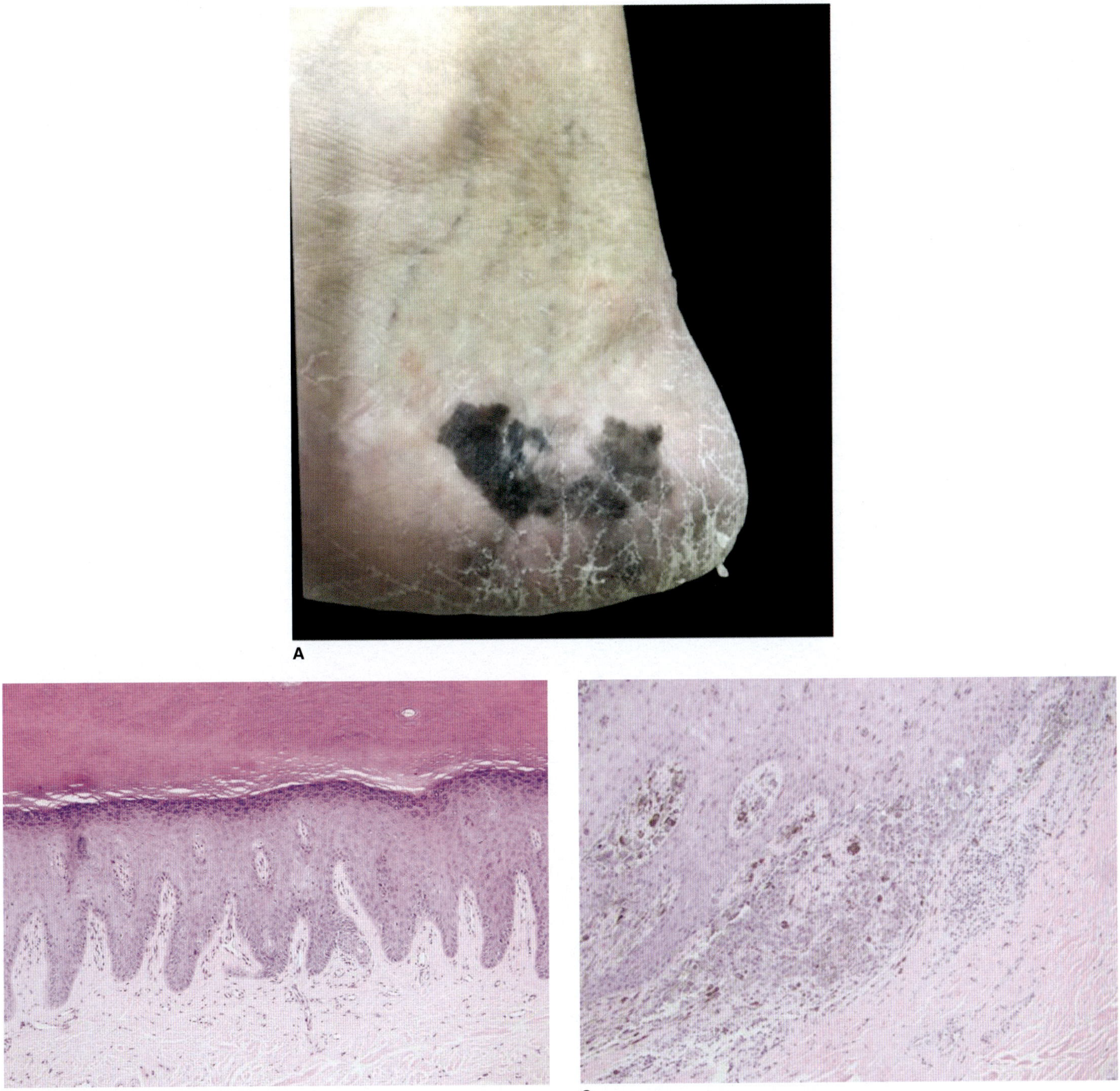

A

B

C

FIGURE 23-9. (A) Acral lentiginous melanoma in situ: asymmetric brown patch with irregular borders and variegated pigmentation on the heel of the foot. **(B)** Acral lentiginous melanoma in situ: low cell density proliferation of single atypical melanocytes along the dermoepidermal junction in early melanoma in situ. **(C)** Acral lentiginous melanoma: higher cell density proliferation of atypical melanocytes with confluent growth and pagetoid spread.

dendrites reach the superficial epidermis and their dendritic processes form webs around basal keratinocytes, (d) pagetoid melanocytes demonstrate an increased nuclear-to-cytoplasm ratio and/or dendritic or pleomorphic morphology and have hyperchromatic nuclei, (e) solitary melanocytes preferentially proliferate in the crista profunda intermedia (ridge pattern), (f) presence of a papillary dermal lymphocytic infiltrate [**Figure 23-9B and C**].[14]

REFERENCES

1. Kanik A. Skin. In: Mills SE, ed. *Histology for Pathologists*. 5th ed. Lippincott Williams & Wilkins; 2020:3-30.
2. Lian C, Murphy G. Histology of the Skin. In: Elder DE. *Lever's Histopathology of the Skin*. 11th ed. Wolters Kluwer Health; 2015:39-154.
3. Arda O, Göksügür N, Tüzün Y. Basic histological structure and functions of facial skin. *Clin Dermatol*. 2014;32(1):3-13.
4. Hood AF, Kwan TH, Mihm MC, et al. Introduction-normal histology of the skin. In: Hood AF, Kwan TH, Mihm MC, et al, eds. *Primer of Dermatopathology*. 3rd ed. Lippincott Williams & Wilkins; 2002:3-15.
5. Bolognia J, Orlow S. Melanocyte biology. In: Bolognia JL, ed. *Dermatology*. 4th ed. Elsevier; 2018:1075-1086.
6. McGrath, J. The structure and function of skin. In: Calonje, E, ed. *McKee's Pathology of the* Skin. 5th ed. Elsevier, 2020:1-34.
7. Wang E, de Berker D, Christiano A. Biology of hair and nails. In: Bolognia JL. *Dermatology*. 4th ed. Elsevier; 2018:1144-1161.
8. He A, Okoye G. Chemical and physical properties of hair: comparisons between Asian, Black, and Caucasian hair. In: Aguh C, Okoye G, ed. *Fundamentals of Ethnic Hair*. Switzerland: Springer; 2017:3-13.
9. Fernandez-Flores A. Regional variations in the histology of the skin. *Am J Dermatopathol*. 2015;37(10):737-754.
10. Miteva M, Tosti A. Pathologic diagnosis of central centrifugal cicatricial alopecia on horizontal sections. *Am J Dermatopathol*. 2014;36(11):859-867.
11. Sperling LC, Sinclair RD, El Shabrawi-Caelen L. Alopecias. In: Bolognia JL, ed. *Dermatology*. 4th ed. Elsevier; 2018:1162-1187.
12. Davis EC, Callender VD. Postinflammatory hyperpigmentation: a review of the epidemiology, clinical features, and treatment options in skin of color. *J Clin Aesthet Dermatol*. 2010;3(7):20-31.
13. Robles-Méndez JC, Rizo-Frías P, Herz-Ruelas ME, Pandya AG, Ocampo Candiani J. Lichen planus pigmentosus and its variants: review and update. *Int J Dermatol*. 2018;57(5):505-514.
14. Darmawan CC, Jo G, Montenegro SE, et al. Early detection of acral melanoma: a review of clinical, dermoscopic, histopathologic, and molecular characteristics. *J Am Acad Dermatol*. 2019;81(3):805-812.

SECTION 4

Cutaneous Disorders

CHAPTER 24

Nuances in Skin of Color

Toni Jenkins
Hope Mitchell

KEY POINTS

- Pigmentation variation is normal in dark-skin people and is not necessarily a sign of disease.
- Uneven skin tone is one of the most common dermatological concerns of people with dark skin.
- Pigmentary demarcation lines (PDLs) are unique marks that show a distinctive line between lighter and darker skin in dark-skin people.
- Hyperpigmentation is a common postinflammatory manifestation in dark skin.
- Acanthosis nigricans is a common dermatologic condition seen in dark skin.
- Hair structure, composition, and cultural practices play an important role in dermatologic conditions affecting the hair and scalp, particularly in Black patients.
- Infants with dark skin tone can have localized hyperpigmentation.

INTRODUCTION

In 2016, Black, Asian, and Hispanic people made up 36.8% of the U.S. population. By 2060, it is estimated that these groups will make up 51.6% of the American population due in large part to the Hispanic population, and the majority of the U.S. population will be non-White.[1] Accurately diagnosing and treating people with dark skin types requires cultural competency and knowledge about differences in disease presentation. Identifying dermatologic conditions in dark-skin people requires the unique ability to recognize nuances in presentation. These nuances revolve around understanding the variations in color presentations of dermatologic conditions on dark skin, hair structure, and cultural self-perceptions of skin and hair health in this population. Reddish-brown or purplish discoloration may represent inflammation or active disease in people with dark skin types in contrast to pink or red tones seen in fair-skinned patients. In addition, knowledge about hair structure and cultural hair practices in Black people can enhance communication and contribute to accurate diagnosis and effective treatment plans and prevent poor outcomes. In some conditions, like melanoma, it is particularly important to be attune to nuances since people tend to present with more advanced and progressive disease. Culturally competent physicians can provide education and quality care to dark-skin patients by bringing awareness to what is a normal presentation versus when they should be concerned.

There is a call to amplify images used to illustrate skin diseases in dark skin types. These images have been sparse in the medical literature and are an integral component of understanding how dermatologic conditions present in people with dark skin types.[2] Dermatologists may readily pick up on inflammatory processes seen within light skin by visualizing redness or erythema as a component of the dermatologic manifestation and by the abundance of images found in the medical literature. However, as an example, rashes can affect all skin types and the inflammatory component may not look red on dark skin types. In fact, rashes may look purplish, reddish-brown, or even be difficult to discern in dark skin tones. It is imperative to advocate for dark skin representation in textbooks and other educational materials to train the next generation of dermatologists.

NORMAL VARIATIONS IN SKIN AND HAIR

Skin serves as a window into the physiology and pathology occurring within. Visual examination provides both opportunity to identify and differentiate important nuances that are normal variants in darker skin as well as diagnose disease.[3] Normal variations in dark skin include findings such as dark pigmentation on the vermillion border around the lips. The melanin present in skin is also located in gum tissue. As a result, dark-skin people may have dark gums as well as hard palate and buccal mucosa [**Figure 24-1**]. Also, this population can have dark pigmentation on the surface of the lips. Adults with dark skin may have pigmented sclera that look yellow or brown; this is another normal variant. Hyperpigmentation in the extensor areas like the knees and elbows can be a normal variation seen in dark skin. The areola in people with dark skin tends to be darker and can present with seborrheic keratosis seen near the nipple.

People with dark skin types can have variations in hair texture and styling practices. For example, some people with dark skin types who have "afro-textured hair" tend to wash their hair once a week or every 2 weeks. Furthermore, dark-skinned people with "afro-textured hair" who report having "permed hair" are describing a process in which the hair has been chemically relaxed or straightened and not chemically curled. Therefore, it is imperative that dermatologists understand the culture of different populations and nuances in hair care practices prior to developing treatment plans. Nails can also have normal variations in this population. People with darker skin can have darker nails or linear streaks in the nails.[4] Longitudinal melanonychia is an example of a physical exam finding that would be concerning in light-skinned patients but is normal in dark-skin patients; pigmented bands may start at the nail bed and extend the length of the nail [**Figure 24-2**].

Pigmentary demarcation lines (PDL) are normal variants in dark skin that can result in sharp distinctive lines seen in these people. Voigt-Futcher lines are an example of PDL that typically extend vertically on the arms and legs [**Figure 24-3**]. They can also be seen along the spine and the abdomen. Another example of PDL is the linea nigra, which is a line from the umbilicus to the mons pubis. The linea nigra typically presents in pregnancy when the line darkens and becomes more apparent, more so in dark-skin people. The linea nigra typically resolves on its own postpregnancy.[5]

Follicular accentuation is a common condition seen in dark-skin people. It can have a goosebump appearance and denote inflammation around the hair follicles. Punctate keratosis of palmar creases is also common in this population as well and presents with skin lesions on the palmar surface [**Figure 24-4**].

PIGMENTARY VARIATION AND DYSCHROMIA

Melanin pigmentation in the skin is responsible for the variation in skin tones. Melanocytes produce melanin within their melanosomes, organelles responsible for synthesis, storage, and transport of melanin. African skin types have the largest melanosomes followed by Indian, Mexican,

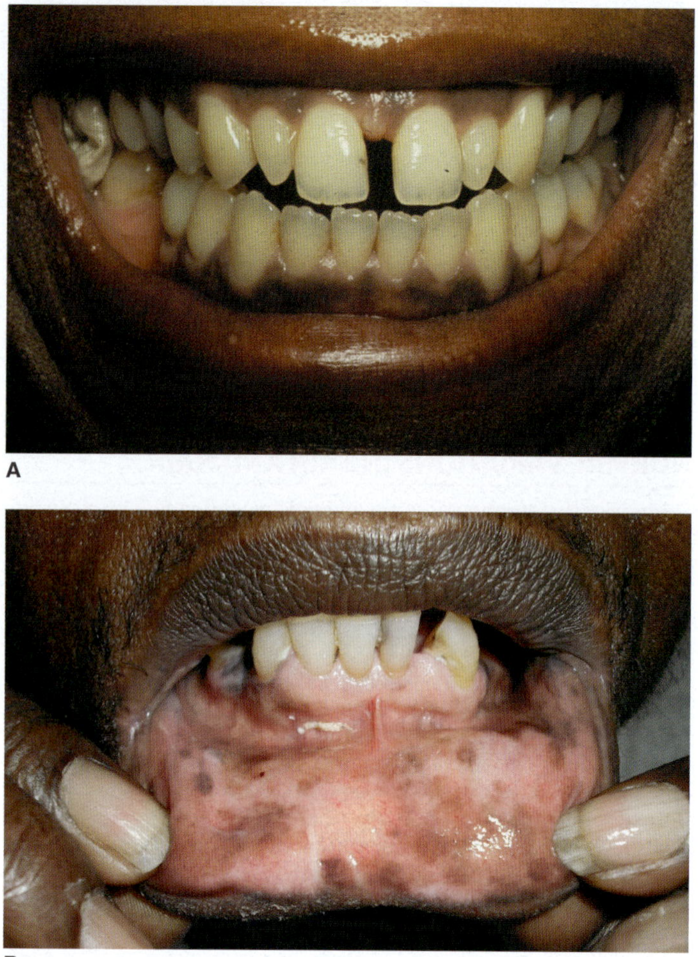

A

B

FIGURE 24-1. Hyperpigmentation demonstrated in the gingiva **(A)** and buccal mucosa **(B)**.

Chinese, and European people.[6] People of all races have the same number of melanocytes; however, people with dark skin types have larger and more numerous melanosomes that interestingly are more sensitive to trauma, heat, and solar radiation. When melanocytes become damaged or unhealthy, skin pigmentation disorders can result. If the body makes too much melanin and releases it into the skin, darker patches result. Dark-skin individuals may require a nuanced approach in the diagnosis and management of some dermatologic conditions.

Dark-skin individuals can present with discoloration in various hues. What may be described as "erythematous" in the medical literature on light skin may appear reddish-brown or look skin-toned and represent an inflammatory process in dark skin [**Figure 24-5A** and **B**]. Hues that are purple, blue, silver, and pink can also be seen in dark skin. Sometimes lesions and dermatologic conditions may not appear with a distinctive color but may present with light or dark patches seen on the skin. Knowing the various nuances in color presentation can aid in building a thorough differential list and diagnosis in dark skin. Dark-skin individuals often present with hyperpigmentation, dyschromia/discoloration, or pigment discoloration and are ultimately concerned about ways to prevent permanent discoloration or scarring often involving their face, back, chest, and arms.

Dyschromias are a category of conditions characterized by uneven pigmentation and may clinically include hyperpigmentation, hypopigmentation, or mottled skin. Uneven skin tone is one of the most common chief complaints seen in darker skin individuals seeking dermatologic care. Even skin tone is an important aspect of the overall aesthetic of skin for dark skin. It is very important to understand the normal variations of skin discoloration in dark skin in order to provide an accurate diagnosis, appropriate education, and proper treatment.

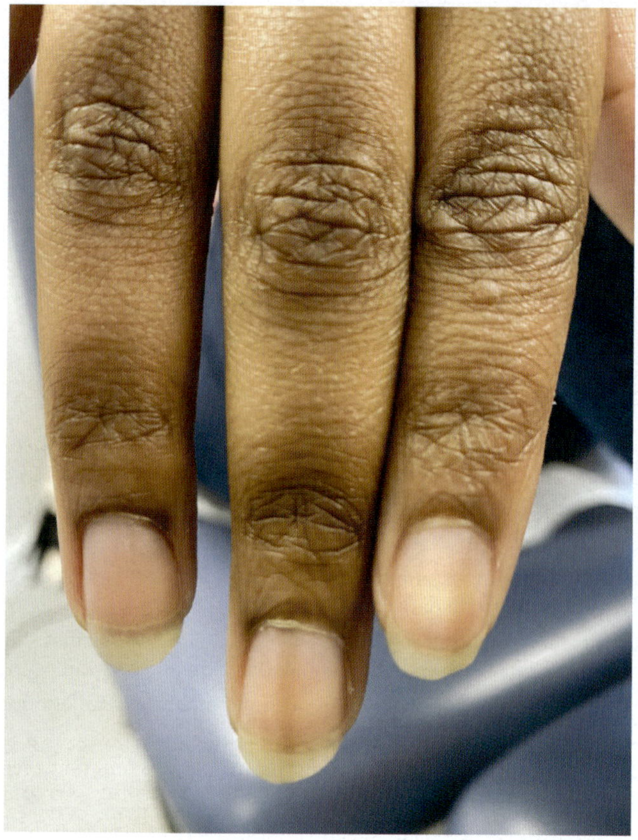

FIGURE 24-2. Pigmented bands seen on the nails of a dark skin patient.

Common causes of hyperpigmentation in dark skin include melasma and postinflammatory hyperpigmentation (PIH) from conditions like acne. Acne in all people tends to present with inflammatory lesions and can result in scarring. Nuances in dark-skin individuals suffering from acne revolve around hyperpigmentation and concurrent scarring.[7]

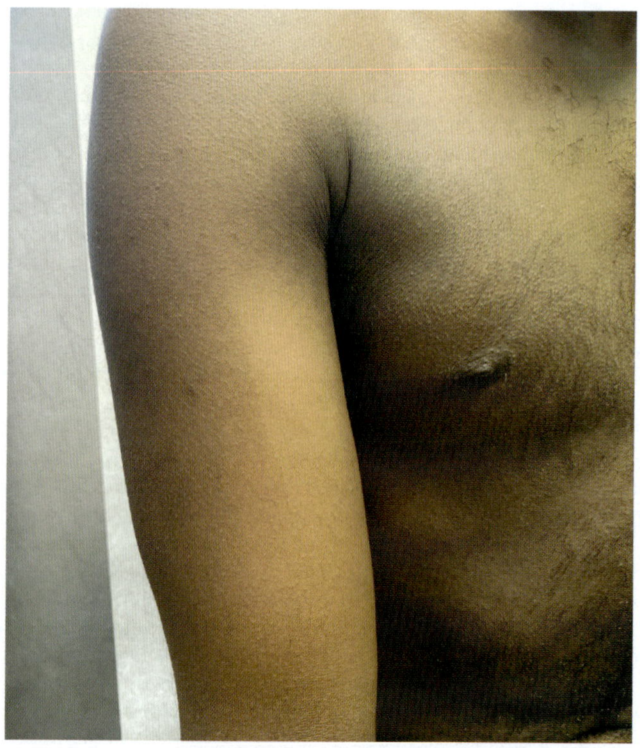

FIGURE 24-3. Pigmentary Demarcation Line (PDL) demonstrated on the arm of a dark skin patient.

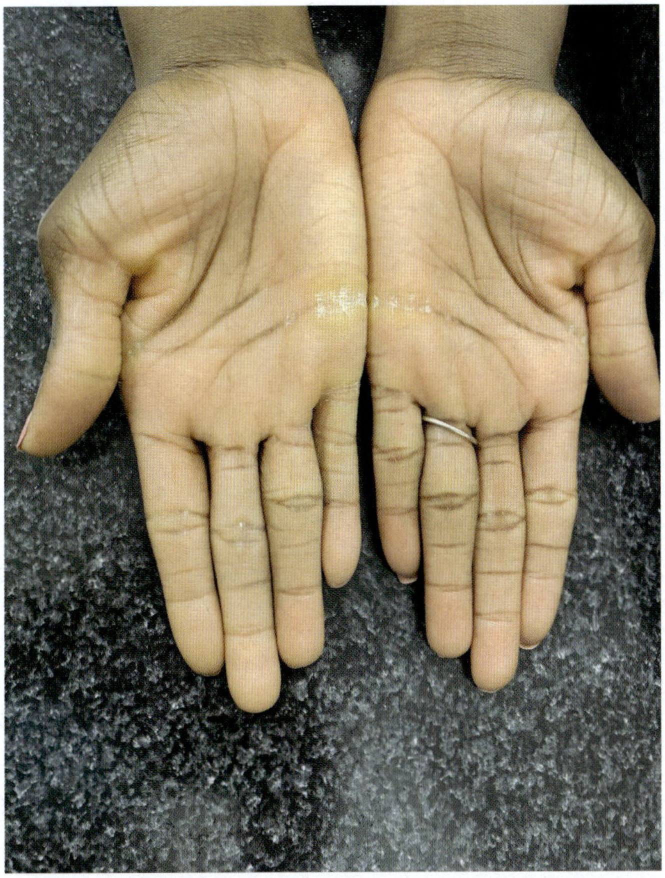

FIGURE 24-4. Punctate keratosis of palmar creases of the hands demonstrated in a dark skin patient.

Dark-skin individuals tend to have a higher incidence of discoloration and usually present with advanced acne progression. Medical literature tends to describe acne mainly as an inflammatory process with erythematous or red papules. Dark-skin patients' acne presentation is marked by reddish-brown hues and hyperpigmentation denoting their inflammatory process. Postinflammatory erythema (PIE) and PIH are common conditions seen during the resolution process of acne. Dark-skin patients typically present with acne-induced PIH and one should prioritize managing this condition to prevent scarring.

People with dark skin types may also present with concerns of hypopigmentation. Hypopigmentation in dark skin tones may indicate xerosis of the skin, may be postinflammatory, or be secondary to underlying disease processes. Some cases of hypopigmentation are easily diagnosed, whereas other manifestations of hypopigmentation may require further investigation (ie, biopsy). Pityriasis alba can result in faint hypopigmented patches on the face and upper extremities and is more commonly seen in children [**Figure 24-6**]. Often caregivers will bring children into the office because they are concerned they may have vitiligo. This warrants proper patient education and assurance. Idiopathic guttate hypomelanosis (IGH) is a benign condition that is asymptomatic. Physical exams on these patients can show hypopigmented macules on sun-exposed regions. Mycosis fungoides (MF), tinea versicolor (TV), and vitiligo are conditions that should be considered when evaluating people with dark skin types that present with hypopigmentation. Vitiligo can be seen in light- or dark-skin patients. It may go unnoticed for years due to it not being readily observable on light skin. In dark-skin patients, vitiligo can present as a conspicuous and advanced condition boldly standing out adjacent to their normal skin tone [**Figure 24-7 A** and **B**].

Pigmentary disorders can take a toll on one's mental health. Some dark-skin individuals utilize social withdrawal to cope, while others fall victim to depression and/or lack of self-confidence. Research shows a relationship between the psychological burden of vitiligo and culture. Understanding the physical and emotional toll that this condition can have on darker skin patients is very important.

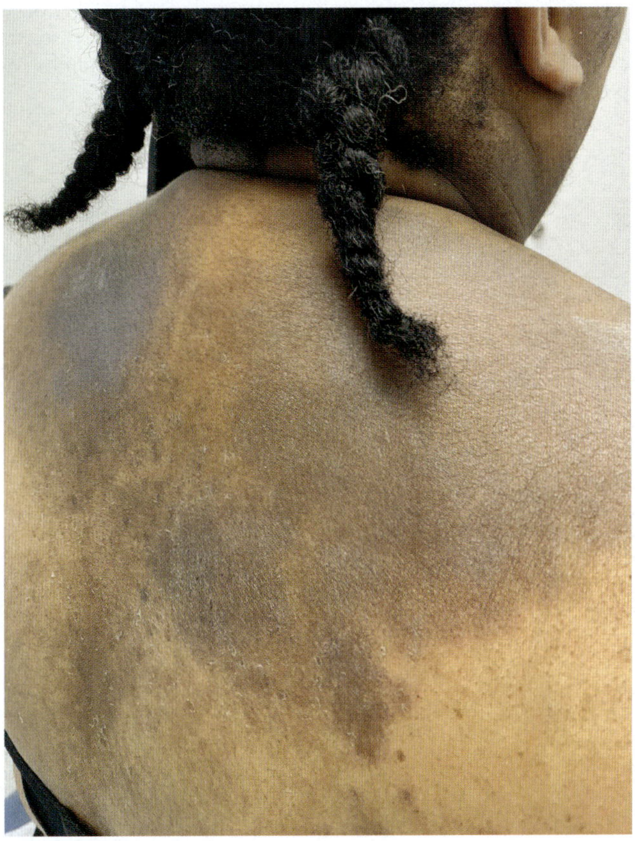

A

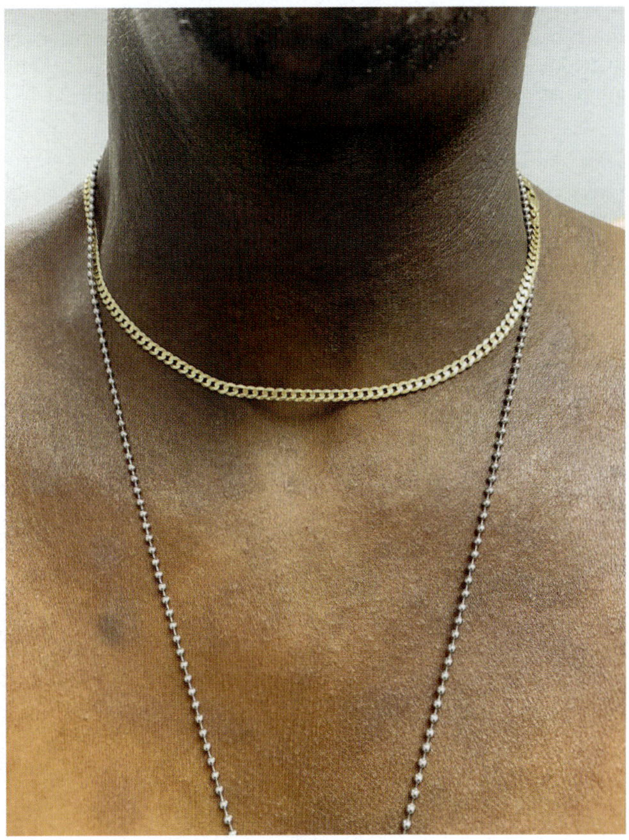

B

FIGURE 24-5. Discoloration seen on the back **(A)** and chest **(B)** of dark skin patients.

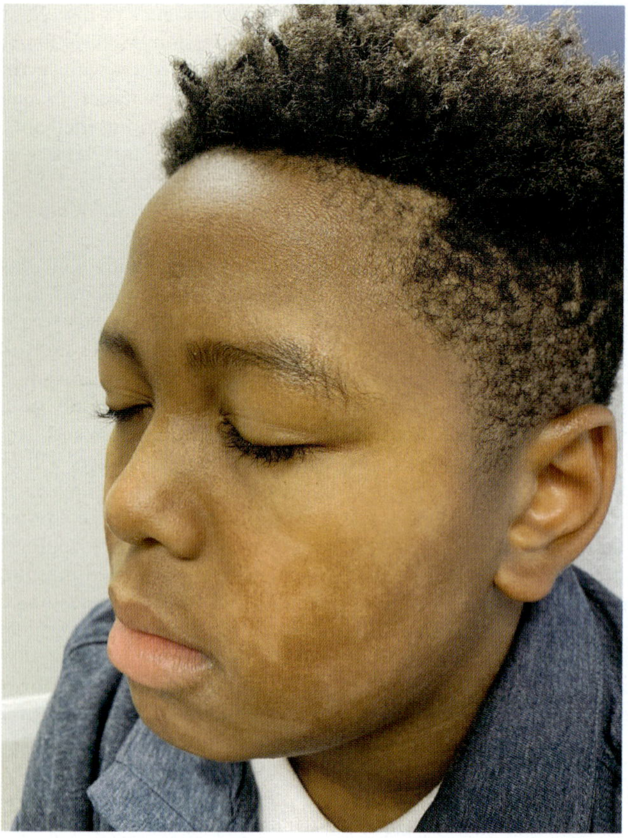

FIGURE 24-6. Pityriasis Alba demonstrated on the face of a dark skin patient.

NUANCES IN COMMON SKIN CONDITIONS IN DARK SKIN

Many studies have evaluated the prevalence of common skin conditions in dark-skin people. Common skin conditions seen in Black, Hispanic, Arab, and South Asian groups in the United States are depicted in **Table 24-1**.

Eczematous dermatitis and acne are the most common skin conditions in people with dark skin. Flares of eczema in dark skin have less pronounced redness than light skin **[Figure 24-8]**. Eczema hues in dark skin may vary from purple to gray and brown. Lichenification represents secondary changes characterized by hyperpigmentation, thickening of the skin, and accentuation of skin creases caused by recurrent rubbing or scratching of the skin **[Figure 24-9]**. In light skin, lichenification can appear with red and pink hues. In dark skin, this same condition can appear dark purple, silver, or with brown hues. Outside of the nuance in color, the overall distribution may differ in dark skin types including more bumps on the torso and dark circles surrounding the eyes. Eczema in dark skin must be managed effectively and efficiently to prevent chronic excessive pigmentation.

A diagnostic nuance particular to acne in dark-skin individuals is the resulting hyperpigmentation. Hyperpigmentation may result from the inflammation of the acneiform lesions themselves or from a person's picking at the lesions. When acne is picked, a condition called acne excorièe, there is a combination of the primary acneiform lesions and secondary excoriation, which can be quite extensive, and in dark skin both result in hyperpigmentation **[Figure 24-10]**. The acne excorièe may result in hypopigmented macules with a hyperpigmented border as opposed to the uniform PIH that occurs secondary to acne that has not been picked. This finding is not as common in light-skin individuals. Picking acne lesions could be an indication of stress, mental anguish, etc. Dark-skin individuals are also more likely to have permanent scarring with picking, making this diagnostic indication an important sign to counsel patients.

Acanthosis nigricans (AN) is a common condition seen in the Hispanic and Black population.[7] Patients may present to the dermatologist with concerns about dark patches on the neck, under the arms, and/or along the inner thighs. **[Figure 24-11]**. Some patients refer to this condition as a "dirty neck." Some try to scrub the discoloration off to no avail. Therefore, health education is important when explaining this diagnosis to patients. Some are not aware that the darkening and thickening of the skin can be a result of insulin resistance. Complete education about AN in the Latinx and African American population will allow them to further explore their risk of diabetes, cardiovascular disease, and polycystic ovary syndrome (PCOS) that are common conditions in these populations.

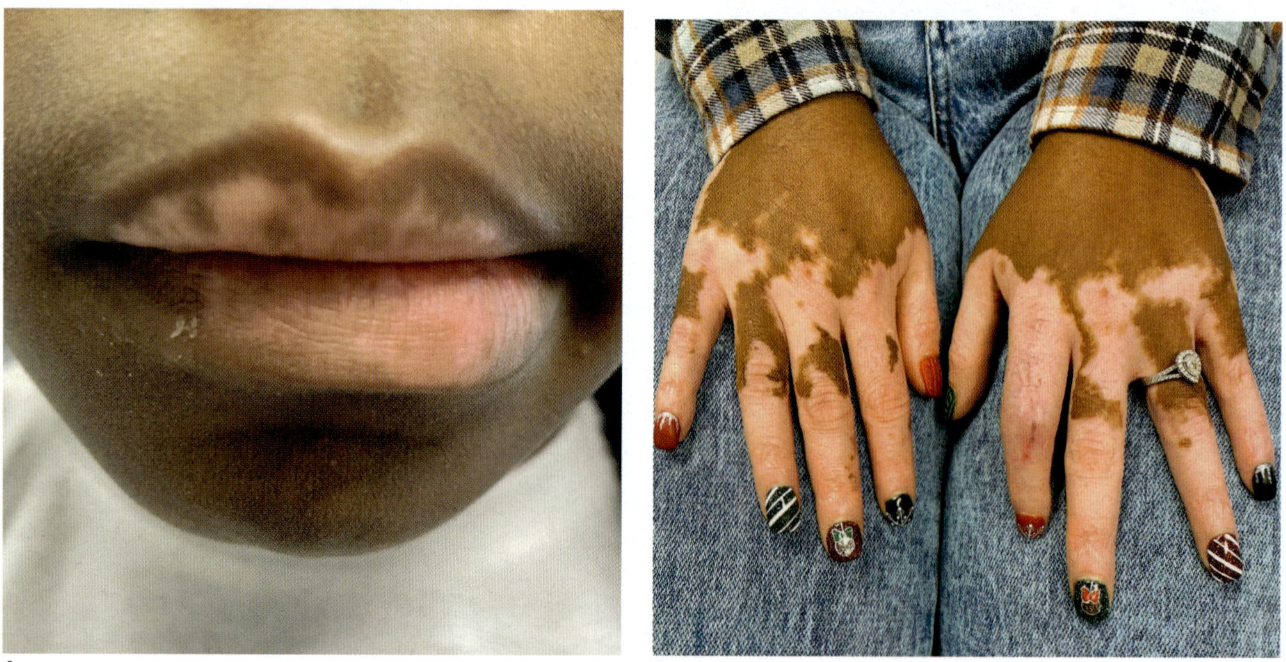

A B

FIGURE 24-7. Vitiligo demonstrated on the lips **(A)** and on the hands **(B)** of darker skin patients.

TABLE 24-1 Common skin conditions reported in Black, Hispanic, Asian, and Arab groups in the United States

Blacks[a]		Hispanics[b]		Arabs[c]		South Asians[d]	
Acne	27.7%	Acne	20.7%	Acne	37.7%	Acne	37.0%
Eczematous dermatitis	23.4%	Eczematous dermatitis	19.3%	Eczematous dermatitis	25.5%	Eczematous dermatitis	22.0%
Pigmentary disorders	9.0%	Photoaging	16.8%	Fungal infection	20.0%	Fungal infection	20.0%
Seborrheic dermatitis	6.5%	Tinea/onychomycosis	9.9%	Condyloma/warts	20.0%	Condyloma/warts	8.0%
Alopecia	5.3%	Melasma	8.2%	Melasma	14.5%	Moles	8.0%
Fungal infections	4.3%	Condyloma/warts	7.1%	Keloid	10.7%		
Condyloma/warts	2.4%	Hyperpigmentation	6%	Psoriasis	4.7%		
Tinea versicolor	2.2%	Seborrheic keratosis	4.5%	Vitiligo	2.0%		
Keloids	2.1%	Acrochordon	4.2%				
Pityriasis rosea	2.0%	Seborrheic dermatitis	3.2%				
Urticaria	2.0%	Alopecia	2.3%				
		Psoriasis	0.8%				

[a]Halder RM, Roberts CI, Nootheti PK. Cutaneous diseases in the black races. *Dermatol Clin.* 2003;21:679-687, ix.

[b]Sanchez MR. Cutaneous diseases in Latinos. *Dermatol Clin.* 2003;21:689-697.

[c]El-Essawi D, Musial J, Hammad A, Lim H. A survey of skin disease and skin-related issues in Arab Americans. *J Am Acad Dermatol.* 2007;56:933-938.

[d]Shah SK, Bhanusali DG, Sachdev A, Geria AN, Alexis AF. A survey of skin conditions and concerns in South Asian Americans: a community based study. *J Drugs Dermatol.* 2011;10:524-528.

Dark-skin individuals have a higher incidence of hirsutism than those with light skin.[8] Hirsutism can cause feelings of embarrassment or social withdrawal and therefore it is important to pay attention to the ways this condition affects people. It occurs most commonly on the face, chest, lower abdomen, and inner thighs **[Figure 24-12]**. Some people are not aware that they have options for treatment. The nuance in diagnosing hirsutism involves the understanding that many people believe it is a part of their genetic heritage and may not know to discuss this condition with a dermatologist, though a provider might notice it at the time of presentation for other concerns. If noted on exam, it is imperative that PCOS be considered. Since hirsutism can be related to modifiable risk factors, it is imperative that one addressed this condition because it can be associated with insulin resistance or diabetes.

Hidradenitis suppurativa (HS) is a condition that can be physically, socially, and emotionally debilitating. It has a higher prevalence in Black people compared to the general population.[9] HS patients can present with nodules or abscesses in intertriginous areas that cause intense pain and affect quality of life **[Figure 24-13]**. Although the higher prevalence in the Black community and the common distribution in the groin, axillary, and other intertriginous locations is well-known, interestingly HS is often misdiagnosed as boils or abscesses and patients may left without adequate education or ongoing management. Delayed or inaccurate diagnosis can cause patients years of mental anguish and a poor

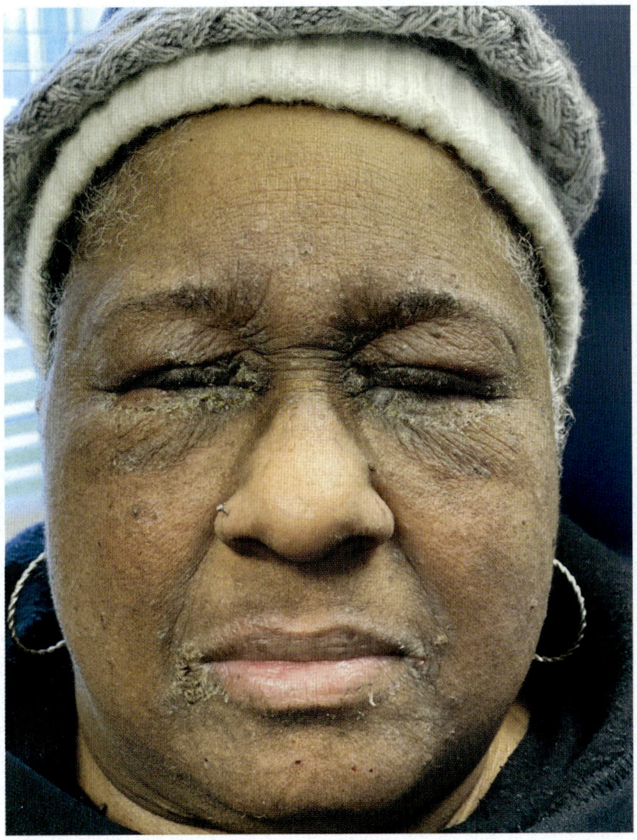

FIGURE 24-8. Eczematous dermatitis demonstrated on the face of a darker skin patients.

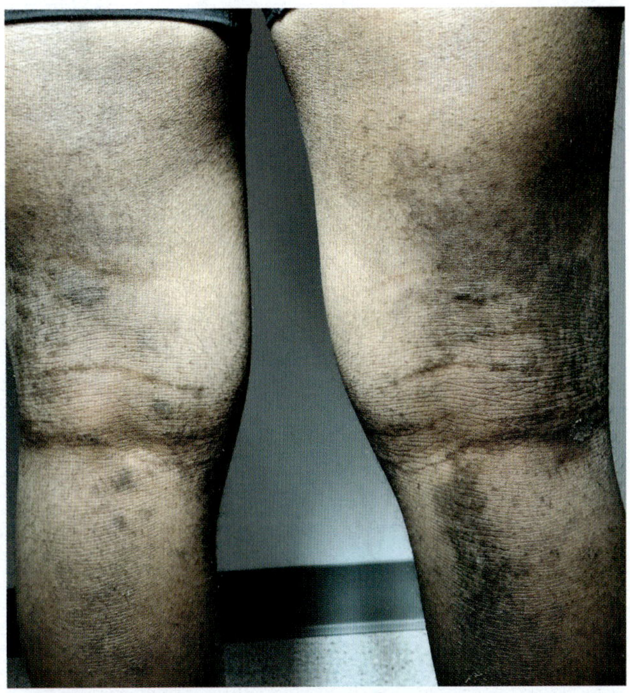

FIGURE 24-9. Eczema demonstrated on the bilateral lower extremities of a darker skin patient.

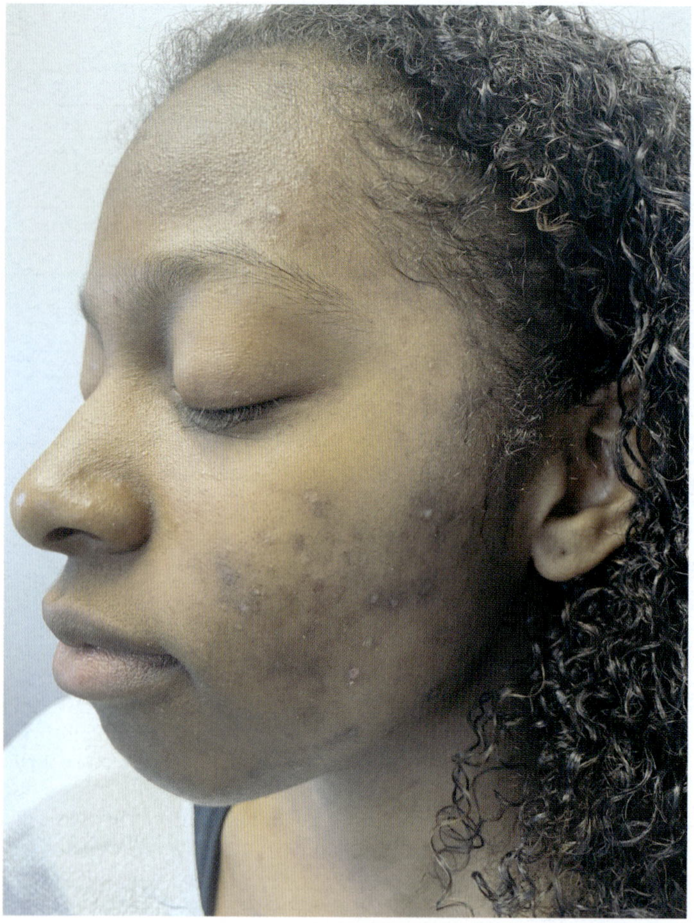

FIGURE 24-10. Acne excorièe demonstrated on the face of a darker skin patient.

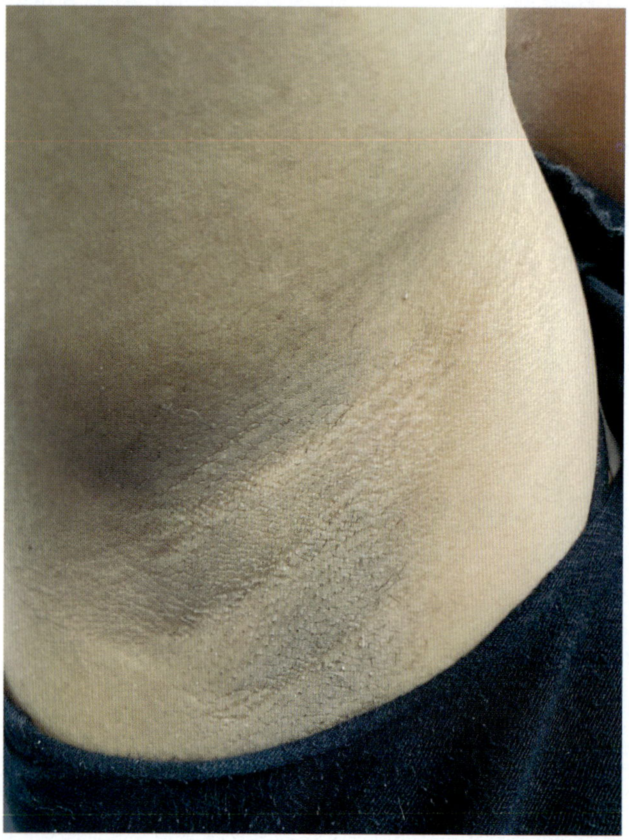

FIGURE 24-11. Acanthosis Nigricans demonstrated in the axilla of a darker skin patient.

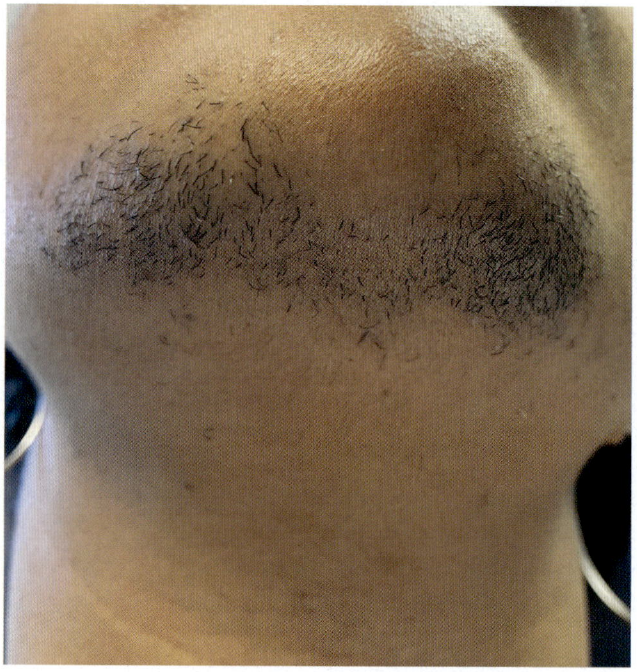

FIGURE 24-12. Hirsutism demonstrated in a darker skin patient.

prognosis.[10] The average diagnostic delay is 7.2 years. If this diagnosis is made early, it saves the patient much distress concerning drastic lifestyle changes and the many challenges of dealing with this disease once it has progressed.[11,12]

HAIR IN THE DARK-SKIN POPULATION

Hair in dark-skin populations carries variations in texture, water composition, and curl pattern. Hair care practices should be considered when developing a dermatologic treatment plan. Hairstyles are often a very important cultural aspect in dark-skin people who have "afro-textured hair." For example, this population may wear confined hairstyles or styles that obstruct the view of the scalp and limit the physical examination and diagnostic process for the dermatologist. It is important to request that patients arrive to their appointments with the hair loose and styled in a manner such that that the dermatologist can perform a complete hair and scalp examination. Readily accessing the scalp allows providers

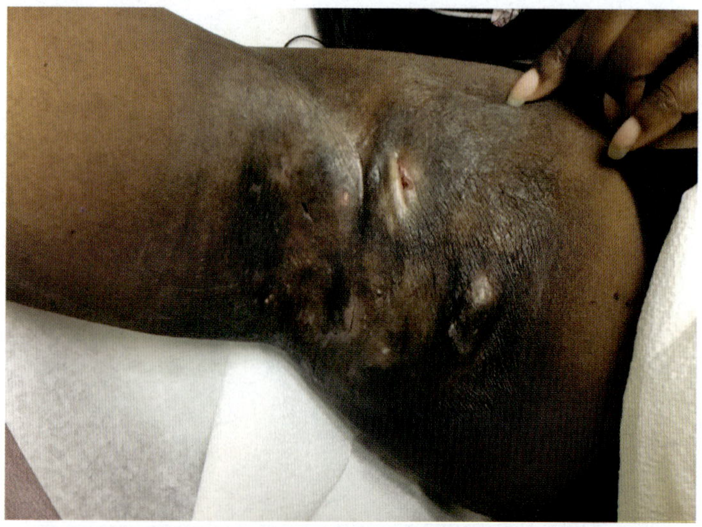

FIGURE 24-13. Hidradenitis suppurativa (HS) demonstrated in the axilla of a darker skin patient. (Courtesy of Chesahna Kindred, MD)

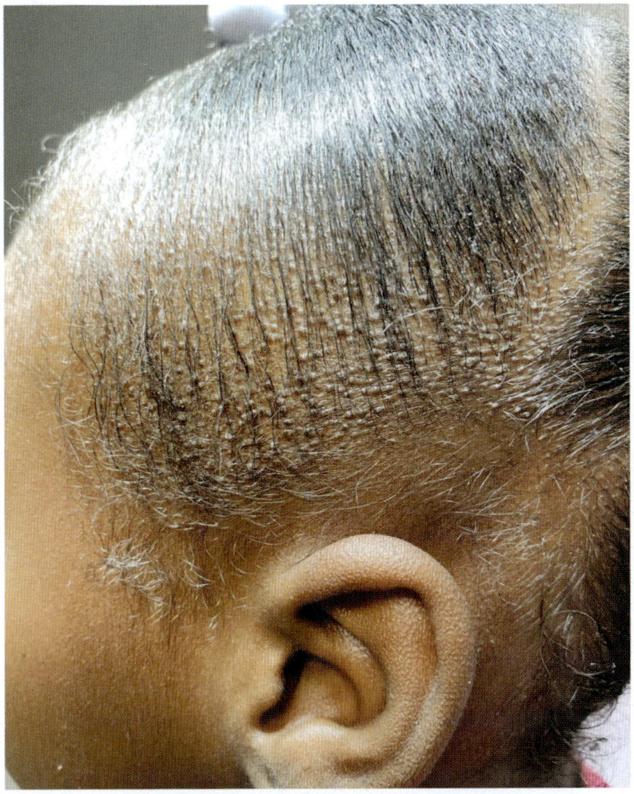

FIGURE 24-14. Traction Alopecia demonstrated in the temporal hairline of a darker skin patient.

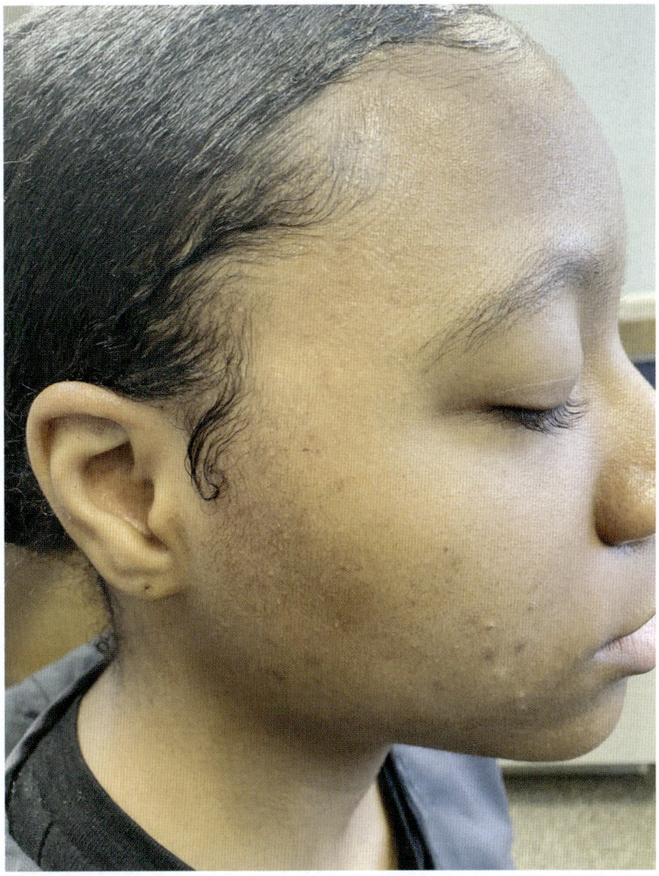

FIGURE 24-15. Hair along the hairline laid down by gel also known as "edges" demonstrated in a dark skin patient.

to fully investigate hair anomalies and scalp diseases. Understanding the cultural nuances in hair care practices can build trust in the patient-provider relationship and improve patient outcomes.

Alopecia affects communities in different ways. One study showed that alopecia leads to higher self-stigmatization than mental disorders.[13] In communities of dark-skin people with "afro-textured hair," there are many braided hairstyles or other cultural hairstyles that involve twisting or putting tension on hair strands. Many of the hairstyles worn by children in this community utilize rubber bands, hair barrettes, or hair beads that stay in place for many days to weeks at a time. This can cause increased tension around the base of the hair shaft leading to traction alopecia.[14] This tightness can result in tension bumps or folliculitis developing near the hairline [**Figure 24-14**]. Shorter hairs along the hairline, also known as "edges," are a very important aspect of the overall aesthetic of a hairstyle in this community. Gels are commonly used to lay down the hairs or "edges" in a wavy pattern along the hairline [**Figure 24-15**]. In addition, extensive brushing of the gel into the hairline to obtain this sleek look is common. This process can also lead to traction alopecia. Treatment plans for both of these styling practices that contribute to traction alopecia include removing hair accessories from the hair at night and counseling in the importance of restructuring hairstyles to prevent hair loss.

The faded hairline in men has a similar level of significance as edges do to women in this population. The nuanced understanding of this cultural practice is knowing the conditions that are related to keeping up this hairstyle that includes pseudofolliculitis barbae (PFB), acne keloidalis nuchae (AKN), and keloids. PFB is a condition that affects the beard area.[15] AKN tends to present at the nape of the neck and can be a result of the curl pattern of the hair or shaving hairstyles[16] [**Figure 24-16**]. Some people may incorrectly believe that either condition results from using "dirty clippers" but this is not the case. Although the exact etiology is unknown, research suggests genetics play a role in a small population. Keloids are more common in dark-skin people and can occur anywhere on the body. The papules resulting from PFB can lead to keloid scarring if the condition is not identified and managed early in its onset.

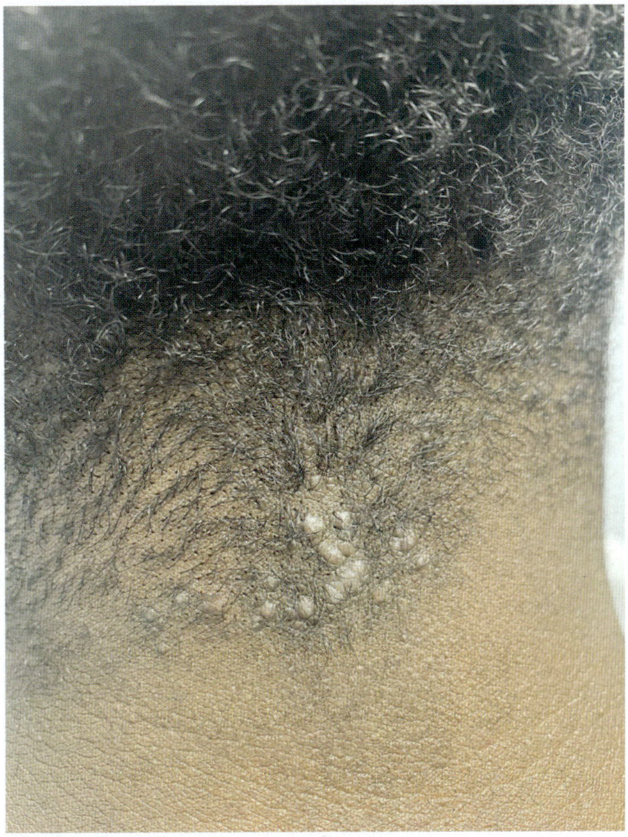

FIGURE 24-16. Acne Keloidalis Nuchae (AKN) demonstrated on the nuchal area of a dark skin patient.

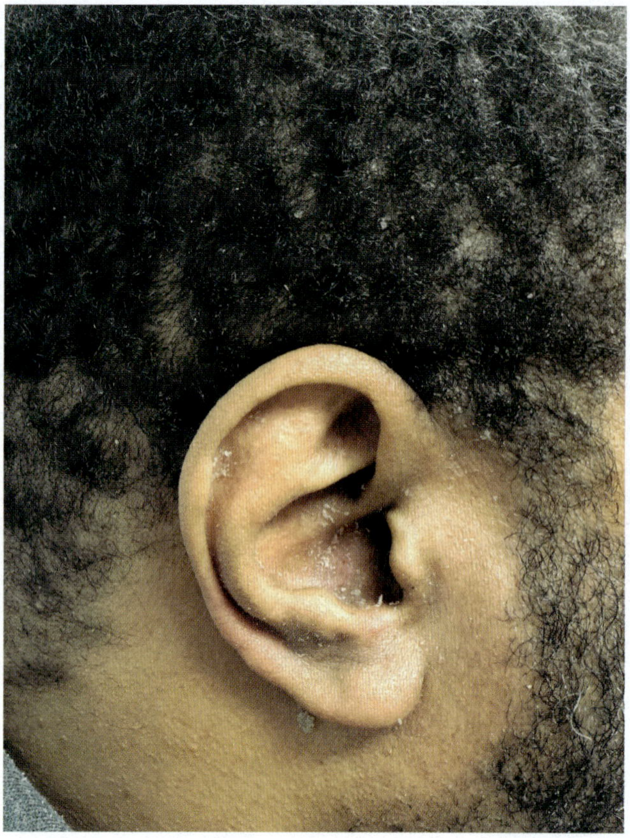

FIGURE 24-17. Seborrheic Dermatitis demonstrated on the ear of a dark skin patient.

Education regarding long-term styling practices and shaving practices is important for people to understand minimizing the risk of causing or exacerbating these conditions. Cultural competence in hairstyle practices is important in the diagnosis and treatment of people with darker skin who have "afro-textured hair."

Seborrheic dermatitis is a dermatologic condition that often results in scaling on the scalp and in the hair[17] [**Figure 24-17**]. People with darker skin who have "afro-textured hair" may use grease or an ointment with a petroleum jelly consistency on their scalp and hair to help with dryness, manageability, and shine. Adding oil to the scalp in any form can worsen this condition. Many of the treatments for seborrheic dermatitis include increased hair washing with specific products. The nuance in treating this condition in Black patients is understanding that Black women often shampoo every 1 to 2 weeks and daily hair washing may not be an attainable treatment option for this population. The treatment regimen that is selected for the patient should be explained in a way that patients are confident their dermatologist knows how to care for their hair type or hair texture.

VARIATIONS IN INFANCY

When infants are born, the ears may show darkening compared to the rest of the body. Ear pigmentation may be an indicator for the future skin tone of the infant. Mongolian spots are commonly seen on dark-skin infants.[18,19] They appear as blue or grayish-blue spots on the back of the infant; most of these will fade completely by adulthood [**Figure 24-18**]. The Nevus of Ota is a common nevus seen in Asian skin. It can present as a bluish-brown hyperpigmentation that is the result of dermal melanocytosis. The hyperpigmentation is distributed along the trigeminal nerve and involves the eye. The nevus of Ito is a similar nevus and is also common in this population. The difference between the two is that the nevus of Ito has no ocular involvement compared to the nevus of Ota, which does. The nevus of Ota and nevus of Ito are mainly diagnosed in infancy and usually resolves around the age of 6.[20]

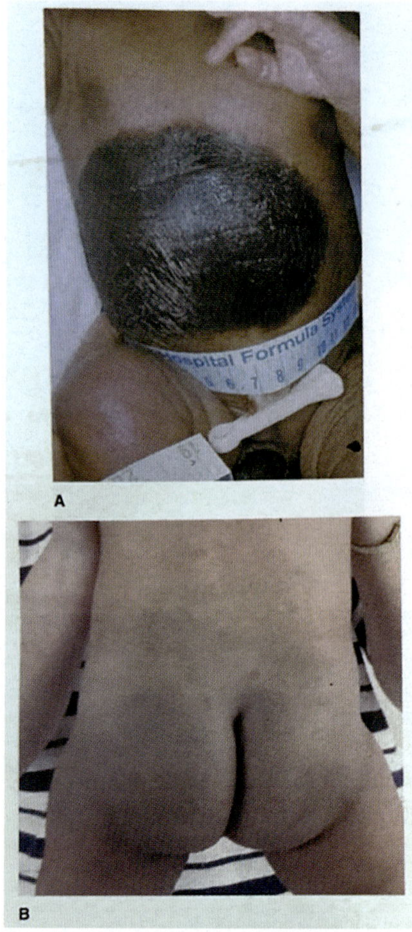

FIGURE 24-18. Mongolian Spots demonstrated on the back of a darker skin patient.

CONCLUSION

It is important to be able to distinguish nuances in dermatology. In order to differentiate pathology from a normal variant, one must comprehend the differences between different skin tones. Normal variants in dark skin evolve from infancy through adulthood. It is imperative that we recognize the signs of pathologic skin findings for darker-skin individuals to accurately diagnose skin conditions and develop appropriate treatment plans.

REFERENCES

1. Vespa J, Medina L, Armstrong DM. Demographic turning points for the United States: population projections for 2020 to 2060 population estimates and projections current population reports. https://www.census.gov/content/dam/Census/library/publications/2020/demo/p25-1144.pdf. Accessed November 16, 2022.
2. Syder NC, Omar D, McKenzie S, Brown-Korsah JB, Taylor SC, Elbuluk N. Gaps in medical education curricula on skin of color in medical school, residency, and beyond: part 1. *J Am Acad Dermatol*. 2023;89(5):885-892.
3. Kelly AP, Taylor SC. *Dermatology for Skin of Color*. New York, NY: McGraw Hill; 2009.
4. Ronger S, Touzet S, Ligeron C, et al. Dermoscopic examination of nail pigmentation. *Arch Dermatol*. 2002;138(10):1327-1333.
5. Jeon C, Agbai O, Butler D, Murase J. Dermatologic conditions in patients of color who are pregnant. *Int J Womens Dermatol*. 2017;3(1):30-36.
6. Alaluf S, Atkins D, Barrett K, Blount M, Carter N, Heath A. Ethnic variation in melanin content and composition in photoexposed and photoprotected human skin. *Pigment Cell Res*. 2002;15(2):112-118.
7. Alexis AF, Sergay AB, Taylor SC, Alexis AF. Common dermatologic disorders in skin of color: a comparative practice survey. *Cutis*. 2007;80(5):387-394.
8. Afifi L, Saeed L, Pasch LA, et al. Association of ethnicity, Fitzpatrick skin type, and hirsutism: a retrospective cross-sectional study of women with polycystic ovarian syndrome. *Int J Womens Dermatol*. 2017;3(1):37-43.

9. Okeke CAV, Perry JD, Simmonds FC, et al. Clinical trials and skin of color: the example of hidradenitis suppurativa. *Dermatology (Basel)*. 2022;238(1):180-184.
10. Okeke CAV, Williams JP, Iwuala CU, et al. What's race got to do with it? CRP levels in immune mediated skin diseases: considerations for hidradenitis suppurativa. *Front Immunol*. 2022;13:847050.
11. Vlassova N, Kuhn D, Okoye GA. Hidradenitis suppurativa disproportionately affects African Americans: a single-center retrospective analysis. *Acta Derm Venereol*. 2015;95(8):990-991.
12. Okeke CAV, Khanna R, Okoye GA, Byrd AS. Assessment of the generalizability of hidradenitis suppurativa microbiome studies: the minimal inclusion of racial and ethnic populations. *J Am Acad Dermatol*. 2022;86(4): e159-e161.
13. Kacar S, Soyucok E, Bagcioglu E, et al. The perceived stigma in patients with alopecia and mental disorder: a comparative study. *Int J Trichology*. 2016;8(3):135-140.
14. Haskin A, Aguh C. All hairstyles are not created equal: what the dermatologist needs to know about black hairstyling practices and the risk of traction alopecia (TA). *J Am Acad Dermatol*. 2016;75(3):606-611.
15. Ogunbiyi A. Pseudofolliculitis barbae; current treatment options. *Clin Cosmet Investig Dermatol*. 2019;12:241.
16. Al Aboud DM, Badri T. *Acne Keloidalis Nuchae Continuing Education Activity*. In: StatPearls. Treasure Island (FL): StatPearls Publishing; 2024.
17. Bs ME, Dlova N, Fcderm M, Ogunleye T, Taylor SC. SPECIAL TOPIC seborrheic dermatitis in skin of color: clinical considerations. *J Drugs Dermatol*. 1924;18(1):24.
18. Gupta D. Mongolian spots: how important are they? *World J Clin Cases*. 2013;1(8):230-231.
19. Wikimedia Commons. File: Giant Mongolian blue spot (1).jpg. 2016. https://commons.wikimedia.org/wiki/File:Giant_mongolian_blue_spot_(1).jpg#file. Accessed November 28, 2022.
20. Agarwal US, Besarwal RK, Gupta R, Agarwal P. Inflammatory linear verrucous epidermal nevus with psoriasiform histology. *Indian J Dermatol*. 2014;59(2):211.

CHAPTER 25

Dermoscopic Patterns of Dermatological Diseases in Skin of Color Individuals

Natalia Jaimes
Alejandra Avila
Antonella Tosti

KEY POINTS

- Dermoscopic patterns seen in nevi differ based on skin color, with individuals of darker skin commonly presenting with smaller dark brown nevi, while those with fair skin often show larger nevi with a light brown to pink color.
- Acral lentiginous melanoma is the most common subtype in individuals with darker skin, and specific dermoscopic patterns such as the parallel ridge pattern could be indicative of acral lentiginous melanoma.
- Squamous cell carcinoma is the most common cutaneous malignancy in Africans and South Asians. Dermoscopic features of this skin cancer subtype may include structureless asymmetric brown areas, blue/gray dots arranged linearly, and coiled vessels.
- In individuals with skin of color, the presence of a perifollicular pigmented network or honeycomb pattern and pinpoint white dots are typical on the scalp.
- Androgenetic alopecia diagnostic criteria are similar across races, but variations such as yellow and white dots and peripilar signs may be more prominent in the skin of color individuals.
- Racial melanonychia is common among individuals with skin of color, with wider and/or darker bands than in lighter-skinned populations. Dermoscopy may reveal a gray or brown-to-black background, with the presence of a pseudo-Hutchinson sign.
- Onychocytic tumors like onychomatricoma and onychocytic matricoma can present with melanonychia, with differences in clinical and dermoscopic features such as perforations in the nail plate and blurred edges in pigmented lesions.

INTRODUCTION

Dermoscopy is a noninvasive, in vivo imaging technique that enables the visualization of structures that are otherwise not visible to the naked eye. Dermoscopy has proven to be a cost-effective tool; it increases the diagnostic accuracy for skin cancer and decreases the number of unnecessary skin biopsies of benign lesions. In addition, dermoscopy is used in other dermatologic infectious and inflammatory disorders, and conditions involving hair and nail.

Skin manifestations and dermoscopic patterns are influenced by different factors, including skin type and color, age, anatomic location, sun-exposure, among others. These variations are due to the diverse color background, reaction patterns (eg, pigmentation and greater affinity for follicles, sclerotic reactions in darker phototypes), and/or dispersion and activation level of melanosomes.[1] This chapter reviews the different dermoscopic patterns of some of the most common dermatological disease in individuals with skin of color (SOC, aka skin type V/VI by the Fitzpatrick skin type (FST) classification system); specifically, melanocytic and nonmelanocytic neoplasms, and hair and nail disorders.

MELANOCYTIC NEOPLASMS

Melanocytic nevi are the primary differential diagnosis of early melanomas. While the clinical morphology of nevi and early melanoma often overlap, dermoscopy has improved the ability to discriminate between the two of them. In general, nevi tend to reveal a symmetric and organized dermoscopic pattern, while melanomas tend to be asymmetric, disorganized, and usually reveal at least one melanoma-specific structure. This section provides an overview of the dermoscopic structures and patterns associated with nevi and melanoma in individuals of SOC.

NEVI

Overall, the first goal when evaluating a melanocytic lesion is to determine whether the lesion is organized or disorganized, and if the lesion adheres to one of the *benign patterns* commonly seen in nevi [**Figure 25-1**]. These benign patterns tend to reveal a symmetric and organized distribution of colors and structures within the lesion.

DERMOSCOPIC PATTERNS FREQUENTLY SEEN IN NEVI ON NONGLABROUS SKIN AMONG INDIVIDUALS WITH SOC

Individuals with darker skin or SOC frequently present with smaller dark brown nevi, whereas individuals with fair skin/FST I and II commonly exhibit larger nevi with a light brown to pink color.[2] The most common dermoscopic patterns encountered in individuals with SOC (ie, FST V-VI)[2] include reticular diffuse, peripheral network with central hyperpigmentation, and homogeneous brown and blue patterns [**Table 25-1**]. Other commonly observed dermoscopic patterns include peripheral network with central globules pattern, and globular pattern including cobblestone pattern, and patterns associated with radial growth (ie, Starburst pattern, and reticular with peripheral globules) [**Table 25-2**].

In general, when performing a skin cancer screening exam and evaluating melanocytic lesions, it is recommended to use the *comparative approach*, in order to determine which is the predominant nevus pattern (aka signature nevus pattern).[6] In the comparative approach, the

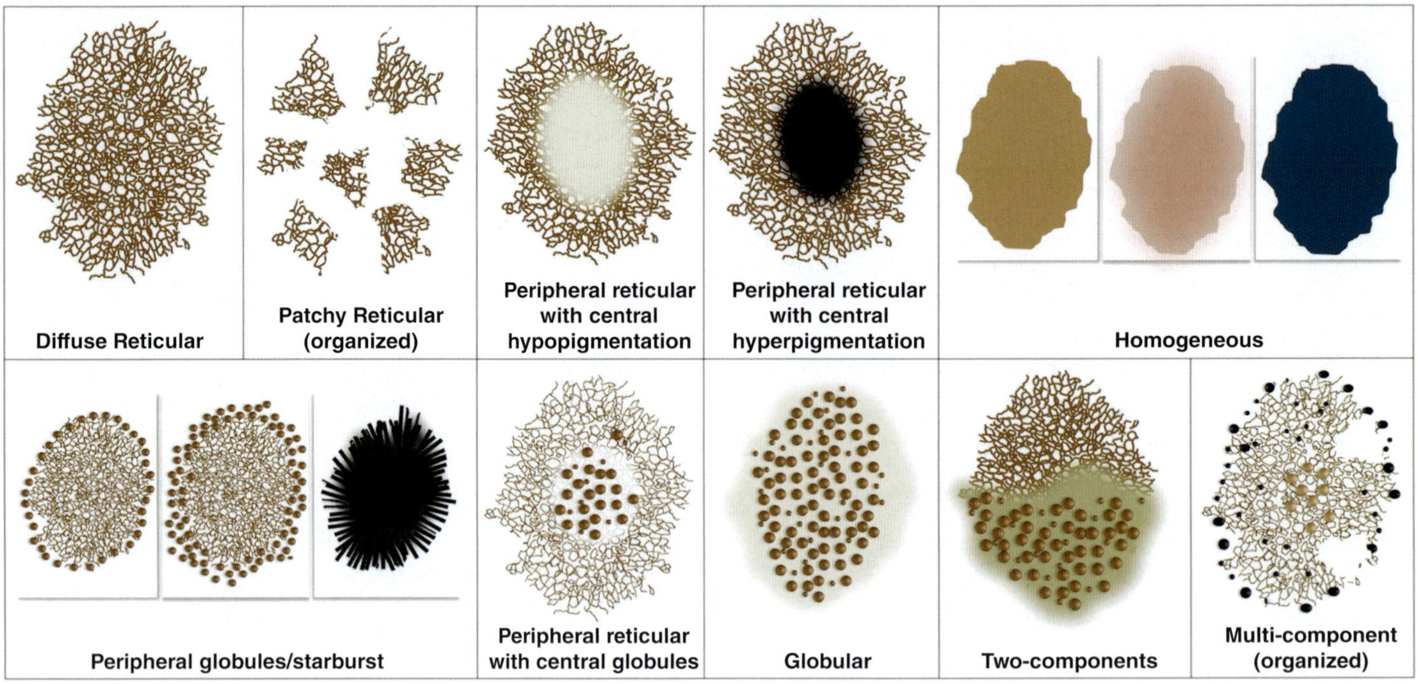

FIGURE 25-1. Nevi patterns.

physician evaluates the nevi of the patient and not only the lesion of concern. The reasoning behind the comparative approach is that nevi in most individuals demonstrate one or two benign patterns.[6] Thus, special attention should be placed on outlier lesions that do not adhere to the predominant nevus pattern, and depending on other contextual factors (eg, age, skin color, past medical history), a skin biopsy should be considered [**Figure 25-2**].[1]

DERMOSCOPIC PATTERNS FREQUENTLY SEEN IN NEVI ON GLABROUS SKIN AMONG INDIVIDUALS WITH SOC

Acral lesions are commonly encountered in individuals with SOC as compared with white/fair-skinned individuals. Therefore, it is essential to understand the anatomy of the palms and soles, in order to identify the *furrows and ridges* of the dermatoglyphics, which are the main sites where the dermoscopic structures are located. On occasion, recognizing the ridges from the furrows can be challenging; thus, knowing some clues can assist in this differentiation: (1) ridges are wider than the furrows; (2) the openings of the eccrine glands are seen as a row of small white dots over the ridges; and (3) the ink test, in which liquid ink is applied directly onto the lesion, highlighting the furrows.[7]

The most common dermoscopic patterns encountered in nevi on palms and soles include the parallel furrow (48% in palms, 40% in soles) [**Figure 25-3**] and latticelike patterns (14% in palms and 15% in soles) [**Figure 25-4**], followed by homogenous pattern in the palms (9%) and fibrillar pattern in the soles (11%) [**Table 25-3**].[8] Other less frequent dermoscopic patterns include globular, reticular, crista-dotted, and peas-in-a-pod.[8]

MELANOMA

Although melanoma is significantly more common in Non-Hispanic Whites as compared to individuals with SOC, melanomas in patients with SOC tend to be diagnosed at more advanced stages and carry a worser

TABLE 25-1 Most common dermoscopic patterns encountered in individuals with SOC (ie, FST V and VI)[2, 3]

Dermoscopic Pattern	Characteristics	Contextual factor
Reticular diffuse pattern	Typical network throughout the lesion [**Figure 25-2C**].	Commonly seen in darker skin, in particular FST IV-V.[3]
Peripheral network with central hyperpigmentation	Typical network at the periphery with a central hyperpigmented area or blotch. Not infrequently, the central blotch is due to accumulation of melanin-laden corneocytes in the stratum corneum (aka black lamella), which can be tape stripped off [**Figure 25-2A, B**].	Lesions displaying an atypical network with hypopigmented areas should raise concern for melanoma.[3]
Homogeneous brown pattern	Nevi in individuals with FST VI commonly reveal dark brown-black to blue-gray homogeneous pattern [Figure 25-3]. A *homogenous brown pattern* consists of a brown color with minimal to no variation in its hues. Although this homogeneous pattern is usually structureless, on rare occasions, few regular dots/globules or fragments of network can be observed within the lesion.	
Homogeneous blue pattern	A homogeneous blue pattern is the hallmark of a blue nevus; it is characterized by a blue color throughout the entire lesion's surface. This color will reveal a steel blue color appearance with minimal variation or hues, especially when visualized with non-polarized light.	Any lesions revealing multiple hues of blue color, the diagnosis of melanoma should be entertained. Also, the contextual factors will be important in lesions that resemble blue nevi, especially in patients with a prior history of invasive melanoma, since on occasions, epidermotropic metastasis can mimic blue nevi.[3]

TABLE 25-2 Other dermoscopic patterns encountered in individuals with SOC

Dermoscopic pattern	Characteristics	Contextual factor
Peripheral network with central globules and *globular pattern including cobblestone pattern*	Brown globules, either in the center of the lesion with a regular network at the periphery or throughout the lesion. Globules are regular, with minimal variation in their size and color. When globules are very large, they can resemble a *cobblestone pattern*.	Overall, these nevi tend to be congenital and are usually found on the head, neck, or torso. Thus, newly acquired lesions with a globular morphology occurring in older individuals, and especially if located on an extremity should raise concern for melanoma.[4]
Starburst pattern	Usually present with symmetric, darkly pigmented streaks at the periphery of the lesion.	Since these nevi are usually in their radial growth phase, **age** is an important contextual factor; thus, any lesion presenting in an older individual should raise concern for melanoma.[5]
Reticular pattern with peripheral globules	Typical network with one peripheral rim of regular brown globules.	Commonly encountered on the torso of younger to middle aged patients, especially with the atypical mole syndrome; thus, older individuals with newly acquired lesions revealing peripheral globules should be viewed with caution, especially if the lesion is located on an extremity, or reveals any melanoma-specific structure.[2,5]

prognosis when compared to the Non-Hispanic White population. Evidence shows that melanomas on nonglabrous skin tend to present with similar clinical and dermoscopic characteristics in patients with lighter skin and SOC. In general, melanomas present as disorganized lesions under dermoscopy, revealing at least one melanoma-specific structure (**Table 25-4**). Yet, the overall pattern will depend on factors such as anatomi location, histopathological subtype, growth phase, history of sun-exposure, among others. This section reviews acral melanoma.

VOLAR MELANOMA

Acral lentiginous melanoma (ALM) is the most common subtype of melanoma seen in African American and Asians individuals. Dermoscopy structures suggestive of acral/volar melanoma, include:

1. The ***parallel ridge pattern (PRP)***, which is the most specific dermoscopic pattern for ALM. The PRP consists of pigmentation located to the ridges [**Figure 25-5 A**]. The presence of a PRP has a diagnostic accuracy of 82% for melanoma, with a sensitivity of 86%, specificity of 99%, a positive predictive value of 94%, and a negative predictive value of 98% for melanoma.[12] However, there are some exceptions to the PRP, including some benign lesions manifesting pigmented ridges; for example, individuals with SOC/darker skin can present with ethnic pigmentation, which usually appears as multiple light brown macules, less than 1cm, with pigment on the ridges or a homogeneous pattern under dermoscopy; also subcorneal hemorrhage, some congenital nevi, and lesions seen in Peutz-Jeghers syndrome or Laugier-Hunziker syndrome can reveal a PRP.
2. ***Homogeneous pattern with multiple shades of brown and/or other colors***, including black, red, white, gray, and blue.[12,13]
3. The ***atypical/irregular fibrillar pattern*** is characterized by lines with increased variability in thickness, spacing and color, and distributed

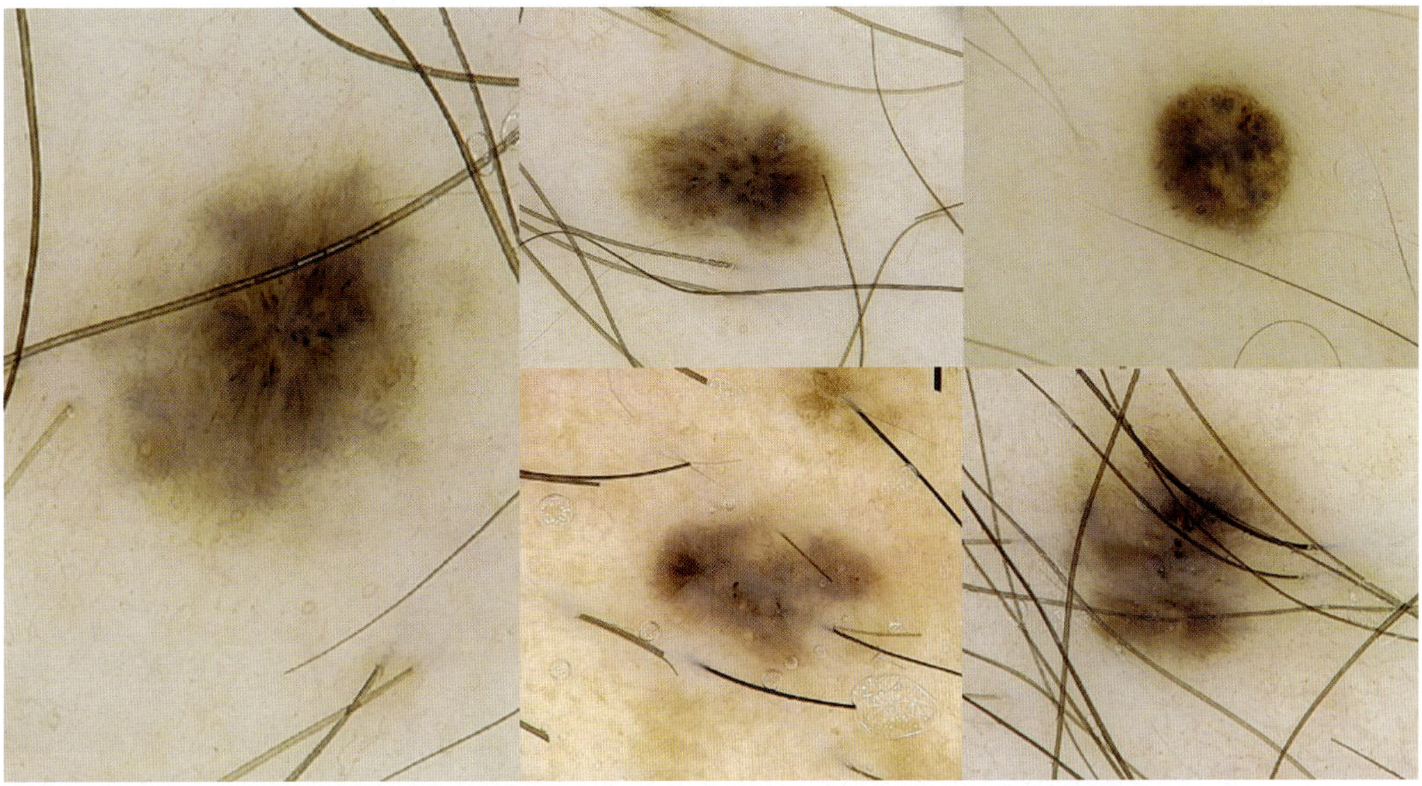

FIGURE 25-2. Nevi in individuals with FST V-VI commonly reveal dark brown-black to blue-gray homogeneous pattern. Since most individuals demonstrate one or two benign patterns as exemplified in the image, the comparative approach is a useful aid to determine which is the predominant nevus pattern (aka signature nevus pattern). Thus, outlier lesions that do not adhere to the predominant nevus pattern, and depending on other contextual factors (eg, age, skin color, past medical history), a skin biopsy should be considered.

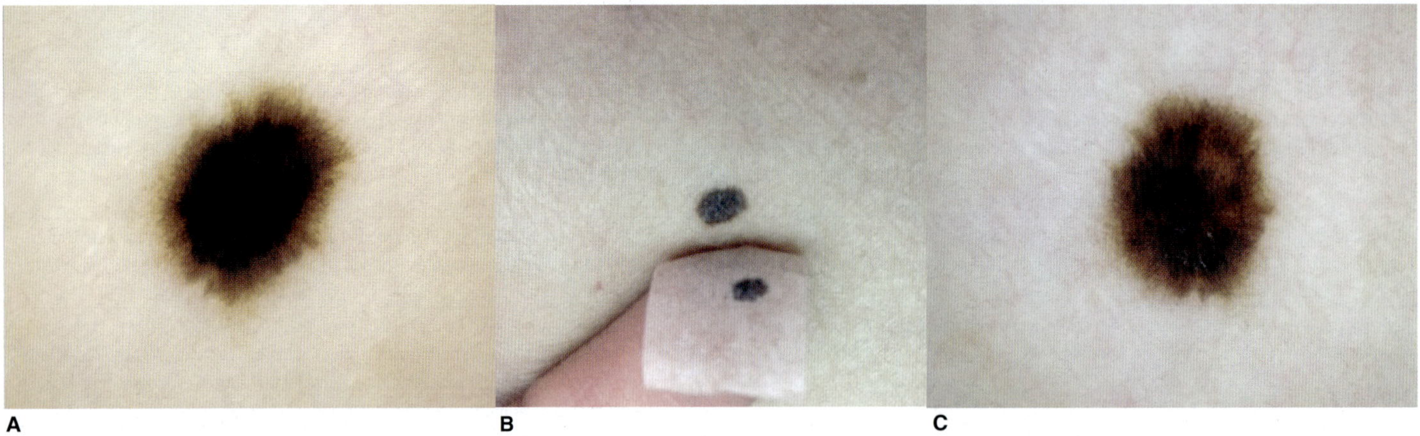

FIGURE 25-3. Common dermoscopic nevi patterns in individuals with skin of color. The peripheral network with central hyperpigmentation **(A)** and reticular diffuse patterns **(C)**. Not infrequently, the central blotch in these nevi is due to the black lamella **(B)**, which corresponds to accumulation of melanin-laden corneocytes in the stratum corneum, and can usually be tape stripped off **(B)**.

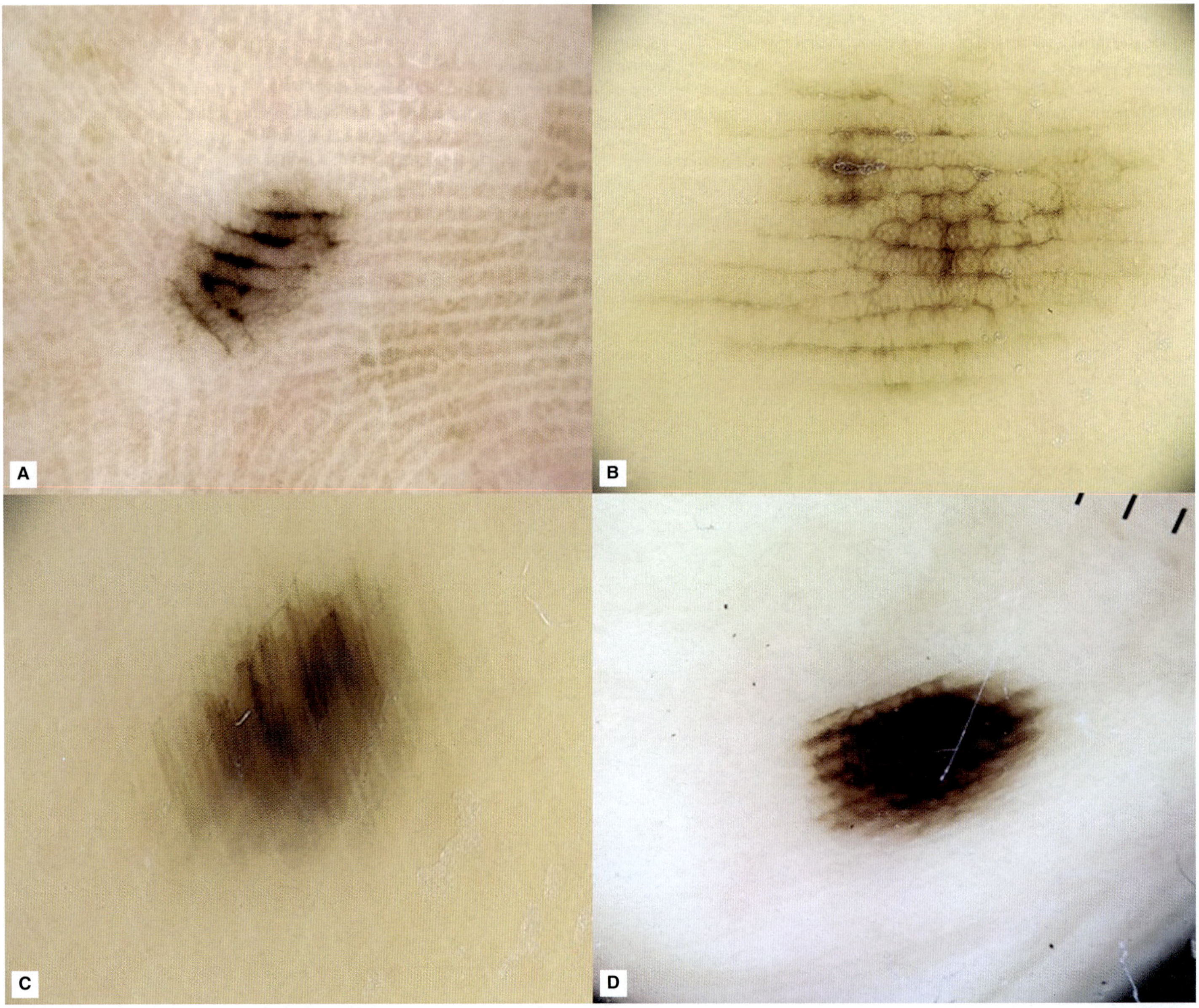

FIGURE 25-4. Common dermoscopic patterns in acral nevi among individuals of skin of color. **(A)** The parallel furrow pattern, the pigmentation is localized to the furrows. **(B)** The lattice-like pattern, the pigmentation is localized to the furrows in combination with pigmented lines that transect over the ridges connecting on furrow to the other. **(C)** The fibrillar pattern consists of multiple thin parallel light-brown lines with minimal variation in thickness and color; and **(D)** the **Homogeneous pattern** demonstrates a uniformly distributed pigment involving the furrows and ridges without any other structures.

TABLE 25-3 Dermoscopic patterns frequently seen in nevi on glabrous skin among individuals with SOC [Figure 25-4]

Dermoscopic pattern	Characteristic	Other
Parallel furrow pattern	Pigment located on the furrows [**Figure 25-4A**].[2-5]	Most nevi display the single line variant (ie, one solid line of pigment on the furrows). However, there are other variants, including the double line, single dotted line, and the double dotted line variants.[10]
Lattice-like pattern	Pigment located on the furrows (i.e., parallel furrow pattern) in combination with pigmented lines that transect over the ridges, connecting one furrow to the other [**Figure 25-4B**].	The lattice-like pattern is commonly encountered on the arch of the foot.
Fibrillar pattern	Multiple parallel thin light-brown thin lines, with minimal variation in thickness and color. The fibrillar pattern is oriented obliquely and appears to cross both the furrows and ridges. It results from the effects of persistent horizontal pressure being applied to the stratum corneum; therefore, it is frequently seen in melanocytic lesions located on weight-bearing parts of the sole [**Figure 25-4C**].[9]	The oblique-view technique is an aid to evaluate those lesions presenting with a fibrillar pattern. This technique attempts to transiently convert the fibrillar pattern into a parallel pattern to help the observer determine if the pigment is originating from the furrows or the ridges. To perform the oblique-view technique, the dermatoscope needs to be in contact mode, in order to apply downward and horizontal pressure that is directed opposite to the normal frictional forces encountered by the lesion.
Homogeneous pattern	Pigment that is uniformly distributed throughout the lesion, and involves the furrows and ridges without other structures [**Figure 25-4D**].[11]	Frequently seen in individuals with SOC more than in White individuals

TABLE 25-4 Dermoscopic melanoma-specific structures

Melanoma-specific structure	Schematic	Definition
Atypical pigment network	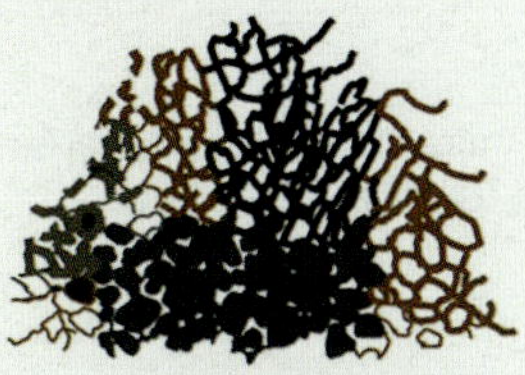	Network with increased variability in color and thickness, and asymmetrically distributed
Negative network	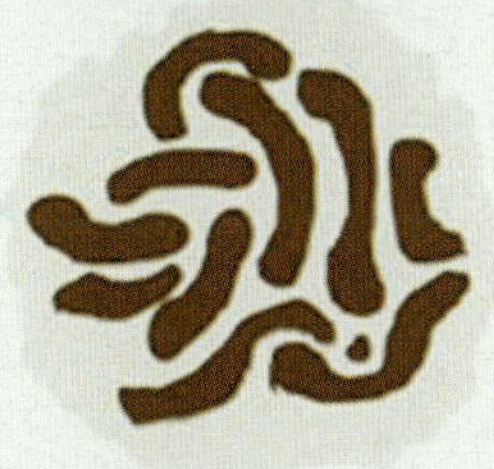	Serpiginous interconnecting broadened hypopigmented lines surrounding elongated and curvilinear globules. Can be seen in Spitzoid lesions, and melanomas, in particular melanomas arising in preexisting nevi
Angulated lines	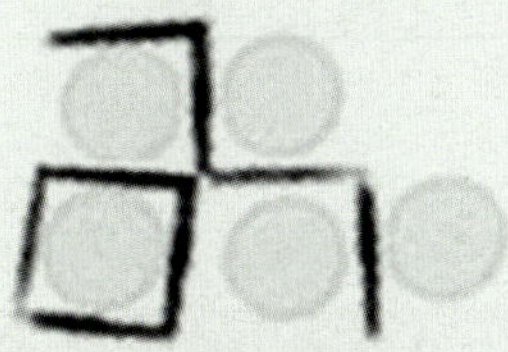	Gray to brown lines that meet at angels creating a zig-zag pattern. These lines can coalesce to form polygons or rhomboids. Mostly seen in melanomas on sun-damaged skin
Atypical globules and/or dots	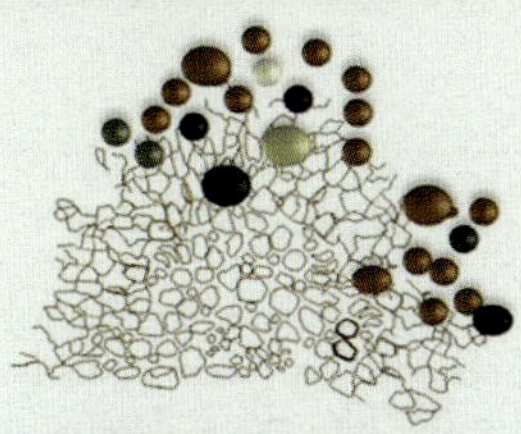	Globules of different size, shape, and/or color. Black or brown dots with heterogeneity in color and off-center distribution
Streaks (ie, pseudopods and radial streaming)	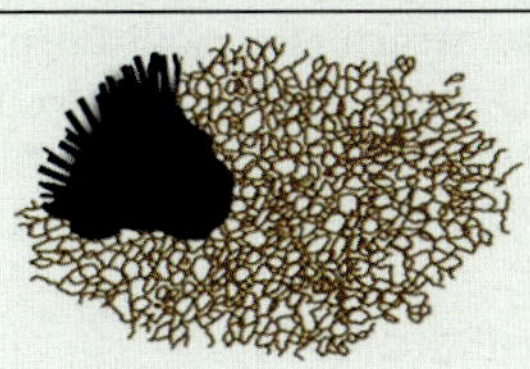	Radial lines with or without bulbous projections at their tips (pseudopods or radial streaming, respectively), focally distributed.

(*Continued*)

TABLE 25-4 Dermoscopic melanoma-specific structures (*Continued*)

Melanoma-specific structure	Schematic	Definition
Irregular blotch	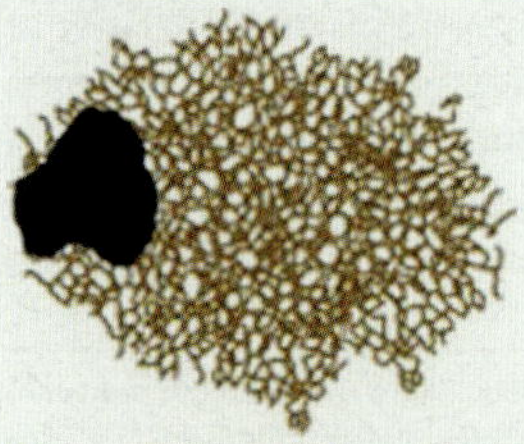	Brown-black-blue structureless area located off-center or multiple blotches within the same lesion.
Regression structures (ie, peppering or granularity, and scar-like depigmentation)	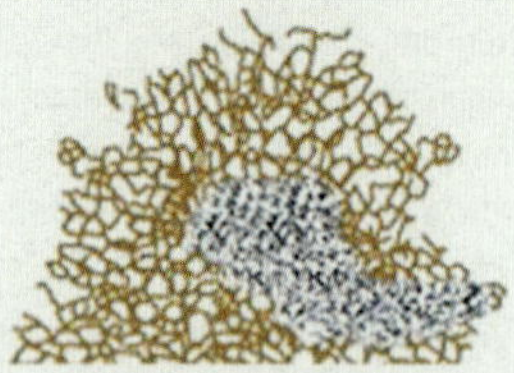	Peppering or granularity, consist of gray fine dots. Scar-like depigmentation, consist of white structureless areas that are lighter than the surrounding skin.
Shiny white structures		Shiny white lines oriented, parallel, and orthogonal to each other. Only seen with polarized light.
Blue-white veil	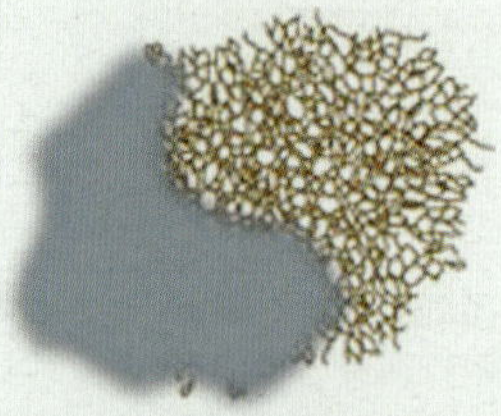	Structureless blue to white area with a "ground-glass haze" appearance. The blue white veil is located over raised areas and does not occupy the entire lesion.
Polymorphous vessels	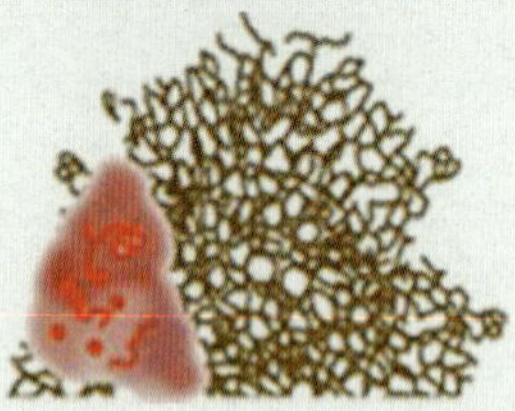	Two or more vessel morphologies within the same lesion. A common combination includes the dotted and linear irregular morphologies.

in a disorganized manner.[13] Lesions revealing a fibrillar pattern on the palms or an irregular fibrillar pattern should raise suspicion for melanoma [**Figure 25-5**].[13]

Any volar lesion not adhering to one of the benign patterns above-described nor revealing any of the aforementioned diagnostic structures should be viewed with caution and management can rely on the maximal diameter of the lesion and age; thus, patients older than 50 years presenting with lesions greater than 7 to 10 mm in diameter should be considered for biopsy, whereas lesions smaller than 7 to 10 mm in diameter can be digitally monitored or, depending on the structures and context, consider a skin biopsy.[14]

Some scoring systems have been created to guide the decision-making process as to whether an acral lesion needs to be biopsied. One of these scoring systems is the BRAAFF checklist,[15] which determines the need for a biopsy based on the presence or absence of specific dermoscopic structures (irregular **B**lotch: +1; parallel **R**idge pattern: +3; **A**symmetry of structures: +1; **A**symmetry of colors: +1; parallel **F**urrow pattern: −1; **F**ibrillar pattern: −1). Skin biopsies are recommended for lesions with scores greater than 1. Nonetheless, more studies are required to establish more accurate conclusions.

NONMELANOCYTIC NEOPLASMS

BENIGN

SEBORRHEIC KERATOSES

Seborrheic keratoses (SK) reveal one or more of the following dermoscopic structures and features: sharply demarcated borders, comedo-like openings, milia-like cysts, cerebriform pattern, fissures and ridges, fingerprint-like structures, moth-eaten border, hairpin vessels with white halo, and network-like structures. Overall, SK in SOC individuals can present as darkly pigmented lesions [**Figure 25-6**] with darker color and less visible hairpin vessels[16].

DERMATOFIBROMA

The classical dermoscopic pattern associated with dermatofibromas (DF) can be seen in individuals with SOC. The typical DF pattern consists of a delicate peripheral pigmented network and central white patch,

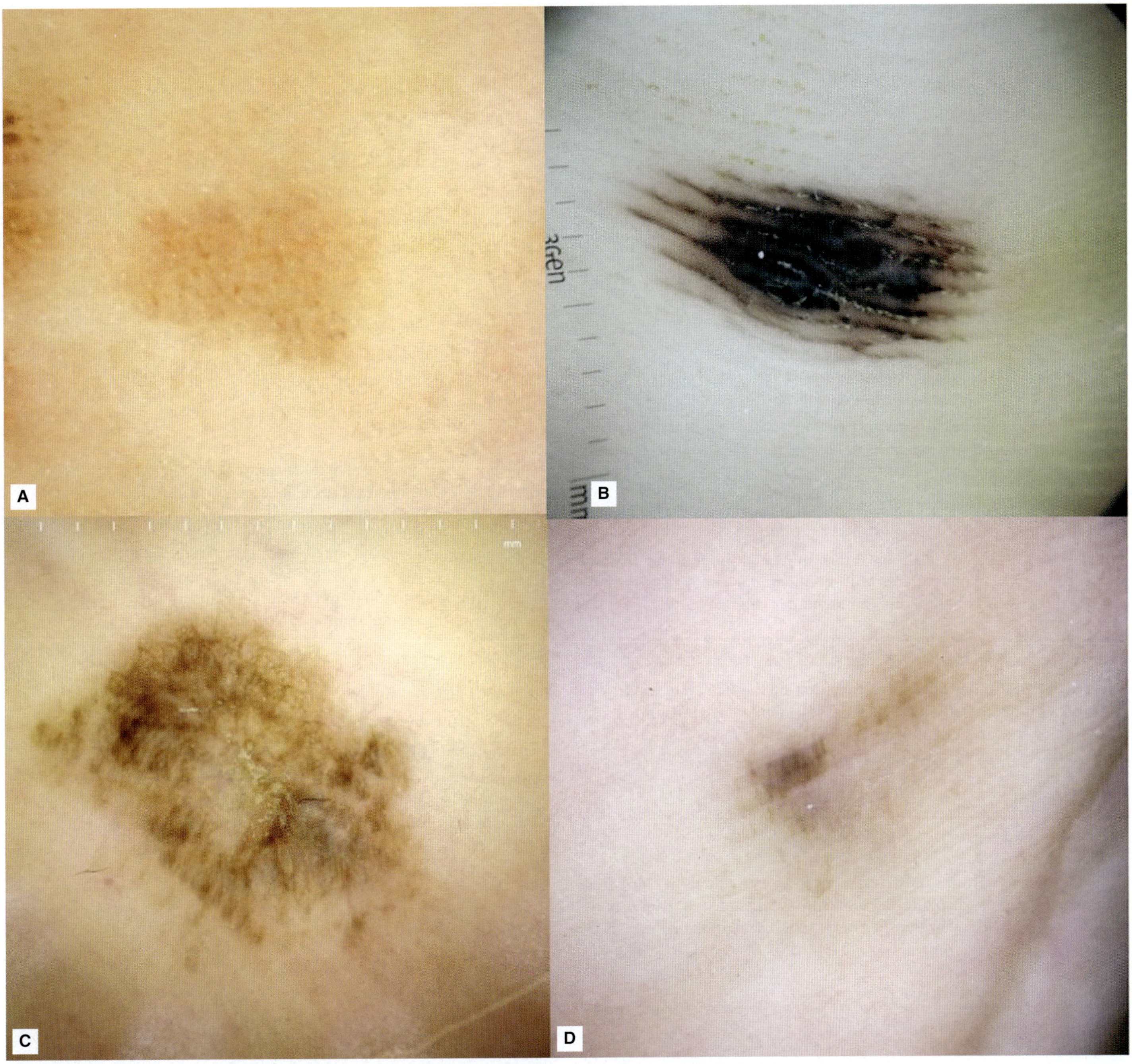

FIGURE 25-5. Dermoscopy images of acral melanomas revealing a parallel ridge pattern (**A** and **B**), which is the most specific dermoscopic pattern for acral lentiginous melanoma; a multicomponent pattern (**B, C**) and an atypical fibrillar pattern (**D**), with lines of different thickness and variability in spacing and color.

which corresponds to pronounced fibrosis within the papillary dermis with hyperpigmented rete ridges at the edge of DF. Other DF patterns that can be seen in patients with FST V and VI include a delicate diffuse pigment network, and a pigment network with pigment encircling follicular openings [**Figure 25-7**].[17]

MALIGNANT

BASAL CELL CARCINOMA

Although basal cell carcinoma (BCC) is more common in patients with fair skin, it can also be seen in patients with SOC. More than 50% of BCCs in non-White individuals, including FST IV and V, are pigmented BCCs, showing leaf-like structures, spoke-wheel-like structures, concentric structures, blue dots/globules/nests,[18] ulceration, and short fine telangiectasias [**Figure 25-8**]. In particular, the presence of ulceration, blue-white color, and arborizing vessels have been associated with nodular BCCs, while leaf-like areas, red-white structureless areas, multiple small erosions, and spoke-wheel areas were associated with superficial BCC.[19]

SQUAMOUS CELL CARCINOMA

Squamous cell carcinoma (SCC) is the most common cutaneous malignancy in Africans and South Asians, representing 30% to 65% of skin cancers. SCC occurs most commonly on sun-exposed sites such as the head and neck in Whites and on sun-protected sites in African Americans, including the anogenital area in 10% to 23% of cases. Common dermoscopic structures include structureless asymmetric brown areas with or without dots, blue/gray dots in a linear arrangement, and coiled vessels.

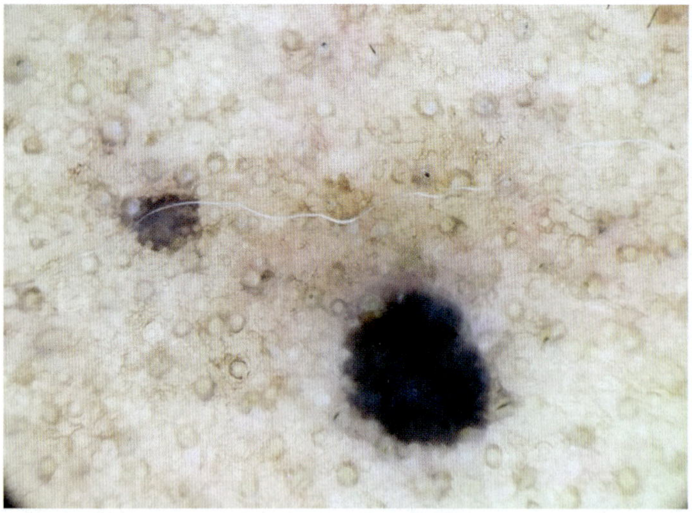

FIGURE 25-6. Seborrheic keratosis in a patient with skin of color. Dermoscopy reveals a darkly pigmented lesion, with regular and well-demarcated borders, and few comedo-like openings; vessels are not visible.

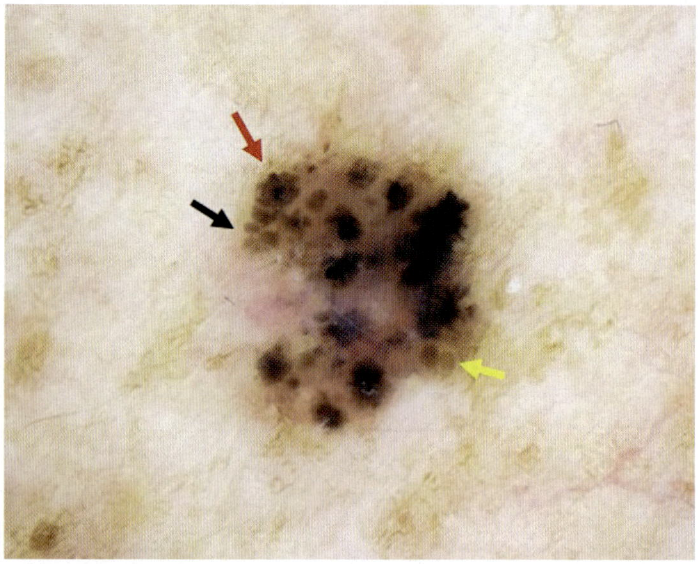

FIGURE 25-8. Pigmented basal cell carcinoma. Dermoscopy demonstrates pigmented structures including leaf-like areas (black arrow), spoke-wheel-like structures (red arrow), and blue-gray ovoid nests (yellow arrow).

Typically, the brown areas are on the periphery of the lesion.[20] Despite these differences, many patients will reveal similar characteristics/patterns to those seen in light-skinned individuals [**Figure 25-9**].

TRICHOSCOPY

Trichoscopy is the dermoscopic evaluation of the hair and scalp; it is noninvasive and cost-efficient. Trichoscopy facilitates the diagnosis and follow-up of hair and scalp disorders. This section reviews some differences in the trichoscopic evaluation of patients with SOC.

PHYSIOLOGICAL CHANGES

DENSITY

Follicular density is lower in African American individuals as compared with Americans of Hispanic descent and Caucasians. A trichoscopy study showed that the hair density means ± SD ranged from 148 ± 25 to 160 ± 27/cm^2 in individuals of African descent, and that the hair density was higher in the frontal than in the occipital scalp.[21]

HAIR FOLLICLE SHAPE

The shape of the hair follicle differs among races and ethnicities[22]:

- Asian patients have round hair shafts emerging from straight follicles.
- Hispanic patients reveal straight hair or elliptical or curled shafts.
- Black patients demonstrate curled hair shafts, which may result in poor flow of sebum across the hair, leading to greater scalp xerosis, more susceptibility to traction alopecia, hair breakage, and ultimately a greater risk for infections.

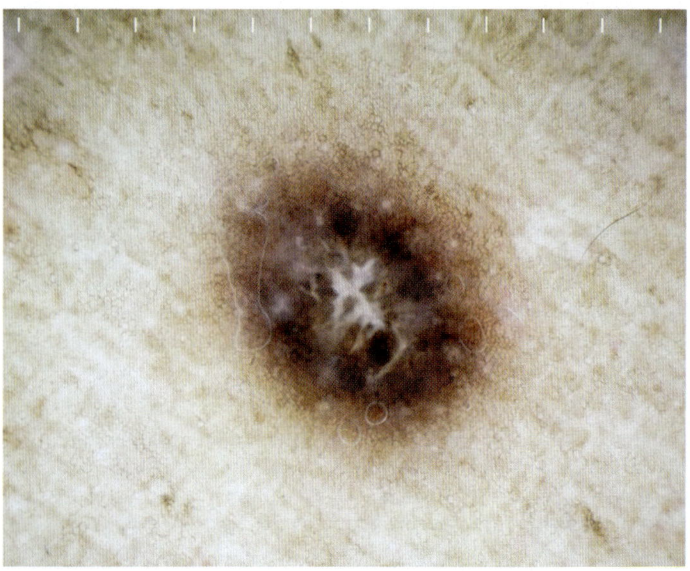

FIGURE 25-7. Dermatofibroma. Dermoscopy reveals a deeply pigment network with pigment encircling follicular openings and central scar-like area.

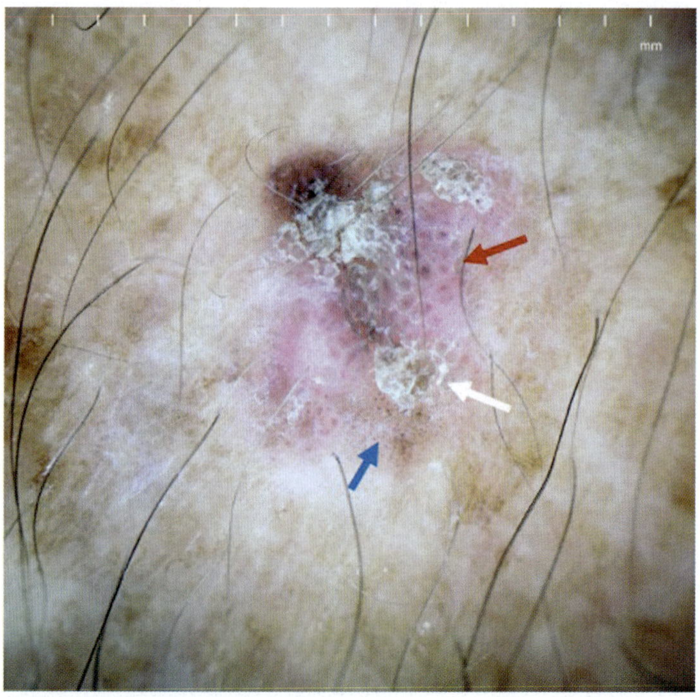

FIGURE 25-9. Pigmented squamous cell carcinoma. Dermoscopy reveals brown dots in a lineal arrangement (blue arrow), coiled vessels (red arrow), and scale (white arrow).

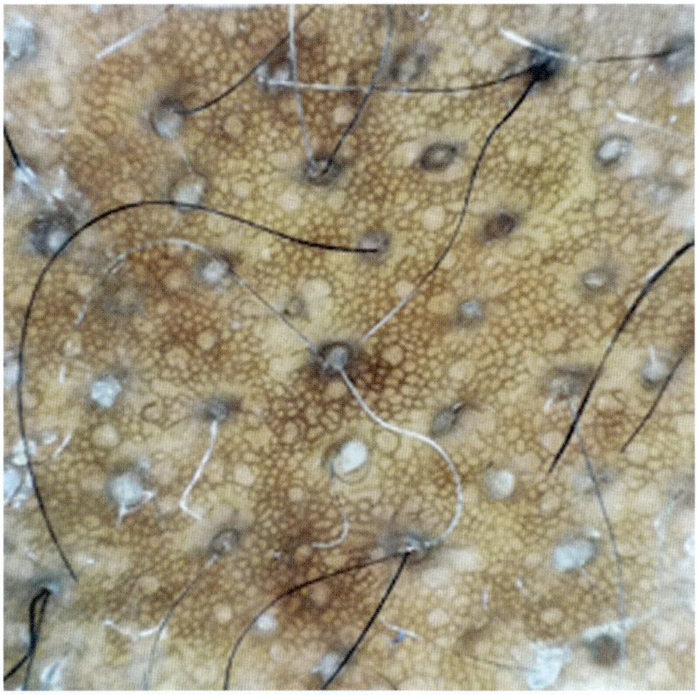

FIGURE 25-10. Pigmented network and pinpoint white dots.

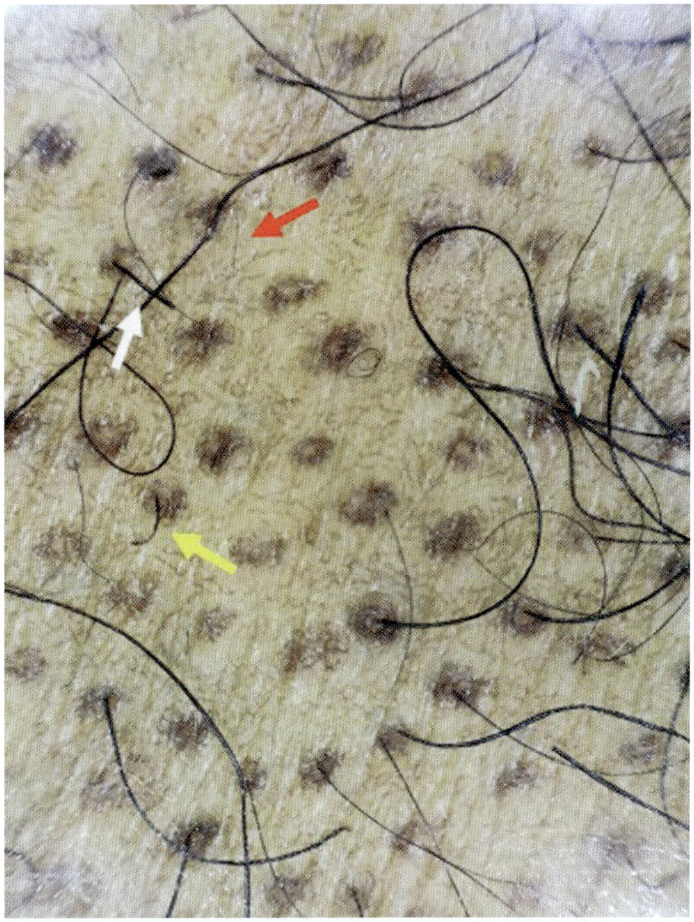

FIGURE 25-11. Alopecia areata. Short vellus hair (red arrow), broken hair (white arrow).

SCALP MORPHOLOGY

A *perifollicular pigmented network or honeycomb pattern* [**Figure 25-10**] is normally visible over the whole scalp. It is formed by pigmented lines (corresponding to pigmented rete ridges) that surround hypochromic areas (fewer melanocytes residing in the supra-papillary epidermis).[23]

Another distinctive feature of the pigmented scalp is the presence of *pinpoint white dots* [Figure 25-10] that are small (0.2-0.3 mm) and regularly distributed between the follicular units. Reflectance confocal microscopy demonstrated that these dots correspond to both the acrosyringium and follicular openings.[23]

Distribution of pinpoint white dots is useful to distinguish nonscarring alopecias, in which they are regularly distributed, from scarring alopecias, in which pinpoint white dots are irregularly distributed and interspersed with white patches.

NONSCARRING ALOPECIA

ANDROGENETIC ALOPECIA

The diagnostic criteria for patients with skin of color is the same as that for White patients: more than 20% variability in hair shaft diameter and presence of short, thin (0.03 mm in diameter), regrowing hairs in the frontal scalp.

Some variations seen in the scalp of individuals with SOC include:

- **Dots.** *Yellow and white dots* in androgenetic alopecia are correlated with the advanced Ludwig and Sinclair stages of hair loss. *White dots* are more visible on SOC scalp due to the degree of pigmentation that allows its easier visualization.[24]
- **Peripilar sign** consists of perifollicular discoloration, which can be brown (31.7%) or white (26.7%).[24] Perifollicular discoloration can be seen in female androgenetic alopecia among patients with SOC (44.3%, 35/79), specifically brown peripilar halo (31.6%, 25/79), which is usually caused by perifollicular lymphocytic infiltration, and white peripilar halo (11.3%, 9/79).
- Predominance of one hair per follicle and presence honeycomb pigmentation.[24,25]

ALOPECIA AREATA

Alopecia areata (AA) has been reported to occur equally among races. Nonetheless, one recent study in the United States found significantly higher odds of AA in African Americans compared with Whites.[26] Common dermoscopic findings in AA include white dots, black dots, short vellus hairs, exclamation mark hair, and broken hair [**Figure 25-11**]. Yellow dots are not commonly seen in patients of African descents but have been reported as a highly sensitive sign for the diagnosis of AA in South Asians including prepubertal patients. This finding should be interpreted with caution since it can also be seen among people who apply oils to their scalp.[27,28]

TINEA CAPITIS

The clinical diagnosis of tinea capitis in dark-skinned scalp can represent a diagnostic challenge as erythema of the scalp is more difficult to appreciate. Corkscrew hairs, which present as irregularly twisted short hairs, are a characteristic sign in patients of African descent [**Figure 25-12**].[23] Other common signs are:

- ***Comma hairs***: short haris that result from cracking and bending of the shaft due to fungal invasion.
- ***Morse code-like hairs***, also known as bar code-like hairs, are due to perforation of shaft by the fungal spores.
- ***Zig-zag hairs*** refer to the structure of hairs that are bent at different angles

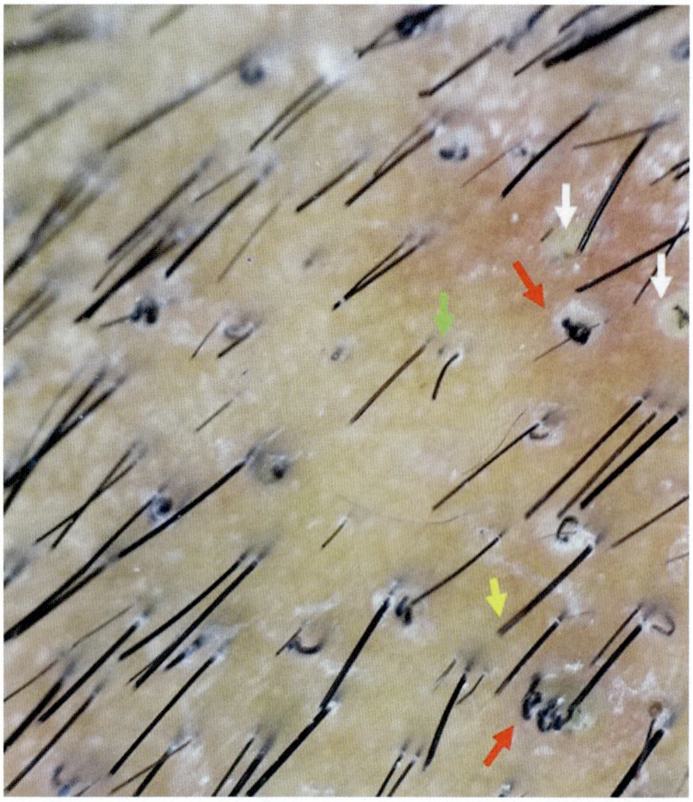

FIGURE 25-12. Tinea capitis. Corkscrew hairs (red arrows), perifollicular pustules (white arrows), and black dot (green arrow).

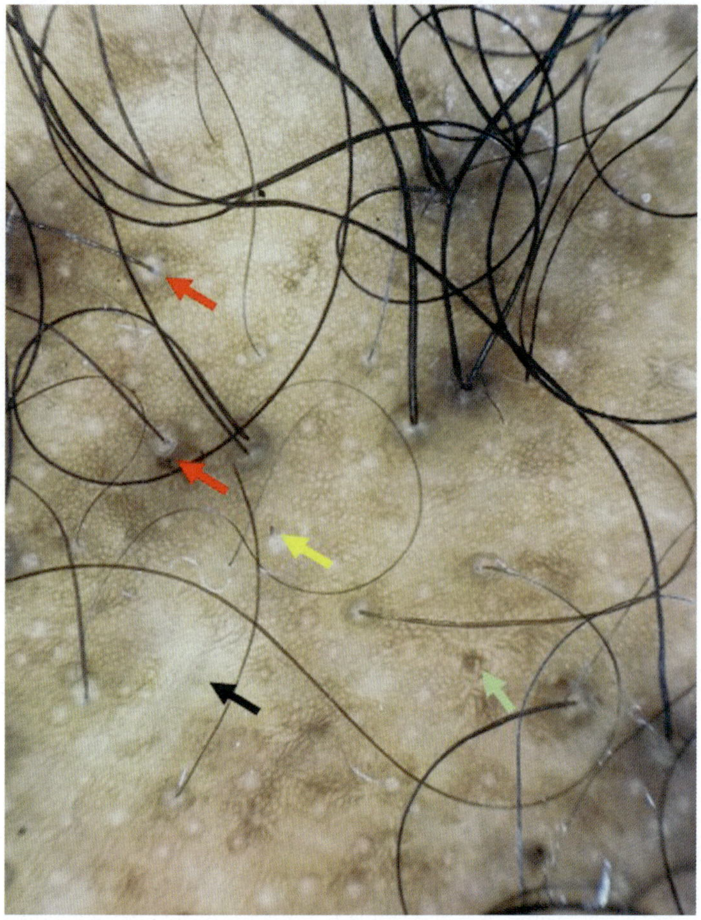

FIGURE 25-13. Central centrifugal cicatricial alopecia. Peripilar gray/white halo (red arrow), which is a suitable site for a scalp biopsy, irregularly distributed pinpoint white dots (yellow arrow) and white patches (black arrow), interfollicular-pigmented asterisk-like brown macules (green arrow).

SCARRING ALOPECIA

CENTRAL CENTRIFUGAL CICATRICIAL ALOPECIA

Central centrifugal cicatricial alopecia (CCCA) is a scarring alopecia regularly seen in African American individuals. Dermoscopy structures suggestive of CCCA, include[29]:

1. Peripilar gray/white halo, which corresponds to the concentric peripilar fibrosis in the affected follicles, and is a specific and sensitive dermatoscopic sign for CCCA.
2. Broken hairs, seen as black dots inside the follicular opening or as short broken shafts, which are a sign of traction.
3. Pinpoint white dots with irregular distribution.
4. Hair shaft variability.
5. White patches, which represent follicular dropout and follicular scarring.
6. Perifollicular erythema.
7. Concentric white perifollicular and interfollicular scales.
8. Interfollicular-pigmented asterisk-like or stellate brown macules.

Dermoscopy is a helpful aid to identify the optimal biopsy site that will ultimately establish the diagnosis. Dermoscopic findings in clinically unaffected and affected sites tend to be similar, thus the suitable site for biopsy must include, one, two, or more hairs surrounded by the peripilar gray-white halo or a broken hair [**Figure 25-13**].[29]

ACNE KELOIDALIS NUCHAE

Individuals with SOC, especially African Americans, are more prone to developing acne keloidalis nuchae, and shaving is considered an important predisposing factor. Dermoscopy allows the visualization of pseudo-folliculitis, which is due to ingrown hairs with extra follicular penetration [**Figure 25-14**]. In advanced stages, dermoscopy reveals the presence of tufted hairs.[30]

TRACTION ALOPECIA

Traction alopecia affects any area of the hair-bearing scalp. Early in its clinical course, trichoscopy reveals signs of repetitive traction, which appears as nonscarring features with perifollicular erythema, regularly distributed pinpoint white dots and preservation of the honeycomb patter*n*[22]. With continued traction, trichoscopy shows signs of scarring alopecia including pinpoint white dots with an irregular distribution and irregular white patches. It is common to observe follicular papules or pustules. Presence of casts [**Figure 25-15A**] around the proximal shaft of the hairs surrounding the patch indicates ongoing traction.[31] In addition, trichoscopy reveals reduced hair density with absence of follicular openings or absence of hairs with preserved follicular openings outlined with brown pigmentation, which correspond to the pigmented basal cell layer of the follicular infundibulum.[32] Recently, Agrawal et al described the "flambeau sign" [**Figure 25-15B**], which corresponds to white linear tracks in continuation with the shaft of hair at one end giving the appearance of a flame or lit torch.[33]

DISCOID LUPUS ERYTHEMATOSUS (DLE)

Patients of color with discoid lupus erythematosus (DLE) have greater probabilities of having scalp involvement compared with other DLE patients.[34] Loss of pigmentation with disruption of the honeycomb pattern, and reduced number or absence of pinpoint white dots are typical and unique features of DLE in the scalp of color. Blue-gray dots arranged in a speckled pattern produced by pigment incontinence are

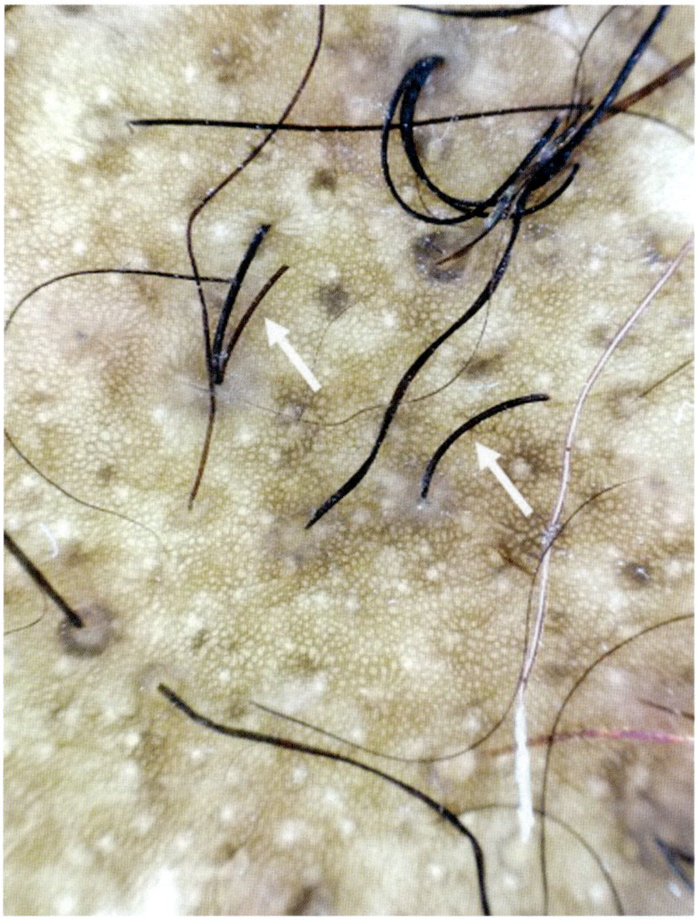

FIGURE 25-14. Acne keloidalis nuchae. Note hair ingrowing with extra follicular penetration (white arrow).

also characteristic.[23] Enlarged tortuous and branching vessels are common, and their presence strongly suggests a diagnosis of DLE. This finding associated with hyperkeratotic follicular scales was 100% specific for the diagnosis of DLE in an Iranian study [**Figure 25-16**].[23]

DISSECTING CELLULITIS

In early stages of the disease, trichoscopy shows signs of nonscarring alopecia with broken hair shafts of variable length, black dots, and enlarged follicular openings filled with a keratotic plug.[35]

LICHEN PLANOPILARIS

The most common trichoscopic features of classic lichen planopilaris in SOC population include irregularly distributed pinpoint white dots that give rise to a starry sky appearance (*starry sky pattern*) and presence of peripilar casts surrounding the hair shafts at their emergency. Other findings include few broken hairs, black dots, and pili torti (flattened hair shafts that twist 180° at irregular intervals).[23]

Furthermore, blue-gray dots around the follicular structures are seen as a "target" pattern. In contrast to DLE, the blue-gray dots target pattern in LPP indicates circular arrangement of melanin around the perifollicular area sparing the interfollicular area.[36]

FRONTAL FIBROSING ALOPECIA (FFA)

Frontal fibrosing alopecia (FFA) also may be misdiagnosed as traction alopecia in Hispanic and Black patients because both conditions occur along the hairline. Trichoscopy of the receding hairline displays absence

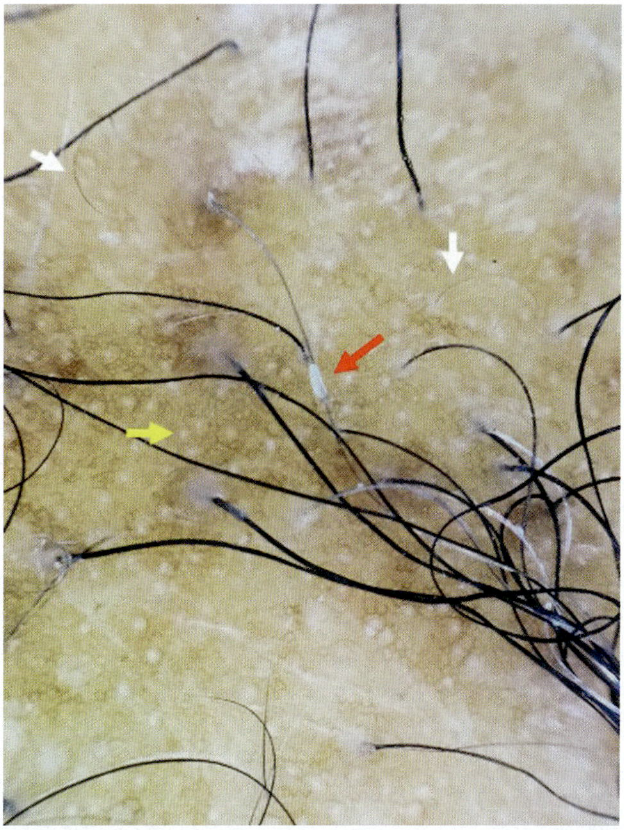

A

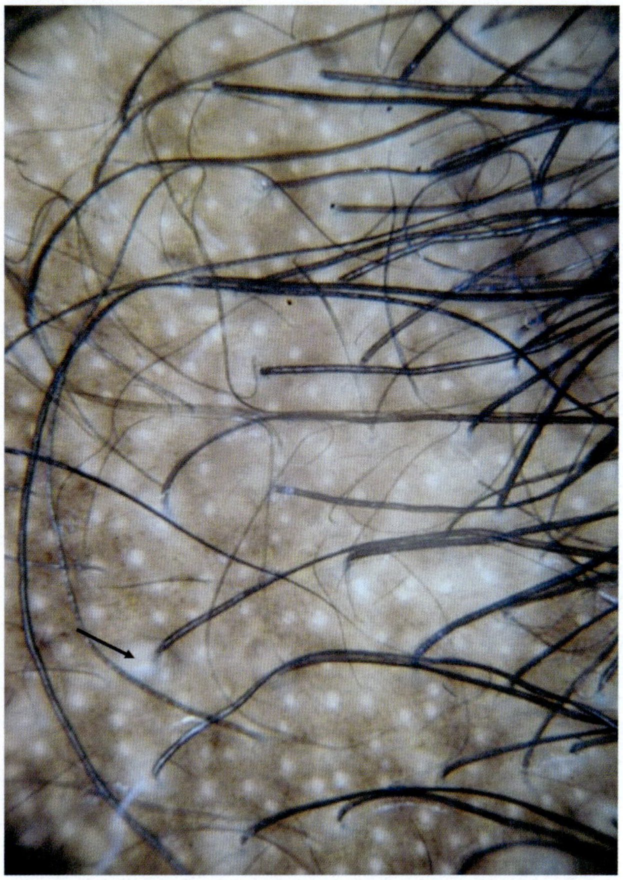

B

FIGURE 25-15. **(A)** Traction Alopecia. Hair casts (red arrow), vellus hair (white arrows), pinpoint white dots (red arrows). **(B)** Flambeau sign.

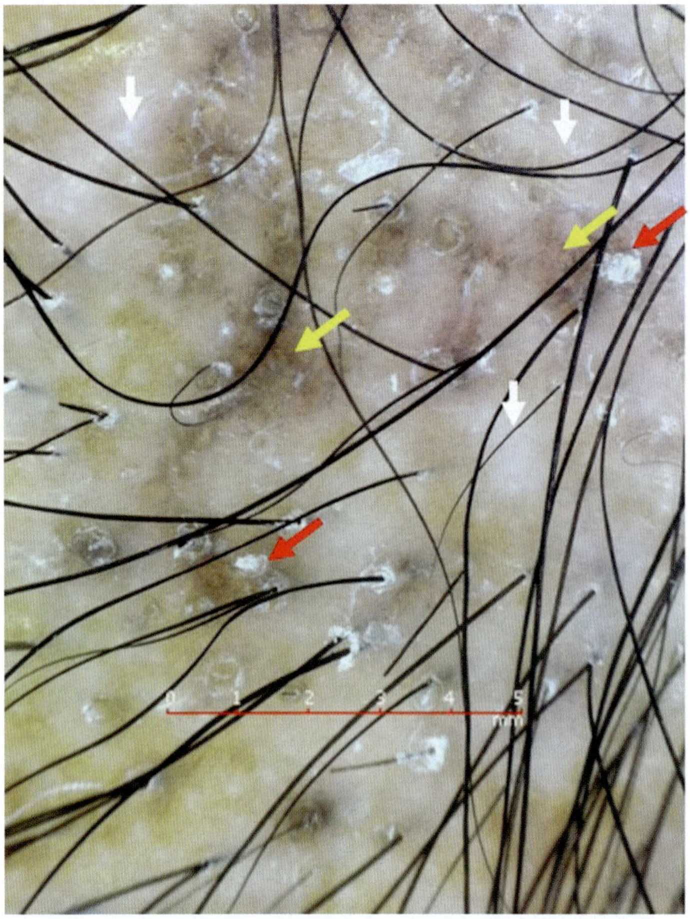

FIGURE 25-16. Discoid lupus erythematosus. Loss of the honeycomb pattern, absence of pinpoint white dots (white arrows), keratin plugs (red arrows), blue-gray dots (yellow arrow) inside the patch of alopecia referred to as "speckles" pattern.

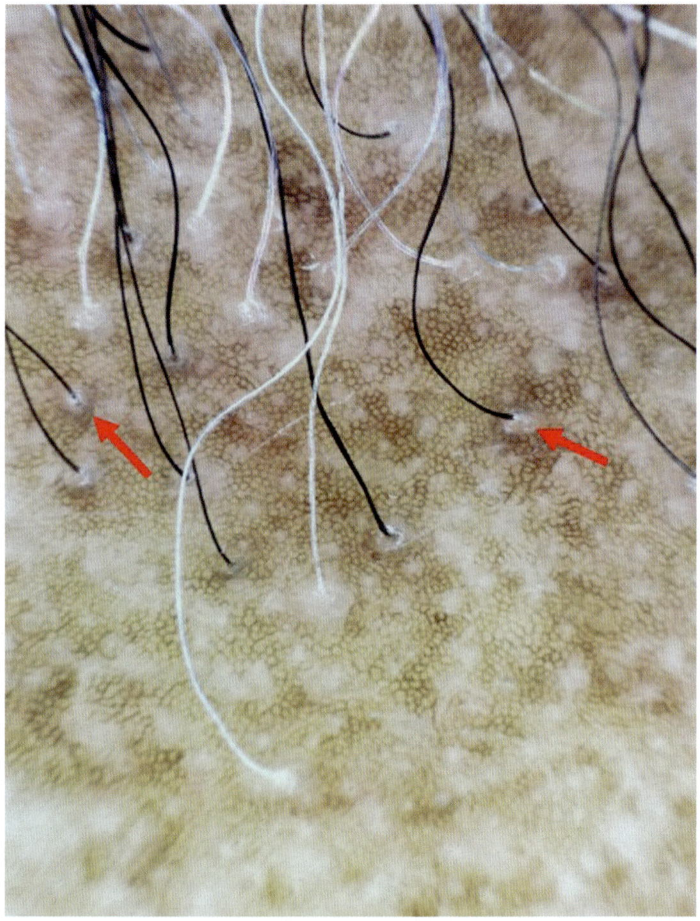

FIGURE 25-17. Frontal fibrosing alopecia. Absence of vellus hairs and peripilar casts. Pinpoint white dots are irregularly distributed.

of vellus hairs and presence of terminal hairs with peripilar casts, which may be subtle or very prominent [**Figure 25-17**]. Black dots, pili torti (flattened hair shafts that twist 180° at irregular intervals), follicular hyperpigmentation, and broken hairs can also be seen.[37]

FOLLICULITIS DECALVANS

Trichoscopic features of folliculitis decalvans change according to the inflammatory activity of the disease.

Saceda-Corralo et al described two groups of features:

Red patterns

- Perifollicular erythema (dilation of the superficial vascular plexus)
- Perifollicular hemorrhages (extravasation of erythrocytes)

Yellow structures

- follicular pustules, yellow tubular scaling and yellow crusts.

All of them represent the neutrophilic inflammatory infiltrate of the disease.[38]

Hair tufting with tufts of more than seven hairs emerging from a common follicular openings is a typical finding [**Figure 25-18**].

OTHER FORMS OF ALOPECIA SEEN IN SOC POPULATION

HAIR BREAKAGE

Hair breakage is the weakening of the hair shaft from root to tip due to excessive styling and straightening. The trichoscopy can be heterogeneous and may include *trichorrhexis nodosa* (segmental increase in the hair diameter like nodules and splitting of their tips) and *trichoptilosis* (longitudinal fractures on the shaft, consisting in the division of the distal end), among other findings [**Figure 25-19**].[39]

ONYCHOSCOPY

Nail unit dermoscopy allows differentiating melanocytic from nonmelanocytic pigmentation, in particular the brown-black nail discolorations due to subungual hematoma, fungal infection, or tumors with secondary pigmentation. When performing dermoscopy on nails, it is important to evaluate the nail plate, hyponychium, proximal and lateral skin folds. In addition, it is useful to use the dermatoscope in the contact mode using ultrasound gel as the liquid interface.

LONGITUDINAL MELANONYCHIA: BENIGN CAUSES

RACIAL MELANONYCHIA

Racial melanonychia is one of the most prevalent nail changes among individuals with FST IV to VI, with a reported prevalence of up to 73%.[40] Racial melanonychia involves multiple nails, and the color tends to be homogeneous gray-brown. Not infrequently, patients with SOC demonstrate wider and/or darker bands as compared to lighter-skin populations.[41] Dermoscopy reveals a gray or brown-to-black background in the European population or FST IV to VI, respectively. During the evaluation of the skin folds, a pseudo-Hutchinson sign (visualization of the nail matrix pigment through the relatively translucent nail folds) [**Figure 25-20**] can be observed in up to 34% of patients with FST IV to VI.

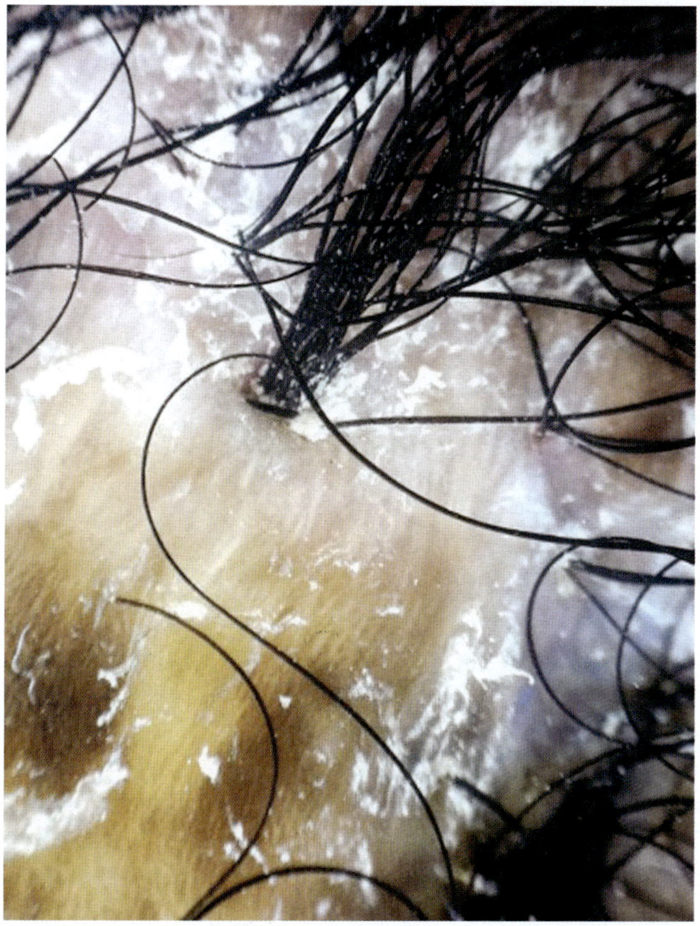

FIGURE 25-18. Folliculitis decalvans. Hair tufting.

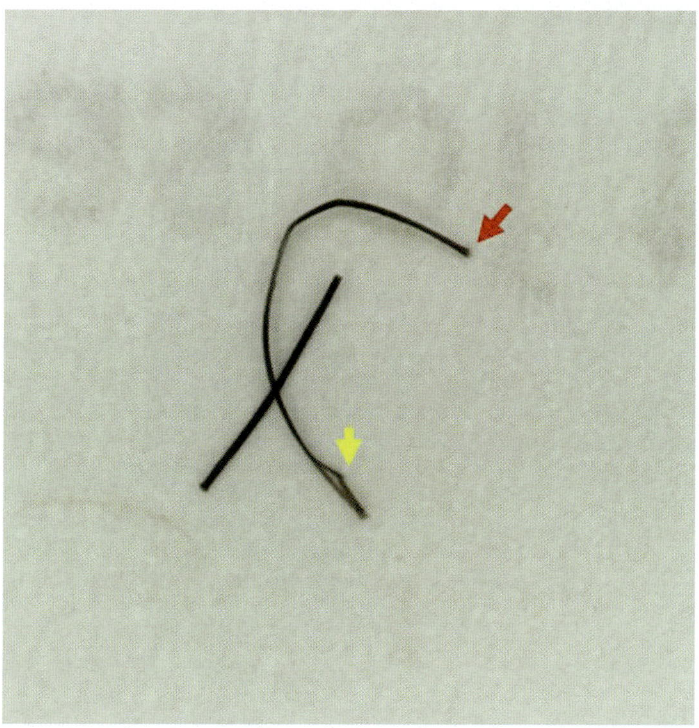

FIGURE 25-19. Hair breakage. Trichoptilosis, longitudinal split in the hair shaft (yellow arrow). Trichorrhexis, segmental increase in the hair diameter and splitting of their tips (red arrow).

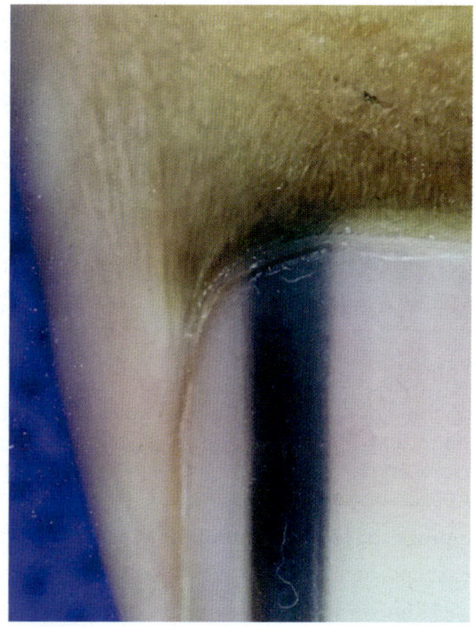

FIGURE 25-20. Pseudo-Hutchinson sign.

MELANOCYTIC HYPERPLASIA

Benign melanocytic proliferations (nevi or lentigo) are among the main causes of longitudinal melanonychia. There are some clinical and dermoscopic characteristics that may help us differentiate these entities from melanoma[42]:

- Lentigo and nevi are often smaller in *size* (less than one-third of the nail width) and tend to be more regular than melanoma
- Melanocytic nevi show a brown to black background with lines that are regular with regard to pattern, coloration, width, spacing, parallelism, and hyponychium pigmentation. Dermoscopic criteria for distinguishing nevi from possible melanoma are not valuable in children, in whom melanocytic nevi often shows dermoscopic irregular patterns of color and lines as well as periungual pigmentation [**Figure 25-21**]. This last one characteristic could be wrongly interpreted due to the

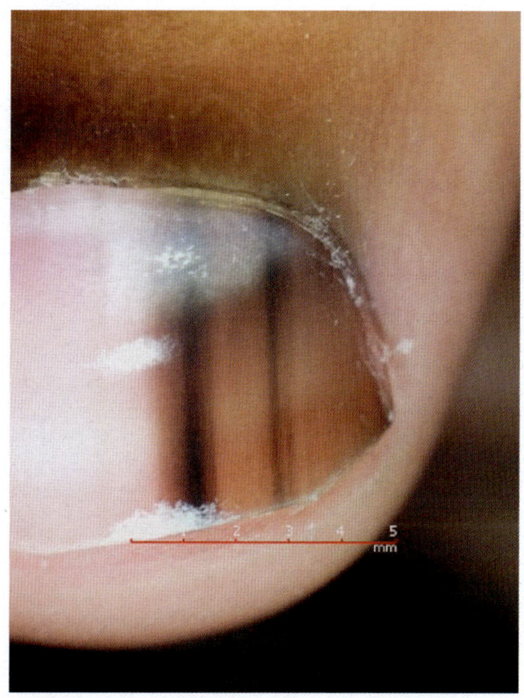

FIGURE 25-21. Nevi in a child. Longitudinal melanonychia with irregular patterns of color and lines as well as periungual pigmentation.

belief that pigmentation of the periungual fold extending from a longitudinal melanonychia (***Hutchinson sign***) is always suggestive of malignancy. On the hyponychium, melanocytic nevi can reveal pigment in a brushy linear fashion, which presents across the skin marking, similar to the dermoscopic features of acquired plantar melanocytic nevus; this phenomenon has been denominated *Benign Hutchinson sign.*[42]

LONGITUDINAL MELANONYCHIA: MALIGNANT CAUSES

NAIL MELANOMA

Although melanoma of the nail unit is a rare condition, it has a higher relative incidence and mortality among the SOC population. Studies show that African American patients have up to 3.5 times higher mortality rate than Caucasian patients.

Clinical findings suggestive of melanoma include[1,43]:

- Longitudinal band covering more than two-thirds of the nail.
- *Hutchison sign*: brown-black pigmentation extending from longitudinal melanonychia into the proximal and lateral nail folds visualized with the naked eye.
- *Triangular shape*: The proximal width of the melanonychia is wider than its distal end. This triangular shape can be seen in rapidly growing tumors, including melanoma [**Figure 25-22**].[13]
- *Nail dystrophy* with complete or partial destruction of the nail plate [**Figure 25-23**].

Dermoscopic structures suggestive of nail melanoma include:

- *Irregular linear pattern*, which consists of an irregular band with multiple longitudinal lines of variable colors and width, as well as irregular spacing between the lines and disruption of the parallelism [Figure 25-23].
- Gray to black pigmented lines over a brown background, with pigmented granules (aka melanin inclusions) [**Figure 25-24**].
- *Micro-Hutchinson sign*: pigmentation on the proximal nail fold or cuticle, only visualized with dermoscopy [**Figure 25-25**]. The micro-Hutchinson sign needs to be differentiated from the pseudo-Hutchinson sign, which occurs when the pigment located in the nail matrix/nail plate is visible through a relatively translucent and normal cuticular skin and which has no diagnostic significance.

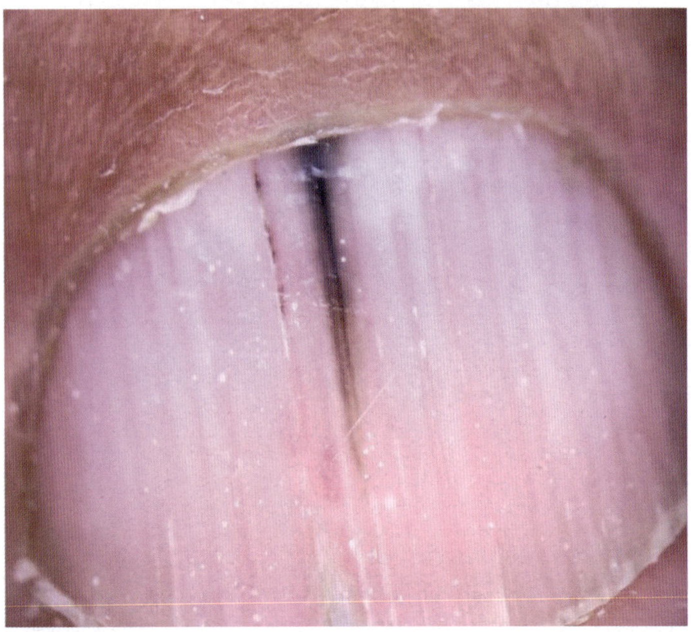

FIGURE 25-22. Nail melanoma. Gray to black pigmented lines with triangular shape.

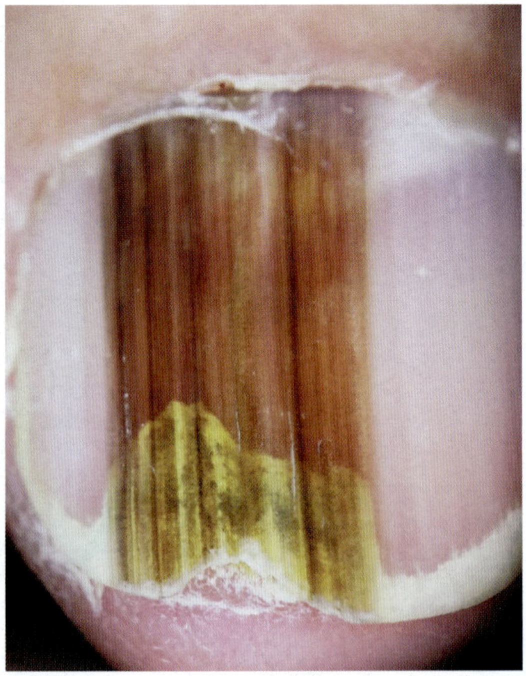

FIGURE 25-23. Nail melanoma. Irregular linear pattern with nail dystrophy.

- Hyponychial pigmentation with any melanoma-specific structure.

Intraoperative evaluation of melanonychia (after removal of nail plate). Four dermoscopic nail matrix patterns have been described:[43]

- Regular gray pattern, characterized by the presence of fine regular grayish lines due to melanocytic activation.
- Regular brown pattern, characterized by regular brown lines. It's most commonly present in benign melanocytic hyperplasia [**Figure 25-26A**].

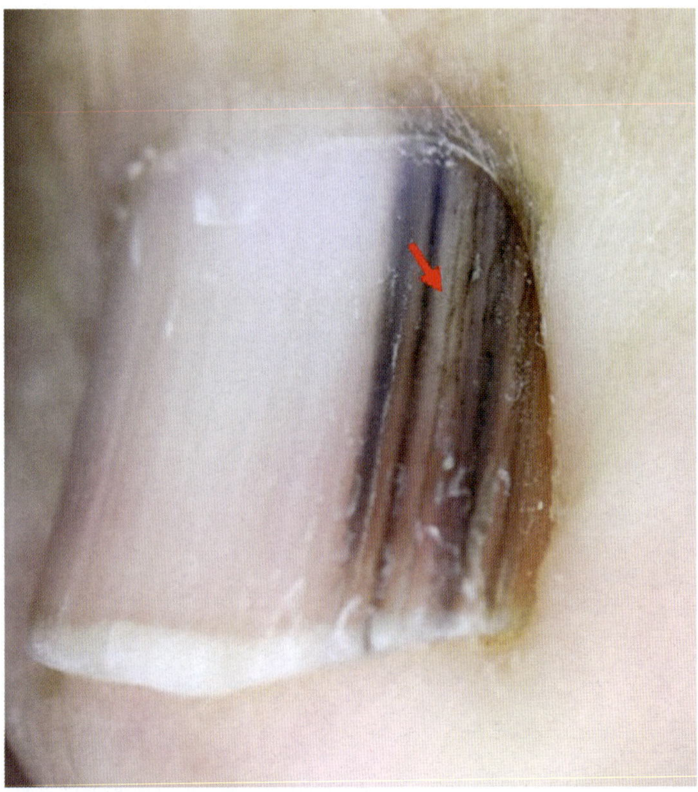

FIGURE 25-24. Nail melanoma. Gray to black pigmented lines over a brown background, with pigmented granules (red arrow).

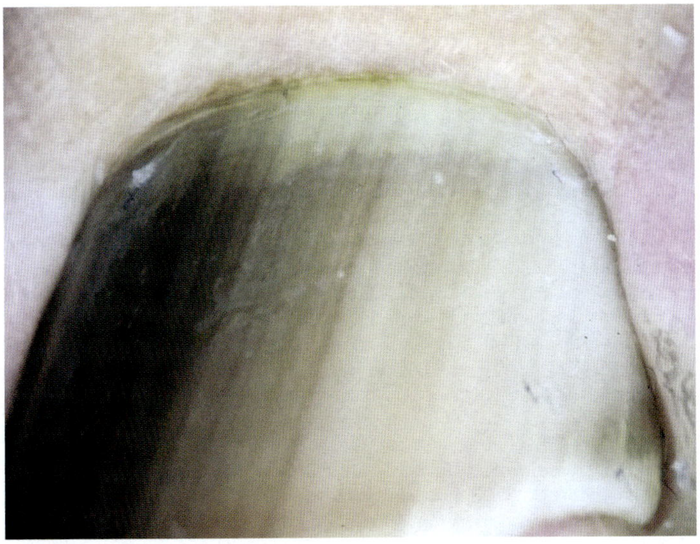

FIGURE 25-25. Micro-Hutchinson sign.

- The regular brown pattern with globules or blotches, characterized by the presence of regular longitudinal brown lines, globules or blotches. They are visualized in melanocytic nevi [**Figure 25-26B**].
- The irregular pattern, characterized by the presence of longitudinal lines of irregular color and thickness, with or without irregular globules or blotches, seen in melanoma [**Figure 25-26C**].

PIGMENTED SQUAMOUS CELL CARCINOMA AND BOWEN'S DISEASE

- Bowen's disease (BD), together with squamous cell carcinoma (SCC), is the most common malignant tumor of the nail unit. Longitudinal melanonychia in the setting of a nail SCC is frequently described in Asians and Black patients.[44] Although this SCC variant seems to be linked to racial origin, Shimizu et al reported the association of HPV-56 in two-thirds of SCC with longitudinal melanonychia.[45]
- Dermoscopy clues for pigmented BD include brown dots in a lineal distribution. It has been suggested that keratinocytes produce high amounts of keratinocyte growth factor and fibroblast growth factor, which leads to an indirect activation of melanogenic transcription factors with the resulting melanonychia [**Figure 25-27**].[46]

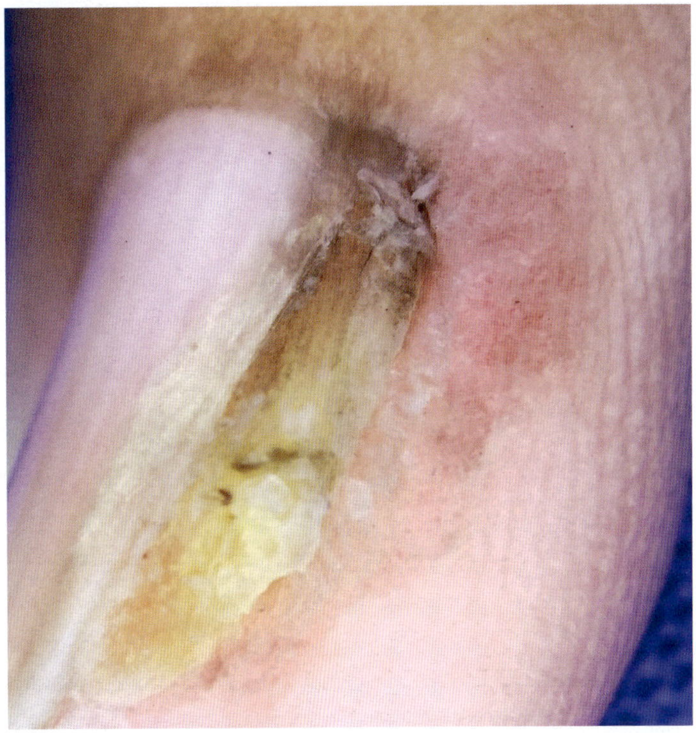

FIGURE 25-27. Pigmented squamous cell carcinoma with coiled vessels, hyperkeratosis, and brown dots in periungual folds.

OTHER PIGMENTED TUMORS

ONYCHOCITYC TUMORS

Onychomatricoma and onychocytic matricoma are neoplasms with matrical differentiation that can present with melanonychia. *Onychomatricoma* displays perforations in the distal portion of the nail plate, hemorrhagic striae, and white longitudinal grooves corresponding to the nail plate channels. Pigmented onychomatricoma has different tones of brown, blurred edges and may have additional coloration (green, yellow) due to mycotic and bacterial infection.

Onychocytic matricoma can present as a subtle localized pachyonychia. Melanonychia in onychocytic matricoma usually has regular

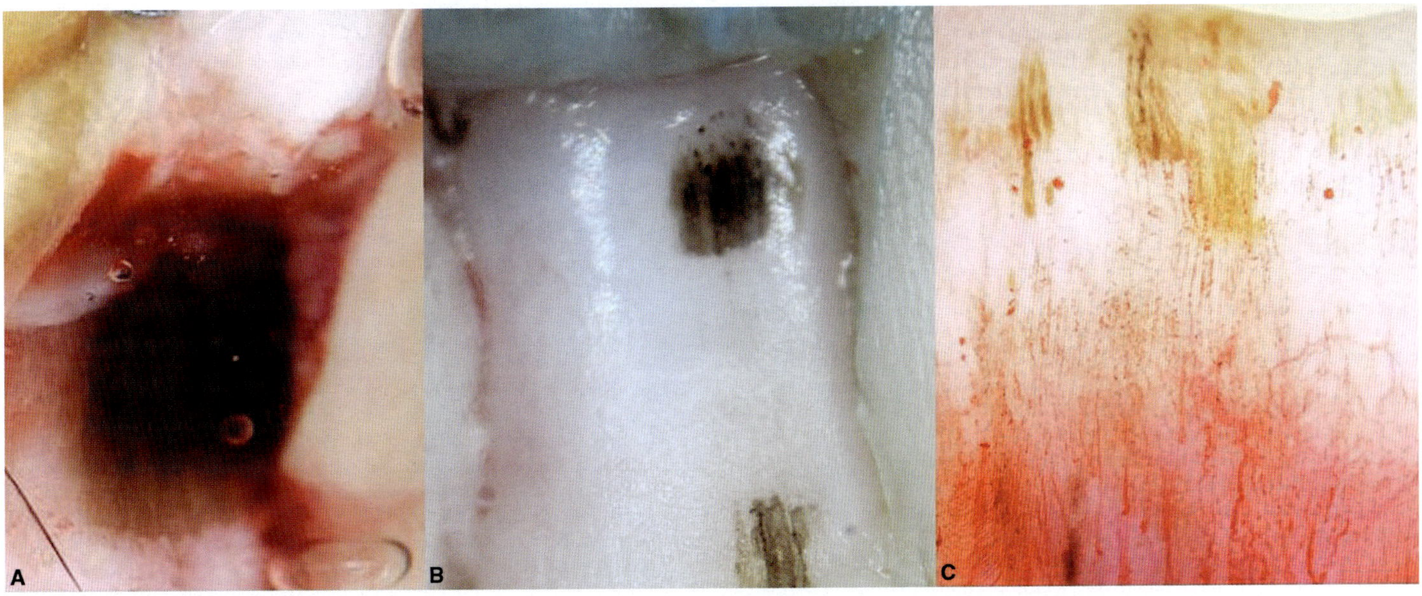

FIGURE 25-26. Intraoperative patterns. **(A)** Regular brown pattern. **(B)** The regular brown pattern with globules or blotches. **(C)** The irregular pattern.

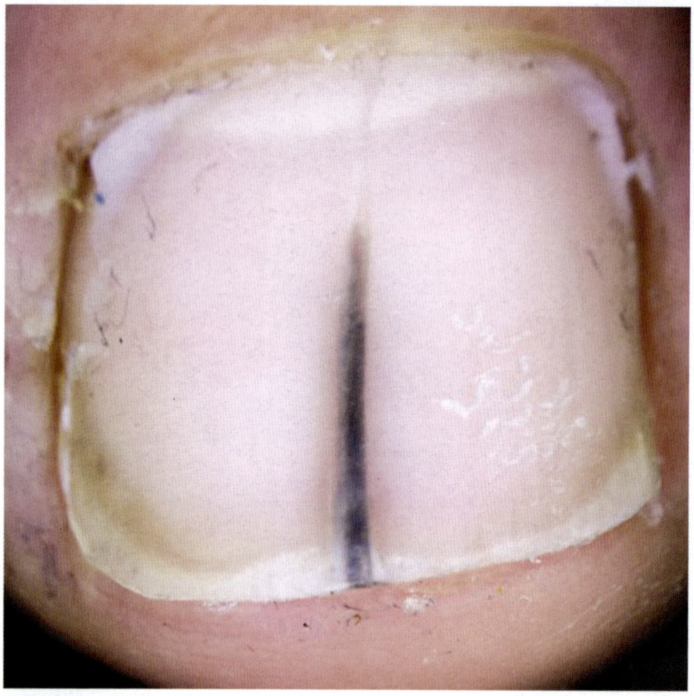

FIGURE 25-28. Onychocytic matricoma.

edges similar to longitudinal melanonychia caused by nevi or melanoma [**Figure 25-28**].[47]

Onychopapilloma can present with melanonychia instead of erytronychia in patients with SOC.[48]

CONCLUSIONS

- The most common dermoscopic patterns in melanocytic nevi among individuals with SOC include reticular diffuse, reticular with central hyperpigmentation, and homogeneous dark brown.
- All benign acral patterns can be seen among individuals with SOC, but the homogenous pattern is more frequently seen among SOC than White individuals.
- A perifollicular pigmented network or honeycomb pattern and presence of pinpoint white dots is a normal finding on the scalp of individuals with SOC.
- Nonscarring alopecia share several diagnostic signs in fair skin and SOC individuals.
- In nonscarring alopecia, the follicular ostium is preserved with the potential for hair regrowth. In scarring alopecia, the hair follicle is irreversibly destroyed due to the destruction of stem cells in the bulge area of the outer root sheath and replaced by white fibrous scar tissue.
- Intraoperative dermoscopy allows a better evaluation of longitudinal melanonychia.

REFERENCES

1. Ezenwa E, Stein JA, Krueger L. Dermoscopic features of neoplasms in skin of color: a review. *Int J Womens Dermatol.* 2021;7(2):145-151.
2. Tuma B, Yamada S, Atallah ÁN, Araujo FM, Hirata SH. Dermoscopy of black skin: a cross-sectional study of clinical and dermoscopic features of melanocytic lesions in individuals with type V/VI skin compared to those with type I/II skin. *J Am Acad Dermatol.* 2015;73(1):114-119.
3. Lallas A, Reggiani C, Argenziano G, Kyrgidis A, Bakos R, Masiero NC. Dermoscopic nevus patterns in skin of colour: a prospective, cross-sectional, morphological study in individuals with skin type V and VI. *J Eur Acad Dermatol Venereol.* 2014;28(11):1469-1474.
4. Zalaudek I, Schmid K, Marghoob AA, et al. Frequency of dermoscopic nevus subtypes by age and body site: a cross-sectional study. *Arch Dermatol.* 2011;147(6):663-670.
5. Reiter O, Chousakos E, Kurtansky N, et al. Association between the dermoscopic morphology of peripheral globules and melanocytic lesion diagnosis. *J Eur Acad Dermatol Venereol.* 2021;35(4):892-899.
6. Argenziano G, Catricala C, Ardigo M, et al. Dermoscopy of patients with multiple nevi: improved management recommendations using a comparative diagnostic approach. *Arch Dermatol.* 2011;147(1):46-49.
7. Uhara H, Koga H, Takata M, Saida T. The whiteboard marker as a useful tool for the dermoscopic "furrow ink test". *Arch Dermatol.* 2009;145(11):1331-1332.
8. Madankumar R, Gumaste PV, Martires K, et al. Acral melanocytic lesions in the United States: prevalence, awareness, and dermoscopic patterns in skin-of-color and non-Hispanic white patients. *J Am Acad Dermatol.* 2016;74(4):724-730.e1.
9. Miyazaki A, Saida T, Koga H, Oguchi S, Suzuki T, Tsuchida T. Anatomical and histopathological correlates of the dermoscopic patterns seen in melanocytic nevi on the sole: a retrospective study. *J Am Acad Dermatol.* 2005;53(2):230-236.
10. Braun RP, Thomas L, Dusza SW, et al. Dermoscopy of acral melanoma: a multicenter study on behalf of the international dermoscopy society. *Dermatology.* 2013;227(4):373-380.
11. González-Ramírez RA, Guerra-Segovia C, Garza-Rodríguez V, Garza-Báez P, Gómez-Flores M, Ocampo-Candiani J. Dermoscopic features of acral melanocytic nevi in a case series from Mexico. *An Bras Dermatol.* 2018;93(5):665-670.
12. Saida T, Miyazaki A, Oguchi S, et al. Significance of dermoscopic patterns in detecting malignant melanoma on acral volar skin: results of a multicenter study in Japan. *Arch Dermatol.* 2004;140(10):1233-1238.
13. Phan A, Dalle S, Touzet S, Ronger-Savlé S, Balme B, Thomas L. Dermoscopic features of acral lentiginous melanoma in a large series of 110 cases in a white population. *Br J Dermatol.* 2010;162(4):765-771.
14. Koga H, Saida T. Revised 3-step dermoscopic algorithm for the management of acral melanocytic lesions. *Arch Dermatol.* 2011;147(6):741-743.
15. Lallas A, Kyrgidis A, Koga H, et al. The BRAAFF checklist: a new dermoscopic algorithm for diagnosing acral melanoma. *Br J Dermatol.* 2015;173(4):1041-1049.
16. Sonagara B, Mehta H, Astik B, Agrawal N. Study of seborrheic keratosis by dermoscopy using polarized and nonpolarized modes. *Indian J Dermatopathol Diagn Dermatol* 2020;7:64-69.
17. Giddens T, Seiverling E, Marghoob A, Usatine R. Absence of central white patch in dermatofibromas presenting in darker skin. *JAAD Case Rep.* 2022;21:63-65.
18. Agbai ON, Buster K, Sanchez M, et al. Skin cancer and photoprotection in people of color: a review and recommendations for physicians and the public. *J Am Acad Dermatol.* 2014;70(4):748-762.
19. Behera B, Kumari R, Thappa DM, Gochhait D, Srinivas BH, Ayyanar P. Dermoscopic features of basal cell carcinoma in dark skin phototype: A retrospective cross-sectional study from South India. *Indian J Dermatol Venereol Leprol* 2023;89:254-60.
20. Yang Y, Lin J, Fang S, Han S, Song Z. What's new in dermoscopy of Bowen's disease: two new dermoscopic signs and its differential diagnosis. *Int J Dermatol.* 2017;56(10):1022-1025.
21. Birnbaum MR, McLellan BN, Shapiro J, Ye K, Reid SD. Evaluation of hair density in different ethnicities in a healthy American population using quantitative trichoscopic analysis. *Skin Appendage Disord.* 2018;4(4):304-307.
22. Imadojemu S, Seykora J. Biology of Hair. Access Medicine. https://accessmedicine.mhmedical.com/content.aspx?bookid=2585§ionid=211764076. Published 2016. Accessed August 28, 2022.
23. Ocampo-Garza J, Tosti A. Trichoscopy of dark scalp. *Skin Appendage Disord.* 2018;5(1):1-8.
24. Tawfik SS, Sorour OA, Alariny AF, Elmorsy EH, Moneib H. White and yellow dots as new trichoscopic signs of severe female androgenetic alopecia in dark skin phototypes. *Int J Dermatol.* 2018;57(10):1221-1228.
25. Zhang X, Caulloo S, Zhao Y, Zhang B, Cai Z, Yang J. Female pattern hair loss: clinico-laboratory findings and trichoscopy depending on disease severity. *Int J Trichology.* 2012;4(1):23-28.
26. Lee H, Jung SJ, Patel AB, Thompson JM, Qureshi A, Cho E. Racial characteristics of alopecia areata in the United States. *J Am Acad Dermatol.* 2020;83(4):1064-1070.
27. Bapu NG, Chandrashekar L, Munisamy M, Thappa DM, Mohanan S. Dermoscopic findings of alopecia areata in dark-skinned individuals: an analysis of 116 cases. *Int J Trichology.* 2014;6(4):156-159.
28. de Moura LH, Duque-Estrada B, Abraham LS, Barcaui CB, Sodre CT. Dermoscopy findings of alopecia areata in an African-American patient. *J Dermatol Case Rep.* 2008;2(4):52-54.
29. Miteva M, Tosti A. Pathologic diagnosis of central centrifugal cicatricial alopecia on horizontal sections. *Am J Dermatopathol.* 2014;36(11):859-867.
30. Chouk C, Litaiem N, Jones M, Zeglaoui F. Acne keloidalis nuchae: clinical and dermoscopic features. *BMJ Case Rep.* 2017;2017:bcr2017222222.

31. Lindsey SF, Tosti A. Ethnic hair disorders. *Curr Probl Dermatol.* 2015;47:139-149.
32. Tosti A, Miteva M, Torres F, Vincenzi C, Romanelli P. Hair casts are a dermoscopic clue or the diagnosis of traction alopecia. *Br J Dermatol.* 2010;163(6):1353-1355.
33. Agrawal S, Daruwalla SB, Dhurat RS. The flambeau sign - a new dermoscopy finding in a case of marginal traction alopecia. *Australas J Dermatol.* 2020;61(1):49-50.
34. Joseph AK, Windsor B, Hynan LS, Chong BF. Discoid lupus erythematosus skin lesion distribution and characteristics in Black patients: a retrospective cohort study. *Lupus Sci Med.* 2021;8(1):e000514.
35. Melo DF, Slaibi EB, Siqueira TMFM, Tortelly VD. Trichoscopy findings in dissecting cellulitis. *An Bras Dermatol.* 2019;94(5):608-611.
36. Duque-Estrada B, Tamler C, Sodré CT, Barcaui CB, Pereira FB. Dermoscopy patterns of cicatricial alopecia resulting from discoid lupus erythematosus and lichen planopilaris. *An Bras Dermatol.* 2010;85(2):179-183. [Published correction appears in *An Bras Dermatol.* 2010;85(4):578.]
37. Yin NC, Tosti A. A systematic approach to Afro-textured hair disorders: dermatoscopy and when to biopsy. *Dermatol Clin.* 2014;32:145-151.
38. Saceda-Corralo D, Moreno-Arrones OM, Rodrigues-Barata R, et al. Trichoscopy activity scale for folliculitis decalvans. *J Eur Acad Dermatol Venereol.* 2020;34(2):e55-e57.
39. Quaresma MV, Martinez Velasco MA, Tosti A. Hair breakage in patients of African descent: role of dermoscopy. *Skin Appendage Disord.* 2015;1:99-104.
40. Astur Mde M, Farkas CB, Junqueira JP, et al. Reassessing melanonychia striata in phototypes IV, V, and VI patients. *Dermatol Surg.* 2016;42(2):183-190.
41. Lee DK, Chang MJ, Desai AD, et al. Clinical and dermoscopic findings of benign longitudinal melanonychia due to melanocytic activation differ by skin type and predict likelihood of nail matrix biopsy. *J Am Acad Dermatol.* 2022;87:792-799.
42. Kawabata Y, Ohara K, Hino H, Tamaki K. Two kinds of Hutchinson's sign, benign and malignant. *J Am Acad Dermatol.* 2001;44(2):305-307.
43. Hirata SH, Yamada S, Enokihara MY, et al. Patterns of nail matrix and bed of longitudinal melanonychia by intraoperative dermatoscopy. *J Am Acad Dermatol.* 2011;65(2):297-303.
44. Williams NM, Obayomi AO, Diaz-Perez JA, Morrison BW. Monodactylous longitudinal melanonychia: a sign of Bowen's disease in skin of color. *Skin Appendage Disord.* 2021;7(4):306-310.
45. Shimizu A, Kuriyama Y, Hasegawa M, Tamura A, Ishikawa O. Nail squamous cell carcinoma: a hidden high-risk human papillomavirus reservoir for sexually transmitted infections. *J Am Acad Dermatol.* 2019;81(6):1358-1370.
46. Chen N, Hu Y, Li WH, Eisinger M, Seiberg M, Lin CB. The role of keratinocyte growth factor in melanogenesis: a possible mechanism for the initiation of solar lentigines. *Exp Dermatol.* 2010;19(10):865-872.
47. d'Almeida LFV, Jeunon T, Leverone AP, Nakamura R. Onychocytic matricoma. *An Bras Dermatol.* 2019;94(2):214-216.
48. Tosti A, Schneider SL, Ramirez-Quizon MN, Zaiac M, Miteva M. Clinical, dermoscopic, and pathologic features of onychopapilloma: a review of 47 cases. *J Am Acad Dermatol.* 2016;74(3):521-526.

CHAPTER 26

Psoriasis

Angad Chadha

KEY POINTS

- Psoriasis occurs worldwide and its prevalence differs among racial groups, likely due to genetic polymorphisms inherent to each group.
- Psoriasis is a chronic inflammatory disease that occurs in genetically susceptible individuals as a result of endogenous or exogenous environmental triggers leading to activation of immunologic circuits and a pathologic interaction between the skin and innate and adaptive immune systems.
- The main clinical subtypes of psoriasis are similar across racial groups, though there are differences in severity of disease, presentation of erythema, and quality of plaques between groups.
- Psoriasis has significant comorbidities such as psoriatic arthritis, cardiovascular disease, metabolic syndrome, and nonalcoholic fatty liver disease. These comorbidities impact patient care, quality of life, and treatment decisions.
- The treatment of psoriasis in the resource-rich setting is the same across racial groups. Certain groups may prefer the use of alternative medicines either in isolation or as a complement to traditional medical therapy.

EPIDEMIOLOGY

The overall average prevalence of psoriasis ranges from 1% to 3% and often varies between geographic and ethnic groups, with White ethnic groups generally having higher prevalence than non-White ethnic groups.[1,2] The National Health and Nutrition Examination Surveys (NHANES) conducted in the United States in 2003-2006 and 2009-2010 revealed a prevalence of 3.7% in White individuals, 2.0% in Black individuals, and 1.6% in Hispanic individuals/others. While some of these differences in psoriasis prevalence may be due to ethnic differences in genetics and environmental exposures, psoriasis prevalence in non-White individuals is likely underestimated due to underdiagnosis and underreporting stemming from decreased healthcare utilization and barriers to care in these patient populations.[3]

There is a dearth of large population-based studies examining the international prevalence of psoriasis. Most data are culled from studies of small subsets of various countries' populations.

Norway reports the highest prevalence of psoriasis in the world (4.8-8.5%), followed by France (5.2%), with rates similar to the United States seen in other European countries such as Denmark (3.7%), Italy (3.1%), United Kingdom (2.2%), and Croatia (1.2%).[4]

Eastern African countries (eg, Kenya, Uganda, Tanzania) report a psoriasis prevalence between 1.9% and 3.5%, while Western African countries (eg, Ghana, Nigeria, Senegal, Mali) report a lower prevalence between 0.025% and 0.9%. This difference is likely attributable to genetic differences between Bantu-speaking Africans in eastern, southern, and central Africa, and non-Bantu-speaking Africans in western Africa. Of note, African Americans are more closely related to the non-Bantu-speaking West Africans, but likely have a higher psoriasis prevalence than this group due to the mixed ancestry of many African Americans. However, it is important to note that with immigration from all over Africa to the United States, the genetic composition of African Americans is ever changing.

Data from Asia show that the prevalence of psoriasis ranges from 0.5% to 2.3% in India, 4% to 5% in Malaysia, and is around 0.4% in Sri Lanka.[5] Studies in Mexico as well as Central/South America have suggested a prevalence of psoriasis around 1.3% to 4.2%.[5]

PATHOGENESIS: TRIGGERS, GENETICS, AND IMMUNOLOGY

Psoriasis is a chronic inflammatory disease that occurs in genetically susceptible individuals as a result of endogenous or exogenous environmental triggers leading to activation of immunologic circuits and a pathologic interaction between the skin and innate and adaptive immune systems. The aberrant inflammation seen in lesional skin leads to rapid keratinocyte proliferation, poor keratinocyte differentiation, and changes in the superficial dermal vasculature, all of which contribute to the clinical and histological features of psoriasis.

TRIGGERS

Numerous external triggers and risk factors for psoriasis have been identified including mechanical stress, air pollutants, vaccination, infections (eg, streptococcal and human immunodeficiency virus), cigarette smoking, and exposure to drugs such as β-blockers, lithium, antimalarials, interferons, imiquimod, and nonsteroidal anti-inflammatory drugs.[6,7]

Ultraviolet radiation can be a trigger for a small subset of patients with photosensitive psoriasis.[8] In the case of external triggers such as mechanical stress, air pollutants, cigarette smoking, and some infections, it is theorized that these triggers induce epidermal damage with subsequent exposure of self-antigens and initiation of an aberrant autoinflammatory cascade leading to the development of psoriasis. The mechanisms behind drug-induced psoriasis are yet to be fully elucidated; it is theorized that β-blockers induce keratinocyte hyperproliferation by decreasing intracellular cyclic adenosine monophosphate (cAMP) concentrations, while lithium induces keratinocyte proliferation and differentiation by interfering with intracellular calcium signaling.[6,7] Influenza vaccine, Bacillus Calmette-Guerin (BCG) vaccine, messenger-RNA (mRNA) vaccines for severe acute respiratory syndrome coronavirus 2 (SARS-CoV-2), and various other vaccines have been implicated in the development or exacerbation of psoriasis in susceptible individuals, likely due to a vaccine-provoked initiation of a T-helper 1 (Th1) and Th17 immune response.[6,9] However, despite this association, the risk of vaccine-associated psoriasis is exceedingly low and the protective benefit of vaccination in these patients, who are often treated with immunomodulatory and immunosuppressive medications, greatly outweighs the risk of this rare phenomenon. Infection-induced psoriasis after streptococcal infection is thought to occur due to cross-reactivity between streptococcal M protein and human keratinocyte antigens.[7]

Intrinsic triggers and risk factors for the development and exacerbation of psoriasis include obesity and mental stress. It is postulated that excess adipose tissue secrets various proinflammatory adipokines such as TNF-α, IL-6, leptin, and adiponectin leading to a low-grade systemic proinflammatory state contributing to the pathogenesis of psoriasis.[6]

GENETICS

Genetics are the main risk factor for the development of psoriasis, as evidenced by the two- to threefold increased risk in monozygotic twins when compared to dizygotic twins.[10] Classic linkage and genome-wide association studies of various populations worldwide have identified many genetic polymorphisms associated with psoriasis, and it is noted that different populations preferentially express different psoriasis susceptibility genes. Some genes have been found to be associated with psoriasis across many different populations, while other genes are associated with psoriasis only for certain populations.

Genome-wide association studies have identified over 80 loci associated with the development of psoriasis.[10] Psoriasis susceptibility gene 1 (PSORS1) is perhaps the strongest such locus and is likely responsible for up to 50% of the genetic predisposition to psoriasis.[11] PSORS1 is located within the major histocompatibility complex (MHC) genes on chromosome 6 and encodes various human leukocyte antigens (HLAs). Within PSORS1, allele HLA-Cw6 was the first allele shown to be significantly associated with psoriasis susceptibility. HLA-Cw6 allele is associated with a strong risk of psoriasis, earlier onset of psoriasis, and guttate psoriasis, particularly in White patients. The percentage of psoriasis patients with HLA-Cw6 ranges from 10% to 77% with higher frequency in White individuals than Asians.[12] However, the HLA-Cw6 allele in non-White patients still correlates with a greater risk of psoriasis and perhaps more severe disease, a pattern that has borne out in Korean, Taiwanese, Pakistani, Indian, and Middle Eastern patients but not in African patients.[12-15] While the HLA-Cw6 allele is highly prevalent in some Black populations, the lower prevalence of psoriasis in Black individuals indicates that interplay between different genes likely leads to development of psoriasis in Black patients.[15] Allele HLA-Cw1 is associated with an increased risk of psoriasis in Middle Eastern and Asian patients.[15] HLA-B46 and HLA-Cw1 are associated with an increased risk in Asian individuals. HLA-A02:07 is strongly associated with psoriasis in Chinese individuals but often absent in Europeans. HLA-C*06:02 is associated with early-onset psoriasis.

Numerous other genes have been implicated in the development of psoriasis. These include genes encoding various molecules involved in innate and adaptive immune system signaling such as NF-κB, CARD14, and various interleukins including IL-12 and IL-23.[1] Additionally, genes in the LCE gene cluster encoding cornified envelope proteins are a susceptibility locus for psoriasis, particularly in non-White patients; the proteins encoded by these genes are important for maintenance of the skin barrier and epidermal differentiation.[1,16]

Psoriatic spondyloarthritis is often associated with HLA-B27, particularly in European patients. HLA-B08 and HLA-B38 have also been implicated.[17] HLA-B51 has been implicated in a few cases of psoriatic arthritis in Japanese patients.[18] Similar to cutaneous psoriasis, numerous other genes encoding various molecules in the innate and adaptive immune system have also been implicated in psoriatic arthritis.

It is worth noting that while certain genetic mutations and alleles confer an increased risk of psoriasis, other mutations and alleles can decrease an individual's risk for psoriasis. For example, HLA-B40 has been shown to decrease the risk of psoriasis in Chinese patients.[1]

Mutations in IL36RN, a gene that encodes a protein called IL-36 receptor antagonist, have been associated with generalized pustular psoriasis (GPP) and are likely found more commonly in patients who present with GPP as an isolated disorder rather than pustular psoriasis in the setting of chronic plaque psoriasis.[19,20] Generalized pustular psoriasis differs from chronic plaque psoriasis due to sustained and aberrant activation of IL-1 and IL-36 signaling in GPP.

IMMUNOLOGY

Knowledge on the immunopathology of psoriasis is constantly evolving. Psoriasis is fundamentally a chronic autoinflammatory disease where pathologic activation of the innate and adaptive immune system results in skin inflammation and keratinocyte hyperproliferation. Numerous cell types, cytokine circuits, and inflammatory pathways have been found to be integral in the development and propagation of psoriasis. These discoveries have led to the development of highly targeted and highly effective medications for the treatment of this disorder.

Key cells involved in the development of plaque psoriasis include keratinocytes, dendritic cells, and T-lymphocytes (including T-helper cells and tissue resident memory T-cells). These cells communicate using a vast array of cytokines including TNF-α, IL-12, IL-17, IL-23, and IFN-γ.

Current theory holds that the inciting stimulus triggering the development of plaque psoriasis starts with distressed epidermal cells releasing peptides and antigens that are then recognized by skin dwelling immature dendritic cells. These molecules include epidermally expressed peptides such as antimicrobial protein LL37, S100 proteins, and β-defensins as well as autoantigens such as melanocyte-derived ADAMTS-like protein 5 and fragments of DNA or RNA from damaged cells.[21] The now-activated plasmacytoid dendritic cells then secrete type I interferons including IFN-α and IFN-β leading to the activation of myeloid dendritic cells that serve as a bridge between the innate and adaptive immune systems. Of note, myeloid dendritic cells can also be directly activated by LL37/RNA complexes.[22] Activated myeloid dendritic cells then secrete TNF-α, IL-6, IL-12, and IL-23 to induce activation and differentiation of T-cells into Th1, Th17, and Th22 cells. These T-cells subtypes secrete psoriatic cytokines such as TNF-α, IFN-γ, IL-17, and IL-22 that act on keratinocytes to induce keratinocyte inflammation, hyperproliferation, and poor differentiation.[23] Chemokines secreted by inflamed keratinocytes (such as CCL20 and CXCL1) attract neutrophils and other inflammatory cells to psoriatic lesions.[21] TNF-α secreted from multiple cell types also serves to increase VEGF expression that encourages angiogenesis in psoriatic lesions.[24]

The inflammatory cascade in psoriasis is often self-perpetuating. IFN-γ secreted by Th1 cells also feeds back to further activate myeloid dendritic cells, thus helping create a positive feedback loop. TNF-α from multiple sources encourages myeloid dendritic cell activation. Keratinocyte inflammation leads to the production of further cytokines, chemokines, and the release of aforementioned peptides (eg, LL37) and nucleic acids that provoke the immune response and perpetuate the inflammatory cascade. Cellular clusters containing mature dendritic cells interacting with T-cells have been found in the dermis of psoriatic skin; this tertiary lymphoid tissue likely further perpetuates the autoinflammatory cascade of psoriasis.[22] There is likely decreased T-regulatory (Treg) cell action in psoriasis, contributing to relatively unchecked inflammation.[25,26]

Generalized pustular psoriasis (GPP) is a distinctive subtype of psoriasis that can present in the setting of preexisting plaque psoriasis or as an independent disorder. In contrast to chronic plaque psoriasis that involves both the innate and adaptive immune systems, GPP presenting as an independent disorder is predominantly characterized by innate immune system activation. While the IL-23/Th17 pathway is the main driver of inflammation in plaque psoriasis, the IL-36 pathway has been implicated in the development of GPP.[27] IL-36 belongs to the IL-1 family and is produced primarily by keratinocytes. Dysregulation of the IL-36 signaling pathway can occur through either constitutive expression of IL-36 or the presence of a faulty IL-36 receptor antagonist. Keratinocytes release IL-36 precursors that undergo processing by neutrophil-derived proteases present in neutrophil extracellular traps (NETs); postprocessing IL-36 is a potent autocrine signal upon the original keratinocytes and induces further IL-36 production by the keratinocytes.[27,28] Dysregulated IL-36 signaling can, therefore, activate a self-perpetuating inflammatory cascade. IL-36 receptor activation in keratinocytes also induces the expression of numerous other cytokines such as IL-1, IL-17, IL-23, and TNF-α as well as chemokines like CXCL1 and CXCL8 (IL-8), the latter of which attracts a large number of neutrophils into the inflammatory milieu.[27,28] This is reflected in the neutrophil-laden clinical picture seen in generalized pustular psoriasis.

Psoriasis relapse after discontinuing treatment is thought to be driven primarily by skin resident memory T-cells (Trm).[23] These cells are nonrecirculating T-cells that are part of the skin-associated lymphoid tissue (SALT) and are meant to mediate rapid, local, protective immunity in the skin when reexposed to previously exposed antigens. They have been shown to persist in clinically resolved psoriasis lesions, and possess factors necessary to independently interact with keratinocytes and produce IL-17.[23]

A small subset of patients on TNF-α-blocking therapies for psoriasis can develop paradoxical worsening of their psoriasis while on treatment. The immunologic underpinnings for this phenomenon may rest in the fact that TNF-α produced in the psoriatic inflammatory cascade acts to mature plasmacytoid dendritic cells and decrease type I interferon production.[29,30] Blocking the action of TNF-α leads to unchecked type I interferon production by plasmacytoid dendritic cells and causes flares of psoriasis.[29,31] Paradoxical psoriasis also seems to operate via a pathway independent of T-cell mediated autoimmunity, perhaps acting via innate lymphoid cells, natural killer cells, and neutrophils. This leads to a general lack of disease memory or recurrent flares after discontinuing anti-TNF-α treatment.[29]

CLINICAL MANIFESTATIONS

Chronic plaque psoriasis accounts for about 90% of all clinical presentations of psoriasis, and this prevalence holds true across different ethnic groups in the United States including Caucasian, Asian, and Hispanic ethnicities.[1,32,33] In lighter skin types, the classic morphology is that of well-demarcated, salmon-pink to erythematous papules and plaques covered in slivery white scale [**Figures 26-1** to **26-3**]. In darker skin types, the plaques are typically less erythematous and feature more hyperpigmentation with violaceous hues and grayish scale; plaques in non-White patients are typically thicker, scalier, more extensive, and create more quality of life issues [**Figures 26-4** to **26-7**].[1,34] Lesions may heal with hypopigmentation or hyperpigmentation; postinflammatory dyschromia is more common in patients with skin of color compared to Caucasian patients. Asian patients may present with a morphology dubbed "small plaque psoriasis" that features numerous smaller plaques similar to guttate psoriasis but with a chronic clinical course.[34] The leading edge of a classic psoriatic plaque is the most active area while the center of a plaque can occasionally clear leading to an annular appearance [**Figure 26-8**]. Characteristic sites of involvement in chronic plaque psoriasis include the extensor hands, elbows, knees, and feet, as well as the scalp, lumbosacral region, and umbilicus; the face is typically spared. Plaques are often symmetrically distributed. Psoriasis can also occur at sites of skin trauma or high pressure, an occurrence known as the Koebner phenomenon. While scalp psoriasis is common across all ethnic groups, it may present more severely in African American patients as a consequence of decreased frequency of hair washing.[1] Hyperkeratotic variants of chronic plaque psoriasis include rupioid and ostraceous psoriasis. Rupioid and ostraceous psoriasis are characterized by intensely hyperkeratotic plaques with either a cone shape or concave shape, respectively [**Figure 26-9**]. The hyperkeratosis is thought to derive from serosanguinous exudate admixed with increased keratinocyte proliferation.[35]

Guttate psoriasis is seen in around 30% of cases of psoriasis; this number is likely somewhat inflated due to the fact that guttate psoriasis often coexists with other clinical subtypes of psoriasis and therefore cases of isolated guttate psoriasis likely have lower prevalence closer to 2%.[1,32,36] Clinically, guttate psoriasis features a rapid onset of innumerable confetti-like pink plaques with silvery scale [**Figure 26-10**]; in darker skin types, the erythema is more subtle and hyperpigmentation or violaceous discoloration may predominate [**Figure 26-11**]. Streptococcal infection is the trigger for a majority of guttate psoriasis, accounting for 50% to

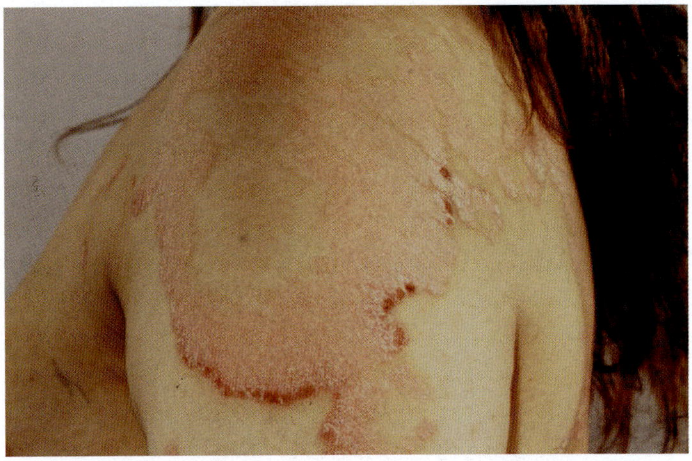

FIGURE 26-1. With lighter skin, like that of this Hispanic patient, the primary psoriatic plaques are salmon-pink or red with silver-white scale.

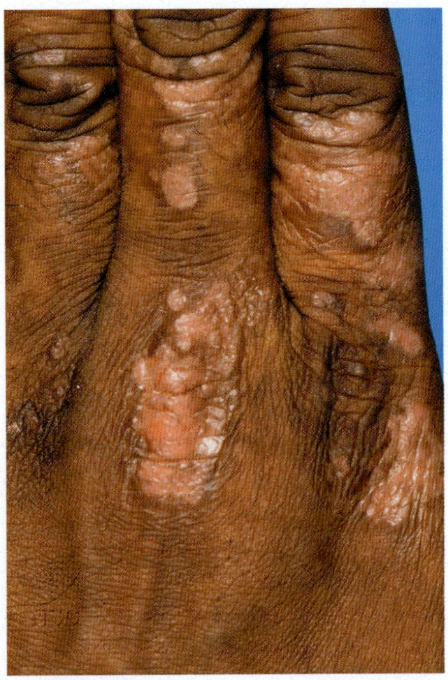

FIGURE 26-2. Chronic plaque psoriasis with well-demarcated salmon-pink papules and plaques on the dorsum of the hand and fingers of an Asian patient. (Courtesy of the National Skin Centre, Singapore.)

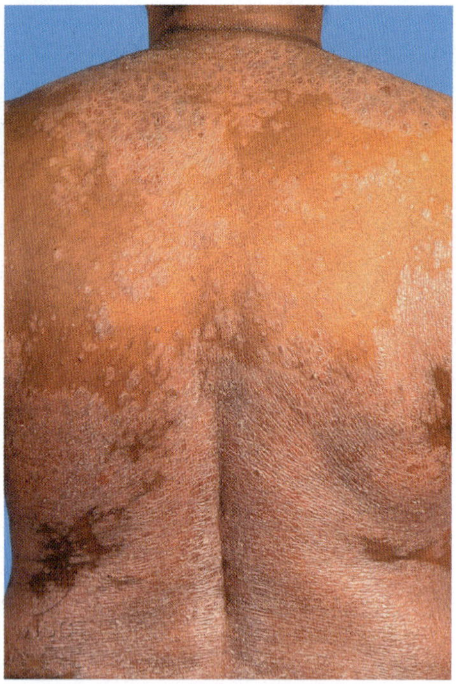

FIGURE 26-3. Chronic plaque psoriasis with extensive well-demarcated salmon pink scaly plaques on the back of an Asian patient. (Courtesy of the National Skin Center, Singapore.)

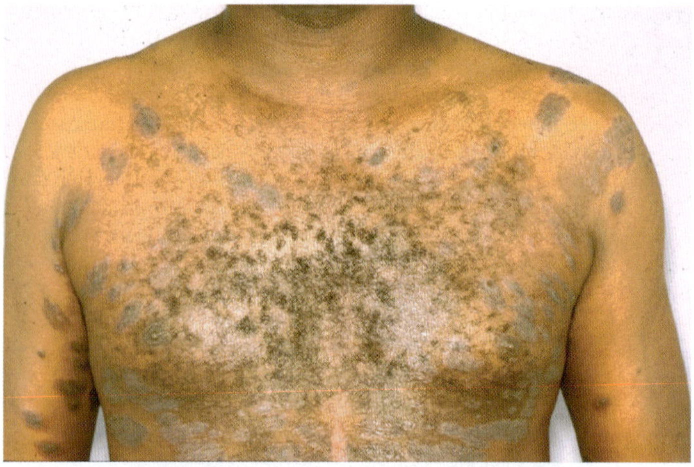

FIGURE 26-4. In patients with darker skin, like this African American patient, the papules and plaques are hyperpigmented to violaceous with gray scale.

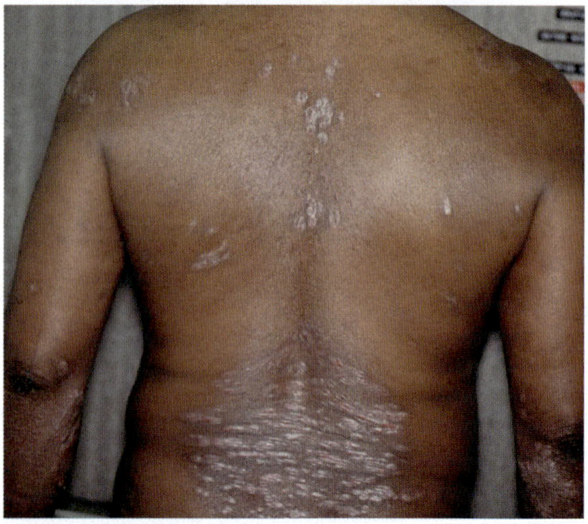

FIGURE 26-5. Well-demarcated pink to violaceous papules and plaques located on the back of an African American patient with psoriasis.

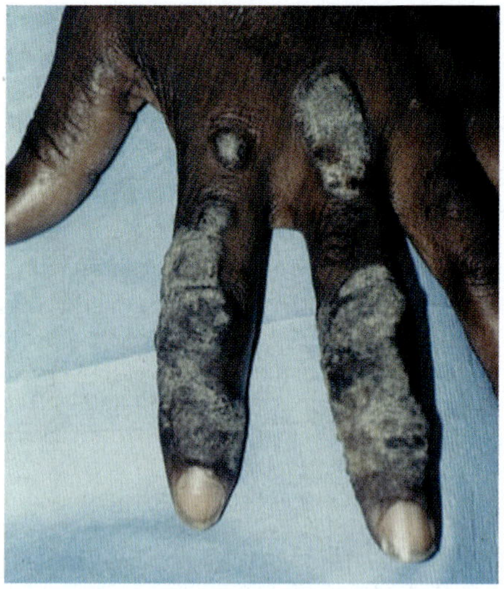

FIGURE 26-6. Thick violaceous plaques with micaceous gray scale on the dorsal fingers of an African American patient with chronic plaque psoriasis.

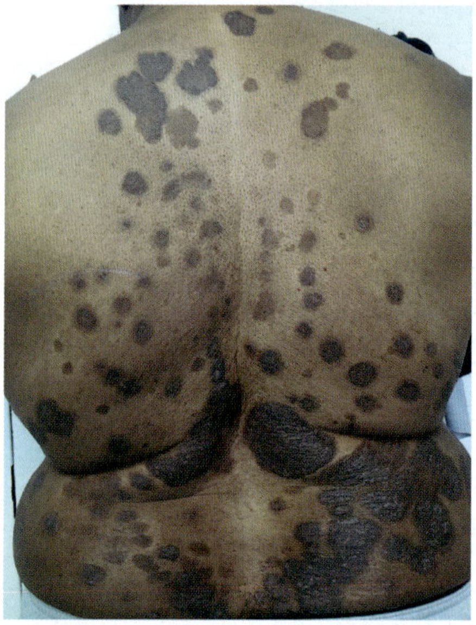

FIGURE 26-7. Extensive hyperpigmented, scaly, well-demarcated plaques of chronic plaque psoriasis on the back of a patient with darker skin. (Reproduced with permission from Kaufman BP, Alexis AF. Psoriasis in skin of color: insights into the epidemiology, clinical presentation, genetics, quality-of-life impact, and treatment of psoriasis in non-White racial/ethnic groups. *Am J Clin Dermatol*. 2018;19(3):405-423.)

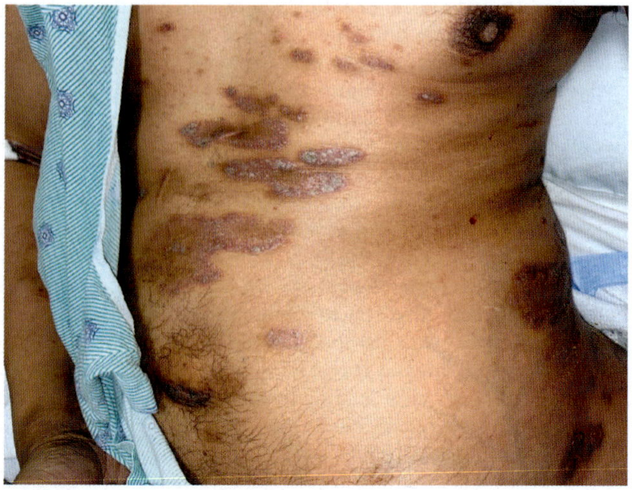

FIGURE 26-8. Psoriatic plaques in a patient with skin of color demonstrating an active leading edge with central clearing and postinflammatory hyperpigmentation.

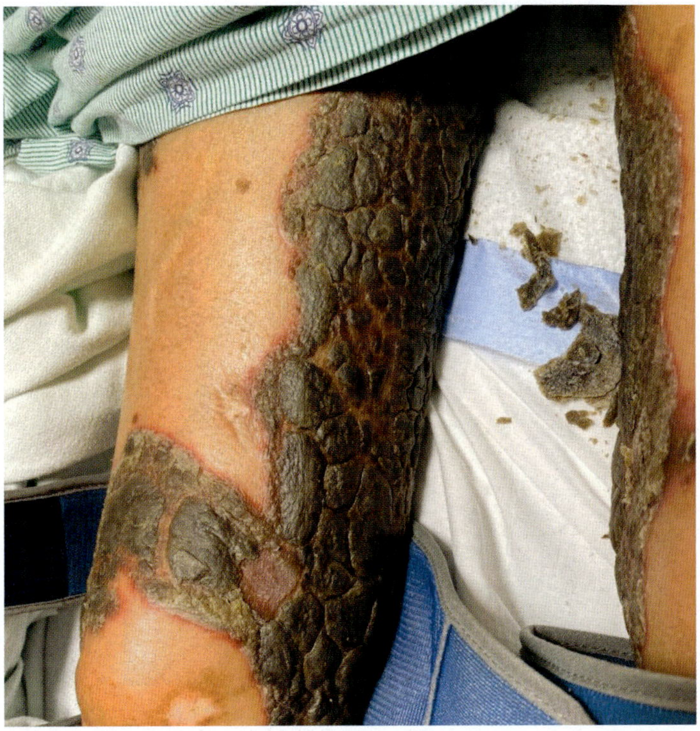

FIGURE 26-9. Rupioid psoriasis with well-demarcated psoriatic plaques with concave hyperkeratotic crusting.

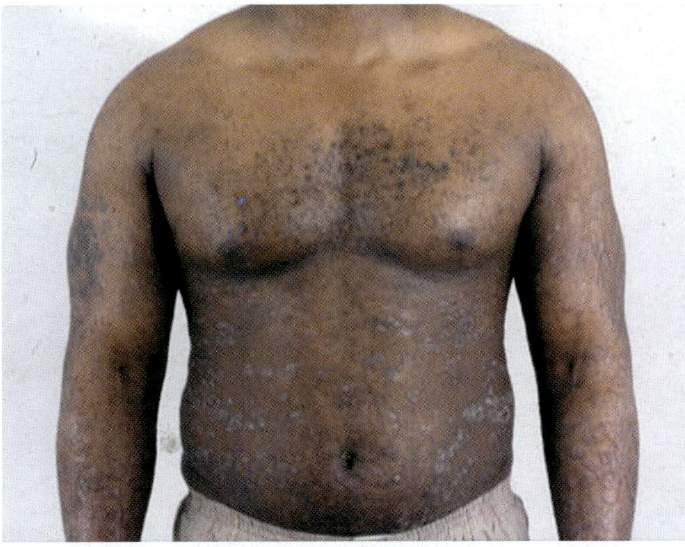

FIGURE 26-11. Guttate psoriasis in a patient with darker skin. Innumerable small, hyperpigmented to violaceous papules and plaques with gray scale.

66% of cases.[10,36] Guttate psoriasis typically remits spontaneously over weeks to months, though up to 40% of patients may progress to having chronic plaque psoriasis.[10,37]

Pustular psoriasis is seen in 1% to 9% of cases of psoriasis and seems to be more prevalent in non-White patients than Caucasian patients.[1,32,38,39] About half of patients with pustular psoriasis also have chronic plaque psoriasis, while the other half have isolated pustular psoriasis.[40] This form of psoriasis is characterized by robust erythema and the presence of sterile pustules. Widespread erythema may be more subtle in patients with darker skin; applying pressure to blanch the skin and examining for resultant color changes can be a clue to the presence of diffuse background erythema [**Figure 26-12**]. Pustular psoriasis can be triggered by abrupt corticosteroid withdrawal, hypocalcemia, pregnancy, infection, or various medications.[36] A few subtypes of pustular psoriasis are recognized. The most severe subtype is acute generalized pustular psoriasis (GPP, formerly von Zumbusch type), characterized by abrupt onset widespread erythematous patches or thin plaques with subsequent rapid development of innumerable submillimeter pustules within the areas of erythema; the pustules can coalesce into larger collections leading to a "lake of pus" appearance and can sometimes take on an annular distribution [**Figure 26-13**]. Patients with acute generalized pustular psoriasis

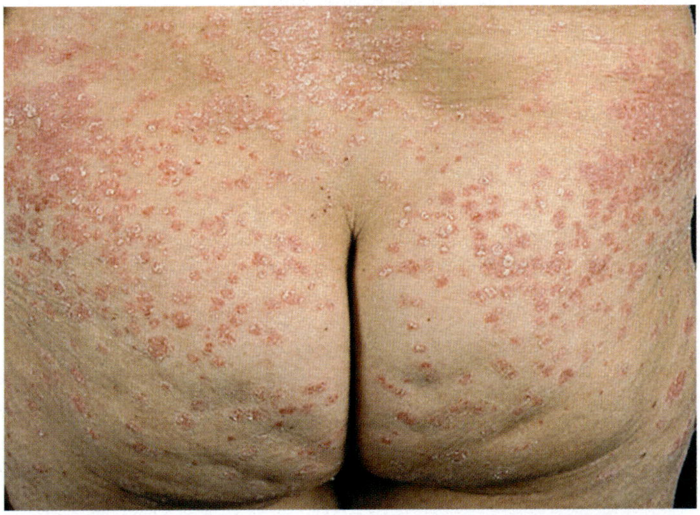

FIGURE 26-10. Guttate psoriasis in a patient with lighter skin. Innumerable small, confetti-like salmon-pink papules with gray scale. (Reproduced with permission from Saavedra AP, Roh EK, Mikailov A. *Fitzpatrick's Color Atlas and Synopsis of Clinical Dermatology*. 9th ed. New York, NY: McGraw Hill; 2023, Figure 3-2.)

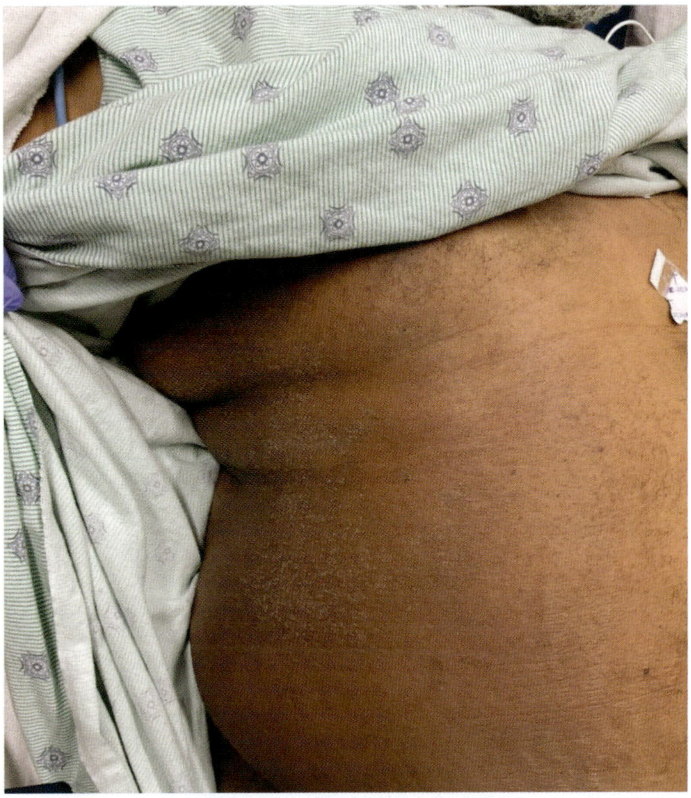

FIGURE 26-12. Diffuse background erythema, scaling, and minute pustules in a patient with darker skin. The difference between erythematous skin (left) and normal skin (right) is apparent but subtle.

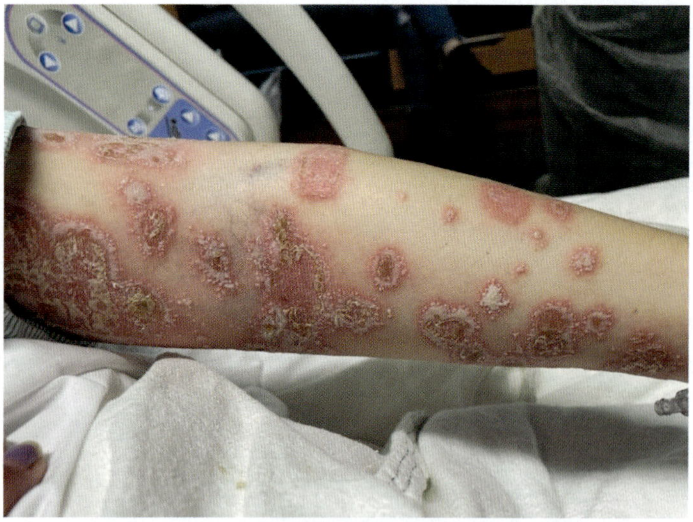

FIGURE 26-13. Generalized pustular psoriasis. Acute onset erythematous patches and edematous plaques studded with innumerable pustules coalescing into larger "lakes of pus" with an annular configuration.

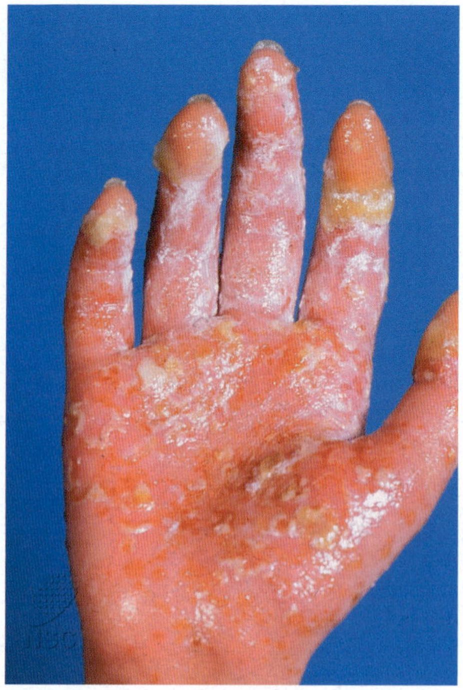

FIGURE 26-15. Palmoplantar pustulosis in an Asian patient with characteristic acral pustulation, erythema, and hyperkeratosis. (Courtesy of the National Skin Centre, Singapore.)

may also have associated fevers, malaise, arthralgias, and ocular abnormalities; rarer extracutaneous manifestations include end-organ damage of the liver or kidney as well as interstitial pneumonitis.[27,38,41] Annular pustular psoriasis is a more subacute presentation of pustular psoriasis that features numerous annular or polycyclic erythematous patches and thin plaques studded with sterile pustules, often developing over the course of weeks to months [**Figure 26-14**]. Localized variants of pustular psoriasis include palmoplantar pustulosis (PPP) and acrodermatitis continua of Hallopeau (ACH). PPP presents with an eruption of pustules on the palms and soles with associated hyperkeratosis and fissuring [**Figure 26-15** to **Figure 26-17**]. ACH is characterized by erythema, pustulation, scaling, hyperkeratosis, and fissuring on one or more digits, often accompanied by features of nail psoriasis as discussed below [**Figure 26-18**].[41]

Other, less common forms of psoriasis include palmoplantar psoriasis, inverse psoriasis, erythrodermic psoriasis, nail psoriasis, and the oral manifestations of psoriasis.

Palmoplantar psoriasis is seen in 4% to 8% of cases of psoriasis, with higher prevalence in Caucasian patients than Asian and Hispanic patients.[32] It is characterized by the presence of well-marginated,

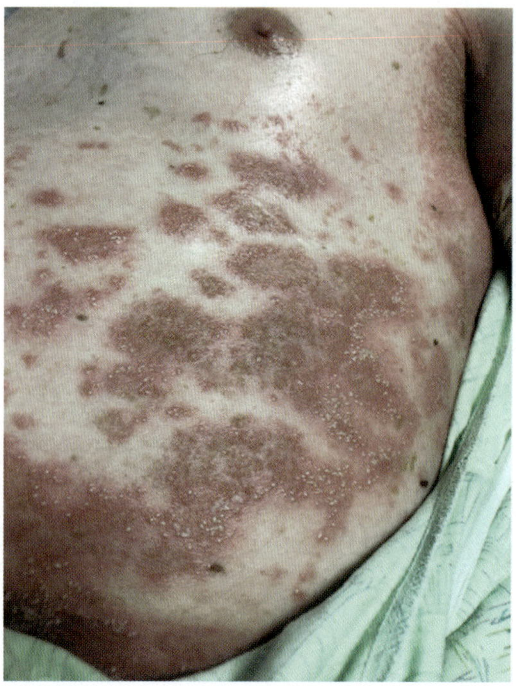

FIGURE 26-14. Annular pustular psoriasis. Subacute onset erythematous annular thin plaques with peripheral pustules and central clearing and hyperpigmentation.

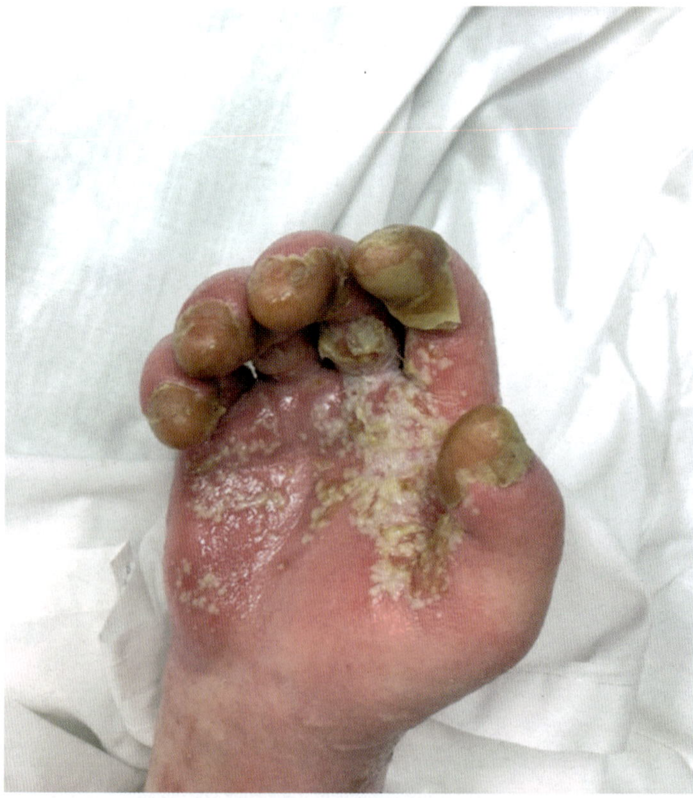

FIGURE 26-16. Palmoplantar pustulosis in a lighter-skinned patient with acral pustulation, erythema, hyperkeratosis, and desquamation.

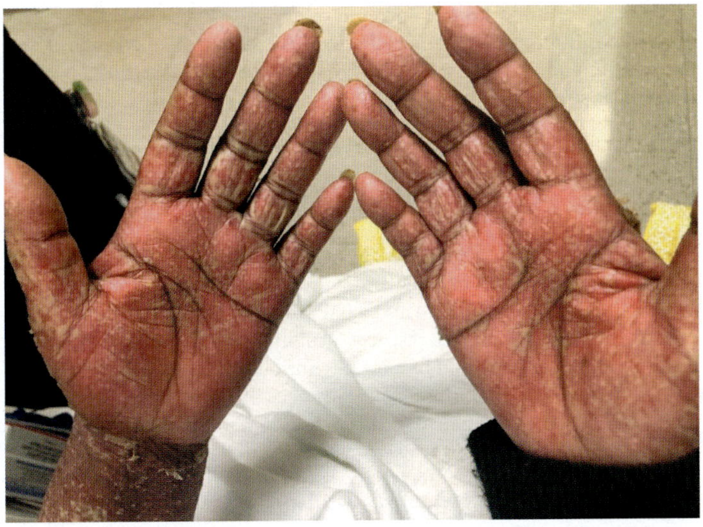

FIGURE 26-17. Palmoplantar pustulosis in a darker skinned patient with acral pustulation and diffuse background erythema.

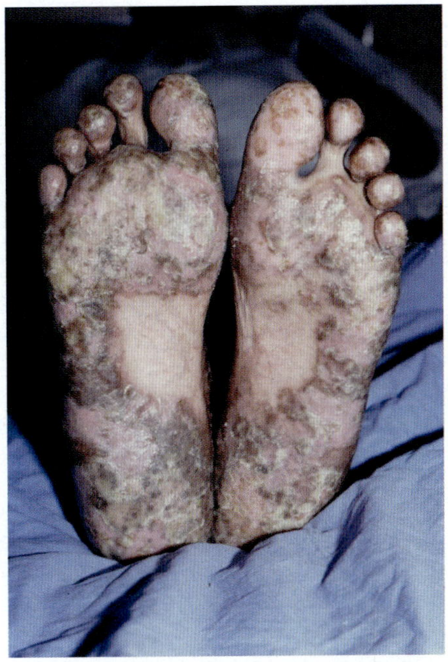

FIGURE 26-19. Palmoplantar psoriasis in a patient with darker skin with well-demarcated violaceous plaques with overlying scale and hyperkeratosis.

hyperkeratotic, scaly, fissured erythematous-to-hyperpigmented plaques on the acral surfaces [**Figure 26-19**]. These plaques often cause functional limitation due to associated pain, often impairing manual dexterity and walking. Palmoplantar psoriasis can occur in isolation or concurrently with other forms of psoriasis such as chronic plaque psoriasis or pustular psoriasis.

Inverse psoriasis is seen in 6% to 10% of cases of psoriasis and often coexists with other subtypes of psoriasis.[32,42] It is characterized by symmetric, shiny plaques in skin folds such as the axillary, inframammary, inguinal, intergluteal, and abdominal pannus folds [**Figure 26-20**]. Lesions of inverse psoriasis tend to lack the characteristic scale seen in chronic plaque psoriasis due to the occlusive, moist environment of the body folds.

Erythrodermic psoriasis is seen in 2% to 5% of the psoriatic population.[10,32] Asian patients are perhaps more likely to present with erythrodermic or pustular psoriasis when compared to their White counterparts.[34] Erythrodermic psoriasis is defined as generalized erythema and scaling affecting at least 75% of body surface area [**Figure 26-21**]. As mentioned previously, erythroderma may be more subtle in patients with darker skin and may present with hyperpigmentation and scaling more so than robust erythema; applying pressure to blanch the skin and examining for resultant color changes can be a clue to the presence of diffuse background erythema. Erythrodermic psoriasis is often accompanied by systemic symptoms such as fever, tachycardia, arthralgia, fatigue, and lymphadenopathy. Peripheral leukocytosis with neutrophilic predominance can be seen. If left untreated, erythrodermic physiology due to generalized cutaneous vasodilation can result in high-output cardiac failure, dehydration, electrolyte imbalances, hypothermia, and sepsis, while chronic severe inflammation can result in anemia and malnutrition. Erythrodermic psoriasis can be seen as a consequence of poorly controlled chronic plaque psoriasis but can also be triggered by the abrupt withdrawal of systemic corticosteroids in a patient with preexisting or undiagnosed psoriasis, as a side effect of various medications (eg, lithium, interferon, β-blockers), and as a consequence of underlying systemic infections.[43,44]

Nail psoriasis is seen in 50% to 80% of patients with cutaneous psoriasis, and in up to 80% of patients with psoriatic arthritis.[45] Psoriatic disease of the nail can involve the nail matrix, nail bed, proximal nail fold, and/

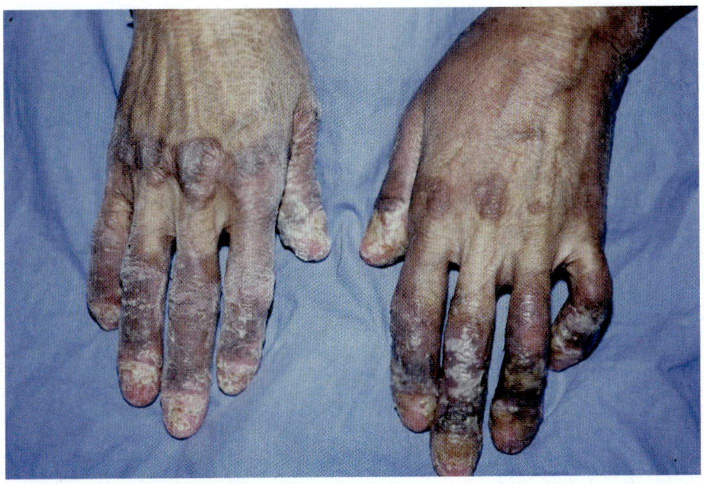

FIGURE 26-18. Acrodermatitis continua of Hallopeau with erythema, edema, pustulation, and erosion of the fingers. There is also concurrent plaque psoriasis on the metacarpophalangeal joints as well as nail psoriasis.

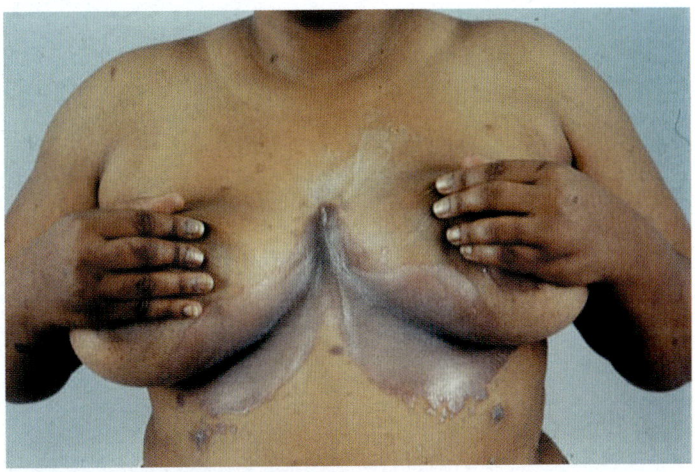

FIGURE 26-20. Inverse psoriasis in a patient with darker skin featuring shiny, well-demarcated violaceous to brown thin plaques without characteristic psoriatic scale.

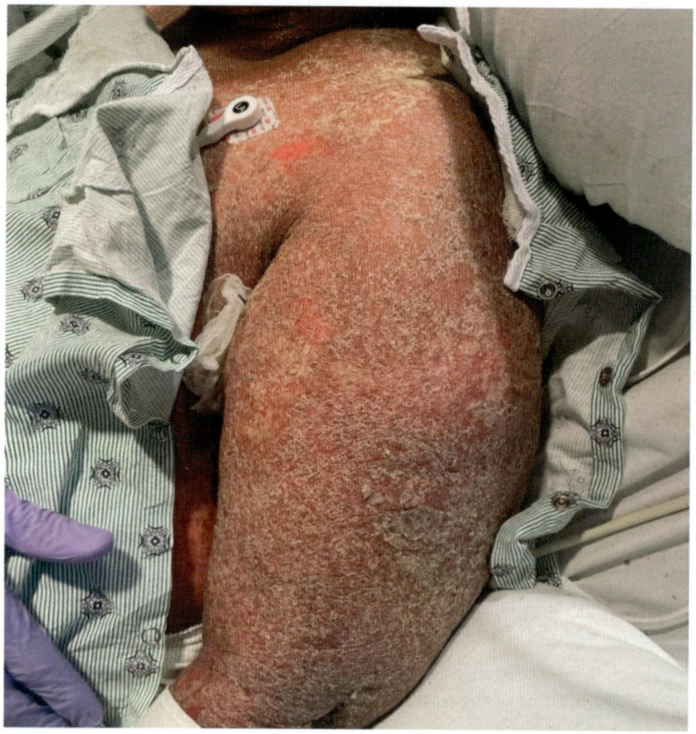

FIGURE 26-21. Erythrodermic psoriasis in a patient with darker skin with generalized erythema and scaling of the entire body surface area.

or hyponychium. Nail matrix disease produces irregular pitting of the dorsal nail plate, nail plate crumbling, and red macules in the lunula.[45] Nail bed disease decreases nail plate adhesion and causes onycholysis, subungual hyperkeratosis, splinter hemorrhages, yellowish patches (so-called oil spots), or reddish macules (so-called salmon spots).[45] Psoriasis of the proximal nail fold can cause psoriatic paronychia with erythema, edema, scaling, and loss of the cuticle.[46]

Oral manifestations of psoriasis are seen in 10% of patients with psoriasis and are usually more prominent during flares of cutaneous psoriasis.[47] The tongue is most frequently involved followed by the buccal and labial mucosa. Annular, white, serpiginous, polycyclic, migratory plaques are the hallmark of oral psoriasis [**Figure 26-22**] and are colloquially dubbed "geographic tongue" or "migratory glossitis." Other, less common manifestations include erythematous patches on the mucosa and fissured tongue. Exfoliative cheilitis may be seen in the setting of erythrodermic psoriasis.

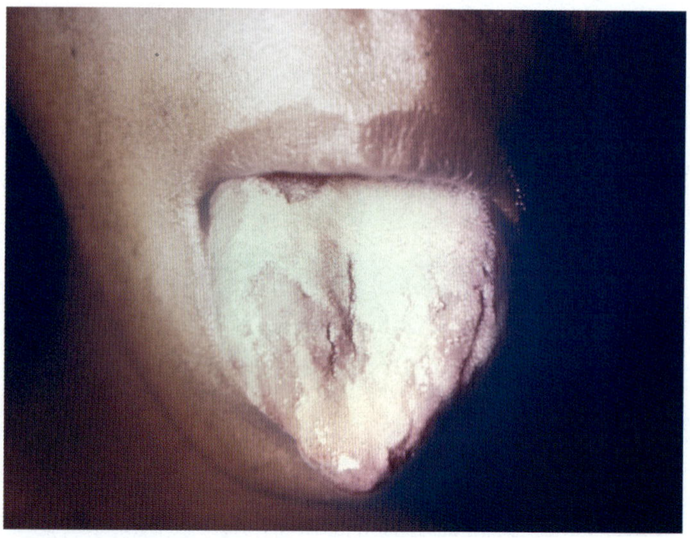

FIGURE 26-22. Geographic tongue seen in psoriasis with annular, white, serpiginous, polycyclic, migratory plaques. (Photo Permission from Centers for Disease Control and Prevention.)

EXTRACUTANEOUS COMORBIDITIES OF PSORIASIS

PSORIATIC ARTHRITIS

Psoriatic arthritis (PsA) is a chronic, immune-mediated, inflammatory arthropathy of the peripheral and axial skeleton that features inflammation of the joints and entheses. It is usually seronegative with negative testing for anti-rheumatoid factor (RF) antibodies and anti-cyclic citrullinated peptide (CCP) antibodies. Psoriatic arthritis is the most common comorbidity seen in patients with psoriasis. The prevalence of psoriatic arthritis in patients with psoriasis is estimated to be 15% to 30%.[48-50] Caucasian patients tend to be affected by psoriatic arthritis 2 to 5 times more frequently than African American patients, despite African American patients traditionally having a higher cutaneous disease burden.[51,52] The prevalence of PsA is also higher in Caucasian patients than in other ethnic groups.[52,53] Data on the correlation between severity of skin and joint disease are conflicting. In most patients, the onset of cutaneous psoriasis precedes the development of psoriatic arthritis by about 7 years. However, in 7% to 15% of patients, psoriatic arthritis can present before or concurrently with the onset of skin disease.[54] The risk of psoriatic arthritis is increased in patients with scalp, nail, and intergluteal psoriasis and nail psoriasis is more common in the PsA population compared to the cutaneous psoriasis population.[55,56] The extensor tendon overlying the distal interphalangeal joint inserts at the terminal phalanx and its enthesis interacts with the nail unit fascia at the proximal nail unit, thus providing evidence of how enthesitis from psoriatic arthritis can give rise to concomitant nail psoriasis.[57]

Psoriatic arthritis can affect the peripheral or axial skeleton. There are five broadly described clinical patterns of PsA which include: (1) asymmetric oligoarthritis of less than five small or large joints, (2) symmetric polyarthritis similar to rheumatoid arthritis, (3) distal arthritis of the distal interphalangeal joints, (4) arthritis mutilans characterized by destructive and deforming arthritis, and (5) sacroiliitis and spondyloarthritis.[58] Patients can have multiple patterns of joint involvement and their pattern of joint involvement may change over the course of their disease. The joint pain of psoriatic arthritis is similar to that of other inflammatory arthritides, often featuring prolonged stiffness and pain after immobilization (eg, upon waking from sleep), pain at entheses, joint swelling and erythema, and dactylitis or "sausage digits" that features diffuse swelling of the tissues between the metacarpophalangeal or metatarsophalangeal joints and interphalangeal joints. Signs of ocular inflammation such as uveitis and conjunctivitis can occur in psoriatic arthritis as in other inflammatory arthritides.

Colleagues in rheumatology should be consulted to assist in the diagnosis and management of psoriatic arthritis. The presence of psoriatic arthritis necessitates the use of systemic anti-inflammatory therapies including traditional disease modifying antirheumatic drugs, small molecule inhibitors, and biologic agents. Goals of therapy center around controlling symptoms, improving quality of life, and preventing irreversible structural damage to the joints.

ATHEROSCLEROTIC DISEASE, METABOLIC SYNDROME, AND NONALCOHOLC FATTY LIVER DISEASE

Psoriasis is associated with an increased risk for the development of atherosclerotic disease including cardiovascular, cerebrovascular, and peripheral vascular disease. Numerous studies have demonstrated that the risk of myocardial infarction and stroke are increased in patients with psoriasis compared to controls.[59] Patients with psoriasis also have higher mortality rates after major cardiovascular events that are independent of traditional cardiovascular risk factors.[59] Psoriasis has been identified as an independent risk factor for coronary artery calcification and the development of high-risk coronary artery plaques, on par with diabetes mellitus and hyperlipidemia.[36]

The pathogenesis of increased atherosclerotic disease in patients with psoriasis is not well understood. There is increased prevalence of risk factors for cardiovascular disease such as obesity, hypertension, smoking, hyperlipidemia, and metabolic syndrome in the psoriasis population, which likely drives some of the atherosclerosis. Psoriasis also creates a state of chronic systemic inflammation that is not just skin limited. It is postulated that increased systemic inflammation in psoriasis can drive insulin resistance, endothelial cell dysfunction, and promote atherosclerosis.[60] This hypothesis is supported by the observation that systemic medications targeted at reducing inflammation from psoriasis tend to ameliorate the risk of cardiovascular events when compared to the use of skin-directed therapies alone (eg, phototherapy or topical medications).[61-64] This trend has been best demonstrated with the use of TNF-α inhibiting agents but has also been seen with other disease modifying antirheumatic medications (eg, methotrexate). Preliminary experimental and clinical data suggest that newer biologics targeted at the IL-23/Th17 axis may also lead to a reduction in atherosclerotic disease and cardiovascular risk.[65-67]

Epidemiologic studies have also supported an increased prevalence of metabolic syndrome in patients with psoriasis.[68,69] Metabolic syndrome is defined as the presence of at least three of the following: elevated waist circumference, elevated blood pressure, elevated fasting glucose, elevated triglycerides, and reduced high density lipoprotein levels (HDL) levels.[70] The pathogenic link between psoriasis and metabolic syndrome is not well-defined; current theories implicate the action of proinflammatory psoriatic cytokines and adipokines on glucose regulation, insulin resistance, endothelial dysfunction, and lipid metabolism. Similarly, epidemiological studies have demonstrated an increased risk of nonalcoholic fatty liver disease (nonalcoholic steatohepatitis) in patients with psoriasis.[71,72] Clinicians should be aware of these associations from a therapeutic standpoint since treatment of psoriasis may involve the use of hepatotoxic medications (eg, methotrexate, acitretin) or medications that cause hypertriglyceridemia (eg, acitretin, cyclosporine).

TREATMENT

The treatment of psoriasis should be the same across all ethnic groups and should take into account the cutaneous burden of the patient's disease as well as patient-specific comorbidities such as the presence of psoriatic arthritis or cardiovascular risk factors. Patient preferences for treatment modality (topical, oral, injectable) also have bearing on choosing the appropriate therapy to ensure adherence to the medication regimen. The psoriasis treatment ladder is best stratified by disease severity and the presence of joint or cardiovascular disease.

Mild psoriasis with limited body surface area involvement and no joint involvement is best treated with topical agents. Mainstays include topical corticosteroids and topical vitamin D analogs (calcipotriene, calcitriol), often in combination. Topical retinoids (tazarotene) and tar preparations may be added for thicker, keratotic plaques. Steroid-sparing topical therapies such as calcineurin inhibitors (pimecrolimus, tacrolimus), phosphodiesterase-4 inhibitors (roflumilast), or an aryl hydrocarbon receptor modulator (tapinarof) may be used if chronic topical therapy is needed for sensitive areas such as the face and body folds or if there is concern for side effects from chronic topical steroid use. The prescriber should ensure use of an appropriate vehicle when prescribing in order to ensure maximum medication adherence, and should take into account patient preferences that can vary by ethnic group. For example, African American patients tend to prefer ointments for the skin and oils for the scalp, while Caucasian patients tend to prefer creams for the body and solutions for the scalp.[73] That said, the prescriber should not make assumptions and patients should always be presented with all vehicle options before making an informed decision as to what will work best for their skin.

Phototherapy can be considered for patients with cutaneous psoriasis who are not interested in topical medications, as an adjunctive therapy in patients who are already using topical medications, or as a first-line therapy in patients with guttate psoriasis or rapidly progressive psoriasis. Narrowband UVB (NB-UVB), broadband UVB (BB-UVB), 308nm excimer laser, and UVA with or without photosensitizing agents have been used successfully in the treatment of psoriasis, though current clinical practice trends in the United States favor NB-UVB and excimer laser over BB-UVB or PUVA.[74] The use of phototherapy for moderate to severe plaque psoriasis has decreased since the advent of small molecule inhibitors and biologics for psoriasis.[36] Patients with skin of color may be hesitant to undergo phototherapy due to unwanted tanning as a side effect. These patients should be counseled that any unwanted tanning will fade with cessation of phototherapy; additionally, suberythemogenic doses of NB-UVB may be as clinically effective as erythemogenic doses in patients with darker skin types and may avoid unwanted tanning.[75]

While there is no consensus on the definition of moderate to severe psoriasis, most clinicians define moderate psoriasis as ranging from 3-5% up to 10% of body surface area and severe psoriasis as anything over 10% of body surface area.[36] Systemic therapies are the cornerstone of treatment for patients with moderate to severe plaque psoriasis, often in conjunction with topical therapies or phototherapy. Systemic therapies can also be used for localized disease involving special areas such as the palms and soles, scalp, and genitals. The presence of psoriatic arthritis or significant cardiovascular risk factors should prompt earlier consideration of systemic therapy in order to treat comorbid joint and cardiovascular disease. The following sections will review oral and injectable treatment options for psoriasis.

The first oral agents used in the treatment of psoriasis were the antifolate medications aminopterin and methotrexate, soon after their discovery in 1947.[76,77] Since then, the armamentarium of oral medications available for the treatment of psoriasis has expanded and includes agents such as antifolates (methotrexate), oral retinoids (acitretin), oral calcineurin inhibitors (cyclosporine), and oral fumarates (dimethyl fumarate). These oral agents generally have ubiquitous intracellular targets leading to a broad spectrum of activity and generally poor selectivity for psoriatic inflammation. These oral medications have vastly different mechanisms of action and safety profiles; their use should be guided by an experienced clinician. Besides cyclosporine, the efficacy of all of these oral treatments is generally lower than that of injectable biologics.[36] Ethnic differences and polymorphisms in transporter genes, HLA alleles, and metabolic proteins may predispose certain patients to better clinical response or increased risk of toxicity to these oral therapies.[1] With the rise of pharmacogenomics, these intrapatient differences will become more clinically actionable and may assist the clinician in selecting the most efficacious and least toxic therapy for a particular patient. The development of small molecule inhibitors and biologic agents specifically targeted at inflammatory circuits preferentially active in the psoriasis pathway has revolutionized the treatment of psoriasis and their use has largely supplanted the use of these broadly active oral medications in the resource-rich setting; however, in settings where cost of treatment is an important consideration, these medications remain a mainstay of psoriasis treatment. Additionally, given its rapid onset of action, cyclosporine remains a cornerstone of therapy in the control of severe, rapidly progressive plaque or pustular psoriasis.

Newer oral therapies include small molecule inhibitors targeting psoriasis inflammatory pathways. These include an oral phosphodiesterase-4 inhibitor (apremilast) and an oral tyrosine kinase 2 inhibitor (deucravacitinib). These therapies have better safety profiles when compared to the traditional oral therapies listed above, but still have poorer efficacy data when compared to most injectable biologic medications.[78,79]

Injectable biologic medications are a heterogeneous group of agents targeted at various cytokines implicated in the inflammatory circuitry of psoriasis. These agents tend to produce dramatic clinical response in most patients and generally have favorable safety profiles. They have also been used in the treatment of erythrodermic psoriasis with excellent results.[43,44] Currently available biologic agents include agents targeting TNF-α (adalimumab, certolizumab, etanercept, infliximab), the shared p40 subunit of IL-12 and IL-23 (ustekinumab), the p19 subunit of IL-23 (guselkumab, risankizumab, tildrakizumab), IL-17A (ixekizumab, secukinumab), IL-17A and IL-17F (bimekizumab), and the IL-17 receptor A (brodalumab). In general, agents targeting IL-23 and IL-17 tend to show better efficacy data for cutaneous psoriasis than those targeting TNF-α.[78,80] In patients with psoriatic arthritis, agents targeting IL-17 and TNF-α tend to show better efficacy data than agents targeting IL-23 or IL-12/23.[81,82] Current evidence suggests that the use of biologics is safe and effective across diverse racial groups.[1] While biologic therapies often show excellent initial response in many patients, some patients experience loss of treatment response over months to years either due to decreasing blood concentrations with stable maintenance doses or due to the development of antidrug antibodies.[10]

The treatment of pustular psoriasis differs slightly from the treatment of other forms of psoriasis. Due to the often-rapid onset and progression of pustular psoriasis, the use of rapidly acting agents is of utmost importance. Traditionally, cyclosporine, acitretin, and methotrexate were employed in the treatment of pustular psoriasis, along with topical therapies. More recently, there has been increased use of biologic agents intended for the treatment of chronic plaque psoriasis, with agents targeting TNF-α and IL-17 showing greater efficacy and more rapid clinical control of pustular psoriasis than those targeting IL-12/23 or IL-23.[83] IL-1 inhibitors such as anakinra, canakinumab, and gevokizumab have been used successfully in the treatment of pustular psoriasis in a few case series.[84] More recently, the release of an IL-36 receptor inhibitor (spesolimab) provided a breakthrough treatment for generalized pustular psoriasis specifically targeted at blocking the overactive IL-36 signaling pathway implicated in this disease.[85]

The use of complementary and alternative medicine (CAM) therapies is common among patients with psoriasis, and may be more common in certain non-Western ethnic groups than in Caucasian patients. Alternative medicine can be used in isolation or as a complement to conventional medical therapies. CAM encompasses traditional Chinese medicine, herbal therapies, dietary supplements, and mind/body interventions. Traditional Chinese medicine often includes blends of topical and oral herbs; of these herbs, *Mahonia aquifolium*, indigo naturalis, and *Campotheca* have shown topical anti-inflammatory benefits when compared to vehicle; however, the lack of standardization of topical preparations of herbal medications makes it difficult to standardize prescription practices for these medications.[86] Topical aloe vera therapy and topical St. John's wort show some efficacy in the treatment of psoriasis, while oral fish oil, oral omega-3 fatty acid, and oral curcumin (turmeric) supplementation have been shown to have anti-inflammatory benefits in psoriasis.[86] While topical vitamin D analogs are a mainstay of psoriasis therapy, oral vitamin D supplementation does not seem to provide benefit at doses that avoid the side effect of hypercalcemia. The use of acupuncture for psoriasis is not supported by the literature.[86,87] Cupping has shown to induce the Koebner phenomenon with local worsening of psoriasis and is therefore not recommended.[87] Stress reduction therapies such as psychotherapy, meditation, and hypnosis have shown benefit in patients who are receptive to those treatment modalities.[86,87] Climatotherapy and balneotherapy, often performed in and near bodies of water that have unique mineral compositions, have been shown to help psoriasis severity.[87] This is likely due to a reduction in patient perceived stress at these locations, anti-inflammatory or keratolytic effects from local minerals in the water, and increased UV exposure at climatotherapy and balneotherapy locations. A gluten-free diet has not shown any benefit in decreasing psoriasis severity, except in patients with concomitant celiac disease.[86]

CONCLUSION

Psoriasis is a worldwide disease with significant morbidity and burden of disease. There are likely genetic differences that underlie the variable prevalence of psoriasis between different racial groups as well as some of the differential treatment responses seen in different patients. The clinical manifestations of psoriasis are largely similar among most populations and, as such, the treatment ladder of psoriasis is also similar. Special care must be given to tailor treatment regimens to the severity of a patient's psoriasis and their underlying comorbidities such as psoriatic arthritis or cardiovascular disease. Prescribers should take into account patient preferences when considering vehicles for topical medications as well as patient preferences for traditional medical therapy and complementary and alternative medical therapies.

REFERENCES

1. Kaufman BP, Alexis AF. Psoriasis in skin of color: insights into the epidemiology, clinical presentation, genetics, quality-of-life impact, and treatment of psoriasis in non-white racial/ethnic groups. *Am J Clin Dermatol.* 2018;19(3):405-423.
2. Boehncke WH, Schön MP. Psoriasis. *Lancet Lond Engl.* 2015;386(9997):983-994.
3. Yadav G, Yeung J, Miller-Monthrope Y, et al. Unmet need in people with psoriasis and skin of color in Canada and the United States. *Dermatol Ther (Heidelb).* 2022;12(11):2401-2413.
4. Rachakonda TD, Schupp CW, Armstrong AW. Psoriasis prevalence among adults in the United States. *J Am Acad Dermatol.* 2014;70(3):512-516.
5. Raychaudhuri SP, Farber EM. The prevalence of psoriasis in the world. *J Eur Acad Dermatol Venereol.* 2001;15(1):16-17.
6. Kamiya K, Kishimoto M, Sugai J, Komine M, Ohtsuki M. Risk factors for the development of psoriasis. *Int J Mol Sci.* 2019;20(18):4347.
7. Lee EB, Wu KK, Lee MP, Bhutani T, Wu JJ. Psoriasis risk factors and triggers. *Cutis.* 2018;102(5S):18-20.
8. Rutter KJ, Watson REB, Cotterell LF, Brenn T, Griffiths CEM, Rhodes LE. Severely photosensitive psoriasis: a phenotypically defined patient subset. *J Invest Dermatol.* 2009;129(12):2861-2867.
9. Wu PC, Huang IH, Wang CW, Tsai CC, Chung WH, Chen CB. New onset and exacerbations of psoriasis following COVID-19 vaccines: a systematic review. *Am J Clin Dermatol.* 2022;23(6):775-799.
10. Griffiths CEM, Armstrong AW, Gudjonsson JE, Barker JNWN. Psoriasis. *Lancet.* 2021;397(10281):1301-1315.
11. Hugh JM, Weinberg JM. Update on the pathophysiology of psoriasis. *Cutis.* 2018;102(5S):6-12.
12. Chen L, Tsai TF. HLA-Cw6 and psoriasis. *Br J Dermatol.* 2018;178(4): 854-862.
13. Chandra A, Lahiri A, Senapati S, et al. Increased risk of psoriasis due to combined effect of HLA-Cw6 and LCE3 risk alleles in Indian population. *Sci Rep.* 2016;6:24059.
14. Rani R, Narayan R, Fernandez-Vina MA, Stastny P. Role of HLA-B and C alleles in development of psoriasis in patients from North India. *Tissue Antigens.* 1998;51(6):618-622.
15. Brown-Korsah JB, McKenzie S, Omar D, Syder NC, Elbuluk N, Taylor SC. Variations in genetics, biology, and phenotype of cutaneous disorders in skin of color - Part I: Genetic, biologic, and structural differences in skin of color. *J Am Acad Dermatol.* 2022;87(6):1239-1258.
16. Zhang XJ, Huang W, Yang S, et al. Psoriasis genome-wide association study identifies susceptibility variants within LCE gene cluster at 1q21. *Nat Genet.* 2009;41(2):205-210.
17. Eder L, Chandran V, Pellet F, et al. Human leucocyte antigen risk alleles for psoriatic arthritis among patients with psoriasis. *Ann Rheum Dis.* 2012;71(1):50-55.
18. Yamamoto T, Yokozeki H, Nishioka K. Psoriasis arthropathy and HLA-B51: report of 5 cases. *J Dermatol.* 2005;32(7):606-610.
19. Capon F. IL36RN mutations in generalized pustular psoriasis: just the tip of the iceberg? *J Invest Dermatol.* 2013;133(11):2503-2504.
20. Sugiura K, Takemoto A, Yamaguchi M, et al. The majority of generalized pustular psoriasis without psoriasis vulgaris is caused by deficiency of interleukin-36 receptor antagonist. *J Invest Dermatol.* 2013;133(11):2514-2521.
21. Grän F, Kerstan A, Serfling E, Goebeler M, Muhammad K. Current developments in the immunology of psoriasis. *Yale J Biol Med.* 2020;93(1):97-110.
22. Lowes MA, Suárez-Fariñas M, Krueger JG. Immunology of psoriasis. *Annu Rev Immunol.* 2014;32:227-255.
23. Tian D, Lai Y. The relapse of psoriasis: mechanisms and mysteries. *JID Innov.* 2022;2(3):100116.
24. Lee HJ, Hong YJ, Kim M. Angiogenesis in chronic inflammatory skin disorders. *Int J Mol Sci.* 2021;22(21):12035.

25. Shi Y, Chen Z, Zhao Z, et al. IL-21 induces an imbalance of Th17/Treg cells in moderate-to-severe plaque psoriasis patients. *Front Immunol.* 2019;10:1865.
26. Hu P, Wang M, Gao H, et al. The role of helper T cells in psoriasis. *Front Immunol.* 2021;12:788940.
27. Marrakchi S, Puig L. Pathophysiology of generalized pustular psoriasis. *Am J Clin Dermatol.* 2022;23(Suppl 1):13-19.
28. Uppala R, Tsoi LC, Harms PW, et al. "Autoinflammatory psoriasis"—genetics and biology of pustular psoriasis. *Cell Mol Immunol.* 2021;18(2):307-317.
29. Conrad C, Di Domizio J, Mylonas A, et al. TNF blockade induces a dysregulated type I interferon response without autoimmunity in paradoxical psoriasis. *Nat Commun.* 2018;9:25.
30. Psarras A, Antanaviciute A, Alase A, et al. TNF-α regulates human plasmacytoid dendritic cells by suppressing IFN-α production and enhancing T cell activation. *J Immunol Baltim Md 1950.* 2021;206(4):785-796.
31. Mylonas A, Conrad C. Psoriasis: classical vs. paradoxical. The yin-yang of TNF and type I interferon. *Front Immunol.* 2018;9:2746.
32. Yan D, Afifi L, Jeon C, Cordoro KM, Liao W. A cross-sectional study of the distribution of psoriasis subtypes in different ethno-racial groups. *Dermatol Online J.* 2018;24(7):13030/qt5z21q4k2.
33. Kaur I, Handa S, Kumar B. Natural history of psoriasis: a study from the Indian subcontinent. *J Dermatol.* 1997;24(4):230-234.
34. McKenzie S, Brown-Korsah JB, Syder NC, Omar D, Taylor SC, Elbuluk N. Variations in genetics, biology, and phenotype of cutaneous disorders in skin of color. Part II: Differences in clinical presentation and disparities in cutaneous disorders in skin of color. *J Am Acad Dermatol.* 2022;87(6):1261-1270.
35. Ip KHK, Cheng HS, Oliver FG. Rupioid psoriasis. *JAMA Dermatol.* 2021;157(7):859.
36. Armstrong AW, Read C. Pathophysiology, clinical presentation, and treatment of psoriasis: a review. *JAMA.* 2020;323(19):1945-1960.
37. Ko HC, Jwa SW, Song M, Kim MB, Kwon KS. Clinical course of guttate psoriasis: long-term follow-up study. *J Dermatol.* 2010;37(10):894-899.
38. Zheng M, Jullien D, Eyerich K. The prevalence and disease characteristics of generalized pustular psoriasis. *Am J Clin Dermatol.* 2022;23(Suppl 1):5-12.
39. Kumar B, Saraswat A, Kaur I. Palmoplantar lesions in psoriasis: a study of 3065 patients. *Acta Derm Venereol.* 2002;82(3):192-195.
40. Löfvendahl S, Norlin JM, Schmitt-Egenolf M. Prevalence and incidence of generalized pustular psoriasis in Sweden: a population-based register study. *Br J Dermatol.* 2022;186(6):970-976.
41. Hoegler KM, John AM, Handler MZ, Schwartz RA. Generalized pustular psoriasis: a review and update on treatment. *J Eur Acad Dermatol Venereol.* 2018;32(10):1645-1651.
42. Jfri A, Leung B, Said JT, Semenov Y, LeBoeuf NR. Prevalence of inverse psoriasis subtype with immune checkpoint inhibitors. *Immunother Adv.* 2022;2(1):ltac016.
43. Carrasquillo OY, Pabón-Cartagena G, Falto-Aizpurua LA, et al. Treatment of erythrodermic psoriasis with biologics: a systematic review. *J Am Acad Dermatol.* 2020;83(1):151-158.
44. Potestio L, Camela E, Cacciapuoti S, et al. Biologics for the management of erythrodermic psoriasis: an updated review. *Clin Cosmet Investig Dermatol.* 2023;16:2045-2059.
45. Bardazzi F, Starace M, Bruni F, Magnano M, Piraccini BM, Alessandrini A. Nail psoriasis: an updated review and expert opinion on available treatments, including biologics. *Acta Derm Venereol.* 2019;99(6):516-523.
46. Haneke E. Nail psoriasis: clinical features, pathogenesis, differential diagnoses, and management. *Psoriasis Auckl NZ.* 2017;7:51-63.
47. Bruce AJ, Rogers RS. Oral psoriasis. *Dermatol Clin.* 2003;21(1):99-104.
48. Mease PJ, Gladman DD, Papp KA, et al. Prevalence of rheumatologist-diagnosed psoriatic arthritis in patients with psoriasis in European/North American dermatology clinics. *J Am Acad Dermatol.* 2013;69(5):729-735.
49. Haroon M, Kirby B, FitzGerald O. High prevalence of psoriatic arthritis in patients with severe psoriasis with suboptimal performance of screening questionnaires. *Ann Rheum Dis.* 2013;72(5):736-740.
50. Reich K, Krüger K, Mössner R, Augustin M. Epidemiology and clinical pattern of psoriatic arthritis in Germany: a prospective interdisciplinary epidemiological study of 1511 patients with plaque-type psoriasis. *Br J Dermatol.* 2009;160(5):1040-1047.
51. Kerr GS, Qaiyumi S, Richards J, et al. Psoriasis and psoriatic arthritis in African-American patients–the need to measure disease burden. *Clin Rheumatol.* 2015;34(10):1753-1759.
52. Ogdie A, Matthias W, Thielen RJ, Chin D, Saffore CD. Racial differences in prevalence and treatment for psoriatic arthritis and ankylosing spondylitis by insurance coverage in the USA. *Rheumatol Ther.* 2021;8(4):1725-1739.
53. Alinaghi F, Calov M, Kristensen LE, et al. Prevalence of psoriatic arthritis in patients with psoriasis: a systematic review and meta-analysis of observational and clinical studies. *J Am Acad Dermatol.* 2019;80(1):251-265.e19.
54. Tillett W, Charlton R, Nightingale A, et al. Interval between onset of psoriasis and psoriatic arthritis comparing the UK Clinical Practice Research Datalink with a hospital-based cohort. *Rheumatol Oxf Engl.* 2017;56(12):2109-2113.
55. Wilson FC, Icen M, Crowson CS, McEvoy MT, Gabriel SE, Kremers HM. Incidence and clinical predictors of psoriatic arthritis in patients with psoriasis: a population-based study. *Arthritis Rheum.* 2009;61(2):233-239.
56. Takata T, Takahashi A, Taniguchi Y, Terada Y, Sano S. Detection of asymptomatic enthesitis in psoriasis patients: an onset of psoriatic arthritis? *J Dermatol.* 2016;43(6):650-654.
57. Gottlieb A, Merola JF. Psoriatic arthritis for dermatologists. *J Dermatol Treat.* 2020;31(7):662-679.
58. Kishimoto M, Deshpande GA, Fukuoka K, et al. Clinical features of psoriatic arthritis. *Best Pract Res Clin Rheumatol.* 2021;35(2):101670.
59. Masson W, Lobo M, Molinero G. Psoriasis and cardiovascular risk: a comprehensive review. *Adv Ther.* 2020;37(5):2017-2033.
60. Boehncke WH. Systemic inflammation and cardiovascular comorbidity in psoriasis patients: causes and consequences. *Front Immunol.* 2018;9:579.
61. Wu JJ, Joshi AA, Reddy SP, et al. Anti-inflammatory therapy with tumour necrosis factor inhibitors is associated with reduced risk of major adverse cardiovascular events in psoriasis. *J Eur Acad Dermatol Venereol.* 2018;32(8):1320-1326.
62. Hugh J, Van Voorhees AS, Nijhawan RI, et al. From the Medical Board of the National Psoriasis Foundation: the risk of cardiovascular disease in individuals with psoriasis and the potential impact of current therapies. *J Am Acad Dermatol.* 2014;70(1):168-177.
63. Wu JJ, Poon KYT, Channual JC, Shen AYJ. Association between tumor necrosis factor inhibitor therapy and myocardial infarction risk in patients with psoriasis. *Arch Dermatol.* 2012;148(11):1244-1250.
64. Wu JJ, Sundaram M, Cloutier M, et al. The risk of cardiovascular events in psoriasis patients treated with tumor necrosis factor-α inhibitors versus phototherapy: an observational cohort study. *J Am Acad Dermatol.* 2018;79(1):60-68.
65. Wang Y, Zang J, Liu C, Yan Z, Shi D. Interleukin-17 links inflammatory cross-talks between comorbid psoriasis and atherosclerosis. *Front Immunol.* 2022;13:835671.
66. von Stebut E, Boehncke WH, Ghoreschi K, et al. IL-17A in psoriasis and beyond: cardiovascular and metabolic implications. *Front Immunol.* 2019;10:3096.
67. von Stebut E, Reich K, Thaçi D, et al. Impact of secukinumab on endothelial dysfunction and other cardiovascular disease parameters in psoriasis patients over 52 weeks. *J Invest Dermatol.* 2019;139(5):1054-1062.
68. Gisondi P, Fostini AC, Fossà I, Girolomoni G, Targher G. Psoriasis and the metabolic syndrome. *Clin Dermatol.* 2018;36(1):21-28.
69. Rodríguez-Zúñiga MJM, García-Perdomo HA. Systematic review and meta-analysis of the association between psoriasis and metabolic syndrome. *J Am Acad Dermatol.* 2017;77(4):657-666.e8.
70. Grundy SM, Cleeman JI, Daniels SR, et al. Diagnosis and management of the metabolic syndrome: an American Heart Association/National Heart, Lung, and Blood Institute Scientific Statement. *Circulation.* 2005;112(17):2735-2752.
71. Ruan Z, Lu T, Chen Y, et al. Association between psoriasis and nonalcoholic fatty liver disease among outpatient US adults. *JAMA Dermatol.* 2022;158(7):745-753.
72. Takeshita J, Grewal S, Langan SM, et al. Psoriasis and comorbid diseases: Epidemiology. *J Am Acad Dermatol.* 2017;76(3):377-390.
73. Fisher EJ, Adams BB. African American and Caucasian patients' vehicle preference for the scalp. *J Am Acad Dermatol.* 2008;58(2 Suppl):S46-S47.
74. Elmets CA, Lim HW, Stoff B, et al. Joint American Academy of Dermatology-National Psoriasis Foundation guidelines of care for the management and treatment of psoriasis with phototherapy. *J Am Acad Dermatol.* 2019;81(3):775-804.
75. Syed ZU, Hamzavi IH. Role of phototherapy in patients with skin of color. *Semin Cutan Med Surg.* 2011;30(4):184-189.
76. Gubner R, August S, Ginsberg V. Therapeutic suppression of tissue reactivity. II. Effect of aminopterin in rheumatoid arthritis and psoriasis. *Am J Med Sci.* 1951;221(2):176-182.
77. Rees RB. Methotrexate vs. aminopterin for psoriasis. *Arch Dermatol.* 1961;83(6):970.
78. Armstrong AW, Puig L, Joshi A, et al. Comparison of biologics and oral treatments for plaque psoriasis: a meta-analysis. *JAMA Dermatol.* 2020;156(3):258-269.
79. Armstrong AW, Gooderham M, Warren RB, et al. Deucravacitinib versus placebo and apremilast in moderate to severe plaque psoriasis: efficacy and safety results from the 52-week, randomized, double-blinded, placebo-controlled phase 3 POETYK PSO-1 trial. *J Am Acad Dermatol.* 2023;88(1):29-39.

80. Van Muijen ME, Thomas SE, Groenewoud HMM, et al. Direct comparison of real-world effectiveness of biologics for psoriasis using absolute and relative psoriasis area and severity index scores in a prospective multicentre cohort. *Acta Derm Venereol.* 2022;102:adv00712.
81. Zhang H, Wen J, Alexander GC, Curtis JR. Comparative effectiveness of biologics and targeted therapies for psoriatic arthritis. *RMD Open.* 2021;7(1):e001399.
82. Ruyssen-Witrand A, Perry R, Watkins C, et al. Efficacy and safety of biologics in psoriatic arthritis: a systematic literature review and network meta-analysis. *RMD Open.* 2020;6(1):e001117.
83. Wang WM, Jin HZ. Biologics in the treatment of pustular psoriasis. *Expert Opin Drug Saf.* 2020;19(8):969-980.
84. Bachelez H. Pustular psoriasis: the dawn of a new era. *Acta Derm Venereol.* 2020;100(3):adv00034.
85. Bachelez H, Choon SE, Marrakchi S, et al. Trial of spesolimab for generalized pustular psoriasis. *N Engl J Med.* 2021;385(26):2431-2440.
86. Elmets CA, Korman NJ, Prater EF, et al. Joint AAD-NPF guidelines of care for the management and treatment of psoriasis with topical therapy and alternative medicine modalities for psoriasis severity measures. *J Am Acad Dermatol.* 2021;84(2):432-470.
87. Timis TL, Florian IA, Mitrea DR, Orasan R. Mind-body interventions as alternative and complementary therapies for psoriasis: a systematic review of the English literature. *Med Kaunas Lith.* 2021;57(5):410.

CHAPTER 27

Pityriasis Rosea

J. Michael
Alberto Bell
Dwana R. Shabazz

KEY POINTS

- Pityriasis rosea (PR) is a self-limiting papulosquamous dermatosis that is found in all Fitzpatrick skin types (I-VI), with some distinct presentations in patients with skin of color.
- Despite its unclear etiology, PR has been associated with drugs (barbiturates, metronidazole, terbinafine, isotretinoin, gold, and clozapine), vaccinations (hemagglutinin 1 neuraminidase 1, COVID-19), and viruses (human herpes virus [HHV]-6, HHV-7, and HHV-8).
- Mainstay of treatment includes medium potency topical corticosteroids for pruritus and, in severe presentations, antiviral therapies can be considered.

INTRODUCTION

Pityriasis rosea (PR) is an acute, self-limiting papulosquamous dermatosis that is thought to have a viral origin. It occurs over a broad age range, most often between the ages of 10 and 35 years, and rarely before the age of 2. The peak occurrence is during the spring and fall seasons. It usually has a classic clinical presentation, is asymptomatic, and undergoes spontaneous resolution in 6 to 10 weeks.

PR is found worldwide without a racial predilection. In an overview of disorders more commonly seen in patients with skin of color, PR was listed as occurring in about 2% of patients[1] [**Table 27-1**]. A more recent epidemiological study using the *All of Us* database of diverse U.S. adults showed similar prevalence of PR among all ethnicities estimating it around 0.2%.[2]

TABLE 27-1 General information on pityriasis rosea
• Occurs in about 0.2-2% of dermatology patients with skin of color.
• Age of onset is usually between 10 and 35 years.
• Resolves spontaneously, typically between 6 and 10 weeks.

The incidence of PR has been decreasing. This may be due to its self-limiting nature, which could result in cases of PR never coming to the attention of a physician. Furthermore, dermatologists are usually the second or third physician a patient sees for the diagnosis and treatment of PR. By this point, the condition has often cleared up and the patient is seeking to determine the cause of the dermatosis, and/or the patient has healed but has been left with postinflammatory dyspigmentation (often in the form of hyperpigmentation).

Because PR may differ clinically in those with skin of color, in comparison with patients who have Fitzpatrick skin types I to III, it is important to highlight the clinical differences. It is also necessary to note the effects of certain treatment options for patients with skin of color.

PATHOGENESIS

Most of the literature points to a viral etiology.[3] Human herpes virus (HHV)-6 and HHV-7 are the two viruses most closely associated with PR, although this correlation is inconclusive.

HHV-6 belongs to the *Roseolovirus* genus and is closely homologous with HHV-7; thus HHV-7 belongs to the same genus. HHV-6 is widespread in the population and persists, often in a latent state, in its hosts' monocytes and bone marrow progenitor cells and as a chronic infection of the salivary glands. [3] It is this infection of the salivary glands that is thought to be the mode of transmission for HHV-6.[3] In support of the close association between the two viruses, it has been reported that an infection with HHV-7 can lead to the reactivation of HHV-6 from latency.[3] HHV-6 causes ballooning and induces apoptosis in the uninfected cluster of differentiation 4 (CD4) T-helper cells.[3] In addition, HHV-6 causes the enhancement of natural killer T-cell activity, the suppression of peripheral blood mononuclear cell proliferation, and the induction of many cytokines.[3]

Approximately 95% of the human population is seropositive for HHV-6. As a result, a positive viral culture for HHV-6 does not necessarily correspond to a clinically relevant infection, due to the large number of asymptomatic carriers.

HHV-7 is also prevalent worldwide. The primary infection of this virus occurs in childhood, but at a later age than HHV-6 infections. HHV-7 shares its mode of infection with HHV-6, by showing a latency in the peripheral blood T-cells and a persistent infection of the salivary glands. HHV-7 is prone to reactivation. Less is known about the pathogenicity of HHV-7, but it is thought to be the primary causative agent of PR, with HHV-6 having a close association. However, there is no definitive proof that these viruses are the pathogenesis of PR.

Both HHV-6 and HHV-7 are associated with a febrile illness and exanthem subitum (roseola infantum), which has a characteristic rash. Although viruses are not a proven cause, patients with PR may experience a fever as a prodrome and a classic exanthem that resolves spontaneously and peaks in the spring and fall. Therefore, this supports a viral etiology [**Table 27-2**].

Many other studies have been done to resolve the controversy regarding the exact cause of PR; however, no definitive conclusions can be drawn.[4-6] This is due to limitations such as their sample size and the fact that they were not randomized controlled studies. For example, a study was done with 34 Kaposi sarcoma–negative, immunocompetent patients with PR. The results of this study showed that HHV-8 was detected by DNA sequencing in 20% of the cases; however, the small sample size is not sufficient to prove that HHV-8 was the definitive causative agent.[6]

Other viruses and their associated vaccines have also been associated with PR. Hemagglutinin 1 neuraminidase 1 (H1N1) has been associated

TABLE 27-2 Observations supporting viral etiology of pityriasis rosea
• The peak occurrence is in spring and fall, which supports a viral origin.
• Human herpes virus (HHV)-6 and HHV-7 are also closely associated.

TABLE 27-3 Drug-induced pityriasis rosea
Drug-induced pityriasis rosea (PR) displays:
• Atypical clinical patterns
• Slower resolution
• Greater resistance to treatment

Drugs that have been reported to induce PR include gold, arsenic, barbiturates, bismuth, captopril, terbinafine, D-penicillamine, interferon-α, metronidazole, isotretinoin, and omeprazole.

with PR.[7] Furthermore, a patient developed PR after receiving the H1N1 vaccine.[8] However, it is still unclear whether H1N1 was the primary cause in these two cases, or whether H1N1 triggered the reactivation of other viral causes.[7] The latter theory is supported by studies carried out in 2009 and 2010 claiming that the skin manifestations of PR are a reactive response, rather than an actual infection of the skin cells.[9,10]

Similar association have been found with COVID-19. The incidence of pityriasis rosea during the SARS-CoV-2 pandemic increased fivefold.[11] Proposed mechanisms underlying the association include SARS-CoV-2 cytokine storm directly resulting in cutaneous inflammation versus SARS-CoV-2 infection acting after a reactivator for other latent viruses including HHV-6, HHV-7, and VSV.[11] SARS-CoV-2 vaccine-related PR and PR-like eruption have also been reported with one systematic review estimating a rate of 1.6% among cutaneous manifestations of the vaccine.[12,13]

There have been reports of several drugs causing PR or rashes that look quite similar to this condition. These reports show that when PR has been induced by medication, it presents in a more atypical pattern, has a longer course, and is more resistant to treatment. Some of the implicated drugs include arsenic, barbiturates, bismuth, captopril, clonidine, D-penicillamine, interferon-α, isotretinoin, metronidazole, gold, omeprazole, and terbinafine[14] [**Table 27-3**].

CLINICAL PRESENTATION

Medical textbooks illustrate a classic cutaneous exanthem of salmon- or rose-colored papules and plaques in PR patients with Fitzpatrick skin types I to III [**Figure 27-1**]. However, in patients with skin of color, the lesions are usually violaceous or gray in color [**Figures 27-2** and **27-3** and **Table 27-4**]. Following a fever, and a respiratory tract infection in some patients, a herald patch, or "mother patch," can arise. This is seen in 50% to 90% of patients with PR [**Figure 27-4** and **Table 27-5**]. About 1 to 2 weeks later, a generalized secondary rash develops, consisting of oval plaques with a collarette scale. The scale usually occurs on the inner border of the plaque and points to the center of the lesion [**Figure 27-5**]. The secondary rash develops along the Langer lines and has been characterized as occurring in a "Christmas tree" distribution on the trunk [**Figure 27-6**] and a "school of minnows" pattern on the flank [**Figure 27-7**]. The sun-exposed areas of the body are seldom involved. In patients with dark skin of color, the lesions are more papular, and the papules often have small necrotic-like centers [**Figure 27-8**]. These patients also have a more follicular accentuation [**Figure 27-9**], and the lesions usually occur in an inverse pattern, involving the face, neck, axilla, groin, and lower abdomen[1] [**Figure 27-10**]. African American children are particularly predisposed to the papular variant, which is also prevalent in Hispanic children [**Figure 27-11**].

Patients with PR can experience pruritus, which occurs occasionally on the palms and is rarely generalized [**Figure 27-12**]. In a study assessing the quality of life in children with PR, the majority of the children were only minimally itchy; thus their school life, other daily activities, and sleep were not greatly affected.[2] PR usually resolves spontaneously in 6 to 10 weeks, although in some instances, it may last for 4 to 5 months.[3] In patients with skin of color, resolution often occurs with postinflammatory hyperpigmentation, although it occasionally results in postinflammatory hypopigmentation. In rare cases, the scalp, eyelids, penis, and oral mucosa are also involved.

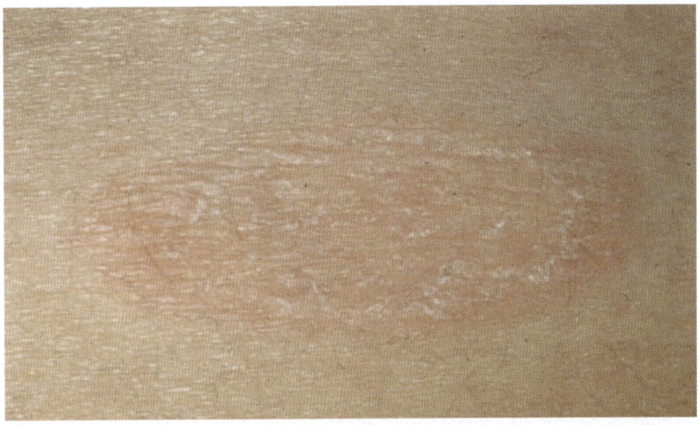

A

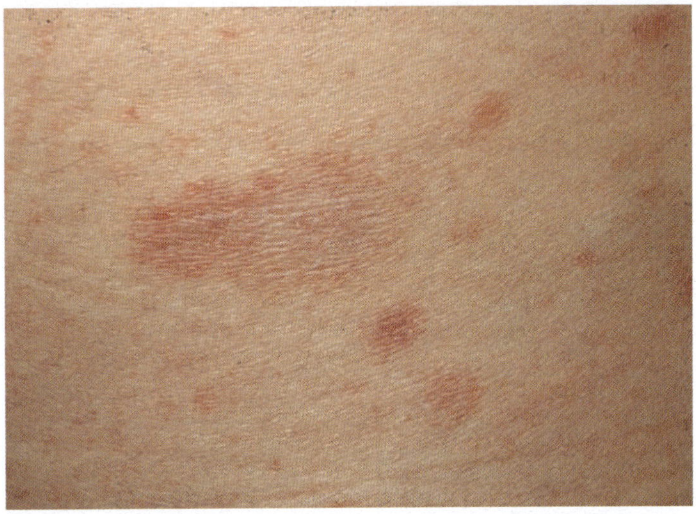

B

FIGURE 27-1. (A) A classic salmon-colored pityriasis rosea lesion. **(B)** Rose-colored pityriasis rosea lesions.

If PR persists beyond 3 months, the diagnosis must be reconsidered. The "Christmas tree" distribution of lesions on the trunk can be confused with ashy dermatosis, other lichenoid reactions, or Kaposi sarcoma, or it can be seen in the setting of human immunodeficiency virus infection. Many annular eruptions may resemble PR, such as pityriasis alba, nummular eczema, seborrheic dermatitis, and tinea. Inverse papular PR can be difficult to distinguish from Gianotti-Crosti syndrome. Secondary syphilis may imitate papular or scaly plaque PR [**Figure 27-13**]; thus, the Venereal Disease Research Laboratory (VDRL) test titer should be checked when considering PR as a diagnosis.

In diagnosing PR, it is important to note that the herald patch may be absent, or it may appear as multiple lesions. The secondary lesions may be located on the extremities with little truncal involvement. Focal lesions may also appear, especially in children. Oral, purpuric, vesicular, and pustular forms of PR are sometimes present in children. The patient's palms and soles may be involved, and it may be difficult to distinguish from secondary syphilis. PR is usually diagnosed clinically. However, in some of the atypical variants, PR may be difficult to diagnose.

PATHOLOGY

The histologic findings of PR are nonspecific. There is a decrease or absence of the granular layer, acanthosis, spongiosis, a superficial dermal infiltrate of lymphocytes, extravasated erythrocytes extending to the epidermis, and parakeratosis. The parakeratosis is often focal and in mounds. In a micropapular variant in patients with dark skin of color,

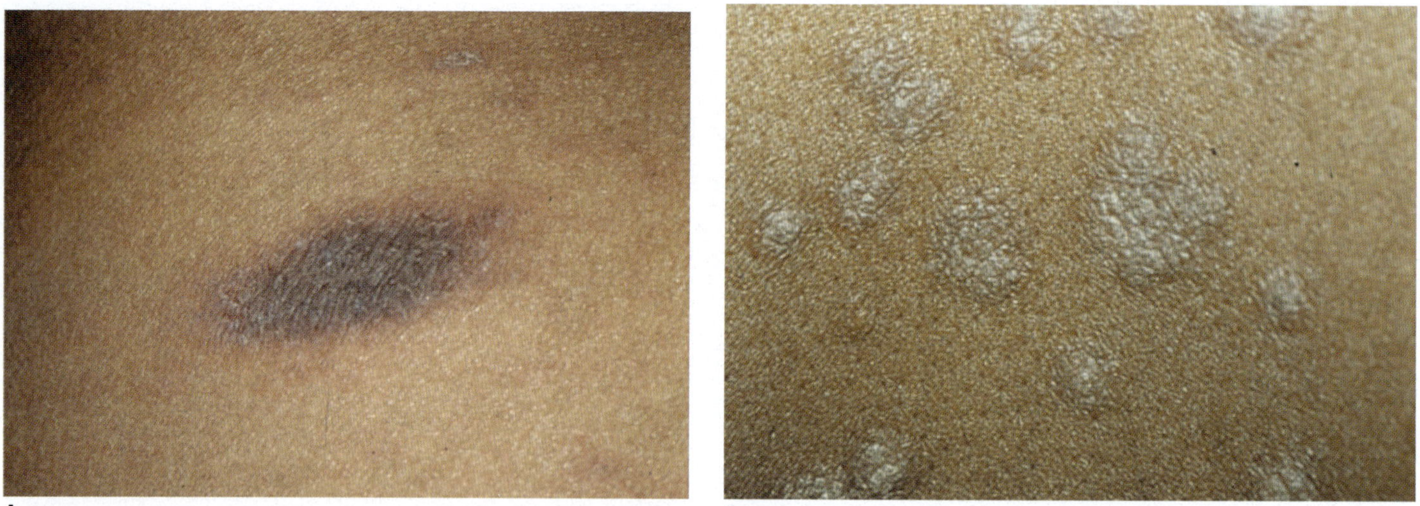

A B

FIGURE 27-2. (A) A violaceous plaque in an African American patient with pityriasis rosea. **(B)** Gray plaques in a pityriasis rosea patient with darker skin of color.

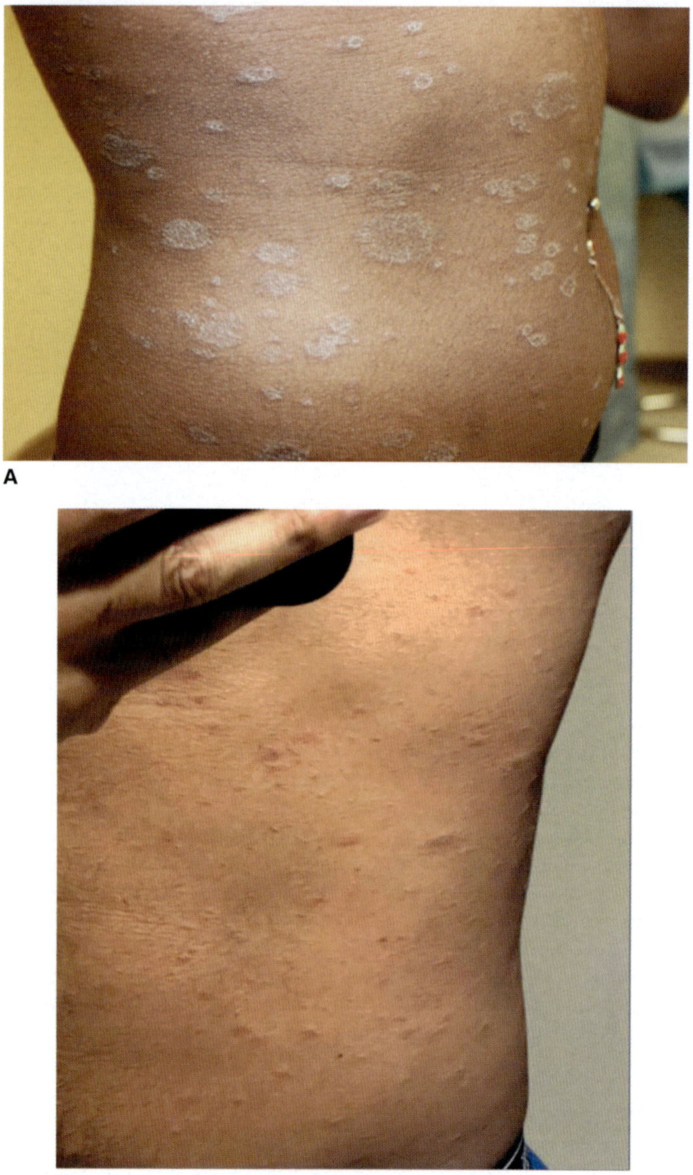

A B

FIGURE 27-3. (A) An African American female patient with pityriasis rosea manifesting as gray plaques on her right abdomen. **(B)** An African American male patient with pityriasis rosea manifesting as violaceous papules and plaques.

TABLE 27-4 Clinical presentation of pityriasis rosea in different Fitzpatrick skin types

Characteristics	I-III	IV-VI
Color of lesions	Rose or salmon	Gray or violaceous
Location	Predominance truncal	Predominance on the extremities
Scale	Collarette scales	Central scales
Special features	Central hyperpigmentation seldom seen	Central necrotic-like hyperpigmentation

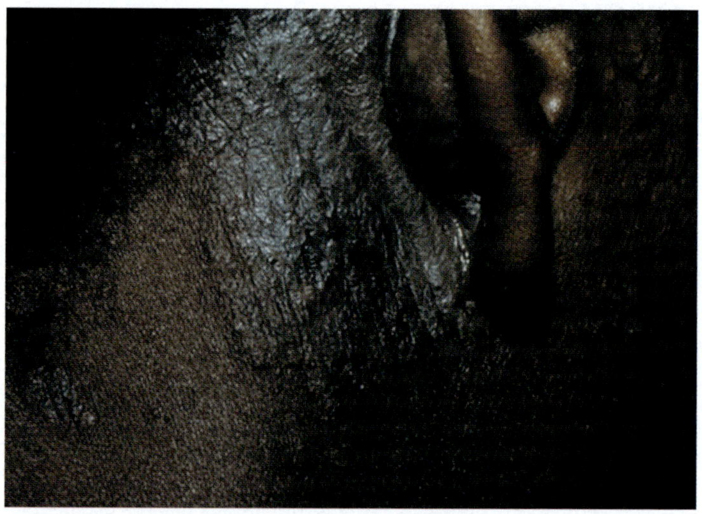

FIGURE 27-4. A violaceous herald patch on the right posterior auricular area.

TABLE 27-5 Clinical features of pityriasis rosea

1. An initial plaque (herald patch) lasts 6-10 weeks, occurs 1-14 days (or longer) before other lesions may appear and heals with postinflammatory hyperpigmentation in darker skin of color.
2. Characteristic individual lesions include collarette scale.
3. Lesions along lines of cleavage may form in a "school of minnows" or a "Christmas tree" pattern.
4. Papules with central necrotic-like hyperpigmentation occur especially on the extremities in children with dark skin of color.

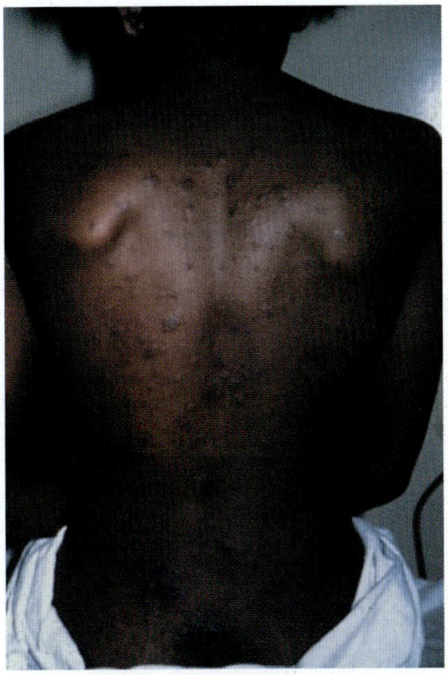

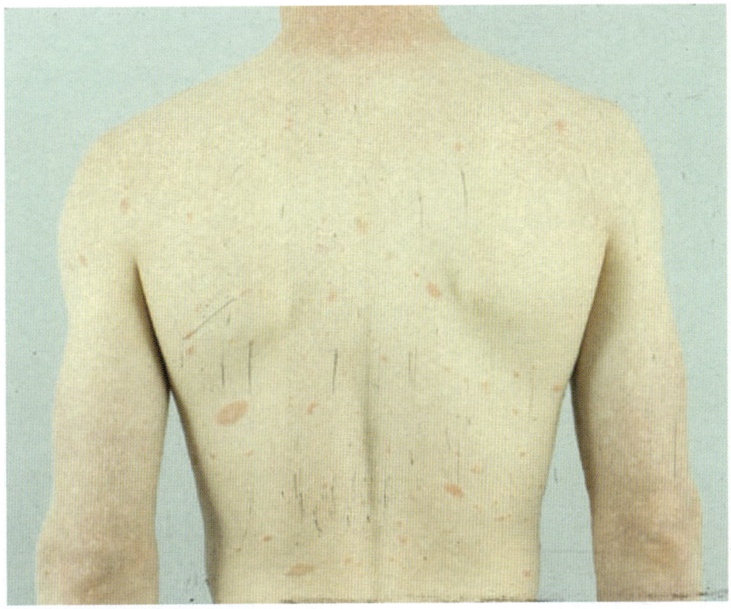

A B

FIGURE 27-5. **(A)** Secondary pityriasis rosea rash with several residual patches with collarette of scale. **(B)** Secondary lesions with several residual herald patches in a Hispanic man. The color is a dark erythema, somewhat intermediate between the rose- or salmon-colored lesions commonly seen in patients with Fitzpatrick skin types I to III, and the violaceous or gray lesion often seen in patients with darker skin of color.

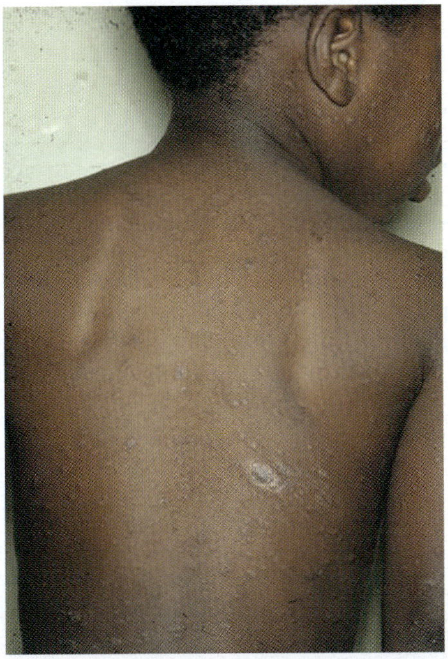

FIGURE 27-6. A "Christmas tree" pattern of pityriasis rosea lesions on the back.

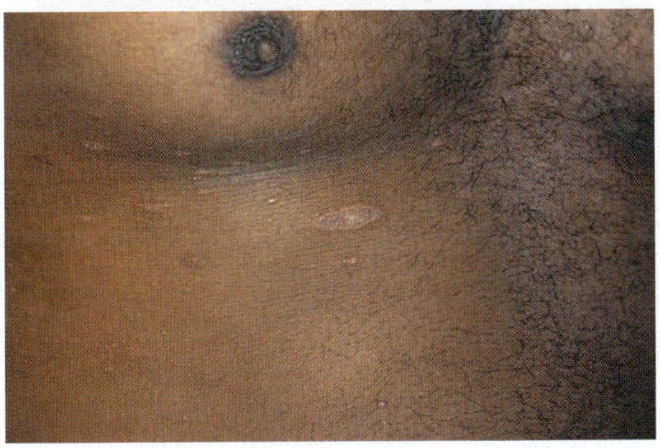

FIGURE 27-7. Pityriasis rosea lesions appearing as a herald patch with narrow linear lesions on the flank chest (the "school of minnows" pattern).

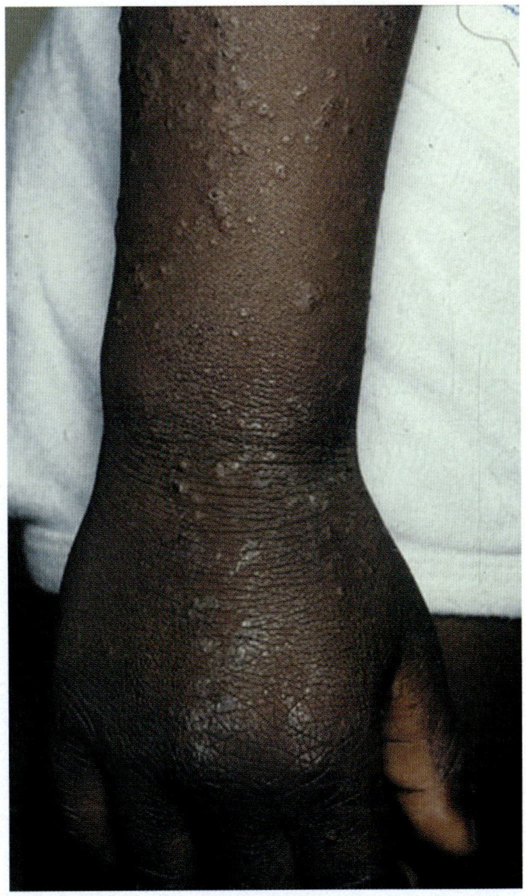

FIGURE 27-8. Papular lesions on the dorsum of the hands and forearms, many with necrotic-like centers.

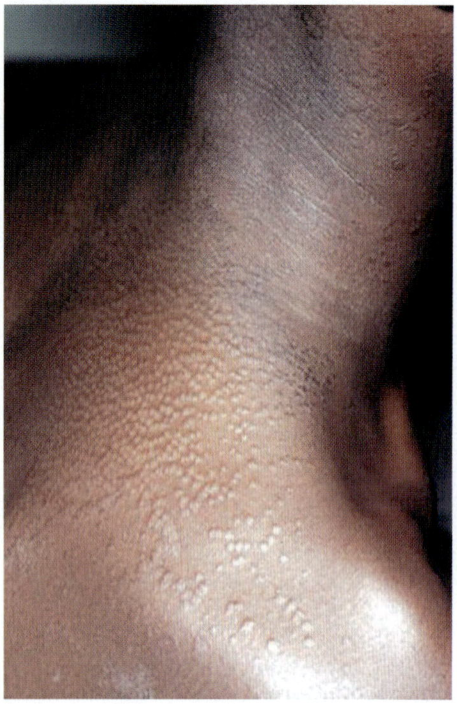

A

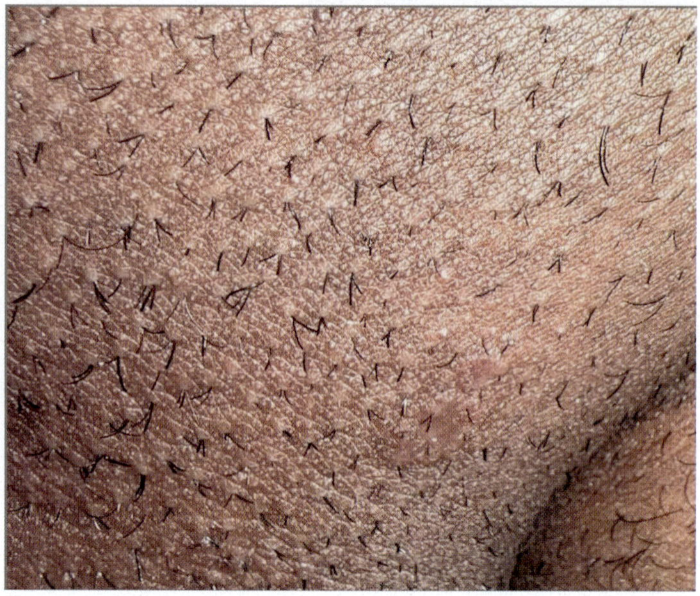

B

FIGURE 27-9. (A) An African American male patient with follicular pityriasis rosea on his right upper back. **(B)** A different African American male patient with follicular pityriasis rosea in the groin area.

there are often triangular mounds of parakeratosis that look tilted with respect to the underlying epidermis.[15] Focal spongiosis occasionally progresses to vesiculation. In older lesions, the perivascular infiltrate is often superficial and deep, with less spongiosis and more epidermal hyperplasia. This makes it difficult to distinguish between psoriasis and lichen planus.[16] More recently, immunohistochemical analysis has suggested a predominantly T-cell-mediated immune response with inflammatory cells in lesional skin staining predominantly CD3, CD4, CD8, and CD45RO and negative CD20 (B-cells).[17]

MANAGEMENT

PR is self-limiting; thus, patient education and symptomatic management of itch often suffice.[18] For symptomatic relief of pruritus, medium-strength topical steroids and/or antihistamines are prescribed. Intramuscular or oral corticosteroids given early may help to prevent postinflammatory hyperpigmentation, especially in patients with skin of color.[19] This usually attenuates the lesions in 2 to 3 weeks, but systemic corticosteroids may exacerbate the other symptoms of PR. In a severe

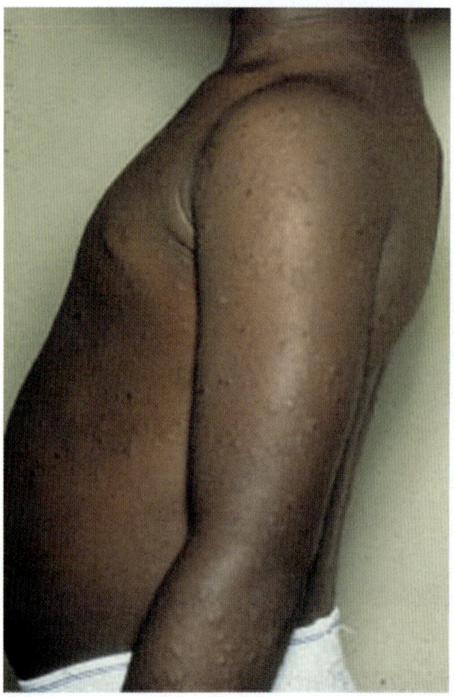

A

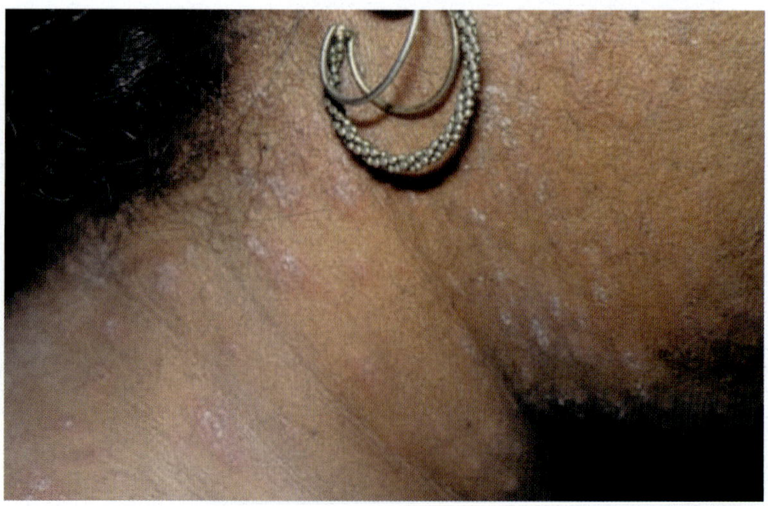

B

FIGURE 27-10. (A) Papules on the arms and chest of a boy with darker skin of color. **(B)** Pityriasis rosea lesions on the face and neck of a woman with darker skin of color.

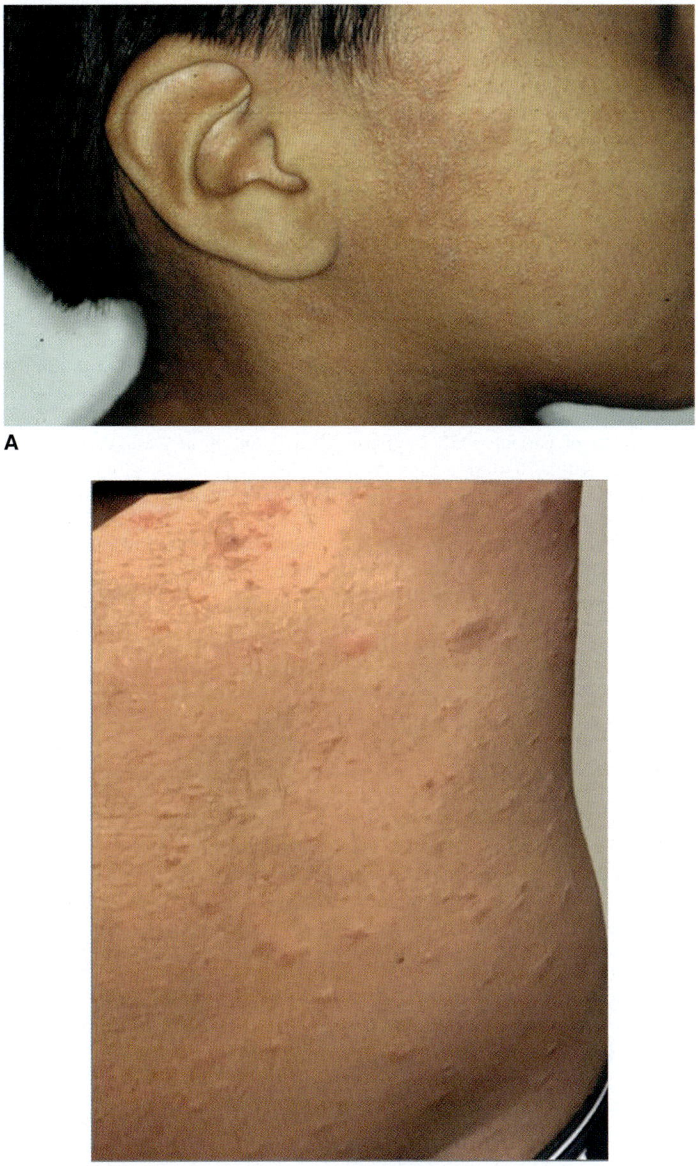

FIGURE 27-11. **(A)** Erythematous papules and plaques on the face and neck of a Hispanic child. **(B)** Erythematous to violaceous papules and plaques on the left abdomen of a young African American male.

vesicular form, PR can be treated with dapsone. Ultraviolet B (UVB) radiation has been shown to decrease the severity of the disease but does not ease the accompanying pruritus.[20] The combination of UVB treatment and a topical corticosteroid may make this mode of therapy more effective. Because UVB can cause postinflammatory hyperpigmentation, it may not be the treatment of choice for patients with skin of color.

Because HHV-6, HHV-7, and HHV-8 have been implicated as potential causes of PR, using antiviral therapy may reduce the severity and duration of the condition. Acyclovir is not the most sensitive agent to treat HHV-6 and HHV-7, but it is the safest. A systematic review and meta-analysis suggests oral acyclovir compared to placebo, vitamins, or no treatment may lead to practioner-rated rash improvement within 2 weeks.[21] Furthermore, the addition of acyclovir to standard care with calamine lotion and oral cetirizine led to a reduction in itch score compared to standard care alone.[21] Although there is debate as to how much acyclovir can be beneficial, given its low side effect profile, consideration should be taken when prescribing this medication in very extensive and/or symptomatic PR cases.[22]

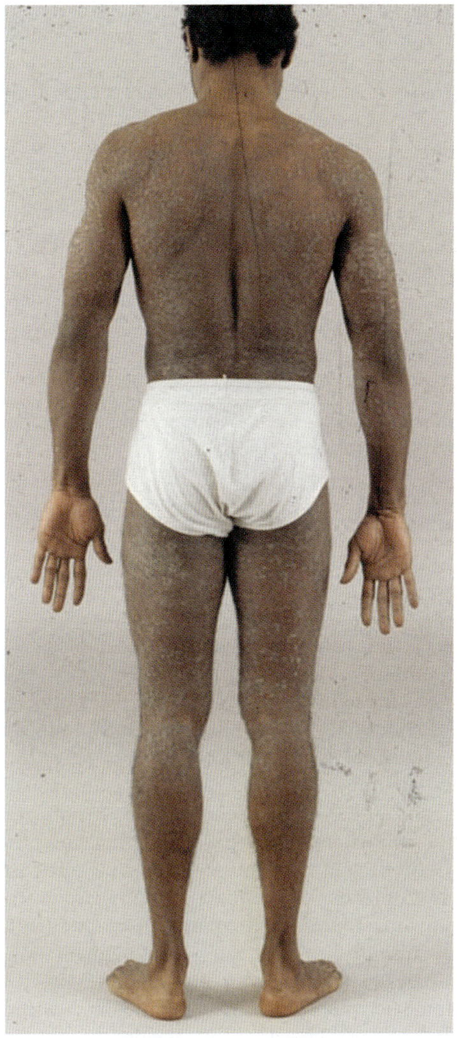

FIGURE 27-12. Generalized pityriasis rosea on the trunk and extremities of a man with darker skin of color.

Macrolide antibiotics have also been used for their nonspecific anti-inflammatory and immunomodulatory effects, but data are limited and conflicting. Erythromycin may help with itch reduction compared to placebo, but other studies found limited benefits.[21,23,24] Trials with azithromycin and clarithromycin found no benefit compared to placebo.[25-27] As a result, these medications are not a definitive therapy for patients with PR [**Table 27-6**].

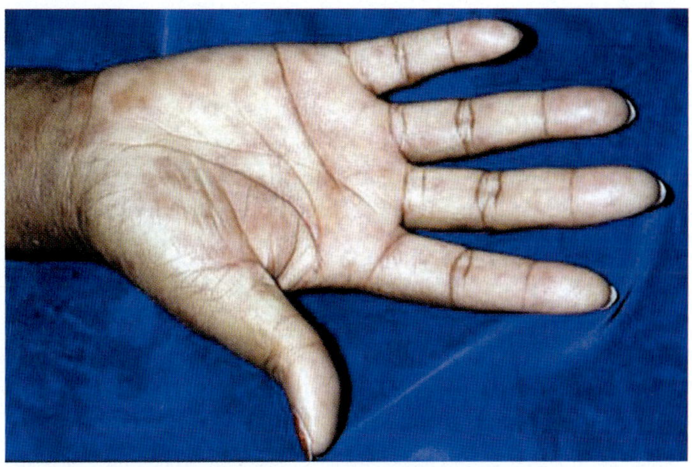

FIGURE 27-13. Palmer lesions of secondary syphilis.

TABLE 27-6 Pityriasis rosea therapy

Treatment	Results/comments
Intramuscular or oral corticosteroids	Attenuates dermatosis but must be used early in the disease process.
UVB radiation and topical treatment	UVB treatment should be used in conjunction with a topical corticosteroid. UVB treatment can cause postinflammatory hyperpigmentation, so it is not optimal for patients with darker skin of color.
Erythromycin, 250 mg qid	Complete clearance is usually achieved in 2 weeks, but there is controversy over its role in the treatment of pityriasis rosea.
Acyclovir	There is a debate over the most effective dosage for acyclovir. It should be considered for extensive and/or symptomatic cases, because it has a low side effect profile.

Note. Pityriasis rosea is self-limiting; therefore, treatment is usually not necessary. When treatment is given, it is often for the symptomatic relief of pruritus.

Abbreviations: qid, four times a day; UVB, ultraviolet B.

CONCLUSION

PR occurs over a wide age range, usually between the ages of 10 and 35 years and is found in individuals with all skin phototypes. PR has some unique features in patients with skin of color, and physicians should be aware of the distinct effects that PR treatment options could have on patients with Fitzpatrick skin types IV to VI.

Due to PR's self-limiting nature, treatment is not usually necessary; however, therapy can be given to relieve symptoms of pruritus. Topical steroids and/or antihistamines are often the first line of treatment. In patients with skin of color, intramuscular or oral corticosteroids given early may help to prevent postinflammatory hyperpigmentation. UVB in conjunction with a topical corticosteroid is another treatment option, but UVB can cause postinflammatory hyperpigmentation, so it is not advised for patients with darker skin of color.

Acyclovir is a new potential PR treatment that is proving to be beneficial. Although there is still a debate over the dosage, acyclovir has minimal side effects and, therefore, should be considered in severe cases of PR. Erythromycin is used to treat PR in some instances; however, physicians should note that studies are not conclusive on the efficacy of this medication.

REFERENCES

1. Halder R, Nootheti P. Ethnic skin disorders overview. *J Am Acad Dermatol.* 2003;48:S143-S148.
2. Joshi TP, Calderara GA, Lipoff JB. Prevalence of pityriasis rosea in the United States: A cross-sectional study using the All of Us database. *JAAD Int.* 2022;8:45-46.
3. Araujo D, Berman B, Weinstein A. Human herpesviruses 6 and 7. *Dermatol Clin.* 2002;20:301-306.
4. Chuh A. The association of pityriasis rosea with cytomegalovirus, Epstein-Barr virus and parvovirus B19 infections: a prospective case control study by polymerase chain reaction and serology. *Eur J Dermatol.* 2003;13:25-28.
5. Parija M, Thappa D. Study of role of streptococcal throat infection in pityriasis rosea. *Indian J Dermatol.* 2008;53:171-173.
6. Prantsidis A, Rigopoulos D, Papatheodorou G, et al. Detection of human herpesvirus 8 in the skin of patients with pityriasis rosea. *Acta Derm Venereol.* 2009;89(6):604-606.
7. Mubki TF, Bin Dayel SA, Kadry R. A case of Pityriasis rosea concurrent with the novel influenza A (H1N1) infection. *Pediatr Dermatol.* 2011;28(3):341-342.
8. Chen J-F, Chiang C-P, Chen Y-F, Wang W-M. Pityriasis rosea following influenza (H1N1) vaccination. *J Chin Med Assoc.* 2011;74(6):280-282.
9. Drago F, Broccolo F, Rebora A. Pityriasis rosea: an update with a critical appraisal of its possible herpesviral etiology. *J Am Acad Dermatol.* 2009;61(2):303-318.
10. Rebora A, Drago F, Broccolo F. Pityriasis rosea and herpesviruses: facts and controversies. *Clin Dermatol.* 2010;28(5):497-501.
11. Borgia F, Li Pomi F, Alessandrello C, Vaccaro M, Pioggia G, Gangemi S. Coronavirus disease 2019 and pityriasis rosea: A review of the immunological connection. *J Dermatol.* 2022;49(10):948-956.
12. Avallone G, Quaglino P, Cavallo F, et al. SARS-CoV-2 vaccine-related cutaneous manifestations: a systematic review. *Int J Dermatol.* 2022;61(10):1187-120.
13. McMahon DE, Kovarik CL, Damsky W, et al. Clinical and pathologic correlation of cutaneous COVID-19 vaccine reactions including V-REPP: A registry-based study. *J Am Acad Dermatol.* 2022;86(1):113-121.
14. Bjornberg A, Tegner E. Pityriasis rosea. In: Freedberg I, Eisen A, Wolff K, et al, eds. *Fitzpatrick's Dermatology in General Medicine.* 6th ed. New York, NY: McGraw-Hill; 2003:445-450.
15. Brady SP. Parakeratosis. *J Am Acad Dermatol.* 2004;50(1):77-84.
16. Ackerman A. *Histologic Diagnosis of Inflammatory Skin Disease.* Philadelphia: Lea & Febiger; 1978.
17. Wang S, Fu L, Du W, Hu J, Zha Y, Wang P. Subsets of T lymphocytes in the lesional skin of pityriasis rosea. *An Bras Dermatol.* 2019;94(1):52-55.
18. Chuh A, Zawar V, Sciallis G, Kempf W. A position statement on the management of patients with pityriasis rosea. *J Eur Acad Dermatol Venereol.* 2016;30(10):1670-1681.
19. Halder RM, Roberts CI, Nootheti PK. Cutaneous diseases in the black races. *Dermatol Clin.* 2003;21(4):679-687.
20. Leenutaphong V, Jiamton S. UVB phototherapy for pityriasis rosea: a bilateral comparison study. *J Am Acad Dermatol.* 1995;33(6):996-999.
21. Contreras-Ruiz J, Peternel S, Jiménez Gutiérrez C, Culav-Koscak I, Reveiz L, Silbermann-Reynoso M de L. Interventions for pityriasis rosea. *Cochrane database Syst Rev.* 2019;2019(10).
22. Rassai S, Feily A, Sina N, Abtahian S. Low dose of acyclovir may be an effective treatment against pityriasis rosea: a random investigator-blind clinical trial on 64 patients. *J Eur Acad Dermatol Venereol.* 2011;25(1):24-26.
23. Sharma PK, Yadav TP, Gautam RK, Taneja N, Satyanarayana L. Erythromycin in pityriasis rosea: A double-blind, placebo-controlled clinical trial. *J Am Acad Dermatol.* 2000;42(2 Pt 1):241-244.
24. Rasi A, Tajziehchi L, Savabi-Nasab S. Oral erythromycin is ineffective in the treatment of pityriasis rosea. *J Drugs Dermatol.* 2008;7(1):35-38.
25. Pandhi D, Singal A, Verma P, Sharma R. The efficacy of azithromycin in pityriasis rosea: a randomized, double-blind, placebo-controlled trial. *Indian J Dermatol Venereol Leprol.* 2014;80(1):36-40.
26. Amer A, Fischer H. Azithromycin does not cure pityriasis rosea. *Pediatrics.* 2006;117(5):1702-1705.
27. Ahmed N, Iftikhar N, Bashir U, Rizvi SDA, Sheikh ZI, Manzur A. Efficacy of clarithromycin in pityriasis rosea. *J Coll Physicians Surg Pak.* 2014;24(11):802-805.

CHAPTER 28 Lichen Planus and Lichen Nitidus

Sara Saheb Kashaf
Victoria Barbosa

KEY POINTS

- Lichen planus (LP) is a T-cell-mediated autoimmune disease that can affect the skin, scalp, mucous membranes, and nails.
- LP has several variants; some forms, such as actinic LP and LP pigmentosus, occur more commonly in patients with skin of color.
- While LP is often self-limited, treatments can reduce the severity and duration of symptoms.
- Lichen nitidus is a rare condition that occurs most commonly in children.
- While lichen nitidus usually appears as flesh-colored papules, it may appear hypopigmented in darker skin tones.
- Lichen nitidus is often self-limited and usually resolves within 1 year.

LICHEN PLANUS

INTRODUCTION

LP is an autoimmune, T-cell-mediated inflammatory disease that can affect the cutaneous skin, scalp, nails, and mucosal surfaces such as the oral mucosa, genitalia, and esophagus. While there are several clinical variants, cutaneous LP lesions most commonly present as itchy, flat-topped, violaceous papules and plaques with overlying reticulated white scale called Wickham's striae (WS). LP has been associated with genetic as well as environmental factors, such as viral infections, medications, and dental materials.[1-3]

When treating patients with skin of color, it is important to recognize that the prevalence of the condition may vary by geographic region, race, and ethnicity, that some variants are more common in skin of color, and that the postinflammatory hyperpigmentation that often results from the primary eruption can be quite distressing to patients. Topical, intralesional, and systemic steroids are the mainstays of treatment, but other options are available for recalcitrant disease.[1]

EPIDEMIOLOGY

LP has an estimated prevalence of 1% in the United States and 0.5% to 1.0% worldwide[1,4] LP affects both men and women, with recent studies demonstrating a female predominance. [4,5] LP is widely considered a disease of the middle-aged, found most commonly in those in their 40s and 50s.[4] This notion is challenged by findings in a U.S.-based cross-sectional study of 788 LP patients by Leasure et al, which found that prevalence peaked in older age groups, with prevalence rates of 0.06% in the 18 to 44 age group, 0.25% in those aged 45 to 54 years, 0.41% in those aged 55 to 64 years, 0.61% in those aged 65 to 74 years, and 0.91% in those aged 75 and older. This study also demonstrated a 3:1 female to male ratio, along with racial and ethnic differences in LP prevalence, with higher rates observed in White (0.45%, 95% CI, 0.41-0.49) and Black (0.42%, 95% CI, 0.36-0.49) populations compared to Hispanics (0.23%, 95% CI, 0.18-0.28).[5] Two recent meta-analyses have estimated the global pooled prevalence of oral lichen planus to be 0.89% and 1.01%, with each study revealing geographic variability.[6,7] Genital LP has been estimated to affect 1% to 2% of the U.S. population.[8] Nail LP was observed in 10% to 15% of patients with cutaneous LP, although it may also occur in the absence of a cutaneous eruption.[9]

ETIOLOGY

LP is an autoimmune disease, the pathogenesis of which is not fully understood. LP is thought to be primarily due to a cell-mediated immune response. One hypothesis is that an internal or external factor, like a virus, medication, or contact allergen, leads to the modification of epidermal self-antigens. This change then triggers the activation of cytotoxic CD8+ T cells. These altered self-antigens cross-react with the normal self-antigens present on basal keratinocytes, leading to the targeting of these cells by T-cells and their subsequent apoptosis.[10] Prior studies have found increased expression of perforin and granzyme B, key components of T-cell cytotoxic activity, in LP lesions. Furthermore, studies have highlighted the potential role of mast cell degranulation and the release of inflammatory mediators in LP. In addition, increased expression of various proteases has been observed in LP lesions. These enzymes are capable of breaking down components of the basement membrane, exacerbating the immune response in LP.[11]

Elevated levels of various cytokines and chemokines, such as IL-5, IL-6, IL-8, IL-9, IL-10, IL-12, IL-17, IL-22, TNF-α, TGF-β, and IFN-γ have been reported in LP lesions or serum of affected patients. Notably, previous studies have observed increased expression of IFN-γ and IL-17 in LP skin lesions, highlighting their potential role in disease. The reported effectiveness of off-label treatments such as JAK inhibitors (eg, tofacitinib) and IL-17 inhibitor secukinumab, along with IL-12/23-targeting ustekinumab and IL-23 inhibitor guselkumab, in improving LP symptoms further supports the roles of IFN-γ, IL-17, and related pathways in LP pathogenesis. Overall, while there have been advances in understanding the cellular and molecular aspects of LP, further research is needed for a more comprehensive understanding of disease pathogenesis.[11]

Various factors have been associated with LP. Genetic susceptibility is thought to play a role in the development of LP, as evidenced by the higher frequency of LP in families, with one study reporting that 10.7% of the affected patients had a family history of disease. The role of genetics is also supported by the overrepresentation in LP patients of certain HLA haplotypes.[3,12-15] A phenome-wide association study of the MHC complex identified six single nucleotide polymorphisms (SNPs), with SNP rs1794275 being the most significant, along with an association with Haplotype *HLA DQB1*05:01*.[16] Interestingly, a meta-analysis exploring the role of the −308 G/A polymorphism in the TNF-α gene found an association with OLP but not with cutaneous LP, suggesting a distinction in the pathogenesis of the two entities.[3,17]

Environmental triggers have also been implicated in the development of LP, such as exposure to certain medications, dental metals, and viral infections.[1] Commonly associated medications include antimalarials, ACE inhibitors, thiazide diuretics, NSAIDs, quinidine, β-blockers, and TNF-α inhibitors.[18,19] However, recurrence of lesions after rechallenging patients with the medication was rare. Furthermore, OLP is associated with contact allergies to metals in dental restorations like mercury, copper, and gold, with prior work reporting resolution of LP lesions after removal of the sensitizing metal.[20,21] LP has also been associated with viral infections, particularly hepatitis C virus (HCV). A meta-analysis investigated 33 studies comparing the seroprevalence of HCV in LP patients and 6 studies reporting the prevalence of LP in patients with HCV infection. This study found a higher prevalence of HCV in LP patients compared to controls and a higher risk (odds ratio 4.85; 95% CI, 3.58-6.56) of HCV seropositivity in LP patients, with these associations varying by geography.[22] Additionally, a systematic review focusing on OLP found a strong association between OLP and HCV infection, with an odds ratio for HCV seropositivity of 6.07 (95% CI, 2.73-13.48), with observed geographical variation in this association.[23] A separate study found the incidence of liver diseases such as hepatitis B and C and liver cirrhosis was higher in LP patients, further supporting a possible association between LP and liver pathology.[24]

CLINICAL PRESENTATION

Cutaneous LP typically presents with the six P's: pruritic, purple, polygonal, planar papules, and plaques [**Figure 28-1**]. Lesions often have an overlying reticulated white scale, or Wickham's striae (WS). In brown skin, lesions may appear more hyperpigmented than violaceous [**Figure 28-2**]. Lesions are typically distributed on the forearms, flexor wrists, dorsal hands, shins, flexor ankles, and lower back but may appear anywhere

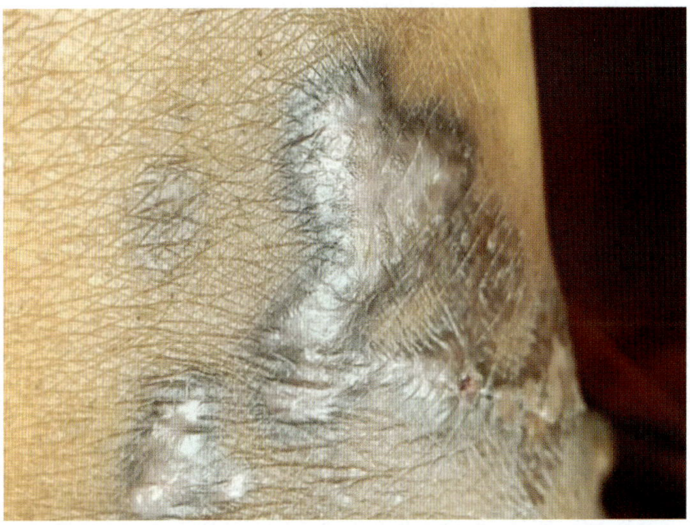

FIGURE 28-1. Classic flat-topped violaceous papules and plaques of lichen planus.

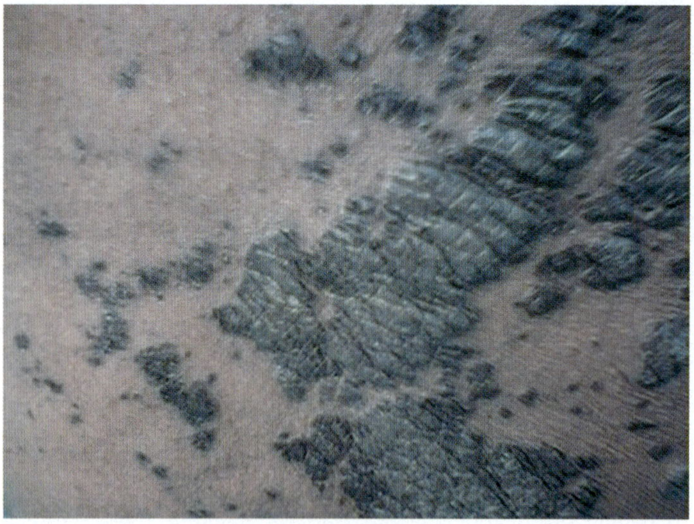

FIGURE 28-2. Lichen planus: hyperpigmented, coalescing polygonal papules and plaques.

on the body. The Koebner phenomenon can be observed in LP, where trauma to the skin triggers the formation of new lesions.[1,3,10]

There are several clinical variants of LP, as listed in **Table 28-1.** Hypertrophic LP typically presents on the anterior lower legs as thickened, hyperkeratotic plaques [**Figure 28-3**]. Ulcerative LP, found between the toes or on the soles of the feet, is characterized by painful, eroded, or ulcerated lesions prone to scarring. LP pigmentosus typically presents as hyperpigmented macules or patches on sun-exposed or flexural areas and is seen more often in skin of color patients.[25] LP pigmentosus inversus is a variant of LP pigmentosus that primarily affects body folds with oval-shaped, brownish-purple macules and patches, often in a linear arrangement. These lesions are usually symmetrical, may cause mild itching, and leave behind thinned, hyperpigmented skin. Actinic LP is also more common in darker skin and manifests as atrophic, hyperpigmented lesions with a rolled edge in sun-exposed areas.[26] These lesions can also result in persistent residual hyperpigmentation even after the rash has cleared, particularly in patients with darker skin tones.[27]

The oral mucosa is involved in over half of LP patients and is sometimes found in the absence of cutaneous lesions.[10] Oral LP (OLP) is most frequently observed on the buccal mucosa [**Figure 28-4**].[28] It presents in various forms, including reticular, erosive, atrophic, bullous, papular, and plaque-like. The most common type is reticular OLP, which presents as bilateral, asymptomatic white lines or lacy WS on the oral mucosa. Other types include atrophic OLP, characterized by atrophic changes and erythema; bullous OLP, presenting with fluid-filled vesicles, often on the lower mucosal lip; and erosive OLP, marked by pain, erythema, erosion, and ulceration.[26,29] A recent meta-analysis demonstrated the rate of malignant transformation in OLP to be 0.44%, with the risk of malignancy increasing with tobacco and alcohol use and HCV infection.[30]

In men, LP may involve the glans penis and display an annular configuration. In women, genital LP often presents with itching, pain, vaginal discharge, or bleeding, and its most common form is erosive LP. Women may experience vulvar or vaginal LP, which can lead to fibrosis, vulvar scarring, or vaginal stenosis if without adequate treatment. Vulvovaginal-gingival syndrome, a specific subtype of LP affecting both oral and genital regions, often results in scarring and is associated with the HLA allele DQB1*0201 in 80% of patients.[31] The association between vulvar LP and vulvar squamous cell carcinoma remains unclear.[32] Differentiating LP from lichen sclerosus (LS) can be challenging, though LS typically does not affect the vagina.[10]

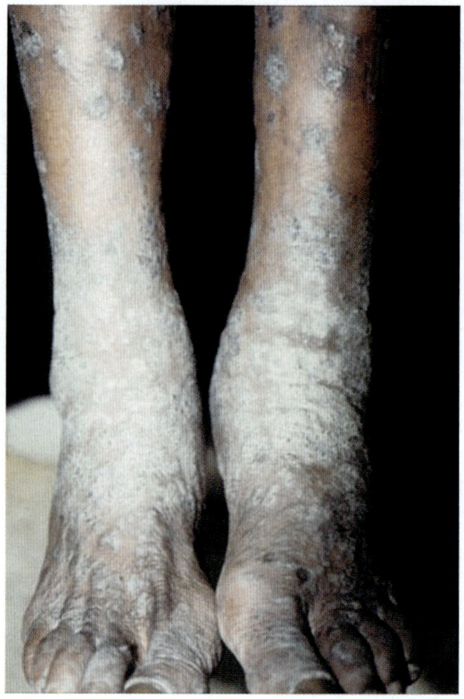

FIGURE 28-3. Hypertrophic lichen planus characteristically involving the shins and ankles.

TABLE 28-1 Clinical variants of lichen planus
Actinic LP
Annular LP
Atrophic LP
Blashkoid LP
Bullous LP
Erpsove LP
Hypertrophic LP
Inverse LP
Lichen planopilaris
Lichen planus pigmentosus
Lichen planus pemphigoides
Linear LP
Lichen planus/lupus overlap
Mucosal LP
Zosteriform LP

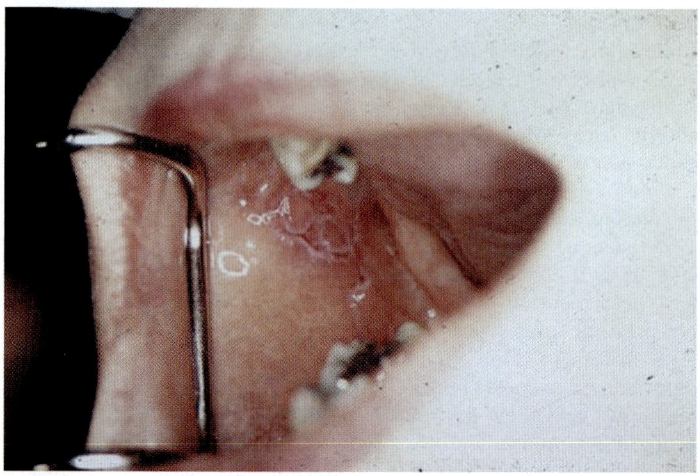

FIGURE 28-4. Oral lichen planus on the buccal mucosa.

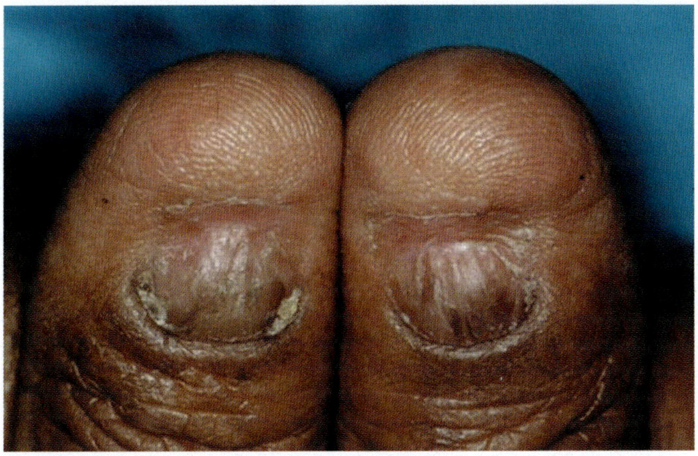

FIGURE 28-5. Pterygium in a patient with lichen planus.

Nail involvement occurs in approximately 10% of patients, often involving multiple nails but not necessarily the adjacent skin. Early symptoms include thinning of the nail plate and longitudinal ridging [**Figure 28-5**].[10] As the disease progresses, it can lead to scarring of the nail matrix, the formation of a dorsal pterygium (the most specific nail finding), chromonychia (nail color changes), subungual hyperkeratosis (nail thickening), rough-textured nails (trachonychia), and in severe cases, total loss of the nail plate.[10,33]

Lichen planopilaris (LPP) is a form of LP that affects the scalp and other hair-bearing areas, often leading to scarring hair loss known as cicatrizing alopecia. This condition is discussed in Chapter 42, the scarring alopecia chapter of this textbook.

Lichenoid drug eruptions typically occur in sun-exposed areas, with a symmetrical and widespread distribution, differing from classic LP. Associated lesions resemble eczema or psoriasis and rarely show Wickham's striae. There can be a delay of several months to a year between starting a medication and the onset of the eruption, making a detailed medication history review essential for diagnosing drug-induced LP.[10,34]

DIAGNOSIS

The diagnosis of LP relies primarily on clinical evaluation. When obtaining a medical history, patients should be asked about symptoms such as pruritus, the presence of oral or genital lesions, and about dysphagia or odynophagia, which could suggest esophageal involvement. Furthermore, it is important to inquire about medications that could cause lichenoid drug eruptions, as these lesions can mimic LP and are clinically and histologically similar.[34] Patch testing may be indicated for OLP. Screening for hepatitis C infection is advised, especially in patients with chronic OLP or if the patient resides in areas where HCV infection is common.[1] Dermosocopy can aid in the diagnosis of LP, with WS visualized exclusively in LP. WS typically appears as pearly white structures with "ferm leaf" projections.[33,35] Biopsy can be used for definitive diagnosis.

HISTOPATHOLOGY

Histopathology of LP is characterized by a dense, lichenoid infiltrate of lymphocytes at the dermal-epidermal junction (DEJ). Vacuolar degeneration of the basal cell layer leads to apoptosis and the formation of Civatte bodies, also known as cytoid bodies. Civatte bodies are necrotic keratinocytes that may be visualized in the epidermis or papillary dermis. The rete ridges may have an irregular "sawtooth" appearance due to irregular acanthosis from chronic inflammation. Max Joseph spaces are subepidermal clefts that may result from the interface inflammation. Damaged basal keratinocytes release melanin, causing melanin incontinence within the underlying dermis. The presence of dermal eosinophils may suggest a drug-induced LP. The epidermis demonstrates hyperkeratosis and "wedge-shaped" hypergranulosis without parakeratosis. Wickham's striae are believed to result from the hypergranulosis. On direct immunofluorescence, LP may demonstrate irregular IgA, IgM, IgG, or C3 deposition and shaggy fibrinogen deposition at the DEJ.[1,3,10]

MANAGEMENT

There are few evidence-based treatment options for LP as there are few randomized controlled trials. Hence, treatment options are largely guided by clinical experience, case studies, and retrospective chart reviews. The treatment approach varies depending on the type of LP, the location of lesions, and the severity of the disease. Of note, drug-induced LP should be considered prior to starting therapy and withdrawal of offending drugs is typically curative. [26]

For cutaneous LP, which is generally self-limiting, the therapeutic focus is on hastening resolution and reducing pruritus. Topical corticosteroids are the first-line treatment for cutaneous LP. Mid- or high-potency medications such as triamcinolone acetonide 0.1% or clobetasol proprionate 0.05% may be used twice daily depending on the location and extent of the lesions. Intralesional triamcinolone 5 to 10 mg/cc may be injected into hypertrophic or recalcitrant lesions of limited distribution [**Figure 28-6A** and **B**].[1,4]

In a review of 444 LP patients by Schwager et al, 30% required one or more nonlocalized forms of therapy. Second-line treatments for more generalized disease include systemic corticosteroids, phototherapy, and retinoids. Systemic corticosteroids can be administered orally or intramuscularly. Prednisone 30 to 60 mg per day can be tapered over 2 to 6 weeks. Alternatively, intramuscular triamcinolone 40 to 80 mg can be administered every 6 to 8 weeks.[1,4] Phototherapy is also an appropriate second-line treatment for generalized cutaneous LP. Pavlotsky et al treated LP patients with phototherapy and found that found 70% of the seven patients receiving ultraviolet B (UVB) therapy had a complete response, and 85% of the patients receiving narrow-band UVB (nb-UVB) had a complete response to treatment.[36] In a retrospective study of 192 LP patients treated with nb-UVB conducted by Dawood et al, 71% showed a significant response, and 74% of these had no recurrence over an average follow-up of 58.7 months. Women and patients with lighter Fitzpatrick phototypes had a more favorable response to treatment.[37] In a study by Schwager et al, narrow-band UVB was one of the most commonly used and effective generalized treatments.[3]

Oral retinoids may be considered as an alternative systemic treatment option. These medications should be accompanied, of course, by adequate contraception for women who can become pregnant. In a double-blind, placebo-controlled trial by Laurberg et al, acitretin, administered at 30 mg/day, significantly improved symptoms in 64% of patients after 8 weeks, compared to improvement in only 13% of patients in the placebo group. In a subsequent 8-week open-phase trial, 83% of patients initially on placebo also showed improvement with acitretin treatment. The drug was generally well-tolerated, with typical retinoid side effects.[38] Prior studies have also supported a potential therapeutic benefit of isotretinoin and tretinoin for cutaneous LP.[39,40]

Several additional treatments have been reported in the literature for the treatment of cutaneous LP, as listed in **Table 28-2.**[3,41] These treatments are considered third-line therapies. Of note, there are reports in the literature of dupilumab as both a cause of and treatment for LP.[42] While more research is needed, JAK inhibitors may offer some promise for treatment. Abduelmula et al reviewed the literature on treatment of LP with four JAK inhibitors: baricitinib, tofacitnib, ruxolitinib, and upadacitinib. Of the 16 patients who received baricitinib, complete resolution was seen in 25% of patients, and partial resolution was seen in 33.3% of patients. Of the 30 people who received tofacitinib, 10% had complete response and 60% had a partial response. Note that 16.7% of the 12 patients who received ruxolitinib achieved complete response, while 83% received partial response. Both of the patients who received upacitibib achieved a complete response. It is important to note that half of the patients in these studies received concomitant treatment with additional agents. This class of medicines will certainly be an area of additional research.[43]

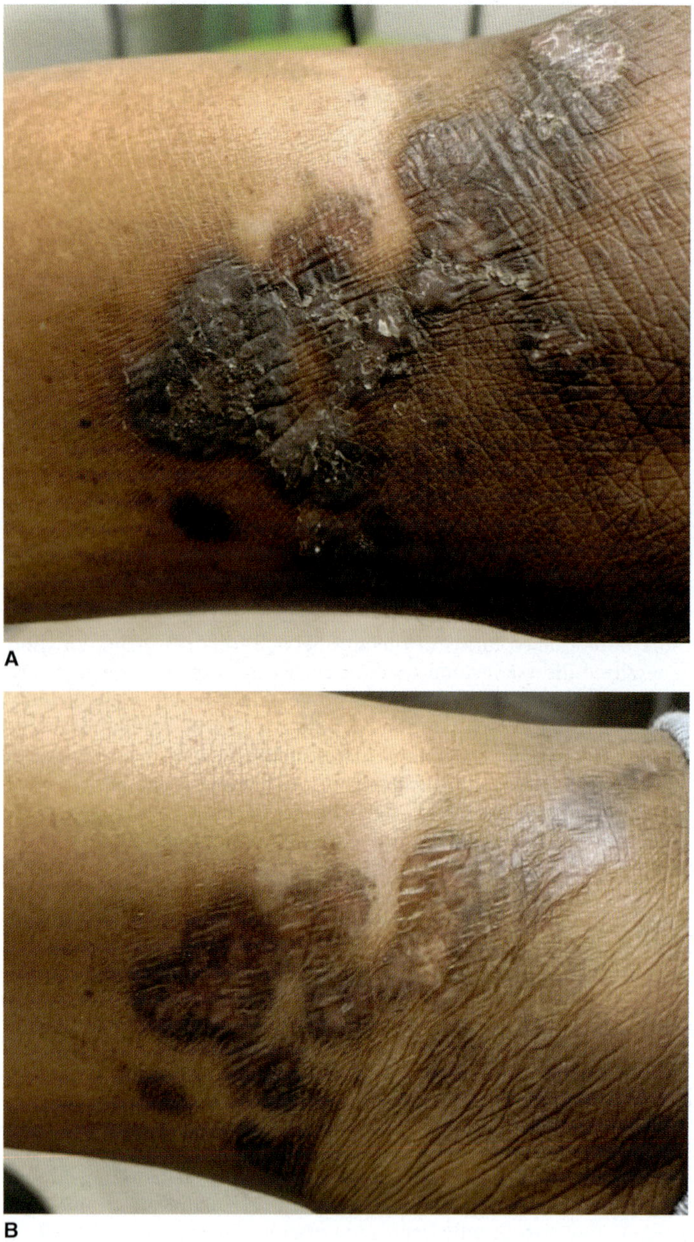

FIGURE 28-6 A and B. Before and after treatment of lichen planus with intralesional triamcinolone. Note the perilesional hypopigmentation secondary to the use of topical corticosteroids.

OLP may take up to 5 years to resolve spontaneously or persist indefinitely. While treatment is not recommended for asymptomatic lesions, painful erosive lesions should be treated and can be managed with topical or oral steroids.[10] Tacrolimus is an alternative topical therapy. In a review of systemic nonsteroid immunomodulators for oral LP, methotrexate and dapsone were the medications with the best evidence for efficacy, with less supporting data for levamisole, hydroxychloroquine, thalidomide, metronidazole, azathioprine, mycophenolate mofetil, and colchicine.[44] Use of topical tacrolimus for nonerosive lesions and apremilast, secukinumab, guselkumab, and JAK inhibitors for erosive oral LP have also been reported. [45]

Treatment of genital LP is similar to that of oral LP, with topical corticosteroids as a first-line treatment and topical tacrolimus as an alternative. These agents may be applied intravaginally if needed. In more severe erosive cases, systemic glucocorticoids such as prednisone 40 to 60 mg per day may be used initially with a 4- to 6-week tape, transitioning to topical therapy for maintenance. There are several case reports

TABLE 28-2 Third-line treatments for cutaneous lichen planus
Acitretin
Adalimumab
Apremilast
Azathioprine
Baribitinib
Cyclosporine
Dapsone
Doxycycline
Dupilumab
Efalizumab
Griseofulvin
Hydroxychloroquine
Low-dose Heparin
Methotrexate
Metronidazole
Mycophenolate mofetil
Ruxolitinib
Sulfasalazine
Thalidomide
Tofacitinib
Upadacitinib

of alternative systemic treatments used for refractory disease, including methotrexate, mycophenolate, minocycline, cyclosporine, trimethoprim-sulfamethoxazole, hydroxychloroquine, and acitretin. Dilator therapy or surgery may be necessary to address adhesions and scarring.[46] Since LP is less common in circumcised men, circumcision may be suggested.[47] Emerging treatments like photodynamic therapy are under study.[48]

In cases of nail LP, treatment aims to reduce pain and minimize scarring. While some studies report use of topical corticosteroids, intramatricial or intramuscular injection is considered first-line therapy, but relapse is common.[26,49]

LICHEN NITIDUS

INTRODUCTION

Lichen nitidus (LN) is an uncommon condition characterized by pinpoint skin-colored papules that are distributed most commonly on the arms, forearms, trunk, and genitalia. It predominantly affects children and young adults. The condition is self-limited and resolves completely, usually within a few months to 1 year. It is often asymptomatic but may be pruritic.[50,51]

EPIDEMIOLOGY

There is limited data on the epidemiology of LN. Historically, there was believed to be no association of LN with any particular sex or race.[50] While a recent study of 17 patients with LN suggested a male predominance, a larger retrospective review of 209 child and adult patients with LN recently demonstrated that patients were more likely to be female. This same study confirmed that LN is more common in Black patients.[51,52]

ETIOLOGY

The etiology of LN is unknown. While there was once speculation that it might be a variant of lichen planus, this has been disproven by immunohistochemical analysis. Some familial cases reported in the literature suggest that genetic factors may play a role.[50]

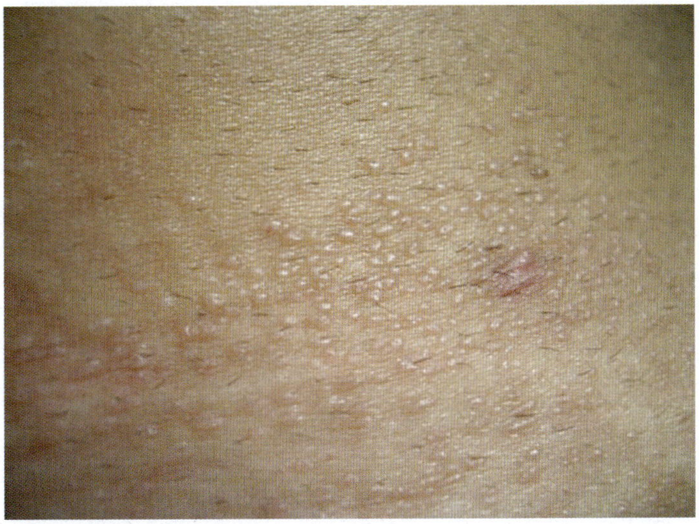

FIGURE 28-7. Lichen nitidus.

CLINICAL PRESENTATION

LN is characterized by a cluster of flesh-colored papules measuring 1 to 2 mm in diameter, although lesions may appear lighter in patients with darker skin [**Figure 28-7**].[50] Areas most commonly involved include the upper extremities, trunk, lower extremities, and genitalia, though 27% of patients in one study had more than one site of involvement.[50,52] In a study by Kundak et al, the mean age of onset was 9 years and the mean duration was 13 months with a range of 1 to 48 months.[51] Oral and nail involvement are uncommon.[50] While LN is usually quite distinct, conditions such as keratosis pilaris, follicular eczema, lichen spinulosis, frictional lichenoid dermatitis, and papular urticaria should be included in the differential.[53,54] Several clinical variants of LN have been reported, including confluent, hemorrhagic, linear, perforating, spinous follicular, vesicular, generalized, and actinic forms.[50]

HISTOPATHOLOGY

While LN is usually a clinical diagnosis, skin biopsy can be used for confirmation. Histopathologically, LN is characterized by an inflammatory infiltrate in the papillary dermis consisting of lymphocytes and histiocytes. Downward extension of the rete ridges surrounds the infiltrate, giving a "ball-in-claw" pattern that spans several dermal papillae. The overlying epidermis exhibits thinning and parakeratosis, with vacuolar degeneration of basal keratinocytes and the formation of cytoid bodies.[50,53]

MANAGEMENT

LN is generally asymptomatic, and the lesions often resolve within 1 year. Treatment is typically reserved for symptomatic cases or when the mere presence of lesions is a concern for the patient or their parents. Oral antihistamines can be used to alleviate itching. Topical corticosteroids or topical calcineurin inhibitors can be used for itching and also to try to shorten the duration of the eruption.[52,55,56] When systemic therapies are required, phototherapy with nb-UVB and oral corticosteroids are often used.[50,57] Additional systemic therapies reported in the literature include cyclosporine, acitretin, isotretinoin, astemizole, itraconazole, and isoniazid.[57,58]

REFERENCES

1. Lehman JS, Tollefson MM, Gibson LE. Lichen planus. *Int J Dermatol.* 2009;48(7):682-694.
2. Solimani F, Forchhammer S, Schloegl A, Ghoreschi K, Meier K. Lichen planus - a clinical guide. *J Dtsch Dermatol Ges.* 2021;19(6):864-882.
3. Tziotzios C, Lee JYW, Brier T, et al. Lichen planus and lichenoid dermatoses: clinical overview and molecular basis. *J Am Acad Dermatol.* 2018;79(5):789-804.
4. Schwager Z, Stern M, Cohen J, Femia A. Clinical epidemiology and treatment of lichen planus: a retrospective review of 2 tertiary care centers. *J Am Acad Dermatol.* 2019;81(6):1397-1399.
5. Leasure AC, Cohen JM. Prevalence of lichen planus in the United States: a cross-sectional study of the All of Us research program. *J Am Acad Dermatol.* 2022;87(3):686-687.
6. Li C, Tang X, Zheng X, et al. Global prevalence and incidence estimates of oral lichen planus: a systematic review and meta-analysis. *JAMA Dermatol.* 2020;156(2):172-181.
7. González-Moles MÁ, Warnakulasuriya S, González-Ruiz I, et al. Worldwide prevalence of oral lichen planus: a systematic review and meta-analysis. *Oral Dis.* 2021;27(4):813-828.
8. Zendell K. Genital lichen planus: update on diagnosis and treatment. *Semin Cutan Med Surg.* 2015;34(4):182-186.
9. Gupta MK, Lipner SR. Review of nail lichen planus: epidemiology, pathogenesis, diagnosis, and treatment. *Dermatol Clin.* 2021;39(2):221-230.
10. Arnold DL, Krishnamurthy K. *Lichen Planus.* Treasure Island (FL): StatPearls Publishing; 2023. https://www.ncbi.nlm.nih.gov/books/NBK526126/.
11. Boch K, Langan EA, Kridin K, Zillikens D, Ludwig RJ, Bieber K. Lichen planus. *Front Med (Lausanne).* 2021;8:737813.
12. Kofoed ML, Wantzin GL. Familial lichen planus. More frequent than previously suggested? *J Am Acad Dermatol.* 1985;13(1):50-54.
13. Luis-Montoya P, Yamamoto-Furusho JK, Vega-Memije E, et al. HLA-DRB1*0101 is associated with the genetic susceptibility to develop lichen planus in the Mexican Mestizo population. *Arch Dermatol Res.* 2007;299(8):405-407.
14. Carcassi C, Cottoni F, Floris L, et al. The HLA-DRB1*0101 allele is responsible for HLA susceptibility to lichen ruber planus. *Eur J Immunogenet.* 1994;21(6):425-429.
15. Lin SC, Sun A. HLA-DR and DQ antigens in Chinese patients with oral lichen planus. *J Oral Pathol Med.* 1990;19(7):298-300.
16. Liu J, Ye Z, Mayer JG, et al. Phenome-wide association study maps new diseases to the human major histocompatibility complex region. *J Med Genet.* 2016;53(10):681-689.
17. Jin X, Wang J, Zhu L, et al. Association between -308 G/A polymorphism in TNF-α gene and lichen planus: a meta-analysis. *J Dermatol Sci.* 2012;68(3):127-134.
18. Asarch A, Gottlieb AB, Lee J, et al. Lichen planus-like eruptions: an emerging side effect of tumor necrosis factor-alpha antagonists. *J Am Acad Dermatol.* 2009;61(1):104-111.
19. Halevy S, Shai A. Lichenoid drug eruptions. *J Am Acad Dermatol.* 1993;29(2 Pt 1):249-255.
20. Dunsche A, Frank MP, Lüttges J, et al. Lichenoid reactions of murine mucosa associated with amalgam. *Br J Dermatol.* 2003;148(4):741-748.
21. Giannetti L, Dello Diago AM, Spinas E. Oral Lichen planus. *J Biol Regul Homeost Agents.* 2018;32(2):391-395.
22. Lodi G, Pellicano R, Carrozzo M. Hepatitis C virus infection and lichen planus: a systematic review with meta-analysis. *Oral Dis.* 2010;16(7):601-612.
23. Shengyuan L, Songpo Y, Wen W, Wenjing T, Haitao Z, Binyou W. Hepatitis C virus and lichen planus: a reciprocal association determined by a meta-analysis. *Arch Dermatol.* 2009;145(9):1040-1047.
24. Wang JH, Hung SJ. Lichen planus associated with hepatitis B, hepatitis C, and liver cirrhosis in a nationwide cohort study. *J Am Acad Dermatol.* 2021;84(4):1085-1086.
25. Mohamed M, Korbi M, Hammedi F, et al. Lichen planus pigmentosus inversus: a series of 10 Tunisian patients. *Int J Dermatol.* 2016;55(10):1088-1091.
26. Le Cleach L, Chosidow O. Clinical practice. Lichen planus. *N Engl J Med.* 2012;366(8):723-732.
27. Irvine C, Irvine F, Champion RH. Long-term follow-up of lichen planus. *Acta Derm Venereol.* 1991;71(3):242-244.
28. Arisawa EA, Almeida JD, Carvalho YR, Cabral LA. Clinicopathological analysis of oral mucous autoimmune disease: a 27-year study. *Med Oral Patol Oral Cir Bucal.* 2008;13(2):E94-E97.
29. van Tuyll van Serooskerken AM, van Marion AM, de Zwart-Storm E, Frank J, Poblete-Gutiérrez P. Lichen planus with bullous manifestation on the lip. *Int J Dermatol.* 2007;46 Suppl 3:25-26.
30. Idrees M, Kujan O, Shearston K, Farah CS. Oral lichen planus has a very low malignant transformation rate: a systematic review and meta-analysis using strict diagnostic and inclusion criteria. *J Oral Pathol Med.* 2021;50(3):287-298.
31. Setterfield JF, Neill S, Shirlaw PJ, et al. The vulvovaginal gingival syndrome: a severe subgroup of lichen planus with characteristic clinical features and a novel association with the class II HLA DQB1*0201 allele. *J Am Acad Dermatol.* 2006;55(1):98-113.

32. Day T, Weigner J, Scurry J. Classic and hypertrophic vulvar lichen planus. *J Low Genit Tract Dis*. 2018;22(4):387-395.
33. Friedman P, Sabban EC, Marcucci C, Peralta R, Cabo H. Dermoscopic findings in different clinical variants of lichen planus. Is dermoscopy useful? *Dermatol Pract Concept*. 2015;5(4):51-55.
34. Halevy S, Shai A. Lichenoid drug eruptions. *J Am Acad Dermatol*. 1993;29(2 Pt 1):249-255.
35. Lallas A, Kyrgidis A, Tzellos TG, et al. Accuracy of dermoscopic criteria for the diagnosis of psoriasis, dermatitis, lichen planus and pityriasis rosea. *Br J Dermatol*. 2012;166(6):1198-1205.
36. Pavlotsky F, Nathansohn N, Kriger G, Shpiro D, Trau H. Ultraviolet-B treatment for cutaneous lichen planus: our experience with 50 patients. *Photodermatol Photoimmunol Photomed*. 2008;24(2):83-86.
37. Dawood M, Sizopoulou C, Greenberger S, Barzilai A, Pavlotsky F. Narrowband ultraviolet B radiation for lichen planus: long-term follow-up of 192 patients. *J Clin Aesthet Dermatol*. 2022;15(4):31-35.
38. Laurberg G, Geiger JM, Hjorth N, et al. Treatment of lichen planus with acitretin. A double-blind, placebo-controlled study in 65 patients. *J Am Acad Dermatol*. 1991;24(3):434-437.
39. Woo TY. Systemic isotretinoin treatment of oral and cutaneous lichen planus. *Cutis*. 1985;35(4):385-386, 390-391, 393.
40. Ott F, Bollag W, Geiger JM. Efficacy of oral low-dose tretinoin (all-trans-retinoic acid) in lichen planus. *Dermatology*. 1996;192(4):334-336.
41. Tziotzios C, Brier T, Lee JYW, et al. Lichen planus and lichenoid dermatoses: conventional and emerging therapeutic strategies. *J Am Acad Dermatol*. 2018;79(5):807-818.
42. Gajraj FA, Zahir J, Adereti C, Gajraj MH. A case report and literature review of the role of dupilumab in the management of lichen planus: cause or treatment? *Cureus*. 2023;15(7):e41274.
43. Abduelmula A, Bagit A, Mufti A, Yeung KCY, Yeung J. The use of Janus kinase inhibitors for lichen planus: an evidence-based review. *J Cutan Med Surg*. 2023;27(3):271-276.
44. Pedraça ES, da Silva EL, de Lima TB, Rados PV, Visioli F. Systemic non-steroidal immunomodulators for oral lichen planus treatment-a scoping review. *Clin Oral Investig*. 2023;27(12):7091-7114.
45. Didona D, Caposiena Caro RD, Sequeira Santos AM, Solimani F, Hertl M. Therapeutic strategies for oral lichen planus: state of the art and new insights. *Front Med (Lausanne)*. 2022;9:997190.
46. Gall R, Navarro-Fernandez IN. *Lichen Planus Erosive Form*. Treasure Island (FL): StatPearls Publishing; 2023.
47. Mallon E, Hawkins D, Dinneen M, et al. Circumcision and genital dermatoses. *Arch Dermatol*. 2000;136(3):350-354.
48. Helgesen AL, Warloe T, Pripp AH, et al. Vulvovaginal photodynamic therapy vs. topical corticosteroids in genital erosive lichen planus: a randomized controlled trial. *Br J Dermatol*. 2015;173(5):1156-1162.
49. Singal A, Gaurav V, Kaur I. Clinical characteristics and management outcomes in isolated nail lichen planus: a retrospective case series. *Indian J Dermatol Venereol Leprol*. 2023;90(3);329-335.
50. Schwartz C, Goodman MB. *Lichen Nitidus*. Treasure Island (FL): StatPearls Publishing; 2023.
51. Kundak S, Çakır Y. Pediatric lichen nitidus: a single-center experience. *Pediatr Dermatol*. 2019;36(2):189-192.
52. Yang K, Lau WC, Lau CB, Pan CX, Kassamali B, Nambudiri VE. Clinicopathologic features of lichen nitidus: a multicenter cohort. *Int J Dermatol*. 2023;62(4):e261-e263.
53. Mahajan SA, Singh S, Kabbannavar YR, Kharkar VD. Clinico-dermatoscopic and histopathological evaluation of a case of generalized lichen nitidus. *Indian J Dermatopathol Diagn Dermatol*. 2022;9(2):64-66.
54. Ochała-Gierek G, Bergler-Czop B, Gierek M. A case report of lichen nitidus and its dermoscopic features. *Postepy Dermatol Alergol*. 2023;40(1):173-175.
55. Park J, Kim JI, Kim DW, et al. Persistent generalized lichen nitidus successfully treated with 0.03% tacrolimus ointment. *Eur J Dermatol*. 2013;23(6):918-919.
56. Farshi S, Mansouri P. Letter: generalized lichen nitidus successfully treated with pimecrolimus 1 percent cream. *Dermatol Online J*. 2011;17(7):11.
57. Do MO, Kim MJ, Kim SH, Myung KB, Choi YW. Generalized lichen nitidus successfully treated with narrow-band UVB phototherapy: two cases report. *J Korean Med Sci*. 2007;22(1):163-166.
58. Rallis E, Verros C, Moussatou V, Sambaziotis D, Papadakis P. Generalized purpuric lichen nitidus. Report of a case and review of the literature. *Dermatol Online J*. 2007;13(2):5.

CHAPTER 29

Atopic Dermatitis and Other Eczemas

Andrew F. Alexis
Ama Alexis

KEY POINTS

- Atopic dermatitis (AD) is a highly prevalent disorder among populations with skin of color.
- Epidemiologic, genetic, immunophenotypic, and clinical variations in populations with skin of color have been reported. Key clinical nuances include erythema presenting with a broader spectrum of hues beyond red; perifollicular, lichenoid, papulonodular morphologies; extensor involvement; and postinflammatory pigment alterations.
- A multi-pronged longitudinal approach that targets AD-related immune and skin barrier dysfunction as well as mechanisms of pruritus is key to reducing the risk of long-term pigmentary and other sequelae of AD in skin of color.

INTRODUCTION

Atopic dermatitis (AD) is a chronic inflammatory skin disorder that is associated with comorbidities and represents a large burden among populations with skin of color. Studies involving populations with skin of color have identified racial/ethnic disparities in prevalence, incidence, persistence, healthcare utilization, access to care or therapies, and enrollment in clinical trials of AD. Racial/ethnic variations in genetic factors and endotypic characteristics of AD have also been reported and these, coupled with socio-environmental factors, may contribute to differences in the clinical presentation and overall burden of AD in skin of color.

EPIDEMIOLOGY AND BURDEN OF DISEASE

Several studies have identified a greater burden of AD on Black populations. In the United States, the prevalence of AD is higher among Black children compared to White children. In the National Survey of Children's Health, a population-based survey of over 100,000 families representing all 50 states, the prevalence among Black children was 15.89% compared to 9.7% among White children.[1] A higher prevalence of AD in Black children compared to White children was also demonstrated in another U.S.-based study, the National Health and Nutrition Examination Survey, where Black children had the highest prevalence when compared to White, Hispanic, or other children.[2] In a study from London, UK, the prevalence of AD by examination of a dermatologist was 16.3% in London-born Black Caribbean children and 8.7% in White children.[3] In a prospective longitudinal cohort study in the United States, AD incidence was significantly higher among non-Hispanic Black children compared to non-Hispanic White children. Persistence of AD from early childhood to mid-childhood was higher in non-Hispanic Black children and Hispanic children compared to non-Hispanic White children.[4] In another U.S. study, the highest AD prevalence and persistence was among urban female or Black children.[5]

In adults, a lower prevalence of AD among non-White populations has been reported in U.S.-based epidemiologic studies, but under-diagnosis/reporting of AD in adult populations with skin of color may contribute to this conflicting finding.[6]

Global epidemiologic studies have identified wide variations in the prevalence of AD across various regions of the world and these data vary by age range and methodology for diagnosing AD.[6-8]

Higher rates of healthcare utilization for AD among populations with skin of color have been reported in several U.S. studies. In a longitudinal cohort study, Black and Hispanic children were almost three times more likely than White children to receive medical care for AD even after adjusting for sociodemographic factors. A higher odds of primary care and emergency visits were seen among Black and Hispanic children compared to White children. Black children with poorly controlled AD were also less likely to see a dermatologist than White children with a similar level of AD control.[9] In another study, Black and Asian/Pacific Islander patients were more likely than White patients to seek medical care for AD. Specifically, AD visits were seen at a two- and sixfold higher visit per capita rate in Black and Asian/Pacific Islander patients compared to White patients, respectively.[10]

Racial/ethnic disparities in the rate of absences from school related to AD have been reported, with higher rates among Black and Hispanic children in the United States. Specifically, Non-Hispanic Black and Hispanic children had a higher adjusted odds of having at least six school absences compared with non-Hispanic White children.[11]

Other racial/ethnic disparities in AD reported in U.S. studies include increased out-of-pocket medical expenses in Black populations,[12] longer hospitalizations among Black children with AD,[13] and less access to frontline prescription therapies in Black patients with AD.[14]

GENETIC FACTORS

Racial/ethnic variations in genetic factors associated with AD have been reported. Most notably, the frequency and type of mutations in genes involved in skin barrier function such as filaggrin (FLG) have been shown to vary between populations of European descent and those of African and Asian ancestry.[15] While the data are limited by methodological biases and other factors, there is evidence to suggest lower frequencies of FLG loss-of-function mutations in populations of African ancestry[16-18] and Asian ancestry[19] compared to populations of European ancestry. These genetic variations do not independently explain differences in prevalence or clinical presentation of AD in patients with skin of color. Beyond filaggrin, a study that investigated whether genes associated with African ancestry are predictive of AD risk or severity in Black/African Americans with AD did not find any association between African genetic ancestry and the above outcomes in this cohort.[20] More research is needed to better understand variations in genetic factors associated with AD across diverse patient populations.

IMMUNOLOGICAL FACTORS

While Th2-activation is a consistent finding across diverse AD populations, racial/ethnic variations in immune response skewing have been reported in AD populations in small studies. In a study of 27 Asian American AD patients of Japanese and Korean ancestry, higher Th17 and Th22 and lower Th1 cytokine expression was noted compared to European American AD controls. This finding has helped support the observation of psoriasiform clinical and histopathological features among East Asian patients with AD.[21] In another study, African American AD patients were found to have an immune response profile with similar Th2/Th22-skewing but reduced Th1 and Th17 expression compared to European American AD patients.[22] Further studies are needed to better elucidate potential racial/ethnic variations in the molecular phenotype of AD across diverse populations.

CLINICAL FEATURES

The clinical presentation of AD in skin of color is distinguished from that in White skin by a number of specific features. Most notably, erythema—the clinical hallmark of inflammation in the skin—may be more subtle or feature a range of hues that are beyond red or pink in richly pigmented skin. While this phenomenon is generally seen across the scope of inflammatory diseases of the skin, it is particularly notable in eczematous conditions. Beyond degrees of redness, erythema in AD patients with skin of color may demonstrate features that are red-brown, dark brown, violaceous, or gray depending on the patient's constitutive skin pigmentation [**Figure 29-1**]. Recognizing these variations and broadening the definition of erythema to include the above hues are paramount in accurately assessing disease severity. For example, reliance on the literal definition of erythema (ie, redness) has been shown to potentially mask severe AD in Black children.[23] Careful examination for other signs such as hyperchromia,[24] edema, skin warmth, papulation, and scale can help to accurately identify the location and extent of active lesions and their overall severity.[8] A patient-oriented scale (Patient-Oriented SCORing for Atopic Dermatitis tool or PO-SCORAD) has been validated for use in Black skin and as such can be a helpful tool in assessing severity of AD in patients with skin of color.[25]

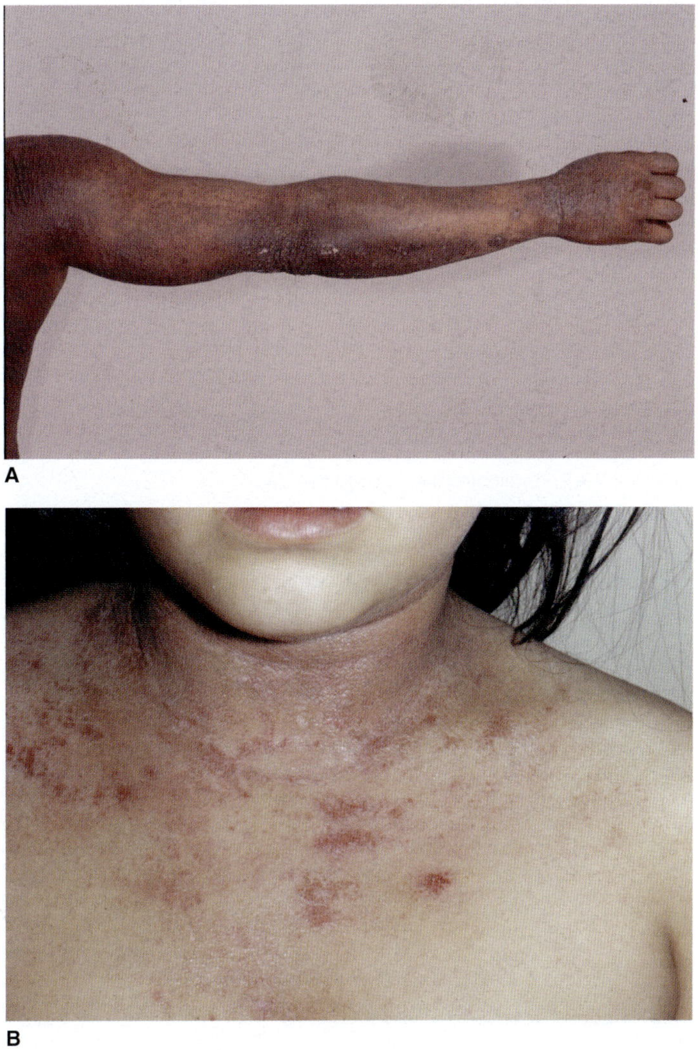

FIGURE 29-1. Atopic dermatitis with **(A)** erythema, lichenification, and focal depigmentation in a patient with darker skin of color compared with **(B)** a Hispanic female with lighter skin of color.

Postinflammatory hyper- and hypopigmentation are of particular concern in AD patients with skin of color. Typically, AD resolves with pigmentary changes that can last several weeks to many months to years [**Figure 29-2**]. To the patient, this dyspigmentation is often of equal or greater concern than the dermatitis itself. Therefore, early recognition and treatment of AD in skin of color is especially important to minimize or prevent long-term postinflammatory pigment abnormalities.

Follicular prominence or perifollicular accentuation is a characteristic presentation of AD in patients of African descent [**Figure 29-3**].[26] In some patients, multiple 1- to 3-mm follicular or perifollicular papules may be the sole feature of AD. In these cases, other characteristic morphologic features of eczema, including lichenification, erythema, crusting, and scale, may be minimal or absent [**Figure 29-4**]. However, lichenification without follicular prominence is also often seen in populations with skin of color as it is in White populations [**Figure 29-5**].

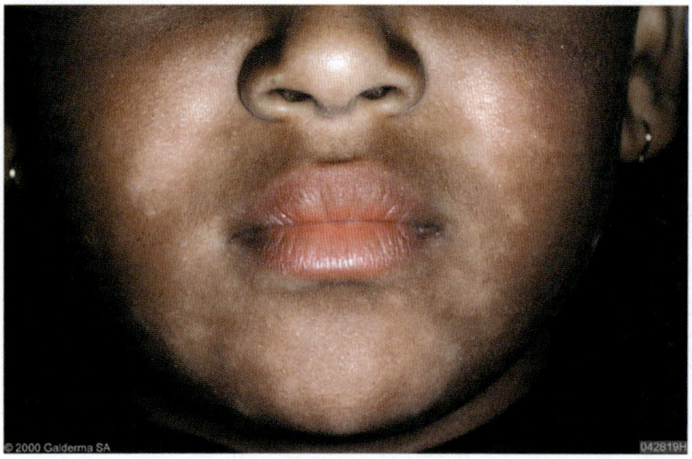

FIGURE 29-2. Postinflammatory hypopigmentation.

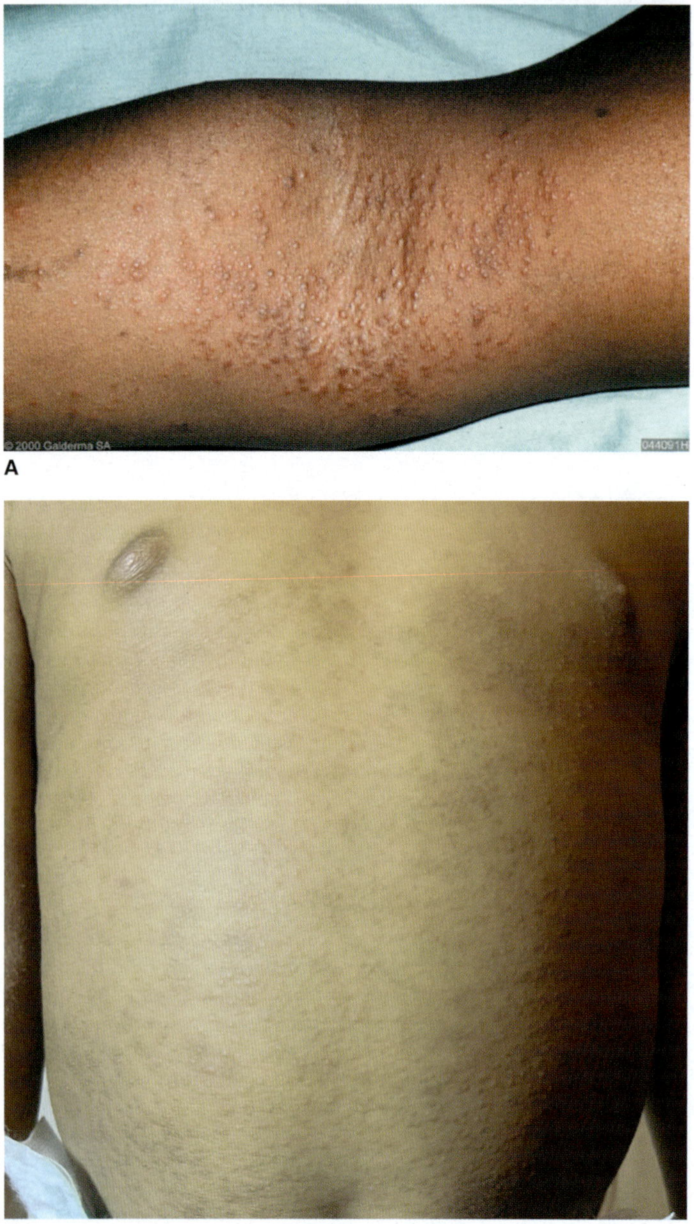

FIGURE 29-3. **(A)** Follicular prominence. **(B)** Perifollicular papules on the trunk of an 18-month-old Black/African American boy.

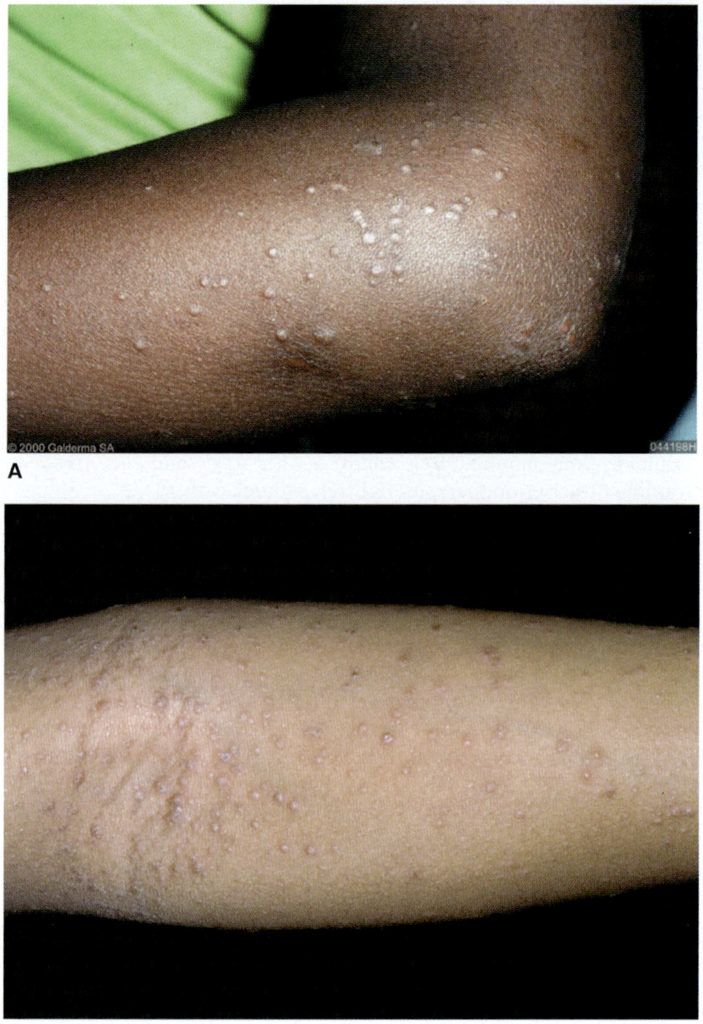

FIGURE 29-4. Discrete papules without lichenification on an **(A)** African American patient and **(B)** Hispanic male. (B: Image appears with permission from VisualDx.)

A lichenoid presentation of AD was reported in 16% of African Americans patients in an inner-city practice and papular lichenoid lesions were seen in 54% of AD patients in a large Nigerian study.[27,28]

Xerosis is a common presenting feature of AD in skin of color. Due to the visual contrast of white/gray scales of dry skin, xerosis tends to be more conspicuous and culturally stigmatizing in populations with skin of color.[8,29] This is most notable in individuals from the African diaspora as well as South Asians with deeply pigmented skin.

Variations in the anatomic distribution of AD across diverse populations have been reported. Extensor involvement is thought to be a common feature of AD in populations with skin of color, most notably, those of African descent, based on a Nigerian study reporting 70.3% of patients having involvement of the extensor surfaces of the joints.[27] Extensor involvement has been reported in several other racial/ethnic/geographic populations and also varies by age [**Figure 29-6**].[6,30-32]

Racial/ethnic variations in disease severity in AD have been reported. In a longitudinal survey of children with AD in the United Kingdom, Black children were found to be almost six times more likely to develop severe AD than White children after adjusting for erythema.[23] In a U.S. study, Black race, lower socioeconomic status, and factors tied to structural racism (such as living in highly segregated communities) were associated with greater AD severity.[33]

Pruritus is the most common symptom associated with AD and in patients with skin of color, pruritus represents a considerable burden. A higher prevalence of pruritus in Black/African American populations has been reported[34] and a clinical presentation of itch-dominant AD[35]

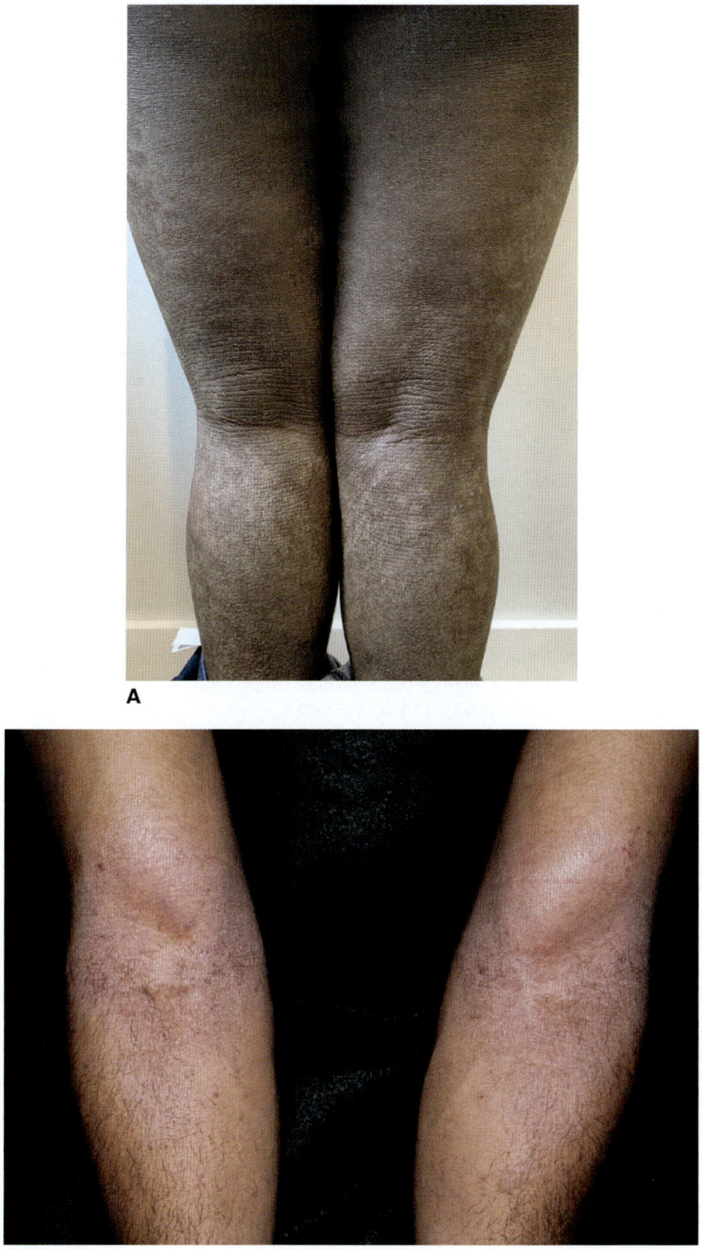

FIGURE 29-5. (A) Severe lichenification on the posterior legs of a 14-year-old Black/African American girl. **(B)** Scaly, lichenified, erythematous plaques in the antecubetal fossae of a Hispanic male. (B: Image appears with permission from VisualDx.)

with less evident morphological signs of AD may also be more common in skin of color.[36]

The clinical nuances of atopic dermatitis in skin of color are outlined in **Table 29-1**.

APPROACHES TO TREATMENT

While the same therapeutic agents are considered safe and effective across the spectrum of racial/ethnic groups and skin phototypes, the approach to managing AD in SOC has some important nuances. Most notably, given that inadequately controlled AD in patients with skin of color is associated with potentially disfiguring and longstanding postinflammatory pigment alteration, the importance of effective longitudinal control of AD is especially paramount in this population. Undertreatment or episodic management of flares (without ongoing preventative measures such as moisturization and noncorticosteroid topical agents, or

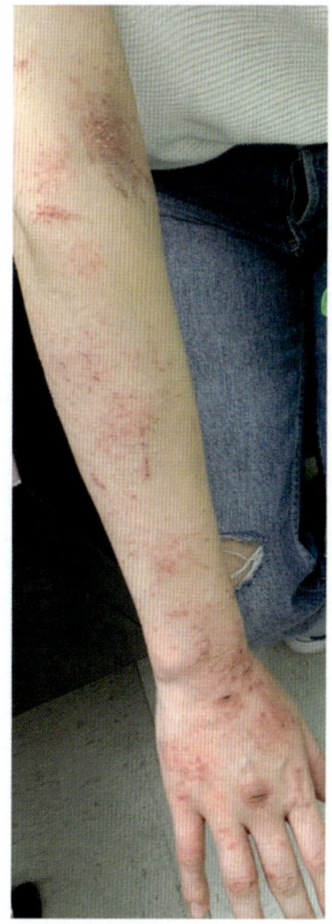

FIGURE 29-6. An East Asian individual with AD involving the extensor surfaces and the antecubital fossa.

in the case of moderate to severe AD, ongoing systemic therapy) carries a higher risk of long-term sequelae including dyspigmentation, prurigo nodularis, and excoriation-related scarring. As such, a multi-pronged longitudinal approach that targets AD-related immune and skin barrier dysfunction as well as pathomechanisms of pruritus comprehensively is ideal. Leveraging the currently available and emerging targeted agents (eg, topical calcineurin inhibitors, topical phosphodiesterase inhibitors, topical and oral JAK inhibitors, and injectable biologic agents) as well as barrier-improving skin care (eg, ceramide-containing moisturizers) allows for highly efficacious therapy across the broad range of disease severities.[8,37,38]

Managing postinflammatory pigment alteration associated with AD is another important nuance in the treatment of AD in patients with skin of color. While effective and long-term treatment of the underlying inflammatory pathways associated with AD ultimately results in improvement of pigmentary sequelae (indirectly), strategies to directly treat dyspigmentation are often considered. The use of topical bleaching agents for postinflammatory hyperpigmentation are limited by potential irritation associated with many active ingredients used in bleaching agents, including, but not limited to, hydroquinone, tretinoin and other retinoids, kojic acid, glycolic acid, and cysteamine. Given the skin

TABLE 29-1 Clinical nuances of atopic dermatitis in skin of color
Erythema may be more subtle and may include red-brown, dark brown, violaceous, or gray hues.
Postinflammatory hyper- and hypopigmentation are frequent sequelae or concomitant features. Pigment changes may be of equal or greater concern to the patient as the AD itself.
Perifollicular accentuation is a common AD morphology in patients with Black skin.
A lichenoid morphology of AD may be more commonly observed in patients with Black skin.
Xerosis is a conspicuous and often culturally stigmatizing feature of AD in darker skin types.
Extensor involvement is more commonly reported.
Itch-dominant AD may be more common.
Chronic excoriation-related dyspigmentation or scarring, and prurigo nodules can result from poorly controlled severe pruritus.

barrier dysfunction and higher risks of irritant dermatitis in patients with AD, the use of potentially irritating agents should be approached with extreme caution, and, if utilized, should be limited to areas on intact skin without clinical evidence of active atopic dermatitis. With the above limitations in mind, topical azelaic acid 15% foam has anecdotally been a well-tolerated topical agent for postinflammatory hyperpigmentation in AD. However, studies for this indication are lacking. Also anecdotally, hydroquinone 4% combined with a low- to mid-potency topical corticosteroid may be considered for persistent hyperpigmented patches that lack clinical signs or symptoms of active eczema/AD. While postinflammatory hypopigmentation is self-limited, resolving with ongoing treatment of AD, phototherapy or, if localized, excimer laser can be considered for severe cases.

Available data and experience pertaining to topical and systemic agents for AD suggest comparable safety and efficacy for AD therapies. However, studies investigating treatments specifically in populations with AD are limited,[39] as are general population studies that compare responses between racial/ethnic groups.[39-42] New studies involving AD treatment of skin of color populations specifically are currently in development and are expected to generate valuable data on the use of biologic agents in AD patients with skin of color.

A key nuance with respect to treatment responses is the risk of corticosteroid-induced hypopigmentation, which tends to be more conspicuous in darkly pigmented skin types. Hypopigmentation is most commonly associated with potent or ultra-potent corticosteroids used for durations greater than 2 weeks or inadvertently applied to perilesional skin. Therefore, effective counseling on the appropriate quantity, site, and duration of application topical corticosteroids is particularly important in patients with skin of color.

Racial/ethnic disparities in access and prescribing patterns related to topical or systemic AD treatments have been reported in U.S. populations and may contribute to the more severe burden of disease experienced by patients with skin of color.[14,43]

OTHER ECZEMAS IN SKIN OF COLOR

Other common eczematous conditions such as nummular eczema, dyshidrotic eczema [**Figure 29-7**], and asteatotic eczema are also seen frequently in skin of color populations. Postinflammatory pigment alterations can be a concomitant feature [Figure 29-7]. Differences in epidemiology, clinical presentation, and responses to treatment for these conditions have not been formally studied but appear to be similar across racial/ethnic groups. Nevertheless, cultural variations in the use of emollients, ointments, astringents, and harsh soaps, as well as frequency of bathing, potentially can lead to differences in prevalence and severity of eczematous conditions in different populations.[29]

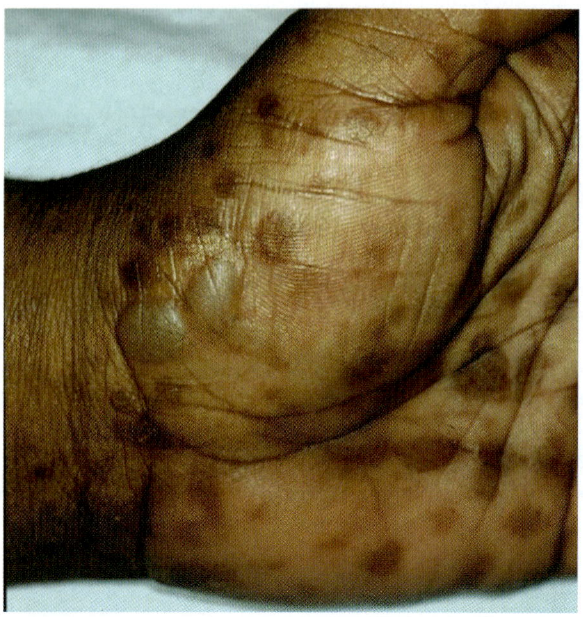

FIGURE 29-7. Dyshidrotic eczema with postinflammatory hyperpigmentation.

REFERENCES

1. Shaw TE, Currie GP, Koudelka CW, Simpson EL. Eczema prevalence in the United States: data from the 2003 National Survey of Children's Health. *J Invest Dermatol.* 2011;131(1):67-73.
2. Fu T, Keiser E, Linos E, et al. Eczema and sensitization to common allergens in the United States: a multiethnic, population-based study. *Pediatr Dermatol.* 2014;31(1):21-26.
3. Williams HC, Pembroke AC, Forsdyke H, Boodoo G, Hay RJ, Burney PG. London-born black Caribbean children are at increased risk of atopic dermatitis. *J Am Acad Dermatol.* 1995;32(2 Pt 1):212-217.
4. Kim Y, Blomberg M, Rifas-Shiman SL, et al. Racial/Ethnic differences in incidence and persistence of childhood atopic dermatitis. *J Invest Dermatol.* 2019;139(4):827-834.
5. McKenzie C, Silverberg JI. The prevalence and persistence of atopic dermatitis in urban United States children. *Ann Allergy Asthma Immunol.* 2019;123(2):173-178.e1.
6. Quan VL, Erickson T, Daftary K, Chovatiya R. Atopic Dermatitis Across Shades of Skin. *Am J Clin Dermatol.* 2023 Sep;24(5):731-751. doi: 10.1007/s40257-023-00797-1. Epub 2023 Jun 19. PMID: 37336869.
7. Mallol J, Crane J, von Mutius E, et al. The International Study of Asthma and Allergies in Childhood (ISAAC) Phase Three: a global synthesis. *Allergol Immunopathol (Madr).* 2013;41(2):73-85.
8. Kaufman BP, Guttman-Yassky E, Alexis AF. Atopic dermatitis in diverse racial and ethnic groups-Variations in epidemiology, genetics, clinical presentation and treatment. *Exp Dermatol.* 2018;27(4):340-357.
9. Wan J, Oganisian A, Spieker AJ, et al. Racial/Ethnic variation in use of ambulatory and emergency care for atopic dermatitis among US children. *J Invest Dermatol.* 2019;139(9):1906-1913.e1.
10. Janumpally SR, Feldman SR, Gupta AK, Fleischer AB Jr. In the United States, blacks and Asian/Pacific Islanders are more likely than whites to seek medical care for atopic dermatitis. *Arch Dermatol.* 2002;138(5):634-637.
11. Wan J, Margolis DJ, Mitra N, Hoffstad OJ, Takeshita J. Racial and ethnic differences in atopic dermatitis-related school absences among US children. *JAMA Dermatol.* 2019;155(8):973-975.
12. Chovatiya R, Begolka WS, Thibau IJ, Silverberg JI. Financial burden and impact of atopic dermatitis out-of-pocket healthcare expenses among black individuals in the United States. *Arch Dermatol Res.* 2022;314(8):739-747.
13. Desai AD, Shah VP, Lipner SR. Racial and economic differences in inpatient pediatric atopic dermatitis: an analysis of the US kids' inpatient database. *Dermatitis.* 2022;33(6S):S139-S141.
14. Bell MA, Whang KA, Thomas J, Aguh C, Kwatra SG. Racial and ethnic disparities in access to emerging and frontline therapies in common dermatological conditions: a cross-sectional study. *J Natl Med Assoc.* 2020;112(6):650-653.
15. Zhu Y, Mitra N, Feng Y, Tishkoff S, Hoffstad O, Margolis D. FLG variation differs between European Americans and African Americans. *J Invest Dermatol.* 2021;141(7):1855-1857.
16. Margolis DJ, Mitra N, Wubbenhorst B, et al. Association of filaggrin loss-of-function variants with race in children with atopic dermatitis. *JAMA Dermatol.* 2019;155(11):1269-1276.
17. Margolis DJ, Mitra N, Gochnauer H, et al. Uncommon filaggrin variants are associated with persistent atopic dermatitis in African Americans. *J Invest Dermatol.* 2018;138(7):1501-1506.
18. Winge MC, Bilcha KD, Lieden A, et al. Novel filaggrin mutation but no other loss-of-function variants found in Ethiopian patients with atopic dermatitis. *Br J Dermatol.* 2011;165(5):1074-1080.
19. Chen H, Common JE, Haines RL, et al. Wide spectrum of filaggrin-null mutations in atopic dermatitis highlights differences between Singaporean Chinese and European populations. *Br J Dermatol.* 2011;165(1):106-114.
20. Abuabara K, You Y, Margolis DJ, Hoffmann TJ, Risch N, Jorgenson E. Genetic ancestry does not explain increased atopic dermatitis susceptibility or worse disease control among African American subjects in 2 large US cohorts. *J Allergy Clin Immunol.* 2020;145(1):192-198.e11.
21. Noda S, Suarez-Farinas M, Ungar B, et al. The Asian atopic dermatitis phenotype combines features of atopic dermatitis and psoriasis with increased TH17 polarization. *J Allergy Clin Immunol.* 2015;136(5):1254-1264.

22. Sanyal RD, Pavel AB, Glickman J, et al. Atopic dermatitis in African American patients is T(H)2/T(H)22-skewed with T(H)1/T(H)17 attenuation. *Ann Allergy Asthma Immunol.* 2019;122(1):99-110.e6.
23. Ben-Gashir MA, Hay RJ. Reliance on erythema scores may mask severe atopic dermatitis in black children compared with their white counterparts. *Br J Dermatol.* 2002;147(5):920-925.
24. Dadzie OE, Petit A, Alexis AF. *Ethnic Dermatology: Principles and Practice.* Chichester, West Sussex: Wiley-Blackwell; 2013.
25. Faye O, Meledie N'Djong AP, Diadie S, et al. Validation of the patient-oriented SCORing for atopic dermatitis tool for black skin. *J Eur Acad Dermatol Venereol.* 2020;34(4):795-799.
26. Weingarten M, Silverberg N. Follicular eczema and accentuation: a survey of published data. *J Am Acad Dermatol.* 2022;87(4):860-862.
27. Nnoruka EN. Current epidemiology of atopic dermatitis in south-eastern Nigeria. *Int J Dermatol.* 2004;43(10):739-744.
28. Allen HB, Jones NP, Bowen SE. Lichenoid and other clinical presentations of atopic dermatitis in an inner city practice. *J Am Acad Dermatol.* 2008;58(3):503-504.
29. Alexis A, Woolery-Lloyd H, Andriessen A, et al. Insights in skin of color patients with atopic dermatitis and the role of skincare in improving outcomes. *J Drugs Dermatol.* 2022;21(5):462-470.
30. Yew YW, Thyssen JP, Silverberg JI. A systematic review and meta-analysis of the regional and age-related differences in atopic dermatitis clinical characteristics. *J Am Acad Dermatol.* 2019;80(2):390-401.
31. Farajzadeh S, Esfandiarpour I, Sedaghatmanesh M, Saviz M. Epidemiology and clinical features of atopic dermatitis in kerman, a desert area of iran. *Ann Dermatol.* 2014;26(1):26-34.
32. Silverberg JI, Margolis DJ, Boguniewicz M, et al. Distribution of atopic dermatitis lesions in United States adults. *J Eur Acad Dermatol Venereol.* 2019;33(7):1341-1348.
33. Tackett KJ, Jenkins F, Morrell DS, McShane DB, Burkhart CN. Structural racism and its influence on the severity of atopic dermatitis in African American children. *Pediatr Dermatol.* 2020;37(1):142-146.
34. Ingrasci G, El-Kashlan N, Alexis A, Yosipovitch G. Chronic itch in African Americans: an unmet need. *Arch Dermatol Res.* 2022;314(5):405-415.
35. Chovatiya R, Lei D, Ahmed A, Chavda R, Gabriel S, Silverberg JI. Clinical phenotyping of atopic dermatitis using combined itch and lesional severity: a prospective observational study. *Ann Allergy Asthma Immunol.* 2021;127(1):83-90.e2.
36. Davis CM, Flohr C, Gupta MR, Koplin JJ. Managing atopic dermatitis in patients with skin of color. *J Allergy Clin Immunol Pract.* 2023;11(5):1376-1383.
37. Boguniewicz M, Fonacier L, Guttman-Yassky E, Ong PY, Silverberg JI. Atopic dermatitis yardstick update. *Ann Allergy Asthma Immunol.* 2023;130(6):811-820.
38. Alexis AF, Woolery-Lloyd H, Andriessen A, Heath C, Han G. INDIVIDUAL ARTICLE: an algorithm for the management of atopic dermatitis in people with skin of color. *J Drugs Dermatol.* 2023;22(8):SF386361s3-SFs10.
39. Eichenfield LF, Lucky AW, Langley RG, et al. Use of pimecrolimus cream 1% (Elidel) in the treatment of atopic dermatitis in infants and children: the effects of ethnic origin and baseline disease severity on treatment outcome. *Int J Dermatol.* 2005;44(1):70-75.
40. Alexis AF, Rendon M, Silverberg JI, et al. Efficacy of dupilumab in different racial subgroups of adults with moderate-to-severe atopic dermatitis in three randomized, placebo-controlled phase 3 trials. *J Drugs Dermatol.* 2019;18(8):804-813.
41. Callender VD, Alexis AF, Stein Gold LF, et al. Efficacy and safety of crisaborole ointment, 2%, for the treatment of mild-to-moderate atopic dermatitis across racial and ethnic groups. *Am J Clin Dermatol.* 2019;20(5):711-723.
42. Mineroff J, Nguyen JK, Jagdeo J. Racial and ethnic underrepresentation in dermatology clinical trials. *J Am Acad Dermatol.* 2023;89(2):293-300.
43. Ahmed F, Takeshita J, Wan J. Differences in prescriptions for systemic medications and nonsteroidal topicals among children with atopic dermatitis. *Pediatr Dermatol.* 2023;40(2):315-319.

CHAPTER 30

Allergic Contact Dermatitis

Walter Liszewski
George Luong

KEY POINTS

- Allergic contact dermatitis (ACD) is a common inflammatory skin condition that results from exposure to exogenous substances.
- ACD is the manifestation of an adaptive immune response (Type IV hypersensitivity), requiring initial sensitization and subsequent re-exposure for elicitation.
- The incidence and severity of ACD are influenced by demographics such as age, ethnicity, and geographic location.
- Studies have found differences in skin structure and physiology in skin of color which may contribute to differences in sensitization.
- Patch testing is the gold standard for diagnosis of ACD. A comprehensive pre-procedure evaluation includes a thorough physical examination and consideration of lifestyle factors such as culture and occupation.
- Due to the challenges of perceiving erythema in skin of color, other qualities such as texture and induration should be used to increase the accuracy of patch testing reads.
- There is a scarcity of research on ACD in skin of color. Additional studies are needed to further identify distinctions in skin of color and to elucidate the fundamental mechanisms that account for these variations.

INTRODUCTION

Contact dermatitis is a common inflammatory skin reaction that results from exposure to exogenous substances. By the nature of its triggering mechanism, the incidence and severity of contact dermatitis can be heavily influenced by demographics such as age, ethnicity, and lifestyle. However, despite the importance of considering these factors when treating patients, there remains a relative lack of specialized medical training for treating contact dermatitis in patients with skin of color. Furthermore, there is a parallel lack of clinical studies specifically investigating contact dermatitis in patients with skin of color [**Figure 30-1**].

There are a limited number of epidemiological studies on contact dermatitis; however, the overall prevalence is estimated to be between 1.7% and 6.3% and appears to be increasing in recent years.[1,2] One contributing factor to the difficulty of determining the

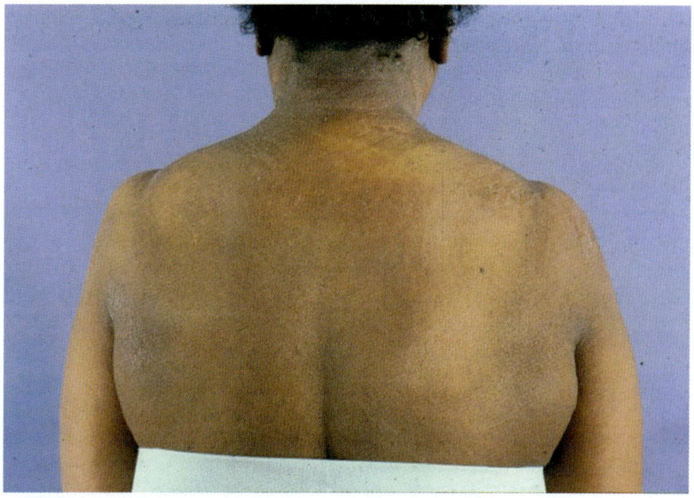

FIGURE 30-1. Contact dermatitis on the back of a female patient with skin of color.

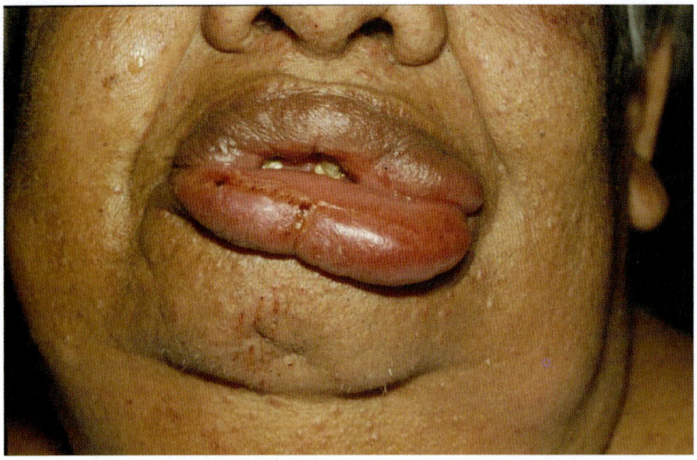

FIGURE 30-2. An allergic immunologic inflammatory response to lip gloss in a patient with skin of color.

true prevalence of contact dermatitis is misdiagnosis as other kinds of dermatitis.[1,3] Contact dermatitis is subdivided into two categories: irritant contact dermatitis (ICD), which comprises about 80% of cases, and allergic contact dermatitis (ACD), which comprises about 20% of cases.[4] Patch testing, first presented by German physician Joseph Jadassohn in 1895, is the gold standard for diagnosis of ACD.[5] In the most recent report of patch test results from the North American Contact Dermatitis Group, 4947 patients were included: 65.4% had at least one positive result and of the 4876 patients with a final diagnosis, 51.2% had a primary diagnosis of ACD and 8.4% had a primary diagnosis of ICD.[6]

ICD is the result of direct damage to the skin due to contact with toxic chemicals or physically abrasive compounds. The damage from irritant activates the innate immune system, causing inflammation. The most common presentation is a well-demarcated, erythematous, dry, scaly rash with possible lichenification. Symptoms of itch and burning sensation are commonly associated with the rash. The causes of ICD can sometimes be personally surmised based on the commonly known or advertised risks of the offending irritants: physical irritants can cause the familiar sensations of mechanical abrasion while chemical irritants such as cleaning agents often have label warnings.

ACD, in contrast to ICD, is caused by an adaptive immune response (Type IV hypersensitivity) that requires an initial exposure for sensitization and subsequent reexposure for elicitation, ultimately resulting in inflammation manifesting as a rash. Classically, ACD can present similarly to ICD as an erythematous, dry, itchy, rash; however, some clues that might help in differentiating the two is that ICD is more often well-demarcated, and symptoms of a stinging or burning sensation can often be relatively greater than pruritus in patients with ICD.[7] Notably, the risk of skin allergens are not as well-labeled as irritants, and thus are more difficult for patients to identify on their own. Additionally, the great variety in possible contact allergens only adds to the challenge of identifying triggers of ACD, thus necessitating formal diagnostic testing [**Figure 30-2**].

Diagnosis of ACD through patch testing involves the loading of small samples of numerous standardized compounds and sometimes personalized testing material into chambers that are then applied to a patient's back, allowed to remain in contact for 2 days, and subsequently removed to allow for a reading of the results. ACD reactions typically present in 48 to 72 hours; thus readings are usually done close to 72 hours after initial application. After allergens are identified, patients are counseled thoroughly to ensure proper avoidance of their allergens. Patient education includes discussion of the chemical properties of their allergens, the relevance of identified allergens to their observed rashes, and recommendations for products that are free of their allergens. With proper avoidance of allergens, significant improvement in the ACD is usually seen within 6 to 8 weeks.

DIFFERENCES IN SKIN PHYSIOLOGY IN SKIN OF COLOR

Fundamentally, the phenotypic difference between skin of color and lighter skin is due to variance in number, size, and distribution of melanosomes (pigment storage units) in the pigment-producing cells (melanocytes) and cells of the epidermis (keratinocytes).[8] However, the primary consequence of these differences are variations in sun-exposure-related and pigmentary skin disorders; in consideration of contact dermatitis specifically, other differences associated with skin of color are more pertinent. Contact dermatitis requires penetration of exogenous substances through the skin barrier to elicit an inflammatory immune response. Thus, variations in genetics, physiology, and anatomy that influence this mechanism can be implicated as reasons for differences in the presentation and diagnosis of ACD in skin of color.

Several studies with small sample sizes have been conducted to study differences in the epidermis in skin of color and have returned inconsistent results. Furthermore, the majority of studies are done in Black individuals, thus they may not be generalizable to other races or ethnicities with skin of color. Nonetheless, it has been well-established by histology that there are no differences in the thickness of the epidermis between fair-skinned individuals and individuals with skin of color.[9,10] However, there are more cell layers in the epidermis of black skin, suggesting a possible unique compactness that may result in a stronger skin barrier.[9,10] Skin of color does in fact appear to have reduced absorption of exogenous substances.[11,12]

Transepidermal water loss (TEWL) measurements are another way of measuring skin barrier integrity; however, results are contradictory across studies.[13,14] In specifically measuring TEWL in the context of skin disruption from tape stripping, it has been found that more tape strips were needed to disrupt the skin barrier in darker skin types and that darker skin types may have higher rates of barrier recovery.[14,15]

Although there remains a need for additional studies, overall, the findings listed above suggest that there is an inherent increased robustness of the skin barrier in skin of color that may hinder the ability of exogenous substances to penetrate. In theory, if this unique quality in fact exists, the prevalence of ACD is skin of color would be expected to be less compared to other populations. However, in the few epidemiological studies that have been done, it appears there is not a significant difference in the prevalence of ACD between White skin and skin of color.[16,17]

DIFFERENCES IN SENSITIZATION RATE IN SKIN OF COLOR

Few experimental studies of the differences in sensitization rate between ethnic groups have been conducted; this is most likely due to the ethical concerns that experiments would require deliberate sensitization but also a subject pool whose environment is restricted to control for other exposures. However, one such study was completed in the early half of the 20th century, which studied the sensitizing effects of 2:4 dinitrochlorobenzene and paranitrosodimethylanilin by conducting four rounds of applying "sensitizing" doses followed by "testing" doses to see if a response was elicited.[18] This study concluded that Blacks were less readily sensitized to paranitrosodimethylanilin but found no difference regarding dinitrochlorobenzene.[18]

Another study investigated the sensitization rates of five chemicals (p-phenylenediamine, monobenzyl ether of hydroquinone, nickel sulfate, penicillin G, and neomycin sulfate) between Caucasians and African Americans.[19] The results were consistent with the aforementioned study with a higher sensitization rate found in Caucasians compared to African Americans.[19] Thus, although experiments studying the differences in sensitization are scarce, these two studies support the theory that patients with skin of color may have resistance to the sensitization required for the development of ACD.

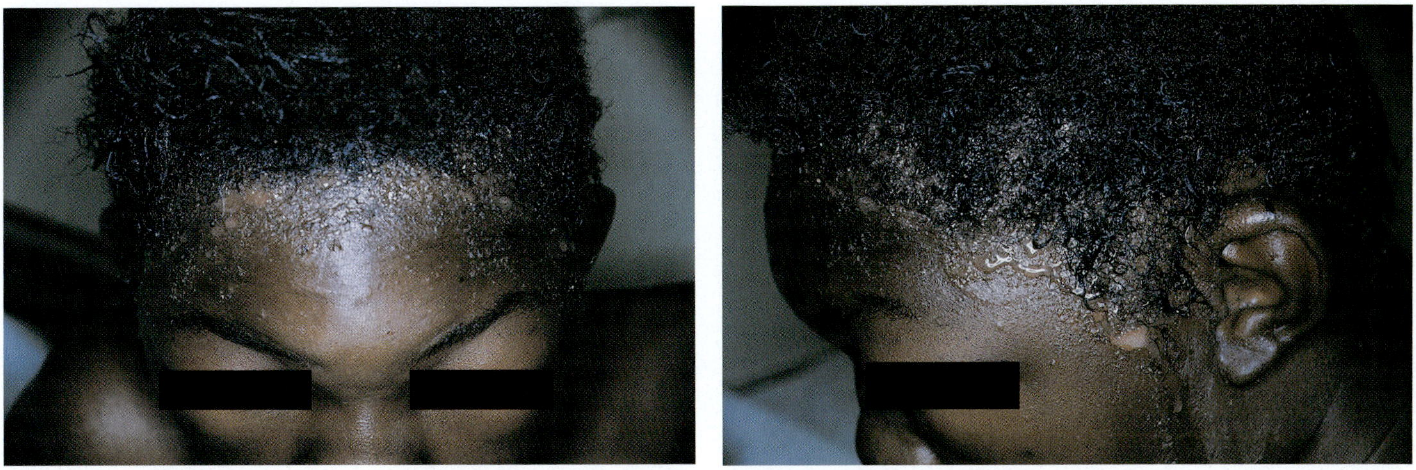

FIGURE 30-3. Contact dermatitis to p-phenylenediamine on the scalp of an African American female with skin type IV to V. **(A)** Front and **(B)** side views.

DIFFERENCES IN COMMON ALLERGY PATTERNS IN SKIN OF COLOR

Multiple studies have investigated differences in the incidence of specific allergies based on ethnic background. One study found that there were differences in the most common allergens, with nickel (II) sulfate hexahydrate, p-phenylenediamine, and methylisothiazolinone/methylchloroisothiazolinone being the most common among African Americans while fragrance mix I or II, nickel (II) sulfate hexahydrate, and balsam of Peru were the most common for White patients.[20] Studies by the North American Contact Dermatitis Group and others echoed some of these findings in analyses of the association of race and ethnicity with patch test results: Blacks had more frequent reactions to p-phenylenediamine, while Whites had higher rates of reactions to fragrances, formaldehyde, and formaldehyde-releaser preservatives [**Figure 30-3**].[21,22]

Considered together, these studies suggest that differences in common allergens do in fact exist between skin types. The root cause of these differences is less clear; however, the authors of these studies and those of others investigating ethnic differences in allergens suggest that these differences can likely be explained by cultural or lifestyle factors.[20-22]

DIAGNOSIS: PATCH TESTING

As the treatment for ACD is unequivocally avoidance of any allergens, the management of ACD is centered around diagnosis. Patch testing is a time-sensitive and involved process, thus a preliminary consult is standard of care to ensure proper allocation of resources and avoid unnecessary burden on patients. Consultations ensure that their presentation is consistent with ACD and is not better explained by another dermatologic condition and also ensure that all appropriate possible allergens are tested [**Figure 30-4**].

CULTURAL CONSIDERATIONS

By the nature of ACD being caused by exposure to exogenous substances, environmental considerations are paramount to proper evaluation of patients and tailoring patch tests to each individual. Fundamentally, demographics naturally have a strong impact on each individual's range of possible exposures to allergens; thus factors such age, gender, ethnicity, location of residence (eg, urban or rural), and occupation should always be considered during patch testing consults.

Race and ethnicity are often closely tied with culture, which in turn can influence many lifestyle choices. Although there are innumerable cultural practices, increased cultural awareness can nevertheless be helpful in evaluating patients for ACD. For example, in Ayurvedic medicine often practiced by East Indians, various topical oils called "thailams" have been shown to be associated with ACD.[23] Black henna tattoos (pseudotattoos) are another unique socioreligious practice that was traditionally practiced by Muslim or Hindu people, but in recent years has become a social trend, regardless of faith or ethnicity.[24] Many current formulations of the dye used in henna tattooing contain p-phenylenediamine and have been associated with increased incidence of ACD.[24] As a final example, studies have also shown that cultural and socioeconomic factors may

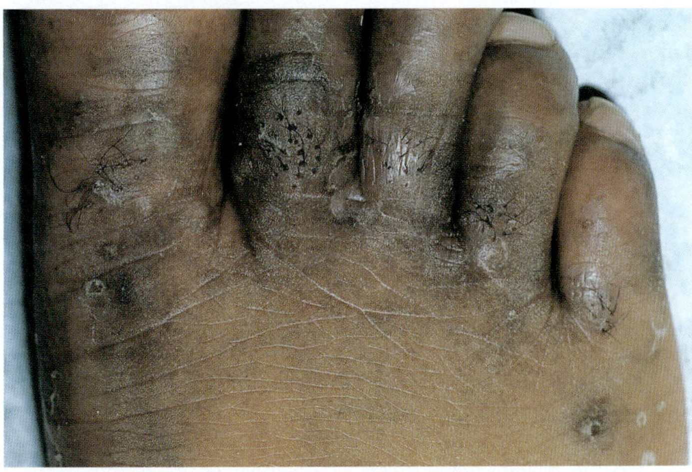

FIGURE 30-4. Contact dermatitis on the dorsum of the toes and foot of an African American male with skin type IV to V.

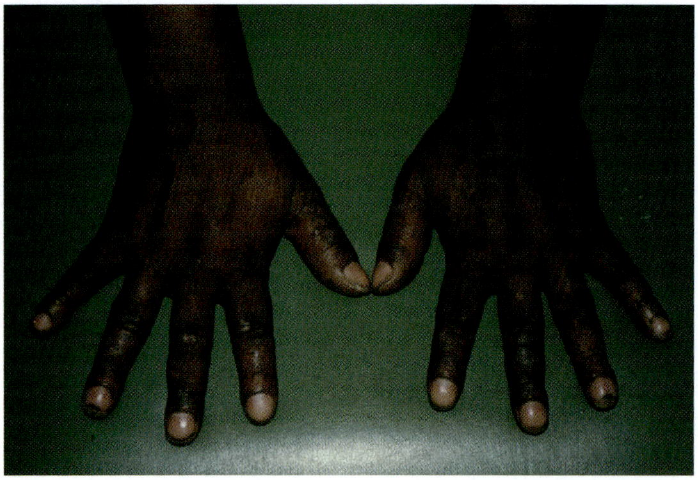

FIGURE 30-5. Irritant contact dermatitis on the dorsum of the hands in an African American cement worker. This occurred as a reaction to the chromium in the cement-manufacturing process.

influence the frequency of body piercings and corresponding incidence of nickel allergy.[25,26]

OCCUPATIONAL CONSIDERATIONS

In addition to cultural influences, occupation undoubtedly also affects people's regular exposure to possible allergens. Contact dermatitis accounts for 90% of all occupational skin diseases.[27] It is well established that certain occupations are associated with particular allergens. Allergies to metal such as cobalt and nickel are the most common occupational allergens and are especially prevalent in the metalworking industry.[27] Another example is that rubber additives such as mercaptobenzothiazoles sensitize workers who regularly use rubber gloves for aseptic purposes such as healthcare or house cleaners.[27] In the realm of hairdressing, professionals may be more likely to develop allergies to ingredients in haircare and styling products such as p-phenylenediamine in hair dyes and cocamidopropyl betaine, a surfactant, in shampoos.[27] Although there may be ethnic differences in predilection for certain occupations, it is much more useful to consider occupation as a risk factor directly rather than try to infer occupational risk factors based on ethnicity or pigmentation of skin [**Figure 30-5**].

THE READ

The physical application of patch tests requires no special considerations in regards to race or ethnicity; however, the reading of the results can present unique challenges. Traditionally, erythema was used an endpoint indicator of positive patch test reactions. However, erythema in skin of color may be less frequently elicited, more difficult to be perceived, and may alternatively take on a more purple coloration, possibly resulting in underdiagnosis.[28] Thus, when reading reactions in skin of color, other clues such as induration and texture are often more helpful in perceiving positive reactions [**Figure 30-6**].[29]

CONCLUSION

ACD is a common skin condition that is acutely affected by endogenous and exogenous factors; therefore, proper evaluation and management requires a thorough history-taking and examination. Current literature suggests that there are inherent differences in susceptibility and allergen patterns between skin of color and lighter skin; however, there remains an overall scarcity of studies specifically studying ACD in skin of color. Additional studies are needed to further identify differences in skin of color and to characterize the underlying mechanisms that explain those differences.

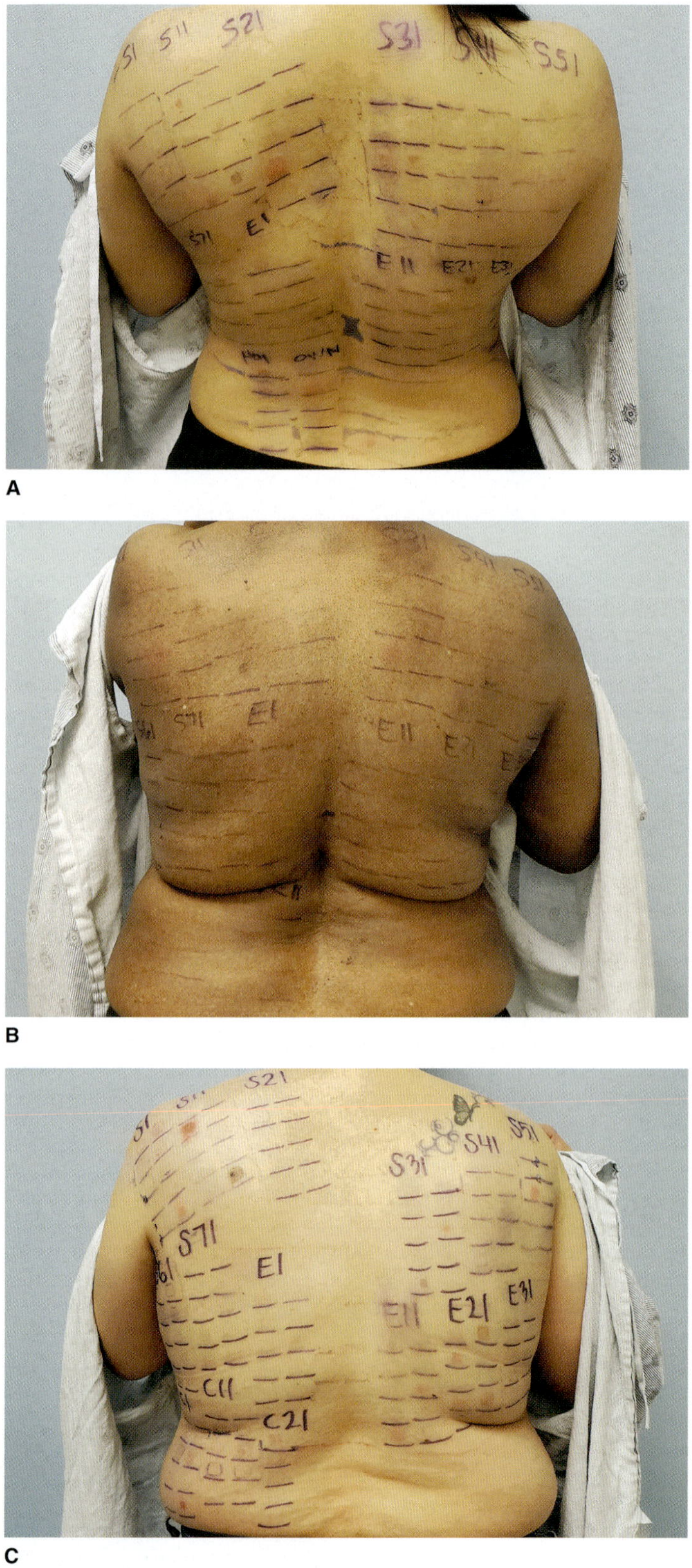

FIGURE 30-6. Photographs of the back and at 72 hours after application of allergens are shown for a self-identified **(A)** Asian, **(B)** Black, and **(C)** Hispanic patient.

REFERENCES

1. Statescu L, Branisteanu D, Dobre C, et al. Contact dermatitis - epidemiological study. *Maedica*. 2011;6(4):277-281.
2. Nguyen SH, Dang TP, MacPherson C, Maibach H, Maibach HI. Prevalence of patch test results from 1970 to 2002 in a multi-centre population in North America (NACDG). *Contact Dermatitis*. 2008;58(2):101-106.

3. Czarnobilska E, Obtulowicz K, Dyga W, Spiewak R. A half of schoolchildren with 'ISAAC eczema' are ill with allergic contact dermatitis. *J Eur Acad Dermatol Venereol.* 2011;25(9):1104-1107.
4. Rubins A, Romanova A, Septe M, Maddukuri S, Schwartz RA, Rubins S. Contact dermatitis: etiologies of the allergic and irritant type. *Acta Dermatovenerol Alp Pannonica Adriat.* 2020;29(4).
5. Wolf R, Orion E, Ruocco V, Baroni A, Ruocco E. Patch testing: facts and controversies. *Clin Dermatol.* 2013;31(4):479-486.
6. DeKoven JG, Silverberg JI, Warshaw EM, et al. North American Contact Dermatitis Group Patch Test Results: 2017-2018. *Dermat Contact Atopic Occup Drug.* 2021;32(2):111-123.
7. Bains SN, Nash P, Fonacier L. Irritant Contact Dermatitis. *Clin Rev Allergy Immunol.* 2019;56(1):99-109.
8. Taylor SC. Skin of color: Biology, structure, function, and implications for dermatologic disease. *J Am Acad Dermatol.* 2002;46(2, Supplement 2):S41-S62.
9. La Ruche G, Cesarini JP. [Histology and physiology of black skin]. *Ann Dermatol Venereol.* 1992;119(8):567-574.
10. Iwuala C, Taylor SC. Structural and functional differences in skin of colour. *Clin Exp Dermatol.* 2022;47(2):247-250.
11. Wedig JH, Maibach HI. Percutaneous penetration of dipyrithione in man: Effect of skin color (race). *J Am Acad Dermatol.* 1981;5(4):433-438.
12. Corcuff P, Lotte C, Rougier A, Maibach HI. Racial differences in corneocytes. A comparison between black, white and oriental skin. *Acta Derm Venereol.* 1991;71(2):146-148.
13. Kompaore F, Marty JP, Dupont C. In vivo Evaluation of the Stratum corneum Barrier Function in Blacks, Caucasians and Asians with Two Noninvasive Methods. *Skin Pharmacol Physiol.* 1993;6(3):200-207.
14. Muizzuddin N, Hellemans L, Van Overloop L, Corstjens H, Declercq L, Maes D. Structural and functional differences in barrier properties of African American, Caucasian and East Asian skin. *J Dermatol Sci.* 2010;59(2):123-128.
15. Reed JT, Ghadially R, Elias PM. Skin type, but neither race nor gender, influence epidermal permeability barrier function. *Arch Dermatol.* 1995;131(10):1134-1138.
16. Epidemiology of Contact Dermatitis in North America: 1972. *Arch Dermatol.* 1973;108(4):537-540.
17. Scott I. Update on Contact Dermatitis and Patch Testing in Patients With Skin of Color. *Cutis.* 2021;108(1).
18. Rostenberg A, Kanof NM. Studies in Eczematous Sensitizations. *J Invest Dermatol.* 1941;4(6):505-516.
19. Kligman AM. The Identification of Contact Allergens by Human Assay. *J Invest Dermatol.* 1966;47(5):375-392.
20. Garg V, Zhan T, Brod BA, Gaspari AA. Patterns of Allergic Contact Dermatitis in African Americans in a Major Metropolitan Area Over a 10-Year Period. *Dermat Contact Atopic Occup Drug.* 2022;33(1):70-79.
21. Deleo VA, Alexis A, Warshaw EM, et al. The Association of Race/Ethnicity and Patch Test Results: North American Contact Dermatitis Group, 1998–2006. *Dermatitis.* 2016;27(5):288-292.
22. DeLeo VA, Taylor SC, Belsito DV, et al. The effect of race and ethnicity on patch test results. *J Am Acad Dermatol.* 2002;46(2, Supplement 2):S107-S112.
23. Kannan RK. Cultural dermatoses: A review. *J Skin Sex Transm Dis.* 2022;4(1):33-39.
24. Le Coz CJ, Lefebvre C, Keller F, Grosshans É. Allergic Contact Dermatitis Caused by Skin Painting (Pseudotattooing) With Black Henna, a Mixture of Henna and p-Phenylenediamine and Its Derivatives. *Arch Dermatol.* 2000;136(12):1515-1517.
25. Rundle CW, Bergman D, Brankov N, Limone B, Jacob SE. The Influence of Cultural Norms on Nickel Allergic Contact Dermatitis Prevalence Data. *Dermatitis.* 2018;29(3):165-166.
26. Schnuch A. Sociology of Nickel Allergy. *Dermatitis.* 2018;29(5):290-291.
27. Sasseville D. Occupational Contact Dermatitis. *Allergy Asthma Clin Immunol Off J Can Soc Allergy Clin Immunol.* 2008;4(2):59-65.
28. Jothishankar B, Stein SL. Impact of skin color and ethnicity. *Clin Dermatol.* 2019;37(5):418-429.
29. Tamazian S, Oboite M, Treat JR. Patch testing in skin of color: A brief report. *Pediatr Dermatol.* 2021;38(4):952-953.

CHAPTER 31

Photosensitivity

Kelly Z. Young
Linna L. Guan
Tasneem F. Mohammad

KEY POINTS

- Photodermatoses can affect individuals of all ages, sexes, and races, including individuals with skin of color.
- A comprehensive history, complete physical exam, and appropriate laboratory testing can aid in diagnosis.
- Pin-head papular eruption is the most common morphology in SOC patients with polymorphous light eruption; this contrast with erythematous urticaria papules and plaques commonly seen in light-skinned patients.
- The mainstay of therapy involves photoprotection, with variations in therapeutic options based on the specific photodermatoses.

INTRODUCTION TO LIGHT, SKIN PIGMENTATION, AND PHOTOSENSITIVITY

Sunlight affects the function, survival, and proliferation of skin cells.[1] It is composed of electromagnetic radiation in the ultraviolet (UV), visible, and infrared wavelengths. Most of the harmful shorter wavelengths, including UVC (<290 nm), are absorbed by the ozone layer and atmosphere.[2] The solar radiation that reaches the earth's surface consists of UVB (290-320 nm), UVA (320-400 nm), visible light (VL, 400-700 nm), and infrared radiation (IR, >700 nm) [**Figure 31-1**].[2] Penetration of UV radiation (UVR) into the skin is dependent on the wavelength, with longer wavelengths penetrating more deeply. While UVB is primarily absorbed in the epidermis and superficial dermis, UVA is capable of reaching deeper into the dermis.[3,4]

The skin reacts to sunlight through absorption, reflection, and scattering of the sun's rays.[2] *Photosensitivity refers to an abnormal or adverse reaction of one's skin to sunlight.*[5,6] Photosensitivity varies with skin pigmentation, which is largely determined by the quantity and quality of melanin pigments.[7] Melanin, which is generated by melanocytes in the basal epidermis and transported to keratinocytes, provides photoprotection through its ability to absorb and scatter UV radiation, transforming UVR into heat.[7,8] Exposure to UVR results in both immediate pigment darkening through modification of existing melanin and delayed tanning through synthesis of new melanin.[4]

There are two chemically distinct types of melanin pigment in the skin: eumelanin and pheomelanin.[8] The brown/black eumelanin is involved in scattering and absorbing UV and scavenging free radicals produced by UV radiation.[8] On the other hand, the yellow/red pheomelanin generates reactive oxygen species (ROS) that increases the skin's susceptibility to DNA damage.[8] Increased ratios of eumelanin to pheomelanin are observed in darker skin types when compared to lighter skin types. These variations in pigmentation likely contribute to differences in photosensitivity.[8] However, other factors play a role in photosensitivity, given the wide variation of erythemal response and photoadaptation within the same skin types and the presence of photodermatoses in more richly pigmented skin.[9]

Photosensitive disorders are categorized as (1) idiopathic photodermatoses, (2) photodermatoses secondary to endogenous agents, (3) photodermatoses secondary to exogenous agents, (4) photoexacerbated dermatoses, and (5) genodermatoses [**Table 31-1**].[10]

INITIAL EVALUATION OF PATIENTS WITH PHOTOSENSITIVITY

When evaluating a patient with photosensitivity, a thorough history should be obtained [**Figure 31-2**]. Emphasis should be placed on symptom onset, duration, factors that improve or worsen symptoms, associated symptoms, and exposure to medications or potential photosensitizers.[3] It is important

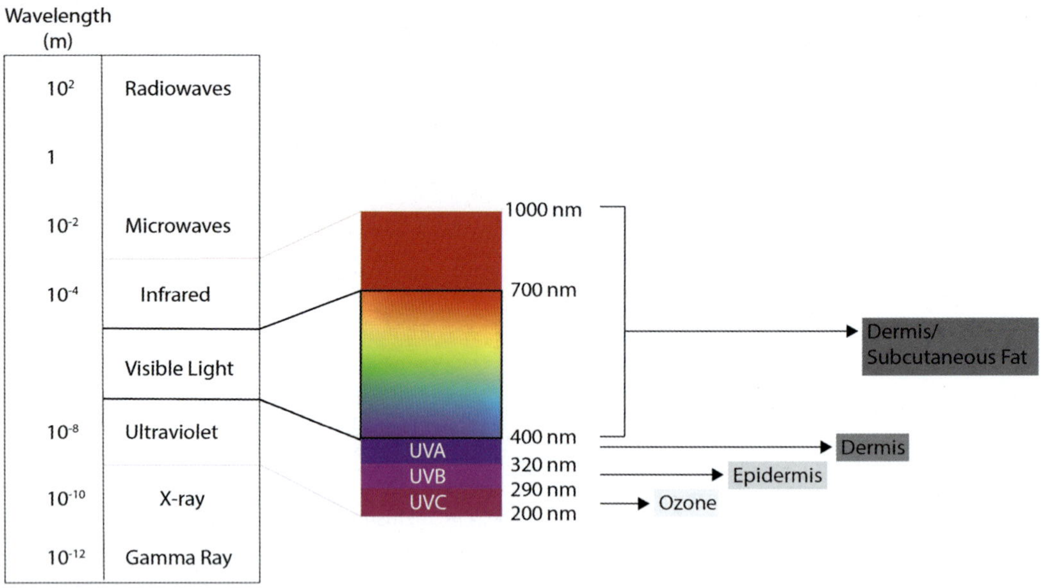

FIGURE 31-1. Electromagnetic spectrum.[3] Sunlight consists of ultraviolet (UV), visible, and infrared light. Most UVC radiation (<290 nm) is absorbed by the ozone layer and atmosphere. UVB radiation (290-320 nm) is primarily absorbed in the epidermis, UVA (320-400 nm) reaches the dermis, and VL (400-700 nm) can reach the dermis and subcutaneous fat.

to ask about sun exposure and the temporal relationship between sun exposure and development of skin findings.[3] Asking about variation of symptoms with seasons (winter vs summer) and whether symptoms are affected by the presence of window glass (since UVB cannot pass through window glass) may help with diagnosis.[3] Additionally, gathering information on family history is important, since some photosensitivity disorders are inherited.[3] Finally, attention should be paid to the age of the patient, as certain diseases present in specific age groups.[3]

On examination, it is important to pay attention to the morphology and distribution of skin lesions. Photosensitivity reactions tend to be the worst on sun-exposed areas, including the forehead, cheeks, nape of the neck, upper back, and extensor arms.[5] Sun-protected areas, such as the nasolabial folds, upper eyelids, postauricular area, submental region, and superior pinna of the ear, are usually spared.[5]

TABLE 31-1 Summary of pediatric photodermatoses

1. **Idiopathic photodermatoses**
Actinic prurigo
Chronic actinic dermatitis
Polymorphous light eruption
Hydroa vacciniforme
Solar urticaria
2. **Photodermatoses secondary to endogenous agents**
Porphyria cutanea tarda
Erythropoietic protoporphyria
X-linked protoporphyria
3. **Photodermatoses secondary to exogenous agents**
Photoallergy
Phototoxicity
Pseudoporphyria
4. **Photoexacerbated dermatoses**
Atopic dermatitis
Darier-White disease
Dermatitis herpetiformis
Herpes simplex infection
Lupus erythematosus
Juvenile dermatomyositis
Pellagra
Psoriasis
Seborrheic dermatitis
5. **Genodermatoses**
Xeroderma pigmentosum
Cockayne syndrome
Trichothiodystrophy
UV light sensitive syndrome
Rothmund-Thomson syndrome
Bloom syndrome
Smith-Lemli-Opitz syndrome
Hartnup disease
Kindler syndrome

Source: Adapted from Chantorn R, Lim HW, Shwayder TA. Photosensitivity disorders in children: part I. *J Am Acad Dermatol.* 2012;67(6):1093.e1-18-quiz1111-2.3.[3]

IDIOPATHIC PHOTODERMATOSES

POLYMORPHOUS LIGHT ERUPTION

Polymorphous light eruption (PMLE) is the most common immunologically mediated photodermatosis, estimated to affect up to 20% of individuals.[11] Colloquially referred to as "sun poisoning" or "sun allergy," PMLE occurs within hours following sun exposure.[12] PMLE is most severe in the spring or early summer and often improves as summer progresses due to photoadaptation or photohardening, a process in which the skin develops increased tolerance to light exposure.[12] Typical onset of PMLE occurs within the first three decades, and affects females more frequently than males.[11] PMLE affects all skin types, with higher prevalence in dark-skinned individuals than fair-skinned individuals.[13,14]

Pathogenesis of PMLE is thought to involve alterations in immune function. In healthy individuals, UV exposure suppresses various T-cell immune pathways in the skin due to appropriate migration of Langerhans cells (LCs).[11] In individuals genetically predisposed to PMLE, changes in the normal migration of LCs result in a lack of immunosuppression after UV exposure.[11] Additionally, prior reports demonstrated that up to 19% of patients with PMLE have antinuclear, anti-SS-A and anti-Ro antibodies.[15] PMLE shares several features with a delayed-type hypersensitivity reaction, suggesting a role of UV-induced photoantigens.[16] The presence of photoantigens combined with the lack of immune suppression causes an immune response, leading to the cutaneous manifestations of PMLE. The action spectrum of PMLE includes both UVA and UVB radiation [**Table 31-2**].

PMLE primarily affects photo-distributed areas, including the upper chest and extensor arms.[11] As the name suggests, there are several morphological variants of PMLE, but the most common form involves pruritic, erythematous, papules, or plaques [**Figure 31-3A**].[12] In darker skin types (Fitzpatrick class IV-VI), the predominant form of PMLE is the

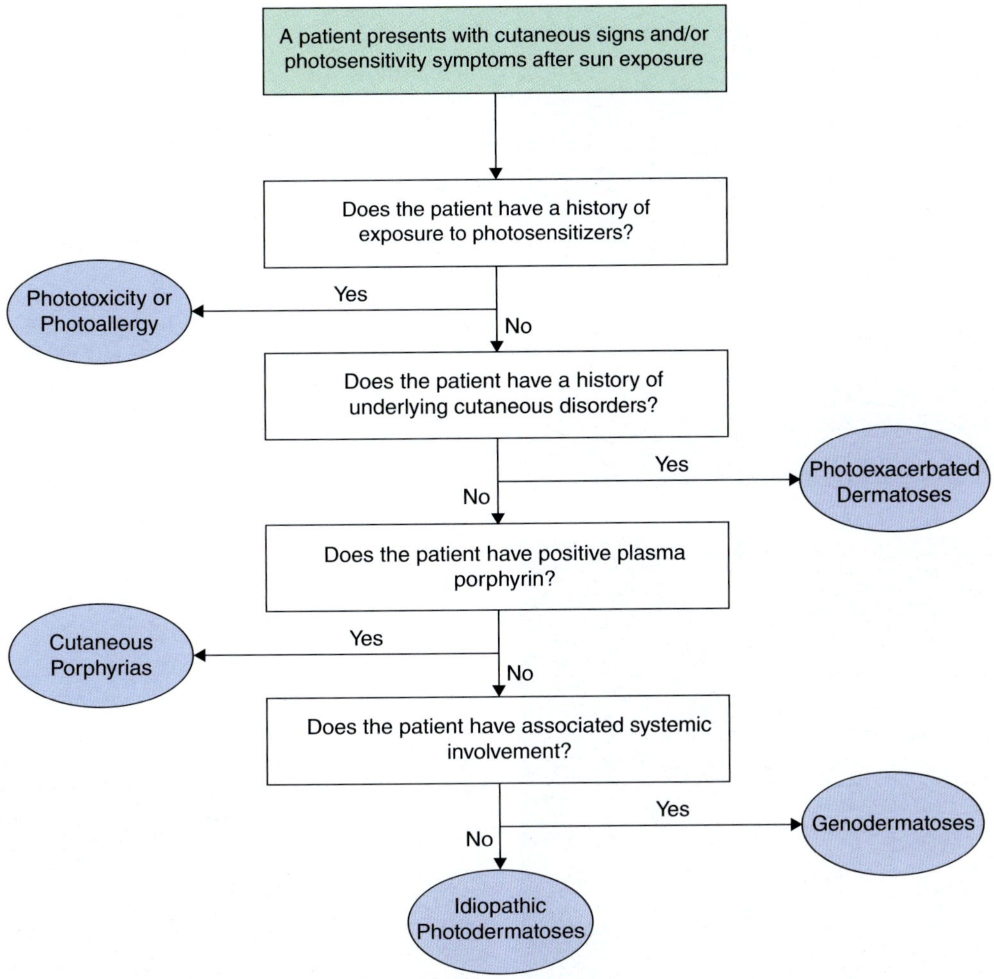

FIGURE 31-2. Diagnostic algorithm for photodermatoses. (Adapted from Chantorn R, Lim HW, Shwayder TA. Photosensitivity disorders in children: part I. *J Am Acad Dermatol.* 2012;67(6):1093.e1–18–quiz1111–2.[3])

pinpoint papular variant, commonly affecting the arms or back of the hands [**Figure 31-3B**].[12] In children, juvenile spring eruption is considered a variant of PMLE and is characterized by localized pruritic erythematous papules, commonly seen in young boys on the superior ears [**Figure 31-3C**].[3] PMLE typically does not affect the face given that it is exposed to some degree of sunlight year-round and is continuously photohardened.[12] This may be different in the era of COVID-19 where masking of the face is common.

TABLE 31-2 Action spectra associated with photodermatoses

Photodermatoses	Action spectrum
Polymorphous light eruption	UVA, UVB
Actinic prurigo	UVA, UVB
Hydroa vacciniforme	UVA, UVB
Chronic actinic dermatitis	UVA, UVB, VL
Solar urticaria	UVA, VL, UVB
Porphyria cutanea tarda	VL
Erythropoietic protoporphyria and X-linked protoporphyria	VL
Xeroderma pigmentosum	UVB, UVA
Cockayne syndrome	UVB, VL
Trichothiodystrophy	UVB
Rothmund-Thomson syndrome	UVA (?)
Smith-Lemli-Opitz syndrome	UVA
Kindler syndrome	UVA, UVB

Source: Reproduced with permission from Nahhas AF, Oberlin DM, Braunberger TL, Lim HW. Recent Developments in the Diagnosis and Management of Photosensitive Disorders. *Am J Clin Dermatol.* 2018;19(5):707-731.[11]

First-line management of PMLE involves patient counseling and sun protection including the use of broad-spectrum sunscreens.[16] For acute or pruritic eruptions, treatments include topical steroids, antihistamines, or oral steroids.[12,16] In-office or less commonly at-home photohardening, where patients are exposed to increasing, sub-erythemal doses of UV light, can be considered in patients with frequent PMLE episodes.[16,17] Additional reported therapies include antimalarials, azathioprine, and cyclosporine.[16] In a small study, calcipotriol was suggested to be effective as a preventative agent in PMLE.[18]

ACTINIC PRURIGO

Actinic prurigo (AP) is a rare, chronic, photosensitive disorder characterized by periods of pruritus and cutaneous eruptions.[11] Symptoms are worst in the spring and can persist through the summer and winter.[19] Typically, onset begins in childhood (around ages 4-8), but adult-onset AP has been reported.[20] AP is more common in females and is more frequently diagnosed in Native American and Mestizo (mixed European and indigenous American) populations, as well as patients with more pigmented skin (Fitzpatrick class IV/V) who live at higher altitudes.[11,21] Although less common, AP can affect Asians and those affected are more frequently males, have adult-onset, and lack mucosal involvement.[20]

The action spectrum of AP includes UVA and UVB radiation [Table 31-2]. Currently, the etiology of AP remains unclear. Studies suggest a potential contribution from delayed hypersensitivity reaction to photo-induced antigens.[11] A strong genetic component is likely, since up to 75% of patients with AP have a positive family history.[20] Furthermore, seminal studies have consistently linked HLA-DR4 polymorphisms to AP.[20]

Patients with AP describe pruritus a few hours following sun exposure followed by the development of symmetric, erythematous papules and nodules in a photodistributed pattern [**Figure 31-4A**].[20] Chronic scratching may result in hemorrhagic crusting and lichenified plaques.[20] Some patients have mucosal involvement of the lips (acute cheilitis; **Figure 31-4B**) or ocular involvement (conjunctivitis and photophobia) with or without cutaneous findings.[20]

Management of AP includes photoprotection, topical and systemic steroids, topical calcineurin inhibitors, phototherapy, and thalidomide.[20] Thalidomide is thought to promote anti-inflammatory effects through alteration of tumor necrosis factor (TNF) and interferon-gamma signaling.[20] Thalidomide, 100 to 200 mg daily, is often effective, even in resistant disease.[11] Once a patient achieves remission, thalidomide may be tapered to maintenance doses.[11] It is important to keep in mind that thalidomide may not be appropriate for all patients given the associated risks of teratogenicity and peripheral neuropathy.[11] Additional therapies, including pentoxifylline, azathioprine, and cyclosporine, have been utilized with variable success.[11]

CHRONIC ACTINIC DERMATITIS

Chronic actinic dermatitis (CAD) is characterized by pruritic eczematous rashes and lichenified plaques on sun-exposed areas.[22] Although

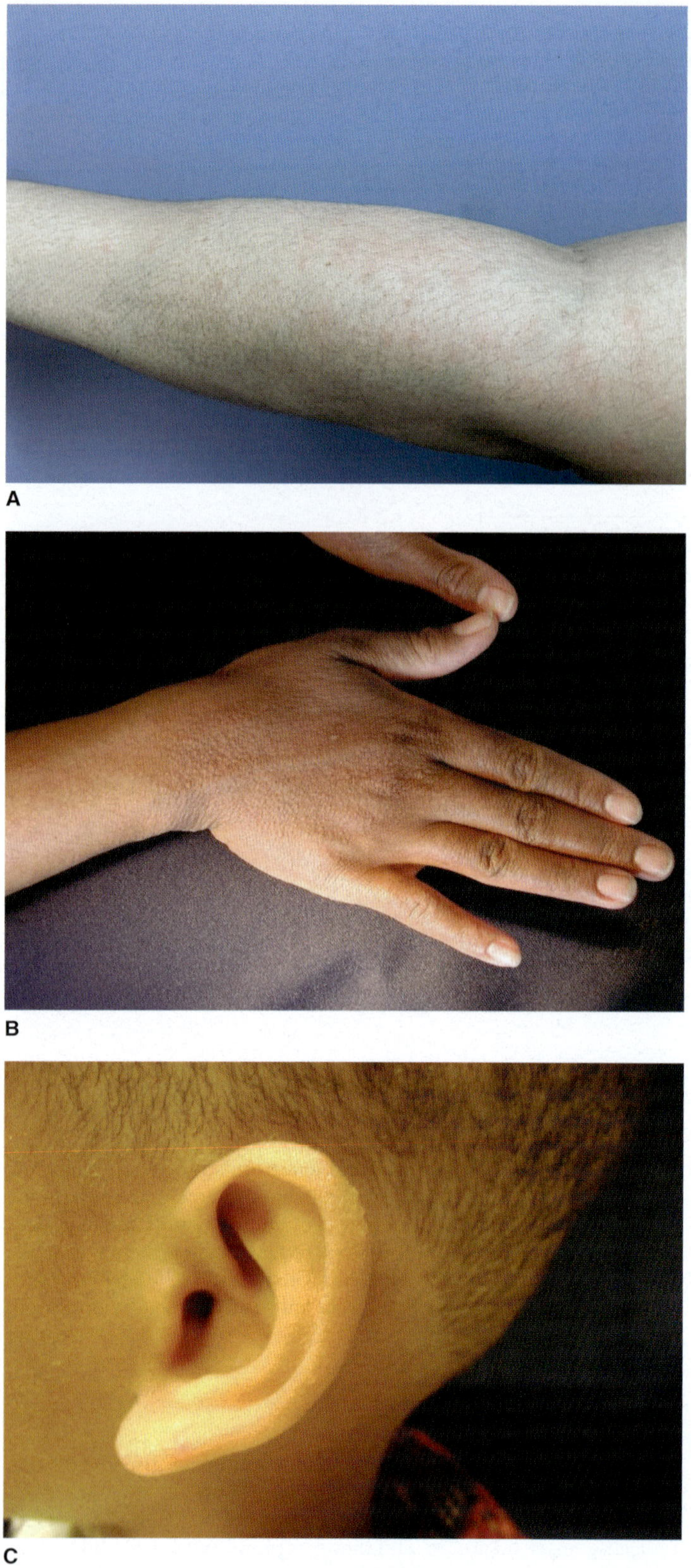

FIGURE 31-3. Polymorphous light eruption (*PMLE*). **(A)** Erythematous papules and plaques, the most common form of PMLE. **(B)** Pinpoint variant of PMLE affecting the dorsum of the hand. **(C)** Erythematous and skin-colored papules on the superior ear, consistent with juvenile spring eruption. (Panels B and C are provided courtesy of Henry W. Lim, MD, Department of Dermatology, Henry Ford Health, Detroit, MI, USA.)

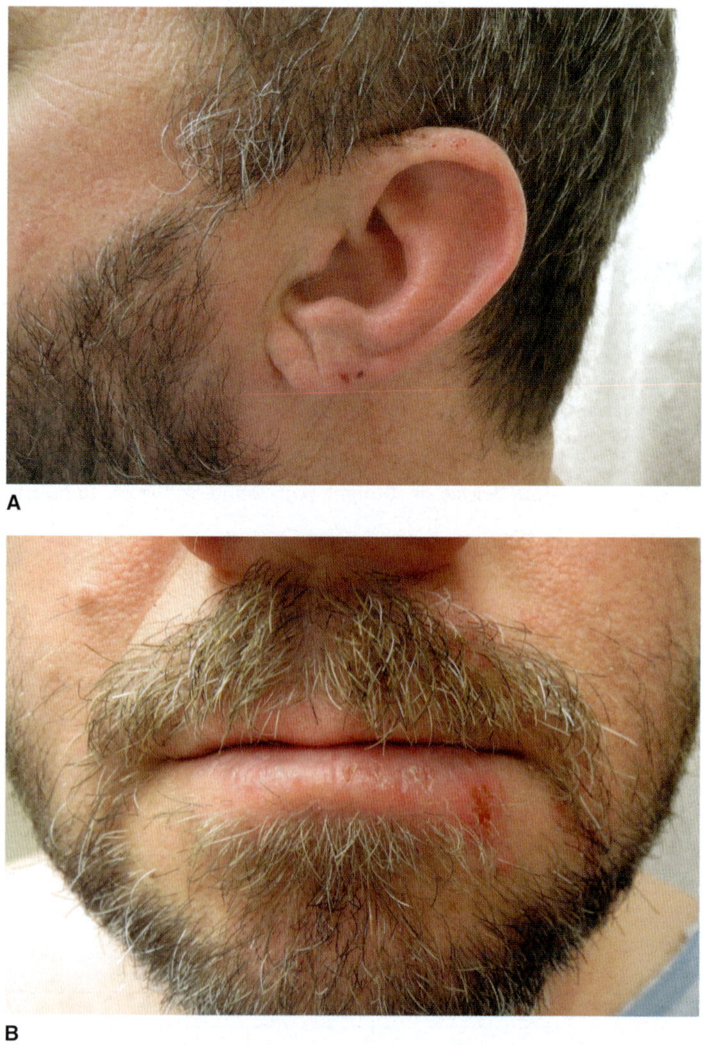

FIGURE 31-4. Actinic prurigo. **(A)** Erythematous papules and erosions of the ear. **(B)** Mucosal involvement of the lips, consistent with acute cheilitis. (Courtesy of Henry W. Lim, MD, Department of Dermatology, Henry Ford Health, Detroit, MI, USA.)

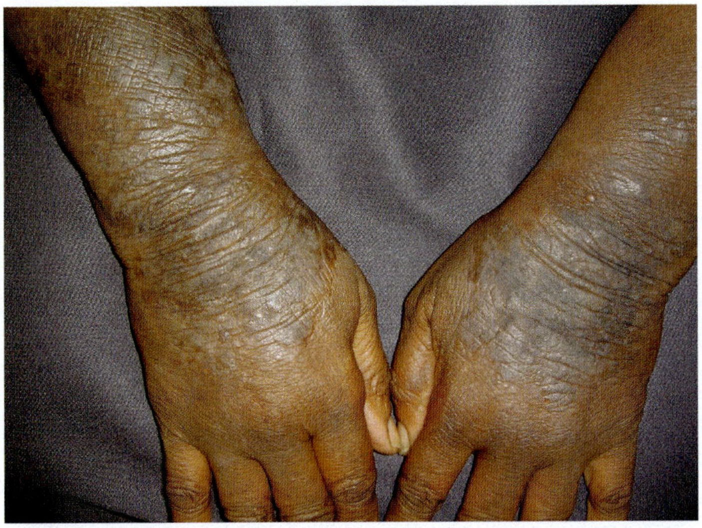

FIGURE 31-5. Chronic actinic dermatitis. Hyperpigmented and lichenified thin plaques of bilateral dorsal hands. (Courtesy of Henry W. Lim, MD, Department of Dermatology, Henry Ford Health, Detroit, MI, USA.)

initial reports focused on CAD in older fair-skinned males, increasing evidence shows that CAD affects patients of all Fitzpatrick skin types and sexes.[23] In patients with more pigmented skin (Fitzpatrick type V-VI), studies suggest a higher prevalence of CAD in females and report onset of disease at younger ages.[11,24] Many patients with CAD have concomitant atopic dermatitis, allergic contact dermatitis, or photoallergy.[25]

Although mechanisms of CAD are not fully understood, most studies suggest an immunologic basis. It is hypothesized that sun exposure generates endogenous allergens, leading to a delayed-type IV hypersensitivity reaction.[11] Alternatively, others have proposed a role of exogenous allergens or sensitizers, such as sunscreen or Compositae, in altering the normal immune response.[11]

Examination often reveals a persistent pruritic, eczematous skin rash with lichenification and fine scale [**Figure 31-5**].[11] CAD lesions localize to sun-exposed areas but may affect nonexposed areas when disease is severe.[11] Patients may notice increased severity of the rash in summer months or with extended periods of sun exposure.[22] Diagnosis generally involves clinical examination, biopsy, and phototesting.[11] Characteristic histopathology findings include epidermal spongiosis, acanthosis, a mixed dermal infiltrate of T-cells, eosinophils, and plasma cells, and lymphocytic exocytosis.[11] The action spectrum of CAD includes UVA, UVB, and VL [Table 31-2].[11]

Management of CAD involves photoprotection and avoidance of potential contact allergens.[11] It is important to screen for sunscreen allergy and if history is suggestive, confirm by patch testing prior to recommending broad-spectrum sunscreens.[26] First-line therapy for active lesions includes topical and/or oral steroids.[11] Additionally, topical calcineurin inhibitors under occlusion, other systemic immunosuppressants (azathioprine, cyclosporine, mycophenolate mofetil), or biologics may be used.[11] In particular, oral tofacitinib[27] and topical tacrolimus under occlusion[28] have demonstrated success in small cohorts of patients with refractory disease.[11] Dupilumab is a human monoclonal antibody that blocks IL4- and IL13-related inflammatory responses that has been approved to treat moderate to severe atopic dermatitis in the United States.[29] Several recent case series support the efficacy of dupilumab in treating CAD.[29,30]

HYDROA VACCINIFORME

Hydroa vacciniforme (HV) is among the more rare, potentially scarring, photodermatoses with an estimated prevalence of 0.34 per 100,000 people.[11] Classically, disease onset occurs in childhood and the course is characterized by intermittent cutaneous flares followed by spontaneous resolution in adulthood.[11] HV is more common in boys and those with lighter skin types.[11,31] Classic HV should be distinguished from Hydroa vacciniforme-like lymphoproliferative disorder, which is a systemic disorder associated with lymphoproliferative disease.[11,20] Workup for lymphoproliferative disease should be considered in the presence of deep or ulcerative skin lesions, involvement of the bone or mucosa, or systemic symptoms.[20]

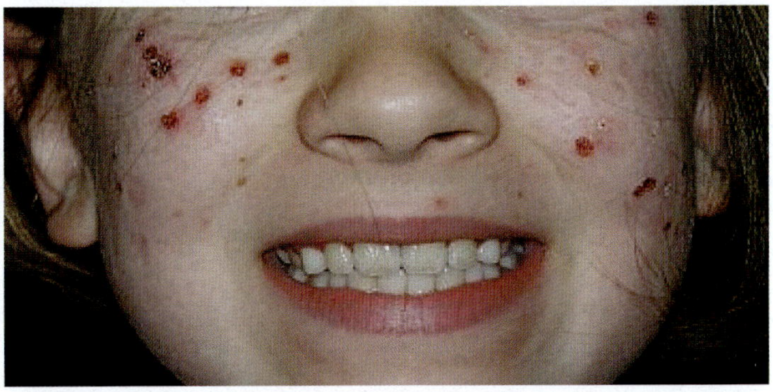

FIGURE 31-6. Hydroa vacciniforme. Papulovesicular and vesiculobullous eruptions on bilateral cheeks with scarring. (Courtesy of Henry W. Lim, MD, Department of Dermatology, Henry Ford Health, Detroit, MI, USA.)

Pathogenesis of HV remains unclear, but studies implicate a role of both UV exposure (UVA, UVB, Table 31-2) and Epstein-Barr virus (EBV) infection in classic HV.[20,32,33] Despite the typical self-limited nature of classic HV, a subset of patients with HV may develop severe, persistent disease. These atypical forms of HV may result from a failure to develop immune tolerance to latent EBV infection, resulting in a heightened response to repetitive UV exposure and abnormal numbers of EBV-positive gamma delta T-cells.[20,33,34]

Clinically, HV is characterized by recurrent crops of papulovesicular lesions or vesiculobullous eruptions in a photodistributed pattern that have the tendency to scar [**Figure 31-6**].[11,33] Management of HV is conservative and primarily involves photoprotection and avoidance of sunlight.[3] Although chloroquine, β-carotene, and phototherapy have shown success in limited cases, no universally effective therapy has yet been identified.[3] In severe cases, systemic steroids may be considered.[3]

SOLAR URTICARIA

Solar urticaria (SU) is characterized by photodistributed urticaria that develop within minutes of sun exposure.[11] Lesions are self-limited and typically resolve within 24 hours.[11] SU has a slight female predominance and most commonly presents in the fourth or fifth decade of life.[11] In a multicenter retrospective study over a 10-year period, SU was found to affect 3.2% of fair-skinned individuals and 0.7% of African American individuals.[23]

Pathogenesis of SU is thought to involve degranulation of mast cells through IgE-mediated hypersensitivity to photo-induced endogenous antigens generated in the skin.[11,35] Type I SU is characterized by IgE antibodies against abnormal chromophores, while Type II is characterized by IgE antibodies against normal chromophores.[35] The action spectra of solar urticaria includes VL, UVA, and UVB radiation [Table 31-2].[35]

SU classically presents with pruritic erythema and wheals in sun-exposed areas [**Figure 31-7**].[35] In rare cases, SU can be associated with anaphylaxis.[11] Since most sunscreens do not adequately cover longer wavelengths, such as those in the visible light or long wavelength UVA spectrum, they are limited in their ability to prevent SU flares.[11] Thus, management primarily involves sun avoidance, symptomatic relief with antihistamines, leukotriene antagonists, topical steroids, and oral steroids.[35] Photohardening is commonly used in mild disease.[11] Recent reports also suggest the utility of omalizumab, a recombinant humanized anti-IgE antibody, in the management of refractory SU.[35]

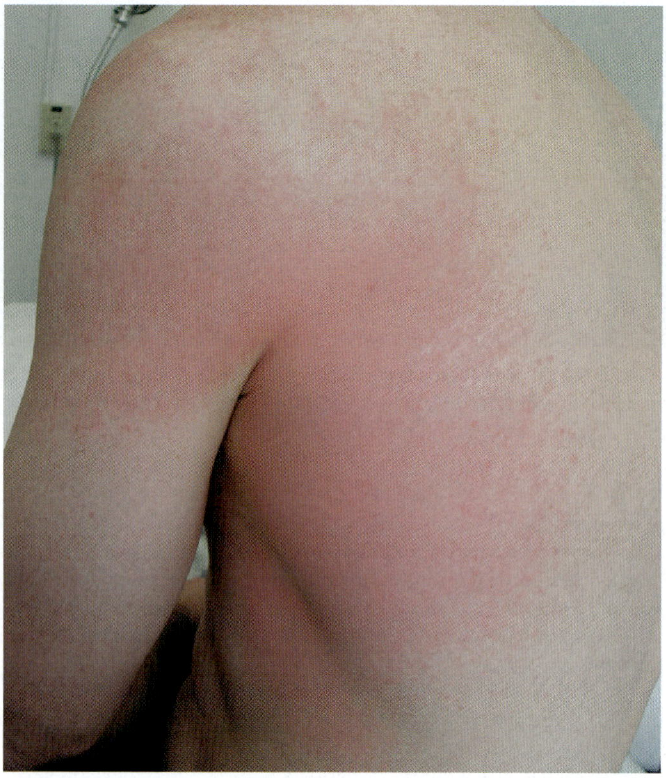

FIGURE 31-7. Solar urticaria. Erythematous wheals on lateral shoulder and trunk. (Courtesy of Henry W. Lim, MD, Department of Dermatology, Henry Ford Health, Detroit, MI, USA.)

PHOTODERMATOSES SECONDARY TO ENDOGENOUS AGENTS

PORPHYRIAS

The porphyrias are a group of disorders characterized by an enzymatic defect in the heme biosynthesis pathway, resulting in the accumulation and oxidation of porphyrinogens and generation of porphyrins.[3] The accumulation of intermediate molecules in the heme pathway results in cutaneous, neurological, and/or hepatic manifestations.[3] There are two broad categories of porphyrias: (1) acute or inducible porphyrias, which cause neurovisceral symptoms, and (2) chronic or cutaneous porphyrias (CP), which are characterized by porphyrin accumulation in the skin, red blood cells, and hepatocytes.[3] Porphyrias may also be classified as hepatic or erythropoietic, determined by the organ in which accumulation of heme precursors is found.[3]

Endogenous porphyrins are photosensitizers, as they can absorb light (commonly 400-405 nm) and cause tissue damage.[3] As this range lies in the visible light spectrum, sunscreens that only protect against UVR are not always beneficial for patients with CP.[3] Patients with CP may present with a wide range of cutaneous symptoms due to differences in water solubility of the various heme precursors.[3] Here, we discuss porphyrias with more prominent cutaneous manifestations including porphyria cutanea tarda, erythropoietic protoporphyria, and X-linked protoporphyria.

Porphyria Cutanea Tarda Porphyria cutanea tarda (PCT) is the most common form of porphyria, caused by a deficiency or decreased activity of the hepatic uroporphyrinogen decarboxylase (UROD) enzyme.[36] Decreased UROD activity results in the accumulation of porphyrinogens in the liver, which are then oxidized to porphyrins.[36] On biochemical examination of plasma, urine, and stool, the classic PCT porphyrin pattern includes elevation of plasma uroporphyrin, urine uroporphyrin and coproporphyrin, and stool, isocoproporphyrin.[37] PCT has a genetic component in roughly 20% of cases, involving mutations in *UROD* or other inherited factors.[36] Onset most commonly occurs during the fifth or sixth decade of life, but PCT may present earlier in hereditary forms.[36] PCT has been associated with alcohol use, hepatitis C, HIV, estrogen exposure, smoking, and mutations in the hemochromatosis gene.[36] Clinically, PCT presents with vesicles, bullae, and blistering on sun-exposed skin [**Figure 31-8A**].[36] However, patients with PCT may also have chronic skin fragility and blistering without direct relation to sun exposure.[3] Histology of vesicles reveal subepidermal bullae with irregular dermal papillae arising from the bullae floor into the cavity (festooning) [**Figure 31-8B**].[3] Management of PCT involves avoidance of aggravating factors (ie, alcohol, estrogen, certain drugs) and photoprotection from visible light.[36] Periodic phlebotomies and deferoxamine may help decrease hepatic iron stores.[36] Additionally, antimalarials such as 100 mg hydroxychloroquine twice a week (to minimize hepatotoxicity) may facilitate urinary excretion of iron and can be effective in treating PCT.[36]

Erythropoietic Protoporphyria Erythropoietic Protoporphyria (EPP) is the most common form of porphyria in children, caused by ferrochelatase gene mutations.[38] EPP is associated with elevated levels of protoporphyrin in the stool, plasma, and red blood cells without increased levels of coproporphyrin.[39] Urine porphyrin levels are typically normal.[39] Clinically, acute flares of EPP present with erythema and edema in sun-exposed areas after minutes to a few hours of sun exposure.[3,38] Cutaneous

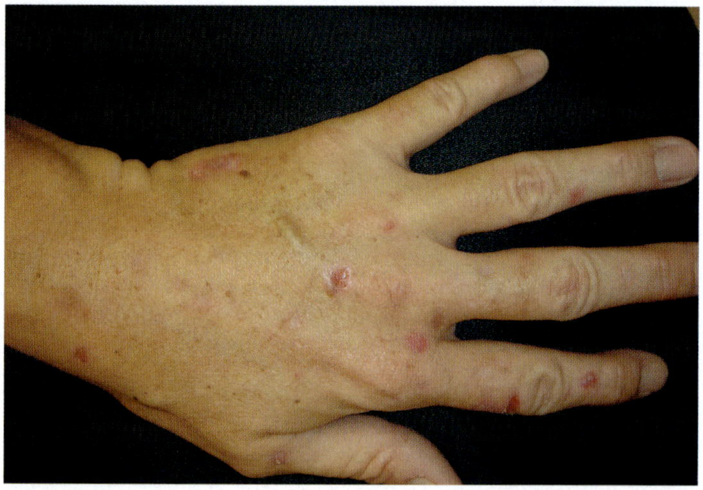

A

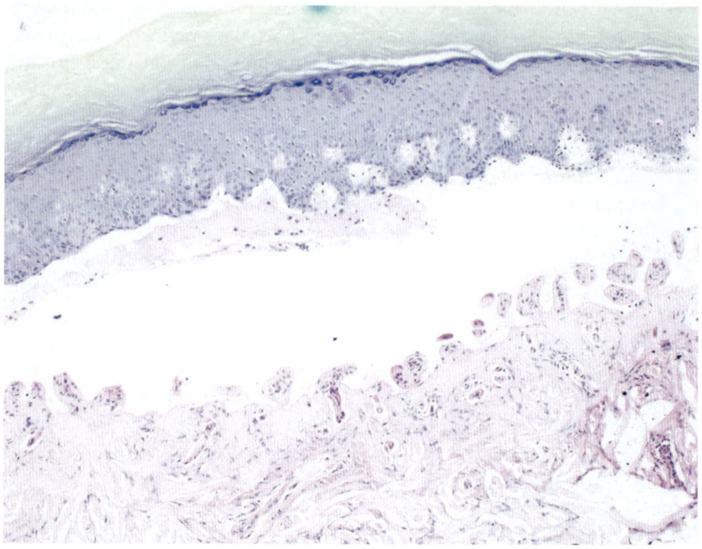

B

FIGURE 31-8. *Porphyria cutanea tarda.* **(A)** Vesicles, bullae, and erosions of the dorsal hand healing with atrophic scars. **(B)** Subepidermal bullae with festooning of the rete pegs. (Courtesy of Henry W. Lim, MD and Marsha Chaffins, MD, Department of Dermatology, Henry Ford Health, Detroit, MI, USA.)

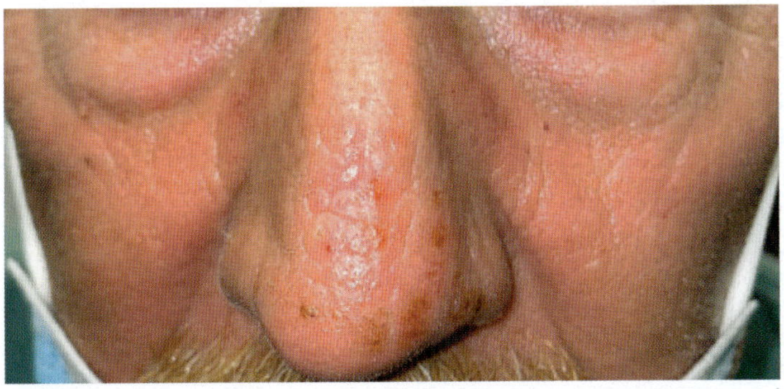

FIGURE 31-9. Erythropoietic protoporphyria. Cobblestone scarring of the nasal bridge.

TABLE 31-3 Summary of drugs commonly implicated in phototoxicity		
Medication class	Systemic agents	Topical agents
Antibiotics	Quinolones, Tetracyclines	
Antifungals	Voriconazole	
Cardiovascular drugs	Amiodarone, Hydrochlorothiazide	
Chemotherapeutic agents	Vemurafenib	
NSAIDs	Naproxen	
Phototoxic agents used in dermatology		Psoralen, Aminolevulinic acid
Psychotropic Drugs	Chlorpromazine	
Plants		Furocoumarins

Source: Adapted from Kim WB, Shelley AJ, Novice K, Joo J, Lim HW, Glassman SJ. Drug-induced phototoxicity: a systematic review. *J Am Acad Dermatol.* 2018;79(6):1069-1075.[48]

findings are typically accompanied by intense pain, burning, stinging, and itching that can last for several days.[3] In contrast to PCT, people with EPP do not classically develop skin fragility and blisters.[38] With chronic disease, cobblestone scarring of the nasal bridge [**Figure 31-9**] and dorsal hands are noted. EPP is associated with liver dysfunction, anemia, vitamin D deficiency, and gallstone formation.[38] Management involves photoprotection with sun avoidance and photoprotective clothing as sunscreen is typically not effective in this condition due to the action spectrum in the VL range.[38] Multiple therapies, such as beta carotene, phototherapy, and cimetidine have been tried for treatment of EPP.[40-42] The most consistently effective therapy is afamelanotide, an implantable alpha-melanocyte-stimulating hormone (α-MSH) analog that promotes eumelanin production. It has been shown to increase pain-free sun exposure in patients with EPP when compared to controls.[38,43] Longer-term studies support that afamelanotide is effective and well-tolerated in patients and has led to significant improvements in quality of life.[38,44] Trials of an oral α-MSH analog are underway and have promising initial results.[45] Novel mechanisms of treatment, including glycine transport inhibitors are also being explored.[46] Regular screening for symptoms of cholelithiasis and lab monitoring for anemia and hepatic dysfunction is recommended.[38] Cholestyramine and liver transplantation may be considered for hepatic complications.[38] Cholecystectomy may be needed for management of cholelithiasis. Bone marrow transplant can be curative but is typically only performed in very severe cases.

X-linked Protoporphyria X-linked protoporphyria (XLP) is caused by gain-of-function mutations of the erythroid-specific ALA synthase gene, *ALAS2,* causing accumulation of erythrocyte protoporphyrin.[38] Affected males tend to present with a more severe form of XLP, but in heterozygous females clinical severity and presentations may vary.[47] XLP shares similar clinical features as EPP, with pain and nonblistering phototoxicity within minutes of sun exposure.[38] Management of XLP is similar to EPP, with afamelanotide currently being the most effective therapeutic option.[38]

PHOTODERMATOSES SECONDARY TO EXOGENOUS AGENTS

PHOTOTOXICITY

Phototoxic reactions are caused by UV exposure to an exogenous agent, typically a drug or its metabolites, which leads to the generation of cytotoxic compounds, ROS, and direct tissue injury.[5] Both topical and systemic agents have been implicated as photosensitizing, and common offenders have been identified in a recent systematic review [**Table 31-3**].[3,5,48] Phototoxic reactions occur within minutes to hours of UV exposure (most commonly to UVB rather than to UVA and VL)[49] and present in sun-exposed areas as erythema, edema, and blistering [**Figure 31-10**].[5,50] Symptoms may include pain, tenderness, burning, and/or prickling.[50] Following phototoxic reactions, patients may observe persistent hyperpigmentation.[50] In dark-skinned individuals, postinflammatory hyperpigmentation is more common and may persist for years.[51] For patients suspected to have phototoxic reactions, phototesting is the diagnostic gold standard, and management includes removal of the offending photosensitizing agent and photoprotection.[5]

PHOTOALLERGY

In contrast to phototoxicity, photoallergy is a cell-mediated delayed hypersensitivity reaction that occurs after initial sensitization to a photoallergen, similar to allergic contact dermatitis.[5] Clinically, photoallergic reactions present with pruritic, papular, and eczematous eruptions 1 to 2 days following reexposure to an offending agent.[52] Mechanisms of photoallergic reactions are complex and involve photo-induced generation of an allergen, oxidative stress pathways, and cutaneous inflammatory responses.[53] During the initial UV exposure, photo-induced allergens bind to endogenous proteins in a process called haptenization.[5] The photoallergens then undergo additional processing by cutaneous LCs that promotes migration of LCs to the lymph nodes.[5,53] Within the lymph nodes, LCs present photoallergen complexes to naïve T cells, resulting in mature photoallergen-specific memory T-cells that play a role in photoallergic reactions in subsequent exposures [**Figure 31-11**].[5,53] Both topical and systemic offenders have been identified [**Table 31-4**].[5] Photoallergens may be detected with photopatch testing, and management involves removal of the offending agent and photoprotection.[5]

PSEUDOPORPHYRIA

Pseudoporphyria is a rare bullous photodermatosis that shares several clinical features with PCT, including skin fragility and blistering in

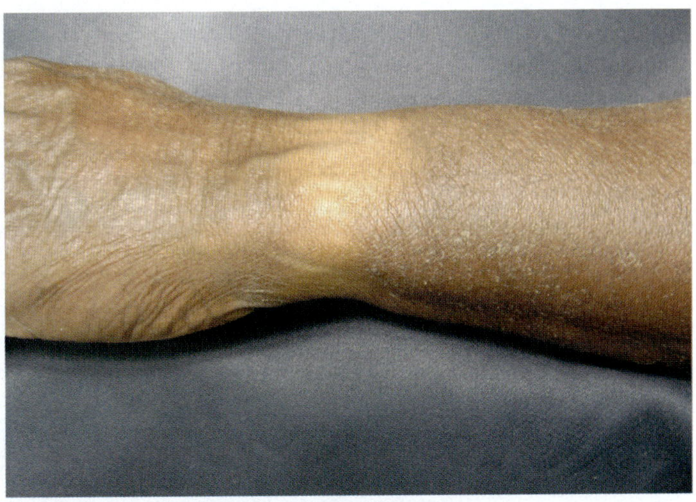

FIGURE 31-10. Phototoxicity. Hyperpigmentation, erythema, and desquamation of wrist from trimethoprim/sulfamethoxazole-induced phototoxicity. (Courtesy of Henry W. Lim, MD, Department of Dermatology, Henry Ford Health, Detroit, MI, USA.)

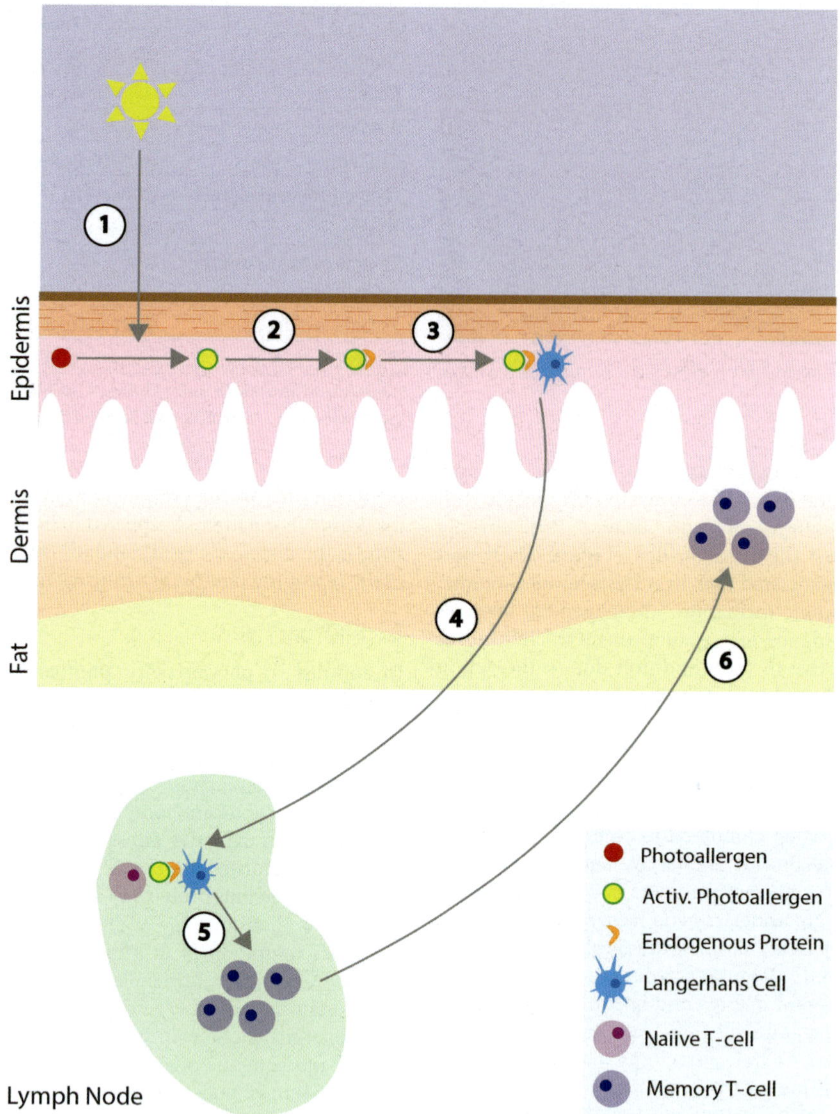

FIGURE 31-11. Proposed mechanism of photoallergy. (1) UV exposure activates an allergen to generate a photoallergen. (2) Photoallergens bind to endogenous proteins in a process called haptenization. (3) The photoallergen-protein complex is recognized by cutaneous Langerhans cells (LCs). (4) The LCs migrate to the lymph nodes. (5) Within the lymph nodes, the LCs present the photoallergen complex to naive T-cells, which generate mature photoallergen-specific memory T-cells. (6) Mature memory T-cells migrate to the skin and induce inflammatory reactions. (Adapted from Guan LL, Lim HW, Mohammad TF. Recognizing photoallergy, phototoxicity, and immune-mediated photodermatoses. *J Allergy Clin Immunol*. 2022;149(4):1206-1209.[5])

TABLE 31-4 Summary of drugs implicated in photoallergy

Medication class	Systemic agents	Topical agents
Antibiotics	Tetracyclines, quinolones, dapsone	Bithionol, chlorhexidine, dibromosalicylanilide, fenticlor, hexachlorophene, tetrachlorosalicylanilide
Antifungals	Griseofulvin	Bromochlorosalicylanilide, buclosamide
Antivirals	Efavirenz	Acyclovir
Cardiovascular drugs	Amiodarone, captopril, diltiazem, enalapril, fenofibrate, hydrochlorothiazide, methyldopa, ramipril, quinidine, simvastatin, valsartan	
Chemotherapeutic agents	Tegafur, vandetanib	
NSAIDs	Aceclofenac, benzydamine, celecoxib, diclofenac, keptoprofen, piroxicam, suprofen, tiaprofenic acid	Benzydamine, diclofenac, ketoprofen, prioxicam
UV Filters		Avobenzone, cinnamates, dibenzoylmethanes, mexenone, ecamsule, octocrylene, oxybenzone, PABA, salicylates, sulisobenzone
Psychotropic drugs	Amitriptyline, chlordiazepoxide, chlorpromazine, clomipramine, citalopram, flupentixol, fluphenazine, fluvoxamine, perazine, paroxetine, perphenazine, sertraline, thioridazine, trifluoperazine	
Others	Quinine, sulfonamides, sulfonylureas	Chlorpromazine, dibucaine, fenofibrate, hydrocortisone, sulfonamides

Source: Adapted from Guan LL, Lim HW, Mohammad TF. Recognizing photoallergy, phototoxicity, and immune-mediated photodermatoses. *J Allergy Clin Immunol.* 2022;149(4):1206-1209.[5]

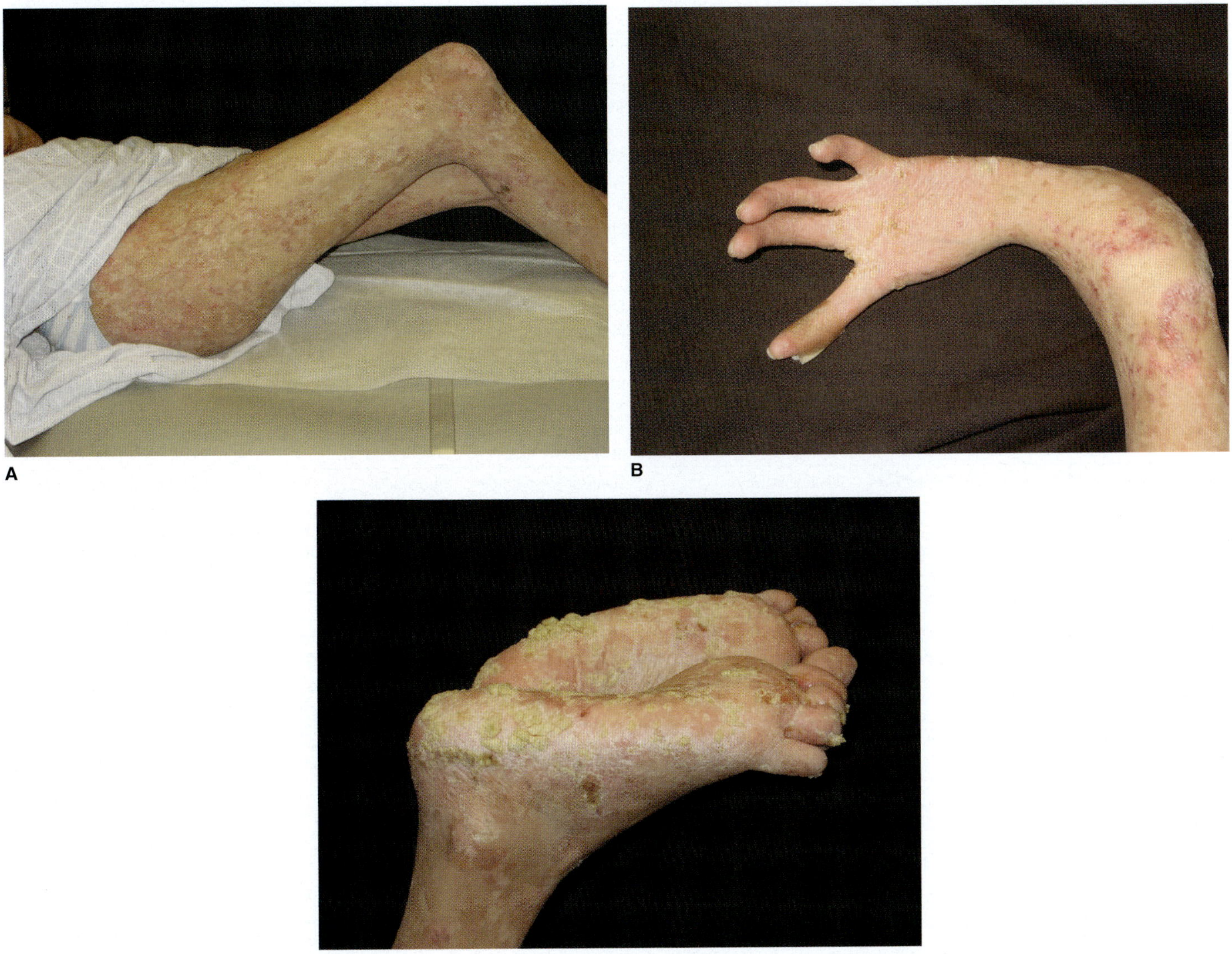

FIGURE 31-12. Rothmund-Thomson syndrome. Erythematous papules, vesicles, atrophic scars, and poikiloderma of thighs (A), wrists (B), and feet (C). Hyperkeratotic papules and plaques on bilateral soles of feet (C). (Courtesy of Tor A Shwayder, MD, Department of Dermatology, Henry Ford Health, Detroit, MI, USA.)

sun-exposed areas.[54,55] However, it is easily differentiated from PCT due to a lack in porphyrin elevation on biochemical analyses.[54,55] In the literature, pseudoporphyria has been linked to chronic renal failure, UVA exposure, and various drugs and substances, including NSAIDs, antibiotics, diuretics, and retinoids, among others.[54,55] These substances may act similarly to porphyrins, becoming photo-activated and contributing to the formation of blisters.[55] Treatment involves discontinuation of the suspected trigger, photoprotection, and avoidance of additional photosensitizing drugs.[55] Additional studies have suggested the efficacy of *N*-acetylcysteine and low doses of antimalarials in treatment of pseudoporphyria.[55]

PHOTOEXACERBATED DERMATOSES

Photoaggravated dermatoses include dermatomyositis, lupus, Darier disease, and pellagra.[56] These are reviewed in depth elsewhere.

GENODERMATOSES CHARACTERIZED BY PHOTOSENSITIVITY

Inherited photodermatoses are associated with defects in DNA repair, including DNA nucleotide excision repair (NER; xeroderma pigmentosum, trichothiodystrophy, Cockayne syndrome), double-strand break repair (Bloom syndrome, Rothmund-Thomson syndrome [**Figure 31-12**]), and alterations in biochemical substances (Smith-Lemli-Opitz syndrome and Hartnup disease).[56] **Table 31-5** reviews select inherited photodermatoses, and their associated action spectra can be found in Table 31-2.

MANAGEMENT OF PATIENTS WITH PHOTOSENSITIVITY

Initial laboratory workup of patients with photosensitivity may include a complete blood cell count and an autoimmune profile.[56] In cases of suspected porphyria, laboratory screening for blood, urine, and stool porphyrins may be performed.[56] Vitamin D levels should be checked to assess for deficiency given that sun avoidance is common in this population. Supplementation should be initiated if necessary.[11] Skin biopsy may be considered if there is diagnostic uncertainty.[56] Evaluation may also involve phototesting, provocative phototesting, or photopatch testing.[11]

Phototesting can confirm photosensitivity and specify the action spectra [Table 31-5]. Phototesting involves exposure of photoprotected areas of skin to increasing doses of UVA, UVB, and VL. During this time, patients with suspected solar urticaria should be monitored shortly after exposure for urticarial response.[11] After 24 hours, patients are assessed for the minimal erythema dosage (MED), defined by the lowest dose of UV radiation that produces perceptible erythema.[11,57] Decreased MED to

TABLE 31-5 Summary of genodermatoses[11]

Hereditary photodermatosis	Inheritance	Associated genes	Cutaneous features	Clinical associations	Proposed pathophysiology	Diagnostics	Management
Xeroderma pigmentosum	AR	*XPA, ERCC3* (*XPB*), *XPC, ERCC2* (*XPD*), *DBB2* (*XPE*), *ERCC4* (*XPF*), *ERCC5* (*XPG*), *ERCC1, POLH* (*XPV*)	Acute blistering and erythema after minimal UV exposure; Poikiloderma on sun-exposed areas before 2 years old; Increased risk of melanoma and nonmelanoma skin cancer; Increased lentigines pigmentary changes	Increased risk of neurologic abnormalities; Occasionally associated with ophthalmologic involvement; Growth abnormalities	Nucleotide Excision Repair	Clinical; DNA repair testing with cultured fibroblasts; Genetic analysis	Photoprotection, Vit D supplementation, Methylcellulose eye drops, Oral isotretinoin
Cockayne syndrome	AR	*ERCC8, ERCC6, ERCC3*	Photosensitivity without pigmentary changes; No increased skin cancer risk	Characteristic facies; Microcephaly; Short stature; Neurological dysfunction; Immature sexual development; Shortened lifespan (avg of 12 years)	Nucleotide Excision Repair	Clinical; Genetic analysis	No effective therapy; Photoprotection; Physical therapy; Gastrostomy tube
Trichothiodystrophy	AR	*XPD, XPB, p8/TTDA, TTDN1*	Photosensitivity	Sulfur-deficient brittle hair; Neuroectodermal defects; Characteristic facies; Short stature; Microcephaly; Intellectual impairment	Nucleotide Excision Repair	Polarizing and light microscopy of hair samples reveal "Tiger Tail" banding of hair shafts	Photoprotection, Emollients
Ultraviolet sensitive syndrome	AR	*ERCC6, ERCC8, UVSSA, CSB*	Photosensitivity; Freckling, Dyspigmentation on sun-exposed areas; No increased risk of skin cancer	No neurologic or developmental abnormalities	Nucleotide Excision Repair	Genetic analysis (normal GG-NER and deficiency of TC-NER of UV-induced cyclobutane pyrimidine dimers)	Photoprotection
Rothmund-Thomson syndrome	AR	*RECQL4*	Photosensitivity; Erythema, swelling, blistering of the face with sparing of the trunk and flexural areas within first few months of age; Poikiloderma within months to years later; Keratotic lesions	Small stature, Radiologic abnormalities, Early onset osteosarcoma, Cataracts; Sparse hair; Hypogonadism; Preserved immune function; Preserved intelligence	Double-strand break repair defect	Clinical; Genetic analysis	Photoprotection; Cataract surgery
Bloom syndrome	AR	*BLM*	Erythema and telangiectasia on sun-exposed areas within the first few weeks of life; Multiple café-au-lait macules	Increased predisposition to all cancers; Lymphoma; Leukemia; Male; Dwarfism; GERD; Recurrent respiratory and GI infections	Double Strand Break Repair Defect	Clinical; Cytogenetics (quadriradial in cultured blood lymphocytes or a greatly increased frequency of sister-chromatid exchanges in cultured cells of any type); Genetic analysis	Photoprotection; Antibiotics; GERD management
Smith-Lemli-Opitz syndrome	AR	*DHCR7*	Photosensitivity	Growth retardation; Mental retardation; Hypospadias; Characteristic facies; Congenital heart defects; GI anomalies; Cognitive and behavioral issues	Biochemical Alterations	Clinical; Elevated 7-DHC; Genetic analysis	Photoprotection; Cholesterol supplementation
Hartnup disease	AR	*SLC6A19*	Pellagra-like skin eruptions; Symmetric erythematous macules that coalesce and scale in sun-exposed areas; Appears in spring/summer; Cutaneous symptoms usually precede neurological symptoms	Cerebellar ataxia, Psychiatric diseases; Gross aminoaciduria	Biochemical alterations	Elevations of neutral amino acids in urine; Plasma amino acids typically normal	Photoprotection; High-protein diet; High doses of oral nicotinic acid or nicotinamide
Kindler syndrome	AR	*FERMT1*	Transient, early-onset photosensitivity; Poikiloderma; Trauma-induced skin blistering; mucosal fragility; Increased cancer risk	Stenosis of the esophagus, vagina, anus, urethra; Colitis; Pseudosyndactyly, conjunctivitis, mandibular abnormalities, Orogenital leukokeratosis	Other; May be associated with oxidative stress, UVB-induced apoptosis, and mitochondrial dysfunction	Clinical; Biopsy reveals poikilodermatous changes; Ultrastructural study identifies duplication of lamina densa; Genetic analysis	Photoprotection

the tested wavelengths is suggestive of a photosensitivity disorder. Provocative phototesting involves repeated irradiation over several consecutive days to determine whether lesions, such as those seen in PMLE and LE, may be induced.[58,59] Photopatch testing is used when photoallergic dermatitis is suspected.[11] Photopatch testing involves placing parallel panels of common photoallergens to two uninvolved areas of skin on the back. After 24 hours, MED is assessed and one of the panels is exposed to UVA while the other is kept unexposed.[11] After 48 hours, both skin sites are examined to identify differences suggestive of photoallergy.[11] If the nonirradiated panel includes a positive read, the most likely contributor is allergic contact dermatitis.[5] If the irradiated panel includes a positive read with concomitant negative read on the nonirradiated panel, the most likely explanation is a photoallergic process.[5]

Determination of MED may vary with skin types, as experience in evaluating erythema in pigmented skin varies. Several studies report increasing MED values in Fitzpatrick skin types II to VI.[60-62] Recent studies have proposed using different phototesting thresholds in different skin types.[61] However, MED values can range significantly within a skin type.[9]

In general, photoprotection is an essential component of management of various photodermatoses.[11] Photoprotection includes behavioral modifications to encourage sun avoidance, such as wearing a wide brim hat, sunglasses, and photoprotective clothing.[11] A letter of medical necessity for patients to obtain tinted windows can also be helpful. Patients should utilize a broad-spectrum sunscreen, with an SPF of at least 30.[5,11] Higher SPF sunscreens may offer additional protection given that most people apply sunscreen at lower concentrations than used in SPF testing.[63,64] Those with photosensitivity to visible light can benefit from VL protection from tinted broad-spectrum sunscreens. Patient counseling should include education about the avoidance of tanning beds and caution around reflective surfaces such as water, snow, and sand.[11] If patients are suspected to have a photodermatosis associated with increased malignancy risk, strict photoprotection and regular cancer screening is encouraged.[11]

As UV radiation exposure generates ROS, antioxidants may be considered in patients with photodermatoses.[65] Topical antioxidants include vitamin C, vitamin E, vitamin A, selenium, silymarin, tea polyphenols, soy isoflavones, among others.[65] When used in combination with UV filters, topical antioxidants may offer additional photoprotection.[65] Recently, studies support the therapeutic potential of *Polypodium leucotomos*, an antioxidant and a photoprotective agent, in photodermatoses such as PMLE.[66]

CONCLUSION

Photodermatoses can affect individuals of all races, ages, and sexes. Prevalence rates and presentations may vary in patients with skin of color, but a comprehensive history, complete physical exam, and appropriate laboratory testing can aid in diagnosis. At this time, the general mainstay of therapy involves photoprotection, with variations in therapeutic options based on the specific photodermatoses. Novel treatment options are in development and may provide additional improvement in symptom relief and quality of life for these patients.

REFERENCES

1. International Agency for Research on Cancer, World Health Organization, United Kingdom. *Solar and Ultraviolet Radiation*. 1992.
2. de Gruijl FR. Skin cancer and solar UV radiation. *Eur J Cancer*. 1999;35(14):2003-2009.
3. Chantorn R, Lim HW, Shwayder TA. Photosensitivity disorders in children: part I. *J Am Acad Dermatol*. 2012;67(6):1093.e1-18.
4. Maddodi N, Jayanthy A, Setaluri V. Shining light on skin pigmentation: the darker and the brighter side of effects of UV radiation. *Photochem Photobiol*. 2012;88(5):1075-1082.
5. Guan LL, Lim HW, Mohammad TF. Recognizing photoallergy, phototoxicity, and immune-mediated photodermatoses. *J Allergy Clin Immunol*. 2022;149(4):1206-1209.
6. Zhao X-Q. [One-stop multi-mode computed tomography in the diagnosis and management of acute intracerebral hemorrhage]. *Zhonghua Yi Xue Za Zhi*. 2012;92(31):2171-2173.
7. Kadekaro AL, Kavanagh RJ, Wakamatsu K, Ito S, Pipitone MA, Abdel-Malek ZA. Cutaneous photobiology. The melanocyte vs. the sun: who will win the final round? *Pigment Cell Res*. 2003;16(5):434-447.
8. Nasti TH, Timares L. MC1R, eumelanin and pheomelanin: their role in determining the susceptibility to skin cancer. *Photochem Photobiol*. 2015;91(1):188-200.
9. Carretero-Mangolis C, Lim HW. Correlation between skin types and minimal erythema dose in narrowband UVB (TL-01) phototherapy. *Photodermatol Photoimmunol Photomed*. 2001;17(5):244-246.
10. Yashar SS, Lim HW. Classification and evaluation of photodermatoses. *Dermatol Ther*. 2003;16(1):1-7.
11. Nahhas AF, Oberlin DM, Braunberger TL, Lim HW. Recent developments in the diagnosis and management of photosensitive disorders. *Am J Clin Dermatol*. 2018;19(5):707-731.
12. Artz CE, Farmer CM, Lim HW. Polymorphous light eruption: a Review. *Curr Derm Rep*. 2019;8(3):110-116.
13. Kerr HA, Lim HW. Photodermatoses in African Americans: a retrospective analysis of 135 patients over a 7-year period. *J Am Acad Dermatol*. 2007;57(4):638-643.
14. Nakamura M, Henderson M, Jacobsen G, Lim HW. Comparison of photodermatoses in African-Americans and Caucasians: a follow-up study. *Photodermatol Photoimmunol Photomed*. 2014;30(5):231-236.
15. Tzaneva S, Volc-Platzer B, Kittler H, Hönigsmann H, Tanew A. Antinuclear antibodies in patients with polymorphic light eruption: a long-term follow-up study. *Br J Dermatol*. 2008;158(5):1050-1054.
16. Lembo S, Raimondo A. Polymorphic light eruption: what's new in pathogenesis and management. *Front Med (Lausanne)*. 2018;5:252.
17. Ling TC, Dawe RS, Gardener E, Rhodes LE. Interventions for polymorphic light eruption. *Cochrane Database Sys Rev*. 2017;2017(10):2-3.
18. Gruber-Wackernagel A, Bambach I, Legat FJ, et al. Randomized double-blinded placebo-controlled intra-individual trial on topical treatment with a 1,25-dihydroxyvitamin D_3 analogue in polymorphic light eruption. *Br J Dermatol*. 2011;165(1):152-163.
19. Pile HD, Crane JS. *Actinic Prurigo*. Treasure Island (FL): StatPearls Publishing; 2022.
20. Adler BL, DeLeo VA. Actinic prurigo and hydroa vacciniforme. *Curr Derm Rep*. 2019;8(2):63-72.
21. Cuevas-Gonzalez JC, Vega-Memíje ME, Borges-Yáñez SA, Rodríguez-Lobato E. Risk factors associated with actinic prurigo: a case control study. *An Bras Dermatol*. 2017;92(6):774-778.
22. Paek SY, Lim HW. Chronic actinic dermatitis. *Dermatol Clin*. 2014;32(3):355-61-viii-ix.
23. Hamel R, Mohammad TF, Chahine A, et al. Comparison of racial distribution of photodermatoses in USA academic dermatology clinics: a multicenter retrospective analysis of 1080 patients over a 10-year period. *Photodermatol Photoimmunol Photomed*. 2020;36(3):233-240.
24. Tan K-W, Haylett AK, Ling TC, Rhodes LE. Comparison of demographic and photobiological features of chronic actinic dermatitis in patients with lighter vs darker skin types. *JAMA Dermatol*. 2017;153(5):427-435.
25. Dawe RS, Ferguson J. Diagnosis and treatment of chronic actinic dermatitis. *Dermatol Ther*. 2003;16(1):45-51.
26. Deleo V. Sunscreen use in photodermatoses. *Dermatol Clin*. 2006;24(1):27-33.
27. Vesely MD, Imaeda S, King BA. Tofacitinib citrate for the treatment of refractory, severe chronic actinic dermatitis. *JAAD Case Rep*. 2017;3(1):4-6.
28. Bhari N, Gupta S. Tacrolimus 0.1% ointment applied under occlusion using cling film clears chronic actinic dermatitis resistant to systemic treatment. *Int J Dermatol*. 2017;56(6):e139-e141.
29. Patel N, Konda S, Lim HW. Dupilumab for the treatment of chronic actinic dermatitis. *Photodermatol Photoimmunol Photomed*. 2020;36(5):398-400.
30. Ali K, Wu L, Lou H, et al. Clearance of chronic actinic dermatitis with dupilumab therapy in Chinese patients: a case series. *Front Med (Lausanne)*. 2022;9:803692.
31. Gupta G, Man I, Kemmett D. Hydroa vacciniforme: a clinical and follow-up study of 17 cases. *J Am Acad Dermatol*. 2000;42(2 Pt 1):208-213.
32. Wang M, Wang S, Yang Q-P, et al. Hydroa vacciniforme-like lymphoma of an adult: a case report with review of the literature. *Diagn Pathol*. 2013;8(1):72-74.
33. Chen C-C, Chang K-C, Medeiros LJ, Lee JY-Y. Hydroa vacciniforme and hydroa vacciniforme-like lymphoproliferative disorder: a spectrum of disease phenotypes associated with ultraviolet irradiation and chronic Epstein-Barr virus infection. *Int J Mol Sci*. 2020;21(23):9314.

34. Hirai Y, Yamamoto T, Kimura H, et al. Hydroa vacciniforme is associated with increased numbers of Epstein-Barr virus-infected γδT cells. *J Invest Dermatol.* 2012;132(5):1401-1408.
35. Snast I, Kremer N, Lapidoth M, et al. Omalizumab for the treatment of solar urticaria: case series and systematic review of the literature. *J Allergy Clin Immunol Pract.* 2018;6(4):1198-1204.e3.
36. Singal AK. Porphyria cutanea tarda: recent update. *Mol Genet Metab.* 2019;128(3):271-281.
37. Frank J, Poblete-Gutiérrez P. Porphyria cutanea tarda–when skin meets liver. *Best Pract Res Clin Gastroenterol.* 2010;24(5):735-745.
38. Balwani M. Erythropoietic protoporphyria and X-linked protoporphyria: pathophysiology, genetics, clinical manifestations, and management. *Mol Genet Metab.* 2019;128(3):298-303.
39. Thapar M, Bonkovsky HL. The diagnosis and management of erythropoietic protoporphyria. *Gastroenterol Hepatol (N Y).* 2008;4(8):561-566.
40. Heerfordt IM, Lerche CM, Wulf HC. Cimetidine for erythropoietic protoporphyria. *Photodiagnosis Photodyn Ther.* 2022;38:102793.
41. Sivaramakrishnan M, Woods J, Dawe R. Narrowband ultraviolet B phototherapy in erythropoietic protoporphyria: case series. *Br J Dermatol.* 2014;170(4):987-988.
42. Warren LJ, George S. Erythropoietic protoporphyria treated with narrow-band (TL-01) UVB phototherapy. *Australas J Dermatol.* 1998;39(3):179-182.
43. Kim ES, Garnock-Jones KP. Afamelanotide: a review in erythropoietic protoporphyria. *Am J Clin Dermatol.* 2016;17(2):179-185.
44. Biolcati G, Marchesini E, Sorge F, Barbieri L, Schneider-Yin X, Minder EI. Long-term observational study of afamelanotide in 115 patients with erythropoietic protoporphyria. *Br J Dermatol.* 2015;172(6):1601-1612.
45. Study to evaluate efficacy, safety, and tolerability of MT-7117 in subjects with erythropoietic protoporphyria or X-linked protoporphyria. ClinicalTrials.gov. https://clinicaltrials.gov/ct2/show/NCT04402489. Accessed March 2, 2025.
46. Halloy F, Iyer PS, Ghidini A, et al. Repurposing of glycine transport inhibitors for the treatment of erythropoietic protoporphyria. *Cell Chem Biol.* 2021;28(8):1221-1234.e1226.
47. Di Pierro E, Granata F, De Canio M, et al. Recognized and emerging features of erythropoietic and X-linked protoporphyria. *Diagnostics (Basel).* 2022;12(1):151.
48. Kim WB, Shelley AJ, Novice K, Joo J, Lim HW, Glassman SJ. Drug-induced phototoxicity: a systematic review. *J Am Acad Dermatol.* 2018;79(6):1069-1075.
49. Mang R, Stege H, dermatitis JKC. *Mechanisms of Phototoxic and Photoallergic Reactions.* Springer, Berlin, Heidelberg; 2006
50. Lankerani L, Baron ED. Photosensitivity to exogenous agents. *J Cutan Med Surg.* 2004;8(6):424-431.
51. Taylor S, Grimes P, Lim J, Im S, Lui H. Postinflammatory hyperpigmentation. *J Cutan Med Surg.* 2009;13(4):183-191.
52. Epstein JH. Photoallergy: a review. *Arch Dermatol.* 1972;106(5):741-748.
53. Kowalska J, Rok J, Rzepka Z, Wrześniok D. Drug-induced photosensitivity-from light and chemistry to biological reactions and clinical symptoms. *Pharmaceuticals (Basel).* 2021;14(8):723.
54. Green JJ, Manders SM. Pseudoporphyria. *J Am Acad Dermatol.* 2001;44(1):100-108.
55. Gil-Lianes J, Luque-Luna M, Morgado-Carrasco D, Aguilera-Peiró P. Pseudoporphyria-a diagnostic challenge: a case series and a proposed diagnostic algorithm. *Photodermatol Photoimmunol Photomed.* 2022;38(6):604-607.
56. Chantorn R, Lim HW, Shwayder TA. Photosensitivity disorders in children: part II. *J Am Acad Dermatol.* 2012;67(6):1113.e1-15-quiz1128-1127.
57. Heckman CJ, Chandler R, Kloss JD, et al. Minimal erythema dose (MED) testing. *J Vis Exp.* 2013;(75):e50175.
58. Das S, Lloyd JJ, Walshaw D, Farr PM. Provocation testing in polymorphic light eruption using fluorescent ultraviolet (UV) A and UVB lamps. *Br J Dermatol.* 2004;151(5):1066-1070.
59. Kuhn A, Sonntag M, Richter-Hintz D, et al. Phototesting in lupus erythematosus: a 15-year experience. *J Am Acad Dermatol.* 2001;45(1):86-95.
60. Wee LK, Chong TK, Quee DK. Assessment of skin types, skin colours and cutaneous responses to ultraviolet radiation in an Asian population. *Photodermatol Photoimmunol Photomed.* 1997;13(5-6):169-172.
61. Welti M, Ramelyte E, Dummer R, Imhof L. Evaluation of the minimal erythema dose for UVB and UVA in context of skin phototype and nature of photodermatosis. *Photodermatol Photoimmunol Photomed.* 2020;36(3):200-207.
62. Gambichler T, Moussa G, Tomi NS, Paech V, Altmeyer P, Kreuter A. Reference limits for erythema-effective UV doses. *Photochem Photobiol.* 2006;82(4):1097-1102.
63. Ouyang H, Meyer K, Maitra P, et al. Realistic sunscreen durability: a randomized, double-blinded, controlled clinical study. *J Drugs Dermatol.* 2018;17(1):116-117.
64. Kim SM, Oh BH, Lee YW, Choe YB, Ahn KJ. The relation between the amount of sunscreen applied and the sun protection factor in Asian skin. *J Am Acad Dermatol.* 2010;62(2):218-222.
65. Chen L, Hu JY, Wang SQ. The role of antioxidants in photoprotection: a critical review. *J Am Acad Dermatol.* 2012;67(5):1013-1024.
66. Berman B, Ellis C, Elmets C. Polypodium leucotomos–an overview of basic investigative findings. *J Drugs Dermatol.* 2016;15(2):224-228.

CHAPTER 32

Amyloidosis

Tiffany Mayo
Sydney A. Weir

KEY POINTS

- Amyloidosis is a spectrum of disorders resulting from abnormal folding and deposition of protein in various organs and tissues of the body.
- Amyloidosis is categorized as primary systemic (AL, AA, hereditary) and localized cutaneous (macular amyloidosis, lichen amyloidosis, nodular amyloidosis, and familiar primary localized amyloidosis) types.
- Lichen amyloidosis more commonly affects individuals with skin of color, particularly individuals of Asian descent.
- Treatments for amyloidosis are not curative and are primarily aimed at alleviating symptoms of pruritus.

INTRODUCTION

The first cases of amyloidosis were reported as early as the 1600s and described patients with "waxy" or "lardaceous" degeneration of the spleen, liver, and kidneys.[1] The substance deposited in these organs was named amyloid after it was incorrectly identified as a starchy material; however, we now know amyloid is an insoluble fibrous protein appearing homogenous and amorphous under light microscopy. When stained with Congo red, amyloid produces a yellow-green birefringence under polarized light.[1] Amyloid is characterized by linear, nonbranching, aggregated fibrils 7.5 to 10.0 nm wide under electron microscopy.[1] These aggregated fibrils are arranged in a meshwork pattern, and each fibril has a β-pleated sheet configuration.[2] Aβ fibrils, naturally occurring types of amyloid, share a common quaternary structure: parallel β-sheet conformation.[3]

Amyloidosis is a spectrum of disorders caused by the abnormal folding and extracellular deposition of proteins in various organs and tissues of the body.[4] Several classifications of amyloidosis exist defined by amyloid protein type. Based on an updated classification system, 36 amyloidogenic proteins in humans have been identified, and there are 18 different systemic and 22 various localized forms of amyloidosis.[5] Localized amyloidosis refers to the deposition of amyloid in one tissue type (commonly the tracheobronchial tree, urinary tract, or skin), not due to an underlying systemic clonal plasma cell disorder.[6] Clinically, it is critical to determine the subtype of amyloidosis to assess whether it is systemic versus localized or sporadic versus hereditary. These factors determine the clinical manifestations and treatability of the disease.[7]

AL and AA amyloidoses, previously known as primary and secondary amyloidoses, respectively, are considered the most common forms of systemic amyloidoses worldwide. AL refers to amyloid derived from immunoglobulin light chain; AL amyloidosis is characterized by kappa or lambda monoclonal light chains, or their fragments, depositing in various tissues.[8] In this subtype, 70% of patients present with renal and cardiac involvement.[7] In contrast, AA refers to amyloid fibrils derived from serum amyloid A (SAA) protein, an acute-phase reactant produced by the liver; AA amyloidosis, secondary to the deposition of SSA proteins in different organs, is typically associated with an underlying chronic inflammatory process.[7,9] This subtype of amyloidosis is more common in developing countries due to the high prevalence of associated infectious diseases. However, AA amyloidosis can also be correlated to autoinflammatory diseases (ie, inflammatory bowel disease).[7]

While hereditary amyloidoses are individually uncommon, the group collectively constitutes approximately 10% of all systemic amyloidoses cases.[7] Hereditary transthyretin (ATTRv) amyloidosis remains the most common hereditary amyloidosis worldwide; mutations in the gene that produces transthyretin, a protein primarily produced by the liver, results in the aggregation of transthyretin monomers into amyloid fibrils.[10] Hereditary ATTRv is autosomal dominant with variable penetrance and age of onset; family history is often lacking.[7] The skin can be variably affected by systemic sporadic or hereditary amyloidosis. The cutaneous signs, which are more indicative of systemic involvement, include hemorrhages, waxy papules that are pruritic and/or hemorrhagic, macroglossia, and lesions resembling scleroderma.[11]

In contrast to systemic amyloidosis, localized cutaneous amyloidosis is characterized by the extracellular deposition of amyloid proteins in the skin without systemic involvement.[12] The major subtypes of localized cutaneous amyloidosis include macular amyloidosis, lichen amyloidosis, nodular amyloidosis, familial primary localized amyloidosis, amyloidosis cutis dyschromia, and secondary localized cutaneous amyloidosis. Macular amyloidosis and lichen amyloidosis are thought to be different clinical manifestations of the same disease, and both types can be seen in the same patient. This coexistent condition is termed biphasic amyloidosis. Secondary cutaneous amyloidosis results from amyloid deposition due to the presence of another primary skin condition. These conditions include sweat gland tumors, dermatofibroma, pilomatrixoma, seborrheic keratosis, basal cell carcinoma, Bowen disease, actinic keratosis, and solar elastosis induced by psoralen and ultraviolet A (PUVA) therapy.[13]

Freudenthal first introduced the term lichen amyloidosis in 1930.[14] Individuals with skin of color, mainly Asian and Southeast Asian, Middle Eastern, and South American individuals, seem to be predisposed to developing localized cutaneous amyloidosis, especially lichen amyloidosis.[15-20]

Lichen amyloidosis is the most common form of primary localized cutaneous amyloidosis (PLCA) and one of the top skin disorders affecting those of Asian ethnicity.[21] The remainder of this chapter will include a discussion of primary localized cutaneous amyloidosis; however, emphasis will be on primary cutaneous lichen amyloidosis, as this form more often affects patients with Fitzpatrick skin types III and IV.

PATHOGENESIS

Many factors have been implicated as possible etiologic factors in primary localized cutaneous amyloidosis [**Table 32-1**].[22-26] In addition to the various disease risks, there are several theories of the pathogenesis. In the lichen and macular types of PLCA, it is thought that the amyloid deposits are derived from keratin intermediate filament proteins.[27] Specifically, degeneration of basal keratinocytes releases cytokeratin that becomes coated with autoantibodies, phagocytosed by macrophages, and enzymatically degraded to form amyloid.[28] Immunohistochemical stains identifying antikeratin antibodies support this theory.[29]

Another theory suggests that lichen amyloidosis is mediated by sweat gland or duct dysfunction. Disturbance to the sweat gland or duct results in the release of sweat into the dermo-epidermal junction triggering an inflammatory response; inflammation then causes damage to the overlying epidermis, which becomes a nidus for amyloid deposition.[27] Additionally, a mutation in the filaggrin (FLG) gene has been identified in certain genetic cases of lichen amyloidosis.[30] FLG mutations in patients of Asian descent have been reported to cause unique ripple-pattern lichen amyloidosis at sites with a predilection for ichthyosis vulgaris.[30] In other types of autosomal dominant PLCA, mutations of the oncostatin M receptor gene and interleukin-31 receptor RA gene have been implicated.[31] Multiple endocrine neoplasia type 2A (MEN2A) has been reported to be rarely associated with cutaneous lichen amyloidosis.[32]

Two other theories of the mechanism of amyloid formation in lichen and macular amyloidosis include the Hashimoto fibrillar body theory of amyloidogenesis and the secretion theory. Hashimoto's fibrillar body theory of amyloidogenesis proposes that epidermal basal keratinocytes are transformed into amyloid proteins from modified colloid bodies.[33] This theory is supported by histologic and ultrastructural studies demonstrating transitional forms between keratinocytes and amyloids and by changes in the antigenic profile from basal keratinocytes to amyloids via colloid bodies.[34-36]

The secretion theory proposes disrupted basal keratinocytes secrete precursor proteins at the epidermal-dermal interface.[37] It has been supported by ultrastructural evidence of a *lamina densa* disruption above the amyloid deposits in lichen amyloidosis and similar electron microscopic evidence of a *lamina densa* disruption in patients with lichen and macular amyloidosis.[35,38]

Regardless of the exact mechanism of amyloid formation, a cycle of chronic pruritis and scratching may contribute to increased amyloid production. Conditions that result in chronic pruritis, such as chronic kidney disease, are considered potential triggers.[39-41]

TABLE 32-1 Possible etiologic factors for primary cutaneous amyloidosis[20,23-25]
Friction from chronic scratching or rubbing
Genetic predisposition
History of atopy
Epstein-Barr virus
Human immunodeficiency virus infection
Environmental factors

CLINICAL PRESENTATION

Lichen amyloidosis is characterized by multiple or rarely generalized firm, discrete, hyperpigmented, and hyperkeratotic, scaly papules that may coalesce to form plaques [**Figure 32-1**]. The lesions tend to have a predilection for the shins, calves, ankles, and dorsa of the feet and thighs.[12] Less commonly, solitary involvement of the scalp or face, specifically the upper lip and nasolabial folds, have been reported.[42,43] Pruritus is a prominent feature of lichen amyloidosis.[12] Additionally, bullous lesions have been described in patients with lichen amyloidosis; however, they are rare and are more commonly found in those with systemic amyloidosis.[31] Lichen amyloidosis may commonly be seen in patients with atopic dermatitis, sarcoidosis, and psoriatic patients receiving PUVA.[39,40,42]

Macular amyloidosis presents as pruritic pigmented macules and/or plaques with a rippled surface [**Figure 32-2**]. The lesions are often seen on the upper back but may occur on the extensor surfaces of the upper extremities. An associated reticulated or rippled pigmentation may also be visible.[12] Macular and lichen amyloidosis typically arises in adulthood.[44] Nodular amyloidosis is typified by grouped or solitary waxy nodules with associated atrophic dermis and telangiectasias.[12]

Dermoscopy of both lichen and macular amyloidosis reveals predominant central hubs of brown and/or white colors, surrounded by brownish pigmentation, and are classified into three primary patterns—fine streaks ("spoke-wheel" pattern), leaf-like extensions, and thick noncircular pedal projections.[45-47] Patterns in nodular amyloidosis are described as atypical with a varying yellow appearance with teardrop-link areas and a homogenous background with serpiginous vessels.[48]

A familial form of primary cutaneous amyloidosis occurs rarely. In all reported cases, inheritance was autosomal dominant. Although most families had skin of color, there have also been reports of families with Fitzpatrick skin types I and II who had this form of amyloidosis.[49-58] Therefore, skin phototypes III and IV may not be a predisposing factor in familial macular and lichen amyloidosis.

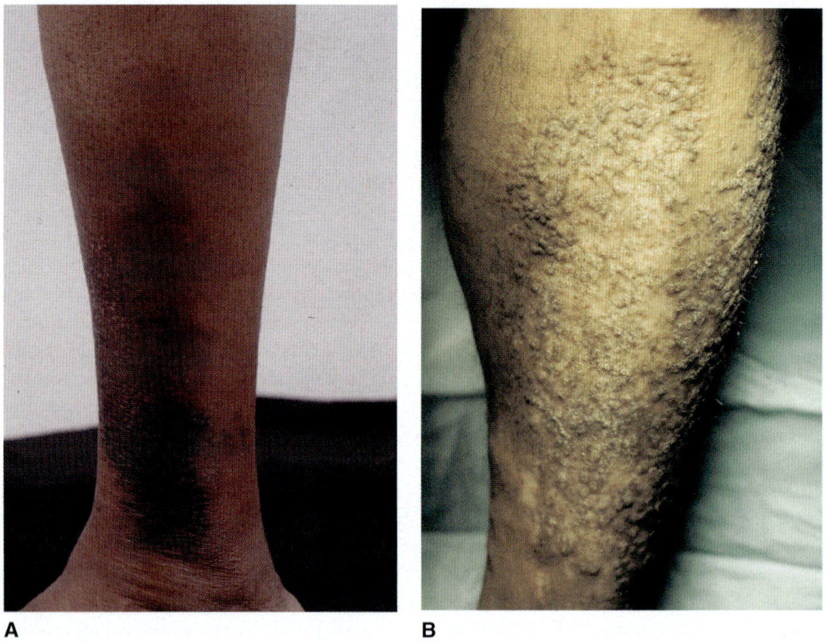

FIGURE 32-1. (A and B) Lichen amyloidosis displaying hyperpigmented and hyperkeratotic scaly papules coalescing into plaques on patients with darker skin of color.

PATHOLOGY

The amyloid deposits are restricted primarily to the papillary dermis mostly in dermal papillae between epidermal rete ridges.[59] The epidermis above the deposits may show acanthosis or thinning and hyperkeratosis. Typically, in macular amyloidosis, the epidermis appears normal.[59] In both macular and lichen amyloidosis, there are often perivascular lymphohistiocytic infiltrate, as well as pigment incontinence [Figure 32-2].

Amyloid deposits can be better visualized using special stains, and Congo red stain is the most effective. When this stain is combined with polarized light, amyloid deposits emit a characteristic apple-green birefringence. Other histologic stains that may also stain amyloid deposits but Congo red is most commonly used [**Figure 32-3**].[60] Additionally, direct immunofluorescence (DIF) may be used in the diagnosis of macular and lichen amyloidosis with a higher sensitivity than Congo Red staining.[61] DIF findings for macular amyloidosis primarily show positivity for IgM and C3 in the papillary dermis, whereas lichen amyloidosis will show positivity for IgM (predominately), C3, and IgA throughout the basement membrane zone.[61,62]

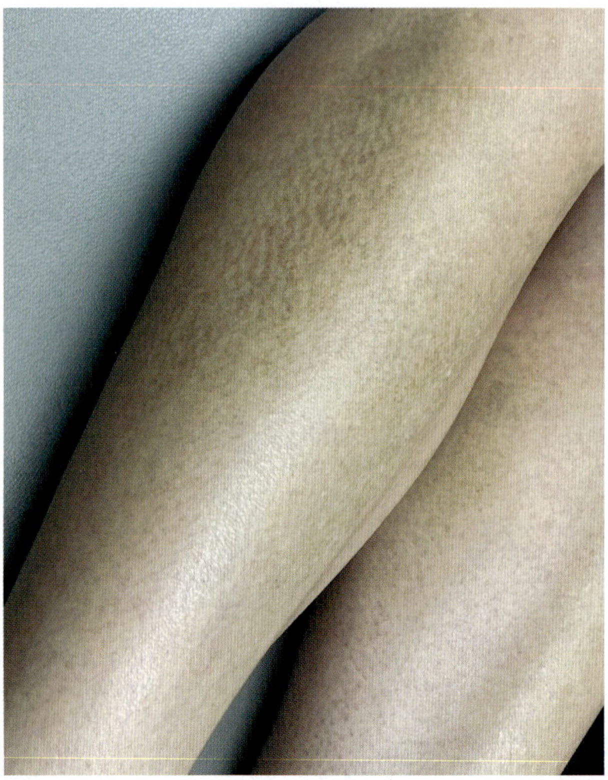

FIGURE 32-2. Macular amyloidosis on leg with characteristic rippled presentation.

TREATMENT

Lichen and macular amyloidosis are chronic skin disorders that rarely show complete response to any single treatment modality. Treatment options aim to alleviate the symptoms of pruritus rather than removing the amyloid deposits [**Table 32-2**]. Possible precipitating and/or aggravating factors, such as chronic friction induced by scratching and rubbing, should be avoided or treated in the case of atopic dermatitis.[12,39]

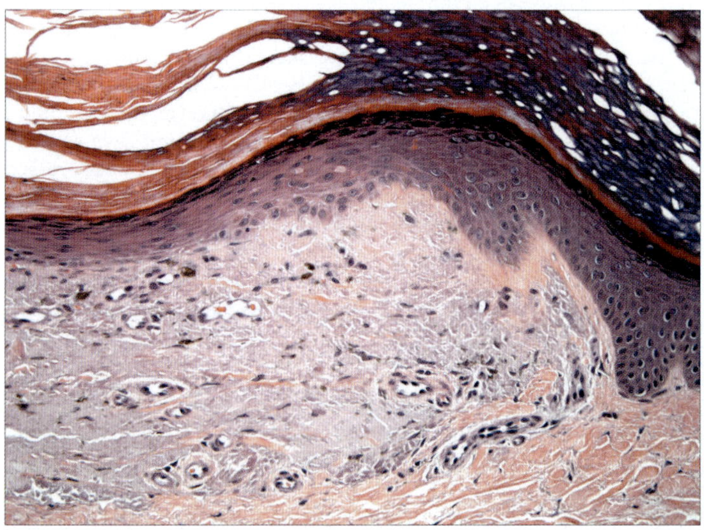

FIGURE 32-3. Using a hematoxylin and eosin stain, this figure shows hyperkeratosis with a thinning of the epidermis. In the papillary dermis, amyloid deposits are seen, as well as a sparse perivascular lymphohistiocytic infiltrate.

TABLE 32-2 Treatment options for primary cutaneous amyloidosis[12,39,40,63-82]

Treat or remove precipitating and/or aggravating factors
Topical corticosteroids (with or without occlusion)
Intralesional corticosteroids
Keratolytic agents
Calcipotriol
Topical tacrolimus
Dimethyl sulfoxide
Phototherapy with narrowband ultraviolet B and photochemotherapy (psoralen with ultraviolet A)
Systemic and topical retinoids
Cyclosporine
Tricholoric acid peels
Dupilumab
JAK inhibitors
Dermabrasion
Laser therapies: Erbium:yttrium aluminum garnet laser Q-switched neodymium-doped yttrium aluminum garnet laser Fractional carbon dioxide laser Ytterbium/erbium laser
Pulsed dye laser
Surgical removal with scapel

In mild cases, topical corticosteroids (with or without occlusion) and intralesional corticosteroids are the first lines of treatment.[12,63,64] The addition of a keratolytic agent, such as urea or salicylic acid, may also be beneficial.[12] It has been shown that calcipotriol can be effective in the treatment of lichen amyloidosis.[64] Tacrolimus has also been reported to have a beneficial effect and may be used as a topical alternative for corticosteroids; 2 months of tacrolimus 0.1% ointment twice daily is associated with improved pruritis and reduced plaque thickness.[65,66] Dimethyl sulfoxide (DMSO) has been known as an effective treatment for both lichen and macular amyloidosis, although some cases are refractory cases.[67,68] Application of DMSO 50% or 100% solutions has been shown to help with pruritus; however, the reported side effects include irritant dermatitis and contact dermatitis/urticaria.[67]

Phototherapy with narrowband ultraviolet B (NB-UVB) and photochemotherapy (PUVA) should be considered in patients who do not respond to topical therapy.[68] Patients with lichen amyloidosis treated with phototherapy may have significant reductions in itch and skin roughness.[69]

Systemic thearpy has been shown to be beneficial but, as is the case with topical therapy, not all patients respond. It has been reported that systemic retinoids, specifically acitretin, have improved the pruritus of lichen amyloidosis and resulted in a flattening of the skin lesions.[70] Cyclosporine has also been shown to be effective and thalidomide has demonstrated benefit in a limited number of cases.[12,40,71-73] More recently JAK inhibitors and dupilumab have been reported to show potential benefit.[39,74-77]

The use of lasers and physical therapies for the effective management of macular and lichen amyloidosis has become increasingly popular. Frequency-doubled Q-switched neodymium-doped yttrium aluminum garnet (Nd:YAG) laser treatment has been used with some success. Additionally, fractional ablative laser CO_2 has proven to be effective in the treatment of lichen and macular amyloidosis after four sessions with or without topical steroids.[78,83,84] Fractional Erbium-Doped Yttrium Aluminum Garnet (Er:YAG) laser offers comparable clinical improvement of macular and lichen amyloidosis with reported low risk of side effects.[85,86] Furthermore, research has found that the combination laser therapy may be more effective than the use of one type alone (ie, Nd:YAG and Er:YAG).[87] Hyperpigmentation may limit the usefulness of lasers, and a test spot should be done prior to treatment. Physical treatment modalities, such as electrodesiccation, dermabrasion, split-thickness skin graft, removal via scalpel, and Trichloroacetic acid chemical peels have also been used with some success.[14,79,80,88] Pain, discomfort, dyspigmentation, and other risks may limit the usefulness of these options.

Potential side effects must be considered when selecting therapies. Less invasive options should be tried before more invasive treatment modalities are pursued.[89] Localized cutaneous amyloidosis is thought to be purely a cutaneous disease. As such, therapy has been directed at relieving the symptoms of pruritus. Despite successful treatment, recurrence is still common.[80,88]

CONCLUSION

Amyloidosis is a condition resulting from abnormal folding and deposition of protein. It can be divided into primary systemic and localized types. Individuals with skin of color appear to have a predisposition for developing localized cutaneous amyloidosis. Macular, lichenoid, and nodular amyloidoses are the most common forms of primary localized cutaneous amyloidosis. Potential treatments range from topical steroids and phototherapy to systemic thearpies, lasers, and surgical options. Treatment options are palliative with most of the potential treatments aimed at alleviating the patients' symptoms of pruritus, rather than removing the amyloid deposits. Therapy may be successful but typically not curative.

REFERENCES

1. Kyle RA. Amyloidosis: a convoluted story. *Br J Haematol.* 2001;114(3):529-538.
2. Toyama BH, Weissman JS. Amyloid structure: conformational diversity and consequences. *Annu Rev Biochem.* 2011;80:557-585.
3. Liu P, Reed MN, Kotilinek LA, et al. Quaternary structure defines a large class of amyloid-β oligomers neutralized by sequestration. *Cell Rep.* 2015; 11(11):1760-1771.
4. Dogan A. Amyloidosis: insights from proteomics. *Annu Rev Pathol.* 2017;12: 277-304.
5. Benson MD, Buxbaum JN, Eisenberg DS, et al. Amyloid nomenclature 2020: update and recommendations by the International Society of Amyloidosis (ISA) nomenclature committee. *Amyloid.* 2020;27(4):217-222.
6. Mahmood S, Bridoux F, Venner CP, et al. Natural history and outcomes in localised immunoglobulin light-chain amyloidosis: a long-term observational study. *Lancet Haematol.* 2015;2(6):e241-250.
7. Picken MM. The Pathology of amyloidosis in classification: a review. *Acta Haematol.* 2020;143(4):322-334.
8. Ryšavá R. AL amyloidosis: advances in diagnostics and treatment. *Nephrol Dial Transplant.* 2019;34(9):1460-1466.
9. Brunger AF, Nienhuis HLA, Bijzet J, Hazenberg BPC. Causes of AA amyloidosis: a systematic review. *Amyloid.* 2020;27(1):1-12.
10. Manganelli F, Fabrizi GM, Luigetti M, Mandich P, Mazzeo A, Pareyson D. Hereditary transthyretin amyloidosis overview. *Neurol Sci.* 2022;43(Suppl 2):595-604.
11. Kumar S, Sengupta RS, Kakkar N, Sharma A, Singh S, Varma S. Skin involvement in primary systemic amyloidosis. *Mediterr J Hematol Infect Dis.* 2013;5(1): e2013005.
12. Weidner T, Illing T, Elsner P. Primary localized cutaneous amyloidosis: a systematic treatment review. *Am J Clin Dermatol.* 2017;18(5):629-642.
13. Breathnach SM. Amyloid and amyloidosis. *J Am Acad Dermatol.* 1988;18(1 Pt 1): 1-16.
14. Wong C-K. History and modern concepts. *Clin Dermatol.* 1990;8(2):1-6.
15. Black M. Amyloid and the amyloidosis of the skin. In: Champion RH, Burton JL, Ebling FJG, eds. *Textbook of Dermatology.* 5th ed. *Oxford: Blackwell scientific Publications.* 1992:2333-2344.
16. Kibbi AG, Rubeiz NG, Zaynoun ST, Kurban AK. Primary localized cutaneous amyloidosis. *Int J Dermatol.* 1992;31(2):95-98.
17. Wong CK. Lichen amyloidosus. A relatively common skin disorder in Taiwan. *Arch Dermatol.* 1974;110(3):438-440.
18. Looi LM. Primary localised cutaneous amyloidosis in Malaysians. *Australas J Dermatol.* 1991;32(1):39-44.
19. Ollague W, Ollague J, Ferretti H. Epidemiology of primary cutaneous amyloidoses in South America. *Clin Dermatol.* 1990;8(2):25-29.

20. Tan T. Epidemiology of primary cutaneous amyloidoses in southeast Asia. *Clin Dermatol.* 1990;8(2):20-24.
21. Ladizinski B, Lee KC. Lichen amyloidosis. *CMAJ.* 2014;186(7):532.
22. Halder RM, Nootheti PK. Ethnic skin disorders overview. *J Am Academy Dermatol.* 2003;48(6 Suppl):S143-S148.
23. Weyers W, Weyers I, Bonczkowitz M, Diaz-Cascajo C, Schill WB. Lichen amyloidosus: a consequence of scratching. *J Am Acad Dermatol.* 1997;37(6): 923-928.
24. Chang YT, Liu HN, Wong CK, Chow KC, Chen KY. Detection of Epstein-Barr virus in primary cutaneous amyloidosis. *Br J Dermatol.* 1997;136(6):823-826.
25. Vaghjimal A, Ahmad H, Soto NE, Mehrein K, Chapnick EK. Lichen amyloidosis in an HIV-infected Patient. A case report and review of the literature. *Acta Derm-Venereol.* 1998;78(5):399.
26. Buezo GF, Peñas PF, Daudén Tello E, Fraga García J, García-Diéz A. Lichen amyloidosus and human immunodeficiency virus infection. *Dermatology.* 1995;191(1):56-58.
27. Shimoda Y, Sato Y, Hayashida Y, et al. Lichen amyloidosus as a sweat gland/duct-related disorder: resolution associated with restoration of sweating disturbance. *Br J Dermatol.* 2017;176(5):1308-1315.
28. Schreml S, Szeimies RM, Vogt T, Landthaler M, Schroeder J, Babilas P. Cutaneous amyloidoses and systemic amyloidoses with cutaneous involvement. *Eur J Dermatol.* 2010;20(2):152-160.
29. Oiso N, Yudate T, Kawara S, Kawada A. Successful treatment of lichen amyloidosus associated with atopic dermatitis using a combination of narrowband ultraviolet B phototherapy, topical corticosteroids and an antihistamine. *Clin Exp Dermatol.* 2009;34(8):e833-e836.
30. Kono M, Nishida K, Takeichi T, Sugiura K, Akiyama M. Ripple-pattern lichen amyloidosis in a case of ichthyosis vulgaris with a novel FLG mutation. *J Eur Acad Dermatol Venereol.* 2017;31(2):e130-e132.
31. Suranagi VV, Siddramappa B, Bannur HB, Patil PV, Davangeri RS. Bullous variant of familial biphasic lichen amyloidosis: a unique combination of three rare presentations. *Indian J Dermatol.* 2015;60(1):105.
32. Malhotra R, Boro H, Shamim SA, Khadgawat R. Multiple endocrine neoplasia type 2A with cutaneous lichen amyloidosis. *BMJ Case Rep.* 2020 Aug 26;13(8):e238423.
33. Kitano Y, Okada N, Kobayashi Y, Tanigaki T, Okano M, Yoshikawa K. A monoclonal anti-keratin antibody reactive with amyloid deposit of primary cutaneous amyloidosis. *J Dermatol.* 1987;14(5):427-429.
34. Hashimoto K. Progress on cutaneous amyloidoses. *J Invest Dermatol.* 1984; 82(1):1-3.
35. Maeda H, Ohta S, Saito Y, Nameki H, Ishikawa H. Epidermal origin of the amyloid in localized cutaneous amyloidosis. *Br J Dermatol.* 1982;106(3):345-351.
36. Black MM, Jones EW. Macular amyloidosis. A study of 21 cases with special reference to the role of the epidermis in its histogenesis. *Br J Dermatol.* 1971;84(3): 199-209.
37. Eto H, Hashimoto K, Kobayashi H, Fukaya T, Matsumoto M, Sun TT. Differential staining of cytoid bodies and skin-limited amyloids with monoclonal anti-keratin antibodies. *Am J Pathol.* 1984;116(3):473-481.
38. Yamagihira M, Kitajima Y, Yaoita H. Ultrastructural observation of the relationship between amyloid filaments and half desmosomes in macular amyloidosis. *J Cutan Pathol.* 1980;7(7):213.
39. Aoki K, Ohyama M, Mizukawa Y. A case of lichen amyloidosis associated with atopic dermatitis successfully treated with dupilumab: a case report and literature review. *Dermatol Ther.* 2021;34(4):e15005.
40. Behr FD, Levine N, Bangert J. Lichen amyloidosis associated with atopic dermatitis: clinical resolution with cyclosporine. *Arch Dermatol.* 2001;137(5): 553-555.
41. Wong CK, Lin CS. Friction amyloidosis. *Int J Dermatol.* 1988;27(5):302-307.
42. Kim Y, Ioffreda MD, Chung CG. Lichen amyloidosis of the scalp and forehead. *Dermatol Online J.* 2017;23(11).
43. Frew JW, Fallah H. Lichen amyloidosis involving the scalp. *Australas J Dermatol.* 2017;58(4):e260-e261.
44. Wang WJ, Chang YT, Huang CY, Lee DD. Clinical and histopathological characteristics of primary cutaneous amyloidosis in 794 Chinese patients. *Zhonghua Yi Xue Za Zhi (Taipei).* 2001;64(2):101-107.
45. Sonthalia S, Agrawal M, Sehgal VN. Dermoscopy of macular amyloidosis. *Indian Dermatol Online J.* 2021;12(1):203-205.
46. Errichetti E, Stinco G. Dermoscopy in general dermatology: a practical overview. *Dermatol Ther (Heidelb).* 2016;6(4):471-507.
47. Zapata-Salazar NA, Garza-Dávila VF, Ocampo-Candiani J, Argenziano G, Chávez-Álvarez S. Dermatoscopic features of lichen amyloidosis: a case report. *Australas J Dermatol.* 2021;62(2):e356-e357.
48. Kaliyadan F, Alkhateeb A, Kuruvilla J, Swaroop K, Alabdulsalam AA. Dermoscopy of primary cutaneous amyloidosis in skin of color. *Dermatol Pract Concept.* 2019;9(3):232-234.
49. Desouza A. Amyloidose cutanea bolhosa familial: observacao de 4 cases. *Rev Hosp Clin Fac Med S.* 1963;18:413-417.
50. Ozaki M. Familial lichen amyloidosis. *Int J Dermatol.* 1984;23(3):190-193.
51. Porto J, Posse F. Amiloidose cutanea genuina familial. *Bol Da Soc Brasil Dermatol E Sif.* 1960;35:102-103.
52. Rajagopalan K, Tay CH. Familial lichen amyloidosis. Report of 19 cases in 4 generations of a Chinese family in Malaysia. *Br J Dermatol.* 1972;87(2):123-129.
53. Vijaya B, Dalal BS, Manjunath GV, Sunila. Primary cutaneous amyloidosis: a clinico-pathological study with emphasis on polarized microscopy. *Indian J Pathol Microbiol.* 2012;55(2):170-174.
54. De Pietro WP. Primary familial cutaneous amyloidosis. A study of HLA antigens in a Puerto Rican family. *Arch Dermatol.* 1981;117(10):639-643.
55. Hartshorne ST. Familial primary cutaneous amyloidosis in a South African family. *Clin Exp Dermatol.* 1999;24(6):438-442.
56. Newton JA, Jagjivan A, Bhogal B, McKee PH, McGibbon DH. Familial primary cutaneous amyloidosis. *Br J Dermatol.* 1985;112(2):201-208.
57. Sagher F, Shanon J. Amyloidosis cutis. Familial occurrence in three generations. *Arch Dermatol.* 1963;87:171-175.
58. Vasily DB, Bhatia SG, Uhlin SR. Familial primary cutaneous amyloidosis. Clinical, genetic, and immunofluorescent studies. *Arch Dermatol.* 1978;114(8): 1173-1176.
59. Molina-Ruiz AM, Cerroni L, Kutzner H, Requena L. Cutaneous deposits. *Am J Dermatopathol.* 2014;36(1):1-48.
60. Yakupova EI, Bobyleva LG, Vikhlyantsev IM, Bobylev AG. Congo red and amyloids: history and relationship. *Biosci Rep.* 2019;39(1).
61. Mehrotra K, Dewan R, Kumar JV, Dewan A. Primary cutaneous amyloidosis: a clinical, histopathological and immunofluorescence study. *J Clin Diagn Res.* 2017;11(8):WC01-WC05.
62. Yadav A, Garg T, Mandal AK, Chander R. Immunofluorescence and immunohistochemistry in macular amyloidosis: an observational study. *Indian Dermatol Online J.* 2017;8(6):499-501.
63. Hashimoto K, Ito K, Kumakiri M, Headington J. Nylon brush macular amyloidosis. *Arch Dermatol.* 1987;123(5):633-637.
64. Khoo BP, Tay YK, Goh CL. Calcipotriol ointment vs. betamethasone 17-valerate ointment in the treatment of lichen amyloidosis. *Int J Dermatol.* 1999;38(7):539-541.
65. Castanedo-Cazares JP, Lepe V, Moncada B. Lichen amyloidosis improved by 0.1% topical tacrolimus. *Dermatology.* 2002;205(4):420-421.
66. Kalkan G, Markoç F, Bas Y. An alternative treatment model: the combination therapy of narrow band ultraviolet B phototherapy and tacrolimus ointment 0.1% in biphasic amyloidosis. *J Pak Med Assoc.* 2014;64(5):579-582.
67. Kobayashi T, Yamasaki Y, Watanabe T, Onoda N. Extensive lichen amyloidosus refractory to DMSO. *J Dermatol.* 1995;22(10):755-758.
68. Ozkaya-Bayazit E, Kavak A, Güngör H, Ozarmagan G. Intermittent use of topical dimethyl sulfoxide in macular and papular amyloidosis. *Int J Dermatol.* 1998;37(12):949-954.
69. Jin AG, Por A, Wee LK, Kai CK, Leok GC. Comparative study of phototherapy (UVB) vs. photochemotherapy (PUVA) vs. topical steroids in the treatment of primary cutaneous lichen amyloidosis. *Photodermatol Photoimmunol Photomed.* 2001;17(1):42-43.
70. Pandhi R, Kaur I, Kumar B. Lack of effect of dimethylsulphoxide in cutaneous amyloidosis. *J Dermatolog Treat.* 2002;13(1):11-14.
71. Teraki Y, Katsuta M, Shiohara T. Lichen amyloidosus associated with Kimura's disease: successful treatment with cyclosporine. *Dermatology.* 2002;204(2):133-135.
72. An Q, Lin J, Zheng S, et al. Dramatic improvement of primary cutaneous amyloidosis with thalidomide. *Eur J Dermatol.* 2011;21(2):270-271.
73. An Q, Zhang L, Zheng S, et al. Thalidomide improves clinical symptoms of primary cutaneous amyloidosis: report of familiar and sporadic cases. *Dermatol Ther.* 2013;26(3):263-266.
74. Chen J, Yang B. Tofacitinib for the treatment of primary cutaneous amyloidosis: a case report. *Dermatol Ther.* 2022;35(4):e15312.
75. Xia D, Xiao Y, Li M, Li W. Refractory cutaneous lichen amyloidosis coexisting with atopic dermatitis responds to the Janus Kinase inhibitor baricitinib. *Dermatol Ther.* 2022;35(9):e15724.
76. Humeda Y, Beasley J, Calder K. Clinical resolution of generalized lichen amyloidosis with dupilumab: a new alternative therapy. *Dermatol Online J.* 2020; 26(12).
77. Zhao XQ, Zhu WJ, Mou Y, Xu M, Xia JX. Dupilumab for treatment of severe atopic dermatitis accompanied by lichenoid amyloidosis in adults: two case reports. *World J Clin Cases.* 2023;11(10):2301-2307.
78. Wang M, Lin Y, Wu W, et al. Treatment of lichen amyloidosis with fractional CO. *Lasers Med Sci.* 2021;36(5):1123-1127.
79. Robinson CG, Jahan-Tigh RR. Successful treatment of lichen amyloidosis with trichloroacetic acid peels. *Dermatol Surg.* 2019;45(6):854-857.

80. Reider N, Sepp N, Fritsch P. Remission of lichen amyloidosus after treatment with acitretin. *Dermatology*. 1997;194(3):309-311.
81. Shoen E, Hou A, Zahn J, Friedman A. Successful treatment of lichen amyloidosis using a fixed combination of halobetasol-propionate and tazarotene lotion. *J Drugs Dermatol*. 2021;20(3):336-337.
82. Zhu Q, Gao BQ, Zhang JF, Shi LP, Zhang GQ. Successful treatment of lichen amyloidosis coexisting with atopic dermatitis by dupilumab: four case reports. *World J Clin Cases*. 2023;11(11):2549-2558.
83. Korbi M, Akkari H, Soua Y, et al. Lichen amyloidosis successfully treated with fractional ablative laser CO. *J Cosmet Laser Ther*. 2019;21(1):1-3.
84. Esmat SM, Fawzi MM, Gawdat HI, Ali HS, Sayed SS. Efficacy of different modes of fractional CO2 laser in the treatment of primary cutaneous amyloidosis: a randomized clinical trial. *Lasers Surg Med*. 2015;47(5):388-395.
85. Fawzy MM, Kamel MM, El Maadawi Z, Hady RA, Osman MA. Fractional erbium-doped yttrium aluminum garnet laser in the treatment of primary cutaneous amyloidosis. *Dermatol Surg*. 2021;47(7):e205-e211.
86. Nahidi Y, Delghandi SR, Kiafar B, Saki A. The therapeutic effects of 1540-nm nonablative fractional erbium laser on macular amyloidosis: a randomized clinical trial. *J Dermatolog Treat*. 2021;32(3):340-344.
87. Nilforoushzadeh MA, Zolghadr S, Heidari-Kharaji M, Alavi S, Mahmoudbeyk M. A comparative study of the efficacy of fractional neodymium-doped yttrium aluminum garnet (Nd: YAG) laser therapy alone and in combination with erbium: YAG laser therapy: tracing and objective measurement of melanin index in macular amyloidosis. *Lasers Med Sci*. 2020;35:1171-1177.
88. Liu HT. Treatment of lichen amyloidosis (LA) and disseminated superficial porokeratosis (DSP) with frequency-doubled Q-switched Nd:YAG laser. *Dermatol Surg*. 2000;26(10):958-962.
89. Harahap M, Marwali MR. The treatment of lichen amyloidosis. A review and a new technique. *Dermatol Surg*. 1998;24(2):251-254.

CHAPTER 33 Keloids

Ariel Knowles
Donald A. Glass II

KEY POINTS

- Keloid disease is a significant clinical problem for patients with skin of color.
- Keloid scars are overgrowths of dense fibrous tissue that develop as a result of a cutaneous injury and invade the healthy tissue in the area surrounding the injury.
- Hypertrophic scars are also overgrowths of fibrous tissue, but in contrast to keloids, they usually stay within the confines of the precipitating cutaneous injury.
- Keloids differ from hypertrophic scars in their metabolic activity and collagen turnover.
- Many theories have been advanced to explain the etiology of keloids, although none have been substantiated. However, it can be said that there is a familial tendency of keloid susceptibility. This hereditary tendency is more common in patients with skin of color.
- Although keloids may be found anywhere on the body, they are seen most commonly on the chest, upper back, shoulders, and earlobes. The torso is the most likely anatomical location for multiple keloid sites. The common development of keloids on the earlobes may be due in part to cultural practices of earlobe piercings.
- Although rare, keloids may develop on the genitalia, palms and soles, and cornea.

INTRODUCTION

Synonyms for Keloids include:

- *Cheloide*
- Keloid disease
- Keloidal scar
- Raised dermal scarring
- Excessive scar tissue
- Abnormal wound healing

Keloids are common, hyperproliferative, reticular, dermal lesions of unknown etiopathogenesis that often occur in genetically susceptible individuals. A keloid scar develops as a result of an overgrowth of dense, fibrous scar tissue that extend beyond the site of the original skin injury. They can result from any sort of trauma (no matter how minor) such as surgical incisions, traumatic wounds, vaccination sites, burns, chickenpox, acne, or even minor scratches. Besides being cosmetically disfiguring, keloids can be both painful and pruritic, affecting a patients' quality of life (QoL).

The few publications on the impact of keloids on QoL establish that keloids can negatively affect QoL.[1-3] Most of these studies include both keloids and hypertrophic scars in their analysis despite a difference in disease process. In contrast to keloids, hypertrophic scars are raised scars that remain confined to the boundaries of the original wound. Additional clinical and histologic characteristics distinguish keloid scars from hypertrophic scars [**Table 33-1**]. However, the medical literature regarding hypertrophic scars and keloid scars is often confusing because many lesions that are keloid-like are mislabeled as hypertrophic scars or vice versa. Additionally, some patients have both kinds of scars caused by some traumatic incident. Clinical studies often lump the two disorders together, thus leading to the dissemination of incorrect information, which is a practical concern when evaluating the therapeutic response.[4,5] Furthermore, the International Classification of Diseases, Tenth Revision, Clinical Modification—more commonly known as ICD-10-CM—also lumps keloids and hypertrophic scars under the same diagnostic code, leading to difficulty in using clinical data to establish the true incidence and prevalence rates of either.

Most of the studies evaluating the effect of keloids on QoL include both keloids and hypertrophic scars in their analysis, thus potentially underestimating the true impact of keloids on QoL. The relationship between keloid symptomatology (eg, pain and itch) and QoL has not been well-characterized. One study has shown that keloids affect QoL as severely as psoriasis, yet the current treatment methods to treat keloids are not as efficacious as psoriasis.[1]

Keloids and hypertrophic scars are thought to be produced by an overgrowth of fibrous tissue, which is always secondary to some form of injury (eg, lacerations, surgical incisions, ear piercings, vaccinations, herpes zoster, acne lesions, folliculitis, insect bites, or burns). There are, however, reports of a small percentage of patients who develop so-called spontaneous keloids—that is, keloids with no known antecedent trauma

TABLE 33-1 A comparison of keloids and hypertrophic scars

Characteristics	Keloids	Hypertrophic Scars
Stays in confines of injury	No	Yes
Precipitated by trauma	Not always	Yes
Growth	For extended period	Regresses in time
Symptomatic	Usually	Usually
Response to treatment	Poor	Good
Sodium	Normal	Decreased
Magnesium	Increased	Decreased
Calcium	Increased	Decreased
Mucinous ground substance	Abundant	Scarce
Fibroblasts	Few	Numerous
Foreign-body reactions	None	Frequent
Luxol fast blue collagen stain	Reddish	Blue
Mast cells	Increased	Increased
Pathogenesis	Unknown	Unknown
Contain myofibroblasts	No	Yes
Alanine transaminase	Increased	Normal

or injury. Whether these are truly spontaneous, or the result of asymptomatic inflammation from processes such as folliculitis, remains unclear. These types of lesions occur most often in patients with a family history of keloids and are usually located in the mid-sternal area. Keloids occur in the second or third decade of life, although they can occur any time between infancy and old age.[6,7]

Hypertrophic scars usually develop rapidly after a cutaneous injury or trauma, whereas keloids develop slowly but continue to enlarge for months to years. In most instances, hypertrophic scars regress with therapy, in contradistinction to keloids, which can be recalcitrant to therapy and/or recur when the therapy is discontinued.

HISTORY

Jean Louis Alibert (1768-1837), one of the principal founders of French dermatology, proposed the world *cheloide* (derived from the Greek *chele*, meaning "crab's claw," and *-oid*, meaning "like") in 1806, which he had originally called *cancroide* [**Figure 33-1**].[8] Alibert later changed the name to *cheloide* to avoid confusion with cancer and its connotations. In 1825, he wrote a chapter entitled, *Les cancroides ou keloids*, using for the first time the word that would be adopted by American, English, and German dermatologists.[9] Even though Alibert was the first to describe the clinical characteristics of keloids, Retz had in 1790, according to Kaposi, already described a cicatricial tumor of the skin, which he thought was of spontaneous origin, under the name *darte de graisse*.[10] In 1835, Hawkins described lesions that may have been keloids, and Macpherson added to the early literature on keloids.[11,12]

The first records description of keloid-like scars appears in the *Edward Smith Surgical Papyrus*: "The existence of swelling on his breast, large, spreading, and hard, touching them is like touching a ball of wrappings."[13]

Also, the Yorubas recorded their awareness of keloid 10 centuries before Alibert and Retz. Omo-Dare described some of these observations on the character and presentations of keloids.[14] The Yorubas knew, for example, that keloids frequently appeared in the same family but that not all members of the family were affected. They knew that there was a time interval between the infliction of the trauma that produced a keloid and the appearance of the lesion. Local customs of facial marking and earlobe perforation were usually performed toward the end of the first week of life. However, if there was a delay in the scarification process, according to a Yoruba saying, facial marks made in adolescence and adult life might then develop into keloids. The Yorubas also knew that once a lesion appeared, it grew and had no effective therapy except when "the Divine Power is suitably appropriated to intervene in bringing about its resolution."[14]

Although animals may form keloid-like scars, they are not good models for studying wound repair because the excessive collagen deposited in animals is reabsorbed when the tissue insult ceases.[15]

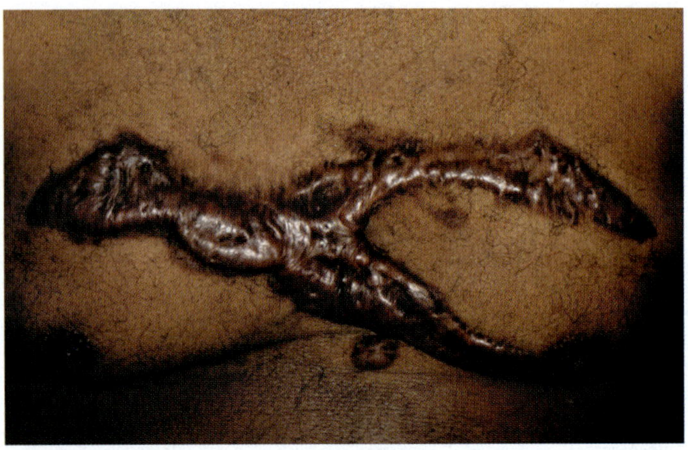

FIGURE 33-1. A crab-like keloid in the mid-sternal region of an African American man. Jean Louis Alibert (1768–1837) proposed the word cheloide (derived from the Greek *chele*, meaning "crab's claw," and *-oid*, meaning "like") in 1806.

TABLE 33-2 Epidemiology
Incidence varies according to population studied
• Low of 0.09% in England
• High of 16% in the Democratic Republic of the Congo
• People with skin of color affected 5-16 times more often than lighter-skinned people
• Asians and Hispanics fall in between these reported incidences
The median age of onset is 22-23 years old
• Onset after puberty
• Young skin more taut due to greater rate of collagen synthesis

EPIDEMIOLOGY

Due to numerous variables, such as the anatomic location, type of trauma, race, age, and gender, the reported incidence of keloids in the general population ranges from a high of 16% in Congolese miners to a low of 0.01% in English Caucasian adults [**Table 33-2**].[4] In general, keloids are thought to occur more frequently in persons with skin of color. In North America, several reports have established a 3× to 7× increased incidence of keloids in Black versus White patients.[16-18]

In Aruba, however, where more than 3% of children have keloids, the children of Polynesian ancestry with keloids outnumber the other dark-skinned children who have keloids. Also, in West Malaysia, the lighter-skinned Chinese appear to be slightly more prone to keloid formation than the darker-skinned Indians and Malays.[19] Arnold et al found that in Hawaii, keloids are five and three times more common in Japanese and Chinese individuals, respectively, than in Caucasians.[20] It has been reported that Europeans living in the tropics are more likely to develop keloids than those living in more temperate zones, although there has been no subsequent documentation of this observation.[21] The question of why people with skin of color develop keloids and hypertrophic scars more often than fairer-skinned individuals has inspired many theories, none of which have been accepted as the sole reason.

The male-to-female incidence has been reported to be equal by some investigators, whereas others have reported that the incidence is greater in females.[22] Cosmon et al found that the average age of patients at the time of initial treatment was 25.8 years, and the median age at onset was 22.3 years in women and 22.6 years in men.[23] Although it is extremely rare, the onset of keloids and hypertrophic scars has been noted in children before their first birthday, as well as in septuagenarians.

ETIOLOGY

TRAUMA

Many theories have been advanced to explain the etiology of keloids [**Table 33-3**]. In most patients, trauma is the main, if not the only, precipitating factor. The trauma may take many different forms, such as simple scratches, abrasions, insect bites, vaccinations, acne papules, chickenpox lesions, surgical procedures, chemical burns, or thermal burns. Because most people sustain cutaneous trauma, especially on the feet, without developing keloids, and because some keloids arise spontaneously on nontraumatized areas, one may summarize that there is most likely another predisposing variable(s) or factor(s) other than trauma that leads to keloid formation.[7,24]

TABLE 33-3 Proposed etiology of keloids
• Trauma
• Skin tension
• Infection
• Endocrine factors
• Genetic predisposition
• Epigenetic factors

INFLAMMATION

It has been postulated that inflammation plays an important role in the pathogenesis of keloids. There are a number of inflammatory cell types found in keloid tissue—T-cells, macrophages, mast cells—and this inflammatory infiltrate persists within keloids. [25-27] Acne and folliculitis can induce keloids without an external traumatic event. Additionally, suppurative keloids can occur, where aseptic inflammation leads to suppuration.[28,29] Several local and systemic anti-inflammatory agents have been used to prevent keloid occurrence or recurrence, including steroids, calcineurin inhibitors, methotrexate, pentoxifylline, and dupilumab.[30,31]

ENDOCRINE FACTORS

Keloid formation has been associated with endocrinologic factors, but there is still no definitive proof that such factors are of major importance. The thymus, parathyroid, ovaries, thyroid, and pituitary glands, alone or in combination, have been incriminated.[32] Acromegalics and pregnant women have demonstrated a marked susceptibility to keloid formation.[33,34]

There seems to be a greater incidence of keloids when hyperpigmentation is associated with hyperthyroidism, pregnancy, or puberty.[33,35] It has been postulated that in all of the preceding conditions, there is an excessive secretion of melanocyte-stimulating hormone (MSH) and the increased sensitivity of melanocytes to MSH. This may explain why people with skin of color, whose melanocytes may be more reactive to MSH, have a higher incidence of keloids than those with lighter skin [**Table 33-5**].[36] Evidence for this supposition is purely circumstantial; keloids are rare on the palms and soles, where the concentration of melanocytes is lower than other skin areas.[37]

Residues of the thymus gland have been reported in several patients with keloids.[38] Other investigators mention that the thymus may be involved in keloid formation, but to date, there has been no proof of this association.[39]

Hyperthyroidism was mentioned as a possible cause of keloid formation by Justice[40] after keloids were induced in hyperthyroid patients by irritating their skin with "excitant pharmacologic substances," the activity of which was slight. Asboe-Hansen[41] reported that young patients who underwent a thyroidectomy for Graves disease were apt to form keloids in the surgical wound, and after the injection of the thyroid extract. Also, it has been reported that hard fibrous patches, which were probably keloids, regressed in a female patient after a unilateral resection of the thyroid gland on that side.[42]

Although Asboe-Hansen[41] reported that the blood calcium level in most patients with keloids was within normal limits, Pautrier and Zorn[43] found an elevated serum calcium concentration of 9 in 12 patients with keloids, each of whom was noted to have elevated calcium levels in all of the keloid tissues. Farndon[44] observed that, during a parathyroidectomy on a patient, if the surgical incision curves down onto the sternum, then keloid formation is more likely.

Pituitary secretions have been held responsible for keloid formation, especially since acromegalics have been reported to have an increased susceptibility of developing keloids. This phenomenon was attributed to the action of growth hormones, which stimulate the formation of new connective tissues, especially collagen fibrils. Keloids seem to be more common in acromegalics and seem to grow more rapidly in pregnancy and puberty, times when there is physiologic hyperactivity of the pituitary gland.[34] The suggestion of pituitary involvement in keloid formation has also been based on the fact that there is an association with increased pigmentation in states of increased pituitary activity (eg, pregnancy and puberty); increased pigmentation is based on an increased production of MSH by the pituitary gland.[34]

Ovarian function has also been associated with keloids: for instance, in the formation of keloids during puberty, the development of keloid growth during pregnancy, and the spontaneous resolution of keloids after menopause.[45] Geschickter and Lewis[46] reported increased estrogen content in keloids, which further supports the ovarian influence, but their findings are somewhat suspect as the results were obtained by assaying an earlobe that had been preserved in formaldehyde for 1 to 3 years. Solomons[47] found that the suppression of the ovaries did not alter keloid growth. In addition, Vargas,[48] attempting to produce uterine fibroids by administering estrogen to monkeys, was not able to produce cutaneous keloids. The observation that scars and keloids tend to grow during pregnancy supports a pituitary-ovarian influence on keloid formation.[34]

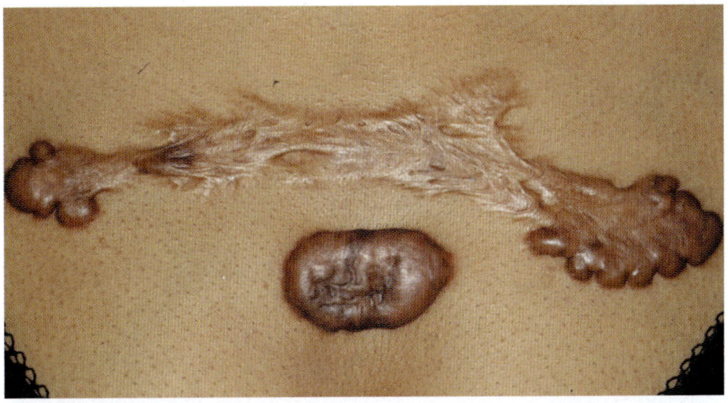

FIGURE 33-2. Keloids in the mid-chest area of an African American woman. Additional evidence favoring the role of androgens in keloid formation is that keloids have a predilection for the chest and upper back, which have an increased rate of dihydrotestosterone metabolism.

Because keloids seldom occur before puberty, the sex hormones may play an important role in their formation. Sex hormone levels have been found to differ between keloids and the clinically normal surrounding skin and between keloids and hypertrophic scars. Personen et al[49] found that the diffusion of progesterone from the culture medium into the tissue is the most effective in keloids, with normal skin being the second most effective; hypertrophic scars and the skin surrounding keloids proved ineffective in taking up progesterone.

Ford et al found that keloids have a high level of androgen binding, whereas estrogen and progesterone receptor binding was essentially undetectable in any of the keloid tissues from males or in the keloid tissues from some females. They also found that the level of androgen binding in the skin adjacent to keloids was elevated, whereas the level in skin adjacent to hypertrophic scars was only 0.1% of that found in keloids.[50]

Mustafa and Abdel-Fattah[34] postulated that estrogen plays a causative role in keloid formation based on a single case of a keloid that enlarged during pregnancy. However, they did not mention that maternal circulating androgens increase during pregnancy, especially in patients carrying a male fetus, nor did they mention the gender of the fetus. Additional evidence favoring the role of androgens is that keloids have a predilection for the chest, upper back, and neck regions, all of which have an increased rate of dihydrotestosterone metabolism [**Figures 33-2** to **33-4**].

A South African study suggests that nutritional inadequacy, most notably the low intake of calcium, may lead to abnormal collagen production

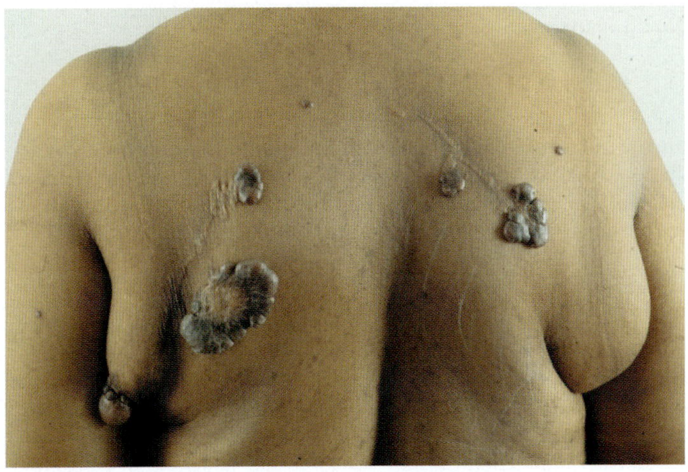

FIGURE 33-3. Keloids on the upper back of an African American woman.

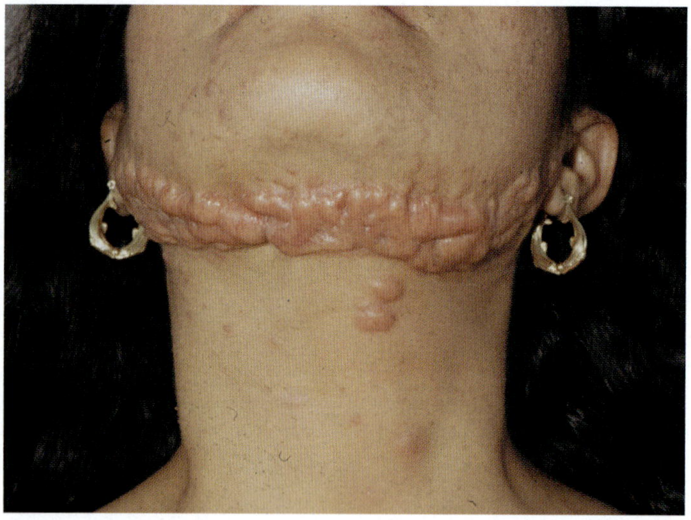

FIGURE 33-4. Keloids on the anterior neck of a Hispanic woman; this area is uncommon for the formation of keloids.

and be a factor in keloid formation.[51] However, malnutrition with protein deficiency seems to decrease fibroplasias.[52,53] Bowesman[54] suggested that adequate nutrition is necessary for keloid formation. Keloid formation is uncommon in patients with acquired immunodeficiency syndrome.[55]

The relationship between hypertrophic scars and hormonal factors is a subject that needs more research to make definitive determinations.[4,56,57]

SKIN TENSION

Increased skin tension has been cited as the reason for keloids occurring after surgery.[22,41,58] Cutting across Langer lines, with a resulting increase in skin tension, has also been suggested. An increased predisposition to developing keloid scars has been observed in certain anatomic sites that are under increased mechanical tension, such as the development of butterfly-shaped keloid scars that occur in the mid-sternal region.[59,60]

Increased skin tension can also cause coiffure keloids, or hairstyle-induced keloids, which form, in a few cases, on the scalp in response to the tightly braided hairstyles. Such hairstyling practices are found in many parts of Africa and are increasing in popularity in the United States and worldwide.[61]

SEBUM

Yagi et al introduced the sebum autoimmune mechanism concept of keloid formation.[62] They postulated that after cutaneous trauma, functioning sebaceous glands may secrete sebum intradermally. The sebum then acts as an antigen, initiating an autoimmune granulomatous response that may lead to keloid formation. These authors cite the virtual absence of keloids on the palms, soles, forehead, and lips, areas that are essentially devoid of sebaceous glands, as further evidence of their theory.

FOREIGN BODY

Some investigators have suggested that it is a foreign-body reaction, or the presence of suture debris or dirt in wounds, that stimulates the formation of keloids and not the trauma itself.[24] Others have also proposed that inert material or natural products such as damaged collagen or keratin are causative stimuli.[63]

CUTANEOUS INFECTIONS

Infections, either bacterial or viral, have been implicated as a contributing factor in the formation of keloids [**Table 33-4**]. One of the earliest opinions was that tubercle bacilli caused keloids.[33] However, in later studies on keloid patients, not one was found to have clinical evidence of tuberculosis, and the number of positive tuberculin reactions was within the normal population range.[33,39] Keloids may appear after chickenpox or herpes zoster infections and after smallpox vaccinations. In the past, there were many inferences that syphilis promoted keloid growth; however, in one study of more than 100 patients with keloids, only one was found to have syphilis.[4,64]

TABLE 33-4 Factors suggesting an association between keloids and melanocytes

- Patients with keloids who developed vitiligo
  - keloids regressed in vitiliginous areas
- May form with secretion of melanocyte-stimulating hormone
  - face, neck, deltoid area
  - presternal area, earlobes

ASSOCIATED COMORBIDITIES

Keloids have traditionally been considered a primarily cutaneous event. However, as research into keloids progresses, systemic medical conditions associated with keloid development are illuminated. Keloids have been associated with cardiovascular comorbidities such as hypertension, atherosclerosis, and coronary stent restenosis.[65-71] Adotama et al[65] highlighted an association between keloids and hypetension and obesity in African Americans. It is possible that the mechanisms underlying keloid pathogenesis may also be involved in the development of these conditions.

There is striking similarity in the appearance of collagen in keloids and leiomyomas. Both keloids and leiomyomas show a decrease in dermatopontin protein.[72,73]

Kwon et al in a study of the Korean National Health Information Database found that among Koreans, patients with atopic dermatitis have a higher risk of keloid development, with coexisting allergic diseases (like asthma, allergic rhinitis, and allergic contact dermatitis) increasing the risk.[74] Both Black and White patients with atopic dermatitis have a higher association with keloids than race-matched healthy controls.[18] Both keloids and atopic dermatitis are mediated by an aberrant Th2-mediated inflammatory response, with increased IL-4/IL-13 signaling.[75,76] Furthermore, mast cells, which play a role in vascular homeostasis as well as innate and adaptive immune responses, are common to both conditions.

Lu et al[77] found an association between keloids and osteoporosis risk in an Asian population. Keloid patients were found to have a 2.64-fold higher osteoporosis risk compared to controls, suggesting keloids to be an early predictor of osteoporosis.

GENETIC FACTORS

Keloids have a definite familial predisposition, especially those with multiple lesions.[4,57,78] Approximately one-third of keloid patients have a first-degree relative with keloids. Also, clinical experience indicates that familial predisposition is more common in dark-skinned individuals. Though both autosomal recessive and autosomal dominant patterns of inheritance have been reported, most commonly the inheritance pattern is autosomal dominant, with incomplete penetrance and variable expressivity.[4] There is linkage identified in families with keloids to chromosomes 2q23 and 7p11.[79]

Bloom also mentioned some studies in the German literature that describe congenital keloids, two cases of which were in identical twins. A study of a Yoruba family found a mutation in the ASAH1 gene segregating with keloids, suggesting ASAH1 may be predisposing to keloid formation. Though functional studies were not performed, the authors postulated that the variant in ASAH1 may lead to decreased ceramide levels and deceased apoptosis in keloid versus normal fibroblasts.[80] Therefore, familial predisposition, high prevalence in certain populations, and frequent occurrence in twins suggest a strong genetic component to keloid susceptibility.[81]

TABLE 33-5 Infections associated with keloids

- Viral infections—higher incidence of keloids after herpes zoster and chickenpox
- Bacterial infections—in the past, tuberculosis and syphilis incriminated; now, no evidence that infections precipitate keloid formation

Numerous approaches have attempted to address and better understand the genetics of keloid scarring, and these include the determination of inheritance patterns, performance of linkage studies, case-control association studies, whole genome gene expression and micro ribonucleic acid (RNA) microarrays, and comparative genomic hybridization studies.[82]

Genome-wide association studies (GWAS) performed in Japanese and Chinese Han populations with keloids, respectively, identified single-nucleotide polymorphisms (SNPs) located at chromosomes 1q41, 3q22.3-23, 15q21.3.[83,84] Admixture mapping of African Americans with keloids also identified a locus at 15q21.2-22.3.[85] Further studies have identified that the SNP at chromosome 15q21.3, rs8032158, is associated with the gene NEDD4. This SNP causes a variant transcript of NEDD4 that results in more inflammation via increased NF-kB and IL-6 signaling.[86] Meanwhile, at locus 1q41, rs1348270, an enhancer-located SNP in strong LD with the GWAS-identified SNP rs873549. rs1348270 is associated with decreased expression of the long noncoding RNA DEIK (down regulated in keloids), which results in increased expression of collagens POSTN and COMP through upregulating BMP2.[87]

Copy number variations (CNVs) in genes have been associated with several human diseases including common skin disorders. CNVs have been found to be present in the genome of keloid patients and may contribute to the development of keloids.[88] In particular, chromosome 6p21.32 (targeting HLA-DRB5) was found to be significantly associated with keloid formation in a Caucasian population ($p < 0.001$). The presence of HLA-DRB5 was associated with the HLA-DRB1*15 status.[88]

Inflammatory responses in keloid patients have pointed to the HLA system as a viable target for investigating disease etiology.[88] Several human leukocyte antigen (HLA) alleles (HLA-DRB1*15, HLA-DQA1*0104, HLA-DQB1*0501, and HLA-DQB1*0503) have been shown to be associated with keloids.[78,89,90] In addition, frequencies of the HLA class I alleles A*01, A*03, A*25, B*07, Cw*08:02, HLA-DQA1, and HLA-DQB1 were analyzed in patients with skin of color, including 165 keloid patients and 119 healthy controls of Jamaican Afro-Caribbean origin. There were no statistically significant differences in allele frequency between the keloid patients and the controls. Additionally, characteristics of the keloid patients, including gender, family history, and multiple- or single-site scarring, did not show any significant allele-disease association.[91] The incidence of keloids in an Italian population was found to be greater in those with HLA-B14 and HLA BW16 antigens, whereas studies by Cohen et al and other researchers have noted a general HLA-A and HLA-B antigen pattern in patients with keloids.[92-95]

CLINICAL FINDINGS

CLINICAL CHARACTERISTICS

There are several clinical findings that distinguish keloids and hypertrophic scars [**Table 33-6**].[57,93,95-97] Although keloids may be found anywhere on the body, they tend to have a regional predilection, which occurs most often on the ears [**Figure 33-5**].[98] The chest, upper back, and shoulders [**Figures 33-6** to **33-8**] have increased skin tension, and keloids in these locations seem to arise with minimal trauma, are usually flatter with broader bases than keloids elsewhere, and respond less favorably to all modes of therapy. Keloids can occur from head to toe and at all locations in between. [**Figures 33-9** and **33-10**]. Keloids on the shoulder and back tend to grow larger compared to keloids elsewhere [**Figure 33-11**]. Abdominal keloids, although rare in men, are common in darker-pigmented women who have had cesarean sections, hysterectomies, or other types of abdominal laparoscopic surgery. Darker-pigmented men who shave tend to develop keloids more often in the facial hair regions than those who do not shave [**Figure 33-12**]. Furthermore, women who pluck or shave unwanted hairs in the jawline and neck region may also develop keloids in these areas. There seems to be greater involvement in the flanks in women than in men [**Figure 33-13**].[99,100]

TABLE 33-6 Clinical findings of keloidal and hypertrophic scars

Keloids	Hypertrophic scars
• Invade clinically normal skin	• Limited to traumatized area
• May continue to grow for the patient's life, often resistant to therapy	• Usually regress spontaneously in 12-18 months
• Erythematous borders indicate continuing growth	• Usually respond to therapy
• Pruritic, painful, burning	• Rarely grow after 2-3 months
	• Usually asymptomatic

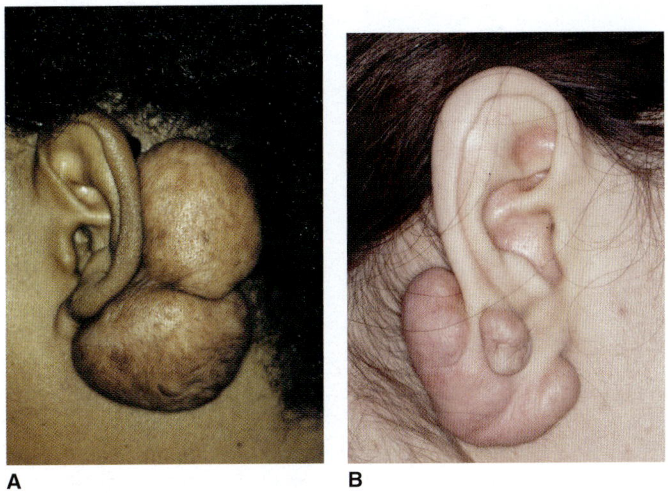

FIGURE 33-5. (A) Two large keloids of the left posterior earlobe of an African American woman. **(B)** Keloids also occur in lighter-skinned patients such as this Hispanic woman.

The areas less commonly associated with the formation of keloids include the face [**Figure 33-14**], neck [Figure 33-4], arms, wrist [**Figure 33-15**], and lower extremities. Mid-sternal lesions are often quite tender [**Figures 33-16** to **33-18**]. Although rare, keloids may develop on the eyelids, genitalia, palms, soles, mucous membranes, tongue, and corneas.[101] Lesions on the extremities can be very taut [**Figures 33-19** to **33-21**].[33] Keloids are rare on the oral mucosa.[4] There have been two known cases of keloids on the penis, one secondary to circumcision and the other from another form of trauma.[102,103] There are some lesions that resemble keloids clinically but that are epidermal cysts of the earlobe, [**Figure 33-22**], lipomas of the earlobe [**Figure 33-23**], and linear xanthomas [**Figure 33-24**].[36]

CLINICAL COURSE AND PROGNOSIS

Keloids present as exaggerated scar tissue growths, extending past the areas of trauma, and once present, tend to continue to enlarge. In contrast, hypertrophic scars are limited to the traumatized area and regress

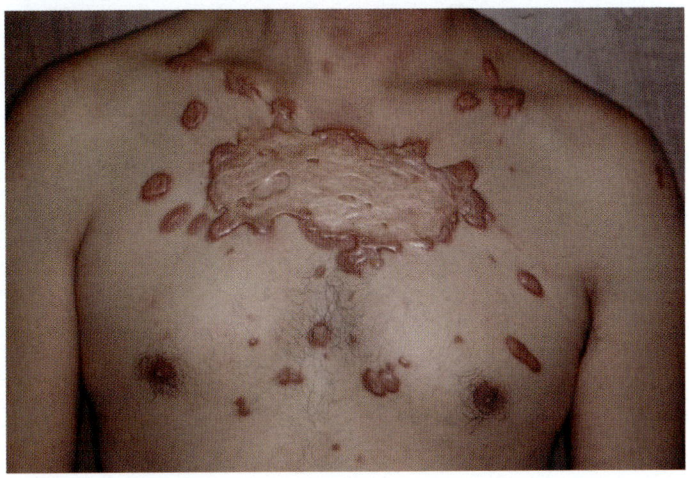

FIGURE 33-6. Regional predilection of keloids on the chest of a lighter-pigmented man.

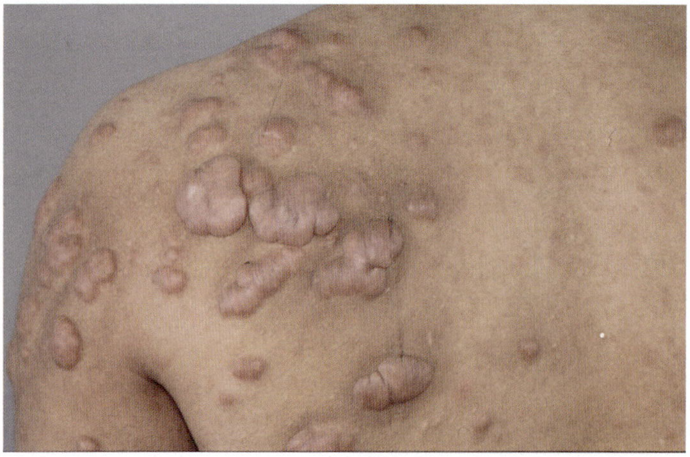

FIGURE 33-7. Regional predilection of keloids on the upper back and shoulders of a Hispanic man.

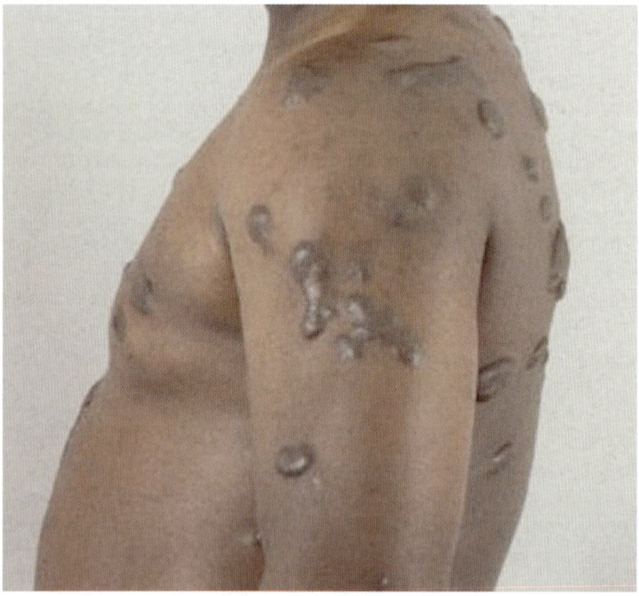

FIGURE 33-8. Regional predilection of keloids on the upper back and shoulders on an African American man.

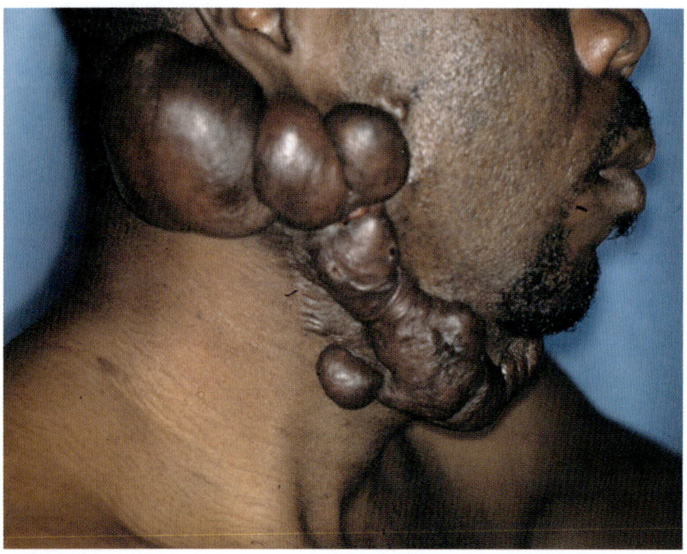

FIGURE 33-9. Large keloid on the head and neck of an African American man.

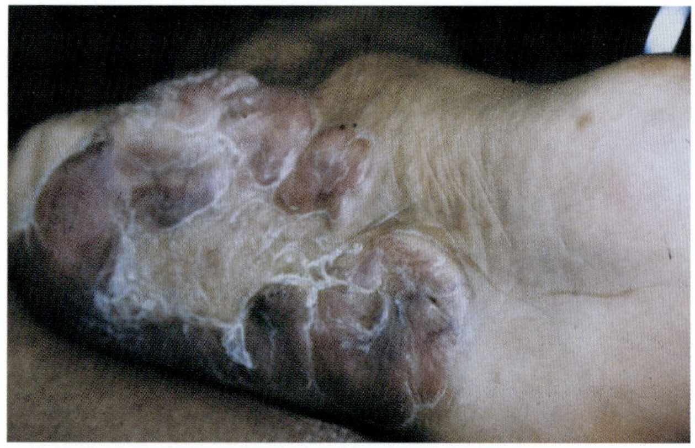

FIGURE 33-10. Keloids on the sole of the left foot; it is uncommon for keloids to occur on the feet.

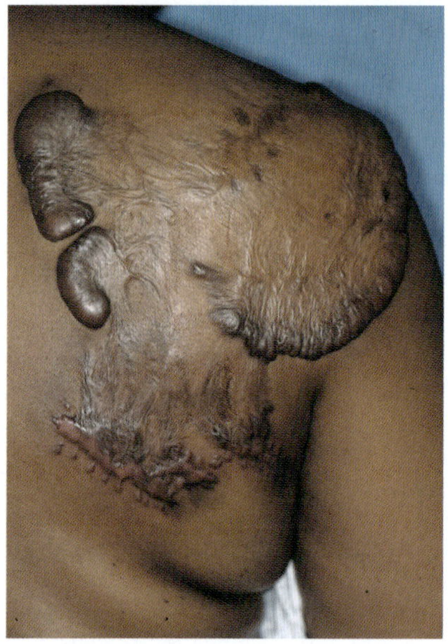

FIGURE 33-11. Keloids on the shoulder and back often grow to be larger than keloids elsewhere. As can be seen in the image, the medial border of the keloid is violaceous, which means that the keloid is still enlarging.

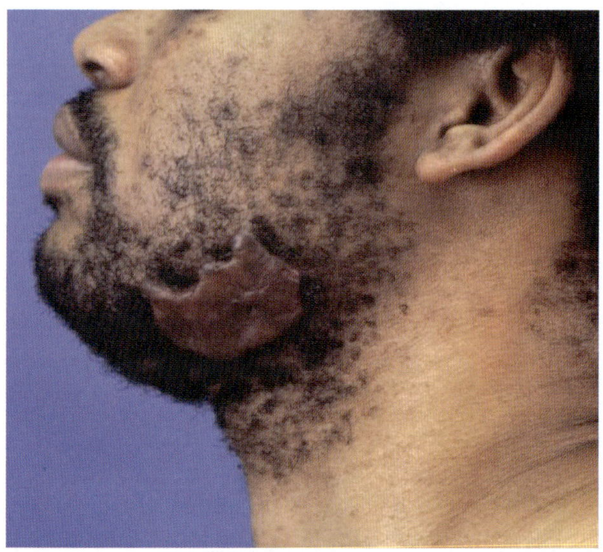

FIGURE 33-12. Darker-skinned African American men who shave can often develop keloids in the beard areas; the coarsely curled hair may act as an irritant in the formation of keloids.

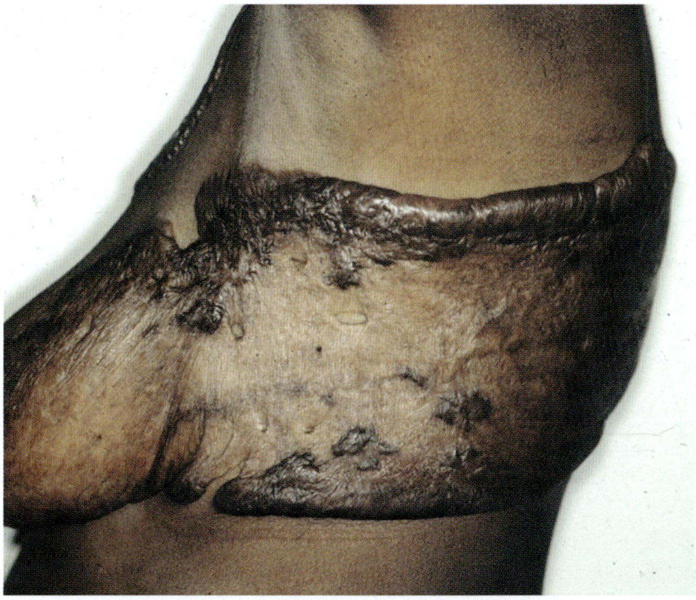

FIGURE 33-13. Keloids on the left flank and breast of an African American woman.

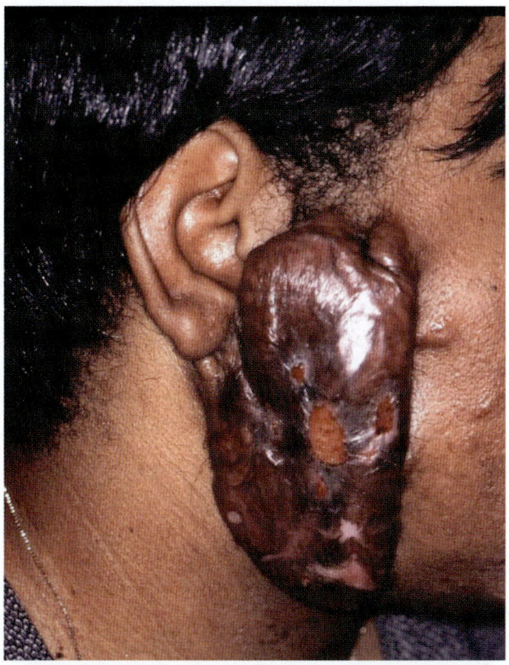

FIGURE 33-14. The face is a less commonly involved area for the formation of keloids.

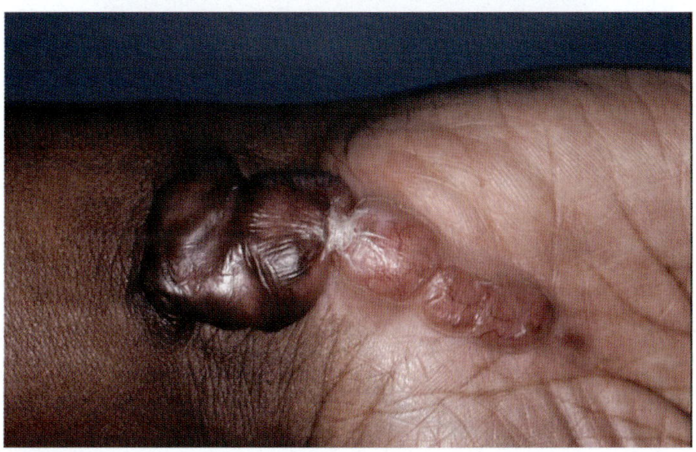

FIGURE 33-15. The wrist is a less commonly involved area for the formation of keloids.

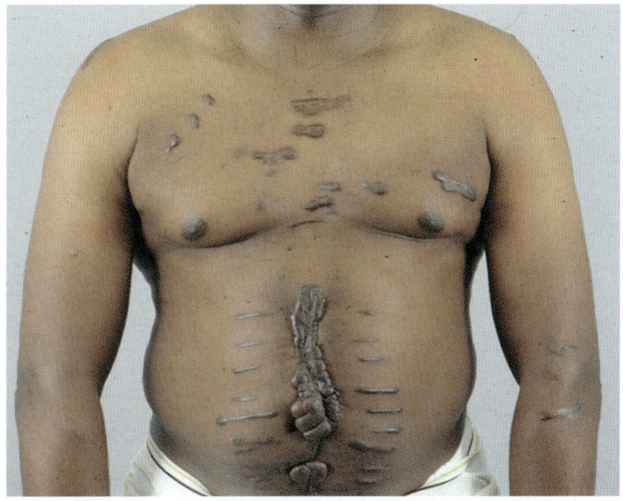

FIGURE 33-16. Chest and abdominal keloids on an African American man; the abdominal keloids were secondary to abdominal surgery.

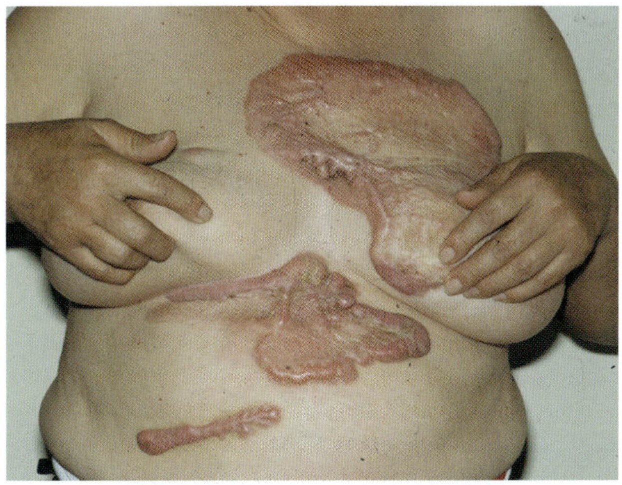

FIGURE 33-17. Chest, breast, and abdominal keloids on a Hispanic woman.

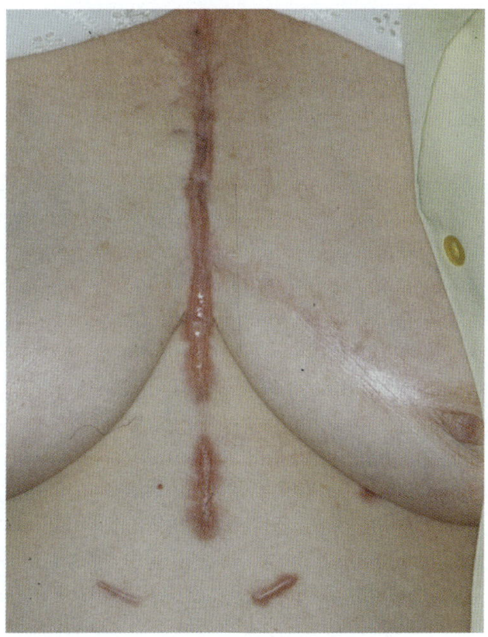

FIGURE 33-18. Keloids on the mid-chest of an Asian American woman, secondary to cardiac surgery.

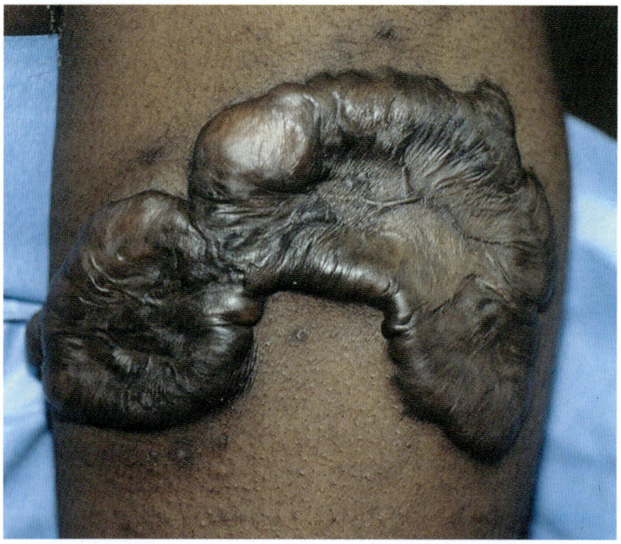

FIGURE 33-19. Keloids on the medial leg of an African American man; extremity lesions are usually quite taut, and this is an uncommon area for the formation of keloids.

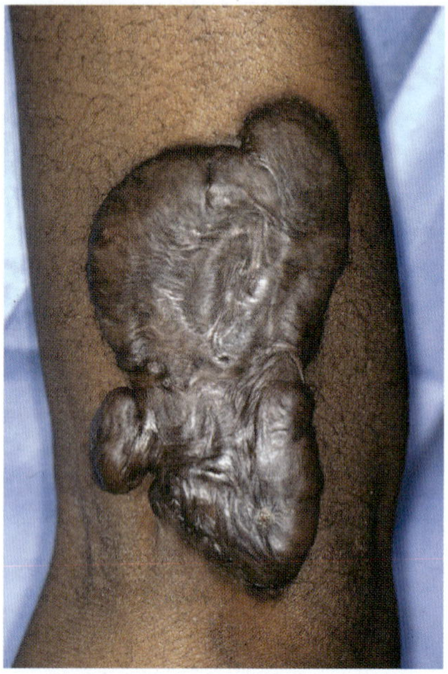

FIGURE 33-20. Proximal right forearm keloids on an African American man; extremity lesions are usually quite taut.

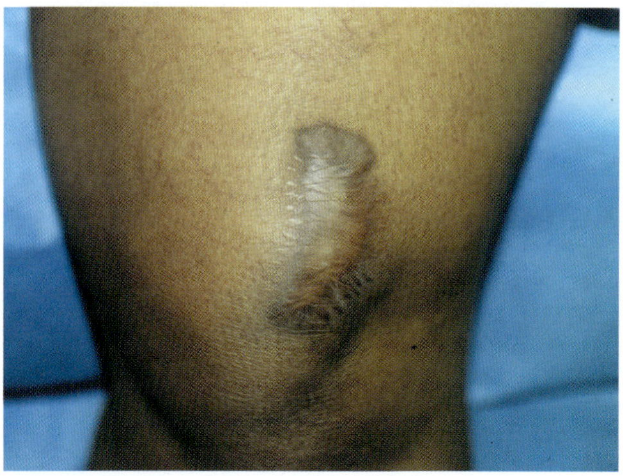

FIGURE 33-21. Keloid of the left thigh of an African American man. This keloid had a reddish center that was biopsied and proved to be sarcoidosis.

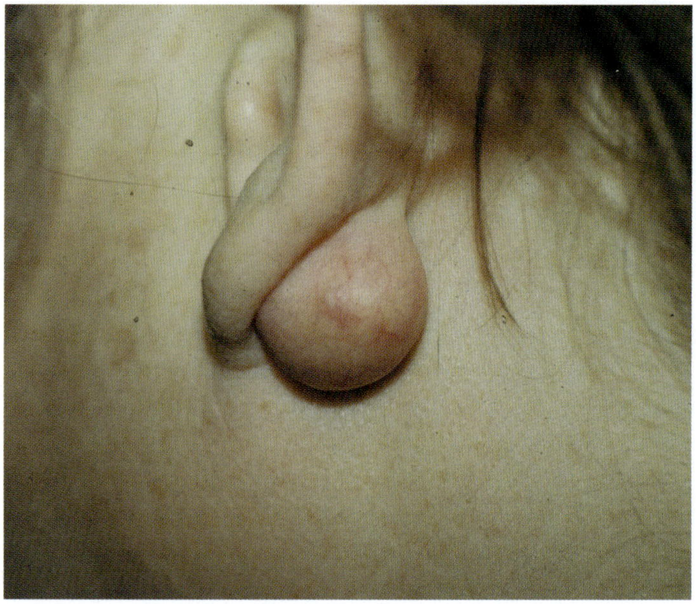

FIGURE 33-22. An epidermal cyst of the left posterior earlobe in a Hispanic woman.

spontaneously in 12 to 18 months [**Figure 33-25**].[104,105] Both types of lesions are usually asymptomatic, but keloids may be tender, painful, and pruritic, or cause a burning sensation. Keloids range in consistency from soft and doughy to rubbery and hard. They project above the level of surrounding skin but rarely extend into the underlying subcutaneous tissue. Even though the overlying epidermis is thinned from pressure, they seldom ulcerate.[99]

Oluwasanmi[21] reported that most keloids occur within a year of the injury or disease that incited their formation, although approximately 20% develop 1 to 24 years after the first recognizable injury. The lag period is usually much shorter in lesions that recur after excision.

Initial lesions are often erythematous, become brownish red and then pale in the center as they age, and are often darker at the outer border. They are usually but not always devoid of hair follicles. Once they are

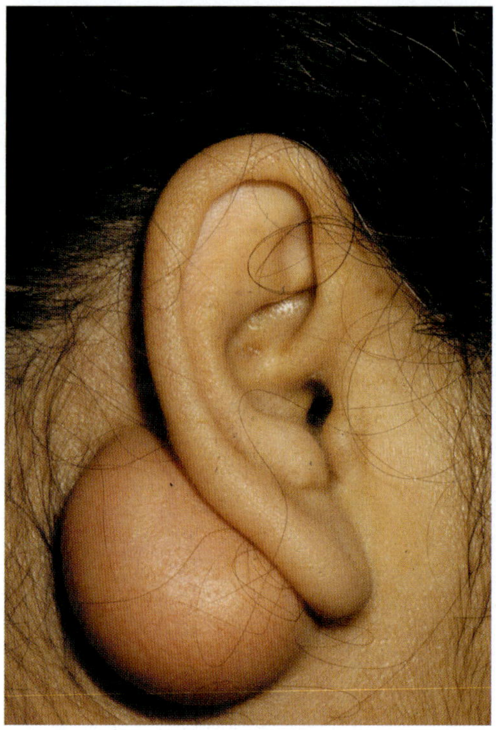

FIGURE 33-23. A lipoma of the right posterior earlobe in a Hispanic woman.

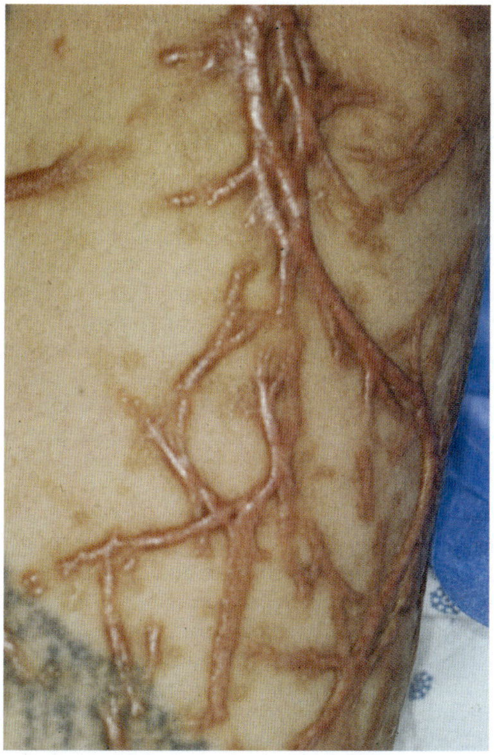

FIGURE 33-24. Linear xanthomas on the back of a Hispanic man.

present, the clinical course varies. Most continue to grow for weeks to months, and others may continue to grow for years. The growth is usually slow, but keloids will sometimes enlarge rapidly, tripling their size in months. Once they stop growing, keloids are usually asymptomatic and remain stable or involute slightly. They rarely regress spontaneously. Spontaneous regression is usually associated with advanced age; it has been reported that one keloid regressed after being present for 40 years.[99]

Keloids may range in size from papules a few millimeters in diameter to football-sized or larger tumors. Those on the ears, neck, and abdomen tend to be pedunculated, whereas those on the central chest and extremities are usually raised with a flat surface, with the base often being wider than the top. Most are round, oval, or oblong with regular margins; however, some have claw-like configurations with irregular borders. Most patients present with one or two keloids, but many patients without a known precipitating trauma have multiple lesions, as do those who develop keloids secondary to acne or chickenpox.[33]

Although keloids are clinically benign (ie, not neoplastic), they can behave in an aggressive manner and are often psychologically and/or socially devastating for patients. Up to 86% of keloid patients experience

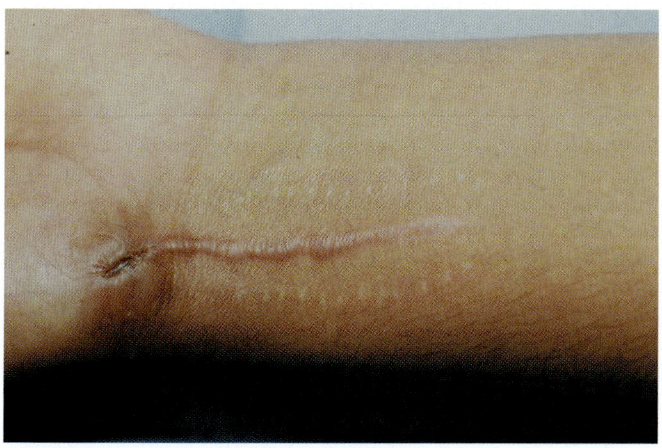

FIGURE 33-25. Linear hypertrophic scar on the wrist.

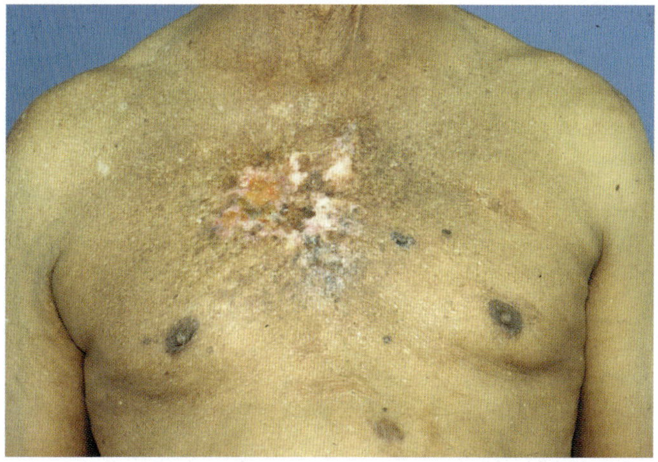

FIGURE 33-26. An African American man who developed squamous cell carcinoma in the mid-chest area, secondary to radiation treatment of a large chest keloid.

keloid-related itch while up to 46% experience keloid-related pain. Itch tends to be felt toward the periphery of the scar while pain tends to occur centrally.[106] Keloids can also be sensitive to touch or pressure, such as chest keloids that are problematic when the patient tries to wear a seatbelt with a shoulder strap (mechanical allodynia).[106] There can also be the sensation of electrical shocks or burning sensation. There are also keloids that have so much inflammation that purulent drainage occurs. Often times bacterial cultures of the purulent exudate are negative or only grow normal skin flora, indicating that these "suppurative keloids" are inflamed but not infected.[28,29] A Turkish study using the Dermatology Life Quality Index (DLQI) showed that keloids affect the quality of life of patients to a degree similar to that of psoriasis.[1]

The malignant transformation of keloids is rare, and reported cases are poorly documented. Most patients had undergone some type of radiation therapy prior to the development of malignancy.[104] Sometimes, keloids are invaded by squamous cell carcinoma. According to Stout,[105] a keloid will never develop into malignant hyperplasia; when a carcinoma does develop within a keloid, it is not a malignant degeneration of the keloid but rather of the overlying epidermis. Thus, no case has yet been reported of an unequivocally malignant change in an unirradiated keloid. Not only do keloids seem to resist malignancy, but they also seem to be spared in most generalized dermatoses [**Figure 33-26**].

PATHOGENESIS

COLLAGEN SYNTHESIS

Electron microscopic studies by Gueft[107] revealed that keloid collagen fibers are thinner and have irregularities of cross-striations, suggesting that keloid collagen is immature.[107] Studies of thermal contraction have demonstrated that, initially, keloid collagen acts like young tissue, which, once formed, proceeds to age the same way as any other newly synthesized collagen.[108]

Harris and Sjoerdsma[109] found that the water content of keloid tissue is uniformly higher than that of the clinically normal skin of the same patients, and there is no correlation between the water content and the age of the lesion. Additional findings were that the soluble collagen content and the alpha-to-beta ratio (single-polypeptide chains: double-peptide chains) are increased in all keloids. The collagen concentration in keloids is normal, but it is lower in recently formed scars. Early hypertrophic scars have the same collagen profile as keloids, whereas those more than 87 months old have the same collagen content as normal skin.[110]

FIBRONECTIN

Fibronectin is a glycoprotein synthesized by fibroblasts and an integral factor in fibroblast aggregation. Kischer and Hendrix[111] found that the immunofluorescence reaction of fibronectin is intense in hypertrophic scars and keloids and reflects exactly the conformation of the nodular structure, especially in the upper and middle reticular dermis. The investigators noted the intense reactivity of fibronectin in the hypertrophic scar and keloid cultures, but little or none in the normal skin cultures, suggesting that fibroblasts cultured from keloids and hypertrophic scars may be synthesizing more fibronectin than those from normal dermis.[110-112]

Keloid formation seems to be a function of the rate of collagen synthesis or degradation, yet does not resemble the conditions involving a change in either collagen synthesis (eg, active scleroderma, pulmonary fibrosis, liver cirrhosis, and synovial tissue proliferation in the inflammatory stages of rheumatoid arthritis) or collagen degradation (eg, cartilage destruction in rheumatoid arthritis, epidermolysis bullosa dystrophica, and hormonal disturbances such as hyperthyroidism, hyperparathyroidism, and Paget disease of bone). Keloids have an exuberance of dermal proliferation composed mostly of bands of collagen that have increased hyaluronic acid (HA) and sulfated glycosaminoglycans.[113]

Keloid lesions have a significantly reduced HA content and also show altered HA organization patterns compared with unscarred skin and normal scars. The levels of tumor necrosis factor-stimulated gene-6 (TSG6), a known HA family molecule, are significantly reduced within keloid lesions compared with the dermis of unscarred skin ($p = 0.017$).[114] An altered expression of hyaluronan synthase and hyaluronidase messenger RNA may affect HA distribution in keloid disease compared with normal skin.[115]

There are 25 types of collagen, of which type I and type III are found in the dermis. The bulk of skin collagen, as well as that of bones and tendons, is type I, which contains two identical alpha chains designated alpha 1 and a third chain called alpha 2. Type III collagen is composed of three chemical features, which are relatively high levels of hydroxyproline and lysine plus some cystine. Type III accounts for more than half of the total collagen in fetal skin but less than 20% in adult skin.[113,116] In light of the preceding, one might surmise that keloids have an increase in type I collagen, especially since this type is more resistant to proteolysis than type III.[117,118] However, studies by Clore et al[119] showed no significant difference in the percentage of type III collagen synthesized by fresh keloid biopsies compared with normal dermis. Likewise, there was no significant difference in the percentage of type III collagen synthesized by keloid fibroblasts compared with normal fibroblasts.[120] However, fibroblasts from different sites in keloid tissue, such as the perilesional site (on the margin) compared with the intralesional and extralesional sites, show differential apoptosis and contraction. Additionally, early versus later cell culture passages display differential collagen expression. Fibroblasts from the growing margin of the keloid scars have a higher production of collagen I and III compared with other lesional sites. Additionally, the temporal extension of the cell passage affects collagen production. Clinically these findings may influence the selection and interpretation of extended cell passages and provide future direction for lesional site-specific therapy in keloid scars.[121]

It has been suggested that the increased collagen accumulation in keloids does not appear to result from increased fibroblast proliferation, because fibroblasts are sparse on the histologic section of older, developing lesions, and the keloid DNA content is the same as in normal dermis. McCoy and Cohen[122] have found that sera from keloid patients do not contain a factor that significantly modifies the in vitro growth kinetics or collagen synthesis of keloid-derived or normal dermal fibroblasts. Other studies by McCoy et al[123] have demonstrated that altered collagen synthesis by keloid fibroblasts is not related to abnormal cell growth. Keloid fibroblasts did not exhibit markedly shortened in vitro life spans compared with normal dermal fibroblasts under routine culture conditions. Under sparse growth conditions, however, the keloid fibroblasts appeared to lose replicative capacities earlier than normal skin fibroblasts.[124] An examination of the collagenase produced by explants from normal skin, hypertrophic scars, and keloids cultured in vitro revealed no significant differences in either the amount of the enzyme produced or in the nature of that enzyme. The principal site of collagenase production in keloid specimens appeared to be, as in normal skin, the upper dermal or epidermal layer, with minimal production occurring in the lower fibrous or nodular areas.[125] On the other hand, an examination of the activity of the enzyme collagen synthesis revealed that it is markedly elevated in both keloids and hypertrophic scars compared with normal scars and normal skin, suggesting that the rate of collagen biosynthesis is increased in both abnormal scar types in vitro.[125] Although collagen synthesis is significantly increased in keloids, collagen degradation (ie, collagenase activity) is also the same or increased compared with that in normal skin and normal scar formation. It would seem as if this increase in collagenase would counterbalance the increase in collagen synthesis. However, Oliver et al[126] found a third factor that influences the collagen production-destruction activity in keloids: tissue α-globulins.[126] Serum α-globulins are known inhibitors of skin collagenase. Patients with keloids have normal serum α-globulins but an increased deposition of the α-globulin α1-antitrypsin and α2-macroglobulin in the keloid tissue. Investigations by Oliver et al[126] postulate that this increased deposition may, in turn, inhibit the activity of collagenase, causing a decrease in the rate of collagen degradation. In addition, these authors found that women taking oral contraceptives had elevated serum levels of α-globulins, a phenomenon that may explain why pregnant women sometimes experience a growth of existing keloids or hypertrophic scars.[126,127] Completing the collagenase-α-globulin picture is the phenomenon of intralesional steroids causing keloids to become smaller. After intralesional triamcinolone acetonide injections, there is usually a reduction in the size of a keloid as well as a significant reduction of the α1-antitrypsin deposits.[128] These findings suggest that α-globulins may be involved in abnormal scar formation and that the triamcinolone acetonide may remove collagenase inhibitors, thereby allowing activation of the collagenase with subsequent breakdown and reabsorption of the excessive collagen.[120]

LABORATORY TESTS

TISSUE CULTURES

In 1935, Tuma[129] published the first report on tissue culture techniques in the study of keloids. Almost 25 years later, Conway et al[130] found three morphologically distinct cell types in keloid tissue cultures. The most abundant was a small, highly spindle-shaped cell with a high metabolic rate, which was called the type I fibroblast. The second type, several times greater in volume with many fine cytoplasmic processes extending from its surface, was called the type II fibroblast. The type II fibroblasts migrated more slowly than type I cells and contained a larger number of mitochondria and larger nuclei. The third cell type appeared to be essentially normal fibroblasts. Conway et al[130] postulated that the type I cell is responsible for the production of the fibrous matrix and the type II cell for absorption of the matrix. This theory is even more plausible in view of the observation that older keloids, both stable and regressing, show a preponderance of cells with abnormally large nuclei (type II fibroblasts) in contrast to recently developed keloids, which usually produce an exuberant growth of type I fibroblasts in tissue culture. Keloid scars contain distinct subpopulations of mesenchymal-like stem cells (MLSCs). Cells positive for CD13, CD29, CD44, and CD90 were found to be significantly higher in the top and middle compartments of keloid scars ($p < 0.05$) compared with the extralesional skin, where cells positive for CD34, CD90, and CD117 (representing hematopoietic stem cells) predominated. A unique population of CD34+ cells (cells positive for CD13, CD29, CD34, CD44, and CD90) were found in keloid scars and in extralesional skin. Fluorescence-activated cell sorting and quantitative polymerase chain reaction analysis showed that many of the mesenchymal stem cell markers were progressively downregulated and all of the hematopoietic stem cell markers were lost during the extended keloid fibroblast culture process.[131] There are distinct subpopulations of hematopoietic and nonhematopoietic cells whereby MLSCs reside in keloid scars, and hematopoietic stem cells accumulate extralesionally. Future therapy for keloids may have to differentially target both stem cell populations to deprive these tumors of their regenerative cell pools.

Mucin-like changes have been demonstrated in keloids. However, the condition is not a true endogenous mucinosis and differs histochemically from cutaneous mucinosis. These patients had previously undergone corticosteroid injections, and the interaction of the steroids within the fibrous tissue probably produced these histologic changes.[132] Other histopathologic findings include one case of keloid calcification and one case of pseudomelanoma.[133,134]

HISTOPATHOLOGY

Because keloids and hypertrophic scars have clinical similarities, histopathologic differentiation between them is difficult.[135] Some investigators claim that no clear distinction can be made between the lesions, whereas others have found definite morphologic differences.[92] Blackburn and Cosman [127] reported that keloids have conspicuous bundles of thick, glassy, faintly refractile, pale-staining collagen—a feature absent from hypertrophic scars. In addition, keloid tissue usually has abundant mucinous ground substance, few fibroblasts, and no foreign-body reactions, whereas hypertrophic scars have scarce mucinous ground substance, numerous fibroblasts, and frequent foreign-body reactions.[136]

Another difference between keloids and hypertrophic scars is that Luxol fast blue stains normal collagen blue and keloid collagens reddish. Keloids that develop in skin defects (eg, burns and cuts) do not have a normal papillary dermis, whereas so-called spontaneous keloids and those that develop from old acne lesions are separated from the epidermis by a fairly normal papillary dermis.[137]

Early forms of fibroblasts persist longer in keloids than in normal scar tissue. In normal wound healing, connective tissue elements regress after the third week, whereas in keloids, fibroblasts proliferate around the neovascular formations to form dense masses of collagen. This process can continue for months to years, thus determining the size of the keloids.[138] Craig et al[139] reported that, in keloid tissue, as in normal skin, mast cells are present only in the dermis and never in the epidermis. However, unlike normal skin, where the mast cells are located primarily around the adnexal tissue in the superficial dermis, keloid mast cells occur throughout the dermis, interspersed among collagen bundles. Although the concentration of mast cells in the keloid dermis is not appreciably different from that in normal skin, the much thicker dermis of a keloid suggests a greater total mast cell number under a given epidermal area.[139] New elastic tissue formation is often a feature of normal scar tissue formation but not of keloids, which are also deficient in or devoid of lymphatics. Normal lymphatic function is associated with the presence of elastic tissue; lymphatics are not able to function without it.[140]

Keloids have an exuberance of dermal proliferation composed mostly of bands of collagen glycosaminoglycans.[24] Chemical analysis shows the activity of α-naphthyl acid phosphatase to be greater in keloids than in normal skin. The enzymes of the Embden-Meyerhof glycolytic pathway, and of other systems relating carbohydrate to amino acid and fatty acid metabolism, are more active in keloids and hypertrophic scars than in normal skin. Because of their high water content, collagen fibrils in keloids are bound to HA until they reach maturity.[24] A significant increase in alanine transaminase is found in keloids but not in hypertrophic scars.[141] Keloids differ from hypertrophic scars in osmotic pressure, metabolic activity, and collagen turnover, as reflected in the local concentrations of sodium, magnesium, and calcium, respectively. Keloids have a higher content of water and soluble collagen than normal skin. They are deficient in lymphatics and associated elastic fibers. These qualities are true of early hypertrophic scars as well, but after 7 months, the two diverge as hypertrophic scars normalize their water and collagen content. Sodium, a measure of osmotic pressure, is normal in keloids and decreased in hypertrophic scars, whereas magnesium, a measure of metabolic activity, is increased in keloids but decreased in hypertrophic scars. Calcium, which reflects collagen metabolism, is increased in keloids and decreased in hypertrophic scars.[142] T-cells and macrophages are increased in keloid scars and are thought to contribute to its pathogenesis. In particular, T-cells, B cells, degranulated and mature mast cells (co-expressing OX40 ligand), and alternative macrophages (M2) are all significantly increased in intralesional and perilesional keloid scar sites compared with normal skin and scar tissue ($p < 0.05$). The increased number and activity of mast cells and M2 may implicate inflammation in the fibrotic process in keloid scar tissue. Additionally, in one study, 15% of keloid cases showed the presence of distinctive lymphoid aggregates called keloid-associated lymphoid tissue (KALT), which resembled mucosa-associated lymphoid tissue.[143]

TABLE 33-7 Keloid preventative measures

- Withhold ear piercing or elective cosmetic surgery from known keloid-formers
- Avoid tattoos
- Close surgical wounds with normal tension
- Avoid making cross-joint spaces
- Avoid mid-chest incisions
- Educate the patient on postoperative care

DIFFERENTIAL DIAGNOSIS

The following are differential diagnoses that could be confused with keloids[144]:

- Hypertrophic scar
- Lipoma
- Dermatofibrosarcoma protuberans
- Dermatofibroma
- Neurofibroma
- Fibromatosis
- Acne keloidalis nuchae
- Sinus histiocytosis with massive lymphadenopathy (Rosai-Dorfman disease)

Keloids are usually distinctive enough not to be confused with other cutaneous lesions, although sometimes hypertrophic scars may be difficult to rule out. As mentioned previously, hypertrophic scars remain within the bounds of the initial injury, are not claw-like, and often regress spontaneously.[39] Allergic contact dermatitis secondary to gold earrings may produce keloid-like lesions on the earlobes, but a histopathologic study of these lesions shows a dense infiltration of lymphoid cells, plus the formation of lymphoid follicles, rather than dense collagen tissue.[96,145-147]

TREATMENT

The first rule of keloid therapy is prevention [**Table 33-7**]. Withhold nonessential cosmetic surgeries from known keloid-formers, close all surgical wounds with minimal tension, make sure that incisions do not cross joint spaces, avoid mid-sternal incisions, and, when making incisions, follow the skin creases if possible. Known keloid-formers should apply pressure with a gradient elastic garment or other apparatus for 4 to 6 months after burns, surgical procedures, or major skin trauma.

No single therapeutic modality is best for all keloids [**Table 33-8**]. The type of therapy depends on the location, size, and depth of the lesion; age of the patient; and past responses to treatment. Treatment can be frustrating for both the patient and the physician. Excision of the lesion is actually the least important part of treatment; the patient's compliance in

TABLE 33-8 Treatment of keloids

- No one therapeutic modality is best for all keloids.
- Standard treatment includes intralesional steroids, surgical excision, pressure, radiation, lasers, cryosurgery, and other medical therapies.
- Polytherapy is more successful than monotherapy.
- Excision alone has a 45-100% recurrence rate.

TABLE 33-9 Intralesional steroid injections

- Inject triamcinolone acetonide (40 mg/mL) with maximum amount of 1-1.5 mL
  - Any dose of triamcinolone acetonide greater than 3 mg/mL may cause hypopigmentation that may last 6-12 months
- Use a small-bore (27- or 29-guage) needle because it does not clog as often as large-bore needles
- Inject where the skin is wrinkled (pinch the skin for more wrinkling)
  - Epidermal-dermal plane is easier to find
  - Atrophy also may occur at injection site(s), usually lasting 6-12 months
  - For preoperative anesthesia and keloid inhibition, inject a mixture of half 40 mg/mL triamcinolone acetonide and half 2% lidocaine
  - Corticosteroids delay wound healing
  - Wait 2-3 weeks before removing sutures, except for the face, where 10 days are sufficient
- Following surgical removal with corticosteroid injections is the most common procedure
  - Wait 2 weeks after suture removal to avoid wound dehiscence
  - Give corticosteroid to postoperative site every 2-3 weeks
- Freeze with liquid nitrogen (N_2) for 10-15 seconds for easier injection
  - Liquid N_2 also provides some anesthesia and edema
- Inject every 2-3 weeks before surgery
  - To ease injection pain, apply 2% lidocaine and 2% prilocaine cream thickly under occlusion 1 hour prior to injection
- Inject inflammatory border surrounding keloid

the postoperative therapy is by far the most important factor.[31] The lack of uniform treatment guidelines, with no foolproof protocol for physicians to follow, is the crux of the problem regarding keloids. In fact, even the optimal time to start treatment is currently unknown.[99]

CORTICOSTEROID INJECTIONS

The treatment of choice for most earlobe keloids, and those in locations other than the mid-sternal region, is corticosteroid injections [**Tables 33-9** to **33-11**]. Corticosteroid injections should be given every 2 to 4 weeks, and at least four times prior to the surgery. Triamcinolone acetonide solution is the most commonly use corticosteroid. The diagnosis and treatment of keloids remain basically the same irrespective of the patient's skin color.[89,148]

Here are a few therapeutic recommendations:

1. Procedures to decrease the pain from injections:
   - Prior to the injection of intralesional steroids, the keloid should be covered with a topical anesthetic such as a eutectic mixture of one-half (2%) lidocaine and one-half prilocaine, to help the patient withstand the pain of the injection. This topical anesthesia should be applied an hour before surgery and occluded with a very thin plastic wrap. The lidocaine does not relieve the initial pain of injection, but does allow multiple injections with minimal discomfort and prevents most postinjection pain.
   - Prior to the injection, the local administration of lidocaine (1%) ± epinephrine as a ring block surrounding the keloid can relive the pain of the steroid injection itself. Though there is some burning/stinging from the local administration, this usually pales in comparison to the pain from the steroid injection itself. In the authors' experience, the local administration of lidocaine ± epinephrine with 30G or 27G needles does not seem sufficient to induce keloidal papules. The topical anesthetic described above can be used prior to the lidocaine ring block to decrease the morbidity of steroid administration, though this must be weighed against the time required to administer these measures.
   - Another way of making steroid injections less painful is to pretreat the keloid with liquid nitrogen, and then allow a 10- to 15-second thaw time. This causes tissue edema, making the injection into the keloid much easier. Allowing more than a 25-second thaw time will often cause hypopigmentation. Triamcinolone acetonide injections in concentrations of 3 mg/mL or higher may also cause hypopigmentation of the injected area for 6 to 12 months; patients need to be informed of this possibility.
2. Needle injection procedure:
   - Because the keloids are often hard, one method of injecting the steroid is to insert the needle deep into the keloid. Slowly remove the needle while injecting the keloid until reaching the dermal–epidermal junction. In this way, the steroid can be injected more easily into the keloid. It is recommended to use a small 27-gauge needle, because larger-bore needles may behave like a punch biopsy.
   - Sometimes the base of the keloid is so fibrotic that it is almost impossible to inject. In these cases, insert a large-bore needle into the keloid, and inject the triamcinolone acetonide solution as the needle is slowly withdrawn.
3. Intralesional steroid mixture for keloid therapy:
   - Triamcinolone acetonide 40 mg/mL can be used for larger keloid lesions, while 20 mg/mL (equal part 40 mg/mL and sterile saline) or even 10 mg/mL can be used to treat hypertrophic scarring.
   - Use a Luer-Lok needle or fixed-needle insulin syringe to prevent the needle from separating from the syringe during the injection. To prevent clogging, use nothing larger than a 27-gauge needle for either dosage of triamcinolone acetonide. The 40 mg/mL dosage sometimes puddles in the injected sites, forming superficial xanthoma-like deposits that may have to be removed for optimal cosmetic results. For easy removal of the steroid, use a small curette, or make a nick in the skin and use a strong suction apparatus.
4. Procedures to prevent leakage/atrophy:
   - The steroid solution is under great pressure and often leaks out. To prevent leaking, paint the area around the needle site with a tincture of benzoin, and cover it with a piece of waterproof tape immediately after withdrawing the needle.
   - Inject only the base of the keloid or the lesion itself, not the surrounding tissue; injecting the surrounding areas may cause normal tissue to atrophy and to result in hypopigmentation, and the keloid

TABLE 33-10 Multiple complications with the use of systemic corticosteroids in the treatment of keloids

- Severe infections
- Hyperglycemia (not usual)
- Edema
- Osteonecrosis
- Myopathy
- Peptic ulcer disease
- Hypokalemia
- Osteoporosis
- Euphoria
- Psychosis
- Myasthenia gravis
- Growth suppression
- Abrupt discontinuation may cause an adrenal crisis

TABLE 33-11 Intralesional interferon-α-2b

- Inject 1 million units per linear centimeter of the postoperative site
- Repeat 1-3 weeks later
- Warn patients about flu-like symptoms
  - Premedicate with 500-1000 mg of acetaminophen
  - Taken every 6 hours in the evening for pain for 2 days
  - 18% recurrence with interferon-α-2b
  - 51-100% recurrence with surgery only

to sink down to the level of surrounding skin without becoming flat or softer.

5. Be sure to inform patients that:
   - The initial injection often produces no visible change in the keloid but may make it softer and alleviate most symptomology.
   - The steroid injections will not narrow the scar, even if it completely flattens.[31,146,149-152]

The effect of corticosteroids on collagen synthesis and degradation is not completely understood, but it is known that corticosteroids seem to work better in early keloids. This may be because only the younger fibroblasts can be induced by steroids to produce collagenase.[153] Older cells appear not to respond to steroids with collagenase production. In addition, cortisol administration in rats causes a rapid disappearance of collagen from the dermis, whereas prednisone, cortisone, and deoxycorticosterone are without effect. This difference indicates that the β-hydroxyl group present in prednisone, cortisol, and triamcinolone acetonide is necessary to exert the effect and may explain why triamcinolone acetonide injections are helpful in reducing the size of keloids.[149-152]

Approximately 50% of patients with keloids are considered nonresponders (or steroid-resistant) with no consensus or indicators in detecting steroid-sensitive patients. In view of the undesirable side effects, uncertainty in timing, and regularity of steroid treatment, it is important to identify responders and nonresponders to target treatment more effectively. Ud-Din et al[154] developed a scar injection pro forma to capture a detailed history, focusing on the symptoms and signs (redness, appearance, contour, texture, distortion, and severity) associated with keloids. The cause, site, number of keloid scars, and scar recurrence were recorded while the lesions were injected on a monthly basis. A detailed description of the response to steroid injection was documented, and photographs were taken. Patients were classified as steroid responders if they showed improvement in symptoms and signs within 3 months. There was a statistically significant correlation between patients with higher contour scores of keloids prior to treatment ($p = 0.013$) and the frequency of injections ($p = 0.003$). Thus, the odds of being a responder were greater for patients with more than one injection and with higher contour scores. This preliminary case series provided early evidence in enabling identification of steroid responders versus nonresponders within a 3-month period.[154] Potentially painful injections, their subsequent side effects, the unnecessary continuation of a redundant therapy, and the need for subsequent follow-ups can all be avoided if keloid nonresponders are not subjected to steroid treatment. Current use of corticosteroid injections is partially beneficial with a significant recurrence rate. Additionally, the efficacy of different steroids, alone or in combination, as opposed to monotherapy in treating keloids remains unclear. Syed and Bayat[155] compared the single and combined efficacy of glucocorticoids—dexamethasone, triamcinolone acetonide, and methylprednisolone—on primary keloid and normal skin fibroblasts at the cellular, protein, and messenger RNA levels in vitro.[155] They demonstrated that cytotoxicity to steroids was dose dependent. Cell spreading, attachment, and proliferation were significantly reduced by methylprednisolone and triamcinolone acetonide, and the migration and invasion properties of the keloid fibroblasts were significantly inhibited by methylprednisolone and triamcinolone acetonide ($p < 0.05$), compared with dexamethasone. Combined treatment with dexamethasone and triamcinolone acetonide, as well as dexamethasone and methylprednisolone, significantly induced apoptosis ($p < 0.05$). In conclusion, this study looked at the efficacy of three well-known steroids on keloid fibroblasts and suggested that a combination of steroids may be superior to using a single steroid in the treatment of keloids.

CHEMOTHERAPEUTIC INJECTIONS

The intralesional injection of chemotherapeutic agent into keloids should be considered in cases recalcitrant to intralesional steroids (ie, steroid nonresponders). These antiproliferative medications work by decreasing the number of fibroblasts and inflammatory cells in the keloids. Older keloids may therefore be less responsive to these medications than newer, actively growing keloids. Injections can be monthly, but the frequency can be increased up to weekly if needed. There is less concern about atrophy, telangiectasias, and hypopigmentation as side effects. However, there may be postinflammatory hyperpigmentation from the medication. In addition, if the medication is injected too superficially, it may affect the overlying keratinocytes in the epidermis leading to shallow ulceration. The antimetabolite 5-fluorouracil (5-FU) disrupts DNA replication and thereby inhibits fibroblast proliferation. It can be used as monotherapy or in combination with other treatments, most commonly intralesional triamcinolone (TAC). Studies have shown superior or noninferior results with IL 5-FU/TAC compared to IL TAC alone.[156-158] Bleomycin has also been shown to be effective in the treatment of keloids.[159,160] With either medication, proper disposal of the unused drug as well as the used syringes/needles is required.

VERAPAMIL INJECTIONS

Verapamil, a calcium channel blocker, was proposed initially for keloid treatment due to its potential to block fibrosis in vitro.[161] However, this treatment has seen quite mixed results, with some studies showing strong efficacy,[162-165] while others show inferiority in efficacy compared to triamcinolone injections.[161,166,167] These conflicting results make future use of intralesional verapamil therapy in keloids quite unclear.

SURGERY

If there is no significant regression of the keloid tissue after four intralesional corticosteroid injections, or if the keloid no longer responds to further injections, surgery is recommended [**Figure 33-27**]. The surgical method differs according to the size and location of the lesions:

1. For keloids with a narrow base (<1 cm in diameter), a simple excision followed by an undermining of the base and closure with interrupted sutures will suffice. Before closure, the base of the operative site should be injected with Kenalog-40 so that the earliest fibroblasts are exposed to steroids. Alternatively, surgical anesthesia can be provided with one-half 2% lidocaine and one-half triamcinolone acetonide (40 mg/mL) mixed together.
2. For posterior pedunculated earlobe keloids, for which cosmetic appearance is not important, shaving followed by pressure hemostasis is a simple and efficient method of removal.
3. For large, nonpedunculated earlobe keloids and keloids with wide bases (>1 cm in diameter) on other parts of the body, removal is more complex. First, a half-moon incision, approximately one-fifth of the size of the lesion, is made from one border onto the part of the keloid with the smoothest and flattest-looking surface. The remaining part of the keloid should then be excised, and the tip of the saved epidermis and superficial dermis carefully dissected from the underlying white

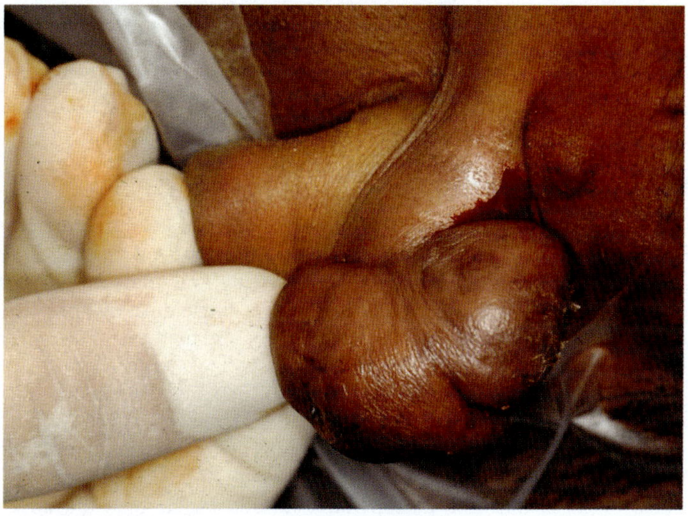

FIGURE 33-27. Surgical removal of an earlobe keloid.

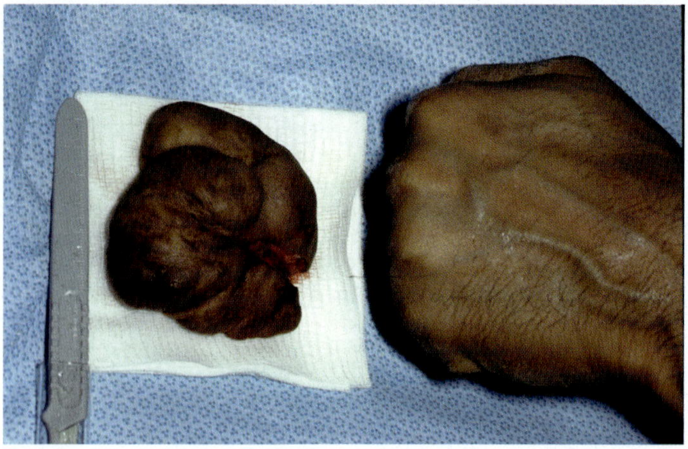

FIGURE 33-28. A surgically removed keloid approximately the size of a man's fist.

glistening fibrous tissue mass. Triamcinolone acetonide (40 mg/mL) should be injected into the base of the surgical site. The overlying skin should then be approximated to the undermined borders of the excision with 6-0 nylon interrupted sutures. The sutures should be left in for 10 to 14 days because earlier removal may cause wound dehiscence. This slow healing is the consequence of the steroid injection. A week after suture removal, the postoperative site should be injected with triamcinolone acetonide (10 mg/mL) every 2 weeks. In most cases, four postoperative injections are sufficient to prevent recurrence [**Figure 33-28**].

4. In patients in whom the overlying skin is not smooth enough to be used as a cover for the excised tissue, a tissue expander may be inserted so that the keloid can be excised and then closed several months later.[99]

Keloid disease is known to show variable clinical behavior in response to surgical excision, and there is no clinicopathologic classification that predicts such varied behavior. A study in 2010 by Tan et al[168] showed the effect of excision margins and other histopathologic characteristics on keloid prognosis. A detailed histopathologic examination of all tissue samples identified keloid border or margin characteristics, which were classified into circumscribed (borders clearly demarcated) and infiltrative (borders not clearly demarcated and not easily definable). The specific histologic findings were correlated with keloid recurrence, which revealed that incomplete peripheral and deep excision margins as well as infiltrative borders were associated with higher 1-year reported recurrence rates ($p < 0.001$, $p < 0.001$, and $p < 0.05$, respectively).[168] This study has provided evidence that incomplete surgical excision is associated with higher recurrence, and this may justify the practice of routine histopathologic reporting of keloid excision margins.

PRESSURE

Another adjunct for preventing recurrence is the use of a pressure gradient garment on the postoperative site for at least 12 hours a day—although 20 hours is preferable—for 4 to 6 months [**Figure 33-29**]. For earlobe keloids, special pressure earrings or devices may be used. The proposed mechanism of action is outlined in **Table 33-12**.[169-171]

RADIATION THERAPY

For patients with mid-chest keloids or a history of keloid recurrence after surgery, radiation therapy is an adjunct modality. A dose of 2.50 Gy is given immediately after surgery, followed by four more treatments at weekly intervals. Other regimens include a single dose of 10 Gy the day after surgery or 3 Gy the day after surgery and then every other day thereafter for a total of three treatments.

Fischer and Storck[172] treated more than 300 patients with radiotherapy alone. In a 20-year follow-up, they found that radiotherapy was most effective when used within the first 5 months of keloid formation. Their total dose ranged from 8 to 24 Gy over a period of 2 to 5 months. They noted better results with postoperative keloids, lacerations, and infections than with scars from burns, scalds, and caustics. More intensive

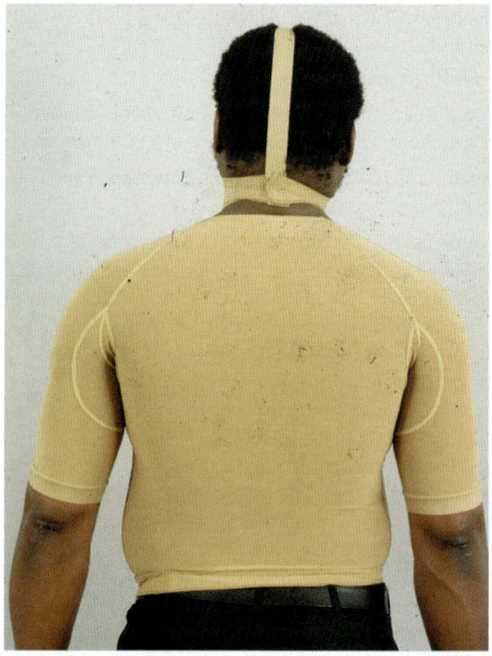

FIGURE 33-29. A pressure-gradient garment that helps to prevent recurrence of treated keloids.

studies by van den Brank and Minty[97] concluded that primary irradiation of early keloids that are still cellular, well-vascularized, and growing may cause some resolution if more than 10 Gy is given. They found no merit in fractionating the doses. When treating older keloids, primary radiation alone failed to cause resolution, although it did relieve symptoms such as pruritus. Doses of 10 Gy or more may cause atrophy of the irradiated area or radionecrosis, leading to more keloid formation.

Additionally, van den Brank and Minty[97] demonstrated that preoperative radiation was unsatisfactory for reducing keloids, and because of the rapid recovery from radiation, there may be superregeneration. Postoperative radiation within 48 hours of surgery was the most effective technique in their series; the optimal dose was between 10 and 15 Gy. They advocated a margin of 0.5 cm of normal skin. This dose caused atrophy of the subcutaneous tissues, which eventually may lead to squamous cell carcinoma.[97]

Other investigators, after protecting the surrounding skin with putty containing bismuth, found that 5 Gy every 5 days, starting on the first postoperative day, for four doses, prevents recurrence.[173,174] Shaffer et al[175] evaluated 13 studies of keloids treated with radiation, with a total of 2225 patients having 2592 keloidal scars. They concluded that although all the studies were retrospective and uncontrolled, it appeared that radiation after surgical excision prevented recurrence of keloidal scars in approximately 75% of patients at a 1-year follow-up. The most frequently used treatment was superficial X-rays of 9 cGy or greater in fractions given within 10 days of surgery.[175]

Young children with keloids either should not be irradiated or, if they are, the metaphyses should be shielded to prevent retardation of bone growth. Even doses of less than 4 Gy may cause growth retardation.[24]

LASER TREATMENT

The Pulse Dye Laser (PDL) was one of the earliest laser interventions used to treat keloids; it targets hemoglobin, making it useful in vascular keloids.[176] While an early case report actually found PDL (585 nm) to

TABLE 33-12 Keloid pressure treatment
• Start pressure garments 1 week after suture removal
• Reduces size and thickness of keloids
• Reduces intralesional mast cells
• Reduces histamine production
• Combine with a class I steroid

result in keloid recurrence after previous flattening, subsequent studies have shown efficacy in keloid treatment.[177] Another study showed us of PDL resulted in a significant decrease in the Vancouver Scar Scale (VSS) score, including improved pain and itch, pliability, and erythema, though hyperpigmentation can be a noted side effect.[178,179]

Abergel et al[180] reported the successful treatment of keloids with the neodymium-doped yttrium aluminum garnet (Nd:YAG) laser. Nd:YAG laser therapy may be combined with intralesional steroids during surgery and every 2 to 3 weeks, with four treatments per week. A study evaluating the 585-nm pulsed-dye laser for the treatment of keloidal scars demonstrated efficacy in reducing subjective symptoms, color, and height of the scars.[181]

More recent work has focused on the use of fractional carbon dioxide (CO_2) laser. CO_2 laser monotherapy (four sessions, 6 weeks apart) was shown to have mixed results in a study of both keloids and hypertrophic scars. While statistically significant reduction of VSS scores was seen (largely because of increased pliability), many patients were not satisfied with this therapy.[182] A case report found that treatment with fractionated CO_2 laser and laser-assisted drug delivery of topical triamcinolone caused scar thinning and visual improvement.[183] CO_2 laser can also be combined with intralesional steroids in a manner similar to that noted for Nd:YAG.

Combination treatment using both triamcinolone as well as 1064 nm Nd:YAG laser reduced height and erythema to a greater degree than triamcinolone monotherapy, and without dyspigmentation.[184] A study comparing Nd:YAG to PDL found neither being statistically superior, though Nd:YAG was more painful.[185] There are case reports of combination laser treatment (eg, PDL and CO_2 laser) and triamcinolone on a keloid that was unresponsive to triamcinolone alone.[186] These results support the use of lasers as an adjunct therapy.

CRYOTHERAPY

In the treatment of keloids, cryotherapy leads to a decrease in inflammation as well as improvement in the organization of dermal collagen. While painful, intralesional therapy is efficacious, especially with newer keloid lesions.[187] One study showed that ear keloids treated with immediate cryotherapy after keloidectomy was 71% effective in flattening of the lesions at a 2 year follow-up. Though there was a 36% recurrence rate after one treatment, 68% of the recurrent lesions achieved flattened after a second treatment.[188] Another study found that hypopigmentation and recurrence after intralesional cryotherapy was more likely to occur in darker Fitzpatrick skin types (types V-VI vs I-II).[189] In comparing intralesional cryotherapy versus spray cryotherapy, spray requires more sessions; both get good results but intralesional seems more effective.[187] For spray cryotherapy, sessions at 2 week intervals seen optimal to maintain results, and may not be ideal as monotherapy in the treatment of thicker keloids.[190] Cryotherapy also can be used an anesthetic in the treatment of keloids; a study using a cryotherapy probe before corticosteroid injections showed a decrease in reported pain that was statistically significant.[191]

FLURANDRENOLIDE TAPE

In contrast to the United States, corticosteroid tapes and plasters are often used as first-line therapy for the treatment of keloids and hypertrophic scars in Japan.[192] In the United States, there is a commercially available formulation that comprises a flurandrenolide-impregnated tape (4 μg/cm^2). The use of a steroid tape/plaster obviates the pain associated with injections. Furthermore, in the pediatric and elderly populations, their thinner skin allows for easier absorption of the medication. Application of the steroid-impregnated tape at least 5 days a week is effective in flattening hypertrophic scars and small keloids, and can be used in combination with corticosteroid injections.[193]

PENTOXIFYLLINE

Pentoxifylline is a methyl xanthine derivative and a nonselective phosphodiesterase inhibitor that has been shown to decrease fibrosis broadly, including radiation-induced fibrosis.[194] In patients with keloids, pentoxifylline is able to halt the progression of keloids as well as the reduce symptomatology (pruritus and pain).[195] Additionally, pentoxifylline has been shown to decrease the post-surgical keloid recurrence risk.[196]

TABLE 33-13 Miscellaneous treatments for keloids

- Silicone gel sheeting, flurandenolide tape, or cosmetic pad
  - Start 1 week after suture removal
- Pentoxifylline (400 mg) 3 times a day
  - Limited success

OTHER TREATMENTS

Silicone gel and other dressings [**Table 33-13**] have been evaluated in 12 studies involving 538 patients with keloidal or hypertrophic scars. Treatment was applied for at least 12 hours. Although most of the studies involved hypertrophic scars, in the one with keloidal scars, 34% of the scars showed flattening after 6 months of continuous gel use.[197]

Ligatures may be used for pedunculated keloids when surgery or corticosteroid injections are either contraindicated or refused by the patient. A 4-0 nonabsorbable suture can be tied tightly around the base of the lesion, and a new one applied every 2 to 3 weeks. The sutures will gradually cut into and strangulate the keloid, eventually causing it to fall off. An interesting past custom in the southern part of the United States was to tie the hair of a horse's mane around the keloid instead of a suture.[99]

Topical tretinoin applied twice a day may alleviate pruritus and other keloid symptoms and may cause various degrees of regression. This method seems to be even more effective when combined with a potent topical steroid.[198]

In addition, there have been small studies or case reports using several other modalities. Ultraviolet A1 radiation has been reported to soften and flatten keloids.[199,200] Onwukwe had success with surgical excision combined with methotrexate. Methotrexate induces folic acid deficiency, resulting in poor collagen formation. Methotrexate (15-20 mg) should be given orally in a single dose every 4 days, starting a week prior to surgery, and continued for 3 to 4 months after the postoperative site is healed.[201]

Oral medications such as asiatic acid, penicillamine, colchicine, and β-aminopropionitrile have been combined with surgical excision to prevent recurrence. Numerous other topical, physical, and systemic modalities have been advocated but have either been unsuccessful or proved less effective than those mentioned earlier.[99,100] Imiquimod is a topical therapeutic agent that behaves as an immune response modulator by inducing interferon-α; interluken-1, interluken-6, and interluken-8; and tumor necrosis factor-α. In a small 13-patient study by Berman and Kaufman,[151] imiquimod cream was applied to the postoperative site daily for 8 weeks, starting immediately after surgery. Some of these patients experienced marked irritation and had to discontinue the medication for 3 to 6 days. Imiquimod should not be used on postoperative incision sites, flaps, grafts, large wounds, and wounds under tension for 4 to 6 weeks because they may splay or dehisce. Also, over half of the patients using imiquimod will develop hyperpigmentation of the treated areas.[150]

A recent study showed that keloid tissue had increased expression of Th2-associated cytokine IL-4R and IL-13, and that an African American patient with atopic dermatitis and concomitant popliteal fossa keloids had substantial keloid regression on dupilumab, an IL4/IL-13 inhibitor.[75] Since this report, there have been conflicting reports as to the efficacy of dupilumab in the treatment of keloids.[202-205] More data including clinical trial results are needed to place dupilumab in the armamentarium for patients with a high keloid burden.

Photodynamic therapy (PDT) uses light to activate a photosensitizer localized in diseased tissues. Two recent case studies and in vitro studies on keloid-derived fibroblasts indicate the potential use of PDT in treating keloids.[206-208] In 2013, Ud-Din et al[209] showed the effect of PDT in 20 keloid patients who were divided into three groups: those with existing keloid scars, those after surgical debulking, and those after total surgical excision. Patients underwent three treatments of PDT at weekly intervals. The methyl aminolevulinate photosensitizer was applied 3 hours prior to the PDT, administered at 37 J/cm^2. Noninvasive measures provided quantitative data for pliability, hemoglobin, melanin, collagen, and flux. Pain and pruritus scores were measured, and patients were monitored for keloid recurrence. All patients had reduced pain and pruritus scores. Hemoglobin flux ($p = 0.032$), collagen ($p = 0.066$), and hemoglobin levels ($p = 0.060$) decreased from week 1 to 3 in all except one patient, and pliability increased significantly ($p = 0.001$). Increases in pliability were significantly related to decreases in flux ($p = 0.001$). Only one patient with a keloid in a stress-prone anatomic location experienced recurrence. None of the other patients showed recurrence at a 9-month follow-up. Minimal side effects were reported. In conclusion, PDT reduces scar formation in keloids, evidenced by decreased blood flow, increased pliability, and decreased collagen and hemoglobin levels. These findings indicate potential utility of PDT in the treatment of keloids.

CONCLUSION

Keloids are benign fibrous growths that potentially can cause significant disfigurement and impacting the quality of life of the patient; they result from an abnormal connective tissue response in certain predisposed individuals. In general, those with greater skin pigmentation form keloids more often than those with less skin pigmentation, but the reason for this difference is not known. Trauma, foreign-body reactions, infections, and endocrine dysfunction have all been proposed as precipitating factors. Keloids are found most commonly on the mid-chest, shoulders, upper back, and earlobes. They extend past the area of trauma and, once present, tend to remain stable. Although sometimes pruritic, painful, or tender, they are usually asymptomatic. Keloids often arise during pregnancy, grow more rapidly during pregnancy, and are more common after puberty. The most common therapeutic approach is a combination of intralesional steroid injections, surgical excision, and pressure devices.

REFERENCES

1. Balci DD, Inandi T, Dogramaci CA, Celik E. DLQI scores in patients with keloids and hypertrophic scars: a prospective case control study. *J Dtsch Dermatol Ges*. 2009;7(8):688-692.
2. Reinholz M, Poetschke J, Schwaiger H, Epple A, Ruzicka T, Gauglitz GG. The dermatology life quality index as a means to assess life quality in patients with different scar types. *J Eur Acad Dermatol Venereol*. 2015;29(11):2112-2119.
3. Poetschke J, Reinholz M, Schwaiger H, Epple A, Gauglitz GG. DLQI and POSAS scores in keloid patients. *Facial Plast Surg*. 2016;32(3):289-295.
4. Datubo-Brown DD. Keloids: a review of the literature. *Br J Plast Surg*. 1990; 43(1):70-77.
5. Atiyeh BS, Costagliola M, Hayek SN. Keloid or hypertrophic scar: the controversy: review of the literature. *Ann Plast Surg*. 2005;54(6):676-680.
6. Bloom D. Heredity of keloids; review of the literature and report of a family with multiple keloids in five generations. *N Y State J Med*. 1956;56(4):511-519.
7. Yedomon GH, Adegbidi H, Atadokpede F, Akpadjan F, Mouto EJ, do Ango-Padonou F. [Keloids on dark skin: a consecutive series of 456 cases]. *Med Sante Trop*. 2012;22(3):287-291.
8. Alibert JLM. *Description des maladies de la peau: Observées à l'Hôspital Saint Louis, et exposition des meilleures méthodes suivies pour leur traitement*. Barrois l'Aîné et Fils, *Brussels*; 1806.
9. Alibert JLM. *Description des maladies de la peau: Observées à l'Hôpital Saint Louis, et Exposition des Meilleures Méthodes Suivies Pour Leur Traitement*. 2nd ed. Auguste Wahlen, *Brussels*; 1825.
10. von Hebra F, Kaposi, M. *On Diseases of the Skin Including the Exanthema*. New Sydenham Society, *London*; 1874.
11. Hawkins C. Cases of warty tumours in cicatrices. *Med Chir Trans*. 1835; 19:19-34.
12. Macpherson J. On tumors of cicatrices. *London Med Gaz*. 1844;35:348.
13. Breasted JH. *The Edwin Smith Surgical Papyrus, Vol 1: Hieroglyphic Translation and Commentary*. University of Chicago Press; 1930.
14. Omo-Dare P. Yoruban contributions to the literature on keloids. *J Natl Med Assoc*. 1973;65(5):367-372 passim.
15. Cohen IK, McCoy BJ. Keloid: biology and treatment. In: Dineen P, Hildick-Smith, G, eds. *The Surgical Wound*. Lea & Febiger, *Paris;* 1981:123-131.
16. Tulandi T, Al-Sannan B, Akbar G, Ziegler C, Miner L. Prospective study of intraabdominal adhesions among women of different races with or without keloids. *Am J Obstet Gynecol*. 2011;204(2):132.e1-4.
17. Young WG, Worsham MJ, Joseph CL, Divine GW, Jones LR. Incidence of keloid and risk factors following head and neck surgery. *JAMA Facial Plast Surg*. 2014;16(5):379-380.
18. Limmer EE, Knowles A, Deng J, Parthasarathy V, Kwatra SG, Glass DA. Atopic dermatitis is associated with an increased risk of keloids: a case-control study. *J Am Acad Dermatol*. 2023;88(5):1177-1179.
19. Alhady SM, Sivanantharajah K. Keloids in various races. A review of 175 cases. *Plast Reconstr Surg*. 1969;44(6):564-566.
20. Arnold HL. Keloids. In: Maddon S, ed. *Current Medical Management*. 2nd ed. Mosby, *London*; 1975:194.
21. Oluwasanmi JO. Keloids in the African. *Clin Plast Surg*. 1974;1(1):179-195.
22. Ketchum LD, Cohen IK, Masters FW. Hypertrophic scars and keloids. A collective review. *Plast Reconstr Surg*. 1974;53(2):140-154.
23. Cosman, B., Crikelair, G.F., Ju, D.M.C., Gaulin, J.C. and Lattes, R. The surgical treatment of keloids. *Plast Reconstr Surg*. 1961;27:335-345.
24. Al-Attar A, Mess S, Thomassen JM, Kauffman CL, Davison SP. Keloid pathogenesis and treatment. *Plast Reconstr Surg*. 2006;117(1):286-300.
25. Ogawa R. Keloid and hypertrophic scars are the result of chronic inflammation in the reticular dermis. *Int J Mol Sci*. 2017;18(3):606.
26. Wang ZC, Zhao WY, Cao Y, et al. The roles of inflammation in keloid and hypertrophic scars. *Front Immunol*. 2020;11:603187.
27. Lee CC, Tsai CH, Chen CH, Yeh YC, Chung WH, Chen CB. An updated review of the immunological mechanisms of keloid scars. *Front Immunol*. 2023;14:1117630.
28. Delaleu J, Duverger L, Shourick J, et al. Suppurative keloids: a complication of severe keloid disease. *Int J Dermatol*. 2021;60(11):1392-1396.
29. Onwukwe MF. The suppurative keloid. *J Dermatol Surg Oncol*. 1978;4(4): 333-335.
30. Limmer EE, Glass DA 2nd. A review of current keloid management: mainstay monotherapies and emerging approaches. *Dermatol Ther*. 2020;10(5):931-948.
31. Viera MH, Amini S, Valins W, Berman B. Innovative therapies in the treatment of keloids and hypertrophic scars. *J Clin Aesthet Dermatol*. 2010;3(5):20-26.
32. Lorber B. Are all diseases infectious? *Ann Intern Med*. 1996;125(10):844-851.
33. Koonin AJ. The aetiology of keloids: a review of the literature and a new hypothesis. *S Afr Med J*. 1964;38:913-916.
34. Moustafa MF, Abdel-Fattah MA, Abdel-Fattah DC. Presumptive evidence of the effect of pregnancy estrogens on keloid growth. Case report. *Plast Reconstr Surg*. 1975;56(4):450-453.
35. Gao FL, Jin R, Zhang L, Zhang YG. The contribution of melanocytes to pathological scar formation during wound healing. *Int J Clin Exp Med*. 2013;6(7):609-613.
36. Diegelmann RF, Bryant CP, Cohen IK. Tissue alpha-globulins in keloid formation. *Plast Reconstr Surg*. 1977;59(3):418-423.
37. Yamaguchi Y, Hearing VJ. Melanocytes and their diseases. *Cold Spring Harb Perspect Med*. 2014;4(5):a017046.
38. Glucksmann A. Local factors in the histogenesis of hypertrophic scars. *Br J Plast Surg*. 1951;4(2):88-103.
39. Garb J, Stone MJ. Keloids: review of the literature and a report of eighty cases. *Am J Surg Pathol*. 1942;58:315-335.
40. Justice J. Beobachtungen und experimente zur ätiologie des keloids. *Arch Dermatol Syph*. 1919;197:274.
41. Asboe-Hansen G. Hypertrophic scars and keloids. Etiology, pathogenesis and dermatologic therapy. *Dermatologica*. 1960;120:178-184.
42. Allan J. The management of keloid in the South African Bantu. *S Afr Med J*. 1954;28:1034-1037.
43. Pautrier L, Zorn R. Calcemie: teneur en calcium de la peau dans les chéloides et les acnés chéloidiennes. *Bull Soc Fr Dermatol Syphiligr*. 1931;38:953-961.
44. Farndon J. Postoperative complications of parathyroidectomy. In: Holzheimer R, Mannick, JA, ed. *Surgical Treatment: Evidence-Based and Problem-Oriented*. Zuckschwerdt, *Munich*; 2001.
45. Myśliwska J, Trzonkowski P, Bryl E, et al. Lower interleukin-2 and higher serum tumor necrosis factor levels are associated with perimenstrual, recurrent, facial herpes simplex infection in young women. *Eur Cytokine Netw*. 2000;11:397-406.
46. Geschickter C, Lewis, D Tumors of connective tissue. *Am J Cancer*. 1935; 25:630-655.
47. Solomons BJ. Keloids and their treatment. *Practitioner*. 1952;168:465-472.

48. Vargas LJ. Attempt to induce formation of fibroids with estrogens in the castrated female Rhesus monkey. *Bull Johns Hopkins Hosp*. 1943;73:23-28.
49. Personen S, Rintala A, Soivio A, et al. On the [4-14C] progesterone metabolism of keloid and hypertrophic scar: a preliminary report. *Scand J Plast Reconstr Surg*. 1976;10:173-176.
50. Ford L, Kind DF, Lagasse LD, et al. Increased androgen binding in keloids: a preliminary communication. *J Dermatol Surg Oncol*. 1983;9:545-547.
51. Louw L, Dannhauser A. Keloids in rural black South Africans. Part 2: dietary fatty acid intake and total phospholipid fatty acid profile in the blood of keloid patients. *Prostaglandins Leukot Essent Fatty Acids*. 2000;63(5):247-253.
52. Edgerton MJ, Hanrahan, EM, Davis, WB. Use of vitamin E in the treatment of keloids. *Plast Reconstr Surg*. 1951;8:224-233.
53. Kobak M, Benditt, EP, Wissler, RM, et al. Relationship of protein deficiency to experimental wound healing. *Surg Gynecol Obstet*. 1947;85:751-756.
54. Bowesman C. *Surgery and Clinical Pathology in the Tropics*. E & S Livingstone, *Edinburgh and London*; 1960.
55. Discussions with Wilbert Jordan, MD, Director of the OASIS Clinic, Los Angeles County Department of Health Services, Martin Luther King Jr. Multi-Service Ambulatory Care Center, Los Angeles, CA.
56. Lee J, Yang, CC, Chao, SC, et al. Histopathological differential diagnosis of keloid and hypertrophic scar. *Am J Dermatopathol*. 2004;26:379-384.
57. Marneros AG, Norris JE, Olsen BR, Reichenberger E. Clinical genetics of familial keloids. *Arch Dermatol*. 2001;137(11):1429-1434.
58. Kelly AP. *An Etiological Update on Keloids*. San Antonio, TX: National Medical Association; 1999.
59. Bayat A, Arscott G, Ollier WE, Ferguson MW, Mc Grouther DA. Description of site-specific morphology of keloid phenotypes in an Afrocaribbean population. *Br J Plast Surg*. 2004;57(2):122-133.
60. Suarez E, Syed F, Alonso-Rasgado T, Mandal P, Bayat A. Up-regulation of tension-related proteins in keloids: knockdown of Hsp27, alpha2beta1-integrin, and PAI-2 shows convincing reduction of extracellular matrix production. *Plast Reconstr Surg*. 2013;131(2):158e-173e.
61. Bayles MA. Coiffure keloids. *Br J Dermatol*. 1972;86(4):415-416.
62. Yagi KI, Dafalla AA, Osman AA. Does an immune reaction to sebum in wounds cause keloid scars? Beneficial effect of desensitisation. *Br J Plast Surg*. 1979;32(3):223-225.
63. Ginarte M, Peteiro C, Toribio J. Keloid formation induced by isotretinoin therapy. *Int J Dermatol*. 1999;38(3):228-229.
64. Fox H. Observations on skin diseases in the American Negro. *J Cutan Dis*. 1908;26:67-79.
65. Adotama P, Rutherford A, Glass DA, 2nd. Association of keloids with systemic medical conditions: a retrospective analysis. *Int J Dermatol*. 2016;55(1):e38-e40.
66. Arima J, Huang C, Rosner B, Akaishi S, Ogawa R. Hypertension: a systemic key to understanding local keloid severity. *Wound Repair Regen*. 2015;23(2): 213-221.
67. Bhavsar S, Nimigan A, Hackam DG, O'Gorman DB, Gan BS, Spence JD. Keloid scarring, but not Dupuytren's contracture, is associated with unexplained carotid atherosclerosis. *Clin Invest Med*. 2009;32(2):E95-E102.
68. Ozdol C, Turhan S, Tulunay C, et al. Association between proliferative scars and in-stent restenosis. *J Cutan Med Surg*. 2007;11(6):206-210.
69. Rutherford A, Glass DA, 2nd. A case-control study analyzing the association of keloids with hypertension and obesity. *Int J Dermatol*. 2017;56(9):e187-e189.
70. Snyder AL, Zmuda JM, Thompson PD. Keloid associated with hypertension. *Lancet*. 1996;347(8999):465-466.
71. Woolery-Lloyd H, Berman B. A controlled cohort study examining the onset of hypertension in black patients with keloids. *Eur J Dermatol*. 2002;12(6):581-582.
72. Catherino WH, Leppert PC, Stenmark MH, et al. Reduced dermatopontin expression is a molecular link between uterine leiomyomas and keloids. *Genes Chromosomes Cancer*. 2004;40(3):204-217.
73. Leppert PC, Catherino WH, Segars JH. A new hypothesis about the origin of uterine fibroids based on gene expression profiling with microarrays. *Am J Obstet Gynecol*. 2006;195(2):415-420.
74. Kwon HE, Ahn HJ, Jeong SJ, Shin MK. The increased prevalence of keloids in atopic dermatitis patients with allergic comorbidities: a nationwide retrospective cohort study. *Sci Rep*. 2021;11(1):23669.
75. Diaz A, Tan K, He H, et al. Keloid lesions show increased IL-4/IL-13 signaling and respond to Th2-targeting dupilumab therapy. *J Eur Acad Dermatol Venereol*. 2020;34(4):e161-e164.
76. Wu J, Del Duca E, Espino M, et al. RNA sequencing keloid transcriptome associates keloids with Th2, Th1, Th17/Th22, and JAK3-skewing. *Front Immunol*. 2020;11:597741.
77. Lu C-C, Qin H, Zhang Z-H, Zhang C-L, Lu Y-Y, Wu C-H. The association between keloid and osteoporosis: real-world evidence. *BMC Musculoskelet Disord*. 2021;22(1):39.
78. Bayat A, Walter JM, Bock O, Mrowietz U, Ollier WE, Ferguson MW. Genetic susceptibility to keloid disease: mutation screening of the TGFbeta3 gene. *Br J Plast Surg*. 2005;58(7):914-921.
79. Marneros AG, Norris JE, Watanabe S, Reichenberger E, Olsen BR. Genome scans provide evidence for keloid susceptibility loci on chromosomes 2q23 and 7p11. *J Invest Dermatol*. 2004;122(5):1126-1132.
80. Santos-Cortez RLP, Hu Y, Sun F, et al. Identification of ASAH1 as a susceptibility gene for familial keloids. *Eur J Hum Genet*. 2017;25(10):1155-1161.
81. Shih B, Bayat A. Genetics of keloid scarring. *Arch Dermatol Res*. 2010; 302(5):319-339.
82. Brown JJ, Bayat A. Genetic susceptibility to raised dermal scarring. *Br J Dermatol*. 2009;161(1):8-18.
83. Nakashima M, Chung S, Takahashi A, et al. A genome-wide association study identifies four susceptibility loci for keloid in the Japanese population. *Nat Genet*. 2010;42(9):768-771.
84. Zhu F, Wu B, Li P, et al. Association study confirmed susceptibility loci with keloid in the Chinese Han population. *PLoS ONE*. 2013;8(5):e62377.
85. Velez Edwards DR, Tsosie KS, Williams SM, Edwards TL, Russell SB. Admixture mapping identifies a locus at 15q21.2-22.3 associated with keloid formation in African Americans. *Hum Genet*. 2014;133(12):1513-1523.
86. Fujita M, Yamamoto Y, Jiang JJ, et al. NEDD4 is involved in inflammation development during keloid formation. *J Invest Dermatol*. 2019;139(2):333-341.
87. Deng CC, Zhang LX, Xu XY, et al. Risk single-nucleotide polymorphism-mediated enhancer-promoter interaction drives keloids through long non-coding RNA down expressed in keloids. *Br J Dermatol*. 2023;188(1):84-93.
88. Shih B, Bayat A. Comparative genomic hybridisation analysis of keloid tissue in Caucasians suggests possible involvement of HLA-DRB5 in disease pathogenesis. *Arch Dermatol Res*. 2012;304(3):241-249.
89. Brown JJ, Ollier WE, Thomson W, Bayat A. Positive association of HLA-DRB1*15 with keloid disease in Caucasians. *Int J Immunogenet*. 2008;35(4-5):303-307.
90. Brown JJ, Ollier WE, Arscott G, Bayat A. Association of HLA-DRB1* and keloid disease in an Afro-Caribbean population. *Clin Exp Dermatol*. 2010;35(3):305-310.
91. Ashcroft KJ, Syed F, Arscott G, Bayat A. Assessment of the influence of HLA class I and class II loci on the prevalence of keloid disease in Jamaican Afro-Caribbeans. *Tissue Antigens*. 2011;78(5):390-396.
92. Cohen IK, McCoy BJ, Mohanakumar T, Diegelmann RF. Immunoglobulin, complement, and histocompatibility antigen studies in keloid patients. *Plast Reconstr Surg*. 1979;63(5):689-695.
93. Laurentaci G, Dioguardi D. HLA antigens in keloids and hypertrophic scars. *Arch Dermatol*. 1977;113(12):1726.
94. Halim AS, Emami A, Salahshourifar I, Kannan TP. Keloid scarring: understanding the genetic basis, advances, and prospects. *Arch Plast Surg*. 2012;39(3):184-189.
95. Mowlem R. Hypertrophic scars. *Br J Plast Surg*. 1951;4(2):113-120.
96. Psillakis JM, de Jorge FB, Sucena RC, Mariani U, Spina V. Water and electrolyte content of normal skin, scars, and keloid. *Plast Reconstr Surg*. 1971;47(3):272-274.
97. Van Den Brenk HA, Minty CC. Radiation in the management of keloids and hypertrophic scars. *Br J Surg*. 1960;47:595-605.
98. Bayat A, Arscott G, Ollier WE, McGrouther DA, Ferguson MW. Keloid disease: clinical relevance of single versus multiple site scars. *Br J Plast Surg*. 2005;58(1):28-37.
99. Kelly AP. Keloids. *Dermatol Clin*. 1988;6(3):413-424.
100. Kelly AP. Update on the management of keloids. *Semin Cutan Med Surg*. 2009;28(2):71-76.
101. Lahav M, Cadet JC, Chirambo M, Rehani U, Ishii Y. Corneal keloids–a histopathological study. *Graefes Arch Clin Exp Ophthalmol*. 1982;218(5):256-261.
102. Körmöczy I. Enormous keloid (?) on a penis. *Br J Plast Surg*. 1978;31(3): 268-269.
103. Parsons RW. A case of keloid of the penis. *Plast Reconstr Surg*. 1966;37(5): 431-432.
104. Perez CA, Lockett MA, Young G. Radiation therapy for keloids and plantar warts. *Front Radiat Ther Oncol*. 2001;35:135-146.
105. Stout AP. Fibrosarcoma the malignant tumor of fibroblasts. *Cancer*. 1948;1(1):30-63.
106. Lee SS, Yosipovitch G, Chan YH, Goh CL. Pruritus, pain, and small nerve fiber function in keloids: a controlled study. *J Am Acad Dermatol*. 2004;51(6):1002-1006.

107. Gueft B. Keloids. *Trans Electron Microsc Soc Am*. 1965;23:5.
108. Rasmussen DM, Wakim KG, Winkelmann RK. Isotonic and isometric thermal contraction of human dermis. II. Age-related changes. *J Invest Dermatol*. 1964;43:341-348.
109. Harris ED, Jr., Sjoerdsma A. Collagen profile in various clinical conditions. *Lancet*. 1966;2(7466):707-711.
110. Tuan TL, DiCesare P, Cheung P, Nimni ME. Keloids and Hypertrophic Scars. In: Nimni ME and Kang AH. *Collagen: Photobiochemistry. CRC Press, Boca Raton*; 1991:125-136.
111. Kischer CW, Hendrix MJ. Fibronectin (FN) in hypertrophic scars and keloids. *Cell Tissue Res*. 1983;231(1):29-37.
112. Kischer CW, Wagner HN, Jr., Pindur J, et al. Increased fibronectin production by cell lines from hypertrophic scar and keloid. *Connect Tissue Res*. 1989;23(4):279-288.
113. Babu M, Diegelmann R, Oliver N. Fibronectin is overproduced by keloid fibroblasts during abnormal wound healing. *Mol Cell Biol*. 1989;9(4):1642-1650.
114. Tan KT, McGrouther DA, Day AJ, Milner CM, Bayat A. Characterization of hyaluronan and TSG-6 in skin scarring: differential distribution in keloid scars, normal scars and unscarred skin. *J Eur Acad Dermatol Venereol*. 2011;25(3):317-327.
115. Sidgwick GP, Iqbal SA, Bayat A. Altered expression of hyaluronan synthase and hyaluronidase mRNA may affect hyaluronic acid distribution in keloid disease compared with normal skin. *Exp Dermatol*. 2013;22(5):377-379.
116. Cohen IK, Keiser HR, Sjoerdsma A. Collagen synthesis in human keloid and hypertrophic scar. *Surg Forum*. 1971;22:488-489.
117. Tuan TL, Nichter LS. The molecular basis of keloid and hypertrophic scar formation. *Mol Med Today*. 1998;4(1):19-24.
118. Bettinger DA, Yager DR, Diegelmann RF, Cohen IK. The effect of TGF-beta on keloid fibroblast proliferation and collagen synthesis. *Plast Reconstr Surg*. 1996;98(5):827-833.
119. Clore JN, Cohen IK, Diegelmann RF. Quantitative assay of types I and III collagen synthesized by keloid biopsyes and fibroblasts. *Biochim Biophys Acta*. 1979;586(2):384-390.
120. Uitto J, Perejda AJ, Abergel RP, Chu ML, Ramirez F. Altered steady-state ratio of type I/III procollagen mRNAs correlates with selectively increased type I procollagen biosynthesis in cultured keloid fibroblasts. *Proc Natl Acad Sci U S A*. 1985;82(17):5935-5939.
121. Syed F, Ahmadi E, Iqbal SA, Singh S, McGrouther DA, Bayat A. Fibroblasts from the growing margin of keloid scars produce higher levels of collagen I and III compared with intralesional and extralesional sites: clinical implications for lesional site-directed therapy. *Br J Dermatol*. 2011;164(1):83-96.
122. McCoy BJ, Cohen IK. Effects of various sera on growth kinetics and collagen synthesis by keloid and normal dermal fibroblasts. *Plast Reconstr Surg*. 1981;67(4):505-510.
123. McCoy BJ, Galdun J, Cohen IK. Effects of density and cellular aging on collagen synthesis and growth kinetics in keloid and normal skin fibroblasts. *In Vitro*. 1982;18(1):79-86.
124. Calderon M, Lawrence WT, Banes AJ. Increased proliferation in keloid fibroblasts wounded in vitro. *J Surg Res*. 1996;61(2):343-347.
125. García-Ulloa AC, Arrieta O. Tubal occlusion causing infertility due to an excessive inflammatory response in patients with predisposition for keloid formation. *Med Hypotheses*. 2005;65(5):908-914.
126. Oliver N, Babu M, Diegelmann R. Fibronectin gene transcription is enhanced in abnormal wound healing. *J Invest Dermatol*. 1992;99(5):579-586.
127. Blackburn WR, Cosman B. Histologic basis of keloid and hypertrophic scar differentiation. Clinicopathologic correlation. *Arch Pathol*. 1966;82(1):65-71.
128. Craig RD. Collagen biosynthesis in normal human skin, normal and hypertrophic scar and keloid. *Eur J Clin Invest*. 1975;5(1):69-74.
129. Tuma W. Quelques experiences sur la culture des keloids humaines in vitro. *Comp Rend Assoc Anatomistes*. 1935;30:507.
130. Conway H, Gillette RW, Findley A. Observations on the behavior of human keloids in vitro. *Plast Reconstr Surg Transplant Bull*. 1959;24:229-237.
131. Iqbal SA, Syed F, McGrouther DA, Paus R, Bayat A. Differential distribution of haematopoietic and nonhaematopoietic progenitor cells in intralesional and extralesional keloid: do keloid scars provide a niche for nonhaematopoietic mesenchymal stem cells? *Br J Dermatol*. 2010;162(6):1377-1383.
132. Santa Cruz DJ, Ulbright TM. Mucin-like changes in keloids. *Am J Clin Pathol*. 1981;75(1):18-22.
133. Redmond WJ, Baker SR. Keloidal calcification. *Arch Dermatol*. 1983;119(3):270-272.
134. Hiss Y, Shafir R. "Pseudomelanoma" in a keloid. *J Dermatol Surg Oncol*. 1978;4(12):938-939.
135. Uitto J, Lichtenstein JR. Defects in the biochemistry of collagen in diseases of connective tissue. *J Invest Dermatol*. 1976;66(02):59-79.
136. Boyce DE, Ciampolini J, Ruge F, Murison MS, Harding KG. Inflammatory-cell subpopulations in keloid scars. *Br J Plast Surg*. 2001;54(6):511-516.
137. Mehregan AH. Pinkus' guide to dermatohistopathology. *Arch Dermatol*. 1987;123(11):1432-1433.
138. Mancini RE, Quaife JV. Histogenesis of experimentally produced keloids. *J Invest Dermatol*. 1962;38:143-181.
139. Craig SS, DeBlois G, Schwartz LB. Mast cells in human keloid, small intestine, and lung by an immunoperoxidase technique using a murine monoclonal antibody against tryptase. *Am J Pathol*. 1986;124(3):427-435.
140. Crockett DJ. Regional keloid susceptibility. *Br J Plast Surg*. 1964;17:245-253.
141. Bhangoo KS, Quinlivan JK, Connelly JR. Elastin fibers in scar tissue. *Plast Reconstr Surg*. 1976;57(3):308-313.
142. King GD, Salzman FA. Keloid scars. Analysis of 89 patients. *Surg Clin North Am*. 1970;50(3):595-598.
143. Bagabir R, Byers RJ, Chaudhry IH, Müller W, Paus R, Bayat A. Site-specific immunophenotyping of keloid disease demonstrates immune upregulation and the presence of lymphoid aggregates. *Br J Dermatol*. 2012;167(5):1053-1066.
144. Halder RM, Roberts CL, Nootheti PK, Kelly AP. Dermatologic disease in blacks. In: Halder, RM, ed. *Dermatology and Dermatologic Therapies in Pigmented Skins. Taylor & Francis Group, Boca Raton*; 2006:405-435.
145. Fisher AA. Allergic dermal contact dermatitis due to gold earrings. *Cutis*. 1987;39(6):473-475.
146. Iwatsuki K, Yamada M, Takigawa M, Inoue K, Matsumoto K. Benign lymphoplasia of the earlobes induced by gold earrings: immunohistologic study on the cellular infiltrates. *J Am Acad Dermatol*. 1987;16(1 Pt 1):83-88.
147. Niessen FB, Spauwen PH, Schalkwijk J, Kon M. On the nature of hypertrophic scars and keloids: a review. *Plast Reconstr Surg*. 1999;104(5):1435-1458.
148. Brown JJ, Ollier W, Thomson W, Bayat A. Positive association of HLA-DRB1*15 with Dupuytren's disease in Caucasians. *Tissue Antigens*. 2008;72(2):166-170.
149. Berman B, Flores F. Recurrence rates of excised keloids treated with postoperative triamcinolone acetonide injections or interferon alfa-2b injections. *J Am Acad Dermatol*. 1997;37(5 Pt 1):755-757.
150. Berman B, Kaufman J. Pilot study of the effect of postoperative imiquimod 5% cream on the recurrence rate of excised keloids. Research Support, Non-U.S. Gov't. *J Am Acad Dermatol*. 2002;47(4 Suppl):S209-S211.
151. Fitzpatrick RE. Treatment of inflamed hypertrophic scars using intralesional 5-FU. *Dermatol Surg*. 1999;25(3):224-232.
152. Bodokh I, Brun P. [Treatment of keloid with intralesional bleomycin]. *Ann Dermatol Venereol*. 1996;123(12):791-794.
153. Houck JC, Sharma VK, Carillo AL. Control of cutaneous collagenolysis. In: Weber G, ed. *Advances in Enzyme Regulation. Pergamon Press, Oxford*; 1970:269-278.
154. Ud-Din S, Bowring A, Derbyshire B, Morris J, Bayat A. Identification of steroid sensitive responders versus non-responders in the treatment of keloid disease. *Arch Dermatol Res*. 2013;305(5):423-432.
155. Syed F, Singh S, Bayat A. Superior effect of combination vs. single steroid therapy in keloid disease: a comparative in vitro analysis of glucocorticoids. *Wound Repair Regen*. 2013;21(1):88-102.
156. Srivastava S, Patil AN, Prakash C, Kumari H. Comparison of intralesional triamcinolone acetonide, 5-fluorouracil, and their combination for the treatment of keloids. *Adv Wound Care (New Rochelle)*. 2017;6(11):393-400.
157. Reinholz M, Guertler A, Schwaiger H, Poetschke J, Gauglitz GG. Treatment of keloids using 5-fluorouracil in combination with crystalline triamcinolone acetonide suspension: evaluating therapeutic effects by using non-invasive objective measures. *J Eur Acad Dermatol Venereol*. 2020;34(10):2436-2444.
158. Sadeghinia A, Sadeghinia S. Comparison of the efficacy of intralesional triamcinolone acetonide and 5-fluorouracil tattooing for the treatment of keloids. *Dermatol Surg*. 2012;38(1):104-109.
159. Khan HA, Sahibzada MN, Paracha MM. Comparison of the efficacy of intralesional bleomycin versus intralesional triamcinolone acetonide in the treatment of keloids. *Dermatol Ther*. 2019;32(5):e13036.
160. Huu ND, Huu SN, Thi XL, et al. Successful treatment of intralesional bleomycin in keloids of vietnamese population. *Open Access Maced J Med Sci*. 2019;7(2):298-299.
161. Danielsen PL, Rea SM, Wood FM, et al. Verapamil is less effective than triamcinolone for prevention of keloid scar recurrence after excision in a randomized controlled trial. *Acta Derm Venereol*. 2016;96(6):774-778.
162. El-Kamel MF, Selim MK, Alghobary MF. Keloidectomy with core fillet flap and intralesional verapamil injection for recurrent earlobe keloids. *Indian J Dermatol Venereol Leprol*. 2016;82(6):659-665.
163. Ahuja RB, Chatterjee P. Comparative efficacy of intralesional verapamil hydrochloride and triamcinolone acetonide in hypertrophic scars and keloids. *Burns*. 2014;40(4):583-588.

164. Margaret Shanthi FX, Ernest K, Dhanraj P. Comparison of intralesional verapamil with intralesional triamcinolone in the treatment of hypertrophic scars and keloids. *Indian J Dermatol Venereol Leprol.* 2008;74(4):343-348.
165. D'Andrea F, Brongo S, Ferraro G, Baroni A. Prevention and treatment of keloids with intralesional verapamil. *Dermatology.* 2002;204(1):60-62.
166. Aggarwal A, Ravikumar BC, Vinay KN, Raghukumar S, Yashovardhana DP. A comparative study of various modalities in the treatment of keloids. *Int J Dermatol.* 2018;57(10):1192-1200.
167. Abedini R, Sasani P, Mahmoudi HR, Nasimi M, Teymourpour A, Shadlou Z. Comparison of intralesional verapamil versus intralesional corticosteroids in treatment of keloids and hypertrophic scars: a randomized controlled trial. *Burns.* 2018;44(6):1482-1488.
168. Tan KT, Shah N, Pritchard SA, McGrouther DA, Bayat A. The influence of surgical excision margins on keloid prognosis. *Ann Plast Surg.* 2010;64(1):55-58.
169. Brent B. The role of pressure therapy in management of earlobe keloids: preliminary report of a controlled study. *Ann Plast Surg.* 1978;1(6):579-581.
170. Lawrence WT. Treatment of earlobe keloids with surgery plus adjuvant intralesional verapamil and pressure earrings. *Ann Plast Surg.* 1996;37(2):167-169.
171. Snyder GB. Button compression for keloids of the lobule. *Br J Plast Surg.* 1974;27(2):186-187.
172. Fischer E, Storck H. X-ray treatment of keloids. *Schweiz Med Wochenschr.* 1957;87: 1281-1285.
173. Arnold HL, Jr., Grauer FH. Keloids: etiology, and management by excision and intensive prophylactic radiation. *Arch Dermatol.* 1959;80:772-777.
174. Borok TL, Bray M, Sinclair I, Plafker J, LaBirth L, Rollins C. Role of ionizing irradiation for 393 keloids. *Int J Radiat Oncol Biol Phys.* 1988;15(4):865-870.
175. Shaffer JJ, Taylor SC, Cook-Bolden F. Keloidal scars: a review with a critical look at therapeutic options. *J Am Acad Dermatol.* 2002;46(2 Suppl Understanding):S63-S97.
176. Srinivas CR, Kumaresan M. Lasers for vascular lesions: standard guidelines of care. *Indian J Dermatol Venereol Leprol.* 2011;77(3):349-368.
177. Shih P-Y, Chen H-H, Chen C-H, Hong H-S, Yang C-H. Rapid recurrence of keloid after pulse dye laser treatment. *Dermatol Surg.* 2008;34(8):1124-1127.
178. Yang Q, Ma Y, Zhu R, et al. The effect of flashlamp pulsed dye laser on the expression of connective tissue growth factor in keloids. *Lasers Surg Med.* 2012;44(5):377-383.
179. Cannarozzo G, Sannino M, Tamburi F, Morini C, Nistico SP. Flash-lamp pulsed-dye laser treatment of keloids: results of an observational study. *Photomed Laser Surg.* 2015;33(5):274-277.
180. Abergel RP, Dwyer RM, Meeker CA, Lask G, Kelly AP, Uitto J. Laser treatment of keloids: a clinical trial and an in vitro study with Nd:YAG laser. *Lasers Surg Med.* 1984;4(3):291-295.
181. Alster TS, Williams CM. Treatment of keloid sternotomy scars with 585 nm flashlamp-pumped pulsed-dye laser. *Lancet.* 1995;345(8959):1198-200.
182. Azzam OA, Bassiouny DA, El-Hawary MS, El Maadawi ZM, Sobhi RM, El-Mesidy MS. Treatment of hypertrophic scars and keloids by fractional carbon dioxide laser: a clinical, histological, and immunohistochemical study. *Lasers Med Sci.* 2016;31(1):9-18.
183. Kraeva E, Ho D, Jagdeo J. Successful treatment of keloid with fractionated carbon dioxide (CO_2) laser and laser-assisted drug delivery of triamcinolone acetonide ointment in an African-American man. *J Drugs Dermatol.* 2017;16(9):925-927.
184. Rossi A, Lu R, Frey MK, Kubota T, Smith LA, Perez M. The use of the 300 microsecond 1064 nm Nd:YAG laser in the treatment of keloids. *J Drugs Dermatol.* 2013;12(11):1256-1262.
185. Al-Mohamady AE-SAE-H, Ibrahim SMA, Muhammad MM. Pulsed dye laser versus long-pulsed Nd:YAG laser in the treatment of hypertrophic scars and keloid: a comparative randomized split-scar trial. *J Cosmet Laser Ther.* 2016;18(4):208-212.
186. Martin MS, Collawn SS. Combination treatment of CO_2 fractional laser, pulsed dye laser, and triamcinolone acetonide injection for refractory keloid scars on the upper back. *J Cosmet Laser Ther.* 2013;15(3):166-170.
187. Mourad B, Elfar N, Elsheikh S. Spray versus intralesional cryotherapy for keloids. *J Dermatolog Treat.* 2016;27(3):264-269.
188. Litrowski N, Boullie MC, Dehesdin D, De Barros A, Joly P. Treatment of earlobe keloids by surgical excision and cryosurgery. *J Eur Acad Dermatol Venereol.* 2014;28(10):1324-1331.
189. van Leeuwen MCE, van der Wal MBA, Bulstra A-EJ, et al. Intralesional cryotherapy for treatment of keloid scars: a prospective study. *Plast Reconstr Surg.* 2015;135(2):580-589.
190. Park TH, Cho HJ, Lee JW, Kim CW, Chong Y, Chang CH, Park KS. Could −79 °C Spray-Type Cryotherapy Be an Effective Monotherapy for the Treatment of Keloid? *Int J Mol Sci.* 2017;18(12), 2536.
191. Wang X, Wu X, Liu K, et al. Topical cryoanesthesia for the relief of pain caused by steroid injections used to treat hypertrophic scars and keloids. *Medicine.* 2017;96(43):e8353.
192. Ogawa R. Effectiveness of corticosteroid tapes and plasters for keloids and hypertrophic scars. In: Teot L, Mustoe TA, Middelkoop E, Gauglitz GG, eds. *Textbook on Scar Management: State of the Art Management and Emerging Technologies.* Springer, *Princeton, NJ.*; 2020:491-496.
193. Ogawa R, Akaishi S, Kuribayashi S, Miyashita T. Keloids and hypertrophic scars can now be cured completely: recent progress in our understanding of the pathogenesis of keloids and hypertrophic scars and the most promising current therapeutic strategy. *J Nippon Med Sch.* 2016;83(2):46-53.
194. Flickinger JC. A radiobiological analysis of multicenter data for postoperative keloid radiotherapy. *Int J Radiat Oncol Biol Phys.* 2011;79(4):1164-1170.
195. Wong TW, Lee JY, Sheu HM, Chao SC. Relief of pain and itch associated with keloids on treatment with oxpentifylline. *Br J Dermatol.* 1999;140(4):771-772.
196. Tan A, Martinez Luna O, Glass DA 2nd. Pentoxifylline for the prevention of postsurgical keloid recurrence. *Dermatol Surg.* 2020;46(10):1353-1356.
197. Mercer NS. Silicone gel in the treatment of keloid scars. *Br J Plast Surg.* 1989;42(1):83-87.
198. Janssen de Limpens AM. The local treatment of hypertrophic scars and keloids with topical retinoic acid. *Br J Dermatol.* 1980;103(3):319-323.
199. Asawanonda P, Khoo LS, Fitzpatrick TB, Taylor CR. UV-A1 for keloid. *Arch Dermatol.* 1999;135(3):348-349.
200. Hannuksela-Svahn A, Grandal OJ, Thorstensen T, Christensen OB. UVA1 for treatment of keloids. *Acta Derm Venereol.* 1999;79(6):490.
201. MF O. Surgery and methotrexate for keloids. *Schoch Lett.* 1978;28:4.
202. Wong AJS, Song EJ. Dupilumab as an adjuvant treatment for keloid-associated symptoms. *JAAD Case Rep.* 2021;13:73-74.
203. Tirgan MH, Uitto J. Lack of efficacy of dupilumab in the treatment of keloid disorder. *J Eur Acad Dermatol Venereol.* 2022;36(2):e120-e122.
204. Luk K, Fakhoury J, Ozog D. Nonresponse and progression of diffuse keloids to dupilumab therapy. *J Drugs Dermatol.* 2022;21(2):197-199.
205. Peterson DM, Damsky WE, Vesely MD. Treatment of lichen sclerosus and hypertrophic scars with dupilumab. *JAAD Case Rep.* 2022;23:76-78.
206. Mendoza J, Sebastian A, Allan E, et al. Differential cytotoxic response in keloid fibroblasts exposed to photodynamic therapy is dependent on photosensitiser precursor, fluence and location of fibroblasts within the lesion. *Arch Dermatol Res.* 2012;304(7):549-562.
207. Nie Z, Bayat A, Behzad F, Rhodes LE. Positive response of a recurrent keloid scar to topical methyl aminolevulinate-photodynamic therapy. *Photodermatol Photoimmunol Photomed.* 2010;26(6):330-332.
208. Sebastian A, Allan E, Allan D, Colthurst J, Bayat A. Addition of novel degenerate electrical waveform stimulation with photodynamic therapy significantly enhances its cytotoxic effect in keloid fibroblasts: first report of a potential combination therapy. *J Dermatol Sci.* 2011;64(3):174-184.
209. Ud-Din S, Thomas G, Morris J, Bayat A. Photodynamic therapy: an innovative approach to the treatment of keloid disease evaluated using subjective and objective non-invasive tools. *Arch Dermatol Res.* 2013;305(3):205-214.

CHAPTER 34

Drug Eruptions

Alana Ferreira
Jeromy Gotschall
Temitayo A. Ogunleye

KEY POINTS

- Cutaneous drug eruptions are among the most common signs of adverse drug reactions.
- Recent pharmacogenetic studies have elucidated that certain HLA genotypes are associated with increased risk of some drug eruptions, and these genotypes may differ in prevalence by race and ethnicity.
- Cutaneous adverse drug reactions can vary greatly in clinical findings and symptoms.
- A systematic approach to identifying drug eruptions including a complete medication history and recognition of reaction patterns on clinical examination are important in determining the causative medication.
- Prompt withdrawal of suspected medications is essential, along with supportive care and case-dependent appropriate treatment.

INTRODUCTION

Cutaneous eruptions are among the most common signs of adverse drug reaction.[1] Drug reactions are estimated to occur with a prevalence of 2% to 3% in hospitalized patients, and up to 1 in every 1000 patients has a serious cutaneous drug reaction.[1-3] Reactions may range from common exanthematous eruptions to life-threatening conditions, and may be limited to the skin or, alternatively, have multiorgan system involvement. In patients with darker skin, clinical findings may be subtle and more challenging to diagnose. In this chapter, we discuss relevant clinical findings in various drug eruptions and some important differences that may be seen in patients with skin of color.

CLINICAL FEATURES IN SKIN OF COLOR

Drug eruptions in skin of color populations differ little in progression, diagnosis, and treatment. Minor differences in clinical presentation may include subtleties in discerning early erythema in drug eruptions, differences in quality of erythema, and the presence of posteruption sequelae. In patients with darker skin tones, initial areas of erythema may be difficult to visualize and may have a darker purple hue. In addition, postinflammatory hyperpigmentation may be a more significant cosmetic issue in patients with skin of color than in lighter populations, even after seemingly mild eruptions.

PHARMACOGENETICS

The emerging field of pharmacogenetics has played a major role in identifying patients and population groups that are at increased risk for developing certain types of adverse cutaneous reactions. For example, pharmacogenetic studies have linked human leukocyte antigen (HLA) B*5701 allele to the abacavir hypersensitivity syndrome. This allele is found in 5% to 7% of White (including Hispanic) populations; 5% to 20% of Indian populations; less than 2% of Chinese, Korean, and Thai populations, and less than 1% of African populations.[4] It is believed that HLA-B*5701 has a high correlation with abacavir hypersensitivity in both Black and White individuals, although its significance in other populations remains unclear.[5-8] While these studies suggest the presence of HLA-B*5701 is necessary for development of abacavir hypersensitivity, it is not sufficient, as 45% of patients who carry HLA-B*5701 do not develop this syndrome.[6]

Recent advances in pharmacogenetics have led to the identification of additional HLA alleles associated with an increased risk of drug eruptions, including HLA-B1502 with carbamazepine-induced Stevens-Johnson syndrome and toxic epidermal necrolysis, and HLA-A3*101 with carbamazepine-induced hypersensitivity reactions.[9] Incorporation of HLA genotyping into clinical practice may inform prescribing practices[10] and subsequently decrease the incidence of adverse cutaneous drug reactions [**Tables 34-1** and **34-2**].[11] The ongoing development of precision medicine approaches to drug therapy, with personalized treatment plans based on genetic makeup, will continue to refine our understanding of drug reactions and minimize the risk of adverse events.

TABLE 34-1 Reported genetic biomarkers for anticonvulsants and allopurinol-induced cutaneous drug reactions

Causative drug	HLA	Population	Cutaneous reaction
Carbamazepine	B*1502 A*3101	Han Chinese (Taiwan) Han Chinese (Hong Kong) Thai Indians	SJS/TEN
Carbamazepine	B*1511	Japanese	SJS/TEN
Phenytoin	B*1502	Han Chinese (Taiwan) Thai	SJS/TEN
Lamotrigine	B*1502	Han Chinese (Taiwan)	SJS
Oxcarbazepine	B*1502	Han Chinese (Taiwan)	SJS
Allopurinol	B*5801	Han Chinese (Taiwan) Thai Caucasians Japanese	SJS/TEN or DRESS SJS/TEN

Abbreviations: DRESS, drug reaction with eosinophilia and systemic symptoms; HLA, human leukocyte antigen; SJS, Stevens-Johnson syndrome; TEN, toxic epidermal necrolysis.

Source: Reproduced with permission from Aihara M. Pharmacogenetics of cutaneous adverse drug reactions. *J Dermatol.* 2011;38:246-254.

PATIENT APPROACH [TABLE 34-3]

EXANTHEMATOUS ERUPTIONS

Exanthematous drug eruptions, also known as morbilliform or maculopapular eruptions, are the most common type of cutaneous drug eruption, accounting for 80% to 90% of drug reactions, followed by urticaria and angioedema.[2,12-14] Morbilliform eruptions typically begin 7 to 14 days after initiation of the causative medication, and the initial presentation may occur even after drug discontinuation. However, in some cases, particularly among individuals who have previously shown sensitivity to the causative drug, morbilliform eruptions can appear as early as 6 to 12 hours after starting treatment. Lesions consist of pink to red macules that coalesce, with involvement of the trunk and subsequent progression peripherally onto the limbs [**Figures 34-1** and **34-2**]. In patients with darker skin hues, redness may be difficult to visualize, with erythema manifesting as a purplish discoloration [**Figure 34-3**]. Mucous membranes are classically spared. Pruritus is a common feature, and low-grade fever may be present. Resolution of the eruption consists of fading erythema and may be followed by scaling or desquamation.

Common causative medications include penicillins, sulfonamides, cephalosporins, nonnucleoside reverse transcriptase inhibitors, antiepileptic medications, and immune checkpoint inhibitors.[1,15] The major differential diagnosis includes a viral exanthem, and the two may be difficult to distinguish.

Drug-viral enhancement of these eruptions, such as that which can occur after treatment of a patient with infectious mononucleosis with penicillins, increases this risk several fold, from a range of 4% to 13% to a range of 60% to 100%.[16] Similar drug-viral interactions occur in patients with human immunodeficiency virus (HIV) who take sulfonamide antibiotics, and Epstein-Barr virus and cytomegalovirus infection have also been linked to increased risk of developing drug-induced exanthem.[17]

The presence of underlying medical conditions, such as liver or renal dysfunction, and concomitant use of multiple medications can increase the likelihood of developing drug-induced exanthems.[18] Patients with immunodeficiencies or autoimmune disorders may also be more susceptible to these reactions.[19] While it is well-established that particular HLA types can increase the risks of severe cutaneous reactions (such as SJS/TEN or DRESS) in response to certain medications, the available information on whether specific HLA alleles are linked to exanthematous drug eruptions remains limited and conflicting.[20,21]

TABLE 34-2 Reported genetic markers for antiretroviral medications

Causative medication	HLA	Population	Cutaneous reaction
Abacavir	B*5701	Caucasian African origin Japanese	Hypersensitivity syndrome
Nevirapine	B*3505	Thai	Hypersensitivity syndrome
	Cw8	Japanese Sardinian	Hypersensitivity syndrome
	B14	Sardinian	Hypersensitivity syndrome

Abbreviation: HLA, human leukocyte antigen.

Source: Reproduced with permission from Aihara M. Pharmacogenetics of cutaneous adverse drug reactions. *J Dermatol.* 2011;38:246-254.

TABLE 34-3 Approach to the patient with suspected drug eruption

Complete history
Date of onset of the eruption
Time interval between drug introduction and skin eruption
Full medication list (discontinued, active) used in last 2 weeks to 6 months, including herbal medications, vitamins, and illicit drugs with start/end dates
Physical examination
All skin; oral, genital, ocular, and anal mucosa; and lymph nodes
Determination of the type of primary lesion and the distribution of lesions
Associated signs and symptoms
Testing and other inquiry
Skin biopsy if indicated
Laboratory evaluations (CBC, CMP, vasculitis and/or connective tissue disease evaluation, etc)
Perform literature search to determine most likely agent(s)
Discontinuation of suspected nonessential medications
Provide appropriate treatment and/or supportive care

Abbreviations: CBC, complete blood count; CMP, complete metabolic panel.

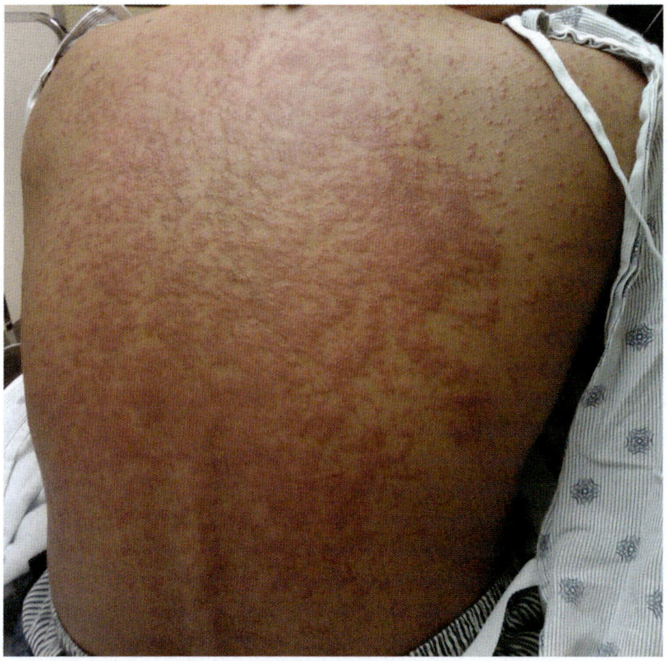

FIGURE 34-1. Morbilliform drug eruption. (Used with permission from Lisa Pappas-Taffer, MD.)

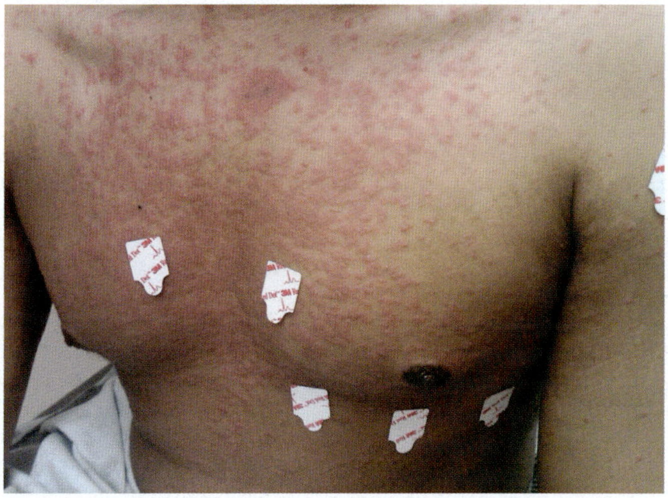

FIGURE 34-2. Morbilliform drug eruption. (Used with permission from Lisa Pappas-Taffer, MD.)

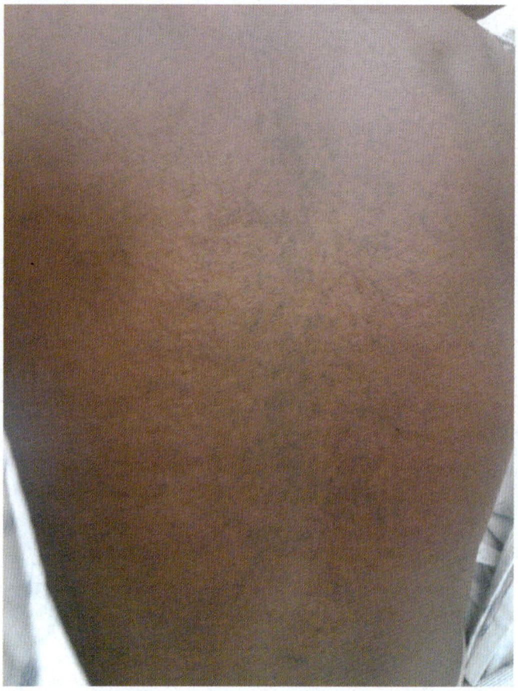

FIGURE 34-3. Morbilliform drug eruption. (Used with permission from Lisa Pappas-Taffer, MD.)

Drug Reaction with Eosinophilia and Systemic Symptoms Hypersensitivity syndrome, or drug reaction with eosinophilia and systemic symptoms (DRESS), is a rare, potentially life-threatening, drug-induced hypersensitivity reaction characterized by a cutaneous eruption, hematologic abnormalities, lymphadenopathy, and/or internal organ involvement. The incidence of this reaction is estimated to be 1 in 1000 to 1 in 10,000 exposures to high-risk drugs such as anticonvulsants. This condition typically begins 2 to 8 weeks after exposure to the suspected medications such as antiepileptic drugs (phenytoin, carbamazepine, phenobarbital), sulfonamides, nevirapine, abacavir, minocycline, or allopurinol, and may continue for several weeks or months after discontinuation of the offending medication. The pathogenesis of DRESS is complex, and may involve a drug-specific immune response and human Herpesviridae reactivation (HHV 6 and 7).[22] In fact, the detection of HHV-6 reactivation has been recently proposed as a diagnostic marker for DRESS.[22]

Fever and a morbilliform eruption are the most common symptoms. Pustular variants rarely occur [**Figure 34-4**]. The face, upper trunk, and extremities are common areas of involvement, with facial edema as a frequent additional finding. Lymphadenopathy is often present, with arthralgia/arthritis sometimes occurring. Visceral involvement can be serious and life-threatening. Hepatitis is the most common visceral involvement, with fulminant hepatitis being a frequent cause of death in these patients. However, almost any organ system may be involved, with reports of thyroiditis, pneumonitis, myocarditis, nephritis, and central nervous system infiltration. As the name indicates, prominent eosinophilia is a characteristic feature. Atypical lymphocytosis may also be seen. Treatment with immunosuppressive therapy for several months is frequently necessary.

Recent advances in understanding the pathogenesis of DRESS have highlighted the role of genetic factors in susceptibility to this syndrome. For example, HLA alleles such as HLA-B*58:01 have been shown to be associated with an increased risk of DRESS in response to allopurinol in Han Chinese, European, Thai, and Korean populations.[23] This finding has potential implications for the development of personalized medicine approaches to minimize the risk of DRESS in particular at-risk populations.

Acute Generalized Exanthematous Pustulosis Acute generalized exanthematous pustulosis (AGEP) is a rare acute febrile drug eruption characterized by sterile non-follicular-based pustules, arising on an erythematous base. It typically begins on the face or intertriginous areas but can generalize within a few hours. Associated signs and symptoms

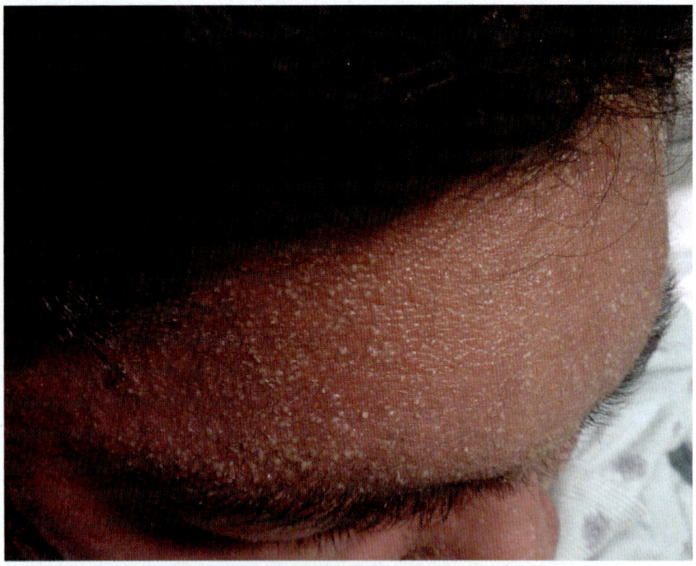

FIGURE 34-4. Pustular variant of drug reaction with eosinophilia and systemic symptoms. (Used with permission from Lisa Pappas-Taffer, MD.)

include lymphocytosis, edema of the face and hands, purpura, vesicles, bullae, erythema multiforme-like lesions, and mucous membrane involvement.[24] AGEP can arise as early as 2 days after starting the offending medication (commonly β-lactam and macrolide antibiotics, calcium channel blockers, and antimalarials) and resolves with generalized desquamation occurring 1 to 2 weeks after the start of the eruption.

The differential diagnosis includes acute pustular psoriasis of von Zumbusch, as well as toxic epidermal necrolysis (TEN) in severe cases. These entities can usually be differentiated via medication history and pathologic findings. The diagnosis of AGEP is based upon the clinical presentation and histologic examination. Management primarily involves prompt withdrawal of the offending medication. Supportive care with liberal emollient use and topical steroids can also be effective in relieving symptoms such as pruritus and skin inflammation. Systemic corticosteroids are generally not utilized, but may be used in severe cases, if deemed necessary. Reexposure to the causative agent should be avoided to avoid recurrence.

FIXED DRUG ERUPTIONS

Fixed drug eruptions (FDE) are a type of cutaneous drug reaction that typically presents with round to oval, dusky red to brown/black macules that may evolve into edematous plaques or bullae [**Figure 34-5**].

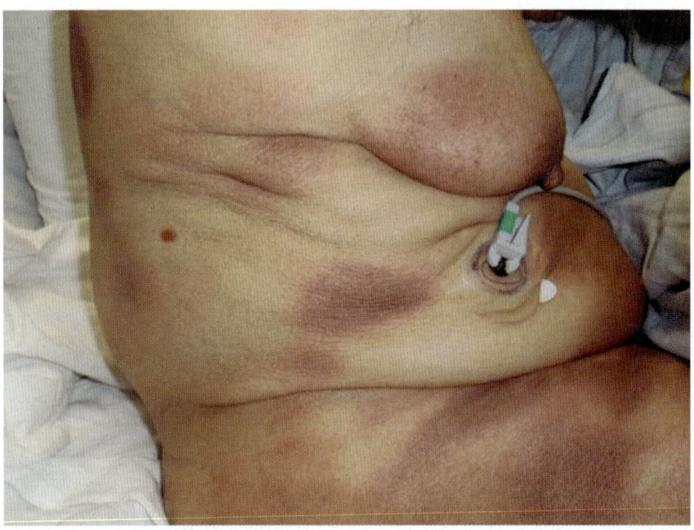

FIGURE 34-5. Fixed drug eruption. (Used with permission from Dr. Temitayo Ogunleye, MD.)

FDE rarely may present with atypical features that mimic other skin diseases such as erythema multiforme, or Stevens-Johnson syndrome/toxic epidermal necrolysis (SJS/TEN). The nonpigmented variant, commonly associated with pseudoephedrine, consists of large erythematous plaques that heal without residual pigmentation. Patients may be asymptomatic or complain of burning, stinging, or pain, especially with mucosal or bullous lesions. Lesions can recur in the same location upon reexposure to the causative medication and can appear within 24 hours of exposure. Antibacterial sulfonamides, antibiotics, nonsteroidal anti-inflammatory drugs, analgesics, and hypnotics are the most frequent causes of FDE.[25-27]

While the typical presentation of FDE is usually straightforward and diagnosis is based on lesion morphology and history, in cases with unusual clinical features, histologic examination of a skin biopsy may be helpful in establishing the diagnosis. Additionally, systemic or topical provocation tests may be used to identify the culprit drug when history is unclear or multiple medications are suspected. The eruption resolves over the course of a few days or weeks, but often leaves residual postinflammatory hyperpigmentation.

OTHER BULLOUS ERUPTIONS

Linear IgA Bullous Dermatosis Linear IgA bullous dermatosis is a rare autoimmune blistering disease typically characterized by the sudden appearance of tense bullae and inflammatory skin lesions in an annular configuration on the trunk and extremities. It can, however, be heterogeneous in its presentation, with morphology mimicking erythema multiforme, bullous pemphigoid, and dermatitis herpetiformis. The condition can affect both children and adults. Most cases of LABD are idiopathic, but drug exposure has been linked to the development of LABD, with vancomycin being the most common culprit, responsible for just under half of all drug-related cases.[28] Other medications that can cause linear IgA bullous dermatosis include captopril and trimethoprim/sulfamethoxazole.[28] For vancomycin-associated cases, mean time to reaction ranges from 2 days to 2 weeks.

Children with LABD may develop widespread annular or arciform blisters that often affect the groin, lower abdomen, and medial thighs. In adults, the annular lesions are less common, and the trunk and extremities are more frequently affected. Mucosal involvement can occur and may result in serious complications such as blindness, airway obstruction, and esophageal strictures.

The diagnosis of LABD is based on the detection of linear deposits of IgA using direct immunofluorescence microscopy of a tissue specimen taken from perilesional skin. Treatment options for LABD are primarily based on case reports and case series, and dapsone is recommended as first-line therapy for both children and adults with LABD.[29] Complete clinical resolution after the discontinuation of the offending drug may only be seen in approximately 50% of cases.[28] When long-term immunosuppression is necessary, a glucocorticoid-sparing agent like mycophenolate mofetil is recommended.[30-32]

Drug-Induced Bullous Pemphigoid Drug-induced bullous pemphigoid (BP) is typified by large, tense bullae on an erythematous base, although the eruption may be polymorphic and mimic other drug-induced diseases such as erythema multiforme/Stevens-Johnson syndrome, fixed drug eruption, porphyria cutanea tarda, and eczematous disorders.[33] The most common drugs implicated in drug-induced BP are furosemide and captopril, among others such as penicillamine, sulfasalazine, and tumor necrosis factor-alpha (TNF-α) inhibitors. Features that may distinguish drug-induced BP from idiopathic BP include younger age and mucous membrane involvement. In addition, overlap of clinical and immunohistologic features of pemphigoid and pemphigus suggest a drug-induced variant.[34-36] Spontaneous remission or resolution after short-term immunosuppressive treatment may also favor drug etiology.[37] However, some cases of drug-induced BP may require prolonged immunosuppressive therapy; it is thought that in these patients, the drug may have triggered the idiopathic form of the disease.

Drug-Induced Pemphigus Drug-induced pemphigus is a rare autoimmune bullous disease that can present with physical findings consistent with either pemphigus vulgaris or pemphigus foliaceus subtypes. Clinical findings congruent with a diagnosis of pemphigus foliaceus are more common than those of pemphigus vulgaris.[37,38] Physical findings may include scaly, crusted erosions on an erythematous base, in a seborrheic distribution, consistent with a diagnosis of pemphigus foliaceus. However, findings of pemphigus vulgaris, including flaccid, fragile blisters occurring on skin and mucosal surfaces, may occur. Pruritus and burning are common complaints in pemphigus foliaceus subtypes, whereas pain is more commonly described in pemphigus vulgaris subtypes, though overlap is common. In some patients with drug-induced pemphigus, direct immunofluorescence (DIF) and indirect immunofluorescence (IIF) studies may be negative. However, ELISA has been found to be positive for desmoglein 1 or desmoglein 3 in all patients with drug-induced pemphigus.[39]

The causative drugs often contain thiol groups (-SH), including penicillamine, captopril, and gold sodium thiomalate, or drugs that contain sulfur in their molecular structure that may be metabolized to form active thiol groups, such as penicillins, cephalosporins, and piroxicam.[40,41] The incubation period to the start of the eruption ranges from 2 weeks to 6 months.[41] Up to 50% of cases may remit spontaneously upon discontinuation of the offending medication, whereas others may require immunosuppressive therapy.

LICHENOID ERUPTIONS

Lichenoid drug eruptions are an uncommon cutaneous adverse effect of several drugs, characterized by a symmetric, papular eruption resembling lichen planus on the trunk and extremities. Purple polygonal plaques scattered on the trunk and extremities are present, although mucous membranes and nails are usually spared [**Figure 34-6A-E**]. The drugs most commonly implicated include angiotensin-converting enzyme (ACE) inhibitors, thiazide diuretics, antimalarials, beta blockers, and checkpoint inhibitors.[42-57] The onset of the eruption may occur several weeks to a year or more after starting the medication.

The diagnosis of lichenoid drug eruption is based on a combination of clinical findings, histologic findings, temporal relationship between drug intake and skin lesions, and resolution upon drug withdrawal and recurrence upon rechallenge. Lichenoid drug eruptions generally resolve spontaneously a few weeks to a few months after discontinuation of the offending drug. However, treatment may be warranted in patients who cannot discontinue the offending drug or have symptomatic or extensive disease.

For patients with limited disease, topical corticosteroids are suggested, while for extensive/symptomatic disease, oral corticosteroids, acitretin, or steroid-sparing medications are recommended. Offending medications may include penicillamine, captopril, and β-blockers, among others. Unlike other drug eruptions, the reaction may begin 2 months to 2 years after beginning the medication. Lichenoid eruptions may require several months or years to resolve, and like lichen planus, often resolve with postinflammatory hyperpigmentation.

DRUG-INDUCED PIGMENTARY CHANGES

Drug-induced pigmentation may occur via several mechanisms, including the induction of melanin production, deposition of drug products in skin, or postinflammatory changes. Hyperpigmentation may be more pronounced in sun-exposed areas, as is seen in reactions caused by amiodarone, chlorpromazine, desipramine, and silver.[58] Amiodarone may cause an overall slate gray discoloration, in addition to golden brown pigmentation in sun-exposed areas. Desipramine has been associated with a slate gray pigmentation, and silver may cause blue-black pigmentation in sun-exposed areas. Clofazimine causes violet-brown to blue-gray discoloration in areas of inflammation and diffuse reddish discoloration of the skin and conjunctivae.

Minocycline is a common cause of pigmentary abnormalities that are divided into four types.[59] Type I is characterized by blue-black discolorations in scars or areas of inflammation, including those from acne [**Figure 34-8**]. Type II consists of blue-gray patches on the anterior legs. Diffuse muddy brown discoloration more prominent in sun-exposed areas typifies type III. Type IV consists of circumscribed blue-gray pigmentation concentrated within acne scars on the back.

Topical hydroquinone is a rare cause of pigmentation in the form of exogenous ochronosis. It manifests as gray-brown or blue-black macules in hydroquinone-exposed regions, typically in sun-exposed regions [**Figure 34-9**]. Risk factors include darker skin, lack of sun protection, skin irritation and vigorous friction, and hydroquinone concentrations greater than 3% for a period longer that 6 months, although there have been reports of exogenous ochronosis with the use of 2% concentrations for less than 6 months.[60,61]

In some cases, drug-induced pigmentation may be associated with photosensitivity reactions. For example, amiodarone, chlorpromazine, and tricyclic antidepressants can cause slate-gray hyperpigmentation due to phototoxicity.

Pigmentary changes induced by chemotherapeutic agents can vary in pattern, distribution, and the involvement of skin, mucous membranes, hair, or nails. These alterations can present as either hypo- or hyperpigmentation areas and may be diffuse, localized, or patterned. Changes in hair color may also occur. Pigmentary alterations are more commonly associated with treatment using signal transduction inhibitors and immunotherapies as opposed to cytotoxic agents. Hypopigmentation and depigmentation are typical manifestations of these therapies. In contrast, hyperpigmentation is more frequently observed due to cytotoxic agent administration. Black patients are disproportionately impacted by immunomodulatory drug-related hyperpigmentation of the skin, as it occurs more than 10 times more frequently among Black patients compared to patients of all other races.[62] Among darker-skinned individuals, hyperpigmentation may be more noticeable on the palms, faces, and soles of the feet. These changes typically occur early during treatment and are often not fully reversible, even after drug cessation.[62]

Discontinuation of the inciting medication halts the progression in most cases, but discoloration, especially in cases of pigment/metal deposition, may take months or years for complete resolution. In many cases, complete spontaneous resolution will not occur. Treatment with laser therapy may be helpful, but early recognition and discontinuation of the offending medication are critically important.

STEVENS-JOHNSON SYNDROME AND TOXIC EPIDERMAL NECROLYSIS

Stevens-Johnson syndrome (SJS)/toxic epidermal necrolysis (TEN) is one of the most serious drug-induced skin reactions. This life-threatening condition is characterized by mucocutaneous necrosis and extensive tenderness, erythema, and skin sloughing. SJS/TEN may be caused by various medications, and early discontinuation of the causative drug is of paramount importance. Commonly associated medications include allopurinol, sulfa medications, NSAIDs, barbiturates, carbamazepine, antiretroviral medications, and antiepileptic drugs such as phenytoin and lamotrigine.

SJS/TEN has an incidence of approximately one to seven cases per million people per year.[3,63] Groups at increased risk include immunocompromised patients, especially those with HIV/AIDS.[64] SJS and TEN typically begin 4 to 28 days after the initiation of the causative agent. Initial symptoms include fever, stinging of eyes, and pain with swallowing that may precede cutaneous symptoms by a few days. Patients then develop erythematous to dusky purpuric, irregularly shaped macules that coalesce to larger patches, starting on the trunk and spreading to the neck, face, and extremities. Spontaneous epidermal detachment may occur, indicative of the full-thickness epidermal necrosis observed on histopathology. Epidermal detachment may also reveal a positive Nikolsky sign when applying tangential pressure on dusky areas of involvement.

Cases are categorized based on the percentage of total body surface area with epidermal detachment: less than 10% body surface area epidermal detachment in SJS, 10% to 30% in SJS/TEN overlap, and greater than

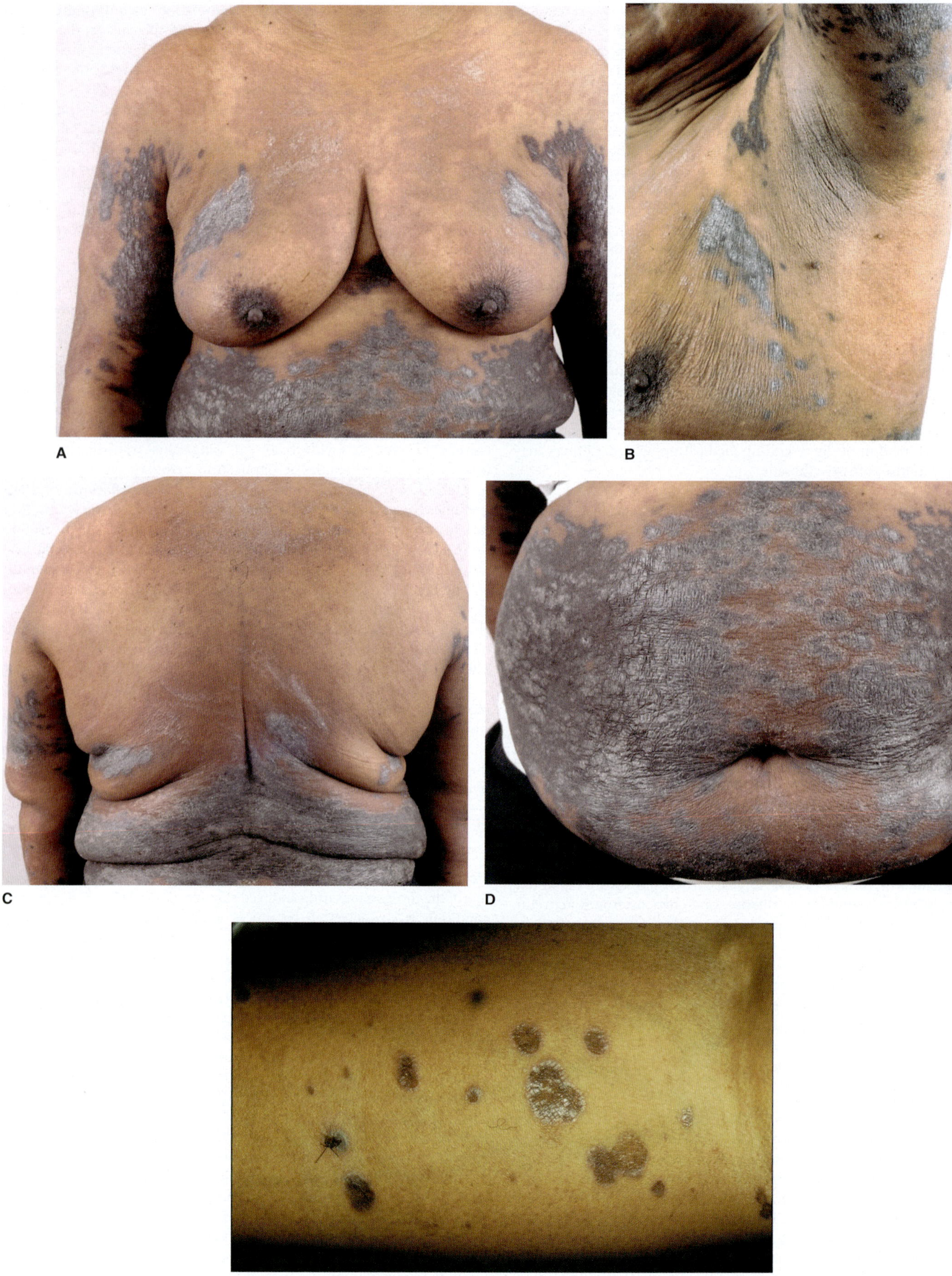

FIGURE 34-6. (A–E) Lichenoid drug eruption. (**E:** Used with permission from William D. James, MD.)

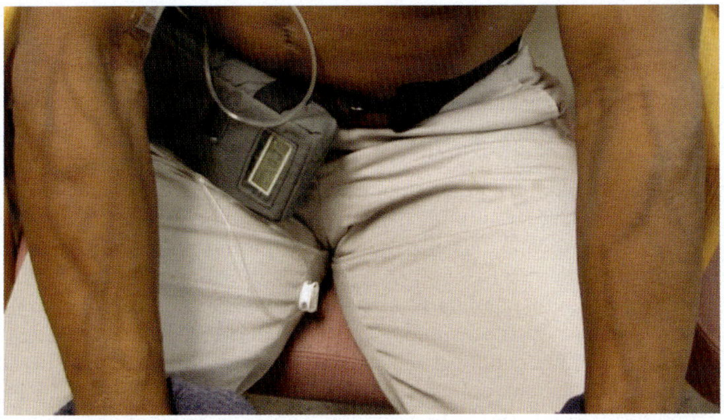

FIGURE 34-7. Supravenous hyperpigmentation secondary to peripheral intravenous fluorouracil treatment. This is thought to be a result of extravasation of the cytotoxic agent, causing epidermal basal hyperpigmentation and dermal melanin incontinence.

30% in TEN. Mucosal involvement is nearly ubiquitous, with painful erosions possible on the lip, oral cavity, conjunctiva, nasal cavity, urethra, vagina, gastrointestinal tract, and/or respiratory tract [**Figures 34-10** and **34-11**].[65] Progression can occur very quickly over the course of a few hours or days with large areas of total body surface involvement.

Mortality rates range from 25% to 50% (average, 25% to 35%) for patients with TEN; the mortality rate is 5% for patients with SJS.[66,67] In patients with TEN, the SCORTEN [**Table 34-4**][68] is a prognostic scoring system that can be used to predict outcome. Immediate discontinuation of the causative medication is crucial, and supportive care is a mainstay of treatment. Immunosuppressive therapy with corticosteroids or intravenous Ig is controversial but can be effective in select cases.[69-73]

Healing of areas of involvement begins in a few days after halting of the process, with complete healing in approximately 3 weeks. Sequelae may include symblepharon, entropion, vaginal synechiae, phimosis, scarring, or dyspigmentation. A multidisciplinary approach to patient care is necessary to decrease morbidity, with consultations from appropriate specialties based on areas of involvement.

CHEMOTHERAPY DRUG REACTIONS

Over the past few decades, remarkable progress in oncology research has expanded and enhanced cancer therapies. Consequently, cancer patients now benefit from more diverse treatment options and improved survival. Despite these advances, the increased utilization of these therapies has resulted in a higher incidence of related cutaneous side effects. While cutaneous side effects are generally not life-threatening, they can considerably impact patients' quality of life.[74]

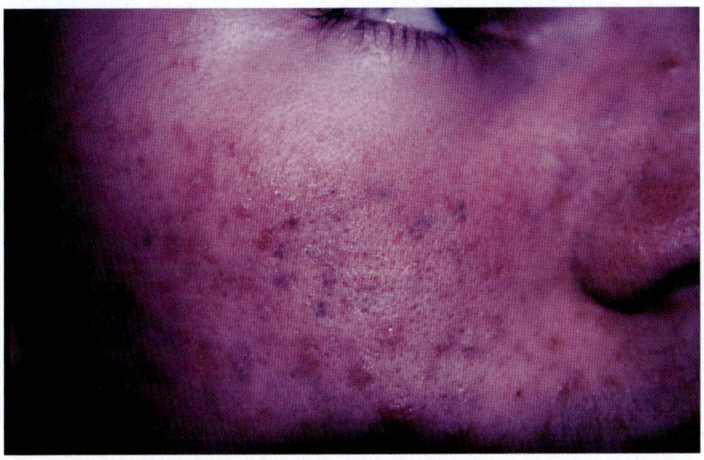

FIGURE 34-8. Minocycline pigmentation within acne scars.

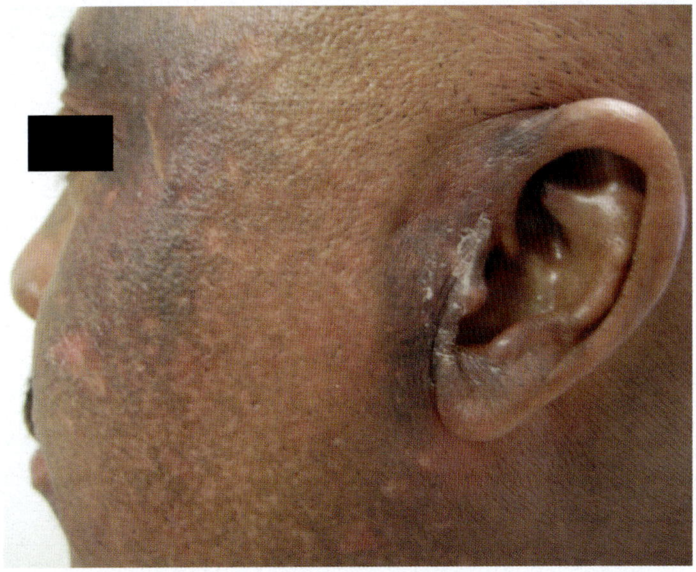

FIGURE 34-9. Exogenous ochronosis. (Used with permission from Lisa Pappas-Taffer, MD.)

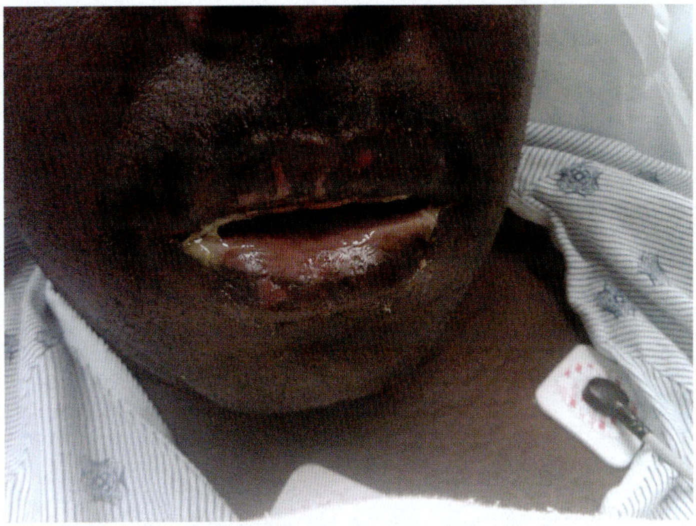

FIGURE 34-10. Oral mucosal involvement in Stevens-Johnson syndrome/toxic epidermal necrolysis. (Used with permission from Lisa Pappas-Taffer, MD.)

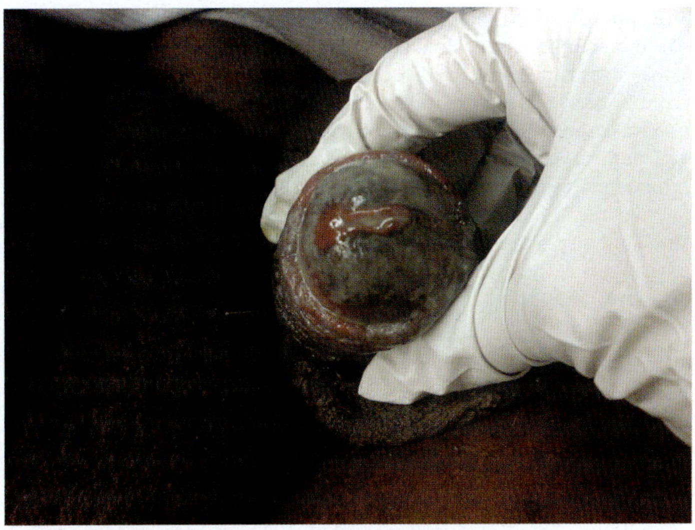

FIGURE 34-11. Genital mucosal involvement in Stevens-Johnson syndrome/toxic epidermal necrolysis. (Used with permission from Lisa Pappas-Taffer, MD.)

TABLE 34-4 SCORTEN: A prognostic scoring system for patients with toxic epidermal necrolysis

Risk factor	0 Points	1 Point
Age	<40	>40
Associated malignancy	No	Yes
Heart rate (bpm)	<120	>120
Total body surface area involvement on day 1	<10%	>10%
Serum urea level (mg/dL)	<27	>27
Serum bicarbonate level (mEq/L)	<20	<20
Serum glucose level (mg/dL)	<250	>250
Number of risk factors (points)	**% Mortality**	
0-1	3.2	
2	12.1	
3	35.8	
4	58.3	
≥5	90	

Source: Bastuji-Garin S et al. SCORTEN: a severity-of-illness score for toxic epidermal necrolysis. *J Invest Dermatol*. 2000;115(2):149-153.

To effectively diagnose and manage chemotherapy-related side effects, healthcare providers must thoroughly understand the general cutaneous reaction patterns linked to patients' medications and the dermatological implications of various cancer treatments. Moreover, providers should be well-acquainted with the diagnostic framework necessary for identifying and confirming the causative agent when a drug reaction is suspected. We propose the following schema to characterize the spectrum of known chemotherapy-associated adverse drug reactions with cutaneous manifestations [**Tables 34-5** and **34-6**].[75]

Extravasation Reactions Extravasation occurs when fluids or medications intended for intravenous administration inadvertently leak into surrounding tissues, causing damage through various mechanisms. The incidence of chemotherapy extravasation is unknown due to a lack of centralized reporting.[76] Early signs of extravasation include discomfort, pruritus, burning, tingling, edema, and erythema at the infusion site. Although these symptoms often present immediately, they can sometimes be delayed by days or weeks [**Figure 34-7**].[77]

Several patient risk factors can contribute to extravasation, such as difficult device insertion, catheter migration, prolonged dwell time, the presence of fibrin sheaths or thrombi, small or fragile veins, patient movement, and the use of specific infusion devices. Implementing proper infusion techniques is essential to prevent extravasation injury from chemotherapy and other infusions.

Approaches to managing extravasation injuries vary depending on the specific agent involved. Cold application is recommended for extravasations of vesicant agents, except for vinca alkaloids and etoposide, which require heat application. Dexrazoxane is advised for anthracycline extravasations with a high risk of tissue ulceration but not for liposomal anthracyclines. High doses of oral glucocorticoids are suggested for oxaliplatin extravasations, while local injections of sodium thiosulfate are recommended for mechlorethamine, bendamustine, dacarbazine, and cisplatin extravasations. Finally, hyaluronidase injections are advised for extravasations with vinca alkaloids and taxanes (paclitaxel, docetaxel).

HAND-FOOT SYNDROME

Hand-foot syndrome (HFS), alternatively known as acral erythema, palmoplantar erythrodysesthesia, Burgdorf syndrome, or toxic erythema of chemotherapy, is a condition characterized by the presence of well-defined, red, swollen plaques on the palms and soles of the feet [**Figure 34-12**]. The choice of chemotherapeutic agent, treatment schedule, and duration of treatment influences the likelihood of developing HFS.[78] HFS is more prevalent among Black patients than White patients.[79-81]

Initial symptoms of HFS typically include numbness, tingling, and burning pain in the palms and soles. These symptoms are often accompanied by erythema, which may or may not present with edema, cracking, and desquamation. In more advanced stages of the condition, blistering and ulceration may occur. It is important to note that in individuals with darker skin tones (Fitzpatrick skin types V-VI), HFS may manifest as macular hyperpigmentation rather than erythema.[78] Limited case studies suggest that HFS may also initially present with acral hyperpigmentation rather than erythema in Black patients.[82] Furthermore, disabling palmar-plantar keratoderma has been observed to develop relatively quickly (within 3-6 months) among Black patients, whereas it is uncommon in White patients.[82] This often progresses to grade 3 HFS, characterized by ulceration and infection, particularly in patients with fragile peripheral vasculature.[6] Diagnosis of HFS is generally based on the patient's medication history and clinical presentation. Skin biopsies are not routinely necessary for diagnosing the condition.

Further research is needed to understand the clinical nuances relating to observed variations in HFS clinical manifestations by race and ethnicity. A different grading system for HFS in non-White patients has been proposed to include: (1) hyperpigmentation of the palms and soles; (2) skin thickening of the palms and soles, accompanied by pain and loss of function; (3) ulceration, dermatitis, or desquamation.[79] This grading system aims to provide a more comprehensive and accurate assessment of HFS in patients of diverse racial and ethnic backgrounds.

Hand-Foot Skin Reaction (HFSR) Hand-foot skin reaction (HFSR) is a distinct dermatologic condition associated with kinase inhibitors, characterized by localized, erythematous, tender, and edematous changes in the hands and feet. HFSR typically manifests as demarcated lesions in areas subjected to pressure or friction, such as the heels, metatarsal heads, or areas affected by shoe wear or manual labor. In contrast to HFS, HFSR is often marked by painful hyperkeratosis, which develops in over 50% of patients after blister formation. Hypertension has been identified as a risk factor for HFSR in patients undergoing treatment with bevacizumab or sorafenib.[83]

Studies have shown that the occurrence of HFSR may predict positive treatment outcomes in specific patient populations, such as those with metastatic renal cell carcinoma or unresectable hepatocellular carcinoma. For example, in a Japanese prospective study of patients with metastatic renal cell carcinoma treated with sorafenib, patients with HFSR had a median progression-free survival of 4.6 months compared to 1.5 months for those without HFSR.[84] In a study conducted in Korea, HFSR predicted long-term survival (>2 years) in patients treated with sorafenib for unresectable hepatocellular carcinoma.[85] Furthermore, the incidence of HFSR appears to vary by race and ethnicity, with a higher prevalence among Asian patients.[86,87] One study found that hand-foot skin reactions are more common in Taiwan than in the West and are an independent predictor of better treatment outcomes.[88]

Neutrophilic Eccrine Hidradenitis Neutrophilic eccrine hidradenitis (NEH) is a condition that can occur in the context of cancers (with or without chemotherapy), infections, and certain medications. In cases related to medication use, patients typically develop a rash 1 to 2 weeks after treatment with the offending agent. The clinical manifestation of NEH is nonspecific, with lesions often presenting as asymptomatic, erythematous, and edematous plaques on the limbs, trunk, and face, including the periorbital region, where coalescing lesions may resemble cellulitis. However, they can also be purpuric and painful, and[89] in some cases, widespread lesions resembling erythema multiforme have been reported.

Diagnosis requires a biopsy, which reveals degenerative vacuolar changes in the secretory coils of the eccrine gland and epithelial necrosis.[90] There is no widely accepted treatment for NEH; supportive care is generally advised.[91,92]

Eccrine Squamous Syringometaplasia Eccrine squamous syringometaplasia (ESS) is associated with chemotherapeutic agents, tumors,

TABLE 34-5 Adverse cutaneous reactions by mechanism of action and examples

Mechanism of action of adverse reaction	Examples	Causative drugs
Cytotoxicity and drug accumulation	Extravasation reactions	Alkylating agents: carmustine, carboplatin, cisplatin, cyclophosphamide, dacarbazine, daunorubicin, melphalan, mechlorethamine, oxaliplatin Antimetabolites: F-5U, gemcitabine Antitumor antimicrobials: bleomycin, dactinomycin, doxorubicin, epirubicin, mitomycin C, mitoxantrone Proteasome inhibitor: bortezomib Spindle inhibitors: docetaxel, etoposide, paclitaxel, topotecan, vinblastine, vincristine
	Hand-foot syndrome	Alkylating agents: cisplatin, cyclophosphamide, temozolomide Antimetabolites: capecitabine, cytarabine, decitabine, 5-fluorouracil (5-FU) Antitumor antimicrobials: doxorubicin, daunorubicin Spindle inhibitors: docetaxel, etoposide, paclitaxel
	Neutrophilic eccrine hidradenitis	Alkylating agents: cisplatin, cyclophosphamide Antimetabolites: cytarabine, decitabine Antitumor antimicrobials: bleomycin, daunorubicin Signal transduction inhibitors: cetuximab, dabrafenib, imatinib, vemurafenib Spindle inhibitors: paclitaxel, topotecan
	Eccrine squamous syringometaplasia	Alkylating agents: busulfan, carmustine, cisplatin, cyclophosphamide, melphalan Antimetabolites: 5-FU, cytarabine, pemetrexed Antitumor antimicrobials: bleomycin, daunorubicin, doxorubicin, mitoxantrone Signal transduction inhibitors: dabrafenib, imatinib, sunitinib, vemurafenib Spindle inhibitors: etoposide, paclitaxel, vincristine
	Pigmentary alterations	Alkylating agents: busulfan, carmustine, cisplatin, cyclophosphamide, mechlorethamine Antimetabolites: 5-FU, capecitabine, pemetrexed Antitumor antimicrobials: bleomycin, dactinomycin, daunorubicin, doxorubicin, mitoxantrone Spindle inhibitor: docetaxel
	Alopecia	Alkylating agents: busulfan, carboplatin, carmustine, cisplatin, cyclophosphamide, mechlorethamine, melphalan, oxaliplatin, procarbazine Antimetabolites: 5-FU, capecitabine, cytarabine, fludarabine, gemcitabine Antitumor antimicrobials: bleomycin, dactinomycin, daunorubicin, doxorubicin, epirubicin, mitomycin C, mitoxantrone Spindle inhibitors: docetaxel, etoposide, paclitaxel, topotecan, vinblastine, vincristine Signal transduction inhibitors: dabrafenib, erlotinib, gefitinib, sorafenib, sunitinib, regorafenib, vemurafenib, vismodegib
	Subacute cutaneous lupus erythematosus	Alkylating agent: cyclophosphamide Antimetabolites: 5-FU, capecitabine, gemcitabine Antitumor antimicrobial: doxorubicin Spindle inhibitors: docetaxel, paclitaxel
Hypersensitivity reactions (HSRs)	Type I	Alkylating agents: carboplatin, cisplatin, cyclophosphamide, chlorambucil, mechlorethamine, oxaliplatin, procarbazine Antimetabolite: cytarabine Antitumor antimicrobials: doxorubicin, epirubicin Immunotherapy: tocilizumab Signal transduction inhibitors: bevacizumab, cetuximab, crizotinib, gefitinib, lapatinib, sorafenib, trastuzumab Spindle inhibitors: etoposide, docetaxel, paclitaxel
	Type II	
	Type III	Alkylating agents: busulfan, cisplatin, oxaliplatin Antimetabolites: 5-FU, capecitabine Antitumor antimicrobial: mitomycin C Signal transduction inhibitors: erlotinib, panitumumab, sorafenib, vemurafenib
	Type IVa	Alkylating agent: mechlorethamine Antitumor antimicrobial: mitomycin C
	Type IVb	Alkylating agent: chlorambucil Immunotherapy: ipilimumab Proteasome inhibitor: bortezomib Signal transduction inhibitors: imatinib, vemurafenib, vismodegib
	Type IVc	Alkylating agents: bendamustine, chlorambucil, cyclophosphamide, mechlorethamine, procarbazine, temozolomide Antimetabolites: capecitabine, cladribine, cytarabine, fludarabine, gemcitabine, pemetrexed Antitumor antimicrobials: bleomycin, dactinomycin, doxorubicin Immunotherapies: ipilimumab,6 mogamulizumab, nivolumab, pembrolizumab Proteasome inhibitors: bortezomib Signal transduction inhibitors: Afatinib, brentuximab, cetuximab, erlotinib, gefitinib, imatinib, panitumumab, regorafenib, sorafenib, sunitinib, vandetanib, vemurafenib Spindle inhibitors: docetaxel, etoposide, paclitaxel

(*Continued*)

TABLE 34-5 Adverse cutaneous reactions by mechanism of action and examples (*Continued*)

Mechanism of action of adverse reaction	Examples	Causative drugs
	Type IVd	Antimetabolites: azacytidine, capecitabine, decitabine, gemcitabine Antitumor antimicrobials: mitoxantrone Immunotherapy: ipilimumab Proteasome inhibitors: bortezomib Signal transduction inhibitors: dabrafenib, dasatinib, imatinib, nilotinib, ruxolitinib, sorafenib, trametinib, vemurafenib Spindle inhibitors: topotecan
Aberrant molecular signaling	Hand-foot skin reaction	Signal transduction inhibitors: axitinib, bevacizumab, brentuximab, cediranib, cabozantinib, erlotinib, pazopanib, regorafenib, sorafenib, sunitinib, vemurafenib
	Papulopustulosis	Signal transduction inhibitors: afatinib, cetuximab, dabrafenib, dacomitinib, dasatinib, dovitinib, erlotinib, gefitinib, lapatinib, necitumumab, panitumumab, pertuzumab, rociletinib, selumetinib, sorafenib, trametinib, trastuzumab, vandetanib
	Pigmentary alterations	Immunotherapies: ipilimumab, nivolumab, pembrolizumab Signal transduction inhibitors: cabozantinib, dasatinib, gefitinib, imatinib, pazopanib, sorafenib, sunitinib, vandetanib, vemurafenib

chronic ulcerations, and other inflammatory disorders. ESS has a nonspecific clinical presentation that overlaps with other chemotherapy-related eccrine gland disorders, including NEH. Erythematous macules, papules, and plaques, which may be localized or disseminated, typically develop several days to weeks after drug administration. A definitive diagnosis of ESS requires a skin biopsy and is characterized histologically by the replacement of cuboidal epithelium lining eccrine ducts and glands with keratinizing squamous cell epithelia. In most cases, ESS resolves spontaneously once the causative agent is removed, and the skin lesions heal without scarring. Topical corticosteroids may be used to manage symptoms, and discontinuing the causative drug may sometimes be necessary.

Alopecia Alopecia is one of the most common adverse side effects of chemotherapy, with its incidence and severity influenced by the drug, dose, duration of treatment, and drug administration route. Chemotherapy-induced alopecia (CIA) usually begins a few days to a few weeks after drug administration and progresses over the next 2 to 3 months. A retrospective, case-control, genome-wide association study of DNA samples from chemotherapy-treated breast cancer patients suggested that the single-nucleotide polymorphism rs3820706 in calcium channel voltage-dependent subunit beta 4 (CACNB4) on 2q23 (among others) was significantly associated with complete CIA (odds ratio 3.71, $p = 8.13 \times 10^{-6}$).[93] According to one study, the risk of permanent CIA may be higher in Black women ($n = 10$) than in White women ($n = 3$). Furthermore, hair loss may be more diffuse in Black women compared to White women.[94,95]

Scalp cooling may be an effective treatment modality for CIA, but there may be differences in use by race and ethnicity.[96] For example, non-White patients are less likely to choose scalp cooling than White patients. Proper counseling by the healthcare team on how to use scalp cooling most effectively with curly hair may reduce these disparities, given that the fit of the cap is an essential factor in the effectiveness of scalp cooling.

Papulopustulosis Papulopustulosis, also referred to as acneiform or acne-like eruption, is a frequent dermatologic side effect of signal

TABLE 34-6 Chemotherapy drugs classification by mechanism of action and examples

Alkylating agents	Alkylsulfonate: busulfan Hydrazine and triazene: dacarbazine, procarbazine, temozolomide Metal salts: carboplatin, cisplatin, oxaliplatin Mustard gas derivatives: bendamustine, carmustine, chlorambucil, cyclophosphamide, mechlorethamine, melphalan
Antimetabolites	Purine analogs: cladribine, fludarabine Pyrimidine analogs: 5-FU, azacitidine, capecitabine, cytarabine, decitabine, gemcitabine Combined mechanism: pemetrexed
Antitumor antibiotics	Anthracyclines: daunorubicin, doxorubicin, epirubicin, mitoxantrone Non-anthracyclines: bleomycin, dactinomycin, mitomycin C
Immunotherapies	CCR4: mogamulizumab CTLA-4: ipilimumab IL-6: tocilizumab PD-1: nivolumab, pembrolizumab
Proteasome inhibitors	Bortezomib
Signal transduction inhibitors	ALK/ROS1: crizotinib, nilotinib BRAF: dabrafenib, vemurafenib CD-30: brentuximab EGFR: afatinib, cetuximab, dacomitinib, erlotinib, gefitinib, necitumumab, panitumumab, pertuzumab, rociletinib JAK: ruxolitinib MEK: selumetinib, trametinib SMO/SHH: vismodegib VEGF: axitinib, cediranib, trastuzumab Multikinase: cabozantinib, dasatinib, dovitinib, imatinib, lapatinib, pazopanib, regorafenib, sorafenib, sunitinib, vandetanib
Spindle inhibitors	Camptothecin analog: topotecan Podophyllotoxin: etoposide Taxanes: docetaxel, paclitaxel Vinca alkaloids: vinblastine, vincristine

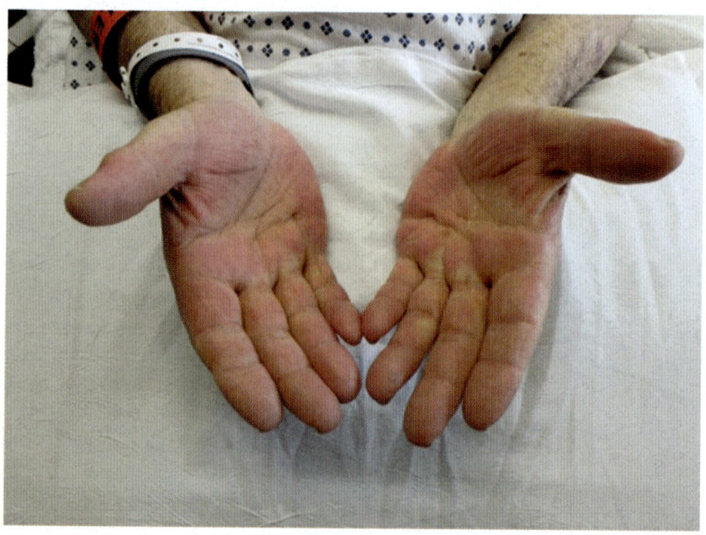

FIGURE 34-12. Erythema of palms in toxic erythema of chemotherapy. (Reproduced with permission from Loscalzo J, Fauci AS, Kasper DL, et al, eds. *Harrison's Principles of Internal Medicine*. 21st ed. New York, NY: McGraw Hill; 2022, Figure 60-2.)

transduction inhibitors, particularly epidermal growth factor receptor inhibitors (EGFRis) and mitogen-activated protein kinase inhibitors, which interfere with keratinocyte function. This condition is characterized by papules and pustules primarily on the face and upper trunk. Comedones are generally absent unless androgens are the underlying cause. Mild to moderate cases may be managed with hydrocortisone (1-2.5% cream), clindamycin (1% gel), or pimecrolimus (1% cream) with the addition of either doxycycline (100 mg, p.o. bid) or minocycline (100 mg, p.o. bid). Severe cases unresponsive to the above may require the administration of oral steroids. Testing for bacterial superinfection should also be performed.[97]

ADDITIONAL SKIN OF COLOR CONSIDERATIONS

Dermatologists and primary care physicians must become more familiar and comfortable with diagnosing adverse cutaneous events in the skin of color. Non-White patients are half as likely to be diagnosed with an adverse cutaneous event following chemotherapy compared to White patients. Still, they are six times more likely to be referred to a dermatologist when a reaction occurs.[98] This disparity likely reflects the need for more preparedness of primary care physicians to recognize dermatologic reactions in patients with skin of color. Furthermore, delays in diagnosis and treatment for patients with skin of color may lead to poorer outcomes for these populations.

TREATMENT FRAMEWORK

General management of cutaneous drug eruptions includes discontinuing the causative medication, symptom management, and, if necessary, administering immunosuppressive therapies. In cases where multiple medications may be implicated in a drug eruption, it is best practice to discontinue all nonessential medications. In mild cases, if the continuation of the suspected medication is necessary and there are no alternative treatment options, the causative drug may be continued with careful symptom management. Topical steroids, antihistamines, and emollients are appropriate treatment modalities for mild eruptions. More severe eruptions may require immunosuppressive therapy, wound care, and additional support. Avoidance of repeat exposure to the causative medication is recommended and is necessary for more severe reactions.

REFERENCES

1. Bigby M, Jick S, Jick H, Arndt K. Drug-induced cutaneous reactions. A report from the Boston Collaborative Drug Surveillance Program on 15,438 consecutive inpatients, 1975 to 1982. *JAMA*. 1986;256(24):3358-3363.
2. Bigby M. Rates of cutaneous reactions to drugs. *Arch Dermatol*. 2001;137(6):765-770.
3. Roujeau JC, Stern RS. Severe adverse cutaneous reactions to drugs. *N Engl J Med*. 1994;331(19):1272-1285.
4. Hughes AR, Mosteller M, Bansal AT, et al. Association of genetic variations in HLA-B region with hypersensitivity to abacavir in some, but not all, populations. *Pharmacogenomics*. 2004;5(2):203-211.
5. Sun HY, Hung CC, Lin PH, et al. Incidence of abacavir hypersensitivity and its relationship with HLA-B*5701 in HIV-infected patients in Taiwan. *J Antimicrob Chemother*. 2007;60(3):599-604.
6. Saag M, Balu R, Phillips E, et al. High sensitivity of human leukocyte antigen-b*5701 as a marker for immunologically confirmed abacavir hypersensitivity in white and black patients. *Clin Infect Dis*. 2008;46(7):1111-1118.
7. Zucman D, Truchis P de, Majerholc C, Stegman S, Caillat-Zucman S. Prospective screening for human leukocyte antigen-B*5701 avoids abacavir hypersensitivity reaction in the ethnically mixed French HIV population. *J Acquir Immune Defic Syndr 1999*. 2007;45(1):1-3.
8. Sadiq ST, Pakianathan M. Uncertainties of routine HLA B*5701 testing in black African HIV cohorts in the UK. *Sex Transm Infect*. 2007;83(3):181-182.
9. Amstutz U, Shear NH, Rieder MJ, Hwang S, Fung V, Nakamura H, Connolly MB, Ito S, Carleton BC; CPNDS clinical recommendation group. Recommendations for HLA-B*15:02 and HLA-A*31:01 genetic testing to reduce the risk of carbamazepine-induced hypersensitivity reactions.
10. Manson LEN, Swen JJ, Guchelaar HJ. Diagnostic test criteria for HLA genotyping to prevent drug hypersensitivity reactions: a systematic review of actionable HLA recommendations in CPIC and DPWG guidelines. *Front Pharmacol*. 2020;11:567048.
11. Aihara M. Pharmacogenetics of cutaneous adverse drug reactions. *J Dermatol*. 2011;38(3):246-254.
12. Stubb S, Heikkilä H, Kauppinen K. Cutaneous reactions to drugs: a series of in-patients during a five-year period. *Acta Derm Venereol*. 1994;74(4):289-291.
13. Kauppinen K, Stubb S. Drug eruptions: causative agents and clinical types. A series of in-patients during a 10-year period. *Acta Derm Venereol*. 1984;64(4):320-324.
14. Crowson AN, Brown TJ, Magro CM. Progress in the understanding of the pathology and pathogenesis of cutaneous drug eruptions: implications for management. *Am J Clin Dermatol*. 2003;4(6):407-428.
15. Hwang SJE, Carlos G, Wakade D, et al. Cutaneous adverse events (AEs) of anti-programmed cell death (PD)-1 therapy in patients with metastatic melanoma: a single-institution cohort. *J Am Acad Dermatol*. 2016;74(3):455-461.e1.
16. Breathnach S, Hintner H. *Adverse Drug Reactions and the Skin*. Wiley, *NY*; 1992.
17. Tohyama M, Hashimoto K. New aspects of drug-induced hypersensitivity syndrome. PubMed. https://pubmed.ncbi.nlm.nih.gov/21342223/. Accessed April 15, 2023.
18. Schaub N, Bircher AJ. Severe hypersensitivity syndrome to lamotrigine confirmed by lymphocyte stimulation in vitro. *Allergy*. 2000;55(2):191-193.
19. Demoly P, Adkinson NF, Brockow K, et al. International consensus on drug allergy. *Allergy*. 2014;69(4):420-437.
20. Shafeng N, Han DF, Ma YF, Abudusalamu R, Ayitimuhan B. Association between the HLA-B*1502 gene and mild maculopapular exanthema induced by antiepileptic drugs in Northwest China. *BMC Neurol*. 2021;21(1):340.
21. Sukasem C, Chaichan C, Nakkrut T, et al. Association between HLA-B alleles and carbamazepine-induced maculopapular exanthema and severe cutaneous reactions in Thai patients. *J Immunol Res*. 2018;2018:2780272.
22. Tohyama M, Hashimoto K, Yasukawa M, et al. Association of human herpesvirus 6 reactivation with the flaring and severity of drug-induced hypersensitivity syndrome. *Br J Dermatol*. 2007;157(5):934-940.
23. Ko TM, Tsai CY, Chen SY, et al. Use of HLA-B*58:01 genotyping to prevent allopurinol induced severe cutaneous adverse reactions in Taiwan: national prospective cohort study. *BMJ*. 2015;351:h4848.
24. Roujeau JC, Bioulac-Sage P, Bourseau C, et al. Acute generalized exanthematous pustulosis. Analysis of 63 cases. *Arch Dermatol*. 1991;127(9):1333-1338.
25. Nnoruka EN, Ikeh VO, Mbah AU. Fixed drug eruption in Nigeria. *Int J Dermatol*. 2006;45(9):1062-1065.
26. Brahimi N, Routier E, Raison-Peyron N, et al. A three-year-analysis of fixed drug eruptions in hospital settings in France. *Eur J Dermatol*. 2010;20(4):461-464.
27. Mahboob A, Haroon TS. Drugs causing fixed eruptions: a study of 450 cases. *Int J Dermatol*. 1998;37(11):833-838.
28. Fortuna G, Salas-Alanis JC, Guidetti E, Marinkovich MP. A critical reappraisal of the current data on drug-induced linear immunoglobulin A bullous dermatosis: a real and separate nosological entity? *J Am Acad Dermatol*. 2012;66(6):988-994.
29. Kenani N, Mebazaa A, Denguezli M, et al. Childhood linear IgA bullous dermatosis in Tunisia. *Pediatr Dermatol*. 2009;26(1):28-33.
30. Farley-Li J, Mancini AJ. Treatment of linear IgA bullous dermatosis of childhood with mycophenolate mofetil. *Arch Dermatol*. 2003;139(9):1121-1124.
31. Talhari C, Mahnke N, Ruzicka T, Megahed M. Successful treatment of linear IgA disease with mycophenolate mofetil as a corticosteroid sparing agent. *Clin Exp Dermatol*. 2005;30(3):297-298.
32. Lewis MAO, Yaqoob NA, Emanuel C, Potts AJC. Successful treatment of oral linear IgA disease using mycophenolate. *Oral Surg Oral Med Oral Pathol Oral Radiol Endod*. 2007;103(4):483-486.
33. Vassileva S. Drug-induced pemphigoid: bullous and cicatricial. *Clin Dermatol*. 1998;16(3):379-387.
34. Troy JL, Silvers DN, Grossman ME, Jaffe IA. Penicillamine-associated pemphigus: is it really pemphigus? *J Am Acad Dermatol*. 1981;4(5):547-555.
35. Velthuis PJ, Hendrikse JC, Nefkens JJ. Combined features of pemphigus and pemphigoid induced by penicillamine. *Br J Dermatol*. 1985;112(5):615-619.
36. Rasmussen HB, Jepsen LV, Brandrup F. Penicillamine-induced bullous pemphigoid with pemphigus-like antibodies. *J Cutan Pathol*. 1989;16(3):154-157.
37. Ruocco V, Sacerdoti G. Pemphigus and bullous pemphigoid due to drugs. *Int J Dermatol*. 1991;30(5):307-312.

38. Brenner S, Bialy-Golan A, Ruocco V. Drug-induced pemphigus. *Clin Dermatol.* 1998;16(3):393-397.
39. Feng S, Zhou W, Zhang J, Jin P. Analysis of 6 cases of drug-induced pemphigus. *Eur J Dermatol.* 2011;21(5):696-699.
40. Wolf R, Tamir A, Brenner S. Drug-induced versus drug-triggered pemphigus. *Dermatologica.* 1991;182(4):207-210.
41. Brenner S, Wolf R, Ruocco V. Drug-induced pemphigus. I. A survey. *Clin Dermatol.* 1993;11(4):501-505.
42. Antiga E, Melani L, Cardinali C, et al. A case of lichenoid drug eruption associated with sildenafil citratus. *J Dermatol.* 2005;32(12):972-975.
43. Brauer J, Votava HJ, Meehan S, Soter NA. Lichenoid drug eruption. *Dermatol Online J.* 2009;15(8):13.
44. Asarch A, Gottlieb AB, Lee J, et al. Lichen planus-like eruptions: an emerging side effect of tumor necrosis factor-alpha antagonists. *J Am Acad Dermatol.* 2009;61(1):104-111.
45. Halevy S, Shai A. Lichenoid drug eruptions. *J Am Acad Dermatol.* 1993;29 (2 Pt 1):249-255.
46. Woo V, Bonks J, Borukhova L, Zegarelli D. Oral lichenoid drug eruption: a report of a pediatric case and review of the literature. *Pediatr Dermatol.* 2009;26(4):458-464.
47. Teraki Y, Shiohara T. Spontaneous tolerance to terbinafine-induced lichenoid drug eruption. *Dermatol Basel Switz.* 2004;208(1):81-82.
48. Bong JL, Lucke TW, Douglas WS. Lichenoid drug eruption with proton pump inhibitors. *BMJ.* 2000;320(7230):283.
49. Van den Haute V, Antoine JL, Lachapelle JM. Histopathological discriminant criteria between lichenoid drug eruption and idiopathic lichen planus: retrospective study on selected samples. *Dermatologica.* 1989;179(1):10-13.
50. De Simone C, Caldarola G, D'Agostino M, Rotoli M, Capizzi R, Amerio P. Lichenoid reaction induced by adalimumab. *J Eur Acad Dermatol Venereol.* 2008;22(5):626-627.
51. Vergara G, Silvestre JF, Betlloch I, Vela P, Albares MP, Pascual JC. Cutaneous drug eruption to infliximab: report of 4 cases with an interface dermatitis pattern. *Arch Dermatol.* 2002;138(9):1258-1259.
52. Powell FC, Rogers RS, Dickson ER. Primary biliary cirrhosis and lichen planus. *J Am Acad Dermatol.* 1983;9(4):540-545.
53. Rotstein E, Rotstein H. Drug eruptions with lichenoid histology produced by captopril. *Australas J Dermatol.* 1989;30(1):9-14.
54. Bauer F. Quinacrine hydrochloride drug eruption (tropical lichenoid dermatitis). Its early and late sequelae and its malignant potential: a review. *J Am Acad Dermatol.* 1981;4(2):239-248.
55. Shi VJ, Rodic N, Gettinger S, et al. Clinical and histologic features of lichenoid mucocutaneous eruptions due to anti-programmed cell death 1 and anti-programmed cell death ligand 1 immunotherapy. *JAMA Dermatol.* 2016;152(10): 1128-1136.
56. Kratzsch D, Simon JC, Ziemer M. Lichen planus-like drug eruption on anti-PD-1 therapy. *J Dtsch Dermatol Ges.* 2017;15(12):1238-1240.
57. Reschke R, Mockenhaupt M, Simon JC, Ziemer M. Severe bullous skin eruptions on checkpoint inhibitor therapy - in most cases severe bullous lichenoid drug eruptions. *J Dtsch Dermatol Ges.* 2019;17(9):942-948.
58. Gould JW, Mercurio MG, Elmets CA. Cutaneous photosensitivity diseases induced by exogenous agents. *J Am Acad Dermatol.* 1995;33(4):551-573; quiz 574-576.
59. Mouton RW, Jordaan HF, Schneider JW. A new type of minocycline-induced cutaneous hyperpigmentation. *Clin Exp Dermatol.* 2004;29(1):8-14.
60. Charlín R, Barcaui CB, Kac BK, Soares DB, Rabello-Fonseca R, Azulay-Abulafia L. Hydroquinone-induced exogenous ochronosis: a report of four cases and usefulness of dermoscopy. *Int J Dermatol.* 2008;47(1):19-23.
61. Bongiorno MR, Aricò M. Exogenous ochronosis and striae atrophicae following the use of bleaching creams. *Int J Dermatol.* 2005;44(2):112-115.
62. Milrod CJ, Blevins F, Hughes D, et al. Incidence of skin hyperpigmentation in Black patients receiving treatment with immunomodulatory drugs. *Blood.* 2021;137(21):2987-2989.
63. Letko E, Papaliodis DN, Papaliodis GN, Daoud YJ, Ahmed AR, Foster CS. Stevens-Johnson syndrome and toxic epidermal necrolysis: a review of the literature. *Ann Allergy Asthma Immunol.* 2005;94(4):419-436; quiz 436-438, 456.
64. Chan HL. Observations on drug-induced toxic epidermal necrolysis in Singapore. *J Am Acad Dermatol.* 1984;10(6):973-978.
65. Hazin R, Ibrahimi OA, Hazin MI, Kimyai-Asadi A. Stevens-Johnson syndrome: pathogenesis, diagnosis, and management. *Ann Med.* 2008;40(2):129-138.
66. Roujeau JC, Guillaume JC, Fabre JP, Penso D, Fléchet ML, Girre JP. Toxic epidermal necrolysis (Lyell syndrome). Incidence and drug etiology in France, 1981-1985. *Arch Dermatol.* 1990;126(1):37-42.
67. Revuz J, Penso D, Roujeau JC, et al. Toxic epidermal necrolysis. Clinical findings and prognosis factors in 87 patients. *Arch Dermatol.* 1987;123(9):1160-1165.
68. Bastuji-Garin S, Fouchard N, Bertocchi M, Roujeau JC, Revuz J, Wolkenstein P. SCORTEN: a severity-of-illness score for toxic epidermal necrolysis. *J Invest Dermatol.* 2000;115(2):149-153.
69. Tripathi A, Ditto AM, Grammer LC, et al. Corticosteroid therapy in an additional 13 cases of Stevens-Johnson syndrome: a total series of 67 cases. *Allergy Asthma Proc.* 2000;21(2):101-105.
70. Schneck J, Fagot JP, Sekula P, Sassolas B, Roujeau JC, Mockenhaupt M. Effects of treatments on the mortality of Stevens-Johnson syndrome and toxic epidermal necrolysis: a retrospective study on patients included in the prospective EuroSCAR Study. *J Am Acad Dermatol.* 2008;58(1):33-40.
71. Prins C, Kerdel FA, Padilla RS, et al. Treatment of toxic epidermal necrolysis with high-dose intravenous immunoglobulins: multicenter retrospective analysis of 48 consecutive cases. *Arch Dermatol.* 2003;139(1):26-32.
72. Mittmann N, Chan B, Knowles S, Cosentino L, Shear N. Intravenous immunoglobulin use in patients with toxic epidermal necrolysis and Stevens-Johnson syndrome. *Am J Clin Dermatol.* 2006;7(6):359-368.
73. Shortt R, Gomez M, Mittman N, Cartotto R. Intravenous immunoglobulin does not improve outcome in toxic epidermal necrolysis. *J Burn Care Rehabil.* 2004;25(3):246-255.
74. Biswal S, Mehta R. Cutaneous adverse reactions of chemotherapy in cancer patients: a clinicoepidemiological study. *Indian J Dermatol.* 2018;63(1):41-41.
75. Haynes D, Ortega-Loayza AG. Adverse cutaneous reactions to chemotherapeutic drugs. *Clin Dermatol.* 2020;38(6):712-728.
76. Reynolds PM, MacLaren R, Mueller SW, Fish DN, Kiser TH. Management of extravasation injuries: a focused evaluation of noncytotoxic medications. *Pharmacother J Hum Pharmacol Drug Ther.* 2014;34(6):617-632.
77. Susser WS, Whitaker-Worth DL, Grant-Kels JM. Continuing medical education. *J Am Acad Dermatol.* 1999;40(3):367-398.
78. Kwakman JJM, Elshot YS, Punt CJA, Koopman M. Management of cytotoxic chemotherapy-induced hand-foot syndrome. *Oncol Rev.* 2020;14(1):442.
79. Saif MW, Sandoval A. Atypical hand-and-foot syndrome in an African American patient treated with capecitabine with normal DPD activity: is there an ethnic disparity? *Cutan Ocul Toxicol.* 2008;27(4):311-315.
80. Saif MW. Capecitabine and hand-foot syndrome. *Expert Opin Drug Saf.* 2011; 10(2):159-169.
81. Saif MW, Seller S, Diasio RB. Atypical toxicity associated with 5-Fluororacil in a DPD-deficient patient with pancreatic cancer. Is ethnicity a risk factor? *JOP.* 2008;9(2):226-229.
82. Narasimhan P, Narasimhan S, Hitti IF, Rachita M. Serious hand-and-foot syndrome in black patients treated with capecitabine: report of 3 cases and review of the literature. *Cutis.* 2004;73(2):101-106.
83. Jain L, Sissung TM, Danesi R, et al. Hypertension and hand-foot skin reactions related to VEGFR2 genotype and improved clinical outcome following bevacizumab and sorafenib. *J Exp Clin Cancer Res.* 2010;29(1):95.
84. Nakano K, Komatsu K, Kubo T, et al. Hand-foot skin reaction is associated with the clinical outcome in patients with metastatic renal cell carcinoma treated with sorafenib. *Jpn J Clin Oncol.* 2013;43(10):1023-1029.
85. Cho YY, Yu SJ, Lee HW, et al. Clinical characteristics of long-term survivors after sorafenib treatment for unresectable hepatocellular carcinoma: a Korean national multicenter retrospective cohort study. *J Hepatocell Carcinoma.* 2021;8:613-623.
86. Sahoo TP, Kaklamani VG, Lokanatha D, et al. A regional subgroup analysis of a multinational, double-blind, randomized, placebo-controlled, phase IIb study evaluating sorafenib (SOR) with paclitaxel (PAC) in patients (pts) with advanced breast cancer (BC). *J Clin Oncol.* 2010;28(15_suppl):1114-1114.
87. Zhang H, Dong B, Lu JJ, et al. Efficacy of sorafenib on metastatic renal cell carcinoma in Asian patients: results from a multicenter study. *BMC Cancer.* 2009;9:249.
88. Huang PW, Chou WC, Shen WC, et al. Hand-foot skin reaction predicts treatment outcome of pazopanib in patients with metastatic soft tissue sarcoma: a multicenter study in the Asian population. *Asia Pac J Clin Oncol.* 2018;14(4):353-360.
89. Thorisdottir K, Tomecki KJ, Bergfeld WF, Andresen SW. Neutrophilic eccrine hidradenitis. *J Am Acad Dermatol.* 1993;28(5, Part 1):775-777.
90. Brehler R, Reimann S, Bonsmann G, Metze D. Neutrophilic hidradenitis induced by chemotherapy involves eccrine and apocrine glands. *Am J Dermatopathol.* 1997;19(1):73-78.
91. Cohen PR, Kurzrock R. Sweet's syndrome revisited: a review of disease concepts. *Int J Dermatol.* 2003;42(10):761-778.
92. Cohen PR. Neutrophilic dermatoses occurring in oncology patients. *Int J Dermatol.* 2007;46(1):106-111.
93. Chung S, Low SK, Zembutsu H, et al. A genome-wide association study of chemotherapy-induced alopecia in breast cancer patients. *Breast Cancer Res.* 2013;15(5):R81.
94. Hrin ML, McMichael AJ. Chemotherapy-induced alopecia in African American women: a literature review demonstrates a knowledge gap. *J Am Acad Dermatol.* 2022;86(6):1434-1435.

95. Masidonski P, Mahon SM. Permanent alopecia in women being treated for breast cancer. *Clin J Oncol Nurs.* 2009;13(1):13-14.
96. Rose L, Schnell PM, Radcliff L, Lustberg M, Dulmage B. Retrospective cohort study of scalp cooling in breast cancer patients. *Support Care Cancer.* 2023;31(2):118.
97. Fabbrocini G, Panariello L, Caro G, Cacciapuoti S. Acneiform rash induced by EGFR inhibitors: review of the literature and new insights. *Skin Appendage Disord.* 2015;1(1):31-37.
98. Thompson LL, Pan CX, Chang MS, Krasnow NA, Blum AE, Chen ST. Impact of ethnicity on the diagnosis and management of cutaneous toxicities from immune checkpoint inhibitors. *J Am Acad Dermatol.* 2021;84(3):851-854.

CHAPTER 35

Cutaneous Sarcoidosis

Christina M. Murphy
Sotonye Imadojemu
Avrom S. Caplan
Misha Rosenbach

KEY POINTS

- Sarcoidosis is a granulomatous disorder that leads to multiorgan dysfunction.
- In the United States, Black Americans are affected by sarcoidosis at a disproportionate rate and experience more disease-related morbidity and mortality.
- Sarcoidosis presents with a variety of cutaneous lesions that may resemble other inflammatory conditions, making it a diagnostic challenge. When sarcoidosis is diagnosed on the skin, prompt systemic evaluation should follow to detect other organ involvement.
- The etiology of sarcoidosis is incompletely understood, though genetics and environmental exposures are known to play a role. Ongoing investigation and emerging therapies are increasing our understanding of the disease.

INTRODUCTION

Sarcoidosis is a granulomatous, multiorgan disease that most commonly affects the lungs followed by the skin.[1,2] The cutaneous lesions of sarcoidosis are often the presenting symptom of this multisystem disease and therefore critical to identify.[3] Cutaneous sarcoidosis can arise at any point relative to internal organ involvement, and for a subset of patients remains the primary impact of the disease. Though sarcoidosis was first described in 1869 and given its name by a Boeck, a Norwegian dermatologist due to its appearance as a benign-sarcoma-like disease, the etiology of this disease remains an area of active investigation.[4] Most researchers agree that the pathogenesis of sarcoidosis begins when a genetically susceptible individual is exposed to an antigen, culminating in a dysregulated immunologic cascade characterized by exaggerated T helper 1 and T helper 17 (T_H1/T_H17) immune responses.[5] This manifests clinically with noncaseating granuloma formation in the lungs, skin, lymph nodes, eyes, heart, and other organs. In the United States, sarcoidosis affects Black Americans at a higher rate and imposes greater burden of disease. On average, patients with skin of color present with more advanced disease and experience poorer outcomes.[6]

INCIDENCE AND PREVALENCE

Sarcoidosis impacts people of all races, ethnicities, ages, and sexes. However, in the United States, incidence and prevalence are consistently reported to be highest in Black Americans.[7,8] A study out of Detroit, Michigan in the 1990s reported an incidence of 35.5 per 100,000 Black compared to 10.9 per 100,000 White Americans, representing nearly a fourfold difference.[7] More recently, analysis of a national healthcare use database from 2009 to 2013 showed significantly higher incidence and prevalence for Black Americans (17.8 and 141.4 per 100,000) compared to White Americans (8.1 and 49.8 per 100,000).[8] In both studies, the highest rate of disease was found in Black females.[7,8]

Disease prevalence also varies by region of the world, from 1 to 5 per 100,000 in Japan,[9] South Korea,[10] and Taiwan[11] to between 120 and 160 per 100,000 in Canada,[12] Sweden,[13] and Switzerland.[14] Sarcoidosis occurs at all stages of life but is most frequent in young and middle-aged adults, with diagnosis peaking at age 30 to 50 in males and 50 to 60 in females.[15] Sarcoidosis is less common in the elderly and rare in children.

PROGNOSIS

Sarcoidosis is a heterogeneous disease with variable extent of organ involvement and severity. Cutaneous lesions occur in up to 30% of reported cases.[2] The prognostic value of specific cutaneous lesions remains largely unclear; however, early detection of cutaneous lesions can hasten diagnosis and allow for prompt systemic evaluation and treatment: in a Spanish study, 17% of patients with sarcoidosis had cutaneous involvement, and in 80% of those cases, skin lesions were present prior or simultaneous to diagnosis of systemic sarcoidosis.[16] Skin disease can be the initial sign of sarcoidosis, and represents an accessible organ for histologic confirmation of suspected sarcoidosis. In some patients, it may be the most profoundly impacted organ, or rarely the only site of disease.

Long-term prognosis generally depends on the degree of systemic involvement. However, there are notable differences in presentation and prognosis based on demographic factors such as race.[17] African Americans and Asian Indians typically have more advanced disease at diagnosis,[18] while asymptomatic cases and Löfgren syndrome (associated with favorable prognosis) are more common in White patients.[19,20] A Case-Control Etiologic Study of Sarcoidosis (ACCESS) enrolled patients within 6 months of diagnosis at multiple centers in a prospective manner, allowing for the study of relationships between demographic factors, socioeconomic status, and barriers to care with severity of disease at presentation.[19,20] ACCESS showed that Black patients tend to experience greater extent of organ involvement and lower FVC% on spirometry at presentation.[20] Black Americans are also more likely to live with chronic cutaneous sarcoidosis, and experience poorer overall outcomes as indicated by age-adjusted, disease-specific mortality.[21-24] Lupus pernio, a chronic, severe type of cutaneous sarcoidosis, is also more common in Black Americans. Interestingly, disease prevalence is reported to be lower in populations of African descent outside the United States, such as in the West Indies and West Africa, suggesting that the higher incidence in Black Americans cannot be attributed to genetics or ancestry alone.[25,26] A French multicenter study including sites in the Caribbean and Indian Ocean isles used hierarchical clustering analysis to describe five phenotypes of sarcoidosis. In this study, African descent was not associated with a statistically significant odds ratio of having the disease.[27]

ETIOLOGY AND PATHOGENESIS

Although sarcoidosis has been studied extensively, its precise etiopathogenesis remains elusive. Sarcoidosis likely develops when a genetically susceptible host is exposed to an antigen, eliciting the formation of noncaseating granulomas. No single causative antigen has been identified, but proposed antigens include bacterial, viral, self, or environmental exposures.[4,28-30] As modern molecular techniques are employed to investigate its pathophysiology, sarcoidosis may prove to represent a group of diseases.

A genetic component to the pathophysiology of sarcoidosis is supported by familial aggregation, association with major histocompatibility complex genes, and genome-wide association studies. Siblings of patients with sarcoidosis are found to have about a fivefold increased risk of developing sarcoidosis.[31] Moreover, a co-twin of an affected identical twin has an 80-fold increased risk of getting sarcoidosis compared with the general population, whereas the risk was increased only by sevenfold in a co-twin of an affected dizygotic twin.[32] Major histocompatibility genes have been studied extensively, and the association of HLA-DQB1 and HLA-DRB1 with the risk of developing sarcoidosis has been confirmed by a host of studies.[33-35] These HLA alleles have even been linked to specific disease phenotypes or disease risk within certain populations. For example, HLA-DRB1 is associated with the development of diastolic dysfunction[34] and Löfgren syndrome[19] as well as sarcoidosis susceptibility in Asian and White patients.[35] In those with skin of color, HLA-DQB1 has been identified to confer increased risk for sarcoidosis.[35] In the United States, African Americans and skin of color groups have been studied to have greater HLA type II diversity compared to those of European ancestry. This enhanced variation in HLA haplotypes is thought to account for some of the racial differences in prevalence, presentation, and course.[35,36]

Non-HLA genes associated with sarcoidosis include *ANXA11*, *BTNL2*, *CCR5*, *COX2*, and *NOTCH4*, and some are enriched within certain ethnic groups.[33] Butyrophilin-like 2 (*BTNL2*) also resides in the MHC class II region on chromosome 6, though variants have a stronger association with sarcoidosis in White Americans than in African Americans.[37] Greater allelic diversity or an antagonistic effect of HLA class II risk alleles on *BTNL2*-associated risk have been hypothesized to explain the attenuated association in African Americans.[37] On the other hand, a nonsynonymous single-nucleotide polymorphism of annexin A11 (*ANXA11*) identified in a German study and validated in two other European populations was investigated in the United States and risk variants were only associated with sarcoidosis in African Americans.[38] Genome analysis performed by the Sarcoidosis Genetic Analysis Consortium (SAGA) found the strongest linkage signal on chromosome 5 among a cohort of African American siblings.[39] Fine-mapping revealed a sarcoidosis susceptibility gene on chromosome 5q11.2 and a gene that provides protective effect on 5p15.2.[40] Recent sequencing of a family with a high prevalence of sarcoidosis identified additional potential genetic contributors, including mutations in *JAK2*.[41]

If encountered by a susceptible host, certain environmental factors are also thought to contribute to development of sarcoidosis. This is supported by the fact that sarcoidosis commonly affects the organs most exposed to the environment, such as the lungs, skin, and eyes. Multiple environmental agents have been reported to increase risk of sarcoidosis, including tree pollen, inorganic particles, insecticides, and molds.[42] Occupational studies have shown associations with U.S. Navy personnel, metalworking, firefighters, and the handling of building supplies.[43,44] In the skin, sarcoidosis has been observed to develop within scars,[45] venipuncture points,[46] tattoos,[47] and injection sites of insulin,[48] anesthetic, or of various cosmetics.[49]

Finally, socioeconomic status plays a role in progression of disease and has been inversely correlated with disease severity. ACCESS demonstrated that lower income, absence of Medicare or private health insurance, and other barriers to care were all associated with increased severity at presentation, as was Black race and female sex.[21]

CLINICAL FINDINGS

The skin is involved in up to 30% of patients with sarcoidosis.[2] Cutaneous sarcoidosis presents with many clinical morphologies and can mimic numerous disease processes, requiring clinicians to maintain a high index of suspicion in evaluating these patients. Clinical findings also vary with chronicity and patient skin color. The skin provides a readily accessible site for biopsy to obtain histologic confirmation of granulomas: "specific" sarcoidosis findings have evidence of noncaseating granulomas on histology, while "nonspecific" lesions do not.

SPECIFIC CUTANEOUS FINDINGS

Papules and Plaques Papules are the most common cutaneous lesion of sarcoidosis. They can be localized or generalized. They are typically firm, red-brown to violaceous, and sometimes have an "apple jelly" appearance that can be detected on diascopy. Plaques tend to be erythematous, infiltrative, and associated with chronic disease and scarring [**Figures 35-1** and **35-2**].[50]

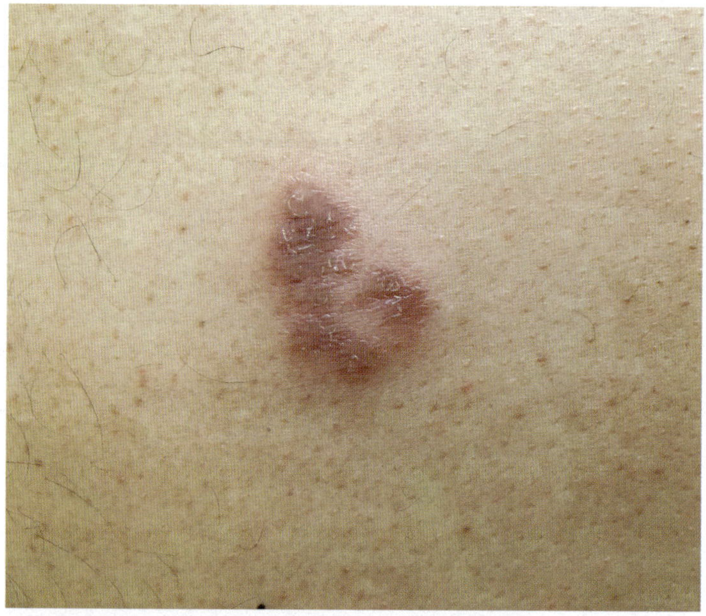

FIGURE 35-1. Violaceous plaque. This erythematous to violaceous flat scaly plaque is a common presentation of cutaneous sarcoidosis.

Lupus Pernio This is a clinical variant of plaque sarcoidosis that presents with brown to violaceous or erythematous plaques or nodules, which may have associated scale [**Figure 35-3**]. Lesions have a predilection for the nose and central face and can be quite disfiguring, even extending to involve the nasal mucosa and septum, sinuses, and upper airway. Lupus pernio is most common in Black American women and portends a more chronic, recalcitrant disease course.[50,51] In the Epidemiology of Sarcoidosis (EpiSarc) study, a hierarchical cluster analysis

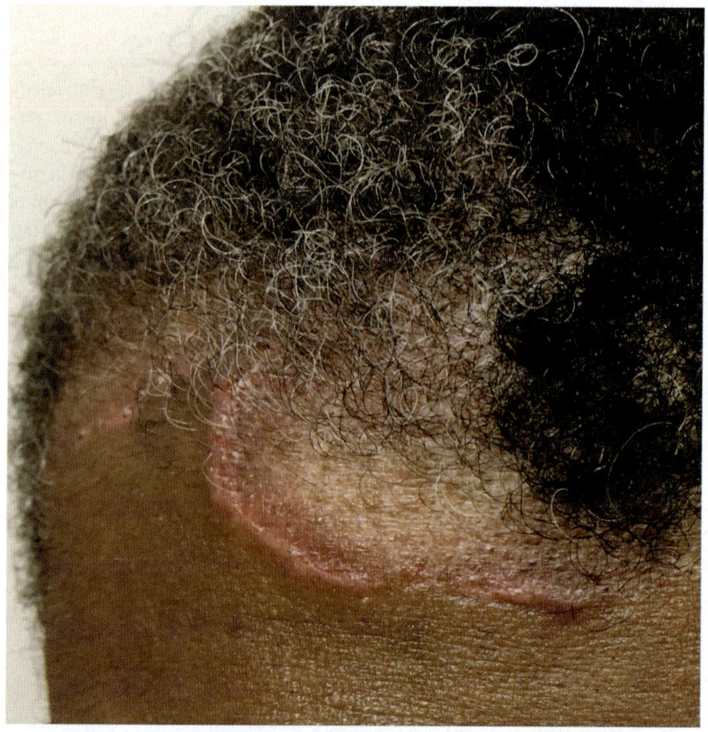

FIGURE 35-2. Annular plaque. Sarcoidosis can sometimes present with annular, or ring-like lesions, which are frequently noted in the scalp. This erythematous annular scaly plaque also has central atrophy and hypopigmentation.

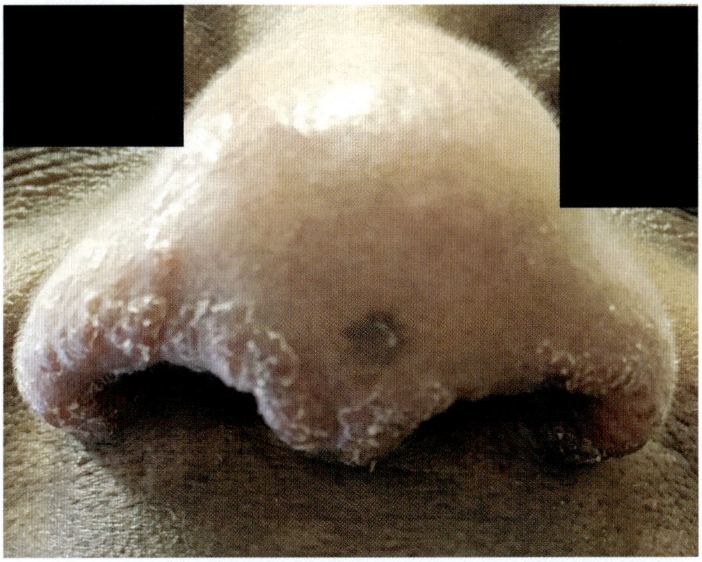

FIGURE 35-3. Lupus pernio. This form of sarcoidosis presents with scaly papules, plaques, and nodules, on the nose and central face, and portends a treatment-resistant, chronic course.

was performed on a French multicenter cohort that identified five distinct phenotypes of extrapulmonary sarcoidosis, including a cluster with lupus pernio that was strongly associated with severe phenotype, more frequent use of TNF inhibitors (41%), and patients received more treatments than with other phenotypes.[27] In the EpiSarc study, lupus pernio was also associated with high frequency of pulmonary fibrosis, ear nose and throat involvement, and bone involvement.[27]

Scar and Tattoo Sarcoidosis Sarcoidal infiltration of tattoos and old scars can cause these regions to become raised and erythematous or violaceous [**Figure 35-4**]. Scar sarcoidosis may occur in patients with acute disease and erythema nodosum, or in cases of chronic sarcoidosis. Granulomas within tattoos may represent a limited, localized hypersensitivity reaction or infection in some cases but can also be a sign of systemic sarcoidosis.[1]

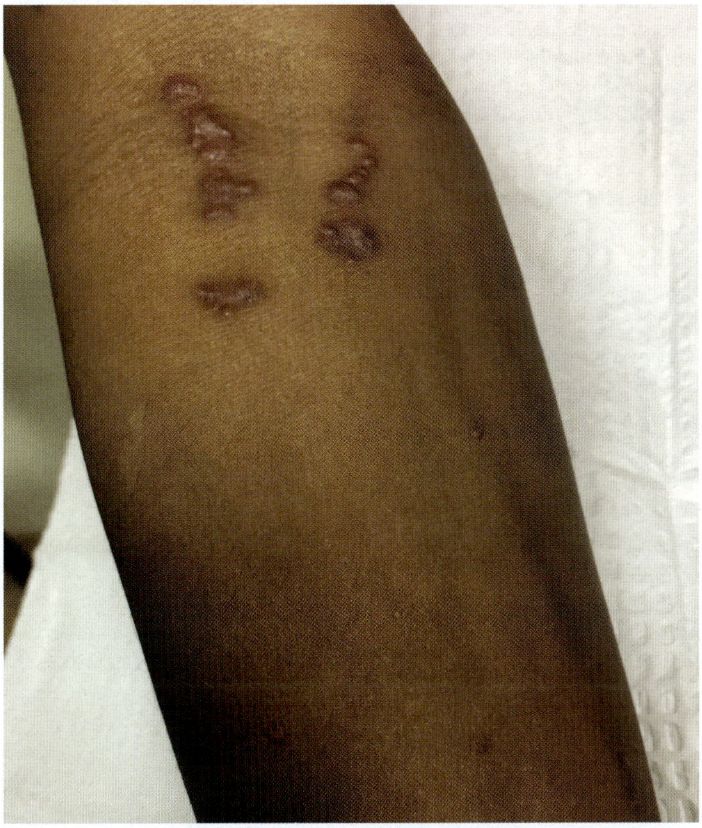

FIGURE 35-4. Scar sarcoidosis. This patient developed sarcoidosis at venipuncture sites, shown here with flesh colored to slightly erythematous papules in the antecubital fossa.

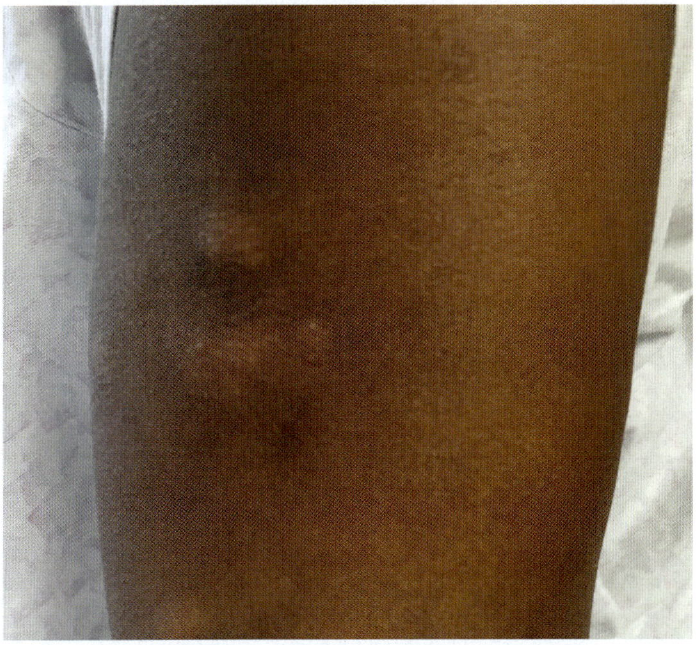

FIGURE 35-5. Hypopigmented sarcoidosis. Sarcoidosis may rarely present with lighter lesions, or hypopigmented sarcoidosis; frequently these lesions have a palpable, dermal component correlating with granulomatous inflammation seen histologically.

Other Specific Findings Less common morphologies include ichthyosiform, hypopigmented [**Figure 35-5**], ulcerative, psoriasiform, lichenoid, or verrucous lesions as well as subcutaneous nodules. Rare manifestations include erythroderma, or involvement of other sites such as mucosal, alopecic, and nail sarcoidosis.

NONSPECIFIC CUTANEOUS FINDINGS

Nonspecific findings of cutaneous sarcoidosis include erythema nodosum, calcinosis cutis, clubbing, erythema multiforme, and prurigo. Sweet syndrome has rarely been reported with sarcoidosis.[52] Other cutaneous findings may result from therapy, such as steroid-induced acne or TNF-inhibitor-induced psoriasis.

Erythema Nodosum Erythema nodosum is a reactive inflammatory panniculitis that presents as tender, red subcutaneous nodules of the anterior legs. It is the most common nonspecific manifestation of cutaneous sarcoidosis, developing in over 20% of patients.[2] Erythema nodosum is associated with fair prognosis and Löfgren syndrome.[2] It is relatively more common in people with Scandinavian ancestry and rare in Black Americans.[2]

Löfgren Syndrome Löfgren syndrome or acute sarcoidosis is the clinical tetrad of erythema nodosum, hilar adenopathy, migratory polyarthralgia, and fever with acute onset. It is associated with favorable prognosis, though patients can experience severe symptoms initially. However, it is typically a self-limiting disease with 90% of patients experiencing resolution of symptoms within 2 years.[19]

DIAGNOSIS

HISTOLOGICAL

The key to histopathologic diagnosis of sarcoidosis is the identification of noncaseating granulomas. However, clinicopathologic correlation is essential as noncaseating granulomas are not exclusive to sarcoidosis. The histologic differential for noncaseating granulomas includes tuberculoid leprosy, cutaneous Crohn disease, Melkersson-Rosenthal, granulomatous rosacea, specific immunodeficiency disorders, silica, beryllium, and zirconium granulomas.[53,54] Foreign body reactions and fungal infections can also contain noncaseating granulomas so specimens should be stained for microorganisms. Examining slides under polarized light can reveal a foreign body, though their presence does not exclude sarcoidosis.[46]

CLINICAL

Sarcoidosis is one of the great imitators and has a wide variety of clinical manifestations, frequently presenting a diagnostic challenge. The differential diagnosis for cutaneous sarcoidosis is broad. Other entities to consider include other granulomatous diseases such as granuloma annulare, necrobiosis lipoidica, and necrobiotic xanthogranuloma, as well as granulomatous secondary syphilis, granulomatous mycosis fungoides, and Blau syndrome. The diagnosis of sarcoidosis is based on a compatible clinical and radiological picture, demonstration of noncaseating granulomas with negative cultures for mycobacteria and fungus, and exclusion of other granulomatous diseases.[55]

Comprehensive evaluation is imperative when patients present with suspected sarcoidosis and in all patients with cutaneous sarcoidosis. Work-up should include thorough patient history and clinical examination, tissue biopsy, imaging, and laboratory evaluation. Basic tests to include are chest radiography, pulmonary function tests, electrocardiogram, tuberculosis assay, ophthalmologic examination, and routine laboratory tests, including calcium levels. A recent study identified a practice gap in the ordering of electrocardiograms among dermatologists who have diagnosed sarcoidosis.[56] Black patients with sarcoidosis are more likely to have cardiac sarcoidosis and extracutaneous sarcoidosis upon diagnosis of cutaneous sarcoidosis than patients in other racial groups.[57] The major organs routinely assessed are the lungs, eyes, liver, and heart; coordination with other specialists is required.

MEASURING DISEASE IMPACT

Currently, there are no adequate biomarkers of disease in sarcoidosis. Angiotensin converting enzyme, vitamin D, chitotriosidase, and adenosine deaminase have been studied without clear evidence of supporting clinical utility.[55,58] Clinical assessment tools can help monitor disease activity and track treatment response. The Cutaneous Sarcoidosis Activity and Morphology Instrument (CSAMI) and the Sarcoidosis Activity and Severity Index (SASI) have both been validated for this purpose in the clinical or research setting.[59-62] Patient-centered and health-related quality-of-life assessments provide tools for clinicians to assess global patient well-being using a standardized method, and direct therapy accordingly.[63]

MANAGEMENT

Initial therapy should be directed toward the most severely affected organ system and cutaneous disease will often improve. Skin-directed therapies should be considered if cutaneous sarcoidosis is the primary impact of disease, or if cutaneous lesions are symptomatic, distressing, or disfiguring. Cutaneous sarcoidosis is treated with both local and systemic drugs; combination therapy is often used. Therapeutic recommendations are based largely on case series data, limited prospective studies, and expert opinion, though more evidence-based therapies are emerging with recent clinical studies [**Table 35-1**].

LOCAL THERAPIES

Topical and intralesional steroids are first-line therapies for cutaneous sarcoidosis. Potent topical steroids, such as clobetasol and halobetasol, may adequately treat mild cutaneous disease and should be applied twice daily until lesions resolve.[64] Intralesional injections of triamcinolone are also effective; direct drug delivery to the dermis where granulomas form is especially useful for infiltrative lesions. Injections of 2.5 to 20 mg/mL (or higher), at 4- to 6-week intervals are effective.[64] Topical and intralesional corticosteroids may lead to skin atrophy and hypopigmentation. Hypopigmentation is more obvious in skin of color and can be distressing to patients, so excessive or prolonged use of topical steroids should be avoided, and patients be made aware of this side effects. Steroid-sparing topicals include tacrolimus and pimecrolimus applied twice daily, or topical retinoids.[65] Recent reports have highlighted potential benefits of topical JAK-inhibitors.[66,67]

SYSTEMIC IMMUNOMODULATORY THERAPIES

The antimalarial drugs hydroxychloroquine and chloroquine are first-line systemic agents used to treat generalized cutaneous disease or refractory localized disease. Use of antimalarials is supported by data from small, uncontrolled studies. A systematic review of studies leading up to 2004 demonstrated favorable response in 82% of patients treated with these drugs.[68] Time to response may be prolonged, and care must be taken with dosing and duration of therapy as ocular toxicity is a known risk. Baseline and routine eye examinations should be performed.

TABLE 35-1 Selected treatments for sarcoidosis, dosing information, and evidence supporting their use

Drug class	Typical dosing	Adverse effects and precautions	Indication
Topical corticosteroids (clobetasol, halobetasol)	Superpotent (class I) twice daily	Hypopigmentation, skin atrophy; Use less potent steroids depending on site	First line
Intralesional corticosteroids (triamcinolone)	2.5-20 mg/mL monthly	Hypopigmentation, skin atrophy	First line (thick lesions)
Antimalarials (hydroxychloroquine, chloroquine)	200-400 mg hydroxychloroquine daily 250-500 mg chloroquine daily	Ocular toxicity (less likely with hydroxychloroquine); Perform baseline and routine ophthalmic exams	First-line systemic for recalcitrant or extensive disease
Tetracycline antibiotics (minocycline, doxycycline)	100 mg twice daily	Minocycline: hyperpigmentation, Doxycycline: nausea, photosensitivity Contraindicated in pregnancy	First-line systemic for recalcitrant or extensive disease
Oral corticosteroids (prednisone)	40-80 mg daily for 4-6 weeks, followed by gradual taper	*Short term*: Gastrointestinal irritation, mood disturbances *Long term*: Osteoporosis, hypertension, acne, hyperglycemia, Cushing syndrome	Internal involvement (cutaneous disease may respond to lower doses)
Antimetabolites (methotrexate)	7.5-25 mg methotrexate weekly	Hepatic and renal toxicity; Avoid other hepatotoxic agents (including alcohol), supplement with folate and monitor bloodwork	First-line immunosuppressive
Biologics (TNF inhibitors: adalimumab, infliximab)	40 mg adalimumab weekly 5 mg/kg infliximab at weeks 0, 2, 6, then q4-6 weeks	Tuberculosis reactivation, infections, lymphoma; Higher dosing required than for typical dermatologic indications	Severe ulcerative refractory disease; lupus pernio

Tetracycline antibiotics are also used as first-line systemic treatment for cutaneous sarcoidosis.[69,70] Minocycline has demonstrated efficacy in larger studies but frequently leads to hyperpigmentation, including within lesions, and most experts start with doxycycline. Other agents supported by evidence from case series and reports include PDE4 inhibitors, isotretinoin, leflunomide, and thalidomide.[71-75]

SYSTEMIC IMMUNOSUPPRESSIVE THERAPIES

Systemic corticosteroids are often used in the management of pulmonary sarcoidosis and are also effective in treating cutaneous disease. Chronic use is associated with significant morbidity, so patients should be prescribed the lowest effective dose. Effective doses range from 40 to 80 mg/day and should be tapered slowly.

Methotrexate is a first-line immunosuppressive agent for patients who have not responded to trials of topical steroids and topical immunomodulatory treatment. Methotrexate, from 7.5 to 25 mg weekly, has been shown to benefit up to 80% of patients.[76,77] A randomized controlled trial of methotrexate in sarcoidosis demonstrated efficacy, though response time was generally at least 6 months.[78] Mycophenolate mofetil and azathioprine are alternative steroid-sparing agents that can be considered if methotrexate fails or is contraindicated, though recent European practice guidelines point out that there is limited data to suggest efficacy for these agents in cutaneous sarcoidosis.[79-81] TNF inhibitors are beneficial in the treatment of severe, refractory sarcoidosis, including lupus pernio. Lupus pernio response rates to traditional treatment is as low as 30%, whereas use of TNF inhibitors can achieve response rates close to 90%.[82] Adalimumab and infliximab are backed by the most clinical data, with efficacy reported in numerous small studies, including randomized controlled trials.[82-88] Etanercept is generally avoided as it has been more frequently associated with the development of cutaneous granulomatous disease.[89,90]

EMERGING THERAPIES

New and emerging treatments for sarcoidosis are under study. Janus kinase (JAK) inhibitors have been reported to treat cutaneous sarcoidosis as well as other granulomatous diseases.[91-96] A recent study showed that oral tofacitinib treatment is associated with improved cutaneous and systemic sarcoidosis, acting predominantly via inhibition of type 1 immunity.[97] Evolving data on the use of these agents offer excitement about the future of sarcoidosis treatment and promise for potential targeted therapies.

REFERENCES

1. James WD, Berger TG, Elston DM, eds. *Andrews' Diseases of the Skin: Clinical Dermatology*. 13th ed. Toronto, Ontario, Canada: Saunders Elsevier; 2020.
2. Yanardağ H, Pamuk ON, Karayel T. Cutaneous involvement in sarcoidosis: analysis of the features in 170 patients. *Respir Med.* 2003;97:978-982.
3. Esteves TC, Aparicio G, Ferrer B, et al. Prognostic value of skin lesions in sarcoidosis: clinical and histopathological clues. *Eur J Dermatol.* 2015;25:556-562.
4. Sharma OP. Sarcoidosis: a historical perspective. *Clin Dermatol.* 2007;25:232-241.
5. Grunewald J, Grutters JC, Arkema EV, et al. Sarcoidosis. *Nat Rev Dis Primers.* 2019;5:45.
6. Iannuzzi MC, Rybicki BA, Teirstein AS. Sarcoidosis. *N Engl J Med.* 2007;357:2153-2165.
7. Rybicki BA, Major M, Popovich J Jr, Maliarik MJ, Iannuzzi MC. Racial differences in sarcoidosis incidence: a 5-year study in a health maintenance organization. *Am J Epidemiol.* 1997;145(3):234-241.
8. Baughman RP, Field S, Costabel U, et al. Sarcoidosis in America. Analysis based on health care use. *Ann Am Thorac Soc.* 2016;13(8):1244-1252.
9. Morimoto T, Azuma A, Abe S, et al. Epidemiology of sarcoidosis in Japan. *Eur Respir J.* 2008;31:372-379.
10. Yoon HY, Kim HM, Kim YJ, et al. Prevalence and incidence of sarcoidosis in Korea: a nationwide population-based study. *Respir Res.* 2018;19:158-153.
11. Wu CH, Chung PI, Wu CY, et al. Comorbid autoimmune diseases in patients with sarcoidosis: a nationwide case-control study in Taiwan. *J Dermatol.* 2017;44:423-430.
12. Fidler LM, Balter M, Fisher JH, et al. Epidemiology and health outcomes of sarcoidosis in a universal healthcare population: a cohort study. *Eur Respir J.* 2019;54:1900444.
13. Arkema EV, Grunewald J, Kullberg S, et al. Sarcoidosis incidence and prevalence: a nationwide register-based assessment in Sweden. *Eur Respir J.* 2016;48:1690-1699.
14. Deubelbeiss U, Gemperli A, Schindler C, et al. Prevalence of sarcoidosis in Switzerland is associated with environmental factors. *Eur Respir J.* 2010;35:1088-1097.
15. Arkema EV, Cozier YC. Sarcoidosis epidemiology: recent estimates of incidence, prevalence and risk factors. *Curr Opin Pulm Med.* 2020;26:527-534.
16. Marcoval J, Mañá J, Rubio M. Specific cutaneous lesions in patients with systemic sarcoidosis. Relationship to severity and chronicity of disease. *Clin Exp Dermatol.* 2011;36:739-744.
17. Judson MA, Boan AD, Lackland DT. The clinical course of sarcoidosis: presentation, diagnosis, and treatment in a large white and black cohort in the United States. *Sarcoidosis Vasc Diffuse Lung Dis.* 2012;29:119-127.
18. Hena KM. Sarcoidosis epidemiology: race matters. *Front Immunol.* 2020;11:537382.
19. Grunewald J, Eklund A. Löfgren's syndrome: human leukocyte antigen strongly influences the disease course. *Am J Respir Crit Care Med.* 2009;179:307-312.
20. Iriarte A, Rubio-Rivas M, Villalba N, et al. Clinical features and outcomes of asymptomatic pulmonary sarcoidosis. A comparative cohort study. *Respir Med.* 2020;169:105998.
21. Rabin DL, Thompson B, Brown KM, et al. Sarcoidosis: social predictors of severity at presentation. *Eur Respir J.* 2004;24(4):601-608.
22. Baughman RP, Teirstein AS, Judson MA, et al. Clinical characteristics of patients in a case control study of sarcoidosis. *Am J Respir Crit Care Med.* 2001;164:1885-1889.
23. Kearney GD, Obi ON, Maddipati V, et al. Sarcoidosis deaths in the United States: 1999-2016. *Respir Med.* 2019;149:30-35.
24. Ogundipe F, Mehari A, Gillum R. Disparities in sarcoidosis mortality by region, urbanization, and race in the United States: a multiple cause of death analysis. *Am J Med.* 2019;132:1062-1068.
25. Coquart N, Cadelis G, Tressières B, et al. Epidemiology of sarcoidosis in Afro-Caribbean people: a 7-year retrospective study in Guadeloupe. *Int J Dermatol.* 2015;54:188-192.
26. Kaloga M, Gbéry IP, Bamba V, et al. Epidemiological, clinical, and paraclinic aspect of cutaneous sarcoidosis in Black Africans. *Dermatol Res Pract.* 2015;2015:802824.
27. Lhote R, Annesi-Maesano I, Nunes H, et al. Clinical phenotypes of extrapulmonary sarcoidosis: an analysis of a French, multi-ethnic, multicentre cohort. *Eur Respir J.* 2021;57(4):2001160.
28. Bindoli S, Dagan A, Torres-Ruiz JJ, et al. Sarcoidosis and autoimmunity: from genetic background to environmental factors. *Isr Med Assoc J.* 2016;18:197-202.
29. Eishi Y. Etiologic aspect of sarcoidosis as an allergic endogenous infection caused by Propionibacterium acnes. *Biomed Res Int.* 2013;2013:935289.
30. Oswald-Richter KA, Beachboard DC, Seeley EH, et al. Dual analysis for mycobacteria and propionibacteria in sarcoidosis BAL. *J Clin Immunol.* 2012;32:1129-1140.
31. Ianuzzi MC. Genetics of sarcoidosis. *Sem Respir Crit Care Med.* 2007;28:15-21.
32. Sverrild A, Backer V, Kyvik KO, et al. Heredity in sarcoidosis: a registry-based twin study. *Thorax.* 2008;63(10):894-896.
33. Spagnolo P, Maier LA. Genetics in sarcoidosis. *Curr Opin Pulm Med.* 2021;27:423-429.
34. Ozyilmaz E, Akilli R, Berk İ, et al. The frequency of diastolic dysfunction in patients with sarcoidosis and its relationship with HLA DRB1* alleles. *Sarcoidosis Vasc Diffuse Lung Dis.* 2019;36:285-293.
35. Rybicki BA, Maliarik MJ, Poisson LM, et al. Sarcoidosis and granuloma genes: a family-based study in African Americans. *Eur Respir J.* 2004;24:251-257.
36. Cox C, David-Allen A, Judson M. Sarcoidosis. *Med Clin North Am.* 2005;89:817-828.
37. Rybicki BA, Walewski JL, Maliarik MJ, Kian H, Iannuzzi MC, ACCESS Research Group. The BTNL2 gene and sarcoidosis susceptibility in African Americans and Whites. *Am J Hum Genet.* 2005;77:491-499.
38. Levin AM, Iannuzzi MC, Montgomery CG, et al. Association of ANXA11 genetic variation with sarcoidosis in African Americans and European Americans. *Genes Immun.* 2013;14:13-18.
39. Iannuzzi MC, Iyengar SK, Gray-McGuire C, Elston RC, Baughman RP, Donohue JF, et al. Genome-wide search for sarcoidosis susceptibility genes in African Americans. *Genes Immun.* 2005;6:509-518.
40. Gray-McGuire C, Sinha R, Iyengar S, Millard C, Rybicki BA, Elston RC, et al. Genetic characterization and fine mapping of susceptibility loci for sarcoidosis in African Americans on chromosome 5. *Hum Genet.* 2006;120:420-430.

41. Fritz D, Ferwerda B, Brouwer MC, van de Beek D. Whole genome sequencing identifies variants associated with sarcoidosis in a family with a high prevalence of sarcoidosis. *Clin Rheumatol.* 2021;40(9):3735-3743.
42. Newman LS, Rose CS, Bresnitz EA, et al. A case control etiologic study of sarcoidosis: environmental and occupational risk factors. *Am J Respir Crit Care Med.* 2004;170:1324-1330.
43. Barnard J, Rose CS, Newman L, et al. Job and industry classifications associated with sarcoidosis in A Case-Control Etiologic Study of Sarcoidosis (ACCESS). *J Occup Environ Med.* 2005;47:226-234.
44. Izbicki G, Chavko R, Banauch GI, et al. World Trade Center "sarcoid-like" granulomatous pulmonary disease in New York City Fire Department rescue workers. *Chest.* 2007;131:1414-1423.
45. Dulguerov N, Vankatova L, Landis BN. Subcutaneous sarcoidosis in a rhinoplasty scar. *BMJ Case Rep.* 2015;2015:bcr2015209337.
46. Marcoval J, Penín RM, Mañá J. Specific skin lesions of sarcoidosis located at venipuncture points for blood sample collection. *Am J Dermopathol* 2018;40:362-366.
47. Marcoval J, Mañá J, Moreno A, et al. Foreign bodies in granulomatous cutaneous lesions of patients with systemic sarcoidosis. *Arch Dermatol.* 2001;137:427-430.
48. Marcoval J, Fanlo M, Penin RM, et al. Systemic sarcoidosis with specific cutaneous lesions located at insulin injection site for diabetes mellitus. *J Eur Acad Dermatol Veneorol.* 2014;28:1259-1260.
49. Marcoval J, Mañá J, Penin RM, et al. Sarcoidosis associated with cosmetic fillers. *Clin Exp Dermatol.* 2014;39:397-399.
50. Marcoval J, Mañá J, Rubio M. Specific cutaneous lesions in patients with systemic sarcoidosis. Relationship to severity and chronicity of disease. *Clin Exp Dermatol.* 2011;36:739-744.
51. Stagaki E, Mountford WK, Lackland DT, et al. The treatment of lupus pernio: results of 116 treatment courses in 54 patients. *Chest.* 2009;135:468-476.
52. Dadban A, Hirschi S, Sanchez M, et al. Association of Sweet's syndrome and acute sarcoidosis: report of a case and review of the literature. *Clin Exp Dermatol.* 2009;34:189-191.
53. Rabinowitz LO, Zaim MT. A clinicopathologic approach to granulomatous dermatoses. *J Am Acad Dermatol.* 1996;35:588-600.
54. Karadağ AS, Parish LC. Sarcoidosis: a great imitator. *Clin Dermatol.* 2019;37:240-254.
55. Crouser ED, Maier LA, Wilson KC, et al. Diagnosis and detection of sarcoidosis. An official American Thoracic Society clinical practice guideline. *Am J Respir Crit Care Med.* 2020;201:e26-e51.
56. Villa-Ruiz C, Lo K, Desai S, Vleugels RA, Imadojemu S. Practice gaps in the evaluation of systemic involvement in patients with cutaneous sarcoidosis presenting to a dermatologist: a retrospective review of 48 patients. *J Am Acad Dermatol.* 2021;85(3):794-796.
57. Kassamali B, Villa-Ruiz C, Kus KJB, et al. Increased risk of systemic and cardiac sarcoidosis in Black patients with cutaneous sarcoidosis. *J Am Acad Dermatol.* 2022;86(5):1178-1180.
58. Bennett D, Cameli P, Lanzarone N, et al. Chitotriosidase: a biomarker of activity and severity in patients with sarcoidosis. *Respir Res.* 2020;21.
59. Rosenbach M, Yeung H, Chu EY, et al. Reliability and convergent validity of the cutaneous sarcoidosis activity and morphology instrument for assessing cutaneous sarcoidosis. *JAMA Dermatol.* 2013;149:550-556.
60. Yeung H, Farber S, Birnbaum BK, et al. Reliability and validity of cutaneous sarcoidosis outcome instruments among dermatologists, pulmonologists, and rheumatologists. *JAMA Dermatol.* 2015;151:1317-1322.
61. Berg SA, Yeung H, English JC. Inter-rater reliability of cutaneous sarcoidosis assessment tools via remote photographic assessment. *Sarcoidosis Vasc Diffuse Lung Dis.* 2017;34:165-169.
62. Noe MH, Gelfand JM, Bryer JS. Responsiveness to change and establishment of the minimal clinically important difference for the cutaneous sarcoidosis activity and morphology instrument. *JAMA Dermatol.* 2020;156:98-99.
63. Saketkoo LA, Russell AM, Jensen K, et al. Health-Related Quality of Life (HRQoL) in sarcoidosis: diagnosis, management, and health outcomes. *Diagnostics (Basel).* 2021;11:1089.
64. Wanat KA, Rosenbach M. Cutaneous Sarcoidosis. *Clin Chest Med.* 2015;36:685-702.
65. Green CM. Topical tacrolimus for the treatment of cutaneous sarcoidosis. *Clin Exp Dermatol.* 2007;32:457-458.
66. Singh K, Wang A, Heald P. Treatment of angiolupoid sarcoidosis with tofacitinib ointment 2% and pulsed dye laser therapy. *JAAD Case Rep.* 2020;1:122-124.
67. Alam M, Fang V, Rosenbach M. Treatment of cutaneous sarcoidosis with tofacitinib 2% ointment and extra virgin olive oil. *JAAD Case Rep.* 2020;9:1-3.
68. Mosam A, Morar N. Recalcitrant cutaneous sarcoidosis: an evidence-based sequential approach. *J Dermatolog Treat.* 2004;15:353-359.
69. Bachelez H, Senet P, Cadranel J, et al. The use of tetracyclines for the treatment of sarcoidosis. *Arch Dermatol.* 2001;137:69-73.
70. 116. Steen T, English JC. Oral minocycline in treatment of cutaneous sarcoidosis. *JAMA Dermatol.* 2013;149:758-760.
71. Zabel P, Entzian P, Dalhoff K, et al. Pentoxifylline in treatment of sarcoidosis. *Am J Respir Crit Care Med.* 1997;155:1665-1669.
72. Baughman RP, Judson MA, Ingledue R, et al. Efficacy and safety of apremilast in chronic cutaneous sarcoidosis. *Arch Dermatol.* 2012;148:262-264.
73. Waldinger TP, Ellis CN, Quint K, et al. Treatment of cutaneous sarcoidosis with isotretinoin. *Arch Dermatol.* 1983;119:1003-1005.
74. Baughman RP, Lower EE. Leflunomide for chronic sarcoidosis. *Sarcoidosis Vasc Diffuse Lung Dis.* 2004;21:43-48.
75. Nguyen YT, Dupuy A, Cordoliani F, et al. Treatment of cutaneous sarcoidosis with thalidomide. *J Am Acad Dermatol.* 2004;50:235-241.
76. Lower EE, Baughman RP. The use of low dose methotrexate in refractory sarcoidosis. *Am J Med Sci.* 1990;299:153-157.
77. Lower EE, Baughman RP. Prolonged use of methotrexate for sarcoidosis. *Arch Intern Med.* 1995;155:846-851.
78. Baughman RP, Winget DB, Lower EE. Methotrexate is steroid sparing in acute sarcoidosis: results of a double blind, randomized trial. *Sarcoidosis Vasc Diffuse Lung Dis.* 2000;17:60-66.
79. Papiris S, Stagaki E, Papadaki G, et al. Mycophenolate mofetil as an alternative treatment in sarcoidosis. *Pulm Pharmacol Ther.* 2019;58:101840.
80. Hamzeh N, Voelker A, Forssén A, et al. Efficacy of mycophenolate mofetil in sarcoidosis. *Respir Med.* 2014;108:1663-1669.
81. Baughman RP, Valeyre D, Korsten P, et al. ERS clinical practice guidelines on treatment of sarcoidosis. *Eur Respir J.* 2021;58(6):2004079.
82. Stagaki E, Mountford WK, Lackland DT, et al. The treatment of lupus pernio: results of 116 treatment courses in 54 patients. *Chest.* 2009;135:468-476.
83. Tu J, Chan J. Cutaneous sarcoidosis and infliximab: evidence for efficacy in refractory disease. *Australas J Dermatol.* 2014;55:279-281.
84. Tuchinda P, Bremmer M, Gaspari AA. A case series of refractory cutaneous sarcoidosis successfully treated with infliximab. *Dermatol Ther (Heidelb).* 2012;2:11-19.
85. Wanat KA, Rosenbach M. Case series demonstrating improvement in chronic cutaneous sarcoidosis following treatment with TNF inhibitors. *Arch Dermatol.* 2012;148:1097-1100.
86. Judson MA. Successful treatment of lupus pernio with adalimumab. *Arch Dermatol.* 2011;147:1332-1333.
87. Pariser RJ, Paul J, Hirano S, et al. A double-blind, randomized, placebo-controlled trial of adalimumab in the treatment of cutaneous sarcoidosis. *J Am Acad Dermatol.* 2013;68:765-773.
88. Baughman RP, Judson MA, Lower EE, et al. Infliximab for chronic cutaneous sarcoidosis: a subset analysis from a double-blind randomized clinical trial. *Sarcoidosis Vasc Diffuse Lung Dis.* 2016;32:289-295.
89. Ishiguro T, Takayanagi N, Kurashima K, et al. Development of sarcoidosis during etanercept therapy. *Intern Med.* 2008;47:1021-1025.
90. González-López MA, Blanco R, González-Vela MC, et al. Development of sarcoidosis during etanercept therapy. *Arthritis Rheum.* 2006;55:817-820.
91. Wei JJ, Kallenbach LR, Kreider M, et al. Resolution of cutaneous sarcoidosis after Janus kinase inhibitor therapy for concomitant polycythemia vera. *JAAD Case Rep.* 2019;5:360-361.
92. Damsky W, Young BD, Sloan B, et al. Treatment of multiorgan sarcoidosis with tofacitinib. *ACR Open Rheumatol.* 2020;2:106-109.
93. Damsky W, Thakral D, Emeagwali N, et al. Tofacitinib treatment and molecular analysis of cutaneous sarcoidosis. *N Engl J Med.* 2018;379:2540-2546.
94. Alam M, Fang V, Rosenbach M. Treatment of cutaneous sarcoidosis with tofacitinib 2% ointment and extra virgin olive oil. *JAAD Case Rep.* 2020;9:1-3.
95. Damsky W, King BA. Treatment of granuloma annulare with tofacitinib 2% ointment. *JAAD Case Rep.* 2019;6:69-71.
96. Damsky W, Singh K, Galan A, et al. Treatment of necrobiosis lipoidica with combination Janus kinase inhibition and intralesional corticosteroid. *JAAD Case Rep.* 2020;6:133-135.
97. Damsky W, Wang A, Kim DJ, et al. Inhibition of type 1 immunity with tofacitinib is associated with marked improvement in longstanding sarcoidosis. *Nat Commun.* 2022;13(1):3140.

CHAPTER 36

Prurigo Nodularis

Viviane Liao
Shawn G. Kwatra

KEY POINTS

- Prurigo nodularis (PN) is an intensely pruritic, chronic inflammatory skin disease that disproportionately affects African Americans.
- The pathogenesis of PN involves both neural and immune dysregulation.
- PN presents as firm, itchy nodules that are often times distributed on the extensor surfaces of the limbs and trunk.
- PN in African American patients frequently presents with firmer and larger nodules that have greater hyperpigmentation compared to those in light-skinned individuals.
- PN often requires systemic treatment with immuno- and neuromodulatory therapies.

INTRODUCTION

PN is a chronic inflammatory skin condition characterized by intensely itchy nodules spread over the extensor surfaces of the limbs and the trunk, always in sites reachable to patients. PN can affect any race or sex, although it is more prevalent in African American patients and primarily occurs in the later decades of life. The itch associated with PN can be extremely debilitating, and breaking the itch-scratch cycle of PN is a key to therapeutic success.[1] Multiple novel therapeutics are in late stage development for PN.

EPIDEMIOLOGY

PN was first described by Hyde and Montgomery in 1909, characterized by nodules spread primarily over the extensor surfaces and intolerable pruritus.[2] The prevalence rate is between 22 and 72 per 100,000 persons.[3,4] PN is slightly more common in females than males and primarily affects patients in their fifth and sixth decades of life, with a median age of 54 years.[3] African American patients were 3.4 times more likely to have PN than White patients in a cross-sectional study of 909 PN patients and were 2.37 times more likely than White patients to be diagnosed with PN in a large study of patients evaluated for itch in the United States.[5,6] African American PN patients also had increased odds of hospitalization as compared to White PN patients, often for cellulitis or sepsis.[7] Another study shows African American PN patients have the highest all-cause mortality compared to PN patients in other racial subcategories, possibly due to exacerbation of racial disparities in social determinants of health, or increased systemic inflammation.[8]

Patients with PN have a significantly higher comorbidity burden than healthy controls.[4] PN is frequently associated with other dermatologic diseases, such as atopic dermatitis, which may be associated with an atopic disposition in those affected [**Figure 36-1**].[5] PN has also been associated with systemic comorbidities including infections, metabolic dysfunction, malignancies, mental health disorders, and others. There is high infectious disease comorbidity burden associated with PN, including hepatitis C, HIV, hepatobiliary, and CNS infections.[5,9] HIV is a common reason for hospital admission among PN patients, and PN patients with concomitant HIV are more likely to be Black than White.[7] Patients with PN also have increased odds of type 1 and 2 diabetes mellitus, hypertension, hyperlipidemia, and obesity, although it is unclear whether metabolic dysregulation contributes to the development of PN or is a result of the systemic inflammation associated with PN.[2,3,5] Associated malignancies include primarily skin and hematologic malignancies, such as basal cell carcinoma, squamous cell carcinoma, and non-Hodgkin lymphoma.[10] PN is also associated with increased rates of anxiety and depression, eating disorders, substance use disorders, self-harm, attention-deficit/hyperactivity disorders, and schizophrenia. Other systemic conditions associated with PN include chronic kidney disease, anemia, chronic obstructive pulmonary disease, coronary heart disease, and cerebrovascular disease.[2,3] In a cross-sectional study, PN patients have also been clustered by distinct patterns of comorbidities, suggesting the existence of PN endotypes characterized by atopic comorbidities, neuropsychiatric comorbidities, overall high comorbidity burden, or chronic and cardiopulmonary comorbidities.[11]

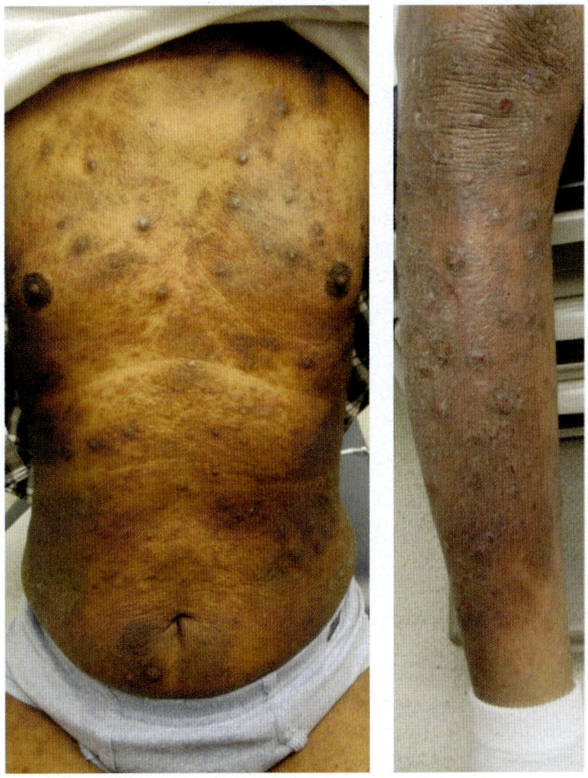

A B

FIGURE 36-1. Prurigo nodularis in the setting of atopic dermatitis.

PATHOGENESIS

While the exact pathogenesis of PN is still not entirely clear, it is understood that PN is associated with both neural and immune dysregulation that contribute to the intractable itch and inflammation characteristic of the condition. While aspects of the pathophysiology of PN are similar to other inflammatory dermatoses, such as atopic dermatitis, cutaneous transcriptomics show that PN features unique fibroproliferative and neurovascular dysregulation.[12]

IMMUNE DYSREGULATION

PN patients show Th2, Th17, and Th22 immune polarization, with elevated levels of associated inflammatory cytokines in the lesional epidermis and the plasma.[13,14] Released by Th2 cells, IL-4, IL-13, and IL-31 are able to both directly activate small-diameter sensory neurons in the skin that signal itch and signal through the JAK-STAT pathway to increase production of pro-inflammatory cytokines and activate eosinophils, mast cells, and fibroblasts.[13] Activated fibroblasts not only contribute to dermal fibrosis but also release periostin, which is elevated in PN, stimulates itch-sensing nerve fibers, and further drives release of inflammatory cytokines.[16] The Th17 and Th22 axes also play important roles in PN, as PN lesions show upregulated expression of Th17 and Th22-related markers.[14] IL-17 induces endothelin-1, a histamine-independent pruritogen, and IL-22 drives epidermal differentiation, cutaneous inflammation, and keratinocyte proliferation that are consistent with histologic findings in PN.[13,14] In addition to these immune axes, vascular endothelial growth factor (VEGF) activity is also shown to be elevated in PN lesions and corresponds to itch severity, contributing to further inflammation at lesional sites.[12]

NEURAL DYSREGULATION

PN is not only driven by immune dysregulation but also neural dysregulation. The dermis of PN patients shows neuronal hyperplasia, while the epidermis shows low nerve fiber density. Repeated scratching and neurotrophins released from mast cells and eosinophils, specifically nerve growth factor (NGF), likely result in neuronal hyperplasia in the dermis. On the other hand, low intraepidermal nerve fiber density may reflect small fiber sensory neuropathy.[17] Cutaneous nerve fibers activated by pruritogens not only signal itch to the brain but also release substance P (SP) and calcitonin gene-related peptide (CGRP), neuropeptides that induce inflammation, vasodilation, and activation of eosinophils and mast cells. Both SP and CGRP have been shown to be upregulated in the dermis of PN lesions, suggesting they are important players in the development of itch and nodules.[13] Activation of mu opioid receptors (MORs) and inhibition of kappa opioid receptors (KORs) on nerve fibers may also contribute to pruritus in PN.[17]

DISEASE ENDOTYPES

The pathogenesis of PN, however, is not homogenous among patients and there are likely different endotypes of PN with differing clinical manifestations. A recent study has pointed to the existence of an inflammatory endotype with high systemic inflammation that is predominantly composed of African American patients and is characterized clinically by more severe itch and lower quality of life. This racial disparity in disease severity may be attributed to differences in socioeconomic status, healthcare access, environmental factors, structural racism, implicit bias, and genetics.[15] On the other hand, patients in that study with levels of inflammatory biomarkers more similar to those of healthy controls had higher rates of myelopathy, suggesting more neural rather than immune dysregulation in that subset.[16] A separate study analyzing the renin-angiotensin-aldosterone system (RAAS) in PN patients also showed African American PN patients had higher levels of RAAS dysregulation and more renal comorbidities, suggesting RAAS abnormalities may be important specifically to this subgroup of PN patients.[17] Analysis of circulating type 2 inflammatory biomarkers also show an atopic subgroup with elevated markers of type 2 inflammation, including IL-13 and periostin.[18] Taken together with the clustering of PN patients by comorbidities, there is a growing body of evidence for the existence of various endotypes of PN that will be clinically useful in targeting treatment for patients.

CLINICAL FEATURES

PN typically presents with firm, nodular lesions symmetrically distributed and grouped on the extensor surfaces of the extremities and trunk [**Figure 36-2**]. The middle upper back is often spared, which is termed the "butterfly" sign [**Figure 36-3**]. Nodules can range from a few millimeters up to 2 cm in diameter and can be flesh-colored, pink, brown, or black [**Figure 36-4**].[2,19] African American patients with PN may have firmer, larger, and darker nodules that are more recalcitrant to treatment [**Table 36-1**].[20] Repeated mechanical scratching or manipulations of the skin due to itch also often leads to thickening, excoriation, and crusting of the nodules, which often leave scars as they heal.[2] Patients can have a few to hundreds of nodules and may also experience burning or stinging pain along with itch at the sites of the nodules and in the intervening skin.[21] Ultimately, the itch, pain, appearance, and stress associated with PN lead to profound negative impacts on quality of life, affecting sleep, mood, and work. In fact, the discomfort associated with PN corresponds to "severe disability" based on the average Ontario Health Utilities Index Mark 3 (HUI3) score in a study of PN patients at a tertiary care center.[22]

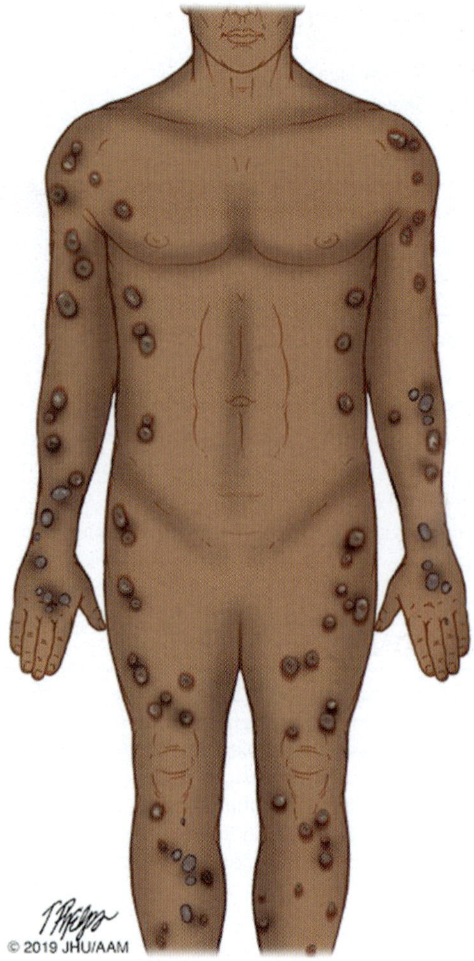

FIGURE 36-2. Typical bilateral distribution of nodules on the extensor limbs and trunk. (Illustration: Tim Phelps © 2019 JHU AAM Department of Art as Applied to Medicine The Johns Hopkins University School of Medicine.)

HISTOLOGY

PN is characterized by a constellation of histological features in the lesional skin. In the epidermis, there is often orthohyperkeratosis, focal parakeratosis, hypergranulosis, and acanthosis. The papillary dermis shows fibrosis with unique vertical streaking of collagen bundles, and increased numbers of fibroblasts and capillaries. The reticular dermis is often fibrotic as well. A perivascular/interstitial inflammatory infiltrate is also present in the dermis, comprising mainly lymphocytes and macrophages but also including neutrophils and eosinophils [**Figure 36-5**].[23]

DIAGNOSIS

PN is a clinical diagnosis, featuring intense pruritus for more than 6 weeks that can be accompanied by burning or stinging. Physical examination will show at least 10 clustered nodules on more than two different extensor surfaces and possibly the trunk, ranging from 0.5 to 2.0 cm.[13] Other conditions to consider may include insect bites, scabies surrepticius, lupus erythematosus, multiple keratoacanthomas, psoriasis, and atopic dermatitis. More rare conditions to consider include pemphigoid nodularis, epidermolysis bullosa, actinic prurigo, hypertrophic lichen planus, and excoriation disorder. As PN often has an associated systemic etiology, including other dermatologic, infectious, neurologic, psychiatric, and metabolic conditions, a thorough laboratory workup is recommended. PN patients should get a complete blood count (CBC) with differential and complete metabolic panel (CMP) with additional tests based on patient risk factors. Additional tests include hemoglobin A1c

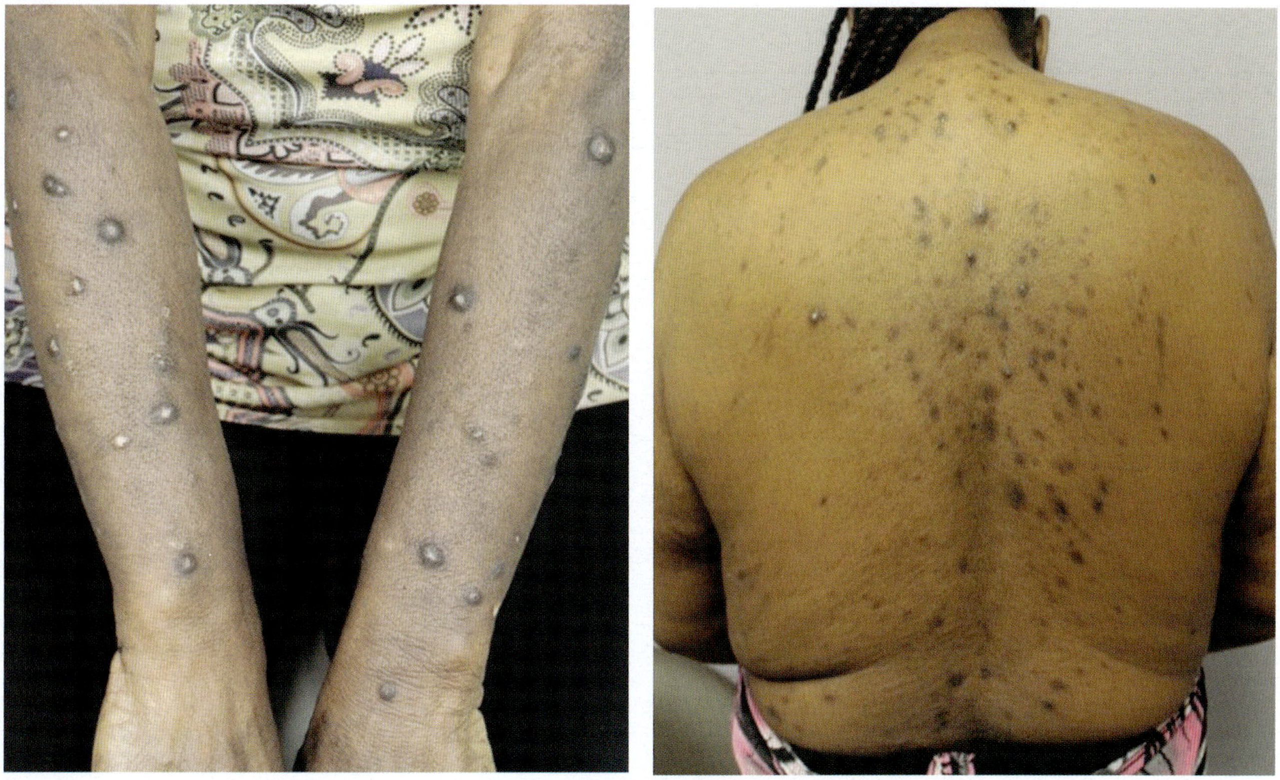

A B

FIGURE 36-3. **(A)** Bilateral distribution of nodules on the extensor forearms. **(B)** Butterfly sign, showing sparing of the upper middle back.

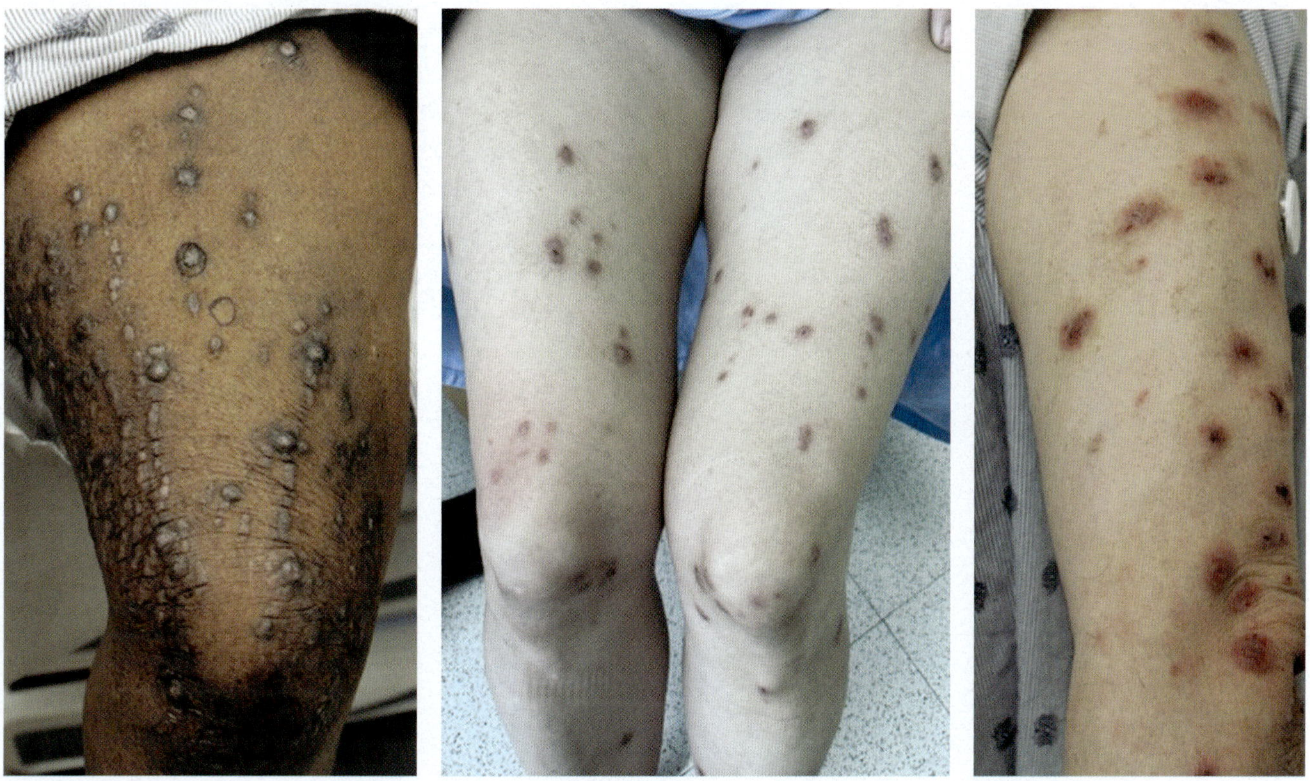

A B C

FIGURE 36-4. Nodules on an **(A)** African American female, **(B)** Hispanic female, and **(C)** Asian male.

TABLE 36-1 Clinical features of PN

Clinical feature	Differences in skin of color
Pruritus lasting greater than 6 weeks	African American patients may experience more severe itch[16]
Nodules spread over at least 2 extensor surfaces and possibly the trunk	Firmer, darker nodules in African American patients
Picking and scratching at nodules	Often times significant hyper- and hypopigmentation of nodules
Pathophysiology based in immune and neural dysregulation	African American patients have greater increased blood systemic inflammation, including elevated C-reactive protein levels and blood eosinophils

(HbA1c), HIV antibody test, hepatitis serologies, and liver, kidney, and thyroid function tests. Skin biopsy with hematoxylin and eosin staining and other tests, including intraepidermal nerve fiber density, imaging studies, stool studies for ova and parasites, iron studies, serum/urine protein electrophoresis, and mood screening may also be useful in further distinguishing PN from other skin conditions and uncovering any systemic etiologies of the condition.[19]

TREATMENT

Current treatment options for PN have variable efficacy and there is currently only one therapy, dupilumab, that is approved by the Food and Drug Administration (FDA) for PN. Dupilumab is a monoclonal antibody that targets the IL-4 receptor through which IL-4 and IL-13 signal through. In phase 3 clinical trials for patients with moderate to severe PN, a clinically significant reduction in itch was elicited in 60% of patients treated with dupilumab as compared to 18% of patients treated with placebo.[24] Some patients, however, are not responsive to dupilumab and continued development of new therapeutics remains critical. Treatment generally targets the neural and immunologic components of PN, but should be individualized based on patient age, comorbidities, disease severity, and tolerance of side effects. Locally acting topical or intralesional agents and phototherapy are commonly used with variable success, but systemic immunomodulating or neuromodulating agents are often required [**Figure 36-6**, **Table 36-2**].[13]

LOCAL TREATMENTS

Although topical treatments are easy to use and generally have lower potential for serious adverse events, they have variable efficacy in treating PN. High-potency topical corticosteroids are most commonly used and block inflammation through immunosuppression. Side effects are mainly limited to skin irritation, but skin atrophy may occur with prolonged use. For increased absorption at specific nodules, occlusive dressings may be used in conjunction with topical corticosteroids. Unna boot is a cost-effective nonmedicated compressive dressing, and flurandrenolide tape is an occlusive tape with topical corticosteroid that may be used. Intralesional corticosteroid injections, usually triamcinolone acetonide, may be used with or without adjunctive cryotherapy for even greater efficacy. Cryotherapy for PN has only been assessed in a few case reports, but it was effective in these reports in reducing pruritus and flattening lesions. Topical calcineurin inhibitors (TCIs), such as pimecrolimus and tacrolimus, are also commonly used and allow for long-term use of a topical immunomodulatory agent without the side effects of topical steroids. They act as immunosuppressants by blocking

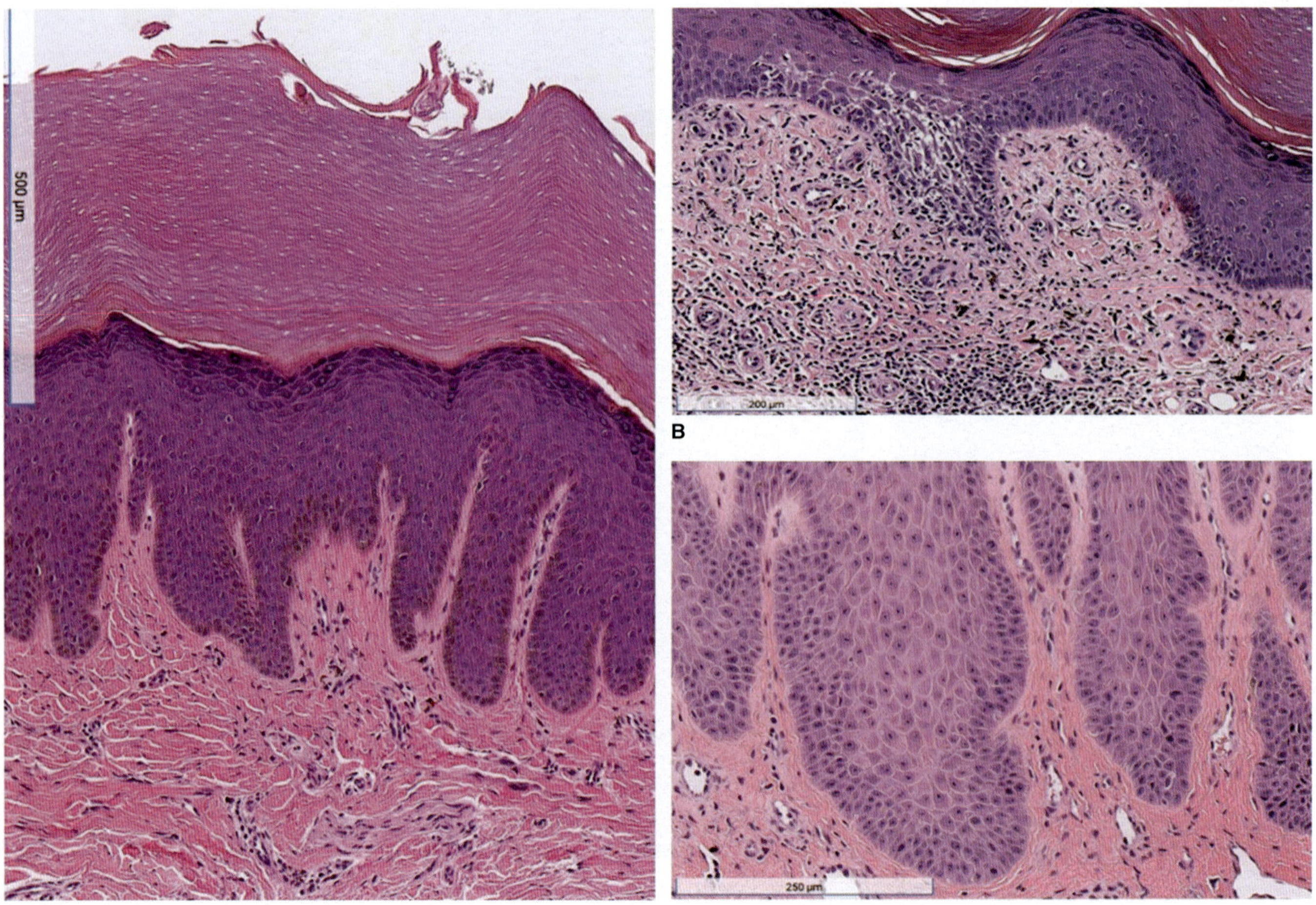

A B C

FIGURE 36-5. Histological findings characteristic of prurigo nodularis. (A) Elongated rete ridges, orthohyperkeratosis, and hypergranulosis (B) dermal lymphocytic infiltrate (C) magnified view showing epidermal acanthosis and vertical streaking of collagen in the papillary dermis.

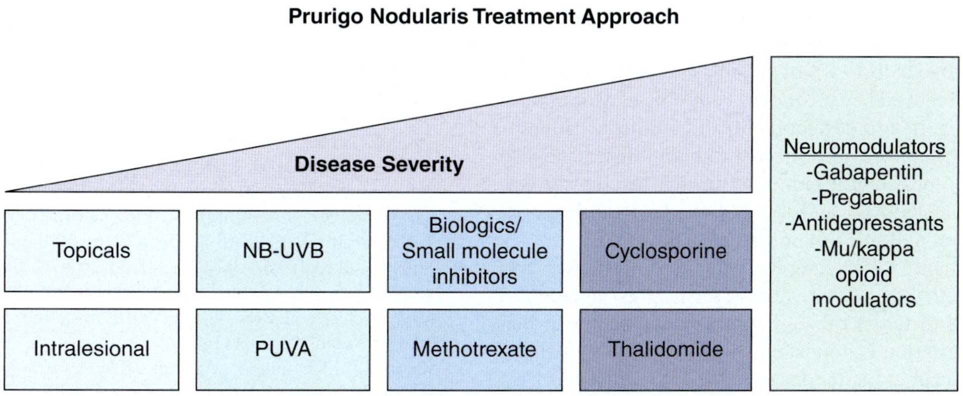

FIGURE 36-6. Prurigo nodularis treatment ladder. *Neuromodulators are unlikely to resolve immune dysregulation but may adjunctively help to reduce itch.

cytokine release and desensitizing the transient receptor potential cation channel subfamily V member 1 (TRPV1) on itch-sensing nerve fibers. Pimecrolimus cream 1% has shown efficacy matching that of hydrocortisone in a randomized controlled trial with 30 patients. Topical calcipotriol, a synthetic form of vitamin D, is also known to reduce levels of inflammatory cytokines and was shown to be more effective than betamethasone valerate in treating prurigo in an intraindividual randomized controlled trial of 10 patients. Less commonly used are local agents that target the neural component of PN, including topical capsaicin and topical anesthetics, such as ketamine, amitriptyline, and lidocaine. Although antihistamines are often used to treat itch, no strong evidence has shown they are effective in treating PN, suggesting histamine is not a major driver of itch in PN.[13,25]

TABLE 36-2 Summary of treatments for PN

Local treatments	Dosing
Corticosteroids	
Betamethasone valerate	0.05% cream or ointment BID
Intralesional triamcinolone acetonide	5-20 mg/mL; 0.05-0.1 mL per lesion
Calcineurin Inhibitors	
Pimecrolimus	1% cream BID
Tacrolimus	0.1% ointment BID
Phototherapy	
Psoralen and UVA (PUVA)	2-3× per week
Narrow-band UVB (NB-UVB)	2-3× per week
Systemic treatments	
Immunomodulatory:	
Methotrexate	15-25 mg PO weekly
Cyclosporine	2.5-5 mg/kg PO daily
Azathioprine	50-200 mg PO daily
Dupilumab	600 mg SC initial dose, then 300 mg SC every other week
Nemolizumab*	0.5 mg/kg SC every 4 weeks
Tofacitinib	5 mg PO BID
Baricitinib	4 mg/day PO
Neuromodulatory:	
Gabapentinoids	
Gabapentin	100-3600 mg/day PO
Pregabalin	75-600 mg/day PO
Antidepressants	
Paroxetine	10-40 mg/day PO
Duloxetine	20-60 mg/day PO
Amitriptyline	10-60 mg/day PO
NK1R Antagonists	
Aprepitant	80 mg/day PO
Thalidomide	50-150 mg/day PO

BID, 2 times daily; PO, per oral; SC, subcutaneous.

*Not FDA approved at time of writing, although successful in late phase 3 trials.

PHOTOTHERAPY

As UV radiation is known to reduce inflammation and has an antipruritic effect, it is frequently used concomitantly with localized topical treatments. Both psoralen plus ultraviolet A (PUVA) and narrowband ultraviolet B (NB-UVB) have been effective in treating PN lesions and itch across many studies, with most studies showing either complete or partial remission in all patients treated with phototherapy. A randomized prospective trial of 22 patients showed that combination therapy using both full-body bath PUVA and targeted 308 nm excimer UVB together is even more effective than PUVA alone in treating PN, requiring 30% less PUVA radiation to achieve remission. Currently, NB-UVB is the more commonly used modality; treatment is given two to three times weekly and generally well-tolerated, with the main side effects being erythema, xerosis, and hyperpigmentation.[25,26]

SYSTEMIC TREATMENTS

As many patients with PN are refractory to localized therapies and phototherapy, systemic therapies are often required. To address immune dysregulation, oral immunosuppressive agents such as cyclosporine, methotrexate, and azathioprine have shown efficacy in treating refractory PN. Cyclosporine, a calcineurin inhibitor, has shown success in treating PN in a few small studies but does require monitoring of blood pressure, renal function, hepatic function, and blood counts as it may have significant side effects. Methotrexate is a purine synthesis inhibitor that is used in low doses for treatment of PN, showing significant improvement in pruritus in 89% of patients after 3 months of treatment in a retrospective study of 39 PN patients. Like cyclosporine, however, it also has significant side effects including nausea, fatigue, anemia, and transaminitis.[13,25] Azathioprine, a purine analog that blocks purine synthesis to target B and T cell proliferation, has also been efficacious in treating chronic pruritus. A case study showed success in treating severe PN in two patients, although recurrence of PN appeared after treatment termination. Adverse events also are common and include transaminitis, gastrointestinal upset, azathioprine hypersensitivity, myelosuppression, and infection.[25]

Monoclonal antibodies represent a promising avenue for targeted treatment, with dupilumab and nemolizumab being the only FDA-approved therapies for PN. Dupilumab targets IL-4 receptor alpha while nemolizumab targets the IL-31 receptor involved in type 2 inflammation. In addition to modulation inflammatory signaling, it also regulates neural development and epithelial differentiation in PN patients, as demonstrated by plasma proteomic analysis of PN patients successfully treated with nemolizumab.[27] In a phase 2 clinical trial with treatment administration at weeks 0, 4, and 8, the primary endpoint of percent change from baseline in peak pruritus score on the numeric rating scale (PP-NRS) at week 4 was −53% in the nemolizumab group as compared to −20.2% in the placebo group. Even 10 weeks after the last dose, patients treated with nemolizumab maintained a 57.9% reduction in PP-NRS from baseline.[28] In a phase 3 trial, nemolizumab patients achieved an itch-free state, defined by PP-NRS less than 2, in 19.7% of patients as compared to 2.2% of placebos at week 4 and met all key secondary endpoints.[29] Modulation of inflammatory signaling, neural development, and epithelial differentiation of two oral JAK inhibitors, tofacitinib and baricitinib, have also been reported to induce meaningful reduction in itch in case studies. Tofacitinib specifically blocks JAK1 and JAK3, while baricitinib blocks JAK1 and JAK2, inhibiting multiple inflammatory pathways.[30]

Other systemic treatments target neural, rather than immune, dysregulation associated with PN. Gabapentinoids, such as gabapentin and pregabalin, are used to target calcium signaling important in itch transmission, although titration is important as sedation is a significant adverse event that may occur at higher dosages that are required to treat pruritus. Antidepressants, including tricyclic and tetracyclic antidepressants, selective serotonin re-uptake inhibitors (SSRIs), and selective norepinephrine reuptake inhibitors (SNRIs), have also been used across small studies to treat the neuropathic aspect of PN. The mechanism of action for antidepressants in treating pruritus, however, has yet to be elucidated and their many side effects should be considered before use. The neurokinin-1 receptor (NK1R) antagonist aprepitant has also been used to treat PN due to its ability to block signaling via the neuropeptide SP, which has been strongly implicated in the pathogenesis of PN. It showed promise in early studies, but ultimately was unable to elicit greater reduction in pruritus than placebo in randomized controlled trials. Finally, thalidomide has been used to effectively treat PN in small studies, eliciting complete improvement in 54% of patients and slight improvement in 31% of patients in a retrospective study of 13 patients. Its significant adverse effects including peripheral neuropathy and teratogenicity, however, should be strongly considered before use.[13,25]

REFERENCES

1. Kwatra SG. Breaking the Itch-Scratch Cycle in Prurigo Nodularis. *N Engl J Med.* 2020;382(8):757-758. doi: 10.1056/NEJMe1916733.
2. Huang AH, Williams KA, Kwatra SG. Prurigo nodularis: epidemiology and clinical features. *J Am Acad Dermatol.* 2020;83(6):1559-1565.
3. Huang AH, Canner JK, Khanna R, Kang S, Kwatra SG. Real-world prevalence of prurigo nodularis and burden of associated diseases. *J Invest Dermatol.* 2020;140(2):480-483.e4.
4. Wongvibulsin S, Sutaria N, Williams KA, et al. A nationwide study of prurigo nodularis: disease burden and healthcare utilization in the United States. *J Invest Dermatol.* 2021;141(10):2530-2533.e1.
5. Boozalis E, Tang O, Patel S, et al. Ethnic differences and comorbidities of 909 prurigo nodularis patients. *J Am Acad Dermatol.* 2018;79(4):714-719.e3.
6. Whang KA, Khanna R, Thomas J, Aguh C, Kwatra SG. Racial and gender differences in the presentation of pruritus. *Medicines.* 2019;6(4):98.
7. Whang KA, Kang S, Kwatra SG. Inpatient burden of prurigo nodularis in the United States. *Medicines.* 2019;6(3):88.
8. Sutaria N, Adawi W, Brown I, et al. Racial disparities in mortality among patients with prurigo nodularis: a multi-center cohort study. *J Am Acad Dermatol.* 2022;86(2):487-490.
9. Sutaria N, Choi J, Roh YS, et al. Association of prurigo nodularis and infectious disease hospitalizations: a national cross-sectional study. *Clin Exp Dermatol.* 2021;46(7):1236-1242.
10. Larson VA, Tang O, Stander S, Miller LS, Kang S, Kwatra SG. Association between prurigo nodularis and malignancy in middle-aged adults. *J Am Acad Dermatol.* 2019;81(5):1198-1201.
11. Wongvibulsin S, Parthasarathy V, Pahalyants V, et al. Latent class analysis identification of prurigo nodularis comorbidity phenotypes. *Br J Dermatol.* 2022;186(5):903-905.
12. Sutaria N, Alphonse MP, Roh YS, et al. Cutaneous transcriptomics identifies fibroproliferative and neurovascular gene dysregulation in prurigo nodularis compared with psoriasis and atopic dermatitis. *J Invest Dermatol.* 2022;142(9):2537-2540.
13. Williams KA, Huang AH, Belzberg M, Kwatra SG. Prurigo nodularis: pathogenesis and management. *J Am Acad Dermatol.* 2020;83(6):1567-1575.
14. Belzberg M, Alphonse MP, Brown I, et al. Prurigo nodularis is characterized by systemic and cutaneous T helper 22 immune polarization. *J Invest Dermatol.* 2021;141(9):2208-2218.e14.
15. Sutaria N, Semenov YR, Kwatra SG. Understanding racial disparities in prurigo nodularis. *J Am Acad Dermatol.* 2022;87(3):e111-e112.
16. Sutaria N, Alphonse MP, Marani M, et al. Cluster analysis of circulating plasma biomarkers in prurigo nodularis reveals a distinct systemic inflammatory signature in African Americans. *J Invest Dermatol.* 2022;142(5):1300-1308.e3.
17. Sutaria N, Marani M, Choi J, et al. Racial differences in dysregulation of the renin-angiotensin-aldosterone system in patients with prurigo nodularis. *J Dermatol Sci.* 2022;105(2):130-136.
18. Parthasarathy V, Cravero K, Deng J, Sun Z, Engle SM, Auxier AN, Hahn N, Sims JT, Okragly AJ, Alphonse MP, Kwatra SG. Circulating plasma IL-13 and periostin are dysregulated type 2 inflammatory biomarkers in prurigo nodularis: A cluster analysis. Front Med (Lausanne). 2022 Dec 6;9:1011142. doi: 10.3389/fmed.2022.1011142.
19. Kwon CD, Khanna R, Williams KA, Kwatra MM, Kwatra SG. Diagnostic workup and evaluation of patients with prurigo nodularis. *Medicines.* 2019;6(4):97.
20. McColl M, Boozalis E, Aguh C, Eseonu AC, Okoye GA, Kwatra SG. Pruritus in black skin: unique molecular characteristics and clinical features. *J Natl Med Assoc.* 2021;113(1):30-38.
21. Aggarwal P, Choi J, Sutaria N, et al. Clinical characteristics and disease burden in prurigo nodularis. *Clin Exp Dermatol.* 2021;46(7):1277-1284.
22. Whang KA, Le TK, Khanna R, et al. Health-related quality of life and economic burden of prurigo nodularis. *J Am Acad Dermatol.* 2022;86(3):573-580.
23. Weigelt N, Metze D, Ständer S. Prurigo nodularis: systematic analysis of 58 histological criteria in 136 patients. *J Cutan Pathol.* 2010;37(5):578-586.
24. Yosipovitch G, Mollanazar N, Ständer S, et al. Dupilumab in patients with prurigo nodularis: two randomized, double-blind, placebo-controlled phase 3 trials. *Nat Med.* 2023;29(5):1180-1190.
25. Elmariah S, Kim B, Berger T, et al. Practical approaches for diagnosis and management of prurigo nodularis: United States expert panel consensus. *J Am Acad Dermatol.* 2021;84(3):747-760.
26. Nakamura M, Koo JY. Phototherapy for the treatment of prurigo nodularis: a review. *Dermatol Online J.* 2016;22(4):13030/qt4b07778z.
27. Deng J, Liao V, Parthasarathy V, et al. Modulation of neuroimmune and epithelial dysregulation in patients with moderate to severe prurigo nodularis treated with nemolizumab. *JAMA Dermatol.* 2023;159(9):977-985.
28. Ständer S, Yosipovitch G, Legat FJ, et al. Trial of nemolizumab in moderate-to-severe prurigo nodularis. *N Engl J Med.* 2020;382(8):706-716.
29. Galderma. Galderma @ WCD 2023: Late-Breaking Phase III Results for Nemolizumab Monotherapy in Prurigo Nodularis Show a Significant Proportion of Itch-Free Patients by Week 4. https://www.galderma.com/news/galderma-wcd-2023-late-breaking-phase-iii-results-nemolizumab-monotherapy-prurigo-nodularis. Accessed August 31, 2023.
30. Pereira MP, Zeidler C, Ständer S. Improvement of chronic nodular prurigo with baricitinib. *J Eur Acad Dermatol Venereol.* 2022;36(6):e486-e488.

CHAPTER 37

Collagen Vascular Diseases

Drew Hicks
Sindhuja Sominidi Damodaran
Hafsa M. Cantwell
Olayemi Sokumbi

LUPUS ERYTHEMATOSUS

KEY POINTS

- Cutaneous lupus erythematosus (CLE) disproportionately occurs more often in patients with skin of color.
- Clinical history, morphologic evaluation, and lesional skin biopsy are required for CLE classification.
- Patients with darker skin may present with subtle pigment changes as a manifestation of their CLE.
- Scarring and dyspigmentation occur more frequently in CLE patients with dark skin.

- Educating skin of color patients on photo-avoidance, use of broad-spectrum sunscreens, and photoprotective clothing is imperative in disease management.
- Cultural competence is key to understanding and addressing the quality-of-life impact of CLE in skin of color patients.

INTRODUCTION

Cutaneous lupus erythematosus (CLE) is a broad group of autoimmune, inflammatory diseases affecting the skin. It is often, but not exclusively, associated with systemic lupus erythematosus (SLE) with the European Alliance of Associations for Rheumatology (EULAR)/American College of Rheumatology (ACR) diagnostic criteria mucocutaneous findings constituting a major component of SLE diagnosis.[1] CLE can be subdivided into three major manifestations: acute cutaneous lupus (ACLE), subacute cutaneous lupus (SCLE), and chronic cutaneous lupus (CCLE) [**Table 37-1**]. Development of CLE is multifactorial and complex. There is evidence that it may be influenced by a myriad of factors including genetic predisposition, age, sex, and environmental triggers such as ultraviolet (UV) radiation and tobacco use.[2] UV radiation is thought to induce keratinocyte damage, causing keratinocyte release of autoantigens and expression of proinflammatory cytokines and chemokines that recruit other immune cells to the skin.[3-7] Smoking is another environmental risk factor that has been linked to CLE, and patients who smoke have increased disease severity and require higher doses of therapeutics for their disease.[8] Genetic risk factors include the human leukocyte antigen (HLA) class II alleles DQA1 and DRB1*16.[9] Additionally, associations between single nucleotide polymorphisms (SNP) in ITGAM, FCGR2A, vitamin D receptor (VDR) gene, and interleukin-6 with susceptibility to cutaneous manifestations have been described.[9] Because approximately 40% of patients with CLE meet diagnostic criteria for systemic lupus erythematosus, care must be taken in diagnosis and management of CLE to monitor for development of systemic symptoms.[10] Patients with skin of color often develop complications of CLE such as postinflammatory hypo/hyperpigmentation and scarring that contributes to a reduced quality of life.[11]

TABLE 37-1 Clinical findings and common clinical mimics of CLE in skin of color

	Clinical findings	Clinical mimics
ACLE		
• Localized	Photo-induced malar erythema sparing nasolabial fold, nonscarring; may result in dyspigmentation	Heliotrope erythema of dermatomyositis (involves the nasolabial fold), seborrheic dermatitis, contact dermatitis, rosacea
• Generalized	Pruritic, photodistributed symmetric macules and papules; may result in dyspigmentation	
SCLE	Erythematous annular plaques with raised border that may be vesicular or crusted; psoriasiform papulosquamous lesions. Photodistributed on V of the upper chest, upper back, upper arms Lesions are nonscarring and resolve with vitiligo-like hypopigmentation Commonly drug-induced	Psoriasis, dermatitis, erythema multiforme, tinea corporis, gyrate erythemas, pemphigus foliaceus, dermatomyositis, cutaneous T-cell lymphoma
CCLE		
• DLE	Discoid plaques with adherent scale; late-stage lesions with peripheral hyperpigmentation, atrophy and central hypopigmentation. Commonly presents on head, scalp, and neck. Rarely, becomes generalized. Significant scarring of lesions, scarring alopecia, and dyspigmentation.	Nummular dermatitis, petaloid seborrheic dermatitis, psoriasis, granuloma faciale, sarcoidosis, vitiligo, cutaneous T-cell lymphoma
• Lupus profundus	Scarring and lipoatrophy most commonly on upper arms, chest, thighs	Dermatomyositis-associated panniculitis, subcutaneous panniculitis-like T-cell lymphoma

Abbreviations: ACLE, acute cutaneous lupus erythematosus; SCLE, subacute cutaneous lupus erythematosus; CCLE, chronic cutaneous lupus erythematosus; CLE, cutaneous lupus erythematosus; DLE, discoid lupus erythematosus.

EPIDEMIOLOGY

Limited population-based research on CLE incidence and prevalence has been conducted to date. A community-based epidemiological inquiry in Olmsted County, MN and of the Swedish National Patient Register found a CLE incidence rate of 4.30 (95% CI, 3.62-4.98) per 100,000 and 4.0 per 100,000, respectively.[12,13] However, these studies are limited by their relatively homogenous populations with limited racial and ethnic diversity.[12,13] Among the University of Texas Southwestern Medical Center CLE registry, of the 244 registered individuals with diagnosed CLE, 51% identified as African American.[14] Patients with skin of color represented approximately two-thirds of those on the registry.[14] A study from New Zealand demonstrating an overall CLE prevalence of 86.0 (95% CI, 78.1-94.7) per 100,000 is notable for finding a sex-adjusted relative risk of 2.47 (95% CI, 3.06-3.67) among the Maori/Pacific population as compared to the European population.[15] This is in concordance with additional observations noting higher rates of SLE and its cutaneous manifestations among people of color than their Caucasian counterparts.[16] Additionally, the phenotype of CLE in African Americans and Hispanics is marked by increased severity with more systemic complications.[17] The disease burden of both SLE and CLE impact female patients much more commonly than males (between 7% and 20% male prevalence in studies conducted worldwide).[16]

CLINICAL PRESENTATION

ACUTE CUTANEOUS LUPUS ERYTHEMATOSUS

Acute cutaneous lupus erythematosus (ACLE) is most often associated with SLE and typically diagnosed in the third decade of life. Although the lesions are classically photoinduced, they persist days after UV-exposure.[18] ACLE can be subdivided into localized ACLE and generalized ACLE. Cutaneous manifestations of the localized form include the characteristic malar erythema (often termed a "butterfly rash") spanning the cheeks and nasal bridge but sparing the nasolabial folds.[18] In skin of color, the erythema may have a violaceous appearance or may present as more subtle brown and dark brown patches [**Figure 37-1**]. The generalized variant is rare and is characterized by photodistributed widespread erythematous macules and papules [**Figure 37-2**]. It is often associated with erythematous or hyperpigmented patches on the dorsal hands that spare the bony prominences of the dorsal distal interphalangeal (DIP), proximal interphalangeal (PIP), and metacarpophalangeal (MCP) joints.[19] Nonspecific cutaneous findings such as mucosal ulcers, Raynaud phenomenon, and diffuse hair loss are also common in ACLE [**Figure 37-3**].[18] Recently, an unusual finding of diffuse melanonychia was reported in a cohort of Black SLE patients in Africa.[20] ACLE often results in postinflammatory dyspigmentation of the affected sites without scarring.[18] Recognition of the subtlety of erythema presentation in dark skin allows for prompt diagnosis of ACLE. Clinical mimics of ACLE include seborrheic dermatitis, dermatomyositis, and photoallergic dermatitis.[18]

SUBACUTE CUTANEOUS LUPUS ERYTHEMATOSUS (SCLE)

Subacute cutaneous lupus erythematous (SCLE) is notable for its photosensitive presentation. SCLE occurs predominantly in Caucasians and is uncommon in Blacks, Koreans, and Chinese.[21] SCLE presents with either an annular polycyclic or psoriasiform papulosquamous morphology.[18] Lesions typically affect sun-exposed regions of the trunk,

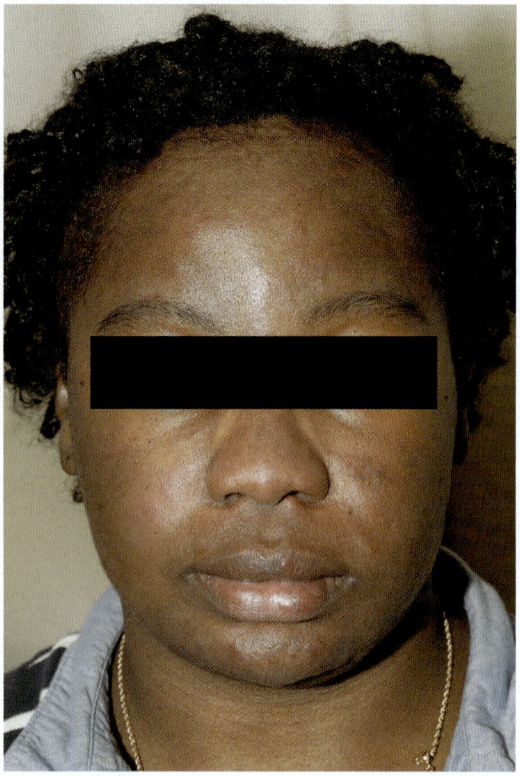

FIGURE 37-1. Black patient with malar rash of ACLE presenting with subtle erythema on cheeks and nose with sparing of the nasolabial folds.

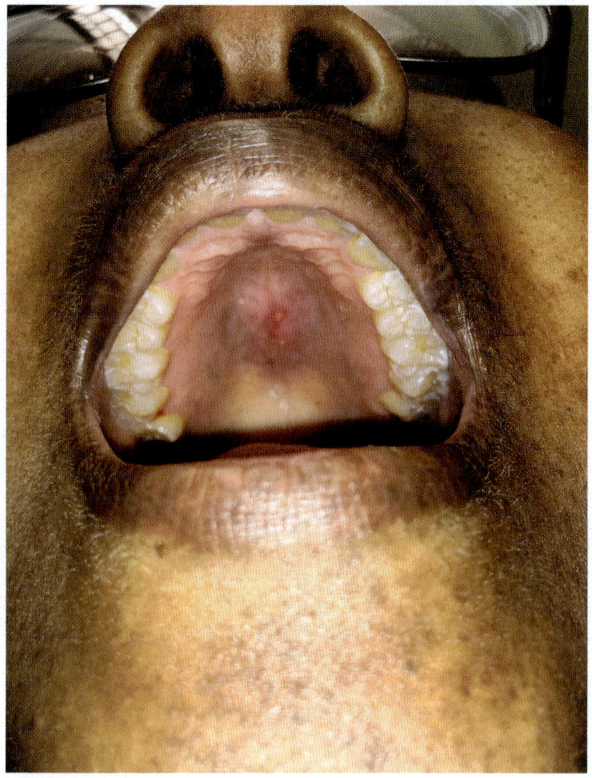

FIGURE 37-3. Ulcer on the hard palate of Black patient with SLE.

neck, and upper extremities and spare the face and lower extremities. The annular subtype typically forms scaly, erythematous plaques with elevated borders and the papulosquamous subtype resembles dermatitic or psoriasiform lesions.[18] The annular variant may present with crusting and vesiculation at the active border of the lesion. Both subtypes typically heal without scarring but marked vitiligo-like hypopigmentation with telangiectasia may occur with resolution.[18] SCLE is associated with anti-Ro/SSA antibodies and approximately 50% of SCLE patients will fulfill ACR criteria for SLE, therefore warranting investigation for systemic disease.[22]

SCLE is estimated to be drug-induced in up to 30% of patients with resolution occurring after discontinuation of the culprit drug.[23,24] Several medications have been implicated including antihypertensives, terbinafine, proton pump inhibitors, and nonsteroidal anti-inflammatory drugs.[25] Clinical mimics of SCLE include psoriasiform dermatomyositis, cutaneous T-cell lymphoma, tinea corporis, and the gyrate erythemas.[18]

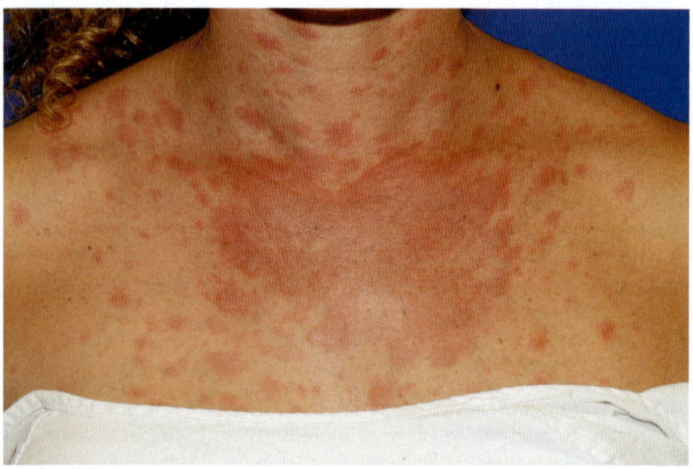

FIGURE 37-2. Photodistributed erythematous papules and plaques of ACLE on the chest of a multiracial female.

CHRONIC CUTANEOUS LUPUS ERYTHEMATOSUS

Chronic cutaneous lupus erythematosus (CCLE) can be subdivided into discoid lupus erythematosus, hypertrophic discoid lupus erythematosus, lupus panniculitis, lupus erythematosus tumidus, and chilblain lupus erythematosus. The discussion will be focused on DLE and lupus panniculitis.

DISCOID LUPUS ERYTHEMATOSUS

Discoid lupus erythematosus (DLE) is the most common form of CCLE.[18] In contrast to ACLE and SCLE, it is rarely associated with systemic disease.[18] It occurs most frequently in females in their fourth and fifth decade of life, and epidemiological studies have demonstrated higher incidence and prevalence in racial and ethnic minority groups, particularly Black individuals.[26] Clinically, it is characterized by erythematous, scaly, coin-like atrophic plaques that are painful on manipulation [**Figure 37-4**].[18] In addition, the lesions often demonstrate follicular dilatation with keratin plugging [**Figure 37-5**].[27] Like other forms of cutaneous lupus, the lesions are triggered by UV exposure and are typically located on face, neck, concha of ears, and head [**Figure 37-6**]. Uncommonly, the discoid lesions may present as hypertrophic or verrucous DLE with severely thickened lesions on the upper extremities and face.[18] A generalized variant of DLE is rare and presents with disseminated discoid lesions [**Figure 37-7**]. Patients with this variant are more likely to progress to SLE.[28] While the DLE plaques may heal, they often result in scarring, scarring alopecia, atrophy, and peripheral hyperpigmentation with central hypopigmentation [**Figures 37-8** and **37-9**]. Black patients experience higher rates of scalp and ear dyspigmentation and scarring alopecia with DLE than non-Black patients.[11] Squamous cell carcinoma has been reported as an infrequent complication of DLE scars years after diagnosis in patients of African descent.[29,30] Therefore, careful attention should be given to a changing longstanding DLE lesion. Clinical mimics of DLE in skin of color include petaloid seborrheic dermatitis, sarcoidosis, granuloma faciale, and cutaneous T-cell lymphoma.[18]

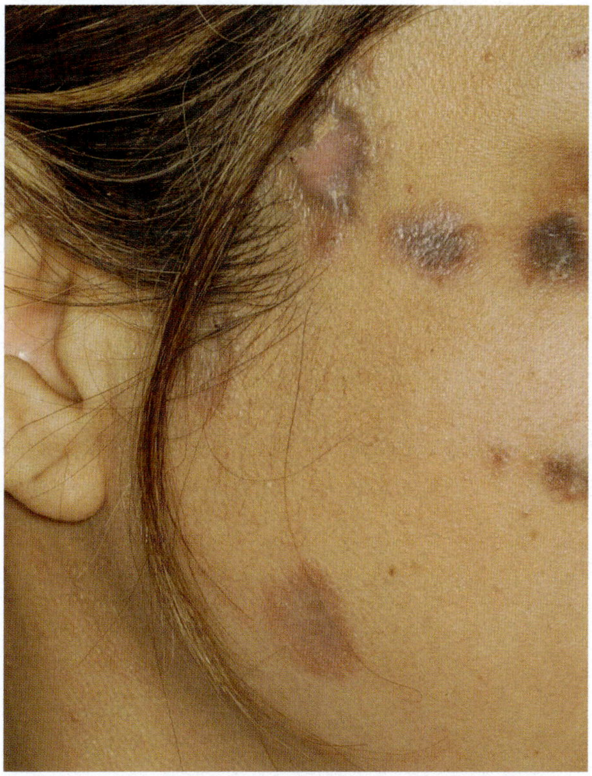

FIGURE 37-4. Coin-like atrophic plaques of DLE with peripheral hyperpigmentation and central hypopigmentation.

LUPUS PANNICULITIS

Lupus panniculitis, sometimes referred to as lupus profundus, is often accompanied by discoid lupus lesions. The clinical findings include subcutaneous nodules in areas of typical areas of body fat accumulation (breasts, thighs, upper arms, and face) that are firm and tender to palpation and resulting in atrophic scarring [**Figures 37-10** and **37-11**].[18] Lupus panniculitis has a clinical course that is chronic in nature with repeated flares and remission.[18]

HISTOPATHOLOGY

Each subtype of CLE has its own distinctive histopathology most often characterized by the presence of vacuolar interface dermatitis, perivascular, periadnexal lymphocytic inflammation, dermal edema, and mucin deposition.[18] These changes can vary depending on the subtype and duration of the LE lesions. ACLE lesions can show subtle inflammation but more edema compared to DLE lesions, which shows dense superficial and deep perivascular and periadnexal inflammation with

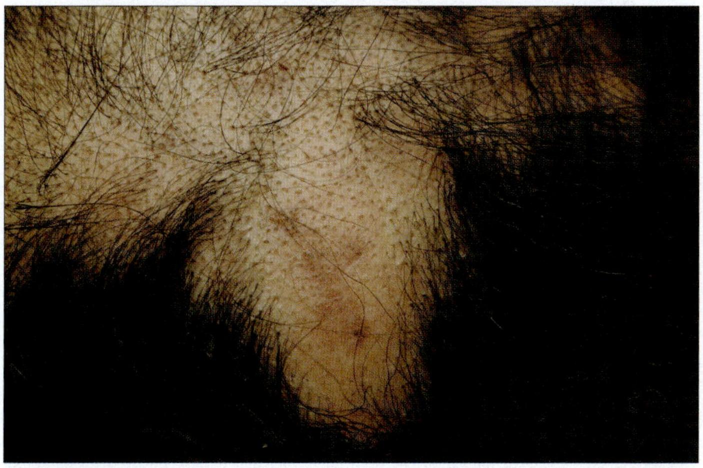

FIGURE 37-5. Scarring alopecia with prominent follicular plugging in patient with end-stage DLE.

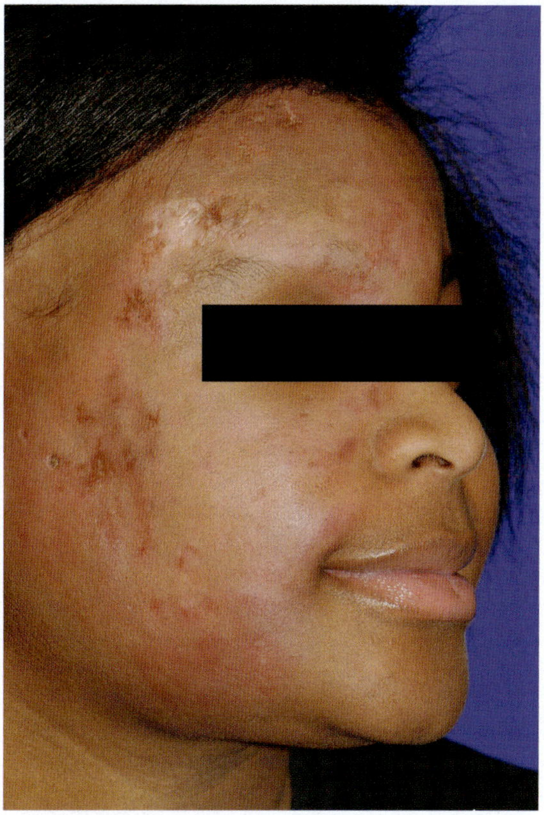

FIGURE 37-6. Erythematous scarring lesions of DLE on the face.

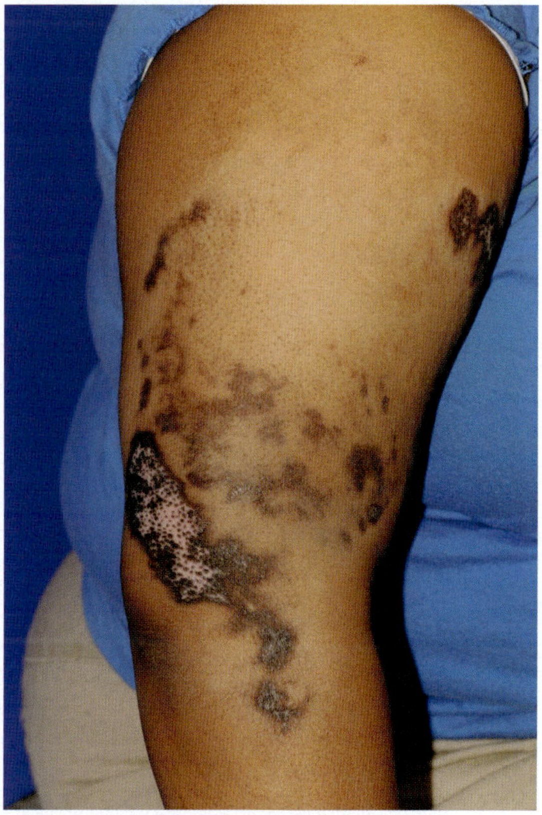

FIGURE 37-7. Generalized scarring lesions of DLE.

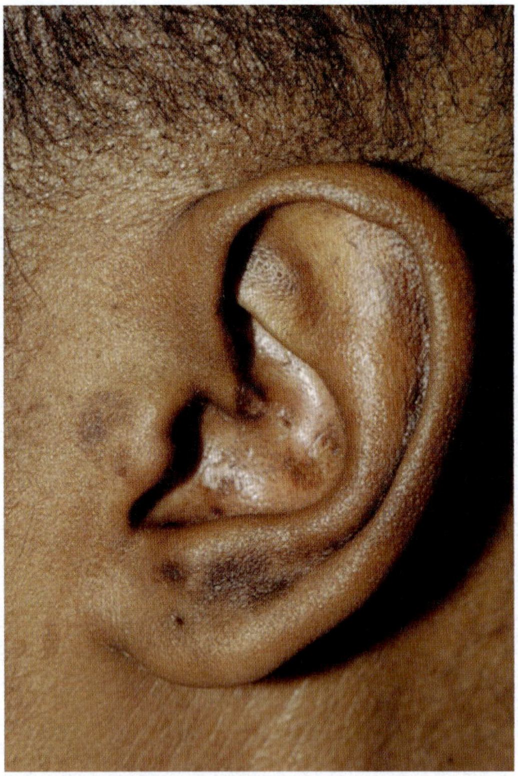

FIGURE 37-8. Scarring lesions of DLE in the conchal bowl of the ear.

prominent follicular plugging and hyperkeratosis [**Figure 37-12**]. SCLE demonstrates an intermediate between the subtle findings of ACLE and the prominent features of DLE. Biopsy from late hyperpigmented plaques in higher Fitzpatrick skin type patients can show pigment incontinence as a prominent feature. Direct immunofluorescence

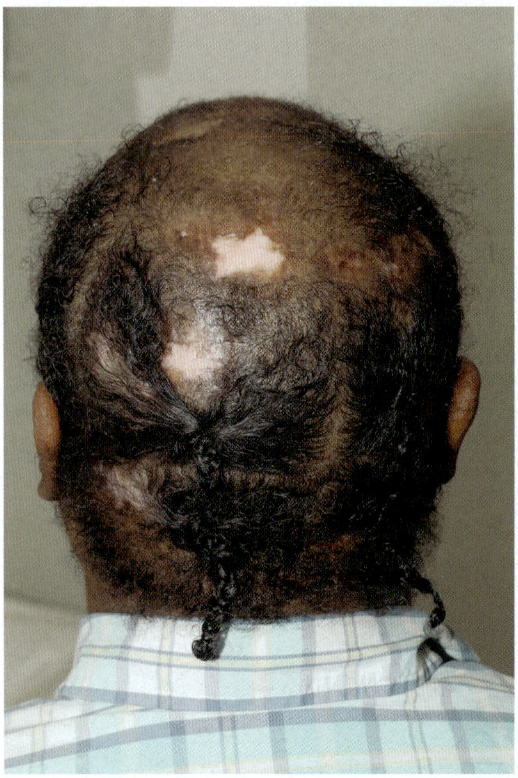

FIGURE 37-9. Scarring plaques of DLE on the scalp with central hypopigmentation and peripheral hyperpigmentation.

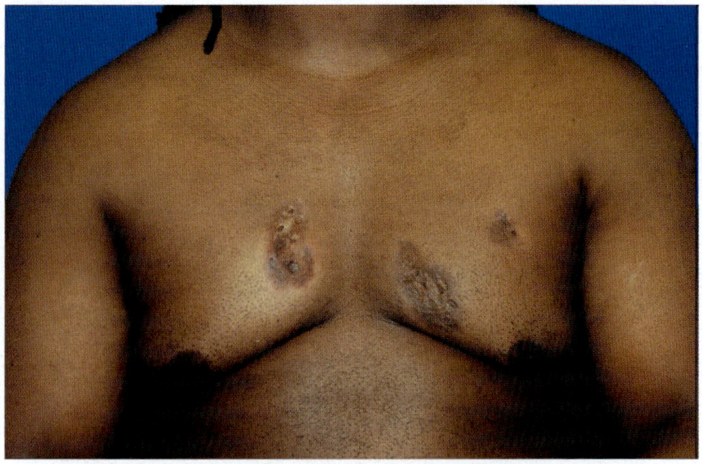

FIGURE 37-10. Subcutaneous atrophy and scarring of lupus on chest of a Black man.

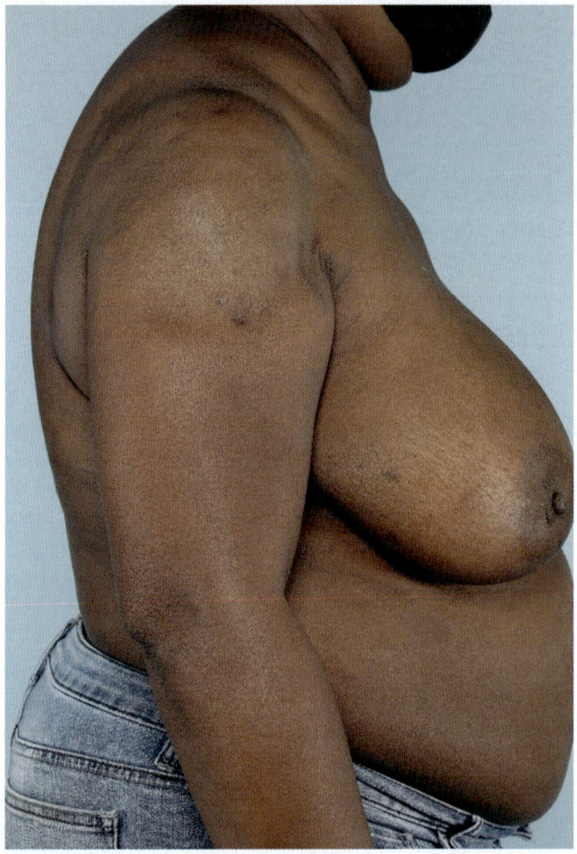

FIGURE 37-11. Subcutaneous atrophic plaques of the upper arm in a Black woman with lupus profundus.

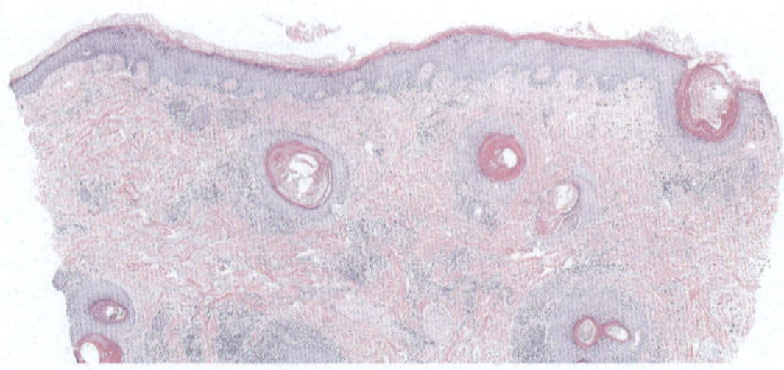

FIGURE 37-12. Vacuolar interface dermatitis, follicular hyperkeratosis with plugging, superficial and deep perivascular and periadnexal lymphocytic inflammation of DLE. This biopsy from the scalp of a Black woman has prominent pigment incontinence.

(DIF) studies show granular band-like deposits of immunoglobulin and complements at the dermal-epidermal junction (lupus band) in greater than 90% of SLE patients.[31] Lupus panniculitis can be challenging to differentiate from subcutaneous panniculitis-like T-cell lymphoma (SPTCL) and may require immunohistochemical stains. Characterized by the presence of lymphocytic lobular panniculitis, lupus panniculitis may or may not show additional findings including interface changes, perivascular and periadnexal inflammation, and hyaline fat degeneration making it challenging to distinguish from SPTCL.[32,33]

EVALUATION AND TREATMENT

Evaluation should begin with thorough history and physical examination as 20% of patients with CLE may progress to SLE.[10] Patients with CLE should be screened at diagnosis and at routine intervals for internal organ involvement. Assessment should be made based on the ACR or Systemic Lupus International Collaborating Clinics (SLICC) diagnostic criteria for SLE.[34] The additional investigation is particularly important in patients of color as they are disproportionately burdened by LE and have a worse outcomes than White patients.[35] In addition, the increased likelihood of renal involvement and progression to systemic disease requires that skin of color patients should be counseled on the importance of reducing risk factors that may be associated with systemic involvement.[36,37]

The significant dyspigmentation following active CLE is challenging to treat. Sun avoidance and full UV protection with clothing, wide-brimmed hats, and broad-spectrum, SPF50 sunscreen is recommended. Sunscreens should be applied prior to sun exposure with some individuals being so photosensitive as to necessitate protection from window glass-filtered sunlight or indoor fluorescent light exposure.[18] In addition, tinted sunscreens with iron oxides with protection against visible light is recommended in dark-skinned patients.[38] Vitamin D supplementation (800-1000 IU daily) should be considered in dark-skinned patients with CLE as this population is especially predisposed to vitamin D insufficiency due to judicious sun-protection.[39] Smoking cessation should also be prioritized, as smoking decreases likelihood of cutaneous improvement in CLE and reduces the efficacy of hydroxychloroquine.[26] Thorough review should be performed to identify culprit drugs in drug-induced lupus erythematosus before beginning therapy; treatment of these cases should begin with discontinuation of the causative drug.[24] Topical steroids are first-line treatment for CLE, with evidence promoting the use of potent or ultra-potent steroids particularly for DLE.[18] Topical tacrolimus and pimecrolimus (calcineurin inhibitors) may be used as a steroid alternative with similar efficacy but with a safer side effect profile. Other topical agents such as tretinoin have been used in case reports with varying success but do not constitute mainstay treatment for CLE.[18]

For CLE in the context of SLE or where more conservative topical treatment has failed, systemic agents should be considered. For ongoing CLE activity, aggressive systemic treatment is required to reduce the risk of scarring and dyspigmentation. Antimalarials such as hydroxychloroquine (5 mg/kg/day) or chloroquine (2.3 mg/kg/day) constitute first-line therapies.[18] Other drugs such as methotrexate (10-25 mg/week), mycophenolate mofetil (1-3 g/day), dapsone (25-200 mg/day), thalidomide (50-100 mg/day), lenalidomide (5-10 mg/day), and acitretin (0.2-1 mg/kg/day) are commonly used, often in combination with antimalarials for difficult to manage disease.[18,26] Biologics such as rituximab and belimumab are currently being researched for use in the management of CLE.[26]

Cultural competence and understanding of hair practices in skin of color patients with scalp lesions is imperative. Gentle hair practices to minimize further scalp damage is recommended. Psychiatry evaluation may be needed to address the psychological burden associated with the profound dyspigmentation and scarring that maybe seen in CLE. Patients may find concealing cosmetics a helpful option to camouflage dyspigmentation.

DERMATOMYOSITIS

KEY POINTS

- Dermatomyositis (DM) presents with violaceous erythema, which may have a subtle presentation in skin of color.
- Due to the subtle appearance of erythema, recognition of additional clinical signs of dyspigmentation, edema, scale, or poikiloderma is imperative in skin of color.
- Diagnosis of DM is primarily clinical; however, histopathology with interface dermatitis can be supportive of a diagnosis.
- Autoantibody testing is beneficial for risk-stratification with positive anti-NXP-2 or anti-TIF-1γ associated with high risk of malignancy.
- Age appropriate and symptom-guided screening is advised in all adult DM patients, with further screening advised in high-risk subtypes.

INTRODUCTION

Dermatomyositis (DM) is an inflammatory myopathy with characteristic accompanying skin findings. It is classified as one of the idiopathic inflammatory myopathies (IIM), which also include polymyositis, inclusion body myositis, and other myositis subgroups.[40] Myopathies typically manifest with symmetric, proximal muscle weakness. Cutaneous findings may occur with or without muscular involvement (amyopathic DM) and may additionally persist after treatment of underlying myopathy. Therefore, rendering a diagnosis of DM primarily relies on recognition of its heterogeneous cutaneous findings. This can be problematic as racial minorities and patients with darker skin tones are significantly underrepresented in the medical literature depicting DM manifestations.[41] The lack of education and inability to recognize the salient features of DM in darker skin tones may lead to diagnostic delay and contribute to the healthcare disparities in DM.[42]

The exact pathogenesis of DM is unknown, though multiple factors such as genetics, immunology, infection, UV radiation, and drugs have been associated with disease development. Previously associated haplotypes that have been reported include HLA DRB1*0301 in African Americans and HLA DQA1*0104 and HLA DRB1*07 in Han Chinese.[43,44] Viral agents such as Coxsackie B, Epstein-Barr virus, parvovirus, polyomavirus, and SARS-CoV-2 have also been observed to trigger DM.[45-47] Medications implicated in drug-induced DM include hydroxyurea, nonsteroidal anti-inflammatory agents, tumor necrosis alpha inhibitors, chemotherapeutic agents, antibiotics, and immune checkpoint inhibitors.[46,48-50]

EPIDEMIOLOGY

Limited population-based research on DM incidence and prevalence has been conducted to date. DM has a bimodal incidence with an adult-onset peak between 40 and 60 years and a pediatric peak between ages 5 and 15 years.[51] A community-based epidemiological inquiry in Olmsted County, MN, found a DM incidence rate of 9.63 (95% CI, 6.09-13.17) per 1,000,000 with an overall prevalence of 21.42 (95% CI, 13.07-29.77) per 100,000, though the study is limited by its relatively homogenous populations with limited racial and ethnic diversity.[52] Female-to-male incidence ratio is generally regarded to be between 2 and 3:1.[53] Additionally, within the United States, significantly more African Americans experience DM at rates of approximately 3 to 4:1 when compared to Caucasians.[54] In a systematic review, hospitalization with a primary diagnosis of dermatomyositis and increased length of stay was found to be associated with African American, Hispanic, Asian, multiracial/other race compared with Whites.[55] Dermatomyositis is associated with increased risk of malignancy in all groups, but those of Asian descent particularly have an increased risk of nasopharyngeal carcinoma.[56]

CLINICAL PRESENTATION

Current classification of DM lacks a skin-focused criteria for patients with skin-predominant DM. Cutaneous findings can be categorized as pathognomonic, characteristic, compatible, less common, rare, recent, and nonspecific [**Table 37-2**].[57] Pathognomonic signs of DM include Gottron papules, Gottron sign, and heliotrope erythema.[57] Gottron sign is characterized by symmetric erythematous macules on extensor surfaces of the hands, elbows, and knees [**Figure 37-13A** and **B**].[57] Gottron papules are scaly violaceous papules and plaques on the bony prominences of the dorsal metacarpophalangeal and intraphalangeal joints [**Figure 37-14A** and **B**].[57] Heliotrope erythema is characterized by violaceous erythema of the upper eyelids often in association with periorbital edema [**Figure 37-15A** and **B**].[57] Erythematous patches are often seen on the mid-face imitating the malar rash of acute LE; however, in contrast to acute LE, DM does affect the nasolabial folds. Characteristic findings include diffuse macular erythema called shawl sign (upper back, posterior neck, and shoulders, V sign [upper chest and anterior neck] and holster sign [lateral thighs and hips]) [**Figures 37-16, 37-17A-C,** and **37-18**].[57] Periungual telangiectasia with dystrophic cuticles and hemorrhagic nail fold infarcts are characteristic and sensitive markers of DM [**Figure 37-19**].[58] Mechanic's hands with thickened, fissuring skin on the sides of fingers and palms is a rare finding in DM that is present more frequently in antisynthetase syndrome or anti-MDA5 DM [**Figure 37-20**].[59] Calcinosis cutis that appears as popcorn-like is a compatible finding that may be observed in pediatric populations but is rarer in adults. Zebra-like erythematous streaks that appear hyperpigmented in skin of color patients represent flagellate erythema, a rare manifestation of DM [**Figure 37-21**]. A rare variant of DM termed "Wong-type DM" presents with diffuse follicular hyperkeratosis that mimics pityriasis rubra pilaris.[60] The erythema of dermatomyositis is typically violaceous and may be more subtle with a hyperpigmented appearance in skin of color, thus necessitating attention to dyschromia, hyperpigmentation, and any poikilodermatous changes in anatomic regions associated with DM [**Figure 37-22**].[61] Other clinical clues may be associated scale, edema (particularly in periorbital region), or ulceration. Digital ulcerations have been associated with anti-MDA5 type of DM that is often associated with underlying vasculopathy and interstitial lung disease [**Figure 37-23**].[62] Treatment refractory pruritus may represent a clue supporting DM over CLE. Similar to CLE, photosensitivity and Raynaud phenomenon may be seen in DM.[57] Significant inflammation associated with DM often results in pronounced dyspigmentation that may mimic systemic sclerosis.

TABLE 37-2 Clinical findings and common clinical mimics of DM in skin of color

	Clinical findings	Clinical mimics
Pathognomonic		
• Gottron papules	Violaceous to hyperpigmented scaly papules on MCP and ICP joints	ACLE on dorsal hands typically spares the MCP and ICP joints
• Gottron sign	Erythematous to hyperpigmented macules and patches on extensor elbows, knees	
• Heliotrope	Periorbital edema of upper lids with hyperpigmentation and gray-brown macules and patches	Malar rash of ACLE spares the nasolabial folds
Characteristic		
• V-sign	Hyperpigmented to hypopigmented, confluent macules and patches on lower anterior neck and upper chest	SCLE, dermatitis, psoriasis, seborrheic dermatitis for scalp involvement in DM, mixed connective disease
• Shawl sign	Violaceous, hyper/hypopigmented macules and patches on upper back, posterior shoulders, back of neck	
• Holster sign	Hyperpigmented patches on hips and lateral thigh	
• Nailfold changes	Periungual telangiectasias, dystrophic cuticles, hemorrhagic nailfold infarcts	
• Scalp	Atrophic, erythematous pruritic plaques	
Compatible		
• Poikiloderma	Hypopigmentation, hyperpigmentation, and atrophy on upper chest, lateral upper arms	Massive edema may be seen in malar rash of ACLE
• Periorbital edema	With or without erythema	
Less common		
• Vesiculobullous/ necrotic/ ulcerative lesions, vasculitis, calcinosis cutis		
Rare		
• Mechanic's hands, flagellate erythema, follicular hyperkeratosis, panniculitis, mucinosis		
Recently described		
• Digital ulceration, ulcerated Gottron papules/sign, hiker's feet		

Abbreviations: DM, Dermatomyositis; ICP, intercarpal phalangeal; MCP, metacarpal phalangeal.

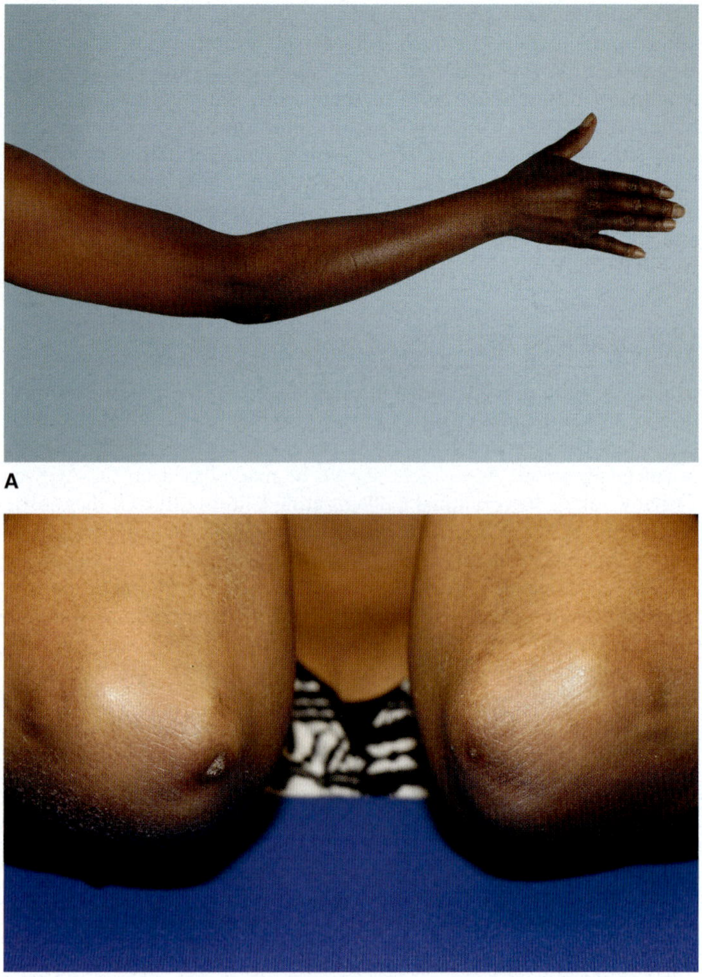

FIGURE 37-13. **(A)** Gottron sign presenting as hyperpigmented patch on the elbow. **(B)** Gottron sign presenting as symmetric crusted papules involving bilateral elbows.

HISTOPATHOLOGY

Although identification of DM relies on primary clinical recognition, histopathology is often beneficial in supporting the diagnosis and excluding mimics. Histopathology findings can be subtle and include: epidermal atrophy, vacuolar interface dermatitis, dermal mucin, mild perivascular mononuclear cell infiltrate, and pigment incontinence [**Figure 37-24**].[63] Although interface alteration is classically seen, there are cases of DM without interface dermatitis.[64] Performing a biopsy of erythematous regions such as the shawl sign

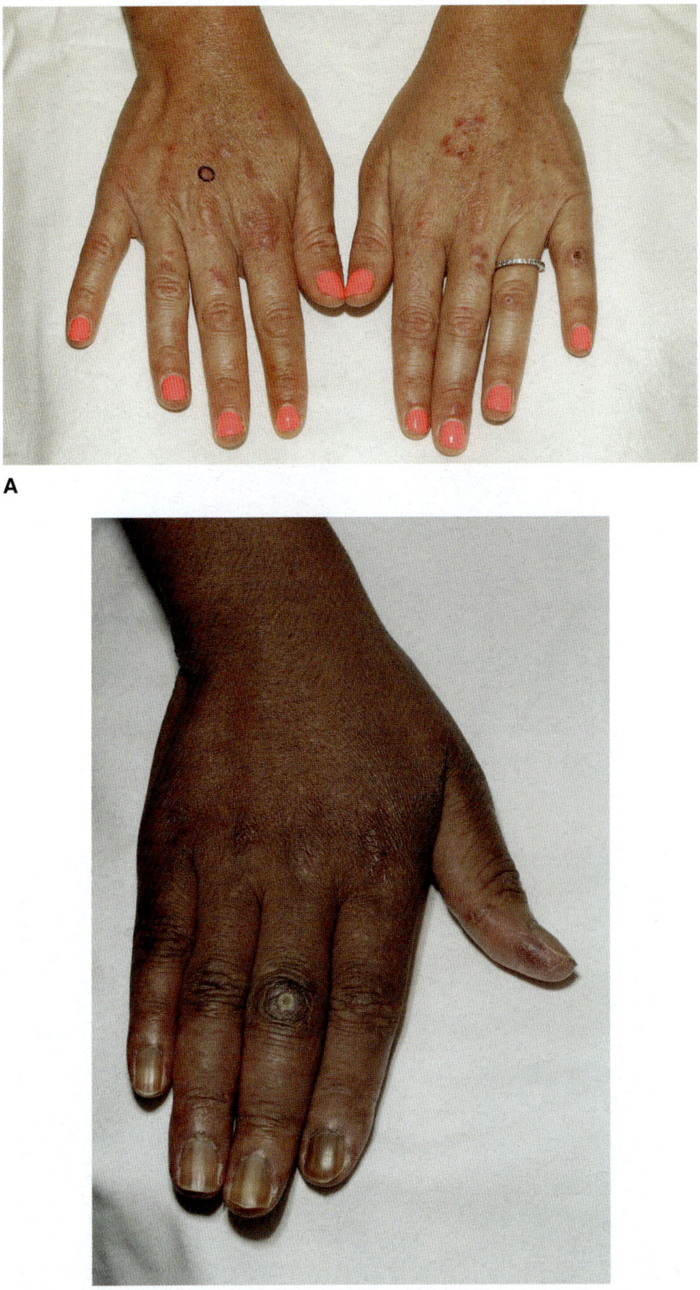

A

B

FIGURE 37-14. **(A)** Hispanic woman with erythematous to violaceous papules on the PIP and MCP consistent with Gottron papules. A crusted ulcerated lesion is present on the left fifth PIP. **(B)** Subtle violaceous papules on the PIP and MCP consistent with Gottron papules. A crusted ulcerated lesion is present on the right third PIP.

or V-sign are likely to have inconclusive and nonspecific findings.[61] Histopathology of DM can be indistinguishable from findings seen in CLE highlighting the significance of clinician familiarity with cutaneous manifestations of DM.

EVALUATION AND TREATMENT

In cases of suspected dermatomyositis after thorough history and physical examination, laboratory evaluation of muscle enzymes and autoantibodies should be pursued.[63] Myositis specific autoantibody (MSA) testing may include anti-Mi2, anti-TIF-1γ, anti-MDA5, anti-NXP2, anti-SAE, antisynthetase syndrome antibodies, and, if clinically deemed appropriate, antinuclear antibody and extractable nuclear antibodies. As above, skin biopsy may be supportive of diagnosis.

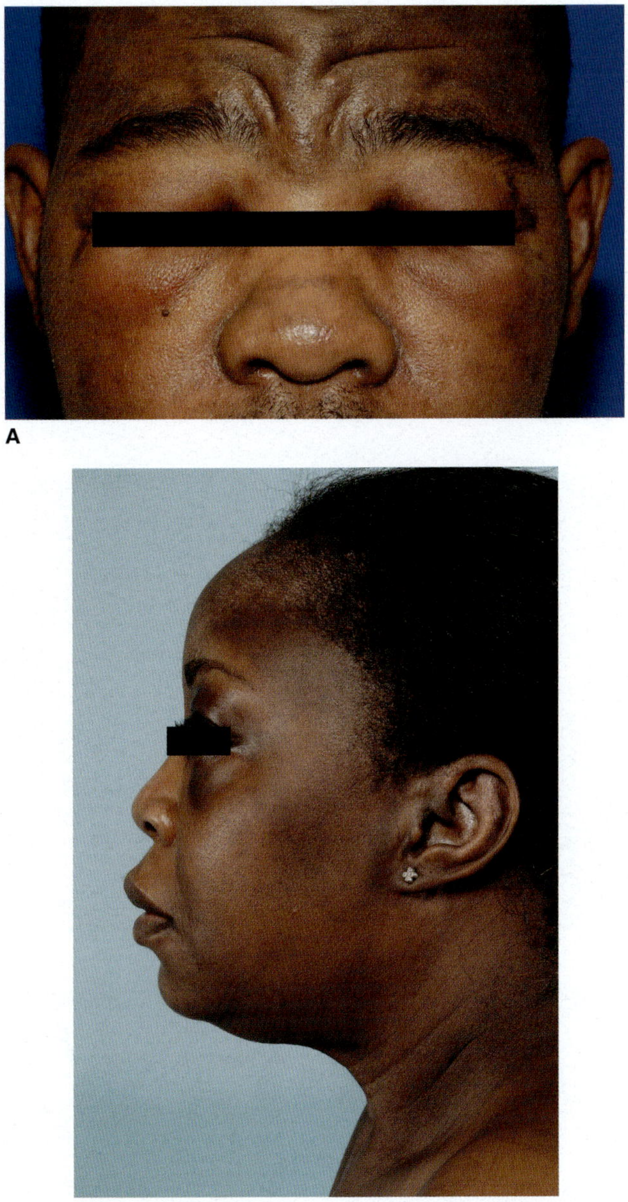

A

B

FIGURE 37-15. **(A)** Heliotrope rash presenting as periorbital edema with violaceous erythema. **(B)** Heliotrope rash with periorbital edema with hyperpigmentation. There is also lateral forehead and preauricular cheek hyperpigmentation.

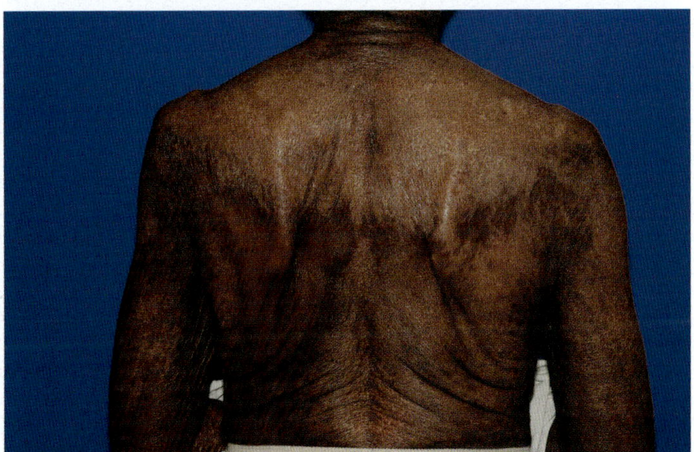

FIGURE 37-16. Shawl sign presenting as prominent hypopigmentation and hyperpigmentation of the upper back in a Black patient.

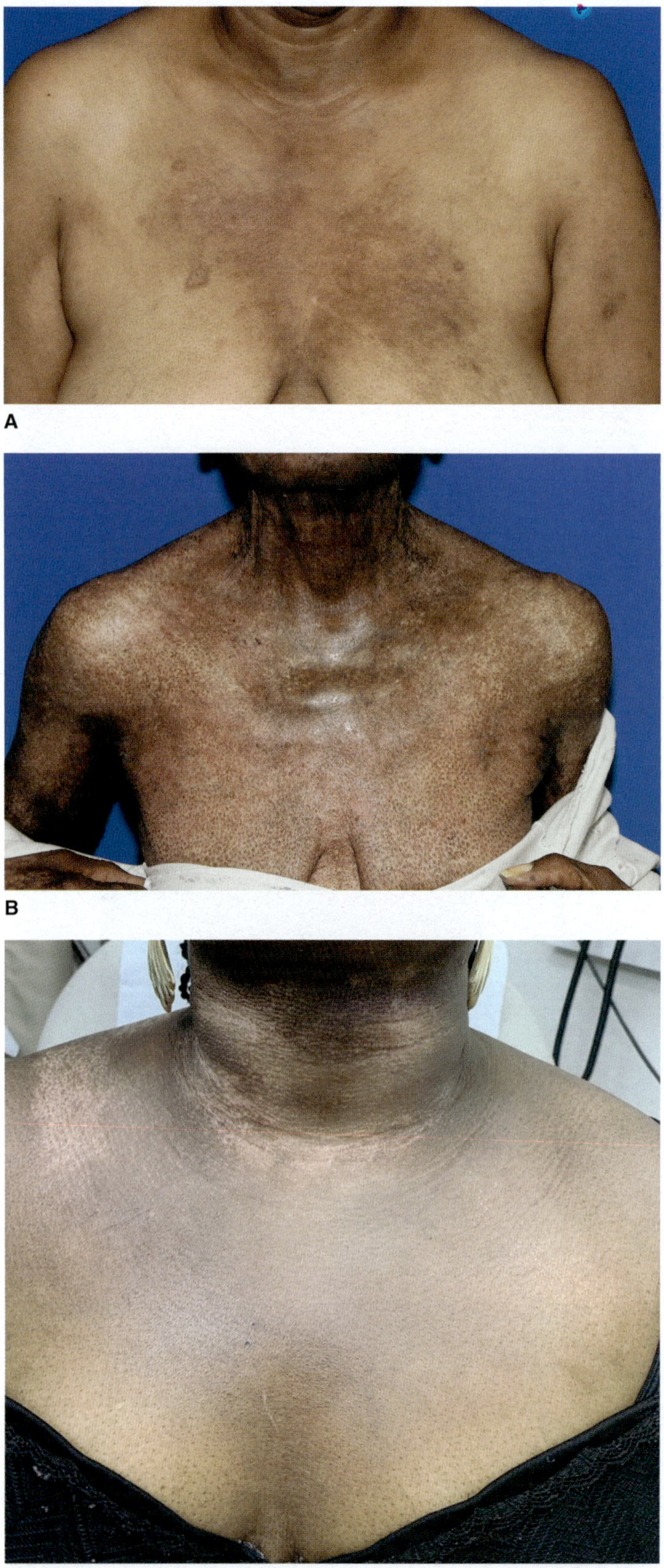

A

B

C

FIGURE 37-17. **(A)** V-sign presenting as photodistributed hyperpigmentation on the upper V of the neck and chest. **(B)** Hyperpigmented patches with diffuse poikiloderma in a V-distribution on the upper chest. **(C)** Hyperpigmented patches with vitiligo-like hypopigmentation as V-sign.

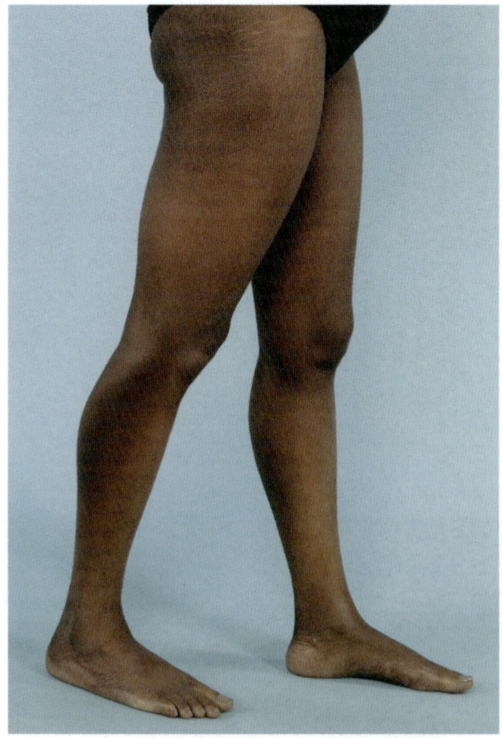

FIGURE 37-18. Holster sign with hyperpigmentation on the lateral aspect of bilateral thighs.

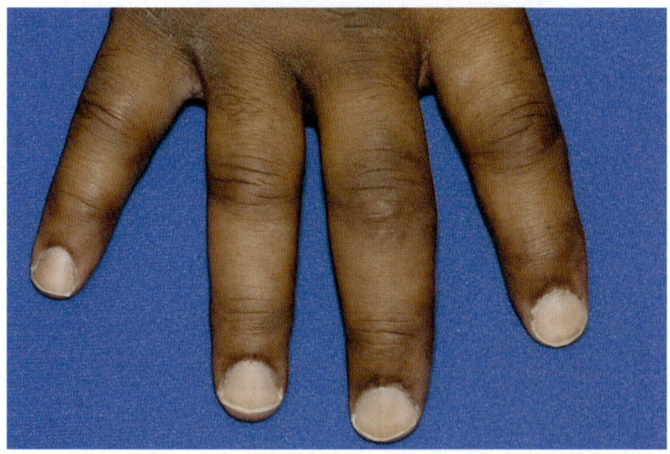

FIGURE 37-19. Ragged cuticles of several fingernails present in DM.

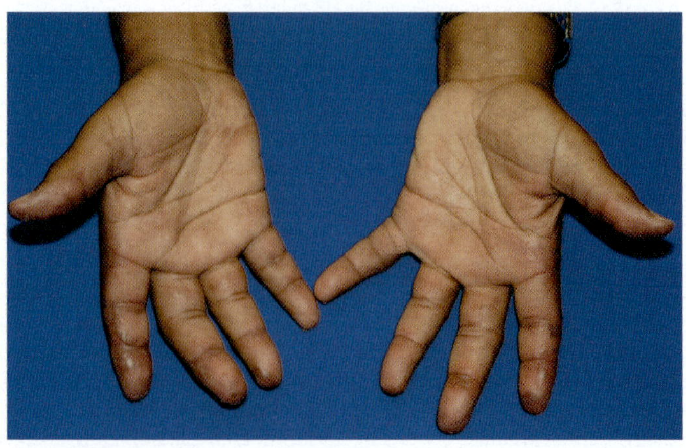

FIGURE 37-20. Scaling, cracking, and fissuring of the tips and sides of the fingers seen in Mechanic's hands of DM.

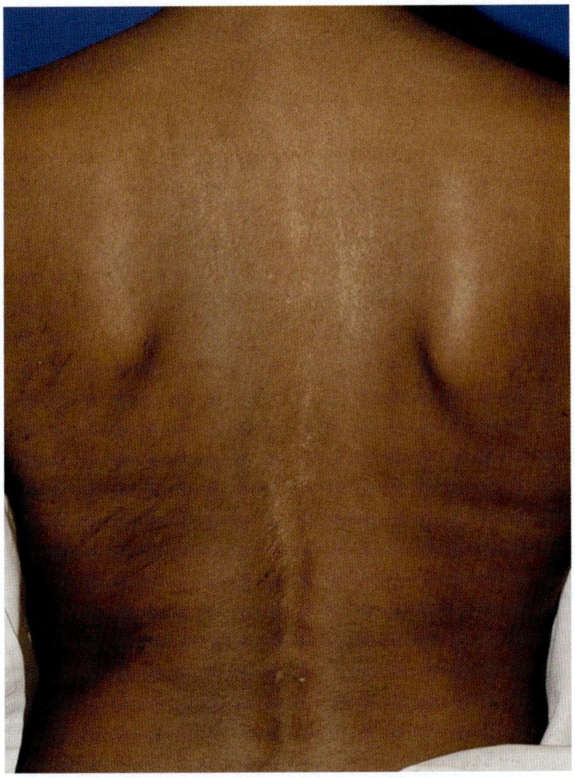

FIGURE 37-21. Hyperpigmented linear streaks of flagellate erythema in DM.

Because of its relation to systemic disease and increased risk of malignancy, careful management and education of DM patients is of utmost priority. Age > 45 at diagnosis, male sex, skin necrosis, periungual erythema, and rapid onset of cutaneous and muscular symptoms are additional risk factors identified for malignancy.[65] Risk of malignancy in DM has been found to be highest in the first 5 years from diagnosis with higher risk in the first year.[66] Thorough evaluation for malignancy is

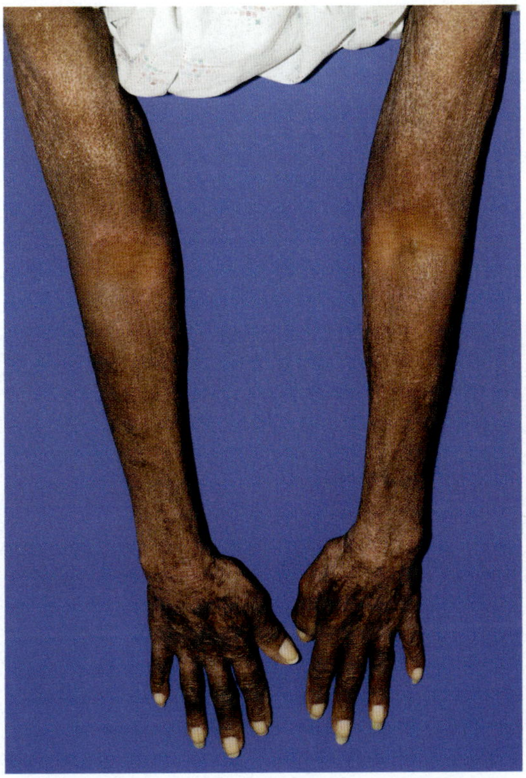

FIGURE 37-22. Vitiligo-like hypopigmentation of the upper arms in DM.

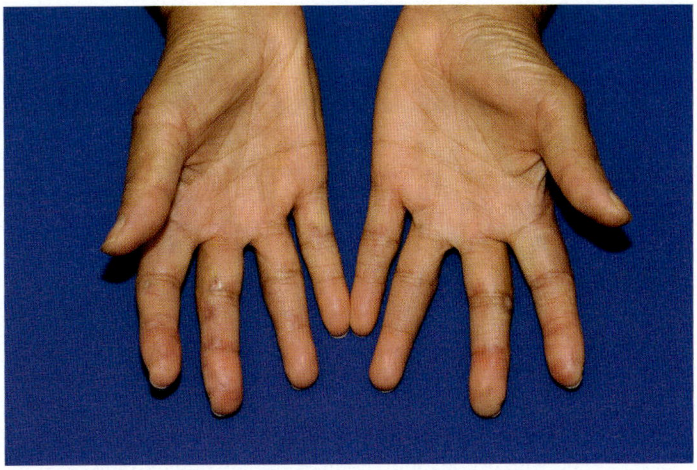

FIGURE 37-23. Digital ulcerations in patient with MDA5-associated DM.

not indicated in juvenile DM.[40,63] In adult DM, MSA profile is beneficial for risk stratification. For adult patients positive for anti-NXP-2 or anti-TIF-1γ, which are high risk for malignancy, thorough evaluation is advised with baseline age-appropriate malignancy screening, symptom directed screening, whole body imaging studies, and esophagogastroduodenoscopy and colonoscopy if not performed as part of remaining evaluation.[63] In these patients with high-risk autoantibodies, annual whole-body imaging is advised for at least the first 5 years from presentation. For other adult patients with DM, age-appropriate screening along with symptom directed screening is advised.[63] In addition to malignancy, all patients should be evaluated for interstitial lung disease (ILD) at the time of initial DM diagnosis; this involves pulmonary function testing (PFT) and assessment of diffusion capacity of the lung for carbon monoxide (DLCO).[67] Patients with symptoms or preliminary tests suggestive of ILD should receive high-resolution CT scans (HRCT).[67] Much like malignancy-associated DM, MSA profiles can help inform a patient's risk for ILD. For instance, anti-MDA5 antibodies are present in at least half of all cases of DM-associated ILD,[68] although it is worth noting that a significant number of myositis patients have ILD without detectable MSAs.[68-70] Early recognition of ILD in patients with DM is paramount, as a subset of patients may have a severe form of ILD termed rapidly progressive ILD (RPILD) that can be fatal in as early as 6 months, the prognosis of which can be improved with early treatment initiation.[71]

Initial treatment with high-dose corticosteroids (1 mg/kg/day) is considered the gold standard for patients with associated myopathy.[40] For cutaneous limited disease, hydroxychloroquine (5 mg/kg/day) is considered a first-line agent. Systemic corticosteroids in conjunction with corticosteroid-sparing immunosuppressive agents (such as methotrexate [10-25 mg/week], mycophenolate mofetil [2-3g/day], and azathioprine [1.5-2.5 mg/kg/day]) are beneficial for patients with systemic disease, severe cutaneous disease, or cutaneous disease refractory to topical or systemic corticosteroids.

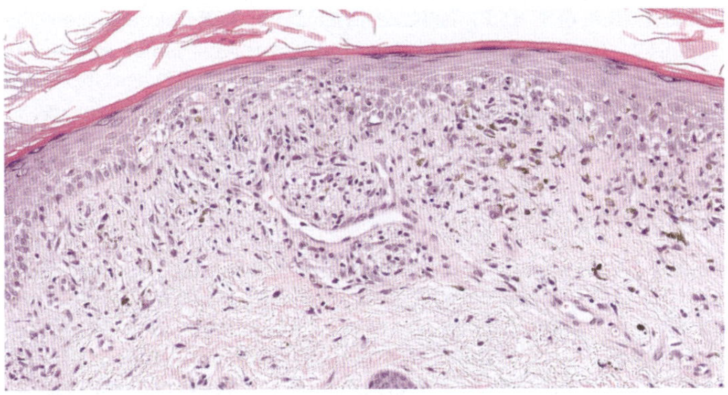

FIGURE 37-24. Subtle vacuolar alteration with necrotic keratinocytes and pigment incontinence from chest of Black woman with DM.

SCLERODERMA

KEY POINTS

- Scleroderma is a broader term that encompasses localized scleroderma (morphea) and systemic sclerosis (SSc).
- Morphea is diagnosed based on clinical and histopathology findings.
- Characterized by indurated asymmetric plaques, morphea tends to resolve after several years.
- SSc is a complex, progressive, and debilitating disease with internal organ involvement.
- Autoantibodies play a crucial role in diagnosis, and management requires a multidisciplinary team.
- SSc affects African American patients at an earlier age, with increased severity and with overall poorer outcomes than other groups.
- Cutaneous changes in SSc are difficult to treat and can cause significant psychological distress in skin of color patients.

INTRODUCTION

Scleroderma is a rare autoimmune connective tissue disorder characterized by chronic skin thickening and induration. Depending on the extent of involvement, scleroderma is divided into two major subtypes: localized (morphea and its variants) and systemic scleroderma (systemic sclerosis, SSc).[72] Several possible inciting factors like genetic predisposition, environmental triggers like silica, vaccinations, trauma, radiation, and autoimmunity have been proposed but the exact etiology for the onset of the disease remains unknown.[72] Autoantibodies play a major role in SSc diagnosis and prognosis. These include anti-topoisomerase I (anti-topo I), anticentromere antibodies (ACA), antibodies to ribonuclear proteins (U1-RNP, U3-RNP, anti-U11/U12 RNP), anti-RNA polymerase III, anti-nucleolar (anti-Th/To), and anti-PM/Scl (myositis overlap).[72,73] Genetically, HLA class-II complexes, HLA-DRB1*01, HLA-DRB1*11, HLA-A*30, and HLA-A*32 have significant association with increased susceptibility to SSc.[72,73] Ethnic differences in severity of SSc has been described, with African Americans and Hispanics showing severe cutaneous and systemic symptoms compared to Caucasians.[74,75] The difference in severity may be related to the underlying genetic predisposition and antibody profile. A case control study on three ethnic groups (African Americans, Hispanics, and Whites) showed HLA-DRB1*08 was more common in African Americans when compared to control matched local group, anti-RNP and anti-U3-RNP antibodies to be higher in African Americans, while ACA antibodies were higher in Whites.[76]

The development of sclerosis in scleroderma is a result of complex interplay between vascular endothelium damage, immune system activation, and fibroblast stimulation.[77] While the exact sequence of events is unclear, it is possible that the endothelial injury is an initial event that results in upregulation of adhesion molecules, release of chemokines, and activation of T- and B-cells.[77] The release of the cytokines, especially TGFβ and IL-4 among others, has shown to play a major role in the recruitment and activation of fibroblasts and their differentiation into myofibroblasts.[77] The activated myofibroblasts then lays down the excess collagen and extra cellular matrix seen in scleroderma.[77]

EPIDEMIOLOGY

Both localized and systemic scleroderma show female predominance, with 2.4 to 4:1 female to male ratio in morphea and 5:1 for systemic scleroderma.[78] Morphea appears to be more common in Whites compared to other ethnicities. A study on 245 adult and pediatric patients with morphea showed higher distribution in White patients (72.7%) compared to combined 27.3% in Hispanics, African American, Asian, and others.[79] Another study on 136 pediatric patients showed similar findings, with higher number of Caucasian patients (82%) compared to other ethnic groups.[78] SSc on the other hand shows significant racial differences in the severity of the disease manifestation in skin of color. A large multicenter cohort study on 1009 African American patients with systemic scleroderma reported a high prevalence of diffuse disease (57%) compared to 37% in cohort of 7000 patients of European ancestry.[80] A study involving 203 patients with systemic sclerosis showed African American ancestry to be an independent association for early pulmonary involvement and significantly higher rates of pulmonary fibrosis.[81] African Americans have been found to have early onset of scleroderma, more frequent systemic involvement, and overall poorer outcomes of the disease than other groups.[80] In one study, African Americans had 21% higher rate of death during follow up as compared to 11% in non-African Americans ($p = 0.005$).[82]

CLINICAL PRESENTATION

LOCALIZED SCLERODERMA

Localized scleroderma is limited to skin and underlying structures (muscle and bone). It is differentiated from SSc by the presence of asymmetric plaques, and absence of Raynaud and systemic involvement.[83] The most common clinical presentation of localized scleroderma is plaque type morphea.[83] Initial lesion presents as asymptomatic or mildly pruritic erythematous, yellowish or violaceous and edematous plaque with characteristic purple border [**Figure 37-25**].[83] The presence of purple border is a sign of underlying inflammation, thereby an indicator of disease activity.[83] In skin of color, the lesions can be hyperpigmented or hypopigmented (**Figures 37-26** and **37-27**). In deeply pigmented skin, when asymptomatic, early edematous stage can go unnoticed until the plaques develop induration and thickening.[84] The induration is better appreciated by palpation of the affected area in comparison to the adjacent skin. At later stages, the lesions develop central atrophy that clinically presents as shiny, thin, and wrinkled skin.[83]

Morphea has several subtypes depending on the distribution and depth of involvement [**Table 37-3**]. Generalized morphea presents as multiple expanding plaques of morphea, usually more than four plaques and can involve multiple anatomical sites.[85] Pansclerotic morphea is a severe and debilitating subtype involving larger body surface area and can affect bones and muscles.[86] It can mimic scleroderma when extensive, but typically spares toes and fingertips and does not have systemic involvement.[85] Linear morphea is commonly seen in children and can extend deep to involve muscle, bone, and joints leading to growth retardation and deformity of the affected limb.[85] Linear morphea of the face and scalp, known as en coup de sabre type, affects forehead and adjacent scalp causing scarring alopecia.[85] Parry Romberg is a severe linear variant that causes

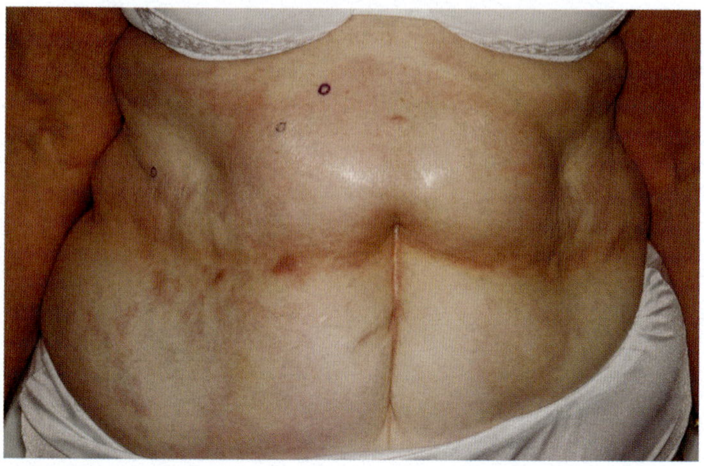

FIGURE 37-25. Erythematous plaque with lilac border in morphea involving the trunk.

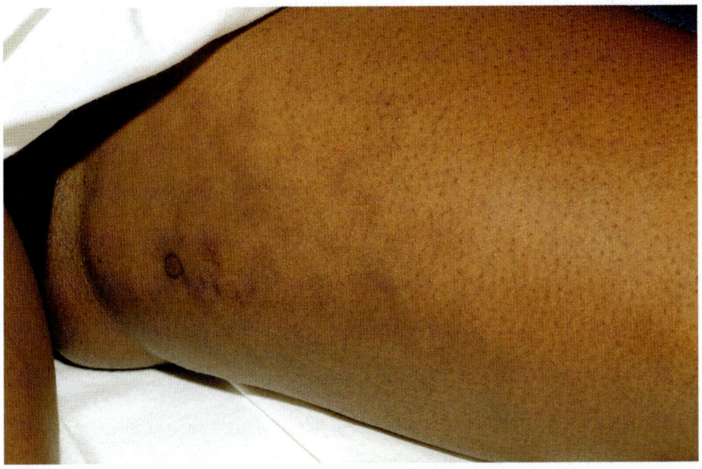

FIGURE 37-26. Hyperpigmented plaque of morphea involving medial thigh.

hemifacial atrophy with involvement of the underlying muscle, cartilage and osseous structures.[83,85] Guttate morphea is characterized by multiple small morphea lesions.[84] Keloidal morphea is clinically indistinguishable from keloids, and morphea profunda has sclerosis primarily of the deeper structures.[87,88] Lichen sclerosus et atophicus can sometimes occur in association with morphea.

SYSTEMIC SCLERODERMA

SSc is a multisystem autoimmune disease of skin and internal organs [**Table 37-4**]. Unlike morphea, the sclerosis of skin in SSc is usually symmetric in nature with accompanying other cutaneous findings of Raynaud phenomenon, telangiectasias, calcinosis, and ulcerations.[89] In limited SSc, sclerosis is limited to the fingers, hands, and face. In diffuse SSc, sclerosis extends beyond forearms to involve trunk and proximal extremities.[89]

Limited SSc is characterized by symmetric skin thickening of hands, extending to the MCP joints, affecting the movement of fingers CREST syndrome. A classic presentation of limited SSc comprises calcinosis cutis, Raynaud phenomenon, esophageal hypomotility, sclerodactyly, and telangiectasia, but variation from this presentation may occur.[90] Raynaud phenomenon is a common early presentation but is not pathognomonic for scleroderma. Typical phases and color changes of Raynaud phenomenon can be hard to appreciate in skin of color. At times, pigmentary changes can be the initial presentation of SSc in skin of color. In the early stages, fingers are puffy and edematous, subsequently leading to thickening and induration [**Figure 37-28A** and **B**].[89] Sclerodactyly and flexure contracture can be seen at later stages [**Figure 37-29**].[89] Digital ulcers are common and are a result of vascular compromise [**Figure 37-30**].[89] In severe cases, infarction and digital gangrene can occur. Matted telangiectasias are frequently seen on the face and extremities.[89] Facial skin may become bound down resulting in expressionless facies and a conspicuous lack of normal age-related wrinkling [**Figure 37-31**].[89] Microstomia, together with a pursed mouth, may be seen.[89]

SSc has been associated with a myriad of pigmentary changes including diffuse hyperpigmentation of the skin, areas of hyper- and hypopigmentation, vitiligo-like depigmentation with perifollicular hyperpigmentation (salt and pepper pigmentation), and reticular pigmentation [**Figure 37-32A-D**].[91] These changes are more prominent in skin of color and can be the initial presenting symptom. Pigmentary changes can also be seen in normal skin not affected by sclerosis.[92] These changes can cause significant psychological distress in skin of color patients.

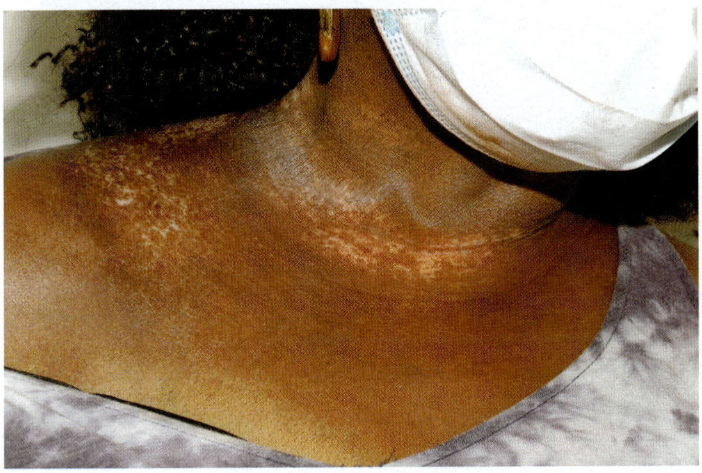

FIGURE 37-27. Hyperpigmented and hypopigmented sclerotic plaque of morphea involving lateral neck and chest.

TABLE 37-3 Types of scleroderma

Localized scleroderma/morphea	Plaque type Generalized Pansclerotic Guttate Linear Bullous Morphea profunda Nodular/keloidal En coup de sabre Parry Romberg
Systemic scleroderma	Limited/CREST Diffuse scleroderma

TABLE 37-4 Cutaneous manifestations of scleroderma

Skin sclerosis • Earliest changes—edema and erythema • Induration and thickening • Taut skin with decreased mobility
Fingers and hands • First affected • Puffy fingers at the early stages, nonpitting edema of the fingertips • Sclerosis of the digits • Sausage shaped digits • Decreased mobility • Flexure contractures • Digital ulcers • Capillary changes of the nail beds. Digital capillaroscopy shows disorganization, dilated capillaries, capillary dropout, hemorrhage • Telangiectasia
Face • Mask-like facies • Pursed lips • Microstomia • Matted telangiectasia • Thin lips and nose • Loss of skin folds with a waxy appearance
Pigmentation • Hyperpigmentation • Hypopigmentation • Salt and pepper pigmentation • Reticular pigmentation
Calcinosis cutis Raynaud phenomenon

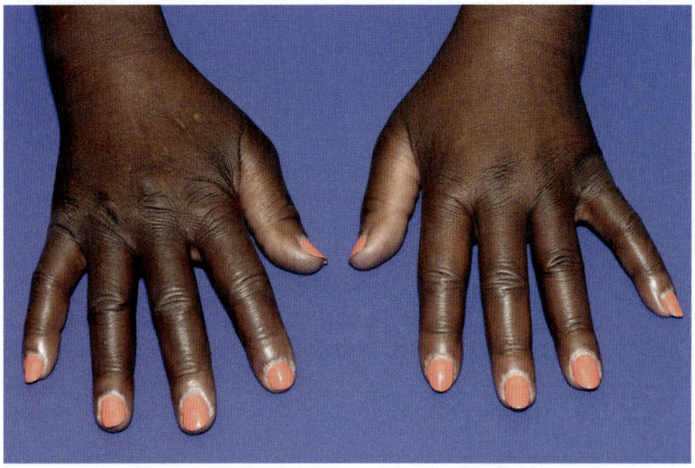

A

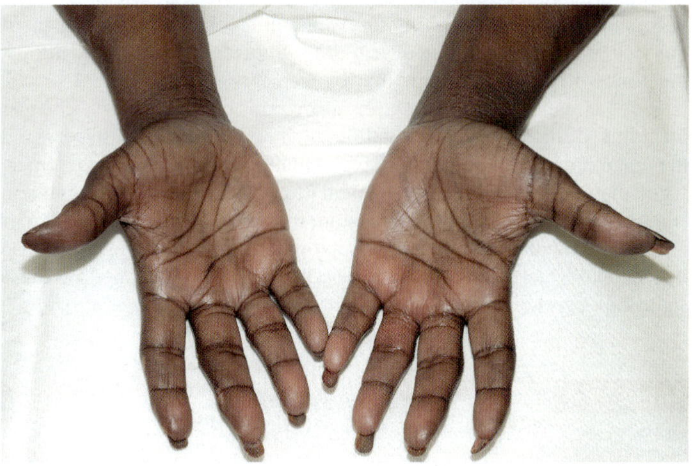

B

FIGURE 37-28. **(A** and **B)** Edematous fingers in a patient with systemic sclerosis.

Diffuse systemic scleroderma shares many of the same signs and symptoms of limited scleroderma but is notable for its progression and systemic organ involvement. Unlike limited systemic scleroderma, skin manifestations may extend beyond the distal extremities to involve proximal limb and trunk.[89] In addition to abovementioned cutaneous findings, internal organ involvement such as pulmonary hypertension, interstitial lung disease, cardiac fibrosis, and renal crisis may be present.[89] This often occurs at an earlier age with faster progression of symptoms

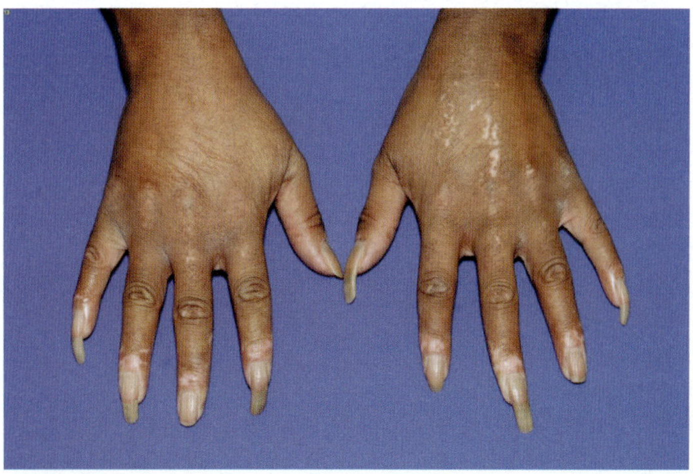

FIGURE 37-29. Sclerodactyly with parrot beak appearance of several fingernails. Vitiligo-like hypopigmentation of the dorsal hands and fingertips.

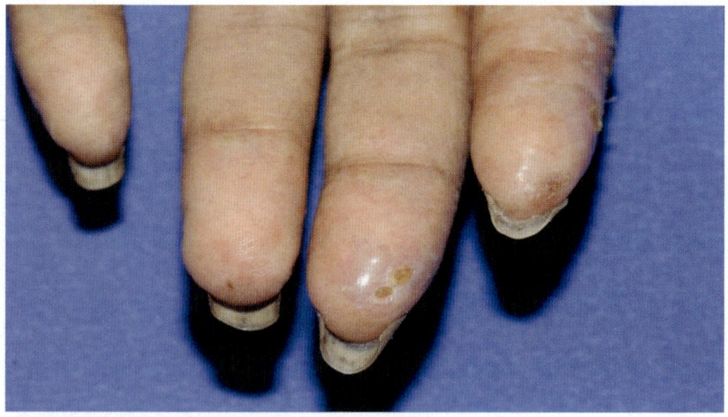

FIGURE 37-30. Digital ulcers involving the pulp of several fingers in scleroderma.

and poorer outcomes in African Americans.[80] Greater reductions in vital capacity, diffusion capacity, greater fibrosis of lung parenchyma, higher prevalence of pulmonary hypertension, and more severe cardiac involvement are common in this patient group.[82] Scleroderma renal crises can be life-threatening, presenting with oliguria, malignant hypertension, and microangiopathic hemolytic anemia.[90]

TREATMENT

Management of morphea depends on the activity, extent of the disease, and presence of any functional impairment. The exact course of the disease is hard to predict but most of the lesions tend to resolve after years.[93] Burnt out lesions can become active after several years of quiescence.[84] Limited cutaneous involvement is usually treated with topical corticosteroids, topical calcineurin inhibitors, topical calcipotriol, and phototherapy (NB-UVB, PUVA, UVA1).[94] Systemic therapy is usually indicated for generalized morphea, linear morphea, and morphea causing functional impairment including risk of contractures, joint mobility,

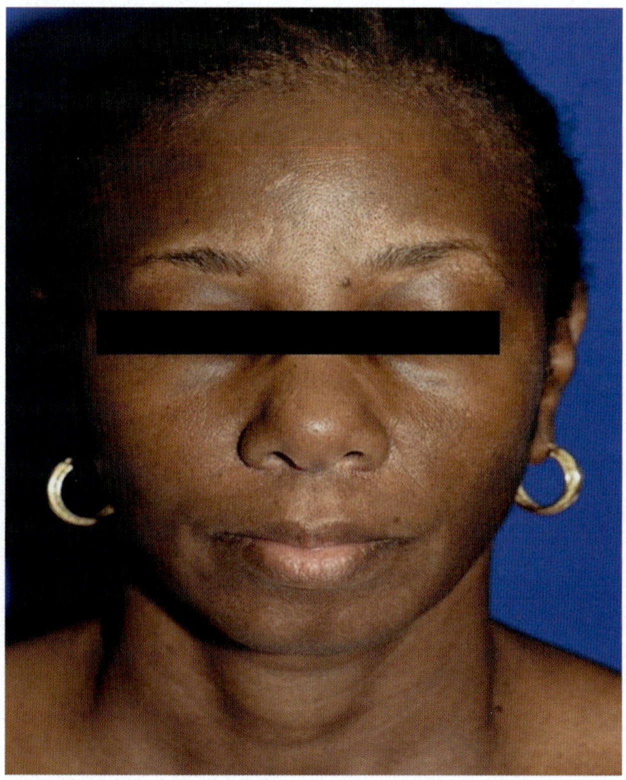

FIGURE 37-31. Expressionless facies with eyebrow hypopigmentation and pursed mouth.

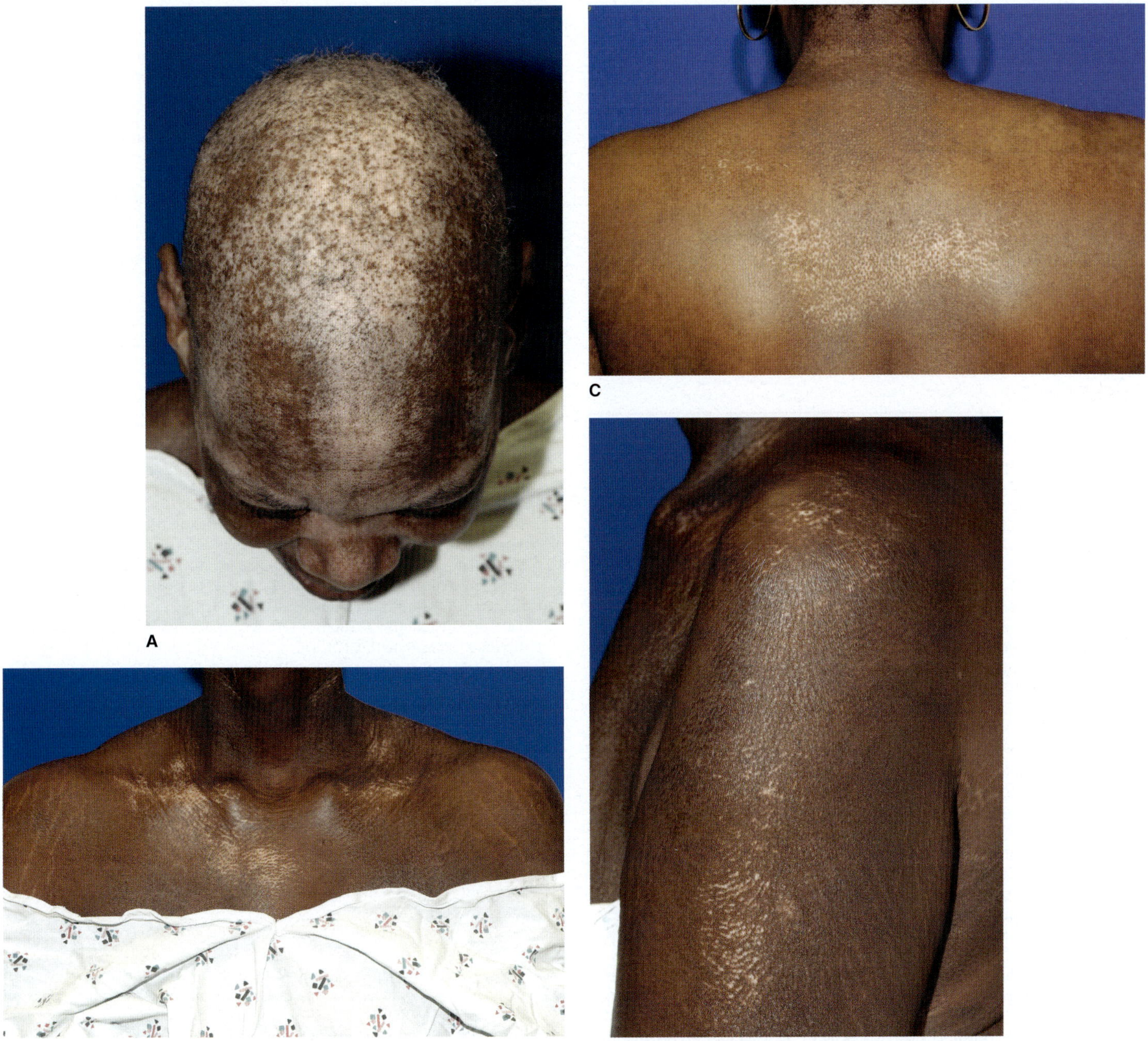

A B C D

FIGURE 37-32. (A-D) Diffuse hyperpigmentation with vitiligo-like depigmentation with perifollicular hyperpigmentation (salt and pepper pigmentation) on scalp, upper arm, chest, and back.

or facial deformity.[93] Methotrexate (15-20 mg weekly) alone or in combination with short course of oral steroids (1mg/kg/day) is usually first-line systemic agent used for morphea.[94] Patients are closely monitored, and treatment modified accordingly. Mycophenolate mofetil (2-3 g/day) can be considered as a second-line treatment.[94] Other systemic options trialed include hydroxychloroquine (5 mg/kg/day; 400 mg/day), cyclosporine (2.5-5 mg/kg/day), extracorporeal photopheresis, and recently tocilizumab (162 mg SC weekly).[86] Combined topical, systemic and phototherapy can be considered in severe cases.

SSc is a complex disease managed by multidisciplinary team. Pulmonary function tests, at-home blood pressure monitoring, and renal function tests should be conducted at regular intervals to monitor disease progression.[89] Gastrointestinal involvement should be assessed with symptom-based investigations and cardiac manifestations should be monitored with echocardiography and electrocardiogram.[89]

For management of Raynaud phenomenon, lifestyle changes should be discussed with the patient including keeping fingers warm, cold avoidance, smoking cessation, and avoidance of vasoconstrictive drugs.[95] For severe Raynaud and vascular complications, pharmacotherapy can be considered including topical nifedipine, topical nitrate, oral calcium channel blockers, phosphodiesterase-5 inhibitors, prostacyclin analogs, and endothelin receptor antagonists.[95,96] Botulinum toxin injection at the base of fingers is an effective treatment for severe Raynaud phenomenon refractory to conventional treatment. For cutaneous calcinosis, treatment options include surgical excision, calcium channel blockers, minocycline, and bisphosphonates.[97-100] Patients are usually co-managed with other specialities. Cutaneous pigmentary changes can be prominent and particularly bothersome in skin of color patients. Treatment is difficult and changes can be permanent. General measures such as strict sun protection using suncreens, UV protective clothing, hats, sunglasses, and sun avoidance during peak hours (10 AM to 2 PM) should be discussed.

For hyperpigmented patches on cosmetically bothersome areas like face, bleaching agents such as hydroquinone cream can be considered. Patients should be warned about the risk of ochronosis with prolonged use.[101] In an open label study involving 12 patients, treatment with topical calcipotriene showed improvement of dyspigmentation that can be considered as an option.[102] While phototherapy is commonly used to treat vitiligo, there is no robust data available for its use in hypopigmented or vitiligo-like patches of scleroderma. A case report on repigmentation following natural sunlight exposure was reported but its role in clinical practice has not been tested widely.[103] Also, use of phototherapy can potentially worsen background hyperpigmentation.[104] Data on the role of lasers in management of dyspigmentation are limited at this time but an area for future exploration. Lasers and light-based devices such as pulsed dye laser and intense pulsed light are used to treat matted telangiectasia of face effectively.[105]

REFERENCES

1. Aringer M, Costenbader K, Daikh D, et al. 2019 European League against rheumatism/American College of Rheumatology classification criteria for systemic lupus erythematosus. *Arthritis Rheumatol.* 2019;71(9):1400-1412.
2. Little AJ, Vesely MD. Cutaneous lupus erythematosus: current and future pathogenesis-directed therapies. *Yale J Biol Med.* 2020;93(1):81-95.
3. Patsinakidis N, Wenzel J, Landmann A, et al. Suppression of UV-induced damage by a liposomal sunscreen: a prospective, open-label study in patients with cutaneous lupus erythematosus and healthy controls. *Exp Dermatol.* 2012;21(12):958-961.
4. Biazar C, Sigges J, Patsinakidis N, et al. Cutaneous lupus erythematosus: first multicenter database analysis of 1002 patients from the European Society of Cutaneous Lupus Erythematosus (EUSCLE). *Autoimmun Rev.* 2013;12(3):444-454.
5. Foering K, Chang AY, Piette EW, Cucchiara A, Okawa J, Werth VP. Characterization of clinical photosensitivity in cutaneous lupus erythematosus. *J Am Acad Dermatol.* 2013;69(2):205-213.
6. Zahn S, Graef M, Patsinakidis N, et al. Ultraviolet light protection by a sunscreen prevents interferon-driven skin inflammation in cutaneous lupus erythematosus. *Exp Dermatol.* 2014;23(7):516-518.
7. Liu Y, Xu M, Min X, et al. TWEAK/Fn14 activation participates in ro52-mediated photosensitization in cutaneous lupus erythematosus. *Front Immunol.* 2017;8:651.
8. Piette EW, Foering KP, Chang AY, et al. Impact of smoking in cutaneous lupus erythematosus. *Arch Dermatol.* 2012;148(3):317-322.
9. Hersh AO, Arkin LM, Prahalad S. Immunogenetics of cutaneous lupus erythematosus. *Curr Opin Pediatr.* 2016;28(4):470-475.
10. O'Brien JC, Chong BF. Not just skin deep: systemic disease involvement in patients with cutaneous lupus. *J Investig Dermatol Symp Proc.* 2017;18(2): S69-S74.
11. Joseph AK, Windsor B, Hynan LS, Chong BF. Discoid lupus erythematosus skin lesion distribution and characteristics in Black patients: a retrospective cohort study. *Lupus Sci Med.* 2021;8(1):e000514.
12. Durosaro O, Davis MD, Reed KB, Rohlinger AL. Incidence of cutaneous lupus erythematosus, 1965-2005: a population-based study. *Arch Dermatol.* 2009;145(3):249-253.
13. Gronhagen CM, Fored CM, Granath F, Nyberg F. Cutaneous lupus erythematosus and the association with systemic lupus erythematosus: a population-based cohort of 1088 patients in Sweden. *Br J Dermatol.* 2011;164(6): 1335-1341.
14. Kunzler E, Hynan LS, Chong BF. Autoimmune diseases in patients with cutaneous lupus erythematosus. *JAMA Dermatol.* 2018;154(6):712-716.
15. Jarrett P, Thornley S, Scragg R. Ethnic differences in the epidemiology of cutaneous lupus erythematosus in New Zealand. *Lupus.* 2016;25(13):1497-1502.
16. Stojan G, Petri M. Epidemiology of systemic lupus erythematosus: an update. *Curr Opin Rheumatol.* 2018;30(2):144-150.
17. Uribe AG, McGwin G, Jr, Reveille JD, Alarcon GS. What have we learned from a 10-year experience with the LUMINA (Lupus in Minorities; Nature vs. nurture) cohort? Where are we heading? *Autoimmun Rev.* 2004;3:321-329.
18. Okon LG WV. Cutaneous lupus erythematosus: diagnosis and treatment. *Best Pract Res Clin Rheumatol.* 2013;27(3):391-404.
19. Uva L, Miguel D, Pinheiro C, Freitas JP, Marques Gomes M, Filipe P. Cutaneous manifestations of systemic lupus erythematosus. *Autoimmune Dis.* 2012; 2012:834291.
20. Koch K, Tikly M. Spectrum of cutaneous lupus erythematosus in South Africans with systemic lupus erythematosus. *Lupus.* 2019;28(8):1021-1026.
21. Sontheimer RD. Subacute cutaneous lupus erythematosus: 25-year evolution of a prototypic subset (subphenotype) of lupus erythematosus defined by characteristic cutaneous, pathological, immunological, and genetic findings. *Autoimmun Rev.* 2005;4(5):253-263.
22. Sontheimer RD, Thomas JR, Gilliam JN. Subacute cutaneous lupus erythematosus: a cutaneous marker for a distinct lupus erythematosus subset. *Arch Dermatol.* 1979;115(12):1409-1415.
23. Lowe GC, Henderson CL, Grau RH, Hansen CB, Sontheimer RD. A systematic review of drug-induced subacute cutaneous lupus erythematosus. *Br J Dermatol.* 2011;164(3):465-472.
24. Lee, Lela A., and Victoria P. Werth. "Lupus Erythematosus." *Dermatology*, edited by Jean L. Bolognia, 5th ed., Elsevier, 2018, pp. 670-688. Amsterdam, Netherlands.
25. Gronhagen CM, Fored CM, Linder M, Granath F, Nyberg F. Subacute cutaneous lupus erythematosus and its association with drugs: a population-based matched case-control study of 234 patients in Sweden. *Br J Dermatol.* 2012;167(2):296-305.
26. Jarrett P, Werth VP. A review of cutaneous lupus erythematosus: improving outcomes with a multidisciplinary approach. *J Multidiscip Healthc.* 2019;12:419-428.
27. Patel P, Werth V. Cutaneous lupus erythematosus: a review. *Dermatol Clin.* 2002;20(3):373-385.
28. McDaniel B, Sukumaran S, Koritala T, Tanner LS. *Discoid Lupus Erythematosus.* StatPearls; 2022. Treasure Island (FL)): StatPearls Publishing.
29. Alsanafi S, Werth VP. Squamous cell carcinomas arising in discoid lupus erythematosus scars: unusual occurrence in an African-American and in a sun-protected area. *J Clin Rheumatol.* 2011;17(1):35-36.
30. Shapera EA, Kim PD. Squamous cell cancer arising in an African American male cheek from discoid lupus: a rare case and review of the literature. *Case Rep Surg.* 2016;2016:9170424.
31. Shetty VM, Subramaniam K, Rao R. Utility of immunofluorescence in dermatology. *Indian Dermatol Online J.* 2017;8(1):1-8.
32. Magro CM, Crowson AN, Harrist TJ. Atypical lymphoid infiltrates arising in cutaneous lesions of connective tissue disease. *Am J Dermatopathol.* 1997;19(5):446-455.
33. Sarantopoulos GP, Palla B, Said J, et al. Mimics of cutaneous lymphoma: report of the 2011 Society for Hematopathology/European Association for Haematopathology workshop. *Am J Clin Pathol.* 2013;139(4):536-551.
34. Tan EM, Cohen AS, Fries JF, et al. The 1982 revised criteria for the classification of systemic lupus erythematosus. *Arthritis Rheum.* 1982;25(11):1271-1277.
35. Babaoglu H, Li J, Goldman D, Magder LS, Petri M. Predictors of predominant Lupus Low Disease Activity State (LLDAS-50). *Lupus.* 2019;28(14):1648-1655.
36. Lea JP. Lupus nephritis in African Americans. *Am J Med Sci.* 2002;323(2): 85-89.
37. Williams EM, Bruner L, Adkins A, et al. I too, am America: a review of research on systemic lupus erythematosus in African-Americans. *Lupus Sci Med.* 2016;3(1):e000144.
38. Dumbuya H, Grimes PE, Lynch S, et al. Impact of iron-oxide containing formulations against visible light-induced skin pigmentation in skin of color individuals. *J Drugs Dermatol.* 2020;19(7):712-717.
39. Word AP, Perese F, Tseng LC, Adams-Huet B, Olsen NJ, Chong BF. 25-Hydroxyvitamin D levels in African-American and Caucasian/Hispanic subjects with cutaneous lupus erythematosus. *Br J Dermatol.* 2012;166(2): 372-379.
40. Ernste FC, Reed AM. Idiopathic inflammatory myopathies: current trends in pathogenesis, clinical features, and up-to-date treatment recommendations. *Mayo Clin Proc.* 2013;88(1):83-105.
41. Babool S, Bhai SF, Sanderson C, Salter A, Christopher-Stine L. Racial disparities in skin tone representation of dermatomyositis rashes: a systematic review. *Rheumatology (Oxford).* 2022;61(6):2255-2261.
42. Lester JC, Taylor SC, Chren MM. Under-representation of skin of colour in dermatology images: not just an educational issue. *Br J Dermatol.* 2019;180(6):1521-1522.
43. O'Hanlon TP, Rider LG, Mamyrova G, et al. HLA polymorphisms in African Americans with idiopathic inflammatory myopathy: allelic profiles distinguish patients with different clinical phenotypes and myositis autoantibodies. *Arthritis Rheum.* 2006;54(11):3670-3681.
44. Gao X, Han L, Yuan L, et al. HLA class II alleles may influence susceptibility to adult dermatomyositis and polymyositis in a Han Chinese population. *BMC Dermatol.* 2014;14:9.
45. Adler BL, Christopher-Stine L. Triggers of inflammatory myopathy: insights into pathogenesis. *Discov Med.* 2018;25(136):75-83.

46. Bax CE, Maddukuri S, Ravishankar A, Pappas-Taffer L, Werth VP. Environmental triggers of dermatomyositis: a narrative review. *Ann Transl Med.* 2021;9(5):434.
47. Holzer MT, Krusche M, Ruffer N, et al. New-onset dermatomyositis following SARS-CoV-2 infection and vaccination: a case-based review. *Rheumatol Int.* 2022;42(12):2267-2276.
48. Dourmishev AL, Dourmishev LA. Dermatomyositis and drugs. *Adv Exp Med Biol.* 1999;455:187-191.
49. Seidler AM, Gottlieb AB. Dermatomyositis induced by drug therapy: a review of case reports. *J Am Acad Dermatol.* 2008;59(5):872-880.
50. Sheik Ali S, Goddard AL, Luke JJ, et al. Drug-associated dermatomyositis following ipilimumab therapy: a novel immune-mediated adverse event associated with cytotoxic T-lymphocyte antigen 4 blockade. *JAMA Dermatol.* 2015;151(2):195-199.
51. Na SJ, Kim SM, Sunwoo IN, Choi YC. Clinical characteristics and outcomes of juvenile and adult dermatomyositis. *J Korean Med Sci.* 2009;24(4):715-721.
52. Bendewald MJ, Wetter DA, Li X, Davis MD. Incidence of dermatomyositis and clinically amyopathic dermatomyositis: a population-based study in Olmsted County, Minnesota. *Arch Dermatol.* 2010;146(1):26-30.
53. Oddis CV, Conte CG, Steen VD, Medsger TA, Jr. Incidence of polymyositis-dermatomyositis: a 20-year study of hospital diagnosed cases in Allegheny County, PA 1963-1982. *J Rheumatol.* 1990;17(10):1329-1334.
54. Cheeti A, Brent LH, Panginikkod S. Autoimmune Myopathies. StatPearls; 2022. Treasure Island (FL): StatPearls Publishing.
55. Kwa MC, Ardalan K, Laumann AE, Silverberg JI. Predictors of hospitalization, length of stay, and cost of care among adults with dermatomyositis in the United States. *Arthritis Care Res (Hoboken).* 2017;69(9):1391-1399.
56. Liu WC, Ho M, Koh WP, et al. An 11-year review of dermatomyositis in Asian patients. *Ann Acad Med Singap.* 2010;39(11):843-847.
57. Bogdanov I, Kazandjieva J, Darlenski R, Tsankov N. Dermatomyositis: current concepts. *Clin Dermatol.* 2018;36(4):450-458.
58. Elmansour I, Chiheb S, Benchikhi H. Nail changes in connective tissue diseases: a study of 39 cases. *Pan Afr Med J.* 2014;18:150.
59. Ang CC, Anyanwu CO, Robinson E, et al. Clinical signs associated with an increased risk of interstitial lung disease: a retrospective study of 101 patients with dermatomyositis. *Br J Dermatol.* 2017;176(1):231-233.
60. Mutasim DF, Egesi A, Spicknall KE. Wong-type dermatomyositis: a mimic of many dermatoses. *J Cutan Pathol.* 2016;43(9):781-786.
61. Kassamali B, Mazori DR, LaChance AH, Christopher-Stine L. Exploring dermatomyositis through an interdisciplinary lens: pearls from dermatology and rheumatology. *Int J Womens Dermatol.* 2021;7(5Part A):576-582.
62. Mehta P, Machado PM, Gupta L. Understanding and managing anti-MDA 5 dermatomyositis, including potential COVID-19 mimicry. *Rheumatol Int.* 2021;41(6):1021-1036.
63. Waldman R, DeWane ME, Lu J. Dermatomyositis: diagnosis and treatment. *J Am Acad Dermatol.* 2020;82(2):283-296.
64. Smith ES, Hallman JR, DeLuca AM, Goldenberg G, Jorizzo JL, Sangueza OP. Dermatomyositis: a clinicopathological study of 40 patients. *Am J Dermatopathol.* 2009;31(1):61-67.
65. Khanna U, Galimberti F, Li Y, Fernandez AP. Dermatomyositis and malignancy: should all patients with dermatomyositis undergo malignancy screening? *Ann Transl Med.* 2021;9(5):432.
66. Qiang JK, Kim WB, Baibergenova A, Alhusayen R. Risk of malignancy in dermatomyositis and polymyositis. *J Cutan Med Surg.* 2017;21(2):131-136.
67. Vij R, Strek ME. Diagnosis and treatment of connective tissue disease-associated interstitial lung disease. *Chest.* 2013;143(3):814-824.
68. Ikeda S, Arita M, Morita M, et al. Interstitial lung disease in clinically amyopathic dermatomyositis with and without anti-MDA-5 antibody: to lump or split? *BMC Pulm Med.* 2015;15:159.
69. Chen Z, Cao M, Plana MN, et al. Utility of anti-melanoma differentiation-associated gene 5 antibody measurement in identifying patients with dermatomyositis and a high risk for developing rapidly progressive interstitial lung disease: a review of the literature and a meta-analysis. *Arthritis Care Res (Hoboken).* 2013;65(8):1316-1324.
70. Schultz HY, Dutz JP, Furukawa F, et al. From pathogenesis, epidemiology, and genetics to definitions, diagnosis, and treatments of cutaneous lupus erythematosus and dermatomyositis: a report from the 3rd International Conference on Cutaneous Lupus Erythematosus (ICCLE) 2013. *J Invest Dermatol.* 2015;135(1):7-12.
71. Kurasawa K, Arai S, Namiki Y, et al. Tofacitinib for refractory interstitial lung diseases in anti-melanoma differentiation-associated 5 gene antibody-positive dermatomyositis. *Rheumatology (Oxford).* 2018;57(12):2114-2119.
72. Dumoitier N, Lofek S, Mouthon L. Pathophysiology of systemic sclerosis: state of the art in 2014. *Presse Med.* 2014;43(10 Pt 2):e267-e278.
73. Peoples C, Medsger TA, Jr., Lucas M, Rosario BL, Feghali-Bostwick CA. Gender differences in systemic sclerosis: relationship to clinical features, serologic status and outcomes. *J Scleroderma Relat Disord.* 2016;1(2):177-240.
74. Gelber AC, Manno RL, Shah AA, et al. Race and association with disease manifestations and mortality in scleroderma: a 20-year experience at the Johns Hopkins Scleroderma Center and review of the literature. *Medicine (Baltimore).* 2013;92(4):191-205.
75. Amoda O, Ravat V, Datta S, Saroha B, Patel RS. Trends in demographics, hospitalization outcomes, comorbidities, and mortality risk among systemic sclerosis patients. *Cureus.* 2018;10(5):e2628.
76. Reveille JD, Fischbach M, McNearney T, et al. Systemic sclerosis in 3 US ethnic groups: a comparison of clinical, sociodemographic, serologic, and immunogenetic determinants. *Semin Arthritis Rheum.* 2001;30(5):332-346.
77. Pattanaik D, Brown M, Postlethwaite BC, Postlethwaite AE. Pathogenesis of systemic sclerosis. *Front Immunol.* 2015;6:272.
78. Christen-Zaech S, Hakim MD, Afsar FS, Paller AS. Pediatric morphea (localized scleroderma): review of 136 patients. *J Am Acad Dermatol.* 2008;59(3):385-396.
79. Leitenberger JJ, Cayce RL, Haley RW, Adams-Huet B, Bergstresser PR, Jacobe HT. Distinct autoimmune syndromes in morphea: a review of 245 adult and pediatric cases. *Arch Dermatol.* 2009;145(5):545-550.
80. Morgan ND, Shah AA, Mayes MD, et al. Clinical and serological features of systemic sclerosis in a multicenter African American cohort: analysis of the genome research in African American scleroderma patients clinical database. *Medicine (Baltimore).* 2017;96(51):e8980.
81. Steen V, Domsic RT, Lucas M, Fertig N, Medsger TA, Jr. A clinical and serologic comparison of African American and Caucasian patients with systemic sclerosis. *Arthritis Rheum.* 2012;64(9):2986-2994.
82. Moore DF, Kramer E, Eltaraboulsi R, Steen VD. Increased morbidity and mortality of scleroderma in African Americans compared to non-African Americans. *Arthritis Care Res (Hoboken).* 2019;71(9):1154-1163.
83. Careta MF, Romiti R. Localized scleroderma: clinical spectrum and therapeutic update. *An Bras Dermatol.* 2015;90(1):62-73.
84. George R, George A, Kumar TS. Update on management of morphea (localized scleroderma) in children. *Indian Dermatol Online J.* 2020;11(2):135-145.
85. Laxer RM, Zulian F. Localized scleroderma. *Curr Opin Rheumatol.* 2006;18(6):606-613.
86. Zhang A, Nocton J, Chiu Y. A case of pansclerotic morphea treated with tocilizumab. *JAMA Dermatol.* 2019;155(3):388-389.
87. Savoia P, Zaccagna A, Bernengo MG. Guess what? Inflammatory disseminated morphea profunda. *Eur J Dermatol.* 1999;9(8):654-656.
88. Labandeira J, Leon-Mateos A, Suarez-Penaranda JM, Garea MT, Toribio J. What is nodular-keloidal scleroderma? *Dermatology.* 2003;207(2):130-132.
89. Sobolewski P, Maslinska M, Wieczorek M, et al. Systemic sclerosis - multidisciplinary disease: clinical features and treatment. *Reumatologia.* 2019;57(4):221-233.
90. Denton CP, Khanna D. Systemic sclerosis. *Lancet.* 2017;390(10103):1685-1699.
91. Chuamanochan M, Haws AL, Pattanaprichakul P. Reticulate hyperpigmentation in systemic sclerosis: a case report and review of the literature. *J Med Case Rep.* 2015;9:219.
92. Pope JE, Shum DT, Gottschalk R, Stevens A, McManus R. Increased pigmentation in scleroderma. *J Rheumatol.* 1996;23(11):1912-1916.
93. Fett NM. Morphea: evidence-based recommendations for treatment. *Indian J Dermatol Venereol Leprol.* 2012;78(2):135-141.
94. Zwischenberger BA, Jacobe HT. A systematic review of morphea treatments and therapeutic algorithm. *J Am Acad Dermatol.* 2011;65(5):925-941.
95. Bolster MB, Maricq HR, Leff RL. Office evaluation and treatment of Raynaud's phenomenon. *Cleve Clin J Med.* 1995;62(1):51-61.
96. Kowal-Bielecka O, Fransen J, Avouac J, et al. Update of EULAR recommendations for the treatment of systemic sclerosis. *Ann Rheum Dis.* 2017;76(8):1327-1339.
97. Mendelson BC, Linscheid RL, Dobyns JH, Muller SA. Surgical treatment of calcinosis cutis in the upper extremity. *J Hand Surg Am.* 1977;2(4):318-324.
98. Robertson LP, Marshall RW, Hickling P. Treatment of cutaneous calcinosis in limited systemic sclerosis with minocycline. *Ann Rheum Dis.* 2003;62(3):267-269.
99. Palamaras I, Kyriakis K. Calcium antagonists in dermatology: a review of the evidence and research-based studies. *Dermatol Online J.* 2005;11(2):8.
100. Rauch L, Hein R, Biedermann T, Eyerich K, Lauffer F. Bisphosphonates for the treatment of calcinosis cutis-a retrospective single-center study. *Biomedicines.* 2021;9(11):1698.
101. Gandhi V, Verma P, Naik G. Exogenous ochronosis after prolonged use of topical hydroquinone (2%) in a 50-year-old Indian female. *Indian J Dermatol.* 2012;57(5):394-395.

102. Cunningham BB, Landells ID, Langman C, Sailer DE, Paller AS. Topical calcipotriene for morphea/linear scleroderma. *J Am Acad Dermatol.* 1998;39(2 Pt 1):211-215.

103. Freiman A, Khanna M, Muhn CY, Billick RC. Ultraviolet autorepigmentation in scleroderma. *J Am Acad Dermatol.* 2003;49(5):960-961.

104. Hassani J, Feldman SR. Phototherapy in scleroderma. *Dermatol Ther (Heidelb).* 2016;6(4):519-553.

105. Goldman MP, Fitzpatrick RE. Pulsed-dye laser treatment of leg telangiectasia: with and without simultaneous sclerotherapy. *J Dermatol Surg Oncol.* 1990;16(4):338-344.

CHAPTER 38

Dermatoses in Africa

Ncoza C. Dlova
Anisa Mosam
Gail Todd
Bwanali Haji Ntaibu Jereni
San Honde
Adebola Ogunbiyi

KEY POINTS

- A diverse array of cutaneous conditions may be encountered in Africa that are often poorly represented in the commonly prescribed dermatology texts. A selection of some of these common and unique local disorders are highlighted.
- Interaction with a large variety of insects is common on the African continent resulting in bites, stings, skin irritation, infestations and systemic disease. The *Paederus* rove beetle causes irritant dermatitis when body fluids contact unprotected skin. Infestations such as myiasis (fly larvae) and tungiasis (sand fleas) are due to parasites invading the normal skin. Schistosomiasis (bilharzia), a water-borne parasitic infection with a snail intermediate host, and African trypanosomiasis a vector-borne parasitic disease transmitted by a bite from infected tsetse flies are systemic infections.
- Practices and habits frequently encountered in African populations including scarification and the role of photoprotection are discussed relative to South African populations.
- Settler colonists introduced founder genodermatoses such as keratolytic winter erythema.
- Some skin conditions appear unique to the continent. Dermatitis cruris pustulosa et atrophicans presents as folliculitis of unknown etiology and is found across central Africa. Onyalai thought to be related to food contaminated by certain fungi may result in outbreaks of hemorrhagic blisters of the mucosa and skin especially in southern Africa.

INTRODUCTION

A diverse array of cutaneous diseases may be encountered in Africa that may be infectious in etiology, related to environmental and climatic factors, or due to dietary or cultural practices. Some of the more unique and sometimes common disorders are highlighted in this section illustrating these etiologies. Schistosomiasis (bilharzia) is a systemic water-borne parasitic infection with a snail intermediate host, while African trypanosomiasis is a systemic vector-borne parasitic disease that is transmitted by a bite from infected tsetse flies. Infestations such as myiasis (fly larvae) and tungiasis (sand fleas) are due to parasites invading the normal skin. Interaction with a variety of insects is common on the African continent resulting in bites and stings. The *Paederus* rove beetle causes irritant dermatitis when body fluids contact unprotected skin. Practices and habits frequent in African populations including scarification and the role of photoprotection are discussed relative to South African populations. Dermatitis cruris pustulosa *et* atrophicans of predominantly tibial skin presents as folliculitis of unknown etiology and is found across central Africa. Onyalai thought to be related to food contaminated by certain fungi may result in outbreaks of hemorrhagic blisters of the mucosa and skin especially in southern Africa. A founder genodermatoses (keratolytic winter erythema) of the extremities described in South African families of Afrikaner descent is found in South Africa.

SUN PROTECTION IN SOUTH AFRICA

In hot, sunny climates as experienced in Durban, South Africa, photoprotective measures are required year-round for prevention of sun burn and pigmentation, irrespective of skin phototype. Indigenous African women, particularly those from rural areas, use local clay material for photoprotection. These women follow a subsistence lifestyle and are outdoors for many hours each day, gardening, fetching wood and water, cooking, and performing other chores. They also lack the means to purchase commercial sunscreen products. Although they typically present with Fitzpatrick Skin Types 5 and 6, for which skin cancer is less common, photoprotection is important to prevent hyperpigmentation disorders such as melasma.

Clay materials are widely used in the pharmaceutical industry for a variety of purposes in oral and topical applications, as excipients and in aesthetic medicine.[1] They have been used since ancient times,[1] so it is not surprising that they form part of the heritage in Southern Africa. Because clay is opaque, it serves as a physical shield against UV and visible light. Two clays are typically used: one white in appearance and the other red. The white clay is known locally as *umcaku* (isiZulu/isiXhosa), and the red as *ibomvu* (isiZulu/isiXhosa).

Clay analysis undertaken by Dlova et al showed that the clays typically used in rural parts of South Africa for UV protection consist chiefly of the mineral kaolinite.[2] Traditionally, clay soils rich in this mineral are widely used in Southern Africa for a variety of medicinal purposes because they exhibit low toxicity. Although the SPF of both clays was found to be low, they do provide some degree of UVA protection. This is an important consideration, since UVA constitutes the greater amount of incident solar radiation and has been implicated in skin cancer. These clays provide a cost-effective, easily available, and culturally appropriate product for rural South African women [**Figure 38-1**]. Although the

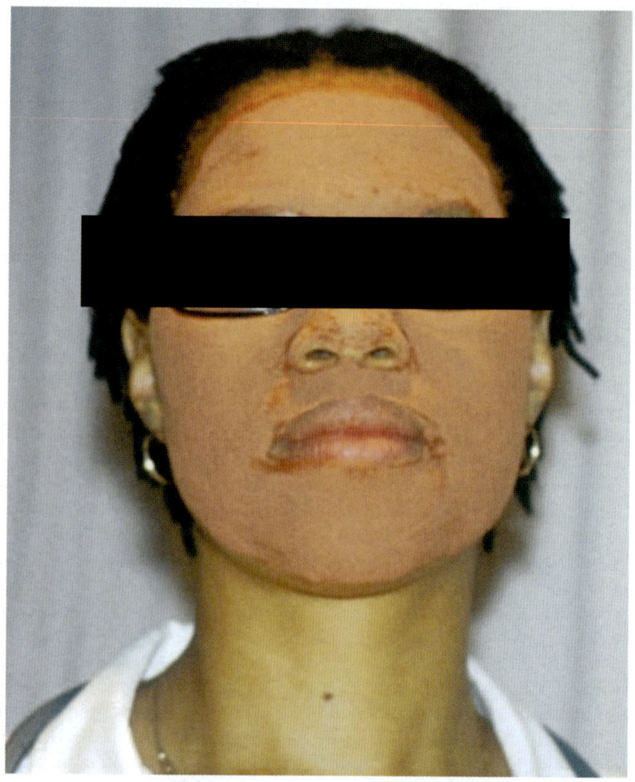

FIGURE 38-1. Red clay (*ibomvu*) used on the face as sunscreen by rural African women.

study did not consider the safety profile of these clays, the indigenous women who had used these clays for decades never reported any cutaneous side effects apart from a residual orange hue on the skin. Given the difficulty in finding suitable photostable and nontoxic organic sunscreen absorbers, greater consideration should be given to the potential of clays as additives for sun-protection creams.

SCARIFICATION AND TRIBAL MARKINGS IN AFRICA

Body modification is a very common form of body adornment and has been performed for a number of reasons in numerous societies. A myriad of ancient as well as current forms of body modifications are in existence. There are a number of reported uses of body and skin modifications including branding, ear shaping, scarification, and tattooing, as well as modern plastic and aesthetic surgery. Of note, body modification, particularly tattooing as compared to scarification, has become increasingly frequent in industrialized countries: approximately one-third of U.S. citizens wear tattoos, with considerable social acceptance. The skin depicts a lot about who we are and demarcates an obvious boundary between ourselves and the environment, conveying and showing signals and messages to those who understand their meaning. Moreover, scarification and tattooing in ethnic groups may demonstrate cultural marks and inscriptions of a person's "social skin."[3] In the anthropology field, the evolution and alteration of skin-associated messages into the informed perception of individuals, communities, ethnic groups, and societies has long been an important issue.[3]

A number of methods are used to create scarification, some through lacerations and cuts of the skin using a variety of instruments like blades, knives, metal, etc. Others make use of fire creating burns and branding, use chemicals and a variety of other techniques. Although the general acceptance of scarification's appears to be waning with time, a number of population groups in Africa, Asia, South America, Australia, and New Zealand still practice skin scarification.

Numerous communicable and noncommunicable complications of scarification have been reported, including hypertrophy, keloids, infections, and sarcoidosis. In Ghana, rapid progression of filarial elephantiasis caused by *Wuchereria bancrofti* has been reported as a risk factor.[4] In rural and traditional villages, unsterile instruments are frequently used for tribal decorations. Unsanitized objects are also applied and massaged into the wounds to enhance wound healing, thus predisposing to both bacterial and viral (HIV, hepatitis) infections.

Interestingly, a number of published works have reported scarification as a common practice predominantly among people of lower socioeconomic status. It has also been recorded that only 10.5% of individuals with scarification would accept scarification or tribal marks if they were requested to do so again.[5]

Numerous indigenous ethnicities in sub-Saharan Africa practice tribal scarring as a common custom. Most of this is performed during early childhood when affected patients have no say in the matter; however, the cosmetic repercussions of scarring in adulthood cannot be underestimated as many more patients seek ways of removing the scars that were inflicted as part of the custom [**Figure 38-2A** and **B**]. As much as we respect culture and individual customs, our recommendations would be to be intentional in educating the communities to use sterile instruments and settings, to obtain consent, and to avoid these in children who have no say at the time [Figure 38-2B and **C**].[6]

OUDTSHOORN DISEASE (KERATOLYTIC WINTER ERYTHEMA)

Oudtshoorn disease is a genodermatosis initially described in 1977 in South African families, linked to inhabitants of the Western Cape.

The disease is transmitted as autosomal dominant, linked to a founder in France, due to a mutation in the intergenic region of chromosome.[7] It presents as erythema on the palms and soles, blisters with centrifugal, cyclic peeling that is usually arrested at the skin creases [**Figures 38-3** and **38-4**]. The history of recurrent waves usually lasts for 6 weeks with precipitating factors being cold, stress, and febrile illness. The pathognomonic histopathologic feature is necrobiosis of the Malpighian layer with absence of the overlying granular layer, scattered vacuolated keratinocytes with formation of a broad band in the epidermis showing ballooning degeneration.[7] The disease is self-limiting and improves with age. Some cases have responded to topical steroids and photodynamic therapy seems to be promising.

TUNGIASIS (SAND FLEA DISEASE)

Tungiasis is one of the neglected tropical diseases, caused by the parasite *Tunga penetrans*. It is prevalent in poor rural communities worldwide, especially sub-Saharan Africa, South America, and the Caribbean. In sub-Saharan Africa, it is prevalent along the coast of Kenya with 11% to 50% of school going children affected. The prevalence in the overall population in the Kilifi County on the Kenyan coast was 25% with 33% of children less than 15-years-of-age affected.[8] The elderly is the other group that have a predilection for infection.[8]

The fleas penetrate under the skin of the feet, specifically the toes, soles, and heels [**Figure 38-5**]. They range in number from less than 10 to several hundred, mature and set up an inflammatory reaction with oedema, erythema, and desquamation. The inflammatory response is directly proportional to the number of penetrating organisms. This causes great discomfort and impairs walking; the abnormal gait often leads to stigmatization. Secondary bacterial infection often complicates the penetration of fleas leading to abscesses and in extreme cases lymphangitis and gangrene. The attempts at removal of embedded fleas with sharp objects like thorns, safety pins, and knives is another cause of secondary bacterial infection as well as a risk factor for HIV and hepatitis B because these objects are used by multiple individuals.[9]

The only treatment is surgical extraction, taking care not to break the body of the flea that creates an inflammatory response. The foot needs to be washed with sterile water and then a topical antibiotic applied. A few other topical therapies have recently shown efficacy, a silicone (dimethicone) gel that kills 98% with a single application by suffocation registered in South America. A combination of coconut and neem oils used in Kenya has shown a 77% response rate when applied twice daily for 7 days.[9]

The main risk factors are walking barefoot, the presence of animals and improper housing, specifically using animal dung to build the floors of homes. Washing of feet daily, using of insect repellants coconut oil products, and wearing closed shoes help to prevent the penetration of fleas. Sealing the floors with low-cost options and regular cleaning to prevent buildup of sand will also prevent larvae from surviving.[9]

SCHISTOSOMIASIS/BILHARZIASIS

Schistosomiasis is a snail borne, fresh water-transmitted neglected tropical disease affecting poor communities in sub-Saharan Africa (SSA) with at least 800 million people at risk, accounting for at least 90% of the global disease burden and 280,000 deaths annually. Schistosomiasis is a public health problem with a high burden of disease in SSA.[10] The WHO has declared 2030 as the goal for interruption in transmission of schistosomiasis. One of the major methods of control has been the mass administration of praziquantel across at-risk communities, especially children who are at highest risk due to contact with water. However, reinfection is always a challenge.

The country with the highest burden in Africa and worldwide is Nigeria, followed by Tanzania and then the Democratic Republic of Congo and Ghana. Morocco, in North Africa, has been successful in transmission interruption with no new cases since 2004.[10]

Schistosomiasis is a snail-borne disease. Two genera of snails (*Bulinus* and *Biomphalaria*) are responsible for the distribution of schistosomes

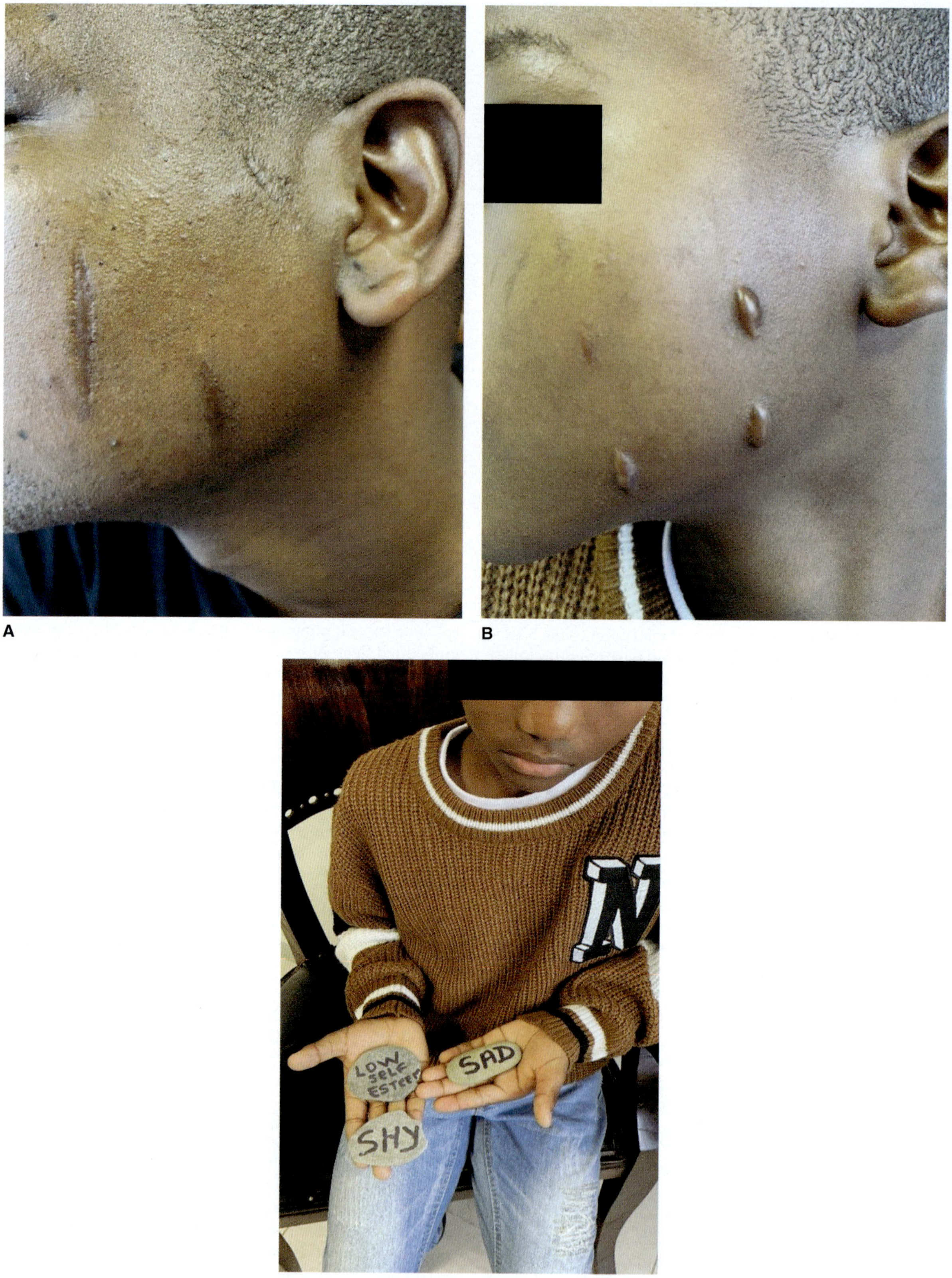

FIGURE 38-2. (A) Father (35 years) with facial scarification that denotes a certain ethnic clan in South Africa. **(B)** Son (6 years) with facial scarification that denotes a certain ethnic clan in South Africa. **(C)** Child displaying with pebbles how the scarification scars that healed with keloids affect him. A novel technique for gauging feelings was used. Feeling options were painted onto flat stones in isiZulu for the child to select those appropriate for him. The English translation of the inscription was on the flip side as shown. *Ukuzenyeza* was the isiZulu translated to low self-esteem.

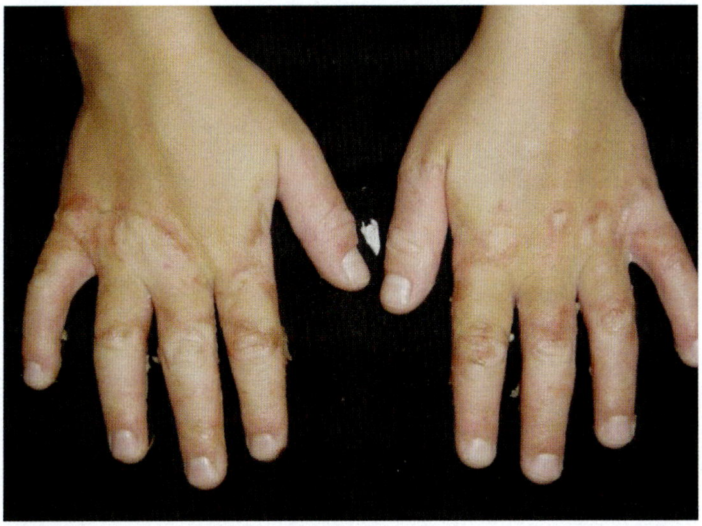

FIGURE 38-3. Oudtshoorn disease (keratolytic winter erythema). Erythema with peeling of the skin on the dorsa of the hands. (Courtesy of Dr. Sian Hartshorne, South Africa.)

in Africa caused by contamination and contact with fresh water. The two main organisms responsible for infection are *Shistosoma mansoni* responsible for intestinal and *Schistosoma haematobium* for urogenital schistosomiasis. The risk factors for the infection are lack of proper sanitation, contact with nonpotable water, and lack of adequate healthcare facilities.[10]

There are three distinct phases of clinical presentation. The first signs are those of itching and cercarial dermatitis that develop on penetration of the cercariae through the skin. The second phase is the development of symptoms of acute schistosomiasis called the Katayama syndrome. These include fever, malaise, weight loss, vomiting, and diarrhea. The third phase is that of chronic schistosomiasis when the eggs are deposited in various tissues, for example, commonly the liver, gastro-intestinal, and urogenital system. Uncommonly, they may be deposited in the CNS and skin [**Figure 38-6**].[10]

Cercariae causing disease in other species may penetrate human skin, resulting in limited pruritic cercarial dermatitis but the organisms do not survive or cause systemic disease.

Despite mass drug administration of praziquantel, reinfection is still a problem. A multi-pronged approach is key with education, destigmatization, access to better sanitation facilities, safe potable water,

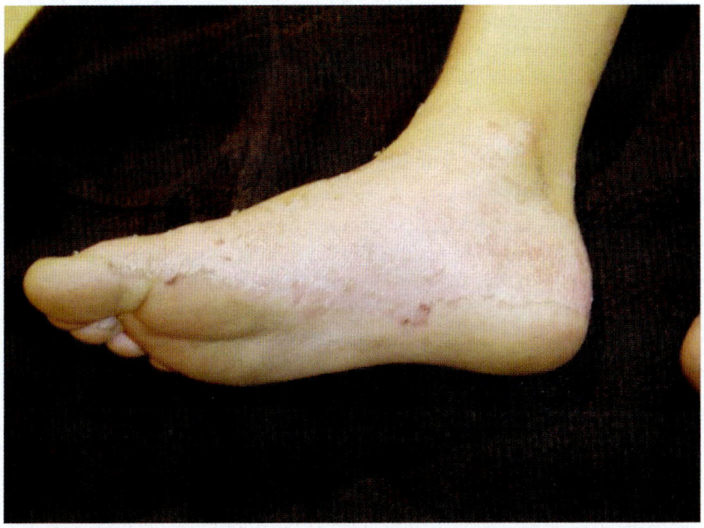

FIGURE 38-4. Oudtshoorn disease (keratolytic winter erythema). Erythema with peeling of the lateral borders and soles of the feet. (Courtesy of Dr. Sian Hartshorne, South Africa.)

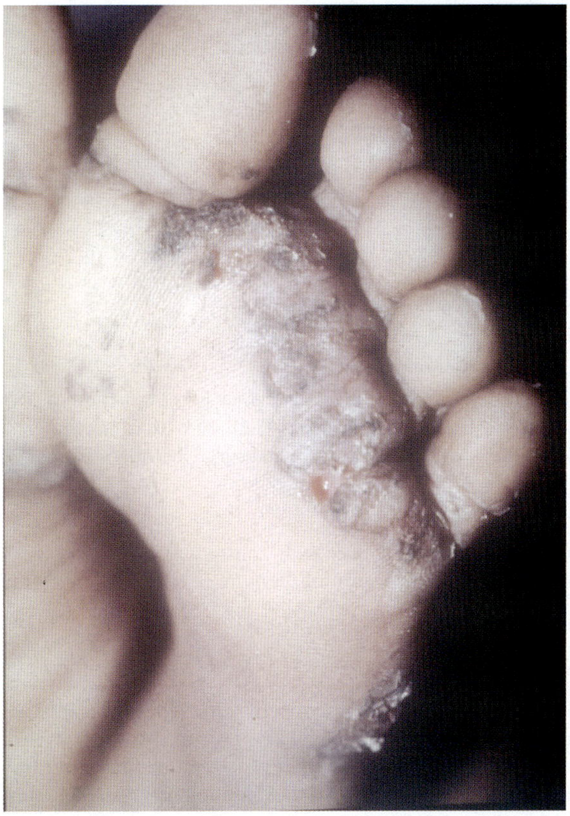

FIGURE 38-5. Papules, erosions, and peeling of the plantar surface of the feet and web spaces, typical of tungiasis. (Courtesy of Dr. Ben Naafs, the Netherlands.)

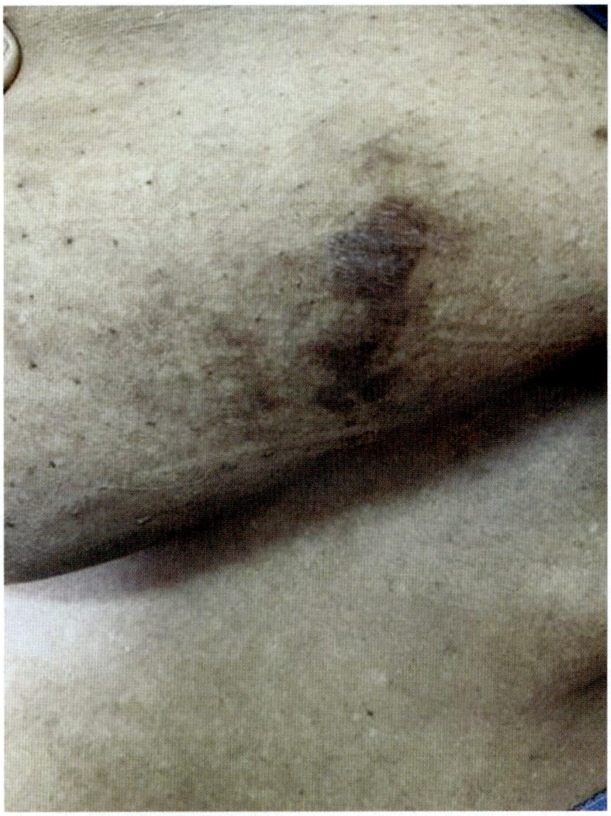

FIGURE 38-6. Hyperpigmented asymptomatic plaque on the breast that revealed schistosomiasis on histology. (Courtesy of Dr. Ndo Ngcobo, Department of Dermatology, University of KwaZulu Natal, Durban, South Africa.)

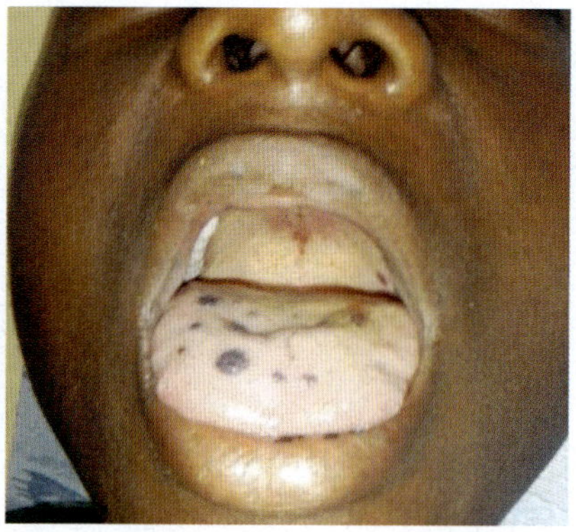

FIGURE 38-7. Hemorrhagic blisters of the tongue, oro-nasopharynx, and skin typical of onyalai. (Courtesy of Dr. San Honde, Illovo Sugar (PLC), Matiki Clinic, Dwangwa Estate, Malawi and Dr Bwanali Haji Ntaibu Jereni, Princess Marina Hospital, University of Botswana.)

and healthcare. All the above, with constant surveillance, are vital to identify areas where intervention is required.[10]

ONYALAI

Onyalai is an acquired thrombocytopenia, first reported in 1904. It occurs predominantly in African populations in central southern Africa. The disease may occur at any age and in both sexes, but it has most frequently been described in young adult males. The etiology is linked to traditional diets and eating sorghum grains contaminated with the mycotoxins of the endophytic fungus *Epicoccum sorghinum*. Onyalai occurs acutely with hemorrhagic blisters and hemorrhages of the oral and nasal mucosa [**Figure 38-7**], but they can occur on any serosal surface or the skin. It is associated with thrombocytopenia and variable anemia, dependent on the amount of blood loss. Hemorrhage from ruptured bullae, epistaxis, or gastrointestinal bleeding may cause hemorrhagic shock and death. The condition may become chronic or relapsing.[11-13] Major differences between onyalai and idiopathic thrombocytopenic purpura are outlined in **Table 38-1**.

Treatment is directed at the prevention of hemorrhagic shock. A variety of targeted therapies including glucocorticoids, intravenous immunoglobulin, chemotherapy, or splenectomy have been used with minimal success.[11,13]

TABLE 38-1 Major differences between onyalai and idiopathic thrombocytopenic purpura (ITP)

Features	Onyalai	ITP
1	Africa between equator and 30° south latitude in endemic malaria area	Ubiquitous
2	Restricted to the black population	All ethnic groups affected
3	Haemorrhagic bullae is the clinical hallmark	Haemorrhagic bullae is the exception
4	Newborns of affected mothers are normal	Newborns of affected mothers may have thrombocytopenia
5	IgM and IgG platelet antibodies in serum	Mainly IgG platelet antibodies in serum
6	Response to corticosteroids: poor	Response to corticosteroids: fair
7	Mortality rates: up to 10% in acute phase	Mortality rate: 1% in acute phase
8	Linked to traditional diet and lifestyle	Not linked to cultural habits
9	Aetiology unknown	May be precipitated by viral diseases

Source: Reproduced with permission from Hesseling PB. Onyalai in Namibia. Clinical manifestations, haematological findings, course and management of 103 patients in the Kavango territory. Trans R Soc Trop Med Hyg. 1987; 81(2): 193-6.[11]

AFRICAN TRYPANOSOMIASIS (SLEEPING SICKNESS)[14-17]

African trypanosomes or Old World trypanosomes are hemoflagellate protozoans of the genus *Trypanosoma*. They cause the neglected tropical disease, human African trypanosomiasis (HAT), a lethal meningoencephalitis if not treated.[14] Two subspecies of trypanosomes, which are morphologically indistinguishable, cause distinct disease patterns in humans. They are transmitted to humans by bloodsucking tsetse flies of the genus *Glossina*. The proportion of tsetse flies, predominantly found in rural areas, that are infected with this parasite is low.

T. brucei gambiense causes the more common chronic West African or Gambian trypanosomiasis with humans as the main reservoir of trypanosomes. *T. brucei rhodesiense* causes the less common acute East African or Rhodesian trypanosomiasis with animals, such as antelope and cattle, as the main reservoir of trypanosomes.

Untreated, three clinical stages for HAT were proposed by McGovern.[15] A primary stage chancre, a secondary hemolymphatic stage, and a tertiary neurologic and central nervous system (CNS) stage.

The primary stage

The initial skin lesion, the *Trypanosomal chancre,* occurs 2 to 3 days after the bite of the infected tsetse fly. Multiplication of the parasites at the inoculation site produces a localized, red, tender, inflammatory nodule that may ulcerate. There are no extracutaneous signs and symptoms.[15]

The secondary stage

After the development of the chancre, organisms spread through lymphatic channels to the bloodstream, inducing lymphangitis and a proliferative enlargement of the lymph nodes and ultimately an intermittent parasitemia. Low-grade intermittent parasitemia with antigenic shifts results in trypanosome localization in small blood vessels causing local vasculitis while high levels of specific and nonspecific antibodies cause immune complex vasculitis and anemia. The *hemolymphatic* phase general symptoms and signs are nonspecific. They include recurrent bouts of fever, lymphadenopathy (posterior cervical lymphadenopathy known as Winterbottom sign in Gambian HAT), hepatosplenomegaly, malaise/fatigue, arthralgia, weight loss, headache, dizziness, and impaired mentation. Cutaneous manifestations include *nonspecific transient, recurring, variable skin rashes (trypanids)*, itch/pruritus, petechiae/purpura, localized edema, acroparesthesia, erythema nodosum, ichthyosis, and icterus.[15]

The tertiary stage

Neurological or meningoencephalic stage-symptoms include a wide constellation of symptoms and signs potentially involving the whole nervous system presenting as mental disturbances, motor system disturbances, sensory system involvement (classically delayed, bilateral pain, out of proportion to mild trauma known as *Kerandel deep delayed hyperesthesia* that results in an obsessive fear of hurting oneself), and abnormal reflexes. Sleep abnormalities, which give the disease its name, include nocturnal insomnia and daytime somnolence, uncontrollable episodes of sleep, and alteration in sleep patterns.

In those with East African trypanosome infections, myocarditis and CNS involvement may result in heart failure, convulsions, and coma with death following in 6 to 9 months. In those with West African trypanosome infections, the disease is more indolent and progresses more slowly. Bouts of fever often persist for years before CNS manifestations gradually appear.

In the terminal stages, the patient develops a lethal intercurrent infection or lapses into a final coma.

There is little evidence of coinfections of African trypanosomes and HIV, both of which cause immunosuppression.

In the febrile traveler, a high level of suspicion is necessary as the symptoms and signs of infection can be atypical manifesting as gastrointestinal disturbances with minimal sleep disturbance and the disease may be rapidly fatal.

TABLE 38-2 Cutaneous manifestations of human African trypanosomiasis (HAT)[14-17]

Although HAT is listed as a neglected tropical disease by the World Health Organisation, it is classified as having no cutaneous features.
This is not correct as characteristic skin lesions are seldom reported.

- A painful *chancre** at the inoculation site heralds infection, typically a large, erythematous, indurated, fixed cutaneous swelling which may ulcerate. Amongst West African HAT patients, the reaction is milder and often overlooked as an insect bite reaction or local cellulitis.
- Characteristic, although rarely reported (less than 10% of cases), evanescent, recurring, macular *trypanid rashes** may be present during the *hemolymphatic stages.* Polycyclic plaques, morbilliform, and urticarial rashes may be haemorrhagic/purpuric.
- Localized intense itching.*
- Localized cutaneous oedema of the hand, feet, or face may be found in the more advanced stages of the illness.
- Delayed, bilateral pain, out of proportion to mild trauma known as *Kerandel deep delayed hyperesthesia** that results in an obsessive fear of hurting oneself.
- Nonspecific features include petechiae/purpura, acroparesthesia, erythema nodosum, ichthyosis, and icterus.

*The most significant manifestations of HAT.

Diagnosis can be made in a person with a travel history to regions of Africa between latitudes 20° north and 20° south [**Table 38-2**].[15] A blood smear should reveal trypanosomes. A lumbar puncture is mandatory. Urgent treatment with input from infectious disease specialists familiar with this disease is necessary. The choice of therapy and HAT outcome depends on the presence or absence of CNS involvement, and the subspecies of trypanosome causing the infection.

There is currently no specific preventative therapy. Tsetse fly bites are painful. Protection against bites is strongly recommended in endemic areas. Wear thick, cotton, long sleeve shirts and trousers possibly impregnated with permethrin. Choose neutral color clothes and avoid bright, dark, or contrasting colors as they attract tsetse flies that bite during the day. The flies are also attracted to moving vehicles and clouds of dust. Regular application of insect repellents is advised.

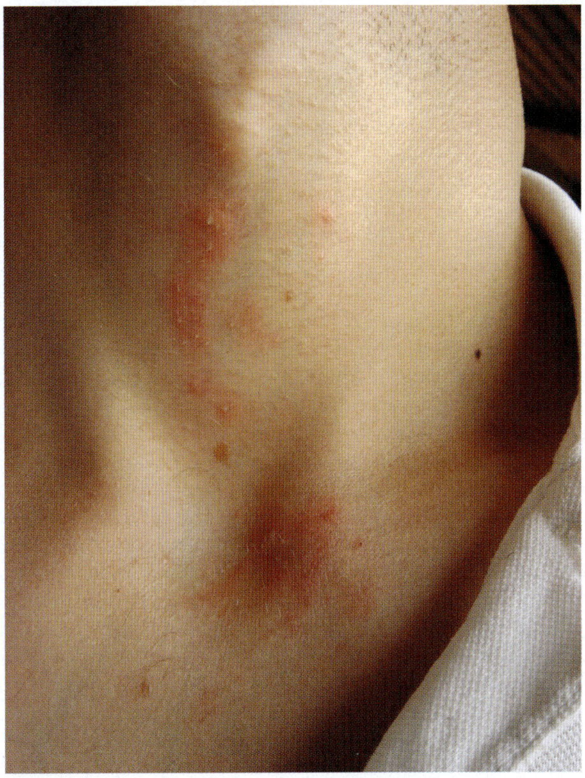

FIGURE 38-9. Linear erythematous, crusted, papular-vesicles on the neck classic of *Paederus* dermatitis. (Courtesy of the University of Cape Town, South Africa.)

PAEDERUS DERMATITIS

Paederus beetles (rove beetles) belong to *Staphylinidae* family of which there are about 622 species with 30 producing vesicants [**Figure 38-8**]. Most beetles have a similar structure; however, the sizes of their body parts, color, and shape may differ, which helps with identification of the various species. They are commonly found in warm and humid settings, with outbreaks occurring yearly.

Beetles are attracted to neon and fluorescent light sources that explains outbreaks in school hostels, military bases, and hospitals. Deforestation and expansion of urban settlements are responsible for the increase of outbreaks in the cities.[18] Reflex brushing of the beetles produce hemolymph, a strong vesicant with epidermolytic properties when touched or brushed on the skin, which can be transferred to distant sites by scratching.

Initial symptoms are pain and stinging at the site followed by pruritus and blistering within 24 hours. Sites typically affected are the exposed parts of the body: face, neck, upper back, and limbs. Distal sites include the genitals, eye, and mucosa. Lesions may be linear, erythematous, papulo-vesicles, "dermatitis linearis" [**Figure 38-9**], or kissing (mirror images) [**Figure 38-10**] that occurs when normal skin is apposed on acutely involved skin.[19]

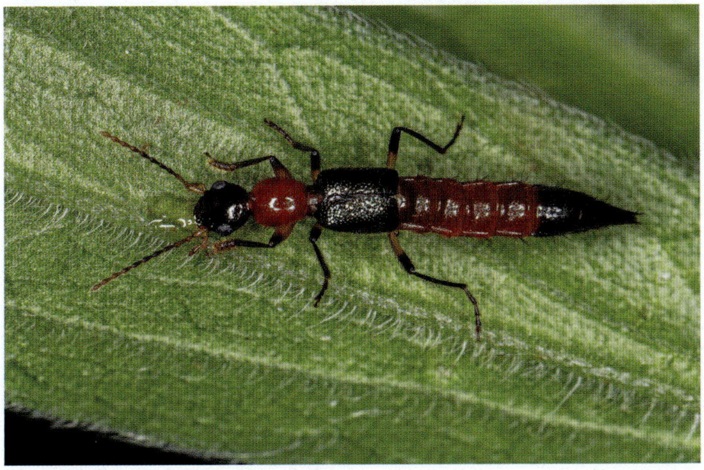

FIGURE 38-8. *Paederus* beetle (rove beetle) the cause of *Paederus* dermatitis. (Used with permission from Vinicius R. Souza/Shutterstock.)

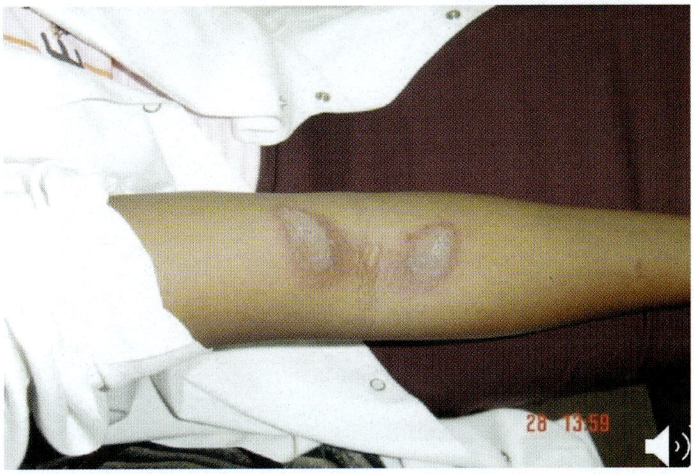

FIGURE 38-10. Mirror image of erythematous, crusted, papular-vesicles lesions, classic of the "kissing lesions" of *Paederus* dermatitis.

Superficial ulceration, crusting, and desquamation are seen in older lesions. The skin usually heals within 3 weeks leaving a transient postinflammatory hyper- or hypopigmentation. Antihistamines, topical corticosteroids, and antibiotics are useful in management. People should be discouraged from sleeping under fluorescent lights without nets in endemic areas.[18]

DERMATITIS CRURIS PUSTULOSA *ET* ATROPHICANS (NIGERIAN SHIN DISEASE)

Dermatitis cruris pustulosa *et* atrophicans (DCPA), also termed Nigerian shin disease, was described by Clark in 1952 and is a form of chronic superficial folliculitis of the lower limbs that was difficult to treat. It is seen mainly in west and central Africa and India. The etiology and pathogenesis of DCPA remain unclear but appear multifactorial. Occlusion from oils, trauma, microorganisms, immunological abnormalities, and individual susceptibility has been implicated. However, restriction of the rash to the legs despite the application of oils to other body sites with terminal hair makes occlusion an unlikely primary causative factor. The occurrence, however, appears to have decreased in the region.

Primarily seen in young adult males, the initial lesions are pustular affecting the hair follicles and normal skin on the anterior and lateral aspects of the legs [**Figure 38-11**]. Strikingly, systemic symptoms are absent even when lesions are extensive and involve the upper limbs and axilla. As the disease progresses, papules and atrophic plaques appear as a result of fibrosis. The skin appears shiny, scaly, and hairless [**Figure 38-12**]. Intensity of pruritus is variable through the course of the disease. Subsequent postinflammatory dyspigmentation is also variable. Currently, there are no clear guidelines for the management of DCPA.[20,21] Avoidance of possible precipitating factors and early use of antibiotics and antiseptics may reduce chronicity of the disease. Spontaneous regression occurs once the terminal hairs in the affected site are destroyed.

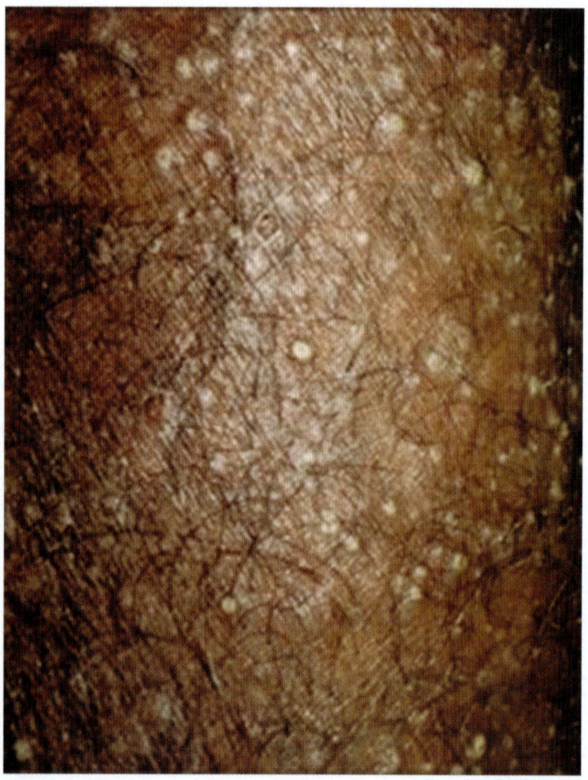

FIGURE 38-11. Numerous, predominantly follicular pustules, on the shin skin in early dermatitis cruris pustulosa *et* atrophicans. (Courtesy of Regional Dermatology Training Centre, Kilimanjaro Christian Medical Centre and Tumaini University Moshi, Tanzania.)

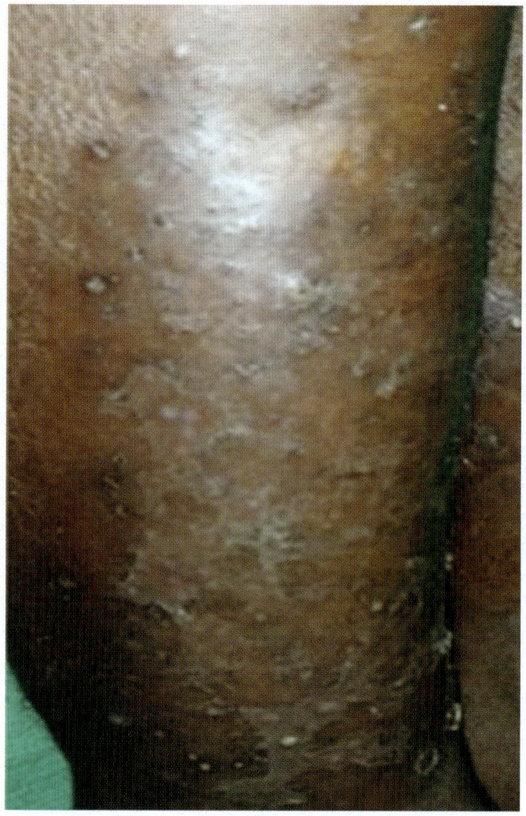

FIGURE 38-12. Atrophic skin with loss of follicular structures in late-stage dermatitis cruris pustulosa *et* atrophicans. (Courtesy of Regional Dermatology Training Centre, Kilimanjaro Christian Medical Centre and Tumaini University Moshi, Tanzania.)

MYASIS

Myiasis is an ectoparasitic infestation of dipterous larva found in tropical, hot humid climate. The larva are obligatory parasites of mammals. *Cordylobia* species are primarily responsible for myiasis in Africa.[22] *Cordylobia anthropophaga* (Tumbu fly or mango fly) is the widest spread species in sub-Saharan Africa.

Children are more frequently affected by disease. The cutaneous presentation that occurs most commonly is the furuncular form, due to the larva of the *Cordilobia anthropophaga*. The wound and creeping dermal forms are less common. The flies lay eggs on clothes hung on lines

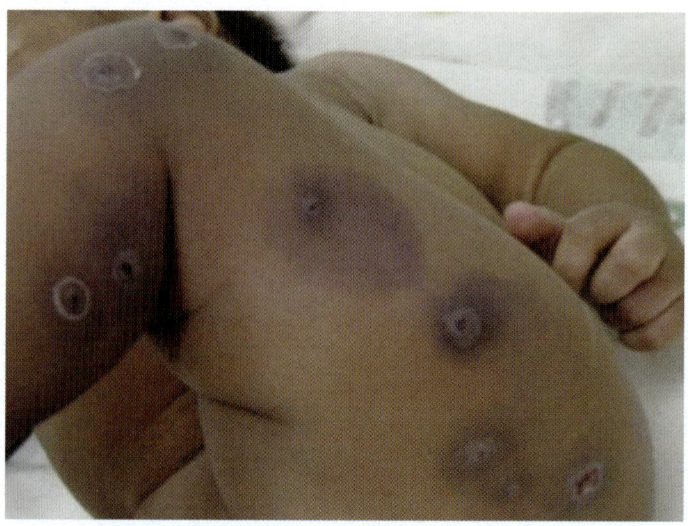

FIGURE 38-13. Multiple furuncular lesions on the thigh and lower leg of a 12-month-old baby.

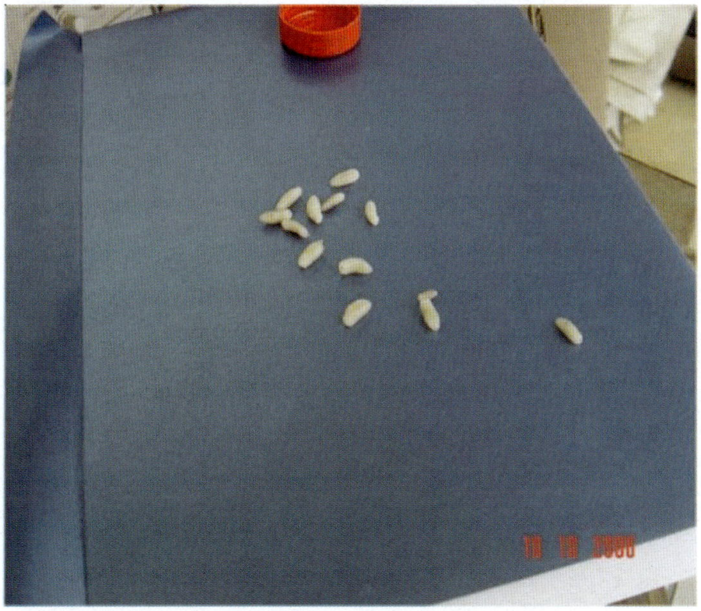

FIGURE 38-14. Larvae of *Cordylobia* fly removed from young girl above.

or spread on the grass in shady areas as heat from direct sunlight may destroy both the eggs and larvae. The warmth from the human body causes the eggs on contaminated clothing to hatch in 1 to 3 days after which the larva penetrates intact skin and continue to develop.

Due to the cutaneous larva, an inflammatory response ensues with pain, itching, and a sensation of movement within the skin. A furuncle or carbuncle with a central pore with fluid draining from the pore develops. The caudal part of the larvae may become visible after the application of oil, which causes the larva to move up to avoid suffocation. Site of predilection in adults and children include the back, buttocks, thighs, and breast that are usually covered by clothing [**Figure 38-13**]. Extensive lesions are associated with fever and regional lymphadenopathy. The growing larva drops on to the ground 8 to 12 days later and pupates.

Wound myiasis occurs when flies lay eggs on an open wound, and migratory myiasis is due to penetration of certain types of the larvae in the lower epidermis producing serpiginous erythematous lesions similar to larva migrans. Diagnosis of cutaneous myiasis is primarily clinical with a history of itching predating a furunculoid-like lesion with a central pore. Dermoscopy is useful in confirming the diagnosis. Treatment involves removal of the larvae [**Figure 38-14**], and prevention of secondary bacterial infection. This can be done by occlusion, surgical removal, or the use of larvicides.

REFERENCES

1. Carretero MI. Clay minerals and their beneficial effects upon human health. A review. *Appl Clay Sci.* 2002;21(3-4):155-163.
2. Dlova NC, Nevondo FT, Mwangi EM, et al. Chemical analysis and in vitro UV-protection characteristics of clays traditionally used for sun protection in South Africa. *Photodermatol Photoimmunol Photomed.* 2013;29(3):164-169.
3. Turner T. The social skin. In: Cherfas J, Lewin R, eds. *Not Work Alone: A Cross-Cultural View of Activities Superfluous to Survival.* London, UK: Temple Smith; 1980:112-140.
4. Dunyo SK, Ahorlu CK, Simonsen PE. Scarification as a risk factor for rapid progression of filarial elephantiasis. *Trans R Soc Trop Med Hyg.* 1997;91(4):446.
5. Babatunde OP, Oyeronke AE. Scarification practice and scar complications among the Nigerian Yorubas. *Indian J Dermatol Venereol Leprol.* 2010;76(5): 571-572.
6. Garve R, Garve M, Türp JC, Fobil JN, Meyer CG. Scarification in sub-Saharan Africa: social skin, remedy and medical import. *Trop Med Int Health.* 2017;22(6):708-715.
7. Ramsay M, Ngcungcu T, Grayson W. Keratolytic winter erythema: an update. *Dermatopathology (Basel).* 2019;26;6(2):126-132.
8. Wiese S, Elson L, Reichert F, Mambo B, Feldmeier H. Prevalence, intensity and risk factors of tungiasis in Kilifi County, Kenya: I. Results from a community-based study. *PLoS Negl Trop Dis.* 2017;11(10):e0005925.
9. Elson L, Feldmeier H, Fillinger U. Tungiasis. *Community Skin Health.* 2022;18(2):19-23.
10. Aula OP, McManus DP, Jones MK, Gordon CA. Schistosomiasis with a Focus on Africa. *Trop Med Infect Dis.* 2021;6(3):109.
11. Hesseling PB. Onyalai in Namibia. Clinical manifestations, haematological findings, course and management of 103 patients in the Kavango territory. *Trans R Soc Trop Med Hyg.* 1987;81(2):193-196.
12. Berman C. Onyalai, an acute form of idiopathic thrombocytopenic purpura. *Am J Clin Pathol.* 1955;25(12):1349-1358.
13. Hesseling PB. Onyalai. *Baillieres Clin Haematol.* 1992;5(2):457-473.
14. Kennedy PG. Clinical features, diagnosis, and treatment of human African trypanosomiasis (sleeping sickness). *Lancet Neurol.* 2013;12(2):186-194.
15. McGovern TW, Williams W, Fitzpatrick JE, et al. Cutaneous manifestations of African trypanosomiasis. *Arch Dermatol.* 1995;131(10):1178-1182.
16. Ezzedine K, Darie H, Le Bras M, Malvy D. Skin features accompanying imported human African trypanosomiasis: hemolymphatic Trypanosoma gambiense infection among two French expatriates with dermatologic manifestations. *J Travel Med.* 2007;14(3):192-196.
17. Tatibouet MH, Gentilini M, Brucker G. Lésions cutanées au cours de la trypanosomiase humaine africaine [Cutaneous lesions in human African trypanosomiasis]. *Sem Hop.* 1982;58(40):2318-2324.
18. George AO, Hart PD. Outbreak of Paederus dermatitis in southern Nigeria. Epidemiology and dermatology. *Int J Dermatol.* 1990;29(7):500-501.
19. Olumide YM. An approach to the patient with skin disease. *Trop Doct.* 1992;22 Suppl 1:7-14.
20. Olumide YM, Odunowo BD, Odiase AO. Regional dermatoses in the African black. III. Pretibial lesions. *Int J Dermatol.* 1991;30(6):425-431.
21. Kaimal S, D'Souza M, Kumari R, et al. Dermatitis cruris pustulosa et atrophicans revisited: our experience with 37 patients in south India. *Int J Dermatol.* 2009;48(10):1082-1090.
22. Pampiglione S, Bettoli V, Cestari G, Staffa M. Furuncular myiasis due to *Cordylobia anthropophaga*, endemic in the same locality for over 130 years. *Ann Trop Med Parasitol.* 1993;87(2):219-220.

Hair, Scalp, and Nail Disorders

SECTION 5

CHAPTER 39

Hair Care Practices: Complications, Treatments, and Prevention

Aditi Gadre
Maria Fernanda Gavazzoni
Crystal Aguh

KEY POINTS

- Curly hair is more fragile than straight or wavy hair.
- Dermatologists should be knowledgeable about the various styling methods of patients with tightly curled hair to recommend practices that will prevent traction alopecia or acquired trichorrhexis nodosa.

Although there are no biochemical differences in hair across racial and ethnic groups, some distinctive characteristics emerge among the major racial groups: Caucasian, Asian, and African.[1] This chapter will outline and discuss hair care practices among these groups—considering Asian hair as typical straight hair, Caucasian hair as typical wavy hair, and African hair as classic curly or kinky hair—with a focus on patients of African descent who are more likely to suffer from alopecia as a result of styling practices.

PHENOTYPE

The shape and diameter of the hair shaft are unique attributes that affect hair health. Straight (Asian) hair fibers have the largest diameter and a round shape, whereas wavy (Caucasian) hair shafts have an intermediate diameter and are less round. Curly or kinky (African) fibers have an ellipsoid or oval cross-sectional fiber and a variable diameter.[2] They also demonstrate variable ellipticity not only among different strands of hair but also within a single hair shaft, forming several narrow-angle twists[3] prone to breakage.[3] African hair also has lower tensile strength than Asian and Caucasian hair, identifying a need for specialized hair care. Porosity is a different factor that impacts the degree of hair swelling and frizz with studies demonstrating that Caucasian hair holds more water content than Asian and African hair. However, it is important to recognize that water content is unrelated to moisturization, which contributes to the smooth quality of hair.[1] Finally, although the hair growth cycle and the number of hairs in the anagen or telogen phase are conserved across racial and ethnic groups, a larger diameter of the hair shaft is associated with more rapid hair growth.[4,5] Studies report the fastest and slowest growth rates among Asian patients and African patients, respectively.[5]

A patient's curl pattern is arguably the most significant feature guiding hair care management as it affects the innate fragility of hair. The Walker system classifies hair by four curl patterns (Types 1-4),[6] whereas the Loussouarn system classifies hair by eight curl patterns (Types I-VIII) across ethnic groups [**Figure 39-1**].[7] As the classification type for both systems increases, the number of waves and propensity for breakage increases, whereas the diameter of curls decreases. It is worth noting that there is considerable variability in the tightness of the curl across the African diaspora, with type V being the most common curl type among African Americans and Caribbeans, while VIII is exceedingly rare; in contrast, types VII and VIII are the most common curl patterns in African countries such as Ghana and South Africa, and type V is noted as occurring very infrequently (see **Table 39-1** for a summary).[7,8] However, a single patient can present with a range of curl patterns, with the tightest curl pattern informing maintenance strategies.

Given the inherent fragility of curly hair, its propensity for tangling, and higher maintenance requirements, many of the preferred hairstyles seen in those with curly hair aim to achieve one of two results: (1) create a straighter formation to enhance moisture retention and manageability; (2) avoid breakage that can occur from overmanipulating the hair by braiding the hair or wearing camouflage styles. Both options can lead to secondary hair loss, but it is important to proceed with this understanding in mind when approaching alternative styling options for patients with curly hair.

HAIR CARE COMPLICATIONS: TRACTION ALOPECIA

Traction alopecia is thinning of the hair in areas exposed to a constant, pulling force [**Figure 39-2**]. A third of Black women are estimated to experience traction alopecia over the course of their lifetime.[9] Although many hairstyles are attributed to the development of traction alopecia, often affecting the frontal scalp hairline, this chapter will focus on four particularly popular styles: dreadlocks, braids, weaves, and wigs.

DREADLOCKS

Dreadlocks, also known as locks or locs, are formed by intentionally twisting and tangling the hair until it "locks" permanently into place [**Figure 39-3**]. Hair can be twisted, braided, or coiled with natural oils or pomades using fingers, palms (a technique called palm rolling), or implements like a crochet hook or latch pin (a technique known as interlocking). A backcombing technique may be preferred for straight hair.[1] Locks are popular because compared to hair worn loosely, they are generally low maintenance, requiring infrequent shampooing and no use of styling tools, with the exception of natural oils for moisturization. Retwisting occurs every 6 to 8 weeks to incorporate new growth, serving as a source of tension against the scalp. Sisterlocks are much smaller than classic dreadlocks, and they are installed in salons by licensed stylists who use a special, looped pin, but due to their small size, patients should be cautioned about heightened risks of traction alopecia upon frequent retwisting.

BRAIDS AND TWISTS

Braids (also called plaits) are a low maintenance hairstyle often worn by women of African descent and exist in innumerable forms, with some of the more common patterns discussed below. They are created by interlocking three or more strands of hair three dimensionally, with or without incorporation of extensions, which are packaged bulks of synthetic or human hairs that are integrated with the existing hair at the scalp [**Figure 39-4**]. Microbraids, which are smaller braids with a diameter of 2 to 4 mm, incorporate smaller amounts of the individual's own hair. Unlike braids and microbraids, cornrow braids lay flat against the scalp, often in a geometric design. Plaits and cornrows are commonly worn underneath wigs or weaves, or on their own, and they can be done with or without added extensions. Use of extensions increases the weight of the braid, and extra twisting of the hair is required to intertwine natural hair with extension hair.

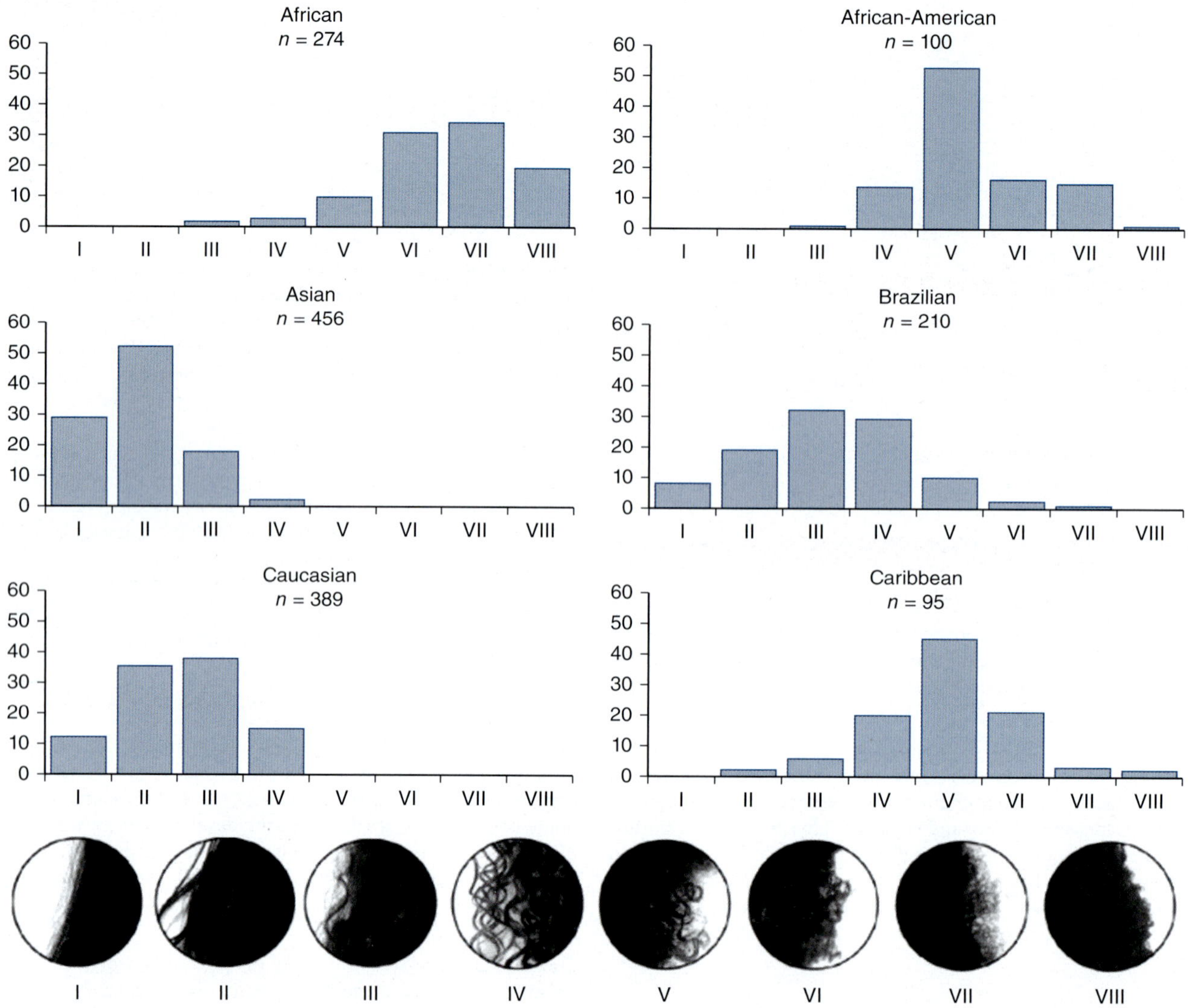

FIGURE 39-1. Significant worldwide variation is seen in curl patterns around the world with curly hair types being particularly diverse among populations of the African diaspora. (Source: Reproduced with permission from Loussouarn G, Garcel A-L, Lozano I, et al. Worldwide diversity of hair curliness: a new method of assessment. *Int J Dermatol.* 2007;46:2-6.)

Twisting of the hair can help to minimize the bulk of thick hair and redefines the hair shaft's natural curl, making the hair more manageable. To form a twist, two pieces of hair are twisted around one another [**Figure 39-5**]. Extensions can also be incorporated to lengthen twists.

WEAVES AND OTHER EXTENSIONS

Many women enjoy using hair weaves and extensions to create the appearance of increased volume or length. Both human and synthetic options are available commercially, although human hair is more expensive. A weave is a type of extension that is sewn with a needle and thread onto plaits or cornrows of natural hair. Other methods for extension attachment include clip-ons or adhesive agents like tape or latex-based bonding glue.[1] Unfortunately, glue can cause allergic contact dermatitis

TABLE 39-1 Hair characteristics among different ethnic groups

Parameter	Asian	Caucasian	Black*
Growth rate (μm/day)[1]	411	367	280
Hair density (hairs/cm^2)[1]	175	226	161
Ellipticity[1]	90% (circular)	75% (less circular)	60% (oval)
Loussouarn Classification[7]	Types I-III	Types I-IV	Types IV-VIII

*Black includes those of the African diaspora, who are of mixed racial heritage; Types IV-VI are relatively more common in these populations than in patients of direct African descent.

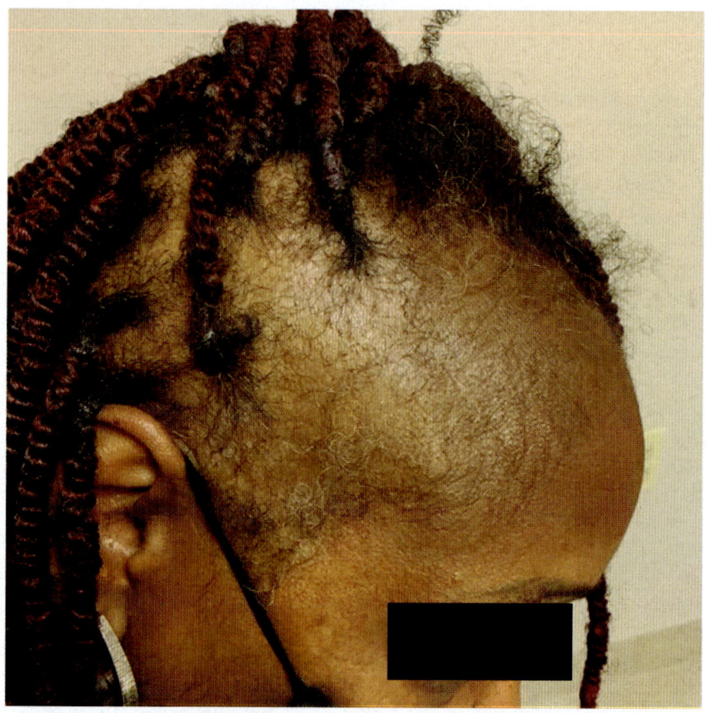

FIGURE 39-2. Traction alopecia.

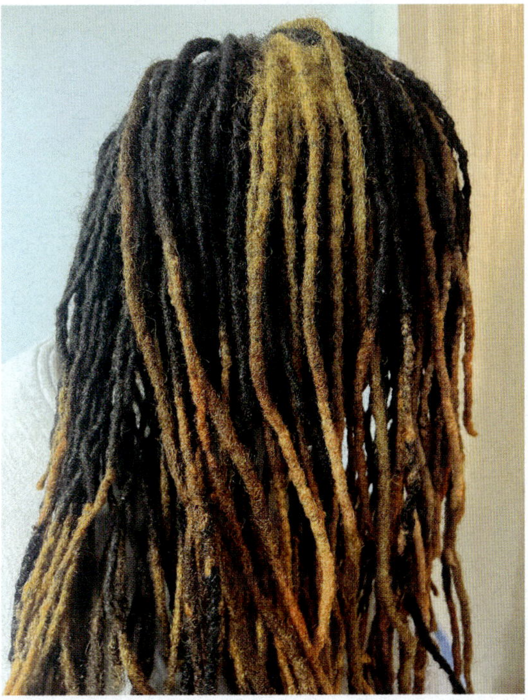

FIGURE 39-3. Dreadlocks.

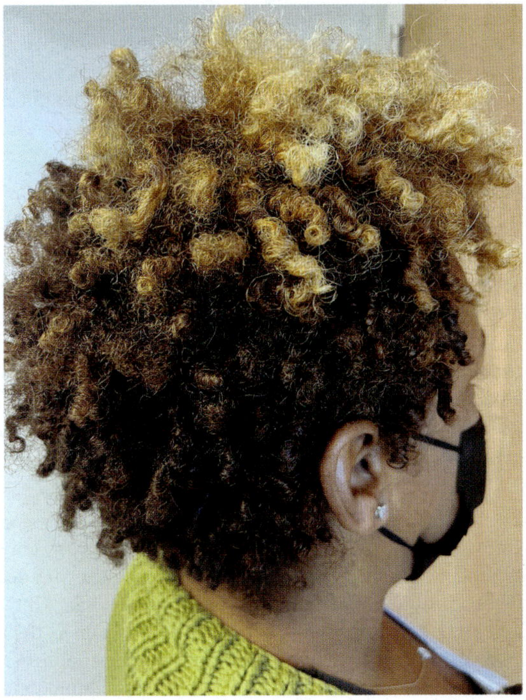

FIGURE 39-5. Twist-out.

as well as hair damage upon removal. The solvents available to ease this process may also lead to irritant contact dermatitis.[10,11] Instead, when installing weaves, it is preferred that individuals first cornrow their own hair, and the weave be attached directly to these braids using a needle and thread (termed a "sew-in" weave). While this can be associated with tension along the hairline, it significantly diminishes the risk of a contact dermatitis reaction.

WIGS

Wigs can be used to reduce the frequency of heat application or chemicals and to cover alopecia. Lace wigs (shafts of hair extensions attached to a lace net wig cap) are becoming increasingly popular among celebrities as well as patients because they allow for convenient and versatile hairstyling. Use of adhesives or glues to place wigs can predispose patients to allergic contact dermatitis and accelerate presentation to end-stage traction alopecia.

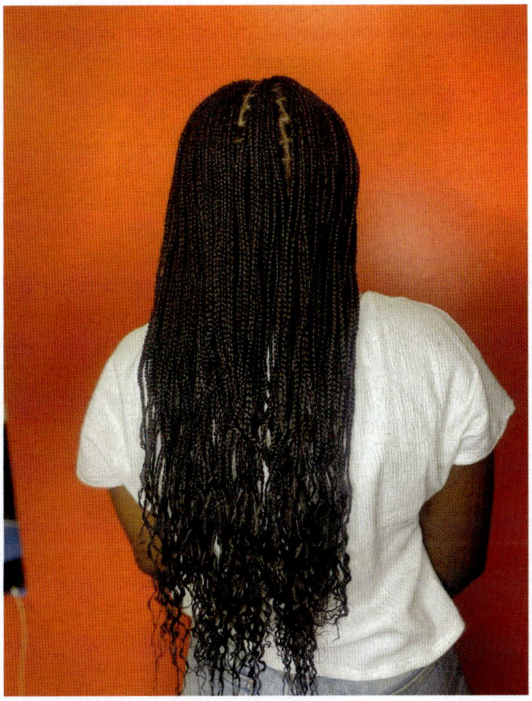

FIGURE 39-4. Braids.

OTHER CULTURAL CONSIDERATIONS

Traction Alopecia in Muslim Women A hijab is a type of headscarf worn by Muslim women to cover hair publicly in front of unrelated males. Methods for securing the hijab range from pinning it underneath the chin or wrapping the hijab at the back of the head. If worn tightly, traction alopecia may occur over time at the frontal or occipital hairline. Alternative methods for securing the hijab or mild loosening that still covers the hair but eases tension can reverse traction alopecia at an early stage.[12]

Traction Alopecia in Sikh Men Practitioners of the Sikh religion, often with ancestral roots in the state of Punjab in India, may make a commitment to avoid cutting their hair. Men tie their hair into a bun at the crown of their scalp that is covered with a turban. Tension from this practice can cause alopecia that impacts the occipital scalp.[13]

TREATMENT AND PREVENTION OF TRACTION ALOPECIA

Traction alopecia presents in three stages: (1) early, which is reversible with avoidance of triggering hairstyles; (2) intermediate, which is responsive to medical therapies; and (3) end-stage, which is irreversible. Classifying patients by severity of disease determines appropriate treatment recommendations. Early-stage patients benefit from reduced frequency of extensions, with a maximum of wear three times a year for 6 to 8 weeks at a time. Patients at this stage should also be encouraged to adhere to healthy hair practices such as regular cleansing to minimize the risk of future damage. As patients continue use of extensions, they progress to an intermediate stage, which is characterized by more widespread, decreased density without overt signs of follicular dropout. At this stage, patients are responsive to minoxidil to encourage growth, or to topical steroids and intralesional triamcinolone injections for alleviating active inflammation. Additionally, patients should be strongly encouraged to eliminate or drastically reduce use of extensions to prevent progression to end-stage disease. At this stage, widespread follicular dropout is noted, necessitating hair transplantation. If hair is natural, it may be easiest to wear the hair short to minimize maintenance [**Figure 39-5**] (see Chapter 100). This is a cosmetic treatment but can be quite effective for patients.

HAIR CARE COMPLICATIONS: ACQUIRED TRICHORRHEXIS NODOSA

Acquired trichorrhexis nodosa (ATN) is a disorder of hair breakage caused by trauma. It often occurs in African hair types due to its fragility and the involvement of damaging hair styling practices, although similar outcomes can be seen in straighter hair that has been subjected to repeated chemical or thermal insults. Etiologies include thermal styling, chemical relaxers, hair coloring, overuse of extensions, and under moisturized hair.

THERMAL STYLING TECHNIQUES

Hair can be straightened by applying heat to modify hydrogen bonds in the hair shaft. This process is achieved by multiple thermal techniques including hot combing, flat ironing, and blow drying. Hot combing involves a brush heated up to 500° F/260°C that is pulled through hair covered in oil or petrolatum-based ointment. Hair can be worn straight for approximately 2 weeks until curls assume their original pattern from perspiration and humidity.[1] Flat ironing [**Figure 39-6**] may be preferred due to improved temperature control, which mitigates the likelihood of thermal burns of the scalp, ears, or neck that can lead to postinflammatory dyspigmentation.[14] To straighten, two metal plates are squeezed together from the root to the tip of the hair [**Figure 39-7**]. A variation of this technique is the "silk press," in which silicone-based products are applied to the hair prior to passing it through a flat iron.[1] Hair pressing should not be done more than twice a week for straight hair, and much less frequently for curly hair. Curly hair should also be properly cleansed and conditioned prior to the application of heat. Damaged caused by heat styling can be minimized by applying a heat protectant styling product prior to use of a heat device. These can be purchased at beauty supply stores.

CHEMICAL RELAXERS/LANTHIONIZATION

Straightening can also be accomplished with chemical relaxers, which permanently alter the hair's natural texture until hair grows out. It is estimated that at least 70% of African American women have used chemical relaxers at least once in their lifetime.[15] Relaxers contain sodium, potassium, or guanidine hydroxides that disrupt the cysteine disulfide bonds between keratin molecules of the hair.[16] Chemical relaxation begins with leaving the relaxer in the hair for approximately 10 to 20 minutes.

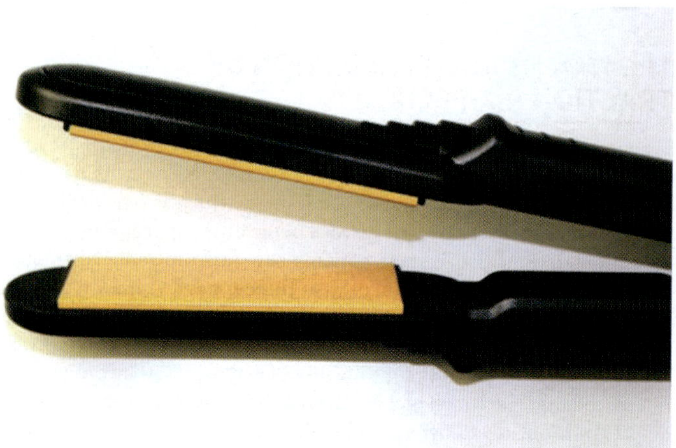

FIGURE 39-6. Flat iron.

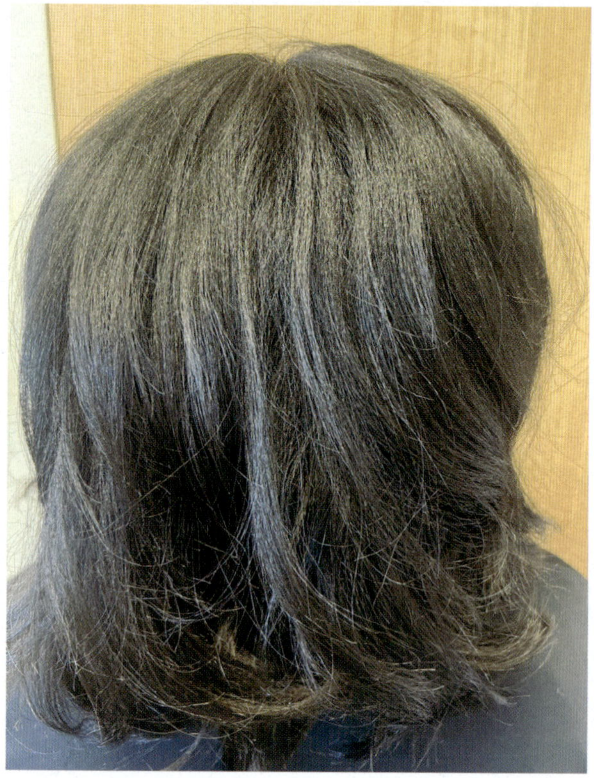

FIGURE 39-7. Thermal styling.

Once combed through and processed, the hair is neutralized with a shampoo that reinstates the normal pH of the hair and conditioned.[17] Finally, retouching occurs at least 6 weeks after relaxation to ensure new hair grows before reapplying relaxer.[14] Sodium hydroxide (lye-based) relaxers are used mainly in salons, whereas other relaxers (non–lye-based) are popular for home use. It is widely believed by stylists and patrons that lye-based relaxers have a better straightening effect. Lye-based relaxers have more irritation potential, yet they are preferred by stylists for perceived relaxer performance. However, recent studies indicate that non–lye-based (guanidine-based) cream-finished products show greater efficacy over lye-based products.[18] One note of caution is that non–lye-based relaxers may deposit minerals that harden hair, leading to severe hair breakage. Additionally, due to lower irritation potential, patients may be more likely to inadvisably extend application time leading to increased breakage and hair shedding. Texturizers have a similar composition to chemical relaxers, but they have a lower percentage of the active straightening ingredient, and they are left on the scalp for less time, weakening fewer disulfide bonds in hair. This reduced contact time contributes to a slightly improved safety profile, and the process creates a manageable, looser curl pattern that some women prefer.[1]

Side effects of relaxation include contact dermatitis, scalp burns, traction alopecia, diffuse hair loss, and formation of abscesses from *Staph aureus*.[1] Many of these side effects occur from improper application of relaxers, and for that reason, application by a professional is recommended. See **Table 39-2** for advice to minimize damage from chemical relaxation and thermal straightening.

HAIR DYES

Dyes are used cosmetically to color the hair, exerting their effect by penetrating the hair shaft. Smaller molecular weights facilitate deeper penetration, which is associated with greater dye permanence. Temporary dyes are unable to enter the cuticle, the outer layer of the hair shaft, whereas semipermanent, demi-permanent, and permanent dyes (listed in order of increasing durability) permeate the cortex, the middle layer. Synthetic permanent dyes require an alkaline pH, often

TABLE 39-2 Hair shaft damage prevention from chemical and thermal straightening

Tips to minimize damage from chemical straighteners[15]
1. Have a professional stylist apply the relaxer.
2. Have the stylist apply a base to the entire scalp before application.
3. Decrease the frequency of touch ups to every 8-10 weeks.
4. Take a relaxer holiday for 2-3 months at a time (weaves or wigs recommended during this break).
5. Have a stylist suggest a chemical-free, natural hairstyle.
Tips to minimize damage from thermal straightening
1. Use temperature-controlled devices or a low/medium setting less than 350°F.[19]
2. Minimize frequency of thermal styling; hot combs should not be used more than once a week.
3. Use a deep conditioner or silicone-based heat protectant prior to styling.

achieved through ammonia, as well as an oxidizing reaction to color hair.[1] Permanent and semipermanent dyes are associated with the highest risk of developing contact dermatitis.[10] Studies suggest that African Americans are more sensitive to paraphenylenediamine (PPD), a known agent in dyes that causes allergic and irritant contact dermatitis,[20] than Caucasian patients.[21] PPD is not found in natural permanent dyes like henna, a flowering plant that can be mixed into a paste and lends a reddish hue to hair.[1]

KERATIN TREATMENTS AND BRAZILIAN BLOWOUTS

Straightening keratin treatment consists of naturally occurring, hydrolyzed keratin that rapidly diffuses into the cortex to react with hair keratin. The amino acids in hydrolyzed keratin are cross-linked to the hair keratin by agents such as formaldehyde or its derivatives, formalin, or methylene glycol.[22] In a salon, the treatment is applied in small sections and followed by heat styling to seal the hydrolyzed keratin onto the hair. The client must wait for at least 72 hours before wetting their hair to avoid reversing the process. Additionally, the hair cannot be pulled back in any way, such as with clips or sunglasses, prior to washing to maintain the hair in a straight formation for as long as possible. To maintain the keratin treatment, only sodium sulfate-free shampoos and hair care products should be used.[1] Out of concern for systemic side effects from formaldehyde, non–formaldehyde keratin-straightening products containing glyoxyloyl carbocysteine, glyoxyloyl keratin amino acids, silicone derivatives, and fatty acids[22] have been introduced with comparable results.[20] New versions of Brazilian Keratin Treatment (BKT), popular in the U.S. and Latin American countries, treat hair with methylene glycol or glyoxylic acid, which release formaldehyde when heated.[23]

BKT for Type 1 and 2 Curls: The Brazilian Experience In Brazil, where BKT is very popular, hair with Type 1 and 2 curls use keratin treatment as monotherapy to diminish frizz. Lye and no-lye relaxers are too potent for those hair types, whereas BKT can align the keratin molecules and close the cuticle scales resulting in smooth, shiny hair. Some patients apply BKT only to hair at the frontal scalp, which is thought to be an "undisciplined" region more prone to frizz. This patient population includes men who have undergone hair transplantation. In Brazil, hair transplant specialists even recommend BKT application for their patients at the affected site to smooth hair. Keratin treatment is applied to Type 1 and 2 curls between one and three times a year; Type 3 and 4 curls require a greater frequency. As a hot iron is applied more than 20 times to each strand of hair, breakage is expected to gradually occur at the distal tips, which are more susceptible to breakage.

BKT for Type 3 and 4 Curls: The Brazilian Experience Curly and kinky hair may take advantage of BKT being applied after the use of a chemical hair straightening product. As BKT is not capable of straightening severely tight curls, it is used after chemical relaxers to add shine to the hair by sealing the cuticles and aligning the keratin molecules. In addition, lubricants present among the ingredients of the treatment can alleviate the protein loss that occurs with the use of chemical relaxers. In daily practice, hair treated with chemical relaxers and BKT looks healthier and shinier than hair treated with chemical relaxers alone. Hair manageability is also improved after the application of a keratin hair treatment. BKT can be performed on the same day of chemical relaxer administration, just after the chemical relaxer is neutralized during blow drying.

DRY, NATURALLY CURLY HAIR

ATN is most common in naturally curly hair. As of the writing of this textbook, "going natural" is meant to signify hair that has not been chemically straightened, and this styling choice has become increasingly popular among those with curly hair. As previously noted, in those with the curliest hair types (Loussouarn Types VI-VIII), risk of breakage is high when the hair is under-moisturized. Severe cases can cause hair to break off at the root diffusely across the scalp, mimicking conditions like central centrifugal cicatricial alopecia. Treatment involves initiation of a healthy hair routine as outlined below.

TREATMENT AND PREVENTION OF ACQUIRED TRICHORRHEXIS NODOSA

A healthy hair care routine can lead to substantial improvements in strengthening the hair shaft to prevent breakage while maintaining moisturization.

CUTTING AND TRIMMING

As African hair grows more slowly and breaks more often than Asian or Caucasian hair,[7] combing increases the number of fractures in the hair shaft at longer lengths. Breakage is also exacerbated by knot formation and the high static charge African hair develops when combed in a dry state.[1] Consequently, combed natural hair can remain short for many years without being cut due to a "steady state" of daily breakage and equivalent new growth.[24] Women may be averse to cutting their hair because of the natural "daily haircut" due to breakage. Counseling patients to trim their hair every 8 to 12 weeks may minimize distal breakage and maximize luster and style maintenance.

CLEANSING

Unlike straight hair, curly or kinky hair is less likely to be coated by moisturizing sebum along the length of the hair shaft, increasing its susceptibility to damage from frequent shampooing. African hair also tends to be dry from low water content retention, leading to a buildup of negatively charged acids. Other cleansing agents targeted to populations with curly hair may contain mild amphoteric detergents, silicone-based materials, and quaternary ammonium compounds that will not aggravate the scalp.[10,25] Anionic surfactant shampoos, which often contain sulfates,[25] should be limited to one to two times per month, and used in situations of excess product buildup as they are extremely effective in removing sebum but harsh on hair. For women with African hair, general shampooing should be performed once every 1 to 2 weeks as increased frequencies are associated with higher rates of damage to the hair shaft. However, the act of cleansing can extend for many hours for a single session due to the need for detangling and moisturizing that is required. As a result, many patients may report washing every 4 to 12 weeks and should be encouraged to increase frequency to weekly to increase opportunities to provide moisture to the hair. Additionally, weekly washing is recommended for conditions such as seborrheic dermatitis, tinea capitis, and psoriasis, which necessitate more frequent washing.[1]

CONDITIONERS

Conditioners mimic natural sebum by increasing hair moisture and decreasing friction, making hair manageable. This minimizes the

TABLE 39-3 Recommendations for type IV to VIII healthy hair care practices

1. Deep condition every week for moisturization.
2. Use leave-in conditioner between 3 and 5 times a week. A "soak and smear" method is recommended.
3. Trim hair every 6 to 8 weeks.
4. Avoid use of extensions, including wigs, to prevent breakage.
5. Establish routine based on tightest curl pattern present.

likelihood of developing trichoptilosis, or split ends, from repetitive trauma. Heavier conditioning products are required to overcome the higher static charge of African hair. Options include rinse-out conditioners, deep conditioners, leave-ins, and protein-containing conditioners.[1] Conditioners, which are positively charged, work best following shampooing, which leaves behind a negative charge along the hair shaft.[26] Patients may report frequent "cowashing," or conditioner-only washing, which enhances moisturization but also leads to cowashing product accumulation, necessitating an occasional shampoo. Protein treatments are especially useful for damaged hair as they have a small molecular weight that can penetrate the hair shaft and increase its strength, but they should be limited to monthly or bimonthly use to prevent a brittle hair texture. A "soak and smear" approach popularized for atopic dermatitis, which consists of applying a thick emollient after soaking skin in water, can be utilized for curly or kinky hair to increase moisture retention. Shampoo and conditioner use is followed by blotting hair with a towel, applying a water-based leave-in conditioner as well as hair oil, and air drying or styling hair. In the media, this is known as the "L.O.C." method, which stands for liquid, oil, and cream.[1] Patients should avoid products that contain high-melting hydrocarbons or are vegetable oil- or petrolatum-based as overuse can lead to pomade acne involving the forehead.[27]

NATURAL VERSUS RELAXED HAIR

Wearing hair naturally can offer significant benefits by avoiding the use of chemicals associated with relaxers, maintaining hair strength, and providing a full appearance, which is desirable if hair is naturally fine. However, the degree of time and effort to moisturize hair as well as the attention required between stylist appointments is substantial. Additionally, for curl types VII to VIII, achieving long length with natural hair is exceedingly difficult as breakage rates are high. For this reason, weighing the pros and cons of loosening the curl with a texturizer or relaxer versus maintaining the curl pattern requires nuance and a discussion of patient styling goals. For example, patients with natural VII to VIII curl types should consider embracing shorter styles when natural, which are easier to moisturize to avoid severe breakage. Regardless of the choice, patients will have to adhere to healthy styling and cleansing choices to obtain optimal outcomes. By adopting healthy hair care practices, both styling options are sustainable. See **Table 39-3** for recommendations.

REFERENCES

1. Aguh C, Okoye GA, eds. *Fundamentals of Ethnic Hair*. Cham: Springer International Publishing; 2017.
2. Franbourg A, Hallegot P, Baltenneck F, Toutaina C, Leroy F. Current research on ethnic hair. *J Am Acad Dermatol*. 2003;48:S115-S119.
3. Robbins CR. *Chemical and Physical Behavior of Human Hair*. Berlin, Heidelberg: Springer Berlin Heidelberg; 2012.
4. saint Olive Baque C, Zhou J, Gu W, et al. Relationships between hair growth rate and morphological parameters of human straight hair: a same law above ethnical origins? *Int J Cosmet Sci*. 2012;34:111-116.
5. Lewallen R, Francis S, Fisher B, Richards J, Li J, Dawson T, et al. Hair care practices and structural evaluation of scalp and hair shaft parameters in African American and Caucasian women. *J Cosmet Dermatol*. 2015;14:216-223.
6. Walker A, Wiltz T, Winfrey O. *Andre Talks Hair!* Simon and Schuster, New York, NY; 1997.
7. Loussouarn G, el Rawadi C, Genain G. Diversity of hair growth profiles. *Int J Dermatol*. 2005;44:6-9.
8. Loussouarn G, Garcel A-L, Lozano I, et al. Worldwide diversity of hair curliness: a new method of assessment. *Int J Dermatol*. 2007;46:2-6.
9. Billero V, Miteva M. Traction alopecia: the root of the problem. *Clin Cosmet Investig Dermatol*. 2018;11:149-159.
10. Draelos ZD. *Hair Care*. CRC Press, Boca Raton, Fl; 2004.
11. Banka N, Bunagan MJK, Dubrule Y, Shapiro J. Wigs and hairpieces: Evaluating dermatologic issues. *Dermatol Ther*. 2012;25:260-266.
12. Malhotra YK. Tractional alopecia among Libyan women. *Arch Dermatol*. 1980;116:987.
13. James J, Saladi RN, Fox JL. Traction alopecia in Sikh male patients. *J Am Board Fam Med*. 2007;20:497-498.
14. McMichael AJ. Ethnic hair update: Past and present. *J Am Acad Dermatol*. 2003;48:S127-S133.
15. Callender VD, McMichael AJ, Cohen GF. Medical and surgical therapies for alopecias in black women. *Dermatol Ther*. 2004;17:164-176.
16. McMichael AJ. Hair and scalp disorders in ethnic populations. *Dermatol Clin*. 2003;21:629-644.
17. Quinn CR, Quinn TM, Kelly AP. Hair care practices in African American women. *Cutis*. 2003;72:280-282, 285-289.
18. Mamabolo T, Agyei NM, Summers B. Cosmetic and amino acid analysis of the effects of lye and no-lye relaxer treatment on adult black female South African hair. *J Cosmet Sci*. 2013;64:287-296.
19. Mirmirani P. Ceramic flat irons: improper use leading to acquired trichorrhexis nodosa. *J Am Acad Dermatol*. 2010;62:145-147.
20. Guerra-Tapia A, Gonzalez-Guerra E. Hair cosmetics: dyes. *Actas Dermo-Sifiliogr*. 2014;105:833-839.
21. DeLeo VA, Taylor SC, Belsito DV, et al. The effect of race and ethnicity on patch test results. *J Am Acad Dermatol*. 2002;46:S107-S112.
22. Weathersby C, McMichael A. Brazilian keratin hair treatment: a review. *J Cosmet Dermatol*. 2013;12:144-148.
23. Pierce JS, Abelmann A, Spicer LJ, et al. Characterization of formaldehyde exposure resulting from the use of four professional hair straightening products. *J Occup Environ Hyg*. 2011;8:686-699.
24. Khumalo NP. African hair morphology: macrostructure to ultrastructure. *Int J Dermatol*. 2005;44:10-12.
25. Diana Draelos Z. The biology of hair care. *Dermatol Clin*. 2000;18:651-658.
26. Gavazzoni Dias MF, Pichler J, Adriano A, Cecato P, de Almeida A. The shampoo pH can affect the hair: myth or reality? *Int J Trichology*. 2014;6:95.
27. Bhate K, Williams HC. Epidemiology of acne vulgaris. *Br J Dermatol*. 2013;168:474-485.

CHAPTER 40 Clinical Assessment of Hair and Hair Loss

Tiffany T. Mayo
Ashley Slack
Valerie D. Callender

KEY POINTS

- Alopecia requires complete clinical assessment and understanding that hair type and cultural practices may impact diagnosis.
- Classifications such as chronic versus acute, diffuse versus focal, and scarring versus nonscarring can assist in the clinical assessment.
- Patients may have more than one type of alopecia.
- Dermoscopy, biopsy, and laboratory assessment are tools that, along with clinical correlation, can assist in developing the correct diagnosis.

INTRODUCTION

Hair-related conditions are a frequent chief concern for skin of color patients. Hair phenotype and hair care practices vary within and between cultures. Language regarding hair type and hair care may also differ between patients and clinicians. For instance, hair type is categorized as African, Asian, and Caucasian in literature, but hair characteristics and concerns can vary significantly within these categories. Patients may also use different language, referring to their hair type based on its curl patterns. Curl pattern characteristics affect the structural properties of hair with tighter curl patterns seen in patients of African descent, being more susceptible to complex knot formation, longitudinal fissures, and breakage.[1] These differences should be taken into consideration when examining the hair as they may affect the overall assessment, diagnosis, and treatment plan.

In addition to this, it is important to consider the impact of alopecia on quality of life. Alopecia has been found to be associated with negative psychosocial outcomes, including anxiety and depression.[2] The impact can be as significant as that of severe psoraisis.[3] Female gender, younger age at onset, and scarring alopecia are factors associated with higher psychosocial burdeon.[2] Early diagnosis and management are critically important for this patient population.

Because of variations in hair phenotype, race discordance can be a source of anxiety for both the patient and clinician during the hair assessment.[4] A survey study found that 68% of African American patients felt their physician did not understand their hair.[5] Similarly, studies have shown dermatology residents and some training programs have decreased confidence and exposure in managing conditions in skin of color patients compared to non-Hispanic White patients.[6,7] A thorough clinical assessment requires openness to understanding cultural practices and cultural humility.

In this chapter, we will discuss how to approach a patient with hair loss, the initial clinical assessment, and differential diagnoses and workup to consider. A particular emphasis will be placed on patients of African descent.

CULTURAL HUMILITY

Hair is beyond cosmetic and can be integrally tied to one's identity. For many people, healthy hair reflects health, youth, and femininity or masculinity, but many cultures also view hair in a unique significant way. For centuries in Africa, hair and hair styles have held spiritual and societal significance. Certain hair styles may have symbolized age, marital status, ethnic identity, geographic origins, community rank, and other social, political, and religious statuses. Historically, hair aesthetics, usually involving a clean neatly braided style, were just as important as having hair.[8] Many current styles and braids worn by people of African descent are redolent of these cultural traditions.

Hair symbolism is also prominent in Asian culture, particularly South Asian culture. Hair style, length, and decisions to cut or shave hair may hold significant religious, societal, or cultural meaning.[9]

Hair style preference not only holds traditional and historic significance, but may also be influenced by social beauty standards, stereotypes, and discrimination. For instance, until recently, many natural Afro-textured hair styles were banned in dress codes, schools, sports, and the workplace. Recently the CROWN (Create a Respectful and Open World for Natural hair) Act of 2022 was introduced and passed by the House of Representatives and several states prohibiting discrimination based on race-based hairstyles.[10] Societal factors may consciously or unconsciously influence personal hair style preferences.[11]

When addressing hair concerns, it is important to consider cultural influences and other factors contributing to a patient's hair care practice. Hair-shaming and/or blaming is not appropriate.[4] Hair may represent the essence of beauty or hold other significant traditional meaning in one's self-identity and should be approached with cultural humility.

APPROACH TO HISTORY

History taking is an opportunity to build rapport, establish trust, and learn important clues to assist in developing a diagnosis and treatment plan. Physicians should sit facing the patient during this portion of the exam. It is recommended to start with an open-ended question, allowing the patient to express their concern(s). Questions related to the onset and duration of hair loss can assist in guiding the differential diagnosis [**Table 40-1**]. In addition to asking "How long have you experienced hair loss," providing a time reference, such as "1 year ago, would you describe your hair density as normal?" may result in a more accurate history. Avoid leading with accusatory questions regarding "tight braids" or "relaxers." This may cause the patient to feel defensive and may hinder the physician's ability to form an appropriate differential diagnosis. Instead, allow the patient adequate time to describe their concern and follow with any remaining questions related to hair styling history.

TABLE 40-1 History questions in alopecia assessment

Questions about alopecia
• How long have you noticed alopecia? Do you feel your hair density was normal 1 year ago? 2 years? 5 years?
• Is alopecia located in one spot or throughout scalp?
• Has alopecia worsened over time or remained stable?
• Has the hair ever regrown?
• Do you feel your hair is thinning, falling out from the root/shedding, or breaking off?
Questions about symptoms
• Have you noticed itch, pain, burning, or stinging in your scalp?
• Have you noticed scale?
Questions about other history/triggering factors
• Has your diet changed recently? Does your diet have limited protein?
• Have you started any new medications?
• Have you had any recent procedures or illnesses?
• Have you had any rapid weight gain or weight loss? Fatigue?

During this portion of the exam, one may consider thinking of the differential diagnosis in terms of scarring versus nonscarring alopecia [**Table 40-2**]. Onset, duration, and character may help determine which category of alopecia the patient is most likely experiencing. The onset of hair loss occurring in the pediatric population is most often nonscarring. Alopecias occurring more commonly in the pediatric age group include alopecia areata, traction alopecia, trichotillomania, loose androgen syndrome, and tinea capitis.[12] Gender can be helpful but should not limit the differential diagnosis. Though nonscarring androgenetic alopecia is common in males, scarring alopecias may also occur, particularly in Black males. For adults, acuity can assist in deciding between scarring and nonscarring hair loss. Scarring alopecias such as central centrifugal cicatricial alopecia (CCCA), lichen planopilaris (LPP), and frontal fibrosing alopecia (FFA) are chronic processes, whereas nonscarring alopecias, such as alopecia areata (AA), acute traction alopecia, and telogen effluvium (TE) may cause noticeable hair loss in a short time period. Characterizing hair loss may also help to focus the differential diagnosis. Decipher between shedding, thinning, and breakage if possible. Shedding may be indicative of TE, whereas breakage, trichorrhexis nodosa, may indicate an extrinsic cause (ie, chemicals, heat, or hair styling technique) or an early sign of CCCA, particularly if focally located in the crown.[13] Other characteristics to consider are relapsing and remitting (nonscarring) versus chronic and expanding (scarring) and diffuse versus localized [**Table 40-3; Figure 40-1**]. Finally, associated symptoms (pain, tenderness, burning, pustules, and pruritus) are important and more often point to an inflammatory scarring process.

Next, information regarding hair loss involving other parts of the body and hair care practices should be obtained. Hair loss beyond the scalp may be caused by alopecia areata, LPP, and thyroid dysfunction. Ask about hair loss involving eyebrows, eyelashes, axilla, pubic region, and extremities. Past hair styling history should be obtained. This may include information regarding chemical dyes, relaxers or perms, tight hairstyles, weaves, braids, and hair adornments or scalp coverings. Hairstyling history is rarely helpful in determining a primary diagnosis beyond traction alopecia and trichorrhexis, but it may provide additional

TABLE 40-2 Differential diagnosis for scarring and nonscarring alopecia[14–18]

Diagnosis	Onset	Location	Clinical findings	symptoms	Dermoscopy findings
Scarring alopecia					
Acne keloidalis nuche (AKN)	Post puberty—throughout middle age	Occipital scalp	Firm follicular papules; keloidal plaques	± Pain, pruritus	Tufted hairs; fibrosis; penetration of hairs into epidermis
Central centrifugal cicatricial alopecia (CCCA)	Young adults—middle aged	Crown of scalp	Round alopecia patch in vertex; ± erythema and/or scale	± Burning, pain, or pruritus in area of hair loss	Loss of follicular ostia; perihilar gray-white halo; erythema; hypo and hyperpigmentation
Discoid lupus erythematosus (DLE)	Young adults	Variable; often multiple isolated patches or plaques	Patches/plaques with erythema, atrophy, follicular plugging, erythema, hypopigmentation, hyperpigmentation, telangiectasias	± burning, pain, or pruritus	Follicular plugging, erythema, hypopigmentation; hyperpigmentation
Dissecting cellulitis of the scalp	Young adult to middle aged	Vertex and occipital scalp; Variable	Boggy purulent nodules, interconnecting abscesses with overlying patchy alopecia	Pain	Enlarged follicular openings; follicular plugging; may resemble AA in early stages
Fibrosing alopecia in patterned distribution (FAPD)	Middle aged	Frontal scalp in FPHL distribution	Decreased hair density in the frontal scalp ± red dots on chest or facial papules	± Pruritus or pain	Hair diameter variability, loss of follicular ostia, perifollicular erythema, peripilar casts
Folliculitis decalvans	Young adults – middle age	Vertex and occipital scalp	Follicular papules, pustules, and crusts Hair tufting	± Pain, pruritus, burning	Tufted hairs (>5 from a single follicular ostia), serum crust, pustules, papules, scale
Frontal fibrosing alopecia (FFA)	Middle age	Frontotemporal hairline	Band-like recession of frontotemporal hairline, few isolated remaining terminal hairs (lonely hairs) ±Loss of eyebrows ±Facial papules	± Pruritus, pain, burning	Loss of follicular ostia; absence of vellus hairs; perifollicular scale, and perifollicular erythema
Lichen planopilaris	Young adults—middle age	Parietal or frontal scalp	Patches of hair loss with irregular borders	± Pruritus, pain, burning	Perifollicular scale, perifollicular erythema, loss of follicular ostia
Nonscarring alopecia					
Alopecia areata	Any age	Variable	Single or multiple patches to complete loss of hair on scalp Diffuse pattern presents with diffuse hair loss similar to telogen effluvium or FPHL ±involvement of brows, lashes, beard, body hair; ±nail pits	Usually asymptomatic	Preserved follicular ostia; exclamation point hairs; broken hairs; black dots
Anagen effluvium	Any age	Variable	Positive hair pull test Tapered fracture of hair shaft Abrupt shedding of most or all of scalp hair	Usually asymptomatic	Black dots; monilethrix-like hairs, exclamation point hairs
Female pattern hair loss (androgenetic alopecia)	Post-puberty throughout adulthood	Diffuse in frontal and vertex scalp	Decreased density in frontal scalp with preservation of anterior hairline; widened midline part	Usually asymptomatic	Miniaturized hair; shaft thickness heterogeneity; preserved follicular ostia
Loose anagen syndrome	Children mostly	Diffuse or occipital scalp	Patches with decreased density	Usually asymptomatic	Nonspecific; dermoscopy of pulled hairs reveals anagen hairs
Male Pattern Hair Loss (androgenetic alopecia)	Puberty throughout adulthood	Bitemporal thinning of frontal scalp, vertex	Decreased density of hair in bitemporal and/or in vertex distribution	Usually asymptomatic	Miniaturized hair; shaft thickness heterogeneity; preserved follicular ostia
Telogen effluvium	Any age	Diffuse	Diffuse thinning without focal areas of alopecia	Usually asymptomatic	Nonspecific
Tinea Capitis	Children mostly; any age	Varies	Rounds patches of alopecia, scales, black dots/broken hairs ± pustules, erythema Cervical lymphadenopathy	± Pruritus, pain	Comma hairs, corkscrew hairs
Traction Alopecia	Children throughout adulthood	Temporal, preauricular regions, and above the ears	Decreased density at the temporal and frontal region of scalp. May spare rim of hairs of the frontal hair line, "fringe sign" ± papules and pustules in acute traction alopecia	± pain or stinging in acute setting	Preservation of vellus hairs and follicular ostia; hair casts Chronic traction alopecia may result in loss of follicular ostia
Trichotillomania	Children and adolescents mostly; any age	Fronto-temporal; Variable	Patch(s) of alopecia with ill-defined borders	Usually asymptomatic	Hairs broken at different lengths; black dots; V-sign; hair powder

TABLE 40-3 Localized versus diffuse alopecia differential diagnosis

	Localized	Diffuse
Scarring	• Acne keloidalis nuche • Central centrifugal cicatricial alopecia • Discoid lupus erythematosus • Dissecting cellulitis • Frontal fibrosing alopecia • Lichen planopilaris	• Fibrosing alopecia in pattern distribution • Folliculitis decalvans
Nonscarring	• Alopecia • Alopecia areata • Tinea capitis • Traction alopecia • Trichotillomania	• Alopecia areata—totalis, universalis, and diffuse types • Anagen effluvium • Androgenetic/FPHL (diffuse involvement in frontal scalp) • Loose anagen syndrome • Telogen effluvium • Alopecia secondary to nutritional deficiency, thyroid or other hormonal imbalance

information to counsel on overall hair and scalp health. Caution should be taken to avoid assuming the hairstyle is related to the patient's alopecia without proper assessment.

Finally, additional history including recent illness or procedure, medical problems, medications, nutritional history, psychosocial history, and family history of alopecia can provide additional context and help develop the differential diagnosis.

THE ASSESSMENT

Before assessing the hair, the patient should be asked to remove any hats, wigs, scarves, or hair ties. The hair should be loose to allow evaluation of the entire scalp. Many patients may feel embarrassed to reveal their hair and should be approached with thoughtfulness and consideration for this portion of the exam [**Table 40-4**].[4] Take a moment to ask permission. A simple question "Do you mind if I examine your hair now?" demonstrates consideration and builds rapport. If the patient is a child or adolescent, ask the patient's care giver to join you when performing the exam, and show the patient the tools you will be using (ie, dermatoscope, cotton tip applicator, culture swab, etc) to decrease anxiety. Examine the patient's hair and scalp with gentle confidence. Hesitation to touch the hair or incomplete examination may cause the patient to feel uncomfortable or perceive the provider as being uncomfortable, especially in cases of race discordance. Consider having the patient sit in a chair if the exam table's height will limit the ability to perform a thorough exam.

A cotton tip applicator may be used to section through the hair to determine if any alopecia patterns or focal locations are readily noticeable. Alopecia localized to the frontal scalp may represent traction alopecia (TA), FFA, or AA. Patchy areas of alopecia throughout the scalp may be caused by AA, discoid lupus, tinea capitis, trichotillomania, syphilitic alopecia, or TA related to chronic tight braids or locs. Papules, pustules, scale, excoriations, and erythema should also be noted during this general assessment of the hair and scalp.

Next, a hair pull test can be done to assess for hair shedding and hair breakage. A bundle of 50 to 60 hairs is pulled from multiple areas of the scalp. Recent findings suggest that two hairs or fewer represent normal hair shed. Greater than two hairs may be indicative of TE or other types of alopecia associated with shedding such as loose anagen syndrome, AA, and anagen effluvium.[19] The hair pull test should be corroborated with history. If hair has been washed within 24 hours, hair pull test may be falsely negative. If the patient has recently had a low maintenance hair style (see Chapter 39), hair pull test can be falsely positive depending on the length of time the hair style was in place prohibiting combing/brushing. Broken hair, trichorrhexis nodosa, during hair pull may be indicative of heat, chemical or physical trauma, underlying medical conditions such as thyroid disorders, or congenital. This can be assessed with the hair card test in which a small white card (or black card for light hair) is placed behind the distal hair shaft to allow for easy assessment of blunted ends, indicative of broken hairs, or tapered ends, new growing hairs [**Figure 40-2A** and **B**].[14]

Separate the hair with a straight midline part from the central frontal hairline to the crown using the cotton tip applicator. Assess the occipital scalp to determine baseline hair density if this area is unaffected. The midline part may help discern less obvious density loss. This is also the ideal position to photograph the scalp. The part width is a useful technique to assess thinning. A part width that widens with decreased density from the crown toward the frontal scalp, also known as "Christmas tree pattern," may indicate female pattern hair loss (FPHL).[20] A part width that widens with decreased density in the crown may be indicative of a scarring alopecia [**Figure 40-3A** and **B**].

Trichoscopy, or dermoscopy of the hair and scalp, is an excellent tool to further assess alopecia (see Chapter 25, Dermoscopic

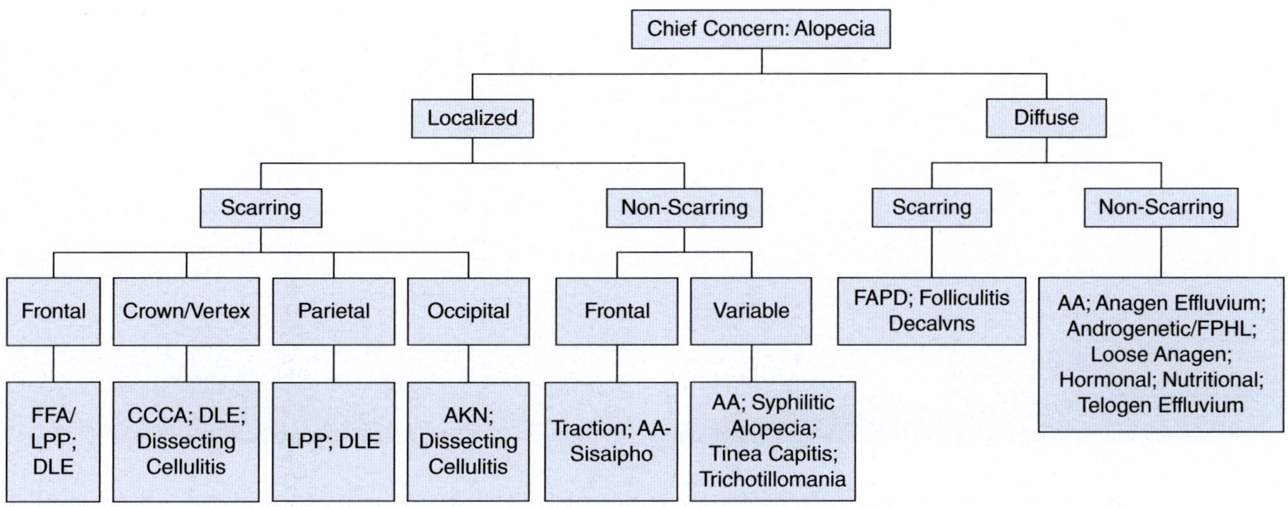

FIGURE 40-1. Differential diagnosis of localized and diffuse alopecias. (Reproduced from Tiffany Mayo, MD.)

TABLE 40-4 Alopecia clinical assessment pearls

Alopecia clinical assessment pearls
The hair assessment • Position patient to allow visualization of entire scalp; consider having patient sit in a chair rather than exam table • A cotton tip applicator or blunt metal probe can be useful to section through hair • Determine baseline density to assess amount of hair loss in area of concern; occipital scalp may serve as baseline in most alopecias
Pediatric patient • Invite the parent/guardian to join you while performing the assessment • Allow patient to see tools such as cotton tip applicator, culture swab, or dermatocope to decrease anxiety
Biopsy anxiety • Utilize vibratory tools while performing injections • Consider scheduling biopsy on separate day to allow patient to mentally prepare
Developing a positive patient-physician relationship • Be open and honest; ask questions • Set expectations upfront but avoid the "nothing can be done" mentality. For instance, focus on goals to preserve remaining hair and address symptoms for severe scarring alopecia
Patient education/counseling • Supplement verbal and written education with photographs of the patient's scalp. Use trichoscopy photos to help patient understand their alopecia. Use before and after photos to assess improvement and encourage patient

Patterns of Dermatological Diseases in Skin of Color Individuals). With a dermatoscope, the scalp should be evaluated for variability in follicle diameter, erythema, scale, dyspigmentation, and hair tufting. It can also help distinguish between scarring and nonscarring alopecia. Diameter variability of 20% is seen in androgenetic alopecia/FPHL.[15] Scarring alopecias are characterized by loss of follicular ostia, scattered white patches, and asterisk-like macules and disruption of the pigment network in darker skin.[21,22] Nonscarring alopecias feature retained follicular ostia and a retained pigment network [**Figure 40-3C** and **D**].

It is not uncommon for patients to present with more than one type of alopecia. For instance, a patient may have both FPHL and scarring alopecia, or FPHL, traction, and scarring alopecia. Biopsy of involved areas along with clinical assessment can determine the cause(s) of alopecia.

It is important to discuss any clinical findings and the plan with the patient. This is a good time to set expectations and goals. At the conclusion of the assessment or biopsy, ensure the patient has access to a mirror and is allowed adequate time to groom before leaving the exam room.

BIOPSY

A scalp biopsy is the gold standard to diagnose the type of alopecia but can be challenging without clinical correlation. Biopsy site should be chosen in an active area with retained hair follicles; usually the peripheral edge is appropriate. A 4-mm punch biopsy is preferred, and 1 to 2 specimens should be obtained. For suspected scarring alopecia, 2 specimen side-by-side allows for both horizontal and vertical sectioning along the length of the hair follicle, which may be helpful in challenging cases. In suspected nonscarring alopecia, one specimen from the frontal scalp and one from the occipital scalp may be useful.[23,24] Additional specimens may be obtained from different sites when more than one alopecia type is suspected, and direct immunofluorescence (DIF) can be obtained if discoid lupus is suspected.[14]

LABORATORY ASSESSMENT

Alopecia can result from systemic processes and nutrient deficiencies. Laboratory work up may include evaluation of thyroid hormones along with iron, vitamin D, and zinc levels.[15] Thyroid hormones are thought to be key regulations of hair follicle cycling. Dysregulation of thyroid hormones results in classic clinical findings including dry brittle hair and loss of lateral eyebrows in hypothyroidism, and fine hair or thinning in hyperthyroidism.[25] Micronutrient deficiencies lack distinguishable hair findings but may be associated with various alopecias. Iron-dependent genes are expressed in the hair follicle bulge region. Fluctuations in serum iron affect expression of these genes, resulting in alteration of the hair cycle.[26,27] In addition, iron is a cofactor involved in DNA synthesis, and its bioavailability can affect rapidly dividing hair matrix cells.[26] The vitamin D receptor plays a role in anagen initiation; deficiency in vitamin D affects hair follicle cycling.[26] Finally, zinc is important in multiple metabolic pathways. It is an inhibitor of hair follicle regression and promotes hair follicle recovery. Zinc deficiency has been associated with telogen effluvium, androgenetic alopecia, and alopecia areata.[28,29] A laboratory workup can help further guide diagnosis and management.

CONCLUSION

Alopecia significantly impacts quality of life and can be challenging for both patient and physician. It requires a thorough clinical assessment in all pediatric and adult patients with hair loss. Differences in hair

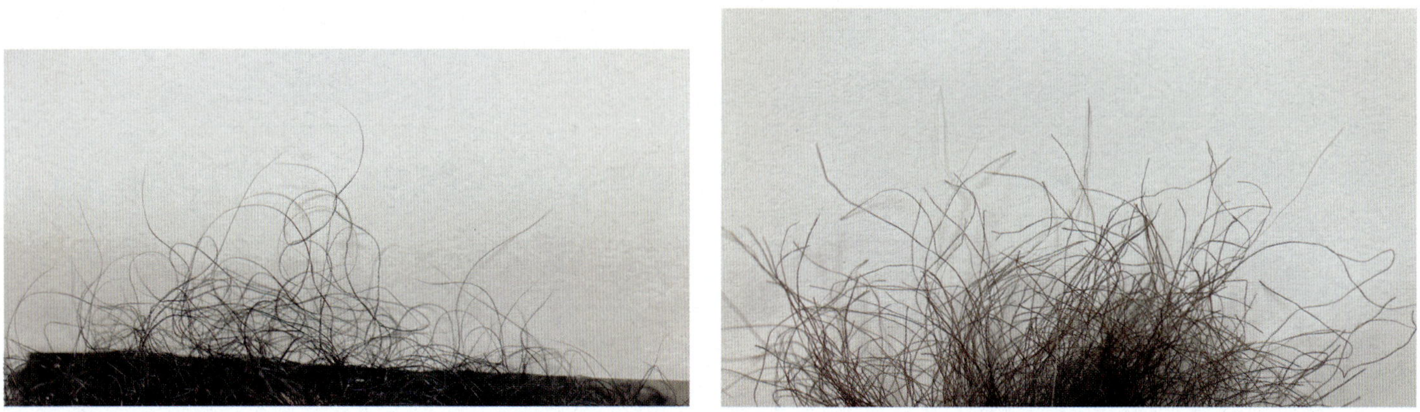

A B

FIGURE 40-2. (A) Hair card demonstrating short hairs with tapered ends, indicative of new growing hairs. **(B)** Hair card demonstrating blunt and fractured ends, indicative of broken hairs. (Reproduced with permission from Tiffany Mayo, MD.)

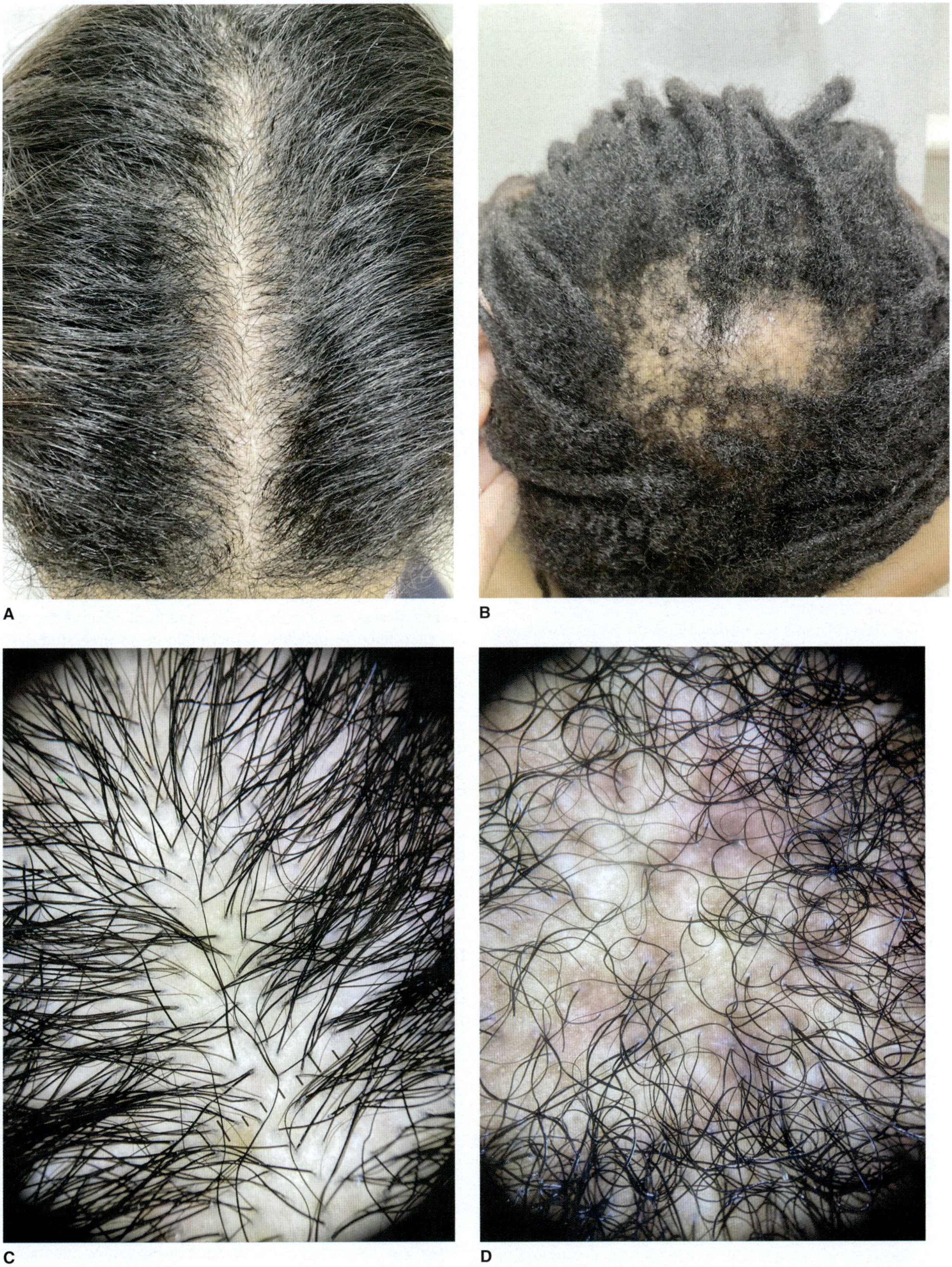

FIGURE 40-3. (A) Nonscarring alopecia. (B) Scarring alopecia. (C) Trichoscopy of nonscarring alopecia. (D) Trichoscopy of scarring alopecia. (Reproduced with permission from Tiffany Mayo, MD.)

type and cultural hair care practices can impact the underlying cause of alopecia. The history is an opportunity to help better understand the patients' concerns in the context of hair care practices and build rapport. The differential diagnosis is vast; however, categories such as chronic versus acute, diffuse versus focal, and scarring versus nonscarring can help arrive quickly and efficiently at an accurate differential diagnosis. Additional tools such as dermoscopy, biopsy, and laboratory assessment can further assist in diagnosing alopecia.

REFERENCES

1. Khumalo NP, Doe PT, Dawber RP, Ferguson DJ. What is normal black African hair? A light and scanning electron-microscopic study. *J Am Acad Dermatol.* 2000;43(5 Pt 1):814-820.
2. Davis DS, Callender VD. Review of quality of life studies in women with alopecia. *Int J Womens Dermatol.* 2018;4(1):18-22.
3. Williamson D, Gonzalez M, Finlay AY. The effect of hair loss on quality of life. *J Eur Acad Dermatol Venereol.* 2001;15(2):137-139.
4. Grayson C, Heath C. An approach to examining tightly coiled hair among patients with hair loss in race-discordant patient-physician interactions. *JAMA Dermatol.* 2021;157(5):505-506.
5. Gathers RC, Mahan MG. African american women, hair care, and health barriers. *J Clin Aesthet Dermatol.* 2014;7(9):26-29.
6. Gupta R, Ibraheim MK, Dao H, Jr., Patel AB, Koshelev M. Assessing dermatology resident confidence in caring for patients with skin of color. *Clin Dermatol.* 2021;39(5):873-878.
7. Nijhawan RI, Jacob SE, Woolery-Lloyd H. Skin of color education in dermatology residency programs: does residency training reflect the changing demographics of the United States? *J Am Acad Dermatol.* 2008;59(4):615-618.
8. Byrd A, Tharps L. *Hair Story: Untangling the Roots of Black Hair in America.* New York, NY: St. Martin's Publishing Group; 2014.
9. Hiltebeitel A, Miller BD, Obeyesekere G, Miller PADWSPBD. *Hair: Its Power and Meaning in Asian Cultures.* Albany, NY: State University of New York Press; 1998.
10. Creating a Respectful and Open World for Natural Hair Act of 2022, H.R. 2116 - 117th Congress(2022).
11. Koval CZ, Rosette AS. The natural hair bias in job recruitment. *Social Psychol Pers Sci.* 2021;12(5):741-750.
12. Goldberg LJ, Castelo-Soccio LA. Alopecia: kids are not just little people. *Clin Dermatol.* 2015;33(6):622-630.
13. Callender VD, Wright DR, Davis EC, Sperling LC. Hair breakage as a presenting sign of early or occult central centrifugal cicatricial alopecia: clinicopathologic findings in 9 patients. *Arch Dermatol.* 2012;148(9):1047-1052.
14. Mubki T, Rudnicka L, Olszewska M, Shapiro J. Evaluation and diagnosis of the hair loss patient: part I. History and clinical examination. *J Am Acad Dermatol.* 2014;71(3):415.e411-415.e415.
15. Gordon KA, Tosti A. Alopecia: evaluation and treatment. *Clin Cosmet Investig Dermatol.* 2011;4:101-106.
16. Griggs J, Trüeb RM, Gavazzoni Dias MFR, Hordinsky M, Tosti A. Fibrosing alopecia in a pattern distribution. *J Am Acad Dermatol.* 2021;85(6): 1557-1564.
17. Larrondo J, McMichael AJ. Scarring alopecia. *Dermatol Clin.* 2023;41(3): 519-537.
18. Rodney IJ, Onwudiwe OC, Callender VD, Halder RM. Hair and scalp disorders in ethnic populations. *J Drugs Dermatol.* 2013;12(4):420-427.
19. McDonald KA, Shelley AJ, Colantonio S, Beecker J. Hair pull test: Evidence-based update and revision of guidelines. *J Am Acad Dermatol.* 2017;76(3):472-477.
20. Olsen EA. The midline part: an important physical clue to the clinical diagnosis of androgenetic alopecia in women. *J Am Acad Dermatol.* 1999;40(1): 106-109.
21. Miteva M, Tosti A. Dermatoscopic features of central centrifugal cicatricial alopecia. *J Am Acad Dermatol.* 2014;71(3):443-449.
22. Ocampo-Garza J, Tosti A. Trichoscopy of dark scalp. *Skin Appendage Disord.* 2018;5(1):1-8.
23. Sperling LC. Scarring alopecia and the dermatopathologist. *J Cutan Pathol.* 2001;28(7):333-342.
24. Tailor A, Asher RG, Craig PJ, Groves RW, Fenton DA, Stefanato CM. The current state of play in the histopathologic assessment of alopecia: two for one or one for two? *J Cutan Pathol.* 2013;40(3):298-304.
25. Mancino G, Miro C, Di Cicco E, Dentice M. Thyroid hormone action in epidermal development and homeostasis and its implications in the pathophysiology of the skin. *J Endocrinol Invest.* 2021;44(8):1571-1579.
26. Yorulmaz A, Hayran Y, Ozdemir AK, et al. Telogen effluvium in daily practice: patient characteristics, laboratory parameters, and treatment modalities of 3028 patients with telogen effluvium. *J Cosmet Dermatol.* 2022; 21(6):2610-2617.
27. St Pierre SA, Vercellotti GM, Donovan JC, Hordinsky MK. Iron deficiency and diffuse nonscarring scalp alopecia in women: more pieces to the puzzle. *J Am Acad Dermatol.* 2010;63(6):1070-1076.
28. Kil MS, Kim CW, Kim SS. Analysis of serum zinc and copper concentrations in hair loss. *Ann Dermatol.* 2013;25(4):405-409.
29. Park H, Kim CW, Kim SS, Park CW. The therapeutic effect and the changed serum zinc level after zinc supplementation in alopecia areata patients who had a low serum zinc level. *Ann Dermatol.* 2009;21(2):142-146.

CHAPTER 41

Aesthetic Assessment of Hair Loss and Aesthetic Treatments

Ogechukwu Opaigbeogu
Cheryl M. Burgess
Valerie D. Callender

KEY POINTS

- Aesthetic therapies for hair loss can be a great option when medical therapies are not an option.
- Types of alopecia are broadly split into two categories: scarring and nonscarring.
- Before suggesting an aesthetic therapy, a thorough history of the factors surrounding the hair loss and previous treatment(s) are needed.
- Along with questions, a thorough assessment of the hair and scalp should be performed.
- Success of an aesthetic therapy will depend on the type of hair loss.
- Aesthetic treatments are available for hair on the scalp, eyebrows, and eyelashes.

When medical therapies for hair loss are not an option or are not able to achieve desired results, there are a multitude of aesthetic therapies that can be offered to patients. A multitude of research studies have shown that hair loss has a negative effect on quality of life especially for women and scarring alopecias.[1] Hair loss is often associated with depression and anxiety. Aesthetic therapies are sometimes the only options available for people with certain types of hair loss, so it is important to know what types of therapies are available and what can be realistically achieved with each type of therapy. Aesthetic therapies might not have as much evidence-based data to support their utility or might be temporary solutions that do not correct the underlying cause of hair loss, so it is important to discuss outcomes and realistic expectations with patients before offering an aesthetic therapy. Not every patient will qualify for every aesthetic therapy.

Below is a guideline for ascertaining if an aesthetic therapy is appropriate and if so which one.

INITIAL VISIT

History questions:

- Before considering therapy, it is best if the patient understands the underlying cause of the hair loss as this will affect which therapy options are suitable. Steps should first be made to properly diagnose the cause of the hair loss (see Chapter 40).
- Determine if the patient is currently experiencing symptoms of pruritis, burning, or tenderness; and if the hair loss is stable or still progressive. Refer to Chapter 40 on guidelines for obtaining a history and assessing the hair to properly diagnose the cause of hair loss.
- Once the underlying cause of hair loss has been discussed and confirmed, it is important to ascertain what the patient's goals are for their hair loss. Does the patient wish to regrow hair or maintain the current density and length or does the patient simply wish to hide the hair loss without much regard to preventing further damage?
- Once goals for the hair have been discussed, it is important to note what medical and over-the-counter therapies have already been tried. If the patient has not used any medical therapies for hair restoration, it would be prudent to start with established medical therapies before trying any aesthetic therapies. It is important to note if the medical treatments were continued for an appropriate length of time and at an appropriate dosage before the patient sought alternative methods.

Assessment during the first visit:

- An assessment of the scalp and hair strands should be performed during the first visit.
  - Be sure to check the scalp for signs of irritation, scaling, flaking, inflammation, and erythema redness.
  - Hair loss scales can be used to quantify the severity of hair loss [**Figures 41-1**][2]
  - Check the density of the hair and note any areas of thinning.
  - Check the length of the strands to see if there are areas of hair breakage.
  - Perform a hair pull test.
  - Check for the fringe sign (TA) or lonely hair sign (FFA)
  - Traction Alopecia and Frontal Fibrosing Alopecia
- Trichoscopy should be performed to get a closer visualization of the hair shaft and scalp morphology (see Chapter 25.)
- High-quality wide-focused and close-up photographs should be taken to help measure progress of hair growth over time [Figure 41-1]. A photo should be taken at the first visit and subsequent visits to monitor treatment progress. Be sure to obtain consent forms for the photos as well.
- Artificial intelligence technology can be used for detailed visualization and taking photographs.

The type of hair loss, history of previous treatments, current symptoms, and hair goals will determine what aesthetic therapies the patient qualifies for. Cost and time commitment will also play a role in determining appropriate therapy as well.

After a detailed history is taken, a hair and scalp assessment has been performed and realistic expectations have been agreed upon, inform the patient about any recommended procedures including pre-op and post-op care, side effects, follow-up appointments, risks, and costs.

It is important to provide verbal and written instructions to the patient, including special instructions and information about hair care after each procedure.

FOLLOW-UP VISITS

Questions for subsequent visits:

1. Any side effects from the chosen treatment?
2. Have you noticed any hair regrowth?
3. Have you develop any new symptoms?
4. Are there any obstacles to completing the current treatment regimen?

Assessment for subsequent visits:

- The scalp and hair should be checked at subsequent visits to assess the presence of clinical signs of scalp inflammation or irritation.

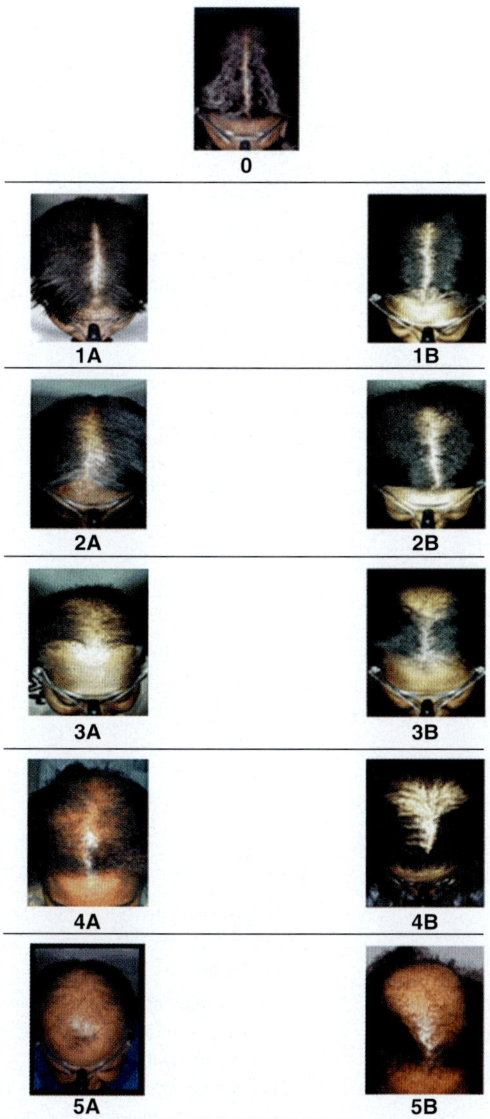

FIGURE 41-1. (Reproduced with permission from Olsen EA, Callender V, Sperling L, et al. Central scalp alopecia photographic scale in African American women. Dermatol Ther. 2008;21(4):264-7.)

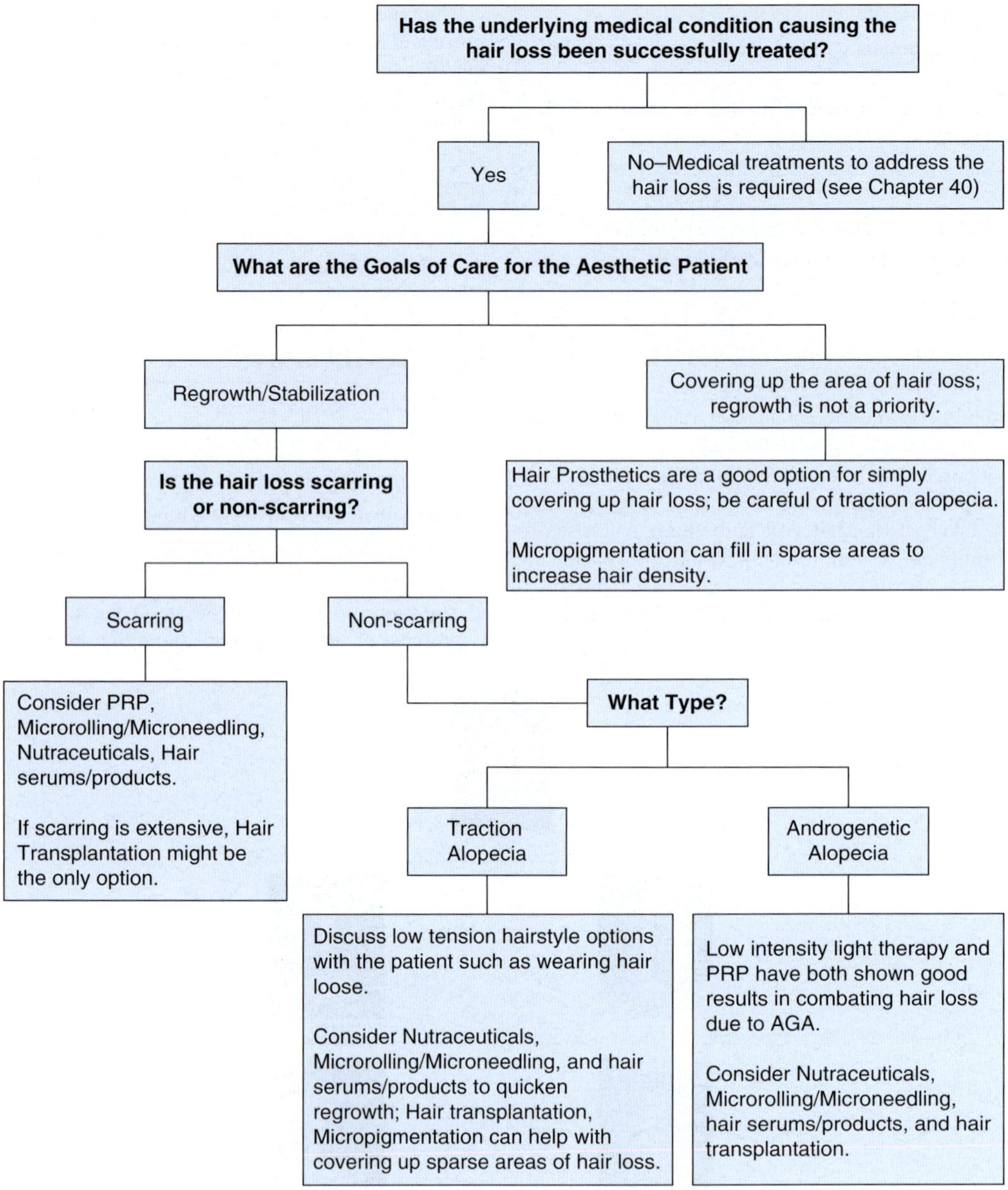

FIGURE 41-2.

- Perform a trichoscopic examination of the scalp to aid in the detection of erythema in skin of color.
- Obtain high-quality wide-focused and close-up photographs to document the success or failure of the procedure.

We have included an algorithm for the aesthetic patient to simplify the approach [**Figure 41-2**]; however, an individualized treatment plan and strategy is recommended [**Table 41-1 to 41-4**].

TABLE 41-1 Types of alopecias, scarring versus nonscarring

Scarring Alopecias ***Not an exhaustive list*** ***(see Chapter 42)***	Nonscarring alopecias (over time these can become scarring) ***Not an exhaustive list*** ***(see Chapter 43)***
Chronic cutaneous discoid lupus erythematosus	Acquired trichorrhexis nodosa, anagen effluvium,
Lichen planopilaris	traction alopecia (TA), and other hair shaft disorders
Central centrifugal cicatricial alopecia (CCCA)	Telogen effluvium
Frontal fibrosing alopecia	Androgenetic alopecia (AGA), male- and female-pattern hair loss[3]
Folliculitis keloidalis	Alopecia areata, totalis, or universalis
Folliculitis (acne) necrotica	Loose anagen syndrome
Erosive pustular dermatosis	Infection

TABLE 41-2 Questions to ask at the Initial Visit

1. What type of hair loss do you have?
   a. If patient has had a scalp biopsy previously, obtain a copy of the pathology report for review.
   b. Be sure to ask about hair loss on the body including eyebrows and eyelashes.
2. How long have you been experiencing hair loss?
3. Is your hair loss stable? Are you trying to regrow or cover up lost hair or are you trying to stop the current loss of hair?
4. Do you have any symptoms, that is, itching, burning, pain, irritation, redness?
5. Are you a smoker or take any illicit drugs?
6. Do you have a history of any allergies, in particular to latex or synthetic hair extensions?
7. What treatments have you used in the past?
   a. Which if any have been successful?
   b. What if any side effects did you experience from treatment?
8. Do you have any other medical history? Do you have any psychological conditions, such as anxiety, depression, etc.
9. Are you on any medications, that is, blood thinners, hypertension medications, hormonal therapy?
10. What is your current hair grooming routine?
    a. How often do you shampoo and condition your hair?
    b. What hair styles do you use? Do you change them frequently?
    c. What oils and hair grooming products do you use? How often do you use them?
11. What are your current hair and hair loss goals?
12. What level of time commitment do you want to designate for treating and managing your hair loss condition?
13. How much are you willing to invest to treat your hair condition?

TABLE 41-3 Aesthetic treatments for hair loss of the scalp

Therapy	Procedure	Good candidate	Not a candidate	Risks/other information
Hair prosthetics	Noninvasive, nonmedical adornments and attachments that can be added to cover areas of hair thinning, add length or thickness to the hair, or cover the entire head. Includes wigs, weaves, toupees, and hair extensions	Any patient with hair loss including scarring and nonscarring alopecia that wishes to cover up hair loss	Improperly applied hair prosthetics can worsen traction alopecia; Patients with active inflammation should address that before applying a hair prosthetic	This method will cover existing hair loss but will not help to regrow hair Methods for applying hair prosthetics may increase hair thinning or loss especially if the style is too tight, uses adhesives, or the natural hair is neglected while covered
Hair serums/products	Oils, butters, creams applied topically to the scalp to promote hair growth and decrease hair loss[4]; common ingredients include rosemary oil, castor oil, Vitamin E oil, argan oil, henna, and Amla oil[5]	Any patient with hair loss including scarring and nonscarring alopecia, hair breakage and seborrheic dermatitis	N/A	Minoxidil and Finasteride are the only FDA-approved hair growth products; Some products may cause allergic reactions or inflammation, pomade acne
Microroller/ microneedling	A device that enters the skin via multiple needle insertions and is thought to increase collagen production and cell turnover; Also used for deeper penetration of topicals so can be used with platelet rich plasma therapy	Any patient with hair loss including scarring and nonscarring alopecias	N/A	Not enough research has been done to show statistical efficacy[12]
Scalp micropigmentation (SMP)	Pigment applied to the scalp to give the appearance of hair	Any patient with hair loss including scarring and nonscarring alopecia who typically wears the hair short or who has small areas of hair loss to conceal	N/A	Will not help with regrowth of hair and will only cover up areas of hair loss
Nutraceuticals	Various oral supplements taken to promote hair growth; common ingredients include biotin and turmeric, ashwagandha, collagen, saw palmetto, and curcumin	Any patient with hair loss including scarring and nonscarring alopecia	Some ingredients may be allergens or interact with other medications so check the ingredients list before taking any nutraceuticals	There is no FDA regulation on nutraceuticals although there have been papers published on efficacy[13]
Low-intensity light therapy (low-level laser therapy)	Red/infrared laser or LED light (600-1200 nm) is directed at areas of hair loss to promote tissue repair and regeneration; Laser light can be applied to small sections using a comb, hood, or cap[6]	Best for AGA, Alopecia areata, and Chemotherapy-induced hair loss	Data on light-therapy in scarring alopecias is limited[10]	Hypertrichosis is a potential side effect
Platelet rich plasma injection (PRP)	Patient's blood is drawn, and plasma is extracted which includes the platelets; these platelets are then injected in the scalp in areas of hair loss/thinning	Best for patients with AGA[7]; few case reports for TA and CCCA[8,9]	Efficacy remains unclear for cicatricial alopecias[11]	Although extremely low, there is a risk for Infection, injury to blood vessels or nerves, and scarring
Scalp microblading/ micropigmentation	Pigment applied to the scalp to give the appearance of hair	Any patient with hair loss of the scalp	N/A	Will not help with regrowth of hair and will only cover up areas of hair loss

(Continued)

TABLE 41-3 Aesthetic treatments for hair loss of the scalp (*Continued*)

Therapy	Procedure	Good candidate	Not a candidate	Risks/other information
Scalp hair transplantation	Intact hair follicles from the patient's donor site are removed either as a strip or individual follicular units (FUE) and inserted into areas with hair loss (recipient site).[14] Multiple transplants may need to be done to achieve desired look. Rejection is less than 5% since graft is autologous	Best for patients with AGA and traction alopecia, and in scarring alopecia that is refractory to other treatments and stable[15]	Active inflammation, itching; No follicles that can be used as donor sites	Hair transplants are typically expensive and are often time intensive;[16] Large amounts of local anesthetic are used to anesthetize the area so headache and pressure can occur. There is also a risk of scarring the donor sites.

TABLE 41-4 Aesthetic treatments for eyelashes/eyebrows

Therapy	Procedure	Good candidate	Not a candidate	Risks/other information
Prostaglandin analogs	This solution is applied to the lash line for 16 weeks during the initiation phase and then every other day during the maintenance phase	Any patients with eyelash loss; Some studies have shown hair re-growth when prostaglandins are used on the scalp and eyebrows[18]	N/A	Once use is stopped, hair loss is likely to return Side effects include eye redness and irritation, darkening of the eyelid, and darkening of the iris. All but darkening of the iris are irreversible if medication is discontinued.
Eyebrow microblading/ micropigmentation	Pigment applied to the eyebrow area to give the appearance of hair	Any patient with hair loss of the scalp	N/A	Will not help with regrowth of hair and will only cover up areas of hair loss
Eyelash hair transplantation	Intact hair follicles from the patient's scalp (donor site) are removed as individual units and then transplanted onto the lash line[17]	Best for patients with eyelash loss due to trauma such as burns or infection; Can also be used for patients with genetically sparse or short lashes	Patients with hair loss due to autoimmune conditions, patients on blood thinners, or who are prone to infection	Eyelash transplants are typically expensive. Because these hairs come from the scalp, they may require trimming and curling to prevent ocular irritation.

REFERENCES

1. Davis DS, Callender VD. Review of quality of life studies in women with alopecia. *Int J Womens Dermatol*. 2018;4(1):18-22.
2. Olsen EA, Callender V, Sperling L, et al. Central scalp alopecia photographic scale in African American women. *Dermatol Ther*. 2008;21(4): 264-267.
3. Nestor MS, Ablon G, Gade A, Han H, Fischer DL. Treatment options for androgenetic alopecia: efficacy, side effects, compliance, financial considerations, and ethics. *J Cosmet Dermatol*. 2021;20(12):3759-3781.
4. Phong C, Lee V, Yale K, Sung C, Mesinkovska N. Coconut, castor, and argan oil for hair in skin of color patients: a systematic review. *J Drugs Dermatol*. 2022;21(7):751-757.
5. Phong C, Lee V, Yale K, Sung C, Mesinkovska N. Coconut, castor, and argan oil for hair in skin of color patients: a systematic review. *J Drugs Dermatol*. 2022;21(7):751-757.
6. Pillai JK, Mysore V. Role of low-level light therapy (LLLT) in androgenetic alopecia. *J Cutan Aesthet Surg*. 2021;14(4):385-391.
7. Gupta AK, Cole J, Deutsch DP, et al. Platelet-rich plasma as a treatment for androgenetic alopecia. *Dermatol Surg*. 2019;45(10):1262-1273.
8. Larrondo J, Petela J, McMichael AJ. Transitory hair growth using platelet-rich plasma therapy in stabilized central centrifugal cicatricial alopecia. *Dermatol Ther*. 2022;35(11):e15798.
9. Alves R, Grimalt R. Platelet-rich plasma and its use for cicatricial and non-cicatricial alopecias: a narrative review. *Dermatol Ther (Heidelb)*. 2020;10(4):623-633.
10. Madu P, Kundu RV. Follicular and scarring disorders in skin of color: presentation and management. *Am J Clin Dermatol*. 2014;15(4):307-321.
11. Svigos K, Yin L, Shaw K, et al. Use of platelet-rich plasma in lichen planopilaris and its variants: a retrospective case series demonstrating treatment tolerability without koebnerization. *J Am Acad Dermatol*. 2020;83(5):1506-1509.
12. Dhurat R, Sukesh M, Avhad G, Dandale A, Pal A, Pund P. A randomized evaluator blinded study of effect of microneedling in androgenetic alopecia: a pilot study. *Int J Trichology*. 2013;5(1):6-11.
13. Ablon G, Kogan S. A six-month, randomized, double-blind, placebo-controlled study evaluating the safety and efficacy of a nutraceutical supplement for promoting hair growth in women with self-perceived thinning hair. *J Drugs Dermatol*. 2018;17(5):558-565.
14. Collins K, Avram MR. Hair transplantation and follicular unit extraction. *Dermatol Clin*. 2021;39(3):463-478.
15. Ekelem C, Pham C, Atanaskova Mesinkovska N. A systematic review of the outcome of hair transplantation in primary scarring alopecia. *Skin Appendage Disord*. 2019;5(2):65-71.
16. Avram MR, Finney R, Rogers N. Hair transplantation controversies. *Dermatol Surg*. 2017;43 Suppl 2:S158-S162.
17. Suchonwanit P, Chanasumon N, Sriphojanart T. Efficacy and safety of bimatoprost 0.01% for the treatment of eyebrow hypotrichosis: a randomized, double-blind, vehicle-controlled study. *Dermatol Surg*. 2019;45(12): 1549-1556.
18. Umar S. Eyelash transplantation using leg hair by follicular unit extraction. *Plast Reconstr Surg Glob Open*. 2015;3(3):e324.

CHAPTER 42 Scarring Alopecia

Robert Hight
Grace Y. Duan
Karina Grullon-Perez
Victoria Barbosa

KEY POINTS

- Scarring alopecias are classified according to the type of inflammatory cells present in each disease state.
- Several forms of scarring alopecia are more common in patients with skin of color, including central centrifugal cicatricial alopecia, chronic cutaneous lupus erythematosus, acne keloidalis nuchae, folliculitis decalvans, and dissecting cellulitis of the scalp.
- Lichen planopilaris and frontal fibrosing alopecia are easily misdiagnosed in skin of color patients and should remain on one's differential diagnosis when evaluating all patients with scarring alopecia.
- Management of these chronic progressive alopecias is challenging; goals include halting progression of scarring and hair loss, trying to achieve some regrowth and alleviation of any associated symptoms.

TABLE 42-1 Scarring alopecia classification

Lymphocytic	Neutrophilic	Mixed
Alopecia mucinosa	Dissecting cellulitis	Acne keloidalis nuchae
Central centrifugal cicatricial alopecia	Folliculitis decalvans	Erosive pustular dermatosis
Chronic cutaneous lupus erythematosus		
Classic pseudopelade of Brocq		
Frontal fibrosing alopecia		
Graham-Little syndrome		
Keratosis follicularis spinulosa decalvans		
Lichen planopilaris		

OVERVIEW

Scarring alopecia, also known as cicatricial alopecia, represents a category of scalp diseases where inflammation results in damage to the follicles, ultimately leading to complete fibrosis and permanent hair loss. Scarring alopecias are categorized by the types of cells that are found in their infiltrate; they may be lymphocytic, neutrophilic, or mixed [**Table 42-1**]. The most common forms of scarring alopecia include central centrifugal cicatricial alopecia (CCCA), lichen planopilaris (LPP), frontal fibrosing alopecia (FFA), chronic cutaneous lupus erythematosus (CCLE), acne keloidalis nuchae (AKN), folliculitis decalvans (FD), and dissecting cellulitis of the scalp (DCS).[1] Of these, CCCA, CCLE, AKN, FD, and DCS are seen disproportionately in people with skin of color (SOC), and particularly in people of African descent with more highly curled hair. Historically, little has been understood about the etiology of these conditions and treatment options were limited. Fortunately, there has been increasing interest in research in alopecia in recent years. Understanding of the pathogenesis of some of these conditions is starting to emerge and there is an expanding armamentarium of treatment options. This chapter reviews the etiology, epidemiology, clinical presentation, and management of these most common forms of scarring alopecia.

CENTRAL CENTRIFUGAL CICATRICIAL ALOPECIA

ETIOLOGY AND EPIDEMIOLOGY

CCCA is a primary lymphocytic scarring alopecia that mainly affects women of African descent. Terminology for the disease has changed since it was first described. In 1968, CCCA was first termed "hot comb alopecia" because of the assumption that permanent hair loss occurred due to the use of a hot comb, the heated metal comb that was often used by Black women for the purpose of straightening their hair.[2] "Hot comb alopecia" was subsequently replaced with the name "follicular degeneration syndrome" in 1992 based on a study that found histological evidence of follicular degeneration that was not tied to the use of the hot comb.[3] In 2000, the name "central centrifugal scarring alopecia" (CCSA) was suggested to reflect clinical and histologic characteristics of the condition. In the subsequent year, CCCA was the term adopted by the North American Hair Research Society (NAHRS) and has been in use ever since.[4]

The etiology of CCCA is not well understood. One study identified that some patients with CCCA have a mutation in the *PADI3* gene that encodes peptidyl arginine deaminase type III, an enzyme that is necessary for normal hair shaft formation.[5] Another study demonstrated upregulation of fibroproliferative genes in CCCA-involved scalp compared to uninvolved scalp in five patients.[6] Other studies have suggested autosomal dominant inheritance and questioned the role of hair care practices, particularly those that place traction on the hair.[7-9] There has been keen interest in whether there is an association between relaxer use and CCCA; studies thus far have produced conflicting results.[10] Clearly more research is needed to better understand this common condition. The prevalence of the condition is not known, but studies in the United States and South Africa estimate the range to be from 2.7% to 16% in Black women.[7] It is uncommon in other populations including Black men and people of other racial backgrounds.

CLINICAL PRESENTATION

CCCA most commonly presents as a patch of alopecia that begins at the crown and expands over time, though it can occur anywhere on the scalp [**Figure 42-1**]. It may be preceded by thinning or breakage before follicle loss is evident clinically. The follicle destruction that ensues leaves the skin smooth and without visible follicular ostia. There may be associated erythema, scale, or papules. While the condition is asymptomatic for some, others may experience scalp discomfort including itching, burning, or tenderness.[11]

The differential for CCCA includes female pattern hair loss (FPHL) and lichen planopilaris (LPP). FPHL is similar to CCCA in that it causes hair loss at the central scalp but is differentiated by the presence of miniaturized follicles rather than the absence of follicles. LPP is a condition that is less common than CCCA but seen in people of all ethnicities and genders, including Black women. Because LPP also favors the crown and results in scarring, it can be challenging to differentiate between the two conditions clinically. Making an accurate diagnosis can be assisted by trichoscopy or by biopsy. Peripilar white-gray halos were observed in 94% of CCCA patients in one study and are considered to be a sensitive and specific finding.[12] Histopathology of CCCA reveals a perifollicular lymphocytic infiltrate that may be accompanied by a mild perivascular infiltrate. Premature desquamation of the inner root sheath is common but not diagnostic as this can be found in other forms of scarring alopecia. Sebaceous epithelium is lost, there is concentric lamellar fibroplasia around the follicles and there is a decrease in the number of hair follicles as viable follicles are replaced by fibrous tracts.[13]

There are emerging data regarding the association of CCCA with other diseases, although several studies have conflicting findings. Conditions that may be associated with CCCA include type 2 diabetes, uterine leiomyomas, hyperlipidemia, vitamin D deficiency, and breast cancer.[10,14,15] The clinician may consider screening CCCA patients for these diseases.

MANAGEMENT

The goals of treatment of CCCA are to slow or stop disease progression, to promote regrowth, and to reduce symptoms. Early diagnosis and initiation of treatment as soon as possible is imperative to maximize the likelihood of successful treatment. Anti-inflammatory treatments used to slow the progression of the disease may include high-potency topical

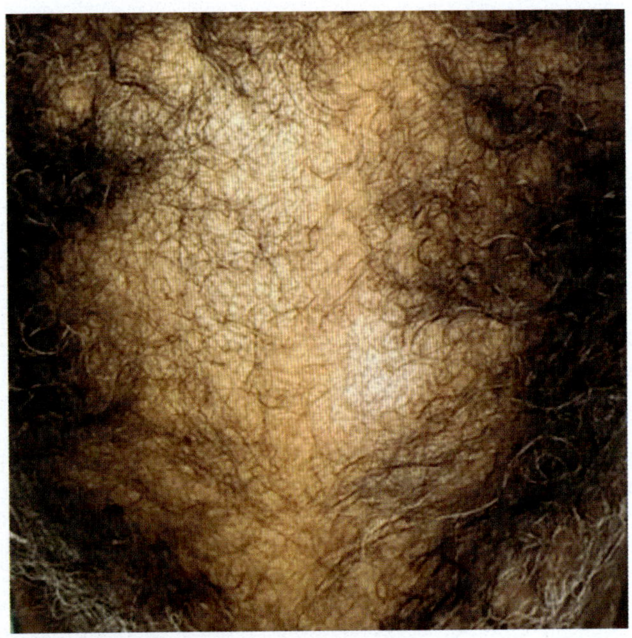

FIGURE 42-1. Central centrifugal cicatricial alopecia.

steroids used up to once daily, intralesional triamcinolone (IL TAC) injections (5-10 mg/mL) spaced at least 4 weeks apart, and the use of oral antibiotics such as doxycycline 100 mg BID for 3 to 4 months. Minocycline may also be used but is less preferable due to its side effect profile. Ketoconazole or ciclopirox shampoo may be helpful to reduce inflammation, relieve itching, and treat flaking if present.[15] Because ketoconazole shampoo can be drying to the hair, it is important to counsel the patient to apply it to the scalp for 3 to 5 minutes but to refrain from lathering the hair with it. For cases that are refractory to standard treatment, hydroxychloroquine, mycophenolate mofetil, cyclosporine, and topical calcineurin inhibitors may be of benefit.[7,15]

Some regrowth is possible for patients depending on the amount and extent of follicle damage. Minoxidil is the first-line treatment to address this goal and may be administered topically or orally.[7] Topical minoxidil 2% solution should be applied twice daily, topical minoxidil 5% solution or foam can be applied just once daily, and higher concentrations of minoxidil can be compounded by a pharmacist although there is no evidence demonstrating increased efficacy of these higher doses, and the risk of scalp irritation can increase with the higher doses. The senior author usually starts oral minoxidil at 1.25 mg daily for women after counseling about risks, benefits, and side effects. Lower doses may be used depending on the patient's other medications and health conditions. Platelet-rich plasma (PRP) injections offer an additional treatment option to stimulate regrowth. Small studies have demonstrated the effectiveness of this procedure. Finally, there is one study of two patients who achieved regrowth with topical metformin 10% cream. If regrowth has not been satisfactory, hair transplantation can be considered in select patients depending on factors such as whether there is sufficient healthy donor site tissue, and only after patients have been stable for at least 1 year.

Grooming modifications such as reducing or discontinuing the use of chemical relaxers, reducing hair styles that cause excessive traction on hair follicles (such as cornrows, braids, and extensions), and minimizing heated styling tools (hot combs, heated dryers, and flat irons) can help to minimize damage to the hair shaft and may decrease the progression of CCCA.

LICHEN PLANOPILARIS

ETIOLOGY AND EPIDEMIOLOGY

Lichen planopilaris (LPP) is a lymphocytic cicatricial alopecia that is thought to result after loss of immune privilege of hair follicle bulge stem cells and subsequent irreversible T lymphocyte-mediated damage. As in lichen planus (LP), cytotoxic CD8+ T cells are thought to be the key players in LPP pathogenesis, while helper CD4+ T cells assist in disease propagation via cytokine secretion. Various molecular mediators have been implicated in LP and lichenoid dermatoses including PPAR-γ, type I interferons, and transcription factor Brn2.[16,17] Further work is required to identify upstream drivers of immune dysregulation in LPP, and to elucidate potential environmental factors influencing their pathogenesis.[17]

LPP is an uncommon condition, with overall prevalence in the United States reported between 0.017%[18] and 0.043%.[19] There is a strong female predominance, with women comprising more than 90% of patients with LPP. It is also reported to be most prevalent among those who identify as White, although LPP may be underdiagnosed in patients with SOC. LPP is most prevalent among people older than 55 years of age, with the typical age of onset between 40 and 70 years. The true median age of onset is difficult to determine given that detection and diagnosis of hair disorders are often delayed.[18,19]

CLINICAL PRESENTATION

LPP classically presents with asymmetric multifocal patches of scarring alopecia most commonly at the parietal and vertex scalp, though it can involve any region. As it progresses, LPP can look very similar to CCCA on examination [**Figure 42-2**]. LPP is often, but not always, associated with sensations of burning, pruritus, pain, or other discomfort. LPP may present independent of or in association with nonscalp cutaneous, ungual, or oral LP. Loss of body hair is often reported by patients. Characteristics of LPP on histopathology include lichenoid perifollicular lymphoid cell infiltration, perifollicular fibrosis, hyperkeratosis, and replacement of hair follicles with fibrous tracts.[20]

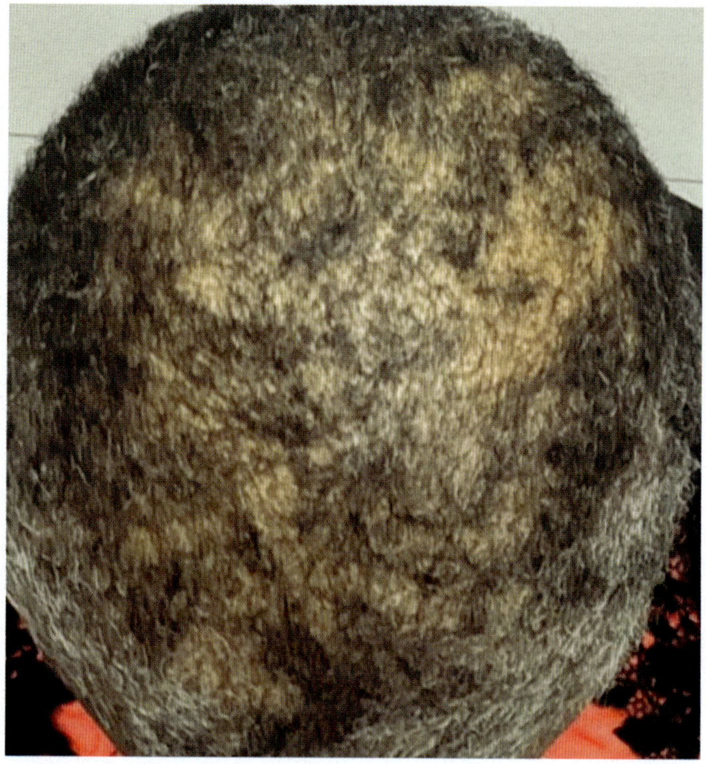

FIGURE 42-2. Lichen planopilaris.

The differential diagnosis for LPP includes CCCA, which is a more common cause of scarring alopecia in Black patients. Trichoscopy may be helpful in distinguishing the two conditions. Loss of follicular openings can be appreciated in both conditions, but CCCA may be distinguished from LPP by the presence of peripilar white-gray halos where blue-gray dots may be seen with LPP. Biopsy may be required for definitive diagnosis.[21]

MANAGEMENT

There are no standard guidelines for treating LPP. A variety of topical, intralesional, and oral medications have been used as monotherapy and in combination; however, the efficacy of these therapies is limited, and patients display variable treatment response and commonly do not achieve long-term remission. Nevertheless, early diagnosis and treatment are critical to preserve existing hair follicles and to reduce symptoms.[21]

Topical treatments used in the management of LPP include high-potency topical steroids, calcineurin inhibitors such as tacrolimus, and minoxidil, and are often chosen as first-line therapy due to their relatively favorable adverse effect profiles. Topical corticosteroids and calcineurin inhibitors help reduce inflammation, pruritus, and burning, while topical minoxidil can be used to improve background hair regrowth. Twice daily application of anti-inflammatory agents is typical, and the frequency of use can be titrated down based on treatment response.[21] Topical minoxidil 5% can be used once a day in women and twice a day in men. Topical minoxidil 2% should be used twice a day in women.

Intralesional glucocorticoids and PRP injections have also been used to treat LPP. Evidence of superiority of intralesional relative to topical glucocorticoids is debated, though there may be improved efficacy when combining the treatment modalities. PRP injections has been trialed in the treatment of other alopecias with promising results, but its use in LPP has not been well-studied.[21]

Oral medications are often used in combination with topical and/or intralesional therapies to treat LPP. Hydroxychloroquine is often the first oral medication utilized with treatment response rate of approximately 50%. Long-term use of hydroxychloroquine is associated with adverse effects including retinal toxicity. This medication should be dosed by weight, ideally not exceeding 5 mg/kg/day up to 200 mg twice daily to minimize this risk, and patients should be followed by an ophthalmologist for the duration of their therapy. Other immunosuppressive medications can be used for refractory cases, including mycophenolate mofetil, cyclosporine, or methotrexate. Short courses of oral glucocorticoid with tapering have been used in severe, refractory or rapidly progressive cases of LPP and yield substantial initial response, but relapse is common. Reports of using 5α-reductase inhibitors finasteride and dutasteride in patients with LPP have been limited. Other oral medications reported in the literature include tetracyclines, low-dose naltrexone, oral retinoids, pioglitazone, and pentoxifilline.[21] There is increased interest in the use of Janus kinase (JAK) inhibitors given the hypothesized role of JAK signaling and interferon production in LPP pathogenesis.[22]

Hair transplantation (HT) has been suggested to improve cosmetic appearance in patients with quiescent LPP. Reports of LPP reactivation following HT should caution clinicians considering the procedure to potential Koebner phenomenon.[2] It is recommended that HT is not attempted until at least 1 to 2 years after cessation of disease activity, though the risk of Koebnerization may persist even after 5 years of remission.[21]

FRONTAL FIBROSING ALOPECIA

ETIOLOGY AND EPIDEMIOLOGY

Frontal fibrosing alopecia (FFA) is a widely believed to be a variant of LPP. A possible hormonal basis for FFA has been hypothesized given that it predominantly affects postmenopausal female patients; however, a direct role of hormones in FFA pathogenesis has not been well-established.[23] Emerging research reveals a potential genetic basis for FFA susceptibility involving players in the IFN-γ pathway, which has an important role in regulating antigen presentation. Recent studies also have implicated the frequent use of sunscreens and other facial products in the development of FFA, although data have been conflicting.[17,22]

The prevalence of FFA is estimated to be about 0.015%. FFA has a stronger female predominance than classic LPP and tends to affect patients who are older (51-70 years) compared to classic LPP (41-50 years).[18] FFA is associated with personal history of autoimmune conditions and a positive family history for FFA.[23]

CLINICAL PRESENTATION

FFA presents distinctly from classic LPP as scarring alopecia that spreads symmetrically along the frontal hairline in a band-like distribution and often progresses to involve the eyebrows and peripheral body hair [**Figure 42-3**].[17] "Lonely hairs" surrounded by alopecic patches can often be identified. Similar to LPP, FFA may be accompanied by scalp pain or pruritus. Classic LPP and FFA share many similar histopathologic characteristics including perifollicular lymphoid infiltration, fibrosis, and hyperkeratosis. A notable difference is that the inflammatory infiltrate in FFA may be less severe than in LPP, although the infiltrate may extend below the isthmus in FFA.[17]

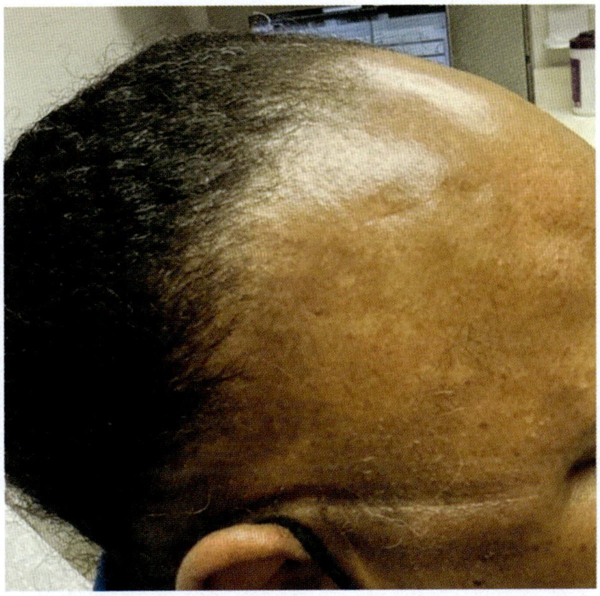

FIGURE 42-3. Frontal fibrosing alopecia.

A recent study suggests that Black patients with FFA may present with hairline recession at a younger age despite a similar duration of hair loss compared to White patients, suggesting faster progression of clinical course in Black patients. Furthermore, there may be greater prevalence of occipital scalp involvement among Black patients with FFA.[24] Another study found that Asian patients with FFA may present asymptomatically more often than White patients, and more commonly display diffuse and pseudo-fringe sign patterns.[23] Black and Asian patients with FFA may also present with higher prevalence of concomitant lichen planus pigmentosus of the face than White patients.[22,24] Association with sunscreen use has been shown; however, no causal relationship has been established nor have the studies focused on patients with SOC.

FFA is often misdiagnosed as traction alopecia in patients with SOC. History of tight hairstyles and the presence of a fringe sign are more suggestive of traction alopecia. The differential diagnosis also includes ophiasis pattern alopecia areata, which is more common in Black patients. It can be distinguished from FFA by the presence of follicular ostia on trichoscopy.[21] However, scalp biopsy may be required for definitive diagnosis.

MANAGEMENT

Treatment options for FFA are similar to those discussed for LPP. There is little research on the management of FFA specifically in patients with SOC, but one systematic review of the literature notes that African American patients may be less responsive to treatment than Asians; where 90% of a cohort of Asian individuals had stabilization or improvement of their disease, a separate study demonstrated just 45.1% of Black patients had stabilization or improvement in their disease with treatment. Of note, Black patients who did show improvement were treated with oral steroids.[25] In terms of other treatment options previously discussed for LPP, it is worth noting that there is one randomized controlled trial that demonstrates equal efficacy between hydroxychloroquine and finasteride for the treatment of FFA.[26] Also, there are case reports of topical tofacitinib 2% cream, topical ruxolitinib 1.5% cream, oral tofacitinib, and oral baricitinib used in combination with dutasteride and other treatments with some success. The efficacy of JAK inhibitors warrants additional study.[27]

CUTANOUS LUPUS ERYTHEMATOSIS

ETIOLOGY AND EPIDEMIOLOGY

While cutaneous lupus erythematosis (CLE) is discussed in more detail elsewhere in this textbook, it bears mentioning here as a cause of scarring alopecia, particularly in patients with SOC. CLE refers to the dermatologic manifestations of lupus erythematosus (LE), an autoimmune condition characterized by circulating autoantibodies, systemic inflammation, and a broad range of symptoms. CLE can be classified into three subtypes based on histology, duration of lesions, laboratory findings, and clinical presentation: acute CLE, subacute CLE, and chronic CLE (CCLE).[28] CCLE is further subdivided into discoid LE (DLE), LE tumidus, LE panniculitis, and chilblain LE. The term CCLE is sometimes used interchangeably with DLE, its most common subvariant that causes scarring alopecia.[29] The pathogenesis of CLE is not fully understood, though current evidence suggests an interplay of genetic, environmental, and immune system factors. CLE subtypes may be associated with certain human leukocyte antigen (HLA) haplotypes; ultraviolet (UV) light exposure has also been implicated in CLE pathogenesis.[29]

Over 75% of patients with SLE have cutaneous manifestations.[30] The incidence of CLE has been reported to be 4.3 per 100,000 with a female predominance and average age of onset of 48.5 years.[29] In DLE, there is higher incidence and prevalence among Black individuals. Black patients may also present with more severe disease earlier in their disease course.[31]

CLINICAL PRESENTATION

DLE presents as coin-shaped, erythematous plaques with hyperkeratosis that develop hyperpigmented borders and central atrophy. The lesions frequently appear on the scalp, face, ears, and extensor arms. Unlike acute and subacute CLE, lesions of CCLE/DLE heal with scarring and dyschromia. Lesions affecting the hair follicles lead to scarring alopecia [**Figure 42-4**].

Histopathological features of all subtypes of CLE include hyperkeratosis, cellular infiltrate at the dermoepidermal junction, and inflammation in perivascular and periadnexal regions. Immunopathology may show deposition of IgG immunoglobulin and C3 complement at the dermoepidermal junction.[29] Characteristically, DLE also exhibits subepidermal basement membrane thickening.[30]

Black patients with DLE are more likely to have scalp involvement compared to non-Black patients with DLE. It is thought the cultural hair care practices may lead to Koebnerization and subsequent scarring alopecia, as in traction alopecia and central centrifugal cicatricial alopecia that also disproportionately affect Black patients.[31] Patients with SOC who have DLE have increased risk for extensive postinflammatory hyperpigmentation and keloid scarring, which can lead to significant psychosocial distress. Patients with SOC are also at increased risk for DLE-associated squamous cell carcinoma.[30]

MANAGEMENT

Consensus guidelines recommend short-term topical corticosteroids as first-line treatment for all CLE lesions; scalp lesions may require more prolonged use. Localized, refractory DLE lesions may be treated with intralesional corticosteroids. Alternatively, calcineurin inhibitors may be used as first-line topical treatment for CLE lesions. In patients with widespread or severe CLE, hydroxychloroquine is the first-line therapy with add-on quinacrine for refractory cases, or add-on systemic corticosteroids with subsequent tapering and maintenance with steroid-sparing agents; long-term maintenance with corticosteroids is not recommended due to risk for adverse effects. The consensus for second-line treatment for refractory CLE includes systemic retinoids, dapsone, low-dose methotrexate, or thalodomide. Third- and fourth-line agents are mycophenolate mofetil and belimumab. For refractory, cosmetically distressing lesions, surgical removal with grafting using full-thickness abdominal skin can be considered in combination with medical maintenance treatment. Other cosmetic options include pulsed-dye laser[28] and tattoo therapy.[30]

Patients should be educated on sun protection and smoking cessation, as these are risk factors associated with higher risk of disease and disease severity. Medications should be reviewed, as drug-induced CLE has been reported, most commonly with anti-TNF biologics, proton pump inhibitors, and terbinafine. Patients should also be advised to avoid cutaneous traumas.[28] CLE is sometimes the first manifestation of systemic lupus erythematosus (SLE), thus patients presenting with CLE should undergo comprehensive assessment to exclude possible systemic involvement. In addition to standard tests, serologic titers of autoantibodies should be obtained.[29] Routine screening for SLE is recommended.[28]

ACNE KELOIDALIS NUCHAE

ETIOLGY AND EPIDEMIOLOGY

Acne keloidalis nuchae (AKN), also known as folliculitis keloidalis, is a common, chronic skin disorder that causes inflammation and scarring of the hair follicles at the occipital scalp. While the etiology of AKN is unknown, there have been several factors hypothesized to play a role in its development. AKN is seen most commonly in men of African descent. This may be due to the coarse, curly nature of the hair compared to people of other racial backgrounds. A hair may penetrate the wall of the follicle before it emerges, or may emerge from the follicle, curl around, and penetrate the skin's surface. These ingrown hairs may lead to an inflammatory response.[32] Other contributing factors may include trauma, friction from shirt collars, androgens, genetic factors, heat and/or bacterial infection. [32,33]

Black males are primarily affected, but Black women and other racial populations have been reported. There is little data on the discussing AKN in women, but several sources have indicated that the ratio of males to females is 20:1.[32] Estimates ranging from 0.7% to 9% of dermatology referrals were in patients of African ancestry.[34]

CLINICAL PRESENTATION

AKN initially presents as dome-shaped follicular papules at the occiput [**Figure 42-5**] and occasionally extends onto the posterior neck and vertex. Pustules may also be present. Papular lesions may coalesce into keloid-like plaques.[33] These lesions can become pruritic, painful, or cosmetically disfiguring that can negatively impact a patient's self-esteem and self-image. If an infection ensues, then there may be findings such as erythema, pain, drainage, odor, suppuration, or fever.[35]

While the diagnosis of AKN is usually a clinical one that can be made without biopsy, histopathology reveals a lymphoytic and neutrophilic

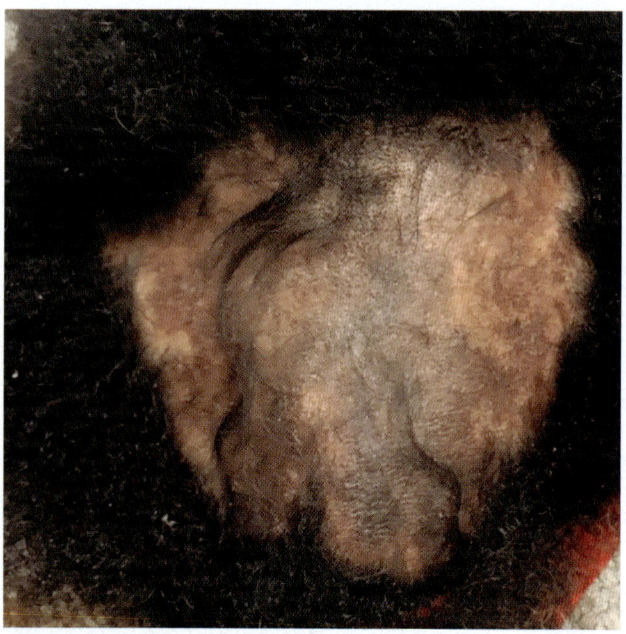

FIGURE 42-4. Discoid lupus erythematosus.

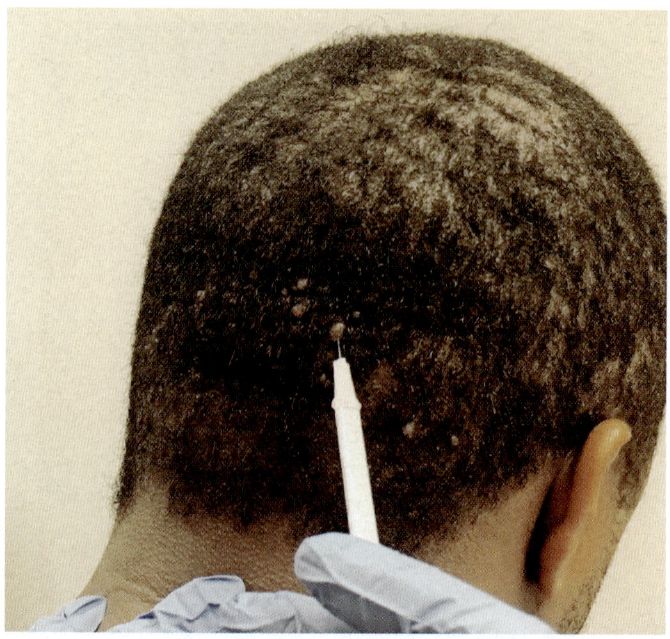

FIGURE 42-5. Acne keloidalis nuchae.

granulomatous inflammation primarily at the lower isthmus of the follicle with some plasma cells higher up. Sebaceous glands and follicles are ultimately destroyed and fibrosis occurs.[36] There are several studies reporting other diseases associated with AKN, including hypothyroidism, hidradenitis supperativa, increased body mass index, systolic hypertension, and metabolic syndrome.[37-40] Patients presenting with AKN should be screened for these other conditions.

MANAGEMENT

The treatment of mild to moderate AKN is centered on reducing inflammation and treating infection if present. Use of intralesional triamcinolone (IL TAC) is the standard treatment. Concentrations of 5 to 40 mg/mL may be used depending on the size of lesions and the patient's response to treatment. Injections can be repeated at 4 week intervals. High-potency topical steroids may be used in place of or in addition to intralesional therapy. If pustules are present, a topical antibiotic such as clindamycin, or oral antibiotics such as doxycycline, clindamycin, or rifampin should be added. Other treatments that have been reported include the use of topical retinoids, isotretinoin, prednisone, and liquid nitrogen cryotherapy.[41]

The more extensive plaques of severe AKN are best managed by surgical intervention. Elliptical excision may be followed by primary closure or the defect can be left to heal by secondary intent. There have been reports of staged exision and excision with staged reconstruction to improve the cosmesis of the excision. Follicular unit excision (FUE) has been reported to treat papular lesions that did not respond to other treatments.[41-44]

Laser epilation with the long-pulsed neodymium-doped yttrium aluminum garnet (Nd:YAG) laser may be helpful in preventing further AKN or in treating the condition. Treatment has also been reported with the 650-microsecond 1064 nm nd:YAG laser and with the erbium:YAG laser. Low-dose radiotherapy has also been reported in recalcitrant cases.[43-48]

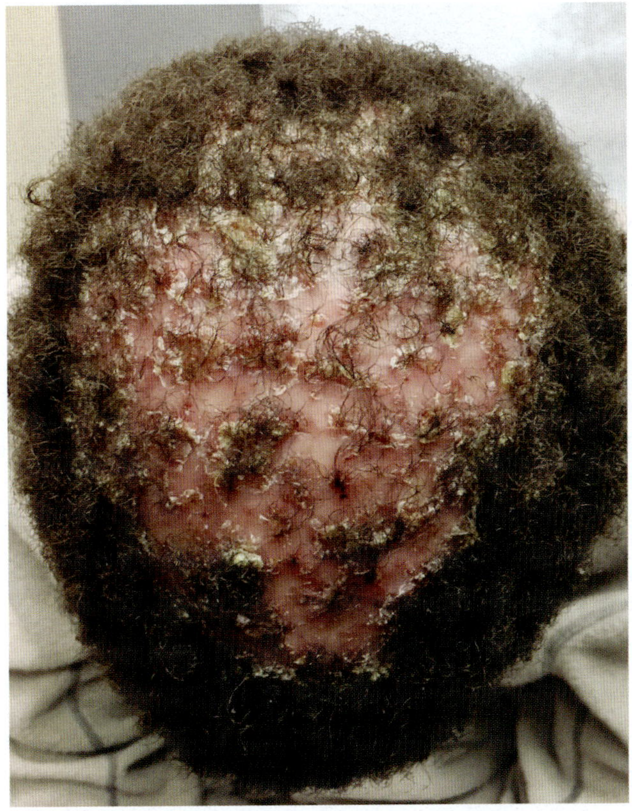

FIGURE 42-6. Folliculitis decalvans. (Comp: authors request that you crop off the border of this image.)

FOLLICULITIS DECALVANS

ETIOLOGY AND EPIDEMIOLOGY

Folliculitis decalvans (FD) is a chronic and relapsing primary neutrophilic cicatricial alopecia, predominantly affecting young and middle-aged adults of both genders; it is seen more commonly in men.[49,50] FD occurs more frequently in African Americans compared to Caucasian patients.[49,51] There are no large multicenter studies that accurately describe the epidemiology of FD. It is estimated that it accounts for approximately 11% of all primary cicatricial alopecia cases.[49] The pathogenesis of FD remains poorly understood, but *Staphylococcus aureus* has been isolated from follicular pustules of untreated patients, and an impaired host immunity to this organism has been proposed.[49-51] Some familial cases of FD have been reported, suggesting a possible genetic predisposition.[49,50]

CLINICAL PRESENTATION

Clinically, FD presents with patches of scarred alopecia, follicular pustules, crusts, and tufted hair. The vertex and occipital scalp are predominantly involved [**Figure 42-6**]. Patients frequently report pain, itching and/or burning sensations along with occasional episodes of spontaneous bleeding.[49-51] Tufted hairs are characterized by multiple hairs emerging from one single dilated follicular orifice and represent a common finding in patients with FD.[49]

The histological features of FD include the presence of a neutrophilic scarring alopecia, with dilated follicular infundibula in combination with intrafollicular and perifollicular neutrophilic infiltrate in early lesions. In advanced lesions, the inflammatory infiltrate may consist of neutrophils, lymphocytes, and plasma cells, and extend into the dermis along with some multinucleated giant cells around naked hair shafts.[49-51] End-stage lesions include fibrous tracts in the area of the former hair follicle and interstitial dermal fibrosis.[49]

MANAGEMENT

FD is a distressing disease for patients, for which there is currently no long-term effective treatment available. Oral antibiotics are widely used due to their anti-inflammatory and antibacterial effects given the role *S. aureus* likely plays in the pathogenesis of FD. Antibiotics most commonly used include doxycycline, clindamycin, rifampin, and azithromycin. Some studies have found that the combination of clindamycin plus rifampin, when effective, achieve a longer remission than doxycycline.[52] Other oral treatment options reported in the literature with variable efficacy include corticosteroids, isotretinoin, acetretin, dapsone, cyclosporine and methotrexate.[49,50,52] Topical treatment may be used as adjunctive therapy, for maintenance, or as a primary therapy in particularly mild cases; options include clindamycin, high-potency topical corticosteroids such as clobetasol, tacrolimus, and antiseptic cleansers. For recalcitrant cases, photodynamic therapy, Nd;YAG laser, tumor necrosis factor-alpha (TNF-α) antagonists, and intravenous immunoglobulin may also be considered as they have shown some success in case reports and case series.[50,52] Relapses are common in this condition so medications may need to be adjusted over time depending on disease activity. Successful hair transplantation surgery has been reported and is an option for some patients.[53] It is important for the patient to know that results are not guaranteed. Ideally, the disease has been quiescent for at least 1 year and there should be no active inflammation on scalp biopsy. To optimize the management of FD, there is a need for randomized control trials to assess the efficacy of the various treatments.

DISSECTING CELLULITIS

ETIOLOGY AND EPIDEMIOLOGY

Dissecting Cellulitis of the Scalp (DCS) is an uncommon, primary neutrophilic scarring alopecia. It predominately affects African American and Hispanic males in the second and third decades of life.[54-56] The incidence of DCS is unknown and it is likely due to underreporting of the disease. DCS can occur in isolation or coexist with acne conglobate (AC), hidradenitis suppurativa (HS), and/or pilonidal cyst in a combination referred to as the "follicular occlusion tetrad."[54] These diseases share a common pathogenic mechanism of abnormalities in keratinization,

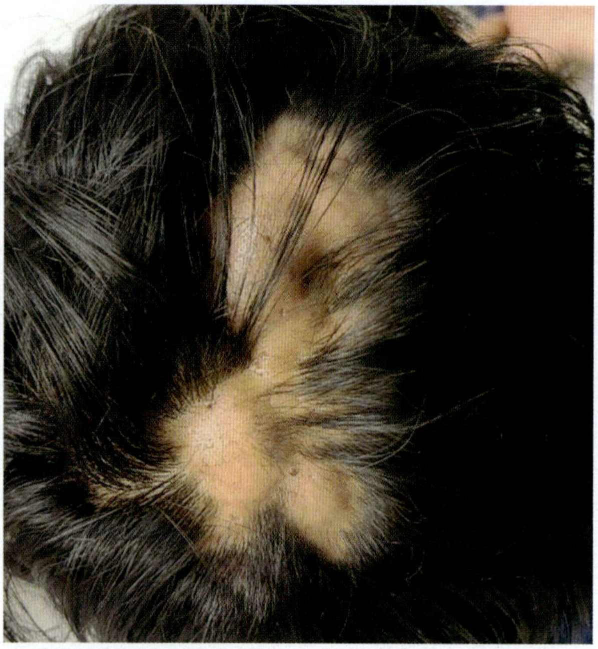

FIGURE 42-7. Dissecting cellulitis.

follicular occlusion, and accumulation of cellular debris, eventually leading to inflammation, follicular rupture, and secondary bacterial infections.[54,55]

CLINICAL PRESENTATION

DCS usually located on the vertex and occipital scalp. It is characterized clinically by painful, boggy scalp nodules and abscesses that interconnect by sinus tracts, and permanent alopecia [**Figure 42-7**]. The histopathology of DCS is characterized by perifollicular inflammation of the reticular dermis extending to the subcutis along with hyperplasia of follicular epithelium and follicle rupture. As the disease progresses, there is development of granulation tissue in the deep dermis and subcutis, and proliferation of the vasculature. In advanced stages, abscesses and sinus tracts form. In the end stage, when the disease is "burned out" and there is absence of active inflammation, dense fibrosis remains in the dermis and superficial fat with scarred alopecia.[57]

MANAGEMENT

Management of DCS is difficult because of the chronic, relapsing, and remitting course. Topical treatments are of limited value, although there are case reports of use of clindamycin gel, isotretinoin gel, and resorcinol 15% with some success.[58] For mild to moderate disease, treatments include systemic antibiotics alone or in combination with topical or intralesional corticosteroids. The most commonly recommended systemic antibiotics are doxycycline, clindamycin, and rifampin. There are also reports in the literature of use of dapsone, azithromycin, ciprofloxacin, and gentamycin with variable success.[55-58] For moderate to severe disease, treatments can include isotretinoin, acitretin, or TNF-α antagonists.[55,56,58] The most used TNF-α antagonist is adalimumab.[55] For refractory cases, surgical excision, photodynamic therapy, Nd:YAG laser therapy, and X-ray epilation may improve symptoms.[56,58] In the future, randomized control trials evaluating the efficacy of these treatment options at various stages of DCS are needed.

CONCLUSION

Caring for patients with scarring alopecia is simultaneously very rewarding but also frustrating. It is rewarding because one is able to care for a person's dermatological condition while also helping them address their underlying feelings about their condition, their overall well-being, and their sense of self-esteem. It's also rewarding because a clinican is sometimes able to achieve improvement in the most unlikely of patients and the physican and patient can both celebrate these victories. Managing alopecia is frustrating because there are more questions than answers regarding etiologies for these conditions, and our treatments do not always offer the efficacy that physicians or patients would prefer. And though the phrase gets repeated too often, it is no less true; more research is needed. In the meantime, early diagnosis and intervention is critical. This means that awareness of scarring alopecia must be raised among people living with hair loss, hairstylists, and primary care physicians so that referrals to a dermatologist can be made in a timely manner. And, it is incumbent upon dermatologists and other providers to have both the knowledge and the cultural humility to treat all patients.

REFERENCES

1. Hordinsky M. Scarring alopecia: diagnosis and new treatment options. *Dermatol Clin*. 2021;39(3):383-388.
2. LoPresti P, Papa CM, Kligman AM. Hot comb alopecia. *Arch Dermatol*. 1968;98(3):234-238.
3. Sperling LC, Sau P. The follicular degeneration syndrome in black patients. "Hot comb alopecia" revisited and revised. *Arch Dermatol*. 1992;128(1):68-74.
4. Herskovitz I, Miteva M. Central centrifugal cicatricial alopecia: challenges and solutions. *Clin Cosmet Investig Dermatol*. 2016;9:175-181.
5. Malki L, Sarig O, Romano MT, et al. Variant PADI3 in central centrifugal cicatricial alopecia. N *Engl J Med*. 2019;380(9):833-841.
6. Aguh C, Dina Y, Talbot CC Jr, Garza L. Fibroproliferative genes are preferentially expressed in central centrifugal cicatricial alopecia. *J Am Acad Dermatol*. 2018;79(5):904-912.e1.
7. Lawson CN, Bakayoko A, Callender VD. Central centrifugal cicatricial alopecia: challenges and treatments. *Dermatol Clin*. 2021;39(3):389-405.
8. Callender VD, Onwudiwe O. Prevalence and etiology of central centrifugal cicatricial alopecia. *Arch Dermatol*. 2011;147(8):972-974.
9. Gathers RC, Jankowski M, Eide M, Lim HW. Hair grooming practices and central centrifugal cicatricial alopecia. *J Amer Acad Dermatol*. 2009;60(4):574-578.
10. Green M, Feschuk A, Valdebran M. Risk factors and comorbidities associated with central centrifugal cicatricial alopecia. *Int J Womens Dermatol*. 2023 21;9(3):e108.
11. Aguh C, McMichael A. Central centrifugal cicatricial alopecia. *JAMA Dermatol*. 2020;156(9):1036.
12. Miteva M, Tosti A. Dermatoscopic features of central centrifugal cicatricial alopecia. *J Am Acad Dermatol*. 2014;71(3):443-449.
13. Whiting DA, Olsen EA. Central centrifugal cicatricial alopecia. *Dermatol Ther*. 2008;21(4):268-278.
14. Brown-Korsah JB, Roche FC, Taylor SC. Association of breast and colorectal cancer in patients with central centrifugal cicatricial alopecia: a retrospective, cross-sectional pilot study. *J Am Acad Dermatol*. 2021;84(3):859-860.
15. George EA, Matthews C, Roche FC, Taylor SC. Beyond the hot comb: updates in epidemiology, pathogenesis, and treatment of central centrifugal cicatricial alopecia from 2011 to 2021. *Am J Clin Dermatol*. 2023;24(1):81-88.
16. Tziotzios C, Lee JYW, Brier T, et al. Lichen planus and lichenoid dermatoses: clinical overview and molecular basis. *J Am Acad Dermatol*. 2018;79(5):789-804.
17. Senna MM, Peterson E, Jozic I, Cheret J, Paus R. Frontiers in lichen planopilaris and frontal fibrosing alopecia research: pathobiology progress and translational horizons. *JID Innov*. 2022;2(3):100113.
18. Trager MH, Lavian J, Lee EY, et al. Prevalence estimates for lichen planopilaris and frontal fibrosing alopecia in a New York City health care system. *J Am Acad Dermatol*. 2021;84(4):1166-1169.
19. Joshi TP, Zhu H, Naqvi Z, Holla S, Duruewuru A, Ren V. Prevalence of lichen planopilaris in the United States: a cross-sectional study of the All of Us research program. *JAAD Int*. 2022;8:69-70.
20. Araoye EF, Thomas JAL, Aguh CU. Hair regrowth in 2 patients with recalcitrant central centrifugal cicatricial alopecia after use of topical metformin. *JAAD Case Rep*. 2020;6(2):106-108.
21. Svigos K, Yin L, Fried L, Lo Sicco K, Shapiro J. A practical approach to the diagnosis and management of classic lichen planopilaris. *Am J Clin Dermatol*. 2021;22(5):681-692.
22. Tziotzios C, Petridis C, Dand N, et al. Genome-wide association study in frontal fibrosing alopecia identifies four susceptibility loci including HLA-B*07:02. *Nat Commun*. 2019;10(1):1150.

23. Panchaprateep R, Ruxrungtham P, Chancheewa B, Asawanonda P. Clinical characteristics, trichoscopy, histopathology and treatment outcomes of frontal fibrosing alopecia in an Asian population: a retro-prospective cohort study. *J Dermatol.* 2020;47(11):1301-1311.
24. Adotama P, Callender V, Kolla A, et al. Comparing the clinical differences in white and black women with frontal fibrosing alopecia. *Br J Dermatol.* 2021;185(5):1074-1076.
25. Hai J, Meyer SN, Agbai ON. Treatment of frontal fibrosing alopecia in Black patients: a systematic review. *Cutis.* 2023;111(4):186-190.
26. Saber M, Farokhshahi M, Fatemi Naeini F, Mohaghegh F, Asilian A. Clinical effectiveness of finasteride versus hydroxychloroquine in the treatment of frontal fibrosing alopecia: a randomized controlled trial. *J Cosmet Dermatol.* 2024;23(2):576-584.
27. Dunn C, Griffith V, Coican A, et al. Janus kinase inhibition for the treatment of refractory frontal fibrosing alopecia: a case series and review of the literature. *JAAD Case Rep.* 2023;40:47-52.
28. Lu Q, Long H, Chow S, et al. Guideline for the diagnosis, treatment and long-term management of cutaneous lupus erythematosus. *J Autoimmun.* 2021;123:102707.
29. Hejazi EZ, Werth VP. Cutaneous lupus erythematosus: an update on pathogenesis, diagnosis and treatment. *Am J Clin Dermatol.* 2016;17(2):135-146.
30. Nozile W, Adgerson CN, Cohen GF. Cutaneous lupus erythematosus in skin of color. *J Drugs Dermatol.* 2015;14(4):343-349.
31. Joseph AK, Windsor B, Hynan LS, Chong BF. Discoid lupus erythematosus skin lesion distribution and characteristics in Black patients: a retrospective cohort study. *Lupus Sci Med.* 2021;8(1):e000514.
32. Ogunbiyi A. Acne keloidalis nuchae: prevalence, impact, and management challenges. *CCID.* 2016;9:483-489.
33. Al Aboud DM, Badri T. Acne Keloidalis Nuchae. In: *StatPearls.* StatPearls Publishing; 2022. Accessed February 20, 2023. http://www.ncbi.nlm.nih.gov/books/NBK459135/.
34. Shapero J, Shapero H. Acne keloidalis nuchae is scar and keloid formation secondary to mechanically induced folliculitis. *J Cutan Med Surg.* 2011;15(4):238-240.
35. Mackay-Wiggan JM, Hussain S. (2021, October 26). *Acne keloidalis nuchae: Management.* UpToDate. Retrieved February 20, 2023.
36. Bernárdez C, Molina-Ruiz AM, Requena L. Histologic features of alopecias: part II: scarring alopecias. *Actas Dermosifiliogr.* 2015;106(4):260-270.
37. Valdman-Grinshpoun Y, Kridin K, Schonmann Y, Cohen AD. Acne keloidalis nuchae and thyroid diseases: a population-based cohort study. *Int J Dermatol.* 2021;60(4):466-470.
38. Kridin K, Patel PM, Jones VA, Damiani G, Amber KT, Cohen AD. Hidradenitis suppurativa is associated with acne keloidalis nuchae: a population-based study. *Arch Dermatol Res.* 2021;313(5):333-337.
39. Saka B, Teclessou JN, Akakpo SA, et al. Acne keloidalis nuchae and hypertension in black subjects: a case-control study. *BMC Res Notes.* 2020;13(1):431.
40. Kridin K, Solomon A, Tzur-Bitan D, Damiani G, Comaneshter D, Cohen AD. Acne keloidalis nuchae and the metabolic syndrome: a population-based study. *Am J Clin Dermatol.* 2020;21(5):733-739.
41. Taylor SC, Barbosa V, Burgess C, Heath C, McMichael AJ, Ogunleye T, Callender V. Hair and scalp disorders in adult and pediatric patients with skin of color. *Cutis.* 2017;100(1):31-35.
42. Curtiss P, Nijhawan RI. Staged excisions for extensive acne keloidalis. *J Am Acad Dermatol.* 2023;89(3):e119-e120.
43. Labib A, Salfity L, Powell B. Acne keloidalis nuchae: a staged reconstruction. *Cureus.* 2021;13(9):e18173.
44. Umar S, Khanna R. Papular acne keloidalis nuchae treatment success using follicular unit excision. *JAAD Case Rep.* 2023;39:96-100.
45. Woo DK, Treyger G, Henderson M, Huggins RH, Jackson-Richards D, Hamzavi I. Prospective controlled trial for the treatment of acne keloidalis nuchae with a long-pulsed neodymium-doped yttrium-aluminum-garnet laser. *J Cutan Med Surg.* 2018;22(2):236-238.
46. Roberts WE, Henry M, Burgess C, Saedi N, Chilukuri S, Campbell-Chambers DA. Laser treatment of skin of color for medical and aesthetic uses with a new 650-microsecond Nd:YAG 1064 nm laser. *J Drugs Dermatol.* 2019;18(4):s135-137.
47. Gamil HD, Khater EM, Khattab FM, Khalil MA. Successful treatment of acne keloidalis nuchae with erbium:YAG laser: a comparative study. *J Cosmet Laser Ther.* 2018;20(7-8):419-423.
48. Umar S, Sila CR. Acne keloidalis nuchae: a role for low-dose radiotherapy. *JAAD Case Rep.* 2021;13:90-93.
49. Otberg N, Kang H, Alzolibani AA, Shapiro J. Folliculitis decalvans. *Dermatol Ther.* 2008;21(4):238-244.
50. Vañó-Galván S, Molina-Ruiz AM, Fernández-Crehuet P, et al. Folliculitis decalvans: a multicentre review of 82 patients. *J Eur Acad Dermatol Venereol.* 2015;29(9):1750-1757.
51. Tan E, Martinka M, Ball N, Shapiro J. Primary cicatricial alopecias: clinicopathology of 112 cases. *J Am Acad Dermatol.* 2004:50:25-32.
52. Rambhia PH, Conic RRZ, Murad A, Atanaskova-Mesinkovska N, Piliang M, Bergfeld W. Updates in therapeutics for folliculitis decalvans: a systematic review with evidence-based analysis. *J Am Acad Dermatol.* 2019;80(3):794-801.e1.
53. Ekelem C, Pham C, Atanaskova Mesinkovska N. A Systematic review of the outcome of hair transplantation in primary scarring alopecia. *Skin Appendage Disord.* 2019;5(2):65-71.
54. Chicarilli ZN. Follicular occlusion triad: hidradenitis suppurativa, acne conglobata, and dissecting cellulitis of the scalp. *Ann Plast Surg.* 1987;18(3):230-237.
55. Gamissans M, Romaní J, López-Llunell C, Riera-Martí N, Sin M. Dissecting cellulitis of the scalp: a review on clinical characteristics and management options in a series of 14 patients. *Dermatol Ther.* 2022;35(8):e15626.
56. Thomas J, Aguh C. Approach to treatment of refractory dissecting cellulitis of the scalp: a systematic review. *J Dermatolog Treat.* 2021;32(2):144-149.
57. Zagelbaum Ward NK, Jun JA, Vecerek N, Donaldson M, Quismorio FP Jr. Dissecting cellulitis of the scalp associated with peripheral and axial spondyloarthritis: report of a case and review of the literature. *Clin Rheumatol.* 2022;41(8):2553-2560.
58. Masson R, Jeong CY, Ma E, et al. Treatments for dissecting cellulitis of the scalp: a systematic review and treatment algorithm. *Dermatol Ther (Heidelb).* 2023;13(11):2487-2526.

CHAPTER 43 Nonscarring Alopecias

Jorge Larrondo
Ivie Obeime
Amy J. McMichael

KEY POINTS

- Although the biochemical composition of human hair is remarkably similar, hair morphology does differ among different racial and ethnic groups.
- Hair shafts in those of African descent and pigmented scalp have unique features that can challenge diagnosis.
- Principal differential diagnoses of nonscarring alopecia include alopecia areata, tinea capitis, trichotillomania, pattern hair loss, and telogen effluvium.

INTRODUCTION

Based on macroscopic characteristics, human hair has traditionally been classified into three major groups (African, Asian, and Caucasian).[1] Although the biochemical composition of hair from all three groups is remarkably similar, hair morphology does differ.[2] For example, African hair shafts are curlier, drier, and more susceptible to chemical and physical damage.[1,2] In addition, it appears elliptical in cross-section, with a high degree of irregularity in the diameter along the hair shaft, with frequent twists and random changes in direction.[1,2]

The association of two or more hair disorders is common in patients of African descent.[2] Also, patients with darker skin color present unique trichoscopic patterns, like a pigmented network reflecting the rete ridge melanocytes surrounding hypochromic areas of the suprapapillary epidermis as well as the visualization of acrosyringeal and follicular openings as small pinpoint white dots regularly distributed.[3] Therefore, a deep understanding and a thorough evaluation will help establish appropriate diagnoses and better outcomes.

ALOPECIA AREATA

EPIDEMIOLOGY, ETIOLOGY, AND PATHOGENESIS

Alopecia areata (AA) is a relapsing-remitting autoimmune disease that leads to patchy or diffuse hair loss. In the United States, the prevalence of the disease ranges from 0.2% to 0.7%.[4] A cross-sectional study utilizing National Alopecia Areata Registry data from 2002 to 2016 suggested that Black patients have greater odds of developing AA.[5] Another retrospective, single-institution study evaluating all Black patients with AA seen over 5 years showed that females were more commonly seen than males, and there was an increased distribution of disease in young patients. Most of these patients had patchy hair loss, seen in 68.2% of patients, followed by the ophiasis pattern (occipitotemporal bandlike hair loss), seen in 15.1% of patients.[6] The disease results from a disturbance in the hair follicle immune privilege that leads to anagen inhibition. While the pathogenesis of AA is linked to autoimmunity, there is still uncertainty of the leading drive to these epidemiologic findings of increased prevalence in Black patients.

CLINICAL FINDINGS

Patchy forms of AA are sharply demarcated, round, smooth, nonscarring patches of alopecia [**Figure 43-1 A**]. Areas of involvement may be mildly inflamed, but they are usually asymptomatic. Typically, the hair pull test may be positive at the periphery of active lesions. Nail involvement in AA is frequent and presents mainly with pitting and trachyonychia.[7] The severity of the nail changes reflects the severity of the disease, with red spots on the lunula as a predictor for severe alopecia.[8] According to the amount and location of hair loss, the following variations can be seen:

- Patchy AA (partial hair loss).
- AA totalis (total loss of scalp hair).
- AA universalis (complete loss of scalp and body hair).
- AA ophiasis pattern.
- AA sisapho (frontotemporal bandlike hair loss).
- Less frequent clinical forms are diffuse AA and AA incognito.

TRICHOSCOPY

Trichoscopy shows a well-preserved pigmentary network and pinpoint white dots regularly distributed. Similar features in Caucasians and Asians may be seen in black scalp patients. These include black dots, broken hairs, circle hairs, and exclamation mark hairs [**Figures 43-1B** and **43-2**].[7] However, yellow dots could be harder to evaluate in higher skin phototypes, giving the appearance of white rather than yellow dots.[9]

HISTOPATHOLOGY

Acute forms of AA can present with peribulbar lymphocytic infiltrate, referred to as a "swarm of bees," increased catagen/telogen count, pigmented casts, and trichomalacia. On the other hand, chronic forms often show miniaturized follicles with significantly decreased terminal:vellus ratio, and mild to none peribulbar inflammation.[7]

DIFFERENTIAL DIAGNOSIS

Patchy AA can mimic tinea capitis (TC) and trichotillomania (TTM). Diffuse forms of AA can be confused with male/female pattern hair loss, syphilis, telogen effluvium, and traction alopecia.

TREATMENT

The treatment goals include controlling the disease progression and stimulating hair regrowth. Therapies used may base on the extent of hair loss, the patient´s age, and the progression velocity. Traditionally, AA treatment consisted of anti-inflammatory therapies, including topical, intralesional, and systemic steroids.[7] For pediatric AA, topical corticosteroids are the preferred first-line treatment, followed by contact immunotherapy.[10] Topical and oral minoxidil have also been used as adjunctive therapy. Immunosuppressants are supplementary to recalcitrant and extensive AA. Methotrexate induced more than 50% hair regrowth in 63% of AA patients. Combined therapy of methotrexate and corticosteroids has shown a higher response than methotrexate alone. Azathioprine has achieved greater than 75% hair regrowth in 43% of recalcitrant AU patients.[7] Recognition of the role of the JAK/STAT pathway in AA has led to the first US Food and Drug Administration (FDA)-approved Janus Kinase (JAK) inhibitor (baricitinib) for severe AA. Baricitinib is an oral, selective, reversible inhibitor of JAK 1 and JAK 2. In the BRAVE-AA1 and BRAVE-AA2 phase 3 trials, all patients had severe

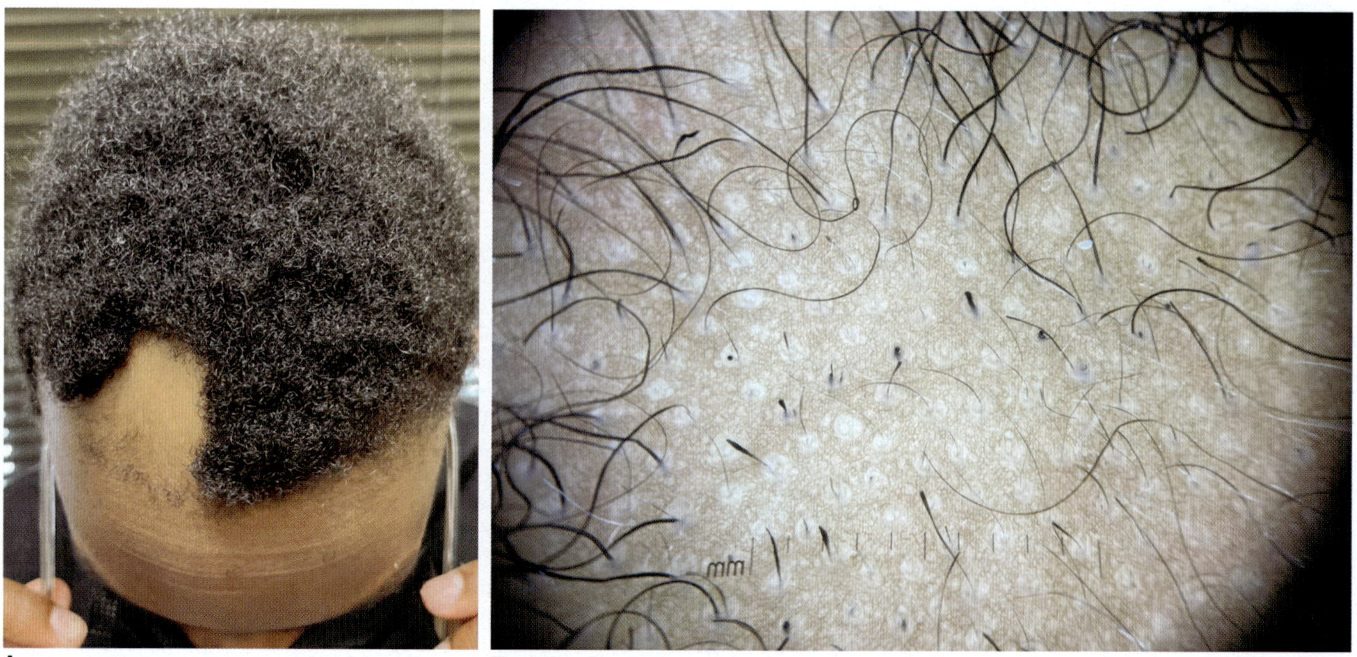

A B

FIGURE 43-1. (A) Clinical presentation of patchy alopecia areata. **(B)** Trichoscopy shows black dots, broken hairs, and exclamation mark hairs. Also, a well-preserved pigmentary network and pinpoint white dots are regularly distributed.

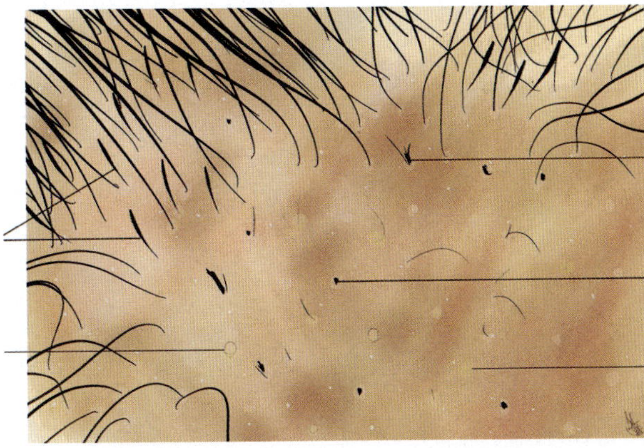

FIGURE 43-2. Illustration of trichoscopic features seen in alopecia areata.

alopecia, and nearly half had AU. In these double-blind, parallel-group, randomized, placebo-controlled trials, 33% of the patient population receiving baricitinib accomplished 80% or more scalp coverage at 36 weeks.[11]

ANDROGENETIC ALOPECIA

EPIDEMIOLOGY, ETIOLOGY, AND PATHOGENESIS

Pattern hair loss is the most common alopecia in men and affects more than 55% of women over 70.[12] This type of hair loss occurs in genetically predisposed individuals secondary to the presence of androgens at the level of the hair follicle. Androgen receptors expressed within the dermal papilla and hair bulb bind testosterone, or dihydrotestosterone (DHT), which binds with a fivefold greater affinity than testosterone. The conversion of testosterone to DHT is mediated by 5α-reductase (types 1 and 2), and DHT is thought to be required for pattern hair loss.[13] Androgen-sensitive hair follicles are located on the frontal and vertex scalp, accounting for the pattern noted in male-pattern hair loss. Although androgens may play a significant role in male-pattern hair loss, their role in female-pattern loss has not been clearly established. Female-pattern hair loss has been described in androgen insensitivity syndromes, and although it can be associated with hyperandrogenic states, it often occurs in women with normal androgen levels.[14] Estrogen signaling modifies androgen metabolism at the follicle and may explain the differences in male- and female-pattern hair loss. The enzyme cytochrome P450 aromatase converts testosterone into estradiol and estrone, reducing testosterone conversion into DHT. This enzyme is found in higher concentrations in the hair follicles of women, particularly in the frontal and occipital scalp. This may explain the preservation of the frontal hairline in women. In addition, women have 40% fewer androgen receptors than men and have 3 to 3.5 times less 5α-reductase than men.[13] There are no studies that describes the prevalence of female pattern hair loss in African American women.

CLINICAL FINDINGS

In men, hair loss usually involves recession of the frontotemporal hairline and nonscarring alopecia of the scalp vertex. Occipital scalp hair is retained. Women typically maintain the frontal hairline, with thinning on the vertex of the scalp, typified by the widening of the central part [**Figure 43-3A**]. The Norwood-Hamilton classification system divides male-pattern hair loss into seven stages according to severity. The Ludwig classification divides female-pattern hair loss into three stages according to severity. African American men may display different hair-loss patterns than Caucasian men. It has been observed that African American men

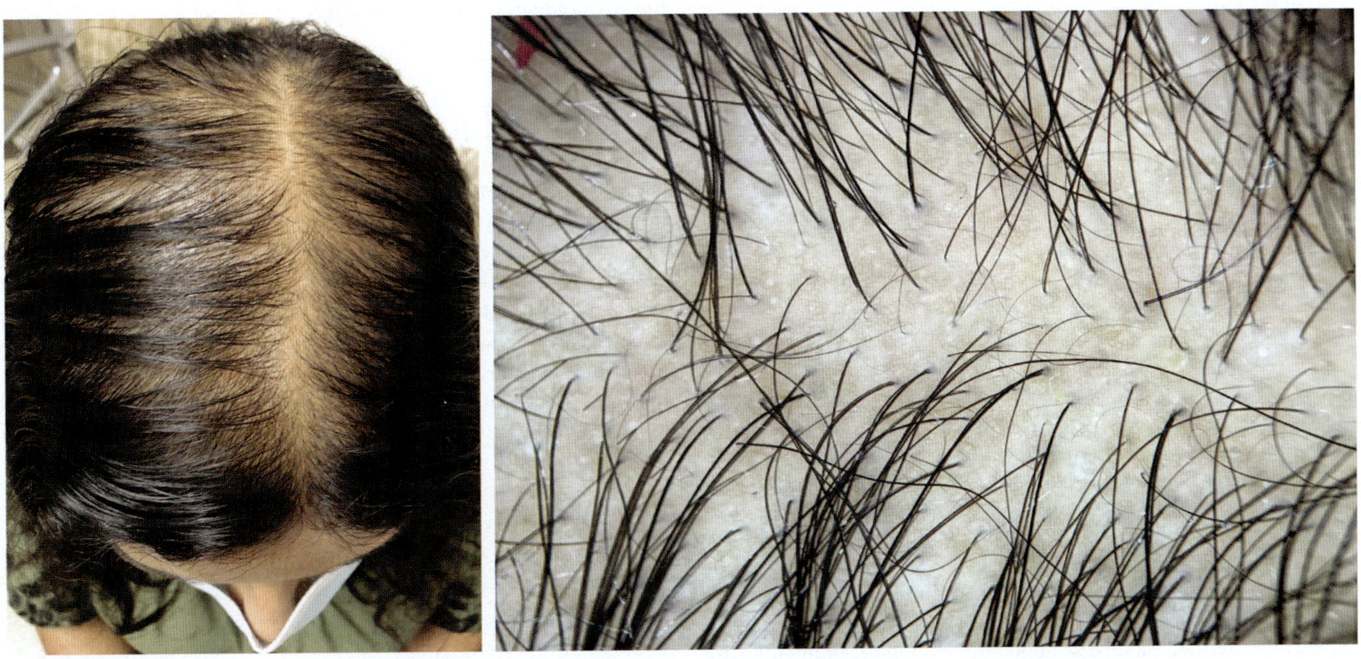

FIGURE 43-3. **(A)** Clinical presentation of female pattern hair loss. **(B)** Trichoscopy shows noticeable variability in hair shaft diameter and thin regrowing hairs in the frontal scalp.

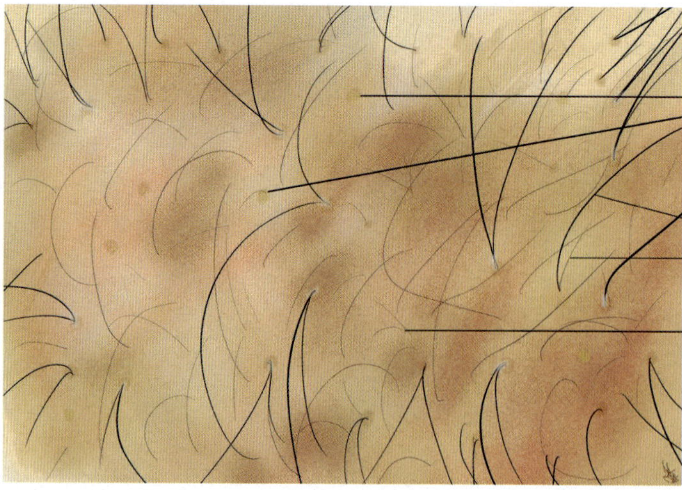

FIGURE 43-4. Illustration of trichoscopic findings seen in androgenetic alopecia.

predominantly exhibit scalp hair loss on the vertex of the scalp. In women with other clinical findings of androgen excess, such as hirsutism, menstrual abnormalities, or severe acne, laboratory analysis of dehydroepiandrosterone (DHEA) sulfate and testosterone may be obtained.

DIFFERENTIAL DIAGNOSIS

Female pattern hair loss can often mimic chronic traction alopecia, chronic telogen effluvium, early forms of central centrifugal cicatricial alopecia, or diffuse AA. Also, among differential diagnoses, fibrosing alopecia in a pattern distribution in both genders must be considered.

TRICHOSCOPY

Although diagnostic criteria remain the same as in Caucasian (>20% variability in hair shaft diameter and thin regrowing hairs in the frontal scalp), the pigmentary network in dark skin is well preserved with regularly distributed pinpoint white dots [Figure 43-3B]. The peripilar sign—a brown peripilar halo corresponding to perifollicular inflammation—has been less reported in the pigmented scalp, possibly due to the difficulty in identifying this feature in dark skin.[9] In addition, other findings, such as a decreased number of hairs per follicular unit and yellow dots, may be observed [**Figure 43-4**].

HISTOPATHOLOGY

There is an increased number of vellus follicles with a decreased terminal:vellus ratio of less than 4:1. A mild increase in the catagen/telogen can be present. Mild to moderate perifollicular lymphocytic inflammation may also be seen.[13]

DIFFERENTIAL DIAGNOSIS

Diffuse AA, chronic telogen effluvium, and fibrosing alopecia in a pattern distribution are the principal differential diagnosis.

TREATMENT

Treatment is sometimes challenging. The FDA has approved topical minoxidil for male- and female-pattern hair loss and oral finasteride (1 mg/day) for male-pattern hair loss. Although supported by regulators in South Korea and Japan, dutasteride 0.5 mg/day for male-pattern hair loss has not been approved by the FDA. In several trials, low-dose oral minoxidil (0.25-5 mg) has shown good safety and efficacy profile.[15] A recent meta-analysis indicates that 0.5 mg/day of oral dutasteride has the highest probability of being the most efficacious treatment, followed by 5 mg/day of oral finasteride, 5 mg/day of oral minoxidil, 1 mg/day of oral finasteride, 5% topical minoxidil, 2% topical minoxidil, and 0.25 mg/day of oral minoxidil.[16] Other used therapies include platelet-rich plasma, low-level laser therapy, and hair restoration surgery.

TRACTION ALOPECIA

EPIDEMIOLOGY, ETIOLOGY, AND PATHOGENESIS

Traction alopecia (TA) is a mechanical form of hair loss caused by prolonged or repetitive tension on the hair, seen most commonly in women of African descent. High-tension hairstyling and the concomitant use of chemicals or heat may increase the risk.[17] Early disease is considered nonscarring and reversible; chronic forms can progress to irreversible hair loss. TA is one of the most prevalent forms of alopecia in patients of color, affecting up to one-third of adult women of African descent.[18]

CLINICAL FINDINGS

A minimally decreased hair density can be seen in early cases. Perifollicular papules and pustules may be present in areas of highest tension. It is helpful to inquire about nocturnal hair care practices because various techniques to maintain hairstyles used while sleeping can generate traction.[19] Marginal traction alopecia usually affects the frontal and temporal scalp leaving a margin of vellus hairs marking the preexisting hairline, also known as the "fringe sign" [**Figure 43-5 A**]. Nonmarginal traction alopecia can occur anywhere throughout the scalp, dictated by the areas of hairstyling with tension.

TRICHOSCOPY

In acute lesions, black dots, broken hairs, and follicular pustules can be seen. The presence of hair casts is a sign of ongoing or persistent traction. In chronic lesions, there is loss of follicular openings, pinpoint white dots or white patches irregularly distributed, and vellus hairs prevailing over terminal hairs [**Figures 43-5B** and **43-6**].[9]

HISTOPATHOLOGY

Acute forms can show an average number of terminal hairs, increased catagen/telogen counts, trichomalacia (distorted hair shafts), and pigmented casts. Chronic forms show fewer hair follicles with follicular dropout. The vellus follicles outnumber the terminal hairs, and sebaceous glands are preserved with minimal inflammation.[20]

DIFFERENTIAL DIAGNOSIS

Acute forms of TA can mimic AA, TC, or TTM. In addition, chronic marginal TA may be confused with frontal fibrosing alopecia, central centrifugal cicatricial alopecia, and female-pattern hair loss.

PREVENTION AND TREATMENT

The clinician must be vigilant regarding the hair care practices of at-risk patients. Minimizing traumatic hairstyling and reducing chemicals and

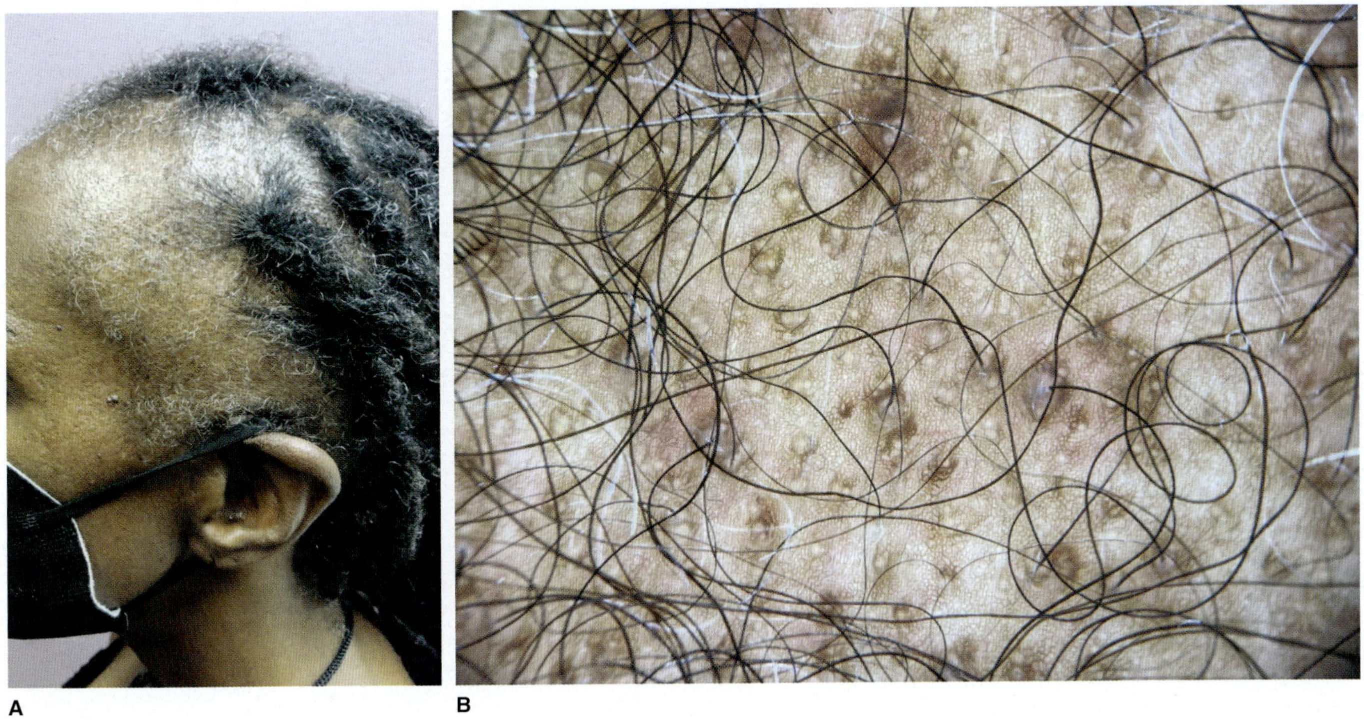

FIGURE 43-5. (A) Clinical presentation of chronic traction alopecia. **(B)** Trichoscopy shows loss of follicular openings, perifollicular erythema, irregularly distributed pinpoint white dots, and increased vellus hairs.

heat are also recommended. Medical treatment for symptomatic cases includes topical and intralesional corticosteroids and topical minoxidil.[21] Also, topical or oral antibiotics can be used, especially in the presence of pustules. Chronic or advanced stages of TA with evidence of scarring alopecia are less likely to respond to medical therapy. Therefore, hair restoration surgery may be an ideal option.[22]

TINEA CAPITIS

EPIDEMIOLOGY, ETIOLOGY, AND PATHOGENESIS

Traction alopecia (TC) describes a scalp and hair dermatophyte infection. Infection may be passed from person to person (anthropophilic) or acquired from animals (zoophilic). The two major causative pathogens in TC are *Trichophyton* (anthropophilic) and *Microsporum* species (zoophilic).[23] TC is an infection affecting Black patients disproportionately in the United States, especially Black children. Although TC is more frequent in children, there has been a recent increase in adults, particularly among African American women.[24] Species differ worldwide by geographic area; *Microsporum canis* is the most frequently reported zoophilic agent, while *Trichophyton violaceum* and *Trichophyton tonsurans* are the principal anthropophilic agents.[25] Species that invade only the inside of the hair shaft are termed endothrix infections, whereas those that invade the outside are responsible for ectothrix infections.

CLINICAL FINDINGS

TC usually presents with areas of scaling and alopecia, with a varying degree of inflammation [**Figure 43-7 A**]. Highly inflammatory lesions or untreated lesions may eventually lead to permanent hair loss. In addition, some cases may associate with cervical lymphadenopathy.

TRICHOSCOPY

Hair shaft abnormalities like comma hairs, corkscrew hairs, black dots, bent hairs, broken hairs, zigzag hairs, and barcode hairs have been described [**Figures 43-7B** and **43-8**].[23] Although none of these features allow for a definitive identification at the genus or species

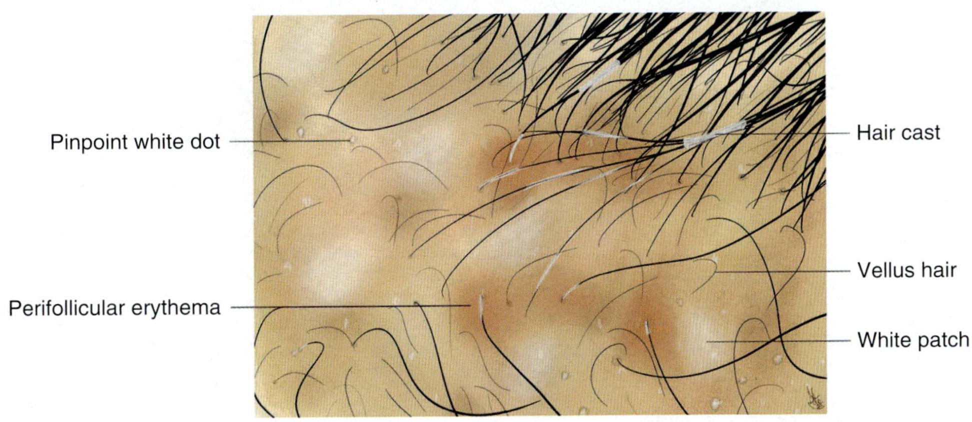

FIGURE 43-6. Illustration of trichoscopic features seen in chronic traction alopecia.

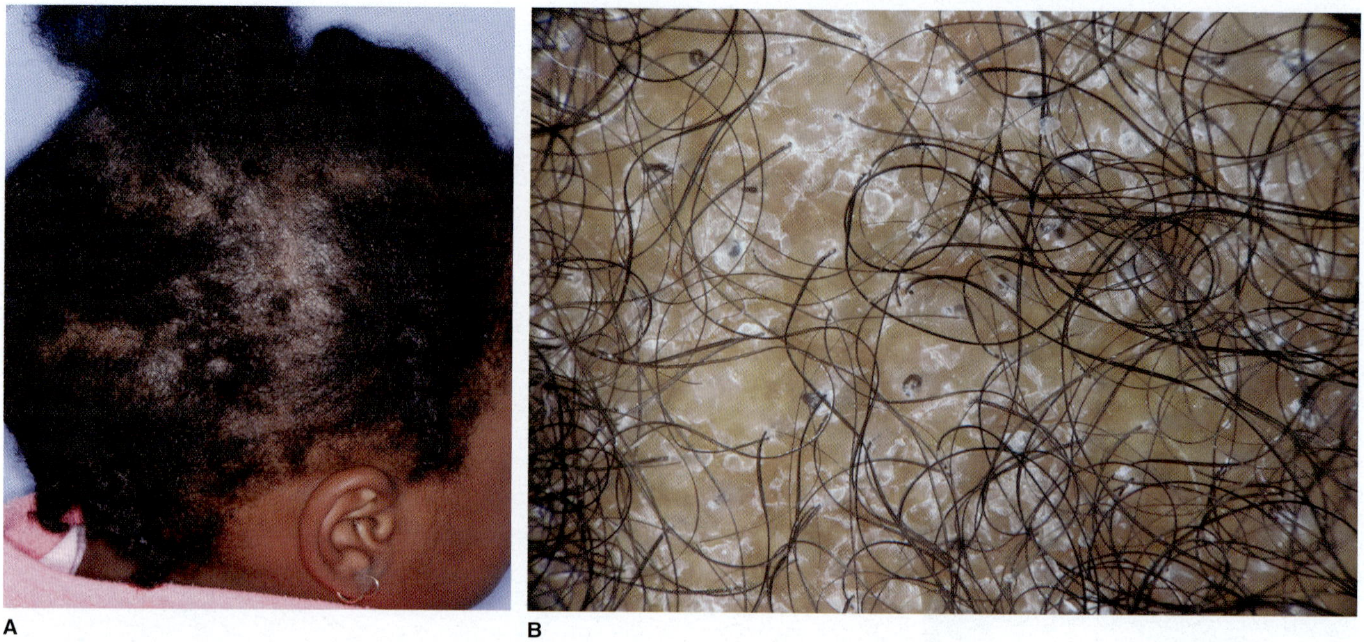

FIGURE 43-7. **(A)** Clinical presentation of tinea capitis. **(B)** Trichoscopy shows scaling, black dots, broken hairs, and comma hairs.

level, a systematic review showed that barcode hairs, zigzag hairs, bent hairs, and diffuse scaling were more suggestive of *Microsporum* TC. Corkscrew hairs were more commonly observed in *Trichophyton* TC.[26]

HISTOPATHOLOGY

In endothrix infection, the common denominator is the presence of spores within the hair shaft. In Black patients, the loaded shafts bend further on the concave side, acquiring a comma shape. In ectothrix infection, the organisms will surround the hair shaft. Inflammatory TC may show a dense mixed cell inflammatory infiltrate of neutrophils, plasma cells, eosinophils, lymphocytes, histiocytes, and granulomas.[23]

DIFFERENTIAL DIAGNOSIS

Noninflammatory TC may resemble AA and TTM. Inflammatory TC may clinically and histologically mimic dissecting cellulitis. Therefore, a complete workup that includes trichoscopy, histology, and potassium hydroxide test or fungal culture should be performed to rule out fungal infections.

TREATMENT

The use of systemic therapy is considered a first-line treatment for TC. Topical agents may serve as adjuvants to prevent the spread of fungal spores. Griseofulvin has been commonly used to treat TC, especially when the causative agent is *M. canis*. Terbinafine is considered first-line therapy, especially for Trichophyton species.[26]

TRICOTILLOMANIA

EPIDEMIOLOGY, ETIOLOGY, AND PATHOGENESIS

TTM is a traumatic alopecia caused by repetitive and compulsive hair pulling and plucking. TTM affects over 11 million Americans, more prominent in females. As of 2007, only 0.5% of all participants included in TTM studies had identified as African American, but this entity does exist in this population.[27] In one study, fewer minority participants reliably improved compared to non-Hispanic White (NHW) participants. This differential response was most clear after the online self-help behavior therapy program, as the NHW participants experienced greater self-reported symptom reduction than the minority participants, while changes in self-reported quality of life and TTM-related disability did

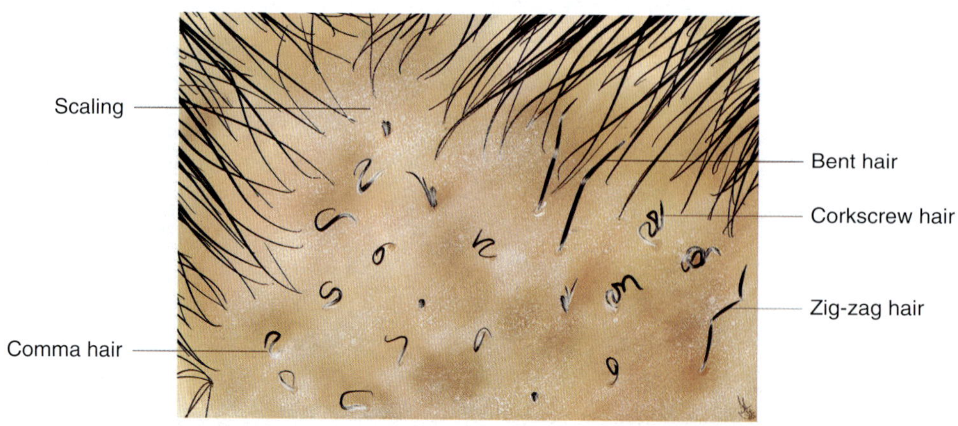

FIGURE 43-8. Illustration of trichoscopic findings seen of tinea capitis.

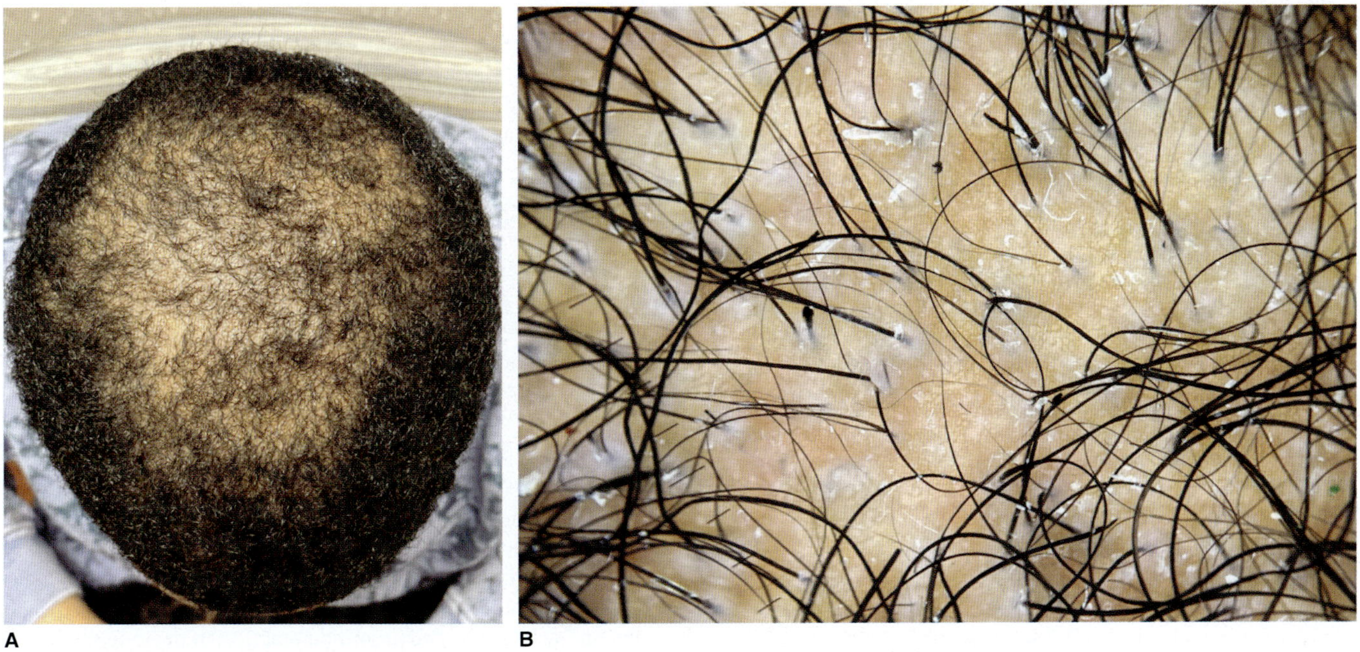

FIGURE 43-9. **(A)** Clinical presentation of trichotillomania. **(B)** Trichoscopy shows black dots and broken hairs at different lengths.

not differ.[28] The etiology is poorly understood and possibly combines genetic, psychological, social, and neurobiological factors. TTM is a highly comorbid disorder, with a concomitant prevalence of psychiatric diseases of up to 80%. The most common conditions are anxiety, major depression, eating disorders, substance misuse, posttraumatic stress disorder, and body dysmorphic disorders.[29]

CLINICAL FINDINGS

Diffuse or bizarre-shaped nonscarring hair loss usually affects the crown or frontoparietal regions [**Figure 43-9 A**]. In addition, broken hairs at different lengths, surrounded by a rim of unaffected hair, can be seen. Eyebrows, upper eyelashes, and pubic area are commonly involved.[29]

TRICHOSCOPY

Hair shafts appear broken at varying lengths or present longitudinal splitting on trichoscopy [**Figure 43-9B**]. Nonspecific features like black dots or broken hairs are usually irregularly distributed. In addition, several signs that correspond to broken hair shafts by the traumatic pulling have been described (flame hairs, tulip hairs, coiled hairs, hook hairs, hair powder, or the V-sign).[9] Among those, the hook hairs represent a particular feature of TTM [**Figure 43-10**].

HISTOPATHOLOGY

Average or slightly decreased number of hair follicles with trichomalacia (abnormal hair shafts in shape and pigmentation). Catagen/telogen shift, perifollicular hemorrhage, and pigmented casts (pigmented fragments of matrical or cortex cells).[20]

DIFFERENTIAL DIAGNOSIS

AA, TC, and traction alopecia are the principal differential diagnosis.

PREVENTION AND TREATMENT

Management is sometimes challenging. A comprehensive therapy can include an interdisciplinary approach with psychotherapeutic and pharmacological alternatives. The current most empirically validated nonpharmacologic treatment is cognitive-behavioral therapy, which seeks to replace the pulling behavior for other activities. Although no medications are specifically approved for TTM, tricyclic antidepressants, selective serotonin reuptake inhibitors, *N*-acetylcysteine, opioid antagonists, and cannabinoid agonists have been described.[29] Though race/ethnicity may not influence TTM symptomatology, there are data to suggest that this variable may influence coping, help-seeking, and other aspects of the disorder.[30]

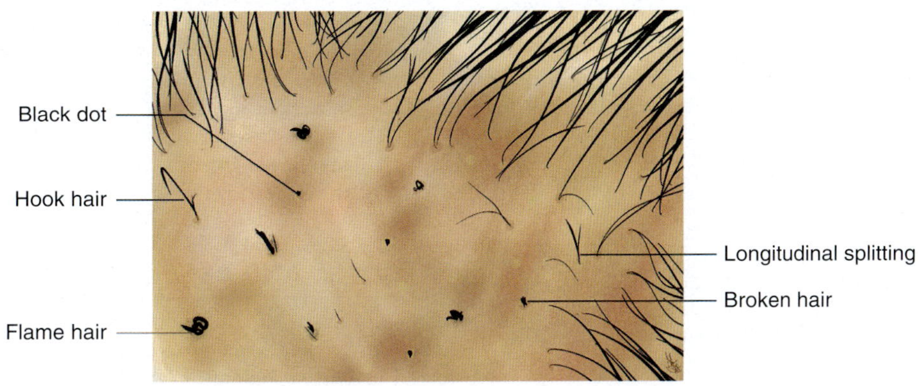

FIGURE 43-10. Illustration of trichoscopic features seen in trichotillomania.

REFERENCES

1. Salam A, Aryiku S, Dadzie OE. Hair and scalp disorders in women of African descent: an overview. *Br J Dermatol.* 2013;3:19-32.
2. Lindsey SF, Tosti A. Ethnic hair disorders. *Curr Probl Dermatol.* 2015;47:139-149.
3. Pirmez R, Tosti A. Trichoscopy tips. *Dermatol Clin.* 2018;36:413-420.
4. Burns LJ, Mesinkovska N, Kranz D, Ellison A, Senna MM. Cumulative life course impairment of alopecia areata. *Int J Trichology.* 2020;12(5):197-204.
5. Lee H, Jung SJ, Patel AB, Thompson JM, Qureshi A, Cho E. Racial characteristics of alopecia areata in the United States. *J Am Acad Dermatol.* 2020;83(4):1064-1070.
6. Feaster B, McMichael AJ. Epidemiology of alopecia areata in Black patients: a retrospective chart review. *J Am Acad Dermatol.* 2022;87(5):1121-1123.
7. Zhou C, Li X, Wang C, Zhang J. Alopecia areata: an update on etiopathogenesis, diagnosis, and management. *Clin Rev Allergy Immunol.* 2021;61(3):403-423.
8. Roest YBM, van Middendorp HT, Evers AWM, van de Kerkhof PCM, Pasch MC. Nail Involvement in alopecia areata: a questionnaire-based survey on clinical signs, impact on quality of life and review of the literature. *Acta Derm Venereol.* 2018;98(2):212-217.
9. Ocampo-Garza J, Tosti A. Trichoscopy of dark scalp. *Skin Appendage Disord.* 2018;5(1):1-8.
10. Barton VR, Toussi A, Awasthi S, Kiuru M. Treatment of pediatric alopecia areata: a systematic review. *J Am Acad Dermatol.* 2022;86(6):1318-1334.
11. King B, Ohyama M, Kwon O, et al. Two phase 3 trials of baricitinib for alopecia areata. *N Engl J Med.* 2022;386(18):1687-1699.
12. Gan DC, Sinclair RD. Prevalence of male and female pattern hair loss in Maryborough. *J Investig Dermatol Symp Proc.* 2005;10(3):184-189.
13. Banka N, Bunagan MJ, Shapiro J. Pattern hair loss in men: diagnosis and medical treatment. *Dermatol Clin.* 2013;31(1):129-140.
14. Cousen P, Messenger A. Female pattern hair loss in complete androgen insensitivity syndrome. *Br J Dermatol.* 2010;162(5):1135-1137.
15. Gupta AK, Talukder M, Williams G. Comparison of oral minoxidil, finasteride, and dutasteride for treating androgenetic alopecia. *J Dermatolog Treat.* 2022;33(7):2946-2962.
16. Gupta AK, Venkataraman M, Talukder M, Bamimore MA. Relative efficacy of minoxidil and the 5-α reductase inhibitors in androgenetic alopecia treatment of male patients: a network meta-analysis. *JAMA Dermatol.* 2022;158(3):266-274.
17. Mirmirani P, Khumalo NP. Traction alopecia: how to translate study data for public education–closing the KAP gap? *Dermatol Clin.* 2014;32:153-161.
18. Khumalo NP, Jessop S, Gumedze F, et al. Hairdressing and the prevalence of scalp disease in African adults. *Br J Dermatol.* 2007;157:981-988.
19. Samrao A, McMichael A, Mirmirani P. Nocturnal traction: techniques used for hair style maintenance while sleeping may be a risk factor for traction alopecia. *Skin Appendage Disord.* 2021;7:220-223.
20. Billero V, Miteva M. Traction alopecia: the root of the problem. *Clin Cosmet Investig Dermatol.* 2018;11:149-159.
21. Uwakwe LN, De Souza B, Tovar-Garza A, McMichael AJ. Intralesional triamcinolone acetonide in the treatment of traction alopecia. *J Drugs Dermatol.* 2020;19(2):128-130.
22. Rogers NE, Callender VD. Advances and challenges in hair restoration of curly Afrocentric hair. *Dermatol Clin.* 2014;32(2):163-171.
23. Miteva M. Hair and scalp infections. In: *Hair Pathology with Trichoscopic Correlations.* Boca Raton, FL: CRC Press; 2022:176-185.
24. Silverberg NB, Weinberg JM, DeLeo VA. Tinea capitis: focus on African American women. *J Am Acad Dermatol.* 2002;46(2 Suppl Understanding):S120-S124.
25. Rodríguez-Cerdeira C, Martínez-Herrera E, Szepietowski JC, et al. A systematic review of worldwide data on tinea capitis: analysis of the last 20 years. *J Eur Acad Dermatol Venereol.* 2021;35(4):844-883.
26. Waśkiel-Burnat A, Rakowska A, Sikora M, Ciechanowicz P, Olszewska M, Rudnicka L. Trichoscopy of tinea capitis: a systematic review. *Dermatol Ther (Heidelb).* 2020;10(1):43-52.
27. Neal-Barnett A, Stadulis R. Affective states and racial identity among African-American women with trichotillomania. *J Natl Med Assoc.* 2006;98(5):753-757.
28. Falkenstein MJ, Rogers K, Malloy EJ, Haaga DA. Race/ethnicity and treatment outcome in a randomized controlled trial for trichotillomania (hair-pulling disorder). *J Clin Psychol.* 2015;71(7):641-652.
29. Melo DF, Lima CDS, Piraccini BM, Tosti A. Trichotillomania: what do we know so far? *Skin Appendage Disord.* 2022;8(1):1-7.
30. Neal-Barnett A, Statom D, Stadulis R. Trichotillomania symptoms in African American women: are they related to anxiety and culture? *CNS Neurosci Ther.* 2011;17(4):207-213.

CHAPTER 44

Seborrheic Dermatitis

Sneha Poondru
Saira Alvi
Roopal V. Kundu

KEY POINTS

- Seborrheic dermatitis is a very common concern in patients with skin of color; it is among the top five dermatological diagnoses in African American patients.
- Various factors may play a role in pathogenesis, including proliferation of Malassezia yeast species and susceptibility of the host's immune system and skin barrier.
- Certain systemic illnesses are risk factors and may be associated with increased severity of seborrheic dermatitis.
- In addition to a scaly appearance, darker skin tones often exhibit hypo- or hyperpigmentation, while underlying erythema may be difficult to appreciate.
- Treatment options and their formulations should be adjusted depending on the hair type and grooming practices of the individual.

Seborrheic dermatitis is a chronic, recurring inflammatory condition that presents as erythematous, hypo- or hyperpigmented patches or plaques with overlying scale, typically on sebum-rich areas of the scalp, face, trunk, and intertriginous areas. While all demographics can be affected, the condition is more common in Black populations.[1] Certain systemic illnesses are associated with increased severity of seborrheic dermatitis, particularly acquired immunodeficiency syndrome (AIDS) and Parkinson disease.[2,3]

Although the exact etiology is unknown, it is theorized that a combination of increased sebaceous gland activity, proliferation of the commensal *Malassezia* yeast species, and susceptibility of the host immune system and skin barrier are involved.[4] Clinically, seborrheic dermatitis is often easily recognized. However, findings may differ based on the Fitzpatrick skin type of the affected individual. In addition to erythema and scaliness, darker skin tones can present with hypo- and hyperpigmentation, which is often a cause of distress. There are various treatment options, but the choice of therapy and its formulation should be further adjusted based on hair grooming practices. Treatment goals include successful control of the symptoms and the clinical manifestations of the disease; however, a cure is typically unattainable as the disease course is remitting and relapsing.

EPIDEMIOLOGY

Seborrheic dermatitis affects 3% to 12% of the general population. Although it can affect individuals of all ages, its incidence peaks in infancy and adulthood between the ages of 40 and 60 years. The male gender and Black populations are more frequently affected than their counterparts.[5] Seborrheic dermatitis is among the five most common dermatological diagnoses observed in African American patients.[6] An increased incidence is found in those with immunodeficiencies, Parkinson disease, chronic alcoholic pancreatitis, familial amyloidosis with polyneuropathy, Down syndrome, eating disorders, and mood disorders.[7-9]

ETIOLOGY AND ASSOCIATED CONDITIONS

Although the exact etiology of seborrheic dermatitis is unknown, several factors have been proposed to play a role: increased sebaceous gland activity, proliferation of the commensal *Malassezia* yeast species, and susceptibility of the host's immune system, skin barrier, and genetics.

Many studies have shown that the quantity of *Malassezia* directly correlates with the severity of seborrheic dermatitis and the locations of lesions.[10] Although *Malassezia* has a role in pathogenesis, it is hypothesized that the mere presence of yeast is insufficient to cause symptoms. In fact, *Malassezia* is the most abundant fungus in healthy skin, and a decrease in *Malassezia* is not always detected in vivo even after resolution of seborrheic dermatitis symptoms with ketoconazole treatment.[11] Additionally, even though *Malassezia* shows increased growth in high temperatures when perspiration increases, the risk of seborrheic dermatitis is highest in cold, dry weather.[12] Therefore, it is proposed that a combination of genetic predisposition and an individual's interactions with the environment—including sebaceous gland activity, epidermal barrier function, and immune reactivity—are required to develop seborrheic dermatitis symptoms.

An abnormal interaction between the host and *Malassezia* leads to an immune response against the fungus and its metabolites. The lipase secreted by *Malassezia* hydrolyzes the lipids from sebum into free fatty acids, which can be inflammatory in certain individuals. Studies have shown that topical application of oleic acid—a *Malassezia* metabolite—did not cause any visible skin changes in healthy control subjects, but it did induce desquamation on the nonlesional skin of those affected by seborrheic dermatitis.[12] This suggests that preexisting epidermal barrier defects, present even in non-lesional skin of those with seborrheic dermatitis, make individuals more susceptible to oleic acid irritation. A recent study also proposed that the presence of the hyphal form of *Malassezia* specifically is pathogenic as it correlated with disease severity.[13]

Seborrheic dermatitis involves an increase in inflammatory interleukins, complement activation, and NK1+ and CD16+ cells. T-cell function is depressed, while natural killer cells and IgA and IgG antibody levels may be increased. However, there is no increase in the total amount of antibodies against *Malassezia*, highlighting that the changes in antibodies are likely not due to the yeast.[2] Immunocompromised individuals, including those with HIV, hepatitis C virus, malignancies, organ transplants, and alcoholic pancreatitis, are at a higher risk of developing seborrheic dermatitis.[8,14] The incidence in HIV-positive patients has been reported to be as high as 83%, with lower CD4-positive T-cell counts associated with more severe disease. It is hypothesized that the immune dysregulation may also alter the skin microbiota, allowing for unopposed *Malassezia* proliferation. In the United States, about 42% of those newly diagnosed with HIV/AIDS are African American and 22% are Latino, therefore it is important to note the significance of skin disease in these communities.[15]

Increased sebum production is also correlated with seborrheic dermatitis symptoms. Males are more likely to be affected than females due to increased sebaceous gland activity by androgens. Likewise, newborns and African Americans are affected at higher rates due to elevated sebum production and larger sebaceous glands.[16] In Parkinson disease, seborrhea is likely due to neuroendocrine dysfunction and increased circulating α-melanocyte–stimulating hormone (α-MSH). Facial immobility in Parkinson disease and other neurological conditions, such as stroke, may also contribute to sebum accumulation. Treatment with levodopa may improve seborrheic dermatitis in those with Parkinson disease by blocking MSH secretion and improving mobility.[9]

Seborrhea-like dermatitis may also develop in those treated with drugs such as cimetidine, chlorpromazine, haloperidol, phenothiazines, interferon alpha, and griseofulvin [**Table 44-1**].[3]

TABLE 44-1 Disorders and drugs commonly associated with seborrheic dermatitis

Chronic alcohol consumption and pancreatitis
Drugs (neuroleptic drugs, griseofulvin, interferon alpha, psoralens)
Eating disorders
Familial amyloidosis with polyneuropathy
HIV/AIDS
Organ transplant
Trisomy 21 genetic disorder
Neurological disorders (Parkinson disease, mood disorders, stroke, epilepsy)

Abbreviations: AIDS, acquired immunodeficiency syndrome; HIV, human immunodeficiency virus.

CLINICAL FEATURES

The clinical features of seborrheic dermatitis depend on age, Fitzpatrick skin type, and the presence or absence of concurrent systemic illnesses.

In adults, clinical findings vary by the location of involvement. The lesions are often present in sebaceous areas, such as the face, scalp, nasolabial folds, glabella, eyelids, eyebrows, ears, postauricular, and skin folds [**Figure 44-1**]. Less scale is appreciated in intertriginous sites, making the lesions appear similar to intertrigo. On the scalp, seborrheic dermatitis can present as dandruff—scaling without inflammation—or greasy, yellow crusts. Hair loss from seborrheic dermatitis is uncommon. In Fitzpatrick skin types IV to VI, the skin is often hypopigmented beneath the scale, but it may also present with hyperpigmentation and underlying erythema that may be difficult to appreciate. Another characteristic finding in patients of color is petal-like patches termed petaloid seborrheic dermatitis. Petaloid seborrheic dermatitis appears as pink or hypopigmented annular coalescing rings with minimal scale [**Table 44-2**]. The associated hypopigmentation may be due to yeast metabolites inhibiting melanocyte tyrosinase function and pigment production. Hypopigmentation typically improves with treatment. Patients with skin of color with recurrent visible hypopigmented lesions or groin involvement were noted to have a more negative quality of life.[17] African American patients can also experience a granulomatous appearance of seborrheic dermatitis.[1,18]

In children, seborrheic dermatitis presents as a yellow or white, thick, greasy scale on the vertex of the scalp termed "cradle cap." In skin of color, "cradle cap" can present with hypopigmentation, scale, and/or erythema. Overlying atopic dermatitis can augment the hypopigmentation. Seborrheic dermatitis in the diaper area of infants is one type of "napkin dermatitis." Unlike adults who tend to have a chronic, unpredictable course, infants with seborrheic dermatitis typically have spontaneous remission of symptoms in 6 to 8 months. Severe and generalized seborrheic dermatitis in infancy may represent Leiner disease, an exfoliative disorder associated with anemia, diarrhea, immunodeficiency, and concomitant infections.[3]

In HIV/AIDS patients, skin involvement is often more extensive and more visibly inflamed. Coexisting blepharitis and occlusion of the meibomian glands can result in scaling and a burning sensation on the eyelids. Axillary, extremity, and groin involvement is often diffuse. Various superinfections, bacterial, fungal, or viral, may also be present.[2]

HISTOPATHOLOGY

Histopathology findings can differ based on whether the disease is acute, subacute, or chronic. Acute and subacute lesions will present with mild to moderate spongiosis, psoriasiform hyperplasia, perivascular lymphocytes and histiocytes, and scale crust around the opening of the hair follicle's infundibulum consisting of orthokeratosis, parakeratosis, and scattered neutrophils. Chronic lesions show the previous characteristics, along with marked superficial blood vessel dilation. Histologically, psoriasis can appear similar to seborrheic dermatitis but is distinguished by the absence of spongiosis and folliculocentric crust. HIV-associated seborrheic dermatitis has distinctive features, such as severe parakeratosis, leukocytoclasia, necrosis of keratinocytes, and superficial perivascular infiltrates of plasma cells.[3,19]

DIFFERENTIAL DIAGNOSIS

Seborrheic dermatitis is typically diagnosed clinically. The differential diagnoses for seborrheic dermatitis include atopic and contact dermatitis, tinea faciei and capitis, psoriasis, scabies, erythrasma, Langerhans cell histiocytosis, rosacea, drug eruption, zinc deficiency,

TABLE 44-2 Clinical patterns of seborrheic dermatitis

Patient group	Pattern/location
Infants	"Cradle cap" and "napkin dermatitis"
Adults	Areas with facial hair (eyebrows, mustache, and eyelid margins)
General	Skin flexures (nasolabial folds, postauricular folds, axillae, and groin)
HIV/AIDS	Extensive involvement with blepharitis and superinfections
Skin of color	Hypopigmentation, hyperpigmentation, "petaloid" seborrheic dermatitis

Abbreviations: AIDS, acquired immunodeficiency syndrome; HIV, human immunodeficiency virus.

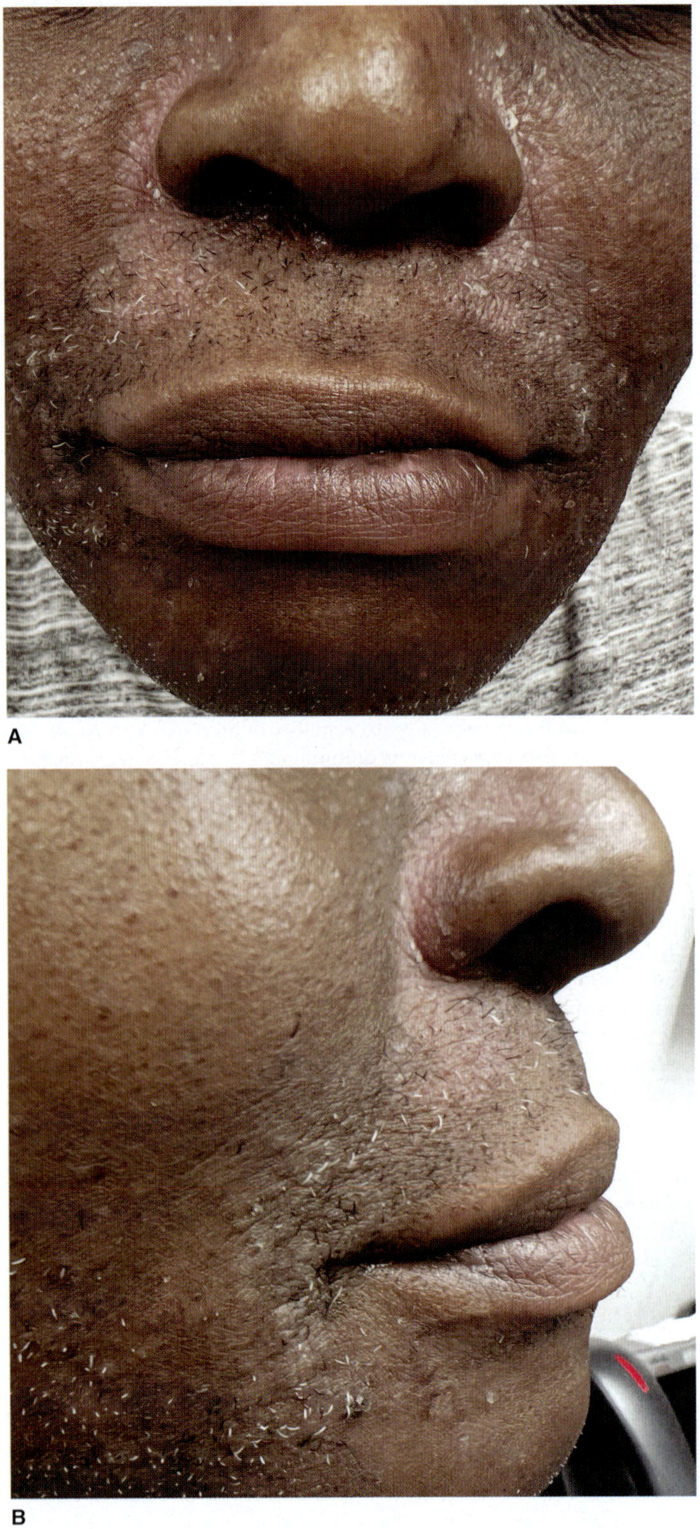

FIGURE 44-1. Male with Fitzpatrick skin type V with annular hypopigmented and erythematous plaques and papules along **(A)** nasolabial folds and **(B)** perioral region.

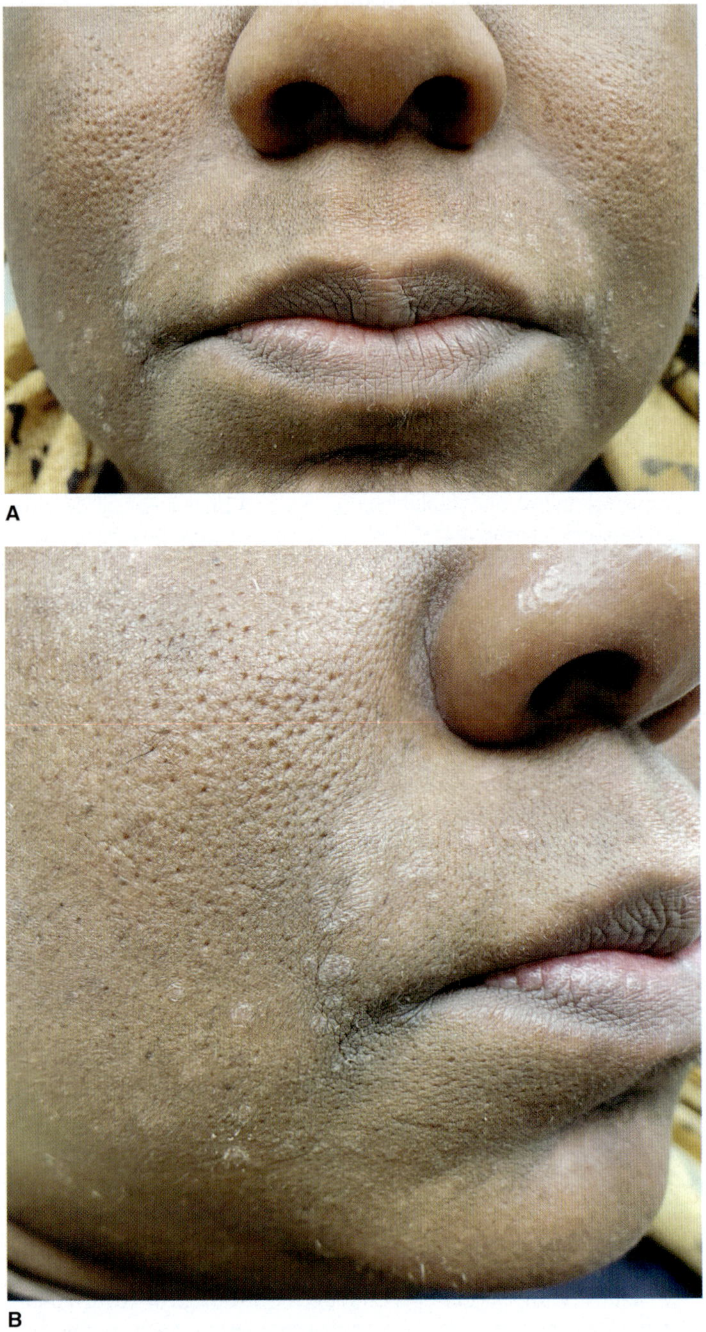

FIGURE 44-2. Annular, scaly erythematous plaques and papules with patches of underlying **(A)** hypopigmentation around the lips and philtrum and **(B)** hyperpigmentation along nasolabial folds, corner of lips, and malar cheek.

and others [**Table 44-3**]. In children with scalp involvement, tinea capitis should be considered, especially the seborrheic type, which is more common than seborrheic dermatitis in Hispanic and African American children.[1] Langerhans cell histiocytosis should be considered in children if there is extensive moist erythematous plaques and petechial lesions of the scalp and intertriginous sites. Although additional history or testing may be required to fully differentiate atopic dermatitis and seborrheic dermatitis, lesions isolated to the diaper region are more consistent with seborrheic dermatitis, while lesions

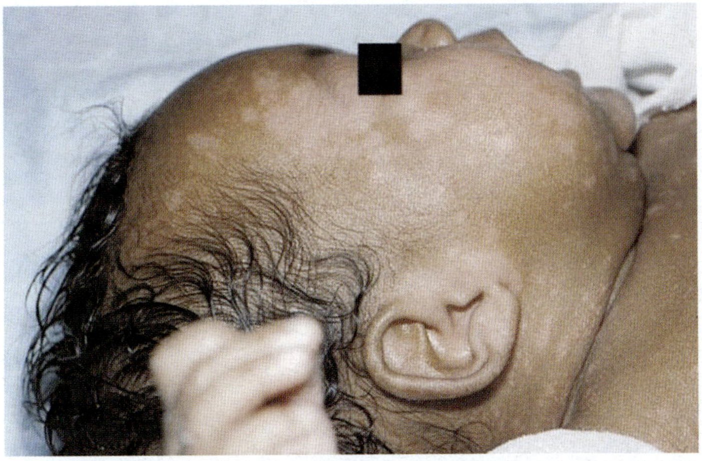

A

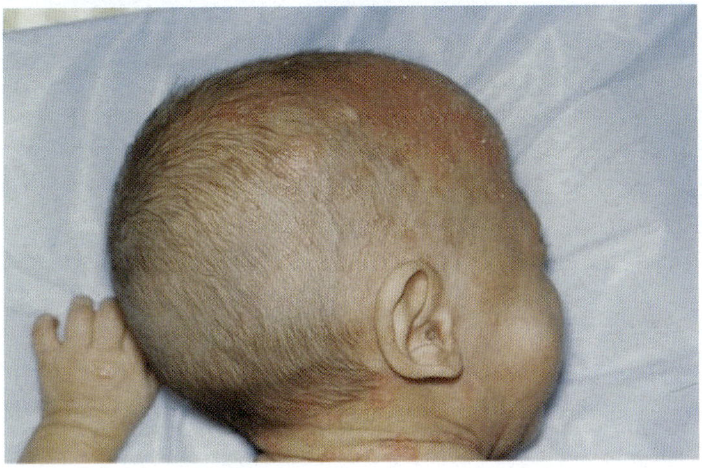

B

FIGURE 44-3. (A) An infant with Fitzpatrick skin type IV with hypopigmented, finely scaled macules. **(B)** An infant presenting with extensive greasy, scaly plaques of "cradle cap."

TABLE 44-3 Differential diagnoses for seborrheic dermatitis and distinguishing features

Diagnosis	Distinguishing features
Contact dermatitis	Distribution pattern consistent with irritant/allergen
Atopic dermatitis	Lesions on the forearms, antecubital/popliteal fossae, and shins while sparing the axillae and nasolabial folds
Tinea capitis, faciei, corporis	Hyphae on KOH cytologic examination, "ringworm pattern"; scaly, red, slightly elevated lesion, central clearing; vesicles with inflammation
Candidiasis	Confined to intertriginous regions and mucous membranes; pseudohyphae on KOH cytologic examination
Impetigo	Thin, fragile vesicles; streptococci or staphylococci infection
Psoriasis	Red, scaling papules coalescing into round/oval plaques on extensor surfaces; inverse variant: sharply defined red patches without scale in intertriginous areas
Pityriasis rosea	"Christmas-tree distribution" pink papules on trunk/extremities; herald patch
Rosacea	Distribution on forehead, cheeks, eyes, nose; erythematous/edematous papules
Langerhans cell histiocytosis (Letterer-Siwe disease)	Moist erythematous plaques and petechial lesions of the scalp and intertriginous sites; histologic specific scaling; fever/systemic symptoms
Erythrasma	Groin, toe webs, axillae distribution; brown-red scaly eruption
Lichen simplex chronicus	Accentuation of skin markings, pruritus, and scratching
Nummular dermatitis	Coin-shaped plaques on extremities, commonly on backs of hands
Secondary syphilis	Influenza like symptoms, adenopathy, copper-colored scaly plaques on palms/soles
Systemic lupus erythematous	Acute: facial butterfly rash; Subacute: papulosquamous, annular lesions on trunk; Discoid: disc-like lesions on face/scalp; Infants: papulosquamous, annular lesions

Abbreviation: KOH, potassium hydroxide.

on the forearms and shins that spare the axillae suggest atopic dermatitis. Scabies should be considered if pruritic lesions are generalized and include the palms and soles. Fungal and bacterial cultures, skin biopsies, and laboratory studies may be performed if necessary.

GROOMING PRACTICES

It is important to be aware of and consider hair type, hair styling, and grooming practices in the management of seborrheic dermatitis.

Many African Americans have textured hair that is inherently dry with reduced moisture content and low tensile strength. The hair's spiral form also makes it more difficult for sebum to be distributed along the hair shaft, leading to increased hair breakage. Thus, those of African ancestry may wash their hair once every 2 weeks on average in order to decrease the hair's loss of moisture and its fragility. Asian hair has the largest diameter and higher tensile strength when compared with African American and white hair. Latino hair can either be textured like African American hair or straight or curly-like white hair. Native American hair is similar to white hair.

African Americans commonly use hair oil, heat sources, and chemical relaxers on their hair. In a recent study, 95% of the African Americans surveyed used chemical relaxers at some point to straighten their hair.[20] Chemical relaxers contain ingredients, such as sodium, guanine, and potassium hydroxide, that work by breaking cysteine disulfide bonds to straighten each strand. This chemical process leads to increased hair breakage when compared to nontreated hair. Heat is also utilized for hair straightening, which requires a heated tool that reaches temperatures greater than 150°F. The straightened hair will revert to original texture when wet. Pomades and oils, which may be applied onto hair for moisture and onto the scalp to reduce scale, may also impact hair washing frequency. However, certain products with high oleic acid content, such as coconut oil, olive oil, and shea butter, can worsen seborrheic dermatitis; several Malassezia species have high lipase activity allowing them to use the applied oils for growth. Thus, use of oils to the hair shaft, not the scalp, is recommended. Additionally, the use of hair gel to keep hairstyles in place can also lead to further product buildup and dryness on the scalp. Gels may contain lanolin, which has the potential to worsen seborrheic dermatitis.[18] Hair may also be bleached or permed with ammonium and hydrogen peroxide. Other methods used to curl the hair include hot curling irons, as well as mousses and gels in combination with heated dryers. All these hairstyles and styling agents may lead to dry hair and increased hair fragility.

In addition to hair grooming practices, hair styling practices in patients of color must also be taken into consideration when treating seborrheic dermatitis. Certain hairstyles more commonly worn by African Americans, such as tight braiding or cornrows, may be maintained for several weeks without washing or releasing tension from the hair. Dreadlocks, now more commonly referred to as "locs," are achieved by allowing the natural hair to twist, knot, and become matted over time. Cleaning the scalp with a clarifying shampoo is recommended. Weaves and hair extensions are also commonly used among this group. Since human or synthetic hair is woven into the base of the natural hair, either by being sewn with a thread or bonded to the scalp with glue, hair extensions may cause scalp irritation and inflammation, contributing to seborrheic dermatitis. Although more studies are needed to fully understand the relationship between hair extensions and seborrheic dermatitis, it is suggested that natural hairstyles may prevent its occurrence.[1] Studies have

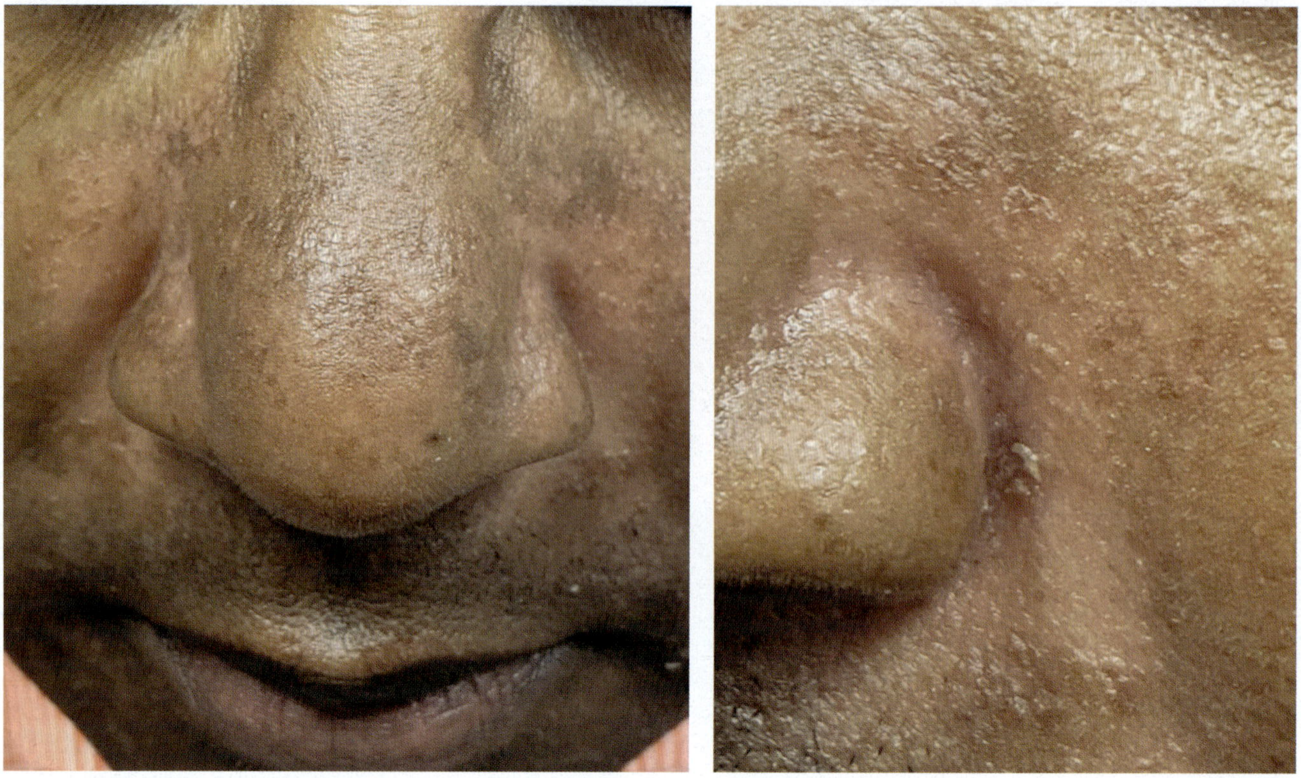

A B

FIGURE 44-4. Thin hypopigmented and erythematous plaques along **(A)** nasolabial folds with **(B)** overlying scale.

not found an association between hair washing frequency and presence of seborrheic dermatitis.[21]

TREATMENT

When treating seborrheic dermatitis in skin of color, it is important to consider hair type, frequency of hair washing, and tendency for hypopigmentation. The goal of treatment is to decrease pruritus, erythema, scale, and postinflammatory dyschromia, as well as maintain remission. Due to the chronic, relapsing nature of seborrheic dermatitis, providing treatment options that align with skin and hair practices can improve compliance and quality of life.

Choosing the correct formulation based on hair type is crucial [**Table 44-4**]. Solutions, sprays, aerosols, lotions, and gels have active ingredients dissolved in alcoholic vehicles that evaporate to leave the active agent on the skin. Since they leave little residue, these agents are generally useful for the natural, nonchemically treated hair of Asians, Native Americans, and Latinos. For African American and chemically treated hair, however, they are often too drying. Thus, focusing on alternative, less drying therapies may increase compliance and treatment success, while preventing hair damage and breakage. African American patients tend to prefer ointments and oil, which are effective at maintaining moisture in natural or chemically treated hair. Foams may be acceptable in chemically straightened hair for individuals who do not wish to use oil-based products.

ANTIFUNGAL

Topical azoles are the mainstay treatment used to decrease inflammation and the burden of *Malassezia*. The most common, ketoconazole 2%, is found as a shampoo, foam, cream, and gel. In a study that evaluated ketoconazole 2% foam and shampoo in African American females, researchers found that both were equally effective at reducing symptoms, but the foam users were more likely to be satisfied.[22] The shampoo can worsen dryness and breakage in chemically treated hair. Thus, it should be advised to limit shampoo use to once weekly followed with moisturizing conditioners. Shampoo should be applied directly to scalp, trying to avoid the hair shaft. Ciclopirox olamine 1%, found as a cream, shampoo, and gel, is a broad-spectrum antifungal with antiinflammatory activity effective for face and scalp seborrheic dermatitis. Terbinafine 1% cream was found to be comparable to ketoconazole 2% cream in terms of efficacy and safety.[23]

CORTICOSTEROIDS

Low to mild potency topical corticosteroids are efficacious in controlling inflammation in seborrheic dermatitis. They can be used as monotherapy or in combination with antifungals. Prolonged use or high doses are discouraged due to adverse effects of skin thinning, atrophy, and hypopigmentation, which may be particularly noticeable in Fitzpatrick skin types IV to VI. Topical ketoconazole 2% treatment showed remission rates similar to that of steroids with lower side effects.[23] Thus, corticosteroids are generally reserved for marked inflammation, acute flares, or failure to resolve with antifungals.

IMMUNOMODULATORS

Tacrolimus ointment and pimecrolimus cream are topical non-corticosteroid immunosuppressants that are effective against seborrheic dermatitis. They may be good options for resistant cases of seborrheic dermatitis and long-term maintenance use without the side effects of steroids, such as skin atrophy. They can safely be used on the face, neck, and intertriginous areas. Tacrolimus ointment applied once to twice weekly in patients with stabilized facial seborrheic dermatitis successfully kept them in remission by controlling erythema, scaling, and pruritus, suggesting its efficacy as maintenance therapy.[24] Pimecrolimus is found as a cream, thus having greater cosmetic acceptability. In a study of African American patients, researchers highlighted improvement in symptoms and hypopigmentation with pimecrolimus cream.[25] Its response rate is comparable to ketoconazole 2% cream and hydrocortisone 1% cream.[23] Case reports have shown successful resolution of symptoms with pimecrolimus after failure with antifungals and steroids.[26] Adverse effects can include burning, tingling, and pruritus. There is a black box

TABLE 44-4 Treatments for seborrheic dermatitis

Medication		Dose/Formulation
Antifungal	Ketoconazole	1% or 2% shampoo, cream, gel, foam
	Ciclopirox	1.5% shampoo, cream, gel, lotion
	Terbinafine	1% cream
Corticosteroids	Hydrocortisone	1% ointment, cream, lotion, gel, foam, spray, solution
	Desonide	0.05% ointment, cream, lotion, gel, foam
	Betamethasone	0.05% lotion
Immunomodulators	Tacrolimus	0.1% ointment
	Pimecrolimus	1% cream
Miscellaneous	Zinc pyrithione	1% or 2% shampoo
	Piroctone	shampoo, cream
	Salicylic acid	3% shampoo
	Coal tar	4% shampoo
	Selenium sulfide	2.5% shampoo, cream
	Sodium sulfacetamide & sulfur	lotion, emollient foam
	Promiseb	cream
	Lithium Succinate	8% ointment or gel
	Benzoyl Peroxide	2.5% wash
	Tea tree oil	N/A
Systemic therapy	Itraconazole	oral
	Prednisone	oral
	Isotretinoin	oral

warning for risk of lymphoma with prolonged use, but there has not been substantial causal evidence in cutaneous use.

OTHER INGREDIENTS

Zinc pyrithione is an antifungal ingredient in many medicated shampoos and conditioners. It comes in a variety of concentrations ranging from 0.25% to 2%. For facial involvement, a 0.25% zinc spray and a 2% zinc cleansing bar are also effective. There is no evidence of tachyphylaxis with long-term zinc-based treatment, so increasing symptoms could be due to lower compliance or progressing disease. Climbazole and piroctone are also antifungal agents found in numerous anti-dandruff shampoos. Researchers found that shampoos containing climbazole and piroctone had similar or better efficacy compared to zinc pyrithione with additional advantages of decreasing wet hair combing force and increasing hair conditioning.[27] Keratolytic agents, such as salicylic acid, coal tar, and selenium sulfide, are found in shampoos that are used in treatment of seborrheic dermatitis. These shampoos may have limited use in those who wash their hair less frequently.

Sodium sulfacetamide and sulfur have antimicrobial and anti-inflammatory properties that make them effective against seborrheic dermatitis. The formulation of 10% sodium sulfacetamide and 5% sulfur is found as a lotion or emollient foam. The scalp foam does not contain alcohol, which allows for less drying and breakage when used on chemically treated hair.

Promiseb is a nonsteroidal cream with anti-inflammatory and antifungal properties. Compared to corticosteroid creams, it has equivalent effects on symptom improvement and increased remission time. A daily regimen of Promiseb cream with episodic use of steroids for flares may be an effective option with less side effects.[28] Lithium succinate is an ointment that limits the growth of yeast and inhibits arachidonic acid, the first step in generating inflammatory leukotrienes and prostaglandins. Benzoyl peroxide, a common acne treatment due to its antibacterial and comedolytic properties, is helpful in seborrheic dermatitis by controlling seborrhea. Tea tree oil has antimicrobial activity that can help with patients looking for alternative treatment options. Mineral oil or petroleum jelly can help loosen crusts and scabs that form on the scalps of infants with cradle cap. This can be combined with a baby shampoo or a low-potency steroid if needed. Seborrheic blepharitis is managed with eyelid hygiene and warm compresses, followed by a topical steroid or antimicrobial agent. Other therapies, such as phototherapy, glycyrrhetinic acid, and mixtures of urea, propylene glycol, and lactic acid, have also been suggested.[23]

Systemic therapy is typically reserved for severe or recalcitrant seborrheic dermatitis. Oral itraconazole is a systemic antifungal with a good therapeutic and safety profile. It has highly lipophilic and keratinophilic properties and is secreted into the sebum, making it an appropriate systemic treatment for seborrheic dermatitis.[29] Prednisone and isotretinoin have also been shown to effective in moderate to severe seborrheic dermatitis.[30]

CONCLUSION

Seborrheic dermatitis is a very common cutaneous disorder in skin of color. In addition to the characteristic scaling of the face and scalp, postinflammatory dyspigmentation is common, which may be particularly disfiguring in those with darker skin. Although various treatment modalities are available, the distinctive hair structure and cultural grooming practices in persons of color determine the suitability and compliance of those therapies. Refraining from shampoos and topical products that dry the hair is important for those who suffer from brittle, low moisture hair. While steroids can be used short-term, medications that avoid potential side effects of atrophy and telangiectasias are preferable, such as antifungal agents and topical calcineurin inhibitors. Finally, topical agents in acceptable vehicles, such as foams, oils, and/or ointments, is important.

REFERENCES

1. Elgash M, Dlova N, Ogunleye T, Taylor SC. Seborrheic dermatitis in skin of color: clinical considerations. *J Drugs Dermatol.* 2019;18(1):24-27.
2. Borda LJ, Wikramanayake TC. Seborrheic dermatitis and dandruff: a comprehensive review. *J Clin Investig Dermatol.* 2015;3(2): doi:10.13188/2373-1044.1000019.
3. Suh DH. Seborrheic dermatitis. In: Kang S, Amagai M, Bruckner AL, et al., eds. *Fitzpatrick's Dermatology*. 9th ed. McGraw Hill Education, New York; 2019. Accessed February 10, 2025. https://accessmedicine.mhmedical.com/content.aspx?bookid=2570&sectionid=210417567
4. Grice EA, Dawson TL, Jr. Host-microbe interactions: malassezia and human skin. *Curr Opin Microbiol.* 2017;40:81-87.
5. Halder RM, Nootheti PK. Ethnic skin disorders overview. *J Am Acad Dermatol.* 2003;48(6 Suppl):S143-S148.
6. Alexis AF, Sergay AB, Taylor SC. Common dermatologic disorders in skin of color: a comparative practice survey. *Cutis.* 2007;80(5):387-394.
7. Bilgili SG, Akdeniz N, Karadag AS, Akbayram S, Calka O, Ozkol HU. Mucocutaneous disorders in children with down syndrome: case-controlled study. *Genet Couns.* 2011;22(4):385-392.
8. Barba A, Piubello W, Vantini I, et al. Skin lesions in chronic alcoholic pancreatitis. *Dermatologica.* 1982;164(5):322-326.
9. Mastrolonardo M, Diaferio A, Logroscino G. Seborrheic dermatitis, increased sebum excretion, and Parkinson's disease: a survey of (im)possible links. *Med Hypotheses.* 2003;60(6):907-911.
10. Tajima M, Sugita T, Nishikawa A, Tsuboi R. Molecular analysis of Malassezia microflora in seborrheic dermatitis patients: comparison with other diseases and healthy subjects. *J Invest Dermatol.* 2008;128(2):345-351.
11. Zani MB, Soares RC, Arruda AC, de Arruda LH, Paulino LC. Ketoconazole does not decrease fungal amount in patients with seborrhoeic dermatitis. *Br J Dermatol.* 2016;175(2):417-421.
12. Akbulut TO, Suslu H, Atci T. Is the frequency of seborrheic dermatitis related to climate parameters? *Sisli Etfal Hastan Tip Bul.* 2022;56(1):91-95.
13. Li J, Feng Y, Liu C, et al. Presence of malassezia hyphae is correlated with pathogenesis of seborrheic dermatitis. *Microbiol Spectr.* 2022;10(1):e0116921.
14. Okada K, Endo Y, Fujisawa A, Tanioka M, Kabashima K, Miyachi Y. Refractory seborrheic dermatitis of the head in a patient with malignant lymphoma. *Case Rep Dermatol.* 2014;6(3):279-282.

15. U.S. statistics. https://www.hiv.gov/hiv-basics/overview/data-and-trends/statistics. Accessed June 11, 2022.
16. Pappas A, Fantasia J, Chen T. Age and ethnic variations in sebaceous lipids. *Dermatoendocrinol.* 2013;5(2):319-324.
17. Moodley N, Hoosen K, Dlova NC. Quality of life in patients with seborrhoeic dermatitis in KwaZulu-Natal, South Africa. *S Afr Med J.* 2016;106:428-428.
18. McMichael AJ. Ethnic hair update: past and present. *J Am Acad Dermatol.* 2003;48(6 Suppl):S127-S133.
19. Park JH, Park YJ, Kim SK, et al. Histopathological differential diagnosis of psoriasis and seborrheic dermatitis of the scalp. *Ann Dermatol.* 2016;28(4):427-432.
20. Coogan PF, Rosenberg L, Palmer JR, Cozier YC, Lenzy YM, Bertrand KA. Hair product use and breast cancer incidence in the Black Women's Health Study. *Carcinogenesis.* 2021;42(7):924-930.
21. Rucker Wright D, Gathers R, Kapke A, Johnson D, Joseph CL. Hair care practices and their association with scalp and hair disorders in African American girls. *J Am Acad Dermatol.* 2011;64(2):253-262.
22. Seborrheic dermatitis of the scalp in populations practicing less frequent hair washing: Ketoconazole 2% foam versus ketoconazole 2% shampoo. Three-year data. *J Am Acad Dermatol.* 2014;70(5):AB54.
23. Borda LJ, Perper M, Keri JE. Treatment of seborrheic dermatitis: a comprehensive review. *J Dermatolog Treat.* 2019;30(2):158-169.
24. Kim TW, Mun JH, Jwa SW, et al. Proactive treatment of adult facial seborrhoeic dermatitis with 0.1% tacrolimus ointment: randomized, double-blind, vehicle-controlled, multi-centre trial. *Acta Derm Venereol.* 2013;93(5):557-561.
25. High WA, Pandya AG. Pilot trial of 1% pimecrolimus cream in the treatment of seborrheic dermatitis in African American adults with associated hypopigmentation. *J Am Acad Dermatol.* 2006;54(6):1083-1088.
26. Cunha PR. Pimecrolimus cream 1% is effective in seborrhoeic dermatitis refractory to treatment with topical corticosteroids. *Acta Derm Venereol.* 2006;86(1):69-70.
27. Schmidt-Rose T, Braren S, Fölster H, et al. Efficacy of a piroctone olamine/climbazol shampoo in comparison with a zinc pyrithione shampoo in subjects with moderate to severe dandruff. *Int J Cosmet Sci.* 2011;33(3):276-282.
28. Bhatia N. Treating seborrheic dermatitis: review of mechanisms and therapeutic options. *J Drugs Dermatol.* 2013;12(7):796-798.
29. Ghodsi SZ, Abbas Z, Abedeni R. Efficacy of oral itraconazole in the treatment and relapse prevention of moderate to severe seborrheic dermatitis: a randomized, placebo-controlled trial. *Am J Clin Dermatol.* 2015;16(5):431-437.
30. de Souza Leão Kamamoto C, Sanudo A, Hassun KM, Bagatin E. Low-dose oral isotretinoin for moderate to severe seborrhea and seborrheic dermatitis: a randomized comparative trial. *Int J Dermatol.* 2017;56(1):80-85.

CHAPTER 45

Pseudofolliculitis Barbae

Annelise Colvin
Hope Mitchell

KEY POINTS

- Pseudofolliculitis barbae (PFB) is a common inflammatory disorder of follicular and perifollicular skin characterized by papules, pustules, and postinflammatory hyperpigmentation.
- It occurs most frequently in men of African descent but can occur in any curly-haired population.
- It is characterized by an inflammatory reaction resulting from close shaving of hair and subsequent follicular wall penetration.
- Diagnosis is clinical.
- The therapeutic objectives for PFB include managing ongoing inflammation and its complications and preventing the development of new lesions.
- Cessation of shaving and/or removal of the involved hair follicles prevents the development of PFB.
- Other treatment options include shaving modification, topical medications, and laser therapy.

BACKGROUND

Pseudofolliculitis Barbae (PFB), colloquially known as "ingrown hairs" and "razor-" or "shaving-bumps," is a chronic, noninfectious inflammatory disorder caused by close shaving of curly hair shafts that grow back into the follicular wall or surrounding skin. While Fox first characterized the appearance of a shaving-induced rash in 1908,[1] the term pseudofolliculitis barbae was coined by Strauss and Kligman in 1956.[2] Most commonly affecting the beard area, it is characterized by an immune-mediated granulomatous foreign body reaction resulting in the development of pruritic papules and pustules that can lead to scarring and postinflammatory hyperpigmentation [**Figures 45-1** and **45-2**].

EPIDEMIOLOGY

The onset of PFB is multifactorial: it is mediated by the combination of the genetically determined curvature of hair follicles combined with an individual's shaving practices. As such, it is most common in men of African descent who shave, affecting approximately 45% to 83% of this population.[3] It is particularly common in men with careers in the military, law enforcement, or other occupations that have stringent and frequent grooming requirements.[4] However, PFB may develop in any population or gender with curly hair and in any areas of frequent hair removal, including the face, chest, axilla, and inguinal regions [**Figures 45-3** to **45-5**]. The age of onset is typically post-pubertal, which coincides with the growth of secondary sexual hair on the face, chest, axilla, and pubic area.[5]

PATHOGENESIS

The onset of PFB is triggered by the transepidermal penetration of sharp-tipped terminal hair shafts following a close shave.[6] PFB is classified as either transfollicular or extrafollicular based on the penetration

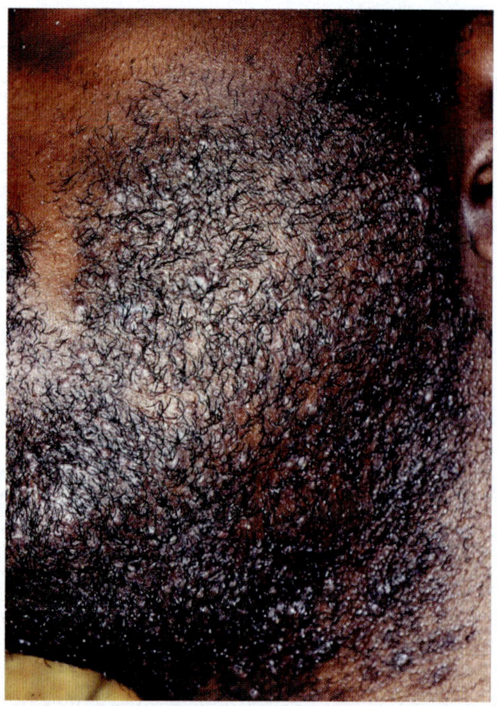

FIGURE 45-1. Profile of a darkly pigmented man with severe/chronic pseudofolliculitis barbae; present are numerous papulopustules, grooving, and postinflammatory hyperpigmentation of the left cheek. (Used with permission from Yvonne Knight, MD, Richmond, VA.)

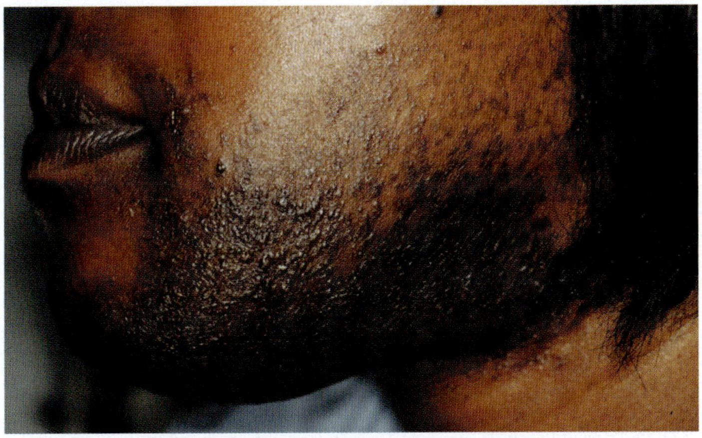

FIGURE 45-2. Moderate pseudofolliculitis barbae of the left cheek in a darkly pigmented woman with postinflammatory hyperpigmentation.

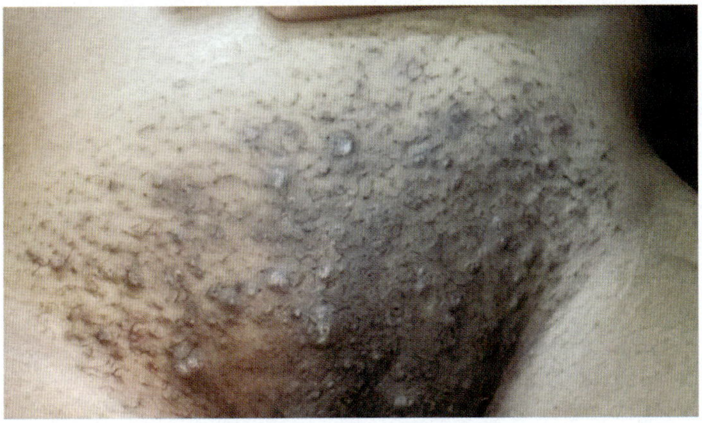

FIGURE 45-3. A female patient with pseudofolliculitis barbae, postinflammatory hyperpigmentation, and scarring due to shaving her suprapubic area.

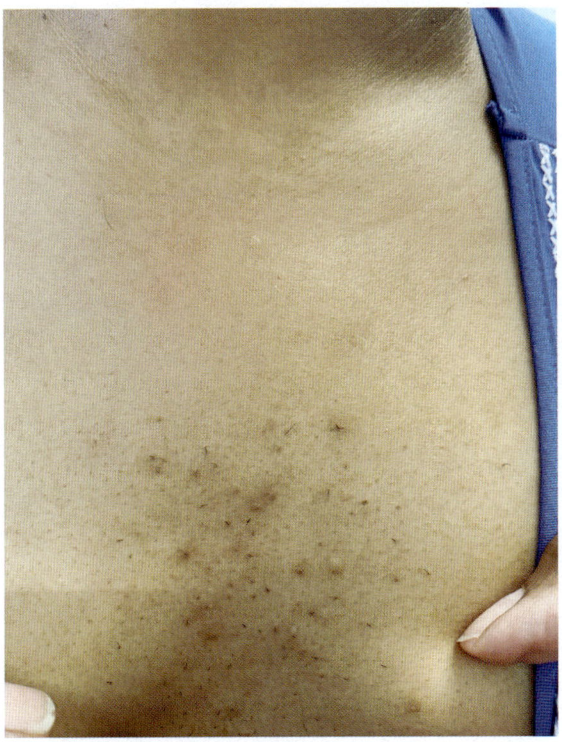

FIGURE 45-4. A female patient with skin of color showing pseudofolliculitis barbae with postinflammatory hyperpigmentation of the chest.

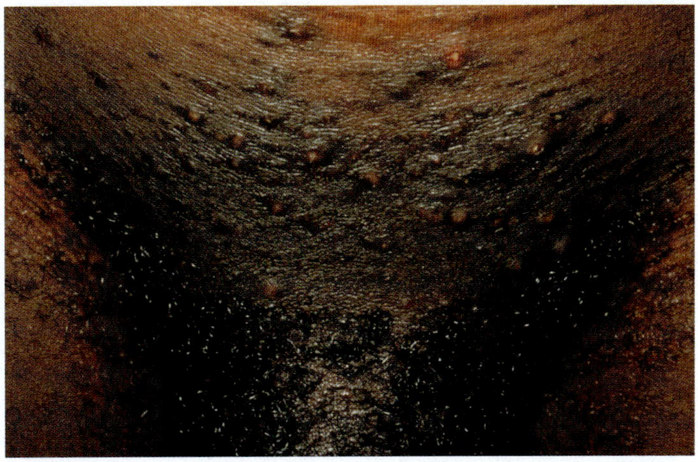

FIGURE 45-5. A darkly pigmented man with pseudofolliculitis secondary to shaving his suprapubic area.

of the hair either through the follicular wall or through the surrounding skin, respectively. The various factors that trigger PFB are discussed in the following sections.

TRANSFOLLICULAR PENETRATION

Transfollicular PFB is defined as penetration by the distal end of sharp-ended hair into the interfollicular skin before exiting the follicular orifice. It is usually caused by hair removal methods that place tension on the hair follicle including skin stretching and the use of multiple-edged razors, whereby one blade pulls the hair out of the follicle while another cuts it. Once the tension is released, the sharp-tipped end of the hair retracts into the follicle below the skin and grows through the follicular wall causing a foreign body reaction. Epilatory practices such as waxing or tweezing the hair can also result in transfollicular PFB by weakening the hair shaft, making it more prone to breakage that results in sharp-tipped hairs.

EXTRAFOLLICULAR PENETRATION

Extrafollicular PFB is defined as the penetration of the epidermis by the distal end of sharp-ended hair after exiting the follicular orifice and reentering the skin 1 to 2 mm away from its emergence. It most commonly affects areas where hair grows at an oblique angle to the skin, such as the anterior neck, whereby the sharp, beveled tips of hair are more easily able to curve back toward the skin and penetrate the epidermis.

In both transfollicular and extrafollicular PFB, the penetration of the epidermis by the hair shaft causes an invagination that simulates a follicle, thus producing the eponymous "pseudofollicle" accompanied by inflammation and microabscesses. This pseudofollicle represents a granulomatous foreign body reaction characterized by the formation of pruritic perifollicular and follicular papules and pustules. Often, the hair continues to grow into the dermis, causing a more severe inflammatory reaction as the epidermis attempts to encapsulate the hair.[7] Once the hair reaches a length of about 10 mm, it is released by spring action from the inflammatory papule, which then tends to resolve without intervention.[6]

HAIR STRUCTURE

The phenotype of tightly curled hair in Black individuals predisposes them to PFB as the hair has a greater tendency to curve back into the skin once cut. In fact, individuals with curly hair are more than 50 times more likely to develop PFB.[8] Further, compared to Caucasian and Asian hair follicles that exhibit a rounder cross-sectional shape, African hair is observed to be elliptic, which causes it to grow at an oblique angle. During shaving, this oblique direction of growth causes the hairs to be cut at an angle, resulting in sharp, pointed hairs that can more easily pierce the skin.[9,10]

GENETICS

A single-nucleotide polymorphism (SNP) in the companion layer-specific keratin K6hf of the hair follicle was found to represent a genetic risk factor for PFB. This SNP, which produces a disruptive Ala12Thr substation in the 1A α-helical segment of K6hf, makes carriers six times more likely to develop PFB. The hair shaft comprised several cellular layers including the outer root sheath (ORS), a thin layer of keratin called the companion layer, and the inner root sheath (IRS). The companion layer and IRS form a functional tissue unit around the hair shaft that serves to guide and stabilize the hair as it grows. The mutation in K6hf is hypothesized to structurally weaken the keratin of the companion layer, thus compromising the integrity of the functional tissue unit and inhibiting its ability to effectively guide the hair to the skin surface. When combined with skin that is mechanically traumatized by shaving, the destabilized, pointed hairs are more likely to become trapped in the hair channel, triggering the development of PFB.[8]

ADDITIONAL RISK FACTORS

Cyclosporin therapy has been reported to cause hyperplastic PFB in renal transplant recipients, hypothesized to be due to a combination of hypertrichosis causing increased shaving, excess granulation tissue, and altered immunity.[11,12] It has also been associated with "Fiddler's neck," a phenomenon of localized lichenification caused by the pressure of a violin against an individual's neck.[13]

CLINICAL FEATURES

The diagnosis of PFB is made clinically, determined by the appearance and location of lesions. PFB presents 1 to 2 days after shaving with erythematous, skin-colored or hyperpigmented papules in a follicular distribution, most commonly accompanied by symptoms of pain and pruritis. Lesions range from 2 to 5 mm in diameter, although they may grow larger, especially when associated with secondary superinfection caused by traumatic nicks in the skin from shaving and excoriations. The most common culprit is *Staphylococcus epidermidis*, which colonizes the skin, but pathogenic microorganisms like *Staphylococcus aureus* have also been identified on culture.[14] The beard and anterior neck area are most commonly affected, hence the term "barbae," due to the frequency of shaving in this region as well as the oblique growth direction and density of the hair follicles in the area. The upper lip region is often spared, likely owing to the fact the hair is less coiled, smaller in diameter, and less likely to grow at an oblique angle [**Figure 45-6**]. In one survey of women with PFB, 41.5% reported a personal or family history of hypertrichosis or hirsutism.[6] Women with PFB are more likely to present with lesions on the chin because hirsute women have a greater density of hair there but may also present with lesions on the anterior neck, chest, pubic area, and cheeks[5] [**Figures 45-7** and **45-8**]. In addition to differences in lesion location, women seek treatment for PFB earlier than men, who seek treatment on average 13 years after onset, and they are more likely to report their condition as severe at presentation (56.1% of women as compared to 30.8% of men).[6] These differences may impact clinical management considerations and psychosocial consequences when treating PFB in men versus women.

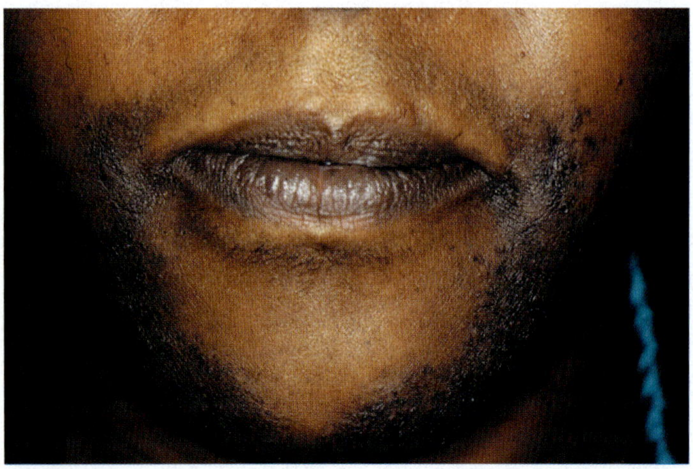

FIGURE 45-6. A female patient showing pseudofolliculitis barbae with postinflammatory hyperpigmentation of the chin and medial cheeks, sparing the upper lip area.

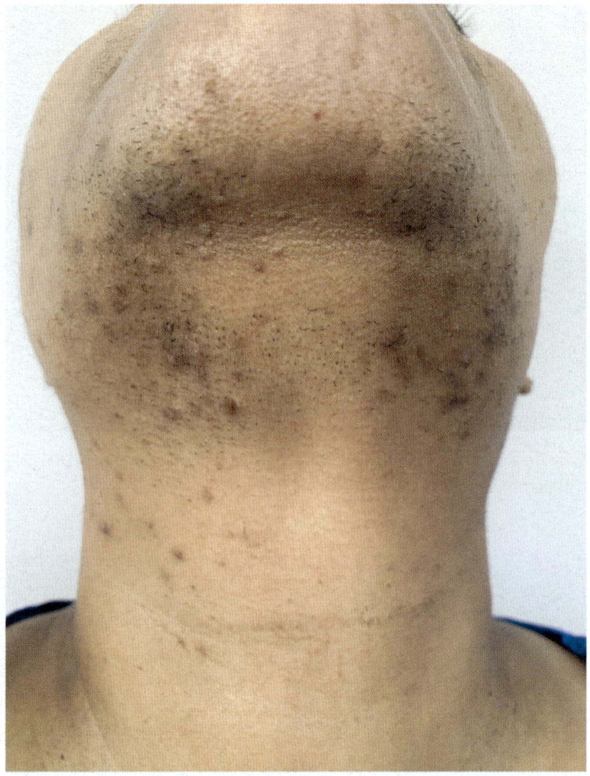

FIGURE 45-7. A female patient with hirsutism showing pseudofolliculitis barbae and postinflammatory hyperpigmentation of the chin and anterior neck.

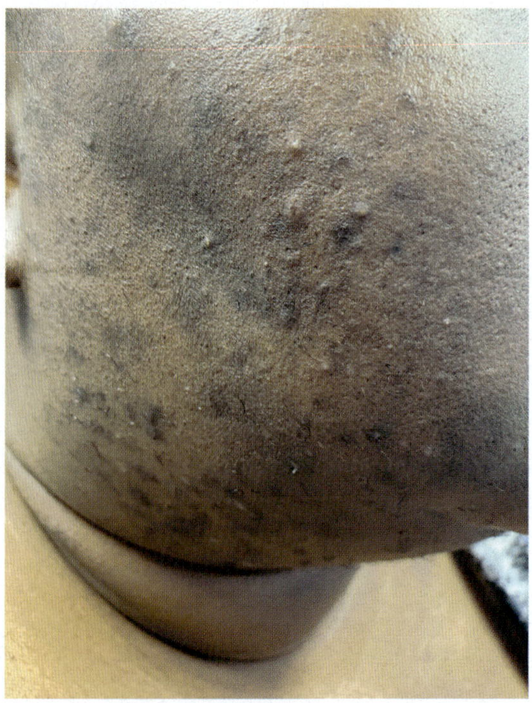

FIGURE 45-8. Profile of a darkly pigmented woman with numerous papulopustules and postinflammatory hyperpigmentation of the right cheek.

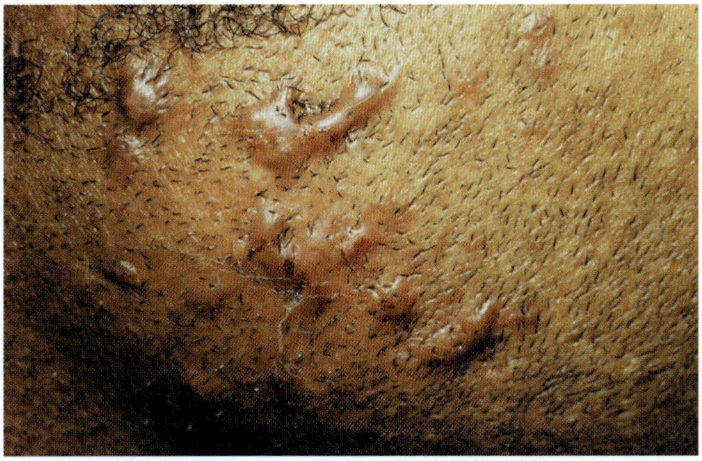

FIGURE 45-9. Small keloids secondary to pseudofolliculitis barbae in a man with skin of color.

COMPLICATIONS

Potential sequelae of PFB include hyperpigmentation, hypertrophic scarring, and rarely, keloid formation [**Figure 45-9**]. Additionally, trapped hairs can grow in parallel causing fine linear depressed scars or grooves in the skin, hindering hair removal with standard shaving techniques[15] [**Figure 45-10**]. Postinflammatory hyperpigmentation is the most common complication of PFB, affecting approximately 90% of patients.[6] Hypopigmented chronic lesions have also been identified in a smaller subset of individuals.[7] These secondary complications are a source of significant morbidity, affecting an individual's self-esteem and quality of life.

DERMOSCOPY

While the diagnosis of PFB is clinical, dermoscopy may be useful adjuvantly in both diagnosis and education of the patient. Dermoscopic findings include U-shaped ingrown hairs beneath a papular lesion, perifollicular hyperkeratosis in older lesions, white areas with scaling, underlying linear bluish pigmentation corresponding to the buried hair shaft, and adjacent erythematous lines indicating aberrant vessels secondary to the inflammatory reaction.[16] Showing patients' dermoscopic images of the PFB lesions has been reported to improve their understanding of its etiology and the principles of treatment, thereby improving patient compliance.[17]

HISTOPATHOLOGY

Histopathologically, PFB is characterized by a foreign body inflammatory reaction to a penetrant, trapped hair. Epidermal penetration typically shows a curled hair invaginating the stratum corneum, accompanied by an inflammatory infiltrate of phagocytic mononuclear leukocytes and polymorphonuclear leukocytes leading to microabscesses. Dermal penetration stimulates a more severe inflammatory response, leading to larger papules and occasionally giant cells and fibrosis. Cultures of PFB lesions are typically sterile or contain only normal skin flora, except for micrococci, but may be positive for pathogenic microorganisms such as *S. aureus* if lesions become secondarily infected.[15]

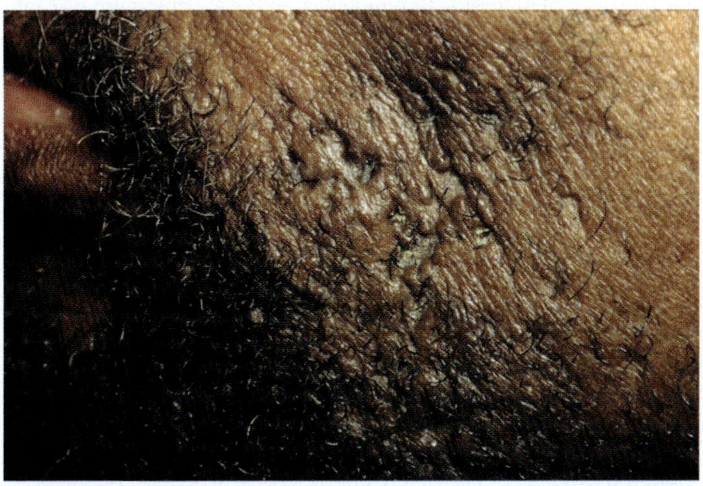

FIGURE 45-10. A darkly pigmented man with hypertrophic scarring and grooving of the left cheek secondary to chronic pseudofolliculitis.

TABLE 45-1 Clinical differential diagnosis of pseudofolliculitis barbae

Diagnosis	Distinguishing clinical features
Acne vulgaris	Presence of comedones; may localize to non-hair-bearing areas
Bacterial folliculitis	Bacterial culture always positive; absence of ingrown hair on dermoscopy
Eosinophilic folliculitis	Upper trunk involvement; immunocompromised (HIV+) host
Impetigo	Honey-colored erosions; positive bacterial culture
Tinea barbae	Confluent lesions and often unilateral; annular, scaly plaques with central clearing and peripheral activity; +KOH microscopy
Traumatic folliculitis (razor burns)	Regresses quickly (1-2 days after shaving)
Sarcoidosis	Multisystem involvement; noncaseating granuloma on biopsy

DIFFERENTIAL DIAGNOSIS

The differential diagnosis for PFB includes conditions causing facial papules [**Table 45-1**]. The absence of ingrown hairs on dermoscopic examination increases the likelihood of alternative diagnoses listed in the above differential.[18]

MANAGEMENT

ACUTE MANAGEMENT

The therapeutic objectives for PFB include managing ongoing inflammation while preventing the development of new lesions. In the acute pustular phase, which is often painful and pruritic, medical intervention is required. The inflammatory reaction can be worsened by microorganisms that enter via defects in the skin barrier. Twice-daily benzoyl peroxide 5%/Clindamycin 1% gel effectively reduces papules by decreasing contamination of normal skin flora and preventing development of secondary infection.[19] If secondary infection is suspected, bacterial cultures of pustules should first be obtained. Systemic antibiotics such as low dose tetracyclines, macrolides, or penicillins may then be initiated. For localized lesions, topical antibiotics such as clindamycin or mupirocin may also be used.[20] For patients with severe inflammation, a limited, 2-week course of low-potency topical corticosteroids such as hydrocortisone valerate or desonide is recommended, as a long-term use is associated with atrophy and hypopigmentation.[21]

TOPICAL THERAPIES

In addition to antibiotics and low-dose corticosteroids, other topical agents include eflornithine hydrochloride cream, chemical peels, skin-lightening agents, and keratolytics such as retinoids, glycolic acid, and salicylic acid [**Table 45-2**].

Topical eflornithine hydrochloride cream has been used in the treatment of PFB in both men and women with Fitzpatrick Skin Types IV and V. It slows the rate of hair growth by inhibiting ornithine decarboxylase, an enzyme required for hair cell division. It has been shown to be most effective in enhancing the rate and degree of hair reduction when combined with long-pulsed Nd-YAG laser.[22,23] Drawbacks include the time required to see improvement, often 2 to 3 months, and the impermanence of the treatment. If treatment is discontinued, PFB can worsen as viable hair follicles become active again. No studies have evaluated the feasibility of long-term treatment following the initial treatment period of 16 weeks.

Keratolytics are thought to improve PFB by reducing the perifollicular hyperkeratosis caused by repeated trauma to the skin. In a study of

TABLE 45-2 Treatment of pseudofolliculitis barbae

Lifestyle			
	Shaving modification	Best used in mild cases	
	Discontinue shaving	Mild cases: 1 month Moderate cases: 2-3 months Severe cases: 3-6 months[9]	PFB may worsen within the first week
	Compresses: warm water, warm saline, Burow's solution	10-15 min 3 times daily	Soothes lesions, reduce drainage, and soften epidermis to allow for release of ingrown hairs
Pharmacologic			
Topical treatment	Low- to mid-potency topical steroids	Daily application for 2 weeks Or one to three times per week	
	Topical antibiotics	Twice daily benzoyl peroxide 5%/ clindamycin 1% gel	Significant reduction in combined papule and pustule counts compared to vehicle[10]
	Topical retinoids	Apply nightly	Significant improvement in clinical lesions and postinflammatory hyperpigmentation Relapse after 2 weeks[11]
	Eflornithine hydrochloride cream	Apply twice daily, rinse off 4 h after application	Decreases the number of hairs and inflammatory papules Eflornithine + laser is more effective than either alone[12,13]
Oral treatment	Systemic antibiotics	Based on bacterial cultures	Can be used if PFB is secondarily infected
	Oral steroids	Prednisone 45-60 mg daily for 7-10 days	May be effective in treatment of recalcitrant disease
Intralesional treatment	Intralesional corticosteroids		
Procedural			
Laser hair removal	Diode laser (800-810 nm) Long-pulse Nd:YAG (1064 mm)	3-7 treatments spaced 4-6 weeks apart	Significant improvement in PFB[14-18] Nd:YAG has the safest profile[19] Lower fluence treatment significantly reduces PFB while mitigating pain, pigmentation alteration, crusting, and blistering[20]
Other procedures	Electrolysis Chemical peels Photodynamic therapy	Glycolic acid[21] Salicylic acid ALA + PDT[22]	

Source: Reproduced with permission from Alexis AF, Kaufman BP. Adnexal Disorders. In: Neelam A. Vashi, Howard I. Maibach, Dermatoanthropology of Ethnic Skin and Hair. Berlin: *Springer*; 2017:359-387.

38 patients with PFB, daily application of 0.05% tretinoin solution was shown to reduce papules in nearly 80% of study patients but worked best in those with milder cases of PFB. Those with chronic, severe disease consisting of large, indolent papules and scarring did not respond well to tretinoin treatment.[24] Glycolic acid, in combination with daily shaving, was also shown to reduce PFB lesions by 60%.[25] In addition to functioning like tretinoin to reduce hyperkeratotic cells, glycolic acid also reduces the curvature of the hair by reducing sulfhydryl bonds in the hair shaft, causing the hair to grow straighter and decreasing the likelihood of trans- and extra-follicular penetration.

Chemical peels containing glycolic or salicylic acid work via the same mechanism, while salicylic acid has the added benefit of reducing inflammation.[26] Cryotherapy in the form of a liquid nitrogen cryospray administered with a 10- to 15-second thaw time may also be used as a light peel. Although it is often discouraged for skin types IV to VI due to the risk of hypopigmentation,[7] chemical peels, as well as azelaic acid and hydroquinone, also work to reduce the postinflammatory hyperpigmentation associated with PFB.[5] Treatment with chemical peels is limited by associated cost as well as the risk of pigmentary dyschromias in patients with darker skin.[5] While effective, no topical therapy can cure PFB and once the treatment is discontinued, papules and erythema recur, especially if prior shaving practices are resumed.

HAIR REMOVAL METHODS

Topical and oral therapies help reduce inflammation, but they do not address the underlying pathophysiology of PFB. Only cessation of shaving or the permanent removal of hair follicles is curative.[21] Thus, discontinuation of shaving for at least a month is recommended to patients as a first-line treatment to prevent new lesions before the sequelae of existing lesions can be addressed. Current ingrown hairs will likely be released within 2 to 6 weeks once they reach 10 mm.[6] However, for many patients, cessation is not a feasible alternative, and they must be counseled that other treatments may control but not cure their PFB. When shaving is necessary or desired, several adjustments to the grooming regimen may help decrease the severity of the condition [**Table 45-3**].

Shaving Warm water, saline, or Burow solution compresses may be applied for 10 to 15 minutes a day to soothe lesions, remove the crust, and soften the epidermis to allow for easier release of ingrown hairs. Electric clippers can be used to remove as much hair as possible without causing irritation. It is recommended to leave a minimum of 1 mm of hair to reduce the chance of trans- and extra-follicular penetration. Then, before shaving, the affected area should be washed with a gentle facial cleanser and a washcloth, soft toothbrush, or polyester sponge may be used to gently free ingrown hairs. A warm compress may also be applied to hydrate the skin and the hair shaft. This works to soften the hairs, thereby making them easier to cut by decreasing the shaving force required and limiting trauma to the epidermis. Shaving cream should also be applied, taking care to avoid letting the lather dry. This helps to moisturize the hair while also providing a protect layer that reduces friction to limit trauma to the epidermis. While previous data suggest single-blade razors are less likely to cause PFB than multi-blade razors, it is most important, regardless of blade number, that the razor is clean and sharp to minimize trauma to the hair shaft. Specific foil-guarded razors made especially for PFB have been reported to significantly decrease PFB lesions.[27] Shaved areas should only be shaved 1 to 2 times with minimal pressure and skin should not be pulled taut to avoid transfollicular penetration and nicks that may cause traumatic or bacterial folliculitis. After shaving, a cool compress may be applied for

TABLE 45-3 Shaving modifications for treatment of pseudofolliculitis barbae

Pre-shave regimen		
	Wash face with water and mild soap-free cleanser	• Washing face softens hairs making them easier to cut • Loosens and reduces the number of trapped and ingrown beard hairs[1]
	Gently rub face in circular motion with a washcloth, cleansing pad, scrub, or brush	• Scrub releases trapped beard hairs[2]
	Apply shaving cream	• Shaving cream creates an antifriction layer and smoother shave[1]
Hair removal practices		
Shaving method	Electric razor	Electric razors that leave 0.5-1 mm of hair are very successful at decreasing PFB[3]
	Single-blade razor versus Multiblade razor	• Single-blade razors are generally recommended; however, recent studies demonstrate that multiblade razors may not exacerbate PFB[4]
	Razors with guards, ie, foil-guarded manual razor	• Guards prevent hair from being cut too close, thereby reducing transfollicular penetration[5,6]
	Chemical depilatories (ie, barium sulfide powder or calcium thioglycolate cream)	• Depilatories are associated with decreased severity of PFB but greater irritant contact dermatitis[7]
Frequency of shaving	Daily versus two to three times per week	• There is no difference in papule or pustule count • Reduced frequency of shaving is associated with a significant reduction in ingrown hairs • Daily shaving is associated with patient perceived better response to treatment and decreased itching[8]
Blade characteristics	Sharp blade	• Use of a sharp blade decreases force of shaving and minimizes trauma to the hair follicle
Direction of shaving	With or against hair growth	• Shaving in the direction of hair growth is generally recommended; however, one study found that men who shaved against the grain had lower papule counts[8]
Postshaving	Aftershave preparation	• Rehydrates and soothes the skin
	Release ingrown hairs (with toothpick or sterile needle)	• Releasing ingrown hairs helps prevent PFB

Source: Reproduced with permission from Alexis AF, Kaufman BP. Adnexal Disorders. In: Neelam A. Vashi, Howard I. Maibach, Dermatoanthropology of Ethnic Skin and Hair. Berlin: *Springer;* 2017:359-387.

5 to 10 minutes followed by the least irritating aftershave preparation. For burning or pruritis, topical hydrocortisone may be applied.

Chemical Depilatories For those desiring hair removal but find shaving too irritating, chemical depilatories such as barium sulfide and calcium thioglycolate are available. They lyse the disulfide bonds in the hair shaft, thereby softening the hair, resulting in a blunt tip less able to penetrate the skin. It is important to patch-test these preparations on a hair-bearing area of the arm before using them on one's face as they can cause irritant and contact dermatitis. These depilatories do not affect existing embedded hair tips. As such, the condition will likely worsen before it improves, which takes several weeks.

Laser Therapy Various laser systems have been successfully used for hair removal to treat PFB, including the neodymium:yttrium aluminum garnet (Nd:YAG 1064 nm) laser, diode 800 to 810 nm, and pulsed alexandrite 755 nm.[28-31] The principal obstacle with laser-mediated hair removal in darker skin types with PFB is not efficacy but rather safety. Most laser treatments target endogenous melanin within the hair follicle and irradiate it with laser light, sufficiently damaging the follicle to achieve severe inhibition or elimination of hair growth. In individuals with significant epidermal melanocytes, laser therapy may inadvertently damage those nonfollicle structures, resulting in permanent dyspigmentation and epidermal damage. This is compounded by the fact that repeated treatments are necessary to maximize hair-growth elimination, usually requiring 3 to 7 sessions for optimal results.[28] These side effects can be mitigated by modifying several light source parameters including spot size, wavelength, pulse width, and epidermal cooling.[32] In any laser system, lower fluences will minimize the risk of thermal transfer between hair follicles, especially in regions like the beard area with increased hair density.[33] Additionally, the amount of absorption of melanin decreases exponentially as wavelengths increase, allowing greater penetration of the longer wavelength to selectively irradiate lower dermal regions of the follicle and target the site of cell proliferation and early hair-shaft differentiation.[33] For this reason, in patients with darker skin, especially Fitzpatrick Skin Types V to VI, the Nd:YAG 1064 nm laser is recommended as its longer wavelength allows for greater epidermal penetration at a lower fluence, giving it the best safety profile while maintaining efficacy.[30] Overall, laser treatment is a safe and effective option for reducing papule formation in patients with PFB, although side effects such as pain, dyspigmentation, scabbing, and scarring may still occur.[30] However, it is important to note that laser treatment is not a permanent solution and would likely require treatment every few months to ensure continued PFB remission.

OTHER TREATMENTS

Additional modalities for hair removal include wax epilation, threading, and mechanical removal via tweezers as well as electrolysis and surgical depilation. Both waxing and tweezing are traumatic hair removal methods that may actually exacerbate transfollicular PFB and as such are not recommended[6]. Although electrolysis and surgical depilation damage the hair follicle, the procedures are expensive and painful and have not proven to be effective in treating PFB. In fact, the straight electrolysis needle may miss the hair bulb in some curved hair follicles, thereby promoting transfollicular penetration and worsening of PFB. There is also a risk of postinflammatory hyperpigmentation at sites of needle entry and keloid formation in predisposed individuals following surgical depilation.[26]

There has been one reported case of PFB in a Caucasian man successfully treated with photodynamic therapy (PDT) in combination with methyl aminolevulinate (MAL) cream as a sensitizer.[34] While MAL-PDT has not been evaluated as a treatment for PFB in darker skin types, it has successfully treated inflammatory acne vulgaris lesions and postinflammatory hyperpigmentation in a patient with type V skin.[35] Therefore, while further investigation is needed, MAL-PDT represents a potential additional adjunctive therapy for PFB.

PSEUDOFOLLICULITIS IN THE MILITARY

The incidence of PFB rose sharply in the 1960s and 1970s when more African Americans entered into the U.S. armed forces and were subjected to the military's "clean-shaven policy." In fact, during the Vietnam War, approximately 6% of dermatology consults were for PFB.[36] Since then, grooming regulations for the military have evolved, notably with the creation of exceptions for shaving called a "shaving waiver" or "shaving profile" in the Army and Air Force and a "shaving chit" in the Navy and Marine Corps.[4] Despite an improvement in grooming regulations, they still present significant obstacles to Black service members. Although available, shaving waivers must be repeatedly renewed, placing an undue burden on individuals with PFB and "systematically draining time away" from their duties compared to colleagues.[37] Moreover, waivers are accompanied by significant social stigma: current policies prohibit shaping one's beard when not shaving, resulting in unkempt facial hair. This may elicit negative perceptions from colleagues and supervisors regarding an individual's professionalism or desire to conform to military standards.[38] While this induces interpersonal conflict, it also results in significant career ramifications. For instance, shaving waivers were found to be associated with a longer time to promotion in the U.S. Air Force and 21.4% of Air Force members with waivers believe it negatively impacted their career.[38,39] This contributes to a fear of harassment or other ramifications, meaning service members are more likely to underreport the severity of PFB or refuse medical help, thereby exacerbating their condition.[40]

CONCLUSION

In conclusion, PFB is a chronic inflammatory disorder that predominantly affects African American patients and can significantly impair one's quality of life. The only permanent cure is cessation of shaving or depilation, but several options exist for managing PFB and a thoughtful use of a combination of therapies may provide the best opportunity for management, especially for individuals that continue shaving.

REFERENCES

1. Fox H. Observations on skin diseases in the Negro. *J Cutan Dis*. 1908;26:67-79.
2. Strauss JS, Kligman AM. Pseudofolliculitis of the beard. *AMA Arch Derm*. 1956;74:533-542.
3. Gray J, McMichael A. Pseudofolliculitis barbae: understanding the condition and the role of facial grooming. *Int J Cosmet Sci*. 2016;38:24-27.
4. Tshudy MT, Cho S. Pseudofolliculitis barbae in the US military, a review. *Mil Med*. 2021;186:e52-e57.
5. Ogunbiyi A. Pseudofolliculitis barbae; current treatment options. *Clin Cosmet Investig Dermatol*. 2019;12:241.
6. Perry PK, Cook-Bolden FE, Rahman Z, et al. Defining pseudofolliculitis barbae in 2001: a review of the literature and current trends. *J Am Acad Dermatol*. 2002;46:S113-S119.
7. Kelly AP. Pseudofolliculitis barbae and acne keloidalis nuchae. *Dermatol Clin*. 2003;21:645-653.
8. Winter H, Schissel D, Parry DA, et al. An unusual Ala12Thr polymorphism in the 1A α-helical segment of the companion layer-specific keratin K6hf: evidence for a risk factor in the etiology of the common hair disorder pseudofolliculitis barbae. *J invest Dermatol*. 2004;122:652-657.
9. Franbourg A, Hallegot P, Baltenneck F, et al. Current research on ethnic hair. *J Am Acad Dermatol*. 2003;48:S115-S119.
10. Raffi J, Suresh R, Agbai O. Clinical recognition and management of alopecia in women of color. *Int J Womens Dermatol*. 2019;5:314-319.
11. Lally A, Wojnarowska F. Hypertrophic pseudofolliculitis in white renal transplant recipients. *Clin Exp Dermatol*. 2007;32:268-271.
12. Lear J, Bourke J, Burns D. Hyperplastic pseudfolliculitis barbae associated with. *Br J Dermatol*. 1997;136:132-133.
13. Lachapelle J-M, Tennstedt D, Cromhaut P. Pseudofolliculitis of the beard and "fiddler's neck". *Contact Dermatitis*. 1984;10(4):247.
14. Laureano AC, Schwartz RA, Cohen PJ. Facial bacterial infections: folliculitis. *Clin Dermatol*. 2014;32:711-714.
15. Madu P, Kundu RV. Follicular and scarring disorders in skin of color: presentation and management. *Am J Clin Dermatol*. 2014;15:307-321.
16. Kaliyadan F, Kuruvilla J, Al Ojail HY, et al. Clinical and dermoscopic study of pseudofolliculitis of the beard area. *Int J Trichol*. 2016;8:40.
17. Chuh A, Zawar V. Epiluminescence dermatoscopy enhanced patient compliance and achieved treatment success in pseudofolliculitis barbae. *Aust J Dermatol*. 2006;47:60-62.
18. Zeichner JA. *Acneiform Eruptions in Dermatology*. Springer, Berlin/Heidelberg, Germany; 2014.
19. Cook-Bolden FE, Barba A, Halder R, et al. Twice-daily applications of benzoyl peroxide 5%/clindamycin 1% gel versus vehicle in the treatment of pseudofolliculitis barbae. *Cutis*. 2004;73:18-24.
20. Lamb A, Yañez GN. Pseudofolliculitis barbae. In: *Acneiform Eruptions in Dermatology*: Springer, New York, NY; 2014:289-294.
21. Alexis A, Heath CR, Halder RM. Folliculitis keloidalis nuchae and pseudofolliculitis barbae: are prevention and effective treatment within reach? *Dermatol Clin*. 2014;32:183-191.
22. Xia Y, Cho S, Howard RS, et al. Topical eflornithine hydrochloride improves the effectiveness of standard laser hair removal for treating pseudofolliculitis barbae: a randomized, double-blinded, placebo-controlled trial. *J Am Acad Dermatol*. 2012;67:694-699.
23. Shokeir H, Samy N, Taymour M. Pseudofolliculitis barbae treatment: efficacy of topical eflornithine, long-pulsed Nd-YAG laser versus their combination. *J Cosmet Dermatol*. 2021;20:3517-3525.
24. Kligman AM, Mills OH. Pseudofolliculitis of the beard and topically applied tretinoin. *Arch Dermatol*. 1973;107:551-552.
25. Perricone N. Treatment of pseudofolliculitis barbae with topical glycolic acid: a report of two studies. *Cutis*. 1993;52:232-235.
26. Bridgeman-Shah S. The medical and surgical therapy of pseudofolliculitis barbae. *Dermatol Ther*. 2004;17:158-163.
27. Alexander A. Evaluation of a foil-guarded shaver in the management of pseudofolliculitis barbae. *Cutis*. 1981;27:534-542.
28. Galadari I. Comparative evaluation of different hair removal lasers in skin types IV, V, and VI. *Int J Dermatol*. 2003;42:68-70.
29. Amer A, Elsayed A, Gharib K. Evaluation of efficacy and safety of chemical peeling and long-pulse Nd: YAG laser in treatment of pseudofolliculitis barbae. *Dermatol Ther*. 2021;34:e14859.
30. Alexis A. Lasers and light-based therapies in ethnic skin: treatment options and recommendations for F itzpatrick skin types V and VI. *Br J Dermatol*. 2013;169:91-97.
31. Leheta TM. Comparative evaluation of long pulse Alexandrite laser and intense pulsed light systems for pseudofolliculitis barbae treatment with one year of follow up. *Indian J Dermatol*. 2009;54:364.
32. Yamauchi PS, Lask GP, Kelly AP. Treatment of pseudofolliculitis barbae with the diode laser. *J Cutan Laser Ther*. 1999;1:109-111.
33. Shander D, Ahluwalia GS. Treatment of pseudofolliculitis barbae. In: *Cosmetics Applications of Laser & Light-Based Systems*: Elsevier, Norwich, NY; 2009:353-367.
34 Diernaes JEF, Bygum A. Successful treatment of recalcitrant folliculitis barbae and pseudofolliculitis barbae with photodynamic therapy. *Photodiagnosis Photodyn Ther*. 2013;10:651-653.
35 Shaundre Terrell B, Daniel Aires M, Eric S. Treatment of acne vulgaris using blue light photodynamic therapy in an African-American patient. *J Drugs Dermatol*. 2009;8:669-671.
36 Gelman AB, Norton SA, Valdes-Rodriguez R, et al. A review of skin conditions in modern warfare and peacekeeping operations. *Mil Med*. 2015;180:32-37.
37 Okonkwo E, Neal B, Harper HL. Pseudofolliculitis barbae in the military and the need for social awareness. *Mil Med*. 2021;186:143-144.
38 Banta J, Bowen C, Wong E, et al. Perceptions of shaving profiles and their potential impacts on career progression in the United States Air Force. *Mil Med*. 2021;186:187-189.
39 Ritchie S, Park J, Banta J, et al. Shaving waivers in the United States air force and their impact on promotions of black/African-American members. *Mil Med*. 2023;188(1-2):e242-e247.
40 Brauner G, Flandermeyer K. Pseudofolliculitis barbae. Medical consequences of interracial friction in the US Army. *Cutis*. 1979;23:61-66.

CHAPTER 46

Nail Disorders

Samantha Jo Albucker
Shari R. Lipner

KEY POINTS

- Longitudinal melanonychia is common in darker skin types, usually as a result of melanocyte activation (racial melanonychia).
- Longitudinal melanonychia that is broad, dark, heterogeneous, with blurred edges, or presents with bleeding or ulceration warrants a biopsy to rule out nail unit melanoma.
- Patients with onychomycosis present with xanthonychia, thickening, onycholysis, and subungual hyperkeratosis.

- Onychomycosis diagnosis requires confirmatory testing, including KOH with microscopy, fungal culture, histopathology, and, if available, polymerase chain reaction.
- Nail psoriasis presents with a combination of nail plate pitting, red spots in the lunula, nail plate crumbling, onycholysis, subungual hyperkeratosis, and splinter hemorrhages.
- Nail lichen planus presents with onychorrhexis, longitudinal melanonychia, onychoschizia, brittleness, and fragility.
- Nail lichen planus may be diagnosed with longitudinal excision and prompt treatment is important to prevent nail loss.
- Nail psoriasis and nail lichen planus may appear as the sole presentation without other dermatologic signs.
- Nail changes with alopecia areata include pitting, trachyonychia, red spots in the lunula, onycholysis, punctuate leukonychia, longitudinal ridging, crumbling, and Beau lines.
- While alopecia areata is prevalent in patients with darker skin types, studies specifically comparing the prevalence of alopecia areata nail changes across ethnoracial groups have not been performed.
- Brittle nail syndrome presents with nail fragility, splitting, and flaking, and may be the result of idiopathic, environmental, or systemic causes.
- Chronic paronychia is defined as nail fold inflammation and is often due to compromise of the protective barrier between the nail plate and nail fold.

Evaluation of nails is important for all patients. There are some nail disorders that are more common in patients with darker skin types, such as longitudinal melanonychia (LM) [**Table 46-1**]. This chapter highlights nail conditions in patients with skin of color (SOC), focusing on melanonychia, nail unit melanoma (NUM), nail psoriasis (NP), nail lichen planus (NLP), nail changes with alopecia areata (AA), brittle nail syndrome (BNS), chronic paronychia, and onychomycosis. We review the etiology, clinical presentation, diagnostic techniques, differentials, treatments of each of these disorders, and differences in patients with SOC when relevant.

PIGMENTARY ONYCHOPATHIES

MELANONYCHIA

Etiology Melanonychia is defined as brown-to-black nail plate discoloration.[1] After activation of nail matrix melanocytes, dendrites transfer melanosomes to differentiating matrix cells, which move distally along the nail plate and transform into nail plate onychocytes.[1] Melanonychia most commonly presents as LM, which is a brown-to-black band starting at the cuticle and extending the length of the nail plate.[1,2]

There are two pathophysiological mechanisms of melanonychia, melanocytic activation and melanocytic hyperplasia. Melanocytic activation, or functional melanonychia, is due to the stimulation of nail matrix melanocytes without an increase in the melanocyte number.[1] LM may be due to physiologic causes, trauma, systemic etiologies, and medications [**Table 46-2**].[1] Overall, 68.7% of melanonychia cases are classified as racial [**Figure 46-1**], 8.5% traumatic, 7.1% fungal, 4.3% mixed, 4.3% squamous cell carcinoma, 5.7% benign melanocytic hyperplasia, and 4.3% NUM.[3] Melanonychia is most prevalent in Fitzpatrick skin types IV, V, and VI.[4] Overall, 77% and nearly 100% of North American Blacks 20 and 50 years old, respectively, present with LM [**Figure 46-2**].[1,4] In the East Asian population, LM presents in 10% to 20% of the population.[4] A cross-sectional prevalence survey examining the prevalence of melanonychia in Chinese populations showed that LM was present in 0.6% of patients ages of 20 to 29 years, and increased to 1.7% in patients 50 years and older.[5] In a cross-sectional analysis that showed inaccuracy of Google reverse image searches for LM, Fitzpatrick Type I/II, III/IV, and V/VI made up 51.7%, 42.5%, and 5.7% of reference images,

TABLE 46-1 Abbreviations

LM	Longitudinal melanonychia
NUM	Nail unit melanoma
NP	Nail psoriasis
NLP	Nail lichen planus
AA	Alopecia areata
BNS	Brittle nail syndrome

TABLE 46-2 Causes of melanocytic activation

Physiologic causes
- Pregnancy
- Racial melanonychia

Local and regional causes
- Carpal tunnel syndrome
- Frictional trauma
- Nail biting
- Onychotillomania
- Occupational trauma

Dermatologic causes
- Amyloidosis
- Basal cell carcinoma
- Bowen disease
- Chronic paronychia
- Chronic radiation dermatitis
- Lichen planus
- Localized scleroderma
- Myxoid pseudocyst
- Onychomatricoma
- Onychomycosis
- Psoriasis
- Subungual fibrous histiocytoma
- Subungual linear keratosis
- Systemic lupus erythematosus
- Verruca vulgaris

Systemic causes
- Acquired immunodeficiency syndrome
- Alkaptonuria
- Endocrine disorders (acromegaly, Addison disease, Cushing syndrome, hyperthyroidism, Nelson syndrome)
- Graft-versus-host disease (lichen planus-type changes accompanied by longitudinal melanonychia)
- Hemosiderosis
- Hyperbilirubinemia
- Nutritional disorders
- Porphyria

Iatrogenic causes
- Drugs
- Electron beam therapy
- Phototherapy
- X-ray exposure

Syndromes
- Laugier-Hunziker syndrome
- Peutz-Jeghers syndrome
- Touraine syndrome

Source: Data from Andre J, Lateur N. Pigmented nail disorders. *Dermatol Clin.* 2006;24(3):329-339.

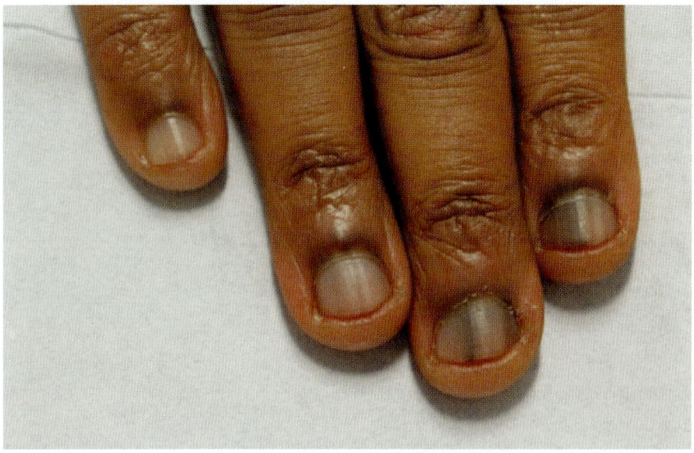

FIGURE 46-1. Racial LM. Patient with Fitzpatrick skin type VI presented with gray-brown longitudinal bands on multiple fingernails. (Reproduced with permission from Lee DK, Chang MJ, Desai AD, Lipner SR. Clinical and dermoscopic findings of benign longitudinal melanonychia due to melanocytic activation differ by skin type and predict likelihood of nail matrix biopsy. *J Am Acad Dermatol.* 2022;87(4):792-799.)

respectively.[6] Therefore, efforts are needed to increase public education on images of LM in diverse skin types.[2]

Melanocytic hyperplasia is defined as an increase in nail matrix melanocytes. It includes lentigo (benign melanocytic hyperplasia without nests), nevus (congenital or acquired melanocytic hyperplasia), and NUM. NUM comprises 0.18% to 2.8% of melanomas in Whites, and up to 23% and 25% of melanomas in Japanese and African Americans, respectively.[1]

Clinical Presentation Patients with LM due to melanocytic activation present with homogenous gray or brown-to-black bands. Bands may be present in one or several digits, and are often found on the first, second, and third fingers, and great toe. The number of bands and band width typically increases with age. NUM may present as an irregular brown-to-black longitudinal band [**Figure 46-3**]. Nail plate splitting, bleeding, or ulceration may be present. Hutchinson sign is defined as pigmentation extending to the nail fold or hyponychium, and typically signifies invasive melanoma.[1]

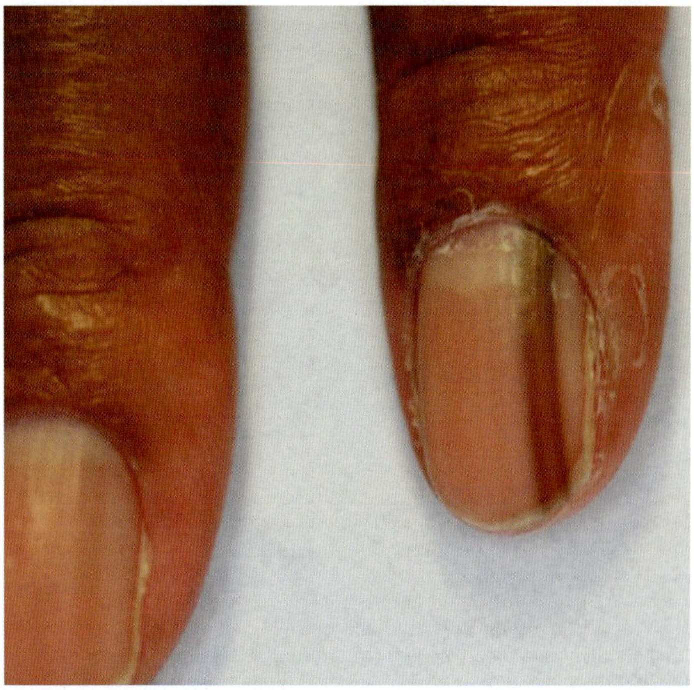

FIGURE 46-2. Benign LM of the right second fingernail in a patient with Fitzpatrick skin type VI, with a band width percentage of 18, prior to nail biopsy. Histopathology showed evidence of a melanotic macule. (Reproduced with permission from Lee DK, Chang MJ, Desai AD, Lipner SR. Clinical and dermoscopic findings of benign longitudinal melanonychia due to melanocytic activation differ by skin type and predict likelihood of nail matrix biopsy. *J Am Acad Dermatol.* 2022;87(4):792-799.)

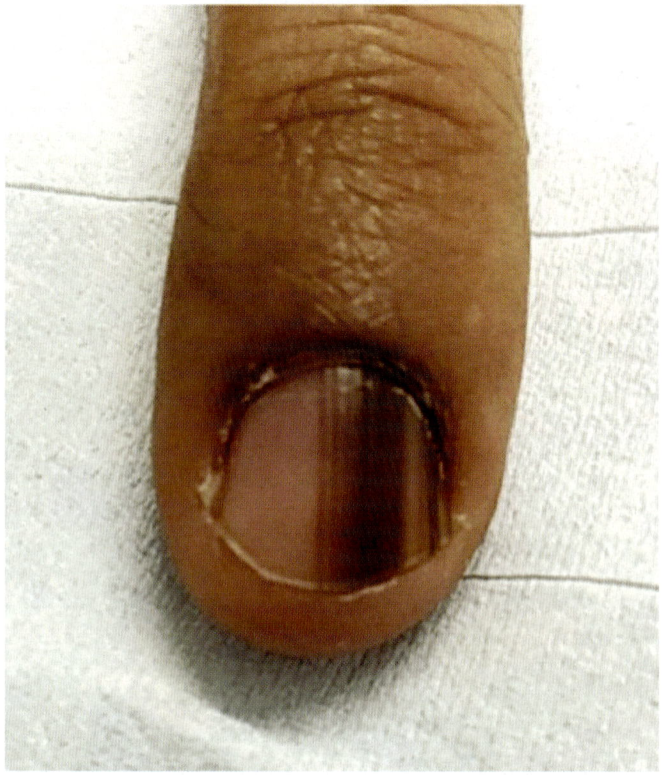

FIGURE 46-3. NUM (6 mm longitudinal brown band) in patient with Fitzpatrick skin type VI. (Reproduced with permission from Dayoung Ko,Clara Oromendia,Richard Scher,Shari R. Lipner. Retrospective single-center study evaluating clinical and dermoscopic features of longitudinal melanonychia, ABCDEF criteria, and risk of malignancy, 2019;80(5): P1272-1283, Figure 1C.)

Diagnosis and Differential Diagnoses Thorough history-taking is important, asking patients about pain, bleeding, duration of the band's appearance, and any changes in width or color. A nail clipping can rule out fungal melanonychia. Dermoscopy is useful to examine color, thickness, spacing, and parallelism.[1] On dermoscopy, melanocytic activation appears as gray background with thin gray parallel lines.[7] Nevi are identified by a brown background with regular lines, while NUM is characterized by a brown background with irregular lines in terms of color, spacing, and width.[1] However, NUM cannot be ruled out without a nail biopsy.

LM that is broad, dark, heterogeneous, with blurred edges, or presents along with nail dystrophy, bleeding, or ulceration warrants a nail unit biopsy. A retrospective cohort study of patients who had nail matrix biopsies for LM showed statistical significance of melanoma versus nonmelanoma with a dichotomizing band width percentage of 40% ($p = 0.047$).[8] Therefore, band width percentage may be a more accurate predicator of nail unit melanoma than band width.[8]

In another retrospective study, 248 cases of benign LM were identified, of which 86 were Fitzpatrick I and II and 162 were III and VI. Compared to I/II, III to VI presented with greater average band width percentage (28.84% vs 18.48%, $p = 0.0125$), lower skin brightness (L^* 45.61 vs L^* 64.90, $p = 0.001$), lower band brightness (L^* 40.40 vs L^* 48.98, $p = 0.001$), and underwent more nail biopsies (22.84% vs 11.62%, $p = 0.032$). Moreover, band darkening and thickening were more common in III and VI than in I/II (21.60% vs 8.13%, $p = 0.0071$).[2]

Differential diagnoses for LM include exogenous pigment, pseudomonas colonization, fungal melanonychia, hematoma, melanotic macule, lentigo, nevus, and NUM.[2]

Treatment NUM is treated with surgery. For melanoma in situ, total excision of the nail apparatus is recommended. For invasive melanoma, amputation of the distal phalanx is required. Adjuvant therapy should be considered for patients with poor prognoses. Sentinel node biopsy is recommended for NUM with Breslow depth greater than 1 mm and for thinner and ulcerated melanomas.[1]

INFLAMMATORY ONYCHOPATHIES

NAIL PSORIASIS

Etiology Up to 90% of patients with cutaneous psoriasis develop NP at some point in their lifetime.[9] A retrospective cross-sectional study of 848 psoriasis patients showed that 51.7% of Hispanics and 54.2% of Asian patients had severe NP, while only 36.6% of Whites had severe NP.[10] In a systemic review of randomized clinical trials for pharmacological treatment of NP, only 35.6% reported race or ethnicity.[11] Proportions of non-White patients enrolled were lower than populations in the 2019 U.S. census (13.4% vs 39.9%) ($p < 0.05$).[11] NP develops due to a combination of genetic, environmental, and immune stressors. There is no correlation of HLA-C0602 with nail and joint disease, though NP is often related to inflammation of tendon and ligament insertion points that bring about enthesitis.[12]

Clinical Presentation Patients with NP typically present with a combination of nail plate pitting, red spots in the lunula, nail plate crumbling, onycholysis, subungual hyperkeratosis, salmon spots, and splinter hemorrhages [**Figure 46-4**].[9] Salmon spots are often dull and red in patients of skin types IV and V.[13]

Diagnosis and Differential Diagnoses Diagnosis of NP is dependent upon history, clinical presentation, dermoscopy, and nail clippings. Joint examination and X-rays of the hands may be obtained to rule out psoriatic arthritis. A nail biopsy is rarely necessary, though may be indicated in more complex cases or when only a single nail is involved to rule out malignancy. Ultrasound may show hyperechoic parts or loss of definition of the nail plates but is not well studied for NP.[9] Differential diagnoses include onychomycosis, eczema, NLP, onychotillomania, or nonspecific onychodystrophy.[9]

Treatment NP is treated based on the number of nails involved and the site of inflammation. If less than three nails are involved and localized to the nail matrix, first-line therapy includes intralesional steroid injections or topical vitamin D and steroids. If less than three nails are involved localized to the nail bed, first-line therapy includes topical steroids and vitamin D or topical steroid monotherapy. If less than three nails are involved localized to both the nail matrix and bed, first-line therapy includes intralesional steroid injections. If more than three nails are involved, topical or systemic treatments with biologic therapies are considered. When NP occurs in the presence of extensive cutaneous diseases and/or psoriatic arthritis, systemic therapy is indicated. In a retrospective study of 4413 systemically treated cutaneous psoriasis patients, the use of biologic agents was lower in Blacks (51.9%) and other racial minorities (46.2%) versus Whites (62.2%) ($p < 0.05$).[10]

Patients with NP are recommended to avoid nail biting or picking, using artificial nails, and wearing high-heeled or narrow-fitting shoes. Patients are counseled to wear cotton gloves during dry work, and cotton gloves under vinyl gloves during wet work.[14]

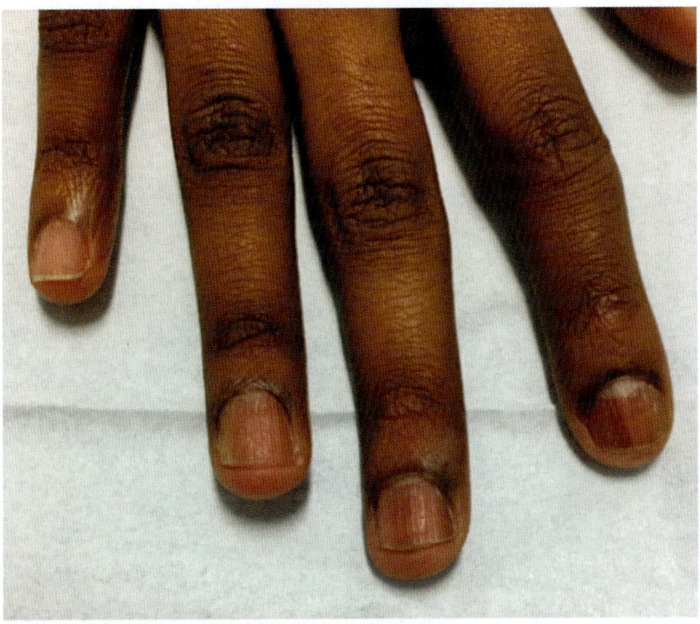

FIGURE 46-4. NP presenting as irregular pitting and onycholysis in a patient with darker Fitzpatrick skin type.

NAIL LICHEN PLANUS

Etiology NLP is an inflammatory nail disorder that occurs in 10% of patients with cutaneous lichen planus or may occur in isolation.[15] It results in permanent onychodystrophy or anonychia in 4% of patients.[15] While the mechanism is not completely understood, it is thought to be due to abnormal toll-like receptor activity in the plasmacytoid dendritic cells, leading to excessive recruitment of CD81 T-lymphocytes and destruction of keratinocytes.[16] There have been no studies to date that show increased prevalence of NLP in particular age, sex, ethnic, or racial groups. However, in a retrospective, open observational study of 26 children with LP over a 10-year period in the United Kingdom, 21 (80%) were Indian.[16,17]

Clinical Presentation Patients with NLP present with onychorrhexis, LM, onychoschizia, brittleness, or fragility [**Figure 46-5 A**].[7] When the nail matrix is affected, patients demonstrate longitudinal ridging, nail plate thinning, splitting, and a red lunula.[16] In a retrospective study of NLP in Asians, longitudinal ridging and fissuring, thinning, melanonychia, and trachyonychia were common clinical presentations.[18] When the nail bed is affected, there is onycholysis, subungual hyperkeratosis and splinter hemorrhages.[16] End-stage NLP presents as anonychia or dorsal pterygium, which represents scarring and is irreversible [**Figure 46-6**].[16]

Diagnosis and Differential Diagnoses NLP is initially diagnosed based on history, clinical examination, and dermoscopy [Figure 46-5B].[18,19] Nail biopsy with histopathology may be required in challenging cases or when only a single nail is involved, since it can look identical to amelanotic melanoma. Longitudinal biopsy is the biopsy method of choice to ensure that nail matrix and bed are sampled.[16] Histopathology will show hyperkeratosis, acanthosis, elongation of rete ridges, lymphocytes in the upper dermis and dermo-epidermal junction, necrosis of the basal layer in the proximal nail fold, and hypogranulosis and absence of the keratogenous zone in the nail matrix.[16] The differential diagnoses of NLP include NP, AA nail changes, lichenoid drug reactions, trauma, onychotillomania, onychophagia, and onychomycosis.[16]

Treatment Similar to NP, treatment for NLP is based according to the number of nails involved and whether there is nail matrix or nail bed disease.[14] If less than three nails are affected involving the nail matrix, first-line therapy includes intralesional or intramuscular triamcinolone acetonide injection, and second-line therapy includes oral acitretin or alitretinoin.[14] If less than three nails are involved with nail bed disease, first-line therapy is intramuscular triamcinolone acetonide injection, and second-line therapy is oral acitretin or alitretinoin.[14] If less than three nails are involved with nail matrix and bed disease, less than three nails are severely involved, or more than three nails are involved, first-line therapy includes intralesional and/or intramuscular triamcinolone acetonide injection, second-line therapy includes oral acitretin or alitretinoin, and third line therapy includes azathioprine, cyclosporine, or mycophenolate.[14] Injections are repeated every 4 to 5 weeks for at least 4 to 6 months.[14] A case report showed clearance of NLP with oral tofacitinib, a Janus kinase 1 and Janus kinase 3 inhibitor, though no clinical trials have been performed.[15] Ultimately, long-term follow-up

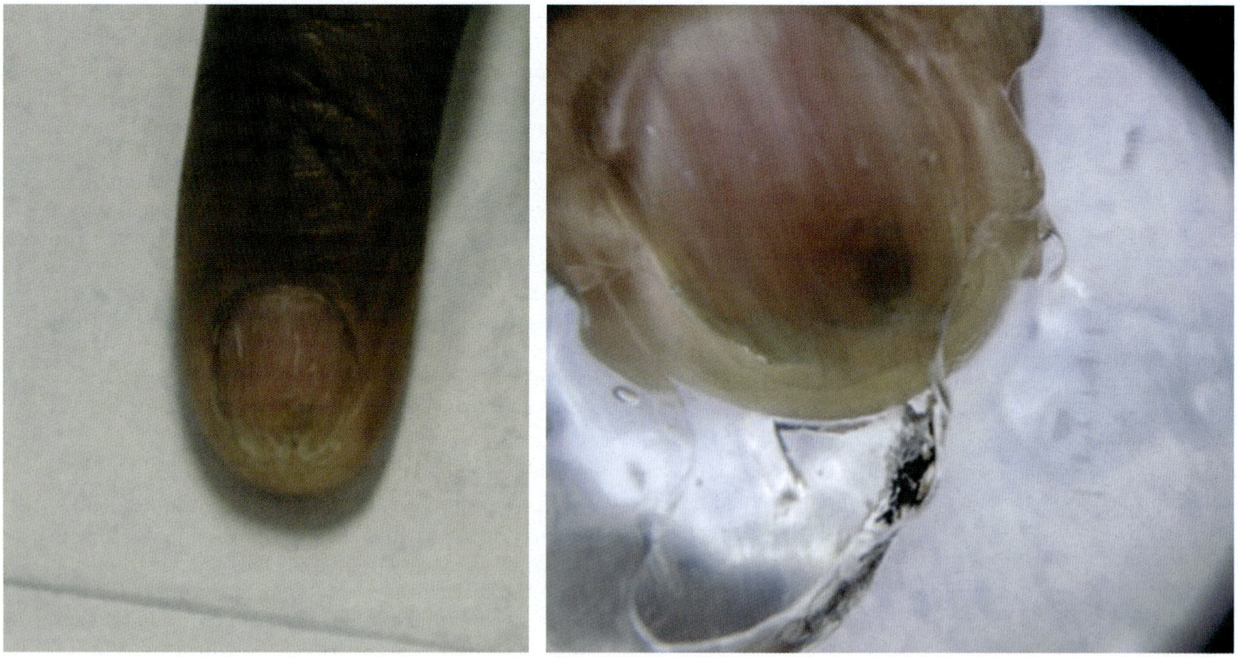

A B

FIGURE 46-5. Patient with NLP of the right fifth fingernail. (A) Patient with Fitzpatrick skin Type VI presenting with onychorrhexis of the nail plate. (B) Dermoscopy shows onychorrhexis and nail plate dyschromia. (Reproduced with permission from Gupta MK, Lipner SR. Review of nail lichen planus. *Dermatol Clin.* 2021;39(2):221-230.)

care for NLP patients is extremely important given high recurrence rates.[15] Moreover, NLP should be treated aggressively to prevent complete nail loss.[15]

NAIL CHANGES WITH ALOPECIA AREATA

Etiology AA is an inflammatory disease causing nonscarring hair loss, with frequent nail findings.[19] It is thought that AA is due to T-cell-mediated autoimmunity targeting hair follicles.[20] In a cross-sectional study of 9340 self-registered AA patients and 2064 non-AA controls, AA was more common in African Americans (OR = 1.92, 95% CI, 1.49-2.47), less common in Asians (OR = 0.44, 95% CI, 0.36-0.54), and no difference in Hispanic/Latinos (OR = 1.05, 95% CI, 0.87-1.28) versus Whites.[20] In a study of AA in the 2007-2016 National Ambulatory Medical Care Survey database, bivariate analysis showed that Latinos versus non-Latinos more often had visits for AA (OR 2.5, CI 95%: 1.1-5.6; $p = 0.03$).[21] There were no significant differences between Asians visiting for AA compared to Whites (OR = 1.6, 95% CI, 0.38-6.7; $p = 0.5$).[21]

Studies comparing the prevalence of AA nail changes across ethnic groups have not been performed. Overall, 30% of patients with AA experience nail changes, including pitting and trachyonychia. Nail changes are more common in women, but trachyonychia is more prevalent in men than women with AA.[22]

Clinical Presentation Patients with nail changes associated with AA often present with pitting and trachyonychia. Other changes include red spots in the lunula, onycholysis, punctuate leukonychia, longitudinal ridging, crumbling, and Beau lines [**Figure 46-7**]. Nail changes are more common in patients with alopecia areata universalis and alopecia areata totalis. In general, nail pits associated with AA are shallow and in a grid-like pattern versus NP, which are deeper and arranged randomly.[22]

Diagnosis and Differential Diagnoses AA nail changes are diagnosed via clinical presentation and thorough history.[22] Dermoscopy is useful

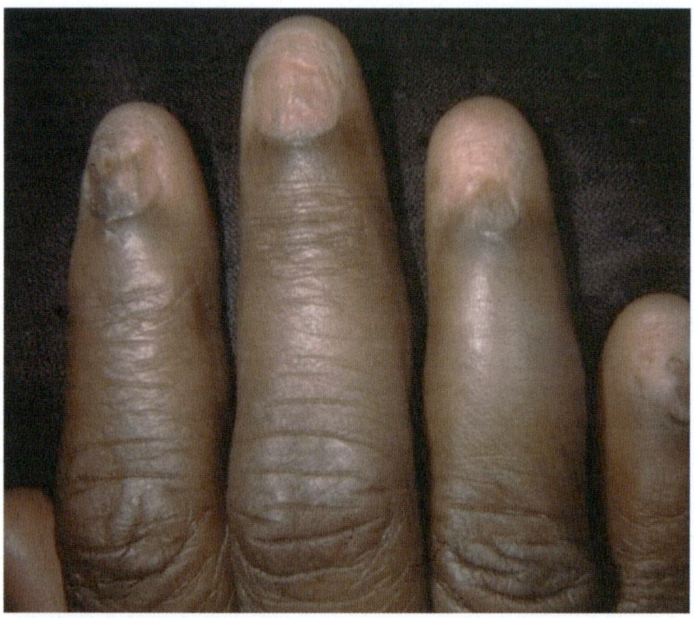

FIGURE 46-6. Patient with Fitzpatrick skin type VI with NLP presenting with dorsal pterygium, nail plate thinning and ridging, and melanonychia in the right second fingernail.

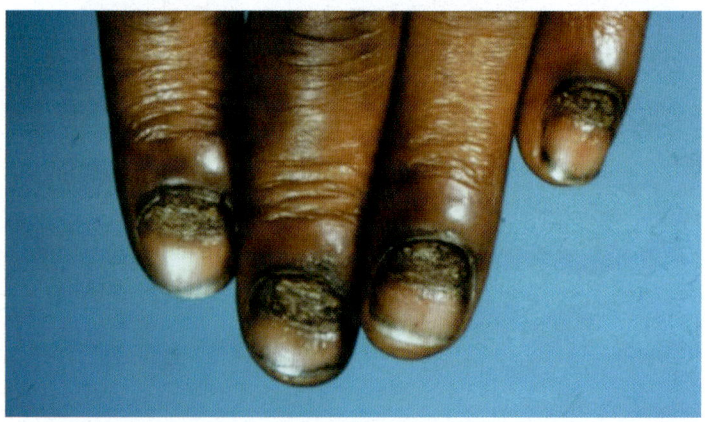

FIGURE 46-7. Proximal nail plate crumbing and mid-nail plate pitting in a patient of Fitzpatrick skin type VI with alopecia areata universalis. (Reproduced with permission from Lipner SR, Scher RK. Alopecia areata. *J Am Acad Dermatol.* 2018;79(1):e9-e10.)

in visualizing subtle pits.[22] A nail clipping is recommended to rule out any infectious processes. Histopathology of nail clippings may show pits lined with parakeratotic cells on the dorsal nail plate.[22] The differential diagnoses consist of NP, NLP, atopic dermatitis, and onychomycosis.[22]

Treatment First-line treatment for AA is topical corticosteroids, such as mometasone furoate 0.1% ointment and betamethasone dipropionate 0.05% ointment. Second-line therapy is intralesional triamcinolone (2.5 mg/mL), which is effective for pitting and trachyonychia. Systemic corticosteroids, such as oral prednisolone (300 mg pulsed monthly), along with intralesional triamcinolone can be used in cases of severe nail changes associated with AA. Tofacitinib has also demonstrated efficacy for AA nail changes.[23] In a study of 23 children with AA-associated trachyonychia, nail appearance improved in most patients at 4-year and 7-year follow-up visits.[22] Hence, it is important to observe and reassure pediatric patients that nail changes associated with AA may resolve spontaneously.[22]

ENVIRONMENTAL ONYCHOPATHIES

BRITTLE NAIL SYNDROME

Etiology BNS is commonly seen in dermatologic practice and may be idiopathic, environmentally driven, or secondary to a pathologic process.[24] Idiopathic brittle nail syndrome is due to the loss of organization and change in chemical composition of the nail, such as dehydration and/or changes in lipid composition.[25] Women, especially those over the age of 50, experience nail fragility twice as frequently as men, perhaps due to weaker intercellular keratinocyte bridges.[26] In addition, as women age, the cholesterol sulfate concentration in the nail plate decreases.[24]

Environmental causes of brittle nail syndrome include frequent contact with water, regular manicures, or trauma to the nail plate.[25] Occupational exposure to chemicals and dishwashing without gloves can dissolve nails' intercellular lipids, thereby damaging the intercellular adhesions.[24] Improper use of manicure tools and frequent use of acrylic gels can also result in brittle nails via intercellular fractures to the nail plate.[24]

Secondary brittle nail syndrome may be due to systemic causes. Deficiencies of vitamins A through E, zinc, iron, and selenium can result in brittle nails.[2] Decreased vascularization due to arteriolosclerosis or Raynaud's disease, and decreased oxygenation due to anemias can cause nail fragility.[24] Inflammatory conditions, such as psoriasis, lichen planus, atopic dermatitis, and AA can cause brittle nails.[25,27] Retinoids, antiretrovirals, antimetabolites, or penicillamine can cause nail weakness.[25]

Clinical Presentation Patients report nail fragility, splitting and flaking, presenting with onychoschizia, lamellar splitting of the nail plate free edge, onychorrhexis, or nail plate longitudinal thickening, thinning, or ridging [**Figure 46-8**].[25] Patients may experience pain or sensitivity when performing activities of daily life, as well as a psychosocial impact due to unpleasant cosmetic appearance.[25] In a cross-sectional survey-based study of 138 adult female patients with BNS, nail fragility was more often reported in Black and mixed-race patients versus White patients (OR = 4.75, CI 95%, 1.36-16.59).[28]

Diagnosis and Differential Diagnoses BNS diagnosis is made based on a careful history and clinical presentation. Nail biopsy is not required. Differential diagnoses include trauma, NP, NLP, and onychomycosis.[24] It is important to rule out any secondary causation for brittle nails, which will affect treatment.

Treatment It is important to treat any underlying cause and offending drugs, if possible, should be discontinued. Once secondary BNS has been ruled out, idiopathic BNS is treated. Patients are instructed to avoid contact with water, wear cotton gloves under rubber gloves when coming into contact with water, minimize the use of nail polish remover, and refrain from using artificial nails and cutting or pushing back the cuticles.[25] Nails should be kept short to limit the area available for dehydration.[25,27] Use of nail strengtheners, lacquers, and moisturizers have been shown some benefit.[25] Some brittle nails may improve with the use of nail hardeners, even though there is potential to inadvertently exacerbate nail weakness and onychoschizia.[27]

CHRONIC PARONYCHIA

Etiology Chronic paronychia is inflammation of the skin surrounding the fingernails or toenails, caused by compromise of the protective barrier between the nail plate and nail fold.[25,29] It may be caused by inadequate treatment of acute paronychia or an inflammatory reaction to irritants.[25] Finger sucking, frequent hand washing, excessive contact with chemicals, nail or cuticle biting, or application of artificial nails predispose to chronic paronychia.[25] Patients with occupations or hobbies that involve frequent contact with water such as swimmers, laundry workers, or dishwashers are more susceptible to chronic paronychia.[25] In a cross-sectional epidemiological study of dermatologic conditions in 226 registered hairdressers in Nigeria, nail disorders comprised 32.74% of occupational dermatologic disorders, with chronic paronychia comprising 64.86% of nail disorders.[30]

Clinical Presentation Patients present with erythema and swelling of the nail folds with retraction of the proximal nail fold [**Figure 46-9**]. There may be discoloration and thickening of the nail plate. Patients may experience pain and tenderness, but pus below the nail fold is a more common feature of acute paronychia. Multiple fingers are usually

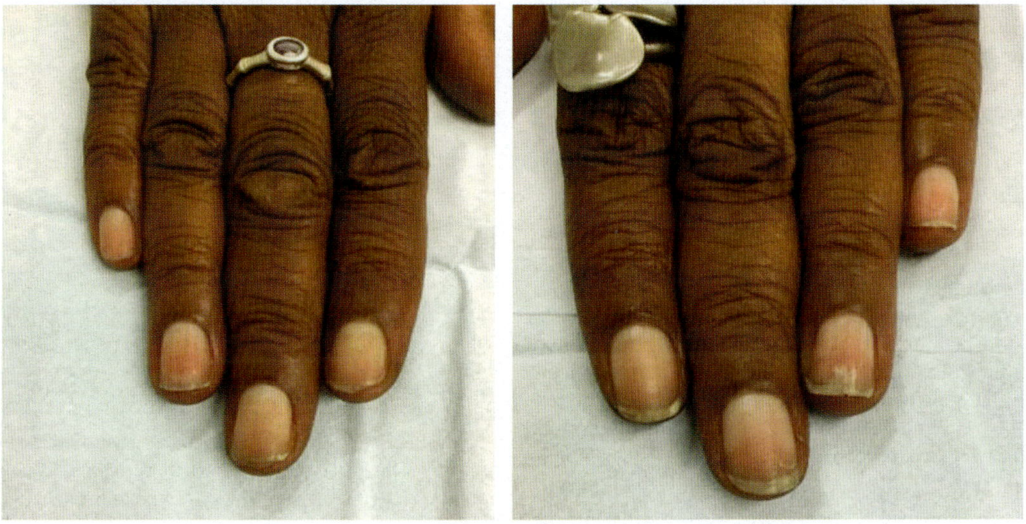

FIGURE 46-8. BNS in a patient of Fitzpatrick type VI showing onychoschizia and nail plate splitting.

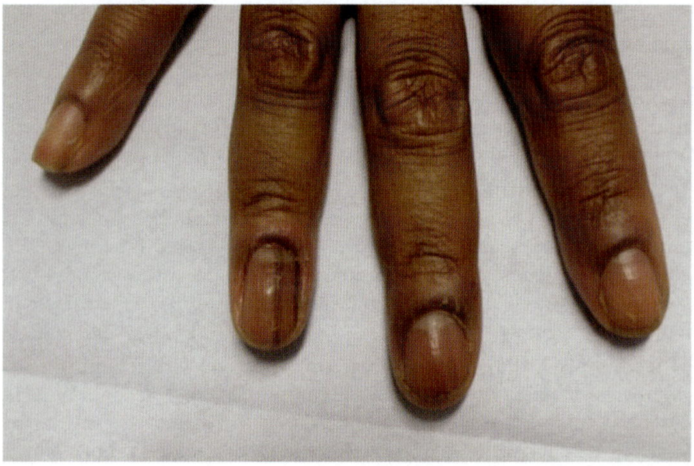

FIGURE 46-9. Chronic paronychia in a patient of Fitzpatrick skin type VI, presenting with edema of the right third and fourth nail folds. Of note, there is also benign LM of the right fourth fingernail.

involved, with the thumb, second and third fingers of the dominant hand being most frequently affected.[25]

Diagnosis and Differential Diagnoses The diagnosis of chronic paronychia is based on thorough patient history and physical examination of the nail units. Differential diagnoses include ingrown fingernail or toenail, NP, and nail changes secondary to atopic dermatitis.[25]

Treatment Treatment for chronic paronychia includes limiting contact with any offending agents. It is important to instruct patients to wear gloves when performing wet work. Patients should refrain from cutting or pushing back cuticles, finger sucking, or obsessive nail picking or biting. First-line medical treatment includes topical corticosteroids and antifungals.[25,29] Intralesional steroids may also be considered in recalcitrant cases.[25]

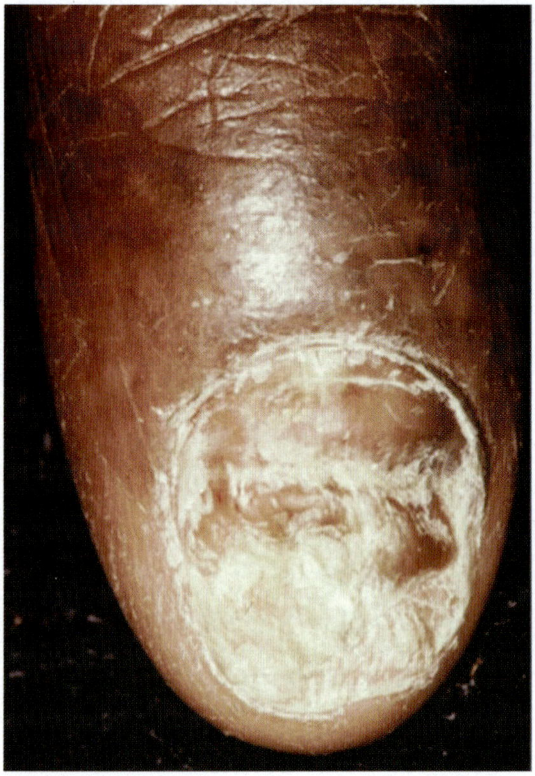

FIGURE 46-10. Onychomycosis with lamellar nail splitting and white patches in the nail plate. (Reproduced with permission from Lipner SR, Scher RK. Onychomycosis: Clinical Overview and Diagnosis. Journal of the American Academy of Dermatology. 2019;80(4):P835-851. photograph courtesy of Dr Robert Baran.)

INFECTIOUS ONYCHOPATHY

ONYCHOMYCOSIS

Etiology Onychomycosis is the most common nail disorder seen clinically, with a worldwide prevalence of 5.5%. Risk factors include trauma, advanced age, diabetes, immunosuppression, tinea pedis, NP, obesity, household contacts with nail fungal infections, and hyperhidrosis. Overall, 60% to 70% of onychomycosis cases are caused by dermatophytes, mostly *Trichophyton rubrum* and *Trichophyton mentagrophytes*, 20% nondermatophyte molds (NDMs), and 10% to 20% yeasts including *Candida* spp.[31]

In a systemic review of race and ethnicity reporting and representation in 182 trials onychomycosis clinical trials, only 17.5% of trials reported on race and/or ethnicity, and only one analyzed treatment outcomes in subgroups. There was an increase in the amount and proportion of non-White participants from 73/1245 (5.9%) (1988-2004) to 1613/8270 (19.5%) (2005-2020). Out of 429 onychomycosis images, only 22.1% were of Fitzpatrick type III/IV and 5.4% were V/VI. Hence, greater effort to display equally representative images in publications is necessary.[32]

Clinical Presentation Patients with onychomycosis may present with yellow nail plate discoloration and thickening, onycholysis, and subungual hyperkeratosis [**Figure 46-10**]. Severe cases may present with crumbling, onychocryptosis, and nail loss. There is often scaling in the interweb spaces and plantar feet. Toenails are affected more often than fingernails, with the great toenail most often involved. In two feet-one hand syndrome, bilateral toenails and fingernails of one hand are affected [**Figure 46-11**]. Patients can experience pain and discomfort with footwear, as well as negative psychosocial impact.[31]

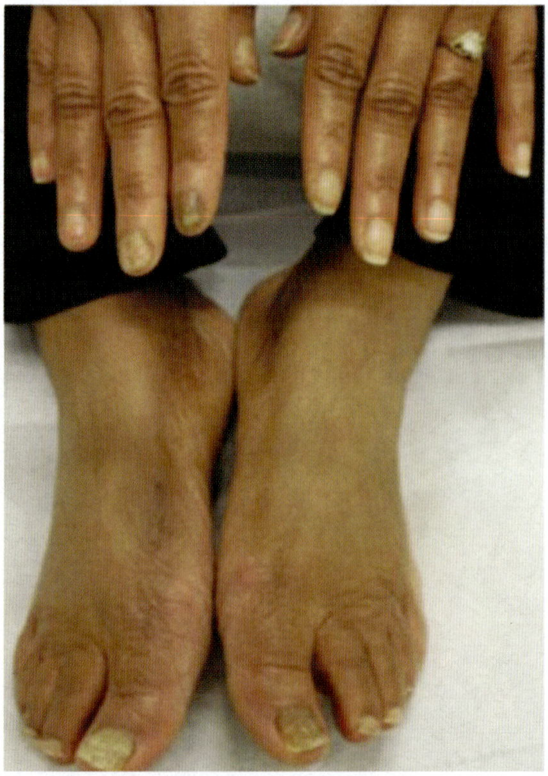

FIGURE 46-11. Two foot-one hand syndrome, involving the bilateral toenails and fingernails of the right hand. (Reproduced with permission from Lipner SR, Scher RK. Onychomycosis: clinical overview and diagnosis. *J Am Acad Dermatol*. 2019;80(4):853-867.)

Diagnosis and Differential Diagnoses Thorough history-taking is important, inquiring about history of tinea pedis, hyperhidrosis of the feet, and any household contacts.[31] Patients should be asked if they are currently taking any antifungals, as treatment can skew results of nail sampling. Dermoscopic findings suggestive of onychomycosis are jagged proximal edges with spikes in the area of onycholysis and longitudinal striae that are rounded proximally and narrow distally.[31] Onychomycosis diagnosis requires confirmatory testing. Options include KOH with microscopy, fungal culture, histopathology, and polymerase chain reaction.[1] The differential diagnoses include NP, NLP, verruca, paronychia, traumatic onycholysis, yellow nail syndrome, exostosis, and squamous cell carcinoma.[31]

Treatment Treating onychomycosis is slow due to nail growth rates.[33] Confirmatory testing before treatment is cost-saving and imperative to avoid misdiagnosis and unnecessary, inappropriate treatment.[31] Oral terbinafine and itraconazole are systemic FDA-approved treatments for onychomycosis. Terbinafine versus itraconazole has higher cure rates and fewer drug-drug interactions. Terbinafine associated side effects include headache, gastrointestinal upset, skin rash, and rarely liver enzyme abnormalities and taste disturbances. Serum transaminases should be checked before starting therapy. Itraconazole is broader spectrum than terbinafine, with efficacy against dermatophyte, NDMs, and yeasts. Side effects include headache, upper respiratory infection, abdominal pain, hypertriglyceridemia, elevated liver enzymes, and rarely hepatic injury and peripheral neuropathy. Topical treatments for onychomycosis include ciclopirox 8% nail lacquer, efinaconazole 10% solution, and tavaborole 5% solution. Recurrences occur in 20% to 25% of cases. Nail avulsion is now rarely performed, because complete cure is unlikely. Devices are not subject to the same stringent requirements for approvals as drugs. Thus, the evidence for laser treatment of onychomycosis is poor and lasers are not currently recommended. Treatment of tinea pedis with either topical or systemic antifungals in patients and household contacts is paramount. Patients are counseled to keep the feet cool and dry, avoid tight-fitting footwear, and cut nails short to avoid nail trauma.[33]

REFERENCES

1. André J, Lateur N. Pigmented nail disorders. *Dermatol Clin.* 2006;24(3):329-339.
2. Lee DK, Chang MJ, Desai AD, Lipner SR. Clinical and dermoscopic findings of benign longitudinal melanonychia due to melanocytic activation differ by skin type and predict likelihood of nail matrix biopsy. *J Am Acad Dermatol.* 2022;87(4):792-799.
3. Dominguez-Cherit J, Roldan-Marin R, Pichardo-Velazquez P, et al. Melanonychia, melanocytic hyperplasia, and nail melanoma in a Hispanic population. *J Am Acad Dermatol.* 2008;59(5):785-791.
4. Astur M de MM, Farkas CB, Junqueira JP, et al. Reassessing melanonychia striata in phototypes IV, V, and VI patients. *Dermatol Surg.* 2016;42(2):183-190.
5. Leung AKC, Robson WmLM, Liu EKH, et al. Melanonychia striata in Chinese children and adults. *Int J Dermatol.* 2007;46(9):920-922.
6. Gao JL, Shoen E, Lipner SR. Inaccuracy of Google reverse image searches for diagnosis of melanonychia: a cross-sectional analysis. *Int J Dermatol.* 2022;61(11):e417-e420.
7. Starace M, Alessandrini A, Brandi N, Piraccini BM. Use of nail dermoscopy in the management of melanonychia: review. *Dermatol Pract Concept.* 2019;9(1):38-43.
8. Ko D, Oromendia C, Scher R, Lipner SR. Retrospective single-center study evaluating clinical and dermoscopic features of longitudinal melanonychia, ABCDEF criteria, and risk of malignancy. *J Am Acad Dermatol.* 2019;80(5):1272-1283.
9. Bardazzi F, Starace M, Bruni F, Magnano M, Piraccini B, Alessandrini A. Nail psoriasis: an updated review and expert opinion on available treatments, including biologics. *Acta Derm Venerol.* 2019;99(6):516-523.
10. Ricardo JW, Lipner SR. Under-representation of racial and ethnic minorities in nail psoriasis randomized clinical trials: a call to action. *J Am Acad Dermatol.* 2022;86(6):e267-e268.
11. Ricardo JW, Qiu Y, Lipner SR. Racial, ethnic, and sex disparities in nail psoriasis clinical trials: a systematic review. *Skin Appendage Disord.* 2022;8(3):171-178.
12. Haneke E. Nail psoriasis: clinical features, pathogenesis, differential diagnoses, and management. *Psoriasis (Auckl).* 2017;7:51-63.
13. Rigopoulos D, Baran R, Chiheb S, et al. Recommendations for the definition, evaluation, and treatment of nail psoriasis in adult patients with no or mild skin psoriasis: a dermatologist and nail expert group consensus. *J Am Acad Dermatol.* 2019;81(1):228-240.
14. Ankad, BS, Bhat Y, Gaikwad SS. Nail disorders in skin of color: approach to onychoscopic diagnosis. *Clin Dermatol Rev.* 2020;4(2):92-101.
15. Kharghoria G, Grover C, Bhattacharya SN, Sharma S. Histopathological evaluation of nail lichen planus: a cross-sectional study. *J Cutan Pathol.* 2021;48(1):11-17.
16. Gupta MK, Lipner SR. Review of nail lichen planus: epidemiology, pathogenesis, diagnosis, and treatment. *Dermatol Clin.* 2021;39(2):221-230. doi:10.1016/j.det.2020.12.002.
17. Balasubramaniam P, Ogboli M, Moss C. Lichen planus in children: review of 26 cases. *Clin Exp Dermatol.* 2008;33(4):457-459.
18. Wechsuruk P, Bunyaratavej S, Kiratiwongwan R, Suphatsathienkul P, Wongdama S, Leeyaphan C. Clinical features and treatment outcomes of nail lichen planus: a retrospective study. *JAAD Case Rep.* 2021;17:43-48.
19. Iorizzo M, Tosti A, Starace M, et al. Isolated nail lichen planus: an expert consensus on treatment of the classical form. *J Am Acad Dermatol.* 2020;83(6):1717-1723.
20. Lee H, Jung SJ, Patel AB, Thompson JM, Qureshi A, Cho E. Racial characteristics of alopecia areata in the United States. *J Am Acad Dermatol.* 2020;83(4):1064-1070.
21. Gonzalez T, Fleischer AB. Reply to: "Racial characteristics of alopecia areata in the United States." *J Am Acad Dermatol.* 2021;84(6):e295-e296.
22. Chelidze K, Lipner SR. Nail changes in alopecia areata: an update and review. *Int J Dermatol.* 2018;57(7):776-783.
23. Yesudian PD, de Berker DAR. Inflammatory nail conditions. Part 2: nail changes in lichen planus and alopecia areata. *Clin Experiment Dermatol.* 2021;46(1):16-20.
24. Van de Kerkhof PCM, Pasch MC, Scher RK, et al. Brittle nail syndrome: a pathogenesis-based approach with a proposed grading system. *J Am Acad Dermatol.* 2005;53(4):644-651.
25. Shemer A, Daniel CR. Common nail disorders. *Clin Dermatol.* 2013;31(5):578-586.
26. Chessa MA, Iorizzo M, Richert B, et al. Pathogenesis, clinical signs and treatment recommendations in brittle nails: a review. *Dermatol Ther (Heidelb).* 2019;10(1):15-27.
27. Lee DK, Lipner SR. Optimal diagnosis and management of common nail disorders. *Ann Med.* 54(1):694-712.
28. Gequelim GC, Kubota CY, Sanches S, et al. Perception of brittle nails in dermatologic patients: a cross-sectional study. *An Bras Dermatol.* 2013;88(6):1022-1025.
29. Relhan V, Bansal A. Acute and chronic paronychia revisited: a narrative review. *J Cutan Aesthet Surg.* 2022;15(1):1-16.
30. Archibong J, Henshaw E, Ogunbiyi A, George A. Occupational skin disorders in a subset of Nigerian hairdressers. *Pan Afr Med J.* 2018;31:100.
31. Lipner SR, Scher RK. Onychomycosis: clinical overview and diagnosis. *J Am Acad Dermatol.* 2019;80(4):835-851.
32. Chang MJ, Qiu Y, Lipner SR. Race reporting and representation in onychomycosis clinical trials: a systematic review. *Mycoses.* 2021;64(8):954-966.
33. Lipner SR, Scher RK. Onychomycosis: treatment and prevention of recurrence. *J Am Acad Dermatol.* 2019;80(4):853-867.

SECTION 6

Follicular, Sebaceous, and Sweat Gland Disorders

CHAPTER 47

Folliculitis

Kim Nichols
Stephanie Smith
Vanesa Kodra

KEY POINTS

- Folliculitis is an inflammatory condition that presents as papules or pustules surrounding the hair follicle.
- Folliculitis can be classified anatomically into superficial versus deep, as well as infectious etiology versus noninfectious etiology.
- Clinically, the classic presentation of folliculitis may vary in light skin tones compared to darker skin tones.
- Although rarely life-threatening, it is important to distinguish when folliculitis may be related to a systemic etiology, such as underlying immunosuppression.
- Treatment for folliculitis depends on the underlying etiology, and may involve topical medications, oral medications, or both.

INTRODUCTION

Folliculitis is an inflammatory disease surrounding the hair follicles and their associated pilosebaceous units. There are multiple different causes of folliculitis, with the most common being an infection, but there are many noninfectious etiologies as well. These include physical and chemical irritants, certain drugs, AIDS, or immunocompromised induced, as well as pseudofolliculitis. In order to further understand the etiology of folliculitis, it is often classified into categories of superficial and deep [**Figure 47-1**]. Superficial folliculitis is when the upper portion of the hair follicle, the follicular infundibulum, is involved. Deep folliculitis is when the inflammation extends into the isthmus and deeper portions of the follicle. In superficial folliculitis, the follicular inflammation is confined, leading to the formation of the characteristic clustered, 1- to 4-mm erythematous papule pustules that typically heal without scarring. This type of folliculitis is usually seen in areas with terminal hair strands. Deep folliculitis is characterized by large, tender erythematous papules or nodules that can scar. The purulent material can extend into the subcutaneous tissue forming a large, deep mass or furuncle. Several infected follicles can coalesce to form a large mass or carbuncle. Both superficial and deep folliculitis can be due to either infectious or noninfectious causes, and some may be hard to distinguish from one another. Therefore, it is important to obtain a detailed history of comorbid conditions, medications, external exposures, in conjunction with appropriate ancillary testing, in order to treat appropriately. Generally, superficial folliculitis is easier to treat than deep folliculitis, and infectious folliculitis responds better to classic treatments than noninfectious causes.[1]

EPIDEMIOLOGY AND PATHOGENESIS

Folliculitis occurs when the hair follicle becomes inflamed, whether that is due to trauma, infection, or occlusion. The pathophysiology is poorly understood, but is thought to be related to epidermal growth factor receptor inhibitors, where inhibition of follicular epidermal differentiation occurs and causes follicular obstruction and subsequent inflammation. Eosinophilic folliculitis has a different etiology than the others and is thought to be autoimmune in nature, affecting the sebocytes or some component of the sebum.

Folliculitis is a very common disorder in children and adults. There are no data to indicate a sexual predilection and it is thought to affect males and females equally. There are a few variants that favor one over the other. For example, folliculitis barbae, eosinophilic folliculitis, folliculitis keloidalis nuchae, and perifolliculitis capitis *abscedens et suffodiens* occur more frequently in males, whereas traction folliculitis occurs more frequently in females. Folliculitis can be seen in persons of all ages, from infancy to the elderly populations; however, *Pityrosporum* folliculitis is much more prevalent in adolescents, likely because of the increased activity of their sebaceous glands.[2]

The overall incidence is increased in individuals who are obese, hirsute, amputees, or immunocompromised, including those undergoing chemotherapy or those with diabetes mellitus, human immunodeficiency virus (HIV) infection, hypogammaglobulinemia, chronic granulomatous disease, or other diseases that suppress the immune system. The most important predisposing factors to the development of folliculitis are occlusion, friction, maceration, topical corticosteroids, and hyperhidrosis. The use of traction, occlusive wigs, and oils predisposes African Americans to folliculitis of the scalp. Pseudofolliculitis and traction folliculitis occur more in African Americans, whereas eosinophilic folliculitis is seen much more in Japanese persons.

Certain drugs have been shown to be of higher risk to cause drug-induced folliculitis, including, but not limited to, topical and systemic steroids, lithium, contraceptives, testosterone, antiepileptics, EGFR-inhibitors, etc. Similarly, folliculitis has been seen following smallpox or anthrax vaccines. Military troops, who are required to get these vaccines prior to deployment, are much more susceptible to these outbreaks. It is thought that EGFR inhibition occurs in 50% to 100% of these patients and is a dose-dependent drug reaction.[3]

The manipulation of the hair strands by shaving, waxing, or plucking can lead to traumatic folliculitis [**Figure 47-2**]. Topical corticosteroids can induce folliculitis, especially when high-potency preparations, ointment vehicles, and occlusion are used. In addition, individuals with some pruritic skin diseases, such as atopic dermatitis, contact dermatitis, arthropod assault, and Darier disease, are prone to develop secondary folliculitis. Folliculitis may also develop in persons with infected abrasions, lacerations, surgical wounds, fistulas, and other breaks in the skin, as well as in those with bacterial infections, such as abscesses.

The infectious folliculitis often occurs more frequently in particular populations or under specific conditions. For instance, because *Staphylococcus aureus* is a normal inhabitant of the anterior nares in approximately 20% of adults, nasal carriers are prone to *S. aureus* folliculitis. *S. aureus* outbreaks are also common in athletes who wear occlusive clothing in hot, humid weather, share towels and athletic equipment, participate in contact sports, and shower in group facilities. *Pseudomonas* folliculitis is caused by colonization of hair follicles with certain strains of *P. aeruginosa* after exposure to contaminated water in hot tubs, whirlpools, swimming pools, water slides, and bathtubs. Gram-negative folliculitis develops in acne patients after prolonged antibiotic treatment. Tinea barbae is a fungal folliculitis that affects the mustache and beard areas of men (usually farm workers) who are exposed to *Trichophyton*-carrying cattle and dogs. This condition, as well as Majocchi granuloma

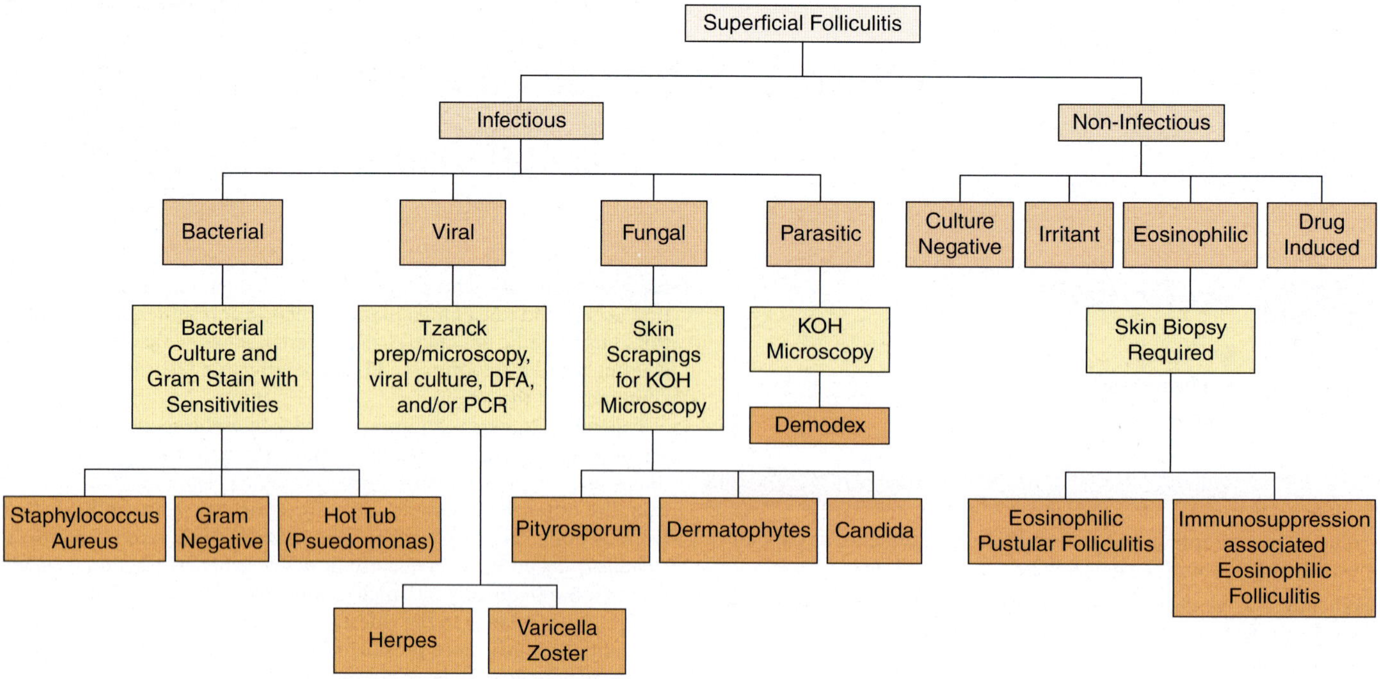

FIGURE 47-1. Superficial folliculitis categorized into infectious versus noninfectious, with explanations on which diagnostic method is best for each.

(caused by *Trichophyton rubrum*), herpetic folliculitis, and molluscum folliculitis, almost always occurs after shaving for both men and women.

SUPERFICIAL FOLLICULITIS

INFECTIOUS

Bacterial

Staphylococcus Aureus The most common type of infectious folliculitis is due to *Staphylococcus aureus*.[4] There is an increased risk in those with diabetes and atopic dermatitis. It is more common in hot and humid weather due to increased sweating. It also occurs more with occlusive clothing, hair removal such as waxing, shaving, or plucking, and the use of topical corticosteroids. Clinically, patients will present with follicular pustules or papules on an erythematous base, usually favoring areas of the body with increased sweat and friction such as the face, trunk, axillae, and buttocks [**Figure** 47-3]. If no pustules are present, there may be a superimposed collarette of scale visible, or the presence of a rim of desquamation around the hair follicles. In skin of color, the erythema of papules and surrounding pustules may be much more subtle, therefore the textural changes of the papules and the pustules may be the only obvious findings. The use of a bright light may help illuminate any subtle color changes present, such as a faint pink hue. Although this is most often diagnosed clinically, the use of a bacterial culture with or without a gram stain may be helpful in confirming the diagnosis. Treatment for *S. aureus* folliculitis depends on if it is localized to one area or widespread. If it is local, the use of a topical antibacterial is appropriate, such as clindamycin 1% lotion, gel, or solution 1 to 2 times a day, mupirocin 2% cream TID for 7 to 10 days. In addition, the patient should use antibacterial soaps, chlorhexidine wash, or benzoyl peroxide 4%, 5%, or 10% wash in the shower daily. Bleach baths twice a week may also be helpful. This involves mixing ¼ cup of household bleach into a half filled, regular size bathtub, and sitting in it for 10 minutes. If the infection is widespread or recurrent, then culture-guided oral antibiotics should be given. If MRSA is not suspected, it is recommended to give dicloxacillin 250 mg po q6h, or cephalexin 250 to 500 mg po q6h for 7 to 10 days. If MRSA is suspected, the following therapies are recommended: doxycycline 100 mg bid for 7 to 10 days, clindamycin 300 to 450 mg q6 to 8 hours for 10 to 14 days, or trimethoprim/sulfamethoxazole (160 mg/800 mg) one double-strength tablet bid for 7 to 14 days. In these recalcitrant cases, a bacterial culture of the patient's nares should be done, for they may be chronic MRSA carriers. In patients who are chronic carriers of MRSA, the use of topical mupirocin 2% ointment should be used twice a day for 5 days to decolonize the nasal passages.[5]

Gram-negative Folliculitis Gram-negative folliculitis, which includes *Klebsiella*, *Enterobacter*, *Escherichia coli*, and *Proteus* spp., is typically seen in acne patients who have been taking long-term antibiotics. Long-term use of antibiotics may alter the nasal normal flora, which allows for Gram-negative organisms to flourish. It is also more prevalent in adult men with oily skin. Clinically, it appears as small follicular pustules or deeper abscesses located in the T-zone and perinasal regions of the face, as a sudden eruption, where their acne was previously controlled with the antibiotics. Bacterial culture and gram stain may be appropriate for isolation of the proper organism. Topical treatments such as benzoyl peroxide or gentamicin are often ineffective, therefore systemic treatments are most commonly used. The best treatment is oral isotretinoin 0.5 to 1.0 mg/kg for 16 to 20 weeks, but if this treatment is contraindicated, the use of oral antibiotics is a second-line choice. Generally, ampicillin 250 to 500 mg q6h or trimethoprim-sulfamethoxazole 160/800 mg q12h may be used, but they are considered suppressive, as flare-ups are often seen once discontinuation of antibiotics occurs.[6]

Hot Tub Folliculitis Hot tub folliculitis is caused by *Pseudomonas aeruginosa* present in the setting of a hot tub, swimming pool, hot springs, or contaminated water in the work place. It also may be caused by objects that are subject to contaminated water, such as loofahs, inflatable swimming pool toys, rubber gloves, and nylon towels. The contamination often occurs because of improper chlorine levels. *P. aeruginosa* may also grow within biofilms in properly chlorinated pools. Patients will present with edematous pink-red follicular papules and pustules that are often pruritic and tender, located on the trunk, buttocks, and extremities. These follicular pustules spare the palms, soles, and face. One key feature of *Pseudomonas* folliculitis is the presence of more peripheral redness, compared to usual folliculitis. If the lesions are not in areas with visible terminal hairs, dermoscopy of vellus hairs may be useful.

History is important in this diagnosis because patients will have been in a contaminated water source 12 to 48 hours prior to eruption. Symptoms may include mild fever, malaise, lymphadenopathy, and leukocytosis. Although rare, breast tenderness may also be present, for both males and females, due to inflammation of Montgomery follicles in the breast.

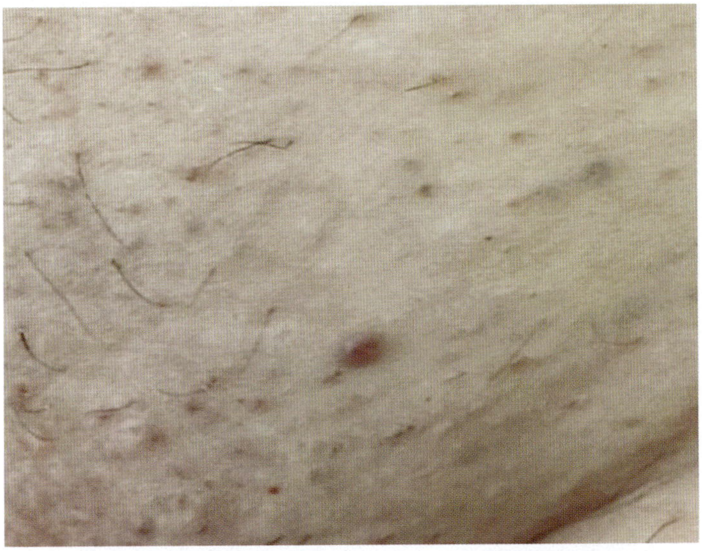

A

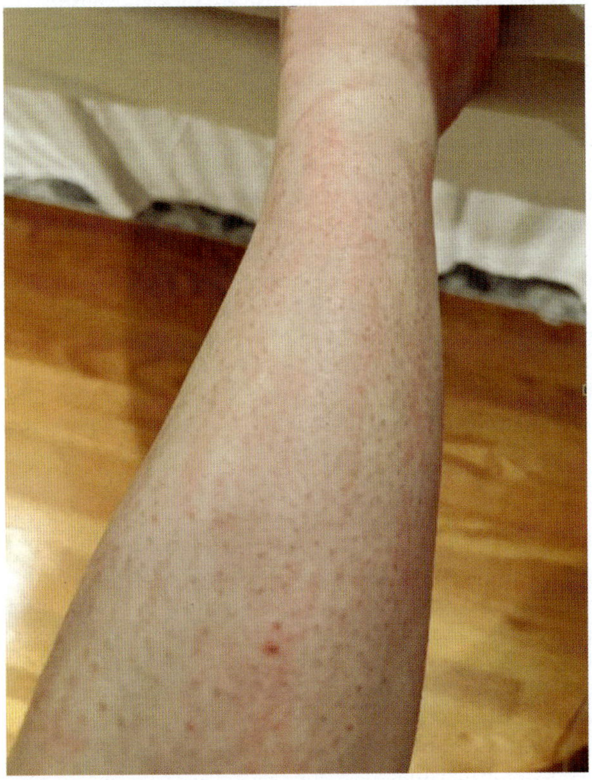

B

FIGURE 47-2. **(A)** Classic folliculitis on the mons pubis. **(B)** Heat-related irritant folliculitis on the lower leg after laser hair removal.

It may be helpful to examine the patient's feet, as this type of folliculitis sometimes occurs concomitantly with *Pseudomonas* hot foot syndrome, where painful plantar nodules are present. Although this type is often self-limited in immunocompetent patients, usually fading within 7 to 14 days without therapy, it may be more serious in immunocompromised patients. Treatment for these cases that are more severe or symptomatic influence topical and oral therapies. Topical treatments such as gentamicin 0.1% cream, povidone-iodine, or 1% acetic acid soaks may be helpful. The standard oral therapy, specifically for immunosuppressed and patients with mastitis or long-standing disease, includes ciprofloxacin 500 mg bid for 10 days. Maintenance of hot tubs with a free chlorine concentration of 1 to 3 mg/L and pH of 7.2 to 7.8 is recommended by the CDC. Adequate drying of sponges and loofahs in between use may also prevent contamination.

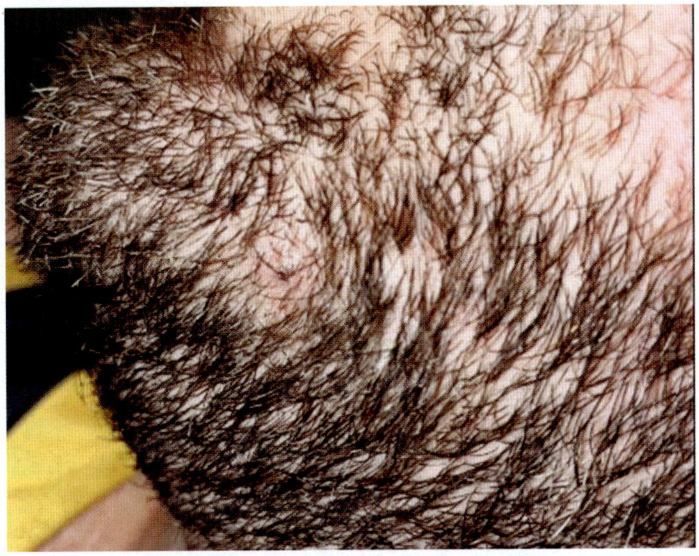

FIGURE 47-3. Pustular folliculitis on a beard after shaving with a razor.

Fungal

Dermatophyte Folliculitis Dermatophyte folliculitis is inflammation of the hair follicles most commonly in the beard area and scalp due to tinea, known as tinea barbae and tinea capitis, respectively. Tinea barbae, also known as barbers itch, presents as inflamed follicular papules and pustules in the loose hairs of the beard area, often unilateral, and may have crusts. It is a localized inflammatory reaction to the dermatophyte, most commonly the species of *Trichophyton*. A potassium hydroxide (KOH) preparation of plucked hairs is helpful in diagnosis, which will show endothrix (fungal spores within hair shafts) if positive for *Trichophyton*, and ectothrix (fungal spores attached to the outside of the hair shaft) if *Microsporum* is present. A KOH preparation of skin scrapings will show typical septate hyphae. A Woods lamp examination may be helpful in diagnosing if the causative agent is *M. canis*, as this will fluoresce under the lamp. If these are all negative, it may be necessary to perform a skin biopsy with periodic acid-Schiff (PAS) stain.

Treatment for dermatophyte folliculitis requires oral medications, as topical antifungals are often ineffective. Oral antifungals include micronized griseofulvin 500 to 1000 mg/day or ultra-micronized griseofulvin 500 to 700 mg/day PO for 4 to 6 weeks. Alternative options include terbinafine 250 mg/day PO for 2 to 4 weeks, fluconazole 200 mg qd for 4 to 6 weeks, or itraconazole 200 mg po bid for 1 week per month for two pulses.[7]

Pityrosporum Folliculitis *Pityrosporum folliculitis* is caused by *Malassezia* spp., and is most likely to occur in young adults, immunocompromised individuals who are on chronic oral prednisone, and those with diabetes. It is more common in areas of warm weather, excessive sebum production, occlusive clothing or topicals, those on antibiotic therapy, and iatrogenic immunosuppression. It is more common in individuals being treated for acne with long-term antibiotic use.[8] It presents as an acute outbreak of monomorphic, erythematous follicular pustules, and papules that are extremely pruritic, often on the chest, back, and shoulders. It can also present on the face, specifically the forehead along the hairline, neck, and scalp. Although it is caused by the same species that causes tinea versicolor, most patients will not present with tinea versicolor. Clinically it can be differentiated from acne, as there will be no comedones or cysts present in *Pityrosporum* folliculitis. Microscopic KOH prep of skin scrapings from the pustules may be used as a diagnostic aid, where abundant yeast is seen [**Figure 47-4**]. Treatment includes topical imidazole antifungal creams—such as ketoconazole, clotrimazole, miconazole, or econazole cream bid × 2 to 4 weeks, ciclopirox cream applied two times a day for 2 to 4 weeks, or selenium sulfide or ketoconazole shampoo used as a wash in the shower qd × 4 weeks. Oral antifungals may be necessary though, as organisms are often deep in the

Method for Initial Evaluation of Superficial Folliculitis

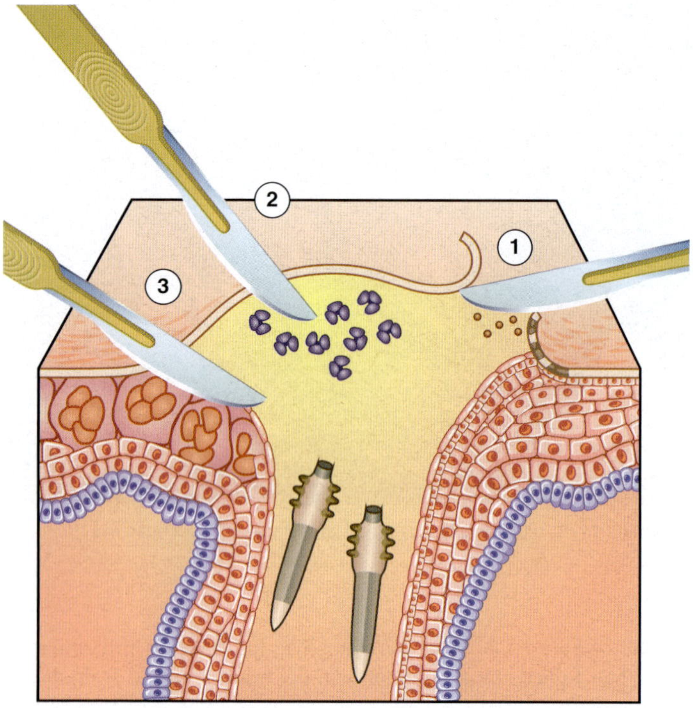

FIGURE 47-4. A visual guide to proper technique of obtaining scrapings from a folliculitis pustule. If considering dermatophytes, *Malassezia* spp., or *Candida* spp., then obtain scrapings from the peripheral scale and the roof of the follicular pustule for KOH (potassium hydroxide) microscopy (1). If considering bacterial etiologies, and depending on the host, the pustular fluid should be sent for gram stain, culture, and sensitivity (2). If considering viral etiologies, the base of the unroofed lesion should be vigorously scraped in order to collect the viral-laden keratinocytes for Tzanck prep/microscopy, viral culture, DFA (direct fluorescent antibody), and/or PCR (polymerase chain reaction) (3). Likewise, if considering *Demodex* folliculitis, scrape the base of the lesion vigorously for KOH microscopy (3). (Reproduced with permission from Bolognia J, Schaffer J, Duncan K, Ko C. Folliculitis. In: *Dermatology Essentials*. Amsterdam: Elsevier; 2014.)

hair follicles. Options include fluconazole 100 to 200 mg/day po for 1 to 3 weeks, or itraconazole 200 mg/day po for 1 to 3 weeks. Relapse is common; therefore, the use of topical agents may need to be continued once oral therapy has been discontinued.

Candida Folliculitis *Candida* folliculitis, which is caused by the organism *C. albicans*, is primarily seen in those who are immunocompromised, diabetic, or patients on antibiotic or steroid therapy. It is more common in febrile patients who are hospitalized or bedridden, lying on their back. It presents as small pustules on an erythematous base at the base of the hair follicle that are pruritic, in intertriginous areas that are moist and occluded. They often present as satellite pustules around intertriginous candidiasis infection of the skin. When *Candida* folliculitis is on the face, it is often difficult to distinguish from tinea barbae, which is why a skin scraping and 10% KOH prep will be helpful in revealing hyphae and pseudohyphae. For mild cases, treatment involves topical azole antifungals, such as miconazole 2% cream bid, or topical nystatin 100,000 units/g cream bid until healing is complete. In severe or recalcitrant cases, oral fluconazole 100 mg/day × 1 week, then qod × 1 month is an appropriate regimen. Alternatively, itraconazole 100 mg bid × 14 days is effective. Patient education is important for proper management and long-term prevention. Patients should be advised to avoid occlusive clothing and keep the skin dry after bathing. Discontinuing antibiotic or steroid therapy may be appropriate, if safe to do so.[9]

Viral

Herpetic Folliculitis Herpetic folliculitis occurs in individuals with a history of recurrent herpes simplex virus. In immunocompetent hosts, individual and grouped follicular pustules and vesicles on an erythematous base will rapidly present on the pubic area of females or face of men after shaving with a blade razor. If vesicles are seen on clinical exam, a viral culture and/or Tzanck smear should be performed. Diagnosis can be confirmed if multinucleated giant cells are seen on Tzanck smear. In immunocompromised individuals, the outbreak will be more widespread or appear in unusual areas. When this happens, it is important to consider VZV as a differential diagnosis, and submit a viral culture, DFA, and/or PCR for further diagnosis. The treatment for herpetic folliculitis requires oral antiviral therapy. Options include Famciclovir 500 mg TID for 5 to 10 days, valacyclovir 500 mg TID for 5 to 10 days, or acyclovir 200 mg five times per day for 5 to 10 days.

Parasitic

Demodex Folliculitis *Demodex* folliculitis, also known as rosacea like demodicosis or papulopustular demodicosis, is inflammation of the pilosebaceous unit due to the presence of the *Demodex* mite. *Demodex* species are the only parasites that are considered a normal component of the skin's microbiome, and it is thought that inflammation occurs when the number of mites surpass a threshold and infiltrate the dermis causing an immune reaction. This type may be associated with immune suppression, but also may occur in those with rosacea flares. On clinical exam, erythematous folliculocentric papules and pustules will be present on the face, often overlying a background of diffuse erythema. Some crusting may be present in long-standing cases. The lesions may be scattered all over the face, or localized to perioral and periocular areas. Generally, more widespread disease is associated with immunocompromised individuals. Identifying the mites can be done in a few different ways, including spin scrapings with KOH, skin scrapings with mineral oil, punch biopsy, or cellophane tape. Cellophane tape should be applied to the affected areas overnight, then visualization of the tape on a microscope slide to identify mites. Topical treatments are generally well tolerated, such as topical 5% permethrin cream, sulfur products such as sodium sulfacetamide 10%/sulfur 5% wash, Metronidazole cream/gel 1%, or dilute camphor oil, applied once a day for 2 to 4 weeks. In long-standing or severe cases, a single dose of ivermectin 200 micrograms po may be more appropriate. Proper hygiene is recommended, including daily facial cleansing to help prevent occurrence. It is important to consider *Demodex* as the culprit in classic folliculitis cases that are resistant to typical bacterial therapies.[10]

NONINFECTIOUS

Culture Negative/Normal Flora Folliculitis Of all folliculitis, this is the most common of all. It appears very similar to *S. aureus* folliculitis, with follicular pustules that are pruritic on the trunk and scalp, but bacterial culture will reveal no growth or only normal flora. Treatment includes topical benzoyl peroxide wash or gel, topical antibiotics such as clindamycin gel, or oral antibiotics (doxycycline, tetracycline) in more severe cases, as these are anti-inflammatory.

Irritant Irritant folliculitis usually occurs due to occlusive materials, such as the application of a topical medication or ointment. It also may be seen on the thighs from the friction of jeans rubbing. It appears as follicular pustules in the specific sites of friction. Treatment involves stopping the inciting agent, applying a topical medication in the same direction as hair growth. The use of a topical mid potency corticosteroid lotion or cream bid × 2 weeks may also calm down inflammation.

Numerous chemical irritants can cause folliculitis, and although engineering and refinery workers experience a greater risk, it is estimated that over 1 million other types of workers in the United States regularly use oils and greases at work. Exposure to these chemicals can lead to occupational acne and folliculitis through mechanical blockage of the pilosebaceous units. The treatment recommendations for chemical-induced folliculitis include the avoidance of occupational irritants, if possible, and frequent cleansing of the skin and washing of oil-soaked uniforms/clothing.

For other workers, folliculitis occurs as a consequence of mechanical irritation. Wherever there is frictional trauma or occlusion, folliculitis can be seen. For example, truck drivers are prone to folliculitis of the buttocks and back, whereas football players have a high incidence of folliculitis underneath their padding and on their posterior scalp and neck, secondary to helmet irritation. Again, it is advised that patients wash their skin frequently and that tight, moist clothing be regularly changed.

Drug Induced Drug-induced folliculitis can occur after many different types of systemic drugs, and usually develops within 2 weeks of starting the culprit. The risk of developing drug-induced folliculitis is proportional to the dose of the drug and the duration of therapy. It is most common in acne-prone patients and age groups. Many common drugs that may cause folliculitis include corticosteroids, androgenic hormones, EGFR inhibitors, iodies, bromides, lithium, isoniazid, and anticonvulsants. On clinical exam, there will be monomorphic erythematous follicular papules and pustules that erupt acutely, and favor the shoulders, upper arms, and trunk. It can be differentiated from acne due to the fact that there will be no comedones. Treatment involved stopping the culprit medication, if possible. Topical medications may be helpful, such as benzoyl peroxide, clindamycin, erythromycin, and topical retinoids. Oral antibiotics may be necessary, such as minocycline, doxycycline, or tetracyclines.

Drug-induced folliculitis is more common in acne-prone patients. It can develop within 2 weeks of starting a new medication, and its appearance and severity are usually dose- and duration-dependent. The eruptions resemble acne with monomorphic erythematous papules and pustules on the chest and back, but comedones are rarely present. Numerous medications have been implicated. Lithium can cause or exacerbate folliculitis, acne, and psoriasis, which are all conditions that are characterized by neutrophilic infiltration. In controlled studies, patients treated with lithium developed more cutaneous reactions than patients on other psychotropics, with a prevalence as high as 45%. Twelve studies have found alarmingly high rates of the use of anabolic steroids by young amateur athletes who take the steroids to improve their performance and by men who want to enhance their physical appearance. The recently introduced tyrosinase kinase and epidermal growth factor inhibitors often cause follicular pustular eruptions of the torso, head, and face. Corticosteroid-induced facial acneiform folliculitis is a problem in individuals with skin of color who use corticosteroids for bleaching purposes. In some patients, the eruption may be prevented with a prophylactic administration of tetracycline antibiotics. For drug-induced folliculitis, discontinuing the medication, if possible, should be the first course of therapy. In addition, topical and oral antibiotics may facilitate more rapid resolution.

Eosinophilic Folliculitis

Ofuji's disease Eosinophilic pustular folliculitis, also known as Ofuji's disease, is not associated with systemic disease and has an unknown etiology. Most cases have been reported in people of Japanese descent, with a slightly more male predominance, and peak incidence around the age of 30. Clinically, a patient will present with recurrent episodes of follicular papulopustules and erythematous patches and plaques with superimposed coalescent pustules, and later with central clearing that leads to figurate lesions. These lesions favor the face, trunk, and upper extremities, occasionally on the palms and soles. Lesions tend to be severely pruritic, and last 7 to 10 days, where they spontaneously resolve, but later relapse. Diagnosis always requires a biopsy, in which the involved follicle will show exocytosis of eosinophils and lymphocytes with or without spongiosis from sebaceous gland and duct to infundibular zone. In the dermis, there will be perifollicular and perivascular eosinophilic and lymphocytic infiltrate. There may be neutrophils seen in more inflamed lesions. Treatment includes topical antipruritics (oatmeal baths, calamine lotion), oral antihistamines (common H1 and H2 blocking agents such as hydroxyzine and doxepin). Cetirizine 20 to 40 mg/day and cyproheptadine 2 to 4 mg/day may also be used, and topical corticosteroids for the relief of pruritus. Oral indomethacin 25 to 75 mg/day has superior effectiveness, and may or may not be combined with systemic steroids, topical indomethacin, topical tacrolimus, or tetracyclines. Second-line treatment included NB-UVB therapy, oral minocycline 100 to 200 mg/day, doxycycline 100 mg/day, corticosteroids, dapsone, or colchicine.[11]

Immunosuppression-Associated Eosinophilic Folliculitis AIDS-associated eosinophilic folliculitis occurs in those with a low CD4 count (<300/mm^3). It is also referred to as immunosuppression-associated eosinophilic folliculitis because it has also been reported in those with lymphoma, leukemias, and stem cell transplant recipients. It is more common in males than females. It has also been reported in sanitation workers in Hong Kong during the COVID-19 pandemic due to the use of protective gear.[12] This type presents as chronic and persistent, very intensely pruritic, dome-shaped follicular papules, with or without pustules. Lesions tend to favor the scalp, face, and upper trunk. The chronicity often leads to prurigo and protracted postinflammatory hyperpigmentation, which is worsened in darker skin phototypes. Skin biopsy is required for proper diagnosis, but other diagnostic tools can be used such as a negative skin culture, CBC that may show eosinophilia and leukocytosis, increased IgE levels, and an HIV test. Since this is chronic and a manifestation of systemic disease, topical and oral antipruritics and corticosteroids are often inadequate at controlling or treating the lesions. Narrow-band UVB therapy may be helpful, as well as topical tacrolimus 0.03% or 0.1%, pimecrolimus cream, or permethrin every night for 6 weeks. Isotretinoin (0.5 to 1 mg/kg/day for 6 to 12 months), acitretin (0.25 to 0.5 mg/kg/day for 4-6 months), metronidazole (250 mg TID × 4 weeks), itraconazole (200 mg qd × 4 to 6 weeks), indomethacin (50 to 75 mg/day), and dapsone (50-200 mg/day for 3 to 6 months) have also been used with variable successes.[13] Ultimately, the best improvement is seen with elevation of CD4 counts with the use of antiretroviral treatment, otherwise known as ART.

DEEP FOLLICULITIS

Deep folliculitis involves the entire hair follicle, causing furuncles (boils), carbuncles, and sycosis. Furuncles are deep-seated erythematous nodules that can enlarge to up to 2 cm and become hard, painful, and fluctuant. Over several days, they may undergo abscess formation, drain pus, and eventually rupture with a gradual diminution of pain and erythema. Furuncles usually evolve from superficial folliculitis in hair-bearing, occluded regions of the body. Carbuncles are red, exquisitely tender masses of coalescing furuncles. They can be associated with fever and malaise and may heal with prominent scarring.1 They most often develop on the neck, back, and thighs. Diagnosis with a gram stain and culture of the furuncle contents, culture of the nares, umbilicus, and perineum for MRSA carriage, and sensitivities on these cultures should be performed. Treatment includes early and adequate drainage via I&D. If surgical drainage is not possible, warm compresses and antibacterial washes with chlorhexidine or triclosan should be advised. Systemic antibiotic therapy should be reserved for recurrent ear canal and nose lesions, as well as lesions not responding to local care. If MSSA is cultured, the initial antibiotic regimen includes dicloxacillin or cephalexin 500 mg four times a day for 10 to 14 days. If MRSA is cultured, antibiotic regimens include TMP-SMX one to two double-strength tabs bid, clindamycin 300 to 450 mg four times a day, or doxycycline 100 mg bid.[14]

PERIFOLLICULOCENTRIC DISORDERS

Perifolliculocentric inflammatory disorders such as acne keloidalis nuchae, PFB, and perifolliculitis capitis *abscedens et suffodiens* (dissecting cellulitis) are not true folliculitis because they involve inflammation surrounding the hair follicles and do not directly involve the hair follicle. They are conditions that are more common in African Americans due to the inflammatory reaction caused by tightly curled hair reentering the perifollicular area. These conditions are discussed in detail in Chapters 36 and 42.

CONCLUSION

Folliculitis is a common skin condition affecting the hair follicle. This condition appears like groups of small-scale pimples around the hair follicles and can be associated with itching, tenderness, inflammation, and can be filled with pus. It is most commonly caused by an infection

TABLE 47-1 Common treatments for infectious folliculitides

Type	Treatment
Bacterial folliculitis	
Staphylococcal aureus	Topical: • Clindamycin 1% lotion, gel, or solution 1-2 times a day • Mupirocin 2% cream TID for 7-10 days • Chlorhexidine wash or benzoyl peroxide 4%, 5%, or 10% wash • Bleach baths twice a week MSSA +: • Dicloxacillin 250 mg po q6h for 7-10 days • Cephalexin 250-500 mg po q6h for 7-10 days MRSA +: • Doxycycline 100 mg bid for 7-10 days • Clindamycin 300-450 mg q6-8 h for 10-14 days • Trimethoprim/sulfamethoxazole (160 mg/800 mg) 1 double strength tablet bid for 7-14 days MRSA colonized carrier: • Topical mupirocin 2% ointment bid for 5 days to the nares in addition to other treatment
Gram negative	First line: • oral isotretinoin 0.5-1.0 mg/kg qd for 16-20 weeks Second line: • ampicillin 250-500 mg q6 h • trimethoprim-sulfamethoxazole 160/800 mg q12 h
Pseudomonas aeruginosa	Mild: • Self-limiting • Gentamicin 0.1% cream, povidone-iodine, or 1% acetic acid soaks 1-2 times a day for 7 days Moderate/severe or immunocompromised: • Ciprofloxacin 500 mg bid for 10 days plus topical
Fungal folliculitis	
Dermatophyte	Oral treatment required: • Micronized griseofulvin 500-1000 mg qd or ultra-micronized griseofulvin 500–700 mg qd for 4-6 weeks • Terbinafine 250 mg qd for 2-4 weeks • Fluconazole 200 mg qd for 4-6 weeks • Itraconazole 200 mg bid for 1 week per month for two pulses
Fungal folliculitis (Cont.)	
Pityrosporum	Topicals: • Topical imidazole antifungal creams—such as ketoconazole, clotrimazole, miconazole, or econazole cream bid for 2-4 weeks • Ciclopirox cream applied bid for 2-4 weeks • Selenium sulfide or ketoconazole shampoo used as a wash in the shower qd for 4 weeks Oral likely required in addition to topical: • Fluconazole 100-200 mg qd for 1-3 weeks • Itraconazole 200 mg qd for 1-3 weeks
Candida	Mild: • Topical azoles such as miconazole 2% cream bid until healing is complete • Topical nystatin 100,000 units/g cream bid until healing is complete Severe/recalcitrant: • Oral fluconazole 100 mg/day for 1 week, then qod for 1 month • Oral itraconazole 100 mg bid for 14 days
Viral folliculitis	
Herpes simplex	Oral antivirals required: • Famciclovir 500 mg TID for 5-10 days • Valacyclovir 500 mg TID for 5-10 days • Acyclovir 200 mg 5 times per day for 5-10 days
Parasitic folliculitis	
Demodex	Mild/Moderate: • Topical 5% permethrin cream • Sulfur products such as sodium sulfacetamide 10%/sulfur 5% wash • metronidazole cream/gel 1% • Dilute camphor oil applied qd for 2-4 weeks Long standing or severe cases: • Single dose of ivermectin 200 micrograms 1 qd one time

qd – once a day
bid – twice a day
tid – three times a day
qod – every other day
q6h – every 6 hours
q12h – every 12 hours

due to normal flora and other bacteria on the skin, but can also be caused by other factors; such as fungus, yeast, HSV, VZV, demodex mites, irritants, chemical agents, medications, physical trauma, or immunosuppression. This condition appears in both children and adults, and is particularly prevalent among those with darker skin of color who are HIV-positive.

Basic self-care measures and prevention is key to treating mild folliculitis. This includes frequent clothing changes, removal of restrictive clothing, washing skin regularly, treatment of hyperhidrosis, using antiperspirant; and the appropriate treatment of skin related conditions. Mild cases of infectious folliculitis should initially be treated with antibacterial soaps and washes. In moderate cases of infectious folliculitis, combining topical antibiotics to antibacterial soaps and washes is recommended. For more severe cases, empirical treatment including oral antibiotics is suggested to avoid worsening of symptoms or permanent scarring. In cases where inflammation extends deeper into the pilosebaceous unit, treatment becomes more difficult and may involve surgical drainage or longer courses of antibiotics. See **Table 47-1** for a list of common treatments for infectious folliculitis.

Pseudomonas folliculitis does not require treatment, however, in some cases, antipruritic treatment is required for the patient's symptoms. The most effective treatment for Gram-negative folliculitis is isotretinoin. However, in cases where it cannot be used, certain Gram-negative bacteria–sensitive antibiotics can be beneficial. *Pityrosporum* folliculitis is treated with an anti-yeast shampoo or cream, and permethrin can be used to treat Demodex folliculitis.

ACKNOWLEDGMENT

Dr. Kim Nichols contributed to this chapter in the second edition and some material from that chapter has been retained here.

REFERENCES

1. Laureano AC, Schwartz RA, Cohen PJ. Facial bacterial infections: folliculitis. *Clin Dermatol.* 2014;32(6):711-714.
2. Winters RD, Mitchell M. Folliculitis. [Updated 2022 May 1]. In: *StatPearls [Internet].* Treasure Island (FL): StatPearls Publishing; 2022 Jan-. https://www.ncbi.nlm.nih.gov/books/NBK547754/
3. Walsh SR, Johnson RP. Vaccinia folliculitis after primary Dryvax vaccination. *Infect Dis Clin Pract.* 2007;15(2):132-134.
4. Bolognia J, Schaffer J, Duncan K, Ko C. Folliculitis. In: *Dermatology Essentials.* Elsevier, Inc; 2014:268-287.

5. Theos KR, Johnson KM, Johnson DW. *Staphylococcus aureus* antibiotic susceptibilities in infections in an outpatient dermatology office on O'ahu. *Hawaii J Med Public Health*. 2019;78(5):163-168.
6. Boni R, Nehrhoff B. Treatment of gram-negative folliculitis in patients with acne. *Am J Clin Dermatol*. 2003;4:273-276.
7. Kuruvella T, Pandey S. Tinea Barbae. In: *StatPearls*. Treasure Island (FL): StatPearls Publishing; September 28, 2021. https://pubmed.ncbi.nlm.nih.gov/33085351/
8. Prindaville B, Belazarian L, Levin NA, Wiss K. Pityrosporum folliculitis: a retrospective review of 110 cases. *J Am Acad Dermatol*. 2018;78(3):511-514.
9. Durdu M, Güran M, Kandemir H, Ilkit M, Seyedmousavi S. Clinical and laboratory features of six cases of Candida and dermatophyte folliculitis and a review of published studies. *Mycopathologia*. 2016;181(1–2):97-105.
10. Elston CA, Elston DM. Demodex mites. *Clin Dermatol*. 2014;32(6):739-743.
11. Nomura T, Katoh M, Yamamoto Y, Miyachi Y, Kabashima K. Eosinophilic pustular folliculitis: a proposal of diagnostic and therapeutic algorithms. *J Dermatol*. 2016;43(11):1301-1306.
12. Chuh A. Eosinophilic folliculitis due to wearing protective gear in citizens volunteering for sanitation services during the COVID-19 pandemic - an original epidemiological, clinical, dermoscopic, and laboratory-based study. *Int J Dermatol*. 2020;59(12):1468-1474.
13. Ellis E, Scheinfeld N. Eosinophilic pustular folliculitis: a comprehensive review of treatment options. *Am J Clin Dermatol*. 2004;5(3):189-197.
14. Atanaskova N, Tomecki KJ. Innovative management of recurrent furunculosis. *Dermatol Clin*. 2010;28(3):479-487.

CHAPTER 48

Acne Vulgaris

Jennifer David
Tatiana Barrera
Sumayah Taliaferro
Valerie D. Callender

KEY POINTS

- Acne vulgaris is a common inflammatory skin condition that affects all ethnicities.
- Acne in skin of color populations is often complicated by postinflammatory hyperpigmentation, postinflammatory erythema, and acne scarring.
- Treatments of acne target the pathogenesis of acne and aim to reduce follicular hyperkeratinization, bacteria, sebum production, and inflammation.
- Treatments must include added considerations to minimize irritation, postinflammatory hyperpigmentation, and hypertrophic scarring.
- Oral agents including antibiotics, retinoids, hormonal and antiandrogen agents are effective for skin of color patients with acne.
- Selective and careful use of laser and procedural modalities are useful adjunctive treatments for acne in skin of color.

INTRODUCTION

Acne vulgaris is a multifactorial skin disorder that affects individuals of diverse ethnic backgrounds. However, when it comes to skin of color (SOC), the impact of acne takes on a distinctive clinical and therapeutic dimension. This chapter aims to shed light on the distinct characteristics and management strategies specific to patients of color. By addressing the epidemiology, pathophysiology, diagnostic challenges, and treatment considerations, we will explore how cultural and genetic factors contribute to the diverse clinical presentations and outcomes of acne vulgaris.

TABLE 48-1 Global incidence and prevalence of acne vulgaris in adult men and women ages 15 to 49 years

	Both sexes	Females	Males
Incidence			
Number of cases (millions) [Rate (per 100,000)]	117 [1585.9]	65.0 [1796]	52.4 [1384.9]
Prevalence			
Number of cases (millions) [Rate (per 100,000)]	231 [3703.3]	129 [3485.9]	103 [2675.9]

Source: https://www.healthdata.org/results/gbd_summaries/2019/acne-vulgaris-level-3-cause

EPIDEMIOLOGY

It is estimated that the global prevalence rate of acne among adults is 3703 per 100,000 [**Table 48-1**].[1] In the United States, acne is the number one reason for which patients with SOC visit a dermatologist, whereas the number one reason why White patients visit a dermatologist is for skin cancer screenings.[2] Acne compromised 34.7% of diagnoses among nearly 17,000 patients with chronic inflammatory skin diseases in the NIH All of Us Research Program who completed the Health Care Access and Utilization Survey.[3] Though not generalizable to the U.S. adult population, this cross-sectional analysis identified that between 40% and 53% of participants with SOC had reported a diagnosis of acne compared to 32% of their White counterparts.[3]

Nevertheless, despite the high prevalence of acne vulgaris in SOC populations—and their predisposition for more severe clinical presentation of active acne lesions, acne scarring, and postinflammatory hyperpigmentation (PIH)—patients from these backgrounds are not only understudied but also underserved as they experience significant barriers to healthcare and unique social determinants of health (SDOH) [**Table 48-2**]. It is estimated that less than 25% of clinical trials for chronic inflammatory skin diseases (CISD) like acne, atopic dermatitis, and psoriasis report race and ethnicity; among those that do, participants with SOC are notoriously underrepresented.[16] Furthermore, U.S. counties that are predominantly SOC experience a paucity of dermatologists: with 75% of predominantly Hispanic/Latinx, 86% of Black/African American, and 100% of Native American counties having not a single dermatologist.[17] Finding a dermatologist can be challenging for the more than one in four Black and Hispanic patients with acne who have Medicaid as their insurance.[4] Even when access to a dermatologist or higher insurance coverage is available, *accessibility* is often lacking in other ways. Patients with SOC are less likely to visit a dermatologist for their acne or receive a prescription for topical retinoids, oral antibiotics, spironolactone, and isotretinoin.[4] Language and literacy can be a major obstacle for those prescribed isotretinoin, as iPledge materials exceed the recommended readability (sixth-grade education level) for patient materials and are only available in English and Spanish, limiting access to patients who speak other languages.[18] Even when SOC acne patients do obtain dermatologic care, data show Black and Hispanic patients with CISD are approximately twice as likely to delay filling their prescriptions due to an inability to afford the cost compared to their White counterparts.[3] Thus, the high prevalence of acne in SOC patients along with their experiences in seeking and obtaining treatment must be understood to provide better quality of care, addressing active lesions, disease sequelae (scars, PIH), and preventive measures.

PATHOPHYSIOLOGY

Following the onset of puberty, the epidermal barrier function changes; depending on acne severity, this can result in up to 50% greater increases of transepidermal water loss (TEWL) in adolescent skin.[19] IGF-1, the principal mediator of growth hormone, increases during puberty, resulting in excess sebum and inflammatory cytokine production.[20] It is postulated that this creates the perfect environment for bacterial proliferation that

TABLE 48-2 Epidemiological data of acne vulgaris among SOC populations

	Frequency and prevalence of acne, PIH, and visits to dermatologist	Lack of representation in research and barriers to care
Black/African American (AA)	• Acne = #1 reason for visit; (9.2%) of all dermatology visits[2] • Conflicting data on whether or not Blacks/AA are more or less likely to see a dermatologist for their acne[3,4] (Of note: Barbieri found 1.20× more likely, but that depended on U.S. geographical location) • Prevalence of acne = 37%[5,6] Blacks PIH = 2 in 3 (65%) Black women.[5,6]	• Statistically lower odds of receiving any type of Rx for acne compared to Whites[4,14] • 1.25-1.35 times more likely to receive Rx for topical medications (eg, topical retinoids, antibiotics) compared to Whites[4] • Less likely to receive Rx for oral medications (eg, antibiotics, spironolactone, OCPs, isotretinoin)[4] • Black females on isotretinoin are significantly more likely to encounter treatment barriers (Rx interruptions and early termination)[15] • Only 16.8% of participant representation in acne clinical trials[16]* • Acne patients with insurance: 26.1% Medicaid; 12.0% Medicare[3]**
Hispanic/Latinx	• Prevalence of acne = 32% Hispanics/Latinx • PIH = 48% of Hispanic/Latinx females • Significantly less likely to see a dermatologist for acne (OR 0.78; 95% CI, 0.70-0.88)[4] • A study evaluating the prevalence of acne among 18-year-old men in Southern Brazil found that light skin color was protective against noninflammatory acne.[7]	• Significantly less Likely to receive Rx for OCPs, tretinoin and dapsone for their acne compared to Whites[4,14] • 23% participant representation in acne clinical trials[16]* • Acne patients with insurance: 28.5% Medicaid; 6.4% Medicare[3]**
Asian/Pacific Islander	• Cross-sectional observational study ($n = 419$): 50% of Indonesian females 20-30 years of age had acne and 71% had PIH[8] • 17 Asian countries were among the countries with the highest (top 10%) increase in acne-associated DALYs.[9] • Scarring and PIH are also major concerns for Asian patients, with one report of seven Asian countries suggesting one in two acne patients who visited a dermatologist had PIH.[6] • Prevalence of scarring among Singapore Chinese: <1% of participants with severe acne/grade 4 scarring[10] • Significantly less likely to see a dermatologist (0.82 OR; 95% CI 0.79-1.06)[4]	• 1.47 times more likely to receive Rx topical antibiotics[4] • Significantly less likely to receive Rx OCPs and oral antibiotics. • Only 1.2% of participant representation acne clinical trials[16]* • Acne patients with insurance: 8% Medicare[3]**
Native American	• Very little epidemiological data on the prevalence of acne among Native Americans • A national survey identified that 79% of participants reported having acne, compared to previous studies showing a 31% prevalence among Native Americans.[5,11] • In a national survey of Native Americans, 55% of participants reported a history of acne scaring.[11]	• Limited access to dermatologists via Native American health system: in that same national survey, 50% of participants endorsed having sought acne treatment by a clinician, but only 1 in 158 had seen a dermatologist for their acne.[11]

Middle Eastern	• Prevalence (approx.) reported in studies conducted in:
	  • Turkey = 61% of 13-18 years old
	  • Iran = 93% of 12-20 years old
	  • Israel = <1%, severe acne in 21-22 years old males[12]
	• 87.2% of Middle Eastern participants (with acne; FST III-VI) reported PIH, with one in two reporting the PIH had been present for at least 1 year.[13]
	• Slightly more likely to see a dermatologist for acne (OR 1.01; 95% CI, 0.94-1.08)[4]
		• Despite their usage of cultural or religious sun-protective clothing, Middle Eastern study participants reported PIH is still clinically present and bothersome.[13]

Abbreviations: AA: African American; CI, confidence intervals; FST, Fitzpatrick skin type; OCP: oral contraceptive pills; OR, odds ratio; PIH, postinflammatory hyperpigmentation, Rx: treatment.

*Among 26 clinical trials that reported race (over 15,000 participants); source: Sevagamoorthy A, Sockler P, Akoh C, Takeshita J. Racial and ethnic diversity of U.S. participants in clinical trials for acne, atopic dermatitis, and psoriasis: a comprehensive review. *J Dermatol Treat*. 2022;33(8):3086-3097.

**Experienced among patients with CISD; source: Nock MR, Barbieri JS, Krueger LD, Cohen JM. racial and ethnic differences in barriers to care among us adults with chronic inflammatory skin diseases: a cross-sectional study of the all of us research program. *J Am Acad Dermatol*. 2023;88(3):568-576.

leads to a disbalance of the skin microbiota. A crucial contributor to the inflammatory nature of acne vulgaris is the commensal bacteria *Cutibacterium acnes* (*C. acnes*), previously known *Propionibacterium acnes* that, along with *Staphylococcus epidermidis*, is known to colonize follicles in both unaffected and acne skin.[6,21] In biopsies of acne skin, *C. acnes* proliferation is visualized as biofilm-like structures that attach to follicle walls, hair shafts, and are contained within the lumen of the spinus granulosum.[22,23] Toll-like receptor 2 (TLR2) present on *C. acnes* have been postulated to promote inflammation via the release of proinflammatory cytokines such as IL-1, IL-8, and GM-CSF.[21] Furthermore, skin biopsies of patients with acne show significantly elevated JAK1 and JAK3 expression ($p < 0.001$), which play key roles in the pathogenesis of CISD.[20]

For the untrained eye, subclinical inflammation may be challenging to identify in SOC patients. However, compared to White patients, the degree of histopathologic inflammation in Black patients far outweighs the clinical appearance of inflammatory lesions.[6,24] Moreover, because the inflammatory process may precede the visible lesion and even the earliest of lesions can show significant macrophagic and neutrophilic infiltration, it is critical that acne treatments in SOC patients target inflammation to prevent permanent scarring and stubborn-to-treat PIH.[25,21] Under histologic inspection, acne lesions can demonstrate an atrophic epidermis and flat DEJ with inflammatory cell aggregates.[26] This inflammatory process then stimulates neighboring melanocytes to overproduce and abnormally deposit melanin,[25] thus resulting in postinflammatory erythema (PIE) and, particularly in darker skin phototypes, PIH.[25] In addition, melanocytes can contribute to the pathogenesis of keloids in patients with SOC by stimulating fibroblast growth and proliferation, augmenting ECM deposition and collagen synthesis, and activating inflammatory signaling pathways such as transforming growth factor-β. This results in a cascade of increased inflammation, scarring,

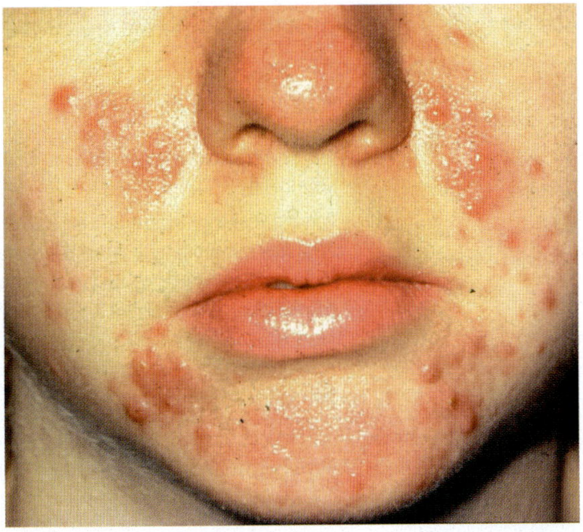

FIGURE 48-1 Acne vulgaris is a common skin disease seen from the preteen years through age 50.

and dyspigmentation in acne patients with darker skin phototypes [**Figure 48-1**].[6]

CLINICAL PRESENTATION

There are various subtypes of acne, of which we have highlighted in **Table 48-3** those that most commonly affect patients of SOC with racial and ethnic backgrounds.

ACNE SEQUELAE IN SKIN OF COLOR

Special considerations of acne in SOC include its propensity to cause scarring, PIH, and PIE [**Figure 48-2**]. Hyperpigmentation is a common sequela of acne in darker skin types. For some patients, it is more bothersome than the acne itself. Acne scarring and keloidal scarring are additional worrisome risks from acne eruptions on the skin, which tend to occur in those with recurrent acne and in ethnic skin.[39] Acne scarring may be classified as erythematous, atrophic, or hypertrophic types. A mix of the different types of scars may occur in the same patient.

ACNE SCARRING

Atrophic or hypertrophic scars occur when the inflammation from an inflamed papule or comedone spills out from the pore and damages surrounding collagen. Healthy tissue is replaced by scar tissue.[40] Timing, duration, and intensity of inflammation correlate with scar formation. It seems that early and prolonged inflammation elevates the risk of scarring. Factors that contribute to extended inflammation and affect scar development include mechanical forces and systemic factors. Hormonal changes during adolescence and pregnancy may affect risk for scarring.[41] High blood pressure levels might even pose an increased risk for keloids.[42] Genetic factors, although not fully elucidated, play a role. While inflammation is preeminent, other factors include levels of matrix metalloproteinases and its inhibitors. Currently, the role of bacteria and the microbiome are being explored as well. Overall, the mixed interplay of numerous factors creates propensity for scarring.

The majority of acne scars are atrophic (80-90%) [**Figure 48-3**]. Categories of atrophic acne scars include ice pick, rolling, and boxcar scars. Ice pick scars are defined by narrow (<2 mm) deep depressions that taper to a narrow base. Most atrophic scars are ice pick type (60% to 70%), V-shaped depressions that extend as far as the deep dermis and subcutaneous layer. Rolling scars, thought to represent 15% to 25% of atrophic scars, refer to wider and more shallow scars with an average measurement of 4 to 5 mm. They often have a sloping edge and form from adhesions of dermis and subcutis. Boxcar scars, representing 20% to 30% of atrophic scars, are rectangular or U-shaped depressions characterized by sharply defined edges, measuring 1 to 4 mm wide. Their sharp edges may dip 0.1 to 0.5 mm deep.[41]

Treatment of atrophic acne scars include chemical peels, particularly salicylic acid, glycolic acid, and trichloroacetic acid (TCA) peels.[43] The TCA cross technique, which offers chemical reconstruction of skin scars, is an effective treatment.[44] Dermabrasion helps clear acne scars, but is not a safe treatment modality in SOC. Surgical treatments include subcision and the punch technique method.[45] Other treatments include microneedling and laser resurfacing.[46] Fractionated laser resurfacing and nonablative 1064 Nd:YAG lasers are considered safer for darker skin types and performing a test spot is highly recommended [**Figure 48-4**]. Fillers, fat transfer, and Platelet rich plasma injections are also used to improve the appearance of acne scars. A combination of these treatments is commonly employed when treating patients for acne scarring, as no one definitive treatment is considered gold standard.[47]

Hypertrophic scars are raised but confined to the size of the injured skin or original wound. In contrast, keloids extend beyond the size of the original wound. Papular acne scars are hypertrophic skin-colored papules that commonly occur on the chin and back [Figure 48-3]. In a study of 416 patients (all FST III or IV), almost all (98%) had atrophic scars, approximately 13% had keloid scars, and 11% had papular scars. Papular scars were significantly more prevalent in patients with keloid scars compared to those without keloid scars.[48]

Experts suggest that keloids and hypertrophic scars form from the same fibrinogenic process of normal wound healing but marked by different degrees of inflammation present during the process. Chronic inflammation that results in hypertrophic and keloidal scars occurs at the level of the reticular dermis.[49] Generally, injuries to the skin causing inflammation more superficially do not cause hypertrophic and keloidal scarring. For this reason, treatment of scars must occur at the subdermal level. Not surprisingly, more successful treatment options for keloids involve controlling inflammation on this plane: intralesional corticosteroid, radiotherapy, and cryotherapy. Topical treatments, while beneficial, often do not penetrate deep enough to effectively treat scars, particularly hypertrophic and keloidal scars [**Figure 48-5**].

Delays in treatment of acne and disease severity increase the risk of scarring. However, acne severity does not always correlate with scarring. Patients with almost clear and mild acne may develop acne scars as well as patients with moderate and severe acne. Scars from acne may lead to profound psychosocial effects. Awareness and recognition of risk factors along with early and persistent treatment may decrease its burden on patients.

POSTINFLAMMATORY HYPERPIGMENTATION

PIH is a known manifestation of cutaneous injury and inflammation and a common complication of acne in SOC [Figure 48-2]. PIH causes significant psychosocial distress in patients. Thus, addressing acne comprehensively in SOC patients calls for thoughtful consideration of this coexisting effect. In PIH, the skin darkens beyond its normal color and is distributed in the same area of the preceding inflammatory skin condition. PIH occurs when inflammatory processes stimulate melanocyte activity. Effects of cytokines and inflammatory mediators include an increase in production of melanin by melanocytes. This results in an overproduction of melanin and irregular accelerated transfer of melanin to keratinocytes. Intense inflammation may also weaken barriers of basal keratinocytes and result in leakage of melanin into the dermis. The free melanin is taken up by dermal melanophages. Histopathology of hyperpigmented skin shows greater amounts of melanin in keratinocytes and in some cases dermal macrophages. Dermal hyperpigmentation often has a blue-gray color and is more resistant to treatment. Naturally, epidermal and dermal PIH exists more in darker skin types due to a greater amount of melanin in the basal layer and more active melanocytes.[50] Treatment with hydroquinone and other tyrosinase inhibitors are mainstays of treatment for PIH.[51]

TABLE 48-3 Acne subtypes common in SOC populations, with their respective clinical presentation, age of onset, distribution, and other considerations among SOC patients

	Clinical presentation	Age onset	Location/distribution of most affected areas	Important factors

Comedonal acne[6,27]	• Most acne lesions are noninflammatory
	• Consists of:
	  • comedones (sebaceous follicles that contain abnormal desquamated corneocytes, lipids, and monofilaments)
	  • open comedones (blackheads; follicles with dilated openings) and closed comedones (white heads; follicle is completely blocked)
		• All ages, including infants and newborns (neonatal and infantile acne)
		• May occur in premenarchal girls, indicating pubarche (onset of puberty)
		• May occur in adult and adolescent females in the late luteal phase of the menstrual cycle
			• Forehead
			• Temples
			• Chin
			• Hairline (ie, pomade acne)
				• May be a precursor of other and/or inflammatory acne lesions
				• Pomade acne is associated with the use of comedogenic hair care products. It presents with closely packed, closed comedones, and small inflammatory papules along the margins of the scalp and forehead. Most observed in patients of African or Asian descent, those with tightly coiled hair, and users of thick oils or waxes as hair products.

Acne vulgaris[6,25,28-31]	• May present with recurrent comedones, papules, pustules, and/or nodules in all skin phototypes. • Treating PIH is often of greater concern in SOC patients with acne vulgaris than treating active lesions[25,28] • Greater acne severity is associated with PIH and keloidal scars in SOC patients[6]	• Incidence peak (among all skin phototypes): 14-17 years (female) versus 16-19 years (male)[29] • Affects approximately 12-22% of U.S. women in their adult life[29]	• Active lesions may vary by gender and age. • In adult women (all phototypes): lower one-third face[29] • Adults >40 years and smokers: frontal and side regions of the face[29] • PIH: jawline and trunk[6]	• Acne lesions, along with their treatments, can result in dyspigmentation in all skin phototypes, but is more common—and harder to treat—in patients with SOC.[30] • Challenge: differentiating PIH (brown-to-violaceous in tone) from erythema associated with active lesions. Tool that may assist clinicians: post-acne hyperpigmentation index (PAHPI)[31]
Hormonal acne (adult female acne)[32]	• May present as acne that does not improve with traditional treatments. • Patient may report trends in worsening, such as around the timing of menses or ovulation	Predominantly affects females >25	• Chin • Jawline	• Postulated that chronic stress in patients with hyperandrogenism can contribute to increased androgen secretion and sebaceous gland stimulation. • Screen for endocrine-related conditions (eg, PCOS, ovarian/adrenal hyperangdrogenism).
Acne rosacea[27,28]	• Less frequently reported: persistent facial erythema • Noncomedonal, acneiform pustules and papules, primarily in the central face • Dry, edematous, and hyperpigmented skin • Thickened nasal and cheek skin • Ocular symptoms: itching, irritation, foreign body sensation, or increased presence of "eye boogers" • Telangiectasias (identified via dermoscopy) • Four subtypes: erythematotelangiectatic (ETR); papulopustular; glandular hyperplastic or phymatous rosacea (most common in SOC); and ocular. • Most important factor in diagnosis is a patient's self-reported history and observations, including flushing, burning, increased warmth, and stinging. These signs may be exacerbated by typical rosacea triggers (heat, stress, spicy foods).	• More commonly identified in women with SOC than men with SOC	• Malar region • Perioral • Periocular	• Reported in up to 10% of darker skin types (FST IV-V), but this may be an underestimation due to failure to recognize erythema against a more pigmented skin phototype.[27] • Inquire about use of skin-lightening products, as these can exacerbate or precipitate rosacea.[27] • Erythema may only be visualized with photography against a blue background or when triggered, such as when pressed against the skin with a slide or glass to visualize redness or blanching. • Due to the presence of papules and pustules, some patients may report a history of being [erroneously] diagnosed and treated for acne with no improvement. Those with positive family histories have a higher genetic predisposition for developing rosacea.
Acne excoriée[32,33]	• Associated with the repetitive scratching, squeezing, picking, or rubbing of skin and/or skin lesions (eg, acne lesions or scars) • Patients may report experiencing an uncontrollable urge to pick at the skin	All ages	• Face • Upper extremities • Areas that a patient's hand can reach. For example, "butterfly pattern" with central clearing on a patient's back due to the physical limitation of reaching behind to pick at the skin	• May be a manifestation of obsessive-compulsive processes (eg, skin picking disorder) or other illnesses (eg, Prader-Willi syndrome) • Increased risk of PIH, scarring, and infection • Treatment should address underlying lesions (acne vulgaris, comedones) and the behavioral aspect (psychologic therapy, physical barriers, etc)

(*Continued*)

TABLE 48-3 Acne subtypes common in SOC populations, with their respective clinical presentation, age of onset, distribution, and other considerations among SOC patients (*Continued*)

	Clinical presentation	Age onset	Location/distribution of most affected areas	Important factors
Acne fulminans (AF)[34,35]	• Rare • Severe, acute, abrupt onset • Large inflammatory lesions (erosions, nodules, plaques, ulcers) with hemorrhagic crusting • Presents with fevers, ulcers, and polyarthritis. • May also include osteolytic bone lesions	• Adolescent males >> females • 2 years duration of acne prior to AF onset	• Face • Chest/Back • Extremities (less common)	• Laboratory findings may include leukocytosis, elevated ESR, transaminases. • Biopsies: neutrophils in epidermis and dermis, as well as around hair follicles • Can be triggered by the usage of anabolic steroids- testosterone. • Associated with patients taking isotretinoin but may arise de novo.
Acne conglobata[32]	• Chronic, severe nodulocystic acne • Deep interconnected polymorphous comedones, nodules, abscesses, and cysts • Lesions drain purulent contents onto the skin.	• Infancy and adulthood • More common in adults	Broad including face, scalp, upper and lower extremities, trunk, axillae, groin, and buttocks.	• High risk for severe PIH and scarring • Has been reported among patients abusing anabolic-androgenic steroids, adalimumab (TNF-α inhibitor), and pyoderma gangrenosum
Steroid-induced acne[36,37]	• Assoc. w/use of skin-lightening products that contain steroids (commonly used by SOC populations) • Patients may use these products to treat their acne-related pigmentation or other dyspigmentary disorders. • Will present w/ new-onset acne or exacerbation of preexisting acne. • May also present with erythema, telangiectasia, hyper/hypo- pigmentation, acneiform eruption, hypertrichosis, rosacea, photosensitivity, and/or skin atrophy.[36,37]	Predominantly affects females in their 20-30s[36,37]	Face	• Skin-lightening products: may contain class I topical steroids that can result in increased comedogenesis[27] • South African study: steroid-induced acne was reportedly the second most commonest subtype of acne (12.7%) seen in tertiary derm clinics.[38] • This highlights the importance of inquiring about the use of steroid use and/or skin-lightening creams or skin care products purchased overseas (where prescription strength steroids can be easily obtained). Patients may not be aware that the products contain steroids. • Treat the underlying PIH (for those using it to lighten skin) and acne (for those using it to treat acne).

PCOS, polycystic ovarian syndrome; PIH: postinflammatory hyperpigmentation; SOC, skin of color.

POSTINFLAMMATORY ERYTHEMA

PIE also results from inflammation of the skin and may become long-standing in some patients [**Figure 48-6**].[52] It may occur as a sequela of an inflammatory skin condition such as acne or trauma of the skin such as a burn. PIE is important to recognize and address as it may persist and become cosmetically unacceptable and progress into PIH.

Sunscreen use is crucial in preventing long-term erythema and hyperpigmentation. Avoiding irritants during treatment of acne and especially after procedures used to treat acne helps to prevent exacerbation of PIE. Treatments employed to reduce PIE include use of topical niacinamide, azelaic acid, metronidazole, topical corticosteroids, topical tranexamic acid, and antioxidants, particularly vitamin C.[53] Topical antihistamines and α-adrenergic blockers (oxymetazoline and brimonidine) are reported in the medical literature to improve PIE.[54,55] Emollients containing ceramides and silicone gels are also reported to minimize erythema. When there is major concern for ensuing hyperpigmentation, cautious treatments with hydroquinone are employed and helpful in

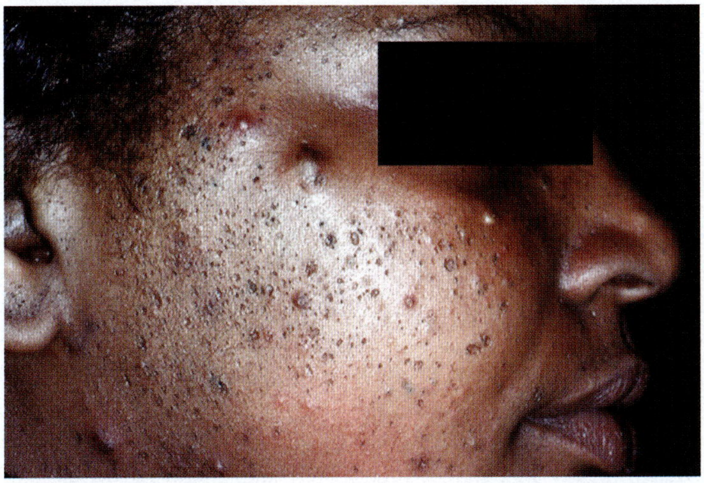

FIGURE 48-2 Papules, ice pick scars, pustules, open comedones, and postinflammatory hyperpigmentation in a patient with acne.

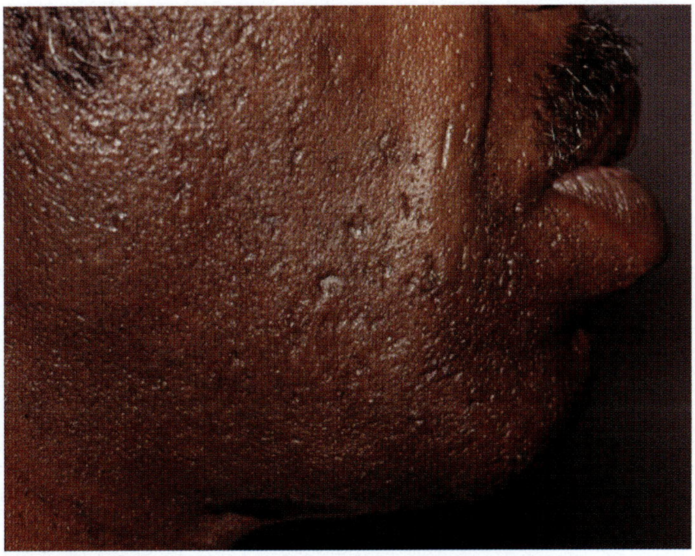

FIGURE 48-3 Postacne scarring in an African American patient.

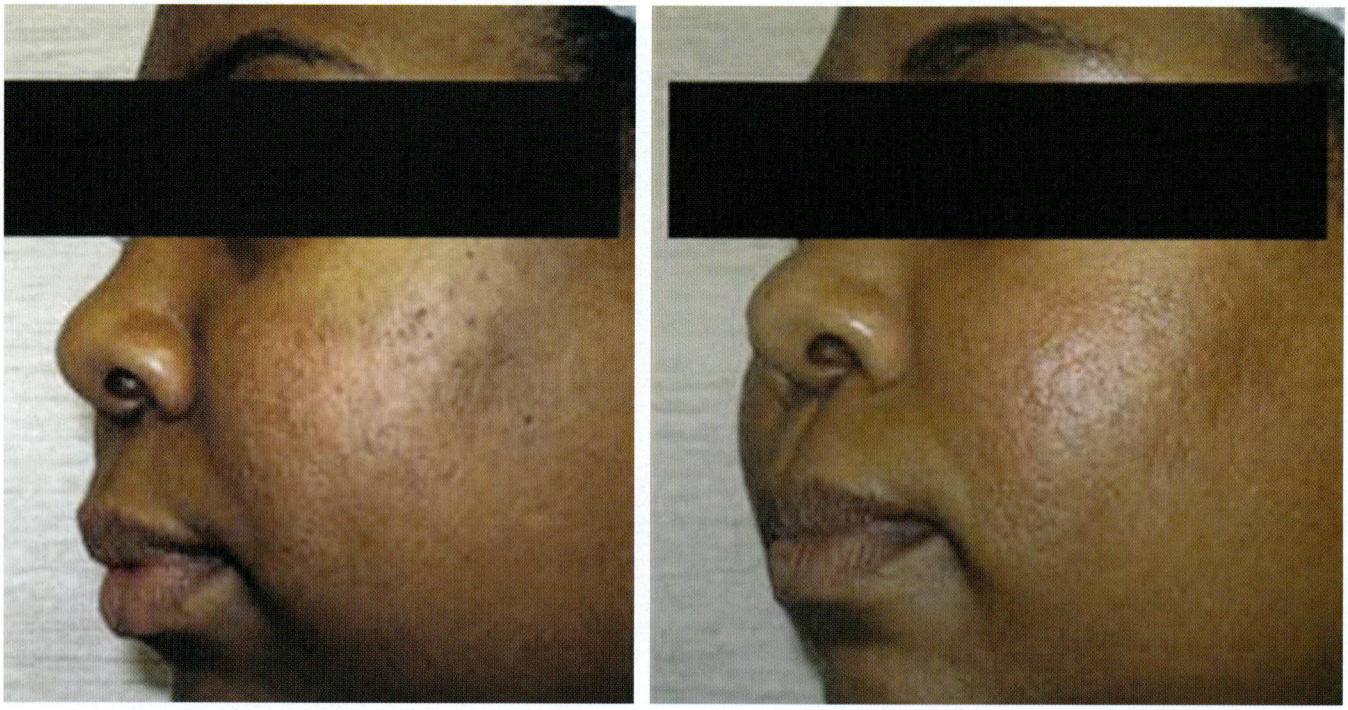

A B

FIGURE 48-4 **(A)** Acne scarring. **(B)** Some improvement after two treatments with a fractionated laser.

some cases. Even under the best care, persistent erythema may develop. Successful use of intense pulse light (IPL) and vascular lasers to treat PIE is well-documented as a treatment option but are of limited use in darker skin types. However, laser treatments such as the 650 microsecond 1064 Nd:YAG and carefully selected fractional laser treatments may yield notable improvements in PIE in darker skin.[56]

TREATMENT

GOAL OF ACNE THERAPY

The goal of acne therapy is to reduce follicular hyperkeratosis, bacteria, sebum production, inflammation, and PIH.[57,58] Treatment regimens for acne vulgaris in SOC patients are similar to those for fair skin patients. In order to achieve these goals, there are many factors one must take into account when selecting the best treatment regimen for each patient, especially if they have deeply pigmented skin. The basic considerations for all patients include the type and severity of acne, location of lesions, current treatments, prior failed treatments, allergies, and pregnancy status. As noted in prior sections, inflammation is the underlying factor involved in the pathophysiology of acne itself and is also the driving force behind the secondary disease processes of PIH, PIE, and scarring. Thus, considering a patient's skin sensitivity and tolerability level is imperative when selecting topical agents for patients of color in order to minimize the risk of inflammation. This may involve opting for gentler formulations (eg, creams over gels), avoiding products with fragrance, selecting lower strength prescription agents, spacing out the frequency of their use, and then gradually increasing both over time.

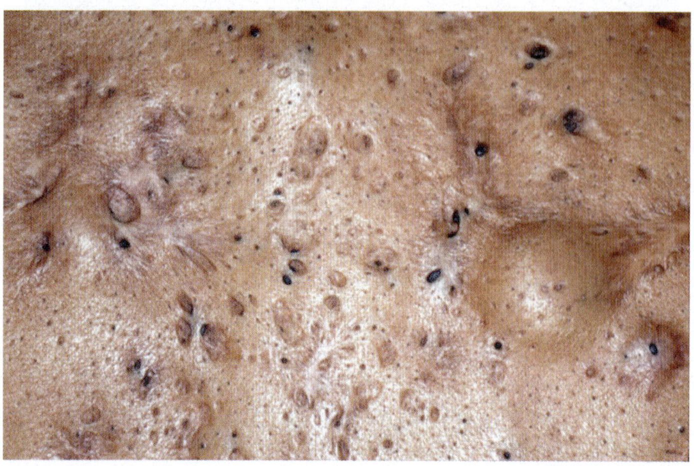

FIGURE 48-5 A patient with acne located on the upper back nodules, cysts, open and closed comedones, and hypertrophic scars can be seen.

Taylor et al has classified SOC into three categories to assist in the selection of topical therapeutic agents[58]:

1. Dry/sensitive → skin with propensity to irritant reactions
2. Normal → skin with minimal propensity to irritant reactions
3. Oily → skin with no propensity to irritant reactions

Selection of appropriate agents may be enhanced by taking skin type into consideration. For example, a patient with dry skin is more likely to experience irritation, secondary to the gel or foam formulation of topical medications, especially during the winter months or in areas of low humidity. Hence, cream formulations are appropriate for this type of patient during the winter months, but a regimen may include a gel formulation during the hot and humid summer months. **Table 48-4** offers a comprehensive review of treatment options, and special considerations to keep in mind when treating SOC.

TREATMENT APPROACHES FOR ACNE VULGARIS IN SKIN OF COLOR PATIENTS

TOPICAL TREATMENTS

Topical treatments play a pivotal role in managing acne vulgaris in patients with SOC. Among the various options available, retinoids have demonstrated efficacy in reducing acne lesions and improving overall skin appearance. When selecting appropriate formulations and concentrations of retinoids for SOC patients, it is essential to consider their potential to cause irritation and PIH. Studies have shown that low-strength retinoid

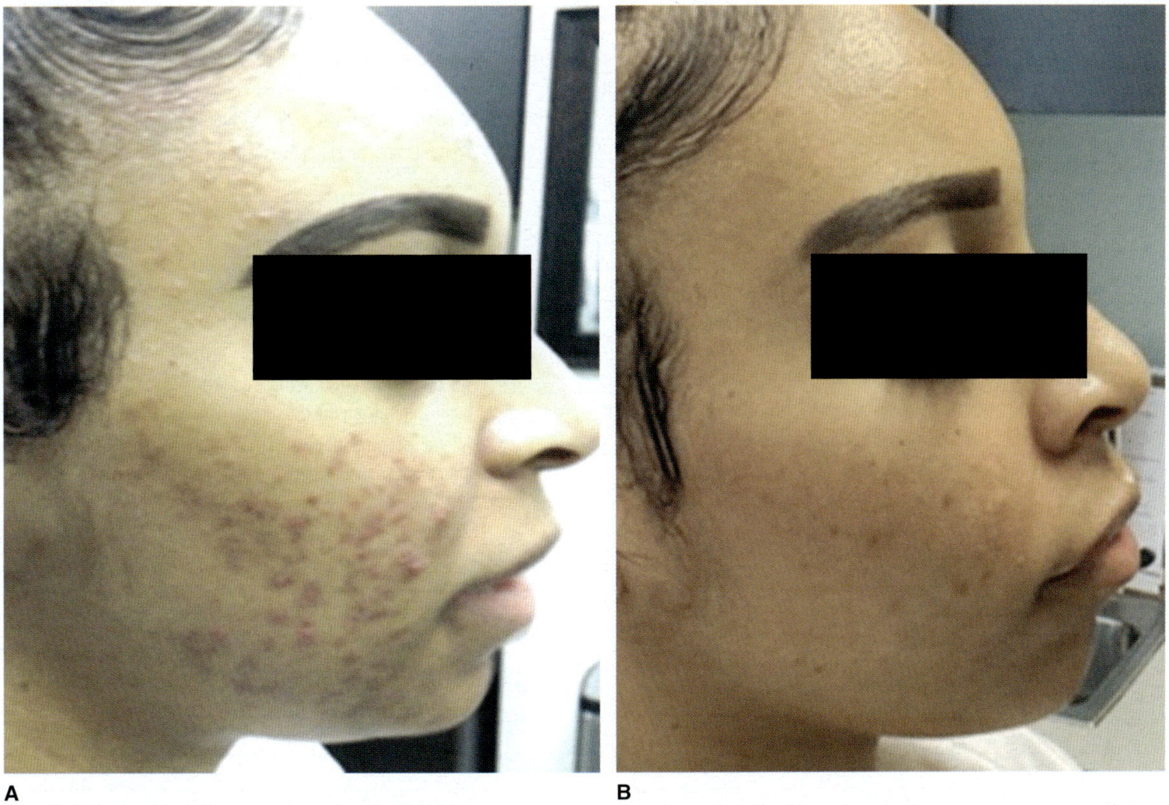

FIGURE 48-6 **(A)** Inflammatory acne with postinflammatory erythema and postinflammatory hyperpigmentation. **(B)** Improvement after treatment with isotretinoin.

TABLE 48-4 Treatment options for acne vulgaris in skin of color

Treatment	Dose and formulation	Level of evidence	Special considerations in skin of color
Topical treatments			
Over-the-counter therapy			
Benzoyl peroxide	2.5-10% wash, bar, gel, foam, lotion, or cream daily or twice daily	I and II	• Provides both antibacterial and comedolytic effects. Its efficacy in managing acne and preventing PIH has been well-documented.[59] • Consider once daily application in the morning to avoid potentiating dryness/irritation if mixed with nightly retinoid.
Adapalene	0.1% gel daily	I and II	• Consider starting every other night and slowly increase as tolerated • Combine with moisturizer to avoid dryness/irritation
Salicylic acid	0.5-2% wash, gel, toner, cream daily or twice daily	I	• Very effective in treating comedonal/pomade acne in skin of color patients • Introduce into regimen as a wash 2-3 times per week, beginning with lowest concentration • Avoid directly mixing with retinoids (ie, use SA wash/cream/toner in the morning only or at nights when taking a break from retinoids)
Azelaic acid	12% cream, serum	III	• Effectively reduce inflammatory and noninflammatory acne lesions.[60] • Generally well tolerated in all skin types • Treats both acne and PIH
Prescription single-agent therapy			
Erythromycin	2% gel, pad, or solution daily	I and II	• Selecting antibiotics with broader spectra, such as clindamycin or erythromycin, can minimize the risk of allergic reactions, while periodic reassessment of treatment response and potential switch to nonantibiotic alternatives should be considered to prevent resistance development
Clindamycin	1% pledget, lotion, solution, or foam daily	I and II	
Minocycline	1.5%, 4% foam	I and II	
Adapalene	0.3% gel daily	I and II	• Consider starting at a low concentration and applying 2-3 nights a week and then slowly increase as tolerated • "Sandwiching" between layers of moisturizers to prevent dryness/irritation • Choosing formulations such as creams, lotions, and aqueous gels with hydrating ingredients may decrease the risk of dry skin and irritation
Tretinoin	0.025%, 0.05%, or 0.1% cream or gel daily or 0.04%, 0.08%, or 0.1% microgel daily	I and II	
Trifarotene	0.005% cream daily	I and II	
Tazarotene	0.045%, 0.05%, or 0.1% cream, gel, or foam	I and II	

(*Continued*)

TABLE 48-4 Treatment options for acne vulgaris in skin of color (*Continued*)

Treatment	Dose and formulation	Level of evidence	Special considerations in skin of color
Dapsone	5% or 7.5% gel daily or twice daily	I and II	• Both topical dapsone 5% and 7.5% gel are effective and safe in treating moderate acne in extensive studies including SOC patients. • Well-tolerated and effective for both inflammatory and noninflammatory lesions
Clascoterone	1% cream	I and II	
Azelaic acid	15%, 20% cream	I and II	Acne and PIH
Prescription fixed-dose combination therapy			
Benzoyl peroxide-erythromycin	5% benzoyl peroxide/3% erythromycin gel daily	I	• These combinations address different aspects of the pathogenesis of acne, including bacterial overgrowth, inflammation, and hyperkeratinization.[59] • The synergistic effect of these agents helps to optimize treatment outcomes while minimizing the risk of adverse events when treating skin of color. • Tolerable formulations such as creams, lotions, and aqueous gels with hydrating ingredients may decrease the risk of dry skin and irritation
Benzoyl peroxide-clindamycin	5% benzoyl peroxide/1% clindamycin gel; 3.75% benzoyl peroxide/1.2% clindamycin; 2.5% benzoyl peroxide/1.2% clindamycin gel	I	
Adapalene-benzoyl peroxide	0.1% adapalene/5% benzoyl peroxide; 0.3% adapalene/5% benzoyl peroxide	I and II	
Tretinoin-benzoyl peroxide	0.1% tretinoin/3% cream	I	
Tretinoin-clindamycin	0.025% tretinoin/1.2% clindamycin gel	I	
Systemic treatments			
Antibiotic agents			
Doxycycline	100 mg daily or twice daily, 20 mg twice daily, or 40 mg daily with delayed release	I and II	• Short-term use (up to 3 months), intermittent dosing, and combination with topical treatments can optimize treatment outcomes while minimizing adverse effects.
Minocycline	100 mg daily or twice daily	I and II	
Tetracycline	500 mg daily or twice daily	I and II	
Serecycline	60 mg, 90 mg, 150 mg once daily	I and II	
Hormonal agents			
Combined oral contraceptives	Ethinyl estradiol-norgestimate daily, ethinyl estradiol-norethindrone daily, or ethinyl estradiol-drospirenone daily	I	• Regulate hormones and sebum production, leading to improved acne outcomes • Regular monitoring for potential side effects, such as venous thromboembolism or changes in blood pressure, is necessary
Spironolactone	25-100 mg daily or twice daily	II and III	• Inhibit androgen receptor binding and reducing sebum production
Retinoid			
Isotretinoin	0.5 mg/kg/day, increasing to 1 mg/kg/day after 1 month	I and II	• A highly effective treatment option for severe and recalcitrant acne vulgaris in patients with SOC. • Consider slower titration to full dose during winter months to avoid excessive dryness and subsequent irritation

*Levels of evidence are classified with the use of the Strength of Recommendation Taxonomy as follows: level I (good quality, patient-oriented evidence [ie, evidence measuring outcomes that matter to patients, including death, complications, symptom abatement, cost reduction, and quality of life]), level II (limited-quality, patient-oriented evidence), and level III (other evidence, including consensus guidelines, opinion, case studies, and disease-oriented evidence [ie, evidence measuring intermediate, physiologic, or surrogate end points that may or may not reflect improvements in patient outcomes]).

formulations, such as adapalene 0.1% or tretinoin 0.025%, can effectively improve acne lesions without significant adverse effects in patients with skin of color.[61] Careful monitoring and gradual titration of retinoid concentrations are recommended to minimize the risk of skin irritation and enhance treatment compliance. Newer aqueous gel formulations and microsphere formulations, which allow for the controlled release of tretinoin, may also lead to less irritation and be better tolerated.[62]

In addition to retinoids, antibiotics are frequently employed as topical treatments in acne management. However, their use should be approached cautiously in SOC patients due to the potential for hypersensitivity reactions and the risk of developing antibiotic resistance. Studies have highlighted the need for balancing the efficacy of antibiotic treatment with sensitivity concerns in this population.[63] Selecting antibiotics with broader spectra, such as clindamycin or erythromycin, can minimize the risk of allergic reactions, while periodic reassessment of treatment response and potential switch to nonantibiotic alternatives should be considered to prevent resistance development.

Azelaic acid has emerged as a versatile treatment option for acne vulgaris in patients with SOC. This dicarboxylic acid exhibits antibacterial and anti-inflammatory properties while simultaneously inhibiting hyperpigmentation. Azelaic acid has been shown to effectively reduce inflammatory and noninflammatory acne lesions, making it a valuable therapeutic choice for patients with SOC.[60] Furthermore, the role of azelaic acid in addressing PIH makes it a preferred option in this population.

Benzoyl peroxide remains a cornerstone in acne treatment for SOC patients, as it provides both antibacterial and comedolytic effects. Its efficacy in managing acne and preventing PIH has been well-documented.[59] However, caution must be exercised to minimize potential irritation, particularly when using higher concentrations. Gradual introduction, short contact therapy, and combination with other agents can optimize its efficacy while reducing adverse effects.

Combination products that incorporate multiple active ingredients, such as benzoyl peroxide with clindamycin or adapalene, offer enhanced treatment efficacy in managing acne vulgaris in patients with SOC. These combinations address different aspects of the pathogenesis of acne, including bacterial overgrowth, inflammation, and hyperkeratinization.[59] The synergistic effect of these agents helps to optimize treatment outcomes while minimizing the risk of adverse events. Individualized selection of combination products based on the severity and type of acne lesions can lead to improved treatment response in SOC patients.

Salicylic acid, a beta-hydroxy acid, has demonstrated effectiveness in addressing comedonal acne, a common presentation in patients with SOC. Its lipophilic properties allow it to penetrate sebaceous follicles and exfoliate the stratum corneum, promoting the resolution of comedones.[64] Salicylic acid can be incorporated into cleansers, toners, and leave-on products, making it a versatile choice for acne management. However, its potential to cause skin irritation and dryness should be considered, and lower concentrations are often recommended in patients with SOC to minimize the risk of PIH.

ORAL TREATMENT OPTIONS

Oral treatments play a crucial role in the management of moderate to severe acne vulgaris in skin of color patients. Antibiotics, such as tetracyclines (eg, doxycycline, minocycline, sarecycline), are commonly prescribed to address the inflammatory component of acne. However, the selection of suitable agents and duration of use should be carefully considered. Tetracyclines have shown efficacy in reducing acne lesions; however, their potential to cause photosensitivity and gastrointestinal side effects must be weighed against their benefits.[65] Short-term use, intermittent dosing, and combination with topical treatments can optimize treatment outcomes while minimizing adverse effects.

Oral contraceptives, particularly those containing ethinyl estradiol and antiandrogenic progestins, offer an additional treatment option for managing acne in skin of color patients, especially in cases related to hormonal imbalances. Oral contraceptives help regulate hormones and sebum production, leading to improved acne outcomes.[66] Selecting appropriate formulations based on the individual's medical history, contraindications, and preferences is crucial. Regular monitoring for potential side effects, such as venous thromboembolism or changes in blood pressure, is necessary when prescribing oral contraceptives.

Isotretinoin, a potent retinoid, represents a highly effective treatment option for severe and recalcitrant acne vulgaris in patients with SOC. Despite concerns about its potential to induce adverse cutaneous reactions, careful assessment of risks and benefits can guide its appropriate use in this population. Several studies have demonstrated the effectiveness of isotretinoin in reducing acne lesions and improving quality of life, including in patients with SOC [Figure 48-6].[67] Close monitoring for potential adverse effects, including dyspigmentation or keloid formation, is essential during isotretinoin therapy in SOC patients.

Spironolactone and other antiandrogen medications are considered valuable options for managing hormonal acne in patients with SOC. These agents work by inhibiting androgen receptor binding and reducing sebum production.[68] Spironolactone has demonstrated efficacy in improving acne outcomes in women. Close monitoring for potential side effects, such as menstrual irregularities or hyperkalemia, is necessary when prescribing antiandrogen medications.

Corticosteroids, when used judiciously and under close medical supervision, can be employed to address inflammatory acne lesions in SOC patients. Intralesional corticosteroid injections are particularly beneficial in managing large, painful nodules or cysts, hastening their resolution and reducing the risk of scarring.[69] However, potential side effects associated with corticosteroid use, such as hypopigmentation or skin atrophy, should be carefully considered, and cautious injection technique is essential to minimize adverse events

COMBINATION AND SEQUENTIAL THERAPY APPROACHES

Combination therapy involving the concurrent use of topical and oral agents can offer improved outcomes in the management of acne vulgaris in SOC patients. By addressing multiple pathogenic factors simultaneously, combination therapy targets different aspects of acne pathogenesis, such as inflammation, bacterial overgrowth, and hyperkeratinization.[70] For example, combining topical retinoids or benzoyl peroxide with oral antibiotics can enhance efficacy while minimizing antibiotic resistance development.[71] Close monitoring of treatment response and potential side effects is essential when employing combination therapy, ensuring an individualized approach to optimize outcomes.

Sequential therapy involves the use of different treatment modalities at different stages of acne management to achieve optimal results. This approach allows for a stepwise escalation or de-escalation of treatment intensity based on the patient's response and disease severity.[72] For instance, starting with topical treatments and then escalating to oral therapies can be effective for moderate to severe acne. Conversely, as acne improves, a gradual step-down approach involving the discontinuation of oral treatments while maintaining topical therapies may be appropriate to maintain remission and minimize potential side effects. Close monitoring and regular follow-up assessments are crucial to guide the appropriate timing of treatment adjustments and ensure sustained improvement.

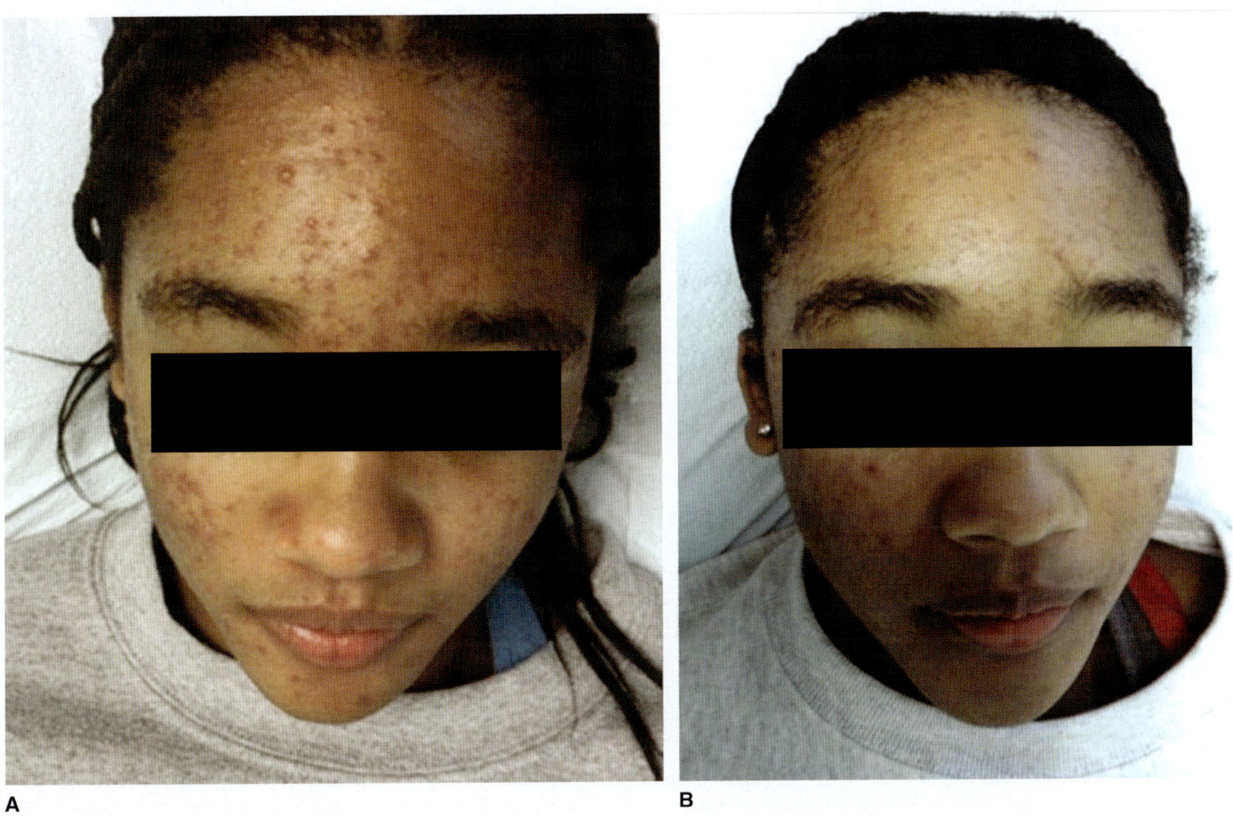

FIGURE 48-7 (A) Acne with PIH and PIE. **(B)** Improvement after TCA chemical peels and laser treatments with 650 microsecond 1064 Nd/YAG laser.

INTEGRATING PROCEDURAL AND LASER-BASED TREATMENTS

Procedural and laser-based treatments offer additional therapeutic modalities for acne management in SOC patients. These procedures can be employed as adjunctive therapies to address specific concerns, such as PIH, acne scarring, or persistent comedonal acne. Chemical peels, microdermabrasion, and fractional lasers are among the options available [Figure 48-4].[62] However, careful consideration of the patient's skin type, potential adverse effects (eg, hyperpigmentation or hypopigmentation), and the experience and expertise of the provider is necessary to ensure optimal outcomes. Integration of procedural and laser-based treatments should be based on individual patient needs and preferences, with an emphasis on minimizing the risk of complications and achieving the desired aesthetic results.

CHEMICAL PEELS

Chemical peels can be useful in acne patients, particularly those with hyperpigmentation and/or scarring [**Figure 48-7**]. Glycolic acid (GA) in concentration of 20% to 70% and salicylic acid (SA) in concentrations of 20% to 30% are used commonly.[73] Superficial chemical peels can accelerate the removal of epidermal melanin and increase the penetration and potentially the efficacy of topical treatments for acne and dyspigmentation.[74] Grimes demonstrated improvement of acne in 67% of patients and in PIH in 80% of patients treated with a series of five salicylic acid peels at 2-week intervals.[75] A study done on Korean patients found that SA peels can also cause lightening of patient's normal skin as well as a decrease in erythema.[76] Another commonly used peel is Jessner solution, which is a combination of resorcinol, salicylic acid, and lactic acid in ethanol, and causes keratolysis by decreasing keratinocytes cohesion. Studies have shown that for acne treatment, Jessner is most effective when used in combination with other peels. Salicylic-mandelic acid (SMA) peels are a combination peel combining SA with mandelic acid, an alpha hydroxy acid that penetrates the epidermis more slowly and uniformly, an advantage for treating sensitive skin patients with severe acne and pigmentary issues.[77] A study done in India on 44 patients (skin types IV-VI) comparing glycolic acid peels with SMA peels found that SMA peels had higher efficacy for most active acne lesions and hyperpigmentation.[77] SMA peels may also be a good alternative option to use in patients who have shown more resistance to other peels. Deeper chemical peels, such as phenol, although potentially more effective than superficial and medium depth peels, should be avoided in darker skin types to avoid dyspigmentation and scarring. Chemical peels should be used conservatively in the SOC population to avoid adverse effects such as PIH and scarring. Physicians should start at the lowest concentration and discontinue use of retinoids 1 week prior to treatment and 1 week after treatment.

CONCLUSION

In conclusion, the treatment of acne vulgaris in SOC patients requires a tailored approach that considers the unique characteristics and challenges of this population. Topical treatments, such as retinoids, antibiotics, azelaic acid, benzoyl peroxide, and salicylic acid, offer effective options for managing acne lesions while minimizing the risk of PIH and adverse effects. Oral treatments, including antibiotics, oral contraceptives, isotretinoin, spironolactone, corticosteroids, and zinc supplements, address systemic factors contributing to acne and can be integrated into treatment regimens when necessary.

Combination therapy and sequential approaches optimize treatment outcomes, and procedural or laser-based treatments serve as valuable adjunctive therapies for specific concerns. By understanding these treatment options and considering the individual patient's needs and preferences, healthcare providers can provide comprehensive and effective acne management for patients of all diverse skin types.

REFERENCES

1. Acne vulgaris — Level 3 cause. Institute for Health Metrics and Evaluation. https://www.healthdata.org/results/gbd_summaries/2019/acne-vulgaris-level-3-cause. Published July 1, 2020. Accessed October 20, 2022.
2. Peck GM, Roberson FA, Feldman SR. Reasons for visits to the dermatologist stratified by race. *South Med J.* 2022;115(10):780-783.
3. Nock MR, Barbieri JS, Krueger LD, Cohen JM. Racial and ethnic differences in barriers to care among US adults with chronic inflammatory skin diseases: a cross-sectional study of the all of us research program. *J Am Acad Dermatol.* 2023;88(3):568-576.
4. Barbieri JS, Shin DB, Wang S, Margolis DJ, Takeshita J. Association of race/ethnicity and sex with differences in health care use and treatment for acne. *JAMA Dermatol.* 2020;156(3):312-319.
5. Perkins AC, Cheng CE, Hillebrand GG, Miyamoto K, Kimball AB. Comparison of the epidemiology of acne vulgaris among Caucasian, Asian, Continental Indian and African American women. *J Eur Acad Dermatol Venereol JEADV.* 2011;25(9):1054-1060.
6. Alexis AF, Woolery-Lloyd H, Williams K, et al. Racial/ethnic variations in acne: implications for treatment and skin care recommendations for acne patients with skin of color. *J Drugs Dermatol JDD.* 2021;20(7):716-725.
7. Duquia RP, Santos I da S dos, Jr H de A, Souza PRM, Breunig J de A, Zouboulis CC. Epidemiology of acne vulgaris in 18-year-old male army conscripts in a south Brazilian city. *Dermatology.* 2017;233(2-3):145-154.
8. Du Y, Doraiswamy C, Mao J, et al. Facial skin characteristics and concerns in Indonesia: a cross-sectional observational study. *Skin Res Technol.* 2022;28(5):719-728.
9. Urban K, Chu S, Giesey RL, et al. Burden of skin disease and associated socioeconomic status in Asia: a cross-sectional analysis from the Global Burden of Disease Study 1990-2017. *JAAD Int.* 2021;2:40-50.
10. Heng AHS, Say YH, Sio YY, Ng YT, Chew FT. Epidemiological risk factors associated with acne vulgaris presentation, severity, and scarring in a Singapore Chinese population: a cross-sectional study. *Dermatology.* 2022;238(2):226-235.
11. Zullo SW, Maarouf M, Shi VY. Acne disparities in Native Americans. *J Am Acad Dermatol.* 2021;85(2):499-501.
12. Heng AHS, Chew FT. Systematic review of the epidemiology of acne vulgaris. *Sci Rep.* 2020;10(1):5754.
13. Abanmi A, Al-Enezi M, Al Hammadi A, Galadari I, Kibbi AG, Zimmo S. Survey of acne-related post-inflammatory hyperpigmentation in the Middle East. *J Dermatol Treat.* 2019;30(6):578-581.
14. Bell MA, Whang KA, Thomas J, Aguh C, Kwatra SG. Racial and ethnic disparities in access to emerging and frontline therapies in common dermatological conditions: a cross-sectional study. *J Natl Med Assoc.* 2020;112(6): 650-653.
15. Charrow A, Xia FD, Lu J, Waul M, Joyce C, Mostaghimi A. Differences in isotretinoin start, interruption, and early termination across race and sex in the iPLEDGE era. *PLoS One.* 2019;14(3):e0210445.
16. Sevagamoorthy A, Sockler P, Akoh C, Takeshita J. Racial and ethnic diversity of US participants in clinical trials for acne, atopic dermatitis, and psoriasis: a comprehensive review. *J Dermatol Treat.* 2022;33(8):3086-3097.
17. Hooper J, Shao K, Feng H. Racial/ethnic health disparities in dermatology in the United States, part 1: overview of contributing factors and management strategies. *J Am Acad Dermatol.* 2022;87(4):723-730.
18. Shao K, Hooper J, Feng H. Racial and ethnic health disparities in dermatology in the United States. Part 2: disease-specific epidemiology, characteristics, management, and outcomes. *J Am Acad Dermatol.* 2022;87(4): 733-744.
19. Marson J, Baldwin H. Supplement article: dysbiosis, (Barrier) dysfunction, and dermatoses: a chicken-and-egg dilemma. *J Drugs Dermatol.* 2022;21(9):SF3502913-SF3502914. Accessed January 21, 2023. https://jddonline.com/articles/supplement-article-dysbiosis-barrier-dysfunction-and-dermatoses-a-chicken-and-egg-dilemma-S1545961622Ssup3X/.
20. Shamloul G, Khachemoune A. An updated review of the sebaceous gland and its role in health and diseases Part 2: pathophysiological clinical disorders of sebaceous glands. *Dermatol Ther.* 2021;34(2):e14862.
21. O'Neill AM, Gallo RL. Host-microbiome interactions and recent progress into understanding the biology of acne vulgaris. *Microbiome.* 2018;6(1):177.
22. Zouboulis CC, Coenye T, He L, et al. Sebaceous immunobiology - skin homeostasis, pathophysiology, coordination of innate immunity and inflammatory response and disease associations. *Front Immunol.* 2022;13:1029818.
23. Dagnelie MA, Corvec S, Timon-David E, Khammari A, Dréno B. Cutibacterium acnes and *Staphylococcus epidermidis*: the unmissable modulators of skin inflammatory response. *Exp Dermatol.* 2022;31(3):406-412.
24. Falder RM, Holmes YC, Bridgeman-Shah S, Kligman AM. A clincohistopathological study of acne vulgaris in black females. *J Invest Dermatol.* 1996;4(106):888.
25. Elbuluk N, Grimes P, Chien A, et al. The pathogenesis and management of acne-induced post-inflammatory hyperpigmentation. *Am J Clin Dermatol.* 2021;22(6):829-836.

26. Ebrahim HM, Artima AY, Elardi A, Mohamed Morsi H. Clinical and histopathological evaluation of different tools for the Subcision of Atrophic Acne Scars. *J Cosmet Dermatol.* 2022;21(3):1127-1134.
27. Maruthappu T, Taylor M. Acne and rosacea in skin of colour. *Clin Exp Dermatol.* 2022;47(2):259-263.
28. Alexis AF, Callender VD, Baldwin HE, Desai SR, Rendon MI, Taylor SC. Global epidemiology and clinical spectrum of rosacea, highlighting skin of color: review and clinical practice experience. *J Am Acad Dermatol.* 2019;80(6):1722-1729.e7.
29. Rocha MA, Bagatin E. Adult-onset acne: prevalence, impact, and management challenges. *Clin Cosmet Investig Dermatol.* 2018;11:59-69.
30. Treating acne in patients with skin of color. Global Academy for Medical Education. https://www.globalacademycme.com/cme/dermatology-skin-disease-education-foundation/acne-and-rosacea-applying-emerging-science-improve/treating-acne-patients-skin-color. Published June 14, 2018. Accessed January 22, 2023.
31. Callender VD, Baldwin H, Cook-Bolden FE, Alexis AF, Stein Gold L, Guenin E. Effects of topical retinoids on acne and post-inflammatory hyperpigmentation in patients with skin of color: a clinical review and implications for practice. *Am J Clin Dermatol.* 2022;23(1):69-81.
32. Greydanus DE, Azmeh R, Cabral MD, Dickson CA, Patel DR. Acne in the first three decades of life: an update of a disorder with profound implications for all decades of life. *Dis Mon.* 2021;67(4):101103.
33. Nemeh MN, Hogeling M. Pediatric skin picking disorder: a review of management. *Pediatr Dermatol.* 2022;39(3):363-368.
34. Bhatia J, Sarin A, Bhatia K. Acne fulminans: a case report and review of literature. *Indian J Paediatr Dermatol.* 2021;22(1):43.
35. Meena M, Mittal A, Khare AK, Gupta LK. Pseudo acne fulminans: an under recognized entity. *Indian Dermatol Online J.* 2018;9(6):462-464.
36. Jain S, Mohapatra L, Mohanty P, Jena S, Behera B. Study of clinical profile of patients presenting with topical steroid-induced facial dermatosis to a tertiary care hospital. *Indian Dermatol Online J.* 2020;11(2):208-211.
37. Al Dhafiri M, Almutairi M, Alutaibi HM, Aldandan HR, Albshr FA, Alkhalifa FS. Attitude toward using the triple combination bleaching formula and related outcomes: a cross-sectional study. *Cureus.* 13(12):e20542.
38. Dlova NC, Mosam A, Tsoka-Gwegweni J. The spectrum and sequelae of acne in black South Africans seen in tertiary institutions. *Skin Appendage Disord.* 2018;4(4):301-303.
39. Liu L, Xue Y, Chen Y, et al. Prevalence and risk factors of acne scars in patients with acne vulgaris. *Skin Res Technol.* 2023;29(6):e13386.
40. Fabbrocini G, Annunziata MC, D'Arco V, et al. Acne scars: pathogenesis, classification, and treatment. *Dermatol Res Pract.* 2010;2010:893080.
41. Holland DB, Jeremy AH, Roberts SG, Seukeran DC, Layton AM, Cunliffe WJ. Inflammation in acne scarring: a comparison of the responses in lesions from patients prone and not prone to scar. *Br J Dermatol.* 2004;150(1):72-81.
42. Arima J, Huang C, Rosner B, Akaishi S, Ogawa R. Hypertension: a systemic key to understanding local keloid severity. *Wound Repair Regen.* 2015;23(2):213-221.
43. Sun C, Lim D. Chemical peels for atrophic acne scarring: evolution of peel types and methods. *Australas J Dermatol.* 2023;64(1):18-27.
44. Chung HJ, Al Janahi S, Cho SB, Chang YC. Chemical reconstruction of skin scars (CROSS) method for atrophic scars: a comprehensive review. *J Cosmet Dermatol.* 2021;20(1):18-27.
45. Lobo Y, Lim DS. Surgical subcision for acne scars: a review of instrumentation. *Dermatol Surg.* 2023;49(4):355-362.
46. Schoenberg E, O'Connor M, Wang JV, Yang S, Saedi N. Microneedling and PRP for acne scars: a new tool in our arsenal. *J Cosmet Dermatol.* 2020;19(1):112-114.
47. Zaleski-Larsen LA, Fabi SG, McGraw T, Taylor M. Acne scar treatment: a multimodality approach tailored to scar type. *Dermatol Surg.* 2016;42(Suppl 2): S139-S149.
48. Lee YJ, Lee CY, Shin MK. A neglected acne scar type: papular acne scars and their correlations with keloid scars. *Dermatol Surg.* 2021;47(10):1347-1351.
49. Ogawa R. Keloid and hypertrophic scars are the result of chronic inflammation in the reticular dermis. *Int J Mol Sci.* 2017;18(3):606.
50. Elbuluk N, Grimes P, Chien A, et al. The pathogenesis and management of acne-induced post-inflammatory hyperpigmentation. *Am J Clin Dermatol.* 2021;22(6):829-836.
51. Davis EC, Callender VD. Postinflammatory hyperpigmentation: a review of the epidemiology, clinical features, and treatment options in skin of color. *J Clin Aesthet Dermatol.* 2010;3(7):20-31.
52. Bae-Harboe YS, Graber EM. Easy as PIE (Postinflammatory Erythema). *J Clin Aesthet Dermatol.* 2013;6(9):46-47.
53. Jakhar D, Kaur I. Topical 5% tranexamic acid for acne-related postinflammatory erythema. *J Am Acad Dermatol.* 2020;82(6):e187-e188.
54. Lee SJ, Ahn GR, Seo SB, Park KY, Kim BJ, Nam Kim M. Topical brimonidine-assisted laser treatment for the prevention of therapy-related erythema and hyperpigmentation. *J Cosmet Laser Ther.* 2019;21(4):225-227.
55. Agamia N, Essawy M, Kassem A. Successful treatment of the face post acne erythema using a topically applied selective alpha 1-Adrenergic receptor agonist, oxymetazoline 1.5%, a controlled left to right face comparative trial. *J Dermatolog Treat.* 2022;33(2):904-909.
56. Alam M, Voravutinon N, Warycha M, et al. Comparative effectiveness of nonpurpuragenic 595-nm pulsed dye laser and microsecond 1064-nm neodymium: yttrium-aluminum-garnet laser for treatment of diffuse facial erythema: a double-blind randomized controlled trial. *J Am Acad Dermatol.* 2013;69(3):438-443.
57. Callender VD. Acne in ethnic skin: special considerations for therapy. *Dermatol Ther.* 2004;17:184-195.
58. Taylor SC, Cook-Bolden F, Rahman Z, Strachan D. Acne vulgaris in skin of color. *J Am Acad Dermatol.* 2002;46:S98-S106.
59. Ebede TL, Arch EL, Berson D. Hormonal treatment of acne in women. *J Clin Aesthet Dermatol.* 2009;2(12):16-22.
60. Woolery-Lloyd HC, Keri J, Doig S. Retinoids and azelaic acid to treat acne and hyperpigmentation in skin of color. *J Drugs Dermatol.* 2013;12(4):434-437.
61. Kircik LH, Draelos ZD, Berson DS. Polymeric emulsion technology applied to tretinoin. *J Drugs Dermatol.* 2019;18(4):s148-154.
62. Alexis AF, Lamb A. Concomitant therapy for acne in patients with skin of color: a case-based approach. *Dermatol Nurs.* 2009;21(1):33-36.
63. Alexis AF, Sergay AB, Taylor SC. Common considerations in cosmetic treatments for black patients. *J Drugs Dermatol.* 2019;18(5): 454-458.
64. Draelos ZD, Elewski BE, Harper JC, Kempiak S, Kircik LH. A new era in acne management: acne treatment today and beyond. *Cutis.* 2010;85(1S):4-11.
65. Bikowski JB. Antibiotic resistance in acne management. *J Drugs Dermatol.* 2009;8(8):798-801.
66. Worret WI, Arp W. Medium-dose isotretinoin for the treatment of acne. *J Am Acad Dermatol.* 2003;49(5):832-836.
67. Taylor SC, Burgess CM, Callender VD, Gottlieb AB. Acne vulgaris and acneiform eruptions. In: *Dermatology for Skin of Color.* McGraw Hill Professional; 2012:183-220.
68. Zaenglein AL, Pathy AL, Schlosser BJ, et al. Guidelines of care for the management of acne vulgaris. *J Am Acad Dermatol.* 2016;74(5):945-973.
69. Grimes PE, Alikhan A, James WD. Acne and rosacea. In: *Fitzpatrick's Dermatology in General Medicine.* 8th ed. McGraw Hill Professional; 2009:719-737.
70. Zeichner JA. Optimizing topical combination therapy for the treatment of acne vulgaris. *J Drugs Dermatol.* 2012;11(3):313-317.
71. Gollnick H, Cunliffe W, Berson D, et al. Management of acne: a report from a Global Alliance to Improve Outcomes in Acne. *J Am Acad Dermatol.* 2003;49(1):S1-S37.
72. Layton AM. The use of isotretinoin in acne. *Dermatoendocrinology.* 2010;2(3):162-169.
73. Davis EC, Callender VD. A review of acne in ethnic skin: pathogenesis, clinical manifestations, and management strategies. *J Clin Aesthet Dermatol.* 2010;3(4):24-38.
74. Coley MK, Alexis AF. Managing common dermatoses in skin of color. *Semin Cutan Med Surg.* 2009;28(2):63-70.
75. Grimes PE. The safety and efficacy of salicylic acid chemical peels in darker racial ethnic groups. *Dermatol Surg.* 1999;25:18-22.
76. Ahn HH, Kim I. Whitening effect of salicylic acid peels in Asian patients. *Dermatol Surg.* 2006; 32:372-375.
77. Garg VJ, Sinha S, Sarkar R. Glycolic acid peels versus salicyclic-mandelic acid peels in active acne vulgaris and post-acne scarring and hyperpigmentation: a comparative study. *Dermatol Surg.* 2009;35:59-65.

CHAPTER 49

Hidradenitis Suppurativa

Alicia Edwards
Jahdonna Isaac
Toni Jenkins
Ginette A. Okoye

KEY POINTS

- Hidradenitis Suppurativa (HS) is a condition characterized by chronic and relapsing inflammation leading to painful purulent nodules, abscesses, and sinus tracts.
- HS can have distressing effects on activities of daily living, work-life, and mental health. These patients require a holistic and interdisciplinary treatment approach.
- African Americans are disproportionately affected by HS and historically underrepresented in HS research.

INTRODUCTION

Hidradenitis suppurativa (HS), also referred to as acne inversa, is a chronic inflammatory skin disease that predominantly affects terminal hair follicles.[1] HS presents as recurrent painful, inflamed nodules, abscesses, and sinus tracts with subsequent fibrotic scarring. These lesions are found in intertriginous areas of the body such as the axillae, inframammary folds, inguinal folds, genital, and gluteal regions. The estimated prevalence of HS varies widely. A recent prevalence estimate of 0.3% to 1.7% was based on pooled data from the United States, Western Europe, Scandinavia, and Australia.[2] However, prevalence data from Africa, Asia, and other parts of the world are lacking, and deserve further study to truly inform the global prevalence of HS.

HS usually presents at or after puberty,[3] and women are more commonly affected than men.[1,4] The pain and purulent drainage associated with HS lesions as well as the movement restrictions from pain and scarring make HS a disabling disease that affects day-to-day functioning. HS is also associated with significant psychosocial comorbidities, including depression, anxiety, and suicidality.[5] While the pathogenesis of HS is not yet completely understood, it is recognized as a multifactorial disease that involves immunologic, hormonal, genetic, environmental, and socioeconomic factors. This pathologic process is thought to begin with hair follicle occlusion. The follicle expands to form a cystic structure that eventually ruptures and spills its contents into the surrounding dermis. These contents, which include naked hair shafts, keratin, and bacteria, contribute to a robust neutrophil-rich inflammatory response leading to perifolliculitis, abscess formation, and destruction of the pilosebaceous unit and nearby structures.[1] The pathogenesis of HS may also involve aberrant signaling in the γ-secretase/Notch pathway that, among other functions, regulates the maintenance of the inner and outer root sheath of the hair follicle.[6] Other contributing elements include a dysregulated proinflammatory cytokine cascade, decreased antimicrobial peptide formation, bacterial colonization, and keratinocyte malfunction.[1,7] Furthermore, growing evidence suggests that HS should not be solely seen as a follicular occlusion disorder but more broadly as an autoinflammatory disease with systemic inflammation being a central feature.[8] This complexity creates many challenges for those engaged in HS research and contributes to the inconsistent results of our current therapeutic options.

HISTORY

In 1854, HS was first described by Aristide Verneuil, a French surgeon and venerologist who published a series of articles on skin tumors arising from sweat glands.[9] His first encounter with this condition was on the corpse of a young patient who had unfortunately died from cachexia. He described numerous scattered eschars and pustules filled with liquid on the intertriginous regions of the groin and buttocks. He notably meticulously depicted cavities connected by channels running within the dermis. Verneuil named this ailment "Hidrosadénite Phlegmoneuse" or *phlegmonous hidradenitis* due to its supposed, though not confirmed, association with sweat glands. In 1889, Sebastiano Giovannini performed the first histopathological study on a specimen revealing an inflammatory process affecting the sweat glands and causing their complete destruction.[9,10] By the 1890s, the notion that HS was a type of folliculitis that could be either generalized or localized to areas like the labia majora, axillae, or perianal skin was adopted by a few scholars.[9] In more modern years, several groups eventually established a common association of follicular hyperkeratosis in HS, acne conglobata, dissecting cellulitis of the scalp and pilonidal cyst thus forming the "follicular occlusion tetrad." With clearer evidence that HS represents a disorder of the pilosebaceous unit rather than of apocrine glands, "hidradenitis suppurativa" has been described as a misnomer by several authors who prefer the term "acne inversa" as more etiologically accurate.[9,11]

EPIDEMIOLOGY

The global prevalence of HS varies widely, ranging from 0.00033% to 4.1%.[12] The most recent prevalence estimate for the United States is approximately 0.1%.[12] Epidemiological data for Australian, Asian, and African populations are limited, with an estimated prevalence of 0.67% in Australia, 0.06% in South Korea, and 0.8% in Ghana, respectively.[13] Many of the epidemiological studies in HS have been performed in countries with a predominantly Caucasian population. Consequently, there are fewer studies on the prevalence of HS in skin of color. In the United States, African American and biracial individuals (ie, people with both Caucasian and African American ancestry) have a threefold and twofold increased prevalence of HS, respectively, compared to Caucasians.[12] In a systematic review analyzing the prevalence of HS in several countries, African Americans had the highest prevalence (1.30%), followed by Caucasians (0.75%), and Hispanic populations (0.07%).[14] Interestingly, based on limited data, the prevalence of HS in people of African descent who live outside the United States seems to be lower than that of African Americans. For example, the prevalence of HS among African immigrants in Spain is only 0.2%,[15,16] and the prevalence of HS in Ghana is closer to 0.67%.[17] Whether these differences are due to environmental factors in the United States or due to differences in access to dermatologic care outside the United States is unknown.

HS is more common in women compared to men at a ratio of almost 3:1.[12] The reasons for this difference have not been elucidated and deserve further study. The prevalence of HS in the pediatric and adolescent populations is increasing, and is also more common in female adolescents.[18,19]

The onset of the disease is typically after puberty, with an average age of onset of 12.5 years old.[19] Yet, the majority of patients are diagnosed in their second or third decade with an average delay in diagnosis of approximately 7 years.[3] This diagnostic delay likely contributes to the higher healthcare utilization and higher-cost care seen in HS.[20,21]

Smoking, obesity, and low socioeconomic status are risk factors for HS,[22,23] and triggers commonly identified by patients include stress, friction, and diet.[24] There are multiple comorbidities associated with HS, including metabolic syndrome, cardiovascular disease, psychiatric comorbidities, and other inflammatory disorders such as inflammatory bowel disease and pyoderma gangrenosum.[25,26]

PATHOGENESIS

Currently, the primary pathogenic event in HS is believed to center around the occlusion of the hair follicle leading to a robust inflammatory response and tissue damage. This follicular occlusion can be the result of a follicular epithelial defect[27] or infundibular hyperkeratosis that creates a follicular-based cyst.[5] When the cyst ruptures and releases its contents into the dermis, this triggers a complex inflammatory cascade with ensuing tissue damage and remodeling. When this process occurs in adjacent follicles, cystic structures may eventually interconnect, forming epithelialized tunnels in the dermis. This process results in the characteristic abscess and sinus tract formation seen in HS.[1,8] The characteristics of the inflammatory milieu seen in HS is multifaceted and still being elucidated. A proposed theory is that the release of cyst content within the dermis prompts neutrophil recruitment, formation of specific inflammasomes (ie, NLRP3) and induces IL-1β.[1] Furthermore, neutrophils are particularly important for the formation of neutrophil extracellular traps or "NETs," which were found to correlate with disease severity and progression in biospecimens predominantly from African American subjects.[28] These web-like complexes made of nucleic acids, cytosolic granules, and other proteins act in response to pathogenic or sterile stimuli to promote innate and adaptive immunity including type I interferon response.[28] Other implicated cells includes T lymphocytes (ie, Th1, Th17), B lymphocytes, plasma cells, macrophage, and dendritic cells that can be found within HS lesions.[1] Pro- and anti-inflammatory mediators including Th17, IL-12, IL-23, TNF-α, IL-10, and others generate an inflammation cascade, whereas the scarring process is mediated in part by matrix metalloprotease-2 and transforming growth factor.[1,29] Alternatively, some authors have postulated a primary autoinflammatory process arising from predisposing factors and subclinical systemic inflammation, then resulting in follicular occlusion and rupture as a sequelae.[8] Furthermore, though HS is not an infectious condition, superimposed bacterial colonization may exacerbate the disease. The purulent exudate from HS lesions can be sterile or contain normal skin flora. However, certain studies have identified the presence of pathogenic bacteria such as *Staphylococcus aureus*, *S. lugdunensis*, *Prevotella* spp., Streptococci, and Actinomycetes, which contribute to biofilm formation and subsequent chronic inflammatory response.[30] There is also mounting evidence revealing a relationship between a disrupted skin or gut microbiome and HS.[30-32]

CLINICAL FEATURES

HS is characterized by recurrent and chronic nodules and draining abscesses occurring in intertriginous, friction-prone, and apocrine-rich areas of the skin. These painful nodules produce purulent and sometimes bloody discharge and scarring ensues. Six different phenotypes of HS have been identified: (1) regular type; (2) frictional furuncle type; (3) scarring folliculitis type; (4) conglobata type; (5) syndromic type; and (6) ectopic type. Few papers postulate a difference between a follicular and inflammatory subtype, the latter being associated with a worse outcome.[1,33] The Hurley system staging is commonly used to establish disease severity: Stage 1 is defined as solitary or multiple lesions without sinus tract formation, Stage 2 is defined as recurrent widely separated abscesses or cyst with scarring and/or sinus tracts, and Stage 3 is defined as multiple interconnected abscesses with extensive scarring and/or sinus tracts over a large anatomic area [**Table 49-1** and **Figure 49-1**]. [4,34]

The prognosis of HS has not been well-studied, and there are no clinical or molecular markers known to predict outcomes. A study consisting of 212 Dutch and Danish patients assessed remission, improvement, unchanged severity, and worsening of HS with observed rates of 39.4%, 31.5%, 20.5%, and 8.7%, respectively.[35] A higher percentage of nonsmoker (40%) and nonobese (45%) patients were able to achieve remission compared to active smokers and obese patients (29% and 23%, respectively).[35] Other pertinent prognostic factors include hormonal fluctuations. A survey of female HS patients found that 76.7% of respondents experienced a worsening of symptoms around the time of menstruation, while 22.2% reported no associated changes.[36] During pregnancy, 36.6% of women noticed an improvement, while 34.8% and 28.7% saw a deterioration or no changes in their condition, respectively.[36] The same study estimated that 39.5% of women experienced worsening of symptoms during menopause and 44.2% had no changes.[36] This contrasts with other reports, suggesting higher rates of remission in postmenopausal women.[37]

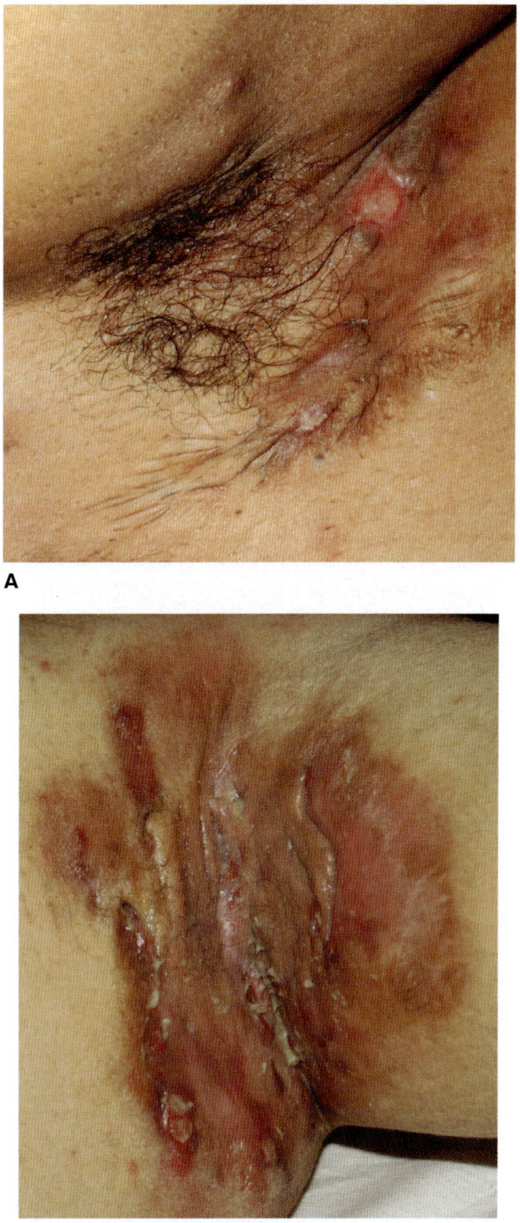

A

B

FIGURE 49-1 Axillary hidradenitis suppurativa illustrating the spectrum of disease severity as measured by Hurley stage. **(A)** Stage II. **(B)** Stage III."

TABLE 49-1 Clinical staging in hidradenitis suppurativa

Stage I	Abscess formation, single or multiple, without sinus tracts and cicatrization.
Stage II	Recurrent abscesses with tract formation and cicatrization. Single or multiple, widely separated lesions.
Stage III	Diffuse of near diffuse involvement, or multiple interconnected tracts and abscesses across entire area.

Source: Reproduced with permission from Randall K. Roenigk, Henry H. Roenigk. Roenigk & Roenigk's *Dermatologic Surgery: Principles and Practice*, Second Edition. New York: M. Dekker; 1996.

HISTOLOGY

Biopsies are not necessary to establish a diagnosis of HS. However, several histopathologic findings are consistent among HS lesions and may help more complex cases. A recent systematic review of 18 studies demonstrated that follicular occlusion, follicular hyperkeratosis, hyperplasia of follicular epithelium, epidermal psoriasiform hyperplasia, and perifolliculitis are the most commonly associated features.[38] Interestingly, there is no defined histologic relationship between HS and sweat glands. When affected, eccrine glands are more involved than apocrine glands but overall these sweat glands behave more like "innocent bystanders"[38] than true pathogenic entities. Immunohistochemical and special stains may be helpful in characterizing the disease as a study found expression of CD3, CD4, CD8, CD68, and CD79 with a CD4:CD8 ratio of 2.1:1 at the terminal follicle.[38,39] The histopathology of HS can vary depending on the stage of disease. Histopathologic mimickers include chronic deep folliculitis, Crohn disease, pyoderma gangrenosum, and even Langerhans cells histiocytosis or folliculotropic mycosis fungoides.[38] Nonetheless, distinguishing HS from other inflammatory conditions involving follicular occlusion and hyperkeratinization can be difficult without appropriate clinicopathological correlation.

DIFFERENTIAL DIAGNOSIS

Early lesions of HS may pose a diagnostic challenge to those unfamiliar with the disease. Without the stigmata of chronicity, one could easily mistake HS lesions for a simple folliculitis, carbuncle, furuncle, or other superficial staphylococcal infection. As lesions evolve, additional differential diagnoses include epidermal inclusion cysts, Crohn disease, syphilis, squamous cell carcinoma (ie, Marjolin ulcer), cutaneous tuberculosis, actinomycosis, or lymphogranuloma venereum.[4] Typical HS lesions in typical HS locations with recurrences (ie, at least two recurrences within 6 months) and/or evidence of chronicity (ie, scarring, contractures, post-inflammatory hyperpigmentation) should raise suspicion for HS and help decipher it from other entities.

TREATMENT

Treatment of HS is complex. Research efforts and awareness have grown tremendously over the past decade, yet consistently effective treatment options are still lacking. First-line treatments include topical antimicrobials such as benzoyl peroxide, chlorhexidine, zinc pyrithione, and clindamycin.[40] Early treatment with laser hair reduction is a promising option that may alter the course of the disease by reducing the development of new lesions through destruction of the pilosebaceous unit and thermal destruction of specific bacterial species.[41,42] Oral antibiotics (specifically doxycycline, minocycline, and clindamycin plus rifampin) and intralesional injections of corticosteroids can ameliorate painful disease flares. Antibiotic courses should not exceed 2 to 3 months at a time,[40] and should be an adjunct to other systemic therapies for patients with frequent flares. Metabolic and hormonal dysregulation can be treated with metformin, oral contraceptive pills, spironolactone, and finasteride. Spironolactone and the oral contraceptive pills that are FDA-approved for the treatment of acne can be particularly useful in patients with polycystic ovarian syndrome (PCOS) or patients who report a history of premenstrual flares.[40] Metformin can be a useful adjunctive treatment in patients who have metabolic syndrome or PCOS. Topical and oral retinoids have been used in patients with concurrent severe acne, but their effect on HS is usually suboptimal. However, patients with the follicular subtype of HS may benefit more than those with the inflammatory subtype of HS. Systemic inflammation has been targeted with systemic corticosteroids, other immunomodulators such as dapsone and colchicine as well as biologics.[40] Adalimumab, a tumor necrosis factor-alpha (TNF-α) inhibitor is currently the only U.S. Food and Drug Administration-approved biologic for the treatment of moderate to severe HS.[40] Several other biologics such as infliximab, ustekinumab, anakinra, secukinumab, and novel molecules (JAK inhibitors, C5a inhibitors, CXC receptors) have shown encouraging preliminary results.[40,43] Despite this momentum, it is worth mentioning that African American populations are still disproportionally underrepresented in clinical trials addressing HS. In a study of 15 recent phase II and III HS clinical trials, 68% of participants identified as Caucasian compared to 14% as of African descent.[44] These results are problematic knowing that African Americans populations are significantly more affected by HS compared to other ethnic groups and have shown increased disease burden and severity.[45,46] This illustrates an imperative need for more diversity in future research endeavors.

Surgical intervention may be unavoidable in advanced and refractory cases. Removal of inflammatory lesions and sinus tracts can be performed via marsupialization, carbon dioxide laser surgery, or traditional wide excisions. In one cohort, recurrence was estimated at 24.4% of patients postoperatively.[47] Initiating biologic therapy before surgery and continuing its use throughout the postoperative period has been shown to be more effective than either treatment alone.[48]

Lifestyle modifications can play a major role in alleviating symptoms. Given the metabolic and cardiovascular comorbidities associated with HS, smoking cessation should be strongly recommended. Additionally, smoking cessation may impact progression of the disease.[49] Additionally, obesity and hyperhidrosis are other known treatable exacerbating factors.[49,50]

Pain management is an important aspect of HS treatment. Topical lidocaine, NSAIDs, acetaminophen, and anticonvulsants such as gabapentin and pregabalin have all been reported with varying efficacy in the literature.[51] Moreover, given the detrimental effects on quality of life, screening for symptoms of depression, anxiety, and suicidality and providing mental health resources to vulnerable patients is essential[25]. Overall, HS is a complex disease requiring multimodal therapies and multidisciplinary care. More research is needed in the epidemiology, pathophysiology, and treatment of HS, and this research should include all of the diverse patient populations that are affected by this devastating disease. The psychosocial impact of HS must not be overlooked. Early diagnosis and treatment are imperative to decreasing the burden of this disease on individuals and society as a whole.

REFERENCES

1. Scala E, Cacciapuoti S, Garzorz-Stark N, et al. Hidradenitis suppurativa: where we are and where we are going. *Cells*. 2021;10(8):2094.
2. Jfri A, Nassim D, O'Brien E, et al. Prevalence of hidradenitis suppurativa: a systematic review and meta-regression analysis. *JAMA Dermatol*. 2021;157(8):924-931.
3. Saunte DM, Boer J, Stratigos A, et al. Diagnostic delay in hidradenitis suppurativa is a global problem. *Br J Dermatol*. 2015;173(6):1546-1549.
4. Jemec GBE, Revuz J, Leyden JJ. *Hidradenitis Suppurativa*. 1. Aufl., Springer-Verlag; 2006: 58-64.
5. Nguyen TV, Damiani G, Orenstein LAV, Hamzavi I, Jemec GB. Hidradenitis suppurativa: an update on epidemiology, phenotypes, diagnosis, pathogenesis, comorbidities and quality of life. *J Eur Acad Dermatol Venereol*. 2021;35(1):50-61.
6. Melnik BC, Plewig G. Impaired Notch-MKP-1 signalling in hidradenitis suppurativa: an approach to pathogenesis by evidence from translational biology. *Exp Dermatol*. 2013;22:172-177.
7. Hotz C, Boniotto M, Guguin A, et al. Intrinsic defect in keratinocyte function leads to inflammation in hidradenitis suppurativa. *J Invest Dermatol*. 2016;136(9):1768-1780.
8. Frew JW. Hidradenitis suppurativa is an autoinflammatory keratinization disease: a review of the clinical, histologic, and molecular evidence. *JAAD Int*. 2020;1(1):62-72.
9. Tilles G. "Verneuil and verneuil's disease: an historical overview". In: *Hidradenitis Suppurativa*. Berlin, Heidelberg: Springer Berlin Heidelberg; 2006:4-10.
10. Sellheyer K, Krahl D. "Hidradenitis suppurativa" is acne inversa! An appeal to (finally) abandon a misnomer. *Int J Dermatol*. 2005;44(7):535-540.
11. Garg A, Kirby JS, Lavian J, Lin G, Strunk A. Sex- and age-adjusted population analysis of prevalence estimates for hidradenitis suppurativa in the United States. *JAMA Dermatol*. 2017;153(8):760-764.
12. Ingram JR. The epidemiology of hidradenitis suppurativa. *Br J Dermatol*. 2020;183(6):990-998.
13. Sachdeva M, Shah M, Alavi A. Race-specific prevalence of hidradenitis suppurativa. *J Cutan Med Surg*. 2021;25(2):177-187.
14. Zouboulis CC, Goyal M, Byrd AS. Hidradenitis suppurativa in skin of colour. *Exp Dermatol*. 2021;30(Suppl 1):27-30.

15. Albares MP, Belinchón I, Ramos JM, Sánchez-Payá J, Betlloch I. Estudioepidemiológico de la patologíacutáneaen la poblacióninmigrante de Alicante. *Actas Dermosifiliogr*. 2012;103:214-222.
16. Hagan PG, Bouazzi D, Nyarko G, et al. Prevalence of hidradenitis suppurativa in Berekum, Ghana. *Br J Dermatol*. 2022;187(4):586-587.
17. Garg A, Lavian J, Lin G, Strunk A, Alloo A. Incidence of hidradenitis suppurativa in the United States: a sex- and age-adjusted population analysis. *J Am Acad Dermatol*. 2017;77(1):118-122.
18. Liy-Wong C, Kim M, Kirkorian AY, et al. Hidradenitis suppurativa in the pediatric population: an international, multicenter, retrospective, cross-sectional study of 481 pediatric patients. *JAMA Dermatol*. 2021;157(4):385-391.
19. Kilgour JM, Li S, Sarin KY. Hidradenitis suppurativa in patients of color is associated with increased disease severity and healthcare utilization: a retrospective analysis of 2 U.S. cohorts. *JAAD International*. 2021;3:42-52.
20. Khanna R, Whang KA, Huang AH, et al. Inpatient burden of hidradenitis suppurativa in the United States: analysis of the 2016 National Inpatient Sample. *J Dermatolog Treat*. 2022;33(2):1150-1152.
21. Kromann CB, Deckers IE, Esmann S, Boer J, Prens EP, Jemec GB. Risk factors, clinical course and long-term prognosis in hidradenitis suppurativa: a cross-sectional study. *Br J Dermatol*. 2014;171(4):819-824.
22. Deckers IE, Janse IC, van der Zee HH, et al. Hidradenitis suppurativa (HS) is associated with low socioeconomic status (SES): a cross-sectional reference study. *J Am Acad Dermatol*. 2016;75(4):755-759.e1.
23. Thompson AM, Fernandez JM, Rick J, et al. Identifying triggers for hidradenitis suppurativa flare: a patient survey. *Br J Dermatol*. 2021;185(1):225-226.
24. Garg A, Malviya N, Strunk A, et al. Comorbidity screening in hidradenitis suppurativa: evidence-based recommendations from the US and Canadian Hidradenitis Suppurativa Foundations. *J Am Acad Dermatol*. 2022;86(5):1092-1101.
25. Sokumbi O, Hodge DO, Ederaine SA, Alavi A, Alikhan A. Comorbid diseases of hidradenitis suppurativa: a 15-year population-based study in Olmsted County, Minnesota, USA. *Int J Dermatol*. 2022;61(11):1372-1379.
26. Danby FW, Jemec GBE, Marsch WC, Laffert M von. Preliminary findings suggest hidradenitis suppurativa may be due to defective follicular support. *Br J Dermatol*. 2013;168:1034-1039.
27. Byrd AS, Carmona-Rivera C, O'Neil LJ, et al. Neutrophil extracellular traps, B cells, and type I interferons contribute to immune dysregulation in hidradenitis suppurativa. *Sci Transl Med*. 2019;11(508):eaav5908.
28. Vossen ARJV, van der Zee HH, Prens EP. Hidradenitis suppurativa: a systematic review integrating inflammatory pathways into a cohesive pathogenic model. *Front Immunol*. 2018;9:2965.
29. Nikolakis G, Liakou AI, Bonovas S, et al. Bacterial colonization in hidradenitis suppurativa/acne inversa: a cross-sectional study of 50 patients and review of the literature. *Acta Derm Venereol*. 2017;97(4):493-498.
30. McCarthy S, Barrett M, Kirthi S, et al. Altered skin and gut microbiome in hidradenitis suppurativa. *J Invest Dermatol*. 2022;142(2):459-468.e15.
31. Ring HC, Thorsen J, Saunte DM, et al. The follicular skin microbiome in patients with hidradenitis suppurativa and healthy controls. *JAMA Dermatol*. 2017;153(9):897-905.
32. Martorell A, Jfri A, Koster SBL, et al. Defining hidradenitis suppurativa phenotypes based on the elementary lesion pattern: results of a prospective study. *J Eur Acad Dermatol Venereol*. 2020;34(6):1309-1318.
33. Hurley H. *Axillary Hyperhidrosis, Apocine Bromhidrosis, Hidradenitis Suppurativa, and Familial Benign Pemphigus: Surgical Approach*. New York, NY: Marcel Dekker; 1989.
34. Kromann CB, Deckers IE, Esmann S, Boer J, Prens EP, Jemec GB. Risk factors, clinical course and long-term prognosis in hidradenitis suppurativa: a cross-sectional study. *Br J Dermatol*. 2014;171(4):819-824.
35. Fernandez JM, Hendricks AJ, Thompson AM, et al. Menses, pregnancy, delivery, and menopause in hidradenitis suppurativa: a patient survey. *Int J Womens Dermatol*. 2020;6(5):368-371.
36. Ingram JR. The epidemiology of hidradenitis suppurativa. *Br J Dermatol*. 2020;183(6):990-998.
37. Smith SDB, Okoye GA, Sokumbi O. Histopathology of hidradenitis suppurativa: a systematic review. *Dermatopathology (Basel)*. 2022;9(3):251-257.
38. von Laffert M, Helmbold P, Wohlrab J, Fiedler E, Stadie V, Marsch WC. Hidradenitis suppurativa (acne inversa): early inflammatory events at terminal follicles and at interfollicular epidermis. *Exp Dermatol*. 2010;19(6):533-537.
39. Alikhan A, Sayed C, Alavi A, et al. North American clinical management guidelines for hidradenitis suppurativa: a publication from the United States and Canadian Hidradenitis Suppurativa Foundations: Part I and II. *J Am Acad Dermatol*. 2019;81(1):76-101.
40. Tierney E, Mahmoud BH, Hexsel C, Ozog D, Hamzavi I. Randomized control trial for the treatment of hidradenitis suppurativa with a neodymium-doped yttrium aluminium garnet laser. *Dermatol Surg*. 2009;35(8):1188-1198.
41. Vossen ARJV, van der Zee HH, Terian M, van Doorn MBA, Prens EP. Laser hair removal alters the disease course in mild hidradenitis suppurativa. *J Dtsch Dermatol Ges*. 2018;16(7):901-903.
42. Świerczewska Z, Lewandowski M, Surowiecka A, Barańska-Rybak W. Immunomodulatory drugs in the treatment of hidradenitis suppurativa-possibilities and limitations. *Int J Mol Sci*. 2022;23(17):9716.
43. Okeke CAV, Perry JD, Simmonds FC, et al. Clinical trials and skin of color: the example of hidradenitis suppurativa. *Dermatology*. 2022;238(1):180-184.
44. Lee DE, Clark AK, Shi VY. Hidradenitis suppurativa: disease burden and etiology in skin of color. dermatology. 2017;233(6):456-461.
45. Ulschmid C, Serrano L, Wu R, Roth GM, Sokumbi O. African American race is a risk factor for severe hidradenitis suppurativa. *Int J Dermatol*. 2023;62(5):657-663.
46. Kohorst JJ, Baum CL, Otley CC, et al. Surgical management of hidradenitis suppurativa: outcomes of 590 consecutive patients. *Dermatol Surg*. 2016;42(9):1030-1040.
47. Bechara FG, Podda M, Prens EP, et al. Efficacy and safety of adalimumab in conjunction with surgery in moderate to severe hidradenitis suppurativa: the SHARPS randomized clinical trial. *JAMA Surg*. 2021;156(11):1001-1009.
48. Macklis PC, Tyler K, Kaffenberger J, Kwatra S, Kaffenberger BH. Lifestyle modifications associated with symptom improvement in hidradenitis suppurativa patients. *Arch Dermatol Res*. 2022;314(3):293-300.
49. Hua VJ, Kuo KY, Cho HG, Sarin KY. Hyperhidrosis affects quality of life in hidradenitis suppurativa: a prospective analysis. *J Am Acad Dermatol*. 2020;82(3):753-754.
50. Savage KT, Singh V, Patel ZS, et al. Pain management in hidradenitis suppurativa and a proposed treatment algorithm. *J Am Acad Dermatol*. 2021;85(1):187-199.

CHAPTER 50

Rosacea in Skin of Color: An Evidence- and Literature-Based Approach to Epidemiology, Pathogenesis, Diagnosis, and Therapy

Justin W. Marson
Hilary E. Baldwin

KEY POINTS

- Rosacea is a chronic condition of the central face believed to be caused by a dysregulated innate and adaptive immune system resulting in chronic inflammation and a hyperreactive cutaneous neurovasculature.
- Individuals with rosacea report significant psychosocial impairment that can interfere with professional and social functioning and quality of life; furthermore, individuals with rosacea are more likely than the general population to also be diagnosed with autoimmune conditions (eg, type 1 diabetes mellitus, celiac disease), inflammatory conditions (eg, sarcoidosis, inflammatory bowel disease), as well as metabolic syndrome and cardiovascular disease among other systemic conditions.
- Although classically associated with lighter skin phenotypes, rosacea in studies has been found to affect up to 2% to 4% of Black, Asian and Pacific Islander, and Hispanic/Latino American population and is likely underdiagnosed given the reliance of the current classification system on phenotypic expressions (eg, the presence or absence of fixed erythema with or without intermittent exacerbations, flushing, and/or telangiectasias).

- Papulopustular-predominant or granulomatous presentations may be more common (than erythematotelangiectatic-predominant rosacea) among patients with skin of color.
- In patients with richly pigmented skin, taking a careful history of symptoms of rosacea to assess the minor/secondary criteria (ie, burning or stinging, edema, dryness, flushing, low tolerance for over-the-counter products, symptom with classic "triggers," family history and/or ocular symptoms) may facilitate diagnosis.
- Assessing erythema in richly pigmented skin can be augmented by having patients identify which areas appear more "red" to them as well as incorporating diascopy and/or dermoscopy to induce blanching of background erythema.
- Treatment regimens for rosacea are largely constructed around the phenotypic presentation (ie, erythema and telangiectasias, papulopustules, phymatous changes, ocular disease) and can include over-the-counter and lifestyle modifications as well as prescription topical, systemic, and procedural therapies across "phenotypic" groupings to best address patient-perceived disease severity and concerns and to minimize any further irritation/inflammation that may drive (postinflammatory) pigmentary alteration.
- Future treatment options can include agents targeting T_H17 axis and anti-CGRP, innate immune system modulators (eg, toll-like receptor 2 inhibitors, synthetic antimicrobial peptides, topical probiotics), as well as use of off-label agents (eg, rifaximin, hydroxychloroquine).
- While there are limited data assessing complementary and alternative medical agents (for primary or adjunctive use), given patients with rosacea may already be at increased risk of contact dermatitis, they should be cautioned against including "natural remedies" in their regimen to prevent additional inflammation and (further) pigment alteration.

INTRODUCTION

Rosacea is a chronic condition of the central face believed to be caused by a dysregulated innate and adaptive immune system resulting in chronic inflammation and a hyperreactive cutaneous neurovasculature.[1,2] Long said to present most commonly in light-skinned women 30 to 50 years of age, recent data show that it is not uncommon in men, different age groups, or in patients with more richly pigmented skin.[3-5] However, since erythema and telangiectasias are hallmarks of the condition, diagnosis may present more of a challenge in patients with darker skin tones. Coupled with a historically low index of suspicion, underdiagnoses and missed diagnoses are common.[5,6] This may lead to delays in diagnoses, poorer quality of life, more advanced disease at the time of diagnosis, and the potential for permanent changes and sight-threatening ocular disease.

It has only been a decade that a discussion of rosacea in patients with skin of color was deemed to be medically important. Consequently, data are still not robust and there remain large gaps in our understanding. In these 10 years, researchers have concluded that there is little difference between skin tones in the etiology, pathophysiology, or response to therapeutic modalities used to treat rosacea. Demographics, diagnostic criteria, the need to avoid iatrogenic hyperpigmentation, and racial disparities that limit access to care remain the quintessential topics of discussion.

Here we will assess through a wide lens advancements in our understanding of rosacea pathogenesis and management and discuss the nuances necessary to manage rosacea in patents with darker skin phototypes with regard to epidemiology and underdiagnosis, diagnostic clues of which to be aware and special considerations in crafting effective therapeutic regimens.

ROSACEA CLASSIFICATION AND CLINICAL RAMIFICATIONS IN PATIENTS WITH SKIN OF COLOR

In 2002, the National Rosacea Society Expert Committee, in an effort to standardize rosacea characteristics for both clinical trials and therapeutic needs, published the first classification of rosacea.[6] Four subtypes were identified: papulopustular (PPR), erythematotelangiectatic (ETR), phymatous (phR), and ocular (OcR) with a variant of granulomatous disease.[6,7] In 2018, the Expert Committee as well as other consensus groups reorganized the classification system recognizing that individual patients rarely fit into the strict categories defined in 2002; there is often significant overlap and patients may transition from one subtype to another over time.[8] Despite these advancements, much of the rosacea literature still relies on subtype classification and although no longer standard of care for diagnosis, these divisions can still provide a framework from which to approach treatment.

TABLE 50-1 Diagnostic criteria for rosacea*

Diagnostic criteria (Presence of ≥1 sufficient for diagnosis)	*Major criteria* (Presence of ≥2 may be diagnostic)	*Secondary criteria*
Fixed erythema affecting central third of the face ± transient, intermittent intensification	**Flushing**	Burning, stinging
Phymatous changes (eg, nose, ears, chin)	Papules, pustules	Edema
	Telangiectasias	Dryness
	Ocular symptoms • scleritis, sclerokeratitis • Lid margin telangiectasia • Conjunctival injection • Spade-shaped corneal infiltrates	Ocular symptoms • Lid margin irregularities • Evaporative tear dysfunction • Honey crusting • Collarette accumulation
		Symptoms of flushing

*Bold underlined criteria comprise the more common signs of rosacea that unfortunately may be more difficult to assess in patients with skin of color.

Adapted from Gallo RL, Granstein RD, Kang S, et al. Standard classification and pathophysiology of rosacea: the 2017 update by the National Rosacea Society Expert Committee. *J Am Acad Dermatol.* 2018;78(1):148-155.

In the new classification system, patients are defined by their phenotypic expressions: the presence or absence of erythema, inflammatory lesions, telangiectasias, ocular changes, phymatous changes, and symptomatology. Diagnostic features include fixed centrofacial erythema and/or phymatous changes. In their absence, the diagnosis of rosacea can also be made by a combination of the major features (eg, flushing, papules, pustules, telangiectasia, and ocular manifestations) as well as minor features (eg, symptoms such as burning, stinging, dryness, edema, and dry gritty sensation of the eyes) [**Table 50-1**].[6]

In patients with richly pigmented skin, the new classification system presents some challenges. If erythema is not evident or if the clinician is inexperienced in detecting erythema in skin of darker hues, this imperative diagnostic feature can be overlooked [**Figures 50-1** to **50-3**]. Two of four major features of flushing and telangiectasias may also be missed; we then rely on the infrequent finding of phymas [**Figures 50-4** and **50-5**], and the variable presence of inflammatory papules and ocular changes to identify rosacea. The diagnosis in darker skin, therefore, often hinges on the presence of symptoms. Taking a careful and thoughtful history that includes exacerbation with common triggers often turns out to be more valuable than the physical exam in patients with skin of color.

EPIDEMIOLOGY AND GENETICS

In the United States, population-based studies have estimated that rosacea may affect upward of 13 to 14 million individuals and as much as 5% of the general U.S. population.[3] In Northern European countries, with a larger more homogenous White population, prevalence may be as high as 10%[3] with at least one German-population study estimating 12% prevalence (9% erythematotelangiectatic-predominant [ETR], and

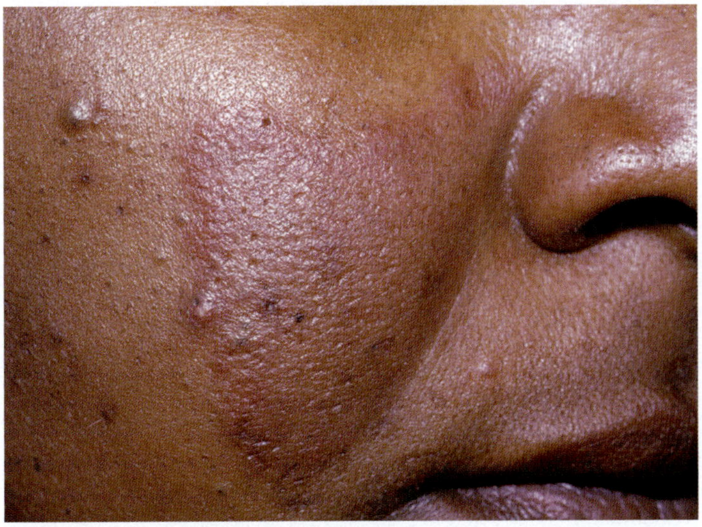

FIGURE 50-1 Mild erythematotelangiectasia-predominant rosacea with sparse papules and pustules. Note faint violaceous appearing erythema and postinflammatory hyperpigmentation. (Image used with permission from VisualDx.)

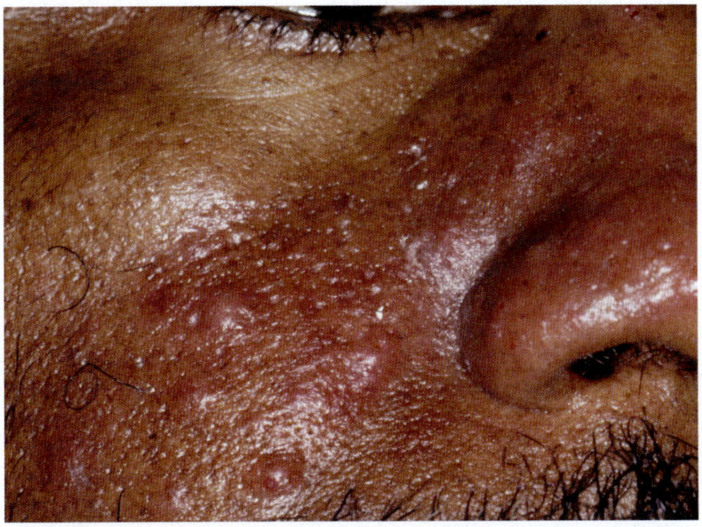

FIGURE 50-2 Predominantly papulopustular rosacea with background erythema. Note classic distribution of papules, pustules, and erythema on the central face. Although more severe, erythema still has a more violaceous tone in more richly pigmented skin and may not be immediately perceptible. (Image used with permission from VisualDx.)

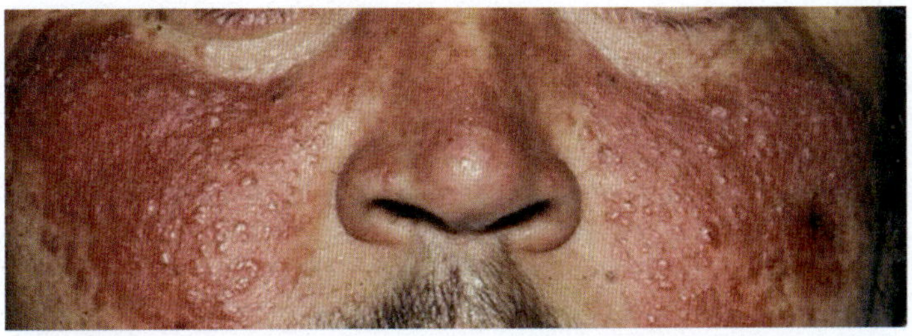

FIGURE 50-3 Severe papulopustular rosacea and background flushing in patient with phototype IV skin. Note slight violaceous hue to erythema and predominant involvement of the central face including nasolabial folds. (Image courtesy of Hilary E. Baldwin, MD.)

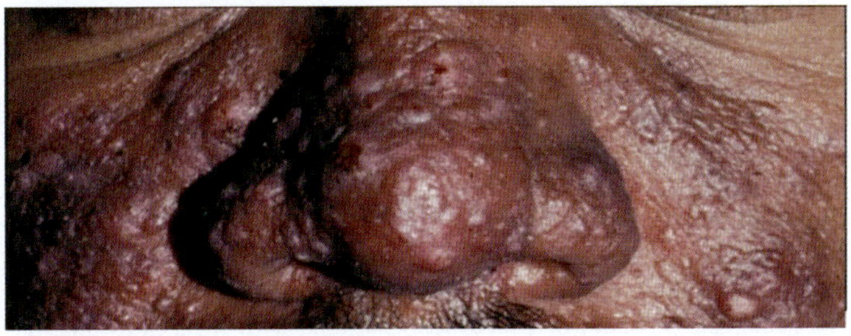

FIGURE 50-4 Early rhinophymatous changes in a patient with rosacea and skin phototype V skin. Note central face erythema appears more violaceous. (Image courtesy of Hilary E. Baldwin, MD.)

3% PPR-predominant rosacea).[9] Twin studies have found up to 46% concordance among identical twins.[10] Gene-wide association studies of individuals of primarily European ancestry have found at least one single-nucleotide polymorphism (SNP) located between genes coding for Human Leukocyte Antigen (HLA)-DRA and BTNL-2 (butyrophilin-like 2, a major histocompatibility complex class 1-associated gene also associated with inflammatory bowel disease and sarcoidosis) as well as three different HLA types (HLA-DRB1*30:01, HLA-DQB1*02:01, HLA-DQA1*05:01) that are also associated with autoimmune and inflammatory conditions including type 1 diabetes mellitus (T1DM), T1DM-associated retinopathy, and celiac disease, demonstrating, at least in White population, a potential genetic predisposition.[11] To the authors' knowledge, similar genetic studies have not focused on non-White populations. Though given the predilection for certain conditions (such as sarcoidosis) for individuals with more richly pigmented skin, there may be additional yet undiscovered genetic correlation among various populations.

A systematic review and meta-analysis of 32 articles capturing 15 different populations estimated the pooled prevalence among the general dermatology outpatient population to be 5.46% and as high as 23.14%.[4] Here, 99% of patients with rosacea in a collective sample size of ~26.5 million were greater than or equal to 31 years old, with a slight prevalence predilection for females (5.41% vs 3.9%). ETR was found to

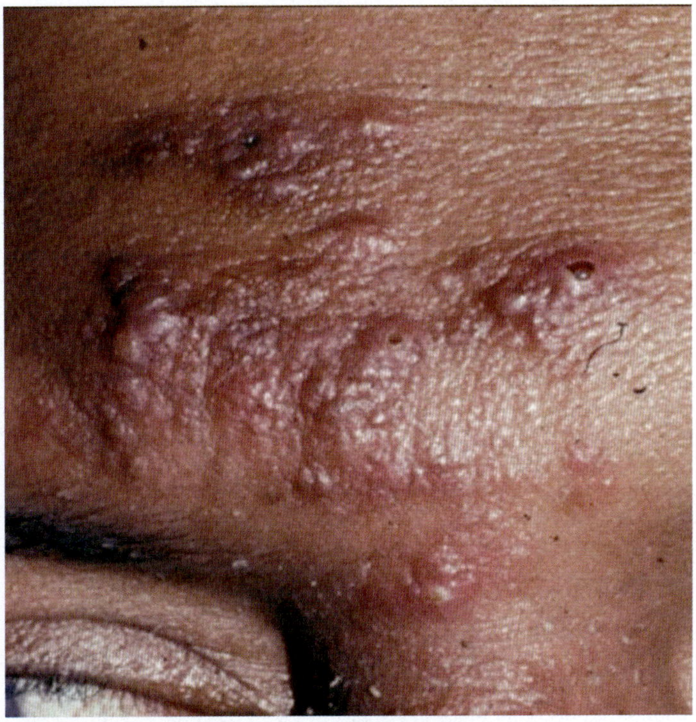

FIGURE 50-5 Forehead of a patient with papulopustular and early granulomatous changes of phymatous rosacea. (Image courtesy of Hilary E. Baldwin, MD.)

be the most prevalent presentation of rosacea (~72-80%) followed by PPR (~18-28%), OcR (6.5-8%), and PhR (4%).[4]

Of note, the sample populations assessed in these older studies were mostly (if not entirely) patients with lighter skin phototypes.[5,6] However, more recent studies have begun to elucidate the impact of rosacea in patients with skin of color.[12] A cross-sectional study of the U.S. National Ambulatory Medical Care Survey found that among all patients diagnosed with rosacea, 3.9% identified as Hispanic/Latino of any race, 2.3% identified as Asian/Pacific Islander, and 2% identified as Black.[13] A retrospective cohort of 168 Korean patients with rosacea found that 56.5% were skin phototype III, 32.7% were IV, and 7.1% were V,[14] while an Estonian case-control study of 440 patients (rosacea, $n = 223$; control, $n = 217$) found that 39% were phototype III and 5.4% phototype IV.[15] A cross-sectional Colombian study found 12% of patients with rosacea had skin phototype V or VI.[16] In a South African case series, while rosacea only comprised 0.2% of patient visits over an 8-year period, all cases were diagnosed in patients with either phototype V ($n = 6$) or VI ($n = 9$) skin.[17]

Another important consideration is that, although ETR may predominate among lighter skin phototypes, this may not be true for darker phototypes, wherein PPR and granulomatous-presentations of rosacea may be more common.[12] As mentioned previously, of the six potential diagnostic or major criteria, three (fixed erythema ± intermittent exacerbations, flushing, telangiectasias) [Table 50-1] may be overlooked in patients with darker skin phototypes, especially if the dermatologist or non-physician clinician has limited training in assessing patients with richly-pigmented skin. While signs of erythema may appear more red-pink in lighter skin phototypes, it may take on a more purple/violaceous to brown hue in the setting of phototype IV to VI skin, which may be mistaken for hyperpigmentation/dyspigmentation.[18] It is currently unclear whether the altered prevalence of rosacea among more richly pigmented populations is a result of protective/provocative factors that increase the likelihood of other rosacea classes such as PPR (eg, ~48.7% of patients in the cross-sectional Colombian study, and 40% to 50% of Korean males and females) or PhR [5,12,14,16,17,19,20] or if these subtler findings, which account for a majority of the necessary diagnostic criteria for rosacea, are more readily overlooked without a high index of suspicion.[12]

COMORBIDITIES AND PATIENT EXPERIENCE/OUTCOMES

In addition to potential association with T1DM, celiac disease, and sarcoidosis, studies, especially among east Asian patients, have found an association with gastrointestinal disease such as inflammatory bowel disease (IBD) (both Crohn disease and ulcerative colitis) irritable bowel syndrome and small intestinal bacterial overgrowth (SIBO).[21,22] Associated neurovasculature changes (discussed below) have also been implicated in other organ systems and may explain increased incidence of migraines in White individuals with rosacea (and vice versa)[23] and potentially cardiovascular disease.[10] Patients with rosacea have also been found to more frequently self-report conditions such as allergies (both food and airborne), respiratory diseases, gastroesophageal reflux disease, hypertension, metabolic syndrome, and urogenital diseases, all of which appear to correlate with worsening rosacea severity.[24]

Patients report significant psychosocial impairment on par with dermatoses such as vitiligo, leg ulcers, and contact dermatitis[25] with upward of 75% of rosacea patients reporting low self-esteem, 70% reporting embarrassment, and 69% feeling frustrated.[5] Those with severe symptoms or signs report rosacea interferes with their professional interactions (88%) and may have caused them to miss work (51%). Approximately 41% also report concurrent anxiety, while 25% report depression associated with decreased quality of life due to symptoms (eg, burning) or cosmetic disfigurement.[5] Furthermore, symptom severity of persistent and episodic flushing correlate with greater social phobia and stress.[26-28] However, these studies were also conducted in primarily (if not exclusively) White populations and likely do not capture (the full extent) of physical and psychosocial comorbidities in patients with more richly pigmented skin.[29]

PATHOPHYSIOLOGY

The pathogenesis of rosacea is thought to comprise a dysregulated innate and adaptive immune system that instigates excessive inflammation and a hyperreactive (cutaneous) neurovasculature coupled with extrinsic/environmental triggers.[30-32] Current data suggest this paradigm may apply to the rosacea pathogenesis across all skin phototypes (however, this too may be limited by diversity of studied populations).

The transcriptome of rosacea-affected skin has increased expression of toll-like receptor 2 (TLR2)[33-35] that regulates expression of vasoactive compounds and antimicrobial peptides such as cathelicidin, which is then processed into the active LL-37 by protease kallikrein 5 (KLK5).[33,36] LL-37 then binds to its lipopolysaccharides (LPS) targets and, via TLR3 and TLR4, can prime and activate the NOD-, leucine-rich repeat, and pyrin domain-containing protein 3 (NLRP3) inflammasome within macrophages[37-39] and recruit neutrophils (seen in PPR and PhR)[35,40] that further generate NADPH-oxidase-derived reactive oxygen species (ROS).[1,35,36] LL37 may also trigger mast cell degranulation, promoting ROS, inflammatory cytokines, and matrix metalloprotease-9 (MMP-9), the latter of which may further convert cathelicidin to LL-37.[39,41] Tetracyclines may reduce inflammation by inhibiting MMP-9 activity given, especially given inconsistent data regarding antimicrobial targets and efficacy at sub-antimicrobial dosing.[42,43] In all rosacea "phenotypes," there is an increase in CD4+ helper T-cell types 1 (T_H1) and type 17 (T_H17) with relevant cytokines (eg, interferon-gamma (IFN-γ); tumor necrosis factor-alpha (TNF-α); IL-12, STAT1, and STAT4; and IL-17A, IL-22, and STAT3, respectively) compared to healthy controls.[35] While PhR shares similar inflammatory markers to PPR and ETR, it is also clinically notable for significant sebaceous gland hyperplasia and fibrosis, both of which may be facilitated by endoplasmic reticulum stress signaling leading to upregulation in type I collagen synthesis and lipogenesis though exact mechanisms are still not yet fully elucidated.[44]

Hyperreactive and persistently dilated blood vessels (associated with persistent and transient exacerbation of facial erythema and telangiectasias) in ETR are thought to be mediated by transient receptor potential vanilloid (TRPV) and ankyrin (TRPA) channels on nerves (and potentially keratinocytes).[1,2] Channel activation ultimately releases vasoactive molecules such as calcitonin gene-related peptide (CGRP), pituitary adenylate cyclase-activating polypeptide (PACAP), substance P, and/or vasoactive intestinal peptide (VIP).[1,2] LL-37 may also upregulate TRPV-4 expression on mast cells decreasing the threshold for degranulation and vasodilation.[45] Frequently reported triggers of ETR such as (but not limited to) ultraviolet exposure, hot and/or cold ambient temperature, culinary spices, exercise, emotional stress/extremes, and alcohol are thought to acutely and chronically exacerbate rosacea severity through these pathways.[2] These external triggers may also upregulate TLR2 found on microglia and astrocytes resulting in neuronal transduction of pain and itch.[44,46] These findings likely translate clinically to the flushing and persistent erythema reported frequently in ETR as well as symptoms of facial burning, itching, and stinging.

These systems are ultimately interconnected in a potentially vicious positive-feedback loop. Vasodilatory peptides such as substance P and CGRP released in response to TRPA-1 and TRPV-1 activation may also stimulate NADPH oxidase activity leading to further ROS-dependent vasodilation.[1] TRP channels may also mediate keratinocyte expression of IL-1 and neuronal response to protease activity thereby augmenting inflammation.[1] In vitro studies moreover suggest that UV-B exposure may upregulate TLR2 and cathelicidin expression and further contribute to ROS production and hypervascularity via endothelial growth factor 2 (EGF2) and fibroblast growth factor 2 (FGF2) and may present an extra and/or alternative pathway by which UVR can exacerbate or influence rosacea severity.[44,47-50]

Importantly, it is unclear how and/or if the pathways described below are generalizable across different Fitzpatrick phototypes, especially given studies that suggest different levels of endothelial (re-)activity and function in response to stimuli based on ethnic backgrounds.[5,12,51-53]

While there are no definitive studies elucidating differences in rosacea pathogenesis among different Fitzpatrick skin types, several studies have noted variances in the epidermal biophysical/mechanical properties between phototypes, which may have theoretical implications for rosacea etiology (and management). Differences in eumelanin and phaeomelanin provide increased UV protection in more richly pigmented skin[54,55] that translates to an estimated sun protection factor (SPF) of ~13.4.[56] Additionally, studies suggest that the cutaneous blood-flow response within microvascular endothelia may have attenuated signaling in patients of Asian and Afro-Caribbean descent compared to White patients, which may be due to genetic variations across populations and also explain in part differential triggers and severity of flushing.[51-53,57] Conversely, data also suggest richly pigmented skin may be more susceptible to extremes in temperature with potentially increased cold-induced vasculature reactivity due to cold and increased retention of infrared (IR) radiation.[56] These factors may alter the likelihood that UVR, IR, and temperature extremes play a role as a triggers for rosacea flares in patients with more richly pigmented skin.

THE MICROBIOME AND EPIDERMAL BARRIER (DYS)FUNCTION

Given the extent to which the innate and adaptive immune systems are dysregulated in rosacea, studies have sought to define triggers/instigators of inflammation with mixed results with special interest afforded to the cutaneous and enteral microbiome.[31,58,59] While microbiome composition can vary with factors such as age,[60,61] gender,[60,61] mucocutaneous anatomic location,[62] geographic location,[60,63,64] climate,[60] and lifestyle,[61,63,64] it is unclear how genetics and race may influence the cutaneous (and enteral) balance.[65,66] Population-based studies have found variations between geographically and culturally distinct populations.[64] However, these findings focused only on bacterial microbiomes and may be confounded by differences in lifestyle and environmental exposures (eg, more urban living among U.S.-based White women compared to more rural living among Tanzanian women).[63] Furthermore, studies have also found shifts in microbiome with transition from nomadic to more settled lifestyle, with a significant decrease in microbiome diversity mirroring that of otherwise healthy U.S.-based study participants.[64] Conversely, a large Chinese-based population study found increased clustering of healthy microbiome samples taken from the palms of Chinese participants, regardless of lifestyle, compared to U.S. and Tanzanian participants.[66] Of note, these studies were done primarily in "healthy" participants; similar studies of dermatoses are infrequent in the literature, especially regarding rosacea.

Despite potential influence from genetic and/or racial backgrounds, several cutaneous microbes have been implicated including Demodex spp. (eg, *D. folliculorum, D. brevis*), *Bacillus oleronius*, *Staphylococcus epidermidis*, and *Cutibacterium acnes*.[67]

Demodex spp. (primarily *D. folliculorum* and D. brevis) are commensal mites that consume sebum within the pilosebaceous units.[68] While studies have demonstrated a long-standing relationship between humans and Demodex spp.,[69] the latter has also been found more frequently in individuals with rosacea than in their healthy age-matched control counterparts (96% vs 74%, $p < 0.01$)[68] while epidemiological studies have found significantly increased Demodex density in patients with PPR compared to healthy controls (36/cm^2 vs ≤5/cm^2).[70] Increased Demodex burden is thought to result in follicular rupture leading to increased expression of LL-37, MMP-9, IL-8, and TNF-α leading to cell-mediated granuloma formation.[68,71] However, in a chicken-and-egg situation, it is unclear if Demodex spp. instigate inflammation or are able to proliferate under these inflammatory changes. Furthermore, different "clades" of *D. folliculorum* have been associated with populations with divergent ancestry with those of European decent having mostly clade D, those of Asian ancestry lacking clade C, while those of African ancestry had a mixture of all clades (A-D).[69] While these clades of *D. folliculorum* appear more static regardless of (change in) geographic regions for at least several generations,[69] it is unclear how this may affect rosacea pathogenesis.

The gram-negative bacterium *B. oleronius* is a commensal of the Demodex mite (and not humans) that has been cultivated from PPR skin.[72] *B. oleronius* has been found to be able to stimulate a macrophage-based response in individuals with rosacea and may also play a role in inflammation in ETR and even OcR via MMP-9, IL-8, and TNF-α.[73-75]

The gram-positive cocci *S. epidermidis* has been cultured from pustules in PPR but not from unaffected skin on the contralateral cheeks of individuals with rosacea.[76] Furthermore, *S. epidermidis* cultured in this manner were more likely to have β-hemolytic activity and secrete virulent factors at higher temperatures that may correlate with cutaneous temperatures overlying excessively dilated facial vascular beds.[77]

Interestingly, the relative decrease in *C. acnes* abundance is also correlated with rosacea.[78,79] When stratified by age, healthy individuals greater than or equal to 60 years old had significantly ($p = 0.018$) less *C. acnes* than healthy individuals less than 60 years old[79] that may contribute in part to rosacea's onset in the fourth and fifth decades of life. Furthermore, cultures from the malar cheeks of individuals with PPR and ETR and healthy controls found significantly ($p < 0.01$) decreased relative abundance of *C. acnes* in individuals with rosacea than their control counterparts.[78]

Microbiome disturbances often go hand-in-hand with epidermal barrier dysfunction (EBD) wherein disruption in one's homeostasis leads to disruption of the other.[59] Signs of EBD include burning, hyperirritability, stinging, and hypersensitivity to topically applied compounds may also be clinical symptoms of rosacea.[80-82] Furthermore, a significantly more alkaline pH and altered surface lipid composition may also predispose individuals with rosacea to common triggers (eg, extreme temperatures, UVR) and an increased risk of allergic/irritant contact dermatitis.[81,83,84] Studies have found localized EBD in the nasolabial folds of individuals with rosacea compared to healthy controls with increased transepidermal water loss (TEWL) (21.1 vs 16.8, $p = 0.127$) and significantly decreased corneal layer hydration(16.5 vs 24.4, $p < 0.001$).[85] These changes may also correlate with rosacea severity wherein independent OTC and prescription topical or systemic monotherapy treatment (with minocycline) of rosacea has been noted to improve EBD.[86-91] Of note, studies have found increased TEWL and decreased stratum corneum hydration (SCH) between White and Black populations.[56,92,93] This may heighten the importance of eliciting symptomatic secondary criteria [Table 50-1] in the diagnosis of rosacea in patients with more richly pigmented skin.

SYSTEMIC MANIFESTATIONS AND INFLAMMATION ASSOCIATED WITH ROSACEA

There is growing, albeit inconsistent, evidence of a cutaneous-enteric axis regarding the microbiome and rosacea.[94] As mentioned previously, several HLA haplotypes have been associated with rosacea and other autoimmune and inflammatory conditions including T1DM, celiac disease, and sarcoidosis.[21] Population studies have also found an association with gastrointestinal disease such as inflammatory bowel disease (IBD) (both Crohn disease and ulcerative colitis) and irritable bowel syndrome, short intestinal bacterial overgrowth (SIBO).[21,22] In a Korean study, patients with IBD had a reciprocated increased risk of also having rosacea.[95] Interestingly, patients with rosacea and SIBO who were treated with rifaximin (a gastrointestinal lumen-limited antibiotic) had not only improvement in their SIBO but also had complete clearance (71.4%) or significant improvement in (21.4%) their rosacea.[22] Other studies have also implicated helicobacter pylori and lesser reported genera of gastrointestinal flora including *Actinomyces, Chloroplast, Corynebacterium, Geobacilus, Gordonia,* and *Vellonella.*[96-98]

DIAGNOSIS AND MANAGEMENT

DIAGNOSTIC PEARLS

A study conducted in a primarily White population found that approximately 47.5% of individuals diagnosed with rosacea during the study had not previously received treatment for it suggesting that even when more commonly expected, rosacea often goes un(der)diagnosed and un(der) treated.

While several risk factors including female sex and central face involvement [Figures 50-1 to 50-3] may hint at rosacea, on an initial patient encounter history is key.[12,20] Here "secondary" criteria such as symptoms of burning or stinging, edema, dryness may suggest epidermal barrier dysfunction associated with rosacea, while a sensation of flushing (ie, a temporary warm sensation over the face) may indicate classic neurovasculature changes associated with ETR.[12,20] As a result, patients may also report low tolerance for common over-the-counter skin care products.[99] Depending on chronicity of disease and how observant patients are of their symptoms, they may also report exacerbation of symptoms with classic triggers including but not limited to UVR, extreme temperatures, spicy food, alcohol, and stress.[12,20] Inquiry into prior treatment of recalcitrant acneiform lesions may also hint at potential PPR, especially in the absence of comedones.[12,20] While not necessarily sensitive or specific for rosacea, given potential genetic predisposition, asking about family history of similar signs and/or symptoms may assist in initial assessment.[12,20] Notably, patients with mixed ancestry may also be at increased risk of inheriting a genetic predisposition to rosacea.[12]

It is also imperative to ask about potential ocular involvement, such as foreign body sensation, itching, irritation, as these symptoms are often preceded by cutaneous disease in over 50% of cases, overlooked even in patient populations with a higher incidence/prevalence of rosacea, and can have severe long-term consequences.[8,31] While the population or cohort/case-control data are limited, case reports have documented severe morbidity including neovascularization, corneal ulcers, transient, and even permanent vision loss with at least one patient previously receiving an enucleation due to long-standing inflammatory changes.[100] Work up for these patients included extensive physical examination and testing (including corneal cultures, RPR and VDRL, ANA, rheumatoid factor, ESR and CRP, CXR) to evaluate potential infectious, autoimmune, and inflammatory conditions because of a low suspicion for oculocutaneous rosacea despite cutaneous findings.[100] Importantly, while rare in the pediatric population, case reports have also noted oculo(cutaneous) rosacea in pediatric patients with richly pigmented skin, further emphasizing the importance of a broad differential and high-degree of suspicion when presented with otherwise characteristic signs and symptoms.[101]

When conducting the physical exam, the authors have found utility in asking patients, "Does your skin look red to you?" and to specifically point out areas that appear abnormal to them. In this way, when compared to their own clinically normal skin, a baseline for erythema and pigmentary changes can be set. Distinguishing different color tones may be facilitated by conducting the exam with good lighting and using a blue-back background to highlight any present erythema.[12,20] More subtle signs of ETR such as telangiectasias and erythema may be better visualized with the aid of dermoscopy or diascopy by inducing localized blanching with applied gentle pressure.[12,20]

As noted before, the presence of papulopustules sans comedones may hint at PPR.[12,20] There is some evidence to suggest a potential increased risk of phymatous changes, most commonly found on/around the nose and cheeks (and rarely chin and ears), in darker skin phototypes.[12,102] While phyma may be more apparent with advanced disease [Figure 50-4], if subtle changes of sebaceous hyperplasia or fibrosis are suspected [Figure 50-5], early detection may be facilitated by comparing patients to previously taken photographs. Finally, if ocular involvement is suspected, a superficial ocular exam should be performed (and referral made to ophthalmology for a more holistic ocular exam).

A diagnosis not considered is a diagnosis not made. While patient background may alter pretest probabilities and a differential diagnosis, rosacea should be considered for any patient presenting with central facial erythema, papules and/or pustules, or other hallmarks of the disease. It is also important not to anchor and consider other central face dermatoses in patients with skin of color, including (but certainly not limited to) seborrheic dermatitis, acne vulgaris, (acute) lupus erythematosus, sarcoidosis, periorificial dermatitis, or steroid acne or acneiform lesions due to other medications.

THERAPEUTIC CONSIDERATIONS AND OPTIONS

Overall, given our current understanding of rosacea pathogenesis, there is little data to suggest material differences in treatment regimens are warranted based on patient skin phototype. As with all patient encounters addressing chronic diseases, managing patient expectations is paramount and time should be taken to provide counseling and education in a manner that aligns with a patient's personal beliefs and treatment goals.[20] Time should be spent in the first visit to address patient's (self-perceived) disease severity (eg, while erythema may be less perceptible in darker skin phototypes, individuals may still find it significantly detracts from their quality of life).[20] Furthermore, there are few key nuances when discussing management options with patients with more richly pigmented skin, primarily related to potential pigment derangements (eg, minimizing irritation and possible dyschromia associated with certain energy-based treatments/devices).

Skin Care and Lifestyle Modification If patients are able to identify triggers (eg, spicy food, alcohol, topical OTC or prescription products, specific foods including marinated meat products or exotic fruit, temperature extremes, UVR, etc) for their condition,[31] they should be advised to minimize or completely avoid them. For newly diagnosed patients or patients with more (sub)acute onset, patients can trial logging potential triggers against symptoms to identify potential lifestyle modifications.

The authors note that no patient encounter for rosacea is complete without adequate discussion of gentle skin care and proper skin hygiene. Given increased propensity for dyspigmentation following resolution of inflammation in patients with skin of color, discussion regarding appropriate general skin care, including avoidance of physical and chemical irritants, is paramount. As patients with rosacea may be at increased risk for contact dermatitis due to EBD, they should be counseled to avoid exfoliants, scrubbing with washcloths, use of scented products, use of alkaline, abrasive, or alcohol-based soaps or cleansers.[12,15,31,58,59,103] Patients should also be counseled on the importance of sun protection and the use of (mineral-based for patients with sensitivity to chemical-based) sunscreen with sun protection factor (SPF) greater than or equal to 30 with either iron oxide or tint to minimize the effects of visible light on pigment changes.[31,104]

Persistent Erythema, Flushing, and Telangiectasias The vasodilation and inflammation that give rise to persistent erythema, flushing, and telangiectasias associated with ETR [Figures 50-1 and 50-2] can be managed with a combination of camouflage, prescription topical vasoconstrictive medications, and energy-based procedures [**Table 50-2**].

Green-tinted foundations and facial cosmetic powders can provide a complementary color tone to mute red pigmentation on top of which patients can then apply a more "true-tone" foundation.[105]

Medical management of vasodilation is best accomplished with either topical brimonidine 0.33% gel or oxymetazoline 1% cream.[12] Topical brimonidine is an α2-adrenergic agonist that has shown efficacy in achieving at least a 2-grade improvement in moderate to severe persistent erythema in skin phototype II to III patients within 3 hours of use (of the 0.5% tartrate gel) and decrease baseline erythema (ie, erythema before topical application) by an average of 1-grade based on clinician's erythema (CEA) and patient's self-assessment (PSA) scores after approximately 3 months of once daily topical application (of the 0.5% tartrate gel).[15,106-109] Though generally well-tolerated, adverse effects can include local skin reactions (eg, burning, stinging, and contact dermatitis)[109] and potential for erythema in areas adjacent to topical application[110] as well as potential for transient "rebound" exacerbation of erythema in an estimated 5% to 20% of patients that may persist up to an additional 12 hours after application.[111,112] Oxymetazoline is an α1-receptor agonist that also demonstrated significant 2-grade improvement in a composite CEA-SSA (subject self-assessment) score for moderate persistent erythema in predominantly phototype II to III patients within 3 hours of application with peak efficacy around hour 6 to 9 that tapered off by hour 12.[113] Of note, additional data from community-based trials suggest oxymetazoline also has efficacy in phototypes IV to VI.[12] A 52-week extension trial demonstrated a similar limited local skin adverse effects

TABLE 50-2 Intervention options based on predominant rosacea phenotype

	Erythematotelangiectatic	Papulopustular	Phymatous	Ocular
Over the Counter				
	Green-tinted foundation			Ω-3 fatty acid
Topical				
	Brimonidine 0.33% gel	Metronidazole 0.75% cream/gel/lotion		Cyclosporine
	Oxymetazoline 1% cream	Ivermectin 1% cream		Ivermectin
		Azelaic acid 15% gel/foam		calcineurin inhibitors
		Sodium sulfacetamide 10%/sulfur 5% cream		
		Minocycline 1.5% foam		
		Microencapsulated benzoyl peroxide 5% cream		
Systemic				
		Doxycycline	Doxycycline	Doxycycline
		Doxycycline modified-release	Doxycycline modified-release	Tetracyclines Azithromycin
		Minocycline	Minocycline	
		Sarecycline	Isotretinoin	
		Isotretinoin	Minocycline, extended-release	
Procedural		Minocycline, extended-release		
	Neodymium-doped yttrium aluminum garnet (Nd:YAG) 1064 nm		Surgical debulking (eg, scalpel, electrosurgery, cryosurgery, dermabrasion)	
			Laser (CO_2, Diode)	
			Nonablative radiofrequency	

to brimonidine with a lower incidence of rebound erythema (~1%) and potential for further improvement based on composite CEA-SSA scores up to 1 year with continual daily usage.[114]

Laser- and light-based treatments may also be used as adjuncts, especially to manage signs and symptoms of ETR, including telangiectasias (which are not affected by topical vasoconstrictors) or PhR.[12,31] While there is some evidence that 585 nm and 595 nm pulsed-dye lasers (PDL) may be safe for darker skin types, especially in conjunction with skin cooling,[115] expert consensus opinion have recommended avoiding PDL in skin phototypes IV to VI and intense-pulsed light (IPL) in phototypes V to VI; for these patients, a neodymium-doped yttrium aluminum garnet (Nd:YAG) microsecond 1064 laser may have a better safety profile.[103] Test spots may also be helpful to assess reaction to energy-based treatment and lower fluences should be considered, especially in patients without prior history of receiving energy-based therapy.[12]

Papules and Pustules Papules and pustules of PPR [Figures 50-2 to 50-4] can be managed with topical and/or oral agents [Table 50-2]. Numerous topical medications have shown efficacy in treating the inflammatory lesions of rosacea and the last decade has seen the introduction of products with improved efficacy and tolerability. Older medications such as metronidazole and azelaic acid have been available since the early 1990s. Metronidazole (0.75% gel/cream, 0.75% lotion, and 1% gel) is well tolerated with minimal application site erythema and scaling and has demonstrated efficacy within 2 to 4 weeks of initiation.[116-120] Azelaic acid is available in 15% gel and foam for the treatment of rosacea. The gel, utilized twice daily, appears to have equal efficacy to metronidazole 1% gel.[121] It typically leads to noticeable improvement within weeks of initiation with maximum efficacy noted within 15 weeks and there may be transient mild to moderate application site burning, stinging, or itching.[119,122-126] In darker skin phototypes, azelaic acid has the additional benefit of treating any postinflammatory hyperpigmentation left after resolution of papules and pustules.[113] Sodium sulfacetamide 10% with sulfur 5% cream has limited data to support its use for this indication and patients should be counseled about potential off-putting scent.[31,127]

Since 2014, we have seen the development and U.S. Food and Drug Administration (FDA) approval of three new topical medications that have improved efficacy and excellent tolerability data. Ivermectin cream 1% was compared to twice daily topical metronidazole 0.75% cream and was found to have greater efficacy at all timepoints in reducing papules and pustules with significant clinical improvement notable within 12 to 16 weeks[121,122,128,129] and may have longer sustained remission of PPR at 36 weeks as well.[130,131]

Recent data demonstrate efficacy for topical minocycline 1.5% foam[132] with no signals regarding dyspigmentation up to 1 year.[34] In parallel phase 3 studies, it demonstrated significant changes as early as week 4.[132,133] Microencapsulated benzoyl peroxide recently (April 2022) received FDA approval with results from parallel, double-blind, vehicle-controlled phase 3 clinical trials demonstrating 70% reduction in inflammatory lesions compared to 38% to 46% for the vehicle by week 12 of the trial with more than 40% reduction in inflammatory lesions as early as week 2.[134-138] Of note, all of these newer therapies have demonstrated excellent tolerability with minimal application site irritation in phase 2 and 3 studies, which should be of utmost importance when creating a topical regimen for richly pigmented skin that avoids iatrogenic hyperpigmentation.[132-134]

Sodium sulfacetamide 10% with sulfur 5% cream and cleanser have limited data supporting their use and patients should be counseled about potential off-putting scent.[31,139,140]

Oral tetracycline antibiotics doxycycline and minocycline dosed 50 to 200 mg daily (with the exception of weight-based extended-release minocycline) are considered a first-line therapy for moderate to severe PPR and have been studied as both monotherapy and in combination with topical medications.[31,141,142] Earlier use may be warranted in patients with darker skin who are experiencing cutaneous irritation with topical medications. Tetracyclines are primarily thought to reduce MMP-9-induced inflammation associated with rosacea.[42,43] Given that rosacea is a chronic inflammatory disorder without evidence of a specific colonizing or virulent microbe, questions have been raised regarding the rationale for the use of full dose antibiotics, especially for long-term usage. With an eye toward being good stewards of antibiotics and in an attempt to maintain doxycycline's anti-inflammatory ability while minimizing antibiotic effect, a "sub-antimicrobial" 40 mg modified release (30 mg immediate release, 10 mg extended release) daily formulation was developed. It demonstrated an absence of antimicrobial/antibiotic selective pressure[143] and similar efficacy to 100 mg dosing with the added benefit of decreased gastrointestinal adverse effects.[31,144-146] Community-based trials have also demonstrated efficacy in the modified-release doxycycline in patients with rosacea who have skin phototypes IV to VI.[147] To date, sub-antimicrobial dosing of doxycycline is the only FDA-approved oral medication for PPR.[148] Combination of "sub-antimicrobial" doxycycline and either topical metronidazole[145,149] or topical ivermectin[150] have demonstrated improved clearance in IGA with the latter also having a noted beneficial effect on erythema and flushing, secondary symptoms (eg, burning and stinging), and ocular symptoms. Recently, a low-dose, extended-release minocycline 40 mg was launched. In a head-to-head comparison trial, the minocycline formulation was found to be superior to MRD in investigator global assessment success and lesion count reduction.[90] In a 16-week, vehicle-controlled study of 60 healthy adults, there was no demonstrable change in the microflora of skin, vagina, stool from baseline to end of trial.[91]

Also with antibiotic stewardship in mind, a pilot study was conducted to investigate the use of the third-generation tetracycline, sarecycline, in rosacea.[151] Sarecycline requires a 16- to 32-fold greater minimum inhibitory concentration (MIC) to be as effective as doxycycline or minocycline against the gram-negative anaerobic species that are primarily found in the gut and induces mutations in *C. acnes* in less than 1 in 10 billion times at 4 to 8 times the MIC.[152,153] An investigator-initiated pilot trial found significant improvement in IGA and reduction in inflammatory lesions at weeks 4, 8, 12 without any significant adverse effects (AEs).[151] It remains to be seen if this full-dose antibiotic causes less ecologic mischief than other tetracyclines in an in vivo setting.

It is important to counsel patients about adverse effects of the tetracycline antibiotic class including tooth discoloration and long-bone growth derangements in children (exposed in utero), risk of pigmentation, vertigo, and rarely a lupus-like syndrome with minocycline, and photosensitivity and gastrointestinal adverse effects of doxycycline.[154]

Patients with severe,[155,156] refractory/recalcitrant,[157,158] and even granulomatous[159] PPR can be trialed off-label on isotretinoin starting at 0.25 mg/kg/day.[122,160] Reports have demonstrated efficacy with doses from 0.1 to 1.0 mg/kg/day.[89,156,161,162] At low daily doses or infrequent dosing, isotretinoin has been shown to improve inflammatory lesions, erythema, and ocular disease and to reduce the volume of phymatous material and halt the progression of phymas (cited as above). iPLEDGE REMS rules and regulations still apply and may be cumbersome considering the need for long-term use. Unlike its use in acne, isotretinoin does not produce a durable response in rosacea and relapses are to be expected. Adverse events with isotretinoin use are well known including but not limited to xerosis, cheilitis, epistaxis, xerophthalmia, myalgia, arthralgia, rare neurologic symptoms such as tinnitus, or laboratory derangements such as hyperlipidemia or elevated serum creatine kinase.[163] Important to note, most isotretinoin adverse effects are dose-dependent; in the authors' experience, patients with rosacea often respond to very low doses of isotretinoin (10 to 20 mg once or twice a week) and thus may be spared from many of the prototypical unwanted outcomes.

Phymatous Changes Early detection and treatment [Table 50-2] of inflammatory phymatous changes [Figures 50-4 and 50-5] offers the best chance at halting disease progression. Here, systemic treatment regimen, namely doxycycline and isotretinoin as prescribed for PPR (see section "Papules and Pustules"), may be efficacious.[31,122] However, once phyma have reached advanced stages of sebaceous hyperplasia and fibrosis, procedural intervention is recommended. Surgical debulking (eg, via scalpel, electrosurgery, cryosurgery, or dermabrasion) and countering may be able to restore shape to the affected areas.[164-168] Energy-based treatments including ablative carbon dioxide lasers and infrared diode lasers have also been used in lighter skin phototypes patients[169-171]; however, patients with darker skin phototypes (ie, V and VI) are at increased risk of scarring and dyspigmentation, especially with ablative lasers.[172] Mild to moderate rhinophyma in patients with darker skin phototype may also be successfully managed with nonablative radiofrequency.[173]

Ocular Disease Ocular rosacea may precede classic cutaneous findings of rosacea in up to 20% of cases and may be found concurrently in up to 50%.[174] Given that rosacea is more frequently overlooked in patients with darker skin phototypes, it is important to inquire about ocular symptoms (including dryness, stinging, burning, foreign body sensation) during each rosacea encounter as not to miss more severe manifestation including keratitis and scleritis.[8]

There is some evidence that increased Ω-3 fatty acid intake and ocular hygiene maintenance (ie, using warm compresses and gentle lid/lash cleansing to express trapped Meibomian gland sebum) may be beneficial.[175,176]

Medical management [Table 50-2] can include topical cyclosporine or oral doxycycline[34] with lesser evidence for oral azithromycin, topical calcineurin inhibitors, and potentially other tetracycline antibiotics.[34,177] Limited evidence also suggests that treatment of adjacent areas and systemic treatment may alleviate inflammation.[34] Sobolewska et al demonstrated that, in a study of 10 patients, application of half pea-size amount of ivermectin 1% cream to closed eyelids and lid margins reduced erythema, ocular symptoms, and evidence of meibomian gland dysfunction.[178]

Clinicians should also have a low threshold for ophthalmology referral, especially if there are signs of corneal ulceration, severe inflammation with a red eye, or worsening or changing vision.

Combination Therapy While we have discussed treatment options as if rosacea is stratified into distinct phenotypes, patients will often present with a spectrum of signs and symptoms (eg, erythema and papules, pustules and telangiectasias, etc). Unfortunately, current prescription regimens do not cover multiple "phenotypes." However, there are no contraindications to combining interventions already approved for rosacea. At least one study has demonstrated that treatment with brimonidine and ivermectin lead to significant and accelerated improvement in both papules and persistent erythema without increase in adverse effects or loss of tolerability.[179] In devising a combination regimen, determining patient priorities (ie, what bothers them the most about their rosacea) and what modalities will promote long-term adherence may ultimately prove more efficacious than what agents are selected.

Therapeutic Pipeline With our increased understanding of the pathogenesis of rosacea, new treatment targets and agents [**Table 50-3**] are continually being developed. Biologic agents targeting the T_H17 axis (namely secukinumab) and an anti-CGRP agent (erenumab) are currently being investigated.[139,180] Agents that modulate the innate immune system including a TLR-2 inhibitor (DMT210 5% gel), a synthetic antimicrobial peptide (omiganan pentahydrochloride), and a topical probiotic (*Nitrosomonas eutropha)* are all under investigation.[181-183] Available medications including rifaximin, which has demonstrated efficacy previously in concurrently treating SIBO and rosacea[22,184] and hydroxychloroquine, which has also demonstrated efficacy but whose long-term use is limited by irreversible retinopathy,[185-187] are also being studied or considered for off-label use.[188]

Alternative and Complementary Medicine While patients may express interest in alternative or complementary approaches to their treatment regimen, they should be counseled that there is limited data on their efficacy. Given patients with rosacea may already be at increased

TABLE 50-3 Therapeutic rosacea pipeline

	Name	Mechanism of action
Biologics		
	Secukinumab	Monoclonal antibody IL-17
	Erenumab	Monoclonal anti-CGRP
Immunomodulators		
	DMT210 5% gel	Anti-TLR 2
	Omigran Pentahydrochloride	Synthetic antimicrobial peptide
	Nitrosomonas eutropha	Topical probiotic
Antibiotic		
	Rifaximin	Intestinal-lumen restricted antibiotic
Other		
	Hydroxychloroquine	unknown

risk of contact dermatitis, they should be cautioned against using even "natural" topical remedies that may induce inflammation and pigment alteration. With that in mind, few small studies have found potential limited evidence for the use of aloe vera, vitamin C, licochalcone, niacinamide, green tea, feverfew, coffeeberry, soy, and oatmeal.[189]

CONCLUSION

Rosacea is a chronic inflammatory dermatosis of the central face that often goes mis- or underdiagnosed in patients with darker skin phototypes. It is important that dermatologists keep rosacea high on the differential for central face dermatosis in patients who may present with primarily "secondary" criteria for diagnosis (ie, facial and/or ocular stinging, burning, sensitivity, etc). Current studies investigating treatment of rosacea in darker skin phototypes is limited and current guidelines are based primarily on standard of care, individual physician experience, and expert consensus. Nuances to care include the importance of emphasizing gentle skin care and proper skin hygiene as well as being cognizant of treatment options that may induce or treat postinflammatory pigment alterations.

REFERENCES

1. Aubdool AA, Brain SD. Neurovascular aspects of skin neurogenic inflammation. *J Investig Dermatol Symp Proc.* 2011;15(1):33-39.
2. Schwab VD, Sulk M, Seeliger S, et al. Neurovascular and neuroimmune aspects in the pathophysiology of rosacea. *J Investig Dermatol Symp Proc.* 2011;15(1):53-62.
3. Elewski BE, Draelos Z, Dréno B, Jansen T, Layton A, Picardo M. Rosacea - global diversity and optimized outcome: proposed international consensus from the Rosacea International Expert Group. *J Eur Acad Dermatol Venereol.* 2011;25(2):188-200.
4. Gether L, Overgaard LK, Egeberg A, Thyssen JP. Incidence and prevalence of rosacea: a systematic review and meta-analysis. *Br J Dermatol.* 2018;179(2):282-289.
5. Rainer BM, Kang S, Chien AL. Rosacea: epidemiology, pathogenesis, and treatment. *Dermatoendocrinol.* 2017;9(1):e1361574.
6. Wilkin J, Dahl M, Detmar M, et al. Standard classification of rosacea: report of the National Rosacea Society Expert Committee on the Classification and Staging of Rosacea. *J Am Acad Dermatol.* 2002;46(4):584-587.
7. Tan J, Almeida LMC, Bewley A, et al. Updating the diagnosis, classification and assessment of rosacea: recommendations from the global ROSacea COnsensus (ROSCO) panel. *Br J Dermatol.* 2017;176(2):431-438.
8. Gallo RL, Granstein RD, Kang S, et al. Standard classification and pathophysiology of rosacea: the 2017 update by the National Rosacea Society Expert Committee. *J Am Acad Dermatol.* 2018;78(1):148-155.
9. Tan J, Schöfer H, Araviiskaia E, et al. Prevalence of rosacea in the general population of Germany and Russia - the RISE study. *J Eur Acad Dermatol Venereol.* 2016;30(3):428-434.
10. Aldrich N, Gerstenblith M, Fu P, et al. Genetic vs environmental factors that correlate with rosacea: a cohort-based survey of twins. *JAMA Dermatol.* 2015;151(11):1213-1219.
11. Chang ALS, Raber I, Xu J, et al. Assessment of the genetic basis of rosacea by genome-wide association study. *J Invest Dermatol.* 2015;135(6):1548-1555.
12. Alexis AF, Callender VD, Baldwin HE, Desai SR, Rendon MI, Taylor SC. Global epidemiology and clinical spectrum of rosacea, highlighting skin of color: review and clinical practice experience. *J Am Acad Dermatol.* 2019;80(6):1722-1729.e7.
13. Al-Dabagh A, Davis SA, McMichael AJ, Feldman SR. Rosacea in skin of color: not a rare diagnosis. *Dermatol Online J.* 2014;20(10):13.
14. Bae YI, Yun SJ, Lee JB, Kim SJ, Won YH, Lee SC. Clinical evaluation of 168 Korean patients with rosacea: the sun exposure correlates with the erythematotelangiectatic subtype. *Ann Dermatol.* 2009;21(3):243-249.
15. Abram K, Silm H, Maaroos HI, Oona M. Risk factors associated with rosacea. *J Eur Acad Dermatol Venereol.* 2010;24(5):565-571.
16. Rueda LJ, Motta A, Pabón JG, et al. Epidemiology of rosacea in Colombia. *Int J Dermatol.* 2017;56(5):510-513.
17. Dlova NC, Mosam A. Rosacea in black South Africans with skin phototypes V and VI. *Clin Exp Dermatol.* 2017;42(6):670-673.
18. Kaufman BP, Guttman-Yassky E, Alexis AF. Atopic dermatitis in diverse racial and ethnic groups-variations in epidemiology, genetics, clinical presentation and treatment. *Exp Dermatol.* 2018;27(4):340-357.
19. Barakji YA, Rønnstad ATM, Christensen MO, et al. Assessment of frequency of rosacea subtypes in patients with Rosacea: a systematic review and meta-analysis. *JAMA Dermatol.* 2022;158(6):617-625.
20. Cices A, Alexis AF. Patient-focused solutions in rosacea management: treatment challenges in special patient groups. *J Drugs Dermatol.* 2019;18(7):608-612.
21. Egeberg A, Weinstock LB, Thyssen EP, Gislason GH, Thyssen JP. Rosacea and gastrointestinal disorders: a population-based cohort study. *Br J Dermatol.* 2017;176(1):100-106.
22. Parodi A, Paolino S, Greco A, et al. Small intestinal bacterial overgrowth in rosacea: clinical effectiveness of its eradication. *Clin Gastroenterol Hepatol.* 2008;6(7):759-764.
23. Wienholtz NKF, Christensen CE, Haugaard JH, et al. Cohort profile: COpenhagen ROsacea COhort (COROCO) and COpenhagen MIgraine COhort (COMICO). *BMJ Open.* 2020;10(8):e039445.
24. Rainer BM, Fischer AH, Luz Felipe da Silva D, Kang S, Chien AL. Rosacea is associated with chronic systemic diseases in a skin severity-dependent manner: results of a case-control study. *J Am Acad Dermatol.* 2015;73(4):604-608.
25. Kini SP, Nicholson K, DeLong LK, et al. A pilot study in discrepancies in quality of life among three cutaneous types of rosacea. *J Am Acad Dermatol.* 2010;62(6):1069-1071.
26. Su D, Drummond PD. Blushing propensity and psychological distress in people with rosacea. *Clin Psychol Psychother.* 2012;19(6):488-495.
27. Elewski BE. Results of a national rosacea patient survey: common issues that concern rosacea sufferers. *J Drugs Dermatol.* 2009;8(2):120-123.
28. Aksoy B, Altaykan-Hapa A, Egemen D, Karagöz F, Atakan N. The impact of rosacea on quality of life: effects of demographic and clinical characteristics and various treatment modalities. *Br J Dermatol.* 2010;163(4):719-725.
29. Shao K, Hooper J, Feng H. Racial and ethnic health disparities in dermatology in the United States. Part 2: disease-specific epidemiology, characteristics, management, and outcomes. *J Am Acad Dermatol.* 2022;87(4):733-744.
30. Buddenkotte J, Steinhoff M. Recent advances in understanding and managing rosacea. *F1000Res.* 2018;7:1885.
31. Marson JW, Baldwin HE. Rosacea: a wholistic review and update from pathogenesis to diagnosis and therapy. *Int J Dermatol.* 2020;59(6):e175-e182.
32. Steinhoff M, Schauber J, Leyden JJ. New insights into rosacea pathophysiology: a review of recent findings. *J Am Acad Dermatol.* 2013;69(6 Suppl 1):S15-S26.
33. Yamasaki K, Kanada K, Macleod DT, et al. TLR2 expression is increased in rosacea and stimulates enhanced serine protease production by keratinocytes. *J Invest Dermatol.* 2011;131(3):688-697.
34. van Zuuren EJ, Arents BWM, van der Linden MMD, Vermeulen S, Fedorowicz Z, Tan J. Rosacea: new concepts in classification and treatment. *Am J Clin Dermatol.* 2021;22(4):457-465.
35. Buhl T, Sulk M, Nowak P, et al. Molecular and morphological characterization of inflammatory infiltrate in rosacea reveals activation of Th1/Th17 pathways. *J Invest Dermatol.* 2015;135(9):2198-2208.
36. Yamasaki K, Di Nardo A, Bardan A, et al. Increased serine protease activity and cathelicidin promotes skin inflammation in rosacea. *Nat Med.* 2007;13(8):975-980.
37. Yoon SH, Hwang I, Lee E, et al. Antimicrobial peptide LL-37 drives rosacea-like skin inflammation in an NLRP3-dependent manner. *J Invest Dermatol.* 2021;141(12):2885-2894.e5.
38. Swanson KV, Deng M, Ting JP. The NLRP3 inflammasome: molecular activation and regulation to therapeutics. *Nat Rev Immunol.* 2019;19(8):477-489.
39. Muto Y, Wang Z, Vanderberghe M, Two A, Gallo RL, Di Nardo A. Mast cells are key mediators of cathelicidin-initiated skin inflammation in rosacea. *J Invest Dermatol.* 2014;134(11):2728-2736.
40. Marks R, Harcourt-Webster JN. Histopathology of rosacea. *Arch Dermatol.* 1969;100(6):683-691.
41. Aroni K, Tsagroni E, Kavantzas N, Patsouris E, Ioannidis E. A study of the pathogenesis of rosacea: how angiogenesis and mast cells may participate in a complex multifactorial process. *Arch Dermatol Res.* 2008;300(3):125-131.
42. Castro MM, Kandasamy AD, Youssef N, Schulz R. Matrix metalloproteinase inhibitor properties of tetracyclines: therapeutic potential in cardiovascular diseases. *Pharmacol Res.* 2011;64(6):551-560.
43. Husein-ElAhmed H, Steinhoff M. Evaluation of the efficacy of subantimicrobial dose doxycycline in rosacea: a systematic review of clinical trials and meta-analysis. *J Dtsch Dermatol Ges.* 2021;19(1):7-17.
44. Melnik BC. Endoplasmic reticulum stress: key promoter of rosacea pathogenesis. *Exp Dermatol.* 2014;23(12):868-873.

45. Mascarenhas NL, Wang Z, Chang YL, Di Nardo A. TRPV4 mediates mast cell activation in cathelicidin-induced rosacea inflammation. *J Invest Dermatol.* 2017;137(4):972-975.
46. Liu T, Gao YJ, Ji RR. Emerging role of Toll-like receptors in the control of pain and itch. *Neurosci Bull.* 2012;28(2):131-144.
47. Niyonsaba F, Kiatsurayanon C, Chieosilapatham P, Ogawa H. Friends or Foes? Host defense (antimicrobial) peptides and proteins in human skin diseases. *Exp Dermatol.* 2017;26(11):989-998.
48. Peric M, Lehmann B, Vashina G, et al. UV-B-triggered induction of vitamin D3 metabolism differentially affects antimicrobial peptide expression in keratinocytes. *J Allergy Clin Immunol.* 2010;125(3):746-749.
49. Bielenberg DR, Bucana CD, Sanchez R, Donawho CK, Kripke ML, Fidler IJ. Molecular regulation of UVB-induced cutaneous angiogenesis. *J Invest Dermatol.* 1998;111(5):864-872.
50. Brauchle M, Funk JO, Kind P, Werner S. Ultraviolet B and H_2O_2 are potent inducers of vascular endothelial growth factor expression in cultured keratinocytes. *J Biol Chem.* 1996;271(36):21793-21797.
51. Petrofsky JS, Alshahmmari F, Lee H, et al. Reduced endothelial function in the skin in Southeast Asians compared to Caucasians. *Med Sci Monit.* 2012;18(1):Cr1-Cr8.
52. Strain WD, Chaturvedi N, Leggetter S, et al. Ethnic differences in skin microvascular function and their relation to cardiac target-organ damage. *J Hypertens.* 2005;23(1):133-140.
53. Yim J, Petrofsky J, Berk L, Daher N, Lohman E. Differences in endothelial function between Korean-Asians and Caucasians. *Med Sci Monit.* 2012;18(6):CR337-CR343.
54. Kaidbey KH, Agin PP, Sayre RM, Kligman AM. Photoprotection by melanin–a comparison of black and Caucasian skin. *J Am Acad Dermatol.* 1979;1(3):249-260.
55. Quevedo WC, Fitzpatrick TB, Jimbow K. Human skin color: origin, variation and significance. *J Hum Evol.* 1985;14(1):43-56.
56. Montagna W, Prota G, Kenney JA. *Black Skin: Structure and Function*/[edited by] William Montagna, Giuseppe Prota, John A. Kenney, Jr. Academic Press; 1993.
57. Rosen T, Stone MS. Acne rosacea in blacks. *J Am Acad Dermatol.* 1987;17(1):70-73.
58. Marson J, Baldwin H. Supplement article: dysbiosis, (Barrier) dysfunction, and dermatoses: a chicken-and-egg dilemma. *J Drugs Dermatol.* 2022;21(9):Sf3502913-sf3502914.
59. Marson J, Bhatia N, Graber E, et al. Supplement article: the role of epidermal barrier dysfunction and cutaneous microbiome dysbiosis in the pathogenesis and management of acne vulgaris and rosacea. *J Drugs Dermatol.* 2022;21(9):Sf3502915-sf35029114.
60. Chen YE, Tsao H. The skin microbiome: current perspectives and future challenges. *J Am Acad Dermatol.* 2013;69(1):143-155.
61. Ying S, Zeng DN, Chi L, et al. The influence of age and gender on skin-associated microbial communities in urban and rural human populations. *PLoS One.* 2015;10(10):e0141842.
62. Costello EK, Lauber CL, Hamady M, Fierer N, Gordon JI, Knight R. Bacterial community variation in human body habitats across space and time. *Science.* 2009;326(5960):1694-1697.
63. Hospodsky D, Pickering AJ, Julian TR, et al. Hand bacterial communities vary across two different human populations. *Microbiology (Reading).* 2014;160(Pt 6):1144-1152.
64. Blaser MJ, Dominguez-Bello MG, Contreras M, et al. Distinct cutaneous bacterial assemblages in a sampling of South American Amerindians and US residents. *ISME J.* 2013;7(1):85-95.
65. Structure, function and diversity of the healthy human microbiome. *Nature.* 2012;486(7402):207-214.
66. Leung MH, Wilkins D, Lee PK. Insights into the pan-microbiome: skin microbial communities of Chinese individuals differ from other racial groups. *Sci Rep.* 2015;5:11845.
67. Holmes AD. Potential role of microorganisms in the pathogenesis of rosacea. *J Am Acad Dermatol.* 2013;69(6):1025-1032.
68. Casas C, Paul C, Lahfa M, et al. Quantification of Demodex folliculorum by PCR in rosacea and its relationship to skin innate immune activation. *Exp Dermatol.* 2012;21(12):906-910.
69. Palopoli MF, Fergus DJ, Minot S, et al. Global divergence of the human follicle mite Demodex folliculorum: persistent associations between host ancestry and mite lineages. *Proc Natl Acad Sci USA.* 2015;112(52):15958-15963.
70. Forton F, Germaux MA, Brasseur T, et al. Demodicosis and rosacea: epidemiology and significance in daily dermatologic practice. *J Am Acad Dermatol.* 2005;52(1):74-87.
71. Bonamigo RR, Bakos L, Edelweiss M, Cartell A. Could matrix metalloproteinase-9 be a link between Demodex folliculorum and rosacea? *J Eur Acad Dermatol Venereol.* 2005;19(5):646-647.
72. Lacey N, Delaney S, Kavanagh K, Powell FC. Mite-related bacterial antigens stimulate inflammatory cells in rosacea. *Br J Dermatol.* 2007;157(3):474-481.
73. Li J, O'Reilly N, Sheha H, et al. Correlation between ocular *Demodex* infestation and serum immunoreactivity to *Bacillus* proteins in patients with Facial rosacea. *Ophthalmology.* 2010;117(5):870-877.e1.
74. O'Reilly N, Bergin D, Reeves EP, McElvaney NG, Kavanagh K. Demodex-associated bacterial proteins induce neutrophil activation. *Br J Dermatol.* 2012;166(4):753-760.
75. O'Reilly N, Menezes N, Kavanagh K. Positive correlation between serum immunoreactivity to Demodex-associated Bacillus proteins and erythematotelangiectatic rosacea. *Br J Dermatol.* 2012;167(5):1032-1036.
76. Whitfeld M, Gunasingam N, Leow LJ, Shirato K, Preda V. Staphylococcus epidermidis: a possible role in the pustules of rosacea. *J Am Acad Dermatol.* 2011;64(1):49-52.
77. Dahl MV, Ross AJ, Schlievert PM. Temperature regulates bacterial protein production: possible role in rosacea. *J Am Acad Dermatol.* 2004;50(2):266-272.
78. Wang R, Farhat M, Na J, Li R, Wu Y. Bacterial and fungal microbiome characterization in patients with rosacea and healthy controls. *Br J Dermatol.* 2020;183(6):1112-1114.
79. Woo YR, Lee SH, Cho SH, Lee JD, Kim HS. Characterization and analysis of the skin microbiota in rosacea: impact of systemic antibiotics. *J Clin Med.* 2020;9(1):185.
80. Misery L, Loser K, Ständer S. Sensitive skin. *J Eur Acad Dermatol Venereol.* 2016;30(Suppl 1):2-8.
81. Crawford GH, Pelle MT, James WD. Rosacea: I. Etiology, pathogenesis, and subtype classification. *J Am Acad Dermatol.* 2004;51(3):327-341; quiz 342-4.
82. Draelos ZD. Facial hygiene and comprehensive management of rosacea. *Cutis.* 2004;73(3):183-187.
83. Baldwin H, Alexis AF, Andriessen A, et al. Evidence of barrier deficiency in rosacea and the importance of integrating OTC skincare products into treatment regimens. *J Drugs Dermatol.* 2021;20(4):384-392.
84. Corazza M, la Malfa W, Lombardi A, Maranini C, Virgili A. Role of allergic contact dermatitis in rosacea. *Contact Dermatitis.* 1997;37(1):40-41.
85. Darlenski R, Kazandjieva J, Tsankov N, Fluhr JW. Acute irritant threshold correlates with barrier function, skin hydration and contact hypersensitivity in atopic dermatitis and rosacea. *Exp Dermatol.* 2013;22(11):752-753.
86. Draelos ZD. Cosmetics in acne and rosacea. *Semin Cutan Med Surg.* 2001;20(3):209-214.
87. Draelos ZD, Green BA, Edison BL. An evaluation of a polyhydroxy acid skin care regimen in combination with azelaic acid 15% gel in rosacea patients. *J Cosmet Dermatol.* 2006;5(1):23-29.
88. Ní Raghallaigh S, Powell FC. Epidermal hydration levels in patients with rosacea improve after minocycline therapy. *Br J Dermatol.* 2014;171(2):259-266.
89. Pelle MT, Crawford GH, James WD. Rosacea: II. Therapy. *J Am Acad Dermatol.* 2004;51(4):499-512; quiz 513-4.
90. Tsianakas A, Pieber T, Baldwin H, et al. Minocycline Extended-Release Comparison with Doxycycline for the Treatment of Rosacea: A Randomized, Head-to-Head, Clinical Trial. *J Clin Aesthet Dermatol.* Dec 2021;14(12):16-23.
91. Sidgiddi S, Bhatia N, Sidgiddi S. 53889 Impact of DFD-29, a Low-Dose Oral Minocycline, on Skin, Gastrointestinal Tract, and Vaginal Microflora in Healthy Adults: A Randomized, Double-Blind, Placebo-Controlled Trial. *Journal of the American Academy of Dermatology.* 2024;91(3):AB52. doi:10.1016/j.jaad.2024.07.214.
92. Berardesca E, Pirot F, Singh M, Maibach H. Differences in stratum corneum pH gradient when comparing White Caucasian and black African-American skin. *Br J Dermatol.* 1998;139(5):855-857.
93. Wesley NO, Maibach HI. Racial (ethnic) differences in skin properties: the objective data. *Am J Clin Dermatol.* 2003;4(12):843-860.
94. Searle T, Ali FR, Carolides S, Al-Niaimi F. Rosacea and the gastrointestinal system. *Australas J Dermatol.* 2020;61(4):307-311.
95. Kim M, Choi KH, Hwang SW, Lee YB, Park HJ, Bae JM. Inflammatory bowel disease is associated with an increased risk of inflammatory skin diseases: a population-based cross-sectional study. *J Am Acad Dermatol.* 2017;76(1):40-48.
96. Marson J, Berto S, Mouser P, Baldwin H. Association between rosacea, environmental factors, and facial cutaneous dysbiosis. *SKIN J Cutan Med.* 2021;5(5):487-495.
97. Nam JH, Yun Y, Kim HS, et al. Rosacea and its association with enteral microbiota in Korean females. *Exp Dermatol.* 2018;27(1):37-42.
98. Zaidi AK, Spaunhurst K, Sprockett D, et al. Characterization of the facial microbiome in twins discordant for rosacea. *Exp Dermatol.* 2018;27(3):295-298.
99. Deng Z, Yan S, Li J, et al. The association between rosacea and the condition of low tolerance to skincare of the facial skin: a case-control study in China. *J Cosmet Dermatol.* 2022;21(3):1171-1177.

100. Browning DJ, Rosenwasser G, Lugo M. Ocular rosacea in blacks. *Am J Ophthalmol.* 15 1986;101(4):441-444.
101. Bass O, Crane D. Case series: underdiagnosis of ocular and oculocutaneous rosacea in an African American pediatric population. *Optom Vis Sci.* 2022;99(6):521-527.
102. Ezra N, Greco JF, Haley JC, Chiu MW. Gnatophyma and otophyma. *J Cutan Med Surg.* 2009;13(5):266-272.
103. Alexis A, Woolery-Lloyd H, Andriessen A, Desai S, Han G, Rodriguez D. Improving rosacea outcomes in skin of color patients: a review on the nuances in the treatment and the use of cleansers and moisturizers. *J Drugs Dermatol.* 2022;21(6):574-580.
104. Lyons AB, Trullas C, Kohli I, Hamzavi IH, Lim HW. Photoprotection beyond ultraviolet radiation: a review of tinted sunscreens. *J Am Acad Dermatol.* 2021;84(5):1393-1397.
105. Draelos ZD. Colored facial cosmetics. *Dermatol Clin.* 2000;18(4):621-631.
106. Layton AM, Schaller M, Homey B, et al. Brimonidine gel 0.33% rapidly improves patient-reported outcomes by controlling facial erythema of rosacea: a randomized, double-blind, vehicle-controlled study. *J Eur Acad Dermatol Venereol.* 2015;29(12):2405-2410.
107. Fowler J, Jarratt M, Moore A, et al. Once-daily topical brimonidine tartrate gel 0·5% is a novel treatment for moderate to severe facial erythema of rosacea: results of two multicentre, randomized and vehicle-controlled studies. *Br J Dermatol.* 2012;166(3):633-641.
108. Fowler J, Jr., Jackson M, Moore A, et al. Efficacy and safety of once-daily topical brimonidine tartrate gel 0.5% for the treatment of moderate to severe facial erythema of rosacea: results of two randomized, double-blind, and vehicle-controlled pivotal studies. *J Drugs Dermatol.* 2013;12(6):650-656.
109. Moore A, Kempers S, Murakawa G, et al. Long-term safety and efficacy of once-daily topical brimonidine tartrate gel 0.5% for the treatment of moderate to severe facial erythema of rosacea: results of a 1-year open-label study. *J Drugs Dermatol.* 2014;13(1):56-61.
110. Gillihan R, Nguyen T, Fischer R, Rajpara A, Aires D. Erythema in skin adjacent to area of long-term brimonidine treatment for rosacea: a novel adverse reaction. *JAMA Dermatol.* 2015;151(10):1136-1137.
111. Routt ET, Levitt JO. Rebound erythema and burning sensation from a new topical brimonidine tartrate gel 0.33%. *J Am Acad Dermatol.* 2014;70(2):e37-e38.
112. Ilkovitch D, Pomerantz RG. Brimonidine effective but may lead to significant rebound erythema. *J Am Acad Dermatol.* 2014;70(5):e109-e110.
113. Kircik LH, DuBois J, Draelos ZD, et al. Pivotal trial of the efficacy and safety of oxymetazoline cream 1.0% for the treatment of persistent facial erythema associated with rosacea: findings from the first REVEAL trial. *J Drugs Dermatol.* 2018;17(1):97-105.
114. Draelos ZD, Gold MH, Weiss RA, et al. Efficacy and safety of oxymetazoline cream 1.0% for treatment of persistent facial erythema associated with rosacea: findings from the 52-week open label REVEAL trial. *J Am Acad Dermatol.* 2018;78(6):1156-1163.
115. Battle EF, Jr., Hobbs LM. Laser therapy on darker ethnic skin. *Dermatol Clin.* 2003;21(4):713-723.
116. Bleicher PA, Charles JH, Sober AJ. Topical metronidazole therapy for rosacea. *Arch Dermatol.* 1987;123(5):609-614.
117. Breneman DL, Stewart D, Hevia O, Hino PD, Drake LA. A double-blind, multicenter clinical trial comparing efficacy of once-daily metronidazole 1 percent cream to vehicle in patients with rosacea. *Cutis.* 1998;61(1):44-47.
118. Dahl MV, Katz HI, Krueger GG, et al. Topical metronidazole maintains remissions of rosacea. *Arch Dermatol.* 1998;134(6):679-683.
119. Elewski BE, Fleischer AB, Pariser DM. A comparison of 15% azelaic acid gel and 0.75% metronidazole gel in the topical treatment of papulopustular rosacea: results of a randomized trial. *Arch Dermatol.* 2003;139(11): 1444-1450.
120. Wolf JE, Jr., Del Rosso JQ. The CLEAR trial: results of a large community-based study of metronidazole gel in rosacea. *Cutis.* 2007;79(1):73-80.
121. van Zuuren EJ, Fedorowicz Z, Carter B, van der Linden MM, Charland L. Interventions for rosacea. *Cochrane Database Syst Rev.* 2015;2015(4): CD003262.
122. van Zuuren EJ, Fedorowicz Z, Tan J, et al. Interventions for rosacea based on the phenotype approach: an updated systematic review including GRADE assessments. *Br J Dermatol.* 2019;181(1):65-79.
123. Bjerke R, Fyrand O, Graupe K. Double-blind comparison of azelaic acid 20% cream and its vehicle in treatment of papulo-pustular rosacea. *Acta Derm Venereol.* 1999;79(6):456-459.
124. Colón LE, Johnson LA, Gottschalk RW. Cumulative irritation potential among metronidazole gel 1%, metronidazole gel 0.75%, and azelaic acid gel 15%. *Cutis.* 2007;79(4):317-321.
125. Thiboutot DM, Fleischer AB, Jr., Del Rosso JQ, Graupe K. Azelaic acid 15% gel once daily versus twice daily in papulopustular rosacea. *J Drugs Dermatol.* 2008;7(6):541-546.
126. Ziel K, Yelverton CB, Balkrishnan R, Feldman SR. Cumulative irritation potential of metronidazole gel compared to azelaic acid gel after repeated applications to healthy skin. *J Drugs Dermatol.* 2005;4(6):727-731.
127. Torresani C, Pavesi A, Manara GC. Clarithromycin versus doxycycline in the treatment of rosacea. *Int J Dermatol.* 1997;36(12):942-946.
128. Trave I, Merlo G, Cozzani E, Parodi A. Real-life experience on effectiveness and tolerability of topical ivermectin in papulopustular rosacea and antiparasitic effect on Demodex mites. *Dermatol Ther.* 2019;32(6):e13093.
129. Stein L, Kircik L, Fowler J, et al. Efficacy and safety of ivermectin 1% cream in treatment of papulopustular rosacea: results of two randomized, double-blind, vehicle-controlled pivotal studies. *J Drugs Dermatol.* 2014;13(3):316-323.
130. Taieb A, Ortonne JP, Ruzicka T, et al. Superiority of ivermectin 1% cream over metronidazole 0·75% cream in treating inflammatory lesions of rosacea: a randomized, investigator-blinded trial. *Br J Dermatol.* 2015;172(4):1103-1110.
131. Taieb A, Khemis A, Ruzicka T, et al. Maintenance of remission following successful treatment of papulopustular rosacea with ivermectin 1% cream vs. metronidazole 0.75% cream: 36-week extension of the ATTRACT randomized study. *J Eur Acad Dermatol Venereol.* 2016;30(5):829-836.
132. Gold LS, Del Rosso JQ, Kircik L, et al. Minocycline 1.5% foam for the topical treatment of moderate to severe papulopustular rosacea: results of 2 phase 3, randomized, clinical trials. *J Am Acad Dermatol.* 2020;82(5):1166-1173.
133. Stein Gold L, Del Rosso JQ, Kircik L, et al. Open-label extension study evaluating long-term safety and efficacy of FMX103 1.5% minocycline topical foam for the treatment of moderate-to-severe papulopustular rosacea. *J Clin Aesthet Dermatol.* 2020;13(11):44-49.
134. Green LJ, Lain E, Prunty T, Rhoades R. Enhancing topical pharmacotherapy for acne and rosacea: vehicle choices and outcomes. *J Clin Aesthet Dermatol.* 2022;15(5):36-40.
135. A study of S5G4T-1 in the treatment of papularpustular rosacea. ClinicalTrials.gov. 2023.
136. Sol-Gel technologies and galderma announce FDA approval of epsolay. April 25, 2022. Accessed November 26, 2022.
137. Leyden JJ. Randomized, phase 2, dose-ranging study in the treatment of rosacea with encapsulated benzoyl peroxide gel. *J Drugs Dermatol.* 2014;13(6):685-688.
138. Bhatia N, Werschler W, Baldwin H, et al. Long-term efficacy and safety of benzoyl peroxide cream, 5%, prepared with microencapsulation in papulopustular rosacea: results from an extension of two phase 3, vehicle-controlled trials. *SKIN J Cutan Med.* 2021;5(1):s25.
139. Efficacy and tolerability of erenumab in the management of persistent redness and flushing in rosacea. ClinicalTrials.gov. 2023.
140. Torok HM, Webster G, Dunlap FE, Egan N, Jarratt M, Stewart D. Combination sodium sulfacetamide 10% and sulfur 5% cream with sunscreens versus metronidazole 0.75% cream for rosacea. *Cutis.* 2005;75(6):357-363.
141. Conde JF, Yelverton CB, Balkrishnan R, Fleischer AB, Jr., Feldman SR. Managing rosacea: a review of the use of metronidazole alone and in combination with oral antibiotics. *J Drugs Dermatol.* 2007;6(5):495-498.
142. Korting HC, Schöllmann C. Current topical and systemic approaches to treatment of rosacea. *J Eur Acad Dermatol Venereol.* 2009;23(8):876-882.
143. Del Rosso JQ. Anti-inflamatory dose doxycycline in the treatment of rosacea. *J Drugs Dermatol.* 2009;8(7):664-668.
144. Del Rosso JQ, Webster GF, Jackson M, et al. Two randomized phase III clinical trials evaluating anti-inflammatory dose doxycycline (40-mg doxycycline, USP capsules) administered once daily for treatment of rosacea. *J Am Acad Dermatol.* 2007;56(5):791-802.
145. Sanchez J, Somolinos AL, Almodóvar PI, Webster G, Bradshaw M, Powala C. A randomized, double-blind, placebo-controlled trial of the combined effect of doxycycline hyclate 20-mg tablets and metronidazole 0.75% topical lotion in the treatment of rosacea. *J Am Acad Dermatol.* 2005;53(5):791-797.
146. Webster GF. An open-label, community-based, 12-week assessment of the effectiveness and safety of monotherapy with doxycycline 40 mg (30-mg immediate-release and 10-mg delayed-release beads). *Cutis.* 2010;86(5 Suppl): 7-15.
147. Alexis AF, Webster G, Preston NJ, Caveney SW, Gottschalk RW. Effectiveness and safety of once-daily doxycycline capsules as monotherapy in patients with rosacea: an analysis by Fitzpatrick skin type. *J Drugs Dermatol.* 2012;11(10):1219-1222.

148. Del Rosso JQ, Brantman S, Baldwin H. Long-term inflammatory rosacea management with subantibiotic dose oral doxycycline 40 mg modified-release capsules once daily. *Dermatol Ther.* 2022;35(1):e15180.
149. Fowler JF, Jr. Combined effect of anti-inflammatory dose doxycycline (40-mg doxycycline, usp monohydrate controlled-release capsules) and metronidazole topical gel 1% in the treatment of rosacea. *J Drugs Dermatol.* 2007;6(6):641-645.
150. Schaller M, Kemény L, Havlickova B, et al. A randomized phase 3b/4 study to evaluate concomitant use of topical ivermectin 1% cream and doxycycline 40-mg modified-release capsules, versus topical ivermectin 1% cream and placebo in the treatment of severe rosacea. *J Am Acad Dermatol.* 2020;82(2):336-343.
151. Rosso JQ, Draelos ZD, Effron C, Kircik LH. Oral sarecycline for treatment of papulopustular rosacea: results of a pilot study of effectiveness and safety. *J Drugs Dermatol.* 2021;20(4):426-431.
152. Moore AY, Del Rosso J, Johnson JL, Grada A. Sarecycline: a review of preclinical and clinical evidence. *Clin Cosmet Investig Dermatol.* 2020;13:553-560.
153. Zhanel G, Critchley I, Lin LY, Alvandi N. Microbiological profile of sarecycline, a novel targeted spectrum tetracycline for the treatment of acne vulgaris. *Antimicrob Agents Chemother.* 2019;63(1). doi:10.1128/aac.01297-18.
154. Graber EM. Treating acne with the tetracycline class of antibiotics: a review. *Dermatol Rev.* 2021;2(6):321-330.
155. Gajardo J. Rosácea severa tratada con isotretinoína oral. [Severe rosacea treated with oral isotretinoin]. *Rev Med Chil.* 1994;122(2):177-179.
156. Hoting E, Paul E, Plewig G. Treatment of rosacea with isotretinoin. *Int J Dermatol.* 1986;25(10):660-663.
157. Erdogan FG, Yurtsever P, Aksoy D, Eskioglu F. Efficacy of low-dose isotretinoin in patients with treatment-resistant rosacea. *Arch Dermatol.* 1998;134(7):884-885.
158. Rebora A. The management of rosacea. *Am J Clin Dermatol.* 2002;3(7):489-496.
159. Rallis E, Korfitis C. Isotretinoin for the treatment of granulomatous rosacea: case report and review of the literature. *J Cutan Med Surg.* 2012;16(6):438-441.
160. Sbidian E, Vicaut É, Chidiack H, et al. A Randomized-controlled trial of oral low-dose isotretinoin for difficult-to-treat papulopustular rosacea. *J Invest Dermatol.* 2016;136(6):1124-1129.
161. Marsden JR, Shuster S, Neugebauer M. Response of rosacea to isotretinoin. *Clin Exp Dermatol.* 1984;9(5):484-488.
162. Plewig G, Nikolowski J, Wolff HH. Action of isotretinoin in acne rosacea and gram-negative folliculitis. *J Am Acad Dermatol.* 1982;6(4 Pt 2 Suppl):766-785.
163. Marson JW, Baldwin HE. Isotretinoin update. *Dermatolog Rev.* 2021;2(6):331-342.
164. Kempiak SJ, Lee PW, Pelle MT. Rhinophyma treated with cryosurgery. *Dermatol Surg.* Mar 2009;35(3):543-545.
165. Abushaala A, Stavrakas M, Khalil H. Microdebrider-assisted rhinophyma excision. *Case Rep Otolaryngol.* 2019;2019:4915416.
166. Sadick H, Goepel B, Bersch C, Goessler U, Hoermann K, Riedel F. Rhinophyma: diagnosis and treatment options for a disfiguring tumor of the nose. *Ann Plast Surg.* 2008;61(1):114-120.
167. Benyo S, Saadi RA, Walen S, Lighthall JG. A systematic review of surgical techniques for management of severe rhinophyma. *Craniomaxillofac Trauma Reconstr.* 2021;14(4):299-307.
168. Kiehlmann MV, Morandi EM, Kühn S, et al. Tangential excision of rhinophyma with the disposable razor blade: simple and cost efficient with aesthetically good results. *J Cutan Aesthet Surg.* 2021;14(1):72-76.
169. Apikian M, Goodman GJ, Roberts S. Management of mild to moderate rhinophyma with a 1,450-nm diode laser: report of five patients. *Dermatol Surg.* 2007;33(7):847-850.
170. Madan V, Ferguson JE, August PJ. Carbon dioxide laser treatment of rhinophyma: a review of 124 patients. *Br J Dermatol.* 2009;161(4):814-818.
171. Tahery J, Zakaria R, Natt RS. Diode laser treatment of rhinophyma. *Clin Otolaryngol.* 2010;35(5):442-444.
172. Fisher GH, Geronemus RG. Short-term side effects of fractional photothermolysis. *Dermatol Surg.* 2005;31(9 Pt 2):1245-1249; discussion 1249.
173. Erisir F, Isildak H, Haciyev Y. Management of mild to moderate rhinophyma with a radiofrequency. *J Craniofac Surg.* 2009;20(2):455-456.
174. Ghanem VC, Mehra N, Wong S, Mannis MJ. The prevalence of ocular signs in acne rosacea: comparing patients from ophthalmology and dermatology clinics. *Cornea.* 2003;22(3):230-233.
175. Odom R, Dahl M, Dover J, et al. Standard management options for rosacea, part 2: options according to subtype. *Cutis.* 2009;84(2):97-104.
176. Tanzi EL, Weinberg JM. The ocular manifestations of rosacea. *Cutis.* 2001;68(2):112-114.
177. Bakar O, Demircay Z, Toker E, Cakir S. Ocular signs, symptoms and tear function tests of papulopustular rosacea patients receiving azithromycin. *J Eur Acad Dermatol Venereol.* 2009;23(5):544-549.
178. Sobolewska B, Doycheva D, Deuter CM, Schaller M, Zierhut M. Efficacy of topical ivermectin for the treatment of cutaneous and ocular rosacea. *Ocul Immunol Inflamm.* 2021;29(6):1137-1141.
179. Gold LS, Papp K, Lynde C, et al. Treatment of rosacea with concomitant use of topical ivermectin 1% cream and brimonidine 0.33% gel: a randomized, vehicle-controlled study. *J Drugs Dermatol.* 2017;16(9):909-916.
180. Kumar AM, Chiou AS, Shih YH, Li S, Chang ALS. An exploratory, open-label, investigator-initiated study of interleukin-17 blockade in patients with moderate-to-severe papulopustular rosacea. *Br J Dermatol.* 2020;183(5):942-943.
181. LLC A. A study to determine safety and efficacy of B244 in subjects with mild to moderate rosacea. ClinicalTrialsgov. 2023; (Identifier NCT03590366) https://www.clinicaltrials.gov/ct2/show/NCT03590366. Therapeutics D. DMT210 topical gel in the treatment of acne rosacea. 11 November, 2024. https://www.clinicaltrials.gov/ct2/show/NCT03003104
182. Maruho Co. L. Study to evaluate the long-term safety of a once-daily omiganan topical gel. ClinicalTrialsgov. 2023; Identifier NCT03590366 (https://www.clinicaltrials.gov/ct2/show/NCT03590366).
183. Maruho Co. L. Study to evaluate the safety and efficacy of a once-daily CLS001 topical gel versus vehicle. ClinicalTrialsgov. 2023; Identifier NCT02576860 (https://www.clinicaltrials.gov/ct2/show/NCT02576860).
184. Weinstock LB, Steinhoff M. Rosacea and small intestinal bacterial overgrowth: prevalence and response to rifaximin. *J Am Acad Dermatol.* 2013;68(5):875-876.
185. Li J, Yuan X, Tang Y, et al. Hydroxychloroquine is a novel therapeutic approach for rosacea. *Int Immunopharmacol.* 2020;79:106178.
186. Wang B, Yuan X, Huang X, et al. Efficacy and safety of hydroxychloroquine for treatment of patients with rosacea: a multicenter, randomized, double-blind, double-dummy, pilot study. *J Am Acad Dermatol.* 2021;84(2):543-545.
187. The Royal College of Ophthalmologists. Clinical Guidelines-Hydroxychloroquine and Chloroquine Retinopathy Monitoring Guideline: recommendations on monitoring. https://www.rcophth.ac.uk/wp-content/uploads/2020/12/Hydroxychloroquine-and-Chloroquine-Retinopathy-Monitoring-Guideline.pdf. Accessed August 9, 2022.
188. S.p.A. A. Safety and efficacy of rifaximin in patients with papulopustular rosacea and positive lactulose breath test. Clinicaltrialsgov. 2022; Identifier NCT03864978 (https://www.clinicaltrials.gov/ct2/show/NCT03864978).
189. Baldwin HE. Integrative management of rosacea. In: Norman R, Shenefelt P, Rupani R, eds. Integrative Dermatology. Oxford University Press. 198 Madison Ave, *New York, NY*, 10016. 2014.

SECTION 7

Neoplasms of the Skin

CHAPTER 51

Benign Skin Neoplasms

Lauren Payne
Adaora Ewulu
Mia Jenkins
Valerie D. Callender

KEY POINTS

- It's important to counsel patients on the commonality and benign nature of these lesions.
- Visualizing dermoscopic features is useful in distinguishing between benign and malignant lesions.
- Physical exam, thorough history, diagnostic imaging, and biopsy are essential for differentiating lipomas from liposarcomas.
- Treatment of benign neoplasms is not necessary and is commonly reserved for irritated lesions or cosmetic satisfaction.
- For the common treatment options of benign lesions (ie, laser, surgical excision, and cryotherapy), the risk of hyper- or hypopigmentation and scarring complications in skin of color should always be considered.
- Most melanocytic nevi will not progress to melanoma. However, patients with darker skin tones and a history of multiple nevi are at a higher risk for developing acral melanomas and should perform periodic self-skin exams using the "ABCDE" guide for melanoma.

ACROCHORDON (AKA SKIN TAG OR FIBROEPITHELIAL POLYP)

Acrochordons, also known as skin tags or fibroepithelial polyps, are benign skin tumors of mesenchymal or ectodermal origin [**Figure 51-1**]. The incidence of these lesions is the same in both males and females, and frequency increases with age.[1] They are grossly described as soft, flesh-colored pedunculated papules, and their size usually does not exceed 5 mm.[1,2] Acrochordons commonly appear on the neck, axilla, groin, eyelid, and inframammary folds of the chest.[3] Uncommonly, they can appear around the genital tract or within the inguinal creases.[2] Common differential diagnoses include filiform warts, seborrheic keratoses, and neurofibromas.[2]

Acrochordons tend to be associated with other medical conditions including obesity, insulin resistance, pregnancy-related hormone imbalances, Birt-Hogg-Dube syndrome, tuberous sclerosis, and polycystic ovarian syndrome (PCOS).[2,3] Treatments include snip excision, cryotherapy, shave excision, and electrodesiccation.[3] However, these treatments can be complicated by the development of neuromas, irritation, removal of normal skin tissue, scarring, and dyspigmentation.[4] Though acrochordons are benign skin lesions that are often isolated in nature, they should not solely be regarded as a separate entity. Patients should also be evaluated for comorbidities such as PCOS, diabetes, or any other form of metabolic syndrome especially if they present with acanthosis nigricans.

LIPOMA

Lipomas are one of the most common mesenchymal tumors of adulthood, and they originate from adipose cells.[5] Solitary lipomas are most common in women while multiple lipomas present most frequently in males.[5] The incidence is 1 per 1000 persons with a peak incidence in the fifth and sixth decades of life.[5] These tumors present as painless, mobile, palpable, well-circumscribed, round/oval subcutaneous nodules that form underneath the skin. Lipomas can range in size anywhere from 1 to 2 mm to greater than 10 cm.[6] If large enough, they have the potential to compress underlying and surrounding muscle and lead to neuropathic pain [**Figure 51-2**].

Lipomas can appear on any part of the body where fat is found but are commonly found on the back, arm, and shoulder.[5] They can also appear on the head and neck.[5] Differential diagnoses include liposarcomas, epidermal inclusion cysts, nodular fasciitis, and sarcoidosis.[5] Lipomas can also be associated with medical conditions including obesity, diabetes, hypercholesterolemia, hereditary multiple lipomatosis, Gardner syndrome, Madelung disease, and Dercum disease.[5]

Treatment options include surgical excision, liposuction, and, when inflamed, intralesional steroid injections although simple excision is the most popular treatment modality.[5] Liposuction is sometimes preferred over surgical excision because it can result in less scarring. The recurrence rate after a surgical excision may be higher than after liposuction if the lipoma is not fully removed.[5] Complications from lipoma treatments include hematoma, bruising, infection, fat embolus, hyperpigmentation from surgical excision or depigmentation, particularly after steroid injections.[5]

Lipomas are often confused with other soft tissue masses. Importantly, dermatologists must distinguish benign lipomas from the painless, large, rapidly growing malignant tumor called liposarcoma. Histologically, these neoplasms can appear very similar, but on microscopic examination, signet rings and atypical fibroblasts are appreciable in liposarcomas.[5] A thorough history, physical exam, diagnostic imaging (CT or MRI), and biopsy are essential for differentiation between these two tumors.[5]

EPIDERMAL INCLUSION CYST

Epidermal inclusion cyst (EIC) is another type of benign neoplasm that can be categorized as primary or secondary in origin. Primary cysts arise from the infundibulum of the hair follicle, and secondary cysts occur after trauma that causes the follicular epithelium to implant within the dermis.[7] EICs are more common in men than women (2:1 ratio), with the most common age range between ages 20 and 30.[7]

EICs typically present as asymptomatic, mobile, subcutaneous nodules underneath the skin with a central, dark punctum.[8] The size of the cysts can be anywhere from a few millimeters to several centimeters, and they have the potential to increase in size over time.[7] The cyst wall has an epidermal-like lining while the cavity is filled with keratohyalin granules, sweat, and oil. EICs can be painful if inflamed, infected, or ruptured, and the development of a keloid may occur in people of color [**Figure 51-3**]. If an inflamed cyst ruptures, foul-smelling, cheesy yellow contents containing keratin and lipid contents can be seen extruding on exam.[7,8] Epidermal cysts can present on any area of the body, though are most common on the face, back, scrotum, and neck.[7] Less common areas include the extremities, trunk, or the back of the ears.[7]

Differential diagnoses include pilar cysts, neurofibromas, lipomas, abscesses, and brachial cleft cysts.[7] Epidermal cysts can be associated with other medical conditions like acne vulgaris, Gardner syndrome, and basal cell nevus syndrome.[7] Surgical excision with a small blade or punch biopsy is the definitive treatment by removing not only the content but also the lining of the cyst. Surgery is not recommended when a cyst is inflamed due to increased risk of infection, incomplete removal,

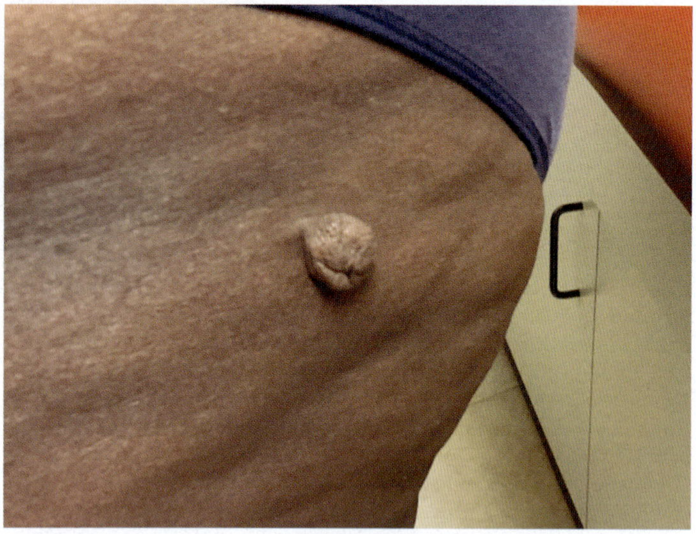

FIGURE 51-1. Large acrochordon on the lateral thigh. (Courtesy of Valerie D. Callender, MD.)

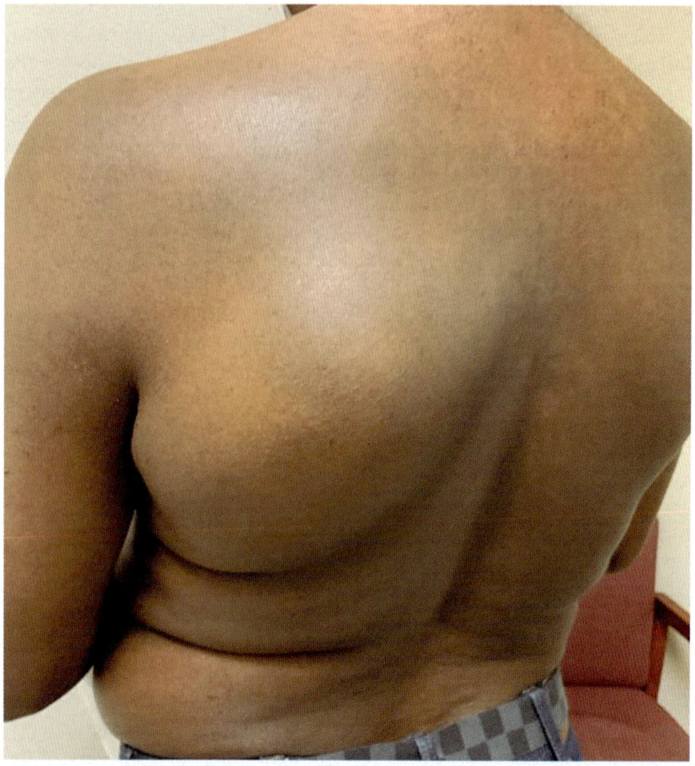

FIGURE 51-2. Large lipoma on the back. (Courtesy of Valerie D. Callender, MD.)

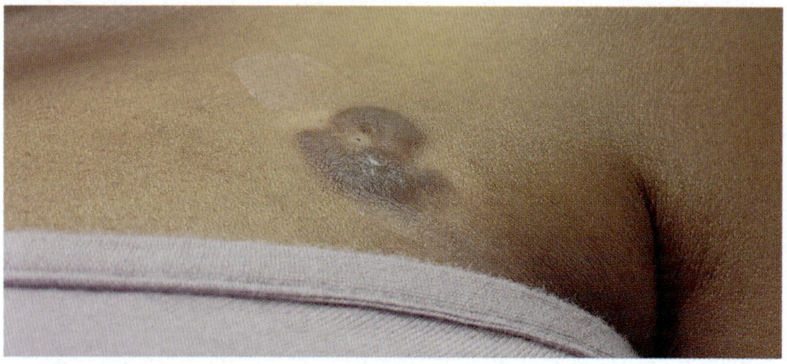

FIGURE 51-3. Epiderma inclusion cyst with a perilesional keloid. (Courtesy of Valerie D. Callender, MD.)

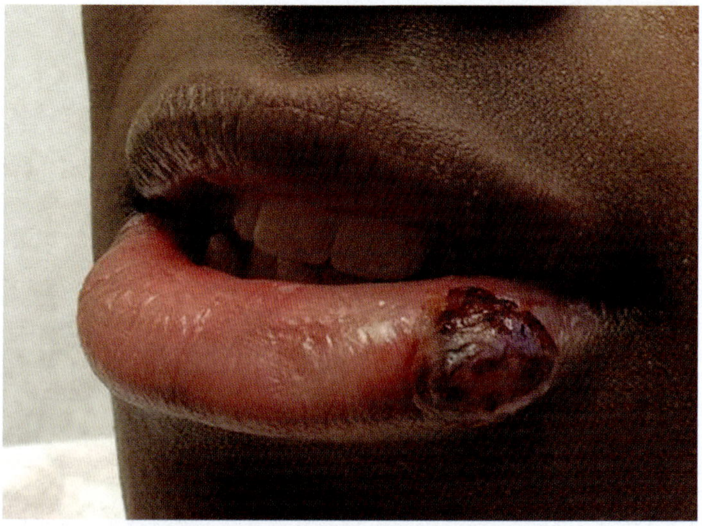

FIGURE 51-4. Pyogenic granuloma on the lower lip. (Courtesy of Valerie D. Callender, MD.)

and chance of recurrence; in that case, intralesional corticosteroid injection to decrease the inflammation is the preferred option. Surgical complications include bleeding, infection, scarring, and dyspigmentation.[7] A fluctuant cyst is often an indication to perform an incision and drainage due to its infectious nature, and oral antibiotics can also be added to reduce the inflammation and/or infection.

PYOGENIC GRANULOMA

Pyogenic granulomas are benign tumors of blood vessels that can present in any age and gender. Clinically, it is described as a solitary, rapidly growing red papule or nodule that often forms after minor trauma to the skin.[9] These neoplasms commonly occur in areas of the body with a prominent vascular supply, so they tend to bleed very easily. They range from a few mm to several cm in size.

Pyogenic granulomas are commonly found in the gingiva, tongue, lips, face, and fingers as these areas of the body have the highest vascularity [**Figure 51-4**].[9] Less commonly, they present in areas of the GI tract or genital area. Kaposi sarcoma, hemangiomas, bacillary angiomatosis, melanoma, warts, and glomus tumors are common differentials that should also be considered.[9,10]

When evaluating a vascular neoplasm, conditions that can be associated with the development of pyogenic granulomas include pregnancy, atopic dermatitis, and psoriasis. These lesions have also been associated with medications including oral contraceptives, retinoids, BRAF inhibitors used to treat melanomas, anti-retroviral (most commonly indinavir), anti-neoplastic, and immunosuppressive agents.[10] Complete excision is the gold standard treatment to prevent recurrence. However, dermatologists also often perform shave removals of these lesions with cauterization of the residual blood vessels at the base of the lesion, minimizing recurrence. Other options for treatment include cryotherapy, pulse dye laser therapy, and CO_2 laser.[10] Treatment complications include lesion recurrence, dyspigmentation, and scar formation.[9] Pyogenic granulomas often have an abrupt onset with high rate of recurrence, so it is important to establish a relationship with a dermatologist who can treat these lesions and send specimens off to the pathology lab for further histopathological evaluation. Pathology is helpful in ruling out other more concerning neoplasms with similar appearance.

BENIGN MELANOCYTIC NEVUS

A benign melanocytic nevus is a nevus that arises from the proliferation of melanocytes and can be categorized as congenital or acquired. Congenital nevi are present at birth, and the acquired

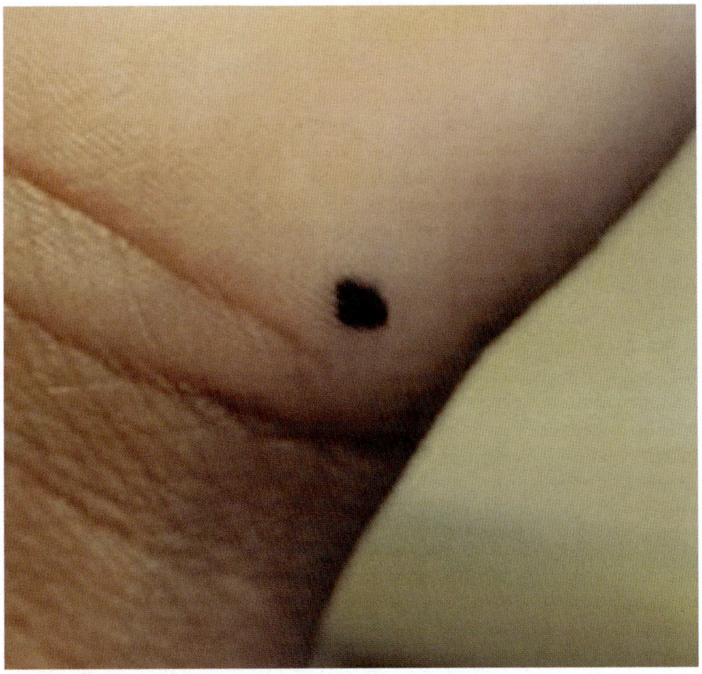

FIGURE 51-5. Nevus on the palm. (Courtesy of Valerie D. Callender, MD.)

form occurs later in life, usually in the first and second decades.[11] The prevalence of nevi increases directly with the degree of skin pigmentation, and they appear more commonly in males than females.[12] Generally, these nevi are gray-black, uniformly-colored, symmetric, flat or raised lesions with diameters that range from 2 to 6 mm [**Figure 51-5**].[11] Acquired melanocytic nevi can be classified into three common sub-groups based on clinical presentation: junctional, compound, and intradermal. Junctional nevi are brown/black macules, compound nevi tend to be more maculopapular with various levels of pigmentation, and intradermal nevi are most often dome-shaped, flesh-colored papules.[13]

In patients with skin types V and VI, melanocytic nevi often have a reticular pattern with central hyperpigmentation.[12] Additionally, relatively large and darkly pigmented nevi are more common in darker skin tones compared to lighter individuals.[12] They most frequently present on the head, neck, and lower extremities. More specifically, in darker skinned patients, these nevi present most commonly on acral sites and less commonly on the face.[14] Cafe-au-lait macules, lentigines, and ephelides should all be included in the differential diagnoses of benign melanocytic nevi. Activating mutations in the BRAFV600E gene have been identified in about 80% of these nevi.[11] Although most melanocytic nevi will never progress to melanoma, 25% to 33% of melanomas arise from nevi, and the risk may be higher in patients with multiple nevi or sun-damaged skin.[11] Patients with darker skin tones are at a higher risk for developing acral melanoma. Other medical conditions in which melanocytic nevi can be present include Noonan syndrome, dysplastic nevus syndrome, and Turner syndrome.

Regarding treatment, surgical excision via shave or punch biopsy is indicated in case of concerning lesions. Once diagnosis is established that the lesion is benign, destruction with laser can be performed for cosmetic treatment. With any treatment, it is important to note that they will all likely leave a scar or area of hyper- or hypopigmentation. There is also the possibility that the nevus may recur if not fully removed.[15] Regular self-examination of nevi on the skin is important. Patients with melanocytic nevi should be educated about the "ABCDE's" of melanoma. They should pay close attention to moles that display asymmetry, irregular borders, discoloration, a diameter greater than 6 mms, or evolution in shape, size, or color. If any of the above characteristics are noted, patients should seek out their dermatologist for additional evaluation and treatment.

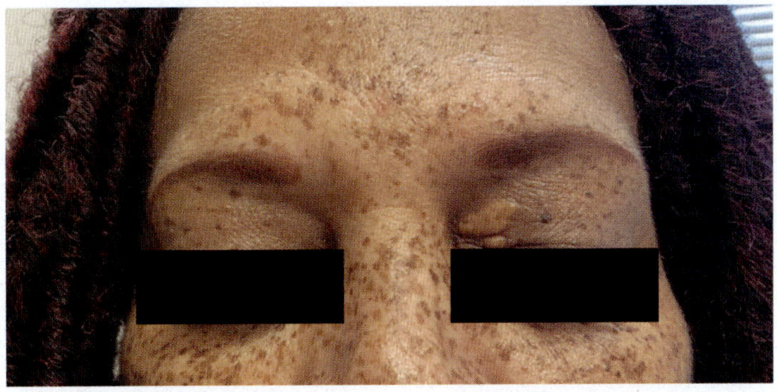

FIGURE 51-6. Ephelides on the face along with a xanthelasma on the left eyelid. (Courtesy of Valerie D. Callender, MD.)

EPHELID (FRECKLE)

Freckles are pigment spots that originate from melanocytes and are most common in children, and tend to become less appreciable in adulthood (inversely associated with age).[16] They are very common in individuals with Fitzpatrick skin types I and II and blond or red-haired individuals, with no gender predominance; however, they can occur in darker skin types [**Figure 51-6**].[16] Clinically, ephelides present as numerous symmetrically distributed light to dark-brown, poorly defined macules ranging from 3 to 10 mm in diameter.[17] Freckles most commonly present in sun-exposed areas such as the face, neck, and chest. Differential diagnoses include simple lentigo, solar lentigo, junctional nevus, and lentigo maligna.[17] A number of genes (ie, MC1R, IRF4, BNC2) have been shown to influence freckle formation.[16] For example, those with red hair are usually homozygous for a variant of the melanocortin-1 receptor (MC1R) gene, hence why they often have more ephelids.[16] Freckles can also be markers of UV damage and therefore, may be a warning sign for an increased risk of melanoma. Though treatment of ephelides is not necessary, some patients desire cosmetic camouflaging or pigment laser treatment that can temporarily lighten the affected skin. Photoprotection can temporarily lighten freckling as well.

SYRINGOMA

Syringomas are benign adnexal neoplasms that originate from intraepithelial luminal cells of eccrine ducts.[18] They are classified into four subtypes: localized, generalized (eruptive), familial, and associated with Down syndrome associated. Syringomas tend to affect middle aged women more than men and can occur at any age though they appear most often after puberty.[19] Clinically, they present as yellow, dark brown, or violaceous dome-shaped medium firm papules ranging from 1 to 5 mm. Commonly syringomas are distributed in the periorbital region around the eyelid margin, though they can also present on the scalp, axilla, abdomen, umbilicus, buttocks, and genital region [**Figure 51-7**].[19] Differential diagnoses include xanthelasma, steatocystoma multiplex, trichoepithelioma, and milia.[18] Treatment isn't necessary, but some patients desire cosmetic therapy due to lesions often appearing in exposed areas. Treatment options include electrodessication, surgical excision, cryotherapy, CO_2 laser therapy, and trichloroacetic acid.[19] Of all the subtypes, eruptive syringomas have the most cosmetic dissatisfaction due to their location, difficult clinical resolution, and risk of dyspigmentation with treatment.

XANTHELASMA

Xanthelasma occurs due to cholesterol-rich deposits found in the reticular dermis, perivascular, or periadnexal regions.[20] These lesions can present in a range of ages with the largest concentration occurring in patients between the age of 30 and 50 and with slight predilection for women. Clinically, xanthelasma palpebrarum presents as semisolid to firm yellow papules, plaques, or nodules on the medial canthus of the

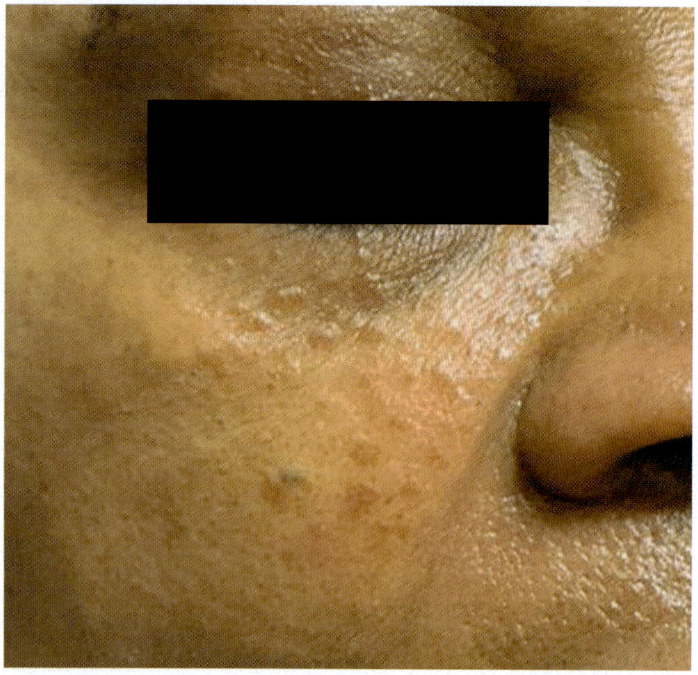

FIGURE 51-7. Syringomas on the face. (Courtesy of Valerie D. Callender, MD.)

upper and lower eyelids [**Figure 51-8**].[20] Xanthelasma palpebrarum can be associated with primary and secondary hyperlipidemia. Primary hyperlipidemia occur due to type II and IV or low high-density lipoprotein, while secondary hyperlipidemia is associated with hypothyroidism, diabetes mellitus, drugs (glucocorticoids, cyclosporine, anabolic steroids, retinoids, estrogens, some antihypertensives, cimetidine, tamoxifen), and diets rich in saturated fats, cholesterol, and alcohol.[20] Differential diagnoses of xanthelasma include syringoma, sebaceous hyperplasia, necrobiotic xanthogranuloma, periorbital xanthogranuloma, and palpebral sarcoidosis. Treatment options include first assessing the underlying condition of hyperlipidemia with lifestyle modifications such as a low-fat diet, regular physical activity, and lipid lowering medications indicated if necessary.[20] Alternative therapies such as surgical excision, laser therapy, chemical trichloroacetic acid, cryotherapy, and radiofrequency are available for treatment of these lesions, though these may not provide satisfactory results. Dyspigmentation is a common sequela with any procedural treatment that is performed.

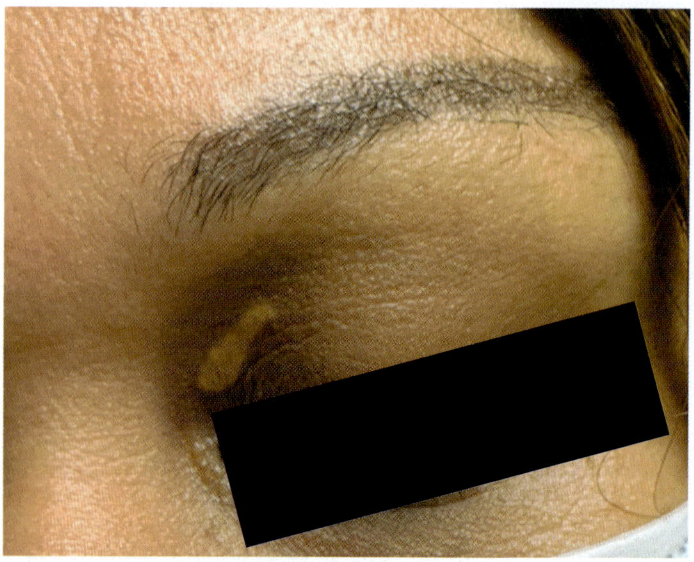

FIGURE 51-8. Xanthelasma on the eyelid. (Courtesy of Valerie D. Callender, MD.)

SEBORRHEIC KERATOSIS

Seborrheic keratoses are one of the most common epidermal neoplasms composed of two keratinocyte components, basaloid cells and squamous monomorphous epithelial cells. The prevalence is consistent among men and women with an increased prevalence with patients over the age of 50.[21] Clinically seborrheic keratoses are described as well-demarcated flesh colored, brown to black waxy, velvety stuck on papules and plaques with a varying range of diameter from a few millimeters to a few centimeters [**Figure 51-9A-D**]. They can appear anywhere on the body but tend to avoid the palms, soles, and mucosal surfaces.[21] Pedunculated seborrheic keratoses are more common in the intertriginous areas. Mutations in *FGFR3* and *PIK3CA* have been found to be associated with the molecular pathogenesis of seborrheic keratoses.[21] Differential diagnoses include basal cell carcinoma, fibroma, Bowen disease, verruca vulgaris, actinic keratosis, verrucous melanoma, and solar lentigo. Treatment is usually reserved for irritated lesions and/or for cosmetic concerns. Treatment options include cryotherapy, curettage with sharp spoon or ring curette, shave excision with scalpel, and cryotherapy. With or without treatment, it is important to counsel patients on the benign nature of the lesions and the likelihood they can increase in size and number over time.

DERMATOSIS PAPULOSA NIGRA

Dermatosis papulosa nigra (DPN) is a common variant of a seborrheic keratosis and has an increased prevalence in persons of African and less commonly, Asian descent.[22] Dermatosis papulosa nigra are epidermal growths that often begin as freckles on the face and neck in adolescence and proceed to grow in size and number with increased age.[22] They are described as dark brown to skin-colored firm papules and can be pedunculated [**Figure 51-10**]. Common locations include face, neck, and trunk but can also occur on the scalp and extremities. DPN lesions are commonly distributed symmetrically in a malar pattern on the cheeks. Mutations in *FGFR3* have been associated with dermatosis papulosa nigra and seborrheic keratoses further indicating similar pathogenesis between the two lesions.[22] Differential diagnosis includes seborrheic keratoses, acrochordons, verrucae, melanocytic nevi, and angiofibromas. Removal is commonly reserved for irritated DPNs only. Treatment options include excision, excision with tenotomy scissors, light curettage, electrodessication, or laser surgery. Patients should be educated on the potential for dyspigmentation and keloid formation of the treated area if they are considering treatment as well as the appearance of new lesions over time.

SEBACEOUS HYPERPLASIA

Sebaceous hyperplasia are proliferations of sebaceous glands commonly found on the cheeks, forehead, and nose of middle to elderly aged adults. Reduced androgens in the older ages cause a slower turnover in sebaceous glands, leading to decrease sebum and hyperplasia of the gland.[23] Though most often occurring on the face, sebaceous hyperplasia lesions can also be found on the lips, nipples, genitals, and the tip of the penis. Lesions are described as 1 to 5 mm round white to yellowish dome-shaped papules with a central umbilication [**Figure 51-11**].[23] Even though sebaceous hyperplasia is common, lesions should be viewed under dermoscopy to distinguish them from basal cell carcinoma. Dermoscopic features of "crown vessels" or nonbranching telangiectasia are a distinct finding in sebaceous hyperplasia.[23] Differential diagnosis includes nevus sebaceous, sebaceous adenoma, sebaceous carcinoma, basal cell carcinoma, molluscum contagiosum, and milia. Treatment options include electrodessication, shave removal, isotretinoin therapy, trichloroacetic acid, cryotherapy, CO_2 laser ablation, electrodessication, erbium or yttrium aluminum garnet laser ablation, and pulsed-dye laser photothermolysis.[23]

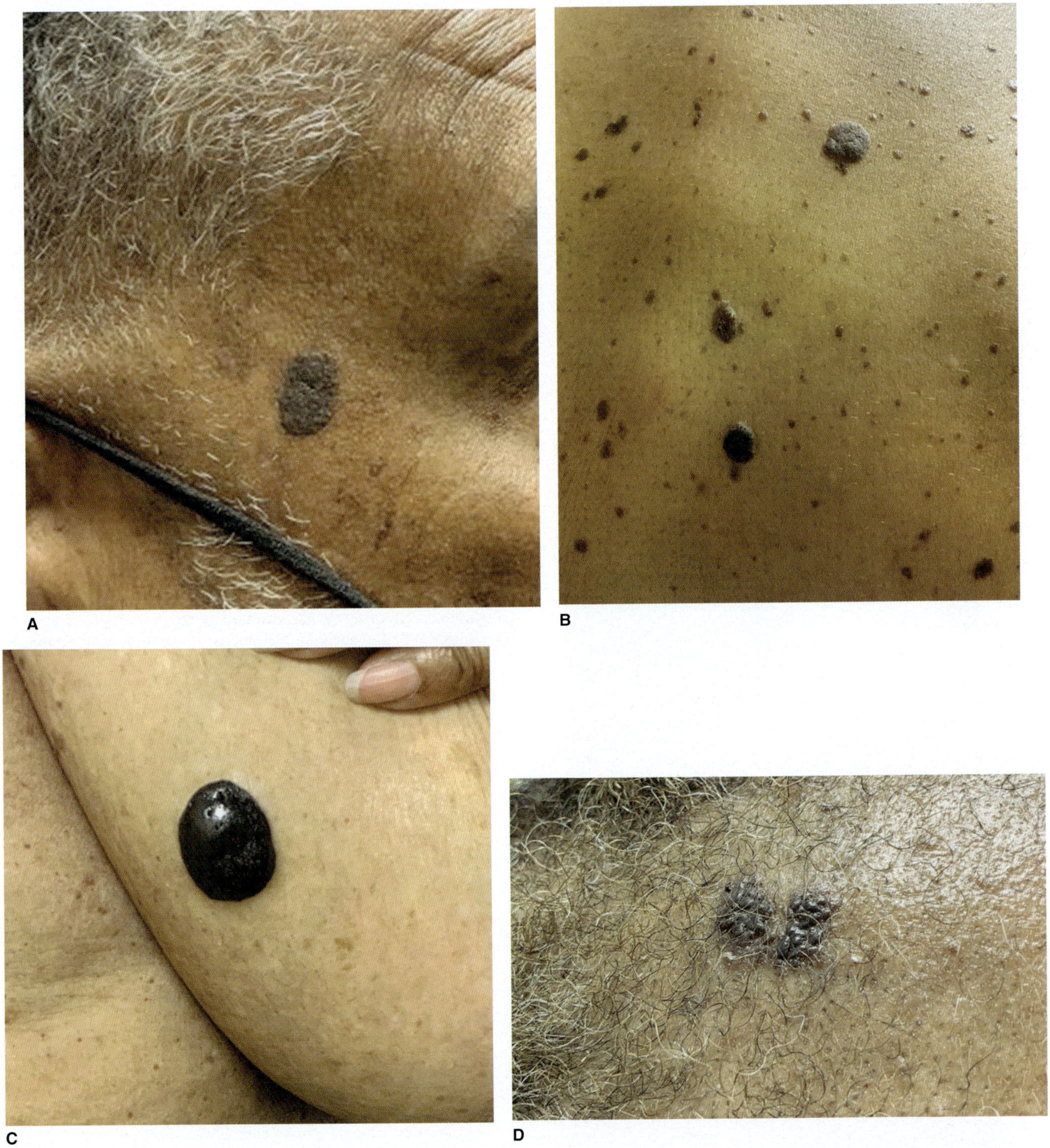

FIGURE 51-9. **(A)** Seborrheic keratosis, a solitary lesion on the face. **(B)** Multiple seborrheic keratoses on the trunk. **(C)** Deeply pigmented nodular seborrheic keratosis on the breast. **(D)** Seborrheic keratosis on the scalp. (Courtesy of Valerie D. Callender, MD.)

DERMATOFIBROMA

Dermatofibromas (DF) are solitary firm dermal proliferations that present as papules, plaques, or nodules ranging in colors from light brown to dark brown [**Figure 51-12**]. Dermatofibromas are commonly found on the lower extremities in areas of prior trauma such as insect bites. They often have a characteristic sign of central dimpling with lateral compression of the lesion. The specific etiology of dermatofibromas is unknown, though a variety of dermatofibroma variants have been characterized, including lichenoid DF, ulcerated DF, keloidal DF, cellular DF, lipidized DF, atrophic DF, hemosiderotic or aneurysmal DF, and fibrous histiocytoma.[24] Differential diagnoses include melanoma, basal and squamous cell carcinoma, morphea, neurofibroma, localized lipoatrophy, and anetoderma. Treatment options include intralesional corticosteroids, cryotherapy, shave removal, punch biopsy, or wide local excision though treatment should be reserved for symptomatic lesions only and less likely for cosmetic concerns.[25]

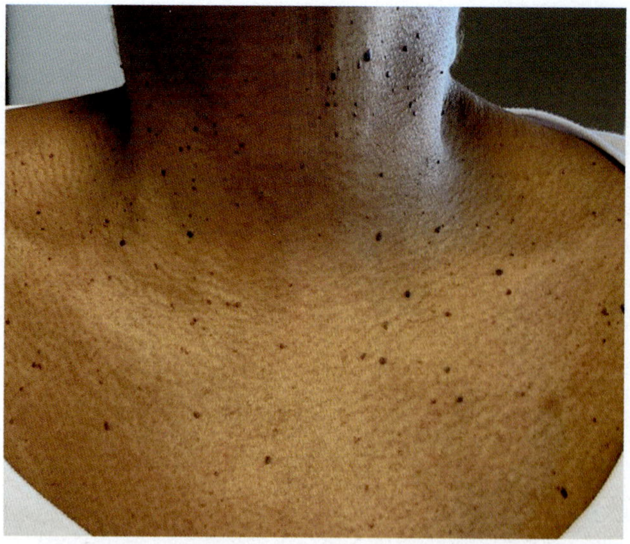

FIGURE 51-10. Dermatosis papulosa nigra on the neck and upper chest. (Courtesy of Valerie D. Callender, MD.)

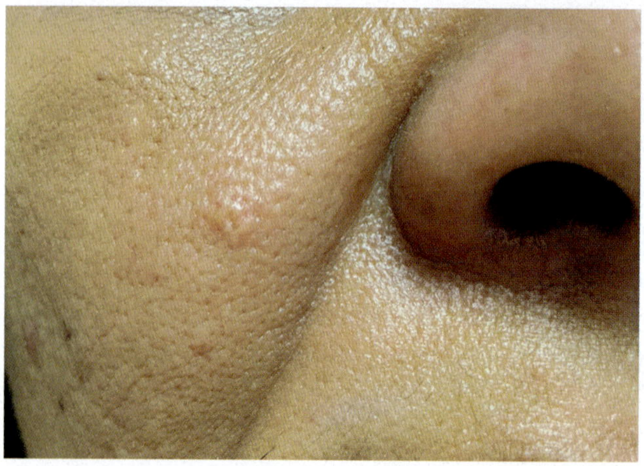

FIGURE 51-11. Sebaceous hyperplasia on the cheek. (Courtesy of Valerie D. Callender, MD.)

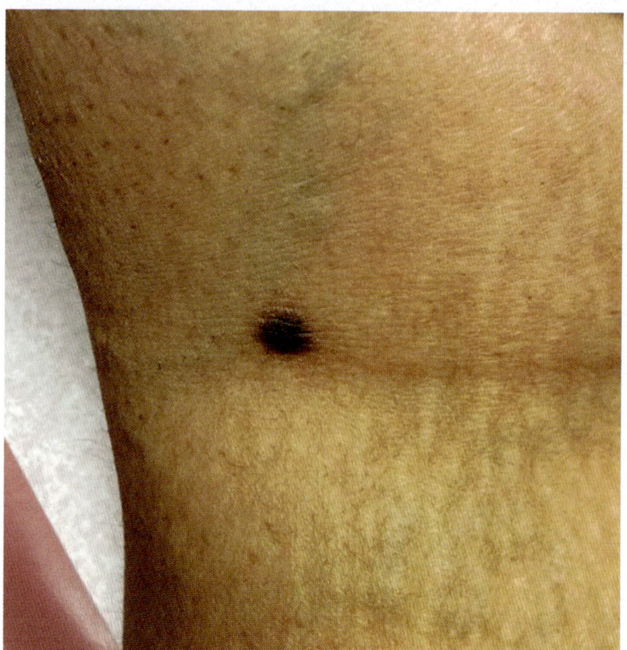

FIGURE 51-12. Dermatofibroma on the leg. (Courtesy of Valerie D. Callender, MD.)

REFERENCES

1. Goldsmith L. VisualDx - acrochordon. VisualDx web site. https://www.visualdx.com/visualdx/diagnosis/acrochordon?diagnosisId=51014&moduleId=17. Accessed Jun 19, 2022.
2. Kurniadi A, Rinaldi A, Yulianti H, Bazar AR, Prasetyawati RD, Tjandraprawira KD. Multiple vulvar giant fibroepithelial polyps: a rare case occurrence. *Case Rep Obstet Gynecol.* 2022;2022:5712925.
3. Belgam Syed SY, Lipoff JB, Chatterjee K. Acrochordon. In: *StatPearls* [Internet]. Treasure Island (FL): StatPearls Publishing; 2024. http://www.ncbi.nlm.nih.gov/books/NBK448169/. Accessed Jun 19, 2022.
4. Pandey A, Sonthalia S. Skin tags. In: *StatPearls* [Internet]. Treasure Island (FL): StatPearls Publishing; 2024. http://www.ncbi.nlm.nih.gov/books/NBK547724/. Accessed Jun 19, 2022.
5. Medina CR, Schneider S, Mitra A, Spears J, Mitra A. Giant submental lipoma: case report and review of the literature. *Can J Plast Surg.* 2007;15(4):219-222. https://www.ncbi.nlm.nih.gov/pmc/articles/PMC2696007/. Accessed June 23, 2022.
6. VisualDx - lipoma. VisualDx web site. https://www.visualdx.com/visualdx/diagnosis/lipoma?diagnosisId=51871&moduleId=101. Accessed June 23, 2022.
7. Weir CB, St. Hilaire NJ. Epidermal inclusion cyst. In: *StatPearls* [Internet]. Treasure Island (FL): StatPearls Publishing; 2024. http://www.ncbi.nlm.nih.gov/books/NBK532310/. Accessed June 23, 2022.
8. Hoang VT, Trinh CT, Nguyen CH, Chansomphou V, Chansomphou V, Tran TTT. Overview of epidermoid cyst. *Eur J Radiol Open.* 2019;6:291-301.
9. Northington ME, Huang CC. Pyogenic granuloma caused by exposed sternotomy wires. *Dermatol Surg.* 2004;30(12 Pt 2):1572-1573.
10. Sarwal P, Lapumnuaypol K. Pyogenic granuloma. In: *StatPearls* [Internet]. Treasure Island (FL): StatPearls Publishing; 2022. http://www.ncbi.nlm.nih.gov/books/NBK556077/. Accessed June 24, 2022.
11. Damsky WE, Bosenberg M. Melanocytic nevi and melanoma: unraveling a complex relationship. *Oncogene.* 2017;36(42):5771-5792.
12. Palicka GA, Rhodes AR. Acral melanocytic nevi: prevalence and distribution of gross morphologic features in white and black adults. *Arch Dermatol.* 2010;146(10):1085-1094.
13. Wang YK, Gao YJ, Liu J, et al. A comparative study of melanocytic nevi classification with dermoscopy and high-frequency ultrasound. *Skin Res Technol.* 2022;28(2):265-273.
14. Tuma B, Yamada S, Atallah ÁN, Araujo FM, Hirata SH. Dermoscopy of black skin: a cross-sectional study of clinical and dermoscopic features of melanocytic lesions in individuals with type V/VI skin compared to those with type I/II skin. *J Am Acad Dermatol.* 2015;73(1):114-119.
15. Sardana K, Chakravarty P, Goel K. Optimal management of common acquired melanocytic nevi (moles): current perspectives. *Clin Cosmet Investig Dermatol.* 2014;7:89-103.
16. Praetorius C, Sturm RA, Steingrimsson E. Sun-induced freckling: ephelides and solar lentigines. *Pigment Cell Melanoma Res.* 2014;27(3):339-350.
17. VisualDx - ephelides. VisualDx web site. https://www.visualdx.com/visualdx/diagnosis/ephelides?diagnosisId=53248&moduleId=101. Accessed June 24, 2022.
18. VisualDx- syringoma [Internet]. [Cited Jul 11, 2022] Available from: https://www.visualdx.com/visualdx/diagnosis/syringoma?moduleId=101&diagnosisId=52371&imgSet=0. Accessed July 11, 2022.
19. Frazier CC, Camacho AP, Cockerell CJ. The treatment of eruptive syringomas in an African American patient with a combination of trichloroacetic acid and CO2 laser destruction. *Dermatol Surg.* 2001;27(5):489-492.
20. Nair PA, Singhal R. Xanthelasma palpebrarum - a brief review. *Clin Cosmet Investig Dermatol.* 2017;11:1-5.
21. Hafner C, Vogt T. Seborrheic keratosis. *J Dtsch Dermatol Ges.* 2008;6(8):664-677.
22. Xiao A, Muse ME, Ettefagh L. Dermatosis papulosa nigra. In: *StatPearls*. Treasure Island (FL): StatPearls Publishing; August 11, 2021.
23. Hogan D, Mohammad S. Sebaceous hyperplasia. *Expert Rev Dermatol.* 2011;6(1):91-96.
24. Ferrari A, Argenziano G, Buccini P, et al. Typical and atypical dermoscopic presentations of dermatofibroma. *J Eur Acad Dermatol Venereol.* 2013;27(11):1375-1380.
25. VisualDx- dermatofibroma [Internet]. [Cited July 31, 2022] Available from: https://www.visualdx.com/visualdx/diagnosis/dermatofibroma?moduleId=101&diagnosisId=51413. Accessed July 31, 2022.

CHAPTER 52

Melanomas

Jordan Lim
Carl V. Washington

KEY POINTS

- Melanoma is the third most common cutaneous malignancy in humans but causes disproportionately more disease-specific morbidity and mortality than all cutaneous malignancies.
- The impact of melanoma varies considerably depending on race, ethnicity, and socio-economic status.
- There is an inverse relationship between the incidence of melanoma and degree of skin pigmentation.
- Acral tumors constitute 40% to 75% of melanomas in African Americans, Asians, and Hispanics, while only 2% to 9% of Caucasians develop acral melanoma.
- Melanoma in skin of color occurs predominantly on the lower extremities, including the palms, soles, and nail units.
- Acral and mucosal melanomas make up the preponderance of melanomas in skin of color patients.
- Melanoma outcomes in skin of color are worse than outcomes in Caucasians, and the reasons are multifactorial.

INTRODUCTION

Malignant melanoma continues to represent a significant contributor of cancer morbidity and mortality in the United States and worldwide. In 2023, an estimated 97,610 adults (58,120 men and 39,490 women) in the United States will be diagnosed with invasive melanoma of the skin.[1] Worldwide, an estimated 324,635 people were diagnosed with melanoma in 2020. The incidence of melanoma in Whites (per 100,000) is 34.7 and 22.1 among White men and women, respectively. By comparison, the male and female incidence was 1.0 and 0.9 among Blacks, and 5.0 among both sexes among Hispanics.[2] While it is true that this disease primarily affects Whites, African Americans (AA) and Hispanics bear a disproportionate share of poor outcomes for melanoma, as well as most cancers.[3] The clinical and socio-economic impact of this disparity is expected to grow as the demographic trends of the U.S. population shift toward a majority-minority status over the next two to three decades. As malignant melanoma has its primary impact on White populations, and to a much lesser degree on AA and other populations with skin of color, it is thus not surprising that the preponderance of clinical studies and public awareness campaigns focus on this population. U.S. Census data about increasing racial heterogeneity underscore the need for research focusing on the clinical and epidemiologic features of melanoma in various populations to understand these differences. While individuals with skin of color bear a disproportionately elevated morbidity and mortality from this disease, there do appear to be gender-specific differences with respect to these measures.[4,5] It is of note that women tend toward better overall survival than men, although the full explanation for these differences is not yet clear.[6] By 2050, Hispanic, African, and Asian Americans will compose 24%, 15%, and 8% of the U.S. population, respectively. Caucasians will compose at most 50% of the population. Between the years 2000 and 2050, these figures represent a population percentage increase of 188% for Hispanics, 71% for African Americans, and 21.3% for Asian Americans, and only 7% for Caucasians.[7] This chapter covers the epidemiology, clinical features, treatment, and prognosis of acral melanoma (AM) in various populations. The findings of our review suggest that the expression of melanoma in skin of color populations is distinct from that in Caucasians and is typified by lower incidence rates, a characteristic anatomic distribution, advanced stage at presentation, and poorer overall prognosis.

From 2011 through 2015, 1795 non-Hispanic Black people were diagnosed with melanomas in the United States, an average of 359 per year (incidence rate, 1.0 per 100,000). Rates are similar for men and women except in the oldest age group (65 or older), and increase with age, with the highest rates among men aged 65 or older (5.5 per 100,000). Half (55.3%) of all melanomas are diagnosed at a localized stage, and women are slightly more likely to be diagnosed at an earlier stages (56.7%) than men (53.6%). Lower extremities, including legs and feet, and subungual areas, are the most common anatomic sites among non-Hispanic Black people.[8] Patterns by anatomic site do not vary widely by sex among African Americans, although a slightly higher percentage of women than men develop melanoma on the lower extremities, and men have a slightly higher percentage of melanoma diagnosed on the head, neck, and trunk. Overall, most diagnosed melanomas demonstrate a nonspecific histology (63.8%). However, among melanomas with a specified histologic subtype, ALM is the most common (16.7%). Finally, more than half (58.7%) of melanoma diagnosed in skin of color occurs among people in the southern United States compared with the Northeast (17.3%), Midwest (13.7%), and West (10.3%). Despite that, studies vary with respect to the significance of sun exposure in skin of color patients. Whites are much more likely than AA and Hispanics to be diagnosed with localized melanoma, while 75% to 78% of non-Hispanic White people are diagnosed with melanoma at a localized stage. Furthermore, 18% of non-Hispanic Black people and 9% of non-Hispanic White people are diagnosed with regional-stage melanoma. More non-Hispanic Black people develop melanoma with distant metastasis (16%) than non-Hispanic White people (5%) or with unstaged melanoma (10%) than non-Hispanic White people (8%). Additionally, ulceration, an independently significant prognostic factor in node-negative cutaneous melanoma patients, is more common in AA (41%) than Caucasians (24%) and is more likely to occur on the lower extremities when present in AA (71.2%) and on the trunk when it develops in Caucasians (31.3%).[8-10] Stage at diagnosis is also significantly associated with race and ethnicity with melanoma diagnosed at stage I for 69% of non-Hispanic Whites, 69% of American Indian/Alaska natives, and 35.4% of non-Hispanic Black women. Surprisingly, in some reports Black women have the highest rates of ulceration and regional lymph node positivity.[11] Of interest among Hispanic patients, tumor distribution varies according to the degree of skin pigmentation: lightly pigmented Hispanics exhibit an anatomic distribution identical to Whites, whereas darkly pigmented Hispanics exhibit a tumor distribution reminiscent of Blacks. Numerous studies report that the most commonly specified histologic subtype on the hands and feet is acral lentiginous melanoma.[12] Although often considered interchangeable, the terms *acral lentiginous melanoma* and *acral melanoma* are not synonymous; acral lentiginous melanoma is a histologic designation, whereas AM is an anatomic designation. AM thus encompasses both acral lentiginous melanoma and other histologic subtypes of melanoma (such as superficial spreading and nodular melanoma) that may arise in acral locations.

EPIDEMIOLOGY

ACRAL MELANOMA

AM occurs on the glabrous skin of the palms, soles, and nail unit. It is the fourth most common subtype, accounting for 2% to 3% of all melanomas. AM is the least common subtype in Caucasians but is the most common melanoma subtype in AA, Asian Americans, and Hispanic populations.[13,14] The observed racial difference on AM prevalence results from the proportionally decreased occurrence of nonacral lesions in certain racial and ethnic populations. Earlier SEER data (1988-2011) demonstrated that AA patients present with AM more commonly (56.1%) than Caucasians (19.1%) for all tumor depths and stages.[9] In a recent review of the SEER Registry, AM was diagnosed in 1724 residents of the 18 SEER Registry areas, compared with 87,442 patients with cutaneous melanoma overall. The age-adjusted incidence rate of AM ranged from 1.6 to 2.4, with an average incidence rate of 2.0 per million person-years.[15]

Incidence rates in AM increase across all races with increasing age and occurs in both men and women. Hispanic Whites had higher incidence rates after the age of 60 compared to other races, but no significant incidence difference with advancing age was seen in non-Hispanic Whites, Blacks, Asian/Pacific Islanders, and Hispanic Whites.[15] Of interest, compared to nonacral subtypes of melanoma, the incidence of AM has remained stable over the past several decades.[16-18]

The unanticipated peculiar epidemiologic pattern of AM and its development on the infrequently sun-exposed sites of the palms and soles have historically suggested an etiologic role other than solar radiation.[19] Recent population-based studies in the United States, however, suggest a positive association between ultraviolet (UV) index and increasing incidence and mortality among Black men ($p < 0.05$), with a nonsignificant association observed among Black women and Hispanics of both sexes.[16,20] Although preliminary, these results suggest that solar radiation may play a greater than expected role in the development of melanoma in darkly pigmented populations. Additional etiologic theories in AM include the effect of long-term chronic trauma on benign acral nevi (given the preponderance of AM on the pressure-bearing heel and ball of the foot)[21]; malignant transformation of unstable foci of acral melanocytes[22]; and the relative paucity of free radical-scavenging melanin on the palms and soles of people with skin of color.[23] None of these explanations appears satisfactory, however, and the pathogenetic sequence of AM should be considered unknown.

SUBUNGUAL MELANOMA

Subungual melanomas (SMs) make up subset of AM and are thus relatively rare. While melanomas of the nail unit occur with equal frequency in all racial groups, SMs are the most common variant of MM among African Americans, Asians, and Hispanics. SM accounts for 75% of melanomas in African populations, 25% in Chinese populations, and 10% in Japanese populations. This variant occurs most commonly in the seventh decade of life for men and the sixth in women. The digits most affected are the great toe, followed by the thumb, with these sites accounting for 75% to 90% of all cases of SMs.[24,25] Hyponychial invasion is an important prognosticator of SM and is associated with invasion depth, metastatic risk, and disease-free survival.[26] SM may also occur in children, although most cases of melanonychia striata in children are associated with benign stable melanocytic proliferations.[27,28]

CLINICAL FEATURES AND DIAGNOSIS

ACRAL MELANOMA

AM in skin of color populations presents most commonly as an asymmetric, enlarging, dark brown or black macule/patch with irregular, notched borders, variegated colors, and a diameter greater than 6 mm [**Figures 52-1** and **52-2**].[29] Although this description echoes the experience in Caucasians, reports in Hispanics highlight the appearance of flecked, gray-white areas in many tumors,[30] whereas reports in Blacks underscore the presence of papillomatous, verrucous, or hyperkeratotic plaques [**Figures 52-3** and **52-4**].[31] In case series reflecting the AM experience in Chinese,[32,33] Japanese,[34] Hispanics,[30] and American[31,35] and African Blacks,[36,37] a significant proportion of tumors present with an unusually large surface area (generally >3 cm in diameter) and with signs of advanced local disease, including pain, crusting, bleeding, and nonhealing ulceration.

In terms of site distribution, case series in skin of color populations report predominance of plantar over palmar melanoma (approximate ratio, 17:1) and of palmoplantar lesions over subungual lesions (approximate ratio, 4:1).[30,32-34,38-40] Among volar lesions, the most common sites on the sole appear to be the heel and the ball of the foot, whereas no site predilection is obvious on the palm.[30,34,36,37,40] Melanoma of mucocutaneous surfaces is also proportionally more common in pigmented than White populations (in which prevalence is <10%). In one series involving African Americans (n = 80), 44% of female subjects developed mucosal melanoma—including lip, palate, nasal, ocular, vulvar, vaginal, cervical, and anorectal surfaces—compared with only 10% of male subjects.[41] Oral, nasal, and ocular melanoma exhibited a favorable prognosis relative to cutaneous melanoma, whereas vulvovaginal and anorectal melanoma showed the worst prognosis. In addition to AM, women of African, and perhaps of other non-European, ancestry may be at increased risk of developing mucosal melanoma.[41]

One challenge in the dermatology of skin of color is the differentiation between benign pigmentation or melanocytic neoplasms and their malignant counterparts. Hyperpigmented macules of the palmoplantar creases, for example, occur in 60% of African American adults and may measure from 2 mm to several centimeters in diameter.[29] Acral nevi are also more common in darker-pigmented races. One series (n = 251) examining African Americans reported an average of eight nevi per patient, with only 2% of the population showing no nevi whatsoever. In this series, darkly pigmented Blacks possessed fewer nevi and exhibited clustering

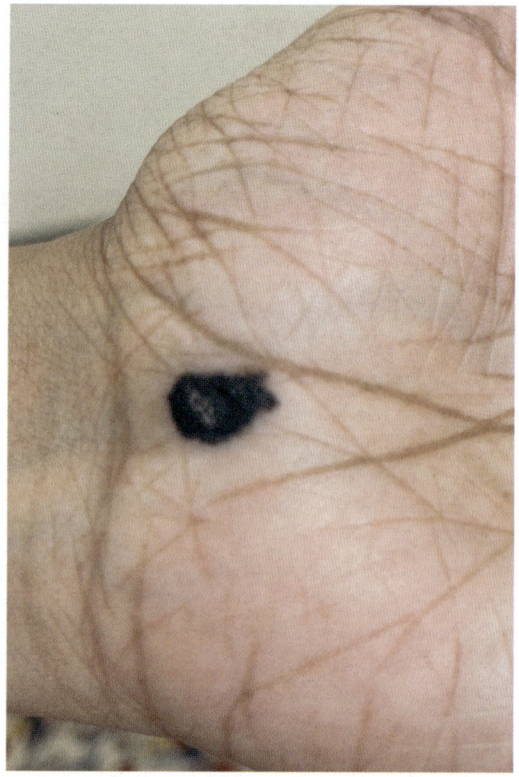

FIGURE 52-1. Acral melanoma. Deeply pigmented asymmetric patch on the proximal palmar surface.

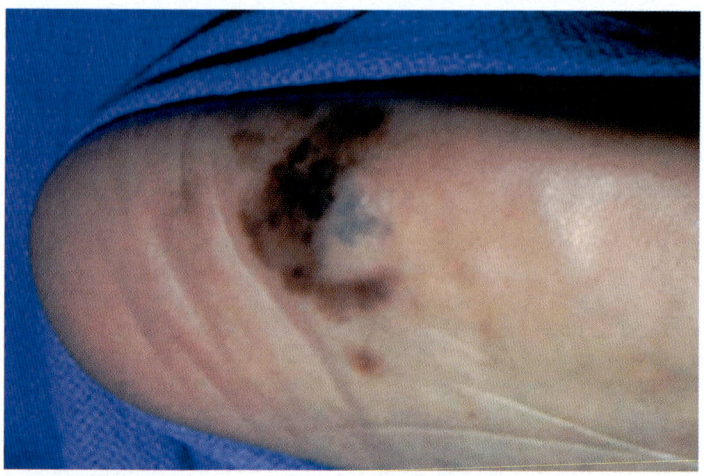

FIGURE 52-2. Acral melanoma. Ill-defined, asymmetric patch with irregular pigmentation on the heel of the foot.

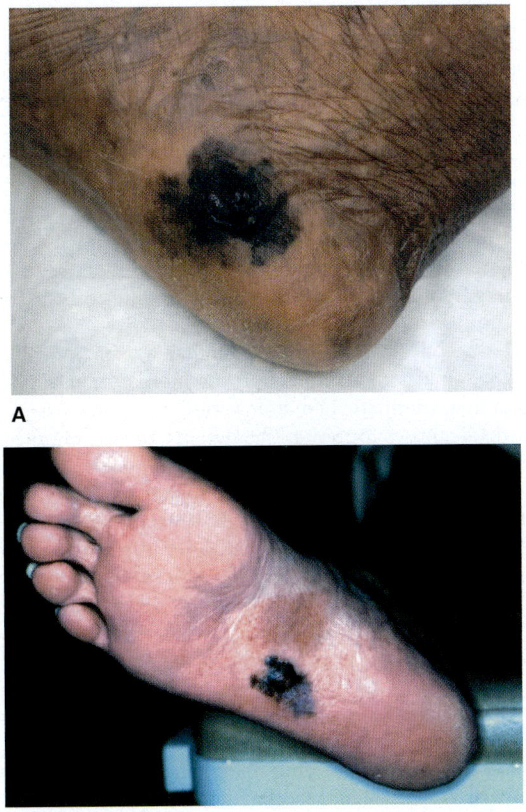

FIGURE 52-3. (A) Advanced acral melanoma. Irregular patch with central verrucous nodule on the heel of a foot. **(B)** Advanced acral melanoma. Long-standing patch with central nodule indicating vertical growth phase.

of their nevi and increased mottled pigmentation on the palmoplantar surface.[40] By contrast, lightly pigmented Blacks possessed more numerous nevi, with a greater proportion scattered over the body and relatively fewer on the palms and soles.[42] A Japanese series (n = 23,165) reported a 3% prevalence of plantar nevi, with a scattered distribution on the sole.[43]

Hyperpigmented macules of the palmoplantar creases, nevi, and mottled hyperpigmentation should not exhibit the classic morphologic features of AM. A diameter 7 mm or greater has been proposed as a screening threshold for plantar melanoma in Asians, although smaller, biopsy-proven AMs have been reported.[44,45] Additional considerations in the differential diagnosis of AM include angioma, hematoma, pyogenic granuloma, ulcer, and digital ischemia. One series of AM (n = 18) reported that 39% assumed the morphology of benign hyperkeratotic dermatoses, including large verruca, calluses, and dermatophyte infections [**Figure 52-5**].[46] This hyperkeratotic AM variant may be associated with diagnostic delay and significantly poorer prognosis.[46-48] Lesions suspicious for melanoma require excisional biopsy or carefully planned incisional biopsy. Shave biopsies should be avoided because the thick stratum corneum of the palms and soles may result in failure to sample deeper, diagnostic pathology.

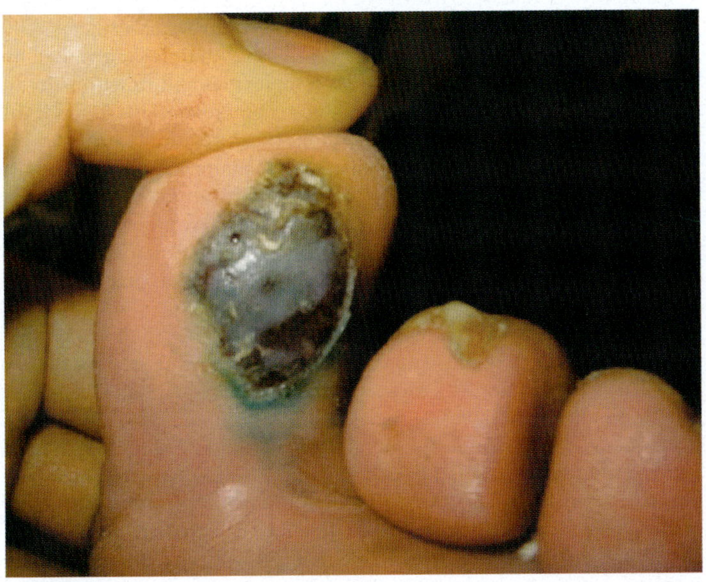

FIGURE 52-4. Advanced acral melanoma. Advanced tumor demonstrating ulceration, crusting, and bleeding.

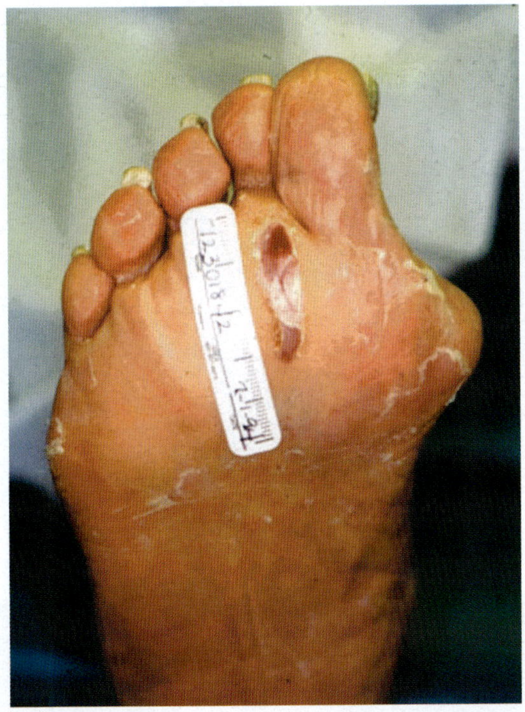

FIGURE 52-5. Acral lentiginous melanoma presenting as a callous. Note pigmentation of the skin along the lateral edge of the hyperkeratotic plaque.

SUBUNGUAL MELANOMA

Tumors arising in the nail bed or nail matrix are classified as SM. It presents clinically as a solitary brown or black longitudinal pigmented band of the nail (melanonychia striata) with irregular borders and variegated colors that increases in width to eventually involve the entirety of the nailbed.[29] It most commonly arises from the nail matrix, and much less commonly the nail bed [**Figure 52-6**]. Hutchinson sign refers to pigment extension to the periungual skin and, when present, may increase the index of suspicion for melanoma [**Figure 52-7**]. Tumor progression to the vertical growth phase results in dystrophy, elevation, and eventually fracture of the nail plate, revealing a friable, ulcerated, and bleeding mass.[32-34,49,50] Among various populations, several studies indicate the predominance of hand over foot lesions, and of the thumbnail and great toenail over the nails of other digits.[32,34,38,50,51] As in AM, the most common histologic pattern is acral lentiginous melanoma.[49-52] The tumor may also arise in children and adolescents, although much less commonly [**Figure 52-8**].

Because misdiagnosis of early SM is common, a Japanese study investigated the clinical features of early SM (Clark level I and early Clark level II) to aid in early detection.[51] Melanonychia striata was the first sign of disease in all cases. Longitudinal pigment streaks, however, are present in approximately 11% of the general population in Japan[53] and in up to 100% of African Americans older than 50 years.[54] The following traits may help differentiate benign pigmented bands from those suspicious for SM in skin of color populations: (1) onset after mid-adulthood,

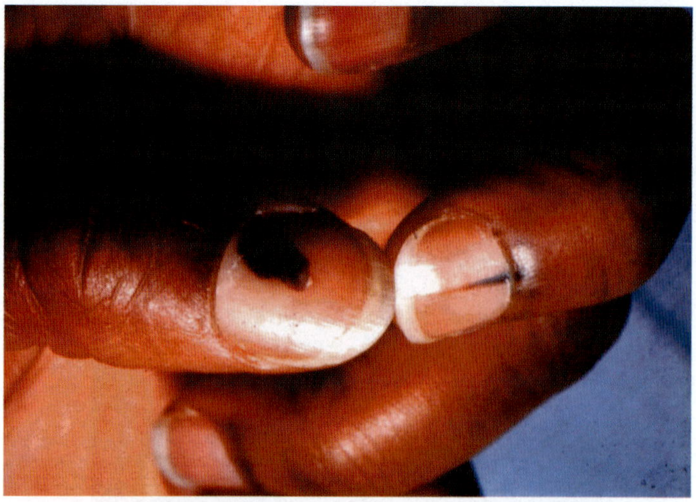

FIGURE 52-6. Early subungual melanoma. Early melanonychia striata of the third digit. Note coincidental subungual hematoma of the thumb.

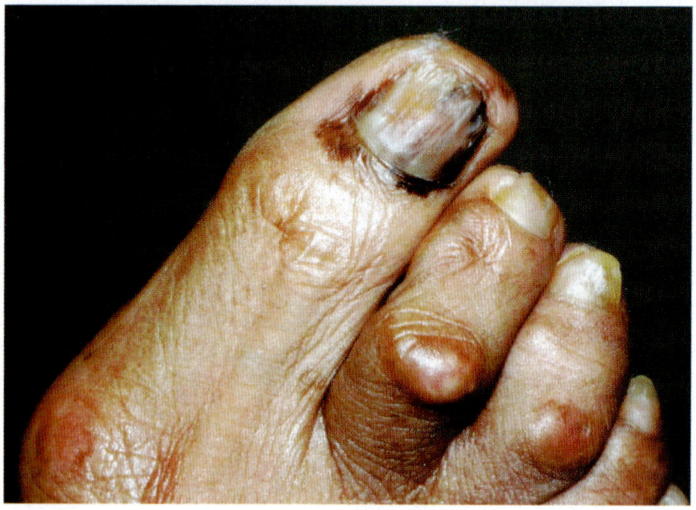

FIGURE 52-7. Subungual melanoma with Hutchinson sign. Subungual melanoma demonstrating pigment extension onto proximal and lateral nail folds, as well as the hyponychium.

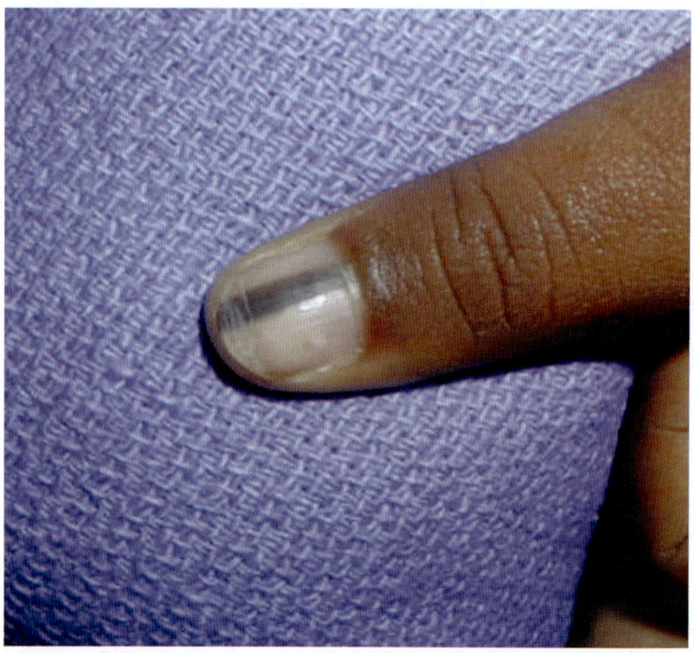

FIGURE 52-8. Subungual melanoma. Deeply pigmented widening melanonychia striata in a child.

(2) diameter greater than 6 mm, (3) variegated brown or homogenously black coloration, and (4) Hutchinson sign.[51] Rapid change may also be added to this list. It is of interest that although Hutchinson sign is traditionally considered a marker of late disease, it was present in all five cases of in situ SM in this series.[51]

Considerations in the differential diagnosis of melanonychia striata include lentigo and melanocytic nevus of the nail matrix or nail bed. Pigment bands of this origin, however, are rarely greater than 4 mm in diameter; however, dysplastic or congenital nevi may attain or exceed this size. Systemic causes of nail pigmentation include Addison disease, Peutz-Jeghers syndrome, and ingestion of 5-fluorouracil, phenothiazines, silver, or arsenic.[51] Additional considerations include pyogenic granuloma, radiodermatitis, onychotillomania, squamous cell carcinoma, epithelioma cuniculatum, porocarcinoma, metastatic bronchogenic carcinoma, traumatic hematoma, and onychomycosis.[54] The most common misdiagnoses for SM are hematoma and onychomycosis. Fortunately, a hematoma will migrate away from the proximal nail fold over a 4-week observation period, and in the case that this movement does not occur, a biopsy may be warranted.[55] In the same way, a 3- to 4-month course of antifungal therapy should yield a reassuring clear plane of nail at the proximal nail fold, and failure to respond to adequate antifungal treatment may warrant reconsideration of the diagnosis.[47]

TREATMENT

ACRAL AND SUBUNGUAL MELANOMA

No randomized studies examining the outcome of AM in skin of color populations exist. Treatment recommendations for subungual and AM rely on the experience of large referral centers. The majority of these studies have been conducted in Caucasian populations, however, which raises the issue of whether they may be generalizable to people with skin of color. Reported standard treatment for AM includes wide excision (WLE), with or without sentinel lymph node dissection (SLND) and adjuvant therapy. Excision on the plantar surface requires the construction of a durable and functional weight-bearing surface that simulates the normal anatomic structures that withstand pressure and shearing forces while simultaneously allowing for satisfactory local disease control.[36] Where possible, preservation of a portion of the heel or ball of the foot to bear pressure while walking and of the fascia of the deep tendons as a base for skin grafting is recommended.[56] Orthotic footwear should routinely be recommended to decrease sheer force and pressure on the graft site. Hyperkeratoses may develop at the interface between graft and normal skin but respond well to mechanical debridement.[57]

Currently, the standard treatment for AM and SM is surgical resection. NCCN guidelines recommend a 0.5-mm to 2-cm margin, as dictated by Breslow depth, and down to fascia.[58] While WLE margins are guided by the NCCN guidelines, acral anatomic complexities and functionality of hands and feet can make achieving these recommendations difficult. In addition, it has been documented that ALM can require larger margins for clearance compared to other subsets of melanoma.[59] As such, the use of comprehensive histologic margin assessment can be considered for ALM. This includes methods such as complete circumferential peripheral and deep margin assessment or Mohs micrographic surgery (MMS), for minimally invasive tumors, with permanent section analysis of the debulk specimen for staging.[58]

MMS for melanoma in its earliest form was published in the 1970s and has since modernized in its approach with use of immunostains and has grown in its utilization.[60-62] Most commonly, this technique is used for in situ or minimally invasive melanomas in cosmetically or physically limiting areas.[58,63] Overall the literature has shown that MMS achieves equivalent or better results when compared to WLE; however, there has yet to be a randomized controlled trial evaluating this outcome and few studies have focused on AM or SM.[64] In a retrospective review of digital melanoma managed with MMS ($n = 62$), 96.5% of cases avoided amputation and achieved a 5- and 10-year melanoma-specific survival (MSS) of 95% and 81.2%, respectively.[65] Since ALMs occur more frequently on the great toe, which contributes to balance, and the thumb, which provides 40% of the hand function, amputating these digits can have a significant impact on quality of life.[65,66] In contrast, after digit sparing surgery for nail MIS, Knackstedt et al found no change in Dermatology Life Quality Index (DLQI) or Disabilities in the arm, shoulder or hand (DASH).[67] In a study of slow Mohs versus WLE for AM in Korean patients, slow Mohs achieved better outcomes for local recurrence, recurrence free survival, and overall survival (OS) when compared to WLE.[68] MMS was also found to yield significantly smaller surgical defects resulting in quicker healing.[68]

While amputation remains a common approach to management of acral and SMs, there has been significant refinement in its use. Since the 1960s, the precise level of amputation for SM has evolved, highlighting the trade-off between preserving hand and foot function versus ensuring local disease control. In the 1990s, a practice changing study by Park and colleagues found that distal amputation was equivalent to proximal amputation and subsequently shifted the approach to more conservative amputation.[69] From that time, many studies have reported similar outcomes for amputation versus WLE. A meta-analysis evaluating these data found that there was no significant difference in local recurrence between amputation and functional/conservative surgery for MIS or minimally invasive nail melanoma.[70] However, when locally advanced disease has bony infiltration, primary amputation is often indicated.[57] Sentinel lymph node biopsy may be offered to patients with tumor thickness greater than 0.8 mm for staging purposes and to inform the decision to embark on adjuvant therapy. Whether choice of amputation level ultimately influences patient survival remains somewhat unclear. A few small studies have reported no survival difference between conservative surgery and amputation; however, there are no large studies validating these results.[38,71]

When reviewing outcomes of adjuvant therapies, including isolated limb perfusion, immunotherapy, interferon-α, and node dissection, it is reasonable to assume that results for SM should be comparable to that observed with AM; however, a precise estimate of outcome is unclear because most studies did not consider SM in a subgroup analysis.[31,37,38,57,72,73]

Surgical excision is preferred for in-transit metastases; however, when not possible, clinical trials and systemic therapy can be considered.[58] If the number of in-transit metastases is limited, isolated limb perfusion, intralesional talimogene laherparepvec (TVEC) and interferon-α are alternatives. One series involving Black patients with stage I AM ($n = 15$) reported a survival benefit of excision and regional limb perfusion compared with excision alone (5-year survival: combined therapy, 72% vs excision, 23%; $p < 0.05$); notably, the results of this approach in Blacks compared favorably to the 5-year survival in Caucasians treated with the same regimen.[31] TVEC has not been widely studied in racial minorities or acral lentiginous melanoma. In one study of 18 Japanese patients with stage IIIB-IVM1c melanoma, of which only 16.7% were ALM, the disease response rate was only 11.1% but consistent with that seen in studies of non-Asian patients.[74] The future of TVEC seems to be in its combination with checkpoint inhibitors, acting as a method to amplify tumor-specific immune response at the primary tumor.[75] Adjuvant interferon-α in metastatic melanoma, typically used for a limited number of in-transit metastases, has consistently shown improved recurrence free survival; however, no improvement in OS.[76,77] A phase II trial in Chinese patients with ALM compared 1 month versus 1 year adjuvant interferon-α and found no difference in recurrence free survival, while OS was not carried out as the median OS was not reached.[78] As such, interferon-α's exact role remains to be elucidated.

As our understanding of the molecular genetics of melanoma improves, current and future therapeutics are targeting specific genetic subtypes. Although few studies have evaluated the molecular genetics of AM, *BRAF* mutations occur less frequently in acral compared to nonacral cutaneous melanoma. *BRAF* mutation frequencies range from approximately 10% to 20% in the acral subtype to greater than 50% in melanomas located elsewhere on the skin.[79-81] BRAF protein is a member of the rapidly accelerated fibrosarcoma (RAF) family of serine/threonine kinases. It is an intermediary component of the mitogen-activated protein kinase (MAPK) pathway, which affects cell growth, survival, and differentiation. In contrast, *KIT* mutations are more frequently observed in acral and mucosal melanomas compared to other cutaneous subtypes.[82] KIT is a transmembrane receptor kinase. When bound to its ligand, activated KIT leads to downstream activation of the MAPK, PI3K-AKT1, and JAK signaling pathways involved in cell development, proliferation, survival, and migration.[83] Such findings imply that BRAF inhibitors may be less useful in AMs, whereas KIT inhibitors may provide benefit.

Several studies have described durable responses with KIT inhibitors such as sorafenib, imatinib, sunitinib, nilotinib, and dasatinib in patients with melanoma harboring *KIT* mutations. The selection of an appropriate KIT inhibitor is dependent on the specific *KIT* mutation present. Certain *KIT* mutations, such as exon 11 and 13 kinase domain mutations, may demonstrate partial imatinib response, whereas exon 17 (D280Y) kinase domain mutation may predict imatinib resistance. In the latter case, sorafenib, a multikinase inhibitor, has been shown to provide 27% reduction in target tumors. Handolias et al reported the palliative effects of KIT inhibitors in a case series wherein four patients received either sorafenib or imatinib depending on the *KIT* mutation present.[84] All patients ($n = 4$) subsequently died from central nervous system (CNS) metastasis. It has been speculated that the progression of CNS disease is explained by the limited penetration of the KIT inhibitors into the brain.[84-88] In a recent systematic review and meta-analysis of metastatic ALM treated with KIT inhibitors, the overall response rate (ORR) was 22% and OS, reported in only one study, was 21.1 months.[89] It should, however, be noted that at least one severe adverse event occurred in 42% of patients.[89] No current head to head comparison trials of KIT inhibitors and checkpoint inhibitors (CPIs) have been published and although cross-trial comparisons should be made with caution, CPI OS has consistently been higher than KIT inhibitors.[89] A potential future direction is combination KIT and CPI therapy; however, minimal data currently exist on this therapy.

CPIs including PD-1 and CTLA-4 inhibitors have become common first-line agents for advanced melanoma; however, in their landmark trials, AM and SM were not stratified as a subgroup.[90,91] As such, a small number of studies have evaluated CPI efficacy in these subtypes. Overall, studies have found better outcomes for ALM since implementation of CPI therapy. AM treated with any CPI regimen has had OS reported between 16 and 31 months compared to the 6- to 12-month range quote prior to CPI therapy.[92-95] For CPI monotherapy, a systematic review and meta-analysis of metastatic ALM from 2010 to 2020 found anti-PD1 to have the highest 12-month OS survival at 53% compared with anti-CTLA-4 at 34%. No large prospective clinical trials are currently published for anti-PD1/CTLA-4 combination therapy in ALM. The largest retrospective cohort study of 325 patients found ORR to be significantly higher for anti-PD1/ipilimumab therapy than anti-PD1 or ipilimumab monotherapy (43% vs 26% vs 15%, respectively).[95] Although the study noted a trend for increased progression-free survival (PFS), there was no significant improvement in PFS for combination therapy versus mono therapy. Most importantly, despite having better initial response to therapy with increased ORR, this did not translate to better OS for those on combination therapy.[95] These findings are contrary to response patterns seen when treating other types of melanomas.[90] Treatment disparity can also be noted when comparing immunotherapy ORRs for ALM versus all melanoma subtypes. In the CheckMate 067 trial where the majority of patients were White and acral subgroup was not specified, ORR to nivolumab monotherapy was 45%, whereas ORR to anti-PD1 therapy in ALM has been reported at only 20% to 26%.[90,95,96] These disparities are also seen when comparing the ORRs for combination therapy and ipilimumab monotherapy (58.3% vs 26% and 19% vs 15%, respectively).[90,95] As such, CPI therapy requires further investigation for its specific use for AM as preliminary studies suggest they may not respond the same as other types of melanoma.

Although deeper understanding of the molecular genetics of melanoma subtypes as well as the genetic differences between racial groups is needed, continued research will add to our fund of knowledge and allow for the development and implementation of more effective, targeted therapies.

PROGNOSIS

Minority populations are diagnosed less frequently with melanoma than White patients but continue to experience worse mortality and morbidity. When compared with nonacral lesions, AMs, more common in skin of color, are associated with higher overall mortality.[38,47] Data from the National Cancer Database (NCDB) (2004-2015) found that ALM was more likely to be diagnosed at a later stage than non-ALM with only 44.6% of ALM patients presenting as stage I versus 63.8% of non-ALM patients. They also found lower 5-year survival for ALM at all stages, with the most pronounced difference in stage III patients. This finding was echoed by a U.S. multicenter substage survival analysis prompting both authors to postulate that management for stage III ALM requires further attention and refinement.[97,98] AM in skin of color populations, however, carries an even graver prognosis when compared with Caucasian populations. Analysis of the California Cancer Registry noted that African Americans, Asians, and Hispanics were significantly more likely to have metastatic disease at diagnosis compared with Whites. Among men, 15% of Hispanics, 13% of Asians, and 12% of Blacks had metastatic disease at diagnosis, compared with only 6% of Whites. Among women, 7% of Hispanics, 21% of Asians, and 19% of Blacks had metastatic disease at diagnosis, relative to only 4% of Whites. These differences are statistically and clinically signficant.[99] Among U.S. Blacks, SEER data (1986-1991) similarly report a threefold increase in the proportion of Blacks diagnosed with distant disease compared with Whites (12% of Blacks vs 4% of Whites).[100] Analysis of the SEER database (1975-2016) found that, for all races, MSS improved over the time period studied. Despite MSS improving over time, minorities continued to experience worse MSS compared to non-Hispanic White (NHW) patients. This disparity was seen across all minorities for localized disease and persisted for regional/distant disease in Hispanic patients.[97] When evaluating OS, White patients had significantly higher median OS followed by Hispanic, Asian, then Black patients.[101]

Many studies involving AM speak to an analogous experience among Blacks, Hispanics, and Asians internationally, characterized by advanced stage at presentation and poor OS. The aggregate experience among U.S. and African Blacks is that AM typically presents as a thick lesion (mean Breslow thickness range, 1.65-7.10 mm),[36,57,101,102] with a high proportion of histologic ulceration and of regional and distant metastases.[32,103] The overall 5-year survival in Blacks is 27% to 59%, whereas a 25% to 70% range was noted for ALM.[4,15,36,57,101,104-107] By contrast, 5-year survival among contemporaneous Whites ranges from 74% to 85% overall and 60% to 89% for ALM, a distinction that attained statistical significance in numerous studies.[4,15,57,101,104-109]

Among U.S. and South American Hispanics, AM similarly presents as a thick tumor (1.5-8.3 mm),[30,101,110] with a high proportion of regional and distant metastases and a 46% to 79% ALM 5-year survival rate.[4,15,101,106,108,110,111] It is of interest that one series in the U.S. Southeast (n = 54) reported a survival advantage of Hispanics over non-Hispanic Whites for both local and regional/distant metastatic disease; these authors suggested that the overall younger age of Hispanic patients may explain this finding.[112] The 5-year survival in AM among Asians and Pacific Islanders ranges from 67% to 85% for ALM and approximately 71% to 77% for all subtypes.[4,15,101,106,107,109] Although much of the historical data for all races denote a large inferior prognostic gap for ALM compared to all subtypes, this seems to be decreasing. Notably, a Korean retrospective review (n = 642) found that AM, accounting for 40% of their cohort, had better OS than non-AM, postulating that greater awareness of ALM risk in Asian populations may have prompted earlier diagnosis by clinicians and patients in their cohort.[113] Future large studies will be required to further elucidate the true trajectory of prognosis of ALM in skin of color.

There is a paucity of data on the comparative survival of skin of color compared with Caucasian populations in SM, and the majority of studies considering prognosis in darker-pigmented individuals consider that of subungual and AM in aggregate. A study by Mejbel et al reported the impact of subungual versus acral location on OS and MSS. While OS at 1, 5, and 10 years was statistically significantly worse for SM (81%, 40%, and 28% vs 94%, 59%, and 38%, p = 0.04 for subungual vs AMs, respectively), no difference was noted for MSS and subungual location was not noted to be an independent poor prognostic factor for OS or MSS. Breslow thickness and LN positivity were the only independent poor prognostic factors for MSS.[114] Although larger prospective studies would benefit solidifying this conclusion, these findings are reassuring and enhance the credibility of previous studies that combined subungual and AM into one category for assessing MSS.

Due largely to diagnostic delay, SM in Whites is associated with poor prognosis. Mean delay ranges from 9 to 23 months in approximately 50% of patients in reported series[54] and is complicated by the high proportion of amelanotic lesions (40% in the Sydney Melanoma Unit database).[50] In White populations, SM is associated with a 55% overall 5-year survival rate (reported range, 16-76%).[50,114] Lesions present at an advanced stage (median thickness, 3.05 mm), with only 20% of subungual tumors presenting at stage I.[50] In one study, no significant difference was noted between 1, 5, and 10 year OS for White and Hispanic patients (92% vs 95%, 57% vs 59%, and 40% vs 32%, respectively).[114] A Japanese study (n = 34) found that 5-year survival rate improved from 53% (1969-1982) to 87% (1981-1993), again citing improved public and provider awareness as a possible cause for the improvement.[115] A U.S. comparative study (n = 11) reported that U.S. Blacks with SM have a 3.5 times higher mortality rate than Caucasians, which remained significant even after controlling for stage and Clark level (suggesting that race may be an independent prognostic factor).[49]

With the data over time persistently reporting that ALM, especially in skin of color population, presents at a later stage, many have investigated the underlying reason to this delay in seeking care. Lower SES, Medicaid insured or uninsured patients are all associated with worse prognosis.[101,116] Since skin of color individuals have significantly higher uninsured rates, authors have suggested that it may be a contributing factor to the racial disparity we see in melanoma outcomes.[101,116] For example, Hispanics represent one of the highest uninsured racial/ethnic groups in the United States at 17.7%, alongside American Indian and Alaska Natives at 18.8%, followed by Blacks at 9.6% and only 5.7% for NHWs.[117] Patient and provider knowledge both contribute to this disparity. In a cross-sectional study by Sanchez et al, it was noted that when surveyed, 39% of patients were unaware of melanoma and these patients were more likely to be categorized as Fitzpatrick III and above.[118] Even further, a study of Korean patients with melanoma found that median time to diagnosis was 6.2 years, possibly highlighting that racial minorities are undereducated by the medical community regarding melanoma.[119] Knowledge-based interventions for those with ethnic skin have found that 3 months after brief counseling, patients retained knowledge on warning signs, self-skin exams, and personal risk.[120] Alongside improving patient-centered knowledge, we must also focus on improving physician knowledge of appropriately diagnosing melanoma in skin of color. It has been demonstrated that these patients are more likely to be misdiagnosed and on average experience a 9-month delay prior to diagnosis, further solidifying that late-stage diagnosis is not simply due to patients delaying seeking care.[121] In another study, it was found that only 44.2% of patients with melanoma were sent for a biopsy upon initial presentation. Even further, 46.5% experienced up to a 3-month delay and 21% experienced up to a 6-month delay until biopsy.[122]

After overcoming the many barriers to diagnosis, there remain many areas of racial disparity in the management of melanoma. Tripathi et al evaluated the NCDB form 2004-2015 and found that Black patients with stage I to III melanoma, when compared to NHW patients, experienced significantly longer delay from diagnosis to definitive surgical management for all insurance types while controlling for sociodemographic factors.[123] When receiving treatment, Black patients with ALM were more likely than NHW patients to be treated with major amputation (10.2% vs 0.6%) regardless of tumor characteristics and sociodemographic factors.[103] These results have been echoed in studies of other databases.[124]

Immunotherapy is also less likely to be provided for Black, low-income, and Medicaid patients.[125] Even if provided, there is limited evidence of immunotherapy's efficacy in SOC patients, especially those with ALM and mucosal melanoma, both of which are more common in this population. Mixed conclusions toward the efficacy of immunotherapy in ALM have been published with some believing that lack of efficacy may be due to lower mutational burden in ALM and mucosal melanoma due to lack of UV exposure leading to a limited immunotherapy response.[126] The limited diversity in pivotal trials, as discussed above, results in our inability to assess if new gold standard immunotherapy is as beneficial for skin of color patients.

The question of whether melanoma is a biologically more aggressive tumor in skin of color populations or whether race in fact serves as a proxy for social, cultural, and economic factors culminating in diagnostic delay and advanced tumor stage is unclear. Conflicting results have been noted in studies done in the U.S. skin of color population, with some studies suggesting that race influences prognosis independent of tumor thickness and stage,[38,127] whereas others report that the prognostic importance of race becomes immaterial in face of regression analyses considering established prognostic indicators, such as Breslow thickness, ulceration, and stage.[35,104] One retrospective study in U.S. Blacks ($n = 79$) examined melanoma outcome over three decades and reported a 35% 5-year survival rate in cohorts diagnosed before 1980, compared with a 49% 5-year survival rate in cohorts diagnosed between 1980 and 1989, reflecting increasing early patient presentation.[104] Earlier melanoma diagnosis and improved survival in more recent decades (1980s to 1990s) were similarly observed in population-based Japanese and Hispanic studies.[39,128] Another study involving 96 African Americans reported that aggressive surgical and adjuvant therapy in those patients with stage I disease amounted to a 78% 5-year survival, which is comparable to the outcome in Caucasian patients.[31] These studies provide encouraging evidence that the poor prognosis historically observed in persons of color may be a greater reflection of diagnostic delay and undertreatment rather than intrinsic tumor aggression and suggest that increased public and clinical awareness of melanoma in skin of color may continue the trend of improved prognosis.

CONCLUSION

As outlined in this chapter, the melanoma experience in people with skin of color is distinct from that in Caucasians and is characterized by decreased incidence, a characteristic anatomic distribution on the acral extremities, advanced stage at presentation, and overall poorer prognosis. Perhaps the most concerning of these features are the advanced presentation and poor survival in these populations from a tumor that is plainly visible and eminently curable in its early stages. Questioning why this occurs is fundamental to any effort to understand and to dismantle racial disparities in healthcare. In relation to dermatology, the concept of race encompasses both skin type and sociocultural beliefs and practices. Although evidence that race may be an independent prognosticator in acral and SM exists,[38,49,127] other studies[21,104] as well as improving survival rates reported in more recent cohorts[39,128] suggest that the poor prognosis historically observed in people with skin of color may be a greater reflection of diagnostic delay rather than intrinsic tumor aggression. In fact, the American Anthropological Association argues in its Statement on Race that modern humans are a relatively homogenous species and that genetic data suggest as much variability between two people of the same racial group as between two people from any two different racial groups.[129] Thus, few biological differences should exist between large populations that are of explanatory relevance.[130,131]

Understanding race as a purely biological variable, divorced from its social and historical context, may oversimplify a public health issue that requires a broad perspective. Access to healthcare is one consideration. One study ($n = 28{,}237$) examining the effects of health insurance on early cancer detection reported a significant positive association between lack of health insurance and Medicaid insurance with late-stage melanoma diagnosis.[132] Socioeconomic variables alone, however, do not account for all racial health disparities; indeed, health inequalities exist even when universal access to healthcare is ensured.[82,131]

Public awareness campaigns that convey the unique features of melanoma in skin of color populations are necessary. Recent studies suggest a deficiency in the knowledge of African Americans and Hispanics regarding melanoma. According to a nationwide survey conducted by the American Academy of Dermatology, 75% of African Americans did not know the meaning of the word melanoma, compared with only 35% of Whites ($p < 0.05$).[133] A recent study in U.S. Hispanics demonstrated less awareness of melanoma, less awareness of skin cancer risk factors, and a decreased risk perception compared with non-Hispanic Whites.[134] Shared beliefs, attitudes, and behaviors may manifest in particular health practices and illness profiles characteristic of a racial or cultural group. One study noted that both cultural and socioeconomic factors were able to account for the discrepancy in breast cancer mortality between African American and Caucasian women in the United States, where neither was sufficient alone.[131] Perspective on such broad determinants of melanoma outcome in people with skin of color and attention to their unique clinical expression are necessary to improve the prognosis for these patients.

REFERENCES

1. Siegel RL, Miller KD, Wagle NS, Jemal A. Cancer statistics, 2023. *CA Cancer J Clin.* 2023;73(1):17-48.
2. SEER Cancer Stat Facts: Melanoma of the Skin. National Cancer Institute: Surveillance, Epidemiology, and End Results Program. Accessed: May 30, 2023. https://seer.cancer.gov/statfacts/html/melan.html.
3. DeSantis CE, Miller KD, Goding Sauer A, Jemal A, Siegel RL. Cancer statistics for African Americans, 2019. *CA Cancer J Clin.* 2019;69(3):211-233.
4. Wu XC, Eide MJ, King J, et al. Racial and ethnic variations in incidence and survival of cutaneous melanoma in the United States, 1999-2006. *J Am Acad Dermatol.* 2011;65(5 Suppl 1):S26-S37.
5. Lam M, Zhu JW, Hu A, Beecker J. Racial Differences in the Prognosis and Survival of Cutaneous Melanoma From 1990 to 2020 in North America: A Systematic Review and Meta-Analysis. *J Cutan Med Surg.* 2022;26(2):181-188.
6. Behbahani S, Maddukuri S, Cadwell JB, Lambert WC, Schwartz RA. Gender differences in cutaneous melanoma: Demographics, prognostic factors, and survival outcomes. *Dermatol Ther.* 2020;33(6):e14131.
7. 2004 Interim National Population Projections. US Census Bureau. Last Revised: December 16, 2021. Accessed: May 30, 2023. https://www.census.gov/data/tables/2004/demo/popproj/2004-int-popproj-summary.html.
8. Culp MB, Lunsford NB. Melanoma Among Non-Hispanic Black Americans. *Prev Chronic Dis.* 2019;16:E79. Published 2019 Jun 20.
9. Mahendraraj K, Sidhu K, Lau CSM, McRoy GJ, Chamberlain RS, Smith FO. Malignant Melanoma in African-Americans: A Population-Based Clinical Outcomes Study Involving 1106 African-American Patients from the Surveillance, Epidemiology, and End Result (SEER) Database (1988-2011). *Medicine (Baltimore).* 2017;96(15):e6258.
10. Higgins S, Nazemi A, Feinstein S, Chow M, Wysong A. Clinical Presentations of Melanoma in African Americans, Hispanics, and Asians. *Dermatol Surg.* 2019;45(6):791-801.
11. Fernandez JM, Bubic BN, Dahak S, et al. Racial and ethnic differences in tumor characteristics and overall survival of women with melanoma: A national cancer database retrospective cohort study. *J Am Acad Dermatol.* 2023;88(3):694-696.
12. Gloster HM Jr, Neal K. Skin cancer in skin of color. *J Am Acad Dermatol.* 2006;55(5):741-764.
13. Cascinelli N, Zurrida S, Galimberti V, et al. Acral lentiginous melanoma. A histological type without prognostic significance. *J Dermatol Surg Oncol.* 1994;20(12):817-822.
14. Ridgeway CA, Hieken TJ, Ronan SG, Kim DK, Das Gupta TK. Acral lentiginous melanoma. *Arch Surg.* 1995;130(1):88-92.
15. Huang K, Fan J, Misra S. Acral Lentiginous Melanoma: Incidence and Survival in the United States, 2006-2015, an Analysis of the SEER Registry. *J Surg Res.* 2020;251:329-339.
16. Pennello G, Devesa S, Gail M. Association of surface ultraviolet B radiation levels with melanoma and nonmelanoma skin cancer in United States blacks. *Cancer Epidemiol Biomarkers Prev.* 2000;9(3):291-297.

17. Dwyer PK, Mackie RM, Watt DC, Aitchison TC. Plantar malignant melanoma in a white Caucasian population. *Br J Dermatol.* 1993;128(2):115-120.
18. Garsaud P, Boisseau-Garsaud AM, Ossondo M, et al. Epidemiology of cutaneous melanoma in the French West Indies (Martinique). *Am J Epidemiol.* 1998;147(1):66-68.
19. Elder DE. Skin cancer. Melanoma and other specific nonmelanoma skin cancers. *Cancer.* 1995;75(1 Suppl):245-256.
20. Hu S, Ma F, Collado-Mesa F, Kirsner RS. UV radiation, latitude, and melanoma in US Hispanics and blacks. *Arch Dermatol.* 2004;140(7):819-824.
21. Bellows CF, Belafsky P, Fortgang IS, Beech DJ. Melanoma in African-Americans: trends in biological behavior and clinical characteristics over two decades. *J Surg Oncol.* 2001;78:10-16.
22. Lewis MG, Johnson K. The incidence and distribution of pigmented naevi in Ugandan Africans. *Br J Dermatol.* 1968;80(6):362-366.
23. Armstrong BK, Kricker A. How much melanoma is caused by sun exposure? *Melanoma Res.* 1993;3(6):395-401.
24. Decker A, Connolly KL, Lee EH, Busam KJ, Nehal KS. Frequency of subungual melanoma in longitudinal melanonychia: a single-center experience. *Dermatol Surg.* 2017;43(6):798-804.
25. Ingkaninanda P, Visessiri Y, Rutnin S. Clinicopathological features and prognostic factors of malignant melanoma: a retrospective analysis of Thai patients in Ramathibodi hospital. *J Med Assoc Thai.* 2015;98(8):820-827.
26. Yoo H, Kim H, Kwon ST, et al. Tumor invasion in the hyponychium is associated with distant metastasis and poor prognosis in subungual melanoma: a histologic landscape of 44 cases. *J Am Acad Dermatol.* 2022;86(5):1027-1034.
27. Cooper C, Arva NC, Lee C, et al. A clinical, histopathologic, and outcome study of melanonychia striata in childhood. *J Am Acad Dermatol.* 2015;72(5):773-779.
28. Goettmann-Bonvallot S, André J, Belaich S. Longitudinal melanonychia in children: a clinical and histopathologic study of 40 cases. *J Am Acad Dermatol.* 1999;41(1):17-22.
29. Rahman Z, Taylor S. Malignant melanoma in African Americans. *Cutis.* 2001;67:403-404.
30. Vaszqez M, Ramos F, Sanchez J. Melanomas of volar and subungual skin in Puerto Ricans. *J Am Acad Dermatol.* 1984;10:39-45.
31. Krementz E, Sutherland C, Carter R, Ryan R. Malignant melanoma in the American Black. *Ann Surg.* 1976;1976:533-542.
32. Collins R. Melanoma in the Chinese of Hong Kong: emphasis on volar and subungual sites. *Cancer.* 1984;54:1482-1488.
33. Lin C-S, Wang W-J, Wong C-K. Acral melanoma: a clinicopathologic study of 28 patients. *Int J Dermatol.* 1990;29:107-112.
34. Seiji M, Takematsu H, Hosokawa M, et al. Acral melanoma in Japan. *J Invest Dermatol.* 1983;80:56s-60s.
35. Bellows C, Belafsky P, Fortgang I, Beech D. Melanoma in African-Americans: trends in biological behavior and clinical characteristics over two decades. *J Surg Oncol.* 2001;78:10-16.
36. Hudson D, Krige J. Plantar melanoma in black South Africans. *Br J Surg.* 1993;80:992-994.
37. Krementz E, Reed R, Coleman W, Sutherland C, Carter R, Campbell M. Acral lentiginous melanoma: a clinicopathologic entity. *Ann Surg.* 1982;195:632-644.
38. Slingluff C, Vollmer R, Seigler H. Acral melanoma: a review of 185 patients with identification of prognostic variables. *J Surg Oncol.* 1990;45:91-98.
39. Black W, Goldhahn R, Wiggins C. Melanoma within a southwestern Hispanic population. *Arch Dermatol.* 1987;123:1331-1334.
40. Panjota E, Llobet R, Roswit B. Melanomas of the lower extremity among native Puerto Ricans. *Cancer.* 1976;38:1420-1423.
41. Muchmore J, Mizuguchi R, Lee C. Malignant melanoma in American black females: an unusual distribution of primary sites. *J Am Coll Surg.* 1996;183:457-465.
42. Coleman W, Gately L, Krementz A, Reed R, Krementz E. Nevi, lentigines, melanomas in blacks. *Arch Dermatol.* 1980;116:548-551.
43. Kukita A, Ishihara K. Clinical features and distribution of malignant melanoma and pigmented nevi on the soles of the feet in Japan. *J Invest Dermatol.* 1989;92:210s-213s.
44. Wong T, Ohara K, Kawashima M, Sober A, Nogita T, Mihm M. Acral lentiginous melanoma (including in situ melanoma) arising in association with naevocellular nevi. *Melanoma Res.* 1996;6:241-246.
45. Saida T, Ishihara K, Tokuda Y. Effective detection of plantar malignant melanoma. *Int J Dermatol.* 1993;32:722-725.
46. Soon S, Solomon A, McAlpine B, Papadoupolous D, Washington C. Acral melanoma mimicking benign disease: the Emory experience. *J Am Acad Dermatol.* 2003;48:183-188.
47. Bennett D, Wasson D, MacArthur J, McMillen M. The effect of misdiagnosis and delay in diagnosis on clinical outcome in melanoma of the foot. *J Am Coll Surg.* 1994;179:279-284.
48. Fortin P, Freiberg A, Rees R, Sondak V, Johnson T. Malignant melanoma of the foot and ankle. *J Bone Joint Surg Am.* 1995;77:1396-1403.
49. O'Leary J, Berend K, Johnson J, Levin L, Seigler H. Subungual melanoma: a review of 93 cases with identification of prognostic variables. *Clin Orthop.* 2000;378:206-212.
50. Quinn M, Thompson J, Crotty K, McCarthy W, Coates A. Subungual melanoma of the hand. *J Hand Surg.* 1996;1996:506-511.
51. Saida T, Oshima Y. Clinical and histopathological characteristics of the early lesions of subungual melanoma. *Cancer.* 1989;63:556-560.
52. Blessing K, Kernohan N, Park K. Subungual malignant melanoma: clinicopathological features of 100 cases. *Histopathology.* 1991;19:425-429.
53. Kawamura T, Nishihara K, Kawasakiya S, Izumi T, Tanaka H. Pigmentatio longitudinalis striata unguium and the pigmentation of the nail in Addison's disease (abstract). *Jpn J Dermatol.* 1958;68:10.
54. Levit E, Kagen M, Scher R, Grossman M, Altman E. The ABC rule for clinical detection of subungual melanoma. *J Am Acad Dermatol.* 2000;42:269-274.
55. Hughes L, Horgan K, Taylor B, Laidler P. Malignant melanoma of the hand and foot: diagnosis and management. *Br J Surg.* 1985;72:811-815.
56. Balch C. Excising melanoma: how wide is enough? And how to reconstruct. *J Surg Oncol.* 1990;44:135-136.
57. Hudson D, Krige J, Subbings H. Plantar melanoma: results of treatment in three populations. *Surgery.* 1998;124:877-882.
58. Referenced with permission from the NCCN Clinical Practice Guidelines in Oncology (NCCN Guidelines®) for Melanoma: Cutaneous V.2.2023. © National Comprehensive Cancer Network, Inc. 2023. All rights reserved. Accessed [May 31, 2023]. To view the most recent and complete version of the guideline, go online to NCCN.org.
59. Zitelli JA, Brown CD, Hanusa BH. Surgical margins for excision of primary cutaneous melanoma. *J Am Acad Dermatol.* 1997;37(3 Pt 1):422-429.
60. Mohs FE. Chemosurgery for the microscopically controlled excision of cutaneous cancer. *Head Neck Surg.* 1978;1(2):150-166.
61. Etzkorn JR, Sobanko JF, Elenitsas R, et al. Low recurrence rates for in situ and invasive melanomas using Mohs micrographic surgery with melanoma antigen recognized by T cells 1 (MART-1) immunostaining: tissue processing methodology to optimize pathologic staging and margin assessment [published correction appears in J Am Acad Dermatol. 2017 Nov 17;:]. *J Am Acad Dermatol.* 2015;72(5):840-850.
62. Siscos SM, Neill BC, Seger EW, Hooton TA, Hocker TLH. The Current State of Mohs Surgery for the Treatment of Melanoma: A Nationwide Cross-Sectional Survey of Mohs Surgeons. *Dermatol Surg.* 2020;46(10):1267-1271.
63. Siscos SM, Neill BC, Seger EW, Rajpara A, Hocker TLH. Practice habits of Mohs surgeons treating melanoma with Mohs surgery: A cross-sectional survey. *J Am Acad Dermatol.* 2021;84(3):833-835.
64. Charalambides M, Yannoulias B, Malik N, et al. A review of Mohs micrographic surgery for skin cancer. Part 1: Melanoma and rare skin cancers. *Clin Exp Dermatol.* 2022;47(5):833-849.
65. Terushkin V, Brodland DG, Sharon DJ, Zitelli JA. Digit-Sparing Mohs Surgery for Melanoma. *Dermatol Surg.* 2016;42(1):83-93.
66. Matsumoto A, Strickland N, Nijhawan RI, Srivastava D. Nail Unit Melanoma In Situ Treated With Mohs Micrographic Surgery. *Dermatol Surg.* 2021;47(1):98-103.
67. Knackstedt TJ, Baltz JO, Wilmer EN, Jellinek NJ. Assessing patient outcomes after digit-sparing en bloc surgery of nail apparatus melanoma in situ using two validated surveys. *J Am Acad Dermatol.* 2020;82(3):746-747.
68. Seo J, Oh Y, Kim SK, Roh MR, Chung KY. Slow Mohs Micrographic Surgery for Acral Melanoma Treatment in Korean Patients. *Dermatol Surg.* 2021;47(2):e42-e46.
69. Park KG, Blessing K, Kernohan NM. Surgical aspects of subungual malignant melanomas. The Scottish Melanoma Group. *Ann Surg.* 1992;216(6):692-695.
70. Jo G, Cho SI, Choi S, Mun JH. Functional surgery versus amputation for in situ or minimally invasive nail melanoma: A meta-analysis. *J Am Acad Dermatol.* 2019;81(4):917-922.
71. Montagner S, Belfort FA, Belda Junior W, Di Chiacchio N. Descriptive survival study of nail melanoma patients treated with functional surgery versus distal amputation. *J Am Acad Dermatol.* 2018;79(1):147-149.
72. Kirkwood J, Strawderman M, Ernstoff M, Smith T, Borden E, Blum R. Interferon alfa-2b adjuvant therapy of high-risk resected cutaneous melanoma: the Eastern Cooperative Oncology Group Trial EST 1684. *J Clin Oncol.* 1996;14:1-3.
73. Kirkwood J, Ibrahim J, Sondak V, et al. High- and low-dose interferon alfa-2b in high-risk melanoma: first analysis of intergroup trial E1690/S9111/C9190. *J Clin Oncol.* 2000;18:2444-2458.
74. Yamazaki N, Isei T, Kiyohara Y, et al. A phase I study of the safety and efficacy of talimogene laherparepvec in Japanese patients with advanced melanoma. *Cancer Sci.* 2022;113(8):2798-2806.

75. Dummer R, Hoeller C, Gruter IP, Michielin O. Combining talimogene laherparepvec with immunotherapies in melanoma and other solid tumors. *Cancer Immunol Immunother.* 2017;66(6):683-695.
76. Eggermont AM, Punt CJ. Does adjuvant systemic therapy with interferon-alpha for stage II-III melanoma prolong survival? *Am J Clin Dermatol.* 2003;4(8):531-536.
77. Jung S, Johnson DB. Management of Acral and Mucosal Melanoma: Medical Oncology Perspective. *Oncologist.* 2022;27(8):703-710.
78. Mao L, Si L, Chi Z, et al. A randomised phase II trial of 1 month versus 1 year of adjuvant high-dose interferon α-2b in high-risk acral melanoma patients. *Eur J Cancer.* 2011;47(10):1498-1503.
79. Curtin JA, Fridlyand J, Kageshita T, et al. Distinct sets of genetic alterations in melanoma. *N Engl J Med.* 2005;353:2135-2147.
80. Maldonado JL, Fridlyand J, Patel H, et al. Determinants of BRAF mutations in primary melanomas. *J Natl Cancer Inst.* 2003;95:1878-1880.
81. Saldanha G, Potter L, DaForno P, et al. Cutaneous melanoma subtypes show different BRAF and NRAS mutation frequencies. *Clin Cancer Res.* 2006;12:4499-4505.
82. Torres-Cabala CA, Wang WL, Trent J, et al. Correlation between KIT expression and KIT mutation in melanoma: a study of 173 cases with emphasis on acral-lentiginous/mucosal type. *Mod Pathol.* 2009;22:1446-1456.
83. Grabbe J, Welker P, Dippel E, Czarnetzki BM. Stem cell factor, a novel cutaneous growth factor for mast cells and melanocytes. *Arch Dermatol Res.* 1994;287:78-84.
84. Handolias D, Hamilton AL, Salemi R, et al. Clinical responses observed with imatinib or sorafenib in melanoma patients expressing mutations in KIT. *Br J Cancer.* 2010;102:1219-1223.
85. Hodi FS, Friedlander P, Corless CL, et al. Major response to imatinib mesylate in KIT-mutated melanoma. *J Clin Oncol.* 2008;26:2046-2051.
86. Lutzky J, Bauer J, Bastian BC. Dose-dependent, complete response to imatinib and temozolomide in patients with metastatic melanoma with a K642E KIT mutation. *Pigment Cell Melanoma Res.* 2008;21:492-493.
87. Woodman SE, Trent JC, Stemke-Hale K, et al. Activity of dasatinib against L576P KIT mutant melanoma molecular, cellular, and clinical correlates. *Mol Cancer Ther.* 2009;8:2079-2085.
88. Minor DR, O'Day S, Kashani-Sabet M, et al. Sunitinib therapy for metastatic melanomas with KIT aberrations. *Proc Am Soc Clin Oncol.* 2010;28:8545.
89. Steeb T, Wessely A, Petzold A, et al. c-Kit inhibitors for unresectable or metastatic mucosal, acral or chronically sun-damaged melanoma: a systematic review and one-arm meta-analysis. *Eur J Cancer.* 2021;157:348-357.
90. Larkin J, Chiarion-Sileni V, Gonzalez R, et al. Five-Year Survival with Combined Nivolumab and Ipilimumab in Advanced Melanoma. *N Engl J Med.* 2019;381(16):1535-1546.
91. Wolchok JD, Chiarion-Sileni V, Gonzalez R, et al. Overall Survival with Combined Nivolumab and Ipilimumab in Advanced Melanoma [published correction appears in N Engl J Med. 2018 Nov 29;379(22):2185]. *N Engl J Med.* 2017;377(14):1345-1356.
92. Klemen ND, Wang M, Rubinstein JC, et al. Survival after checkpoint inhibitors for metastatic acral, mucosal and uveal melanoma. *J Immunother Cancer.* 2020;8(1):e000341.
93. Atkins MB, Hsu J, Lee S, et al. Phase III trial comparing concurrent biochemotherapy with cisplatin, vinblastine, dacarbazine, interleukin-2, and interferon alfa-2b with cisplatin, vinblastine, and dacarbazine alone in patients with metastatic malignant melanoma (E3695): a trial coordinated by the Eastern Cooperative Oncology Group. *J Clin Oncol.* 2008;26(35):5748-5754.
94. Shoushtari AN, Munhoz RR, Kuk D, et al. The efficacy of anti-PD-1 agents in acral and mucosal melanoma. *Cancer.* 2016;122(21):3354-3362.
95. Bhave P, Ahmed T, Lo SN, et al. Efficacy of anti-PD-1 and ipilimumab alone or in combination in acral melanoma. *J Immunother Cancer.* 2022;10(7):e004668.
96. Cho KK, Cust AE, Foo YM, Long GV, Menzies AM, Eslick GD. Metastatic acral melanoma treatment outcomes: a systematic review and meta-analysis. *Melanoma Res.* 2021;31(5):482-486.
97. Qian Y, Johannet P, Sawyers A, Yu J, Osman I, Zhong J. The ongoing racial disparities in melanoma: An analysis of the surveillance, epidemiology, and end results database (1975-2016). *J Am Acad Dermatol.* 2021;84(6):1585-1593.
98. Kolla AM, Vitiello GA, Friedman EB, et al. Acral lentiginous melanoma: a United States multi-center substage survival analysis. *Cancer Control.* 2021;28:10732748211053567.
99. Cress R, Holly E. Incidence of cutaneous melanoma among non-Hispanic whites, Hispanics, Asians and Blacks: an analysis of the California Cancer Registry data, 1988-93. *Cancer Causes Control.* 1997;8:246-252.
100. Howlander N, Nonne AM, Krapcho M, et al. SEER Cancer Statistics Review, 1975-2009. Bethesda, MD: National Cancer Institute; 2012.
101. Behbahani S, Malerba S, Samie FH. Racial and ethnic differences in the clinical presentation and outcomes of acral lentiginous melanoma. *Br J Dermatol.* 2021;184(1):158-160.
102. De Wet J, Tod B, Visser WI, Jordaan HF, Schneider JW. Clinical and pathological features of acral melanoma in a South African population: a retrospective study. *S Afr Med J.* 2018;108(9):777-781. Published 2018 Aug 28.
103. Carter TM, Strassle PD, Ollila DW, Stitzenberg KB, Meyers MO, Maduekwe UN. Does acral lentiginous melanoma subtype account for differences in patterns of care in Black patients? *Am J Surg.* 2021;221(4):706-711.
104. Crowley N, Dodge R, Vollmer R, Seigler H. Malignant melanoma in black Americans: a trend toward improved survival. *Arch Surg.* 1991;126:1359-1365.
105. Byrd K, Wilson D, Hoyler S, Peck G. Advanced presentation of melanoma in African Americans. *J Am Acad Dermatol.* 2004;50:21-24.
106. Yan BY, Barilla S, Strunk A, Garg A. Survival differences in acral lentiginous melanoma according to socioeconomic status and race. *J Am Acad Dermatol.* 2022;86(2):379-386.
107. Cormier JN, Xing Y, Ding M, et al. Ethnic differences among patients with cutaneous melanoma. *Arch Intern Med.* 2006;166(17):1907-1914.
108. Bradford PT, Goldstein AM, McMaster ML, Tucker MA. Acral lentiginous melanoma: incidence and survival patterns in the United States, 1986-2005. *Arch Dermatol.* 2009;145(4):427-434.
109. Zhang J, Yun SJ, McMurray SL, Miller CJ. Management of nail unit melanoma. *Dermatol Clin.* 2021;39(2):269-280.
110. Lino-Silva LS, Zepeda-Najar C, Salcedo-Hernández RA, Martínez-Said H. Acral lentiginous melanoma: survival analysis of 715 cases. *J Cutan Med Surg.* 2019;23(1):38-43.
111. Duarte CA, Flórez JP, López HG, Meneses MX, de Vries E. Survival of acral lentiginous melanoma in the National Cancer Institute of Colombia. *J Eur Acad Dermatol Venereol.* 2017;31(3):438-442.
112. Feun L, Raub W, Duncan R, et al. Melanoma in a southeastern Hispanic population. *Cancer Detect Prev.* 1994;18:145-152.
113. Lim Y, Lee J, Lee DY. Is the survival rate for acral melanoma actually worse than other cutaneous melanomas? *J Dermatol.* 2020;47(3):251-256.
114. Mejbel HA, Torres-Cabala CA, Milton DR, et al. Prognostic significance of subungual anatomic site in acral lentiginous melanoma. *Arch Pathol Lab Med.* 2021;145(8):943-952.
115. Kato T, Suetake T, Sugiyama Y, Tabata N, Tagami H. Epidemiology and prognosis of subungual melanoma in 34 Japanese patients. *Br J Dermatol.* 1996;134(3):383-387.
116. Harvey VM, Oldfield CW, Chen JT, Eschbach K. Melanoma disparities among US Hispanics: use of the social ecological model to contextualize reasons for inequitable outcomes and frame a research agenda. *J Skin Cancer.* 2016;2016:4635740.
117. Census bureau releases new report on health insurance by race and Hispanic origin. United States Census Bureau. Published: November 22, 2022. Accessed: May 31, 2023.
118. Sanchez DP, Maymone MBC, McLean EO, et al. Racial and ethnic disparities in melanoma awareness: a cross-sectional survey. *J Am Acad Dermatol.* 2020;83(4):1098-1103.
119. Roh MR, Kim J, Chung KY. Treatment and outcomes of melanoma in acral location in Korean patients. *Yonsei Med J.* 2010;51(4):562-568.
120. Kundu RV, Kamaria M, Ortiz S, West DP, Rademaker AW, Robinson JK. Effectiveness of a knowledge-based intervention for melanoma among those with ethnic skin. *J Am Acad Dermatol.* 2010;62(5):777-784.
121. Sondermann W, Zimmer L, Schadendorf D, Roesch A, Klode J, Dissemond J. Initial misdiagnosis of melanoma located on the foot is associated with poorer prognosis. *Medicine (Baltimore).* 2016;95(29):e4332.
122. Redi U, Marruzzo G, Lovero S, Khokhar HT, Lo Torto F, Ribuffo D. Acral lentiginous melanoma: a retrospective study. *J Cosmet Dermatol.* 2021;20(6):1813-1820.
123. Tripathi R, Archibald LK, Mazmudar RS, et al. Racial differences in time to treatment for melanoma. *J Am Acad Dermatol.* 2020;83(3):854-859.
124. Collins KK, Fields RC, Baptiste D, Liu Y, Moley J, Jeffe DB. Racial differences in survival after surgical treatment for melanoma. *Ann Surg Oncol.* 2011;18(10):2925-2936.
125. Haque W, Verma V, Butler EB, Teh BS. Racial and socioeconomic disparities in the delivery of immunotherapy for metastatic melanoma in the United States. *J Immunother.* 2019;42(6):228-235.
126. Krauthammer M, Kong Y, Ha BH, et al. Exome sequencing identifies recurrent somatic RAC1 mutations in melanoma. *Nat Genet.* 2012;44(9):1006-1014.
127. Reintgen D, McCarty K, Cox E, Seigler H. Malignant melanoma in black American and white American populations. *JAMA.* 1982;248:1856-1859.
128. Kuno Y, Ishihara K, Yamazaki N, Mukai K. Clinical and pathological features of cutaneous malignant melanoma: a retrospective analysis of 124 Japanese patients. *Jpn J Clin Oncol.* 1996;26:144-151.

129. Overby MM. AAA tells feds to eliminate "race." *Anthropol Newslett.* 1997;38:1-5.
130. Dressler W. Health in the African-American community: accounting for health inequalities. *Med Anthropol Q.* 1993;7:325-345.
131. Lannin D, Mathews H, Mitchell J, Swanson M, Swanson F, Edwards M. Influence of socioeconomic and cultural factors on racial differences in late-stage presentation of breast cancer. *JAMA.* 1998;279:1801-1807.
132. Roetzheim R, Pal N, Tennant C, et al. Effects of health insurance and race on early detection of cancer. *J Natl Cancer Inst.* 1999;91:1409-1415.
133. Anonymous. Survey of knowledge of and awareness about melanoma—United States, 1995. *MMWR.* 1996;45:346-349.
134. Pipitone M, Robinson J, Camara C, Chittineni B, Fisher S. Skin cancer awareness in suburban employees: a Hispanic perspective. *J Am Acad Dermatol.* 2002;47:118-123.

CHAPTER 53

Squamous Cell Carcinoma

Norhan Shamloul
Algin Garrett

KEY POINTS

- Squamous cell carcinoma (SCC) is the most common skin cancer in Black and Indian patients and the second most common in Chinese and Japanese patients.
- Most SCCs in people with skin of color occur in non–sun-exposed areas and have more atypical presentations leading to delayed diagnosis and potential for metastasis.
- SCC that occurs in sun-exposed skin has its origin in loss of the organized control of epidermal keratinocyte differentiation secondary to DNA damage as a direct result of ultraviolet light.
- The factors that are responsible for developing skin cancers in non–sun-exposed areas are unknown.
- Areas of chronic inflammation, chronic ulceration, and scarring are predisposed to the development of SCC and result in higher mortality.

INTRODUCTION

Most of the information regarding nonmelanoma skin cancer in skin of color reported in the U.S. literature focuses on disease incidence primarily in the African American population. The information is reported in the context of case reports or incidence studies from small groups. Information regarding the incidence of nonmelanoma skin cancer in other racial or ethnic groups, including Native Americans, Asians, and Hispanics, is sparse. The groups of people that constitute people with darker skin of color have grown considerably. Considering the changing demographics of the United States, to keep meaningful and accurate data, prospective research should recognize the population changes that are occurring. Larger population studies should be performed involving people with skin of color, which represents multiple ethnic and racial groups. U.S. Census information predicts that by the year 2050, the Caucasian population will be less than 50% of the total population. This figure will continue to decline during the ensuing decades of continued immigration and assimilation in the United States.

MELANIN AND PHOTOPROTECTION

The reduced incidence of skin cancer in people with skin of color has been attributed to various factors. Montagna and Carlisle[1] have studied racial differences in melanin activity, fibroblast activity, and hair distribution on skin that may help to account for the reduced frequency of skin cancer in people with skin of color. Melanin, which is synthesized in melanosomes, is a known photoprotector in both animals and humans. It essentially creates a shield from the sun by absorbing and deflecting ultraviolet (UV) radiation.[2] The basal cell layer melanocyte is responsible for the production of melanin. There is no racial difference in the number of melanocytes.[3] The number of melanocytes may vary from one individual to the other and in different anatomic regions.[4] The variations in color that can be seen in individuals are attributed to the size and aggregation of melanosomes in the melanocyte and keratinocyte. The increased number and dispersion of stage IV melanosomes provide a measure of photoprotection.[2] Racial differences, as well as sun exposure, can affect the melanosome grouping. In African Americans with dark skin, melanosomes are large and nonaggregated, whereas in fair-skinned African Americans, melanosomes are both large and nonaggregated as well as smaller and aggregated. Sun exposure has also been shown to change the pattern of melanosome distribution in Asian and Caucasian skin.[4,5] In addition to the role of melanin in photoprotection, the compactness or density of the keratinocyte layers also provides a measure of photoprotection.[6] The African American population is composed of a heterogeneous group with various shades of skin color; all the factors listed combine to provide an average sun protection factor of approximately 13.4.[2]

The relative safety from some of the effects of the sun is demonstrated by the comparatively low incidence of skin cancer in African Americans. However, there are changes that occur in melanin-laden skin that suggest that skin of color is not immune to photodamage. Kotrajaras and Kligman[7] demonstrated epidermal atypia and atrophy and both dermal collagen and elastin damage. The presence of these changes, which may be consistent with either damage from long-wavelength UV or infrared radiation, suggests that melanin may be an efficient filter for shorter-wavelength UV radiation.

INCIDENCE

Primary carcinoma of the skin is the most common form of cancer diagnosed in the United States. Even though skin cancer is considered the most common form of cancer, the incidence in people with skin of color is reported as rare. McCall and Chen[8] reported a surprisingly high incidence of squamous cell carcinoma (SCC) in older African American females and suggest that the incidence may be higher than previously reported. The incidence of SCC involving the skin in Caucasian patients has been reported to be approximately 100 per 100,000 in women and 150 per 100,000 in men.[9] The incidence in African Americans is reported to be approximately 3.4 per 100,000.[10] There are very few incidence reports of skin cancer among other groups. Koh et al[11] report on the trends and differences of skin cancers in Chinese, Malays, and Indians living in Singapore. The incidence rate for SCC was 3.2 per 100,000 in men and 1.8 per 100,000 in women. The incidence rate for basal cell carcinoma (BCC) was 6.4 per 100,000 in men and 5.8 per 100,000 in women. Ichihashi et al[12] reported on age-adjusted incidence rates of BCC and solar keratosis in 4736 people in Kasai City. Two BCCs, 36 solar keratoses, and no SCCs were diagnosed in the group. It appears at least in the Asian population that BCCs are more common than SCCs.

SCC is the most commonly diagnosed skin cancer in African Americans.[13,14] Bang et al[15] reported that 34.1% of 126 African American patients were diagnosed with SCC, whereas 30.2% of the group was diagnosed with BCC. Fleming et al[16] reported on a small series of 58 African Americans with skin cancer. Thirty-eight cases of SCC and seven cases of BCC were diagnosed. Unlike BCCs, which occur commonly on sun-exposed skin, most SCCs in people with skin of color develop in non–sun-exposed areas. In a series reported by Howard University in 1988, 65% of the patients diagnosed with SCC had leg involvement, and 15% were diagnosed with anal SCC.[14] SCC involvement of the penis and scrotum also has been reported to occur in African Americans.[17-19]

PATHOGENESIS

The pathogenesis of SCC that occurs in sun-exposed skin has its origin in loss of the organized control of epidermal keratinocyte differentiation secondary to DNA damage as a direct result of UV light. The factors that are responsible for developing skin cancers in non–sun-exposed areas are unknown. Areas of chronic inflammation, chronic ulceration, and scarring are predisposed to the development of SCC. In these settings, normal cell differentiation and apoptosis of abnormal cells are altered, eventually producing the clonal expansion of a malignant cell line. The altered role of the *p53* gene in its response to cytotoxic stress may imperil the normal keratinocyte and predispose high-risk lesions to develop SCC.[20,21]

RISK FACTORS

The development of SCC has been linked to natural UV radiation exposure. UVB is known to cause skin cancer. PUVA photochemotherapy used to treat chronic skin diseases such as psoriasis has been shown to increase the risk of nonmelanoma skin cancer.[22] As mentioned previously, most SCCs in people with skin of color occur in non–sun-exposed areas [**Figure 53-1**]; however, when SCC does occur in a sun-exposed area, the anatomic distribution is similar to that in Caucasians [**Figure 53-2**]. SCC develops in the following clinical settings in African Americans: chronic inflammation or scarring, burns, chronic infections, leg ulcers, albinism [**Figure 53-3**], lesions of chronic discoid lupus erythematosus [**Figure 53-4**], chronic radiation exposure [**Figure 53-5**], and uncommonly, vitiligo[14,23] [**Table 53-1**]. SCC can also manifests as cutaneous horns and scrotal ulcers. Chronic scars represent a significant risk for SCC and result in a higher rate of mortality.[24] In fact, chronic inflammatory and scarring disorders account for 20% to 40% of SCC in African Americans, making them the greatest predisposing factor for this entity.[25] Hubbell et al[18] reported on 175 cases of SCC involving the penis in darker skin of color patients. These authors reported a 15.4% overall mortality.

Human papilloma virus (HPV) has been increasingly recognized for its role in development of SCC. When evaluating nonmelanoma skin cancers in nonwhite organ transplant recipients, Pritchett et al found that 66.7% of Hispanic patients and 85.7% of Black patients with SCC had a positive history of HPV, including subtypes 16 and 18 in the groin.[26] Interestingly, this association with HPV was not identified in Asian transplant recipients.

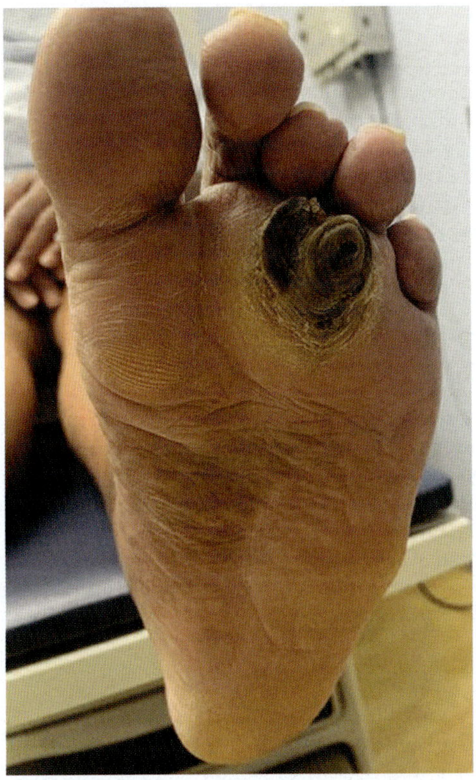

FIGURE 53-1. Squamous cell carcinoma in non–sun-exposed area of a Hispanic female.

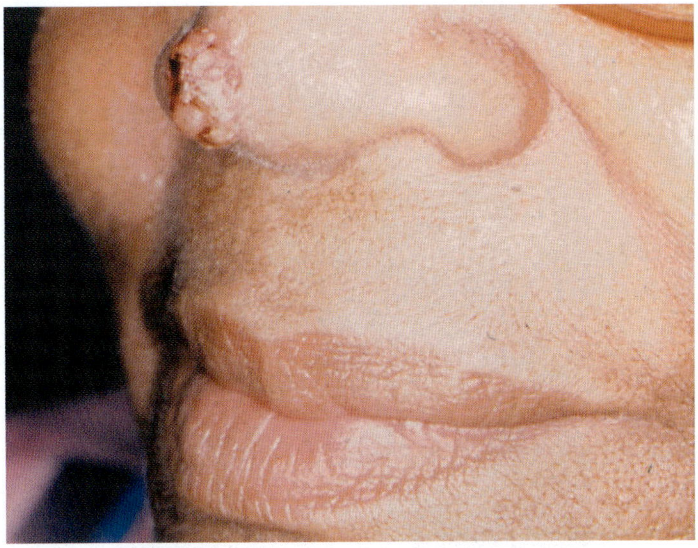

FIGURE 53-2. Squamous cell carcinoma on nasal tip of an African American female.

Actinic keratoses (AKs) are diagnosed more commonly in fair-skinned people and represent the most common precursor lesion for SCC on sun-exposed skin. AKs are rarely seen in African Americans and are diagnosed not infrequently in fair-skinned Asians.[11] In individuals who develop AKs, there is up to a 10% risk of developing SCC.[20]

SCC in African Americans is generally considered to be a more aggressive disease with a poorer prognosis. Mora et al[24] reported an 18.4% mortality in 163 African Americans diagnosed with SCC of the skin. In their series, the face and leg were the most common sites of involvement. Fleming et al[16] reported a mortality rate of 29% in their series of African Americans with SCC. Weinstock reported SCC as the skin cancer that is the major cause of death in African Americans. Not all reported series regarding SCC in AKs demonstrate comparatively decreased survival rates. Singh et al[27] reported on a series of 215 patients in a case-control

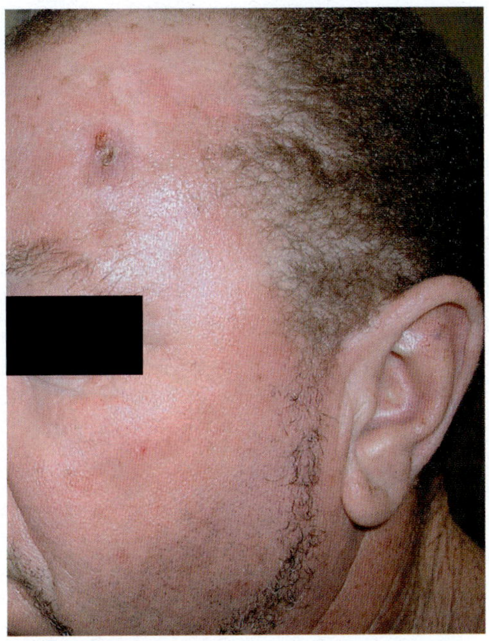

FIGURE 53-3. Squamous cell carcinoma in an albino African American male.

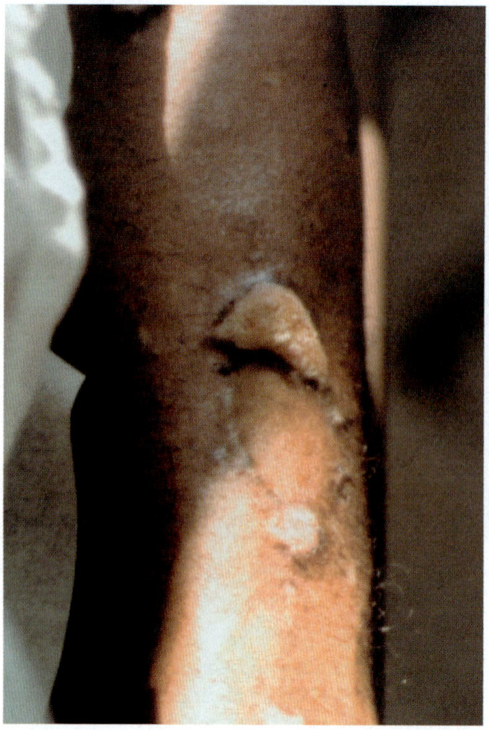

FIGURE 53-4. Squamous cell carcinoma arising in chronic discoid lupus lesions.

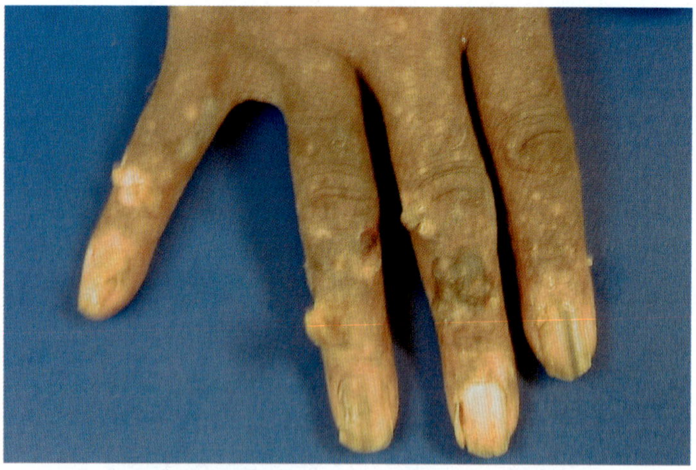

FIGURE 53-5. Squamous cell carcinoma in areas of chronic radiation exposure.

TABLE 53-1 Risks factors for developing squamous cell carcinoma

- Chronic leg ulcers
- Chronic nonhealing wounds
- Discoid lupus erythematosus
- Lichen planus
- Ultraviolet radiation
- Vitiligo (rare)
- Ionizing radiation
- Oculocutaneous albinism
- Nevoid basal cell nevus syndrome
- Organ transplantation
- Acquired immunodeficiency syndrome
- Scrotal ulcers

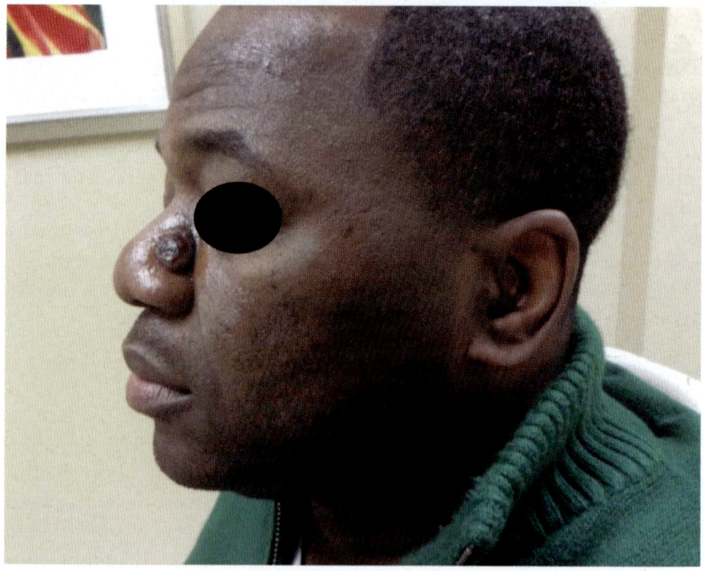

FIGURE 53-6. Keratoacanthoma on the nasal side wall of an African American male.

study in which the presentation, course, and outcome of head and neck skin cancer in African Americans were studied. They showed that head and neck skin cancer is similar with regard to presentation and distribution in White, Latin American, and African American patients. The study also showed that the cancers may be less aggressive in African Americans with appropriate treatment.

Several factors may contribute to the overall poor mortality and morbidity related to SCC in people with skin of color. The diagnosis is usually made at an advanced stage, possibly because of decreased accessibility to the healthcare system. In some instances, for unknown reasons, SCC has a more aggressive course in African Americans than in Caucasian patients with comparable disease. Often when the diagnosis of SCC is made, other associated diseases coexist and may make management of the advanced skin cancer more difficult.

KERATOACANTHOMA

Keratoacanthoma is indistinguishable histologically from SCC [**Figure 53-6**]. Generally, it represents an epithelial tumor that grows rapidly over a period of approximately 6 weeks. The lesion may last for several weeks and then involute spontaneously. It usually appears as a solitary lesion and generally presents as a nodule with a crater-like center with a keratin plug. The lesion is rarely reported in people with skin of color.[28]

SQUAMOUS CELL CARCINOMA IN SITU AND BOWEN'S DISEASE

SCC in situ histologically represents involvement of the entire epidermal thickness with pleomorphic keratinocytes, which is seen in diseases such as Bowen disease and erythroplasia of Queyrat.[14] Bowen disease presents as an erythematous solitary patch or plaque that may resemble eczema or psoriasis[29] [**Figure 53-7**]. Pigmented Bowen disease represents a pigmented form of SCC in situ and occurs in about 1.7% of all SCCs, but its frequency is increased in Black men particularly in intertriginous areas and on the lower extremities.[30,31]

PROGNOSIS

Invasive SCC arising in areas of sun exposure [**Figure 53-8**] has a better prognosis than SCC that arises in non–sun-exposed areas. Aggressive behavior and local metastases occur more frequently in SCC arising in

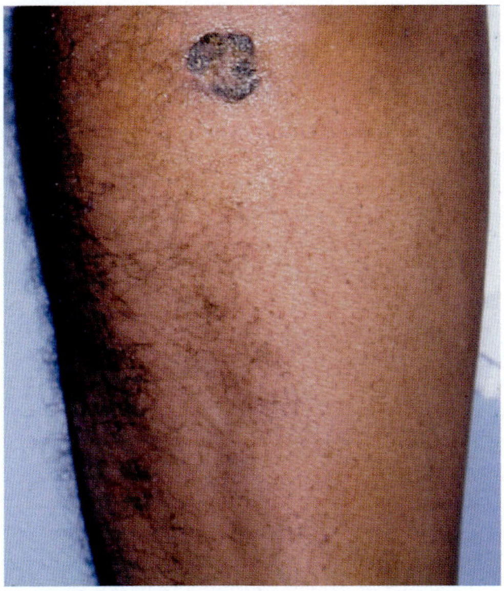

FIGURE 53-7. Bowen disease resembling a psoriatic plaque.

non–sun-exposed areas.[16,18] SCC of the nail bed has been reported to develop in African Americans and may be more common in females [**Figure 53-9**]. Bowen disease of the digits resembles verrucae or chronic paronychia and has been associated with human papillomavirus types 16 and 18.[29,32] SCC involving the mucosal skin has a greater tendency to metastasize and recur. Perianal SCC can arise in preexisting lesions such as perianal warts [**Figure 53-10**]. Anogenital lesions also can develop de novo [**Figure 53-11**].

SCC that presents in preexisting areas of disease such as a chronic leg ulcers or hidradenitis suppurativa or in areas of chronic scars may resemble the underlying disease. Such areas may appear not to respond to therapy or develop nonhealing ulcers or erosions. Invasive SCC can present as plaques, papules, and ulcers with induration. SCC should be excluded in the appropriate setting in which any of the preceding circumstances exist.

DIAGNOSIS AND THERAPY

SCC in an African American is potentially very aggressive and raises the possibility of an associated disease. Therefore, a detailed history and physical examination should be undertaken, and a biopsy of the suspicious lesion should be performed. The history should assess the duration of the lesion and history of prior treatment for preexisting skin cancer or preexisting skin disease. If indicated clinically, any evidence for immune deficiency should be evaluated. A physical examination should be performed for local evaluation of the tumor and to assess the patient for the presence of lymphadenopathy.

The type of biopsy performed should be determined by the characteristics of the lesion. A shave biopsy can be performed on a relatively thin or superficial lesion. Thicker, more indurated plaques or tumors require a deeper punch or excisional biopsy.

Staging of cutaneous SCC is an important step and allows for prognostic value based on numerous risk factors. High-risk features for SCCs include tumor size greater than 2 cm, perineural invasion, and tumor invasion

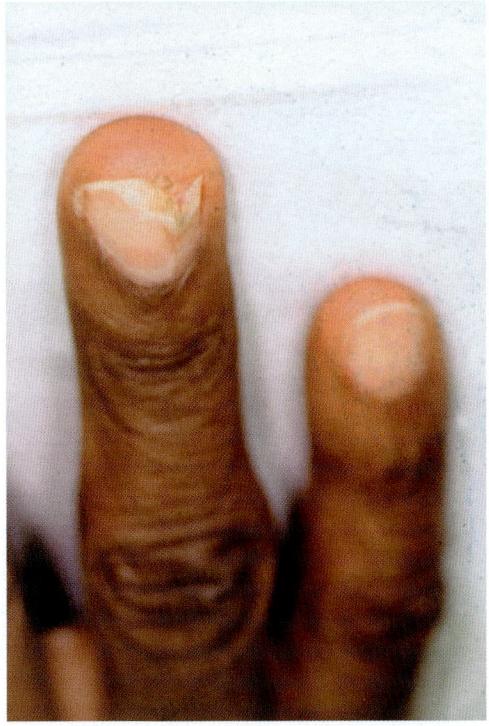

FIGURE 53-9. Squamous cell carcinoma of the nail bed of an African American female.

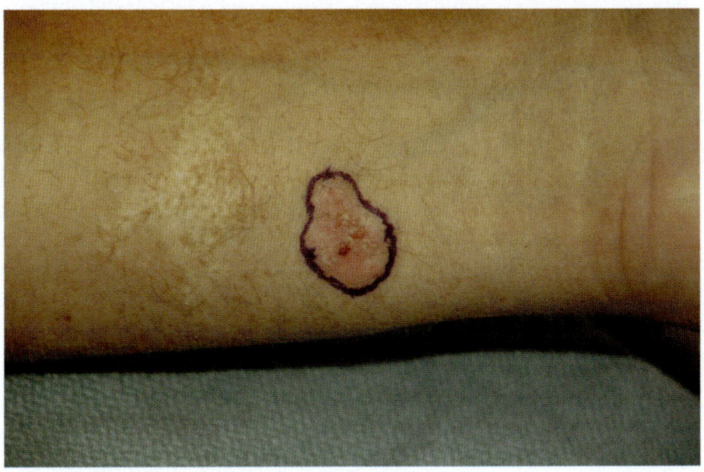

FIGURE 53-8. Squamous cell carcinoma on the arm.

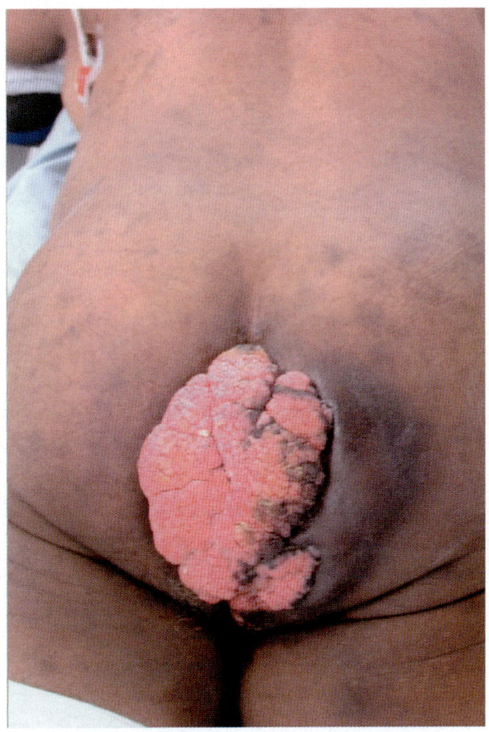

FIGURE 53-10. Perianal SCC arising in a perianal wart in an African American patient.

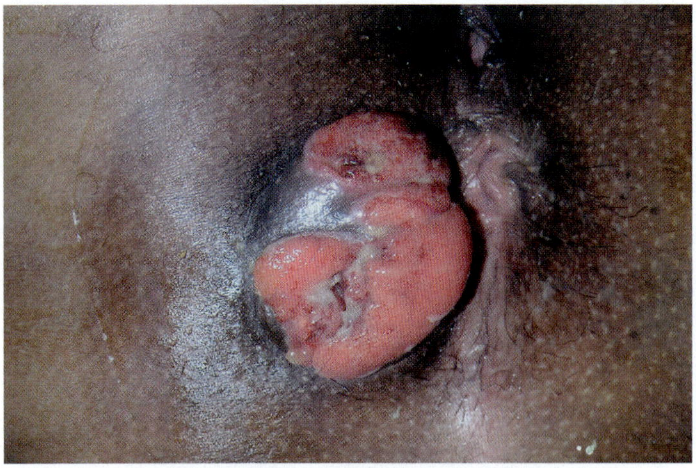

FIGURE 53-11. De novo SCC in an African American patient with HIV.

beyond the subcutaneous fat based on both the Brigham and Women's Hospital (BWH) and American Joint Committee on Cancer (AJCC). The BWH staging system includes poorly differentiated histology as an additional high-risk feature. Staging allows physicians to make decisions regarding additional testing such as sentinel lymph node biopsies, imaging, and more recently molecular testing to determine risk of metastasis of SCC.

The type of therapeutic intervention is determined by the histologic type of SCC, size of the tumor, location of the tumor, and presence or absence of metastatic disease [**Table 53-2**]. In thin lesions such as Bowen disease, a number of therapeutic options could be considered including cryotherapy, 5-fluorouracil, and electrodessication and curettage. The carbon dioxide laser has shown efficacy in the management of severe actinic cheilitis and in the treatment of superficial BCC, Bowen disease, and thin SCCs.[33,34] Additionally, photodynamic therapy and 5-fluorouracil have proven to be efficacious in treating thin or superficial SCC in patients who wish to avoid surgical excision.[35] Interferon-α and imiquimod both have been used in the management of SCCs. Intralesional interferon has been used to treat both SCC and BCC and has shown approximately an 80% cure rate in selected BCCs. The use of imiquimod in the management of BCCs has been approved recently, but its use in the treatment of SCC is currently under study. Imiquimod does appear to be as effective in selected lesions as it is in the treatment of BCC[36] but is not currently an approved drug for the treatment of cutaneous SCC.

For patients who have localized disease, excisional surgery and Mohs micrographic surgery are the primary forms of treatment. Aggressive management of the tumor is indicated because of the potential for SCC in people with skin of color to be more aggressive and have a higher rate of recurrence. Blumenthal et al found that Mohs micrographic surgery defect sizes were 17% larger in Hispanic and Latino patients when compared to non-Hispanic white patients.[37] Additionally, they found that defect sizes of SCC were 80% larger than BCC defects among Hispanic patients as compared to 25% larger in non-Hispanic Whites, highlighting the more aggressive nature of SCCs in patients with skin of color.[37]

If excisional surgery is undertaken, the tumor should be removed with adequate margins. The margins of the excision should be examined completely for evidence of residual disease. For tumors that are in cosmetically sensitive areas and that are considered high risk, Mohs micrographic surgery may be indicated. Large tumors involving the perianal region or tumors in areas of scarring or chronic ulceration require a wide local excision, often with complex repair.

TABLE 53-2 Treatments available for squamous cell carcinoma

Medical	Surgical
5-Fluorouracil	Cryosurgery
Photodynamic therapy	Electrodesiccation and curettage
Imiquimod	Carbon dioxide laser
Interferon	Excision
Radiation therapy	Mohs micrographic surgery
Cemiplimab	

Radiation therapy is used both as a primary form of therapy and as adjuvant therapy in the management of SCC, particularly of the head and neck. As adjuvant therapy, radiation is used when lymph nodes are positive, for the presence of perineural disease, and when residual disease is suspected after an excision or when clear margins are not established.

Immunotherapy treatments have emerged as promising therapies for locally advanced or metastatic SCC. Cemiplimab, an anti-programmed cell death 1 monoclonal antibody was approved for treatment of cutaneous SCC in 2018 and has helped revolutionize the therapeutic landscape for this cancer in advanced stages.

PATIENT PERSPECTIVES AND KERATINOCYTE SKIN CNCER

Patients with skin of color often have greater morbidity and mortality than Caucasians from keratinocyte carcinoma (KC), and African Americans in particular have higher cancer mortality than any other group in the United States.[38-40] Despite this, it has been shown in large studies that perception of skin cancer risk, along with other cancers, remains low in darker-skinned populations such as African Americans, Hispanics, and Asians.[41] In the Health Information National Trends Survey, African American and Hispanic patients were more likely to state that their risk of SCC was low, that behaviors do not lead to increased skin cancer risk, and that there is not much that can be done to lower skin cancer risk. Although it is accurate to state that the incidence of skin cancer is lower in these groups, it is not accurate to state that behavior modification cannot change skin cancer risk. Reduced exposure to UV radiation, scarring, trauma, and inflammation, all of which predispose to skin cancer, particularly in patients with skin of color, can reduce the incidence of skin cancer. Further, it is well established that use of sunscreen can prevent KC, especially SCC.[40] However, Summers et al[42] studied the patterns of sunscreen use in various populations and found that patients with skin of color had a lower likelihood of wearing sunscreen, even if they had a propensity for severe sunburn.[39] This could serve as a point for further education of skin cancer risk in these patient groups. Currently, it has been shown that of patients included in national dermatology screening and education programs over the past 15 years, only 1.2% have been patients with skin of color. Additionally, educational advertisements regarding skin cancer and sunscreen use are five times more common in magazines directed at patients with Caucasian skin.[42,43] Socioeconomic status and education level have also been shown to correlate with cancer risk, along with increased risk of KC and larger KCs. Further, lower skin cancer screening rates correlate with lower screening for other cancers, such as breast and colon, in patients with lower socioeconomic status and education levels.[39] As the number of people of color increases in the United States, it will become increasingly important to modify existing perceptions and understanding of skin cancer in this patient population to improve our ability to detect early disease and begin appropriate treatment in a timely.

REFERENCES

1. Montagna W, Carlisle K. The architecture of black and white facial skin. *J Am Acad Dermatol.* 1991;24(6 Pt 1):929-937.
2. Kaidbey KH, Agin PP, Sayre RM, Kligman AM. Photoprotection by melanin–a comparison of black and Caucasian skin. *J Am Acad Dermatol.* 1979;1(3):249-260.
3. Starkco RS, Pinkus H. Quantitative and qualitative data on the pigment cell of adult human epidermis. *J Invest Dermatol.* 1957;28:33-45.
4. Toda K, Pathak MA, Parrish JA, Fitzpatrick TB, Quevedo WC, Jr. Alteration of racial differences in melanosome distribution in human epidermis after exposure to ultraviolet light. *Nat New Biol.* 1972;236(66):143-145.
5. Olson RL, Gaylor J, Everett MA. Skin color, melanin, and erythema. *Arch Dermatol.* 1973;108(4):541-544.

6. Freeman RG, Cockerell EG, Armstrong J, Knox JM. Sunlight as a factor influencing the thickness of epidermis. *J Invest Dermatol.* 1962;39:295-298.
7. Kotrajaras R, Kligman AM. The effect of topical tretinoin on photodamaged facial skin: the Thai experience. *Br J Dermatol.* 1993;129(3):302-309.
8. McCall CO, Chen SC. Squamous cell carcinoma of the legs in African Americans. *J Am Acad Dermatol.* 2002;47(4):524-529.
9. Gray DT, Suman VJ, Su WP, Clay RP, Harmsen WS, Roenigk RK. Trends in the population-based incidence of squamous cell carcinoma of the skin first diagnosed between 1984 and 1992. *Arch Dermatol.* 1997;133(6):735-740.
10. Scotto, J., Fears, T. R., Fraumeni, J. F., National Cancer Institute, Fred Hutchinson Cancer Research Center., & United States. Department of Health and Human Services. (1983). *Incidence of nonmelanoma skin cancer in the United States.* U.S. Dept. of Health and Human Services, Public Health Service, National Institutes of Health, National Cancer Institute.
11. Koh D, Wang H, Lee J, Chia KS, Lee HP, Goh CL. Basal cell carcinoma, squamous cell carcinoma and melanoma of the skin: analysis of the Singapore Cancer Registry data 1968-97. *Br J Dermatol.* 2003;148(6):1161-1166.
12. Ichihashi M, Naruse K, Harada S, et al. Trends in nonmelanoma skin cancer in Japan. *Recent Results Cancer Res.* 1995;139:263-273.
13. Roenigk RK, Ratz JL, Bailin PL, Wheeland RG. Trends in the presentation and treatment of basal cell carcinomas. *J Dermatol Surg Oncol.* 1986;12(8):860-865.
14. Halder RM, Bang KM. Skin cancer in blacks in the United States. *Dermatol Clin.* 1988;6(3):397-405.
15. Bang KM, Halder RM, White JE, Sampson CC, Wilson J. Skin cancer in black Americans: a review of 126 cases. *J Natl Med Assoc.* 1987;79(1):51-58.
16. Fleming ID, Barnawell JR, Burlison PE, Rankin JS. Skin cancer in black patients. *Cancer.* 1975;35(3):600-605.
17. Rippentrop JM, Joslyn SA, Konety BR. Squamous cell carcinoma of the penis: evaluation of data from the surveillance, epidemiology, and end results program. *Cancer.* 2004;101(6):1357-1363.
18. Hubbell CR, Rabin VR, Mora RG. Cancer of the skin in blacks. V. A review of 175 black patients with squamous cell carcinoma of the penis. *J Am Acad Dermatol.* 1988;18(2 Pt 1):292-298.
19. McDonald MW. Carcinoma of scrotum. *Urology.* 1982;19(3):269-274.
20. Salasche SJ. Epidemiology of actinic keratoses and squamous cell carcinoma. *J Am Acad Dermatol.* 2000;42(1 Pt 2):4-7.
21. Glogau RG. The risk of progression to invasive disease. *J Am Acad Dermatol.* 2000;42(1 Pt 2):23-24.
22. Nijsten TE, Stern RS. The increased risk of skin cancer is persistent after discontinuation of psoralen+ultraviolet A: a cohort study. *J Invest Dermatol.* 2003;121(2):252-258.
23. Halder RM, Bridgeman-Shah S. Skin cancer in African Americans. *Cancer.* 1995;75(2 Suppl):667-673.
24. Mora RG, Perniciaro C. Cancer of the skin in blacks. I. A review of 163 black patients with cutaneous squamous cell carcinoma. *J Am Acad Dermatol.* 1981;5(5):535-543.
25. Davis DS, Robinson C, Callender VD. Skin cancer in women of color: epidemiology, pathogenesis and clinical manifestations. *Int J Womens Dermatol.* 2021;7(2):127-134.
26. Pritchett EN, Doyle A, Shaver CM, et al. Nonmelanoma skin cancer in nonwhite organ transplant recipients. *JAMA Dermatol.* 2016;152(12):1348-1353.
27. Singh B, Bhaya M, Shaha A, Har-El G, Lucente FE. Presentation, course, and outcome of head and neck skin cancer in African Americans: a case-control study. *Laryngoscope.* 1998;108(8 Pt 1):1159-1163.
28. Heyl T, Morrison JG. Keratoacanthoma in a Bantu patient. *Br J Dermatol.* 1975;93(6):699-700.
29. Preston DS, Stern RS. Nonmelanoma cancers of the skin. *N Engl J Med.* 1992;327(23):1649-1662.
30. Ezenwa E, Stein JA, Krueger L. Dermoscopic features of neoplasms in skin of color: a review. *Int J Womens Dermatol.* 2021;7(2):145-151.
31. Cavalleiro de Macedo Mota AN, Piñeiro-Maceira J, de Fatima Guimaraes Scotelaro Alves M, Mateus Tarazona MJ. Pigmented Bowen's disease. *An Bras Dermatol.* 2014;89(5):825-827.
32. Alam M, Ratner D. Cutaneous squamous-cell carcinoma. *N Engl J Med.* 2001;344(13):975-983.
33. Karrer S, Szeimies RM, Hohenleutner U, Landthaler M. Role of lasers and photodynamic therapy in the treatment of cutaneous malignancy. *Am J Clin Dermatol.* 2001;2(4):229-237.
34. Tantikun N. Treatment of Bowen's disease of the digit with carbon dioxide laser. *J Am Acad Dermatol.* 2000;43(6):1080-1083.
35. Morton CA, Whitehurst C, McColl JH, Moore JV, MacKie RM. Photodynamic therapy for large or multiple patches of Bowen disease and basal cell carcinoma. *Arch Dermatol.* 2001;137(3):319-324.
36. Mackenzie-Wood A, Kossard S, de Launey J, Wilkinson B, Owens ML. Imiquimod 5% cream in the treatment of Bowen's disease. *J Am Acad Dermatol.* 2001;44(3):462-470.
37. Blumenthal LY, Arzeno J, Syder N, et al. Disparities in nonmelanoma skin cancer in Hispanic/Latino patients based on Mohs micrographic surgery defect size: a multicenter retrospective study. *J Am Acad Dermatol.* 2022;86(2):353-358.
38. Wingo PA, Bolden S, Tong T, Parker SL, Martin LM, Heath CW, Jr. Cancer statistics for African Americans, 1996. *CA Cancer J Clin.* 1996;46(2):113-125.
39. Gloster HM, Jr., Neal K. Skin cancer in skin of color. *J Am Acad Dermatol.* 2006;55(5):741-760; quiz 761-744.
40. Weinstock MA. Nonmelanoma skin cancer mortality in the United States, 1969 through 1988. *Arch Dermatol.* 1993;129(10):1286-1290.
41. Buster KJ, You Z, Fouad M, Elmets C. Skin cancer risk perceptions: a comparison across ethnicity, age, education, gender, and income. *J Am Acad Dermatol.* 2012;66(5):771-779.
42. Summers P, Bena J, Arrigain S, Alexis AF, Cooper K, Bordeaux JS. Sunscreen use: non-Hispanic blacks compared with other racial and/or ethnic groups. *Arch Dermatol.* 2011;147(7):863-864.
43. Alexis AF, Rossi AM. Skin cancer in skin of color. *Cutis.* 2012;89(5):208-211.

CHAPTER 54

Basal Cell Carcinoma

Norhan Shamloul
Algin Garrett

KEY POINTS

- Keratinocyte skin cancers represent an underrecognized health concern in people of color. Basal cell carcinoma (BCC) is the second most common skin cancer diagnosed in people of color.
- In Caucasians, BCC typically presents with a rolled border, telangiectasias, and an erosion, but in people of color, the most common presentation consists of pigmented papules and nodules.
- Because BCCs are often pigmented, they can be mistaken for seborrheic keratoses, nevocellular nevi, or malignant melanomas.
- BCCs commonly present on the head and neck, but they may also appear in unusual locations such as the groin, scrotum, perianal region, and feet.
- A common misconception among many patients and even some physicians is that darker pigmentation affords complete protection from skin cancer development. Thus, it is important to do a complete skin examination in people with skin of color to ensure that a BCC is not overlooked.
- The approach to treating skin cancers in people with skin of color should not be different from treating patients with lighter skin.

INTRODUCTION

Basal cell carcinoma (BCC) is the most common malignancy found in humans. Its growth is driven by a distinct and well-defined biochemical pathway that has led to new insights into management and treatment. Although BCC does not have significant metastatic potential, it can lead to local destruction and disfigurement and present challenges in management, if unrecognized or untreated. While BCC has been described as uncommon in patients with skin of color, it remains the most common skin cancer in Hispanic, Japanese, and Chinese patients and the second most common skin cancer in Blacks and Asian Indians.[1-4] Furthermore, patients with skin of color may be more likely to have greater morbidity and mortality associated with BCC than Whites.

THE FITZPATRICK PHOTOTYPE SYSTEM

The Fitzpatrick phototype system (FPS) is a subjective skin-type classification based on an individual's reaction to sun exposure and ethnicity.[5] Although it is widely used by dermatologists to classify patients with skin of color, it was initially developed for fair-skinned patients to gauge sun sensitivity.[6] Patients with skin of color are commonly classified as FPS 4 through 6 and thus less likely to burn or develop skin cancers, but this is often inaccurate given the heterogeneity of complexions within groups of mixed ancestry such as Hispanics and African Americans.[6] Thus it is important for clinicians to recognize the limitations of the FPS when assessing the risks of sun exposure and development of BCC in individuals with skin of color.

INCIDENCE

The incidence of BCC in patients with skin of color varies with racial or ethnic group. BCC represents 65% to 75% of skin cancers in Caucasians, 20% to 30% of skin cancers in Asian Indians, 12% to 35% of skin cancers in African Americans,[1,3,7-9] and 2% to 8% of skin cancers in African Blacks.[10,11] Beckenstein and Windle,[12] in a series from 1995, found that 1.8% (5 of 276) of skin cancers in African Americans were BCCs. The series by Fleming et al[5] noted that 12% (7 of 58) of all skin cancers in African Americans were BCCs. The study by Halder and Bang[1] from Howard University showed that 28.8% (38 of 103) of African American patients with skin cancer had a BCC. Altman et al[13] reported that 2.5% of all skin cancers in African Americans are BCCs.

The incidences of BCC per 100,000 population have been reported in non-Black patients as follows: Chinese men (6.4), Chinese women (5.8), Japanese (15-16.5), Japanese residents of Kauai, Hawaii (29.7), Japanese residents of Okinawa (26.1), New Mexican Hispanic women (113), New Mexican Hispanic men (171), southeastern Arizona Hispanic females (50), southeastern Arizona Hispanic males (91), Caucasian men (250), Caucasian women (212), and Caucasians in Kauai, Hawaii (185-340) [**Table 54-1**].[1,2,14-19] Although BCC occurs less commonly in patients with skin of color compared with Caucasians, it remains an important and common diagnosis in patients with skin of color.

PATHOGENESIS

Important insights into the pathogenesis of BCC have led to the development of novel targeted therapies for advanced BCC. BCC formation is driven by mutations in the sonic hedgehog (SHH) pathway, a signaling molecule that classically organizes dorsoventral limb patterning in vertebrates. In its native role, SHH binds to and inhibits patched (PTCH), a transmembrane protein receptor that functions as a tumor suppressor protein. PTCH inhibits the actions of smoothened (SMO), which subsequently activates GLI. GLI acts a nuclear transcription factor for several growth genes, which lead to unrestricted growth and tumorigenesis. Mutations in PTCH and SMO have been shown to be associated with the basal cell nevus syndrome and in sporadic BCCs. Mutations in PTCH have also been associated with esophageal squamous cell carcinoma, trichoepitheliomas, and transitional cell carcinomas of the bladder.[20] Sporadic PTCH mutations can be induced by ultraviolet radiation (UVR), but this effect is mitigated in patients with skin of color due to melanin photoprotection. In addition to PTCH mutations, point mutations in the *TP53* gene occur in at least 50% of cases of BCC and represent the second most common genetic alteration in this skin cancer.[21] A small number of BCCs possess mutations in the *CDKN2A* locus.[22]

TABLE 54-1 Incidence of basal cell carcinoma in non-Black patients

Ethnicity	Incidence (per 100,000)
Chinese men	6.4
Chinese women	5.8
Japanese	15-16.5
Japanese residents of Kauai, Hawaii	29.7
Japanese residents of Okinawa	26.1
New Mexican Hispanic women	113
New Mexican Hispanic men	171
Southeastern Arizona Hispanic females	50
Southeastern Arizona Hispanic males	91
Caucasian men	250
Caucasian women	212
Caucasians in Kauai, Hawaii	185-340

TABLE 54-2 Uncommon locations of basal cell carcinomas

- Ankle
- Buttock
- Cervix
- Groin
- Nipple
- Plantar surface of the foot
- Scrotum
- Vulva

RISK FACTORS

BCC is primarily related to sustained, intensive exposure to UVR in all patients and occurs mainly on sun-exposed areas. In patients with skin of color, the effects of UVR are abrogated by the presence of melanin in the skin, which provides photoprotection. The incidence of BCC in patients with skin of color on sun-exposed and non–sun-exposed sites varies, and BCCs have appeared in unusual locations in both Caucasians and people with skin of color [**Table 54-2**].[12,13,23-26] Some studies suggest that the incidence of BCC on covered sites is the same for African Americans and Caucasians, whereas others demonstrate a higher percentage of BCCs on non–sun-exposed areas in African Americans as compared to those same areas in Caucasians. It has also been shown that 70% to 90% of BCCs occur on sun-exposed areas in African Americans, Japanese, and Asian Indians who develop BCC.[1] Halder and Bang[1] suggest that BCCs occur more often in sun-exposed areas, such as the head and neck [**Figures 54-1** and **54-2**]. However, Lesher et al[27] note in their

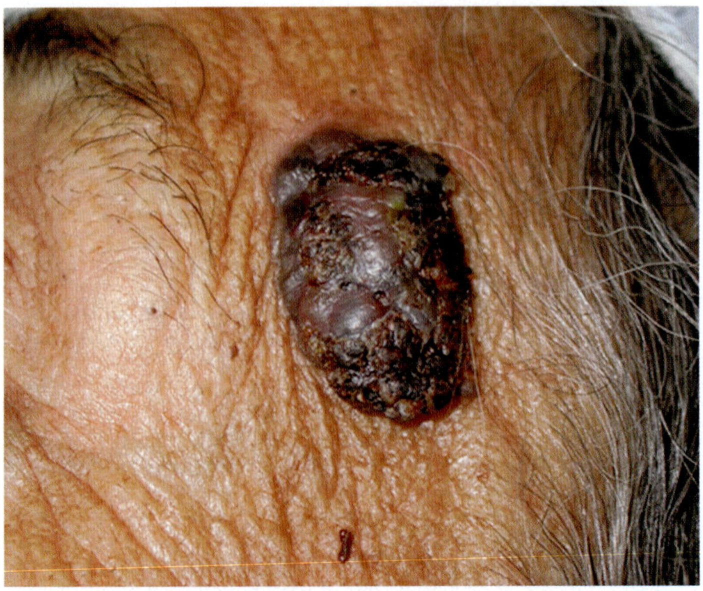

FIGURE 54-1. Pigmented BCC on the left temple of an African American female.

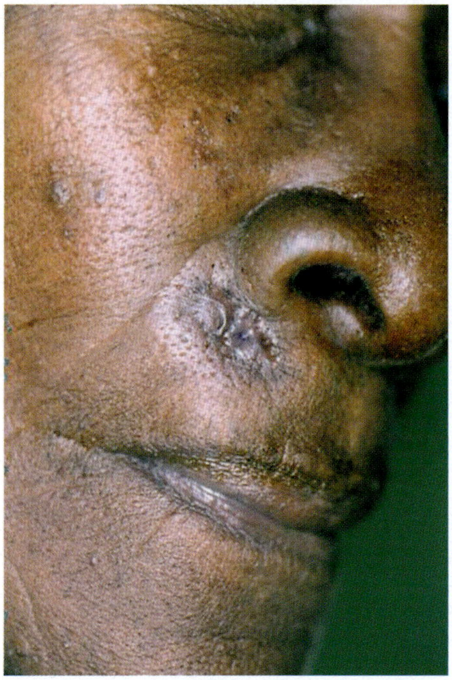

FIGURE 54-2. Pigmented BCC on the right upper cutaneous lip of an African American female.

series that 10% of BCCs in Caucasian patients occurred in covered, non–sun-exposed areas, whereas 24% of BCCs in African American patients occurred in covered, non–sun-exposed areas. Abreo and Sanusi[28] found that 88% (38 of 45) of BCCs occurred in the head and neck region of African American patients. In the series by Fleming et al,[7] it was found that 54.5% (6 of 11) of BCCs diagnosed in African American patients were on covered, non–sun-exposed areas.

Overall, the data suggest that BCCs occur with greater frequency in the sun-exposed areas in people with skin of color. However, there is also evidence that a tumor may arise in covered, non–sun-exposed areas as well.

In addition to UVR, there are reports of BCCs developing in areas of chronic discoid lupus erythematosus lesions, areas previously treated with radiation, and stasis ulcers.[29,30] However, the effects of radiation are much greater in irradiated Caucasian patients, as compared to African American patients. Thermal and physical traumas, such as burns, have also been demonstrated to be important risk factors in the development of BCC in Asian Indians specifically, along with scarring and sun exposure.[3] Vitamin D has recently been examined for its role in cutaneous carcinogenesis. Although vitamin D deficiency is linked to skin cancer in vitro and in mouse models, the role of vitamin D in human skin cancer development is unclear, with studies showing both positive and neutral associations between vitamin D deficiency and skin cancer.

Genetic syndromes can also contribute to the development of BCC in patients with skin of color. Gorlin syndrome (also known as nevoid BCC syndrome), oculocutaneous albinism, and xeroderma pigmentosum occur in skin of color populations.[31-34] These syndromes are associated with an increased incidence of all types of skin cancers, including BCCs. Hall et al[31] commented that less than 5% of cases of Gorlin syndrome occur in people with skin of color. Martin and Waisman[34] reported a case of an African American man with Gorlin syndrome who presented with his first BCC at age 77. Therefore, it may be prudent to look for other diagnostic criteria if one suspects Gorlin syndrome in a person of color (ie, palmar pits, frontal bossing, and odontogenic cysts). People with skin of color with oculocutaneous albinism are most likely to have type II oculocutaneous albinism, which is the expression of a mutation in the *P* gene.[35] Abreo and Sanusi[28] reported an albino patient with 12 separate primary BCCs. Itayemi et al[36] discussed an albino patient with a BCC metastasis to the cervical lymph nodes in their series. In the skin of color population, it is important to consider conditions predisposing a patient to develop BCC[37] [**Table 54-3**].

TABLE 54-3 Syndromes with genetic predisposition for developing basal cell carcinoma
Nevoid basal cell carcinoma syndrome (Gorlin syndrome)
Oculocutaneous albinism
Xeroderma pigmentosum

Some other important risk factors for the development of BCC in individuals with skin of color include immunosuppression in organ transplant recipients and HIV. The incidence of BCC increases 10-fold in organ transplant recipients.[38]

CLINICAL FEATURES AND DIAGNOSIS

The diagnosis of BCC in patients with skin of color is made clinically and via pathology. Reports suggest that a clinical diagnosis of BCC is more difficult than a histopathologic one. Altman et al[13] commented that a BCC in people with skin of color may be misdiagnosed clinically as seborrheic keratosis, nevocellular nevus, or malignant melanoma. Halder and Bang[1] also remarked that a BCC may be confused for a nevus sebaceous. Beckenstein and Windle[12] reported a BCC that was initially misdiagnosed as a fungal infection. While about 5% of BCCs are pigmented in White individuals, more than 50% are pigmented in non-Whites.[6] Hispanics, even those with fair skin, have a high incidence of pigmented BCC [**Figures 54-3 and 54-4**]. The pigmentation in Asian individuals is described as having a brown to glossy black appearance. Dermoscopy can be a useful tool to aid in the diagnosis of BCC in individuals with skin of color. One study found that the most common dermoscopic features in BCCs of patients with skin of color were maple leaf-like areas, blue-white veils, ulceration, and short fine telangiectasias.[39]

A biopsy is the best and most definitive diagnostic test for a presumed BCC. The histologic types of BCC in people with skin of color are similar to those seen in people with lighter skin. Various reports confirm the occurrence of nodular, morpheaform, superficial, adenoid, nodulocystic, and sclerosing types of BCC[13,27,28,40] [**Figure 54-5**]. The ulcerative type is discussed in many of the series and case reports concerning BCC in people with skin of color and is suggestive of a more aggressive course.[1,13,27]

PROGNOSIS

A BCC excised with clear surgical margins provides an excellent prognosis. Complications arise when there is delay in diagnosis, resulting in locally aggressive tumor expansion or even metastasis. In contrast to

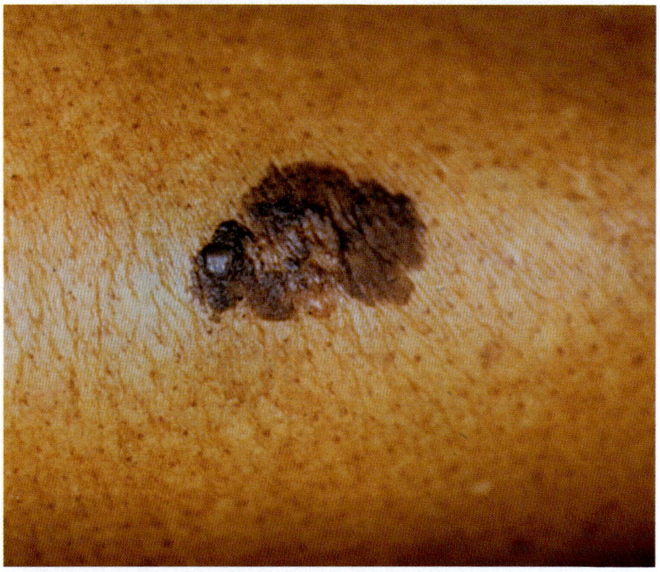

FIGURE 54-3. Pigmented BCC on the lower leg of an African American male.

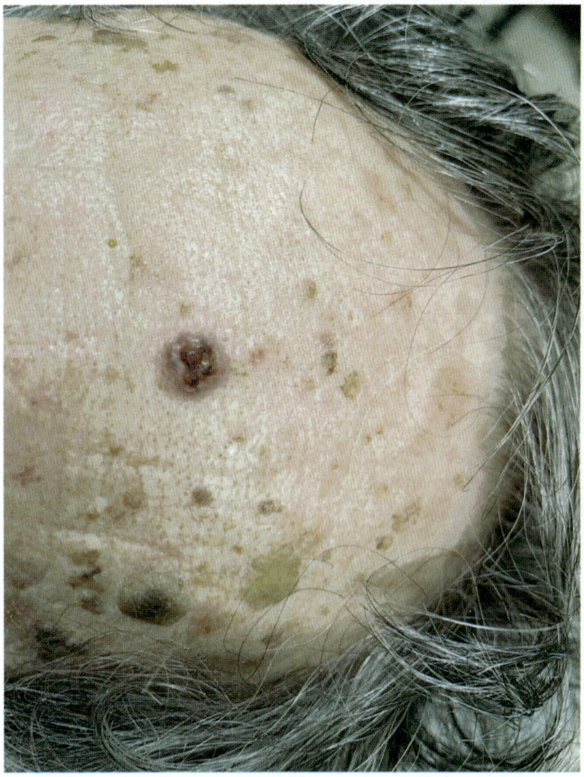

FIGURE 54-4. Pigmented BCC in a fair-skinned Hispanic woman.

SCC, BCC is not associated with increased morbidity in Blacks compared with Caucasians, although case reports and series have described more aggressive BCC behavior in patients with skin of color.[1] Itayemi et al[36] in Nigeria reported that BCCs are most aggressive in people with skin of color. They reported two cases of tumors that were locally aggressive and destructive to the underlying bony structures. Some studies claim that being African American is an independent risk factor for metastasis of BCCs.[41] In the case report of Beckenstein and Windle, [12]a BCC was described as arising within a giant ulcer and spreading locally to the underlying vasculature. Distant metastasis from BCCs of the scalp to cervical lymph nodes has been reported by Itayemi et al.[36] Lanehart et al[30] have reported a metastasis to the ipsilateral upper thigh from a primary tumor in a stasis ulcer. Recurrence of BCC in people with skin of color has not been widely reported in the literature.

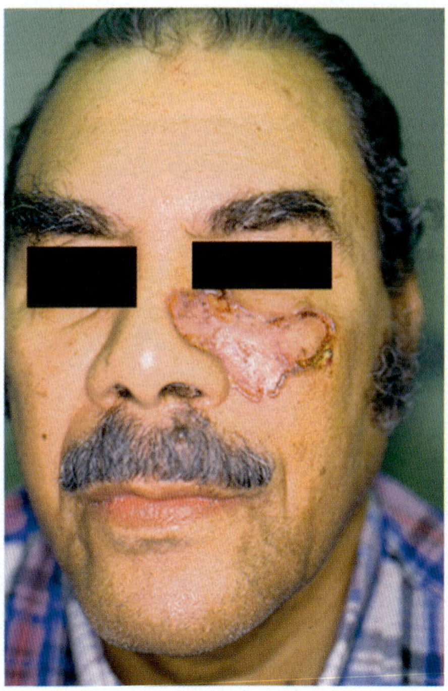

FIGURE 54-5. Sclerosing BCC in an African American male.

TABLE 54-4 Concurrent second primary malignancies
Squamous cell carcinoma of the lung
Breast cancer
Cervical cancer
Prostate cancer
Uterine cancer

SPECIAL CONSIDERATIONS

The occurrence of a BCC or even multiple BCCs in a person with darker skin of color should be reason for pause. Mora and Burris[6] noted in their series of 128 patients that 16.8% of patients with a BCC had a second primary malignancy elsewhere. Altman et al[13] found that one patient in their five-patient series had a second primary malignancy. In particular, women of color with BCC have been shown to be at increased risk for malignancy, particularly breast cancer. The authors suggested various mechanisms, such as abnormal DNA repair capacity, *p53* mutations, or higher levels of transurocanic acid in darker skin of color patients compared with Caucasian patients. Transurocanic acid is a photoreceptor that might induce immunosuppression, leading to decreased cancer surveillance and more rapid tumorigenesis.[42-47] **Table 54-4** lists the types of concurrent malignancies reported. SCC of the lung was the most frequently reported second primary malignancy in the series by Mora and Burris.[8] Therefore, it may be appropriate to perform an age-appropriate cancer screening on any patient who has at least one BCC.

TREATMENT AND COUNSELING

The approach to a person with skin of color should not be different than that for a patient with light skin.[24] Management of a BCC should focus on complete extirpation of the tumor. Surgical techniques available to the practitioner include electrodesiccation and curettage, cryosurgery, excisional surgery with clear surgical margins, and Mohs micrographic surgery.[12,27,40,46] Other modalities in the treatment of BCC include photodynamic therapy, topical imiquimod, and laser surgery.[47] Newer modalities include targeted molecular therapy in the form of vismodegib, a small-molecule analog of the PTCH protein, which functions to inhibit SMO and thus decrease growth of the tumor. Vismodegib is currently approved for adults with metastatic BCC or with locally advanced BCC that has recurred following surgery or who are not candidates for surgery or radiation. More studies would be required to determine the efficacy of vismodegib in skin of color patients. Continued monitoring is essential because recurrence has been reported in up to 37.5% of patients in a series by Ademiluyi and Ijaduola.[32]

In addition to treatment, patients should be counseled on appropriate monitoring and prevention methods once diagnosed with a BCC. Photoprotection such as seeking shade, sun-protective clothing, and broad-spectrum sunscreen use should be encouraged. Patient education on clinical signs of BCC such as nonhealing or bleeding lesions may help facilitate early diagnosis and treatment of this malignancy.

RESEARCH

Future research into the relationship between vitamin D and cutaneous malignancies in individuals with skin of color may be helpful in guiding counseling for patients. Small studies have been conducted on genetic susceptibility to BCC due to *GATA3*, *PTCH/PTCH1*, and *TP53* mutations in Hispanic and Asian populations, respectively. Unfortunately, due to small sample sizes, the results are not generalizable and further research is warranted. Additionally, the relationship between BCC and other internal malignancies has not been fully explored and may provide useful insight into disease pathogenesis.

REFERENCES

1. Halder RM, Bang KM. Skin cancer in blacks in the United States. *Dermatol Clin.* 1988;6(3):397-405.
2. Koh D, Wang H, Lee J, Chia KS, Lee HP, Goh CL. Basal cell carcinoma, squamous cell carcinoma and melanoma of the skin: analysis of the Singapore Cancer Registry data 1968-97. *Br J Dermatol.* 2003;148(6):1161-1166.
3. Dhir A, Orengo I, Bruce S, Kolbusz RV, Alford E, Goldberg L. Basal cell carcinoma on the scalp of an Indian patient. *Dermatol Surg.* 1995;21(3):247-250.
4. Kikuchi A, Shimizu H, Nishikawa T. Clinical histopathological characteristics of basal cell carcinoma in Japanese patients. *Arch Dermatol.* 1996;132(3):320-324.
5. Sharma VK, Gupta V, Jangid BL, Pathak M. Modification of the Fitzpatrick system of skin phototype classification for the Indian population, and its correlation with narrowband diffuse reflectance spectrophotometry. *Clin Exp Dermatol.* 2018;43(3):274-280.
6. Hogue L, Harvey VM. Basal cell carcinoma, squamous cell carcinoma, and cutaneous melanoma in skin of color patients. *Dermatol Clin.* 2019;37(4): 519-526.
7. Fleming ID, Barnawell JR, Burlison PE, Rankin JS. Skin cancer in black patients. *Cancer.* 1975;35(3):600-605.
8. Mora RG, Burris R. Cancer of the skin in blacks: a review of 128 patients with basal-cell carcinoma. *Cancer.* 1981;47(6):1436-1438.
9. White JE, Strudwick WJ, Ricketts WN, Sampson C. Cancer of the skin in Negroes. A review of 31 cases. *JAMA.* 1961;178:845-847.
10. Shapiro MP, Keen P, Cohen L, Murray JF. Skin cancer in the South African Bantu. *Br J Cancer.* 1953;7(1):45-57.
11. Oluwasanmi JO, Williams AO, Alli AF. Superficial cancer in Nigeria. *Br J Cancer.* 1969;23(4):714-728.
12. Beckenstein MS, Windle BH. Basal cell carcinoma in black patients: the need to include it in the differential diagnosis. *Ann Plast Surg.* 1995;35(5):546-548.
13. Altman A, Rosen T, Tschen JA, et al. Basal cell epithelioma in black patients. *J Am Acad Dermatol.* 1987;17(5 Pt 1):741-745.
14. Ichihashi M, Naruse K, Harada S, et al. Trends in nonmelanoma skin cancer in Japan. *Recent Results Cancer Res.* 1995;139:263-273.
15. Naruse K, Ueda M, Nagano T, et al. Prevalence of actinic keratosis in Japan. *J Dermatol Sci.* 1997;15(3):183-187.
16. Harris RB, Griffith K, Moon TE. Trends in the incidence of nonmelanoma skin cancers in southeastern Arizona, 1985-1996. *J Am Acad Dermatol.* 2001;45(4):528-536.
17. Chuang TY, Reizner GT, Elpern DJ, Stone JL, Farmer ER. Nonmelanoma skin cancer in Japanese ethnic Hawaiians in Kauai, Hawaii: an incidence report. *J Am Acad Dermatol.* 1995;33(3):422-426.
18. Munyao TM, Othieno-Abinya NA. Cutaneous basal cell carcinoma in Kenya. *East Afr Med J.* 1999;76(2):97-100.
19. Miller DL, Weinstock MA. Nonmelanoma skin cancer in the United States: incidence. *J Am Acad Dermatol.* 1994;30(5 Pt 1):774-778.
20. Johnson RL, Rothman AL, Xie J, et al. Human homolog of patched, a candidate gene for the basal cell nevus syndrome. *Science.* 1996;272(5268):1668-1671.
21. Rady P, Scinicariello F, Wagner RF, Jr., Tyring SK. p53 mutations in basal cell carcinomas. *Cancer Res.* 1992;52(13):3804-3806.
22. Stacey SN, Sulem P, Masson G, et al. New common variants affecting susceptibility to basal cell carcinoma. *Nat Genet.* 2009;41(8):909-914.
23. Galinski AW. Plantar basal cell carcinoma: a case report. *J Foot Surg.* 1980;19(1):34-35.
24. McDonald MW. Carcinoma of scrotum. *Urology.* 1982;19(3):269-274.
25. Powers CN, Stastny JF, Frable WJ. Adenoid basal carcinoma of the cervix: a potential pitfall in cervicovaginal cytology. *Diagn Cytopathol.* 1996;14(2): 172-177.
26. Morimoto SS, Gurevitch AW. Pedunculated pigmented basal-cell carcinoma on the buttock of a black man. *J Dermatol Surg Oncol.* 1985;11(2):115-117.
27. Lesher JL, Jr., d'Aubermont PC, Brown VM. Morpheaform basal cell carcinoma in a young black woman. *J Dermatol Surg Oncol.* 1988;14(2):200-203.
28. Abreo F, Sanusi ID. Basal cell carcinoma in North American blacks. Clinical and histopathologic study of 26 patients. *J Am Acad Dermatol.* 1991;25(6 Pt 1): 1005-1011.
29. Walther RR, Grossman ME, Troy JL. Basal-cell carcinomas on the scalp of a black patient many years after epilation by x rays. *J Dermatol Surg Oncol.* 1981;7(7):570-571.
30. Lanehart WH, Sanusi ID, Misra RP, O'Neal B. Metastasizing basal cell carcinoma originating in a stasis ulcer in a black woman. *Arch Dermatol.* 1983;119(7):587-591.
31. Hall J, Johnston KA, McPhillips JP, Barnes SD, Elston DM. Nevoid basal cell carcinoma syndrome in a black child. *J Am Acad Dermatol.* 1998;38(2 Pt 2): 363-365.
32. Ademiluyi SA, Ijaduola GT. Occurrence and recurrence of basal cell carcinoma of the head and neck in Negroid and albinoid Africans. *J Laryngol Otol.* 1987;101(12):1324-1328.
33. Kulkarni P, Brashear R, Chuang TY. Nevoid basal cell carcinoma syndrome in a person with dark skin. *J Am Acad Dermatol.* 2003;49(2):332-335.
34. Martin S, Waisman M. Basal cell nevus syndrome in a black patient: report of a case and review of the literature. *Arch Dermatol.* 1978;114(9):1356-1357.
35. Okulicz JF, Shah RS, Schwartz RA, Janniger CK. Oculocutaneous albinism. *J Eur Acad Dermatol Venereol.* 2003;17(3):251-256.
36. Itayemi SO, Abioye AA, Ogan O, Daramola JO, Oluwasanmi JO. Aggressive basal cell carcinoma in Nigerians. *Br J Dermatol.* 1979;101(4):465-468.
37. Frank W, Morris D. Large basal cell carcinoma in a black patient. *Plast Reconstr Surg.* 1995;96(2):493-494.
38. Marzuka AG, Book SE. Basal cell carcinoma: pathogenesis, epidemiology, clinical features, diagnosis, histopathology, and management. *Yale J Biol Med.* 2015;88(2):167-179.
39. Behera B, Kumari R, Thappa DM, Gochhait D, Srinivas BH, Ayyanar P. Dermoscopic features of basal cell carcinoma in skin of color: a retrospective cross-sectional study from Puducherry, South India. *Indian J Dermatol Venereol Leprol.* 2021:1-7.
40. Schwartz RA, Vickerman CE, Phelan JT, et al. Mutilating sclerosing basal cell epithelioma. *J Surg Oncol.* 1979;12(2):131-135.
41. Jahan-Tigh RR, Alston JL, Umphlett M. Basal cell carcinoma with metastasis to the lung in an African American man. *J Am Acad Dermatol.* 2010;63(4):e87-89.
42. Troyanova P, Valerianova Z, Danon S. Clinical stages of cutaneous malignant melanoma in Bulgaria. *Neoplasma.* 2000;47(4):257-260.
43. Frisch M, Melbye M. New primary cancers after squamous cell skin cancer. *Am J Epidemiol.* 1995;141(10):916-922.
44. Rosenberg CA, Greenland P, Khandekar J, Loar A, Ascensao J, Lopez AM. Association of nonmelanoma skin cancer with second malignancy. *Cancer.* 2004;100(1):130-138.
45. Norval M. Effects of solar radiation on the human immune system. *J Photochem Photobiol B.* 2001;63(1-3):28-40.
46. Singh B, Bhaya M, Shaha A, Har-El G, Lucente FE. Presentation, course, and outcome of head and neck skin cancer in African Americans: a case-control study. *Laryngoscope.* 1998;108(8 Pt 1):1159-1163.
47. Geisse J, Caro I, Lindholm J, Golitz L, Stampone P, Owens M. Imiquimod 5% cream for the treatment of superficial basal cell carcinoma: results from two phase III, randomized, vehicle-controlled studies. *J Am Acad Dermatol.* 2004;50(5):722-733.

CHAPTER 55 Cutaneous T-Cell Lymphoma

Supriya Rastogi
Jessica B. Brown-Korsah
Ellen J. Kim

KEY POINTS

- Cutaneous T-cell lymphoma (CTCL) refers to a group of non-Hodgkin lymphomas that primarily involve the skin, of which mycosis fungoides (MF) is the most common form.
- Black patients are more likely to present at more advanced stages and have poorer outcomes.
- Hypopigmented and hyperpigmented MF are predominantly CD8+ diseases that can present with hypopigmented or hyperpigmented patches and plaques, respectively, and have a favorable prognosis.

- Skin-directed therapies for CTCL include topical agents, phototherapy, and radiation (localized and total skin electron beam) therapy.
- Systemic therapies for CTCL include interferons, retinoids such as bexarotene, methotrexate, extracorporeal photopheresis, monoclonal antibodies, histone acetylase inhibitors, and other intravenous systemics, several of which can be used together as part of multimodality therapy.

INTRODUCTION

Patients with skin of color comprise a substantial subset of cutaneous T-cell lymphoma (CTCL) patients. CTCL is a diverse group of non-Hodgkin lymphomas that primarily involve the skin but may involve the lymph nodes, peripheral blood, and other organs. Mycosis fungoides (MF) and Sézary syndrome (SS) make up the majority of CTCL. Skin lesions may be challenging to detect in darker skin, thus Black patients can go undiagnosed for years which contributes to poor health outcomes. Understanding the variety of presentations of MF/SS in patients with skin of color is paramount for earlier disease detection. Multiple skin-directed and systemic therapies are used to manage symptoms, pruritus, prevent infection, and improve overall quality of life.

ETIOLOGY

MF is characterized by infiltration of activated and malignant CLA+ CCR4+ T-cells into the skin with heterogeneous clinical presentation.[1] Despite numerous recent CTCL genomic studies demonstrating mutations in various apoptosis/cell cycle, T-cell signaling, NF-kB, JAK/STAT, and epigenetic pathways, no driver, causative mutations have been identified as yet, thus the etiology of MF/SS remains unknown. MF is a malignancy of skin-resident effector memory T-cells (CCR4+ and CLA+) that are usually CD4+, though CD8+ and other immunophenotypes (CD4-CD8-, CD4+CD8+) can be seen. In contrast, SS cells have been characterized by a phenotype of central memory T-cells (CCR7+, CD27+, and L-selectin+).[2]

In early-stage MF (IA-IIA), the patient's immune system can control tumor outgrowth via the adaptive immune responses. Early-stage skin lesions are characterized by infiltration of malignant T-cells surrounded by reactive immune cells such as CD8+ T-cells and T-helper 1 (Th1) cells. This results in cell-mediated antitumor responses and secretion of cytokines such as interferon-α (IFN-α) and IFN-γ. Signal transducer and activator of transcription 4 (STAT4) expression and interleukin-12 (IL-12) signaling via JAK2/TYK2 maintains the Th1 helper milieu.[2]

The exact mechanism for tumor progression in CTCL is unknown. However, cellular immune responses are suppressed in advanced-stage disease (IIB-IVB) as Th2 phenotype becomes prominent with increased expression of cytokines (IL-4, IL-5, IL10) and Th2 markers (GATA3). JAK/STAT pathway mutations resulting in persistent activation of STAT5 and STAT3 may also contribute to Th2 differentiation and tumor progression.[1,2]

External factors and environmental pollution may play a role in CTCL pathogenesis in some. Nonrandom clustering of CTCL cases has been reported worldwide and within families.[3] In a 2016 systematic review and meta-analysis, the relative risk between glyphosate use, an agent used in pesticides, and non-Hodgkin lymphoma was 1.3.[4] However, a causal relationship could not be established between glyphosate use and MF. There have also been several reports of CTCL with known Agent Orange exposure.[5]

EPIDEMIOLOGY

According to Wong et al, there are likely around 3000 new cases of CTCL each year in the United States. Since there is no cure and median survival is around 12 to 18 years, there is a gross estimate of 25 to 50,000 people in the United States living with CTCL.[6] The incidence of CTCL is estimated to be 0.64 to 0.87/100,000 person-years in the United States, which is higher than in Europe (0.29–0.39/100,000 person-years).[7]

A systematic review and meta-analysis comprising 16,953 patients with CTCL from 15 countries worldwide found that MF/SS accounted for 65% of CTCL in North America and Asia, 85% in South America, and 73% in Europe. Asian studies reported a higher frequency of rare CTCL subtypes, such as NK/T-cell lymphoma or subcutaneous panniculitis-like lymphoma. There was a stable 3% of patients with SS worldwide. Of note, only one study from South America was included and no studies from Africa were included in this meta-analysis.[7]

Regarding demographics, per SEER data 1973-2002, the male-to-female incidence ratio of MF was 1.9:1, with the highest number of cases occurring between 60 and 69 years old. Incidence was higher among Black race compared to other races.[8] A cohort study examining 566 patients between the years 1990 to 2020 found the male-to-female ratio to be 1.1:1 and the median (SD) age to be 55 (16.4) years. Twelve (2.1%) were Asian, 257 (45.4%) were Black, 4 (0.8%) were Hispanic, 284 (50.2%) were White, and 9 (1.6%) were unknown/undeclared.[9]

HEALTH DISPARITIES IN CTCL

Several studies have revealed higher stage at presentation and poorer outcomes associated with Black race[10] with exact cause unknown but is most likely multifactorial. In a retrospective analysis of 4495 MF patients within the U.S. National Cancer Database, Black individuals experienced a significantly shorter overall survival than White individuals, adjusting for sociodemographic factors, treatment received, and clinical characteristics (stage, Charlson-Deyo Score, and regional lymph node status).[11] In a retrospective cohort study of 566 patients with MF/SS diagnosed between 1990 and 2020, self-reported non-Hispanic Black race was associated with increased progression rates to a higher TNMB stage compared to non-Black race. Among patients younger than 60 years without hypopigmented MF, Black race was associated with poorer outcomes, after adjusting for cancer stage and large-cell transformation.[9]

Differences in the receipt of treatment may also play a role. In a study of 65 patients with stage III or IV disease, Black patients were less likely to be treated with extracorporeal photopheresis (ECP) for their MF than White patients. Moreover, ECP was less likely to be discussed with Black patients when compared to White patients. When ECP was discussed as a treatment option, there was no significant difference in ECP use.[12]

In an MF registry of 440 patients treated within the Henry Ford Health System, Medicaid insurance was a significant independent predictor of progression and shorter progression-free survival. Patients on Medicaid also experienced longer median diagnostic delays (5-6 years vs 3-4 years). The impact of Medicaid on outcomes among patients with MF may indicate difficulties in accessing timely treatment and potential bias within the health system.[13] Understanding the role health disparities may play in the poorer prognosis of Black patients and individuals on Medicaid with MF may ultimately create targeted interventions.

CLINICAL PRESENTATION

Classically, MF presents in sun-protected areas on the skin. MF patches present as pink to violaceous macules and patches, sometimes with hyper- or hypopigmentation, and slight scale [**Figure 55-1**]. Plaques are dusky red and scaly and may be round, oval, serpiginous, or arciform in shape [**Figure 55-2**]. Lesions can have varying levels of pruritus. Clinical presentations are polymorphous and depend on skin type. Espinosa et al performed a retrospective chart review of patients with biopsy-proven MF/SS and compared the clinical manifestations of patients with Fitzpatrick skin types I to III to those with skin types IV to VI. They found that patients with skin of color (Fitzpatrick skin types IV-VI) who have MF/SS are more likely to present with lichenification, silver hue, and hyperpigmentation than those with Fitzpatrick skin types I to III, who more commonly present with erythema and poikiloderma. Additionally,

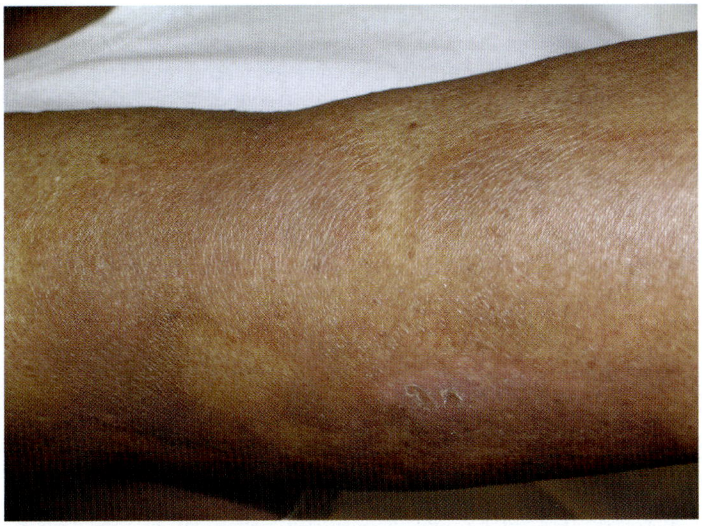

FIGURE 55-1. Mycosis fungoides patches in an Asian MF patient.

erythema may appear violaceous. Lack of recognition of erythema may lead to delayed diagnosis and inadequate treatment.[14] If plaques occur in hair-bearing skin, alopecia may result and can be associated with follicular mucinosis on biopsy. Distribution ranges from solitary, isolated lesions to generalized involvement covering most of the skin surface area. More advanced diseases can present in the form of tumors. Tumors of MF generally arise from a preformed plaque or erythematous skin [**Figure 55-3**] and represent the loss of infiltrate of atypical mononuclear cells in the epidermis (epidermotropism) and extension into the deep dermis. These tumors can ulcerate and may become secondarily infected, a common cause of morbidity.[15]

Generalized erythroderma in MF/SS may present with diffuse hyperpigmentation rather than erythema in skin of color [**Figure 55-4**] and is usually accompanied by extreme pruritus, scaling, and palmoplantar keratoderma [**Figure 55-5**]. The skin may be lichenified or atrophic.

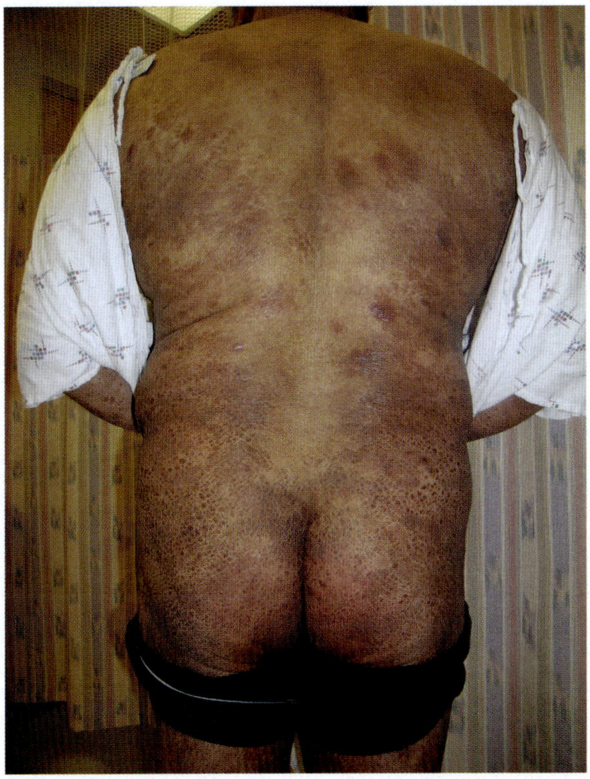

FIGURE 55-2. Mycosis fungoides patches and plaques in a Black MF patient.

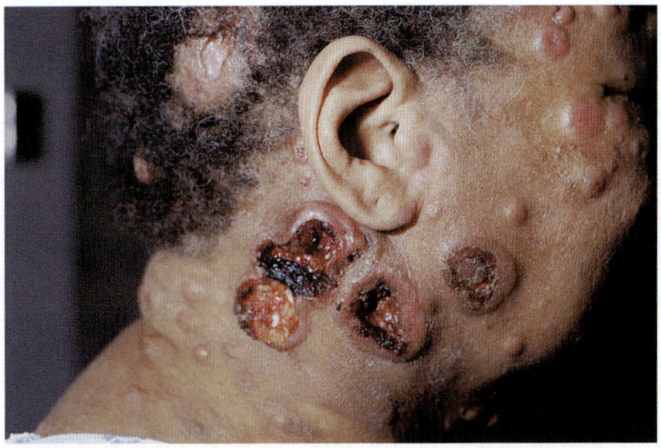

FIGURE 55-3. Ulcerating mycosis fungoides tumors in a Black patient with nodal disease (stage IVA2).

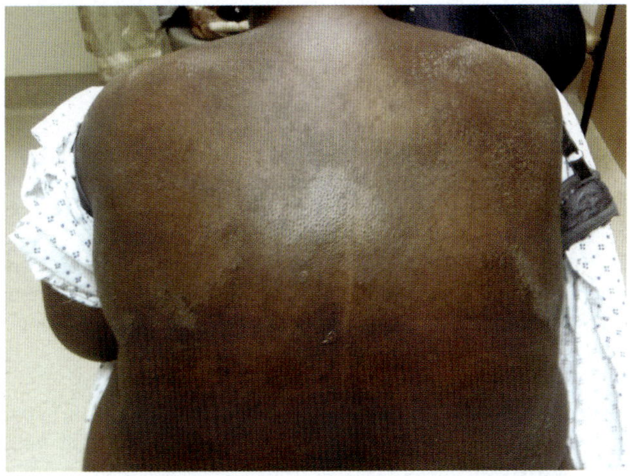

FIGURE 55-4. Black patient with Sezary syndrome with erythroderma presenting as generalized hyperpigmentation.

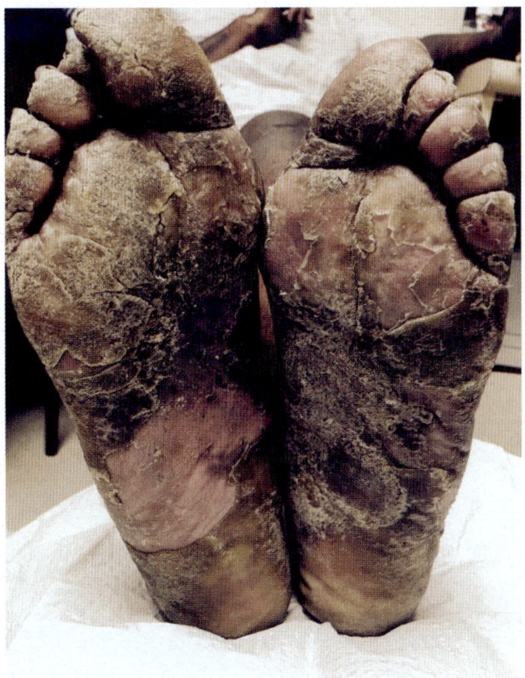

FIGURE 55-5. Plantar keratoderma in a Black patient with Sézary syndrome.

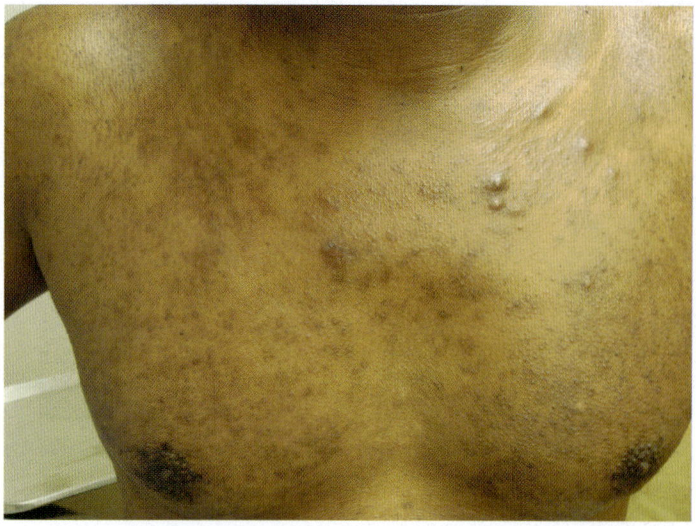

FIGURE 55-6. Folliculotropic mycosis fungoides papules on the chest of a Black patient.

Plaques and tumors of MF also may be present on the background erythema. Advanced stages of CTCL may involve lymph nodes, peripheral blood, bone marrow, or other organs. Extensive skin involvement (generalized patch/plaque, tumor, erythroderma) is a risk factor for developing extracutaneous skin disease. SS presents with generalized erythroderma, lymphadenopathy, and circulating abnormal lymphoid cells (Sézary cells) in the peripheral blood.[15]

There are several variants of MF to be aware of, such as folliculotropic [**Figure 55-6**], poikilodermatous, hypopigmented, and hyperpigmented MF.[16] The latter two occur more often in patients with skin of color.

HYPOPIGMENTED MYCOSIS FUNGOIDES

Hypopigmented MF is a unique clinical entity distinct from the hypopigmentation observed in resolving MF or MF associated with poikiloderma [**Figure 55-7**]. The onset of disease is earlier than with classic MF, with some reporting a median age of 16.5 to 32.2 years (range 4-57 years).[17,18] One study analyzed data from 20 patients with hypopigmented MF in an urban center in the United States. Fifteen patients were African Americans, three were African, one was Hispanic, and one was Afro-Caribbean.[17] Hypopigmented lesions can be the only manifestation of MF, or they can be associated with erythematous plaques or tumors.

Most patients demonstrate an immunophenotype with CD8 predominance, whereas classic MF has CD4 predominance. Hypopigmented MF usually has an indolent course that responds well to topicals (steroids, topical chemotherapy) and/or phototherapy.[19]

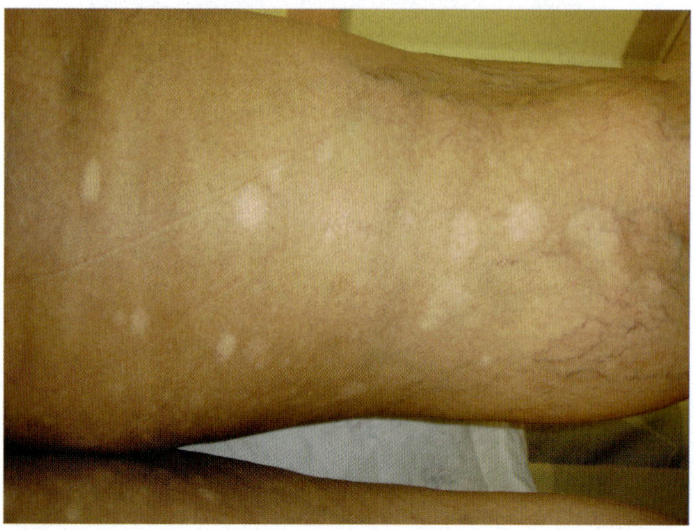

FIGURE 55-7. Hypopigmented patches of mycosis fungoides on the thighs of a Latinx patient.

Repigmentation is common in patients who receive treatment. Rodney et al noted that 8 of the 14 patients achieved repigmentation of all affected skin, a negative skin biopsy, and no clinical disease activity for at least 3 months of treatment with phototherapy, topicals, or a combination of the two. None of the 20 patients diagnosed as Stage 1A-1B disease progressed to advanced stages or died from causes related to hypopigmented MF after an average follow-up of 5.9 years (range 8 months to 14 years).[17] Ten-year survival of patients with hypopigmented MF has been reported to be 100%, compared to 51.8% in patients without hypopigmented MF.[9]

HYPERPIGMENTED MYCOSIS FUNGOIDES

Hyperpigmented MF has been gaining recognition as a rare variant of MF with a predilection for patients with skin of color. Of note, hyperpigmented MF is not to be confused with postinflammatory hyperpigmentation caused by MF. In a case series of hyperpigmented MF, seven of the eight patients were skin of color. Clinical presentation included hyperpigmented patches and plaques. More than half endorsed pruritus, with a few patients presenting with more typical manifestations of MF in addition to hyperpigmented lesions. The median age of diagnosis was 43 years (range 19-69 years), and half were female. Diagnosis took an average of 6.25 years (range 1-14) from initial disease onset. Five of the eight patients demonstrated CD4-CD8+ immunophenotype, while two had CD4-CD8- and one had CD4+CD8- immunophenotype. All patients received skin-directed therapies without evidence of disease progression after a mean follow-up of 3.8 years.[20]

Another study investigating patterns among 14 patients with hyperpigmented MF illustrated similar findings. While some patients presented with hyperpigmented patches/plaques in isolation, others had concomitant hypopigmentation, poikiloderma, ichthyosiform plaques, and purpuric patches. An immunophenotype favoring CD8 positivity was again demonstrated. Most were treated with skin-directed therapies, except for two who necessitated oral acitretin. After a median follow-up of 57 months (range 1-252 months), none developed large cell transformation nor blood involvement. As hypopigmented MF is also associated with a favorable prognosis, these conclusions highlight that MF with altered pigmentation has at least a comparable prognosis to other MF subtypes.[21]

DIFFERENTIAL DIAGNOSIS

MF can imitate many different skin diseases. The differential diagnosis includes atopic dermatitis, psoriasis, drug reactions, photodermatitis, parapsoriasis, neurodermatitis, nummular dermatitis, contact dermatitis, and tinea corporis. Hypopigmented MF can mimic vitiligo, tinea corporis, tinea versicolor, pityriasis alba, postinflammatory hypopigmentation, progressive macular hypomelanosis, idiopathic guttate hypomelanosis, sarcoidosis, and leprosy. Hyperpigmented MF can be confused for postinflammatory hyperpigmentation, fixed drug eruption, pigmented contact dermatitis, lichenoid dermatitis, erythema dyschromicum perstans (ashy dermatosis), cutaneous amyloidosis, atrophoderma of Pasini and Pierini, and idiopathic eruptive macular hyperpigmentation. In patients who present with erythroderma, the differential diagnosis includes atopic dermatitis, contact dermatitis, drug eruption, erythrodermic psoriasis, pityriasis rubra pilaris, and paraneoplastic disease.[16]

DIAGNOSIS AND STAGING

MF/SS are classified using the TNMB classification [**Table 55-1**].[22] In 2021, the International Society for Cutaneous Lymphomas (ISCL), the United States Cutaneous Lymphoma Consortium (USCLC), and the Cutaneous Lymphoma Task Force of the European Organization for Research and Treatment of Cancer (EORTC) addressed updates to diagnosis and staging. Preferably, all patients with primary cutaneous lymphoma should have a biopsy performed. Before performing a biopsy,

TABLE 55-1 ISCL/USCLC/EORTC-modified staging of PCLs

MF/SS				
Skin (T)	T_0[a]	Absence of clinically suspicious lesions		
	T_1	Patches, plaques, or papules <10% BSA	T_{1A}	Patch only lesions
			T_{1B}	Plaque/papule +/− patch lesions
	T_2	Patches, plaques, or papules ≥10% BSA	T_{2A}	Patch only lesions
			T_{2B}	Plaque/papule +/− patch lesions
	T_3	One or more tumors ≥1 cm diameter		
	T_4	Confluence of erythema covering ≥80% BSA[b]		
Nodes (N)[c]	N_0	No clinically abnormal LN; no biopsy necessary		
	N_1	N_{1A}	Pathology Dutch grade 1 or NCI LN 0-2: clone negative **or equivocal**	
		N_{1B}	Pathology Dutch grade 1 or NCI LN 0-2: clone positive **and identical to skin**	
	N_2	N_{2A}	Dutch grade 2, NCI LN3: clone negative **or equivocal**	
		N_{2B}	Dutch grade 2, NCI LN3: clone positive **and identical to skin**	
	N_3[c] (lymphoma)	N_{3A}	Dutch grade 3-4, NCI LN4: clone negative **or equivocal**	
		N_{3B}	Dutch grade 3-4, NCI LN4: clone positive **and identical to skin**	
	N_X	Clinically abnormal peripheral or central lymph node but no pathologic determination of representative LN. **Other surrogate means of determining involvement may be determined by Tri-Society consensus**		
Viscera (M)	M_0	No visceral involvement		
	M_{1a}	**BM only involvement**	**Clone positive and identical to skin**	
			Clone negative or indeterminate	
	M_{1b}	**Non-BM visceral involvement**	**Clone positive and identical to skin**	
			Clone negative or indeterminate	
	Mx	Visceral involvement is neither confirmed nor refuted by available pathologic **or imaging assessment**		
Blood (B)[d]	B_0	B_{0A}	Clone negative **or equivocal**	Absence of significant blood involvement
		B_{0B}	Clone positive **and identical to skin**	
	B_1	B_{1A}	Clone negative **or equivocal**	Low blood tumor burden
		B_{1B}	Clone positive **and identical to skin**	
	B_2	B_{2A}	Clone negative **or equivocal**	High blood tumor burden
		B_{2B}	Clone positive **and identical to skin**	
	Bx	**Bx_A**	**Clone negative or equivocal**	**Unable to quantify blood involvement according to agreed-upon guidelines**
		Bx_B	**Clone positive and identical to skin**	

Based on Olsen E, et al. *Blood.* 2007;110(6): 1713-1722; Olsen EA, et al. *J Clin Oncol.* 2011;29(18): 2598-2607; and Kim YH et al. *Blood*. 2007;110(2):479-484. Changes or confirmation of staging are noted in bold in table above and in further description below. Options for characterizing clonality further by designation as A (clone negative or equivocal) and B (clone positive and identical to skin) are presented. If a clone in LN or viscera is detected but different from that identified in the skin, another concurrent lymphoproliferative process should be considered.

[a] T_0 is used for clinical trials in order to track clearance of lesions in the skin compartment. No patient with PCL at time of diagnosis should be T_0.

[b] Patients with both erythroderma and tumors may be designated as $T_4(T_3)$.[7] The BSA of 80% is used to define erythroderma in MF/SS at study entry, but any decrease in BSA during the study does not affect the entry classification.

[c] Abnormal LNs are those now > 1.5 cm LDi according to the Lugano classification and confirmed by imaging. The pathological findings of a representative abnormal LN may apply to all abnormal lymph nodes.

[d] Blood staging for MF/SS is defined currently as B_0 = <250/μL of $CD4^+/CD26^-$ or $CD4^+/CD7^-$ cells, B_1 = does not meet criteria for B_0 or B_2, and **B_2 = ≥1000/μL of $CD4^+/CD26^-$ or $CD4^+/CD7^-$ cells or other aberrant population of lymphocytes identified by flow cytometry.** It is expected that patients with high blood tumor burden (B_2) will have a clone in the blood that is identical to that in the skin. Nonidentical T-cell clones are often detected in peripheral blood with increasing age and are of unknown clinical significance.

patients should undergo a 2-week washout period from treatment (systemic or skin-directed therapy) to enhance the ability to make a diagnosis.[22] Biopsy of the lesion may yield nonspecific results for months or years before a definitive diagnosis can be made. Even when initial biopsies are negative, repeated biopsies should be performed in patients suspected of having MF. On histology, skin biopsies suggestive of MF reveal a bandlike infiltrate involving the papillary dermis that consists of mononuclear cells with hyperchromatic, cerebriform nuclei without spongiosis. In addition, there is an infiltrate of atypical mononuclear cells in the epidermis (epidermotropism) that can form an intraepithelial aggregate known as a Pautrier microabscess [**Figure 55-8**].[16]

On physical exam, patients should undergo a skin assessment with palpation of the liver, spleen, and peripheral nodal groups. The Modified Severity Weighted Assessment Tool (mSWAT) is a validated tool used to assess body surface involvement of MF/SS weighted by skin lesion type (patch = 1, papule/plaque = 2, tumor = 4). Lymph nodes are considered abnormal if greater than 1.5 cm in longest diameter or are firm, fixed, or rubbery.[22]

Typically, imaging is reserved for T2a disease or above and may include PET-CT or CT scans with contrast of the neck, chest, abdomen, and pelvis.[22] Additionally, staging can include T-cell gene rearrangement (TCR)/polymerase chain reaction (PCR) to evaluate for clones in the skin. Flow cytometry, TCR/PCR, or high-throughput sequencing (next-generation sequencing) can detect a malignant clonal population in the blood. Multiplex/heteroduplex PCR amplification of the TCR V gamma chain is commonly used to detect T-cell clones in patients with CTCL. However, this method may have a high false-negative rate in early-stage disease and can be positive in benign inflammatory

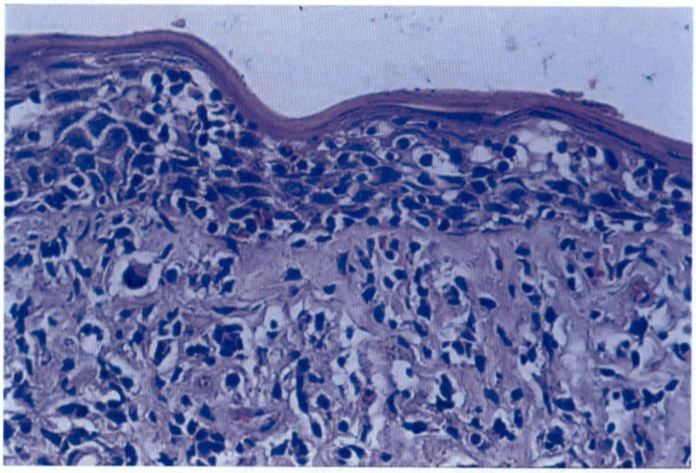

FIGURE 55-8. Histopathology of patch/plaque stage mycosis fungoides showing multiple atypical lymphoctytes in the papillary dermis and epidermotropism. Note the small aggregates of lymphocytes in epidermis (Pautrier microabscesses).

dermatoses.[23] High-throughput TCR sequencing (HTS) may provide another option to aid in diagnosing patients with cutaneous lymphoma. In a study of 46 CTCL skin lesions, HTS of the TCRB CDR3 regions (the third complementarity determining regions of T-cell receptor beta) identified expanded T-cell clones in all lesional CTCL samples. Among 39 patients with clinically confirmed CTCL, HTS demonstrated T-cell clones in 100% of the samples, compared to clonal identification in 70% of samples via TCR gamma PCR.[23] HTS can distinguish between definitive CTCL from reactive and indeterminate histology. In a study of 100 biopsies that were clinically concerning for CTCL, 25 biopsies were placed into each of four categories: "definitive CTCL," "atypical lymphoid infiltrate, concerning for CTCL," "atypical lymphoid infiltrate, favor reactive," or "reactive lymphoid infiltrate." HTS in the skin was highly specific, which may help reduce false-positive results. HTS in blood was more specific than flow cytometry and TCR PCR in blood.[24] HTS may be a useful diagnostic tool in conjunction with the patient's presentation, history, and histopathology.

TREATMENT

SKIN-DIRECTED THERAPIES

Skin-directed therapy includes topical therapy (corticosteroids, retinoids, imiquimod, chemotherapy), phototherapy, and radiation therapy. Topical corticosteroids are first-line therapy and may also be used as adjunctive treatment. Topical retinoids (bexarotene and tazarotene) and imiquimod are useful for localized skin disease treatment but may cause significant irritation or inflammation that may require adjusting application frequency. Topical chemotherapy (nitrogen mustard/mechlorethamine, carmustine) may be used for localized or generalized skin disease. While nitrogen mustard powder suspended in water was widely used in the past, the currently available form is 60 gm gel; because of its high cost, it may be cost-prohibitive for wide-spread disease. Side effects include contact dermatitis in approximately 20% of patients generally within the first 6 months of use, and potential bone marrow suppression with carmustine if used over large skin body surface area.[19] Previously, there was concern about increased risk of nonmelanoma skin cancer development with long-term use of topical chemotherapy but a more recent longitudinal study did not show this.

A widely used skin-directed therapy is phototherapy. Narrowband (NB)-UVB (311 to 313 nm) is currently the most used form given ease of administration, good availability, and compared to PUVA, lower risk of actinic damage. However, because UVA used in PUVA does penetrate deeper into the skin compared to NB-UVB, PUVA should be strongly considered for patients with darker skin type and/or thicker lesions.[19]

PUVA photochemotherapy requires oral 8-methoxypsoralen, which becomes activated by ultraviolet A radiation (330-365 nm) and then inhibits DNA and RNA synthesis by forming thymine adducts. During the clearing phase, treatment is given three times per week, followed by a maintenance phase that ranges from once a week to once a month. Side effects include nausea and actinic damage.[19] PUVA availability has decreased over the past decade.

Localized radiation therapy can be used for targeted treatment and is considered first-line treatment for tumors. Total skin electron beam therapy (TSEBT) is an effective treatment for generalized skin disease (refractory plaques/tumors, erythroderma) and a low-dose regimen has a favorable side effect profile when compared to conventional dose regimen used in the past (30-36 Gy). Side effects include fatigue, radiation dermatitis, alopecia, nail ridging or loss, lower leg edema, xerosis, and ocular irritation; most are reversible with low dose regimens. TSEBT can lead to complete response rates of 97% in patients with T1 disease and has been reported to result in 82% cutaneous and 55% peripheral blood improvement for T4 disease with B1/B2 involvement. TSEBT may be utilized as a part of a multimodality regimen as there is a high relapse rate if no adjuvant therapy is subsequently given.[25]

Assessing treatment response in skin of color can be challenging, particularly given postinflammatory hypo- or hyperpigmentation that can occur more frequently in skin of color with any CTCL treatment. Identification of scale, lichenification, silver hue, and violaceous erythema is critical to assessing residual disease activity. Familiarity with these morphologic features, serial clinical photographs, and surveillance biopsies may aid in assessing patients' clinical response.[14] It is also critical to adequately counsel patients about expectations during/after CTCL treatment as postinflammatory dyspigmentation can take months/years to fully resolve.

SYSTEMIC THERAPIES

Systemic therapies are utilized in refractory early stage and most advanced stage MF/SS patients. Selection is based on disease stage as per treatment guidelines (National Comprehensive Cancer Network in the United States) but patient comorbidities, tempo of disease, and presence of histologic large cell transformation, access, and treatment center preferences also contribute. Oral bexarotene is a retinoid that selectively binds the retinoid X receptors (RXR) leading to apoptosis of malignant cells and inhibition of Th2 cytokine production. Disease resistant to bexarotene may be due to loss of RXR expression on malignant T-cells. The main side effects are hyperlipidemia and central hypothyroidism, which occur in almost all patients and require anti-lipid agents and thyroid replacement therapy upon initiation of bexarotene. Retinoid A receptor retinoids can also be used in CTCL and include acitretin, as well as isotretinoin that is particularly effective for folliculotropic MF.[19,26]

IFN-α and IFN-γ are commonly used agents in treating MF/SS. IFN-α has been effective in 80% of early-stage patients and 70% of patients with SS. IFN-α is produced by dendritic cells and stimulates CD8+ T-cells and NK cells, resulting in an antitumor response. IFN-γ is produced by CD8+ T-cells and NK cells and activates dendritic cells and macrophages to enhance apoptosis of cancer cells.[26] Side effects include fever, chills, myalgias, weight loss, depression, leukopenia, thrombocytopenia, and abnormal liver function tests but are less common with low doses. IFN-γ is less likely to cause cognitive decline, depression, and neuropathy, and is thus more tolerable for older patients. The only formulation of IFN-α currently available in the use is the pegylated IFN-α, administered once weekly.

ECP is a systemic therapy for CTCL patients with blood involvement. Leukocytes are collected and exposed extracorporeally to 8-methoxypsoralen and UVA and then returned to the patient. The reinfused cells stimulate a selective immune response against the malignant cells. This therapy is performed on 2 consecutive days every 2 to 4 weeks, after which maintenance therapy is given less often. Recent studies have found response rates to be 33% for partial response (>50% skin improvement) and 41% for near-complete response (>90% skin improvement).

Patients recently diagnosed and with near-normal CD8 counts are appropriate treatment candidates.[26] ECP is often used in conjunction with other systemic therapies such as IFN-α and IFN-γ, oral bexarotene, TSEBT, and/or mogamulizumab as part of multimodality therapy with synergistic effect resulting from activation of different arms of the immune response to enhance long-term responses.

Targeted therapies include histone deacetylase inhibitors (vorinostat, romidepsin) that affect gene expression. They have been shown to cause cultured cancer cells to undergo arrest of growth, terminal differentiation, and apoptosis. Pralatrexate, an analog of methotrexate, disrupts vital enzymes in the gene synthesis of rapidly proliferating cancer cells, is another systemic agent used to treat refractory or advanced MF/SS.

Mogamulizumab is a novel monoclonal antibody directed against C-C chemokine receptor 4 (CCR4). In Phase 3 MAVORIC clinical trial, mogamulizumab treatment led to significantly greater progression-free survival compared to vorinostat. The overall global response rate of mogamulizumab was 35%, and 44% had a skin compartment response. In the vorinostat group, overall global response rate was 6% with 22% in the skin compartment response. Mogamulizumab is best used in patients with blood involvement and exhibits a median time to response of 1.1 months (1.0-1.2) in blood, 3.0 months (1.9-4.7) in skin, and 3.3 months (2.8-6.8) in lymph nodes. Notably, one side effect of mogamulizumab is a dermatitis, which can be difficult to distinguish from the cutaneous manifestations of the original disease and requires biopsy for diagnosis.[27]

Brentuximab vedotin (BV) is an anti-CD30 antibody-drug conjugate originally approved for relapsed/refractory Hodgkin lymphoma and systemic anaplastic large-cell lymphoma. The pivotal ALCANZA clinical trial compared brentuximab versus methotrexate or bexarotene in CTCL. At a median follow-up of 22.9 months, the BV group had 56.3% objective global response rate that lasted at least 4 months compared to 12.5% in the physician's choice group (who received methotrexate or bexarotene). Seventy-seven percent of patients in the brentuximab group experienced a 50% or greater reduction in their mSWAT compared to 41% in the physician's choice group. The average CD30 expression across all biopsy samples for patients was between 3% and 100%, suggesting that even with minimal CD30 expression, brentuximab can still be effective.[28] Brentuximab has also proven effective in patients with high Sézary counts.[29] The most common adverse effect is peripheral sensory neuropathy that limits long-term use.

Pembrolizumab, an immunoglobulin G4 anti-PD-1 monoclonal antibody, was utilized in a phase II open label clinical trial for refractory MF/SS patients. The overall response rate was 38% with two complete responders. At 1 year, the overall survival and progression-free survival were 95% and 65%, respectively. Programmed death-ligand 1 expression did not significantly differ between responders and nonresponders. The most common adverse event among patients with SS (54%, 8 out of 15) was worsening erythema and pruritus. However, symptoms resolved with supportive management and topical corticosteroids within 12 weeks without discontinuing the drug.[30]

There are emerging therapies for CTCL, including topical hypericin photodynamic therapy (PDT) for early-stage patch and plaque MF. According to the FLASH study, after 6 weeks of treatment, hypericin PDT was more effective than placebo with an index lesion response rate of 40% in patients who received two cycles of treatment.[31] Another emerging treatment is a monoclonal antibody targeting KIR3DL2, which is an inhibitory receptor found on natural killer (NK) cells and may be abnormally expressed on the surface of SS cells. KIR3DL2 has been proposed to be added to the ISCL/EORTC criteria for initial diagnosis of SS and B2 staging.[32] Recombinant IL-12 has also been cited to improve the immune dysregulation of CTCL in advanced-stage patients, although clinical development for CTCL is still in progress. Moreover, the success of Chimeric Antigen Receptor (CAR) T-cells in B-cell malignancies has been the impetus to evaluate the use of CAR T-cells in CTCL, which are currently being evaluated in clinical trials.[26]

Systemic chemotherapy can be used in advanced-stage patients with rapid tempo or refractory disease. Single-agent therapy can induce remission but relapses are common.[19] Agents showing the best results include methotrexate, pralatrexate, cyclophosphamide, cisplatin, etoposide, fludarabine, deoxycoformycin, bleomycin, doxorubicin, vincristine, and vinblastine. Nonmyeloablative allogeneic stem cell transplant is also considered for younger patients with high risk, advanced disease.

THERAPIES FOR PRURITUS

Pruritus is one of the most significant symptoms experienced by patients with erythrodermic MF/SS. Some tools used to quantify itch and the impact of itch on patients' quality of life include the Visual Analogue Scale (VAS) and Skindex-29. The VAS is a scale used to assess the presence of itch and intensity ranging from 0 (none) to 10 (worst imaginable). Skindex-16 and 29 are validated instruments designed to measure health-related quality of life in dermatological patients within the previous 4 weeks.[33]

The cytokine IL-31 has been implicated in the pathogenesis of itch among patients with CTCL. HDAC inhibitors have decreased pruritus and circulating IL-31 expression in patients. The majority of IL-31-producing malignant T-cells also express CCR4, which suggests mogamulizumab may improve pruritus among patients with CTCL with accompanying blood involvement.[34]

According to a 2021 systematic review, HDAC inhibitors such as romidepsin, vorinostat, quisinostat, and belinostat were most used for pruritus. Gabapentin and mirtazapine are oral therapies that have successfully reduced pruritus among patients with CTCL, but no studies on their clinical efficacy have been performed. Aprepitant, a neurokinin-1 antagonist, is another oral medication that effectively reduces pruritus within a short time (hours to days). Of note, patients who did not experience disease response from some therapies achieved relief from their pruritus.[34] Therefore, these agents may have a clinical benefit beyond disease response.

ACKNOWLEDGMENTS

The authors would like to thank Halliday Craige McDonald, Sharif Currimbhoy, and Amit G. Pandya for their contributions to the previous editions of this chapter.

REFERENCES

1. Durgin JS, Weiner DM, Wysocka M, Rook AH. The immunopathogenesis and immunotherapy of cutaneous T cell lymphoma: pathways and targets for immune restoration and tumor eradication. *J Am Acad Dermatol.* 2021;84(3):587-595.
2. Bobrowicz M, Fassnacht C, Ignatova D, Chang YT, DImitriou F, Guenova E. Pathogenesis and therapy of primary cutaneous T-cell lymphoma: collegium internationale allergologicum (CIA) update 2020. *Int Arch Allergy Immunol.* 2020;181(10):733-745.
3. Ghazawi FM, Alghazawi N, Le M, et al. Environmental and other extrinsic risk factors contributing to the pathogenesis of cutaneous T cell lymphoma (CTCL). *Front Oncol.* 2019;9(APR):1-8.
4. Chang ET, Delzell E. Systematic review and meta-analysis of glyphosate exposure and risk of lymphohematopoietic cancers. *J Environ Sci Heal - Part B Pestic Food Contam Agric Wastes.* 2016;51(6):402-434.
5. Del Guzzo CA, Kojadinovic A, Vinnakota RR, et al. Antibiotics and imiquimod for cutaneous T-cell lymphoma in veterans: a patient population with agent orange exposure. *Oncologist.* 2021;26(9):727-e1488.
6. Wong HK, Mishra A, Hake T, Porcu P. Evolving insights in the pathogenesis and therapy of cutaneous T-cell lymphoma (mycosis fungoides and Sezary syndrome). *Br J Haematol.* 2011;155(2):150-166.
7. Dobos G, Pohrt A, Ram-Wolff C, et al. Epidemiology of cutaneous t-cell lymphomas: a systematic review and meta-analysis of 16,953 patients. *Cancers (Basel).* 2020;12(10):1-14.
8. Criscione VD, Weinstock MA. Incidence of cutaneous T-cell lymphoma in the United States, 1973-2002. *Arch Dermatol.* 2007;143(7):854-859.
9. Allen PB, Goyal S, Niyogusaba T, et al. Clinical presentation and outcome differences between black patients and patients of other races and ethnicities with mycosis fungoides and Sézary syndrome. *JAMA Dermatol.* 2022;158(11):1293-1299.

10. Hinds GA, Heald P. Cutaneous T-cell lymphoma in skin of color. *J Am Acad Dermatol.* 2009;60(3):359-375.
11. Su C, Nguyen KA, Bai HX, et al. Racial disparity in mycosis fungoides: an analysis of 4495 cases from the US National Cancer Database. *J Am Acad Dermatol.* 2017;77(3):497-502.e2.
12. Agi C, Kuhn D, Chung J, Zampella J, Hinds G. Racial differences in the use of extracorporeal photopheresis for mycosis fungoides. *J Dermatolog Treat.* 2015;26(3):266-268.
13. Buechler CR, Sagher E, Tisack A, et al. Contribution of socioeconomic risk factors within a diverse mycosis fungoides cohort from Detroit, Michigan. *J Am Acad Dermatol.* 2022;87(4):897-900.
14. Espinosa ML, Walker CJ, Guitart J, Mhlaba JM. Morphology of mycosis fungoides and Sézary syndrome in skin of color. *Cutis.* 2022;109(3):3-7.
15. Querfeld C, Guitart J, Kuzel TM, Rosen ST. Primary cutaneous lymphomas: a review with current treatment options. *Blood Rev.* 2003;17(3):131-142.
16. Hodak E, Amitay-Laish I. Mycosis fungoides: a great imitator. *Clin Dermatol.* 2019;37(3):255-267.
17. Rodney IJ, Kindred C, Angra K, Qutub ON, Villanueva AR, Halder RM. Hypopigmented mycosis fungoides: a retrospective clinicohistopathologic study. *J Eur Acad Dermatology Venereol.* 2017;31(5):808-814.
18. Shi HZ, Jiang YQ, Xu XL, et al. Hypopigmented mycosis fungoides: a clinicopathological review of 32 patients. *Clin Cosmet Investig Dermatol.* 2022;15:1259-1264.
19. Jawed SI, Myskowski PL, Horwitz S, Moskowitz A, Querfeld C. Primary cutaneous T-cell lymphoma (mycosis fungoides and Sézary syndrome): Part II. Prognosis, management, and future directions. *J Am Acad Dermatol.* 2014;70(2):223.e1-223.e17.
20. Pavlovsky L, Mimouni D, Amitay-Laish I, Feinmesser M, David M, Hodak E. Hyperpigmented mycosis fungoides: an unusual variant of cutaneous T-cell lymphoma with a frequent CD8+ phenotype. *J Am Acad Dermatol.* 2012;67(1):69-75.
21. Jung JM, Lee MY, Won CH, Chang SE, Lee MW, Lee WJ. Hyperpigmented mycosis fungoides: a retrospective and comparative analysis with other subtypes of mycosis fungoides. *Leuk Lymphoma.* 2022;63(7):1598-1606.
22. Olsen EA, Whittaker S, Willemze R, et al. Primary cutaneous lymphoma: recommendations for clinical trial design and staging update from the ISCL, USCLC, and EORTC. *Blood.* 2022;140(5):419-437.
23. Kirsch IR, Watanabe R, O'Malley JT, et al. TCR sequencing facilitates diagnosis and identifies mature T cells as the cell of origin in CTCL. *Sci Transl Med.* 2015;7(308).
24. Rea B, Haun P, Emerson R, et al. Role of high-throughput sequencing in the diagnosis of cutaneous T-cell lymphoma. *J Clin Pathol.* 2018;71(9):814-820.
25. Elsayad K, Susek KH, Eich HT. Total skin electron beam therapy as part of multimodal treatment strategies for primary cutaneous T-cell lymphoma. *Oncol Res Treat.* 2017;40(5):244-252.
26. Weiner DM, Durgin JS, Wysocka M, Rook AH. The immunopathogenesis and immunotherapy of cutaneous T cell lymphoma: current and future approaches. *J Am Acad Dermatol.* 2021;84(3):597-604.
27. Kim YH, Bagot M, Pinter-Brown L, et al. Mogamulizumab versus vorinostat in previously treated cutaneous T-cell lymphoma (MAVORIC): an international, open-label, randomised, controlled phase 3 trial. *Lancet Oncol.* 2018;19(9):1192-1204.
28. Prince HM, Kim YH, Horwitz S, et al. Brentuximab vedotin or physician's choice in CD30-positive cutaneous T-cell lymphoma (ALCANZA): an international, open-label, randomised, phase 3, multicentre trial. *Lancet.* 2017;390(10094):555-566.
29. Lewis DJ, Haun PL, Samimi SS, et al. Brentuximab vedotin for relapsed or refractory Sézary syndrome. *JAMA Dermatology.* 2021;157(3):317-321.
30. Khodadoust MS, Rook AH, Porcu P, et al. Pembrolizumab in relapsed and refractory mycosis fungoides and Sézary syndrome: a multicenter phase II study. *J Clin Oncol.* 2020;38(1):20-28.
31. Kim EJ, Mangold AR, Desimone JA, et al. Efficacy and safety of topical hypericin photodynamic therapy for early-stage cutaneous T-cell lymphoma (mycosis fungoides): the FLASH phase 3 randomized clinical trial. *JAMA Dermatology.* 2022;158(9):1031-1039.
32. Roelens M, de Masson A, Ram-Wolff C, et al. Revisiting the initial diagnosis and blood staging of mycosis fungoides and Sézary syndrome with the KIR3DL2 marker. *Br J Dermatol.* 2020;182(6):1415-1422.
33. Serrano L, Martinez-Escala ME, Zhou XA, Guitart J. Pruritus in cutaneous T-cell lymphoma and Its management. *Dermatol Clin.* 2018;36(3):245-258.
34. Farrah G, Spruijt O, McCormack C, Buelens O, Lazarakis S, Prince M. A systematic review on the management of pruritus in patients with cutaneous T-cell lymphoma. *Itch.* 2021;6(2):e55-e55.

SECTION 8

Pigmentary Disorders

CHAPTER 56

Disorders of Facial Hyperpigmentation

Nicole C. Syder
Nada Elbuluk

KEY POINTS

- Disorders of hyperpigmentation that occur primarily on the face or that include the face are common particularly in skin of color and, due to their visibility, can have profound effects on quality of life.
- There is often a wide and overlapping list of differential diagnoses for disorders of facial hyperpigmentation, making it important to determine the correct diagnosis to inform appropriate management.
- Evaluation of facial melanoses involves a thorough clinical examination, detailed history, good lighting as well as Wood's lamp, dermoscopy, biopsy, and laboratory workup when needed.
- Treatment of facial hyperpigmentation can be extremely challenging, with sun protection being essential and some disorders being chronic and progressive or even recalcitrant to treatment. Combination therapies are often utilized and can be done safely and efficaciously in darker skin types.

INTRODUCTION

Facial hyperpigmentation, also referred to as facial melanoses, can result from a variety of conditions and is more commonly seen in skin of color (SOC) individuals with Fitzpatrick skin types III to VI. Hyperpigmentation is one of the most common reasons why patients of color seek dermatologic treatment.[1-3] In addition to posing diagnostic and therapeutic challenges, many of these conditions can have profound effects on quality of life (QoL). This chapter will provide a comprehensive overview of facial hyperpigmentation and important considerations regarding these conditions in SOC populations.

POSTINFLAMMATORY HYPERPIGMENTATION

Patients with postinflammatory hyperpigmentation (PIH) will typically present with light to dark brown macules or patches on various areas of the skin following an exogenous or endogenous insult to the skin [**Figures 56-1** and **56-2**]. Though it can occur in all skin types, it is more common and visible in SOC individuals.[4] It similarly affects both men and women across all ages. Various studies have demonstrated that PIH can be associated with profound psychological effects including decreased QoL and overall self-esteem.[1,4,5] It is important to note that PIH can last for many months to years, even with appropriate treatment.[4]

PIH results from an increase in melanocytic activity leading to melanogenesis and increased melanin production in response to an insult to the skin.[6] The pathogenesis involves the oxidation of arachidonic acid leading to the production of eicosanoids that are involved in cell signaling. Leukotriene D_4, leukotriene C_4, thromboxane B_2, prostaglandin E_2, histamine as well as reactive oxygen species can be released during the inflammatory response, resulting in the proliferation of melanocytes and the increase in melanogenesis.[4] The insult can be from an exogenous injury or from an endogenous inflammatory cutaneous condition. The extent of injury can affect the degree of melanogenesis and if the melanin deposition occurs in the epidermis and/or dermis. Histopathologic features of this condition can include increased melanin concentration in the epidermis, melanophages in the upper layer of the dermis, and lymphohistiocytes around blood vessels in the dermal papilla.[1] Dermoscopic findings, although not well described in the current literature, may include light to dark brown or blue pigment deposition.[7]

The treatment of PIH begins with removing the trigger that is perpetuating the cycle of inflammation. This first step is paramount to adequately treating PIH when the source is endogenous. Hydroquinone (HQ) and retinoids along with combinations of the two, with or without steroids have been considered gold standards of treatment.[8] Numerous other topical lightening agents have been used including azelaic acid, glycolic acid, salicylic acid, arbutin, kojic acid, licorice extracts, niacinamide, and vitamin C.[9] There are also oral and procedural therapies that can be used either as monotherapy or in combination with topical treatments.[8] The current evidence to support systemic agents for the treatment of PIH is limited, but tranexamic acid has demonstrated efficacy in limited studies.[8]

Procedural therapies including lasers and pulsed light therapy have been used with varying efficacy, often adjunctively with topical therapies. A systematic review found that the most extensively studied laser was the Q-switched (QS) ND:YAG laser that demonstrated favorable results in the treatment of PIH in various trials.[10] Other lasers included the QS ruby laser and CO_2 fractional laser; however, some studies demonstrated no improvement or worsening of the PIH following therapy. The picosecond lasers including the 755 nm alexandrite have also been found to be a safe and efficacious treatment modality for PIH in SOC.[11] The picosecond lasers may be a more favorable alternative to QS lasers in patients with SOC. Microneedling has also been shown to be a safe and efficacious treatment modality. A few studies have shown that microneedling in combination with Rucinol and sophora-alpha serum, triple combination creams, or tranexamic acid resulted in overall improvement in hyperpigmentation.[12] Chemical peels, particularly superficial peeling agents, and dermabrasion have also demonstrated similarly varying levels of benefit in the treatment of PIH.[8] As with all procedural-based therapies, caution should be taken with conservative settings (ie, low fluence, longer pulse duration, lower treatment density) and performing of test spots when treating patients of darker skin phototypes to avoid any new or worsening PIH. Sun protection is critical in the management of PIH and is a cornerstone of any regimen to prevent worsening of the pigmentation. Further studies using validated outcome measures are also needed to evaluate best treatment outcomes for PIH. The postacne hyperpigmentation index (PAHPI) is one such scale developed in recent years as a validated outcome measure for assessing the efficacy of therapies in those with acne-induced PIH.[11]

LICHEN PLANUS PIGMENTOSUS

Lichen planus pigmentosus (LPP) is a variant of lichen planus that presents with gray to dark brown or blue ill-defined macules and patches typically on photo-exposed areas such as the temples, forehead, neck, and upper extremities. It can be pruritic and most commonly presents in middle-aged individuals with darker skin phototypes (III-VI), phototype IV being the most common.[13-15]

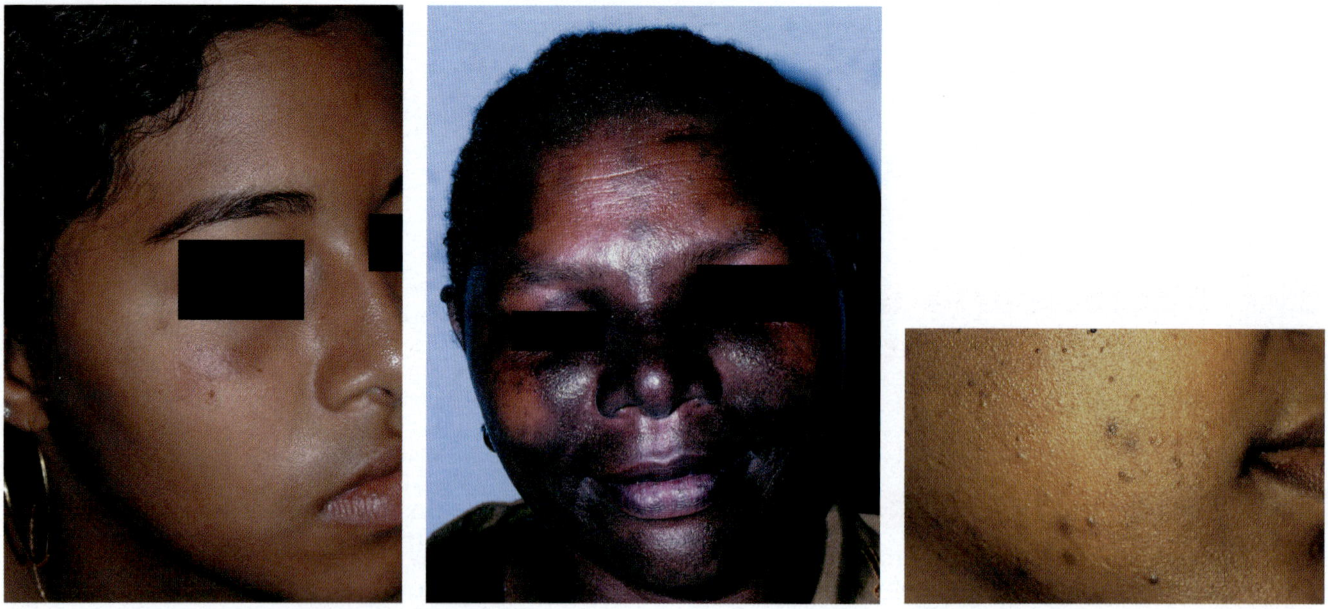

A B C

FIGURE 56-1. Postinflammatory hyperpigmentation (PIH) (A) PIH from acne in a woman with skin type V. (B) PIH on the face of a woman with skin type VI. (Used with permission of Dr. Barbara J. Leppard.) (C) PIH on the cheek of a Hispanic woman with skin type IV.

The cause of lichen planus pigmentosus has not been fully elucidated; however, it has been shown to be associated with hepatitis C infection, ultraviolet exposure, mustard oil, and amla oil.[16] It has also been found to be associated with endocrinopathies such as type 2 diabetes, thyroid disease, and dyslipidemia at 38%, 22%, and 50%, respectively.[17] Differential diagnoses include erythema dyschromicum perstans, drug-induced pigmentation, pigmented contact dermatitis, argyria, and PIH.[18]

LPP can occur in association with frontal fibrosing alopecia (FFA) and facial papules, particularly in women of color. A study from Durban, South Africa reported on 24 cases of LPP preceding FFA by an average of 14 months. The study found that all patients not only presented with LPP and concomitant frontotemporal hair loss but several also exhibited facial papules on the forehead and cheeks, another finding associated with FFA.[19]

There are various patterns of LPP including blaschkoid, inverse, reticular, diffuse, blotchy, annular, gyrate, linear, perifollicular, and zosteriform.[20] LPP-inversus (LPPI) is a rare pattern that typically manifests as medium to dark brown to brown-gray patches affecting intertriginous areas, primarily the axillae. On histopathology, vacuolar degeneration of the basal cell layer coupled with perivascular or lichenoid type infiltrate, superficial dermal melanophages, pigmentary incontinence, and keratinocyte apoptosis is evident in active LPP.[16] A biopsy from older areas of LPP may show lymphocytic infiltrate, melanophages in the superficial dermis, an atrophic, effaced epidermis, and mild vacuolar changes with necrotic keratinoctyes.[16,18] On dermoscopy, patterns that can be seen include pseudonetwork, speckled dots, uniform dotted, dots in circles, and overlapping patterns of these.[7] Rhomboidal structures, erythema, follicular asymmetry, telangiectasias, and decreased vellus hairs may also be evident.

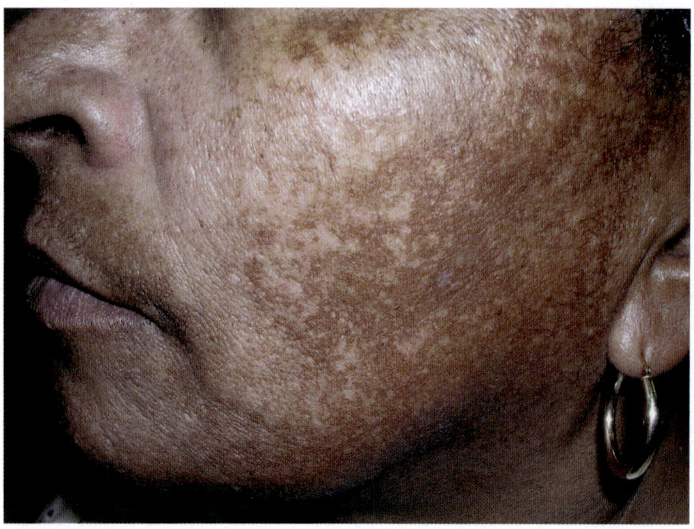

FIGURE 56-2. Melasma of the cheek in a patient with skin of color.

LPP can be difficult to treat, chronic and progressive. Many studies exploring efficacious treatment options have small sample sizes and relatively low levels of evidence.[14] Treatment includes topical, oral, and/or procedural therapies. Hydroquinone (HQ) is a commonly used topical agent, sometimes in conjunction with azelaic acid, retinoids, corticosteroids, kojic or glycolic acid.[20] Oral therapy such as low-dose isotretinoin and hydroxychloroquine have shown efficacy in several studies.[21-23] Chemical peels including modified phenol peels have been used safely and effectively to improve the hyperpigmentation from LPP.[24] Various lasers have also been studied in the management of LPP. A nonrandomized prospective study found that 5 to 6 sessions of 1064 nm Q-switched Nd-YAG (QSNYL) laser was effective in initiating significant clearance.[25] Picosecond lasers have also been successfully used in combination with topical tacrolimus and oral hydroxychloroquine in the treatment of LPP.[23] As with other disorders of hyperpigmentation, diligent use and reapplication of tinted sunscreens containing iron oxides is essential.

ERYTHEMA DYSCHROMICUM PERSTANS

Erythema dyschromicum perstans (EDP) is a rare type of acquired dermal macular hyperpigmentation.[26] It is also commonly known as ashy dermatosis though some have considered these terms to be separate entities. In this chapter, they will be considered as the same entity. The hallmark of early EDP is erythema around the border of pigmented macules or patches.[27] It is important to note, however, that a study found that only ~17.3% of EDP cases presented with the characteristic erythematous halo.[28] Middle to late stage EDP presents with symmetric brown or gray-brown to blue macules and patches most commonly on the proximal extremities, neck, and trunk and uncommonly occurs on the face. Facial presentation alone should raise concern for lichen planus pigmentosus.[26] It can occur at any age and the prevalence is the same between males and females.[26] It has been found to be more common in Latin America and in adults with Fitzpatrick skin type III and IV.

The etiology of EDP is largely unknown, but it is widely accepted that genetic and environmental factors play a significant role. Associations include viral infection, ammonium nitrate, X-ray contrast, parasitic infection, omeprazole, oral antimicrobials, and benzodiazepines.[29] Histopathologic findings of active EDP include interface dermatitis with basal vacuolization, pigment incontinence, and perivascular mononuclear infiltrates. Older areas of EDP, pathology may show epidermal atrophy, apoptotic keratinocytes, and moderate pigmentary incontinence.[30] Dermoscopic findings may reveal either a diffuse or linear distribution of pinpoint gray dots on a blue/gray background.[7] Differential diagnosis includes lichen planus pigmentosus, lichenoid drug eruption, idiopathic eruptive macular hyperpigmentation, urticaria pigmentosa, drug-induced pigmentation, and postinflammatory hyperpigmentation.[18,27]

In prepubescent children, EDP may self-resolve within 2 to 3 years. In adults, it can be progressive and persistent.[29] No one treatment has proven to be particularly effective in treating this condition, but patients have demonstrated improvement in pigmentation with various topical, oral, and procedural therapies including combination therapies. Topical treatments utilized include corticosteroids, calcineurin inhibitors, HQ, and tretinoin. Topical tacrolimus 0.1% ointment applied to the face, neck, upper trunk, and extremities twice daily for 3 months with no concurrent treatment demonstrated significant improvement with no recurrence after 1 year.[31] Oral treatments include dapsone (100 mg daily), clofazimine (100 mg every other day), isotretinoin (<0.5 mg/kg), pentoxifylline, macrolides, minocycline, and tranexamic acid.[27,32] In terms of procedural therapies, a systematic review and meta-analysis found that narrowband UVB phototherapy was also effective with few side effects.[33] Nonablative fractional laser in combination with topical tacrolimus has also been shown to be an effective combination therapy.[27]

MELASMA

Melasma is a common acquired melanosis in which patients present with light to dark brown macules and reticulated patches that are typically bilateral[34] [**Figure 56-2**]. It most commonly occurs on the face and has the following distributions: centrofacial, malar, and mandibular.[35] Melasma can be epidermal, dermal, or mixed.[36] Extrafacial melasma that is less common can also occur on the forearms, neck, back, and sternum.[37] It is more commonly seen in women but can also present in men, with women being affected nine times more than their male counterparts.[34] Those with extrafacial melasma are typically postmenopausal women on supplementary forms of estrogen with risk factors that include a personal history of facial melasma, and/or a family history of either facial or extrafacial melasma.[38]

Melasma can occur in all skin types but is more common in individuals with SOC, with a prevalence of 9% to 30% among Latin American populations, 40% among South-East Asian and South Asian populations, and 13.4% to 15.5% prevalence among Arab-American populations.[39] Melasma can have a significant impact on the QoL of affected individuals, especially when it is recalcitrant to treatment.[40] It can affect self-esteem as well as promote anxiety and depressive disorders. The Melasma Quality of Life Score (MelasQoL) is the only validated instrument to evaluate QoL related to melasma.[41]

Melasma has been found to be associated with hormonal exposure that can include pregnancy, a history of oral contraceptive use and/or hormone replacement therapy.[34] Genetic factors, ultraviolet (UV), and visible light exposure have also been found to play a role in the etiology of melasma. Approximately half of affected individuals report a family history of melasma. Differential diagnosis includes ephelides, solar lentigines, Hori nevi, nevus of Ota, Riehl melanosis, toxic melanoderma, ochronosis, frictional melanosis, and PIH.[42]

Wood's lamp evaluation for melasma can help reveal if it is epidermal, dermal, or mixed and therefore can help predict response to treatment modalities as well.[42] Histopathologic analysis typically reveals an increase in melanin in either the epidermis, dermis, or both. Inflammation is minimal or completely absent.[34] Melanogenesis is increased, but whether or not there is a quantitative increase in melanocytes is still debated.[43] Dermoscopic findings include a pseudonetwork pattern sparing adnexal openings.[7] Brown globules, dots, and annular and arcuate structures can sometimes also be seen. Evolving research has demonstrated that the pathogenesis of melasma also includes gene regulation abnormalities, keratinocyte, and mast cell involvement, as well as increased vascularization and disruption of the basement membrane. The number of mast cells in melasma-affected skin is higher than in unaffected skin, and these mast cells also contribute to hypervascularization, a key finding in melasma.[43]

Treatment of melasma is made more challenging as it can be exacerbated by exposure to UV-B (290-320 nm), UV-A (320-400 nm), and visible light (400-700 nm), all of which can induce the production of α-melanocyte-stimulating hormone, corticotropin, interleukin 1, and endothelin 1 and contribute to increased melanin production.

Melasma does not have a cure but has many treatments to improve it and keep it in remission. Treatment for melasma first and foremost requires diligent sun protection with the use of an SPF 30+, broad spectrum, tinted sunscreen that helps blocks UV and visible light. An evidence-based review concluded that HQ monotherapy and triple combination cream (hydroquinone, tretinoin, and corticosteroid) were the most effective and largely studied topical therapies for melasma.[40] Though hydroquinone is the most widely used depigmenting agent, adverse effects include irritant dermatitis and ochronosis with prolonged use. Risk for ochronosis can vary based on percentage and time frame used. These risks have also led to the creation of many non-hydroquinone-containing alternatives.[44] Nonhydroquinone lightening agents used for melasma include glycolic acid, arbutin, retinoids, licorice extracts, azelaic acid, niacinamide, kojic acid, vitamin C, cysteamine, malassezin, salicylic acid, and silymarin.[9,45,46]

Procedural therapies such as chemical peels and laser/light therapies are also used in treating melasma, often adjunctively with topical regimens. Chemical peels used for melasma include glycolic acid, mandelic acid, trichloroacetic acid, salicylic acid, tretinoin peels, and combination peels like Jessner.[40,47] Lasers and light-based therapies used for melasma include pulsed-dye laser, QS-Nd:YAG laser, intense pulsed light (IPL), picosecond lasers, and fractional CO_2 lasers. A procedure referred to as "laser toning," a multipass technique, with a low-fluence QS-Nd:YAG has been a common treatment option for melasma; however, one notable adverse effect associated with this procedure is mottled hypopigmentation.[40,48] This along with rebound melasma are two risk factors for the treatment of melasma with lasers and lights.[40]

The intradermal application of platelet-rich plasma (PRP) has also been shown to be effective in a few studies for the treatment of melasma.[49] The impact of PRP on melasma is related to growth factors in the platelets that play a significant role in inhibiting melanogenesis.[50] Oral tranexamic acid (TA; 250-325 mg once to twice daily), an antifibrinolytic agent originally indicated for menorrhagia, has also shown efficacy in recent years in treating melasma. TA has also been studied topically in 2% to 5% formulations and as an intradermal injection at varying concentrations.[40,51] Prior to initiation, patients must still be screened for contraindications to TA use including renal dysfunction, malignancy, current anticoagulant therapy, and cardiovascular disease.[52] Oral TA as adjuvant therapy can be helpful in preventing rebound melasma. Further studies on long-term effects of oral TA on melasma are necessary.

Continued studies are being conducted to evaluate the success of melasma treatments. Two of the validated indices that have been used in many studies to measure melasma severity and response to treatment include the Melasma Area and Severity Index (MASI) and the modified MASI score.[53] The new modified MASI score (mMASI) includes an expanded more comprehensive, scoring system to the original MASI.[53]

RIEHL MELANOSIS (PIGMENTED CONTACT DERMATITIS)

Riehl melanosis (RM), also commonly referred to as pigmented contact dermatitis, is an acquired allergic contact dermatitis.[54] In 1917 and at the time of World War I, dermatologist Dr. Gustav Riehl identified various individuals with facial pigmentation and attributed it to war-time food substitutes. "Riehl melanosis" eventually became a popular term during the years between the first two world wars to describe a facial melanosis that was caused by an external chemical agent. Affected individuals typically present with brown to violaceous scaly macules and patches on the face and other photo-exposed sites.[54] Pruritus, erythema, and edema can occur before the hyperpigmentation manifests. It is most commonly seen in young to middle-aged women with darker skin phototypes. Many cases have been reported in Japan, as well as in South Africa, South America, India, and Europe.[54]

The causes of RM can vary significantly as it is typically triggered by one or more of several different allergens.[55] Cosmetic allergens include aniline dyes, pigments containing phenyl-azo-e-naphthol, hydroperoxides of limonene, henna, and ricinoleic acid, a bactericidal agent.[56] Perfume allergens include but are not limited to lemon oil (a photosensitizer allergen), benzyl-salicylate, hydroxycitronellal, jasmine absolute, eugenol, cinnamic derivatives, and lavender oil. Common ingredients in textile and occupational agents can also be allergens.

Understanding of the pathogenesis of RM remains limited. Histopathologic studies have found increased dermal expression intensities of stem cell factor, c-kit, epidermal, and dermal ET-1.[57] Histopathology depicts increased melanin pigment in the epidermis and/or dermis with a significant increase in the number and activity of melanocytes. Basal cell liquefaction, epidermal spongiosis, and pigmentary incontinence is also present.[58] Dermoscopy will likely show a pseudonetwork with gray dots and globules, as well as telangiectatic vessels with erythema.[7] Other more unique features may include slight scale, follicular keratotic plugs, and perifollicular hyperpigmented halos. Differential diagnosis includes melasma, LPP, EDP, Addison disease, frictional melanosis, allergic contact dermatitis, berloque dermatitis, ochronosis, poikiloderma of Civatte, and idiopathic eruptive macular pigmentation.[59,60]

Patch testing is recommended in the diagnostic workup of RM. It should include standard series, cosmetic series, fragrance series, as well as all of the patient's topical products. Photopatch testing can also be considered.[54] A treatment regimen for RM begins with identifying and completely eliminating the causative agent. There are no standardized therapies for RM, but topical lightening agents such as retinoids, ascorbic acid, hydroquinone, niacinamide, glycolic acid, and azelaic acid can be beneficial.[9] Superficial to medium chemical peels including trichloroacetic acid or glycolic acid can be paired with a topical regimen for synergistic effect.[54] Light-based and laser therapies with intense pulsed-light, low-fluence QS-Nd: YAG lasers, or 755-nm and 1064-nm picosecond lasers have also been shown to be effective procedural options.[54]

EXOGENOUS OCHRONOSIS

Exogenous ochronosis (EO) is considered a challenging and at times irreversible pigmentary disorder that typically arises after extended and continuous use of phenolic acids often for greater than 1 year. It primarily occurs in response to use of topical hydroquinone-containing skin-lightening products.[61]

EO presents with dark brown to blue-black macules, patches, papules, plaques, and/or nodules typically on the face where the culprit product has been applied [**Figure 56-3**]. The clinical grading scheme for EO consists of grades I to V. Grade I consists of faint macular pigmentation, while grade II presents as more of macular stippling or small caviar-like papules. Grade III is characterized by dark deposits and papules, grade IV manifests as colloidal milia that are 1 mm or larger in size, and grade V is consistent with keloid-like nodules and cysts.[62] EO has no predilection for men or women and patients with darker skin are the most affected group, as they tend to utilize hydroquinone-containing products at a higher frequency.[62]

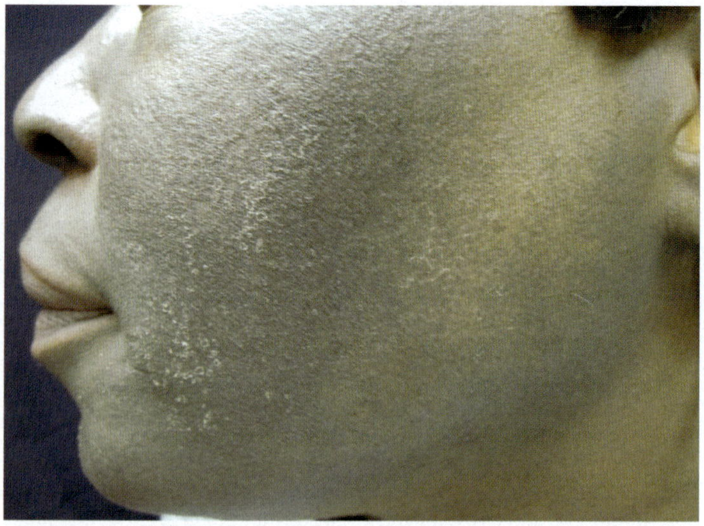

FIGURE 56-3. Exogenous ochronosis in a woman with skin of color.

The etiology of EO is largely related to high and unknown concentrations of long-term topical exposure to phenols such as carbolic acid, picric acid, resorcinol, and hydroquinone.[61] Hydroquinone has been the most heavily implicated phenol in the cause of EO. The characteristic histologic findings include yellow-brown "banana-shaped" collagen pigment deposits in the papillary dermis.[63] Dermoscopic findings consist of brown, black, or blue-gray globular, annular, or arciform structures.[7] The obliteration of follicular openings, along with telangiectasias, and structureless areas in a scattered configuration may also be seen. Differential diagnosis includes nevus of Ota, PIH, drug-induced pigmentation, pigmented contact dermatitis, maturational hyperpigmentation Hori nevi, and melasma.[64,65]

Treatment for EO is extremely difficult and often unsuccessful. The most effective approach is complete prevention by limiting the use of causative phenolic acids, particularly hydroquinone. Use of such products should also be done under the supervision of a board-certified dermatologist. Individuals with other pigmentary disorders that are likely to be treated with hydroquinone-containing products are most at risk of developing EO. A literature review found that most cases were the consequence of lower percentage HQ creams (1-2%) compared to HQ 3% to 4%.[62] This finding demonstrates that lower concentrations applied for long periods or with an increased frequency of use can be higher risk factors for EO.

Mixed responses with mild improvement have been demonstrated with topical treatments such as retinoic acid monotherapy or low potency topical corticosteroids.[66] Procedurally, dermabrasion has been used as well as various laser therapies. The latter include the QS alexandrite, QS Nd:YAG, and picosecond lasers that have been used to target the ochronotic pigment with minimal side effects.[67,68] Fractional nonablative picosecond lasers starting at 532 and 1064 nm have been successful in improving ochronosis and skin texture.[68] Other light-based modalities such as IPL have also been used with improvement.[69]

ACTINIC LICHEN PLANUS

Actinic lichen planus (LP) is considered a photosensitive variant of lichen planus. Affected individuals can vary in presentation predominantly in sun-exposed sites with classic lichenoid papules, annular hyperpigmented plaques, white pin-point, coalescent papules, as well as diffuse facial erythema.[70]

It is most commonly seen in individuals of Middle Eastern, African, or South Asian descent. It often presents in the third decade of life, but there have been some cases of affected children.[71] The cause of actinic LP is thought to be multifactorial, including genetic factors and subtropical climates. Sunlight exposure seems to be a significant triggering factor. In some patients, phototests with repeated irradiations with UV-B on consecutive days have also been shown to induce these lesions, thus reinforcing the role of sunlight exposure in this condition.[70] The exact pathogenesis of actinic LP has not been entirely elucidated, but because most patients with actinic LP come from certain geographic regions, it is postulated that genetic as well as environmental factors may contribute.[72]

Histopathology demonstrates apoptotic keratinocytes with a band-like lymphocytic infiltrate and histiocytes. Vacuolar alterations and pigmentary incontinence are also evident.[70] Differential diagnosis includes granuloma annulare, discoid lupus erythematosus, fixed drug eruption, and secondary syphilis.[73] Treatment for actinic lichen planus is mainly based on case reports, but a universal theme is the importance of sun-protective measures. A few successes have been achieved with the use of hydroxychloroquine, intralesional glucocorticoids, and acitretin.[74]

LENTIGINES AND EPHELIDES

Solar lentigines and ephelides, colloquially referred to as sun spots and freckles, respectively, are very common conditions of facial hyperpigmentation. Solar lentigines appear as light brown to dark brown macules in sun-exposed areas, while ephelides are typically small (1-2 mm) light brown to red brown macules in a similar distribution[75] [**Figures 56-4** and **56-5**]. Solar lentigines typically accumulate with age and are quite common after age 50 mainly in skin types I and III, while ephelides tend to appear within the first 2 to 3 years of age with sun exposure mainly in skin types I and II.[75]

Genetics determine the eventual development of ephelides over the course of one's lifetime and are induced by sun exposure.[75] Solar lentigines are also induced by sun exposure but are not genetically predetermined and are typically an indication of photodamage. The pathogenesis of these conditions has not been thoroughly explored; however, a study concluded that FGFR3 and PIK3CA mutations are involved in the pathogenesis of solar lentigines.[76] It has been speculated that UV exposure induces these mutations. It has been concluded that additive genetic effects explain ~91% of the variance in ephelide counts and that environmental effects are less impactful.[75] Genes associated with the development of ephelides include *MC1R*, *IRF4*, *ASIP*, *TYR*, and *BNC2*.

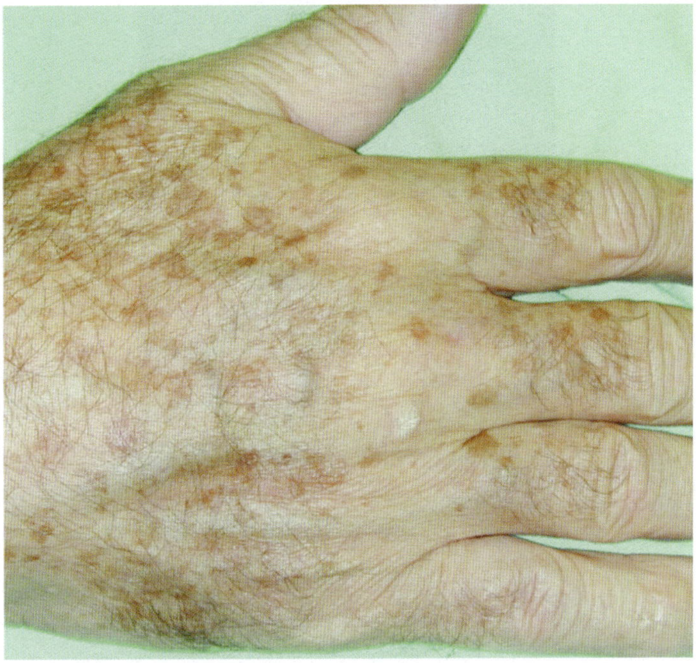

FIGURE 56-5. Solar lentigines on the dorsal hand.

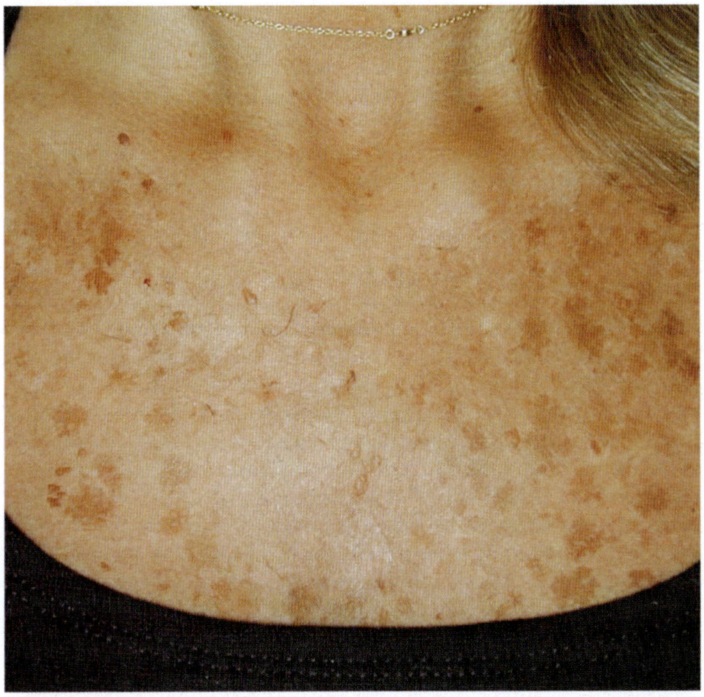

FIGURE 56-4. Solar lentigines on the chest of a patient who had early and intense sun exposure.

Both solar lentigines and ephelides have a hyperpigmented basal layer and elongated epidermal ridges on histology.[75] In both conditions, melanocyte number is increased, but melanocyte size is larger with more dendrites in ephelides, while size remains normal in lentigines. Melanosome number and size are increased in ephelides but normal in lentigines.[75] Dermoscopy of solar lentigines reveal irregular but well-defined borders, akin to "moth-eaten edges."[7] A pigment network may be present. Ephelides tend to look very similar on dermoscopy, with "moth-eaten borders" and homogenous pigmentation.

Treatments for solar lentigines and ephelides include topical creams, cryotherapy, chemical peels, and laser therapy.[77] Topical agents used include retinoids, HQ, and imiquimod cream.[78] Cryopeeling and trichloroacetic acid have been used, with cryopeeling producing the faster, more superior improvement.[79] Cryopeeling is the process of using cryotherapy diffusely on the surface of the skin, particularly in photo-damaged areas to promote cell turnover and desquamation.[80] Additional peels used for the treatment of solar lentigines and ephelides include retinoic acid, glycolic acid, and lactic acid.[81]

Lasers used include argon, 532 nm QS-Nd:YAG, QSRL (Q-switched ruby laser), QSAL (Q-switched alexandrite laser), long-pulsed alexandrite lasers, and nonablative picosecond lasers.[82] A study compared the use of the QS-Nd:YAG laser and fractional carbon dioxide laser for the treatment of solar lentigines and found the QS-Nd:YAG laser to be superior, with the caveat of longer healing times and increased discomfort with treatment.[83] Combination treatments of topical and procedural modalities have also been found to be efficacious.[84] Posttreatment topical lightening agents including retinoids have also been used for maintenance treatment. Diligent sunscreen use is also an essential component of treatment and prevention.

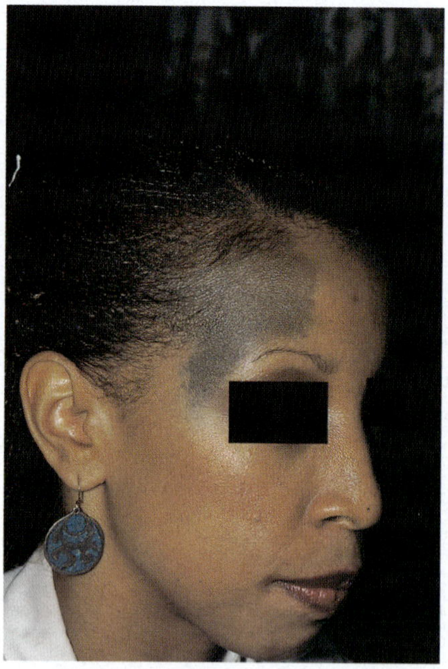

FIGURE 56-6. Nevus of Ota on the right forehead of an African American woman.

NEVUS OF OTA AND NEVUS OF ITO

Nevus of Ota, a periocular dermal melanocytosis, is a benign, typically unilateral, melanosis involving dark brown to blue-gray macules and patches along the distribution of the trigeminal nerve, particularly the ophthalmic V1 and maxillary V2 divisions.[85] Affected individuals may also present with a blue-gray pigmentation of the eye and its adnexa [**Figures 56-6** and **56-7**]. It is most common among females of Asian and African descent. The melanosis will most often be present at birth, but it can also appear during periods of increased hormonal activity such as puberty or pregnancy. Of note, although not on the face, nevus of Ito is also a dermal melanocytosis but involves the distribution of the posterior supraclavicular nerves and the lateral cutaneous brachial nerves of the shoulder.

The etiology of these conditions is unclear, but one proposed hypothesis is that melanocytes fail to migrate from neural crest cells to the basal layer of the epidermis.[85] With this failure of migration, the dermis contains excessive melanocytes. Although there is an increased number of melanocytes in the dermis, malignant degeneration is rare and the prognosis for these conditions is favorable. Histopathology reveals superficially concentrated, spindle-shaped or dendritic, pigmented melanocytes. Differential diagnoses for nevus of Ota and nevus of Ito include lentigo, blue nevi, cutaneous melanoma, melasma, ochronosis, and congenital dermal melanocytosis.[86,87]

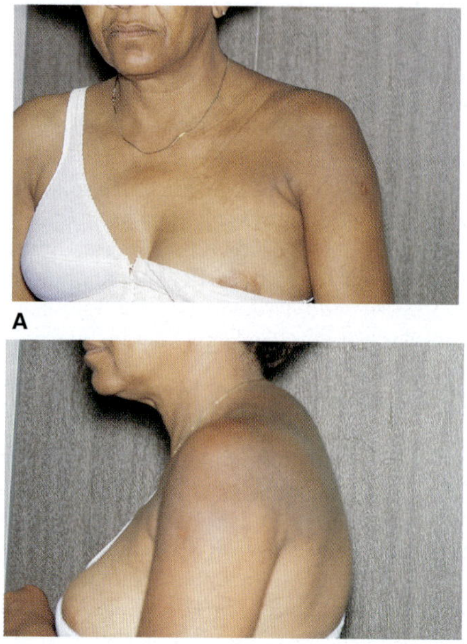

A

B

FIGURE 56-7. Nevus of Ito along **(A)** the left shoulder and **(B)** the upper back.

A 10-year retrospective study found that early treatment of nevus of Ota improved outcomes.[88] The initiation of laser treatment before the age of 5 years lead to a significant improvement in therapeutic outcomes with a low risk of recurrence or adverse effects. QS and picosecond lasers are considered the gold standard for the treatment of Nevus of Ito and Nevus of Ota; however, they should be used with caution and conservative settings in patients with darker skin phototypes as they work by photothermal and mechanical destruction of melanocytes and could lead to hyper/hypopigmentation. A longer wavelength, lower fluence, and longer pulse duration can be used for patients with darker skin types to reduce the risk of epidermal damage and PIH.[82]

HORI NEVI

Hori nevi is a facial dermal melanocytosis presenting with speckled light to dark brown or brown-gray macules on the zygomatic regions of the face, bilaterally.[89] It most commonly affects middle-aged, East Asian females.[72]

Various factors have been considered in the pathogenesis of Hori's nevi such as the relocation of follicular bulb melanocytes or the reactivation of dermal melanocytes already present in the affected areas, which could occur as a consequence of various factors such as dermal inflammation, ultraviolet irradiation, or hormonal disturbance.[90] Diagnosis can be made clinically but biopsy can be done in cases of uncertainty to confirm the diagnosis.[90]

Treatment options include procedural therapies such as dermabrasion and lasers. Selective photothermolysis through lasers such as the QSRL 694 nm, QS Nd:YAG (532 and 1064 nm), QSAL 755 nm, and now picosecond lasers are considered among the most efficacious treatment options for Hori nevi. A systematic review concluded that QSAL, QS:NYL, ER:YAG, QSRL, and CO_2 lasers were more commonly used for the treatment of Hori nevi, and dermabrasion was less popular because it was a more invasive and crude process.[90] A split-faced single-blinded randomized study found that when compared to the alexandrite 755-nm nanosecond laser (QSAL), the 755-nm picosecond laser achieved higher patient satisfaction rates and lower rates of PIH.[90] Additionally, combination laser therapies such as fractional nonablative Er:YAG and QS Nd:YAG 1064 nm laser treatments can work synergistically to produce favorable results with few adverse effects.

MATURATIONAL DYSCHROMIA

Maturational dyschromia or maturational hyperpigmentation (MH) is a more recently coined entity presenting with dark brown to gray macules and patches with ill-defined borders on the lateral forehead and/or zygomatic region of the face.[91] To date, it has been mainly described in Black and South Asian patients. Associations include adult-onset, obesity, lack of cutaneous symptoms, and predilection for occurring on the patient's most common sleeping side.[91] It has been postulated that MH may be a cutaneous marker of metabolic syndrome due to the presence of hyperinsulinemia and fasting hyperglycemia in many affected patients. Differential diagnosis includes frictional melanosis, facial acanthosis nigricans, melasma, nevus of Ota, and PIH.

The pathogenesis of MH is currently not well understood, but chronic sun exposure is felt to be involved, with obesity and diabetes serving as predisposing factors. Histopathology may reveal proliferation of melanocytes in the dermis and epidermis, papillomatous epidermal proliferation, and minimal or absent dermal inflammation.[91] Patients with this condition should be referred for workup of metabolic syndrome. Treatments for MH are similar to the topical and procedural treatments detailed for melasma earlier in this chapter.

PERIORBITAL MELANOSIS

Periorbital melanosis (POM) is a very common condition in which individuals present with bilateral periocular or semi-circular brown or dark-brown macules and patches.[92] The inferior eyelid is most often affected, but the entire periocular skin may also be involved [**Figure 56-8**]. This condition has no increased predilection for males or females and is most commonly seen in individuals with darker skin phototypes. There are multiple causes of POM including physiologic causes, inflammatory conditions, advanced age, genetics, facial anatomy, systemic conditions, and sun exposure.[93] Additionally, the underlying vasculature of the infraorbital skin combined with the thinness of the lower eyelids can also contribute to the Tyndall effect. This can cause a darkened blue to blue gray appearance of the skin in those with lighter skin and a violaceous to dark brown appearance in darker skin types. Physiologic causes include fatigue and chronic lack of sleep. Aging can lead to infraorbital hollowing that can increase the darkened appearance of the skin. Inflammatory processes such as atopic or allergic dermatitis can also contribute to POM through the formation of allergic shiners and lichenification of infraorbital skin.[92] Less common causes include systemic diseases such as Addison disease, hereditary blood disorders, and disorders of the liver.[93]

The pathogenesis of this condition and treatment options depends on the cause of the pigmentation.[93] When the cause is related to increased melanin deposition, topical lightening agents such as hydroquinone, retinols, α-arbutin, azelaic acid, and kojic acid can be used.[94] Chemical peels such as ferulic acid peels, lactic acid peels, and glycolic acid peels formulated for the periocular area can also be quite effective in improving periorbital hyperpigmentation.[95] If the POM is secondary to facial anatomy including infraorbital hollowing that can increase with aging, treatment with hyaluronic acid fillers can be used safely and effectively with excellent cosmetic results.[96] Inflammatory conditions such as atopic dermatitis or contact dermatitis should be appropriately treated with topical anti-inflammatory treatments such as calcineurin inhibitors or topical steroids and patients should be advised to avoid rubbing the area that can contribute to lichenification and darkening. When POM is secondary to systemic diseases, the underlying systemic condition must be treated.

POST-CHIKUNGUNYA HYPERPIGMENTATION

Post-Chikungunya hyperpigmentation is cutaneous manifestation of Chikungunya fever in which affected individuals present with centrofacial freckle-like macules with diffuse hyperpigmentation on the face and extremities.[97] Patients may also present with significantly concentrated dark brown macules or patches on the nose a few weeks following the Chikungunya fever, termed "Chik-sign." This discoloration can persist for 6 months or longer.[98]

Chikungunya fever is a viral infection that is endemic on the Indian subcontinent, in African, Southeast Asia, the Pacific, and sub-tropical regions of the North and South America.[97] It is caused by an arbovirus and transmitted from the Aedes mosquito.

It is currently theorized that the hyperpigmentation may be caused by increased intraepidermal melanin dispersion or retention triggered by the virus.[98] The presence of hyperpigmentation in this characteristic distribution on the nose could be beneficial in retrospectively diagnosing chikungunya fever. Regarding treatment, one case report demonstrated that 4 weeks of topical hydroquinone use was effective in decreasing hyperpigmentation.[97] Sun protection is also integral to any treatment regimen for this condition.

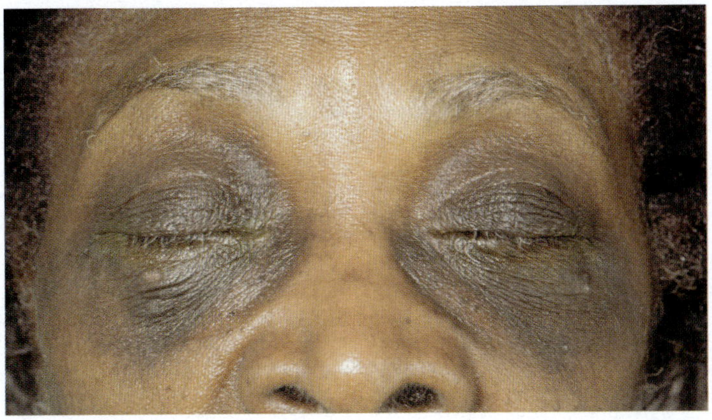

FIGURE 56-8. Periorbital hyperpigmentation in a woman of color.

CONCLUSION

As presented in this chapter, there are a myriad of conditions that can cause varying levels of facial hyperpigmentation. Many of these conditions occur disproportionately in SOC individuals and can have significant impact on the QoL of those affected. Facial hyperpigmentation can pose diagnostic and therapeutic challenges. In addition to diligent photoprotection, combination therapies are often needed to achieve adequate improvement. Patients should be advised on prognosis and that many of these conditions and their associated treatments may take prolonged periods to see improvement. Some conditions may also wax and wane or have relapses. Continued research on the risk factors and pathogenesis of these conditions as well as safe and effective treatment options will be important for obtaining optimal treatment outcomes and increased QoL for affected individuals.

REFERENCES

1. Naik P. Getting to the core of contemporary therapies for post-inflammatory hyperpigmentation. *J Drugs Dermatol.* 2022;21(3):276-283.
2. Davis EC, Callender VD. Postinflammatory hyperpigmentation: a review of the epidemiology, clinical features, and treatment options in skin of color. *J Clin Aesthetic Dermatol.* 2010;3(7):20-31.
3. Lawrence E, Al Aboud KM. Postinflammatory hyperpigmentation. In: *StatPearls.* StatPearls Publishing; 2022. http://www.ncbi.nlm.nih.gov/books/NBK559150/. Accessed August 15, 2022.
4. Kaufman BP, Aman T, Alexis AF. Postinflammatory hyperpigmentation: epidemiology, clinical presentation, pathogenesis and treatment. *Am J Clin Dermatol.* 2018;19(4):489-503.
5. Akinboro AO, Ezejiofor OI, Olanrewaju FO, et al. The impact of acne and facial post-inflammatory hyperpigmentation on quality of life and self-esteem of newly admitted Nigerian undergraduates. *Clin Cosmet Investig Dermatol.* 2018;11:245-252.
6. Anvery N, Christensen RE, Dirr MA. Management of post-inflammatory hyperpigmentation in skin of color: a short review. *J Cosmet Dermatol.* 2022;21(5):1837-1840.
7. Krueger L, Saizan A, Stein JA, Elbuluk N. Dermoscopy of acquired pigmentary disorders: a comprehensive review. *Int J Dermatol.* 2022;61(1):7-19.
8. Chaowattanapanit S, Silpa-archa N, Kohli I, Lim HW, Hamzavi I. Postinflammatory hyperpigmentation: a comprehensive overview: treatment options and prevention. *J Am Acad Dermatol.* 2017;77(4):607-621.
9. Syder NC, Elbuluk N. Going beyond hydroquinone: alternative skin lightening agents. *Cutis.* 2022;109(6):302-304.
10. Agbai O, Hamzavi I, Jagdeo J. Laser treatments for postinflammatory hyperpigmentation: a systematic review. *JAMA Dermatol.* 2017;153(2):199-206.
11. Levin MK, Ng E, Bae YSC, Brauer JA, Geronemus RG. Treatment of pigmentary disorders in patients with skin of color with a novel 755 nm picosecond, Q-switched ruby, and Q-switched Nd:YAG nanosecond lasers: a retrospective photographic review. *Lasers Surg Med.* 2016;48(2):181-187.

12. Nautiyal A, Wairkar S. Management of hyperpigmentation: current treatments and emerging therapies. *Pigment Cell Melanoma Res.* 2021;34(6):1000-1014.
13. Abdel-Naser MB. The color of skin: gray diseases of the skin, nails, and mucosa. *Clin Dermatol.* 2019;37(5):507-515.
14. Syder N, Sicco K, Gutierrez D. Updates in therapeutics for lichen planus pigmentosus. *J Drugs Dermatol.* 2022;21(3):324-330.
15. Robles-Méndez JC, Rizo-Frías P, Herz-Ruelas ME, Pandya AG, Ocampo Candiani J. Lichen planus pigmentosus and its variants: review and update. *Int J Dermatol.* 2018;57(5):505-514.
16. Feng H, Gutierrez D, Rothman L, Meehan S, Sicco KL. Lichen planus pigmentosus. *Dermatol Online J.* 2018;24(12).
17. Lichen planus pigmentosus in patients with endocrinopathies and hepatitis C - ClinicalKey. https://www-clinicalkey-com.libproxy1.usc.edu/#!/content/journal/1-s2.0-S0190962212018579. Accessed August 16, 2022.
18. Ghosh A, Coondoo A. Lichen planus pigmentosus: the controversial consensus. *Indian J Dermatol.* 2016;61(5):482-486.
19. Dlova N c. Frontal fibrosing alopecia and lichen planus pigmentosus: is there a link? *Br J Dermatol.* 2013;168(2):439-442.
20. Al-Rqobah D. Lichen planus pigmentosus: an overview. 2019;26:13.
21. Muthu SK, Narang T, Saikia UN, Kanwar AJ, Parsad D, Dogra S. Low-dose oral isotretinoin therapy in lichen planus pigmentosus: an open-label non-randomized prospective pilot study. *Int J Dermatol.* 2016;55(9):1048-1054.
22. Shah P, Ugonabo N, Liebman TN. A case of recalcitrant lichen planus pigmentosus treated by oral isotretinoin. *JAAD Case Rep.* 2020;6(9):812-814.
23. Wu CY, Lin FL. A successful combination therapy of tacrolimus, hydroxychloroquine and picosecond laser for lichen planus pigmentosus. *Australas J Dermatol.* 2019;60(4):e336-e337.
24. Sonthalia S, Vedamurthy M, Thomas M, et al. Modified phenol peels for treatment-refractory hyperpigmentation of lichen planus pigmentosus: a retrospective clinico-dermoscopic analysis. *J Cosmet Dermatol.* 2019;18(5):1479-1486.
25. Shah DSD, Aurangabadkar DS, Nikam DB. An open-label non-randomized prospective pilot study of the efficacy of Q-switched Nd-YAG laser in management of facial lichen planus pigmentosus. *J Cosmet Laser Ther Off Publ Eur Soc Laser Dermatol.* 2019;21(2):108-115.
26. Wang RF, Ko D, Friedman BJ, Lim HW, Mohammad TF. Disorders of hyperpigmentation. Part I. Pathogenesis and clinical features of common pigmentary disorders. *J Am Acad Dermatol.* 2023;88(2):271-288.
27. Nguyen K, Khachemoune A. Ashy dermatosis: a review. *Dermatol Online J.* 2019;25(5):13030/qt44f462s8.
28. Numata T, Harada K, Tsuboi R, Mitsuhashi Y. Erythema dyschromicum perstans: identical to ashy dermatosis or not? *Case Rep Dermatol.* 2015;7(2):146-150.
29. McNally MA, Farooq S, Brown AE, Rees A, Hsu S, Motaparthi K. Annular lichenoid diseases. *Clin Dermatol.* 2022;40(5):466-479.
30. Rutnin S, Udompanich S, Pratumchart N, Harnchoowong S, Vachiramon V. Ashy dermatosis and lichen planus pigmentosus: the histopathological differences. *BioMed Res Int.* 2019;2019:1-9.
31. Mahajan VK, Chauhan PS, Mehta KS, Sharma AL. Erythema dyschromicum perstans: response to topical tacrolimus. *Indian J Dermatol.* 2015;60(5):525.
32. Wang F, Zhao YK, Wang Z, Liu JH, Luo DQ. Erythema dyschromicum perstans response to isotretinoin. *JAMA Dermatol.* 2016;152(7):841-842.
33. Leung N, Oliveira M, Selim MA, McKinley-Grant L, Lesesky E. Erythema dyschromicum perstans: a case report and systematic review of histologic presentation and treatment. *Int J Womens Dermatol.* 2018;4(4):216-222.
34. Basit H, Godse KV, Al Aboud AM. Melasma. In: *StatPearls*. StatPearls Publishing; 2022. http://www.ncbi.nlm.nih.gov/books/NBK459271/. Accessed June 20, 2022.
35. Achar A, Rathi SK. Melasma: a clinico-epidemiological study of 312 cASES. *Indian J Dermatol.* 2011;56(4):380-382.
36. Syder NC, Elbuluk N. The history of melasma: its roots and evolution. *Dermatol Rev.* 2023;4:5-11.
37. O'Brien TJ, Dyall-Smith D, Hall AP. Melasma of the forearms. *Australas J Dermatol.* 1997;38(1):35-37.
38. Ritter CG, Fiss DVC, Borges da Costa J a. T, de Carvalho RR, Bauermann G, Cestari TF. Extra-facial melasma: clinical, histopathological, and immunohistochemical case-control study. *J Eur Acad Dermatol Venereol.* 2013;27(9):1088-1094.
39. Sangha AM. Dermatological conditions in SKIN OF COLOR-melasma: topical and systemic management. *J Clin Aesthetic Dermatol.* 2022;15(3 Suppl 1):S17-S19.
40. McKesey J, Tovar-Garza A, Pandya AG. Melasma treatment: an evidence-based review. *Am J Clin Dermatol.* 2020;21(2):173-225.
41. Pollo CF, Miot LDB, Meneguin S, Miot HA. Development and validation of a multidimensional questionnaire for evaluating quality of life in melasma (HRQ-melasma). *An Bras Dermatol.* 2018;93(3):391-396.
42. Handel AC, Miot LDB, Miot HA. Melasma: a clinical and epidemiological review. *An Bras Dermatol.* 2014;89(5):771-782.
43. Rajanala S, Maymone MB de C, Vashi NA. Melasma pathogenesis: a review of the latest research, pathological findings, and investigational therapies. *Dermatol Online J.* 2019;25(10):13030/qt47b7r28c.
44. Charoo NA. Hyperpigmentation: looking beyond hydroquinone. *J Cosmet Dermatol.* 2022;21(10):4133-4145.
45. Grimes P, Bhawan J, Howell M, et al. Histopathological changes induced by malassezin: a novel natural microbiome indole for treatment of facial hyperpigmentation. *J Drugs Dermatol.* 2022;21(2):141-145.
46. Desai S, Hartman C, Grimes P, Shah S. Topical stabilized cysteamine as a new treatment for hyperpigmentation disorders: melasma, post-inflammatory hyperpigmentation, and lentigines. *J Drugs Dermatol.* 2021;20(12):1276-1279.
47. Sarkar R, Arsiwala S, Dubey N, et al. Chemical peels in melasma: a review with consensus recommendations by Indian pigmentary expert group. *Indian J Dermatol.* 2017;62(6):578-584.
48. Shah SD, Aurangabadkar SJ. Laser toning in melasma. *J Cutan Aesthetic Surg.* 2019;12(2):76-84.
49. Acar A, Ozturk A, Sokmen N, Unal I, Ertam Sagduyu I. Evaluation of platelet-rich plasma efficacy in melasma. *J Cosmet Laser Ther Off Publ Eur Soc Laser Dermatol.* 2022;24(1-5):36-39.
50. Acar A, Ozturk A, Sokmen N, Unal I, Ertam Sagduyu I. Evaluation of platelet-rich plasma efficacy in melasma. *J Cosmet Laser Ther.* 2022;24(1-5):36-39.
51. Baghaie H, Shukla K, Stone J, Breik O, Munn Z. Effectiveness of prophylactic tranexamic acid versus placebo or no intervention for reducing blood loss in healthy patients undergoing orthognathic surgery: a systematic review protocol. *JBI Evid Synth.* 2023;21(2):430-440.
52. Bala HR, Lee S, Wong C, Pandya AG, Rodrigues M. Oral tranexamic acid for the treatment of melasma: a review. *Dermatol Surg.* 2018;44(6):814-825.
53. Pandya AG, Hynan LS, Bhore R, et al. Reliability assessment and validation of the Melasma Area and Severity Index (MASI) and a new modified MASI scoring method. *J Am Acad Dermatol.* 2011;64(1):78-83, 83.e1-2.
54. Daadaa N, Ben Tanfous A. Riehl melanosis. In: *StatPearls*. StatPearls Publishing; 2022. http://www.ncbi.nlm.nih.gov/books/NBK557437/. Accessed February 19, 2022.
55. Shenoi SD, Rao R. Pigmented contact dermatitis. *Indian J Dermatol Venereol Leprol.* 2007;73(5):285-287.
56. Kwong HL, Lim SPR. Pigmented contact dermatitis in the axillae caused by hydroperoxides of limonene. *JAAD Case Rep.* 2020;6(6):476-478.
57. Woo YR, Park HE, Jeong SW, Park HJ. Melanogenic properties and expression profiles of melanogenic paracrine molecules in Riehl's melanosis. *Int J Mol Sci.* 2020;21(5):E1695.
58. Kim SM, Lee ES, Sohn S, Kim YC. Histopathological features of Riehl melanosis. *Am J Dermatopathol.* 2020;42(2):117-121.
59. Satter EK. Riehl melanosis (pigmented contact dermatitis) differential diagnoses. Riehl emedicine. https://emedicine.medscape.com/article/1119818-differential. Accessed October 31, 2022.
60. Sujay Khandpur UK. Pigmented contact dermatitis. *J Pigment Disord.* 2015;2(10).
61. Ramia de Cap M, Parisi X, Tahan SR. Exogenous ochronosis associated with dimethoxytolyl propylresorcinol (UP302). *J Dermatol.* 2021;48(7):e312-e313.
62. Qorbani A, Mubasher A, Sarantopoulos GP, Nelson S, Fung MA. Exogenous ochronosis (EO): skin lightening cream causing rare caviar-like lesion with banana-like pigments; review of literature and histological comparison with endogenous counterpart. *Autopsy Case Rep.* 2020;10(4):e2020197.
63. Ewulu A, Gaufin M, Cardis MA. Blue-black hyperpigmented patches on the cheeks. *JAAD Case Rep.* 2022;19:81-83.
64. Bhattar PA, Zawar VP, Godse KV, Patil SP, Nadkarni NJ, Gautam MM. Exogenous ochronosis. *Indian J Dermatol.* 2015;60(6):537-543.
65. Luke M, David A G. Exogenous ochronosis with use of low potency hydroquinone in a Caucasian patient. *J Dermatol Res Ther.* 2015;1(1).
66. Simmons BJ, Griffith RD, Bray FN, Falto-Aizpurua LA, Nouri K. Exogenous ochronosis: a comprehensive review of the diagnosis, epidemiology, causes, and treatments. *Am J Clin Dermatol.* 2015;16(3):205-212.
67. Bellew SG, Alster TS. Treatment of exogenous ochronosis with a Q-switched alexandrite (755 nm) laser. *Dermatol Surg Off Publ Am Soc Dermatol Surg Al.* 2004;30(4 Pt 1):555-558.

68. Méndez Baca I, Al-Niaimi F, Colina C, Anuzita A. A case of ochronosis successfully treated with the picosecond laser. *J Cosmet Dermatol.* 2019;18(5):1322-1325.
69. Ceglio WW, Careta MF, Patriota R, Torezan LA. Exogenous ochronosis successfully treated with the combination of intense pulsed light and fractional CO2 laser. *An Bras Dermatol.* 2023;98(1):138-140.
70. Munera-Campos M, Castillo G, Ferrándiz C, Carrascosa JM. Actinic lichen planus triggered by drug photosensitivity. *Photodermatol Photoimmunol Photomed.* 2019;35(2):124-126.
71. Ashraf R, Aggarwal D, Bhattacharjee R, Radotra BD, De D. Dyschromic actinic lichen planus. *Int J Dermatol.* 2022;61(6):e223-e225.
72. Murao K, Tamaki M, Kinoshita H, Kubo Y. Case of actinic lichen planus: the second Japanese case. *J Dermatol.* 2019;46(8):e304-e305.
73. Meads SB, Kunishige J, Ramos-Caro FA, Hassanein AM. Lichen planus actinicus. *Cutis.* 2003;72(5):377-381.
74. Kim GH, Mikkilineni R. Lichen planus actinicus. *Dermatol Online J.* 2007;13(1).
75. Praetorius C, Sturm RA, Steingrimsson E. Sun-induced freckling: ephelides and solar lentigines. *Pigment Cell Melanoma Res.* 2014;27(3):339-350.
76. Hafner C, Stoehr R, van Oers JMM, et al. FGFR3 and PIK3CA mutations are involved in the molecular pathogenesis of solar lentigo. *Br J Dermatol.* 2009;160(3):546-551.
77. Ortonne JP, Pandya AG, Lui H, Hexsel D. Treatment of solar lentigines. *J Am Acad Dermatol.* 2006;54(5 Suppl 2):S262-271.
78. Di Bartolomeo L, Guarneri F, Moretti G. Treatment of solar lentigo with imiquimod 3.75% cream: a dermoscopic study. *J Cosmet Dermatol.* 2022;21(11):6487-6489.
79. Abd Elazim NE, Makboul R, Botros SN, Awad SM. Cryopeeling versus trichloroacetic acid peeling in the treatment of solar lentigines: effect on epidermal Langerhans cells. *Dermatol Ther.* 2020;33(3):e13288.
80. Deonizio JMD. Cryopeeling. In: Abramovits W, Graham G, Har-Shai Y, Strumia R, eds. *Dermatological Cryosurgery and Cryotherapy.* Berlin: Springer; 2016:185-189.
81. Usuki A, Ohashi A, Sato H, Ochiai Y, Ichihashi M, Funasaka Y. The inhibitory effect of glycolic acid and lactic acid on melanin synthesis in melanoma cells. *Exp Dermatol.* 2003;12 Suppl 2:43-50.
82. Polder KD, Landau JM, Vergilis-Kalner IJ, Goldberg LH, Friedman PM, Bruce S. Laser eradication of pigmented lesions: a review. *Dermatol Surg Off Publ Am Soc Dermatol Surg Al.* 2011;37(5):572-595.
83. Vachiramon V, Panmanee W, Techapichetvanich T, Chanprapaph K. Comparison of Q-switched Nd: YAG laser and fractional carbon dioxide laser for the treatment of solar lentigines in Asians. *Lasers Surg Med.* 2016;48(4):354-359.
84. Borelli C, Fischer S. [Chemical peeling for treatment of melasma, pigmentary disorders and hyperpigmentation : indications, effectivity and risks]. *Hautarzt Z Dermatol Venerol Verwandte Geb.* 2020;71(12):950-959.
85. Agarwal P, Patel BC. Nevus Of Ota And Ito. In: *StatPearls.* StatPearls Publishing; 2022. http://www.ncbi.nlm.nih.gov/books/NBK560574/. Accessed June 20, 2022.
86. Hindawi. Nevus of Ota with rare palatal involvement: a case report with emphasis on differential diagnosis. https://www.hindawi.com/journals/crid/2011/670679/. Accessed September 9, 2022.
87. Nevi of Ota and Ito differential diagnoses. https://emedicine.medscape.com/article/1058580-differential. Accessed October 31, 2022.
88. Achavanuntakul P, Manuskiatti W, Wanitphakdeedecha R, Jantarakolica T. Early treatment initiation improves outcomes in nevus of Ota: a 10-year retrospective study. *Am J Clin Dermatol.* 2022;23(1):105-114.
89. Zhong Y, Huang L, Yan T, Chen Y, Yang B, Man MQ. Both age and disease duration are associated with clinical phenotype of Hori's nevus in Chinese: a retrospective analysis of 497 cases. *Clin Cosmet Investig Dermatol.* 2021;14:65-71.
90. Kaur H, Sarma P, Kaur S, et al. Therapeutic options for management of Hori's nevus: a systematic review. *Dermatol Ther.* 2020;33(1):e13167.
91. Sonthalia S, Sarkar R, Neema S. Maturational hyperpigmentation: clinicodermoscopic and histopathological profile of a new cutaneous marker of metabolic syndrome. *Pigment Int.* 2018;5(1):54.
92. Ramakrishnan S, Hegde SP, Shenoy MM, Pinto M, M Iqbal AA, Amin VB. A cross-sectional study on clinico-dermoscopic features of periorbital melanosis in a tertiary care hospital. *J Cosmet Dermatol.* 2021;20(9):2917-2923.
93. Noble A, Greenstein J, Husain A, Zielinski M, Hahn B. Periorbital melanosis. *Am J Emerg Med.* 2017;35(2):380.e1-380.e2.
94. Sawant O, Khan T. Management of periorbital hyperpigmentation: an overview of nature-based agents and alternative approaches. *Dermatol Ther.* 2020;33(4):e13717.
95. Dayal S, Sangal B, Sahu P. Ferulic acid 12% peel: an innovative peel for constitutional type of periorbital melanosis-comparing clinical efficacy and safety with 20% glycolic peel and 15% lactic peel. *J Cosmet Dermatol.* 2020;19(9):2342-2348.
96. Nanda S, Bansal S, Lakhani R. Use of Hyaluronic acid fillers in treatment of periorbital melanosis induced by tear trough deformity: anatomical considerations, patient satisfaction, and management of complications. *J Cosmet Dermatol.* 2021;20(10):3181-3189.
97. Sil A, Biswas SK, Bhanja DB, Das S, Panigrahi A. Post-chikungunya hyperpigmentation. *Postgrad Med J.* 2021;97(1143):60.
98. Chakraborty U, Biswas P, Chandra A, Pal J, Ray AK. Chik sign: post-chikungunya hyperpigmentation. *QJM Mon J Assoc Physicians.* 2021;114(2):137-138.

CHAPTER 57

Disorders of Hyperpigmentation

Linna L. Guan
Iltefat Hamzavi
Tasneem F. Mohammad

KEY POINTS

- Disorders of hyperpigmentation can be congenital or acquired and can be due to increased melanin production and deposition, increased number of melanocytes, increased melanocyte activity, and/or accumulation of pigmented by-products or foreign bodies in the skin.
- Acquired disorders of hyperpigmentation include acanthosis nigricans, confluent and reticulate papillomatosis, prurigo pigmentosa, drug-induced hyperpigmentation, and other systemic causes of hyperpigmentation.
- Congenital causes of hyperpigmentation include pigmentary demarcation lines, familial progressive hyperpigmentation, reticulate acropigmentation of Kitamura, Dowling-Degos disease, dermatopathia pigmentosa reticularis, dyskeratosis congenita, and incontinentia pigmenti.
- Treatment of hyperpigmentation can be challenging particularly due to the effects of both UV and visible light on pigment induction that can be mitigated through use of broad spectrum, tinted sunscreens of at least SPF 30 daily.

INTRODUCTION

Melanocytes are neural-crest-derived cells that regulate normal pigmentation of the skin. While the density of melanocytes is roughly similar among individuals, differences in the number, size, composition, and distribution of melanin-containing granules called melanosomes contribute to variation in skin pigmentation.[1] There are two types of melanin, the brown/black eumelanin and the red/yellow pheomelanin. Both types of melanin are derived from tyrosine, but deviation in this pathway, namely the addition of a thiol-containing conjugate, differentiates pheomelanin from eumelanin. In addition to differences in color, pheomelanin, due to its conjugation of either cysteine or glutathione, is more photolabile and can produce free radicals that cause DNA damage.[1] Therefore, higher pheomelanin to eumelanin ratios in melanosomes not only contributes to lighter skin color but also increases skin cancer risk. After melanin is packaged into melanosomes, these melanosomes are delivered to its surrounding keratinocytes where most of the skin pigment resides to protect against ultraviolet radiation (UVR).

Disorders of hyperpigmentation are common and can be due to a variety of different causes including increased melanin production and deposition, increased number of melanocytes, increased melanocyte activity, and accumulation of pigmented byproducts or foreign bodies in the skin.[2] These disorders can affect various parts of the body and can be congenital or acquired. This chapter will focus on disorders of hyperpigmentation predominantly affecting the body while disorders of facial hyperpigmentation will be discussed in Chapter 56.

ACQUIRED DISORDERS OF HYPERPIGMENTATION

ACANTHOSIS NIGRICANS

Acanthosis Nigricans (AN) is characterized by asymptomatic symmetric tan to brown velvety plaques typically involving the skin folds of the neck, axilla, and groin [**Figure 57-1**].[3] In darker phototypes, AN lesions can appear dark brown to black. Thicker lesions can be verrucous and/or papillomatous. Less commonly, AN presents on the face, areolae, conjunctivae, lips, and buccal mucosa.[4] Biopsy demonstrates hyperkeratosis and epidermal papillomatosis but minimal acanthosis. AN affects individuals across all age groups and ethnicities but are more commonly found in Native American, African American, Hispanic, and Caucasian populations.[4]

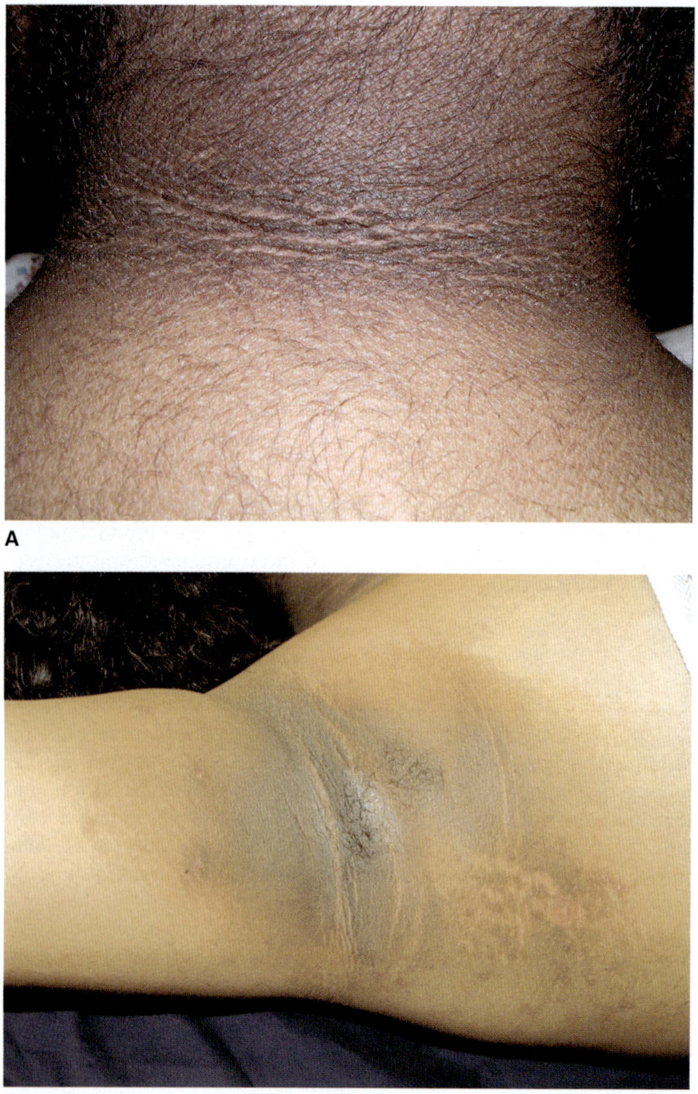

A

B

FIGURE 57-1. Acanthosis nigricans involving the **(A)** posterior neck in a black individual **(B)** axilla of a 11-year-old Black child. (Courtesy of Henry W. Lim, MD and Tor A. Shwayder, MD, Department of Dermatology, Henry Ford Health, Detroit, MI, USA.)

There are various subtypes of AN, the most common being obesity-related AN. Due to the association of insulin resistance in those with obesity-related AN, it is important to recognize this entity and perform appropriate screening for metabolic syndrome and type 2 diabetes mellitus. It is hypothesized that increased insulin levels promote insulin-like growth factor 1 (IGFR1), which stimulates keratinocyte and dermal fibroblast proliferation.[5] Other drugs that increase insulin levels such as systemic steroids, insulin, oral contraceptive pills, and estrogen may also contribute to AN.[4]

Paraneoplastic or malignant AN is a much less common subtype of AN. It is most frequently associated with adenocarcinoma of the stomach or other gastrointestinal and genitourinary malignancies. In comparison to obesity-related AN, the onset of paraneoplastic AN is more rapid, associated with weight loss rather than obesity, and can have more extensive and striking features. It can sometimes present in conjunction with tripe palms, or velvety ridges of the palms.[6] Early recognition of this subtype can have a profound impact on patient survival.

Treatment of AN primarily focuses on addressing the underlying etiology such as weight reduction, treatment of underlying malignancy, or stopping offending medications. Topically, retinoids such as tretinoin, adapalene, and tazarotene are the first-line treatment and have been successful at improving lesions of AN in small clinical studies and case reports.[4,7] Combination of a topical retinoid with ammonium lactate 12% has also been shown to be helpful.[4] Other topical treatments that have been reported with variable success include topical vitamin D analogs and keratolytics. Procedurally, favorable results have been seen with long-pulsed alexandrite laser, CO_2 laser, and trichloroacetic acid (TCA) peels. Systemically, insulin sensitizers such as metformin and alpha-lipoic acid may be considered. Although oral retinoids have shown some benefit in reduction of AN, the large doses and long treatment courses required limit their utility.[4]

CONFLUENT AND RETICULATED PAPILLOMATOSIS

Confluent and reticulated papillomatosis (CARP) is a benign disorder of hyperpigmentation resembling acanthosis nigricans but is characterized by hyperpigmented mildly scaly macules coalescing into reticulate patches on the medial neck, chest, and back that spread centrifugally.[8] Involved areas can be pruritic but are often asymptomatic [**Figure 57-2**]. Histologically, CARP is similar to AN and features hyperkeratosis, acanthosis, and papillomatosis. Other more subtle features that suggest a role of abnormal keratinization in this disorder include increase of transition cell layer, involucrin expression, and lamellar granules in the stratum granulosum.[8] Additionally, increased melanosomes can be seen, accounting for clinical hyperpigmentation.

CARP affects all racial groups and age groups, but tends to appear after puberty. It presents more frequently in those with endocrine abnormalities such as diabetes mellitus and thyroid disease and screening may be warranted if clinical suspicion for either is high. Superficial bacterial and fungal infections have also been implicated for the development of CARP; however, very limited evidence supports this theory.[8,9]

Various agents have been utilized for the treatment of CARP. Tetracyclines, with minocycline being the most frequently used, have shown success with approximately 80% of those treated achieving complete or partial resolution within 51.8 days.[9] Although less commonly used, other antibiotics such as amoxicillin and azithromycin demonstrated similar success rates. Other therapies that have been reported to be successful at treating CARP include topical vitamin D derivatives and oral and topical retinoids. However, evidence is limited by the small size of the cohorts.[9] Development of CARP has previously been attributed to *Malassezia* species, but the limited treatment success with oral and topical antifungals treatment suggests otherwise.[9] It is important to counsel patients that CARP can recur after cessation of therapy and may require multiple treatment courses.

PRURIGO PIGMENTOSA

Prurigo pigmentosa (PP), also known as Nagashima disease, is a rare dermatologic condition that presents with severely pruritic papules and

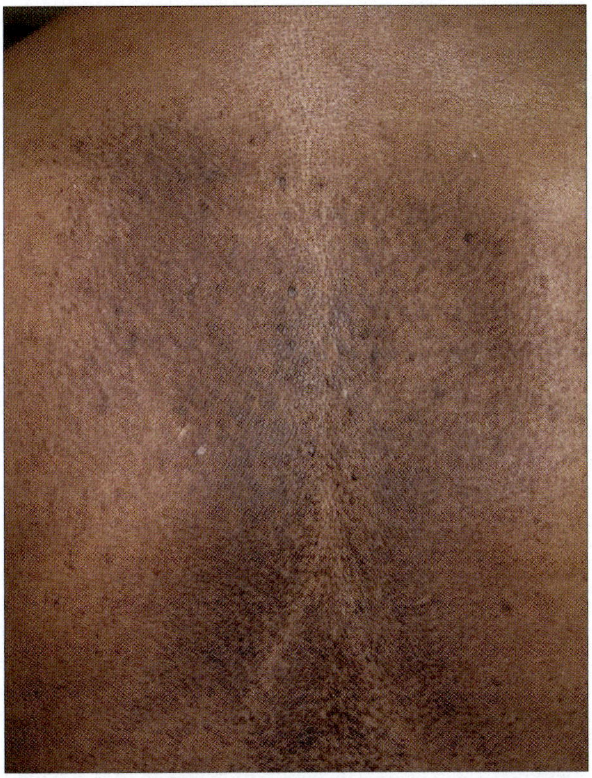

A

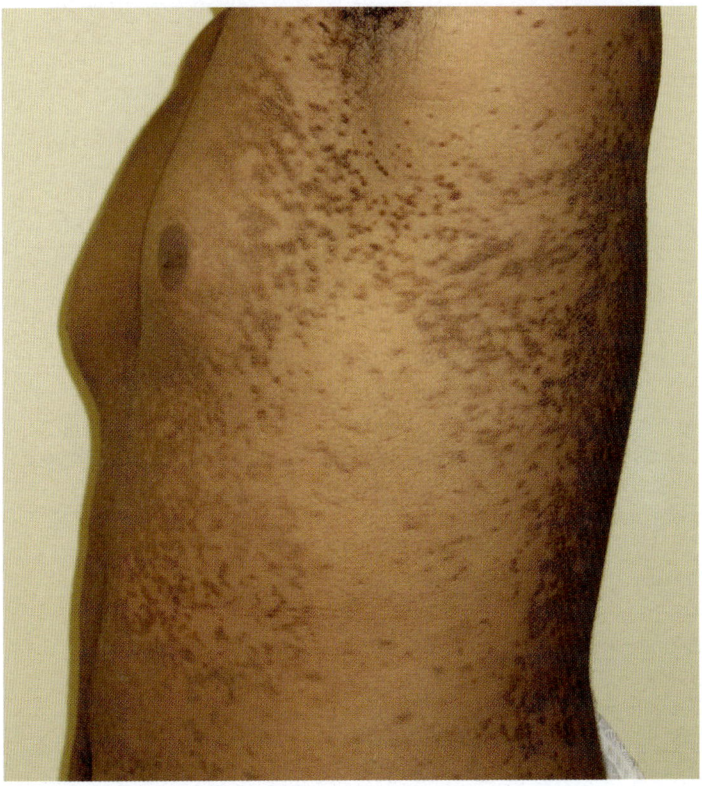

B

FIGURE 57-2. Confluent and reticulate papillomatosis (A) on the chest (B) more diffusely on chest, back, and axilla. (Courtesy of Henry W. Lim, MD and Tor A. Shwayder, MD, Department of Dermatology, Henry Ford Health, Detroit, MI, USA.)

papulovesicles that eventually resolve with tan to dark brown macules and reticulate patches.[10] It favors the neck, chest, and back similar to CARP but often presents with different morphologic stages at one time. The histologic features of PP vary depending on the stage. Early disease is characterized by papillary edema, hyperkeratosis, and neutrophil predominance while late disease presents with scale crust, hyperkeratosis, presence of melanophages in the dermis, and lymphocyte predominance.[10,11] Progression from early to late stage typically occurs over the course of few days to a week.

PP primarily affects young, East Asian women in their 20s but cases in men and individuals of other ethnicities have also reported.[10-12] Although the pathophysiology of PP is unknown, it is associated with ketogenic diet, weight loss, anorexia nervosa, excessive exercise, and the summer months when sweating and heat may play a role in exacerbating this condition.[12] Given these associations, it is suspected that ketosis may contribute to development of PP, but further studies are warranted.

The treatment of choice for PP is minocycline at a dose of 100 to 200 mg daily and patients typically improve within 2 weeks of initiation.[10-12] Doxycycline and dapsone have also been used but are less effective than minocycline. Although the pruritus and papulovesicles resolve shortly after treatment, it is important to note that hyperpigmentation can persist for months to years and recurrences are not uncommon.[10,11]

DRUG-INDUCED HYPERPIGMENTATION

Over 50 drugs have been implicated in the development of hyperpigmentation.[13] It has been suggested that 20% of all cases of acquired hyperpigmentation can be attributed to medications.[13] Drug-induced hyperpigmentation can affect the skin, mucosal surfaces, and nails. Drugs implicated include but are not limited to antimalarials, antimicrobials, cardiovascular agents, chemotherapeutic agents, and heavy metals.[2,13-16] The color of affected skin (ie, brown, gray, blue), distribution of hyperpigmentation (ie, facial, acral, photodistributed, widespread), and duration of hyperpigmentation in relationship to medication initiation can all provide clues into the causal agent. Minocycline is a commonly used antibiotic in dermatology known to cause distinct hyperpigmentation. There are four types of minocycline-induced hyperpigmentation. Type I typically involves the face with blue-black pigmentation occurring within scars. Type II is characterized by blue-gray pigmentation on the shins and forearms [**Figure 57-3**]. Type III occurs on sun-exposed skin with muddy brown hyperpigmentation and type IV occurs on the back with blue-gray hyperpigmentation within scars. Diltiazem is another well-reported cause of drug-induced hyperpigmentation and typically presents with reticulate slate blue to gray or brown pigmentation in photodistributed regions [**Figure 57-4**]. **Numerous other medications can cause hyperpigmentation and present with unique features** [**Table 57-1**]. The mainstay of treatment for drug-induced hyperpigmentation is cessation of the offending agent and photoprotection.[16]

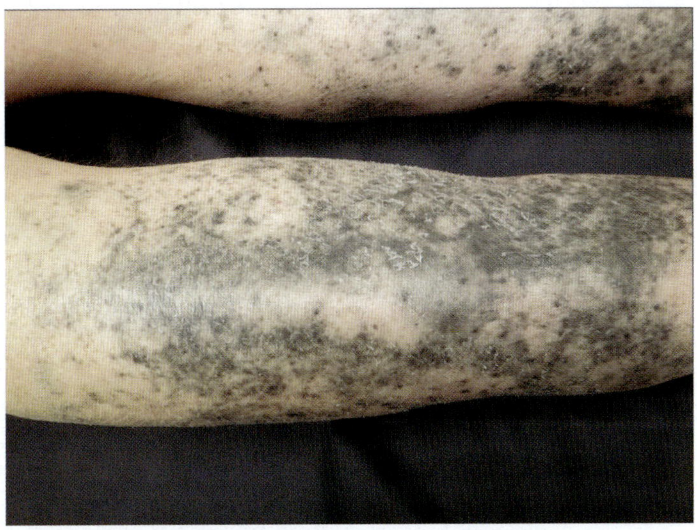

FIGURE 57-3. Blue-gray hyperpigmentation on the shins due to minocycline (Type II minocycline-induced hyperpigmentation). (Courtesy of Henry W. Lim, MD, Department of Dermatology, Henry Ford Health, Detroit, MI, USA.)

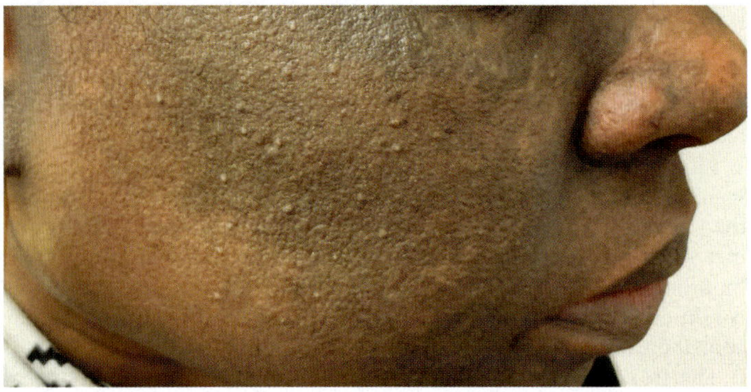

FIGURE 57-4. Diltiazem-induced hyperpigmentation of the face in a Black female.

Q-switched and picosecond lasers have also been tried with varying success.[17,18]

SYSTEMIC CAUSES OF HYPERPIGMENTATION

Hyperpigmentation can be a sign of systemic disease. Endocrinopathies such as Addison disease and hyperthyroidism can increase melanin production while the hyperpigmentation in hemochromatosis is due to increased deposition of ferrous pigment and hemosiderin, along with increased melanin.[19-21] Hyperpigmentation may be the first presenting sign of these disorders and if systemic disease is suspected, additional laboratory screening should be performed with referral to the appropriate specialists.

Addison disease, or chronic primary adrenal insufficiency, is a disorder leading to adrenocortical insufficiency. Due to lack of negative feedback of cortisol production on the hypothalamic-pituitary-adrenal (HPA) axis, the hypothalamus increases production of adrenocorticotropic hormone (ACTH) along with its precursor, proopiomelanocortin.[22] Since proopiomelanocortin is cleaved into ACTH and melanocyte-stimulating hormone (MSH), both levels are increased in Addison disease. MSH then circulates to epidermal melanocytes where it stimulates increased production of melanin.[15,19,22] Hyperpigmentation is typically diffuse but may be more prominent in photodistributed regions simulating the effects of tanning [**Figure 57-5**]. In darker phototypes, it is often helpful to compare with prior photos as pigmentation can be widespread and difficult to discern from an individual's natural skin color. Prior sites of trauma, areas of chronic pressure, the axillae, perineum, areolae, palmar creases, and mucous membranes can also be involved. Longitudinal melanonychia may be noted.[15,19] Addison disease can be diagnosed by a short cosyntropin (synthetic ACTH) stimulation test but elevated ACTH and electrolyte abnormalities may provide clues to this condition.[19] Glucocorticoid replacement is the primary treatment of Addison disease and leads to improvement of hyperpigmentation.[19,22]

There are many causes of hyperthyroidism, with Graves disease being the most common. Hyperpigmentation due to hyperthyroidism can be localized to the face or generalized. When compared to Addison disease, the mucous membranes are less likely to be hyperpigmented.[19,23] Similar to Addison disease, hyperpigmentation can be widespread and present as diffuse "tanning" making it difficult to discern from patient's natural skin color. Therefore, comparison to prior photos can be helpful in making the diagnosis. The pathophysiology of hyperpigmentation

TABLE 57-1 Topical and systemic agents associated with hyperpigmentation[2,13,15,16]

Agent	Distribution of hyperpigmentation	Color	Other features
Antimalarials			
• Chloroquine/ hydroxychloroquine	Pretibial, face, oral mucosa (hard palate), nails; after years, can be diffuse, especially in photodistributed regions	Blue-gray to dark purple	Hyperpigmentation eventually resolves, may take months to years
• Quinacrine	Diffuse and uniform, may involve conjunctiva	Lemon-yellow	Attributed to direct tissue staining of drug
Antimicrobials			
• Clofazimine	Diffuse, may affect conjunctiva	Dark brown to reddish- blue	When used for treatment of leprosy, lesional skin may be preferentially involved
• Levofloxacin	Hands, extensor forearms, shins, and neck	Blue-gray	Similar to type II minocycline induced-hyperpigmentation with involvement of the hands, extensor forearms, shins, and neck
• Minocycline	Type I—face, within scars	Blue-black	Due to iron-containing pigment granules ± melanin
	Type II—shins and forearms	Blue-gray	Due to iron and melanin- containing pigment granules; association with cumulative doses of 70-100 g
	Type III—sun-exposed skin	Muddy brown	Due to increased melanin; association with cumulative doses of 70-100 g, may persist indefinitely
	Type IV—back within scars	Blue-gray	Due to melanin and calcium
Antidepressants and antipsychotics			
• Phenothiazines	Photodistributed; face, extremities, nail beds, sclera, cornea and lens	Violet, purple-gray, metallic	Chlorpromazine is the most common causative agent of the phenothiazines
• Tricyclic antidepressants (amitriptyline, desipramine, and imipramine)	Photodistributed	Brown to blue/slate gray	Amitriptyline causes increased melanin; desipramine and imipramine cause melanin-drug complexes
Antiretrovirals			
• Emtricitabine	Dorsal hands and palms	Brown	Increased melanin
• Zidovudine	Palms and soles, nails	Violaceous to brown	Nail involvement can be diffuse, involve longitudinal streaking, and/or lunula and be blue, gray, or brown
Cardiovascular agents			
• Amiodarone	Photodistributed; face, nose, and ears; mucous membranes	Slate gray, blue-gray, purple	After at least 6 months of therapy; due to lipofuscin deposition
• Diltiazem	Photodistributed; face, chest, neck, and forearms	Slate blue, gray, brown	Reticulate; onset of 6-11 months after initiation; due to increased melanin

(*Continued*)

TABLE 57-1 Topical and systemic agents associated with hyperpigmentation[2,13,15,16] (Continued)

Agent	Distribution of hyperpigmentation	Color	Other features
Chemotherapeutic agents			
• 5- Fluorouracil	Diffuse; palms, soles, and oral mucosa Serpentine supravenous presentation with infusion	Brown	Due to phototoxic reaction resulting in PIH; can be serpiginous along veins in case of infusion
• Bleomycin	Trunk, extremities, face	Brown	Flagellate hyperpigmentation
• Busulfan	Generalized	Brown	Resembling Addison disease, increase pigmentation in palmar creases
• Carmustine	Areas of topical application	Brown	
• Cyclophosphamide/ifosfamide	Diffuse, can involve mucosa, teeth, and nails	Brown	
• Dactinomycin	Generalized	Brown	
• Doxorubicin	Diffuse or localized overlying small joints, palms, soles, and oral mucosa	Brown	Can also have longitudinal or transverse melanonychia
• Hydroxyurea	Back, and over pressure points; nails	Brown	Nails can have longitudinal, transverse or diffuse melanonychia ± lunular pigmentation
• Imatinib	Palatal and dental	Brown	Typically results in hypopigmentation
• Mechlorethamine (nitrogen mustard)	Generalized	Brown	May be more prominent in lesional skin
• Methotrexate	Photodistributed	Brown	May be preceded by eczema or appear in prior eczematous patches; has also been reported in sun-exposed areas
• Sunitinib	Facial, nail, hair	Yellow	Resolves within few weeks of drug discontinuation
Heavy metals			
• Arsenic	Any site, predilection for groin and areola	Bronze	May be associated with hypopigmentation to give "rain drop on a dusty road" appearance
• Bismuth	Diffuse; oral mucosa	Gray	Darkening of the tongue due to bismuth subsalicylate reacting with bacteria producing hydrogen sulfide
• Gold (chrysiasis)	Photodistributed, periorbital	Blue-gray	Permanent, spares oral mucosa; caution needed with Q-switched ruby laser treatments as it can induce local pigmentation in treated areas
• Iron	Site of infusion	Blue-gray to brown	Due to extravasation of iron infusions
• Lead	Gingival	Brown	Blue line at gingival margin can occur—"lead line"
• Mercury	Predilection for eyelids and skin folds when used topically	Slate-gray	Due to granules of mercury within macrophages
• Silver (Argyria)	Diffuse, more prominent in photodistributed areas	Slate-gray	Silver deposits in BMZ and around eccrine glands; can be seen in burn wounds with silver sulfadiazine application
Prostaglandin analogs			
• Bimatoprost/ Latanoprost	Periocular, iris	Brown	Used for glaucoma or induction of eyelash growth
Others			
• Afamelanotide	Diffuse, more prominent in photodistributed areas	Brown or bronze	Analog of α-MSH, used in treatment of EPP
• Hydroquinone	Areas of topical application	Blue-black	Associated with prolonged use, resulting in exogenous ochronosis; histology demonstrates characteristic yellow-brown "banana-like" structures
• Oral contraceptive pills	Face, sun-exposed extremities	Brown	Associated with melasma, Possible role of estrogen in induction of melanocytes

αMSH, α-melanocyte-stimulating hormone; BMZ, basement membrane zone; EPP, erythropoietic protoporphyria; PIH, postinflammatory hyperpigmentation.

in hyperthyroidism has not been well characterized. However, many theories exist, including increased production of ACTH to compensate for accelerated cortisol degeneration and increased TSH receptors on melanocytes.[24] It has also been proposed that hemosiderin deposition due to increased capillary fragility may play a role in hyperthyroidism-related hyperpigmentation, but this finding has not been consistently reported.[23,24] Workup includes laboratory evaluation of serum thyroid stimulating hormone (TSH), triiodothyronine (T3), and thyroxine (T4). Other diagnostic tests may include antithyroglobulin levels and radioactive iodine uptake tests. Although it is prudent to treat the underlying hyperthyroidism, unlike the hyperpigmentation in Addison disease, hyperpigmentation associated with hyperthyroidism does not always respond to treatment of primary disease.

Hemochromatosis can be hereditary or acquired and is due to a buildup of iron, either due to an inherent autosomal-recessive error in iron metabolism (hereditary) or chronic iron overload (acquired) commonly due to frequent blood transfusions.[20,21] Excessive circulating of iron can cause oxidative damage to various organs and result in the classic tetrad of hepatic cirrhosis, diabetes mellitus, skin hyperpigmentation, and cardiac failure. Hyperpigmentation is typically diffuse and ranges from slate-gray to bronze. It can be accentuated in photo-exposed and traumatized skin. Metallic gray pigmentation of the eyelids has also been reported.[20] Biopsy of hyperpigmented skin will demonstrate increased dermal hemosiderin deposition but also increased basal melanin. However, the mechanism of hypermelanosis has not been well elucideated.[21] Laboratory studies show elevations in ferritin, iron, and transferrin

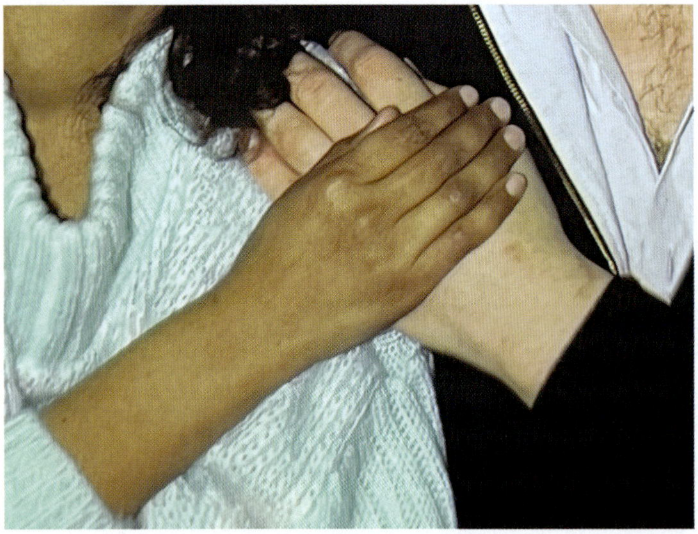

FIGURE 57-5. Hand of woman with Addison disease (left) who was previously the same phototype as her husband (right) (Courtesy of Tor A. Shwayder, MD, Department of Dermatology, Henry Ford Health, Detroit, MI, USA.)

saturation. Genetic studies to evaluate for mutations in the HFE gene can be helpful in cases of hereditary hemochromatosis.[21] Treatment is aimed at reduction of circulating iron and can include cessation of iron supplementation and phlebotomy.

CONGENITAL DISORDERS OF HYPERPIGMENTATION

PIGMENTARY DEMARCATION LINES

Pigmentary demarcation lines (PDL), also known as Futcher lines, Voight lines, or Ito lines, are benign physiologic transition points between hyperpigmented dorsal and lighter ventral surfaces.[15,25] As the name suggests, they appear as lines on the skin with a hyperpigmented region on one side contrasting with a hypopigmented region on the other [**Figure 57-6**]. PDLs typically appear before puberty and persist throughout adulthood.[2] They are more commonly found in darker phototypes with a prevalence of 70% in Black adults and 10% in White adults.[26] Although the exact pathogenesis of PDL is unknown, it has been hypothesized but not substantiated that they developed in utero due to compression on developing nerves.[25]

There are five major subtypes of PDL: Type A—involving the upper limbs with variable trans-pectoral extension; Type B—involving lines along the lower limb; Type C—involving lines on the medial chest with abdominal extension; Type D—involving posteromedian demarcation; and Type E - involving symmetric, hypopigmented macules on the chest.[2,15,25] PDLs have also been reported on the face.[27] PDL typically persists but spontaneous regression over may years may occur. Pregnancy can exacerbate PDL, particularly for type B. No treatment is needed for these normal skin findings. For those who are cosmetically displeased by these findings, Q-switched alexandrite laser, glycolic peels, and a combination of hydroquinone, dexamethasone, and tretinoin may be tried; however, recurrences can occur.[25]

FAMILIAL PROGRESSIVE HYPERPIGMENTATION

Familial progressive hyperpigmentation (FPH) or familial progressive hyperpigmentation and hypopigmentation (FPHH) is a rare autosomal dominant disorder characterized by diffuse and progressive hyperpigmentation starting at birth or infancy.[28-30] Areas of hypopigmentation and ash-leaf-like macules may also be present. It is classically thought to be due to an upregulating mutation in the *KITLG* gene that encodes a ligand of c-KIT, an important regulator of skin pigmentation.[15] However, a recent report detailing the lack of *KITLG* mutations in a Chinese family with distinctive findings of FPH suggests that mutations in other genes may also produce similar phenotypes.[30] FPH can be associated with developmental delay and mental deficiency, therefore, appropriate guidance and counseling can be beneficial to children with this disorder. Currently there are no approved treatments for FPH, but a recent report detailing skin lightening of a patient with FPH on imatinib, a protein-tyrosine kinase inhibitor, raises the possibility of targeted therapies in the future.[31]

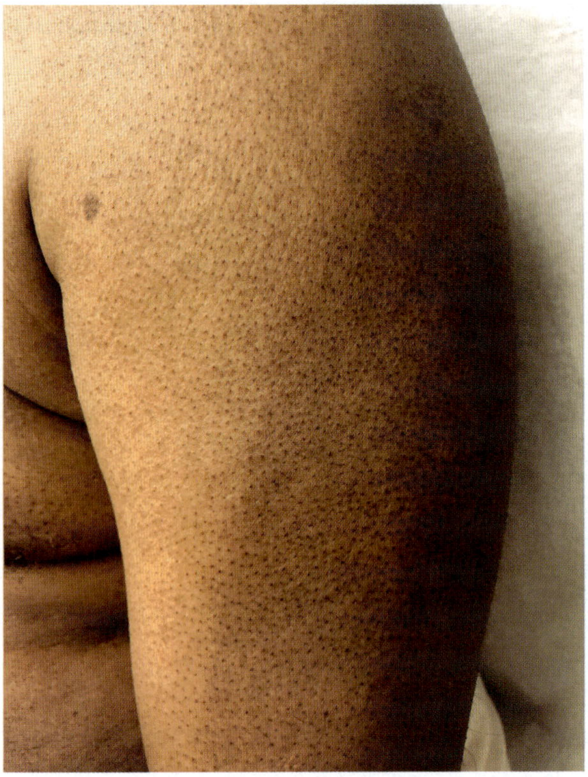

FIGURE 57-6. Pigmentary demarcation lines on the arm. (Courtesy of Henry W. Lim, MD, Department of Dermatology, Henry Ford Health, Detroit, MI, USA.)

RETICULATE ACROPIGMENTATION OF KITAMURA

Reticulate acropigmentation of Kitamura (RAPK) is a rare autosomal dominant disorder that was initially described in Japanese individuals but has since been seen in other ethnicities.[15,32,33] It typically presents with hyperpigmented and hypopigmented, angulated, and slightly atrophic macules in a reticulate pattern on the dorsal hands and feet in the first two decades of life.[15,33] These macules progressively darken and extend toward proximal extremities during adulthood and can spontaneous resolve by the time an individual is in their seventies. Pigmented palmar pits may also be present.[34] RAPK is due to a mutation in the *ADAM10* gene that encodes a zinc metalloprotease with various biological functions.[33,35] There are currently no treatments for RAPK.

DOWLING-DEGOS DISEASE

Dowling-Degos disease (DDD) is characterized by progressive red to dark brown macules and hyperkeratotic papules coalescing into reticulate patches in intertriginous and flexural areas such as the axilla, groin, neck, and inframammary folds.[15,36] In darker skin types, lesions can appear violaceous to black. It typically begins in the axilla and over time begins to involve other skin folds. Cases of generalized DDD have also been reported.[37] Comedone-like lesions, facial pitted scars, and red papules may be present. DDD is typically asymptomatic but can become pruritic when exacerbated by heat, sweat, or friction.[36] Galli-Galli disease is a subtype of DDD characterized by acantholysis.

DDD is autosomal dominant and typically presents in the adulthood with an average age of onset in the 30 to 40s. There are no racial or gender predilections for this disorder. Many genes involved in melanosome transfer, melanocyte differentiation, and keratinocyte differentiation have been implicated in this disorder including *KRT5*, *POFUT1*, *POGLUT1*, and *PSENEN*.[36] It is associated with epidermoid cysts and hidradenitis suppurativa that can also affect the intertriginous areas.[15,36] There are currently no standard treatments for DDD and use of topical treatments have been largely ineffective. Laser devices such as Er:YAG and CO_2 have shown some success in resolving clinical lesions.[36]

DERMATOPATHIA PIGMENTOSA RETICULARIS

Dermatopathia pigmentosa reticularis (DPR) is a rare autosomal dominant ectodermal dysplasia featuring the triad of reticulate brown to gray-brown macules, noncicatricial alopecia, and mild onychodystrophy.[38,39] Hyperpigmentation presents in childhood and is typically generalized with a predilection for the trunk over the extremities, reticulate in quality, and persists throughout adulthood. Other associations with this disorder include adermatoglyphia, sweat gland dysfunction, palmoplantar hyperkeratosis, and nonscarring blisters on acral surfaces.[40] Pterygium of the nail may also form.

DPR is due to a mutation in *KRT14* that increases apoptotic activity in the keratin 14 expressing basal layer.[38] This disorder is allelic to Naegeli-Franceschetti-Jadassohn syndrome (NFJS) and shares many of the same features, but in contrast to DPR, NFJS presents with dental abnormalities but not alopecia.[15,38] Furthermore, the hyperpigmentation in NFJS does not typically persist into adulthood. There are no treatments for DPR, but symptomatic patients may benefit from keratolytics, emollients, or topical steroids.

DYSKERATOSIS CONGENITA

Dyskeratosis congenita (DKC) is a disorder of defective telomere maintenance that presents with the triad of reticulated hyperpigmentation, nail dystrophy, and oral leukoplakia.[15,41] The reticulate brown pigmentation in DKC typically develops in the first decade of life [**Figure 57-7 A**] and may be associated with hypopigmented macules, telangiectasias, epidermal atrophy, and poikiloderma. Nail dystrophy initially presents with nail ridging and onychoschizia but can eventually result in pterygium formation [Figure 57-7B]. The oral leukoplakia of DKC is premalignant and presents in adolescence, therefore it is necessary to examine the oral cavity in those with DKC.[15,41] Other dermatologic findings include adermatoglyphia, palmoplantar hyperkeratosis, hyperhidrosis, premature graying, scalp or eyelash hair loss, epiphora, and lash irritation/blepharitis.[42] Extracutaneous manifestations include bone marrow failure (most common), squamous cell carcinomas and other malignancies, pulmonary fibrosis, liver cirrhosis, developmental delay, short stature, avascular necrosis of the femoral head, esophageal or urethral stenosis, cryptorchidism, male hypogonadism, and immune dysfunction.[15]

There are at least 11 gene mutations linked to DKC including but not limited to *DKC1* (most common, X-linked recessive inheritance), *TINF2*, *TERC*, *TERT*, and *RTEL1*. Given the assortment of genes involved in this disorder, the inheritance pattern and phenotype of this disease can vary widely. DKC has been known to exhibit autosomal dominant, autosomal recessive, and X-linked recessive inheritance, along with de novo mutations.[42] Severe mucocutaneous phenotypes have been associated with worse prognosis than those with milder phenotypes.[42] Early diagnosis of this disorder and access to multidisciplinary care are prudent given the high rates of morbidly and mortality in DKC.

INCONTINENTIA PIGMENTI

Incontinentia pigmenti (IP) is an X-linked dominant genodermatosis that presents with different morphologies at different stages of disease along the lines of Blaschko. It is characterized by four, often overlapping, stages: Stage I—vesiculobullous; Stage II—verrucous; Stage III—hyperpigmented; and Stage IV—hypopigmented or atrophic.[43,44] Nearly 98% of all individuals with IP develop Stage III at some point in their lives. This stage can overlap with other stages and typically appears as distinctive whorls and streaks of brown to slate-gray patches following the lines of Blaschko [**Figure 57-8**].[43] It frequently affects the trunk,

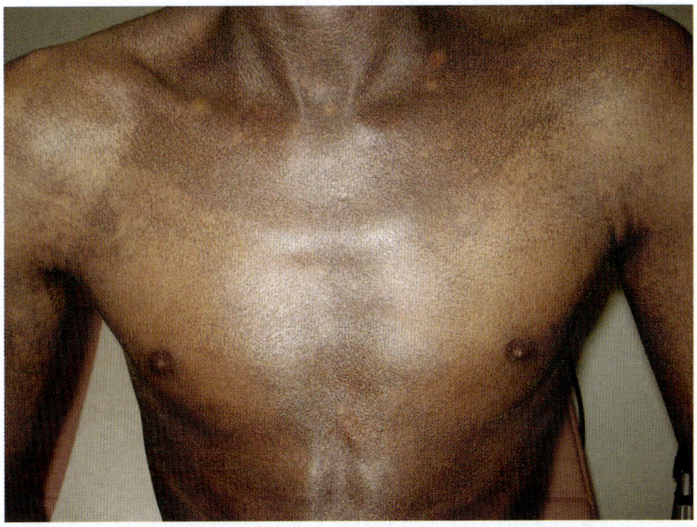

A

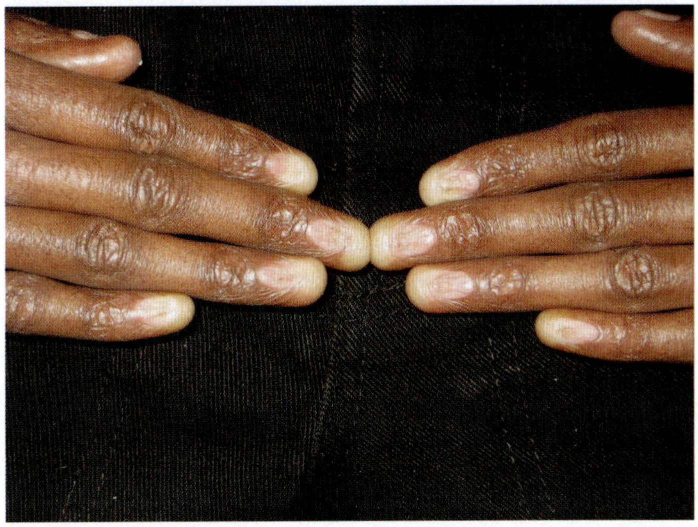

B

FIGURE 57-7. Dyskeratosis congenita presenting with **(A)** reticulate hyperpigmented patches with hypopigmented macules **(B)** pterygium of the fingernails. (Courtesy of Tor A. Shwayder, MD, Department of Dermatology, Henry Ford Health, Detroit, MI, USA.)

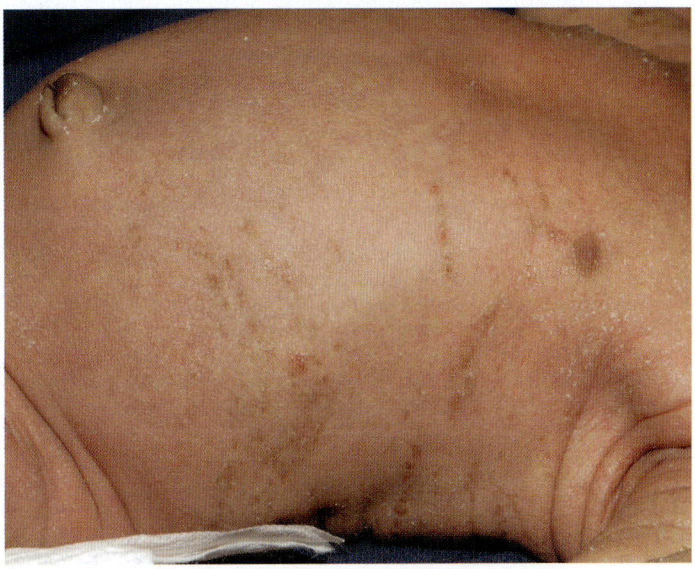

FIGURE 57-8. Blaschkoid hyperpigmentation in an infant with stage 3 incontinentia pigmenti. (Courtesy of Tor A. Shwayder, MD, Department of Dermatology, Henry Ford Health, Detroit, MI, USA.)

nipples, axilla, and groin and gradually fades in late childhood to adolescence.[15] Other features of this disorder include abnormal hair and nails, neurodevelopmental anomalies, dental anomalies, nipple and breast anomalies, ocular anomalies, palatal anomalies, and history of multiple male miscarriages in the family.[44] However, there is a wide range of phenotypical expressivity within the disorder.

IP is most commonly due to an inherited X-linked dominant mutation in the *IKBKG* (previously known as *NEMO*) gene. However, 10% to 20% of patients presenting with clinical findings of IP have no identifiable *IKBKG* pathogenic variant.[44] Additionally, although females are the most frequently affected, there have been many reports of male patients with clinical features of IP, some of whom demonstrate post-zygotic mosaicism for the *IKBKG* gene.[45] This suggests that IP is a genetically heterogeneous disorder and counseling of patients and families must be multidisciplinary in nature, individualized, and tailored to the patients' presentation.

CONCLUSION

Disorders of hyperpigmentation are common and often very distressing to those who are affected. A thorough clinical examination evaluating color, distribution, and pattern of hyperpigmentation along with assessment of other associated features can be helpful in properly diagnosing disorders of hyperpigmentation. When appropriate, additional workup and engagement of a multidisciplinary teams should be initiated for those with systemic disease.

Treatment of hyperpigmentation can be challenging, but the effects of both UV and visible light on pigment induction can be mitigated by using a broad spectrum, tinted sunscreen of at least SPF 30 daily.[46] Additionally, the use of oral antioxidants such as *Polypodium leucotomos* as well as sunscreens containing topical antioxidants have also shown to increase protection against UV- and visible light-induced pigment darkening.[46] Various lightening agents and procedures such as chemical peels and laser therapy have been used for certain disorders of hyperpigmentation, but it is important to discuss the potential of postinflammatory hyperpigmentation and paradoxical skin darkening prior to proceeding with any treatment, particularly in patients with darker skin colors.

REFERENCES

1. Lin JY, Fisher DE. Melanocyte biology and skin pigmentation. *Nature.* 2007;445(7130):843-850.
2. Wang RF, Ko D, Friedman BJ, Lim HW, Mohammad TF. Disorders of hyperpigmentation. Part I. Pathogenesis and clinical features of common pigmentary disorders. *J Am Acad Dermatol.* 2023;88(2):271-288.
3. Schwartz RA. Acanthosis nigricans. *J Am Acad Dermatol.* 1994;31(1):1-19; quiz 20-22.
4. Das A, Datta D, Kassir M, et al. Acanthosis nigricans: a review. *J Cosmet Dermatol.* 2020;19(8):1857-1865.
5. Hirt PA, Castillo DE, Yosipovitch G, Keri JE. Skin changes in the obese patient. *J Am Acad Dermatol.* 2019;81(5):1037-1057.
6. Valejo Coelho MM, Prokop J, Fernandes C. Acanthosis Nigricans Maligna. *JAMA Dermatol.* 2019;155(9):1069.
7. Treesirichod A, Chaithirayanon S, Chaikul T, Chansakulporn S. The randomized trials of 10% urea cream and 0.025% tretinoin cream in the treatment of acanthosis nigricans. *J Dermatolog Treat.* 2021;32(7):837-842.
8. Scheinfeld N. Confluent and reticulated papillomatosis : a review of the literature. *Am J Clin Dermatol.* 2006;7(5):305-313.
9. Mufti A, Sachdeva M, Maliyar K, et al. Treatment outcomes in confluent and reticulated papillomatosis: a systematic review. *J Am Acad Dermatol.* 2021;84(3):825-829.
10. Beutler BD, Cohen PR, Lee RA. Prurigo pigmentosa: literature review. *Am J Clin Dermatol.* 2015;16(6):533-543.
11. Zeng X, Li L, Cui B n. Prurigo pigmentosa: a clinical and histopathological study of nine Chinese cases. *J Eur Acad Dermatol Venereol.* 2016;30(10): 1794-1798.
12. Seol JE, Cho GJ, Park SH, Kim H. Prurigo pigmentosa: an institutional retrospective study of 24 patients. *Australas J Dermatol.* 2021;62(1):70-72.
13. Nahhas AF, Braunberger TL, Hamzavi IH. An update on drug-induced pigmentation. *Am J Clin Dermatol.* 2019;20(1):75-96.
14. Scherschun L, Lee MW, Lim HW. Diltiazem-associated photodistributed hyperpigmentation: a review of 4 cases. *Arch Dermatol.* 2001;137(2):179-182.
15. Chang MW. Disorders of hyperpigmentation. In: *Dermatology.* 4th ed. Amsterdam: Elsevier; 2018.
16. Dereure O. Drug-induced skin pigmentation. Epidemiology, diagnosis and treatment. *Am J Clin Dermatol.* 2001;2(4):253-262.
17. Hamid RN, Yang RG. Treatment of imipramine-induced hyperpigmentation with quality-switched ruby and picosecond lasers. *JAAD Case Rep.* 2021;17:12-17.
18. Wee SA, Dover JS. Effective treatment of psychotropic drug-induced facial hyperpigmentation with a 755-nm Q-switched alexandrite laser. *Dermatol Surg.* 2008;34(11):1609-1612.
19. Jabbour SA. Cutaneous manifestations of endocrine disorders: a guide for dermatologists. *Am J Clin Dermatol.* 2003;4(5):315-331.
20. Chacon AH, Morrison B, Hu S. Acquired hemochromatosis with pronounced pigment deposition of the upper eyelids. *J Clin Aesthet Dermatol.* 2013;6(10):44-46.
21. Gorbatsch S, Helmstädter V, Hartschuh W. Irregular, blotchy hyperpigmentation of the left nose, cheek and eyelid. *J Dtsch Dermatol Ges.* 2020;18(1):50-54.
22. Tong CV, Ooi XY. Addison's disease presenting with hyperpigmentation. *BMJ Case Rep.* 2021;14(8):e245610.
23. Banba K, Tanaka N, Fujioka A, Tajima S. Hyperpigmentation caused by hyperthyroidism: differences from the pigmentation of Addison's disease. *Clin Exp Dermatol.* 1999;24(3):196-198.
24. Song X, Shen Y, Zhou Y, et al. General hyperpigmentation induced by Grave's disease: a case report. *Medicine (Baltimore).* 2018;97(49):e13279.
25. Zieleniewski Ł, Schwartz RA, Goldberg DJ, Handler MZ. Voigt-Futcher pigmentary demarcation lines. *J Cosmet Dermatol.* 2019;18(3):700-702.
26. James WD, Carter JM, Rodman OG. Pigmentary demarcation lines: a population survey. *J Am Acad Dermatol.* 1987;16(3 Pt 1):584-590.
27. Sarma N, Chakraborty S, Bhattacharya SR. Acquired, idiopathic, patterned facial pigmentation (AIPFP) including periorbital pigmentation and pigmentary demarcation lines on face follows the lines of Blaschko on face. *Indian J Dermatol.* 2014;59(1):41-48.
28. Kato M, Yagami A, Tsukamoto T, Shinkai Y, Kato T, Kurahashi H. Novel mutation in the KITLG gene in familial progressive hyperpigmentation with or without hypopigmentation. *J Dermatol.* 2020;47(6):669-672.
29. Wang T, Li H, Dong Y, Hu M, She Q, Deng Y. Familial progressive hyperpigmentation: a family resurvey and ultrastructural skin investigation. *J Cutan Pathol.* 2017;44(11):948-950.
30. Zeng L, Zheng XD, Liu LH, et al. Familial progressive hyperpigmentation and hypopigmentation without KITLG mutation. *Clin Exp Dermatol.* 2016;41(8):927-929.
31. Rosés-Gibert P, Piqueres T, Martínez de Lagrán Álvarez de Arcaya Z. Familial progressive hyperpigmentation: skin lightening due to imatinib. *Med Clin (Barc).* 2022:S0025-7753(22)00373-6. Published online August 4.
32. Woodley DT, Caro I, Wheeler CE. Reticulate acropigmentation of Kitamura. *Arch Dermatol.* 1979;115(6):760-761.
33. Kono M, Akiyama M. Dyschromatosis symmetrica hereditaria and reticulate acropigmentation of Kitamura: an update. *J Dermatol Sci.* 2019;93(2):75-81.
34. Pathania YS, Razmi TM, Radotra BD, Kumaran SM. Pigmented palmar pits in reticulate acropigmentation of Kitamura. *Indian Dermatol Online J.* 2020;11(1):108-110.
35. García-Arpa M, Franco-Muñoz M, Flores-Terry MA, Ramos-Rodríguez C. Reticulate acropigmentation of Kitamura and nevus of Ito. *Actas Dermosifiliogr.* 2017;108(7):675-677.
36. Stephan C, Kurban M, Abbas O. Dowling-Degos disease: a review. *Int J Dermatol.* 2021;60(8):944-950.
37. Wu YH, Lin YC. Generalized Dowling-Degos disease. *J Am Acad Dermatol.* 2007;57(2):327-334.
38. Datta A, Gupta N, Pradhan S, Bandyopadhyay D. Dermatopathia pigmentosa reticularis. *Indian J Dermatol.* 2019;64(2):149-151.
39. Heimer WL, Brauner G, James WD. Dermatopathia pigmentosa reticularis: a report of a family demonstrating autosomal dominant inheritance. *J Am Acad Dermatol.* 1992;26(2 Pt 2):298-301.
40. Brar BK, Mehta V, Kubba A. Dermatopathia pigmentosa reticularis. *Pediatr Dermatol.* 2007;24(5):566-570.
41. AlSabbagh MM. Dyskeratosis congenita: a literature review. *J Dtsch Dermatol Ges.* 2020;18(9):943-967.
42. Ward SC, Savage SA, Giri N, et al. Beyond the triad: Inheritance, mucocutaneous phenotype, and mortality in a cohort of patients with dyskeratosis congenita. *J Am Acad Dermatol.* 2018;78(4):804-806.

43. Berlin AL, Paller AS, Chan LS. Incontinentia pigmenti: a review and update on the molecular basis of pathophysiology. *J Am Acad Dermatol.* 2002;47(2):169-187; quiz 188-190.
44. Wang R, Lara-Corrales I, Kannu P, Pope E. Unraveling incontinentia pigmenti: a comparison of phenotype and genotype variants. *J Am Acad Dermatol.* 2019;81(5):1142-1149.
45. Fusco F, Fimiani G, Tadini G, Michele D, Ursini MV. Clinical diagnosis of incontinentia pigmenti in a cohort of male patients. *J Am Acad Dermatol.* 2007;56(2):264-267.
46. Yeager DG, Lim HW. What's new in photoprotection: a review of new concepts and controversies. *Dermatol Clin.* 2019;37(2):149-157.

CHAPTER 58

Disorders of Hypopigmentation

Sarah Gonzalez
Nada Elbuluk

KEY POINTS

- Disorders of hypopigmentation occur from a variety of causes including inflammatory, infectious, and neoplastic.
- These conditions can cause significant psychological, social, and emotional distress to those affected.
- Certain disorders of hypopigmentation are more prevalent in individuals of color.
- Awareness of how these conditions present in skin of color is important in providing appropriate diagnoses, prognostic expectations, and for devising appropriate therapeutic plans.

INTRODUCTION

Disorders of dyspigmentation that include those of hypopigmentation are the third most common reason individuals with skin of color (SOC) seek treatment from a dermatologist.[1] Hypopigmentation refers to the lightening of the skin due to a decrease in melanin content, which can be from a variety of causes.[1,2] Disorders of hypopigmentation can vary in location, presentation, distribution, and onset. They also can have various etiologies including inflammatory, infectious, and neoplastic. Some of these conditions are more common in individuals with SOC.[1] These conditions can affect quality of life and carry emotional and psychological burden that can be heightened in SOC due to the contrast of affected to normal skin.[1] Accurate and early recognition of these conditions as well as appropriate and timely treatment are important in optimizing treatment outcomes and improving quality of life.

SEBORRHEIC DERMATITIS

EPIDEMIOLOGY

Seborrheic dermatitis (SD) is a benign, chronic, inflammatory disorder arising on body sites with abundant sebaceous glands including the scalp, glabella, eyebrows, nasolabial folds, paranasal skin, cheeks, beard-covered areas, the upper chest, back, and skin flexures.[3] In the United States, an estimated 50 million Americans have seborrheic dermatitis.[4] Studies conducted in the United States and China have demonstrated that prevalence of SD differs by racial/ethnic group, 81% to 95% in African Americans, 66% to 2% in Whites, and 30% to 42% in Chinese.[5] Incidences in African Americans and West Africans have been reported to be 6.5% and 2.9% to 6%, respectively.[3] A study by Alexis et al revealed that SD is the fifth common dermatologic diagnosis in people with SOC in the United States.[6] There is a predilection of SD in men and a bimodal age distribution.[7] Infantile seborrheic dermatitis that appears on the scalp, also known as "cradle cap," may present as early as 2 weeks of age, with peak incidence at 3 months.[8] In infants, the retroauricular scalp, external ear, neck, and diaper region may also be affected.[9]

CLINICAL FEATURES

The archetypal presentation of seborrheic dermatitis in lighter skin types are erythematous patches with overlying greasy yellow hyperkeratotic scale in areas replete with sebaceous glands.[3] Background erythema is not as easily appreciated in individuals with darker skin who tend to present with hypopigmentation with less overlying scale [**Figure 58-1A-B**].[3,10] Individuals with darker skin may have a form of SD known as "petaloid SD" consisting of fused pink to hypopigmented polycyclic patches with subtle scaling.[3] Understanding the different presentations of SD in lighter and darker skin is not only important for accurately diagnosing the condition but also for assessing disease severity and deciding on the appropriate treatment regimen.

DIAGNOSIS

The diagnosis of SD is clinical, based on SD's classic morphology and pattern; however, dermoscopy may be useful to differentiate scalp psoriasis from SD.[8] On dermoscopy, SD can show arborizing vessels and atypical red vessels while scalp psoriasis can show red dots and globules, twisted loops, and glomerular vessels.[8]

A skin biopsy is not necessary but can be done in cases where the diagnosis is not clear. Histopathology may vary on whether the stage of the

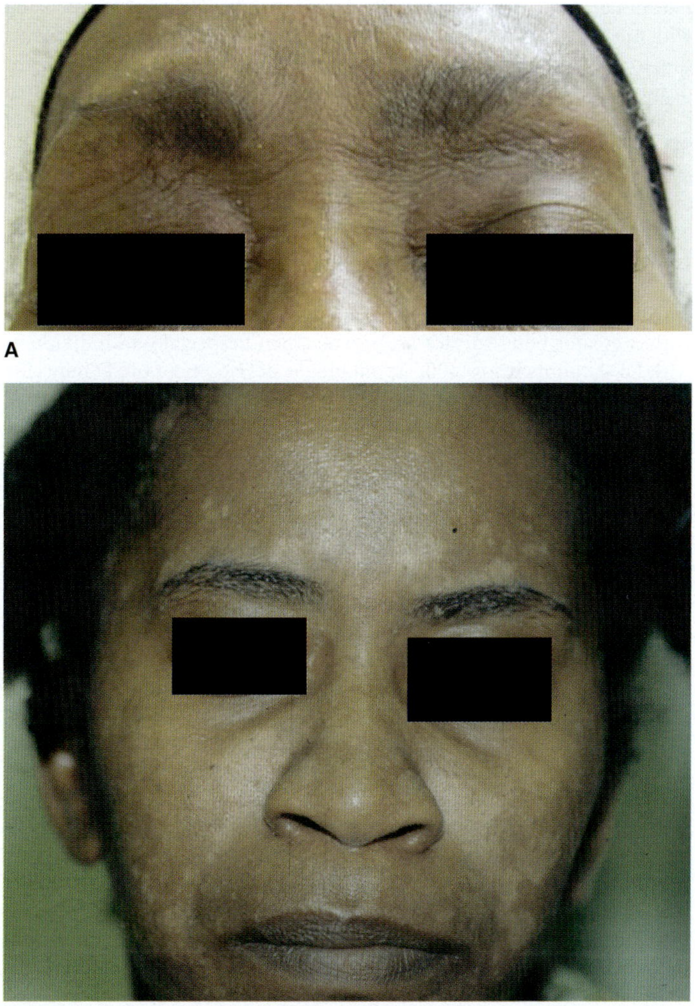

A

B

FIGURE 58-1. (A) Facial seborrheic dermatitis. Adult female with fine scaly plaques on the eyebrows and eyelids. **(B)** Postinflammatory hypopigmentation. Hypopigmented macules coalescing into patches in a seborrheic distribution secondary to prior seborrheic dermatitis.

SD is acute, subacute, or chronic. Acute and subacute changes can include mild spongiotic dermatitis with psoriasiform hyperplasia, folliculocentric crust with neutrophils scattered at the tips of the follicular aperture, orthokeratosis with focal parakeratosis, and superficial perivascular lymphohistiocytic infiltration.[8] Chronic SD can show dilated superficial vessels with exaggeration of the features seen in acute and subacute SD.[8] Potassium hydroxide (KOH) scraping can differentiate SD from tinea or demonstrate concomitant *Malassezia* (*also known as Pityrosporum*) folliculitis.[8]

DIFFERENTIAL DIAGNOSIS

Some of the common differential diagnoses for SD, include tinea capitis, psoriasis, atopic dermatitis, contact dermatitis, rosacea, erythrasma, and vitiligo.[3]

PATHOGENESIS

The evolution of SD can be attributed to propagation of the commensal yeast *Malassezia*, an individual's chemical sebum makeup, and host immune response.[3] Two species of *Malassezia* in particular have been implicated in SD, *Malassieza globose* and *Malassieza restricta*.[7] Sebum is composed of triglycerides and esters, which further break down into diglycerides, monoglycerides, and free fatty acids.[7] During times of stress, increased sebum is produced, which has been noted to trigger or exacerbate SD.[7]

ETIOLOGY AND ASSOCIATIONS

Hormonal changes that stimulate sebaceous glands may be associated with SD in infants and adolescents.[7,11] Sebum excretion is high in infants due to the transfer of maternal sex hormones, resolving after the withdrawal of these maternal hormones and reappearing at puberty when sebaceous glands are most active.[7,11] Furthermore, the predilection of SD in males can be attributed to their elevated androgen levels.[4] However, this hypothesis does not explain the reappearance of SD in adults around the age of 50.[7,11] Stress and anxiety have also been associated with SD as well as neurologic disorders including cerebrovascular incidents, epilepsy, cerebral trauma, and Parkinson disease.[7] In these populations as well as in individuals with HIV, SD can have a more severe and widespread presentation.[7] Incidence in individuals with HIV is 30% to 83% with a greater body surface area involvement, especially in individuals with CD4 counts below 400.[7] Spontaneous development of SD may clue physicians into testing for HIV. In individuals with HIV, improvement of SD is seen with antiretroviral treatment.[7]

TREATMENT

As SD is a chronic disease that can wax and wane in severity, acute and maintenance treatment are needed. Elimination of the yeast, inflammatory abatement, and reduction in production of sebum are the targets of treatment.[7] Traditional topical treatments consist of shampoos containing antifungal ingredients including, selenium sulfide, ketoconazole, and zinc pyrithione.[3,7] Leave on topical treatments include topical imidazoles, topical calcineurin inhibitors, and topical steroids.[3] For scalp involvement, the treatment plan should consider hair type and hair washing frequency. Those with drier hair textures and scalps may prefer their prescriptions in an ointment and/or oil vehicle, while those with oily scalps may prefer a solution-based prescription.[3] The Cochrane collaboration conducted a review of studies using antifungals in the treatment of SD and found that treatment with ketoconazole had a similar remission rate to that of steroids with a side effect profile that was 44% lower than that of steroids.[7,12] The reported side effects included erythema, pruritus, burning, and aloepcia.[12] Rates of relapse were highest in participants using placebo at 47%, compared to those using ketoconazole 2% shampoo once every 2 weeks (31%), and in participants who used ketoconazole 2% shampoo once weekly (19%).[12] Treatment of scalp seborrheic dermatitis should always take into consideration hair type, frequency of hair washing, and prescription vehicle preference. Individuals with SOC presenting with SD-associated hypopigmentation on their face and/or body should be reassured that the hypopigmentation can take longer to resolve even after appropriate treatment has been provided.

TINEA VERSICOLOR

EPIDEMIOLOGY

Tinea versicolor (TV) also known as pityriasis versicolor (PV) is a fungal infection caused by the species *Malassezia globosa and Malassezia furfur*.[2,13] Tinea versicolor typically impacts teenagers and young adults but can also develop in children.[14] Onset is typically during puberty and most often triggered by hyperhidrosis and warm climates.[14] TV is frequently observed in tropical environments as well as during the summer season.[14] Other factors that may increase the risk of TV are endocrinopathies, oral contraceptives, decreased cellular immunity, or topical application of oily substances.[2] Twin studies demonstrate that there may also be a genetic component to TV.[15] There is no consensus as to whether or not there is a predilection of TV in individuals with SOC with several studies showing that tinea versicolor affects people of all racial and ethnic backgrounds and climates equally.[13] Males, regardless of their ethnicity, may have a higher prevalence of tinea versicolor due to increased sebaceous activity.[13]

CLINICAL FEATURES

TV is most commonly located on the neck, trunk, and proximal upper extremities [**Figure 58-2A-C**]. More rarely, TV can also arise on the face and neck.[13] In those with lighter skin, TV may appear as salmon colored to pink scaly macules and patches.[14] In individuals with SOC, TV generally appears as hypopigmented macules with a fine overlying scale that can evolve into larger, confluent, irregular-shaped patches.[13,14] Less commonly in SOC, TV presents as hyperpigmented dark brown scaly macules and patches.[13] Diffuse presentation on the face or lower extremities should raise concern for systemic conditions such as HIV, Parkinson, and a compromised immune system that could present in those on systemic steroids, those suffering from malnutrition, or those with solid organ transplants.[2,15,16]

DIAGNOSIS

The diagnosis can typically be made clinically but a KOH preparation can confirm tinea with the classic "spaghetti and meatballs" appearance of hyphae and spores.[13] A Wood's lamp may also aid in the diagnosis. The source of fluorescence is a fluorochrome known as pityrialactone produced by the fungus *Malassezia*.[17] Under Wood's lamp, pityrialactone emits a yellow-orange fluorescence from the affected skin.[17] Scaling of tinea also becomes more prominent with scratching or stretching of the skin.[18] Dermoscopic features of TV include fine white scaling in skin furrows and a faint brown pigmented network [**Table 58-1**].[19,20]

A biopsy is not necessary but in cases of recalcitrant disease or atypical presentation, a biopsy can be done for confirmation. A fungal stain is applied to establish the presence of hyphae and spores.[21] Histopathology demonstrates yeast and hyphae in the stratum corneum, slight hyperkeratosis and acanthosis, little or no inflammation, and is PAS positive.[22] In darker skin, the biopsy can demonstrate a thicker stratum corneum with more tonofilaments in the granulosum as well as isolated melanosomes.[13]

DIFFERENTIAL DIAGNOSIS

The common differential diagnoses for tinea versicolor includes seborrheic dermatitis, pityriasis rosea, vitiligo, erythrasma, pityriasis alba, secondary syphilis, progressive macular hypomelanosis, and hypopigmented mycosis fungoides.[13]

PATHOGENESIS

TV is considered both melanopenic and melanocytopenic.[1] The fungus *Malassezia* is a benign, chronic member of the skin's normal

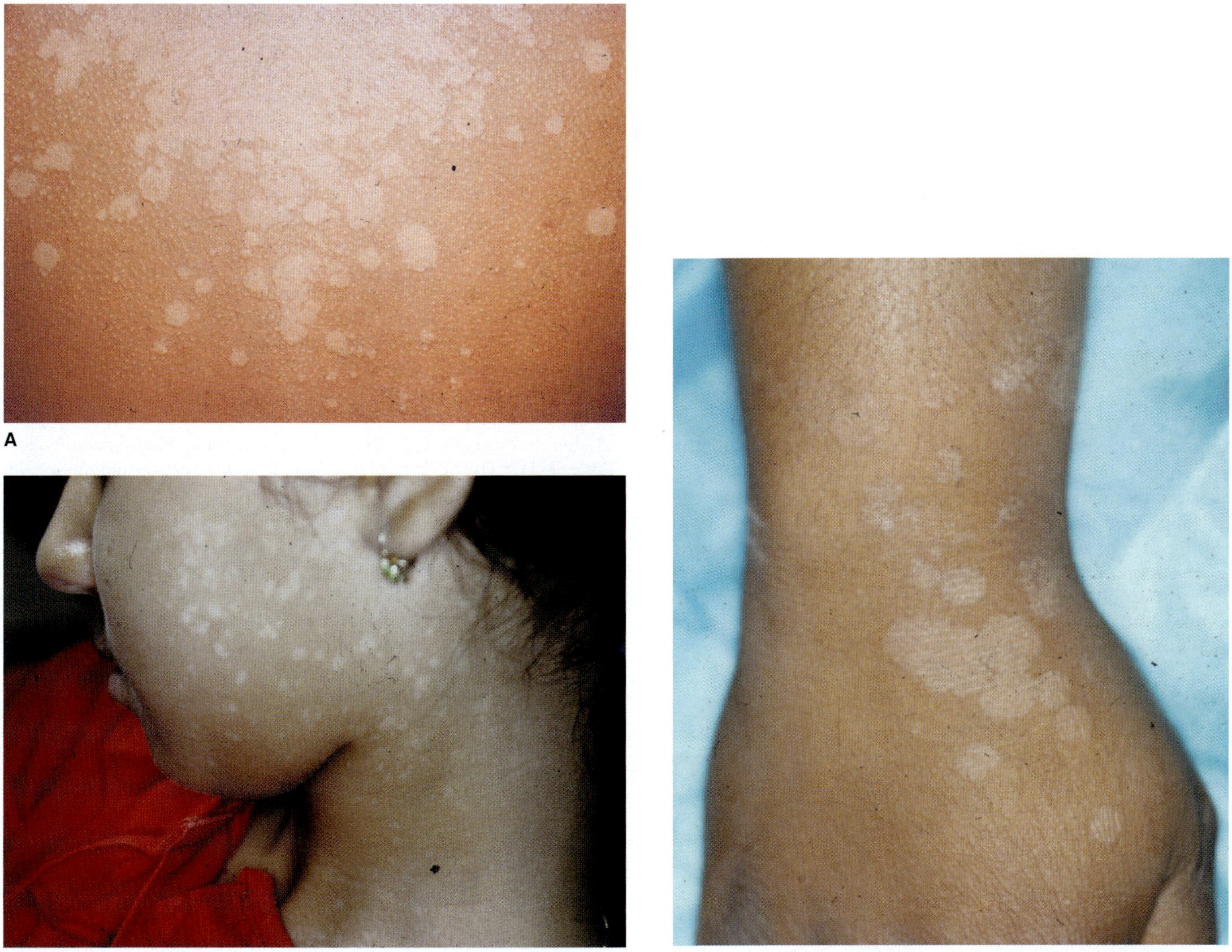

A

C

B

FIGURE 58-2. (A) Tinea versicolor. Hypopigmented scaly macules and patches on the dorsal hand. **(B)** Tinea versicolor. Confluent hypopigmented scaly macules and patches on the trunk. **(C)** Tinea versicolor. Hypopigmented macules along the lateral face and neck of a young woman.

flora.[15] The yeasts are lipophilic, therefore oily preparations, or excess production of sebum in puberty, facilitate the yeast formation of *Malassezia*. Ultraviolet (UV) exposure leads to the production of azelaic acid. In vitro, azelaic acid inhibits tyrosinase and impairs melanocytes, which most likely is the agent responsible for hypochromia in vivo.[1,15]

TREATMENT

The treatment of TV can involve topical and/or oral treatments. Topical antifungal shampoos used include those containing imidazoles (ie, ketoconazole 2% shampoo), selenium sulfide, and zinc-pyrithione.[2,14] Topical leave on treatments include selenium sulfide lotion, ketoconazole cream,

TABLE 58-1 Dermoscopy findings of disorders of hypopigmentation

Pigmentary disorder	Background color	Scale color and distribution	Vessel type and arrangement	Pigment network	Diagnostic clues
Tinea versicolor	White to white-brown	White, diffuse, in perifollicular lines	Not present	Faint brown	Scales are "double edged"
Idiopathic guttate hypomelanosis	White	Not present	Linear and branching	Loss of pigment network	Variant patterns of margins
Pityriasis alba	White to white-brown	White; Diffuse	Not present	Light brown	Margins are ill-defined
Pityriasis rosea	Yellow-orange	Yellow-white; patchy and peripheral	Dotted in patchy arrangement		Jagged edges, collarette of scale
Progressive macular hypopigmentation	Brown to brown-white	Minimal scale only on cleavage lines	N/A	Broken reticulate pigment	Scale limited to cleavage lines
Pityriasis lichenoides chronica	Yellow to yellow-orange	Brown and central	Varies linear and dotted; areas of milky red	Orange-yellow structureless regions, brown dots and globules	

terbinafine, clotrimazole, bifonazole, and miconazole.[2,14,23] More severe, widespread, or recalcitrant cases have been effectively treated with varying regimens of oral antifungal medications: 200 mg of oral ketoconazole for 10 days, itraconazole 200 mg daily for 5 to 7 days, reaching a minimum cumulative dose of 1000 mg, or oral fluconazole 300 mg once weekly for 2 to 4 weeks.[13,24] Oral ketoconazole should be used with caution due to the risk of fulminant hepatitis.[2] Recurrence of TV is common, occurring within 1 year in 60% of patients; however, recurrence may be circumvented with maintenance use of an antifungal shampoo.[2] In individuals with repeat infections or those who are immunocompromised, a 1-month dose of 400 mg prophylactic oral itraconazole has shown to be efficacious.[13,25]

IDIOPATHIC GUTTATE HYPOMELANOSIS

EPIDEMIOLOGY

Idiopathic guttate hypomelanosis (IGH) is a benign skin condition that is often acquired and commonly found in adults and the elderly.[26] It is characterized by multiple, round or oval hypopigmented macules that typically appear on photo-exposed areas such as the pretibial legs and extensor forearms.[26] The prevalence of IGH tends to increase with age with a prevalence of 87% in individuals over the age of 40.[27] There is a nearly equal distribution of cases between women (56%) and men (54%), with women being diagnosed at a younger age likely due to earlier presentation for dermatology consultations.[27]

CLINICAL FEATURES

IGH consists of painless well-defined hypopigmented to depigmented macules most commonly on the upper and lower extremities [**Figure 58-3**].[26] Rarely does IGH appear on the face or trunk.[26,27] IGH macules do not change in size over time but can increase in number with age.[26,27] IGH can be seen among all skin colors but is more noticeable in SOC. [28,29] The initial presence of this condition can sometimes be a source of psychological distress for affected individuals and can be mistaken for vitiligo.

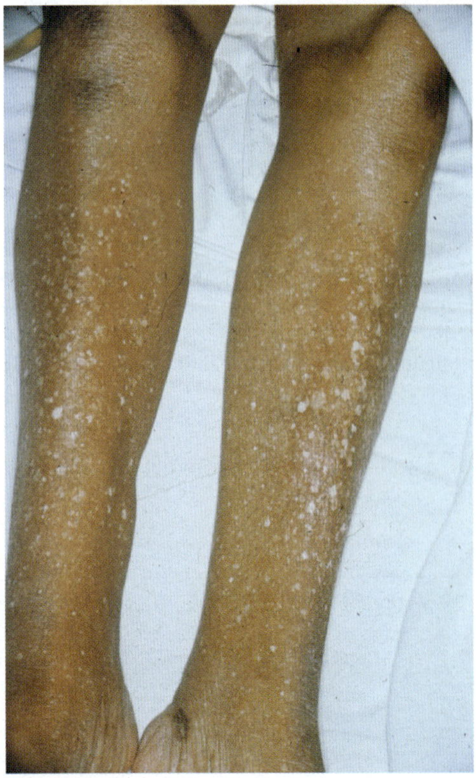

FIGURE 58-3. Idiopathic guttate hypomelanosis. Numerous discrete hypopigmented macules on the bilateral anterior lower extremities.

DIAGNOSIS

The diagnosis can be made clinically but in unclear cases, a biopsy can confirm diagnosis. A biopsy will demonstrate hyperkeratosis, a thin epidermis with flat rete ridges, decreased number of epidermal melanocytes.[30] Histopathology of skin grafts from patients with IGH and control patients demonstrated a higher accumulation of melanin in the basement layer of patients with IGH compared to the control group.[31] Other histopathological features of IGH biopsy include thickened orthokeratotic basket weave stratum corneum, decreased or absent 3,4 dihydroxyphenylalanine (DOPA)-positive epidermal melanocytes within the basal layer of the epidermis, and reduced melanocytes at the dermal-epidermal junction.[32,33] Another characteristic that may be unique to IGH are "skip areas" in which there is alternating loss of melanin in the basal layer.[32]

Using dermoscopy, IGH shows absence of pigment and a white glow [Table 58-1].[34] The margins of IGH have four different variants: ameboid, petaloid, feathery, and nebuloid.[34] Pseudopod extensions are observed in the periphery of the ameboid variant, feather-like fibers in the feathery pattern, and leaf-like extensions in the petaloid variant.[34] The nebuloid pattern is distinguished from the other patterns with its indistinct borders, closely resembling guttate vitiligo.[34] Clinical correlations with the dermoscopy patterns of IGH have been found. Those with a feathery pattern tend to be younger, while those with an amoeboid, nebuloid, or petaloid pattern tend to be older.[26] A study from 2021 found the nebuloid pattern to be seen in individuals with longer duration of IGH, while the petaloid pattern was detected in those with shorter duration of IGH.[26] This contrasts an earlier study, where feathery patterns were seen in individuals with longer duration of IGH and nebuloid patterns in those with shorter duration of IGH.[26]

DIFFERENTIAL DIAGNOSIS

The differential diagnoses for IGH is broad; however, arguably the most important from which to distinguish is vitiligo given the differences in prognosis.[33] Other conditions to consider in the differential include pityriasis alba, tinea versicolor, guttate morphea, progressive macular hypomelanosis, eruptive hypomelanosis, hypopigmented flat verruca, hypopigmented seborrheic dermatosis, pityriasis lichenoides chronica, Darier disease, vitiligo, lichen sclerosus, atrophie blanche, and postinflammatory hypopigmentation.[26,30,33]

PATHOGENESIS

The pathogenesis of IGH remains unclear.[27,29] However, it appears to be associated with aging degeneration, chronic sun exposure, local trauma, oxidative stress, autoimmune processes, genetics, and inhibition of melanogenesis.[26,27]

TREATMENT

There is currently no gold standard treatment for IGH and spontaneous repigmentation has not been reported. Patients should be reassured about the benign nature of the condition. Given the implication of UV exposure in the pathogenesis of IGH, diligent sun protection is recommended. Many treatments have been tried for IGH with varying success.[21] These attempted topical treatments include steroids, phenol, retinoids, prostaglandin analogues, and calcineurin inhibitors.[2,21,26] Procedural treatments that have been used as monotherapy or in combination with topical therapies include cryotherapy, nonablative fractional photothermolysis, fractional photothermolysis, excimer, chemical peels, microneedling, dermabrasion, intralesional steroids, and surgical mini-grafting.[2,21,26] A randomized, controlled, single-blinded study demonstrated results consistent with prior studies, a singular 5-second cycle of cryotherapy resulted in repigmentation up to 4 months posttreatment.[35] Caution should be used with cryotherapy treatment in SOC due to risk of leukoderma.[1,2,30] Transdermal infusion of 5-fluorouracil into IGH macules has shown successful repigmentation in some cases.[2,21,26,36]

PITYRIASIS ALBA

EPIDEMIOLOGY

Pityriasis alba (PA) is self-resolving eczematous disorder that is more common in children and adolescents with a predominance in Fitzpatrick skin type IV to VI, including children of Hispanic and Asian descent.[1,14] Ninety percent of cases occur in children younger than 12 years.[37]

CLINICAL FEATURES

On examination, PA presents with round to oval-shaped, hypopigmented patches with ill-defined margins and little to none overlying scale [**Figure 58-4**].[14] PA is more common on the face and upper extremities, more visible in darker skin types, and more visible in summer months.[1] There are three common variations of PA: classic, extensive, and pigmenting.[1,38] Classic PA is the most common form seen in school-aged children.[38] Initially, the affected area can appear as red macules or patches, which then fade away after a few weeks and result in poorly defined white patches with scale.[1] Although PA typically does not cause any discomfort, some patients may experience mild itching or burning.[1] PA usually appears symmetrically on the cheeks and can vary in size from 5 to 30 mm.[1] On occasion PA presents on the upper extremities.[1] The arms may show more pronounced involvement around the hair follicles.[1] Extensive PA has extensive and symmetric body surface area involvement, presenting as many round, nonscaly hypopigmented patches on the trunk.[1] Some authors consider the extensive variant of PA to be a separate entity from the classical variant as extensive PA lacks preceding erythema and patients report no history of atopy.[1] Pigmenting PA is the least common variant of PA that has currently only been seen in non-SOC individuals.[38] Pigmenting PA appears as blue-tinted macules secondary to melanin deposition in the dermis, surrounded by a scaly ring of depigmentation.[1,38]

DIAGNOSIS

The diagnosis can be made clinically and can be supported by dermoscopy, Wood's lamp, KOH, and a biopsy if needed. KOH will be negative while Wood's lamp will lack fluorescence.[39] These findings differentiate PA from vitiligo, which does fluoresce and in which edges tend to be sharply demarcated.[39]

Faint brown pigment within white structureless areas that have central scaling and ill-defined margins are features of PA on dermoscopy [Table 58-1].[39] Biopsy can be used in unclear cases to rule out other conditions and will show nonspecific findings including chronic spongiotic dermatitis with an interruption of the melanin pigment along the basal layer.[1]

DIFFERENTIAL DIAGNOSIS

The differential diagnosis for PA includes atopic dermatitis, contact dermatitis, leprosy, discoid eczema, delusional tinea, nevus anemicus, pityriasis rosea, tinea corporis, nummular eczema, pityriasis lichenoides chronica, and vitiligo.[39]

PATHOGENESIS

Numerous mechanisms have been proposed as to the pathogenesis of PA.[1] The leading mechanism implicates atopic dermatitis with a resulting hypomelanosis after resolution of the inflammatory process.[1] The impaired transfer of pigment from melanocytes to keratinocytes may be responsible for the hypopigmentation.[1] Xerosis is often linked with both PA and atopic dermatitis, which can occur due to frequent bathing and hot showers, leading to reduced water retention capacity in the stratum corneum.[1] PA has also been associated with nutritional deficiencies, such as low levels of zinc, magnesium, ferritin, hemoglobin, and copper, a cofactor for the enzyme tyrosinase, required for melanin synthesis.[1,40]

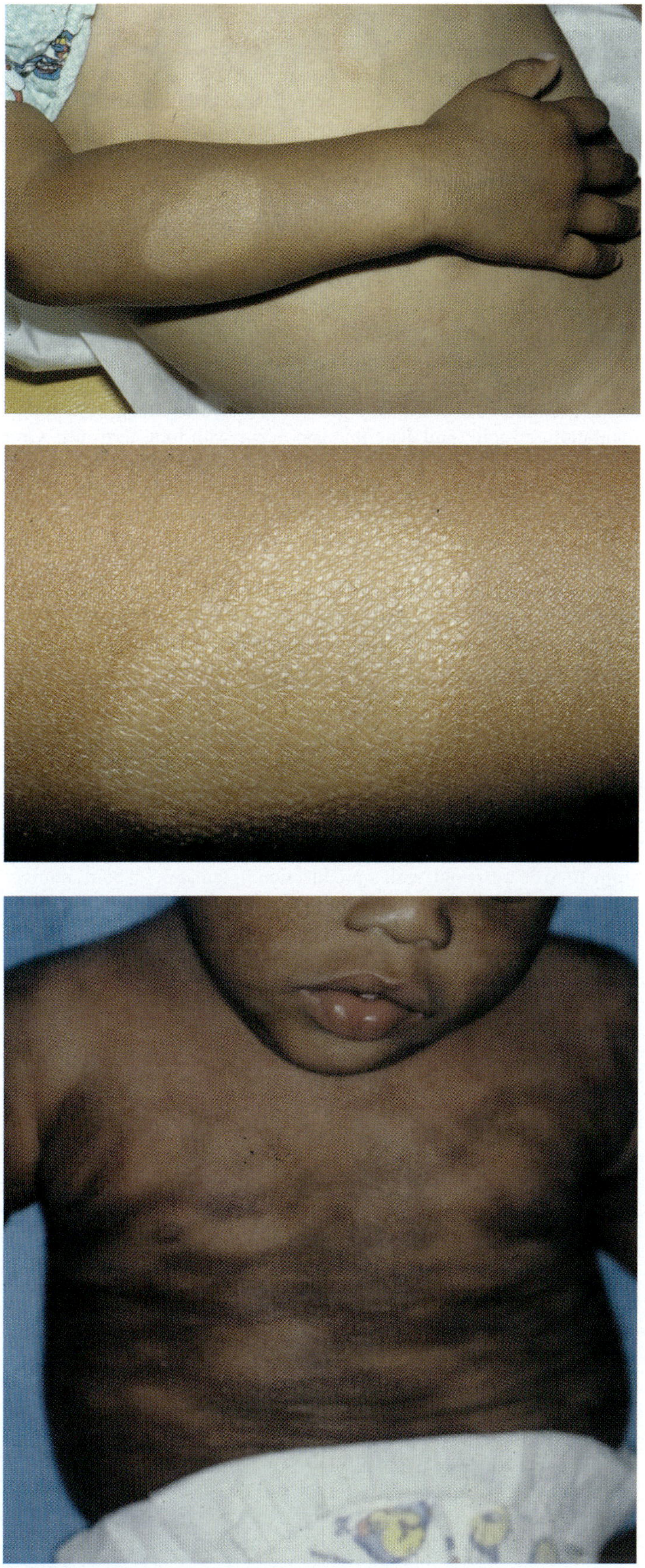

FIGURE 58-4. Pityriasis alba. Large discrete hypopigmented nummular patch on the dorsal forearm. Close-up of hypopigmented patch on the dorsal forearm of an infant. Numerous hypopigmented patches diffusely scattered on the anterior trunk of a baby.

TREATMENT

PA is self-limiting and reassurance should be provided to affected individuals and their parents. Despite the self-liming nature of PA, treatment may be considered in individuals with darker skin due to the obvious contrast of involved and uninvolved skin. Emollients such as petroleum jelly and ammonium lactate may alleviate the associated dryness and inflammation.[1] Treatment modalities include topical steroids, calcineurin inhibitors, tar emulsions, and phototherapy.[1] Tar emulsions are melanogenic without the need for UV light. Twice daily application is recommended, and these are available as a 6% cream or 5% liquor carbonis detergens, either as an acid mantle cream vehicle or combined with a mild-potency steroid.[1] With topical steroids, the potency of the steroid must be considered, with mild potency for the face and medium for the body. In addition to its melanogenic property, the topical steroids alleviate the inflammation and pruritus associated with PA.[1] Overuse of steroids should be avoided as to prevent the adverse effects of hypopigmentation, atrophy, and acne that can occur with long-term use. Oral psoralen plus UVA (PUVA) can be considered for more widespread disease in adults. Narrowband ultraviolet B (NB-UVB) therapy two to three times per week is another alternative.[1] Application of 1% tacrolimus ointment twice daily in Fitzpatrick skin type III and IV and twice daily 1% pimecrolimus cream in Fitzpatrick skin type IV and V have also shown positive results.[1,41] Affected individuals should be advised that after resolution of PA, affected areas may remain hypopigmented for a longer period of time before baseline pigmentation returns.

PITYRIASIS ROSEA

EPIDEMIOLOGY

Pityriasis rosea (PR) is a self-limiting disease with an incidence of 0.5% to 2% that is typically seen in adolescents and young adults, ranging from 10 to 35 years old, with a predilection in females.[42,43] Some sources indicate that PR may disproportionately affect POC; however, a recent cross-sectional study using the *All of Us* database demonstrates similar prevalence among all races and ethnicities.[44,45]

CLINICAL FEATURES

PR can appear differently across skin colors.[44,45] PR begins with the archetypal "herald patch" that has a slow enlargement with new patches appearing over 3 weeks and lasting for up 6 to 8 weeks, in 80% of patients.[42,43] However, compared to adults, children have a shorter interval between the initial herald patch and the emergence of subsequent patches, on average 4 days compared to 2 weeks in adults.[45] Duration of the disease also tends to be shorter in children than in adults by several weeks.[45] On the trunk, the secondary patches have been described as forming a "Christmas tree" pattern along Langer's lines of cleavage.[42,43,45] In lighter skin, the patches tend to be pink to salmon-colored with scaly borders, while in patients with SOC the patches can be brown, gray, or violaceous with less overlying scale or central hyperpigmentation [**Figure 58-5A-C**].[45] PR often resolves with postinflammatory hyperpigmentation. Individuals with darker skin can also have a papular or papulovesicular presentation of PR. While PR tends to affect trunk and proximal extremities, it occurs less commonly on the face, neck, and scalp.[45] However, in individuals with SOC, especially children, PR can be more extensive and is often found on the face, neck, and scalp.[45] PR can be associated with prodromal symptoms, such as, headache, malaise, lymphadenopathy, arthralgia, fever, and nausea.[42,45]

Aside from classic PR, atypical variants arise in 20% of cases.[42,43,46] Hypopigmented PR is more common in individuals with dark skin and presents with hypopigmented patches at the onset of active disease.[42] Although, PR tends to be a benign disease, in pregnant individuals, PR is associated with increased risk of fetal loss and premature birth.[47] This may be due to an association with human herpesvirus 6 (HHV-6) and human herpes virus 7 (HHV-7).[47]

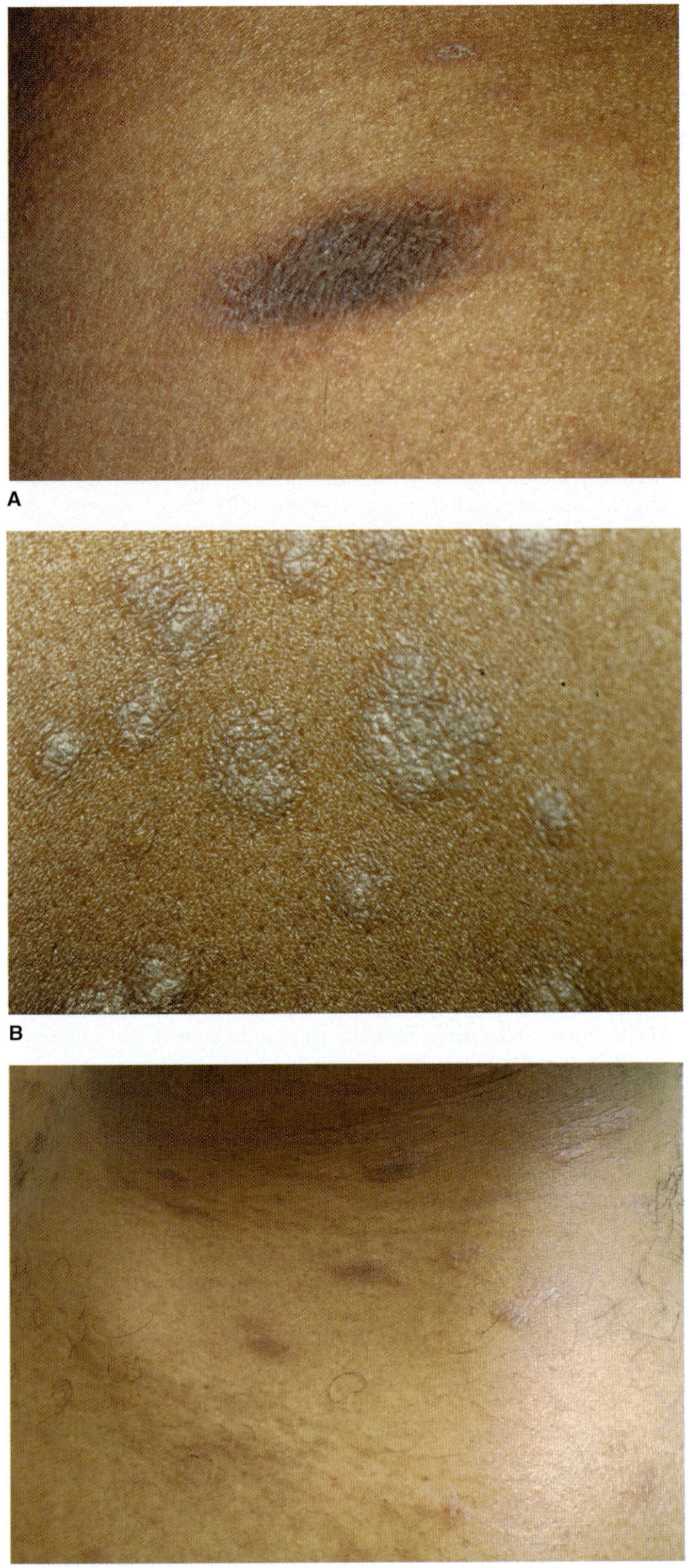

FIGURE 58-5. **(A)** Pityriasis rosea. Violaceous plaque with peripheral rim of erythema. **(B)** Pityriasis rosea. Gray thin scaly plaques. **(C)** Pityriasis rosea. Small red-brown plaques with overlying scale on the superior anterolateral trunk of a Fitzpatrick type IV adult. (Courtesy of Henry W. Lim, MD. Detroit, MI, USA.)

DIAGNOSIS

A diagnosis can often be made clinically but a biopsy can be done in uncertain cases. A biopsy of PR will show subacute spongiotic dermatitis, dispersed erythrocytes, dyskeratosis, and lymphocytes in the perivasculature.[48] On dermoscopy, PR has a yellow-orange background, vessels appear dotted with irregular and peripheral arrangement, scales are yellow-white and/or white-gray, with patchy, peripheral, and collarette distribution [Table 58-1].[49]

DIFFERENTIAL DIAGNOSIS

The differential for PR includes small plaque parapsoriasis, lichen planus, guttate psoriasis, pityriasis lichenoides chronica, secondary syphilis, subacute cutaneous lupus erythematosus, and dermatophytosis.[42,45]

PATHOGENESIS

The exact cause of PR is still unknown, but studies have suggested that it is linked to the reactivation of HHV-6 and HHV-7.[47]

TREATMENT

Treatment is not necessary for PR as the disease is self-limiting; however, patients may seek treatment for pruritus including emollients, topical steroids, and antihistamines.[42,48] Acyclovir has shown to be therapeutic in some cases.[42,45] A randomized controlled trial of acyclovir in patients with PR demonstrated a statistically significant reduction in lesional score and pruritus in those receiving acyclovir 400 mg three times per day for 7 days.[50] Treatment of pregnant patients is still being investigated but acyclovir, which is deemed safe in pregnancy, may be considered beneficial.[47] Macrolides were previously used to treat PR but have recently shown to be ineffective.[42]

POST INFLAMMATORY HYPOPIGMENTATION

EPIDEMIOLOGY

Postinflammatory hypopigmentation is a common pigmentary disorder and consequence of cutaneous inflammation from exogenous or endogenous causes.[1] This natural physiological reaction is more apparent and concerning in people with darker skin tones, and it is responsible for a considerable proportion of visits to dermatologists.[1] The potential causes are vast, including inflammatory conditions such as atopic dermatitis, seborrheic dermatitis, pityriasis lichenoides chronica, lichen planus, lichen striatus, arthropod bites, psoriasis, sarcoidosis, immune-mediated conditions as well as infections, drugs, chemicals, and procedures.[1,51]

CLINICAL FEATURES

It can occur in all skin types but is much more common and apparent in darker skin.[29] The common presentation consists of asymptomatic, hypopigmented macules or patches, with the size and distribution consistent with the areas in which the preceding inflammatory process occurred [**Figure 58-6A-B**].[29] It can also be seen concurrently in individuals with an ongoing inflammatory process that is in different stages.[51]

DIAGNOSIS

The diagnosis can be made clinically if there is a known history of inflammation or trauma to the affected site. A Wood's lamp can aid in differentiating depigmented areas from those that are hypopigmented with the latter appearing accentuated without fluorescence. Under a Wood's lamp, it may appear more visible but will not accentuate as brightly as a disorder of depigmentation.[21] Wood's lamp findings shows no accentuation of the hypopigmentation.[1] This can help in distinguishing postinflammatory hypopigmentation from tinea versicolor, which exhibits a yellow-orange fluorescence under the lamp, and from progressive macular hypomelanosis, which emits red fluorescence.[1,51]

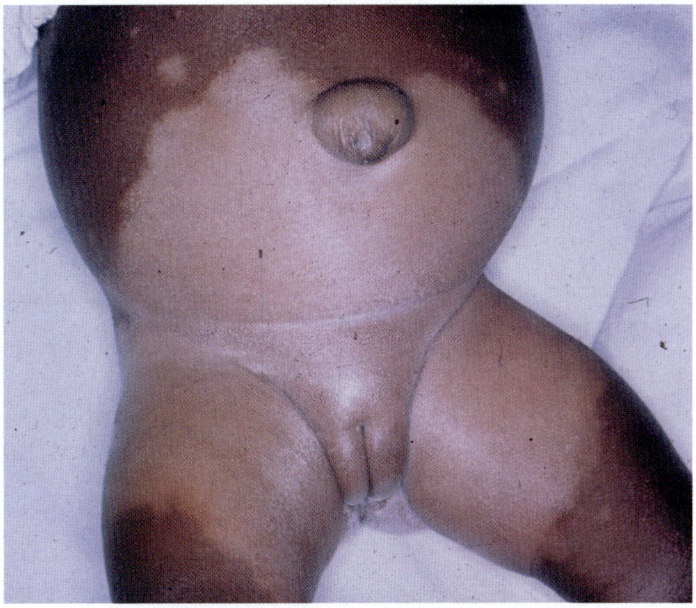

A

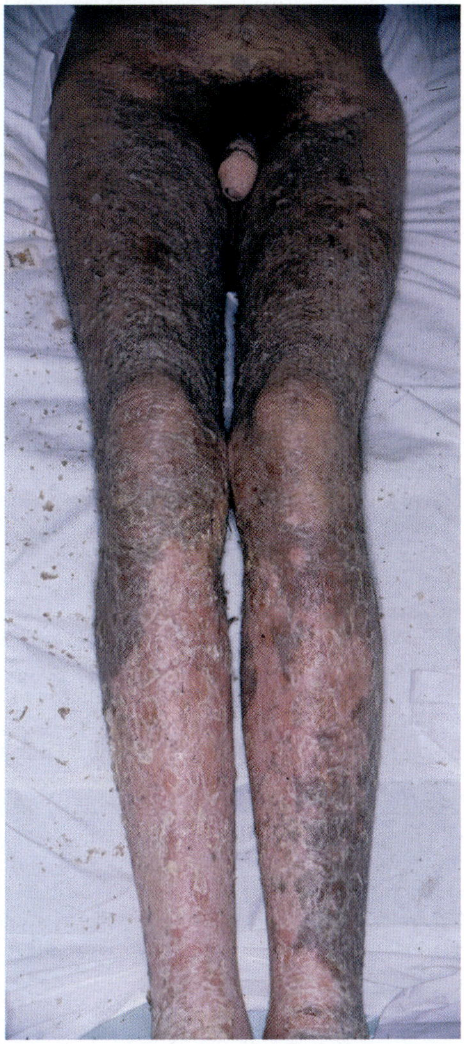

B

FIGURE 58-6. (A) Postinflammatory hypopigmentation. Large confluent hypopigmented patch secondary to a diaper dermatitis in an infant. **(B)** Postinflammatory hypopigmentation. Hypopigmented large plaques along the knees and anterior shins secondary to widespread psoriasis.

The dermoscopic findings will exhibit characteristics similar to the inciting inflammatory process.[20] For example, in pityriasis lichenoides, nondotted vessels/orangish structureless areas may be observed, while dotted vessels are observed in guttate psoriasis, and star-like depigmentation may be seen in prurigo nodularis.[20] These findings can help in retrospectively diagnosing the condition.[20]

A biopsy is also nonspecific and demonstrates reduced epidermal melanin, a spectrum of lymphohistiocytic infiltration, and melanophages in the upper dermis.[1,51] Despite nonspecific biopsy findings, a biopsy may be useful in differentiating from diseases such as hypopigmented mycosis fungoides, sarcoidosis, and hypopigmented leprosy in which these diseases only exhibit hypopigmentation.[51]

DIFFERENTIAL DIAGNOSIS

The differential diagnosis includes pityriasis alba, progressive macular hypomelanosis, tinea versicolor, hypopigmented sarcoidosis, hypopigmented mycosis fungoides, hypopigmented leprosy, drug-induced hypopigmentation, and tumor of the infundibulum (infundibulomatosis).[51]

PATHOGENESIS

Because individuals tend to have a varied response to cutaneous inflammation or trauma, the term "individual chromatic tendency" was coined as a theory to why some individuals respond with either hypo- or hyperpigmentation.[51] This theory supports a genetic component to chromatic tendency that is inherited in an autosomal dominant fashion. Furthermore, the theory suggests that some individuals have weak melanocytes that are easily damaged and therefore predispose them to hypopigmentation. In contrast, individuals with stronger melanocytes are inclined to develop hyperpigmentation in response to the insult. In cases of hypopigmentation, growth factors and cytokines that act on melanocytes, fibroblasts, and keratinocytes are simultaneously released during the inflammatory processes leading to derangements in melanogenesis.[51] Though melanocytes may not be destroyed, melanogenesis may be interrupted. However, in cases of severe inflammation, melanocytes may even be destroyed.[51]

TREATMENT

The management depends on treatment of the underlying cause that generally leads to a gradual improvement of hypopigmentation.[1] Topical treatment options include steroids and calcineurin inhibitors that can be helpful in treating active inflammatory processes in hopes of preventing PIH if treated early and sufficiently.[1] Other treatment modalities include cosmetic cover-up products and NB-UVB phototherapy; however, the use of phototherapy needs to be done with caution as it might induce tanning of the surrounding skin, hence making the hypopigmentation be more obvious. NB-UVB phototherapy can be given twice weekly, with starting doses ranging from 100 to 200 mJ/cm^2 and increasing gradually by 10% to 20% with each treatment, with consideration of the patient's skin type and tolerability.[52] Oral PUVA has been used for more widespread postinflammatory hypopigmentation, with oral 8-methoxsalen given at a dose of 0.4 to 0.5 mg/kg and treatments administered twice weekly.[1] Treatment is continued until minimal asymptomatic erythema occurs. Skin grafting is also an option, however, with varying degrees of success.[1]

The degree of repigmentation depends on the severity of the hypopigmentation. Moderate hypopigmentation may resolve in weeks to months, whereas severe hypopigmentation may take years or in some cases can be permanent.[51]

PROGRESSIVE MACULAR HYPOMELANOSIS

EPIDEMIOLOGY

Progressive macular hypomelanosis (PMH) is a benign condition commonly seen in young women of color originating from tropical backgrounds and individuals with darker skin.[1,53]

CLINICAL FEATURES

PMH appears as symmetric, nonscaly, nonpruritic hypopigmented macules coalescing into larger patches on the anterior and posterior trunk [**Figure 58-7**].[34,53] Other less commonly affected sites are the upper extremities, neck face, and buttocks.[53]

DIAGNOSIS

The diagnosis of PMH is typically clinical.[53] A Wood's lamp examination may aid diagnosis and will show accentuation of affected areas with a follicular orange to red fluorescence on affected skin secondary to the production of coproporphyrin III by *Cutibacterium acnes* (*C. acnes*).[1,17,45,53] A KOH test will yield negative results. Dermoscopy demonstrates ill-defined whitish areas that lack scale, or if scale is present it tends to be confined to cleavage lines.[34,54] Background reticular pigment may also be appreciated [Table 58-1]. A biopsy can be done when the diagnosis is uncertain, demonstrating a normal appearing dermis, reduced epidermal melanin without a change in number of melanocytes and less commonly lymphohistiocytic infiltration of the dermis.[29,53]

DIFFERENTIAL DIAGNOSIS

The differential for PMH includes vitiligo, leprosy, hypopigmented mycosis fungoides, pityriasis alba, tinea versicolor, tuberculoid leprosy, PIH, hypopigmented mycosis fungoides, and hypopigmented sarcoidosis.[1,29]

PATHOGENESIS

C. acnes is thought to be involved in the pathogenesis of PMH and is thought to disrupt melanogenesis resulting in hypopigmentation.[1] PMH tends to lack any preceding inflammatory symptoms including pruritus or pain.[1]

TREATMENT

There is no gold standard of treatment for PMH but treatment typically involves control of *C. acnes*.[53] Topical steroids and topical and systemic antifungals have not been successful.[1] Improvement has been seen with topical clindamycin and benzoyl peroxide wash used along with ultraviolet therapy including PUVA or NB-UVB.[29,55] A 14-week randomized study with 45 patients demonstrated better efficacy with benzoyl peroxide 5% at night, clindamycin 1% in the morning, and UVA phototherapy three times per week compared to fluticasone 0.05% at night and UVA phototherapy three times weekly.[56] A 15-year-old Indian-American female presenting with 3 years of PMH was treated with the same regimen: once daily benzoyl peroxide 5%, 1% clindamycin lotion, and NB-UVB three times per week with complete resolution after 3 months.[57] Sixteen patients with PMH received NB-UVB one to two times per week with reported repigmentation rate greater than 90% in 56.2% of individuals with a relapse rate of 31%.[58] A retrospective analysis, in 108 patients,

FIGURE 58-7. Progressive macular hypomelanosis. Discrete hypopigmented macules on the trunk of a Latina woman. (Used with permission from Marcia Ramos-e-Silva, School of Medicine and University Hospital, Federal University of Rio De Janeiro, Brazil.)

comparing twice weekly NB-UVB to topical antimicrobials, clindamycin or benzoyl peroxide, demonstrated resolution within an average of 8.5 months in 38% of those treated with antimicrobials without relapse.[59] Resolution was reached in 2.5 months in 90% of patients treated with NB-UVB with a relapse rate of 6%. These authors recommend a combination of topical clindamycin, benzoyl peroxide wash, and NB-UVB to treat PMH.[59]

Oral medications have also been used. Oral isotretinoin 10 mg daily for 3 months has shown sustained remission at 10 months.[2,29] Because *C. acnes* is thought to be associated with the pathogenesis of PMH, tetracyclines, doxycycline, and minocycline, have been trialed due to the known efficacy of tetracyclines against *C. acnes* due to their anti-inflammatory profile that results in cytokine inhibition and decreased chemotaxis of neutrophils.[2,60] A pilot study of 11 patients receiving minocycline 100 mg daily for 3 months demonstrated repigmentation in all patients.[60,61] Oral lymecycline, a tetracycline with better pharmacokinetics and less side effects at 300 mg daily in combination with 5% benzoyl peroxide, demonstrated a 90% improvement in 83% of patients.[2,60]

SEBORRHEIC PATTERNED MACULAR HYPOPIGMENTATION

CLINICAL FEATURES

Seborrheic patterned macular hypopigmentation (SPMH) is a newly named entity that was previously described as hypochromic vitiligo or vitiligo minor. It is characterized by hypopigmented macules in a seborrheic distribution on the scalp, face, nose, chest, and/or back.[62] It has been seen more commonly in individuals with SOC.[62,63]

In 2021, SPMH was described in a case series of 14 middle-aged patients with SOC who all had a similar clinical presentation.[62] Prior to this, SPMH was described in a case series of 24 patients with Fitzpatrick skin types V and VI in 2014.[63] At that time, it was described as hypochromic vitiligo and was seen exclusively in those with dark skin.[63]

DIAGNOSIS

The work-up of this condition should involve a biopsy from involved and uninvolved skin. A biopsy will show scattered dermal melanophages with overall retained presence of melanocytes along the dermoepidermal junction.[62] The latter findings help to rule out a diagnosis of vitiligo.[62]

DIFFERENTIAL DIAGNOSIS

The differential diagnosis includes inflammatory, infectious, or neoplastic causes of hypopigmentation, such as PIH, seborrheic dermatitis, tinea versicolor, pityriasis lichenoides chronica, atopic dermatitis, leprosy, vitiligo, and cutaneous T-cell lymphoma.[62,63] SPMH will remain stable over time without inflammation and there is absence of fluorescence on Wood's lamp.[63] Leukotrichia was not seen in any of the patients.[63]

PATHOGENESIS

The pathogenesis remains unclear; however, suggested theories include melanocyte senescence or an unknown inflammatory insult, leading to loss of pigment.[62]

TREATMENT

There is no current consensus on treatment for this condition. Various treatments have been tried with inconsistent success including topical calcineurin inhibitors, topical steroids, antifungals, antibiotics, and NB-UVB.[62]

HYPOPIGMENTED MYCOSIS FUNGOIDES

EPIDEMIOLOGY

Mycosis fungoides is a type of cutaneous T-cell lymphoma (CTCL) compromising 54% of CTCL cases.[64] Typically primary cutaneous lymphomas are rare in children. However hypopigmented mycosis fungoides (HMF) is common in children, accounting for 58% to 91% of MF in children.[65-67] HMF is the most common subtype of mycosis fungoides in those of African ancestry, exhibits an early onset of disease and a predominance of CD8+ T-cells.[66,68,69] Individuals of South Asian, Middle Eastern, and Hispanic descent may also be affected.[69] There are few reports in non-SOC populations.[69]

CLINICAL FEATURES

MF has three stages, patch, plaque, or tumor, that are based off the disease progression. HMF is a variant of the patch-stage MF and was initially described as hypochromic MF in 1973.[70] In this subtype, the majority of patches are hypopigmented with fine overlying scale with a predilection for sun-protected areas of the trunk, extremities, and the buttocks, in a "bathing suit" pattern, usually sparing the face [**Figure 58-8A-D**].[66,69] In some individuals, there may also be subtle background erythema [Figure 58-8E]. Macules and patches vary in shape and are typically round, or oval, and can have irregular borders.[66]

Staging for HMF follows tumor-node-metastasis (TNM) staging system. Based on TNM staging, an individual with stage IA has less than 10% BSA involvement.[71] Individuals that are stage IB have more than 10% BSA involvement.[71] Stage IIA has about 10% BSA involvement with palpable lymphadenopathy.[71] Stage IIB has cutaneous tumors and palpable lymphadenopathy.[71]

DIAGNOSIS

Studies have shown that the time frame from disease to diagnosis may be anywhere from 5 to 9 years.[66] The delayed diagnosis has proven to be a challenge and highlights the importance for providers to recognize HMF as a cause of hypopigmentation.[66] Early diagnosis is essential to decrease morbidity and mortality associated with the disease.[72] Treatment of stage I HMF results with health outcomes similar to individuals without HMF.

Individuals may initially present with an eczematous or psoriasiform dermatitis and are often misdiagnosed as having eczema. Individuals may also have undergone prior treatment with topical anti-inflammatories and/or phototherapy. Those on treatment should have biopsies repeated after the cessation of these treatments since they can modify the biopsy findings.[2,68] Multiple biopsies may sometimes be necessary to ascertain the correct diagnosis. Histology findings of HMF are similar to other MF variants. Findings that may be unique to individuals with darker skin have not been identified. Histology findings include lymphocytic infiltration, lymphocytic epidermotropism, lymphocytes with "cerebriform" nuclei, psoriasiform epidermal hyperplasia or normal appearing epidermis, vacuolar enhancement of the dermoepidemal junction, dyskeratotic keratinocytes, follicular tropism, and melanin incontinence.[73] Pautrier miroabscesses, common in MF, are less often seen in HMF.[73] Epidermotropism of CD4+ T-cells is more often seen in MF; however, epidermotropism of CD8+ T cells is prominent in HMF.[67,69,73]

DIFFERENTIAL DIAGNOSIS

The differential diagnosis for HMF includes lichen planus pigmentosus inversus, inflammatory vitiligo, PMH, digitate dermatoses, actinic reticuloid, pityriasis lichenoides chronica, pityriasis alba, leprosy, pityriasis versicolor, PIH, and hypopigmented sarcoidosis.[70,72]

PATHOGENESIS

Several theories exist as to the pathogenesis of HMF. One theory is that abnormal neoplastic cells lead to destruction of melanocytes and disrupt melanogenesis.[73] Other theories suggest an aberration in the transfer of melanosomes from melanocytes to keratinocytes or defective morphology of melanocytes.[73] This latter theory can be explained by the observed reduced quantity of melanosomes in keratinocytes and a regular amount of melanosomes in melanocytes.[53]

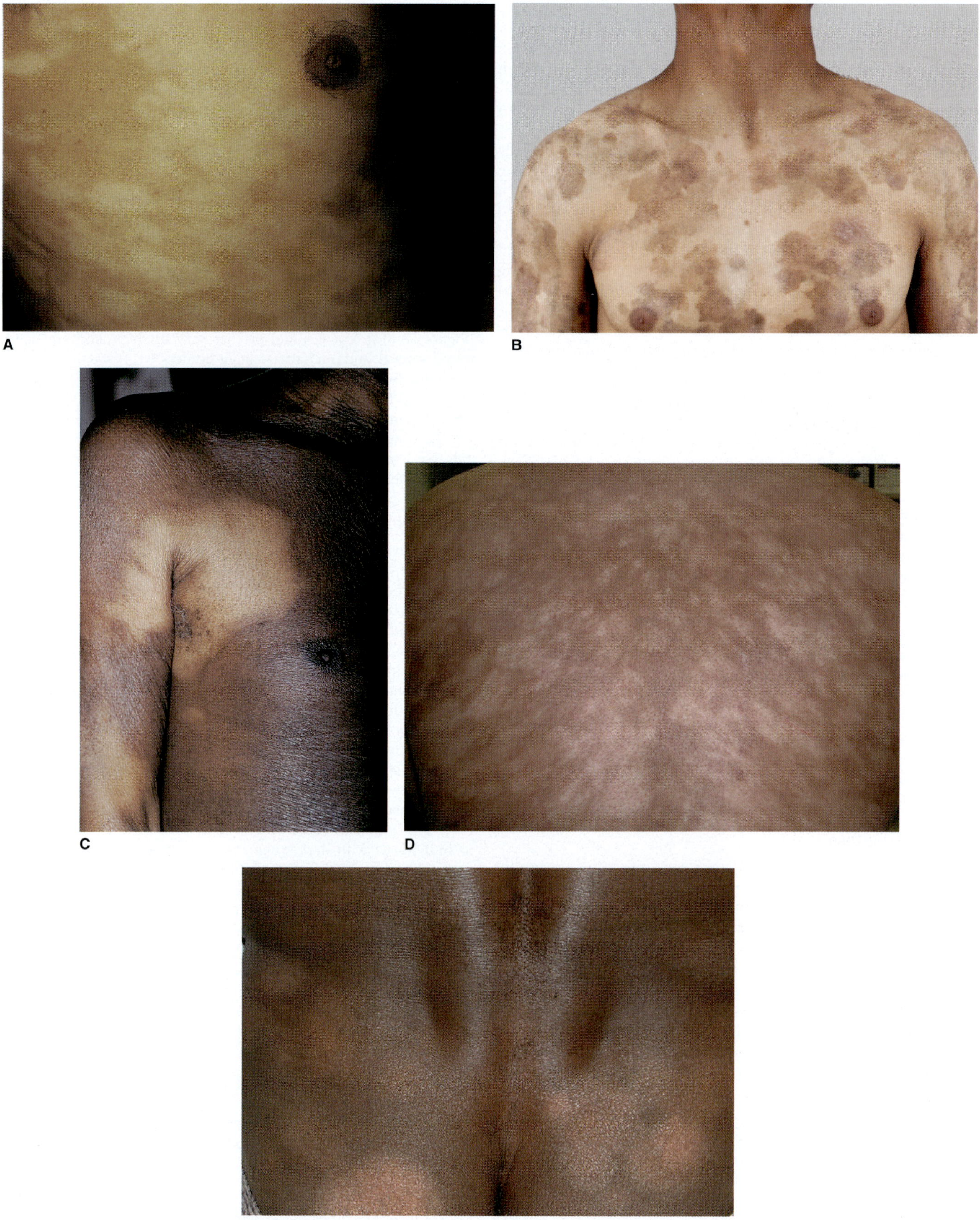

FIGURE 58-8. (A) Hypopigmented mycoses fungoides. Hypopigmented patches with irregular borders along the right chest and flank. **(B)** Hypopigmented mycoses fungoides. Stage IB (plaque-stage) dark brown scaly patches and plaques on the anterior trunk. **(C)** Hypopigmented mycoses fungoides. Stage III, erythroderma represented by dark red-brown confluent patches on the anterior neck and trunk. **(D)** Hypopigmented mycoses fungoides. Hypopigmented macules and patches on the back of a Fitzpatrick type IV individual. (Hypopigmented mycosis fungoides on back of a skin type IV individual. (Courtesy of Henry W. Lim, MD, Detroit, MI, USA.) **(E)** Hypopigmented mycosis fungoides. Light pink to brown hypopigmented patches and thin scaly plaques on the lumbar region. (Hypopigmented mycosis fungoides on the lower back of a skin type V individual.) (Courtesy of Henry W. Lim, MD, Detroit, MI, USA.)

TREATMENT

Treatment depends on disease stage. Treatment modalities that have been used with moderate to good success are PUVA, NB-UVB, topical nitrogen mustard, and topical steroids.[66] Classic MF in individuals with SOC often is associated with a poorer prognosis compared to Whites; however, there is a good prognosis with HMF in SOC.[66] HMF is treated conservatively, using topical steroids and/or NB-UVB phototherapy in stages I and II.[71] Topical nitrogen mustard is useful for areas not responding to phototherapy or on body sites difficult to treat with phototherapy; however, the high cost of this medication has made it cost prohibitive for most patients.[71]

PITYRIASIS LICHENOIDES CHRONICA

EPIDEMIOLOGY

Pityriasis lichenoides chronica (PLC) is a papulosquamous T-cell lymphoproliferative disorder. PLC presents in children and adults but most commonly presents in children 20% of the time.[74] There is controversy over whether there is a predilection in men.[74] Average age of onset is 6.5 years of age with some rare cases reporting onset in infancy.[74] PLC tends to favor the fall and winter seasons.[75]

CLINICAL FEATURES

In lighter skin, PLC presents with central scaly erythematous papules and plaques. PLC tends to resolve with hyperpigmentation or hypopigmentation.[74] However, in individuals with darker skin, PLC presents as hypopigmented scaly papules and plaques, pink-brown to red-brown in color, often resolving with postinflammatory hypopigmentation.[76] It is more commonly seen on the trunk and extremities and can last from months to years.

Variants of pityriasis lichenoides include pityriasis lichenoides et varioliformis acuta (PLEVA). PLEVA is characterized by sudden onset of recurrent crops of erythematous macules and patches, becoming vesicular, hemorrhagic, and crusted.[74] Varioliform scarring may occur in PLEVA but is not common in PLC.[74]

DIAGNOSIS

PL is often diagnosed clinically; however, characteristic biopsy findings can confirm the diagnosis.[74] The biopsy findings for PLEVA will demonstrate a wedge-shaped perivascular infiltrate of lymphocytes and leakage of red blood cells into the epidermis.[74] Epidermal changes such as vesiculation and ulceration may be seen with PLEVA but are absent in PLC.[74] PLC has milder vacuolar changes at the dermoepidermal junction and a less dense lymphocytic infiltrate.[74]

There are no specific laboratory abnormalities associated with PL, although some patients may have high erythrocyte sedimentation rates.[74]

The dermoscopy findings of individuals with skin types III to IV are similar to the findings in individuals with lighter skin: yellow to yellow-orange background color with central scaling in varying degrees of color of white-gray, yellow-white, and brown [Table 58-1].[49] However, the dermoscopy findings in skin types V and VI have diffuse to focal brown pigmentation without any yellow-orange background color and scales are predominantly peripheral.[19]

DIFFERENTIAL DIAGNOSIS

The differential diagnosis for PLEVA is distinct than those for PLC. The differential for PLEVA includes arthropod bites, leukocytoclastic vasculitis, and viral exanthems.[75] The differential for PLC includes guttate psoriasis, lichen planus, papular pityriasis rosea, varicella, small plaque parapsoriasis, lymphomatoid papulosis, erythema multiforme, leukocytoclastic vasculitis, secondary syphilis, and hypopigmented mycosis fungoides.[75,76]

PATHOGENESIS

Two proposed pathogenic mechanisms include an inflammatory reaction to an infection or an immune response secondary to viral antigens or a T-cell lymphoproliferative response.[74,76] A preceding infection has been associated in 30% of cases.[74] PLC secondary to antibiotics or acetaminophen have also been reported.[74]

Conditions to which PLC is associated are alopecia area, type I autoimmune hepatitis, aphthous stomatitis, pharyngitis, adenitis syndrome, periodic fever, common variable immunodeficiency, and idiopathic thrombocytopenic purpura.[74]

TREATMENT

There are currently no FDA-approved treatments for treating PLC. In a retrospective and observational analysis of individuals with Fitzpatrick skin types III and IV with diffuse PLC treated with erythromycin and class I topical steroids had partial response.[77] Four participants out of 11 treated with NB-UVB achieved complete response after a mean number of 91 sessions, and seven achieved partial response after a mean number of 28 sessions.[77] Systemic therapy in the form of methotrexate (15-20 mg weekly) have been used successfully to suppress disease activity.[77] A case report of a 45-year-old man with history of diabetes and hypertension was started on adalimumab 40 mg for recalcitrant psoriasis.[78] He subsequently developed adalimumab-induced PLC and was treated with methotrexate 15 mg weekly and observed resolution of PLC within 6 weeks.[78] Due to a potential infectious trigger preceding PLC, antibiotic agents such as tetracycline, minocycline, and erythromycin are often considered.[79]

PLC is self-limiting, lasting weeks to months, but relapse is common, with symptoms lasting months to years.[74] Children tend to have a longer disease course than adults, therefore it is imperative to consider the side effect profile of systemics.[74,77] The risk of malignant transformation is controversial; however, there are case reports of childhood PL evolving into CTCL.[74] Affected individuals should be made aware of the prognosis and low risk of malignant transformation.

HYPOPIGMENTED SARCOIDOSIS

EPIDEMIOLOGY

Cutaneous manifestations of sarcoidosis present in about 20% of cases of sarcoidosis and are the initial presentation in one-third of the cases.[80] Cutaneous sarcoidosis appears to have an increased female to male ratio and bimodal age distribution.[81] In the United States, the highest annual incidence of sarcoidosis is in African Americans.[80] Hypopigmented sarcoidosis is an uncommon variant of cutaneous sarcoidosis that is more prevalent in SOC.[80,82]

CLINICAL FEATURES

Cutaneous sarcoidosis has a breadth of morphologies that include papules, plaques, nodules, which can also be annular, angiolupoid, psoriasiform, atrophic, ulcerative, ichthyosiform indurated, and/or hypopigmented. Forms of sarcoidosis include lupus pernio, Darier-Roussy, erythema nodosum, and Löfgren syndrome.[83] A prospective study investigated the cutaneous manifestations of sarcoidosis in Black South Africans.[82] The predominant morphology was nodular followed by plaques. Nodules appeared mostly on the face, especially in the periocular area.[82] Plaques appeared mostly on the trunk and extremities, with induration, with smaller nodules overlying.[82] Hypopigmented macules and infiltrative plaques frequently appear on the extremities.[81]

DIAGNOSIS

A biopsy can show noncaseating granulomas with superficial and deep perivascular infiltrate of multinucleated giant cells with cytoplasmic inclusions (ie, asteroid bodies, Schaumann bodies, or birefringent crystalline fragments of calcium oxalate).[83] Uncommon findings are necrosis, foreign particles, granulomas in periadnexal or interstitial regions, concomitant lichenoid and granulomatous infiltrate, or epidermal changes.[83] Histopathology of the various cutaneous manifestations of sarcoidosis are very similar.[80] The reason for the various cutaneous manifestations of sarcoidosis sharing the same histopathological findings is not well understood.[80]

Diascopy produces a yellowish-brown, "apple jelly" color in cutaneous sarcoidosis.[81] This finding is not specific nor pathognomonic for sarcoidosis but provides a noninvasive diagnostic method. However, this physical finding is better elicited in individuals with lighter skin.

DIFFERENTIAL DIAGNOSIS

The differential diagnosis for hypopigmented sarcoidosis includes PIH, pityriasis alba, PLC, HMF, tinea versicolor, leishmaniasis, syphilis, pinta, leprosy, vitiligo, IGH, and chemical leukoderma.[81]

PATHOGENESIS

The etiology of sarcoidosis is not well understood. A complex immune response in genetically susceptible individuals with exposure to appropriate environmental factors has been proposed.[83]

TREATMENT

The first-line treatment for cutaneous sarcoidosis is intralesional or systemic steroids in combination with nonsteroidal systemic treatments such as methotrexate and antimalarials.[84] Cutaneous sarcoidosis refractory to treatment has shown success with infliximab as well as adalimumab.[84] Relapse of cutaneous sarcoidosis may be experienced with cessation of infliximab treatment.[84] Treatment with golimumab, ustekinumab, and rituximab have shown conflicting results.[84]

TUMOR OF FOLLICULAR INFUNDIBULUM

CLINICAL FEATURES

Tumor of the follicular infundibulum (TFI) is a rare, benign, adnexal growth with various presentations.[85,86] TFI commonly presents as a solitary, head and neck keratotic papule in the elderly.[87] TFI can present in less common variations, where multiple or eruptive forms of irregularly shaped macules and papules, or depressed papules, can be observed.[87] These variations may appear as skin-colored, erythematous, or hypopigmented.[87] Rarely, TFI appears on the extremities, buttocks, and vulva.[87]

After the initial discovery, TFI was described as a solitary head and neck tumors in the elderly.[86] In contrast to younger patients, the multiple, eruptive variant is seen, with symmetric hypopigmented macules, papules, or atrophic plaques with irregular borders on the face, neck, upper trunk.[85,86] In a subset of patients, TFI may have a predilection for the posterior calves.[85,86]

DIAGNOSIS

Because of the varying presentations, a biopsy is required for definitive diagnosis.[86] Histopathology demonstrates a platelike proliferation of connecting pale keratinocytes without atypia, interconnecting the epidermis and follicular structures.[86] The monomorphic tumor cells with small, round to oval nuclei are glycogen-filled, staining PAS positive.[86] Peripheral palisading and a network of elastic fibers surrounding the base of the tumor are also observed.[87] The multiple variant of TFI exhibits decreased melanin in lesional epithelium compared to interlesional epithelium, contributing to the observed clinical hypopigmentation.[87]

DIFFERENTIAL DIAGNOSIS

The differential diagnosis for TFI is broad including seborrheic keratosis, basal cell carcinoma (BCC), fibroepithelioma of Pinkus, trichilemmoma, actinic keratosis, trichoblastoma, acne vulgaris, atrophic lichen planus, lichen sclerosus, discoid lupus erythematosus, tinea versicolor, pityriasis alba, vitiligo, tuberculoid leprosy, and idiopathic guttate hypomelanosis.[87]

PATHOGENESIS

The etiology of TFI is unknown but is associated with diseases such as Cowden, sebaceous nevus, Schöpf-Schulz-Passarge syndrome, squamous cell carcinoma, actinic keratosis, epidermal cysts, nevus sebaceous, and malignant melanoma.[85,87] Cowden syndrome is linked to a genetic mutation in a tumor suppressor called phosphatase and tensin homolog (PTEN), resulting in an upregulation of cell proliferation and cell cycle progression, while apoptosis is suppressed.[86] It is believed that UV-induced PTEN mutations may cause TFI, potentially explaining their tendency to occur in sun-exposed skin and their occasional association with other malignancies, such as BCC.[86]

TREATMENT

There are a few treatments for TFI and most with minimal efficacy. Treatment with topical keratolytics and steroids have had minimal success.[88] Treatment with long-term etretinate has had partial resolution.[88] In some cases, cryotherapy has shown to have favorable results, but it is not recommended in SOC due to risk of adverse effects such as hypopigmentation.[86,89] Curettage and excision are considered curative; however, scarring may result with less than favorable cosmetic outcomes.[88]

CONCLUSION

Disorders of hypopigmentation can manifest in individuals of all skin colors, and although many of the conditions are benign, the stark contrast between involved and uninvolved skin can make these disorders particularly distressing for people of color. Additionally, presentation of these disorders may appear with variations that are unique to SOC, which are not seen in people with lighter skin. To prevent misdiagnosis or delay in diagnosis, it is crucial to be able to identify the variations that occur in individuals with darker skin. In some cases, further investigation is required to explore the possibility of an underlying condition. Achieving repigmentation can involve various treatments and can take significant time, therefore it is important to also provide proper counseling on prognosis and treatment guidelines.

REFERENCES

1. Rodney IJ PJ, Hexsel D, Halder RM. Disorders of hypopigmentation. In: Kelly A, Taylor SC, Lim HW, Serrano A, eds. *Taylor and Kelly's Dermatology for Skin of Color*. 2nd ed. New York, NY: McGraw Hill; 2016.
2. Saleem MD, Oussedik E, Picardo M, Schoch JJ. Acquired disorders with hypopigmentation: a clinical approach to diagnosis and treatment. *J Am Acad Dermatol*. 2019;80(5):1233-1250 e10.
3. Elgash M, Dlova N, Ogunleye T, Taylor SC. Seborrheic dermatitis in skin of color: clinical considerations. *J Drugs Dermatol*. 2019;18(1):24-27.
4. Adalsteinsson JA, Kaushik S, Muzumdar S, Guttman-Yassky E, Ungar J. An update on the microbiology, immunology and genetics of seborrheic dermatitis. *Exp Dermatol*. 2020;29(5):481-489.
5. Borda LJ, Wikramanayake TC. Seborrheic dermatitis and dandruff: a comprehensive review. *J Clin Investig Dermatol*. 2015;3(2).
6. Alexis AF, Sergay AB, Taylor SC. Common dermatologic disorders in skin of color: a comparative practice survey. *Cutis*. 2007;80(5):387-394.
7. de Avelar Breunig J, Couto MOR. Seborrheic dermatitis. In: Bonamigo RR, Dornelles SIT, eds. *Dermatology in Public Health Environments: A Comprehensive Textbook*. Berlin: Springer International Publishing; 2018:429-447.
8. Suh DH. Seborrheic dermatitis. In: Kang S, Amagai M, Bruckner AL, et al, eds. *Fitzpatrick's Dermatology*, 9th ed. New York, NY: McGraw Hill Education; 2019.
9. Poindexter GBMD, Burkhart CNMD, Morrell DSMD. Therapies for pediatric seborrheic dermatitis: [1]. *Pediatr Ann*. 2009;38(6):333-338.
10. Chatrath S, Bradley L, Kentosh J. Dermatologic conditions in skin of color compared to white patients: similarities, differences, and special considerations. *Arch Dermatol Res*. 2022;315:1089-1097.
11. Gupta AK, Bluhm R. Seborrheic dermatitis. *J Eur Acad Dermatol Venereol*. 2004;18(1):13-26; quiz 19-20.
12. Okokon EO, Verbeek JH, Ruotsalainen JH, Ojo OA, Bakhoya VN. Topical antifungals for seborrhoeic dermatitis. *Cochrane Database Syst Rev*. 2015;(5): Cd008138.

13. Kallini JR, Riaz F, Khachemoune A. Tinea versicolor in dark-skinned individuals. *Int J Dermatol.* 2014;53(2):137-141.
14. Maymone MB, Watchmaker JD, Dubiel M, Wirya SA, Shen LY, Vashi NA. Common skin disorders in pediatric skin of color. *J Pediatr Health Care.* 2019;33(6):727-737.
15. Mendez-Tovar LJ. Pathogenesis of dermatophytosis and tinea versicolor. *Clin Dermatol.* 2010;28(2):185-189.
16. Varada S, Dabade T, Loo DS. Uncommon presentations of tinea versicolor. *Dermatol Pract Concept.* 2014;4(3):93-96.
17. Dyer JM, Foy VM. Revealing the unseen: a review of Wood's Lamp in dermatology. *J Clin Aesthet Dermatol.* 2022;15(6):25-30.
18. Tey HL. Approach to hypopigmentation disorders in adults. *Clin Exp Dermatol.* 2010;35(8):829-34.
19. Errichetti E, Ankad BS, Sonthalia S, et al. Dermoscopy in general dermatology (non-neoplastic dermatoses) of skin of colour: a comparative retrospective study by the International Dermoscopy Society. *Eur J Dermatol.* 2020;30(6):688-698.
20. Errichetti E, Stinco G. Dermoscopy in general dermatology: a practical overview. *Dermatol Ther (Heidelb).* Dec 2016;6(4):471-507.
21. Saizan AL, Elbuluk N. Pigmentary disorders. In: Soutor C, Hordinsky MK, eds. *Clinical Dermatology: Diagnosis and Management of Common Disorders.* 2nd ed. New York, NY: McGraw Hill Education; 2022.
22. Nurmohamed S, Tan B, Burgin S. Tinea Versicolor. In: Goldsmith LA, ed. *VisualDx.* VisualDx; 2023.
23. Gupta AK, Foley KA. Antifungal treatment for pityriasis versicolor. *J Fungi.* 2015;1(1):13-29.
24. Leung AK, Barankin B, Lam JM, Leong KF, Hon KL. Tinea versicolor: an updated review. *Drugs Context.* 2022;11.
25. Faergemann J, Gupta AK, Al Mofadi A, Abanami A, Shareaah AA, Marynissen G. Efficacy of itraconazole in the prophylactic treatment of pityriasis (tinea) versicolor. *Arch Dermatol.* 2002;138(1):69-73.
26. Buch J, Patil A, Kroumpouzos G, et al. Idiopathic guttate hypomelanosis: presentation and management. *J Cosmet Laser Ther.* 2021;23(1-2):8-15.
27. Juntongjin P, Laosakul K. Idiopathic guttate Hypomelanosis: a review of its etiology, pathogenesis, findings, and treatments. *Am J Clin Dermatol.* 2016;17(4):403-411.
28. Rodney IJ, Halder RM. Disorders of hypopigmentation and depigmentation. In: Kelly AP, Taylor SC, Lim HW, Serrano AMA, eds. *Skin of Color.* Berlin: Springer; 2013:161-179.
29. Hadi A, Elbuluk N. Common conditions in skin of color. *Semin Cutan Med Surg.* 2016;35(4):184-190.
30. Ugonabo N, Iwuala C, Oyerinde O, Burgin S. Idiopathic guttate hypomelanosis. In: Goldsmith LA, ed. *VisualDx.* VisualDx; 2023.
31. Rani S, Kumar R, Kumarasinghe P, et al. Melanocyte abnormalities and senescence in the pathogenesis of idiopathic guttate hypomelanosis. *Int J Dermatol.* 2018;57(5):559-565.
32. Joshi R. Skip areas of retained melanin: a clue to the histopathological diagnosis of idiopathic guttate hypomelanosis. *Indian J Dermatol.* 2014;59(6):571-574.
33. Brown F, Crane JS. Idiopathic guttate hypomelanosis. *StatPearls [Internet].* StatPearls Publishing; 2021.
34. Ankad BS, Koti VR. Dermoscopic approach to hypopigmentary or depigmentary lesions in skin of color. *Clin Dermatol Rev.* 2020;4(2):79.
35. Laosakul K, Juntongjin P. Efficacy of tip cryotherapy in the treatment of idiopathic guttate hypomelanosis (IGH): a randomized, controlled, evaluator-blinded study. *J Dermatol Treat.* 2017;28(3):271-275.
36. Kaya T, Yazici A, Tursen U, Ikizoglu G. Idiopathic guttate hypomelanosis: idiopathic or ultraviolet induced? *Photodermatol Photoimmunol Photomed.* 2005;21(5):270-271.
37. Toychiev A, Mirzoeva M, Davis N, Islamova J, Osipova S. Pityriasis alba: possible associations with intestinal helminths and pathogenic protozoa. *Int J Clin Pract.* 2020;74(2):e13441.
38. Fenner J, Silverberg NB. Skin diseases associated with atopic dermatitis. *Clin Dermatol.* 2018;36(5):631-640.
39. Givler DN, Basit H, Givler A. Pityriasis alba. *StatPearls.* StatPearls Publishing; 2022.
40. Khafagy GM, Nada HR, Rashid LA, El-Samanoudy SI, Abd El-Sattar EM. Role of trace elements in pityriasis Alba. *J Trace Elem Med Biol.* 2020;59:126422.
41. De Klotz CMC, McKinley-Grant L, Lugo-Somolinos A. Pityriasis alba. In: Goldsmith LA, ed. *VisualDx.* VisualDx; 2023.
42. Urbina F, Das A, Sudy E. Clinical variants of pityriasis rosea. *World J Clin Cases.* 2017;5(6):203-211.
43. Litchman G, Nair PA, Le JK. Pityriasis rosea. *StatPearls.* 2022.
44. Joshi TP, Calderara GA, Lipoff JB. Prevalence of pityriasis rosea in the United States: a cross-sectional study using the All of Us database. *JAAD Int.* 2022;8:45-46.
45. Okoji UK, Agim NG, Heath CR. Features of common skin disorders in pediatric patients with skin of color. *Dermatol Clin.* 2022;40(1):83-93.
46. Tantanasrigul P, Wichaidit M, Kullavanijaya P. Acral pityriasis rosea: a rare variant of pityriasis rosea. *Dermatol Rep.* 2021;13(1):9081.
47. Heymann WR. Probing pityriasis rosea in pregnancy. *J Am Acad Dermatol.* 2021;85(6):1413.
48. Shi CR, Burgin S. Pityriasis rosea. In: Goldsmith LA, ed. *VisualDx.* VisualDx; 2023.
49. Jindal R, Chauhan P, Sethi S. Dermoscopic characterization of guttate psoriasis, pityriasis rosea, and pityriasis lichenoides chronica in dark skin phototypes: an observational study. *Dermatol Ther.* 2021;34(1):e14631.
50. Das A, Sil A, Das NK, Roy K, Das AK, Bandyopadhyay D. Acyclovir in pityriasis rosea: an observer-blind, randomized controlled trial of effectiveness, safety and tolerability. *Indian Dermatol Online J.* 2015;6(3):181-184.
51. Vachiramon V, Thadanipon K. Postinflammatory hypopigmentation. *Clin Exp Dermatol.* 2011;36(7):708-714.
52. Grimes PE, Bhawan J, Kim J, Chiu M, Lask G. Laser resurfacing-induced hypopigmentation: histologic alterations and repigmentation with topical photochemotherapy. *Dermatol Surg.* 2001;27(6):515-520.
53. Rao M, Young K, Jackson-Cowan L, Kourosh A, Theodosakis N. Post-inflammatory hypopigmentation: review of the etiology, clinical manifestations, and treatment options. *J Clin Med.* 2023;12(3):1243.
54. Chatterjee M, Neema S. Dermoscopy of pigmentary disorders in brown skin. *Dermatol Clin.* 2018;36(4):473-485.
55. Wang RX, Hawkes JE, Burgin S. Progressive macular hypomelanosis. In: Goldsmith LA, ed. *VisualDx.* VisualDx; 2023.
56. Relyveld GN, Kingswijk MM, Reitsma JB, Menke HE, Bos JD, Westerhof W. Benzoyl peroxide/clindamycin/UVA is more effective than fluticasone/UVA in progressive macular hypomelanosis: a randomized study. *J Am Acad Dermatol.* 2006;55(5):836-843.
57. Leonard N, Krueger S, Rashighi M. Successful treatment of progressive macular hypomelanosis. *Dermatol Rep.* 2020;12(2):8509.
58. Kim MB, Kim GW, Cho HH, et al. Narrowband UVB treatment of progressive macular hypomelanosis. *J Am Acad Dermatol.* 2012;66(4):598-605.
59. Thng ST, Long VS, Chuah SY, Tan VW. Efficacy and relapse rates of different treatment modalities for progressive macular hypomelanosis. *Indian J Dermatol, Venereol Leprol.* 2016;82:673.
60. Cavalcanti SMdM, Querino MCD, Magalhães V, França ERd, Magalhães M, Alencar E. The use of lymecycline and benzoyl peroxide for the treatment of progressive macular hypomelanosis: a prospective study. *An Bras Dermatol.* 2011;86:813-814.
61. Almeida ARTd, Bedani TP, Debs EAF, Ferreira JAD. Estudo piloto para avaliar a eficácia da minociclina no tratamento da hipomelanose macular progressiva (HMP). *Surg Cosmet Dermatol.* 2009;1(1):25-28.
62. Krueger L, Saizan AL, Meehan SA, Ezzedine K, Hamzavi I, Elbuluk N. Seborrheic macular hypopigmentation: a case series proposing a new pigmentary disorder. *J Eur Acad Dermatol Venereol.* 2022;36(5):e361-e362.
63. Ezzedine K, Mahé A, van Geel N, et al. Hypochromic vitiligo: delineation of a new entity. *Br J Dermatol.* 2015;172(3):716-721.
64. Bradford PT, Devesa SS, Anderson WF, Toro JR. Cutaneous lymphoma incidence patterns in the United States: a population-based study of 3884 cases. *Blood.* 2009;113(21):5064-5073.
65. Domínguez-Gómez MA, Baldassarri-Ortego LF, Morales-Sánchez MA. Hypopigmented mycosis fungoides: a 48-case retrospective series. *Australas J Dermatol.* 2021;62(3):e419-e420.
66. Rodney IJ, Kindred C, Angra K, Qutub ON, Villanueva AR, Halder RM. Hypopigmented mycosis fungoides: a retrospective clinicohistopathologic study. *J Eur Acad Dermatol Venereol.* 2017;31(5):808-814.
67. Gameiro A, Gouveia M, Tellechea Ó, Moreno A. Childhood hypopigmented mycosis fungoides: a commonly delayed diagnosis. *BMJ Case Rep.* 2014;2014:bcr2014208306.
68. Wong V, Tan B, Burgin S. Cutaneous T-Cell Lymphoma. In: Goldsmith LA, ed. *VisualDx.* VisualDx; 2023.
69. Martínez Villarreal A, Gantchev J, Lagacé F, et al. Hypopigmented mycosis fungoides: loss of pigmentation reflects antitumor immune response in young patients. *Cancers (Basel).* 2020;12(8).
70. Kim JC, Kim YC. Hypopigmented mycosis fungoides mimicking vitiligo. *Am J Dermatopathol.* 2021;43(3):213-216.
71. Keehn CA, Belongie IP, Shistik G, Fenske NA, Glass LF. The diagnosis, staging, and treatment options for mycosis fungoides. *Cancer Control.* 2007;14(2):102-111.
72. Hinds GA, Heald P. Cutaneous T-cell lymphoma in skin of color. *J Am Acad Dermatol.* 2009;60(3):359-375; quiz 376-8.

73. Furlan FC, Sanches JA. Hypopigmented mycosis fungoides: a review of its clinical features and pathophysiology. *An Bras Dermatol.* 2013;88(6): 954-960.
74. Geller L, Antonov NK, Lauren CT, Morel KD, Garzon MC. Pityriasis lichenoides in childhood: review of clinical presentation and treatment options. *Pediatr Dermatol.* 2015;32(5):579-592.
75. Schieke SM, Wood GS. Parapsoriasis and pityriasis lichenoides. In: Kang S, Amagai M, Bruckner AL, et al, eds. *Fitzpatrick's Dermatology.* 9th ed. New York, NY: McGraw Hill Education; 2019.
76. Wallace EB, Burgin S. Pityriasis lichenoides chronica. In: Goldsmith LA, ed. *VisualDx.* VisualDx; 2023.
77. Cuellar-Barboza A, Cardenas-De La Garza JA, Villarreal-Villarreal CD, et al. Efficacy of phototherapy in pityriasis lichenoides chronica of dark skin: a retrospective study from a tertiary center in Mexico. *Dermatol Ther.* 2018;31(6):e12734.
78. Martínez-Peinado C, Galán-Gutiérrez M, Ruiz-Villaverde R, Solorzano-Mariscal R. Adalimumab-induced pityriasis lichenoides chronica that responded well to methotrexate in a patient with psoriasis. *Actas Dermosifiliogr.* 2016;107(2):167-169.
79. Bellinato F, Maurelli M, Gisondi P, Girolomoni G. A systematic review of treatments for pityriasis lichenoides. *J Eur Acad Dermatol Venereol.* 2019;33(11):2039-2049.
80. Haimovic A, Sanchez M, Judson MA, Prystowsky S. Sarcoidosis: a comprehensive review and update for the dermatologist: part I. Cutaneous disease. *J Am Acad Dermatol.* 2012;66(5):699.e1-18; quiz 717-8.
81. Fernandez-Faith E, McDonnell J. Cutaneous sarcoidosis: differential diagnosis. *Clin Dermatol.* 2007;25(3):276-287.
82. Jacyk WK. Cutaneous sarcoidosis in black South Africans. *Int J Dermatol.* 1999;38(11):841-845.
83. Karadağ AS, Parish LC. Sarcoidosis: a great imitator. *Clin Dermatol.* 2019;37(3):240-254.
84. Dai C, Shih S, Ansari A, Kwak Y, Sami N. Biologic therapy in the treatment of cutaneous sarcoidosis: a literature review. *Am J Clin Dermatol.* 2019;20(3):409-422.
85. Haddad N, Oliveira Filho J, Reis MJ, Michalany AO, Nasser Kda R, Corbett AM. Tumor of follicular infundibulum with unique features. *An Bras Dermatol.* 2014;89(6):964-966.
86. Sorensen EP, Rosman IS, Sternhell-Blackwell K. Eruptive tumors of the follicular infundibulum in photo-exposed skin. *JAAD Case Rep.* 2018;4(4):330-332.
87. Raef H, Burgin S. Tumor of follicular infundibulum. In: Goldsmith LA, ed. *VisualDx.* VisualDx; 2023.
88. Cardoso JC, Reis JP, Figueiredo P, Tellechea Ó. Infundibulomatosis: a case report with immunohistochemical study and literature review. *Dermatol Online J.* 2010;16(1):14.
89. Kolenik SA III, Bolognia JL, Castiglione Jr FM, Longley BJ. Multiple tumors of the follicular infundibulum. *Int J Dermatol.* 1996;35(4):282-284.

CHAPTER 59

Disorders of Depigmentation

Maggi Ahmed
Pearl Grimes

KEY POINTS

- Disorders of depigmentation are common among skin of color individuals. These conditions are most disfiguring for those with darker skin types given the contrast between the depigmented patches and an individual of color's baseline skin color.
- Vitiligo is among the most common disorders of depigmentation and while not more common in skin of color, it is more visible, which can amplify the psychosocial impact of vitiligo.
- The therapeutic objectives for vitiligo include both stabilization and repigmentation. Vitiligo therapies include topical steroids, topical calcineurin inhibitors, topical Janus kinase (JAK) inhibitors, calcipotriol, phototherapy, antioxidants, and surgical therapies.

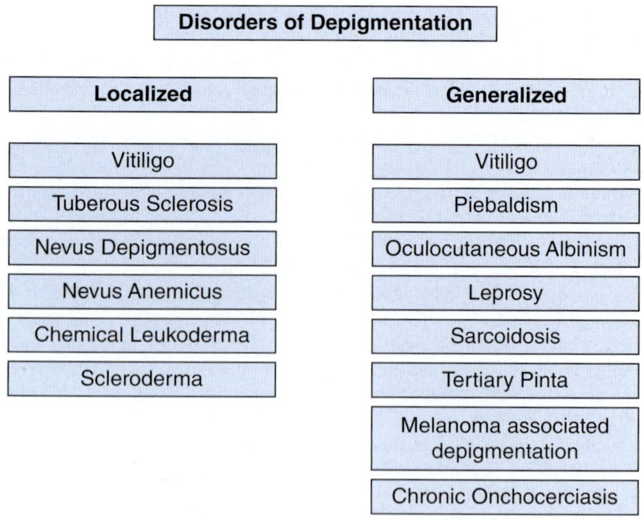

FIGURE 59-1. Localized and generalized disorders of depigmentation.

- In addition to several vitiligo-associated conditions, there are numerous other disorders of depigmentation including albinism, piebaldism, infectious conditions including onchocerciasis, tertiary pinta and leprosy, and neoplastic presentations such as melanoma-associated leukoderma.

INTRODUCTION

Disorders of depigmentation are frequently encountered diagnoses in dermatology including in the skin of color population. These conditions often have devastating effects on the quality of life of affected individuals. Depigmented areas often present as porcelain white patches that may coexist with patches of hypopigmented skin depending on the condition.[1] These clinical features may be caused by a loss or absence of melanocytes or defects in the transfer of melanin from melanocytes to keratinocytes. Common depigmentation disorders will be discussed in further detail in this chapter [**Figure 59-1**].

VITILIGO

INTRODUCTION

Vitiligo is characterized by areas of depigmented skin resulting from the loss of epidermal melanocytes. Given the stark contrast between the depigmented patches and normal skin, this disease is most disfiguring in those with darker skin [**Figure 59-2**]. Vitiligo is one of the most psychologically devastating skin diseases, and the psychological effects are

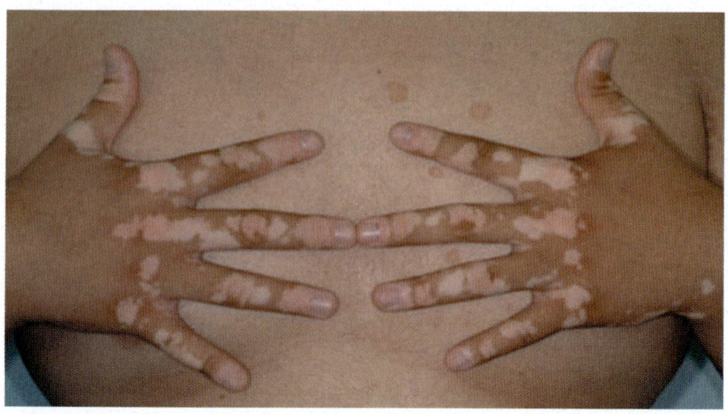

FIGURE 59-2. An individual with extensive vitiligo involvement of the dorsal hands and fingers.

influenced and exacerbated by social perceptions of skin disfigurement and irregularities in skin color.[2] Patients with vitiligo often experience low self-esteem, isolation, job discrimination, stigmatization, depression, and embarrassment in social and sexual relationships.[3]

EPIDEMIOLOGY AND CLINICAL MANIFESTATIONS

The prevalence of vitiligo varies from 0.1% to 3% in various populations worldwide.[4] The onset may occur at any age; however, the peak incidence is during the second and third decades of life. One-fourth of patients with vitiligo are children. Fifty percent of patients develop the disease by age 20. Although females are affected more often than males, the disease shows no racial or socioeconomic predilection. Vitiliginous lesions are typically asymptomatic, depigmented macules and patches that have no clinical signs of inflammation, although, at times, inflammatory vitiligo with erythematous borders has been reported. Hypopigmented and depigmented areas may coexist on the same person. Occasionally, the depigmented patches are pruritic, particularly in actively spreading and inflammatory vitiligo. The areas of depigmentation vary in size from a few millimeters to many centimeters and their borders are usually distinct. Trichrome patches are observed most often in individuals with darker skin. These patches are characterized by zones of white, light-brown, and normal skin. Depigmented hairs (leukotrichia) are often present in lesional skin. Significant leukotrichia suggest a loss of the follicular melanoblast reservoir. This loss can negatively impact repigmentation. In addition, there is a high incidence of premature graying of scalp hair in those with vitiligo and in their families. The vitiliginous patches can remain stable, or they can progress slowly for many years. Only in rare cases do individuals undergo almost complete spontaneous depigmentation in a few years.

Vitiligo is currently classified into two broad categories based on distribution. These include nonsegmental and segmental. Subtypes among patients with nonsegmental vitiligo include the acral, acrofacial, and localized disease. The nonsegmental pattern is characterized by symmetric depigmented macules or patches occurring in a random distribution. Acral or acrofacial vitiligo consists of depigmented macules confined to the extremities or the face and extremities, respectively. A subcategory of the acrofacial type is the lip-tip variety, in which vitiligo is confined to the lips and distal tips of the digits [**Figure 59-3**]. The generalized and acrofacial varieties are the most common. Segmental vitiligo occurs in a quasi-dermatomal distribution, in which the areas of depigmentation usually stabilize within a year and rarely spread beyond the affected anatomical area. Segmental vitiligo is the least common subtype of vitiligo, which commonly affects the face and commonly begins in childhood.[5]

Melanocytes of the eye, ear, and leptomeninges may also be involved in vitiligo. In one study, depigmented areas of the retinal pigment epithelium and choroid were found in 39% of subjects.[6] These asymptomatic lesions did not interfere with visual acuity. However, another study reported a significantly lower incidence of ocular abnormalities.[7] The most common comorbidities associated with vitiligo include Hashimoto thyroiditis, Graves disease, alopecia areata, and type 1 diabetes mellitus, several of which are also autoimmune condition [**Table 59-1**].

PATHOGENESIS

The predominant finding in the depigmented areas of vitiligo is an absence of epidermal melanocytes.[8] The precise cause of the loss of these epidermal melanocytes is unknown. Light microscopic and ultrastructural studies have revealed vacuolar degeneration of basal and parabasal keratinocytes and dermal lymphohistiocytic infiltrates.[9,10] Genetic, autoimmune, neural, biochemical, autocytotoxic, and melanocyte detachment mechanisms, as well as viral infections and oxidative stress, have been proposed to explain the pathogenesis of vitiligo. Current research documents an autoimmune mediated destruction of melanocytes in vitiligo.[11,12]

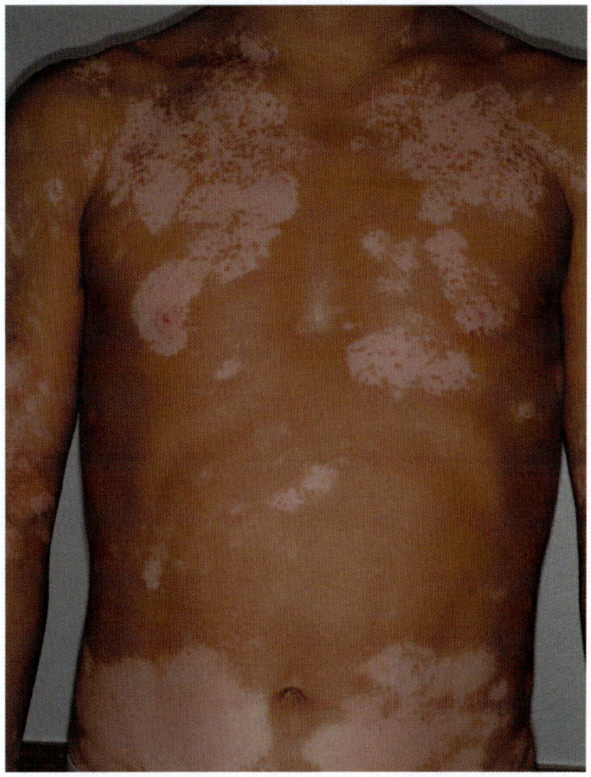

FIGURE 59-3. Generalized areas of depigmentation on the chest, abdomen, and arms with areas of follicular repigmentation of an individual with vitiligo.

Genetic studies support a non-Mendelian inheritance pattern for vitiligo and suggest that vitiligo is a multifactorial, polygenic disorder.[13-15] Between 20% and 30% of vitiligo patients report the condition in their first- and second-degree relatives. The disease has been associated with specific genetic polymorphisms, such as human leukocyte antigen (HLA)-DR4, -Dw7, -DR7, -DR1, -B13, -Cw6, -DR53, and -A19; however, haplotypes may vary considerably within the populations studied.[13,14] A genome-wide linkage scan was performed in 71 Caucasian multiplex families with vitiligo.[15] The linkage was assessed using multipoint nonparametric linkage analysis. The autoimmunity susceptibility locus located on chromosome 1p31 showed a highly significant linkage, suggesting that it is a major susceptibility locus for individuals with Fitzpatrick skin types I to III. The additional signals on chromosomes 1, 7, 8, 11, 19, and 22 meet the genome criteria for a suggestive linkage. Genetic studies also vary between the populations being evaluated. Studies in Chinese families show linkage evidence to chromosome 4q13-q21, in contrast to data in Caucasian families.[16] These findings support significant genetic heterogeneity for vitiligo in different racial populations. The *NLRP1* gene (previously known as *NALP1*) on chromosome 17p13 was identified as the principal regulator of the innate immune system. The *NLRP1* gene encodes the NACHT (neuronal apoptosis inhibitor protein, major histocompatibility complex class 2 transcription activator, incompatibility locus protein from *Podospora anserina*, and telomerase-associated protein) domain leucine-rich repeat protein 1, which contributes to a group of epidemiologically associated autoimmune diseases, including

TABLE 59-1 Common vitiligo comorbidities

Hashimoto thyroiditis	Diabetes mellitus
Alopecia areata	Graves disease
Pernicious anemia	Rheumatoid arthritis
Systemic lupus erythematosus	Addison disease
Inflammatory bowel disease	Multiple sclerosis

vitiligo.[17] Other candidate genes reported to affect vitiligo susceptibility include *HLA*, *ACE*, *CAT*, *FOXD3*, *ESR1*, *COMT*, *PTPN22*, *PDGFRA*, *C12orf10*, *MITF*, *KIT*, *XBP1*, *FAS*, and *COX2*.[8,13,14,18]

Cytomegalovirus DNA was demonstrated in the involved and uninvolved skin of individuals with vitiligo. No viral DNA was detected in the normal skin of matched control subjects.[19] A herpes simplex viral infection has been reported to trigger vitiligo in the Smyth line chicken animal model for vitiligo.[20] A recent study identified varicella zoster mature virions, varicella zoster antigen, and syncytia formation in patients with segmental vitiligo.[21] These findings suggest that some cases vitiligo may be triggered by a viral infection.

The neural theory was suggested in the last decades and was supported by several clinical, biochemical, and ultrastructural observations.[22] These observations include the occurrence of segmental vitiligo; the demonstration of lesional autonomic dysfunction, such as increased sweating; and the demonstration of nerve ending-melanocyte contact. The last observation is rare in normal skin. Most recently the pathogenesis of segmental vitiligo has been mostly explained by neurohormonal theory for the last century. This mainly was based on mischaracterization of segmental vitiligo in a dermatomal distribution and commonly following the trigeminal nerve distribution. However, recent studies have shown that segmental vitiligo patterns of depigmentation rarely follow a dermatome but correlate best with mosaic skin disorders. This suggests that segmental vitiligo may be influenced by postzygotic somatic mutations in developing melanocytes during embryologic development, a process called somatic mosaicism.[23]

Abnormalities in the melanocortin system have been implicated in the pathogenesis of vitiligo. Defects in the melanocortin system reported in vitiligo include low α-melanocyte-stimulating hormone (α-MSH) plasma levels,[24] reduced α-MSH levels in melanocytes,[25] decreased prohormone convertases 1 and 2 (PC1 and PC2) expression in melanocytes,[25] increased melanocortin-1 receptor gene (MC1R) and MC4R messenger ribonucleic acid (mRNA) expression in nonlesional skin, decreased pro-opiomelanocortin (POMC) mRNA expression in lesional skin,[26] and other defects.[27]

Several studies suggest that oxidative stress may be the initial event in the destruction of melanocytes.[28,29] A defective recycling of tetrahydrobiopterin, an increased production of hydrogen peroxide, and decreased catalase levels have been demonstrated in the affected skin of those with vitiligo.[28,29] In addition, lesional catecholamine biosynthesis and release are increased. Peripheral blood studies of patients with vitiligo have shown low catalase and glutathione levels, whereas superoxide dismutase and xanthine oxidase are elevated.[30] Oxidative stress may contribute to melanocyte destruction in susceptible individuals, causing DNA damage as well as protein and lipid peroxidation. Recent studies suggest that oxidative stress may cause the aberrant immune responses observed in vitiligo. Reactive oxygen species can cause apoptosis and the release of neoantigens, which serve as autoantigens that initiate humoral and cell-mediated immune responses.[28]

The self-destruction hypothesis proposes that melanocytes may be destroyed by the phenolic compounds formed during the synthesis of melanin.[22] In vivo and in vitro studies have demonstrated the destruction of melanocytes by phenols and catechols. In addition, industrial workers who are exposed to catechols and phenols may develop depigmented patches. Several environmentally ubiquitous compounds containing catechols, phenols, and sulfhydryls can induce hypopigmentation, depigmentation, or both. These compounds are encountered most often in industrial chemicals and cleaning agents. The possible mechanisms for altered pigment production by these compounds include melanocyte destruction via free radical formation, inhibition of tyrosinase activity, and interference with the production or transfer of melanosomes.[30]

Current studies document immune mechanisms in the pathogenesis of vitiligo and further suggests that vitiligo shares common linkages with other autoimmune diseases.[31,32] Historically, vitiligo has been reported in association with a number of autoimmune endocrinopathies and diseases. Thyroid disorders, in particular Hashimoto thyroiditis and Graves disease, are associated most commonly with vitiligo.[5] Other associated disorders include type 1 diabetes mellitus, alopecia areata, pernicious anemia, rheumatoid arthritis, autoimmune polyglandular syndrome, and psoriasis.[33] A survey of 2624 vitiligo probands in North America and the United Kingdom found that the prevalence of six autoimmune disorders was significantly increased in vitiligo probands and first-degree relatives.[5] These diseases included vitiligo, pernicious anemia, Addison disease, systemic lupus erythematosus, thyroid diseases (predominantly hypothyroidism), and inflammatory bowel disease. In a retrospective study of 1487 patients with vitiligo followed over a 10-year period, there was a statistically significant higher prevalence of hypothyroidism, multiple sclerosis, rheumatoid arthritis, idiopathic thrombocytopenic purpura, seronegative arthritis, pernicious anemia, myasthenia gravis, inflammatory bowel disease, lymphoma, and systemic lupus erythematosus. Rates of comorbid autoimmune diseases varied by race and sex.[34]

Many humoral and cell-mediated immune aberrations have been reported in vitiligo patients. Numerous studies have documented an increased frequency of organ-specific autoantibodies in these patients.[35] Antithyroid (thyroglobulin, thyroid microsomal, and thyroid peroxidase), gastric parietal cell, and antinuclear antibodies are the most associated autoantibodies that have been documented. Vitiligo patients who have organ-specific autoantibodies, unassociated with an overt autoimmune disease, have an increased risk of developing a subclinical or overt autoimmune disease.[35] The presence of antibodies to surface and cytoplasmic melanocyte antigens in the sera of vitiligo patients lends additional support for the autoimmune pathogenesis for this disease.[36,37] These antibodies can induce the destruction of melanocytes grown in the culture by complement-mediated lysis and antibody dependent cellular cytotoxicity.[36,37] In addition, melanocyte antibodies, when passively administered to nude mice grafted with human skin, have a destructive effect on melanocytes within the skin graft.[38] Notably less common are antibodies targeting tyrosinase, tyrosinase-related proteins 1 and 2, melanocyte protein 17 (also known as glycoprotein 100 [gp100]), and melanin-concentrating hormone 1, which have been reported in vitiligo patients.[37] The transcription factors SOX9 and SOX10 have been identified as melanocytic autoantigens in autoimmune polyendocrine syndrome and idiopathic vitiligo.[39]

Recent studies provide additional insights into the role of cell-mediated immunity in the destruction of melanocytes, suggesting that cytotoxic T-lymphocytes may play a significant role in melanocyte destruction in vitiligo.[40,41] Numerous activated cytotoxic T-lymphocytes have been reported in the perilesional area of vitiliginous skin, often in apposition to disappearing melanocytes.[40] These infiltrating lymphocytes are predominantly cytotoxic cluster of differentiation 8-positive (CD8+) lymphocytes that express skin homing receptors (such as the cutaneous leukocyte-associated antigen receptor). Melanocyte-specific CD8 T-cells have been shown to mediate the destruction of melanocytes in human vitiligo skin.[42] In addition, other studies have demonstrated the presence of increased numbers of circulating CD8+ cytotoxic lymphocytes. These lymphocytes are reactive to the melanosomal proteins melan-A/melanoma antigen recognized by T-cells 1, gp100, and tyrosinase in HLA-A2-positive patients with vitiligo.[43]

In a recent study, patients with vitiligo had higher circulating T-cell counts compared to control subjects.[42] Compared with patients with stable vitiligo, the patients with active vitiligo had higher CD8+ T-cell counts and a significantly reduced CD4+:CD8+ ratio. Compared with control subjects, those with generalized vitiligo showed a significant decrease in their regulatory T-cell (Treg) percentage and counts, along with a significant reduction in FOXP3 expression. The Treg cell percentage and counts were significantly reduced in patients with active generalized vitiligo, compared with those whose disease was stable. These findings give further credence to aberrant T-cell formation in vitiligo.

Several investigations have also addressed the role of peripheral blood and lesional cytokine expression in the pathogenesis of vitiligo. Elevated levels of serum soluble interleukin (IL)-2 receptor, IL-6, and IL-8, and elevated lesional tissue levels of IL-2 have been reported in vitiligo patients.[44] These findings correlate with an increased level of

T-cell activation. In biopsies of lesional, perilesional, and healthy skin, there were significantly lower levels of expression for the granulocyte colony-stimulating factor and stem cell factor reported in vitiliginous skin, but the expression of IL-6 and tumor necrosis factor-α (TNF-α) was increased in lesional skin.[45] Granulocyte colony-stimulating factor, basic fibroblast growth factor, and stem cell factor are paracrine cytokines secreted by keratinocytes. These paracrine cytokines stimulate melanogenesis and melanocyte proliferation, whereas IL-6 and TNF-α inhibit melanocyte proliferation and melanogenesis.[46] Together these findings suggest that keratinocyte function is also impaired in vitiliginous skin.

A subsequent report demonstrated an increased expression of TNF-α and interferon-γ in the lesional and adjacent healthy skin of patients with vitiligo, when compared with the skin of matched control subjects.[47] After 6 months of treatment with a twice-daily application of tacrolimus, a topical immunomodulator, there was a significant depression in the level of TNF-α expression in the lesional and adjacent healthy skin compared with baseline levels. This observation suggests that the suppression of TNF-α may be associated with the repigmentation of vitiliginous lesions.[47]

In the past decade, new studies have documented the specific role of interferon gamma and the Janus kinase signal transducer and activator of transcription (JAK-STAT) pathway as key factors in mediating the destruction of melanocytes in vitiligo. The JAK-STAT pathway is utilized by cytokines to transmit signals from the cell membrane to the nucleus. Upon engagement of extracellular ligands, intracellular JAK proteins become activated and phosphorylates STAT proteins, which dimerize and then translocate into the nucleus to directly regulate gene expression and transcription of IFN-γ- dependent chemokines, including CXCL9 and CXCL10. These chemokines promote the recruitment of autoreactive CD8+ T cells that promote melanocyte killing.[48,49]

Whether these immunologic aberrations are primary or secondary events in the destruction of melanocytes in vitiligo remains controversial. Nevertheless, regardless of which event is primary, many of the most effective therapies for vitiligo work via suppression or modulation of the immune response.

DIFFERENTIAL DIAGNOSIS

Other disorders characterized by depigmentation may occasionally clinically mimic vitiligo.[3] These include piebaldism, nevus depigmentosus, nevus anemicus, postinflammatory depigmentation or hypopigmentation, pityriasis alba, pityriasis versicolor, hypopigmented mycosis fungoides, discoid lupus erythematosus, scleroderma, and sarcoidosis. Therefore, in some instances, a skin biopsy may be necessary to substantiate a vitiligo diagnosis.

LABORATORY EVALUATION

In view of the association of vitiligo with a myriad of other autoimmune diseases, the routine baseline evaluation of a patient should include a thorough history and physical examination. Laboratory tests to considering checking include a complete blood count, erythrocyte sedimentation rate, comprehensive metabolic panel, thyroid stimulating hormone, and autoantibody tests (ie, antinuclear antibodies, thyroid peroxidase, and parietal cell antibodies) and vitamin D level.[27]

TREATMENT

The therapeutic objectives for vitiligo should include both the stabilization of the disease and repigmentation. Repigmentation can be accomplished medically or surgically in patients with localized stable lesions. The choice of repigmentation therapies should be predicated on multiple factors including the age of the patient, the body surface area affected (severity), and the activity or progression of the disease. Many studies document enhanced repigmentation in patients with darker skin color. The disease can be divided into four stages: limited (<10% involvement) moderate (10-25% involvement), moderately severe (26-50% involvement), and severe (>50% involvement).[3]

Commonly used medical therapies for vitiligo include topical and systemic steroids, topical and systemic JAK inhibitors, topical calcineurin inhibitors, narrowband ultraviolet B (NB-UVB) phototherapy, psoralen with ultraviolet A (PUVA), targeted phototherapy, nutritional vitamin supplementation, and calcipotriol[8,33] [**Tables 59-2 and 59-3**].

TABLE 59-2 Vitiligo repigmentation therapies and mechanisms of action

Treatment	Mechanism of action
Corticosteroids	Immunosuppressive, anti-inflammatory, antimitogenic
Calcineurin inhibitors	Immunosuppressive, inhibition of T-cell activation
Narrowband UVB phototherapy	Stimulation of melanocyte growth factors; Immunosuppressive, T-cell apoptosis
JAK inhibitors (emerging)	Immunosuppressive; block JAK- STAT signaling/ decreases proinflammatory cytokines
Afamelanotide (emerging)	Synthetic analogue of alpha MSH; increases melanocyte proliferation and melanogenesis; immune modulation

STEROIDS

Mid- to high-potency topical corticosteroids are used as a first-line treatment in those with limited forms of vitiligo.[3,5,27,33] Topical corticosteroids usually produce optimal results (up to 75% repigmentation) on areas with greater sun exposure, such as the face and neck, on more recent lesions, and for individuals with darker skin.[27] The response from topical corticosteroid use is poor in acral areas of the body. Prolonged use of steroids is not recommended; however, short-term use is safe and is an effective treatment in both children and adults. A short course of oral prednisone (0.5-1 mg/kg/day) for 1 to 2 weeks or a course of intramuscular triamcinolone acetonide injections (40 mg for 2-3 months) is often extremely helpful for stabilizing rapid progressive vitiligo. Oral minipulse using 2 to 4 mg of dexamethasone on 2 consecutive days per week for 6 to 12 weeks can be effective for stabilizing progressive vitiligo.[50,51]

Low-potency topical steroids are usually ineffective for patients with vitiligo. Topical mid- to high-potency steroids can be used safely for 2 to 3 months and then interrupted for 1 month or tapered to low-potency preparations. Patients must be monitored closely for topical steroid side effects, which include skin atrophy, telangiectasias, hypertrichosis, acneiform eruptions, and striae.[52] Lower potency and medium-potency (class III) classes of topical corticosteroids, such as mometasone furoate and methylprednisolone aceponate, have an increased benefit-to-risk ratio with fewer side effects.[27] Topical fluticasone propionate has a low

TABLE 59-3 Vitiligo therapies based on disease severity

Localized/limited	Moderate/ severe	Recalcitrant localized	Recalcitrant severe
Topical steroids	Narrowband UVB Phototherapy	Autologous grafting: Sheet grafts, Punch grafts, Split thickness	Depigmentation: monobenzone
Calcineurin inhibitors Vitamin D analogs	Oral PUVA Systemic Corticosteroids	Autologous grafting: Melanocyte cultures, Epidermal suspensions, Suction blisters	755-nm Alexandrite laser Q-switched ND:Yag
Targeted phototherapy: excimer Laser Topical PUVA	JAK inhibitors	5-fluouracil/microneedling	Cryotherapy
Antioxidants/ supplements	Antioxidants/ supplements	Antioxidants/supplements	Antioxidants/ supplements

potential for inducing local and systemically adverse effects.[53] Since the introduction of topical immunomodulators, topical steroids are used less frequently in vitiligo patients.[54]

TOPICAL CALCINEURIN INHIBITORS

Topical calcineurin inhibitors such as tacrolimus and pimecrolimus offer several advantages in treating vitiligo [**Figure 59-4**]. These agents are extremely well tolerated in children and adults and can be used for longer periods without evidence of atrophy or telangiectasias, which are commonly associated with long-term steroid use. This is a significant advantage in treating a chronic disease such as vitiligo. A comparison of the efficacy of topical calcineurin inhibitors and topical steroids in the treatment of vitiligo showed shorter time frame from the start of treatment to the onset of repigmentation with topical calcineurin inhibitors compared to topical steroids (2.4 months compared to 3.3 months, respectively).[54]

Tacrolimus affects T-cell and mast cell functions, and inhibits the synthesis and release of proinflammatory cytokines and vasoactive mediators from the basophils and mast cells through inactivating calcineurin by binding to cytoplasmic immunophilins.[55,56] Multiple studies have demonstrated its efficacy and safety for the treatment of atopic dermatitis.[47,57] A 24-week study assessed the efficacy and safety of tacrolimus ointment, at 24 weeks, 89% of the patients achieved varying levels of repigmentation, with a statistically significant decrease in their overall disease severity scores. Adverse events were minimal throughout the study.[47] Other studies have corroborated these results.[57,58] A recent randomized, double-blind study of 42 patients assessed the efficacy and safety of tacrolimus 0.1% for the treatment of facial vitiligo. Therapeutic success was achieved in 65% of tacrolimus-treated patients versus 0% of vehicle-treated patients at week 24.[59] In a chart review of 101 patients diagnosed with vitiligo, topical tacrolimus was found to be efficacious in all skin colors and more effective for the treatment of vitiligo in skin of color.[60] Children and teenagers aged 2 to 15 years were treated with tacrolimus 0.03%, whereas individuals aged 16 years or older were treated with tacrolimus 0.1% ointment applied twice daily.[60]

Pimecrolimus, which has a mechanism of action similar to tacrolimus, can also induce repigmentation.[58] The efficacy of pimecrolimus and clobetasol was compared in a right/left prospective study that focused on treating symmetric vitiligo; the two agents had comparable rates of repigmentation.[61] As with tacrolimus, pimecrolimus induces maximal repigmentation in the sun-exposed areas. There is an increased risk of skin cancer among transplant recipients who have been treated with systemically administered tacrolimus, given the induction of immunosuppression.[62] Topical tacrolimus, however, has not been associated with systemic immunosuppression or an increased risk of skin and other malignancies in clinical studies.[63] In light of the reports documenting an increase in skin cancers and lymphomas in animal models, tacrolimus and pimecrolimus currently have "black box" warning labels.[64] These animal studies should be interpreted with caution, given the massive oral dosages used in animals. The labeling of these agents recommends that they should not be used in combination with UV light therapy and that appropriate photoprotective precautions should be taken.

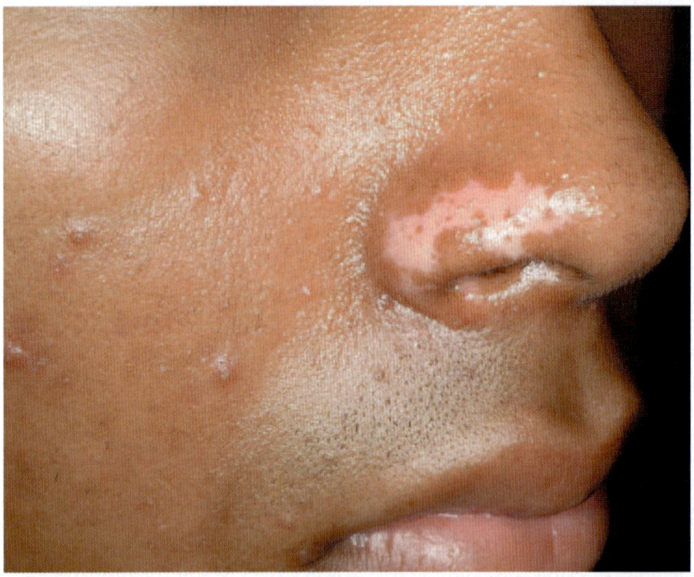

A

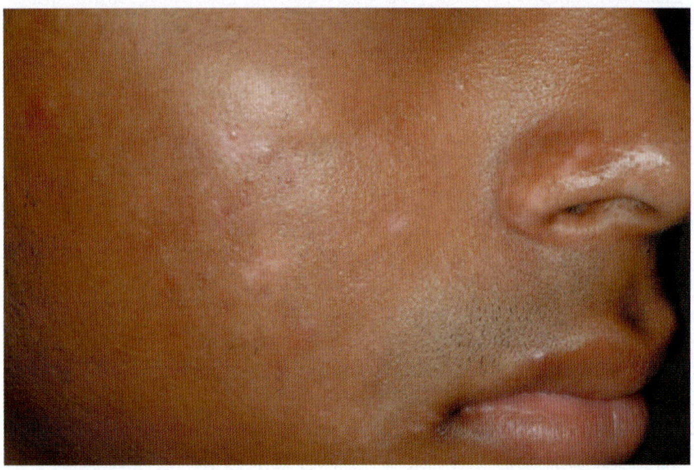

B

FIGURE 59-4. **(A)** Patch of facial depigmentation from vitiligo on the right nasal ala of a patient with skin of color. **(B)** The same patch with significant repigmentation after 3 months of treatment with topical tacrolimus.

NARROWBAND ULTRAVIOLET B

Historically, topical, and systemic PUVA was the "gold standard" for repigmenting vitiligo; however, PUVA-induced repigmentation rates vary considerably.[65] In addition, the adverse effects can be substantial, including phototoxicity and gastrointestinal irritation. Oral PUVA also requires the patient to use ocular protection for 12 to 24 hours following treatment. Given the comparable efficacy of narrowband ultraviolet B (NB- UVB) phototherapy and its lack of systemic adverse effects, it has emerged as a first-line treatment of choice for those with vitiligo [**Figure 59-5**]. NB-UVB involves the use of UV lamps with a peak emission of around 311 nm.[66] These shorter wavelengths provide higher energy fluences and induce less cutaneous erythema. NB-UVB induces local immunosuppression and apoptosis; stimulates the production of melanocyte-stimulating hormones, basic fibroblasts, growth factor, and endothelin-1; and increases melanocyte proliferation and melanogenesis. The first major study of NB-UVB in patients with vitiligo compared its efficacy with that of topical PUVA.[67] The study showed that significantly enhanced repigmentation was achieved in patients treated with NB-UVB compared with those treated with topical PUVA. The adverse effects were minimal in the group treated with NB-UVB in contrast with the increased phototoxicity observed in the those treated with topical PUVA. Subsequent studies have further confirmed the efficacy of NB-UVB and documented enhanced repigmentation rates when compared with PUVA phototherapy for vitiligo[68,69] [**Figure 59-6**]. The major advantages of NB-UVB include an established safety profile in both children and adults and a lack of systemic toxicity. NB-UVB does not require patients to use eye protection beyond the treatment exposure time. There have been no studies that have documented an increase in squamous cell carcinomas, basal cell cancers, or malignant melanomas in vitiligo patients treated with either PUVA or NB-UVB. This is in contrast with reports documenting an increase in squamous cell carcinomas and melanomas in psoriasis patients treated with PUVA.[70] Lifetime prevalence of melanoma and nonmelanoma skin cancer (NMSC) in patients with nonsegmental vitiligo were compared with control subjects

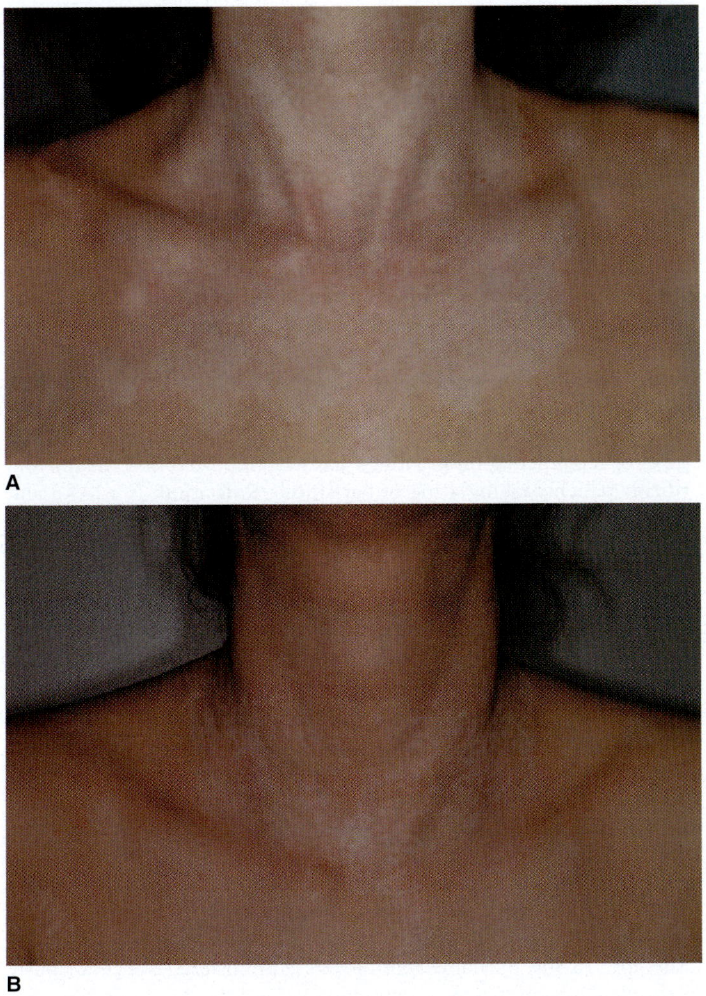

FIGURE 59-5. **(A)** An individual with depigmented patches from vitiligo on the anterior neck and chest. **(B)** Visible repigmentation of the same patches after 30 sessions of narrow-band ultraviolet B phototherapy treatment sessions.

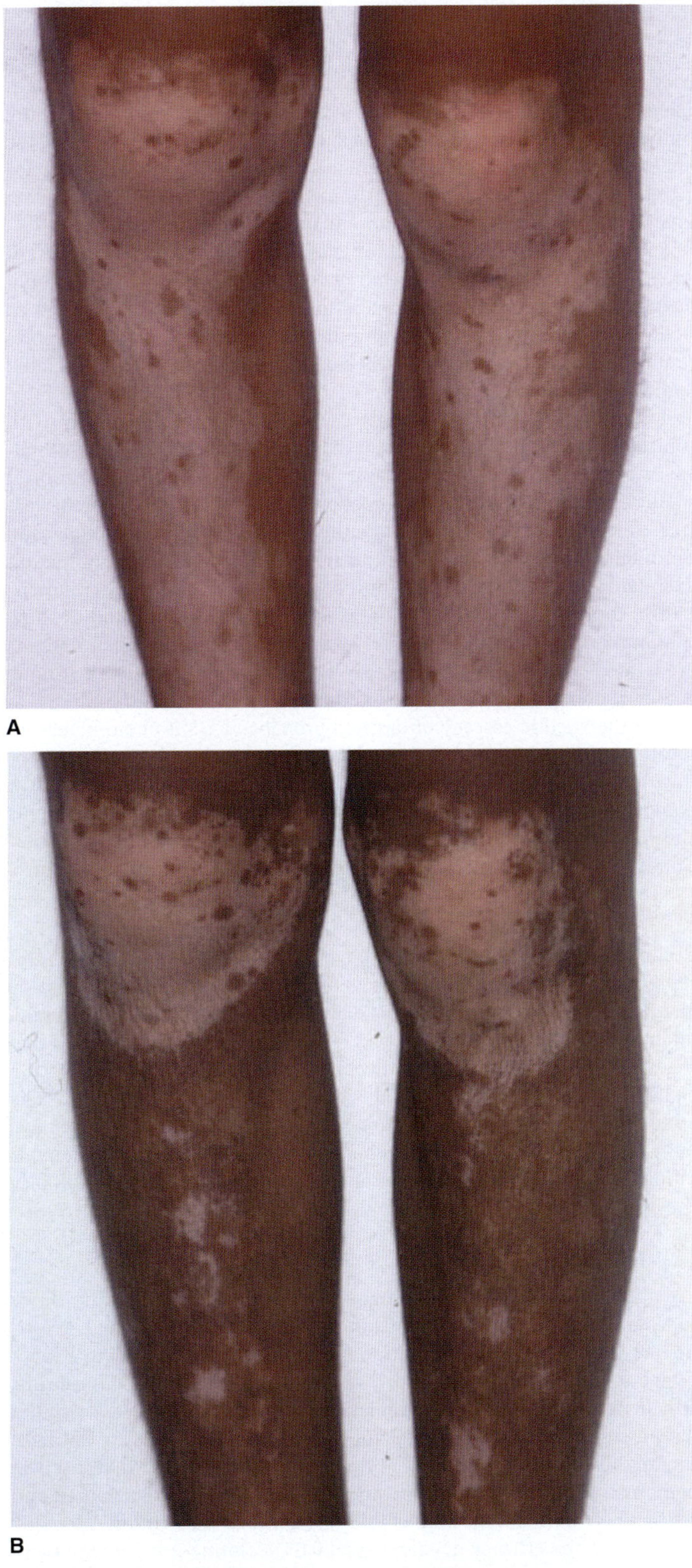

FIGURE 59-6. An individual with skin of color with depigmented vitiligo patches on the anterior knees and shins. **(A)** Before treatment with narrow-band ultraviolet B therapy and **(B)** after 26 treatment sessions.

without vitiligo in a retrospective, comparative cohort survey. It showed that patients with vitiligo had a threefold lower probability of developing melanoma and nonmelanoma skin cancers.[71] A recent cohort study enrolled 60,321 vitiligo patients, and showed that NB-UVB phototherapy was not associated with an increase in the risk of nonmelanoma skin cancer or melanoma in patients with vitiligo. However, the risk of actinic keratosis increased significantly for those who had undergone 200 sessions or more of NB-UVB phototherapy.[72]

Data from 1307 eligible survey questionnaires revealed that patients with vitiligo had a threefold lower probability of developing melanoma and NMSC. The patients who were treated with NB-UVB and PUVA did not show dose-related trends of an increased age-adjusted lifetime prevalence of melanoma or NMSC. A functional color yeast assay demonstrated overexpression of a functioning wild type p53 protein in both the depigmented and healthy pigmented epidermis of patients with vitiligo compared with healthy control subjects.[73] This wild type p53 overexpression may explain the possible low risk of skin cancers in patients with vitiligo. However, long-term follow-up studies are needed to fully assess the risks of NB-UVB. The additive effect of tacrolimus ointment 0.1% applied once daily combined with NB-UVB in the treatment of vitiligo was recently evaluated in a randomized double-blind trial.[74] A total of 40 patients with stable symmetrical vitiligo were treated with tacrolimus ointment 0.1% on one side of their body and a placebo ointment on the other side. Whole-body NB-UVB was administered two or three times weekly for at least 3 months. In 27 patients, significant improvement was seen on the areas of vitiligo treated with tacrolimus. The results showed that combination therapy with NB-UVB and tacrolimus ointment 0.1% was more effective for patients than UVB treatment alone. This effect was dependent on the total dose of tacrolimus applied and was correlated with the number of topical tacrolimus applications, but not the number of UVB treatments.

TARGETED PHOTOTHERAPY

Targeted phototherapy systems have also demonstrated improved efficacy for the treatment of localized vitiligo.[8] These units deliver high-intensity light only to the patient's affected areas while avoiding exposure of the healthy skin and lowering the cumulative UVB dose. In 1999, the effectiveness of UVB radiation micro therapy was first reported for repigmentation of segmental vitiligo in a small series of eight patients.[75] Five of these patients achieved more than 75% repigmentation.

Subsequent investigations have also documented the benefits of excimer laser systems and targeted phototherapy units.[76,77] The excimer laser produces monochromatic radiation at a wavelength of 308 nm. An open-label pilot investigation using the excimer laser in vitiligo reports that 87% of affected areas that received all 12 treatments demonstrated some repigmentation.[76]

Targeted phototherapy systems can also work synergistically with topical therapies. Several studies have assessed the efficacy of combination treatment with an excimer laser and tacrolimus ointment or topical methoxsalen.[77] In a study of eight patients with vitiligo, the subjects were treated with an excimer laser and either topical tacrolimus or a placebo ointment.[77] In the study, 50% of the areas treated with the combination excimer laser and topical tacrolimus achieved 75% or greater repigmentation, compared with 20% for the placebo group. Several studies show that maximal results are achieved with the excimer laser when patients are treated two or three times weekly. Optimal repigmentation is usually achieved on a patient's face, neck, and trunk areas.[78,79]

The therapeutic efficacy of targeted broadband UVB phototherapy in localized vitiligo is good but limited.[80] There is a lack of evidence to support the superior efficacy of excimer lasers compared with NB-UVB. A comparison made in a pilot study of 23 vitiligo patches in eight patients showed both superior effectiveness and earlier appearance of repigmentation with 308 nm excimer laser treatment than with NBUVB treatment.[81]

VITAMINS

Preliminary open-label studies have documented stabilization and repigmentation in vitiligo patients who have been treated with high-dose vitamin supplementation, including daily doses of ascorbic acid (1000 mg), vitamin B_{12} (1000 µg), and folic acid (1-5 mg).[82,83] Data have showed that ingestion of 60 mg of *Ginkgo biloba* twice daily was associated with a significant improvement in total vitiligo area severity index.[84] Orally administered *Polypodium leucotomos* also appears to provide adjunctive benefits in treating vitiligo.[85] Another study showed that oral supplementation of *Polypodium leucotomos* and NB-UVB phototherapy enhance the extent of repigmentation.[86]

VITAMIN D ANALOGS

Calcipotriol is a synthetic analogue of vitamin D_3. Vitamin D_3 binds to vitamin D receptors in the skin, affecting melanocyte and keratinocyte growth and differentiation. It also inhibits T-cell activation.[87] Melanocytes are thought to express 1α-dihydroxy vitamin D_3 receptors, which may have a role in stimulating melanogenesis. Several studies have assessed the efficacy of calcipotriol in combination with UV light therapy in those with vitiligo.[87,88] Some have shown that when used in combination with UV light exposure, calcipotriol is a well-tolerated and efficacious treatment for both children and adults with vitiligo.[87-89]

Recently, the efficacy of calcipotriol 0.05% ointment was reported in combination with clobetasol in a series of 12 patients with vitiligo.[90] A total of 83% of patients responded to treatment with an average 95% repigmentation of their affected areas. A further study showed that calcipotriene 0.005%/betamethasone dipropionate 0.05% ointment used twice daily for at least 12 weeks was effective and well tolerated in the treatment of 31 patients.[89] The responsiveness was greater in patients at a progressive phase than in those at a stable phase.[89]

EMERGING THERAPIES

Topical JAK inhibitors are novel treatments for vitiligo with promising results.[52] Inhibiting JAK-STAT signaling downregulates the secretion of IFN-γ and various chemokines secreted by keratinocytes, and subsequently decrease recruitment of CD8+ T cells that are responsible for the melanocyte killing.[91]

Ruxolitinib 1.5% (Opzelura) cream was approved by the FDA in July 2022. It is a topical Janus kinase (JAK 1 and 2) inhibitor approved for the treatment of nonsegmental vitiligo in adult and pediatric patients 12 years of age and older.[92]

Other JAK inhibitors include tofacitinib, a JAK (1 and 3) inhibitor. Orally administered 5 to 10 mg doses once or twice a day have shown to be effective in treating vitiligo. Side effects from the oral treatments include infections, cancer, and cytopenia, therefore a topical version may therefore be preferred. A small trial has tested a topical tofacitinib cream in treating vitiligo by including 11 patients and showed positive results. Liu and colleagues have shown that treating vitiligo with tofacitinib may require concomitant light exposure.[93]

Baricitinib (Olumiant) is another oral JAK (1 and 2) inhibitor. A case report of repigmentation in vitiligo has been reported in a rheumatoid arthritis patients taking 4 mg of baricitinib. Ritlecitinib is a JAK3 and tyrosine kinase inhibitor. A recent study assessed the efficacy and safety of oral ritlecitinib for the treatment of active nonsegmental vitiligo. A total of 364 patients were treated in the dose-ranging period. Oral ritlecitinib was effective and well tolerated over 48 weeks in patients with active nonsegmental vitiligo.[91]

Nonimmunomodulatory treatments in vitiligo include afamelanotide, a potent and longer-lasting synthetic analogue of naturally occurring α-MSH, which is a novel intervention for reduced α-MSH in patients with vitiligo.[25,94] Afamelanotide is delivered as a subcutaneous bioresorbable implant that promotes melanocyte proliferation and melanogenesis. The efficacy and safety of afamelanotide for treatment of vitiligo was assessed in a randomized multi-center trial for those 18 years or older with Fitzpatrick skin phototypes (SPTs) III to VI and a confirmed diagnosis of nonsegmental vitiligo that involved 15% to 50% of total body surface area. Patients were randomized to combination therapy ($n = 28$) versus NB-UVB monotherapy ($n = 27$). After 1 month of NB-UVB phototherapy, 16 mg of afamelanotide was administered subcutaneously to the combination therapy group monthly for 4 months while NB-UVB phototherapy continued; the other group continued to receive NB-UVB monotherapy. A combination of afamelanotide implant and NB-UVB phototherapy resulted in clinically apparent, statistically significant superior and faster repigmentation compared with NB-UVB monotherapy. The response was more noticeable in patients with SPTs IV to VI.[94]

Prostaglandin E2 (PGE2) is another novel and potentially beneficial treatment for localized stable vitiligo. PGE2 controls the proliferation of melanocytes through stimulant and immunomodulatory effects. In a consecutive series, repigmentation occurred in 40 of 56 patients with stable vitiligo treated with translucent PGE2 0.25 mg.[95] The patients applied the PGE2 gel twice daily for 6 months. The mean onset of repigmentation was 2 months. The response was excellent in 22 of 40 patients, with complete repigmentation observed in eight patients. The patients with a disease duration of 6 months showed the most significant response. Repigmentation occurred the earliest in the face and scalp.[95] Bimatoprost, a topical prostaglandin, is associated with hyperpigmentation of periocular skin caused by increased melanogenesis. In a study by Narang, 10 patients were treated with bimatoprost 0.03% ophthalmic solution twice daily for 4 months. Of the 10 patients, 3 had 100% repigmentation, 3 had 75% to 99% repigmentation, and 1 had 50% to 75% repigmentation. The best responses were observed on the face.[102]

It has been shown that the inducible heat shock protein 70 (HSP70i), a molecular link between stress and the resultant immune response, causes an inflammatory dendritic cell phenotype and is essential for depigmentation in vitiligo mouse models.[96] However, a mutant HSP70i (HSP70iQ435A) behaved differently by binding human dendritic cells and reducing their activation in a mouse model. Mice expressing a transgenic, melanocyte-reactive T-cell receptor treated with HSP70iQ435A-encoding DNA months before spontaneous depigmentation did not develop vitiligo. HSP70iQ435A used therapeutically in another rapid depigmentation model led to a 76% recovery of pigmentation and prevented the relevant T-cell populating of mouse skin. Ex vivo treatment of human skin with HSP70iQ435A prevented the shift from the quiescent to the effector T-cell phenotype associated with vitiligo.[96]

DEPIGMENTATION

Since the 1950s, monobenzylether of hydroquinone (MBEH), or monobenzone, has been used as a depigmenting agent for patients with extensive vitiligo. In general, MBEH causes permanent destruction of melanocytes and induces depigmentation locally and remotely from the sites of application. Hence the use of MBEH for other disorders of pigmentation is contraindicated. Depigmentation is a viable therapeutic alternative in individuals with over 50% cutaneous depigmentation who have demonstrated recalcitrance to repigmentation or in those with extensive vitiligo who have no desire to undergo repigmentation therapies.[3] The major side effects of MBEH therapy are irritant dermatitis and pruritus, which usually respond to topical and systemic steroids. Other side effects include severe xerosis, alopecia, and premature graying. Additional depigmenting agents are 4-methoxyphenol and 88% phenol.[97] Alternatively, procedural therapies may be used for depigmentation, such as Q-switched ruby and alexandrite lasers or cryotherapy. Second-line agents such as imatinib mesylate, imiquimod, and diphencyprone are also used. Experimental agents currently under investigation include phenol derivatives, melanoma vaccines, interferon-γ, and busulfan.[97]

SURGICAL APPROACHES

Surgical therapies have been used for vitiligo for the past three decades. Recently, substantial advances have been made in the techniques and protocols for harvesting and transplanting melanocytes. Surgical therapies remain viable options for patients with localized areas of depigmentation that have failed to respond to medical intervention.[98,99] The major advantage of transplantation procedures is the transfer of a reservoir of healthy melanocytes to the depigmented skin, allowing for proliferation and migration of the transplanted melanocytes into areas of depigmentation. Transplantation procedures are contraindicated for anyone with a history of hypertrophic scars or keloids. Surgical therapies are either tissue grafting techniques that entail the transfer of the intact skin piece or cellular grafting techniques that entail further processing of the skin into a fluid suspension. Tissue grafts include autologous suction-blister grafts, punch grafts, split-thickness grafts, hair follicle grafts, while cellular grafts include, noncultured melanocyte-keratinocyte suspensions, cultured autologous melanocyte, cultured epidermal suspensions, and hair follicle outer root sheath suspension [**Figure 59-7**].[100]

A recent systematic review and meta-analysis assessed surgical interventions for vitiligo. A total of 117 studies and 8000 patients were included.[101] The rate of repigmentation of greater than 90% for surgical interventions was 45.76% for punch grafting, 72.08% for thin skin grafting, 61.68% for suction blister grafting, 47.51% for noncultured epidermal cell suspension, 36.24% for noncultured follicular cell suspension, and 56.82% for cultured epidermal cell suspension. The rate of repigmentation of greater than 50% after any surgical intervention was 81.01%. The best responses were in patients of younger age, segmental vitiligo, nonacral, and joint areas.[102] A study that included 117 patients assessed the influences of age, site of lesion, and type of disease on transplantation outcomes.[103] In this series, the best results were achieved for patients younger than 20 years of age and patients with segmental vitiligo. The grafting site did not significantly affect the outcome. In most instances, tattooing or micropigmentation should be avoided given the risk of koebnerization and oxidation of the tattoo pigment causing further dyschromia.

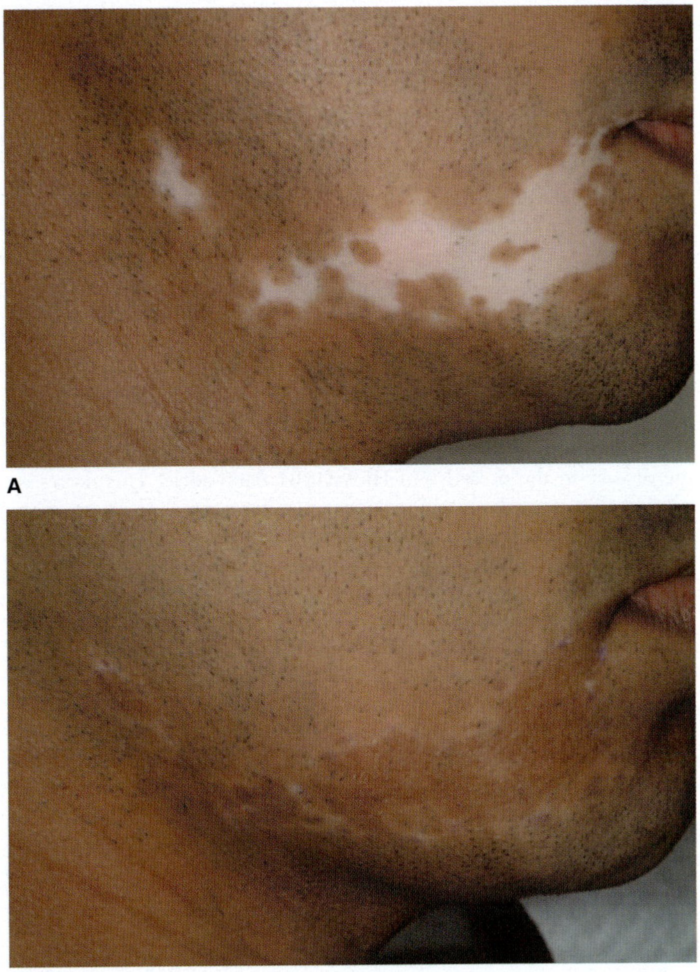

A

B

FIGURE 59-7. A young man with segmental vitiligo of the face **(A)** before grafting and **(B)** 3 months after autologous 1 mm punch grafting.

CONCLUSION

Vitiligo is a pigmentary disorder with an equal incidence in all skin types. Due to the contrast between the affected areas and normal skin, this condition is most disfiguring in those with darker skin of color but can be psychologically devastating for all skin colors. The objectives for vitiligo treatment should include both the stabilization of the disease and the repigmentation of the vitiligo. Typically used medical therapies for vitiligo include topical and systemic steroids, topical calcineurin inhibitors, topical JAK inhibitors, NB-UVB phototherapy, PUVA, targeted phototherapy, nutritional vitamin supplementation, and calcipotriol.

Topical calcineurin inhibitors are a common first-line vitiligo treatment modality. These agents have proven to be very effective and can be used for long periods without substantial adverse effects. NB-UVB phototherapy is currently the initial treatment of choice for moderate to severe vitiligo. This therapy has comparable efficacy to PUVA, and one of its major advantages is its established safety profile. Vitamin supplementation has been found to cause stabilization and repigmentation when administered in high doses. Calcipotriol (a synthetic analogue of vitamin D_3) in combination with UV light therapy is also a well-tolerated and effective treatment for cases of limited localized vitiligo.

Depigmentation and surgical therapies are viable treatment options for patients with severe or recalcitrant vitiligo. For the last 25 years, surgical therapies have been used as a form of vitiligo treatment, and recently, there has been significant progress in the area of harvesting and transplanting melanocytes. Studies have reported the benefits of split-thickness grafting and epidermal suction blister grafting, as well as the transplantation of autologous melanocyte cultures and epidermal suspensions containing mix of epidermal cells including melanocytes and keratinocytes.

VITILIGO-ASSOCIATED DISEASES

VOGT-KOYANAGI-HARADA DISEASE

Vitiligo is part of a condition known as Vogt-Koyanagi-Harada disease (VKHD), or also called Alopecia-poliosis-uveitis-vitiligo-deafness-cutaneous-uveo-oto syndrome. It is rare syndrome that usually begins in the third decade of life but has been reported in children. VKHD is more common in females and tends to be more prevalent among people with skin of color, especially Asians, Hispanic, and Native American populations. In the United States, the incidence of VKHD is approximately 1.5 to 6 per one million patients, while in Japan the annual incidence is approximately 800 new patients each year.[104]

The exact etiology of VKHD is unknown; however, an autoimmune-mediated pathogenesis is likely. Current studies suggest that the disease is a Th1 lymphocyte-mediated destruction of melanocytes caused by a viral trigger in the context of an underlying genetic predisposition for the disease in the presence of HLA-DRB1*0405 allele. This drives an autoimmune granulomatous response against normal tissue in many body systems (mainly pigmented structures), including the meninges, eyes, inner ears, skin, and hair, leading to meningeal irritation, chronic uveitis, dysacusia, poliosis, alopecia, and vitiligo.[105]

Affected individuals can present with bilateral symmetrical skin depigmentation along with a rapid loss of vision, a granulomatous pan uveitis, and neurological manifestations including headache, nausea, and vertigo.[106] The classic treatment of VKHD is a high-dose systemic corticosteroids that must be initiated promptly, either by oral prednisone (1-1.5 mg/kg/day) or intravenous methylprednisolone (1000 mg daily, over 3 days). A maintenance therapy is highly recommended with a slow taper of oral corticosteroids over a period of 6 months. Immunoglobulin (IVIg) therapy is a potential treatment of VKHD that is under clinical trials. However, more research is necessary to determine its long-term safety and effectiveness.[104]

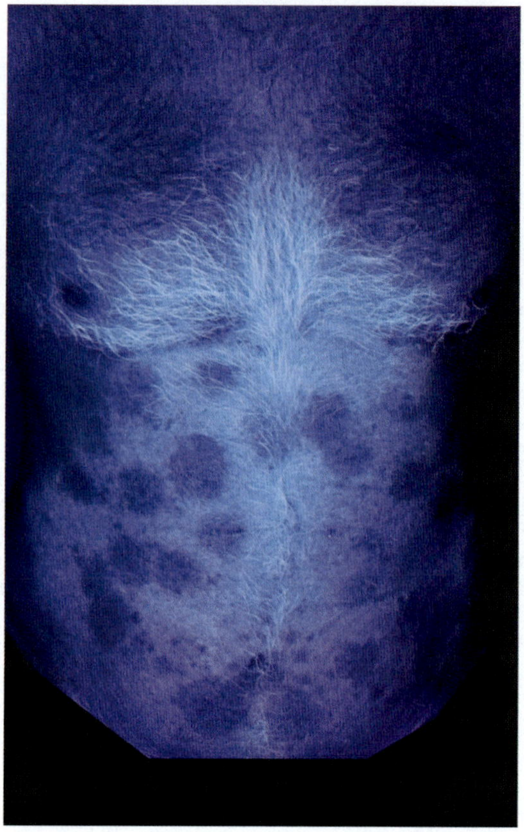

FIGURE 59-8. An individual with piebaldism with depigmented patches on the anterior chest and abdomen. Notice the islands of normal skin color pigmentation.

ALEZZANDRINI SYNDROME

Alezzandrini is a similar but rarer syndrome characterized by unilateral vitiligo, poliosis, and deafness. It was first described in 1959, by Casala and Alezzandrini in a patient who had unilateral vitiligo, poliosis, deafness, and pigmentary retinitis with subsequent visual changes hyperacusis. The exact etiology of Alezzandrini syndrome remains unknown. Viral triggers leading to autoimmune-mediated destruction of melanocytes have been suggested. Melanocytes in the skin, retina, uvea, cochlea, and vestibular labyrinth may be involved. Clinically, Alezzandrini syndrome presents with unilateral gradual loss of vision, followed by ipsilateral facial vitiligo and poliosis several years later. Ipsilateral hypoacusis may also develop. Bilateral deafness has been reported in one patient.[107]

Alezzandrini syndrome can be related to Vogt-Koyanagi-Harada (VKH) syndrome, as they have common cutaneous and ocular signs. Unlike VKHD, patients with Alezzandrini have unilateral rather than bilateral facial vitiligo and lack the meningeal signs. Patients with Alezzandrini syndrome are treated topically for their vitiligo, and systemic steroid may be utilized for the uveitis.[107]

OTHER DISORDERS OF DEPIGMENTATION

PIEBALDISM

Piebaldism is a congenital autosomal dominant genetic disorder. It is caused by mutation in c-KIT proto-oncogene that results in defective melanocytes migration. Clinically, piebaldism manifests as congenital midline and ventral patches of depigmented skin with central islands of normal pigmentation [**Figure 59-8**]. Moreover, there is a characteristic white forelock (poliosis) that presents in 90% of the patients. The lesions fluorescent under Wood's lamp examination and skin biopsy will show a complete absence of melanocytes. Given the autosomal dominance mode of inheritance, patients classically have positive family history, which helps in establishing the diagnosis. The skin depigmentation in piebaldism is permanent and stable. Surgical transplantation of healthy melanocytes from unaffected areas of skin is the main treatment option in piebaldism.[108]

OCULOCUTANEOUS ALBINISM

Oculocutaneous Albinism (OCA) is a congenital genetic, autosomal recessive disorder that is characterized by abnormal melanin biosynthesis and transport within melanosomes. OCA, of which there are four types of OCA, affects the melanocytes of skin, hair follicles, and eyes [**Table 59-4**]. Clinically, in addition to the variable pigmentary dilution of the skin, hair, and eyes, there are frequently associated ocular manifestations in the form of photophobia, nystagmus, with reduced visual acuity. Once the diagnosis is established, sun protection is the mainstay in managing OCA patients due to their high susceptibility to develop skin cancers. Patients also benefit from efforts to improve visual acuity, including corrective lenses and high contrast magnifiers.

TUBEROUS SCLEROSIS

Tuberous sclerosis (TS) is a congenital autosomal dominant genetic multisystem disorder that manifests with benign hamartomas. Common manifestations include angiofibromas mainly on the central part of the face, in addition to seizures, mental retardation, cardiac rhabdomyoma, and renal angiomyolipoma. Characteristically, 40% to 90% of the patients will have an ash leaf that presents as one or more depigmented patches located mainly on the trunk or extremities. Ash leaf patches are stable and do not expand with time. Diagnosis can be made in the context of the characteristic TS constellation of features.[109]

NEVUS DEPIGMENTOSUS

Although nevus depigmentosus (ND) is a congenital localized skin disorder, it may not be obvious at birth and may present later in life,

TABLE 59-4 Types of oculocutaneous albinism

Type	Mutation	Description
OCA1a	TYR gene (completely absent)	White skin Generalized (near-universal) absence of pigmentation at birth. White hair that becomes light yellow over time Amelanotic and pink nevi Severe photosensitivity Increased risk of SCC Gray blue irides markedly reduced visual acuity
OCA1b	TYR gene (decreased to <10% of normal level)	Absence of pigmentation of skin/hair at birth but over time, develop some pigmentation. Amelanotic or pink nevi Milder ocular complications compared to OCA1a. Has a temperature sensitive variant where tyrosinase functions at low temperatures, leading to hair pigmentation at cooler anatomic sites (mainly extremities) and white hairs in warmer sites (trunk, intertriginous zones
OCA2	OCA2 (P gene; pink-eyed dilution)	Most common subtypes Common in Africans population Variable pigmentary dilution Pigmented nevi and lentigines Light brown hair Gray tan irides
OCA3	TYRP1 gene	Africa and New Guinea Reddish-bronze skin and red hair color Blue brown irides
OCA4	SLC45A2 (MATP gene)	Very rare 25% of the OCA cases in Japan Variable pigmentary dilution

often during early childhood. Clinically it is characterized by a unilateral solitary patch, with jagged borders, that is hypopigmented rather than depigmented, hence making the name a misnomer. Under Wood's lamp, the lesions exhibit an off-white accentuation without fluorescence. Since it is a nevus, ND usually remains stable in shape and size over years, with only proportional expansion with the child's growth. Electron microscopy examination shows reduction in melanosomal content of lesional melanocytes and keratinocytes, with more immature and aggregated melanosomes in lesional keratinocytes. Melanocyte numbers are normal; however, the transfer of melanosomes to keratinocytes is defective. Moreover, reduced tyrosinase activity was noted in lesional skin compared to control indicated by reduced DOPA oxidase reaction. Surgical transplantation of melanocytes is the main treatment option.[110]

NEVUS ANEMICUS

Nevus anemicus is another congenital skin disorder that can present with a patch that is paler than the surrounding skin. It is not a true nevus but rather a pharmacologic one. The etiopathogenesis is from sustained vasoconstriction in the skin because of localized hypersensitivity of the cutaneous blood vessels to the circulating catecholamines. The diagnosis can be made clinically by diascopy. Histologically, the melanocytes as well as vasculature of the nevus is normal when stained with hematoxylin-and-eosin and with alkaline-phosphatase. The defect, therefore, may be at the motor end plate or at the smooth muscle effector cell of arterioles.[111]

SCLERODERMA

Scleroderma is an autoimmune disease characterized by fibrosis of cutaneous tissues and visceral organs. The chronic cutaneous inflammation of scleroderma may affect melanocyte function. Pigment alterations in this disease can present as diffuse hyperpigmentation with accentuation in the photo-exposed parts of the body, or more commonly presents as localized areas of hypopigmentation or depigmentation associated with palpable skin induration.[112] Such alteration in pigmentation is more evident in patients with dark complexion as higher levels of melanin correlate with increased postinflammatory depigmentation. Clinically, the depigmented patches usually have preserved perifollicular pigmentation that gives the depigmented patches a characteristic dotted appearance classically described as "salt and pepper" that is considered a cutaneous clue for the diagnosis of systemic sclerosis.[113]

The etiopathogenesis of scleroderma is mainly chronic inflammatory process with an associated microvascular dysfunction and immune dysregulation. Histologically the salt and pepper pattern of scleroderma is explained by the loss of the epidermal melanocytes in the interfollicular region but not the hair follicle melanocytes, with associated variable degrees of epidermal and dermal atrophy. Moreover, there is a significant reduction of FXIIIa in the papillary dermis1 and CD341 cells in the reticular dermis, with a localized increase in FXIIIa1 cells within the areas of fibrotic skin. Scleroderma is a progressive disease, so early diagnosis and prompt medical treatment is of paramount importance to prevent the disfiguring fibrotic sequelae of the disease. Treatments are generally most effective if started early in the course of the disease.[114]

CHEMICAL LEUKODERMA

Chemical irritation can induce skin depigmentation or hypopigmentation known as chemical leukoderma. Leukoderma is defined as an acquired depigmentation that is caused by the cutaneous application of specific chemicals that destroy the epidermal melanocytes. Culprit chemical compounds are mainly aromatic and aliphatic derivatives of phenol and catechol, common examples are monobenzyl ether of hydroquinone and para-tertiary butyl phenol. Diagnosis of chemical leukoderma is clinical, depends mainly on the history of exposure to the reagent, with a sign of depigmented areas confined to the primary site of the chemical's contact. A recent study has shown that patches were limited to the contact area in 73.7% of the enrolled subjects but had spread to remote areas in 26.3% of the subjects. Confetti macules were seen in 89% and associated pruritus was reported in 21.8%. Common associated products included hair dye, deodorant and spray perfume, detergent, cleansers, adhesive binders, rubber chappal, black socks and shoes, eyeliner, lipliner, rubber condoms, lipstick, fur toys, toothpaste, and insecticides. Response to treatment was better when chemical leukoderma was not associated with coexisting vitiligo.[115]

CHRONIC ONCHOCERCIASIS

Onchocerciasis is a tropical disease secondary to an infection transmitted by *Onchocerca volvulus*, a filarial nematode, that is transmitted to humans through the bite of a female blackfly. Geographically, blackflies are found near fast-flowing rivers and streams in the intertropical zones. It is prevalent in sub-Saharan Africa, Latin America, and Yemen. According to the WHO, onchocerciasis persists also in the Amazon region of Brazil and Venezuela; Around 18 million are currently infested with onchocerciasis; four million of which have a skin involvement.[116]

Multiple bites by the female black flies are usually required for infestation with the microfilaria that results in chronic skin, eye, and neurological disease. Depigmentation skin involvement is associated with HLA subtypes DQA1*0501 and DQB1*0301. Clinical manifestations of onchocerciasis are due to inflammatory responses to dying microfilariae. Cutaneous manifestations vary according to the stage of the disease; early cutaneous manifestations are usually in the form of intensely pruritic papular eruption, subcutaneous nodules over bony prominences, with persistent eosinophilia and painless lymphadenopathy. Late cutaneous manifestations are in the form of skin depigmentation, also called leopard skin, with associated islands of normal pigmented skin around the hair follicles. Onchocercal depigmentation is nonpruritic and often symmetrically affects the shin of the tibia.

Diagnosis is highly suspected by the occurrence of the clinical manifestation in the endemic areas. Confirmation of the diagnosis is through identifying the adult worms with a light microscopy in the biopsied subcutaneous nodules or by identifying the microfilariae by microscopical examination of skin snips mainly from the anterior tibia and iliac crests. Polymerase chain reaction (PCR) can also be used to amplify the larval DNA in mild cases when larvae cannot be detected microscopically. Antibodies against *O. volvulus* can also be detected in blood samples—however, it is not reliable in distinguishing between past and present infection. Screening for *L. loa* coinfection is highly recommended to detect any associated subclinical coinfection that may result in life-threatening encephalitis.

Prevention is a golden role in the management of the infection. No vaccine is available to prevent the occurrence of onchocerciasis. However, effective strategies in preventing the infection include vector control using insect repellents to eliminate blackflies as DDT, wearing long-sleeved shirts and pants, and wearing permethrin-impregnated clothing, which are helpful in minimizing the chances of infection while visiting or residing in the endemic areas. Treatment is systemic by using oral ivermectin (150 ug/kg one dose every 3 months), which kills the microfilariae but not the adult worm, followed by doxycycline (200 mg/day) for 4 to 6 weeks. Patients may develop edema, itching, and/or tender lymphadenopathy within the first 24 hours of initiating the systemic treatment. If such reaction develops, a short course of oral prednisone taper starting with 40 mg/day for 5 days is warranted.[117] New agents being studied in treating onchocerciasis to kill the adult worm include suramin and moxidectin.[113]

TERTIARY PINTA

Tertiary Pinta is also a tropical infectious disease caused by infection with *Treponema carateum* and can manifest with skin depigmentation during its late stage. Despite major efforts to eradicate treponemal disorders, it remains endemic in tropical areas such as Mexico, Brazil, Colombia, and the Caribbean islands. Unlike onchocerciasis that necessitate vector for the transmission of infection, pinta is transmitted via direct skin or mucus membrane contact. Clinically, it is relatively benign, mild, and nonprogressive disease that only affects the skin (unlike other treponemal infections like syphilis and yaw that have systemic involvement). Primary pinta, which occurs within 2 weeks of the infection, manifests with itchy papules with lymphadenopathy. Secondary pinta that occurs within 6 months to 3 years of the infection manifests with widespread papules with scaling and dyspigmentation. Nevertheless, atrophic skin depigmentation is the main manifestation of tertiary pinta with the most involved anatomical sites being the palms, wrists, elbows, and ankles.[118] Histopathological examination of skin biopsy reveals reduction of the melanin of the basal layer with predominantly perivascular lymphocytic infiltrate. Serology is crucial in the diagnosis but cannot differentiate between different treponemal species. Parenteral penicillin is the treatment of choice for patient and their close contacts to decrease the chances of the transmission of infection. Single intramuscular dose of penicillin G benzathine is recommended (600,000 units for patients less than 10 years of age and 1.2 million units for patients > 10 years of age). Alternative antibiotics such as tetracycline and erythromycin may also be effective. Affected areas of skin become noninfectious within the first day of initiating the treatment. However, the late pigmentary changes are challenging and frequently persist.[119]

LEPROSY

Leprosy is caused by infection of the skin and superficial nerves by a bacteria called *Mycobacterium leprae*. Based on the patient's cell-mediated immunity status, leprosy can be tuberculoid or lepromatous (in patients with strong vs weak cell-mediated immunity, respectively). Tuberculoid leprosy may present with hypopigmented patches that are infiltrative in nature and characterized by hypoesthesia and loss of the hair overlying the patches. In skin of color individuals, the patches are typically hypopigmented, whereas in lighter skin the patches can be more erythematous. In endemic areas, diagnosis can be suspected clinically by demonstrating a decrease in the sensation of the affected patches using pin or cotton tip testing. Establishing the cutaneous leprosy diagnosis needs a confirmation with a dermatopathological examination of skin biopsy that will show caseating granulomas with acid fast bacilli (*M. leprae*). Leprosy is treated by multidrug therapy, which is a combination of antimicrobial drugs, dapsone, and rifampin, with clofazimine needed for some types of the disease. Duration of multidrug therapy also varies according to the disease subtype, with shorter duration needed for tuberculoid leprosy and longer duration for lepromatous leprosy.[120]

MELANOMA TREATMENT-ASSOCIATED DEPIGMENTATION

Skin depigmentation in melanoma patients can be a side effect of melanoma treatment, specifically immunotherapy with checkpoints inhibitors (anti-PD1/PDL-1, anti-CTLA-4), interleukin 2, or interferon-α. Nevertheless, skin depigmentation can occur spontaneously in patients with melanoma. It is clinically indistinguishable from vitiligo. The Vitiligo Global Issue Consensus Conference has agreed to consider it a distinct entity from vitiligo.[121]

Loss of pigmentation in melanoma can have multiple clinical phenotypes. It may surround the primary melanoma in the form of eccentrically placed depigmented halo and may also occur in different locations away from the primary melanoma.[122]

The etiology of skin depigmentation observed in individuals with melanoma is primarily an immunologic response mediated through activated T-lymphocytes against proteins derived from the malignant melanocytes including antigens encoded by tumor-specific mutated genes as well as melanocytic differentiation antigens that are expressed by all melanocyte lineages including the normal melanocytes. The later explains the attack of the activated T-lymphocytes against normal melanocytes, and the subsequent occurrence of depigmentation on skin areas away from the primary melanoma. The inability to accurately distinguish normal unaltered antigens from tumor antigens demonstrates the potential association between depigmentation, resulting from destruction of normal melanocytes, and melanoma regression, resulting from destruction of malignant melanocytes in the melanoma patients.[123,124] Remarkably, the literature elaborates a more favorable prognosis for the melanoma individuals who develop such immune-mediated depigmentation. A retrospective study showed a significant higher survival than the expected survival according to the thickness of the associated primary melanoma.[124]

CONCLUSION

Numerous disorders of depigmentation exist that can be physically disfiguring and emotionally distressing to affected individuals. These conditions are visibly more apparent in skin of color due to the greater color contrast. A detailed history, careful examination, and thorough work-up are of paramount importance in identifying the correct diagnosis. Barriers to equitable healthcare plus a lack of medical education about disorders of depigmentation across skin colors can make obtaining an accurate diagnosis along with starting early and effective treatments more challenging. Many disorders of depigmentation benefit from early and at times sustained therapeutic intervention along with psychological and emotional support to those affected.

REFERENCES

1. Lerner AB. Book review "Biological perspectives on human pigmentation". *N Engl J Med.* 1992;327(7):504.
2. Grimes PE. Disorders of pigmentation. *DeckerMed Medicine.* Published online 2012.
3. Porter J., Tschopp J, Martinon F, Burns K. The psychological effects of vitiligo: response to impaired appearance. In: *Vitiligo.* Blackwell Science Ltd; 2008:97-100.
4. Alkhateeb A, Fain PR, Thody A, Bennett DC, Spritz RA. Epidemiology of vitiligo and associated autoimmune diseases in Caucasian probands and their families. *Pigment Cell Res.* 2003;16(3):208-214.

5. Grimes PE, Billips M. Childhood vitiligo: clinical spectrum and therapeutic approaches. In: Hann KS, Nordlund JJ, *Vitiligo: A Monograph on the Basic and Clinical Science*. 1st ed. Oxford, London: Blackwell Science Ltd.; 2000. 61-8.
6. Albert DM, Wagoner MD, Pruett RC, Nordlund JJ, Lerner AB. Vitiligo and disorders of the retinal pigment epithelium. *Br J Ophthalmol.* 1983;67(3): 153-156.
7. Cowan CL Jr, Halder RM, Grimes PE, Chakrabarti SG, Kenney JA Jr. Ocular disturbances in vitiligo. *J Am Acad Dermatol.* 1986;15(1):17-24.
8. Grimes PE. New insights and new therapies in vitiligo. *JAMA.* 2005;293(6):730-735.
9. Montes LF, Abulafia J, Wilborn WH, Hyde BM, Montes CM. Value of histopathology in vitiligo. *Int J Dermatol.* 2003;42(1):57-61.
10. Le Poole IC, Das PK. Microscopic changes in vitiligo. *Clin Dermatol.* 1997;15(6):863-873.
11. Frisoli ML, Essien K, Harris JE. Vitiligo: mechanisms of pathogenesis and treatment. *Annu Rev Immunol.* 2020;38:621-648.
12. Bergqvist C, Ezzedine K. Vitiligo: a review. *Dermatology.* 2020;236(6):571-592.
13. Majumder PP, Das SK, Li CC. A genetical model for vitiligo. *Am J Hum Genet.* 1988;43(2):119-125.
14. Nath SK, Majumder PP, Nordlund JJ. Genetic epidemiology of vitiligo: multilocus recessivity cross-validated. *Am J Hum Genet.* 1994;55(5):981-990.
15. Fain PR, Gowan K, LaBerge GS, et al. A genomewide screen for generalized vitiligo: confirmation of AIS1 on chromosome 1p31 and evidence for additional susceptibility loci. *Am J Hum Genet.* 2003;72(6):1560-1564.
16. Chen JJ, Huang W, Gui JP, et al. A novel linkage to generalized vitiligo on 4q13-q21 identified in a genomewide linkage analysis of Chinese families. *Am J Hum Genet.* 2005;76(6):1057-1065.
17. Jin Y, Mailloux CM, Gowan K, et al. NALP1 in vitiligo-associated multiple autoimmune disease. *N Engl J Med.* 2007;356(12):1216-1225.
18. Jin Y, Andersen G, Yorgov D, et al. Genome-wide association studies of autoimmune vitiligo identify 23 new risk loci and highlight key pathways and regulatory variants. *Nat Genet.* 2016;48(11):1418-1424.
19. Grimes PE, Sevall JS, Vojdani A. Cytomegalovirus DNA identified in skin biopsy specimens of patients with vitiligo. *J Am Acad Dermatol.* 1996;35(1):21-26.
20. Erf GF, Bersi TK, Wang X, Sreekumar GP, Smyth JR Jr. Herpesvirus connection in the expression of autoimmune vitiligo in Smyth line chickens. *Pigment Cell Res.* 2001;14(1):40-46.
21. Gauthier Y, Lepreux S, Cario-Andre M, et al. Varicella-zoster virus in actively spreading segmental vitiligo skin: Pathological, immunochemical, and ultrastructural findings (a first and preliminary study). *Pigment Cell Melanoma Res.* 2023;36(1):78-85.
22. Gauthier Y, Cario Andre M, Taïeb A. A critical appraisal of vitiligo etiologic theories. Is melanocyte loss a melanocytorrhagy? *Pigment Cell Res.* 2003;16(4):322-332.
23. Taïeb A, Morice-Picard F, Jouary T, Ezzedine K, Cario-André M, Gauthier Y. Segmental vitiligo as the possible expression of cutaneous somatic mosaicism: implications for common non-segmental vitiligo. *Pigment Cell Melanoma Res.* 2008;21(6):646-652.
24. Pichler R, Sfetsos K, Badics B, Gutenbrunner S, Auböck J. Vitiligo patients present lower plasma levels of α-melanotropin immunoreactivities. *Neuropeptides.* 2006;40(3):177-183.
25. Graham A, Westerhof W, Thody AJ. The expression of α-MSH by melanocytes is reduced in vitiligo. *Ann N Y Acad Sci.* 2006;885(1):470-473.
26. Kingo K, Aunin E, Karelson M, et al. Gene expression analysis of melanocortin system in vitiligo. *J Dermatol Sci.* 2007;48(2):113-122.
27. Taïeb A, Picardo M, VETF Members. The definition and assessment of vitiligo: a consensus report of the Vitiligo European Task Force. *Pigment Cell Res.* 2007;20(1):27-35.
28. Dell'Anna ML, Maresca V, Briganti S, Camera E, Picardo M, Falchi M. Mitochondrial impairment in peripheral blood mononuclear cells during the active phase of vitiligo. *J Invest Dermatol.* 2001;117(4):908-913.
29. Picardo M, Grammatico P, Roccella F, et al. Imbalance in the antioxidant pool in melanoma cells and normal melanocytes from patients with melanoma. *J Invest Dermatol.* 1996;107(3):322-326.
30. Dell'Anna ML, Picardo M. A review and a new hypothesis for non-immunological pathogenetic mechanisms in vitiligo. *Pigment Cell Res.* 2006;19(5): 406-411.
31. Marchioro HZ, de Castro CCS, Fava VM, Sakiyama PH, Dellatorre G, Miot HA. Update on the pathogenesis of vitiligo. *An Bras Dermatol.* 2022;97(4):478-490.
32. Richmond JM, Frisoli ML, Harris JE. Innate immune mechanisms in vitiligo: danger from within. *Curr Opin Immunol.* 2013;25(6):676-682.
33. Njoo MD, Westerhof W. Vitiligo. Pathogenesis and treatment. *Am J Clin Dermatol.* 2001;2(3):167-181.
34. Hadi A, Wang JF, Uppal P, Penn LA, Elbuluk N. Comorbid diseases of vitiligo: a 10-year cross-sectional retrospective study of an urban US population. *J Am Acad Dermatol.* 2020;82(3):628-633.
35. Betterle C, Caretto A, De Zio A, et al. Incidence and significance of organ-specific autoimmune disorders (Clinical, Latent or only Autoantibodies) in patients with vitiligo. *Dermatology.* 1985;171(6):419-423.
36. Naughton GK, Eisinger M, Bystryn JC. Detection of antibodies to melanocytes in vitiligo by specific immunoprecipitation. *J Invest Dermatol.* 1983;81(6):540-542.
37. Ongenae K, Van Geel N, Naeyaert JM. Evidence for an autoimmune pathogenesis of vitiligo. *Pigment Cell Res.* 2003;16(2):90-100.
38. Gilhar A, Pillar T, Eidelman S, Etzioni A. Vitiligo and idiopathic guttate hypomelanosis. Repigmentation of skin following engraftment onto nude mice. *Arch Dermatol.* 1989;125(10):1363-1366.
39. Hedstrand H, Ekwall O, Olsson MJ, et al. The transcription factors SOX9 and SOX10 are vitiligo autoantigens in autoimmune polyendocrine syndrome type I. *J Biol Chem.* 2001;276(38):35390-35395.
40. Ogg GS, Rod Dunbar P, Romero P, Chen JL, Cerundolo V. High frequency of skin-homing melanocyte-specific cytotoxic T lymphocytes in autoimmune vitiligo. *J Exp Med.* 1998;188(6):1203-1208.
41. Ghoneum M, Grimes PE, Gill G, Paul Kelly A. Natural cell-mediated cytotoxicity in vitiligo. *J Am Acad Dermatol.* 1987;17(4):600-605.
42. Harris JE, Harris TH, Weninger W, Wherry EJ, Hunter CA, Turka LA. A mouse model of vitiligo with focused epidermal depigmentation requires IFN-γ for autoreactive $CD8^+$ T-cell accumulation in the skin. *J Invest Dermatol.* 2012;132(7):1869-1876.
43. Mandelcorn-Monson RL, Shear NH, Yau E, et al. Cytotoxic T lymphocyte reactivity to gp100, MelanA/MART-1, and tyrosinase, in HLA-A2-positive vitiligo patients. *J Invest Dermatol.* 2003;121(3):550-556.
44. Caixia T, Hongwen F, Xiran L. Levels of soluble interleukin-2 receptor in the sera and skin tissue fluids of patients with vitiligo. *J Dermatol Sci.* 1999;21(1):59-62.
45. Moretti S, Spallanzani A, Amato L, et al. New insights into the pathogenesis of vitiligo: imbalance of epidermal cytokines at sites of lesions. *Pigment Cell Res.* 2002;15(2):87-92.
46. Imokawa G. Autocrine and paracrine regulation of melanocytes in human skin and in pigmentary disorders. *Pigment Cell Res.* 2004;17(2):96-110.
47. Grimes PE, Morris R, Avaniss-Aghajani E, Soriano T, Meraz M, Metzger A. Topical tacrolimus therapy for vitiligo: therapeutic responses and skin messenger RNA expression of proinflammatory cytokines. *J Am Acad Dermatol.* 2004;51(1):52-61.
48. Rashighi M, Agarwal P, Richmond JM, et al. CXCL10 is critical for the progression and maintenance of depigmentation in a mouse model of vitiligo. *Sci Transl Med.* 2014;6(223):223ra23.
49. Richmond JM, Bangari DS, Essien KI, et al. Keratinocyte-derived chemokines orchestrate T-cell positioning in the epidermis during vitiligo and may serve as biomarkers of disease. *J Invest Dermatol.* 2017;137(2):350-358.
50. Chavez-Alvarez S, Herz-Ruelas M, Raygoza-Cortez AK, et al. Oral mini-pulse therapy in vitiligo: a systematic review. *Int J Dermatol.* 2021;60(7):868-876.
51. Kanwar AJ, Mahajan R, Parsad D. Low-dose oral mini-pulse dexamethasone therapy in progressive unstable vitiligo. *J Cutan Med Surg.* 2013;17(4):259-268.
52. Whitton ME, Pinart M, Batchelor J, Lushey C, Leonardi-Bee J, González U. Interventions for vitiligo. *Cochrane Database Syst Rev.* 2010;(1):CD003263.
53. Korting HC, Schöllmann C. Topical fluticasone propionate: intervention and maintenance treatment options of atopic dermatitis based on a high therapeutic index. *J Eur Acad Dermatol Venereol.* 2012;26(2):133-140.
54. Choi CW, Chang SE, Hana BAK, et al. Topical immunomodulators are effective for treatment of vitiligo. *J Dermatol.* 2008;35(8):503-507.
55. Tharp MD. Calcineurin Inhibitors. *Dermatol Ther.* 2002;15(4):325-332.
56. Kang S, Lucky AW, Pariser D, Lawrence I, Hanifin JM. Long-term safety and efficacy of tacrolimus ointment for the treatment of atopic dermatitis in children. *J Am Acad Dermatol.* 2001;44(1):S58-S64.
57. Travis LB, Weinberg JM, Silverberg NB. Successful treatment of vitiligo with 0.1% tacrolimus ointment. *Arch Dermatol.* 2003;139(5):571-574; discussion 573.
58. Mayoral FA, Gonzalez C, Shah NS, Arciniegas C. Repigmentation of vitiligo with pimecrolimus cream: a case report. *Dermatology.* 2003;207(3):322-323.
59. Seneschal J, Duplaine A, Maillard H, et al. Efficacy and safety of tacrolimus 0.1% for the treatment of facial vitiligo: a multicenter randomized, double-blinded, vehicle-controlled study. *J Invest Dermatol.* 2021;141(7):1728-1734.

60. Silverberg JI, Silverberg NB. Topical tacrolimus is more effective for treatment of vitiligo in patients of skin of color. *J Drugs Dermatol.* 2011;10(5):507-510.
61. Coskun B, Saral Y, Turgut D. Topical 0.05% clobetasol propionate versus 1% pimecrolimus ointment in vitiligo. *Eur J Dermatol.* 2005;15(2):88-91.
62. Woodle ES, Thistlethwaite JR, Gordon JH, et al. A multicenter trial of FK506 (tacrolimus) therapy in refractory acute renal allograft rejection. A report of the Tacrolimus Kidney Transplantation Rescue Study Group. *Transplantation.* 1996;62(5):594-599.
63. Arellano FM, Wentworth CE, Arana A, Fernández C, Paul CF. Risk of lymphoma following exposure to calcineurin inhibitors and topical steroids in patients with atopic dermatitis. *J Invest Dermatol.* 2007;127(4):808-816.
64. Ormerod AD. Topical tacrolimus and pimecrolimus and the risk of cancer: how much cause for concern? *Br J Dermatol.* 2005;153(4):701-705.
65. Grimes PE. Psoralen photochemotherapy for vitiligo. *Clin Dermatol.* 1997;15(6):921-926.
66. Parrish JA, Jaenicke KF. Action spectrum for phototherapy of psoriasis. *J Invest Dermatol.* 1981;76(5):359-362.
67. Westerhof W, Nieuweboer-Krobotova L. Treatment of vitiligo with UV-B radiation vs topical psoralen plus UV-A. *Arch Dermatol.* 1997;133(12): 1525-1528.
68. Yones SS, Palmer RA, Garibaldinos TM, Hawk JLM. Randomized double-blind trial of treatment of vitiligo: efficacy of psoralen-UV-A therapy vs Narrowband-UV-B therapy. *Arch Dermatol.* 2007;143(5):578-584.
69. Njoo M, Bos J, Westerhof W. Treatment of generalized vitiligo in children with narrow-band (TL-01) UVB radiation therapy. *J Am Acad Dermatol.* 2000;42(2):245-253.
70. Nijsten TEC, Stern RS. The increased risk of skin cancer is persistent after discontinuation of psoralen ultraviolet a: a cohort study. *J Invest Dermatol.* 2003;121(2):252-258.
71. Teulings HE, Overkamp M, Ceylan E, et al. Decreased risk of melanoma and nonmelanoma skin cancer in patients with vitiligo: a survey among 1307 patients and their partners. *Br J Dermatol.* 2013;168(1):162-171.
72. Bae JM, Ju HJ, Lee RW, et al. Evaluation for skin cancer and precancer in patients with vitiligo treated with long-term narrowband UV-B phototherapy. *JAMA Dermatol.* 2020;156(5):529-537.
73. Schallreuter KU, Behrens-Williams S, Khaliq TP, et al. Increased epidermal functioning wild-type p53 expression in vitiligo. *Exp Dermatol.* 2003;12(3):268-277.
74. Nordal EJ, Guleng GE, Rönnevig JR. Treatment of vitiligo with narrowband-UVB (TL01) combined with tacrolimus ointment (0.1%) vs. placebo ointment, a randomized right/left double-blind comparative study. *J Eur Acad Dermatol Venereol* . 2011;25(12):1440-1443.
75. Lotti TM, Menchini G, Andreassi L. UV-B radiation microphototherapy. An elective treatment for segmental vitiligo. *J Eur Acad Dermatol Venereol.* 1999;13(2):102-108.
76. Spencer JM, Nossa R, Ajmeri J. Treatment of vitiligo with the 308-nm excimer laser: a pilot study. *J Am Acad Dermatol.* 2002;46(5):727-731.
77. Kawalek AZ, Spencer JM, Phelps RG. Combined excimer laser and topical tacrolimus for the treatment of vitiligo: a pilot study. *Dermatol Surg.* 2004;30(2):130-135.
78. Hadi S, Tinio P, Al-Ghaithi K, et al. Treatment of vitiligo using the 308-nm excimer laser. *Photomed Laser Surg.* 2006;24(3):354-357.
79. Hofer A, Hassan AS, Legat FJ, Kerl H, Wolf P. Optimal weekly frequency of 308-nm excimer laser treatment in vitiligo patients. *Br J Dermatol.* 2005;152(5):981-985.
80. Akar A, Tunca M, Koc E, Kurumlu Z. Broadband targeted UVB phototherapy for localized vitiligo: a retrospective study. *Photodermatol Photoimmunol Photomed.* 2009;25(3):161-163.
81. Hong SB, Park HH, Lee MH. Short-term effects of 308-nm xenon-chloride excimer laser and narrow-band ultraviolet B in the treatment of vitiligo: a comparative study. *J Korean Med Sci.* 2005;20(2):273.
82. Montes LF, Diaz ML, Lajous J, Garcia NJ. Folic acid and vitamin B12 in vitiligo: a nutritional approach. *Cutis.* 1992;50(1):39-42.
83. Bhattacharya SK, Dutta AK, Mandal SB, Chatterjee A. Ascorbic acid in vitiligo. *Indian J Dermatol.* 1981;26(3):4-11.
84. Szczurko O, Shear N, Taddio A, Boon H. Ginkgo biloba for the treatment of vitilgo vulgaris: an open label pilot clinical trial. *BMC Complement Altern Med.* 2011;11:21.
85. Nestor M, Bucay V, Callender V, Cohen JL, Sadick N, Waldorf H. Polypodium leucotomos as an Adjunct Treatment of Pigmentary Disorders. *J Clin Aesthet Dermatol.* 2014;7(3):13-17.
86. Pacifico A, Damiani G, Iacovelli P, et al. NB-UVB plus oral Polypodium leucotomos extract display higher efficacy than NB-UVB alone in patients with vitiligo. *Dermatol Ther.* 2021;34(2):e14776.
87. Parsad D, Saini R, Verma N. Combination of PUVAsol and topical calcipotriol in vitiligo. *Dermatology.* 1998;197(2):167-170.
88. Kullavanijaya P, Lim HW. Topical calcipotriene and narrowband ultraviolet B in the treatment of vitiligo. *Photodermatol Photoimmunol Photomed.* 2004;20(5):248-251.
89. Xing C, Xu A. The effect of combined calcipotriol and betamethasone dipropionate ointment in the treatment of vitiligo: an open, uncontrolled trial. *J Drugs Dermatol.* 2012;11(10):e52-e54.
90. Travis LB, Silverberg NB. Calcipotriene and corticosteroid combination therapy for vitiligo. *Pediatr Dermatol.* 2004;21(4):495-498.
91. Qi F, Liu F, Gao L. Janus kinase inhibitors in the treatment of vitiligo: a review. *Front Immunol.* 2021;12:790125.
92. Sheikh A, Rafique W, Owais R, Malik F, Ali E. FDA approves Ruxolitinib (Opzelura) for Vitiligo Therapy: A breakthrough in the field of dermatology. *Ann Med Surg.* 2022;81:104499.
93. Liu LY, Strassner JP, Refat MA, Harris JE, King BA. Repigmentation in vitiligo using the Janus kinase inhibitor tofacitinib may require concomitant light exposure. *J Am Acad Dermatol.* 2017;77(4):675-682.e1.
94. Grimes PE, Hamzavi I, Lebwohl M, Ortonne JP, Lim HW. The efficacy of afamelanotide and narrowband UV-B phototherapy for repigmentation of vitiligo. *JAMA Dermatol.* 2013;149(1):68.
95. Kapoor R, Phiske MM, Jerajani HR. Evaluation of safety and efficacy of topical prostaglandin E_2 in treatment of vitiligo. *Br J Dermatol.* 2009;160(4): 861-863.
96. Mosenson JA, Zloza A, Nieland JD, et al. Mutant HSP70 reverses autoimmune depigmentation in vitiligo. *Sci Transl Med.* 2013;5(174):174ra28.
97. Thappa D, Gupta D, Kumari R. Depigmentation therapies in vitiligo. *Indian J Dermatol Venereol Leprol.* 2012;78(1):49.
98. van Geel N, Ongenae K, De Mil M, Haeghen YV, Vervaet C, Naeyaert JM. Double-blind placebo-controlled study of autologous transplanted epidermal cell suspensions for repigmenting vitiligo. *Arch Dermatol.* 2004;140(10):1203-1208.
99. Chen YF, Yang PY, Hu DN, Kuo FS, Hung CS, Hung CM. Treatment of vitiligo by transplantation of cultured pure melanocyte suspension: analysis of 120 cases. *J Am Acad Dermatol.* 2004;51(1):68-74.
100. Falabella R, Barona MI. Update on skin repigmentation therapies in vitiligo. *Pigment Cell Melanoma Res.* 2009;22(1):42-65.
101. Ju HJ, Bae JM, Lee RW, et al. Surgical interventions for patients with vitiligo. *JAMA Dermatol.* 2021;157(3):307.
102. Njoo MD, Spuls PI, Bos JD, Westerhof W, Bossuyt PMM. Nonsurgical repigmentation therapies in vitiligo. *Arch Dermatol.* 1998;134(12).
103. Gupta S, Kumar B. Epidermal grafting in vitiligo: influence of age, site of lesion, and type of disease on outcome. *J Am Acad Dermatol.* 2003;49(1):99-104.
104. Moorthy RS, Inomata H, Rao NA. Vogt-Koyanagi-Harada syndrome. *Surv Ophthalmol.* 1995;39(4):265-292.
105. Vasconcelos-Santos DV, Sohn EH, Sadda S, Rao NA. Retinal pigment epithelial changes in chronic Vogt-Koyanagi-Harada disease: fundus autofluorescence and spectral domain-optical coherence tomography findings. *Retina.* 2010;30(1):33-41.
106. Saleem MD, Oussedik E, Schoch JJ, Berger AC, Picardo M. Acquired disorders with depigmentation: a systematic approach to vitiliginoid conditions. *J Am Acad Dermatol.* 2019;80(5):1215-1231.e6.
107. Gupta M, Pande D, Lehl SS, Sachdev A. Alezzandrini syndrome. *Case Rep.* 2011;2011:bcr0420114052.
108. Agarwal S, Ojha A. Piebaldism: a brief report and review of the literature. *Indian Dermatol Online J.* 2012;3(2):144-147.
109. Hake S. Cutaneous manifestations of tuberous sclerosis. *Ochsner J.* 2010;10(3):200-204.
110. Hewedy ESS, Hassan AM, Salah EF, et al. Clinical and ultrastructural study of nevus depigmentosus. *J Microsc Ultrastruct.* 2013;1(1):22-29.
111. Fleisher TL, Zeligman I. Nevus anemicus. *Arch Dermatol.* 1969;100(6): 750-755.
112. Zhu JL, Black SM, Chen HW, Jacobe HT. Emerging treatments for scleroderma/systemic sclerosis. *Fac Rev.* 2021;10:43.
113. Singh A, Ambujam S, Varghese A, Vishranth SP, Sadanandan N. Salt-and-pepper appearance: a cutaneous clue for the diagnosis of systemic sclerosis. *Indian J Dermatol.* 2012;57(5):412-413.
114. Madu PN, Syder N, Elbuluk N. Postinflammatory hypopigmentation: a comprehensive review of treatments. *J Dermatolog Treat.* 2022;33(2): 704-708.
115. Ghosh S, Mukhopadhyay S. Chemical leucoderma: a clinico-aetiological study of 864 cases in the perspective of a developing country. *Br J Dermatol.* 2009;160(1):40-47.

116. Antinori S, Parravicini C, Galimberti L, et al. Is imported onchocerciasis a truly rare entity? Case report and review of the literature. *Travel Med Infect Dis.* 2017;16:11-17.
117. Klarmann-Schulz U, Specht S, Debrah AY, et al. Comparison of doxycycline, minocycline, doxycycline plus albendazole and albendazole alone in their efficacy against onchocerciasis in a randomized, open-label, pilot trial. *PLoS Negl Trop Dis.* 2017;11(1):e0005156.
118. Farnsworth N, Rosen T. Endemic treponematosis: review and update. *Clin Dermatol.* 2006;24(3):181-190.
119. Lupi O, Madkan V, Tyring SK. Tropical dermatology: bacterial tropical diseases. *J Am Acad Dermatol.* 2006;54(4):559-578; quiz 578-580.
120. Shereef PH, Thomas M. Hypopigmented macules in leprosy–a histopathological and histochemical study of melanocytes. *Indian J Lepr.* 1992;64(2):189-191.
121. Ezzedine K, Lim HW, Suzuki T, et al. Revised classification/nomenclature of vitiligo and related issues: the Vitiligo Global Issues Consensus Conference. *Pigment Cell Melanoma Res.* 2012;25(3):E1-E13.
122. Hale EK, Konstadt JW. Melanoma-associated leukoderma. *Dermatol Online J.* 2003 Oct;9(4):20. PMID: 14594593.
123. Kirkin AF, Dzhandzhugazyan K, Zeuthen J. The immunogenic properties of melanoma-associated antigens recognized by cytotoxic T lymphocytes. *Exp Clin Immunogenet.* 1998;15(1):19-32.
124. Rodríguez-Cuevas S, López-Chavira A, Zepeda del Río G, Cuadra-García I, Fernández-Diez J. Prognostic significance of cutaneous depigmentation in Mexican patients with malignant melanoma. *Arch Med Res.* 1998;29(2):155-158.

CHAPTER 60

Diseases of Oral Mucosa Part 1: Normal Anatomy, Benign, Premalignant, and Malignant Lesions

Sara D. Ragi
Mayra Buainain De Castro Maymone
Neelam A. Vashi

KEY POINTS

- Oral mucosal lesions may be poorly recognized and underdiagnosed in patients with skin of color.
- The presentation of oral mucosal lesions may vary in color, location, distribution, and appearance in patients with skin of color.
- Most oral mucosal lesions are diagnosed based on the clinical presentation alone, although histopathologic evaluation is often required to make a definitive diagnosis.
- Here we include salient information about the etiology, epidemiology, clinical features, histopathology, and treatment/management of common oral mucosal lesions with an emphasis on skin of color.

INTRODUCTION

The oral mucosa ranges from white to pink to red-purple in individuals with lighter skin tones while in individuals with darker skin tones, the oral mucosa can be brown to black. Differences in the appearance of the oral mucosa or oral lesions can vary based on the degree of keratinization, thickness, vascularization, melanocytic activity, number of melanocytes, and degree of pigmentation of the submucosal/mucosal tissue. Therefore, it is important to recognize the clinical presentation of oral cavity lesions in patients with skin of color. During dermatologic visits with oral complaints, the mouth/oral cavity and lips should be thoroughly inspected together with a full body skin examination (see Chapter 20 for a review oral anatomy). Furthermore, during the medical interview, a thorough family and personal history regarding lesions of the mouth and lip regions should be obtained. A comprehensive list of medications, occupation, and environmental exposures should also be gathered. Finally, histopathologic examination should be considered to confirm the diagnosis of oral lesions. Many diseases of the oral cavity correlate with diseases observed in the cutaneous skin; however, differences exist between these mucosal versus cutaneous lesions.

This chapter will discuss oral diseases or conditions that may be encountered in the dermatology clinic [**Table 60-1**]. Recognition of these oral conditions in patients with skin of color is necessary to facilitate early diagnosis and interventions and impact healthcare disparities within dermatology.

NORMAL VARIANTS

LEUKOEDEMA

Leukoedema is a benign thickening of the oral mucosal epithelium caused by the accumulation of fluid.[1] The etiology and pathophysiologic mechanisms of oral leukoedema are presently unknown.[1] Oral leukoedema is characterized by asymptomatic, symmetric white-gray mucosal changes most commonly occurring on the buccal mucosa, floor of the mouth, or palatopharyngeal tissues [**Figure 60-1**].[1,2] Oral leukoedema disproportionately affects individuals with skin of color. In particular, there is a higher prevalence in Black/African Americans and Latine/Hispanic individuals.[1,2] It has been reported that approximately 70% to 90% of African American adults, and 50% of African American children may be affected by oral leukoedema.[1,2] Furthermore, the most common oral lesion in Mexico was reported to be leukoedema. Due to the widespread occurrence of leukoedema, it is considered a variant of normal oral mucosa owing to intra- and extracellular imbibition. Upon stretching the mucosa, leukoedema characteristically diminishes. This feature helps distinguish it from leukoplakia or morsicatio buccarum. There are currently no therapeutic recommendations for oral leukoedema as treatment is not indicated.[3]

TORI

Tori are bony exostosis protruding from the midline hard palate into the mouth (torus palatinus) or arising from under the tongue (torus mandibular) [**Figure 60-2**]. Tori can be flat, nodular, lobular, or spindle-shaped.[4,5] While there is a hereditary component, tori tend to appear more frequently during middle age of life. For torus palatinus (TP), females are disproportionately affected in addition to individuals from the Middle East.[4,5] The overall prevalence is 9.5% to 26.9%, although the prevalence range in ethnic groups is wider with 0.9% in Vietnamese individuals and 33.8% in African Americans affected. The etiology of tori is unclear although the most widely accepted theory supports mainly environmental factors related to occlusal stress or functional response to superficial injuries. Bruxism (grinding), nutrient deficiencies and excess have also been hypothesized as causes of oral tori with excess vitamin D or calcium possibly contributing to their formation.

The differential diagnoses of tori include squamous cell carcinoma and adenoid cystic carcinoma. Squamous cell carcinoma is softer than tori and mucous membranes are usually ulcerated.[4,5] Adenoid cystic carcinoma may arise from the minor salivary gland over the hard palate and is distinguished from TP as it is not midline.[4,5] Non-midline suspected tori should be biopsied in order to exclude highly lethal adenoid cystic carcinoma.

Histologically, tori are characterized by a compact structure similar to that of normal bone with a slightly spongier structure with marrow spaces.[4,5] Treatment of tori are not always necessary. Removal may be due to the need for prosthetic treatment or a source of autogenous cortical bone for grafts in periodontal surgery.[4,5]

TABLE 60-1 Oral diseases or conditions

	Characteristic	Oral condition
Normal variants	Benign	• Leukoedema
		• Tori
		• Physiologic oral pigmentation[a]
Nonpigmented ("White") lesions	Benign	• Hereditary benign intraepithelial dyskeratosis
		• Focal epithelial hyperplasia/Heck disease
		• Actinic prurigo[b] (AP)
	Premalignant	• Oral submucous fibrosis
		• Actinic cheilitis
	Malignant	• Squamous cell carcinoma
Pigmented lesions	Benign	• Postinflammatory hyperpigmentation
		• Melanotic macule
		• Melanoacanthoma
		• Smoker's melanosis
		• Systemic disorders associated with oral pigmented lesions
		• *Laugier-Hunziker syndrome*
		• *Peutz-Jeghers syndrome (PJS)*[c]
	Malignant	• Oral melanoma
		• Oral Kaposi sarcoma

[a]Discussed under "Pigmented Oral Lesions" section.

[b]While considered benign regarding risks of malignancy, the quality of life of AP patients may be adversely affected by the cosmetic appearance of AP rash, restriction of outdoor activity, and severe pruritis.

[c]While melanocytic macules in PJS are not associated with malignant transformation, PJS patients require routine cancer surveillance/screenings and consistent observation by a gastroenterologist.

NONPIGMENTED ("WHITE") ORAL LESIONS

BENIGN

Hereditary Benign Intraepithelial Dyskeratosis Hereditary benign intraepithelial dyskeratosis (HBID) is a rare autosomal dominant disorder of the conjunctiva, cornea, and oral mucosa occurring predominantly in individuals of the American Indian Haliwa-Saponi tribe (in North Carolina) and descendants of these individuals. Cases have also been reported in Italy, England, Germany, and Brazil.[2] The prevalence of HBID is <1/1,000,000.[6,7] While the exact etiology of HBID is unknown, HBID has been linked to a genetic duplication in the chromosome 4q35 segment of DNA.[6,7] Additionally, missense mutations in M77T on the *NLRP1* gene, chromosome 17p13.2, have been implicated in HBID cases.[6,7]

HBID is characterized by bilateral elevated white to grayish epithelial plaques on the exposed conjunctiva, sometimes with encroachment on the cornea. Bilateral conjunctival hyperemia may give the appearance of red or bloodshot eyes. Oral mucosal manifestation include white, spongy plaques of the buccal mucosa, tongue, or lips.[6,7] HBID is typically not present at birth and symptoms begin starting in early childhood with a waxing and waning pattern throughout the life course.[6,7] Histopathologically, oral HBID plaques are characterized by acanthosis, dyskeratosis, and parakeratosis within the stratified squamous epithelium.[6,7] Additionally, hallmark dyskeratotic cells in HBID exhibit a dense cytoplasm and pyknotic nuclei. A chronic, stromal mild to moderate lymphocytic inflammatory response is present.[6,7]

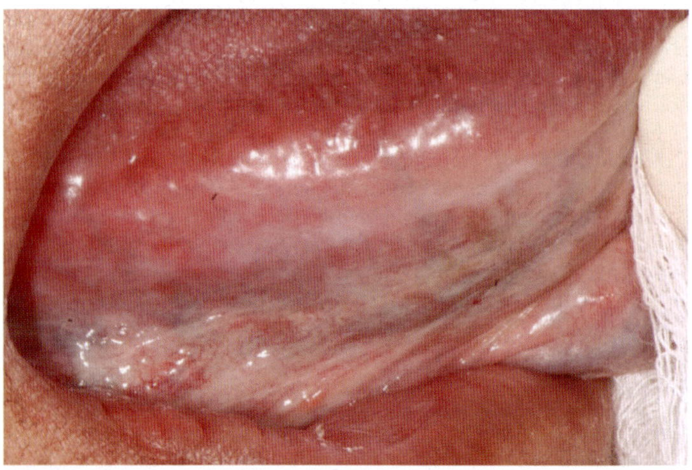

FIGURE 60-1. Leukoedema of lateral tongue.

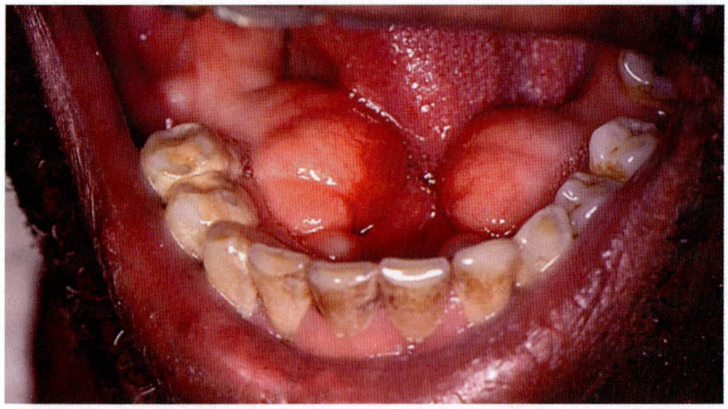

FIGURE 60-2. Mandibular tori.

Differential diagnoses of HBID include hereditary mucoepithelial dyskeratosis, white sponge nevus, and Darier-White disease.[6,7] HBID of the oral mucosa may present similarly to white sponge nevi due to clinical features including painless, diffuse, folded, and spongy white plaques.[6,7] Treatments for hereditary benign intraepithelial dyskeratosis include management with topical corticosteroids and systemic immunosuppression.[6,7] Topical treatments have not been shown to significantly reduce plaque size and systemic treatment typically offers only minimal improvement.[6,7] Routine slit lamp biomicroscopy with slit lamp photography is warranted in patients with ocular manifestations in order to monitor progression of plaques and corneal neovascularization.[6,7]

Focal Epithelial Hyperplasia/Heck Disease Focal epithelial hyperplasia (FEH), also known as Heck disease or multifocal epithelial hyperplasia (MEH), is a rare, benign, oral condition associated with infection by human papillomavirus type 13, 32, or both. Coinfection with HPV16 and HPV18, among others HPV types, has also been reported.[8] FEH is characterized by 0.2 to 3 cm, whitish to mucosal-colored, soft, papular, or nodular elevated lesions in the oral cavity and is typically asymptomatic but can grow to a size that restricts the functionality of the mouth [**Figure 60-3**].[2,8] Diagnosis of FEH is based on clinical and histopathologic

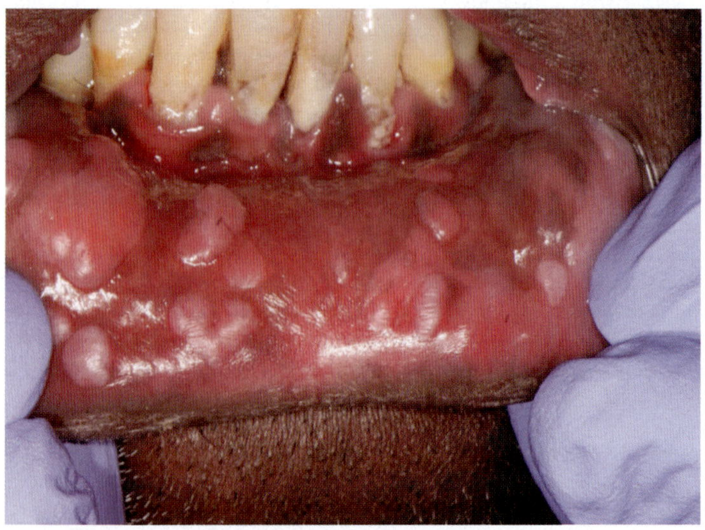

FIGURE 60-3. Heck disease or focal epithelial hyperplasia.

examination.[2,8] PCR or DNA sequencing may be used to identify the specific HPV genotype present.[2,8] Differential diagnoses include condyloma acuminata, verruca vulgaris, papilloma, irritation fibroma, and Cowden syndrome.[8] FEH affects individuals from 3 to 92 years of age, with a higher rate in children and younger people (average age 23.1 years), and disproportionately affects females (with a 3:4 male-to-female ratio).[8] The prevalence of Heck disease is much greater in Indigenous populations around the world with a high prevalence reported among the Indigenous Greenlanders from Nanortalik (19.4%) and in the children of the Mexican Nahuatl (32.3%).[8] FEH has also been associated with low socioeconomic status; families living close together or living in nonmetropolitan location; sharing of food and personal objects, such as utensils or toothbrushes; and inadequate hygiene conditions.[8] Finally, a specific allele of the human leukocyte antigen (HLA), HLA-DR4, was connected to an increased frequency of FEH in small study cohort.[8]

Histologically FEH lesions are characterized by koilocytosis with clear cytoplasm, epithelial hyperplasia with acanthosis and parakeratosis, widened and thickened rete ridges, ballooning degeneration, and mitosoid bodies (cells in which the nuclear DNA has fragmented, resulting in a cell that appears as if it is undergoing mitosis).[8] Oral antiviral drugs and prophylactic vaccination with Gardasil (targeting nine strains of HPV) or other HPV vaccines may prevent FEH.[8] FEH may be treated using imiquimod cream (5%), local cryotherapy with liquid nitrogen application, cauterization, surgical resection, ablative laser treatment, laser excision, and 80% trichloroacetic acid.[8] The prognosis of Heck disease is good based on the fact that most lesions remit spontaneously.[8]

Actinic Prurigo Actinic prurigo (AP) is a rare form of idiopathic photodermatosis.[9] It has a strong underlying genetic etiology, and is commonly observed in American Indians of North, Central, and South America.[9] AP may be explained by an autoimmune pathogenesis as the human leukocyte antigen DR4 (HLA-DR4) allele variant is present in 90% of cases and in particular the DRB1*0407 subtype is observed in 60% of cases.[9-11] Chronic UV irradiation/light exposure may also cause the development of AP via a delayed type-IV hypersensitivity reaction to ultraviolet A and B (UVA and UVB) radiation.[9-11]

AP most commonly presents in the early spring as sunlight increases and becomes stronger.[9-11] Patients present with pruritic papulonodular lesions primarily affecting sun-exposed regions, although lesions are not restricted to sun-exposed areas. Severe cases of AP may result in excoriations, skin thickening, scarring, hypopigmentation, or hyperpigmentation. The face (zygomatic arches, nasal bridge, lower lip, and conjunctiva) is most commonly affected. Cheilitis is a commonly observed hallmark finding of AP. Presentations may include exudative lesions and yellowish adherent crusting in acute lesions [**Figure 60-4**] or irregular lichenification and hyperpigmentation in more chronic lesions. Differential diagnoses of cheilitis in AP includes actinic cheilitis, frictional cheilitis, granulomatous cheilitis, and contact cheilitis.[9-11]

It is important for physicians to obtain a comprehensive history and physical examination in order to properly diagnose AP.[10,11] In cases where AP is suspected, diagnosis may be confirmed by skin photo-testing, histologic evaluation, or genetic testing for the HLA DR4 allele variant. Furthermore, laboratory tests or immunofluorescence studies may be used to rule out systemic lupus erythematosus and other photodermatoses.[9-11] The histopathology of AP is characterized by hyperkeratosis, spongiosis, and acanthosis in the epidermis with lymphocytic perivascular infiltration in the dermis. Lip biopsy may reveal lymphoid germinal centers located in the lamina propria. Other histologic findings include the infiltration of eosinophils and mast cells into the underlying mucosa of lesions corresponding to delayed type-IV hypersensitivity reactions.

Treatment for AP may consist of sun-avoidance alone.[10,11] Other treatments for AP include topical corticosteroids, nonsedating antihistamines for itch relief, and systemic therapies including antimalarial medications, tetracyclines, systemic corticosteroids, cyclosporine, and photochemotherapy with psoralen and ultraviolet A (PUVA).[9-11] Thalidomide has also been a documented therapy for severe refractory cases of AP although the side effect profile of thalidomide (peripheral neuropathy and teratogenicity) makes this treatment less than ideal. The prognosis of AP is good; however, it is important to educate and counsel patients on preventative measures including avoiding sun exposure, using sun protection when outdoors, and raising awareness about the complications of AP. The quality of life of AP patients may be adversely affected by the cosmetic appearance of AP rash, restriction of outdoor activity, and severe pruritis.[9-11]

PREMALIGNANT

Oral Submucous Fibrosis Oral submucous fibrosis (OSMF) is a chronic disorder that produces scarring, tissue fibrosis, and precancerous lesions of the oral mucosa (and in some cases pharyngeal mucosa).[12] A number of risk factors have been reported, including genetic predisposition (individuals with HLA-A10, HLA-B7, and HLA-DR3 phenotypes), chewing or smoking tobacco, and drinking alcohol,[13-15] but consumption of areca/betel nut products is a major one. OSMF primarily occurs in the Western Pacific basin, South Asia, and Southeast Asian regions in populations that chew the betel nut and approximately 600 million people chew betel.[12-14] The prevalence of OSMF is increasingly growing from 0.16% in 1967 to 10.8% in 1998.[12-14] Over 5 million individuals are affected by OSMF globally.[12-14] OSMF develops insidiously presenting with burning sensations and vesicular stomatitis.[12-14] Later in the disease, course, symmetrical fibrosis of the cheeks, lips, tongue, or palate ensues.[12-14] Fibrosis at these sites may appear white [**Figure 60-5**] and become firm, restricting the opening and mobility of the mouth, tongue, and/or palate. Epithelial atrophy, erythroplakia, or leukoplakia may result and development of carcinoma may occur in up to 7% to 8% of cases. Additionally, esophageal fibrosis and conductive hearing loss

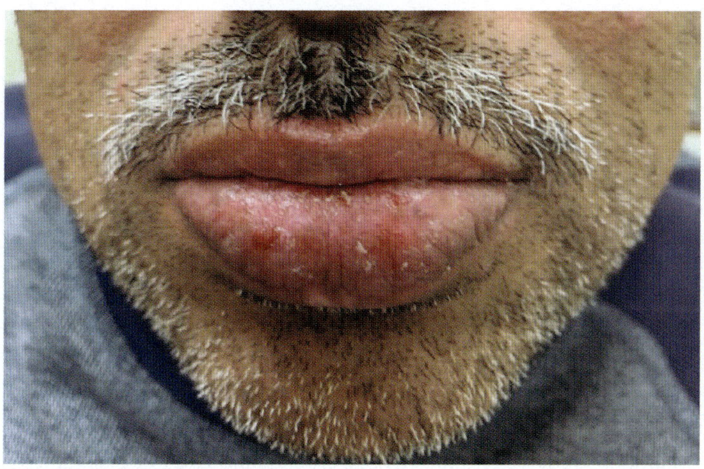

FIGURE 60-4. Actinic prurigo of the lower lip.

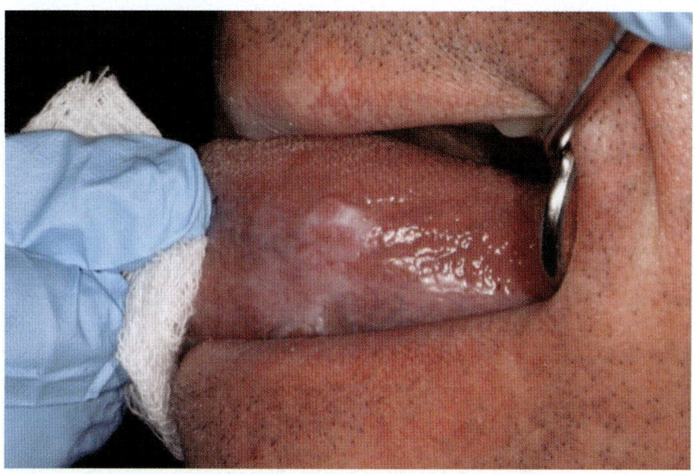

FIGURE 60-5. Oral submucosal fibrosis of the lateral tongue with reticular blanching and alpable, whitish fibrous bands.

may occur if the palatal or paratubal muscles become affected. Tightening of the buccal, palatal, or lingual mucosa may result in trismus.[12-14]

OSMF is diagnosed based on clinical and histological features.[12-14] Histologically, OSMF initially includes mixed inflammation, edema, and large fibroblasts and later collagen bundles with early hyalinization and plasma cells, occasionally resembling lichenoid mucositis. Differential diagnoses of OSMF include amyloidosis, generalized fibromatosis, oral manifestations of scleroderma, oral lichen planus, and/or anemia. Diagnosis may be confirmed by biopsy and through lab work with coexisting anemia often present.[12-14]

Treatments for OSMF include antifibrotic, anti-inflammatory, anti-oxygen radical drug therapy, and surgery in cases at later stages with trismus.[12-14] Steroids, which are anti-inflammatory, are used in early stages of disease including intralesional dexamethasone injections. Hyaluronidase, chymotrypsin, collagenase, pentoxifylline, nylidrin hydrochloride, iron, and lycopene may be used as well. The most effective interventions for OSMF are prevention efforts. Malignant transformation in OSMF may result in squamous cell carcinoma of the esophagus or oral mucosa. The upregulated expression of transforming growth factor-α (TGF- α) and epidermal growth factor receptor (EGFR) in OSMF may be prognostic indicators for malignant transformation.[12-14]

Actinic Cheilitis Actinic cheilitis (AC) is a precursor lesion of squamous cell carcinoma.[16,17] AC is similar to actinic keratoses as actinic cheilitis is a premalignant lesion most commonly of the lower lip along the vermillion border caused by chronic sun or UV radiation exposure.[16,17] Chronic UV exposure damages the tumor suppressor gene *p53* causing uncontrolled replication of defective cells.[16,17] The incidence rate of AC in the United States is currently unknown. The prevalence of actinic cheilitis is greatest among White individuals and in locations closer to the equator where there is greater UV exposure. Men are more likely to be affected than women. Independent risk factors for AC include lighter skin tones, skin pigmentation disorders (ie, albinism), being over the age of 60 years, working outside for over 25 years, spending more than 4 hours per day in the sun, and having a history of nonmelanoma skin cancer.[16,17]

AC presents on physical exam as well-demarcated, persistent white/erythematous thickening, sandpapery papules, fissures, or plaques with scale on the lower lip.[16,17] Additionally, there may be diffuse, multifocal, or heterogeneous lesions with xerosis, scales, hyperkeratotic areas, mottled appearance, atrophy, or demarcation of the vermillion border.[16,17] The differential diagnosis of AC is lichen planus of the lip, squamous cell carcinoma, basal cell carcinoma, malignant melanoma, herpes, inflammatory disorders (eczema, leukoplakia, cheilitis granulomatosa), or lip xerosis with chronic irritation.[16,17] The diagnosis of AC is made by skin biopsy and histopathologic examination.[16,17] The histologic features of AC are variable thickening or atrophy of the lip, partial thickness epidermal dysplasia, solar elastosis, and inflammation in the dermis.[16,17]

Treatment of ACs is difficult and there are no clear guidelines.[16,17] Treatment options include surgical procedures (vermilionectomy, cryotherapy, laser ablation and Mohs surgery), conservative modalities (topical treatment with imiquimod, 5-fluorouacil, diclofenac, ingenol mebutate), and photodynamic therapy. Early diagnosis and treatment are essential for a good prognosis for AC due to the high rate of transformation into invasive SCC.[16,17] Clearance/progression of AC lesions may be evaluated clinically, dermoscopically, or histologically.

MALIGNANT

Squamous Cell Carcinoma Squamous cell carcinoma of the lip and oral cavity, referred to as oral squamous cell carcinoma (OSCC), represent the most common form of nonmelanoma head and neck cancer in the world with 350,000 new cases occurring every year worldwide and 15,000 to 20,000 new cases in the United States annually.[18-20] The highest incidence of OSCC is in South Central Asia and regions of Oceania that have an incidence of 12.9 to 21.2 cases per 100,000 for men and 4.5 to 12 cases per 100,000 for women.[18] In North America, the incidence of OSCC is 6.3 cases per 100,000 for men and 2.4 cases per 100,000 for women.[18] The male to female ratio of OSCC is 2:1 and the incidence increases with age (most cases arise in the sixth to eight decade of life).[18]

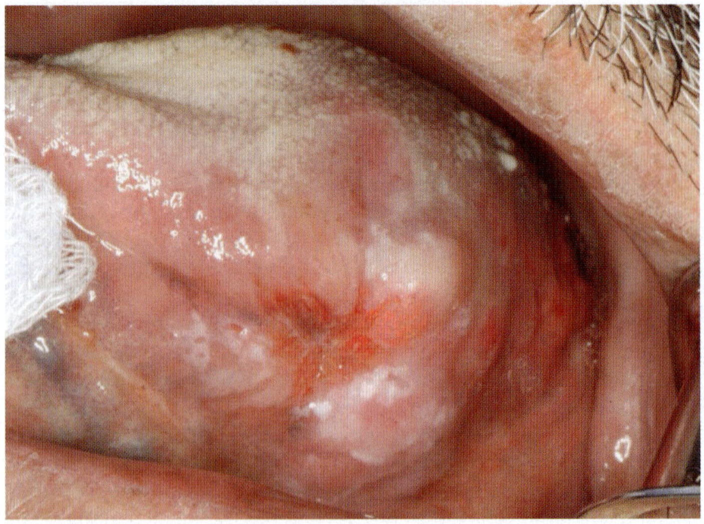

FIGURE 60-6. Squamous cell carcinoma of the left lateral tongue.

The etiology of OSCC is multifactorial and risk factors include systemic diseases, radiation, sun exposure, tobacco use (including smokeless [Shammah] consumption and water pipe [Shishsa] smoking), alcohol consumption, premalignant oral lesion viruses (human papillomavirus), sexually transmitted diseases, immunosuppression, betel quid or Khat chewing, and genetic syndromes (Fanconi anemia and Howel-Evans syndrome).[18-20] Additionally, 1.1% of individuals with oral lichen planus subsequently develop OSCC.[18,19]

Most commonly affected anatomical locations for OSCC include the posterior lateral border of the tongue, followed by the floor of the mouth, soft palate, gingiva, buccal mucosa, and the hard palate.[18-20] The clinical appearance of OSCC presents as white to erythematous lesions that are painless unless they are ulcerated to exophytic tumor masses [**Figure 60-6**].[19] On the lips, OSCC presents as ulcerative lesions known as actinic cheilosis. The differential diagnosis of OSCC includes actinic keratosis (cheilitis), lichen planus, condyloma/verrucous carcinoma, traumatic ulcerative granuloma, leukoplakia, erythroplakia, proliferative verrucous leukoplakia, traumatic ulcer, lobular capillary hemangioma, amelanotic melanoma, fungal infections, and malignant salivary gland or soft tissue tumors.[19] Tissue biopsy and histopathologic examination is the gold standard for diagnosing OSCC.[19] The histology of OSCC depends on the stage/phase of the lesion from preneoplastic damage to the ultimate development of cancer. The histopathology of OSCC used to grade epithelial dysplasia includes both cytological (cell and nuclear pleomorphism, increased or abnormal mitotic figures) and architectural changes (loss of polarity, disturbed maturation from basal to squamous cells, basal cell hyperplasia, and bulbous drop shaped rete pegs).[18-22] On physical examination, it is important to examine any nonhealing ulcerative lesions of the lip or oral cavity and biopsy these lesions for histopathologic analysis. Furthermore, patients should be evaluated for regional cervical lymphadenopathy. OSCC must be graded based on the degree of dysplasia, ranging from mild dysplasia to severe dysplasia and from carcinoma in situ to invasive carcinoma.

Staging of OSCC is based on imaging, including computed tomography (CT) and magnetic resonance imaging (MRI).[19] Both modalities rely on intravenous contrast to distinguish malignancy from the surrounding tissue.[19] Positron Emission Tomography (PET)/CT is an imaging modality used to evaluate locoregional disease as well as distant metastases. OSCC is staged using the American Joint Committee on Cancer TNM staging system. This system includes size of the tumor (and depth of invasion), involvement of adjacent structures, and regional neck metastases based on physical examination and imaging. The National Comprehensive Cancer Network (NCCN) guidelines recommend surgical resection of the primary tumor with adjuvant therapy as determined by the pathologic condition for the lip or oral cavity SCC (ie, radiotherapy or chemoradiotherapy).[21] The prognosis of OSCC is dependent on the TNM staging system and histopathology of tumors.[21] The prognosis for cutaneous lip SCC is promising with a 95% 5-year overall survival due to low cervical node metastatic rate of 2% to 5%. Mucosal lip SCC has a 5-year survival rate of 85% to 95% for stage I and II, while stage III and IV mucosal lip SCC has a 5-year survival rate of 40% to 70%.[21] Oral cavity cancers of all stages have a 5-year survival rate of 60% to 65%. Racial/ethnic differences in prognosis have been reported using national-level data. Compared to other ethnoracialized groups, Black patients demonstrate poorer survival for OSCC largely attributed to differences in stage, insurance, and residential segregation.[21,22]

PIGMENTED ORAL LESIONS

PHYSIOLOGIC ORAL PIGMENTATION

Physiologic oral pigmentation (POP) is genetically determined by the number and size of melanosomes and the type of melanin (eumelanin, or pheomelanin) that is present.[23-25] POP may also result due to an underlying disease process, age, or environmental factors such as smoking, hormones, systemic medications, and ingested pigments from foreign bodies including metals and drugs.[23-25] Melanin pigmentation of the oral mucosa is variable with individuals who have darker skin having more frequent oral pigmentation than individuals with lighter skin.[23,25] The color of oral pigmentation depends on the quantity and depth of the pigment as superficial pigmentation appears brown while deeper pigmentation appears black or blue.[23,24] Individuals with skin of color are more commonly affected by physiological pigmentation, and Black patients are most frequently affected. The prevalence of POP has not been fully elucidated, but a South African study revealed that the overall prevalence of physiological oral melanin pigmentation in the ethnically mixed study population was 42% with 54% of Black patients affected compared to 16% of Indians and 21% of White individuals. Additionally, female to male ratio was 1.2:1.[25]

Physiologic oral pigmentation is diagnosed clinically and presents as patchy or uniform pigmentation most commonly affecting the gingiva although any location in the oral cavity may be affected.[23-25] Microscopically POP shows increased melanin in the basal cell layer, occasional incontinent melanin, and melanin in the upper region of the lamina propria within melanophages or as extracellular melanin particles.[23] The microscopic features of POP are similar to those in melanotic macules and smoker's melanosis.[24] Clinically, POP mimics Addison disease, neurofibromatosis, oral melanotic macules, oral mucosal melanoma, drug-induced oral mucosal pigmentation, and Kaposi sarcoma. Physiologic oral pigmentation requires no treatment.

BENIGN

Postinflammatory Hyperpigmentation Oral postinflammatory pigmentation (OPIH) is similar to cutaneous postinflammatory pigmentation.[26,27] OPIH is caused by a reactive increase in melanin deposition in the basal layer of the epidermis and superficial connective tissue in response to chronic inflammation.[26,27] OPIH occurs most commonly in individuals with darker skin tones and has been associated with inflammation, oral lichen planus, pemphigus, Steven-Johnson syndrome, and graft versus host disease.[26,27] Clinically, OPIH presents as slate-gray and/or blue-black pigmentation. OPIH may be diffuse or localized depending on the type of inflammation present.[26,27] Pigmentation typically fades over the course of months. Histologically, OPIH is characterized by increased epidermal melanin and melanin-laden macrophages in the superficial connective tissue.[26,27] Treatment for OPIH has included laser therapy (low-fluence Q-switch Nd:YAG).[26,27]

Melanotic Macule Oral melanotic macules present as small, well-circumscribed, brown to black lesions most commonly located on the vermillion border of the lips and gingiva, followed by the palate and buccal mucosa.[24] The age range of those affected by oral melanotic macules includes those from 4 to 98 years of age (mean 43.7 years of age) with the peaks of age-frequency distribution in the fifth decade for women (40.0%) and after the sixth decade for men (35.3%).[28] Females are disproportionately affected by oral melanotic macules (with a female:male ratio of 1.9:1).[28] The histopathology of oral melanotic macules includes the in situ increased production of melanin by basal melanocytes with normal morphological features and melanin pigment in melanophages in the upper lamina propria.[28] Although oral melanotic macules are known to be benign, rare cases of malignant transformation into primary oral malignant melanoma have been reported and therefore it is important to diagnose, evaluate, and promptly rule out oral malignant melanoma given the aggressive behavior and poor prognosis.[28,29] Biopsy is typically obtained in order to differentiate melanotic macules from other similarly appearing benign oral melanocytic lesions or oral mucosal malignant melanoma. The differential diagnosis of oral melanotic macules include amalgam tattoos, physiologic pigmentation, melanoacanthoma, melanoma, nevus or blue nevus, varix (venous lake), Peutz-Jeghers syndrome, Carney complex, drug-induced pigmentation, Kaposi sarcoma, and Laugier-Hunziker syndrome, among others.[28,29] Oral melanotic macules are benign lesions and therefore treatment is not necessary although lesions may be removed if deemed cosmetically unacceptable by the patient.

Melanoacanthoma Oral melanoacanthoma (OMA) are benign pigmented lesions with variable clinical presentations and histopathological features.[30-32] OMA are rare with fewer than approximately 100 cases reported since 1978.[31] OMA may occur at any point during the life course, although the median age of diagnosis is 35 years. OMA is mostly seen in patients with darker skin tones and more frequently affect younger females.[30-32] The etiology of OMA is unknown; however, chronic chemical or local trauma that stimulates melanocyte activity/oral pigmentation has been reported to cause OMA.[30-32] Chemical irritants that may cause trauma in OMA include hydrogen peroxide (in mouthwashes), silver amalgam (in dental restoration), and petroleum derivatives (found in toothpaste and mouthwash) including sodium lauryl sulfate, phenolphthalein, nitrophenol, chlorophenol, phenylenediamine sulfate, amine fluorideco, and cocamidopropyl betaine.[30-32] Local factors documented include dental prothesis, chronic trauma to cheeks, dental implant surgery, and teeth whitening strips. OMA is also known to be associated with systemic conditions known as hyperthyroidism and Addison disease.

OMA clinically manifests as new or existing dark spots in the mouth that are typically brown/black, well-circumscribed, flat/raised, asymptomatic solitary lesions, and may possibly be accompanied by pain, burning, or itching.[30-32] The most commonly affected sites include the buccal mucosa, palate, lips, gingiva, and tongue. The clinical presentation of OMA is nonspecific and may mimic carcinomas, neuroendocrine tumors, sarcomas, lymphomas, and other oral pigmented lesions including Peutz-Jeghers syndrome, amalgam tattoo, oral melanoma, Laugier-Hunziker syndrome, etc.[30-32] A thorough oral examination and full body skin examination should be performed; in addition, histopathology and/or immunohistochemical staining are often required for diagnosis.[30-32] OMA lesions exhibit radial growth and then may stabilize and spontaneously regress.[30-32] Treatment includes incisional biopsies, surgical excision with a negative margin, argon plasma coagulation, cryotherapy, curettage, or topical application of fluorouracil 5%.[30-32] The prognosis of OMA is good given that there is no known risk of malignant transformation.

Smoker's Melanosis Smoker's melanosis (SM) is a benign condition characterized by increased pigmentation of the oral mucosa that occurs in response to cigarette use or pipe smoking.[33,34] While the prevalence of SM is currently unknown in the United States, a study in Sweden reported SM in 21.5% of smokers and another study in Nigeria reported a prevalence 6%.[33,34] The etiology of such lesions are thought to be caused by noxious chemicals in cigarette smoke or heat stimulating melanocytes to produce melanin in an effort to protect the mucosa.[33,34] Melanin is thought to bind to compounds in tobacco smoke including nicotine and benzopyrene.[33,34] Smoker's melanosis presents as multiple light brown to dark brown/black macules with lighter versus darker lesions depending on the duration and amount of tobacco smoking that occurred.[33,34] SM most commonly affects the anterior labial mandibular gingiva, buccal mucosa, lip, hard palate, or tongue.[34] Microscopically, SM reveals melanin production in the basal layer of the epithelium, and incontinent melanin and melanophages may be observed in the superficial connective tissue.[34] Histopathologically, SM is identical to that observed in physiologic pigmentation and melanotic macules. Clinical presentation and smoking history typically leads to a diagnosis of SM although a biopsy may be performed to exclude melanoma.[34]

SM requires no treatment; however, counseling regarding smoking and associated health risks is recommended.[33] Smoking cessation may lead to fading of the lesions and cosmetic treatments for the hyperpigmentation include surgical excision or laser ablation.[34] SM lesions may worsen or recur if smoking continues after prior cessation.

Laugier-Hunziker Syndrome Laugier-Hunziker syndrome (LHS) is considered an acquired, benign hyperpigmentation disorder that includes macular hyperpigmentation of the oral mucosa, nail (longitudinal melanonychia), and acral sites.[35,36] LHS presents as macular lesions less than 5 mm in diameter and has no systemic effects or malignant potential.[35,36] The etiology of LHS has been hypothesized to be related to a functional alteration of melanocytes that increases melanosome synthesis and resultant transport to the basal cell layers.[35,36] Additionally, LHS may rarely be caused by sporadic mutations and/or inherited in an autosomal dominant pattern, therefore it is important to take a thorough family history in individuals presenting with hyperpigmented lesions of the oral mucosa.[35,36] LHS has a higher prevalence in Asian populations, specifically in patients of Chinese descent and cases have also been reported to occur in France and Italy.[35,36] LHS also exhibits a female predominance. Diseases associated with LHS include esophageal melanocytosis, actinic lichen planus, hypocellular bone marrow, and thrombocytopenia. The histopathology of lesions includes epithelial acanthosis and increased pigmentation in the basal layer with few dermal melanophages due to accumulation of melanin in basal keratinocytes. Electron microscopy shows mature melanosomes within keratinocytes and melanophages.[35,36]

Differential diagnoses of LHS include lichen planus, Smoker's melanosis, postinflammatory hyperpigmentation, Addison disease, Peutz-Jeghers syndrome, McCune-Albright syndrome, Cronkhite-Canada syndrome, LEOPARD syndrome, Carney syndrome, Bandler syndrome, and hyperpigmentation in advanced acquired immunodeficiency syndrome (AIDS).[35,36] Treatments for LHS, including cryotherapy, Q-switched Nd:YAG laser, Q-switched alexandrite laser, erbium:YAG laser, CO_2 laser, and diode laser, are solely cosmetic in order to address the hyperpigmented appearance of lesions.[35,36] Although cosmetic treatments for LHS exist, lesions typically respond poorly to therapy and exhibit a high rate of recurrence. Sun avoidance may prevent recurrence of LHS lesions.

Peutz-Jeghers Syndrome Peutz-Jeghers syndrome (PJS) is an autosomal dominant disorder caused by germline mutations in the STK11/LKB1 tumor suppressor genes causing gastrointestinal (GI) hamartomatous polyposis and increased risk of neoplasms.[34,37] The incidence of Peutz-Jeghers syndrome is estimated as 1 in 25,000 to 300,000 births.[34] PJS has an equal male and female incidence, and all ethnic groups are affected.[37]

Classic cutaneous manifestations of PJS include mucocutaneous pigmented macules and hamartomatous GI polyps.[34,37] The initial presentation of PJS typically occurs as bowel obstruction due to intussusception from hamartomatous polyps in the GI tract and cutaneous manifestations commonly present after birth with the first oral pigmentation typically occurring during the first year of life.[34,37] Physical examination in PJS reveals pigmented mucocutaneous dark blue, brown to black macules distributed most commonly over the lips, perioral areas, buccal mucosa, eyes, nostrils, fingertips, palms, soles, and perianal regions [**Figure 60-7**].[34,37] Macules may become less noticeable throughout the life course with the exception of lesions of the buccal mucosa that persist throughout the life course.

The diagnosis of PJS is dependent on having two positive criteria out of three criteria including (1) family history, (2) multiple dark blue to brown macules on the mucous membranes and skin, and (3) hamartomatous intestinal polyps.[34,37] PJS is a member of the hamartomatous polyposis syndrome family and has clinical overlap with Bannayan-Riley-Ruvalcaba syndrome and Cowden syndrome. A differential diagnosis of PJS also includes Laugier-Hunziker syndrome.[34,37]

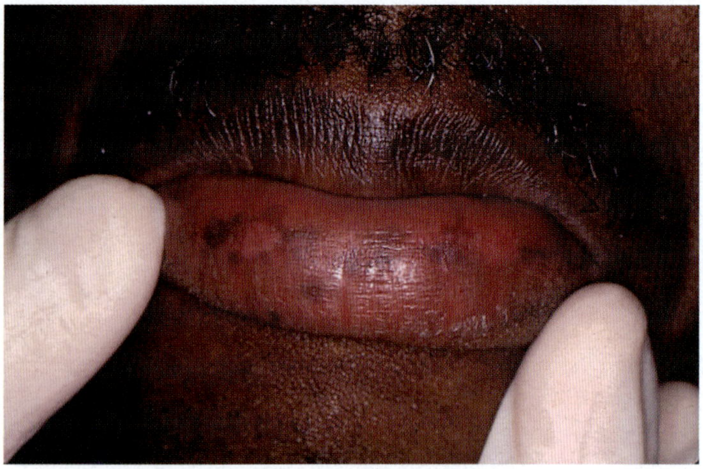

FIGURE 60-7. Peutz-Jeghers syndrome.

Melanocytic macules in PJS are not associated with malignant transformation; however, PJS patients require routine cancer surveillance/screenings and consistent observation by a gastroenterologist.[34,37] Cutaneous manifestations of PJS may be treated by laser therapy.

MALIGNANT

Oral Melanoma Primary oral mucosal melanoma (POMM) represents 0.2% to 8% of all melanomas and 1% to 2% of all oral malignancies.[38,39] The incidence of oral melanoma has remained stable over time. Oral melanoma increases with age, specifically in the fourth and seventh decade of life, with the average age of occurrence at 60.[38,39] Gender differences in oral melanoma have not been reported although select studies have indicated a female predominance.[38,39] Individuals of color are disproportionately affected by oral melanoma, in particular, the neoplasm is more common in Japan and Africa than in Western countries.[38-40] The incidence rate of POMM is highest for Asian men and in the Japanese population oral melanoma represents 7.5% of all melanomas as compared to 1% in White individuals.[38-40]

POMM do not share the environmental risk factor of ultraviolet radiation that is seen in cutaneous melanomas.[38-40] Further, the pathomechanisms of POMM have not been elucidated. Hypothesized risk factors include mechanical trauma, infection, tobacco, ingested or inhaled carcinogens, although no association has been proven. Several case reports have indicated that POMM transform from benign oral pigmentation into primary oral melanoma, although a specific precursor lesion has not been established and most oral melanomas arise de novo from apparently normal mucosa.[38,39] Transformed melanocytes exhibit aberrant expression of the c-kit/stem cell factor pathway, endothelin receptor type B/endothelin pathway, Wnt/β-catenin pathway, and cell-adhesion molecules. Increased expression of c-kit in atypical melanocytes has been reported to correlate with increased activating mutations implicating the proto-oncogene KIT in the development of POMM.[38,39] Increased expression of bcl-2, p53, and loss of p16 expression have also been reported as possible early events in the development of POMM via disruptions in the G1/S phase and prevention of cell death.[38,39]

Oral melanomas primarily affect the hard palate and maxillary alveolus and may appear as black, brown, white, gray, purple, or red lesions that are asymmetric and/or irregularly shaped [**Figure 60-8**].[40] POMM may or may not include a radial growth phase. About 30% of all oral melanomas are amelanotic. Often satellite lesions are present surrounding the primary tumor and the surface of POMMs may be macular, ulcerated, or nodular. There are typically three discrete parts of POMMs, including a nodular component affecting the central part, a flat/elevated deep brown-black pigmented plaque, and a light brown macular component.[38-40] Amelanotic melanomas of the oral mucosa may be difficult to diagnose as they lack a radial growth phase and may resemble benign tumors or squamous cell carcinoma.[38-40]

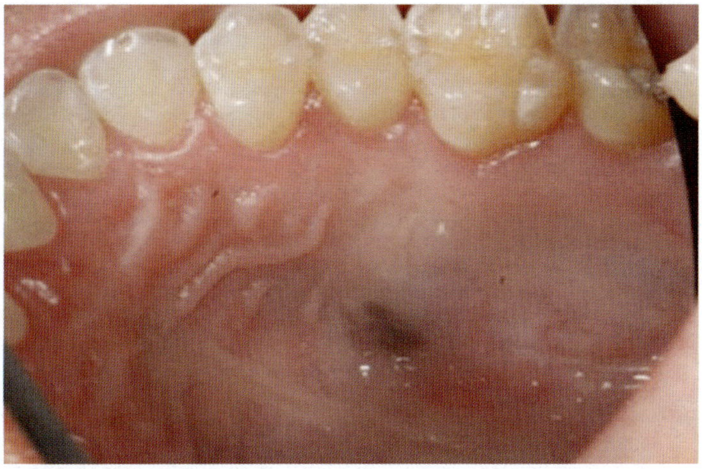

FIGURE 60-8. Oral melanoma.

Given their location and lack of early signs/symptoms, POMM may be difficult to diagnose and therefore diagnosis occurs at later stages.[38-40] Diagnosis is based on clinical and dermoscopic findings and then confirmed by histopathologic examination. Diagnostic criteria include demonstration of clinical and microscopic tumor in the oral mucosa, junctional activity in the oral mucosa, and lack of another primary site.[40] Dermoscopically, POMM is characterized by irregular diffuse pigmentation with a pseudo-network, with regression structures and a blue-whiteish veil.[38,39] Other characteristic features of oral melanoma include irregular jagged borders, asymmetrically pigmented rete ridges, and variably sized granules. Differential diagnoses of oral mucosal melanoma include oral melanotic macule, smoking-associated melanosis, medication-induced melanosis, melanoplakia, pituitary Cushing syndrome, postinflammatory pigmentation, melanoacanthoma, melanocytic nevus, blue nevus, spitz nevus, Addison disease, Peutz-Jeghers lesions, amalgam tattoo, Kaposi sarcoma, oral metastatic disease, monocytic leukemia, physiologic pigmentation, and heavy metal intoxication.

Treatments for oral mucosal melanoma include surgery, radiation, chemotherapy, and immunotherapy.[38-40] Chemotherapy treatments include dacarbazine, platinum analogs, nitrosoureas, and immunotherapy with IL-2. Individuals possessing c-kit gene mutation may benefit from treatment with Imatinib, those with BRAF V600E mutation-positive metastatic melanoma may be treated with vemurafenib and dabrafenib, and finally ipilimumab may be used for metastatic mucosal melanoma as it is targeted against programmed death 1 (PD1). The prognosis of POMM is typically very poor given that patients are often diagnosed at late stages of this disease at which point regional and distant metastases have already occurred. The outcomes for POMM are dependent upon tumor cell morphology, thickness of the tumor, cervical lymph node metastasis, and the anatomic location. Loss of p16 protein expression and abnormal expression of p53 indicate a poorer prognosis. Overall, the 5-year relative survival for mucosal melanomas of the head and neck is 25.5%.

Oral Kaposi's Sarcoma Kaposi sarcoma (KS) is an endothelial multicentric mucocutaneous neoplasm. Caused by human herpes virus 8 (HHV8), KS can present in one of four major forms, including classic KS (common in those individuals of Mediterranean descent), endemic KS (common in parts of Africa), iatrogenic (or post-transplant) KS, and epidemic KS (or acquired immunodeficiency syndrome or AIDS-related).[41,42] KS lesions of the oral cavity occur in all subtypes although the oral cavity is more frequently involved in the epidemic KS form.[42]Approximately 22% of patients with human immunodeficiency virus (HIV) and KS have oral mucosal lesions as the initial presenting site, and 71% of epidemic KS cases may involve the oral mucosa in addition to dermal and visceral sites.[41]

Oral KS (OKS) may affect any part of the oral cavity, but most commonly affects the hard and soft palate, gingiva, and dorsal tongue. Other sites of OKS include the masseter muscle, uvula, and oropharynx. OKS may be solitary or include multiple sites.[42] Lesions may vary in size and shape, and several lesions may coalesce to involve a large quadrant of dentition.[42] OKS progresses from patches to plaques to nodular forms and this progression is associated with worsening of immunosuppression and may occur with pain, bleeding, ulceration, or superinfection.[42] Exophytic OKS may also result in impaired tooth mobility, disfigurement, and poor mastication.[42] OKS at early stages may have erythematous or ecchymotic patches that progress to papular, nodular, or exophytic forms, and lesions vary from brownish red to bluish purple in color [**Figure 60-9**].[42] Violaceous hues may be difficult to see in patients with darker skin types.[43] OKS must be diagnosed by oral biopsy.[42]

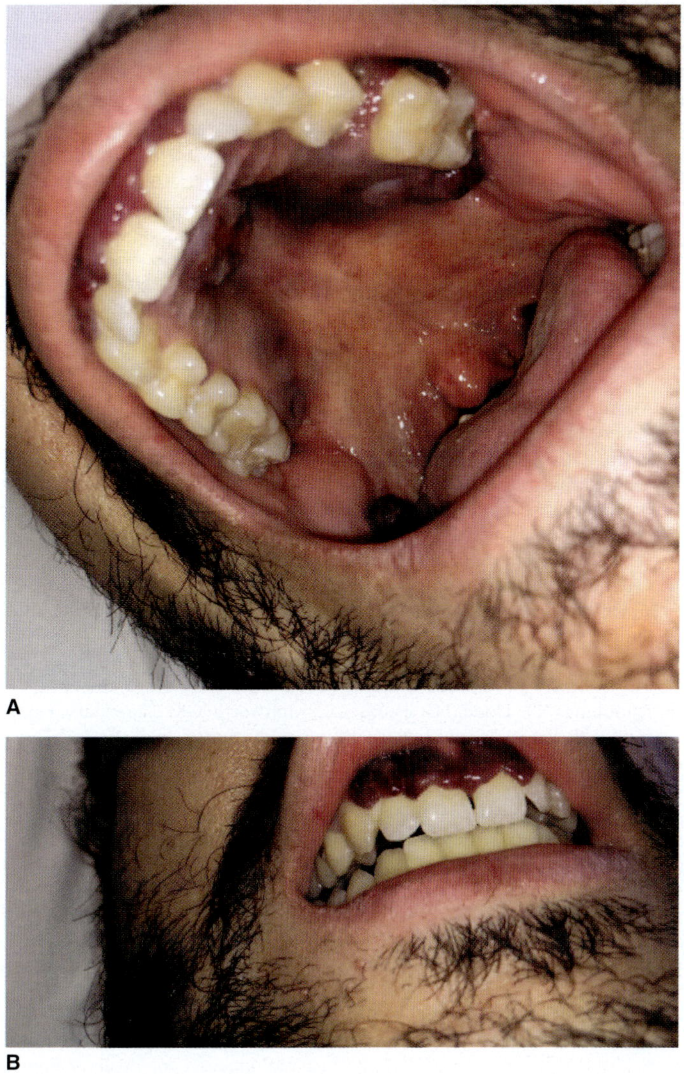

FIGURE 60-9. Oral Kaposi's sarcoma with hard palate **(A)** and gingival involvement **(B)**. Courtesy of Dr. Cristina Thomas.

Differential diagnoses of OKS depend on early versus late stage lesions with early OKS clinically mimicking thermal trauma, atrophic candidiasis, erythroplakia, ecchymosis, and hematomas while late OKS (that is papular or nodular) may clinically resemble oral nevi, pyogenic granulomas, hemangiomas, lymphangiomas, angiosarcoma, Kaposi-like hemangioendothelioma, and bacillary angiomatosis.[42] Differential diagnoses of palatal or gingiva OKS includes melanoma, lymphoma, pyogenic granuloma, peripheral giant cell granuloma, odontogenic abscess, or gingival enlargement secondary to medications or hematologic malignancies.[42]

Histopathological features of OKS is characterized by a mixture of proliferating spindle cells, inflammation, incomplete vascular slits, and extravasated erythrocytes.[42] Treatment for OKS includes highly active antiretroviral therapy (HAART), which if taken for 6 months results in involution of KS lesions in approximately 50% of patients. Despite an overall decline in the incidence of KS among persons living with HIV related to HAART, national data between 2001 and 2018 suggest increasing incidence among young Black men, especially in the South. Causes are multifactorial but likely related to known parallel increases in HIV infection among young Black men who have sex with men in the South, higher levels of poverty and HIV-related stigma, lower rates of preexposure prophylaxis uptake, and lack of access to medical care in the South.[44,45] Other therapies for OKS include intralesional chemotherapy, cryosurgery, and radiation.[43]

REFERENCES

1. Martin JL. Leukoedema: an epidemiological study in white and African Americans. *J Tenn Dent Assoc.* 1997;77:18-21.
2. Pinna R, Cocco F, Campus G, et al. Genetic and developmental disorders of the oral mucosa: epidemiology; molecular mechanisms; diagnostic criteria; management. *Periodontol 2000.* 2019;80:12-27.
3. della Vella F, Lauritano D, Lajolo C, et al. The pseudolesions of the oral mucosa: differential diagnosis and related systemic conditions. *Appl Sci.* 2019;9:2412.
4. García-García AS, Martínez-González JM, Gómez-Font R, Soto-Rivadeneira A, Oviedo-Roldán L. Current status of the torus palatinus and torus mandibularis. *Med Oral Patol Oral Cir Bucal.* 2010;15:e353-e360.
5. Usatine RP, Smith MA, Chumley HS, Mayeaux EJ, eds. *The Color Atlas of Family Medicine.* 2nd ed. New York, NY: The McGraw Hill Companies; 2013.
6. Cummings TJ, Dodd LG, Eedes CR, Klintworth GK. Hereditary benign intraepithelial dyskeratosis: an evaluation of diagnostic cytology. *Arch Pathol Lab Med.* 2008;132:1325-1328.
7. Bui T, Young JW, Frausto RF, et al. Hereditary benign intraepithelial dyskeratosis: report of a case and re-examination of the evidence for locus heterogeneity. *Ophthalmic Genet.* 2016;37:76-80.
8. Bendtsen SK, Jakobsen KK, Carlander AF, Grønhøj C, von Buchwald C. Focal epithelial hyperplasia. *Viruses.* 2021;13.
9. Plaza JA, Toussaint S, Prieto VG, et al. Actinic prurigo cheilitis: a clinicopathologic review of 75 cases. *Am J Dermatopathol.* 2016;38:418-422.
10. Pile HD, Crane JS. Actinic prurigo. In: *StatPearls.* StatPearls Publishing; 2022.
11. Ross G, Foley P, Baker C. Actinic prurigo. *Photodermatol Photoimmunol Photomed.* 2008;24:272-275.
12. Scully C. Challenges in predicting which oral mucosal potentially malignant disease will progress to neoplasia. *Oral Dis.* 2014;20:1-5.
13. Gupta S, Jawanda MK. Oral submucous fibrosis: an overview of a challenging entity. *Indian J Dermatol Venereol Leprol.* 2021;87:768-777.
14. Wollina U, Verma SB, Ali FM, Patil K. Oral submucous fibrosis: an update. *Clin Cosmet Investig Dermatol.* 2015;8:193-204.
15. Xu H, Lyu FY, Song JY, et al. Research achievements of oral submucous fibrosis: progress and prospect. *Biomed Res Int.* 2021;2021:6631856.
16. Muse ME, Crane JS. Actinic cheilitis. In: *StatPearls.* StatPearls Publishing; 2022.
17. Vasilovici A, Ungureanu L, Grigore L, Cojocaru E, Şenilă S. Actinic cheilitis - from risk factors to therapy. *Front Med (Lausanne).* 2022;9:805425.
18. Howard A, Agrawal N, Gooi Z. Lip and oral cavity squamous cell carcinoma. *Hematol Oncol Clin North Am.* 2021;35:895-911.
19. Bugshan A, Farooq I. Oral squamous cell carcinoma: metastasis, potentially associated malignant disorders, etiology and recent advancements in diagnosis. *F1000Res.* 2020;9:229.
20. Maymone MBC, Greer RO, Kesecker J, et al. Premalignant and malignant oral mucosal lesions: clinical and pathological findings. *J Am Acad Dermatol.* 2019;81:59-71.
21. Yu AJ, Choi JS, Swanson MS, et al. Association of race/ethnicity, stage, and survival in oral cavity squamous cell carcinoma: a SEER study. *OTO Open.* 2019;3:2473974x19891126.
22. Harris JA, Hunter WP, Ji YD, Hanna GJ. Effects of racial residential segregation on oral squamous cell carcinoma prognosis and survival. *Oral Oncol.* 2021;119:105364.
23. Feller L, Masilana A, Khammissa RA, et al. Melanin: the biophysiology of oral melanocytes and physiological oral pigmentation. *Head Face Med.* 2014;10:8.
24. Gondak RO, da Silva-Jorge R, Jorge J, Lopes MA, Vargas PA. Oral pigmented lesions: clinicopathologic features and review of the literature. *Med Oral Patol Oral Cir Bucal.* 2012;17:e919-924.
25. Masilana A, Khammissa RAG, Lemmer J, Feller L. Physiological oral melanin pigmentation in a South African sample: a clinical study. *J Investig Clin Dent.* 2017;8.
26. Anvery N, Christensen RE, Dirr MA. Management of post-inflammatory hyperpigmentation in skin of color: a short review. *J Cosmet Dermatol.* 2022;21:1837-1840.
27. Maghfour J, Olayinka J, Hamzavi IH, Mohammad TF. A focused review on the pathophysiology of post-inflammatory hyperpigmentation. *Pigment Cell Melanoma Res.* 2022;35:320-327.
28. Shen ZY, Liu W, Bao ZX, Zhou ZT, Wang LZ. Oral melanotic macule and primary oral malignant melanoma: epidemiology, location involved, and clinical implications. *Oral Surg Oral Med Oral Pathol Oral Radiol Endod.* 2011;112:e21-e25.
29. Kahn MA, Weathers DR, Hoffman JG. Transformation of a benign oral pigmentation to primary oral melanoma. *Oral Surg Oral Med Oral Pathol Oral Radiol Endod.* 2005;100:454-459.
30. Aljanobi HA, Alshuyukh MH, Husain MS, Alqahtani WM. Multifocal intraoral melanoacanthomas: two case reports and a literature review. *Cureus.* 2022;14:e26946.
31. Jimenez M, Brizuela M. Oral melanoacanthoma. In: *StatPearls.* StatPearls Publishing; 2022.
32. Lakshminarayanan V, Ranganathan K. Oral melanoacanthoma: a case report and review of the literature. *J Med Case Rep.* 2009;3:11.
33. Rosebush MS, Briody AN, Cordell KG. Black and brown: non-neoplastic pigmentation of the oral mucosa. *Head Neck Pathol.* 2019;13:47-55.
34. Ko E Panchal N. Pigmented lesions. *Dermatol Clin.* 2020;38:485-494.
35. Nayak RS, Kotrashetti VS, Hosmani, JV. Laugier-Hunziker syndrome. *J Oral Maxillofac Pathol.* 2012;16:245-250.
36. Aboobacker S, Gupta G. Laugier-Hunziker syndrome. In: *StatPearls.* StatPearls Publishing; 2022.
37. Wu M, Krishnamurthy, K. Peutz-Jeghers syndrome. In: *StatPearls.* StatPearls Publishing; 2022.
38. Warszawik-Hendzel O, Słowińska M, Olszewska M, Rudnicka L. Melanoma of the oral cavity: pathogenesis, dermoscopy, clinical features, staging and management. *J Dermatol Case Rep.* 2014;8:60-66.
39. Feller L, Khammissa RAG, Lemmer J. A review of the aetiopathogenesis and clinical and histopathological features of oral mucosal melanoma. *ScientificWorldJournal.* 2017;2017:9189812.
40. Meleti M, Vescovi P, Mooi WJ, van der Waal I. Pigmented lesions of the oral mucosa and perioral tissues: a flow-chart for the diagnosis and some recommendations for the management. *Oral Surg Oral Med Oral Pathol Oral Radiol Endod.* 2008;105:606-616.
41. Schwartz RA, Micali G, Nasca MR, Scuderi L. Kaposi sarcoma: a continuing conundrum. *J Am Acad Dermatol.* 2008;59:179-206; quiz 207-178.
42. Fatahzadeh M, Schwartz RA. Oral Kaposi's sarcoma: a review and update. *Int J Dermatol.* 2013;52:666-672.
43. Bradford PT. Skin cancer in skin of color. *Dermatol Nurs.* 2009;21:170-177, 206; quiz 178.
44. Suk R, White DL, Knights S, et al. Incidence trends of Kaposi sarcoma among young non-Hispanic black men by US regions, 2001-2018. *JNCI Cancer Spectr.* 2022;6(6):pkac078.
45. HIV in the Southern United States. 2019.

CHAPTER 61

Diseases of the Oral Mucosa Part 2: Reactive Processes, Infections, and Other Miscellaneous Disorders

Benjamin Gallo Marin
John McDowell
Cathy M. Massoud

KEY POINTS

- Identification of benign and reactive oral findings is fundamental to delivering effective patient care.
- Recognition of oral infections and oral manifestations of systemic infection is imperative for prompt initiation of appropriate antimicrobial therapy.

- Comprehension of adverse drug reactions and inflammatory dermatoses that impact the oral mucosa is necessary to guide differential diagnoses, workup, and management.

BENIGN AND REACTIVE FINDINGS

GEOGRAPHIC TONGUE

Geographic tongue, also known as benign migratory glossitis and lingual erythema migrans, is a common benign and self-limited condition that has a prevalence of 1% to 2% in the general population.[1] This condition is most often seen in White and Black people, without predilection for age group or sex.[1]

Benign migratory glossitis represents an idiopathic inflammatory process that results in loss of the filiform papillae on the dorsal surface tongue, although rarely there may be involvement of the labial and palatal mucosa.[1] While the exact etiology of geographic tongue remains to be elucidated, it has been postulated that some cases may be a variant of pustular psoriasis.[2] Geographic tongue has been associated with numerous conditions including anemia, psoriasis, hormonal dysregulation, diabetes mellitus, stress, allergy and atopy, reactive arthritis, and Down syndrome.[1]

Examination of the dorsal and lateral tongue reveals migrant, map-like oval red areas that are demarcated by well-defined scalloped white rims [**Figures 61-1** and **61-2**].[3] Patients are generally asymptomatic, although fissured tongue may accompany this condition and result in pain and a burning sensation. Triggers include consuming alcohol and spicy or acidic foods.[3] Although the physical appearance of geographic tongue is striking, it does not require further investigation aside from consideration of comorbid conditions. When asymptomatic, reassurance and avoidance of triggers are sufficient. To manage discomfort, topical corticosteroids, topical tacrolimus, and local anesthetics may be considered.[1]

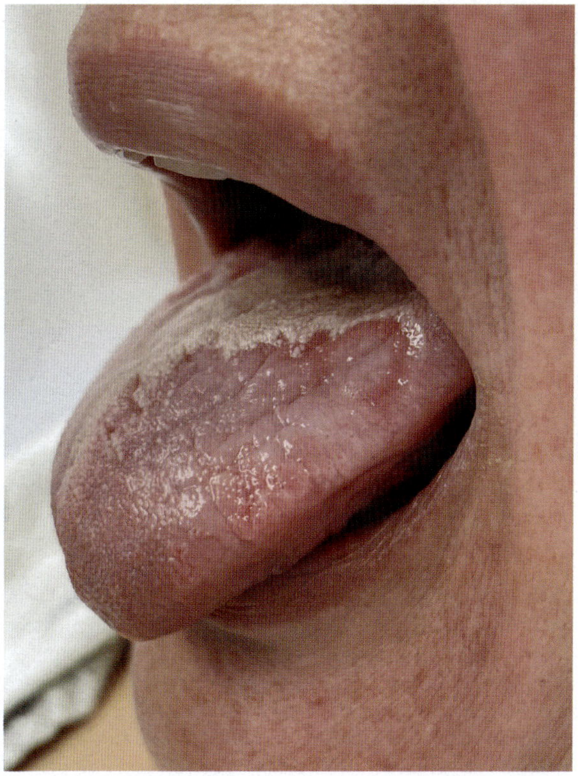

FIGURE 61-2. Geographic tongue: migratory, centrifugally expanding sharply demarcated white plaque with central depapillation.

AMALGAM TATTOO

Amalgam tattoos are generally asymptomatic black, gray, or blue macules on the oral mucosa and often present proximal to teeth that have undergone dental filling procedures [**Figure 61-3**]. Amalgam is a substance that contains tin, silver, mercury, and other metals, and it may diffuse into the adjacent oral mucosa during a dental procedure.[4] Although currently regarded as a common finding, the prevalence of amalgam tattoos is unknown and with the use of newer substances used for dental fillings, these lesions may be seen less frequently in the future.

Obtaining a thorough dental history is important to aid in diagnosis. Management of amalgam tattoos only requires reassurance. However, in the setting of a metal allergy, treatment may be offered to patients including surgical excision, Q-switch ruby laser, and Q-switch alexandrite laser.

Amalgam tattoos may mimic other hyperpigmented lesions including melanocytic nevi, oral melanotic macule, oral melanoacanthoma, and melanoma.[4] In cases of diagnostic uncertainty, such as if a lesion is detected distant from a tooth that has been restored, a biopsy should be considered.[4] Histopathology of amalgam tattoos shows scattered pigmented granules in the superficial dermis and subcutaneous tissue. The use of infrared spectroscopy to differentiate amalgam tattoos from melanocytic neoplasm in tissue samples has been recently studied.[5]

BLACK HAIRY TONGUE

Black hairy tongue, also known as lingua villosa nigra, is an acquired condition that presents as a black plaque anterior to the circumvallate papillae on the dorsal tongue [**Figure 61-4**]. The anterior one-third of the tongue is spared. The lack of mechanical stimulation to the tongue results

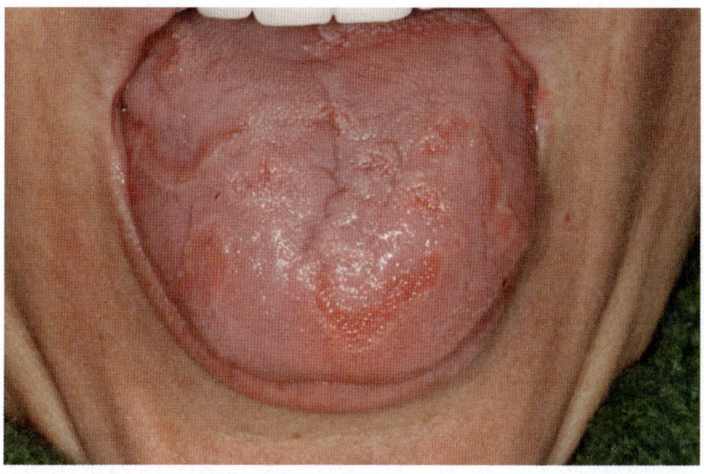

FIGURE 61-1. Geographic tongue: striking arciform pink patches with heaped white borders.

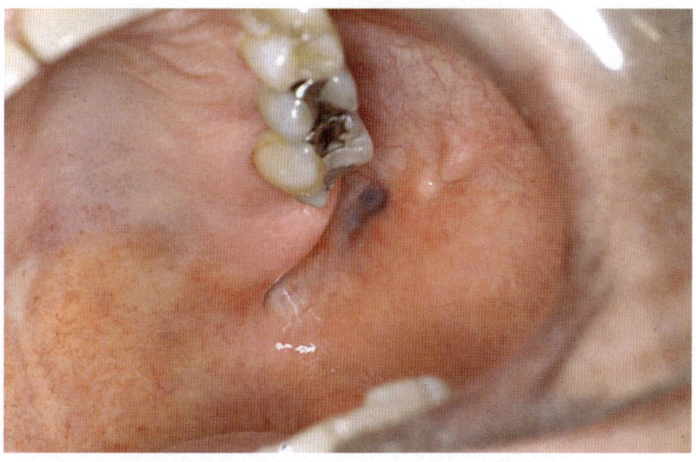

FIGURE 61-3. Amalgam tattoo: blue gray macule of the left posterior buccal mucosa adjacent to the alveolar ridge.

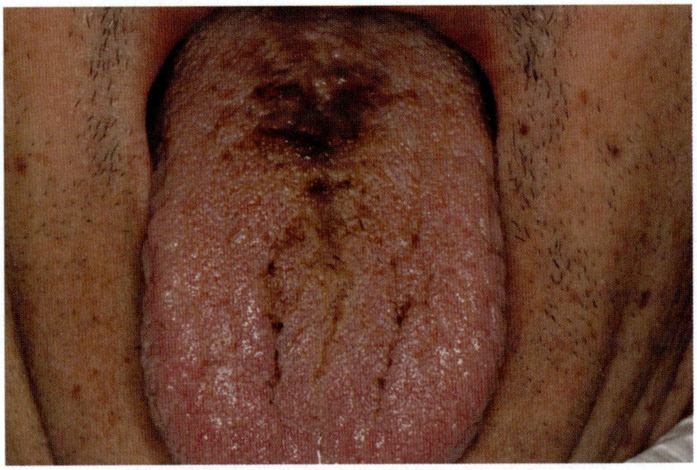

FIGURE 61-4. Black hairy tongue: dorsal tongue plaque with coalescing filiform brown-black projections sparing the distal tongue.

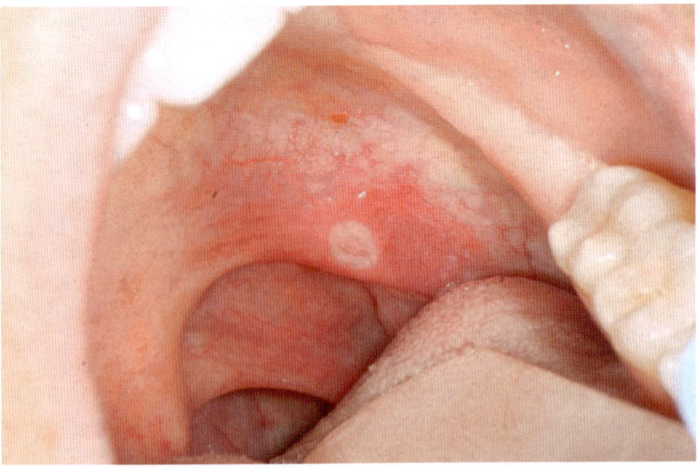

FIGURE 61-6. Aphthous ulcer: yellow-white well demarcated circular ulcer with fibrin base on the left tonsillar pillar.

in inadequate desquamation and accumulation of keratinized cells.[6] Dermoscopy demonstrates elongated dermal papillae with pigmented keratin that give the appearance of hairy outgrowths.[6,7] Filiform papillae with a length greater than 3 mm is diagnostic.[7] Biopsy shows hyperkeratosis with marked parakeratosis at the tips of the filiform papillae.[6]

This conditions is associated with poor oral hygiene, oxidizing mouthwashes, smoking, consumption of coffee, tea, and pureed diets, xerostomia, trigeminal neuralgia, immunosuppression, oral infections, oral tetracycline therapy, history of radiation and stem cell transplant, and neuropsychiatric conditions that restrict masticaction.[7] Treatment includes implementation of oral hygiene and risk factors avoidance.[6,7]

MORSICATIO BUCCARUM AND MORSICATIO LINGUARUM

These are frictional keratosis that result from the habit of chewing one's cheek (morsicatio buccarum) or tongue (morsicatio linguarum).[8] The condition has a predilection for people who are experiencing stressful situations and neuropsychiatric patients. Of note, patients are often unaware of the behaviors that lead to symptoms. It presents as shredded and irregular buccal and or tongue mucosa that may be painful [**Figure 61-5**]. Biopsy is often not indicated for diagnosis. Treatment involves making patients aware of the destructive habit and habit-reversal therapy. Acrylic prostheses that cover the biting surfaces of teeth and protect the oral mucosa and tongue can also be recommended.[8]

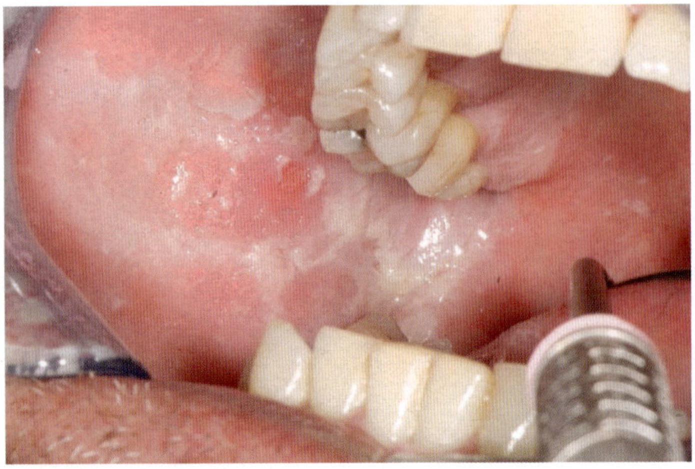

FIGURE 61-5. Morsicatio buccarum: linear white plaques with dental cusp impressions along the buccal mucosa.

RECURRENT APHTHOUS STOMATITIS

Recurrent aphthous stomatitis (RAS) often begins at adolescence and affects 25% of the general population, most often women and nonsmokers.[9] The most common form of this condition is minor aphthous stomatitis, seen in approximately 80% of people with RAS, which consists of oral mucosal ulcers less than 10 mm in diameter that heal within 2 weeks without scarring.[9] Major aphthous stomatitis is a severe form of RAS that presents with oral mucosal ulcers greater than 1 cm in diameter and usually take over 2 weeks to heal with scarring. The least common variant of RAS presents with herpetiform lesions, which are small, grouped ulcerations that coalesce into larger ones.

The lesions of RAS present as shallow, well-defined oval or round ulcers with a necrotic center and yellow-gray pseudomembrane surrounded by erythema [**Figure 61-6**]. These lesions tend to be painful that compromise the ability to eat, swallow, and speak.

The etiology of RAS remains unclear. However, both hereditary and environmental factors have been associated with RAS. Notable associations include history of oral and dental trauma, micronutrient deficiencies (vitamin B_6, vitamin B_{12}, folate, zinc, or iron), stress, smoking cessation, sensitivity to food preservatives (such as cinnamaldehyde and benzoic acid), and hormonal fluctuations related to menstruation and contraception.[9] Of note, there is no data to support that correction of iron or vitamin deficiencies results in ulcer resolution and prevention of further episodes of ulceration.[9] Recent reports have also linked RAS to β-blocker therapy.[10] Systemic conditions that may be linked to RAS include human immunodeficiency virus infection, inflammatory bowel disease, celiac disease, MAGIC syndrome (mouth and genital ulcerations with inflamed cartilage), and PFAPA syndrome (periodic fever, aphthous ulcers, pharyngitis, and adenitis). Recent investigations have posited that elevated saliva levels of tumor necrosis factor-alpha can serve as a useful diagnostic marker for RAS.[11]

Treatment decisions should be determined by the severity of pain and frequency of ulcer episodes. In the absence of an identifiable underlying etiology that could account for RAS, treatment is aimed at reducing inflammation and discomfort.[9] Avoidance of oral trauma is important and patients can be recommended to refrain from consuming hard foods such as toast and chips and switch to soft bristle toothbrushes. Topical corticosteroids (ie, clobetasol gel or triamcinolone compounded in Orabase 2-4 times daily), topical anesthetics (such as lidocaine gel and compounded oral rinses with antihistamine, aluminum hydroxide, and magnesium hydroxide), and protective bioadhesives can be used. Mouthwashes with antimicrobials, specifically those containing chlorhexidine gluconate and triclosan, which inhibit bacterial plaque formation, can be beneficial in accelerating healing.[9] Other treatments include 5% amlexanox paste, with early treatment resulting in decreased ulceration size, pain, and duration.[9] For severe case, use of oral corticosteroids and thalidomide are common.[9]

INFECTIOUS ORAL DISEASE

ORAL HERPES SIMPLEX VIRUS

Herpes simplex virus Type 1 (HSV-1) is the most common cause of oral herpetic infections. HSV-2 accounts for a minority of oral herpes simplex infections and coinfection is possible.[12] HSV is an enveloped double-stranded DNA virus that is transmitted through direct contact, typically via saliva. HSV etymology is derived from the ancient Greek *herpein*, meaning "to creep." This neurotropic virus undergoes latency in the trigeminal ganglion with subsequent anterograde axonal transport to mucocutaneous surfaces during reactivation.

HSV-1 epidemiology in the United States continues to evolve. HSV-1 prevalence has significantly decreased (from 58.94% in 1999-2000 to 47.8% in 2015-2016), yet continues to demonstrate variable trends according to age, sex, race, and Latine/Hispanic origin.[13] HSV-1 prevalence increases with age (27% at 14-19 years vs 59.7% at 40-49 years) and is higher among females compared to males (50.9% vs 45.2%). Notably, HSV-1 epidemiologic trends highlight racial and ethnic disparities, and specifically health inequities, in the United States.[14] HSV-1 seropositivity was highest among Mexican-American persons (71.7%), compared to non-Hispanic Black (58.5%), non-Hispanic Asian (55.7%), and non-Hispanic White (36.9%) persons.[13]

Primary oral HSV infection is usually asymptomatic, yet primary herpetic gingivostomatitis may manifest as coalescing painful punched out erosions of the lips, tongue, buccal mucosa, palate, and gingivae [**Figure 61-7**].[12] Fever, malaise, anorexia, and less frequently headache and cervical lymphadenopathy may occur.[12] Recurrent HSV-1 favors keratinized sites such as the vermillion lips (herpes labialis), yet a multitude of mucosal morphologies have been described. Agminated vesicles and subsequent punched out ulcers on an erythematous base may arise at any mucosal site involved during primary infection [**Figures 61-8** and **61-9**]. Less commonly, phlegmonous glossitis may occur. This entity refers to moist circular thick yellow-brown plaques punctuating the dorsal tongue in the setting of herpes simplex infection [**Figure 61-10**]. In contrast to typical clinical findings, the herpetic erosions of phlegmonous glossitis are typically not agminated. Additionally, recurrent oral HSV infection may present as herpetic geometric glossitis or exquisitely painful thin linear fissures along the median dorsal tongue with peripheral extensions or cross-hatching.[15] Both immunocompromised and immunocompetent patients may demonstrate these uncommon morphologies.

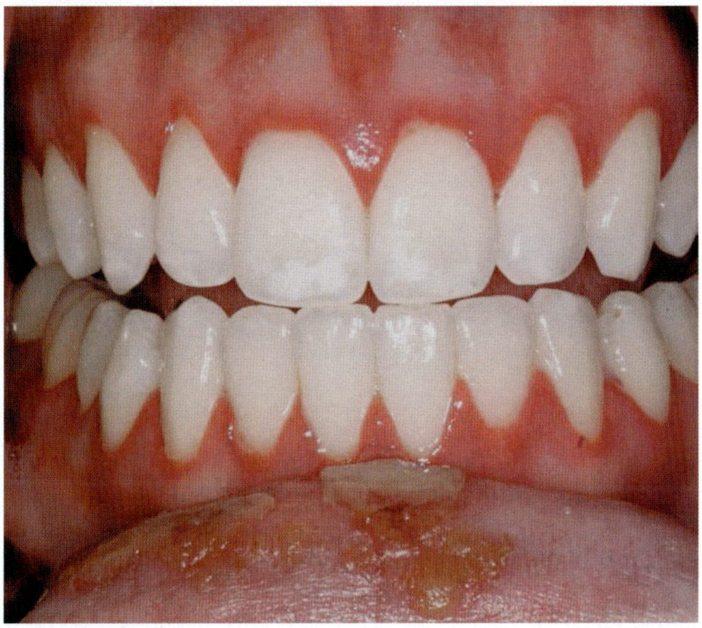

FIGURE 61-7. Primary herpetic gingivostomatitis: injection, focal erosion and ulceration of the gingiva with grouped crusted erosions on an erythematous base of the lower mucosal lip.

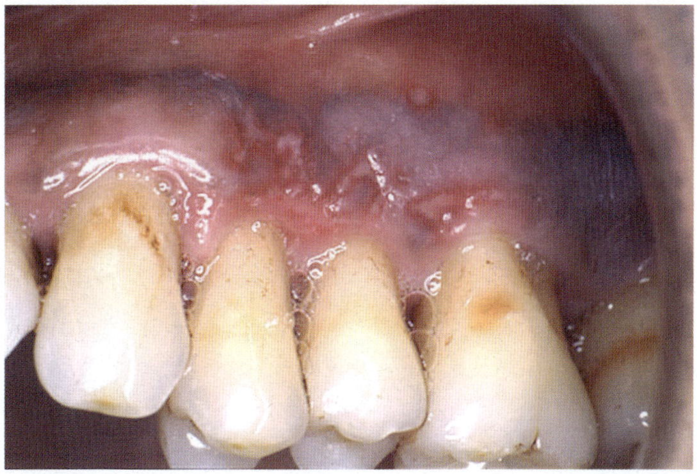

FIGURE 61-8. Recurrent intraoral herpes simplex virus: coalescing punched out erosions with erythematous borders of the gingiva.

Various potential triggers of HSV recurrence include ultraviolet radiation, fever, stress, upper respiratory infection, surgery/trauma, menstruation, chemotherapy, and immunosuppression.[12] Preceding mucositis such as that caused by severe adverse cutaneous drug reactions (toxic epidermal necrolysis or generalized bullous fixed drug eruption) may also predispose patients to experience a recurrent oral HSV flare. Asymptomatic viral shedding may occur in nearly 10% of cases, yet is higher in the setting of immunocompromise or oral surgery.

The differential diagnosis of oral HSV includes aphthous ulcers, erythema multiforme, infectious mononucleosis, and pemphigus. HSV polymerase chain reaction (PCR) swab analysis may be performed from the base of a lesion for confirmation. In the setting of atypical morphologies or negative PCR testing, biopsy may be performed. Diagnostic histologic findings within infected keratinocytes include multinucleation, molding (of nuclei), and margination (of chromatin). Immunohistochemical staining with HSV-specific glycoproteins may be performed in challenging cases with keratinocyte necrosis with nonspecific nuclear degeneration.

Dosing and duration of systemic antiviral therapy is dependent on HSV severity and patient immune status. In patients with multiple recurrent herpes simplex infections in a year, implementation of prophylactic treatment measures may be considered [**Table 61-1**].[16] To date, no approved vaccines exist for HSV-1 or HSV-2.

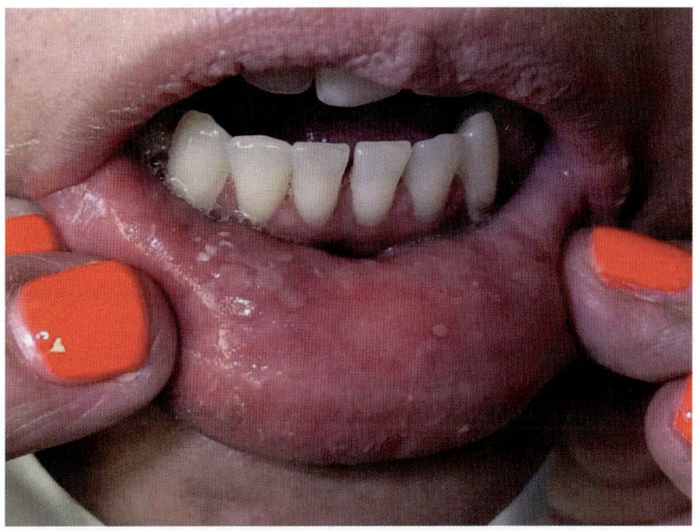

FIGURE 61-9. Herpes labialis and *Candida*: agminated punched out erosions with erythematous borders of the lower mucosal lip in the setting of systemic immunosuppression. Admixed moist white papules of the lateral lower mucosal lip represent concurrent *Candida* infection.

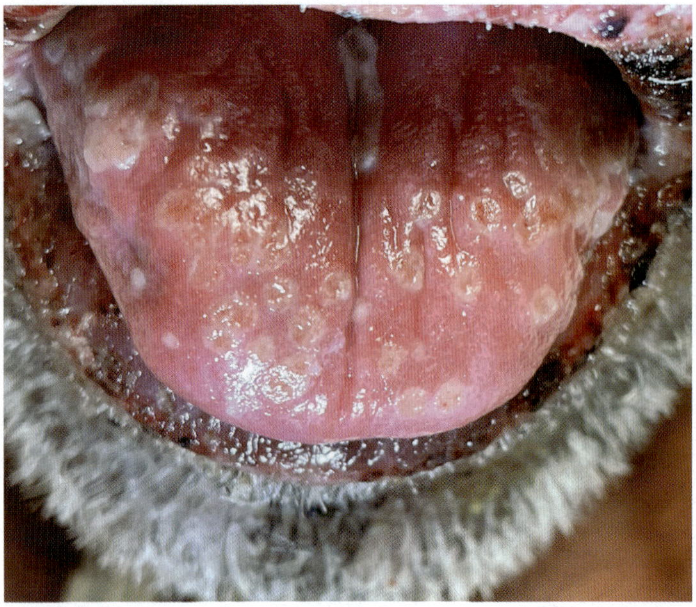

FIGURE 61-10. Phlegmonous (herpetic) glossitis: punctate erosions with yellow-white raised borders studding the dorsal tongue. HSV-1 reactivation occurred in the setting of a biopsy proven generalized bullous fixed drug eruption responsible for the denuded mucosal lips with hemorrhagic crusting.

TABLE 61-1 Herpes labialis prophylaxis[16,17]

Intervention	Dosing	Duration	Outcome
Systemic antivirals	valacyclovir per PO *500 mg daily*	4 months	Significantly reduced number of recurrences (60% of patients with no flares)
	valacyclovir PO *1000 mg daily*	6 months	Significant reduction in recurrence incidence
	acyclovir PO *400 mg twice daily*	4 months	Significant reduction (53%) in number of clinical recurrences
Topical antivirals	acyclovir 5% cream *four applications per day*	4 months	No reduction in number of patient-reported clinical recurrences; significantly reduced average duration of recurrences
Sunscreen	lip balm *sun protective factor 15*	n/a (episodic)	Unclear (protected against recurrences from experimental ultraviolet radiation, yet did not significantly protect against sunlight)
	lip balm *sun protective factor 30 dual layer application reapply after eating/drinking/swimming*		New data (2019) suggest significant protection against sunlight induced recurrences
Low-energy laser	Low energy gallium-aluminum-aresnide laser phototherapy *3 to 4.5 J/cm²; 780 nm; 60 mW 30 treatment points one session/week*	10 weeks	Significant decrease in lesion size and average edema, yet no effect on number of recurrences and pain
Hypnotherapy	symptom-oriented hypnotherapy, and hypnotherapy to improve stress management, and coping with aversive emotions *1 session/week*	5 weeks	Significantly reduced frequency and symptom intensity of recurrences

PO, by mouth.

ORAL CANDIDIASIS AND ANGULAR CHEILITIS

Candida is a commensal dimorphic yeast found in the oral flora of up to 55% of adults.[18] Pathogenic oropharyngeal candidiasis occurs in response to a variety of factors. Risk factors for oropharyngeal candidiasis include dentures, corticosteroids (systemic or mucosal topicals), autoimmune blistering disorders, antimicrobials, radiotherapy, immunosuppression, and diabetes.[18,19] Additionally, neutralizing autoantibodies directed against T-helper 17 cell cytokines have been implicated in impaired epithelial antifungal activity. These autoantibodies are pathogenic for chronic mucocutaneous candidiasis in the setting of autoimmune polyendocrinopathy syndrome type I (APCED) or thymomas.[20] Oropharyngeal candidiasis is most commonly caused by *Candida albicans*. Other causative species are reported (*C. dubliniensis, C. glabrata, C. kefyr, C. krusei, C. parapsilosis, C. stellatoidea,* and *C. tropicalis*) and coinfection is possible.

Oral candidiasis presents as white (pseudomembranous candidiasis, hyperplastic candidiasis) or erythematous (acute/chronic atrophic candidiasis, median rhomboid glossitis) mucosal morphologies. Pseudomembranous candidiasis or thrush is defined by easily removable white plaques of the buccal mucosa, tongue, palate, or pharynx [**Figure 61-11**]. In contrast, hyperplastic candidiasis presents as adherent translucent papules or white plaques with a predilection for the buccal mucosa and oral commissures.[18] Acute atrophic candidiasis manifests as red patches of the palatal, buccal, or tongue surfaces. Chronic atrophic candidiasis may present as petechiae, focal erythema, or papillomatous hyperplasia. The acute form commonly presents after systemic antibiotics and the chronic form is associated with denture use.[18] Median rhomboid glossitis is less common and is caused by asymptomatic atrophy of filiform papillae on the central dorsal tongue.

Angular cheilitis involves the oral commissures and is also referred to as angular stomatitis or perlèche (derived from the French *pourlècher*, meaning "to lick one's lips").[21] Angular cheilitis is a clinical morphology defined by unilateral or bilateral maceration and erythema that may progress to crusted fissures and ulcers. Candida infection is widely recognized as a causative organism, yet noninfectious etiologies such as irritant and allergic contact dermatitides are more commonly implicated.[20] Micronutrient deficiencies have also been implicated, and other infectious etiologies include *Staphylococcus aureus, B-hemolytic streptococci,* and HSV.[18,19]

Diagnosis of mucosal candidiasis may be clinical, yet fungal swab cultures, potassium hydroxide (KOH) preparations, or biopsy may provide

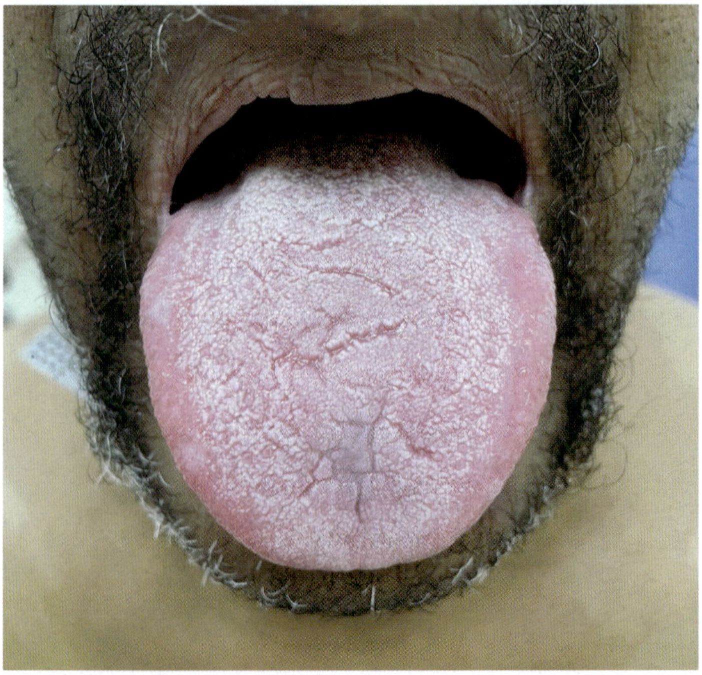

FIGURE 61-11. Oral candidiasis (pseudomembranous): asymptomatic thin white removable plaques of the dorsal tongue.

TABLE 61-2 Oropharyngeal candidiasis treatments[18]

Infection Quality	Medication/Dose	Duration
Mild	clotrimazole troche (lozenge) *10 mg five times daily* miconazole tablet (mucoadhesive) *50 mg once daily* nystatin oral suspension *100,000 U/mL, 4–6 mL, four times daily* nystatin pastilles (lozenges) *200,000 U, four times daily*	1-2 weeks
Moderate to severe	fluconazole per os (PO) *100 to 200 mg daily*	1-2 weeks
Recalcitrant	itraconazole solution *200 mg once daily*	Variable duration according to response
	voriconazole PO *200 mg twice daily*	–
	amphotericin B deoxycholate oral suspension *100 mg/mL four times daily*	–
	posaconazole suspension *400 mg twice daily* *Then, 400 mg daily*	3 days Then, 28 days maximum
Chronic	fluconazole PO *100 mg three times per week*	Continuous (but may result in resistance)
Denture-related	Antifungal therapy as above and regular denture cleaning	

PO, by mouth.

confirmation. KOH analysis as well as Periodic-acid Schiff (PAS) stained histologic sections will demonstrate pseudohyphae or yeast forms. Treatment of oropharyngeal candidiasis is dependent on disease severity and ranges from antifungal troches/pastilles/lozenges and buccal mucosal tablets to oral rinses as well as systemic antifungals [**Table 61-2**].[19] First-line therapy for mild oropharyngeal candidiasis is oral topical therapy (miconazole mucoadhesive dissolvable tablet daily or clotrimazole troche/lozenge five times a day or nystatin oral suspension four times a day). Topical imidazole antifungals creams such as twice daily miconazole 2%, ketoconazole 2%, or clotrimazole 1% are effective for management of *Candida*-induced angular cheilitis. Miconazole and clotrimazole creams also demonstrate antistaphylococcal action.

HAND-FOOT-MOUTH DISEASE

Hand-foot-and-mouth disease (HFMD) is caused by single-stranded RNA viruses of the *Picornaviridae* family, including various enterovirus A and coxsackie strains.[22] HFMD was first noted in 1948 and more recently, nonclassical infections due to coxsackie A6 virus were first reported in 2008. Exposure to children, poor hygiene, and shared dormitories (college or military) are risk factors for HFMD.

HMFD is characterized by painful ovoid erosions and ulcers of the oropharynx and tongue. Accompanying palmoplantar erythematous to hyperpigmented macules, thin papules, or gray-white ovoid vesicles are typical. A low-grade fever may accompany initial skin lesions. Subsequent palmoplantar desquamation occurs in more than half of patients.[22] Onychomadesis may occur more than 1 month after infection.

HFMD is a clinical diagnosis, yet biopsy may be performed in atypical presentations, such as in the adult population. Histopathology demonstrates spongiosis, keratinocyte dyskeratosis/necrosis favoring the upper Malpighian/spiny layer, and neutrophil exocytosis.[23] Dermal edema, lymphocyte predominant inflammation, erythrocyte extravasation, and vasculitic changes have been described.

HMFD is almost always self-limited with clinical findings resolving within 2 weeks. Management consists of isolation and supportive measures. Neurologic or cardiopulmonary complications may rarely result in death in extraordinary cases, and absence of oral lesions has been associated with more severe cases. Notably, a susceptible genetic background is thought to contribute to severe cases; single-nucleotide polymorphisms of inflammatory cytokines and chemokines have been reported in patients of Chinese descent with severe infections.[22] HFMD vaccines have been developed against various strains, yet further efforts are needed to provide broader simultaneous coverage against multiple strains.

ORAL SYPHILIS

Syphilis continues to impact health worldwide and syphilis infection rates have recently increased significantly in the United States. Syphilis is a sexually transmitted infection caused by the spirochetal bacterium *Treponema pallidum*. Primary and secondary syphilis infection rates increased 11.2% from 2018 to 2019, and total reported syphilis cases increased 74% since 2015.[24] Disparities in rates of reported syphilis cases are recognized; non-White patients made up 40% of the 2019 U.S. population, yet represented 66% of primary and secondary syphilis cases.[24] More specifically, Black women and men and notably men who have sex with men (MSM) are at increased risk of syphilis.[25] As with other sexually transmitted infections, these disparities are influenced by the multifactorial intersection of social determinants of health, and barriers to health care experienced by communities that have been marginalized.

Improving recognition of this curable disease is one means of addressing health disparities, and may start with improving representation in the medical literature. Oral manifestations of syphilis are recognized in all races, yet in a recent literature review of acquired oral syphilis, non-White patients are estimated to account for only 5% of published cases ($n = 247$).[26]

Syphilis is the "great masquerader" and its heterogeneous manifestations span primary, secondary, and tertiary clinical stages. Oral lesions are most commonly reported in males (M:F 3.7:1)[26] and in patients between 20 and 49 years of age, though any age may be affected. Nearly two-thirds of patients with oral findings present with a single lesion. The lips, dorsoventral tongue, and palate are most frequently affected, followed by the lateral tongue [**Figure 61-12**] and buccal mucosa.[27] The tonsillar pillars, vestibule, gingival/alveolar mucosa, oral commissures, and floor of mouth may be involved.[26,27] Primary syphilis is defined by an asymptomatic chancre at the site of transmission; when present on the lip, the chancre favors the upper lip in males and the lower lip in females. Secondary syphilis occurs weeks to months after the primary chancre. Gray-white mucous patches are the predominant oral lesion, yet macules, papules, nodules, and ulcers are also recognized.[26] Despite being recognized as a manifestation of syphilitic infection, split papules of the oral commissure

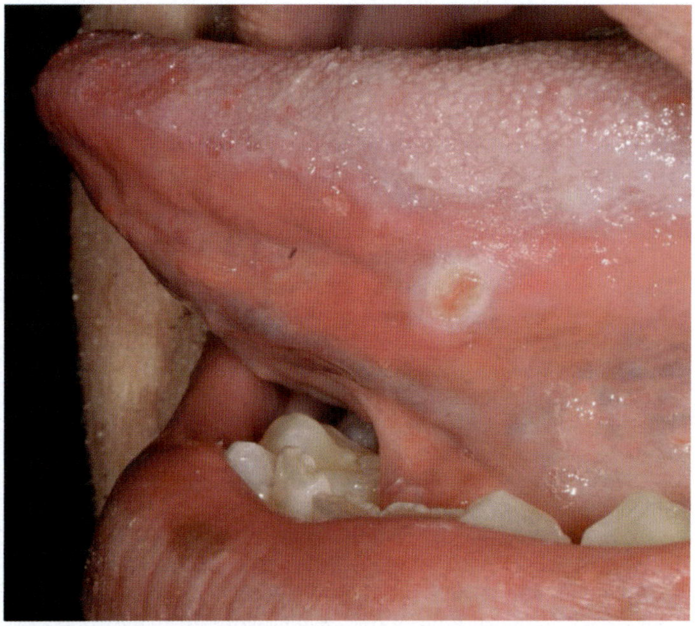

FIGURE 61-12. Primary syphilis (chancre): left lateral tongue circumscribed ulcer with yellow base and white macerated rim.

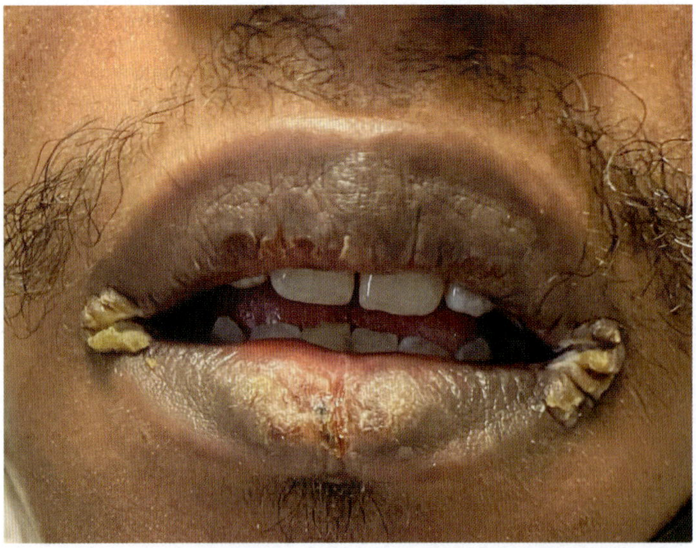

FIGURE 61-13. Secondary syphilis: hyperkeratotic yellow brown papules with central moist fissure of the bilateral oral commissures. (Reproduced with permission from Alshaikh H, Aleisa A, Forcucci J. Cutaneous eruption in an immunocompromised patient. *Cutis.* 2022;110(4):179, 182-183.)

are less frequently reported [**Figure 61-13**]. Over 20% of patients with secondary oral syphilis reported accompanying pain or burning sensation. Tertiary stage may present in the oral mucosa as noduloulcerative gummas, palatal perforations, or atrophic glossitis.[26]

Differential diagnoses include leukoplakia, aphthous ulcers, squamous cell carcinoma, granular cell tumor, lichen planus, and less common infectious etiologies such as deep fungal infection, leishmaniasis, or tuberculosis. Parenteral penicillin G remains the gold standard therapy for syphilis with dose and duration dependent on the stage of disease.

ORAL MANIFESTATIONS IN THE SETTING OF CORONAVIRUS DISEASE 2019

In early 2020, the World Health Organization declared coronavirus disease 2019 (COVID-19) a pandemic. COVID-19 is caused by a novel coronavirus, severe acute respiratory syndrome coronavirus 2 (SARS-CoV-2), which gains entry to host cells via human angiotensin-converting enzyme II (ACE2). ACE2 expression is highly increased in the oral mucosa, making this site vulnerable to COVID-19 pathology.[28] Oral manifestations of COVID-19 may be underreported due to lack of a focused oral examination and comprehension of oral sequelae is evolving. A large retrospective review (n = 64,876) found ulcerations, fungal infections, glossitis, lingual depapillation, and geographic tongue to be the most common oral findings in the setting of COVID-19.[29] A single cross-sectional study (n = 666) found transient anterior lingual papillitis, tongue edema, and aphthous stomatitis to be the three most common oral findings attributed to SARS-CoV-2 infection.[30]

Painful herpes-like ulcerations are a recognized oral manifestation of COVID-19 and demonstrate a predilection for the dorsal tongue.[31] The hard palate and labial mucosa may also be involved. Other reported morphologies include erythematous macules, erosions, vesiculobullae, erythema multiforme-like, and petechiae. Tongue predilection may be explained by higher ACE2 expression in tongue epithelial cells compared to other oral sites such as buccal or gingival mucosa.[28] Similarly, high ACE2 receptor expression has been identified in salivary gland epithelium and direct SARS-CoV-2 invasion of these cells has been proposed to induce edema and salivary inflammation, likely contributing to widespread reports of COVID-19-associated xerostomia.[31]

Oral lesions may resolve quickly within a few days or may persist for a few weeks.[31] Management of oral manifestations includes supportive measures such as topical diphenhydramine and viscous lidocaine as well as consideration of topical or systemic corticosteroids.

OTHER MISCELLANEOUS DISORDERS

ORAL FIXED DRUG ERUPTION

Fixed drug eruption (FDE) is one the most common types of adverse cutaneous drug reactions and may account for over 20% of cases.[32] Any systemic agent may be implicated, including rare reports of quinine exposure from tonic water flavoring.[33] FDE limited to the oral mucosa is less common, yet recognition of this entity is warranted to distinguish FDE from various mimickers.

Oral mucosal FDE lesions are generally bullous/erosive [**Figure 61-14**]; aphthous ulcers are also recognized, and least commonly, erythematous patches of the inner lip mucosa or dorsal tongue. Over 20% of patients may present with an isolated bullous/erosive lesion, typically on the hard palate or dorsal tongue.[34] FDE of the lip may be more likely to demonstrate the characteristic circumscribed ovoid hyperpigmented patches [**Figure 61-15**]. Histopathology of FDE classically reveals an acute stratum corneum, vacuolar interface dermatitis, and subjacent perivascular lymphocytic inflammation with admixed melanophages; however, in the oral mucosa, melanophages may be rare or absent.[34]

Misdiagnosis is common, and in one review (n = 61), over 30% of cases were initially attributed to Behcet disease or menstruation-triggered herpes simplex virus; in the latter, nonsteroidal inflammatory use for dysmenorrhea was identified as the causative agent.[34] The differential may also include erythema multiforme, oral syphilis, and autoimmune blistering disorders. Generalized bullous FDE may mimic toxic epidermal necrolysis, as both may present with full-thickness labial mucosal desquamation [**Figures 61-16** and 61-10]. Clinical suspicion and same site recurrence with medication reexposure are key to a diagnosis of FDE. Management relies on drug cessation.

ORAL LICHEN PLANUS

Oral lichen planus (LP) is observed in about half of patients with cutaneous LP and it has a predilection for women. It is most often seen in adults between the ages of 40 and 70 years; however, cases in childhood have been documented.[35] Oral LP presents most commonly on the oral buccal mucosa with a bilateral distribution, but involvement of the lips, tongue, and plate is possible.[36] The condition is chronic with characteristic relapsing and remission.

There are six subtypes of oral LP: reticular, papular, plaque, atrophic, erosive, and bullous [**Figures 61-17** and **61-18**]. The reticular subtype is the most common form of oral LP, presenting as usually asymptomatic white striae on the buccal mucosa. The second most common form is erosive oral LP, which is characterized by painful erosions covered in yellow-gray pseudomembranes and surrounded by white striae

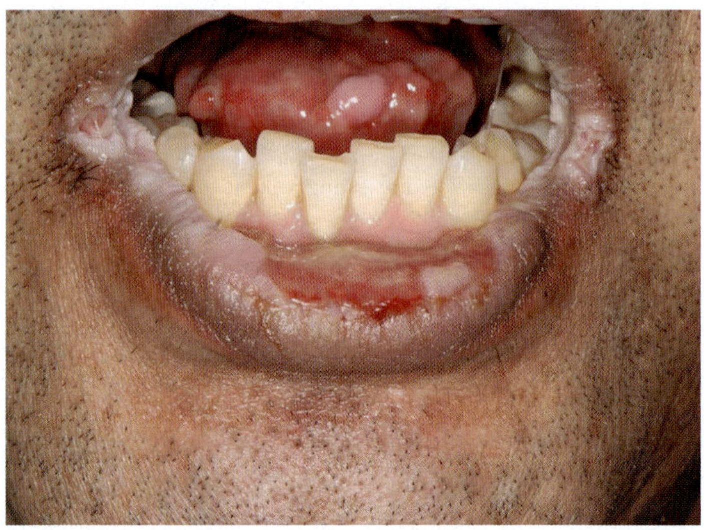

FIGURE 61-14. Fixed drug eruption (ulcer): bullous fixed drug eruption resulting in subsequent lower mucosal lip ulceration.

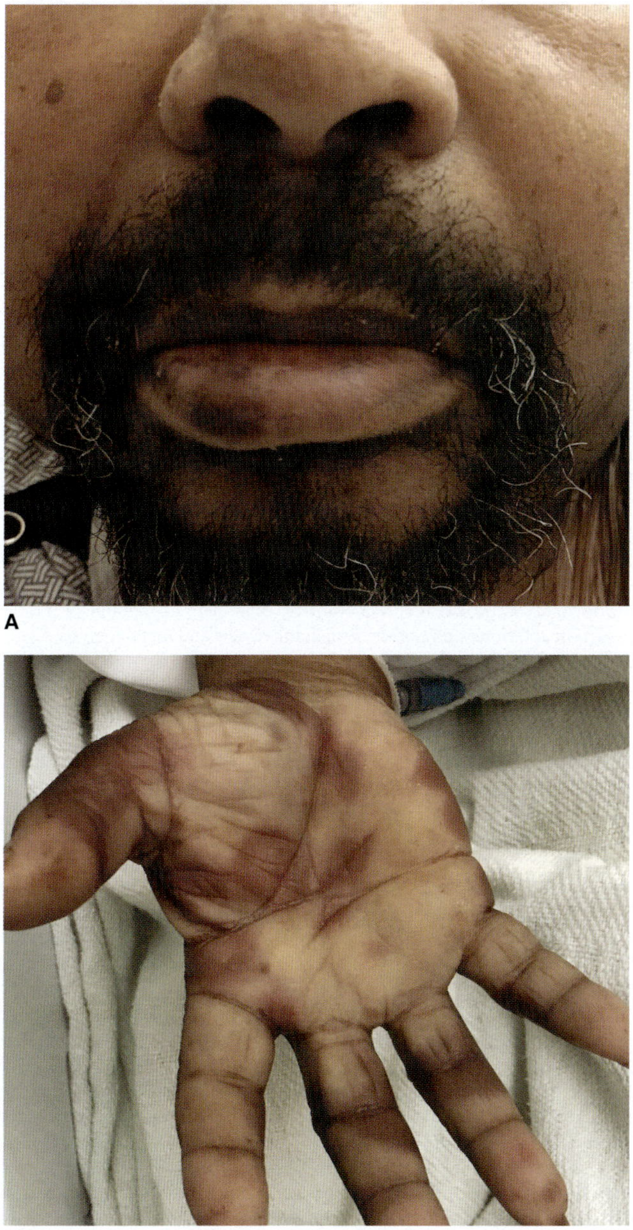

FIGURE 61-15 (A) Fixed drug eruption (oral): ovoid red-brown hyperpigmented patches of the right lower mucosal lip and vermillion border with underlying labial edema; a smaller hyperpigmented ovoid patch is also present on the right upper lateral mucosal lip. **(B)** Fixed drug eruption (cutaneous): coalescing red-brown patches with focal dusky centers of the right palm and volar fingers.

[**Figure 61-19**]. These patients experience aggravation of pain upon exposure to acidic foods. Papular oral LP appears as white painless papules. Plaque-like oral LP is usually seen in the setting of cigarette use and presents as asymptomatic white plaques on the buccal mucosa and dorsal tongue; this form of oral LP can resemble leukoplakia. The most infrequent variant is bullous LP, which presents with flaccid bullae that, upon rupture, leave behind painful erosions.

The etiology of oral LP remains elusive; however, this condition is considered to represent a T-cell-mediated inflammatory process in response to a trigger. Studies have described various potential triggers including hepatitis C virus infection (HCV), implantation of restorative dental materials (such as amalgam, composite, cobalt, and dental acrylics), acute and chronic graft-versus-host disease, and treatment with systemic drugs (including NSAIDs, beta blockers, ACE inhibitors, diuretics, oral hypoglycemics, sulfonylureas, dapsone, antimalarials,

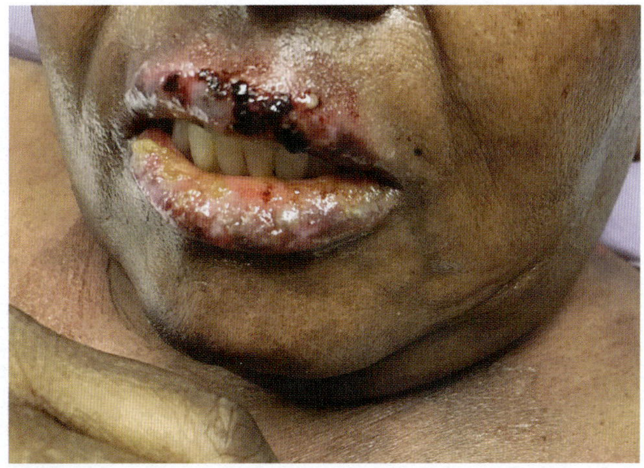

FIGURE 61-16. Toxic epidermal necrolysis (TEN): serohemorrhagic and impetiginized crust overlying fully denuded lip mucosa in a patient with biopsy proven TEN. Upper chest skin demonstrated positive Nikolsky sign. Note the full thickness desquamation with surrounding dusky hyperpigmentation of the left posterior base of neck.

penicillamine, and antiretrovirals for HIV).[37] Repetitive oral trauma has also been described as a factor in the development of oral LP.[37] Grinspan syndrome refers to the association between oral LP, hypertension, and diabetes mellitus. However, it has been postulated that this triad does not represent a true syndrome and instead reflects an oral LP that results from medications used to treat hypertension and diabetes.[37]

Oral LP can be diagnosed clinically, but biopsy may be important to distinguish this diagnosis from dysplasia and malignancy. Histopathological findings of oral LP include liquefactive necrosis of basal cells, colloid bodies, saw-toothed rete ridges, and hyperkeratosis.[37]

Treatment for asymptomatic oral LP is not indicated, but close follow-up is necessary given that these lesions may undergo malignant transformation. Risk factors for malignant transformation of oral LP that have been proposed include erosive and ulcerative oral LP, tongue lesions,

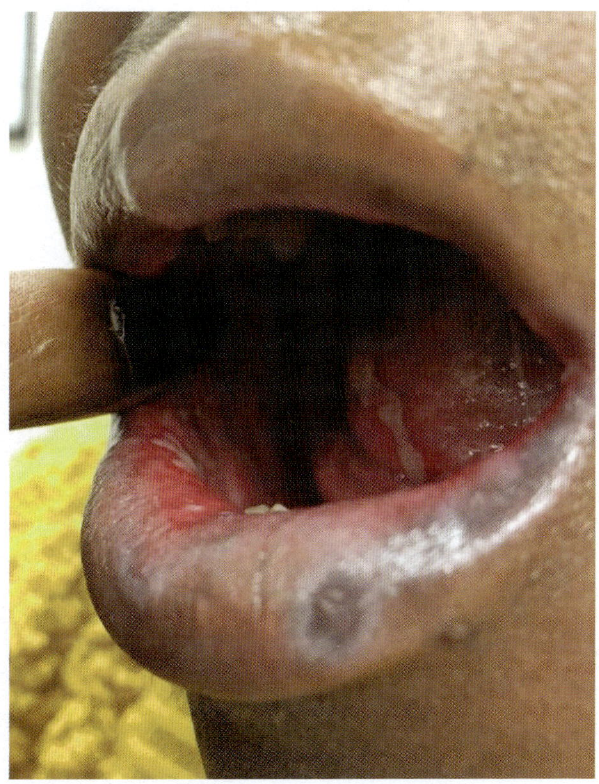

FIGURE 61-17. Erosive lichen planus: erythematous ulcer of the lower mucosal lip and distal lateral tongue with focal fibrin. Accompanying gray-white ovoid plaque of the lower lateral lip.

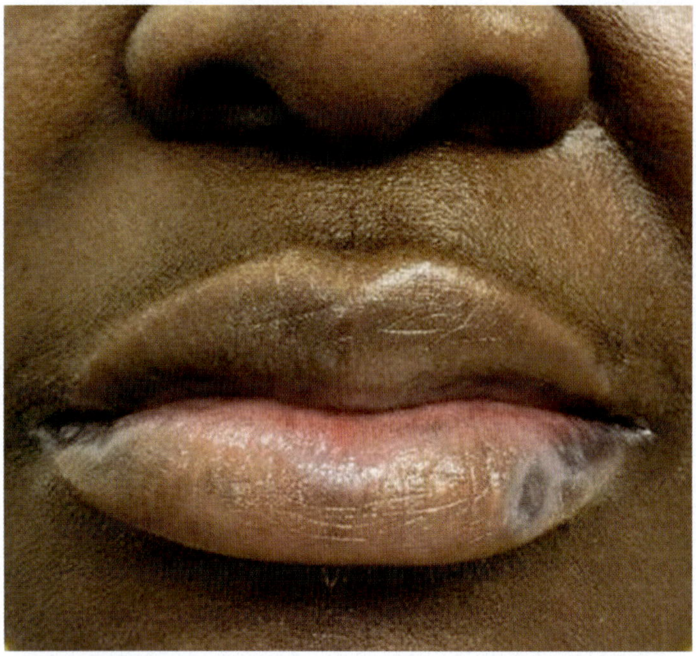

FIGURE 61-18. Oral lichen planus: Coalescing dark gray and white thin plaques of the lateral lips in a patient with biopsy-proven oral lichen planus.

female sex, appearance of lesions in the sixth or seventh decade of life, and *C. albicans* superinfection.[37] For painful lesions, use of local anesthetics, topical corticosteroids, and topical calcineurin inhibitors is common. Treatment options for severe cases include oral corticosteroids and oral mycophenolate mofetil. Newer treatment strategies under investigation range from low intensity laser therapy, aloe vera, and oral curcuminoids.[37]

BEHCET DISEASE

Behcet disease (BD) is a relapsing and remitting condition that presents with oral aphthous stomatitis, painful genital ulcers, anterior uveitis and nongranulomatous uveitis, arthritis, and enthesitis (also see Chapter 82 for further discussion of BD).[38] Accompanying erythema nodosum may also be present. Patients with BD may have a higher risk for vascular thrombosis and aneurysms from vasculitis. The disease is commonly seen in people from regions along the Silk Road (eg, Turkey). Genetically, BD is strongly associated with human leukocyte antigen B51. The diagnosis is often made clinically, although an elevated erythrocyte sedimentation rate (ESR) and C-reactive protein (CRP) level may be supportive. Treatment of a flare Behcet disease is largely supportive, usually with a course of NSAIDs.[38]

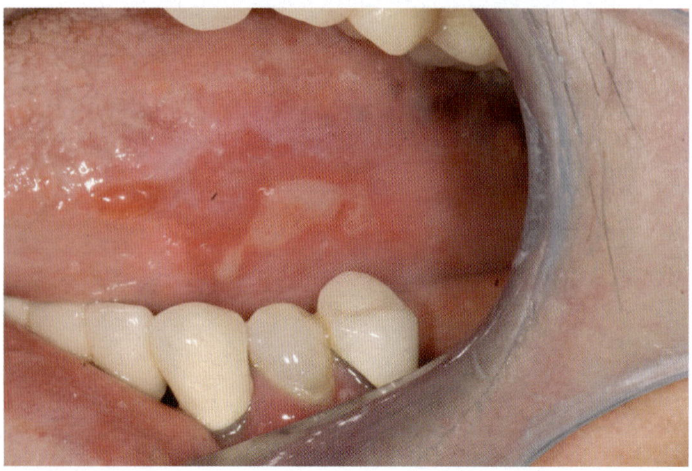

FIGURE 61-19. Erosive lichen planus: circumscribed ulcer with yellow base and erythematous borders of the left lateral tongue in a patient with biopsy-proven erosive lichen planus.

REFERENCES

1. Jacob CN, John TM, R J. Geographic tongue. *Cleve Clin J Med.* 2016;83(8):565-566.
2. Sadlier M. Acrodermatitis continua of Hallopeau and geographic tongue are variants of pustular psoriasis. *JAAD Case Rep.* 2018;4(3):277.
3. Varoni E, Decani S. Images in clinical medicine: geographic tongue. *N Engl J Med.* 2016;374(7):670.
4. Bhatia S, Kohli S, Selvadurai SS. Tattoo in the oral cavity. *Am J Med.* 2021;134(6):e390-e391.
5. Laimer J, Henn R, Helten T, et al. Amalgam tattoo versus melanocytic neoplasm - differential diagnosis of dark pigmented oral mucosa lesions using infrared spectroscopy. *PLoS One.* 2018;13(11):e0207026.
6. Wang X, Yang S, Wang Y. Image gallery: black hairy tongue in a patient receiving enteral feeding. *Br J Dermatol.* 2019;181(4):e91.
7. Jayasree P, Kaliyadan F, Ashique KT. Black hairy tongue. *JAMA Dermatol.* 2022;158(5):573.
8. Cam K, Santoro A, Lee JB. Oral frictional hyperkeratosis (morsicatio buccarum): an entity to be considered in the differential diagnosis of white oral mucosal lesions. *Skinmed.* 2012;10(2):114-115.
9. Scully C. Aphthous ulceration. *N Engl J Med.* 2006;355(2):165-172.
10. Suda T, Fujii H. Beta blocker-induced recurrent aphthous stomatitis. *Intern Med.* Published online August 20, 2022.
11. Surboyo MDC, Boedi RM, Hariyani N, et al. The expression of TNF-α in recurrent aphthous stomatitis: a systematic review and meta-analysis. *Cytokine.* 2022;157:155946.
12. Arduino PG, Porter SR. Herpes simplex virus type 1 infection: overview on relevant clinico-pathological features. *J Oral Pathol Med.* 2008;37(2):107-121.
13. McQuillan G, Kruszon-Moran D, Flagg EW, Paulose-Ram R. Prevalence of herpes simplex virus type 1 and type 2 in persons aged 14-49: United States, 2015-2016. *NCHS Data Brief.* 2018;(304):1-8.
14. Krieger N. Discrimination and health inequities. *Int J Health Serv.* 2014;44(4):643-710.
15. Mirowski GW, Goddard A. Herpetic geometric glossitis in an immunocompetent patient with pneumonia. *J Am Acad Dermatol.* 2009;61(1):139-142.
16. Chi CC, Wang SH, Delamere FM, Wojnarowska F, Peters MC, Kanjirath PP. Interventions for prevention of herpes simplex labialis (cold sores on the lips). *Cochrane Database Syst Rev.* 2015;(8):CD010095.
17. Mazzarello V, Ferrari M, Piu G, Pomponi V, Solinas G. Do sunscreen prevent recurrent herpes labialis in summer? *J Dermatolog Treat.* 2019;30(2):179-182.
18. Millsop JW, Fazel N. Oral candidiasis. *Clin Dermatol.* 2016;34(4):487-494.
19. Pappas PG, Kauffman CA, Andes DR, et al. Clinical practice guideline for the management of candidiasis: 2016 update by the Infectious Diseases Society of America. *Clin Infect Dis.* 2016;62(4):e1-e50.
20. Kisand K, Bøe Wolff AS, Podkrajsek KT, et al. Chronic mucocutaneous candidiasis in APECED or thymoma patients correlates with autoimmunity to Th17-associated cytokines. *J Exp Med.* 2010;207(2):299-308.
21. Park KK, Brodell RT, Helms SE. Angular cheilitis, part 1: local etiologies. *Cutis.* 2011;87(6):289-295.
22. Esposito S, Principi N. Hand, foot and mouth disease: current knowledge on clinical manifestations, epidemiology, aetiology and prevention. *Eur J Clin Microbiol Infect Dis.* 2018;37(3):391-398.
23. Kimmis BD, Downing C, Tyring S. Hand-foot-and-mouth disease caused by coxsackievirus A6 on the rise. *Cutis.* 2018;102(5):353-356.
24. CDC. Sexually transmitted disease surveillance, 2019. Centers for Disease Control and Prevention. Published April 12, 2022. https://www.cdc.gov/std/statistics/2019/default.htm. Accessed September 4, 2022.
25. Amerson EH, Castillo Valladares HB, Leslie KS. Resurgence of syphilis in the US—USPSTF reaffirms screening guidelines. *JAMA Dermatol.* 2022;158(11):1241-1243.
26. Schuch LF, da Silva KD, de Arruda JAA, et al. Forty cases of acquired oral syphilis and a review of the literature. *Int J Oral Maxillofac Surg.* 2019;48(5): 635-643.
27. Thums MA, Koth VS, Figueiredo MAZ, Cherubini K, Salum FG. Oral manifestations of syphilis: an epidemiological study in southern Brazil. *Aust Dent J.* 2021;66(3):289-294.
28. Xu H, Zhong L, Deng J, et al. High expression of ACE2 receptor of 2019-nCoV on the epithelial cells of oral mucosa. *Int J Oral Sci.* 2020;12(1):8.
29. Amorim dos Santos J, Normando AGC, Carvalho da Silva RL, et al. Oral manifestations in patients with COVID-19: a 6-month update. *J Dent Res.* 2021;100(12):1321-1329.
30. González AN, Nuño González A, Magaletskyy K, et al. Are oral mucosal changes a sign of COVID-19? A cross-sectional study at a field hospital. *Actas Dermo-Sifiliográficas (English Edition).* 2021;112(7):640-644.

31. Halboub E, Al-Maweri SA, Alanazi RH, Qaid NM, Abdulrab S. Orofacial manifestations of COVID-19: a brief review of the published literature. *Braz Oral Res.* 2020;34:e124.
32. Lee AY. Fixed drug eruptions. *Am J Clin Dermatol.* 2000;1(5):277-285.
33. Lonsdale-Eccles E, Wallett A, Ward AM. A case of fixed drug eruption secondary to quinine in tonic water presenting to a sexual health clinic. *Sex Transm Infect.* 2014;90(5):356-357.
34. Özkaya E. Oral mucosal fixed drug eruption: characteristics and differential diagnosis. *J Am Acad Dermatol.* 2013;69(2):e51-e58.
35. Cascone M, Celentano A, Adamo D, Leuci S, Ruoppo E, Mignogna MD. Oral lichen planus in childhood: a case series. *Int J Dermatol.* 2017;56(6):641-652.
36. Nogueira PA, Carneiro S, Ramos-e-Silva M. Oral lichen planus: an update on its pathogenesis. *Int J Dermatol.* 2015;54(9):1005-1010.
37. Alrashdan MS, Cirillo N, McCullough M. Oral lichen planus: a literature review and update. *Arch Dermatol Res.* 2016;308(8):539-551.
38. Davatchi F. Behçet's disease. *Int J Rheum Dis.*

CHAPTER 62

Genital Lesions in Men

Wilce Gonzalez
Christine Olagun-Samuel
John G. Zampella

KEY POINTS

- Genital diseases in men can result from a variety of infectious, inflammatory, neoplastic, or mechanical etiologies.
- Manifestations of genital skin diseases in skin of color may present with characteristics that may differ from those in historical educational paradigms.
- Skin diseases involving the genitalia, including syphilis, HSV, and hidradenitis suppurativa, disproportionately impact patients from historically marginalized communities, including Black and Hispanic/Latine patients.
- Black and Hispanic/Latino males suffer from worse prognosis in penile squamous cell carcinoma.
- Coinfection of HIV with other sexually transmitted infections is higher in Black and Hispanic/Latino men who have sex with men and these patients should be considered for preexposure prophylaxis.
- A detailed history (including sexual history), physical exam, and judicious use of diagnostic tests are extremely valuable in diagnosing genital diseases in patients with skin of color.

INTRODUCTION

Many dermatoses affect the male genitalia and have similar morphologies making definitive clinical diagnosis challenging. The appearance of genital lesions may diverge from classic presentation on other body parts. Skin of color (SOC) adds an additional layer of complexity as signs of inflammation may present with a purple to hyperpigmented color. Red and pink hues, which are commonly taught to be inflammatory features, may not be identifiable and are less likely in skin of color.[1]

Lackluster educational paradigms contribute to knowledge gaps in identifying genital diseases in SOC and may contribute to diagnostic bias and poorer health outcomes in patients with SOC.[2] Diagnostic modalities such as dermoscopy can aid in diagnoses but there is limited literature on dermoscopic characteristics of genital diseases in SOC. To diagnose genital skin diseases, utilization of diagnostic tools including skin scrapings, biopsy, serologic testing, and cultures for micro-organisms, among others should be emphasized. A patient's history including sexual history, chronicity of the lesions, and symptoms are often essential in making a diagnosis. Performing a total body skin exam may reveal cutaneous clues to genital lesions on other skin surfaces. Evaluating patients in the context of population health, including the impact of systemic inequities on the social determinants of health (also see Chapter 11), may point to additional risk factors, preventative measures, and interventions that optimize healthcare outcomes.

EXAMINING THE GENITALS

Genital exams can be awkward for providers and patients alike and many dermatologists forgo the genitals in total body skin exams. However, this is to patients' detriment as a thorough evaluation of male patients' genitalia can be helpful in diagnosing skin dermatoses, infections, or malignancies. To examine the genitals, start by making the patient comfortable and provide appropriate positioning and gowning. Providers should explain each step of the exam. The genitalia should be maneuvered in various directions so that all areas of the penis, scrotum, and perineum can be adequately surveyed, including retraction of the foreskin. It may be helpful to have the patient perform the various movements of the genitals. When the exam is completed, explaining exam findings will help patients feel more comfortable and utilizing words that do not carry any judgmental connotations is essential (ie, "normal" rather than "good"). A list of normal variants and benign lesions for the male genitals can be found in **Table 62-1**.

TABLE 62-1 Normal variants and benign lesions

Lesion	Morphology	Etiology
Seborrheic keratoses	Epidermal tumor common in elderly; well-demarcated rounded appearance	Benign proliferation of immature keratinocytes
Syringoma	Brown-pink or yellow papules. In skin of color often presents as asymmetric on the penile shaft	Sweat gland neoplasm; Can require drainage if infected
Epidermoid cyst/sebaceous cyst	Genital growths that develop in hair follicles of sebaceous glands	Sebaceous glands are filled with keratin, fibrous tissue and serosanguineous fluid
Median raphe cyst	Flesh-colored, mobile subcutaneous papule or nodule. May be single or multiple. [**Figure 62-1**]	Cystic structure forming along the embryonic fusion plane known as the median raphe
Pearly penile papules	Flesh colored, monomorphic papules located on the corona of the penis [**Figure 62-2**]	Benign outgrowths of fibrous tissue of unknown etiology
Angiokeratomas	Purple to violaceous papules often found on the scrotum [**Figure 62-3**]	Benign vascular proliferations
Ectopic sebaceous glands (Tyson glands, Fordyce spots)	Flesh-colored to yellow, monomorphic papules located near the frenulum or on the shaft of the penis	Proliferations of normal sebaceous glands in the genital skin
Mucosal lentigines	Hyperpigmented, evenly pigmented macules that can be single or multiple on the penis or scrotum	Normal variant associated with basilar hyperpigmentation
Acrochordon/skin tag	Flesh colored, pedunculated papules	Benign fibrous polyps that may result from friction and associated with systemic diseases such as diabetes mellitus.
Scrotal calcinosis	White to yellow, 1-10 mm firm dermal nodules, typically found on the scrotum.	Generally thought to be caused by idiopathic calcification of scrotal cysts. Patients generally have normal serum calcium.

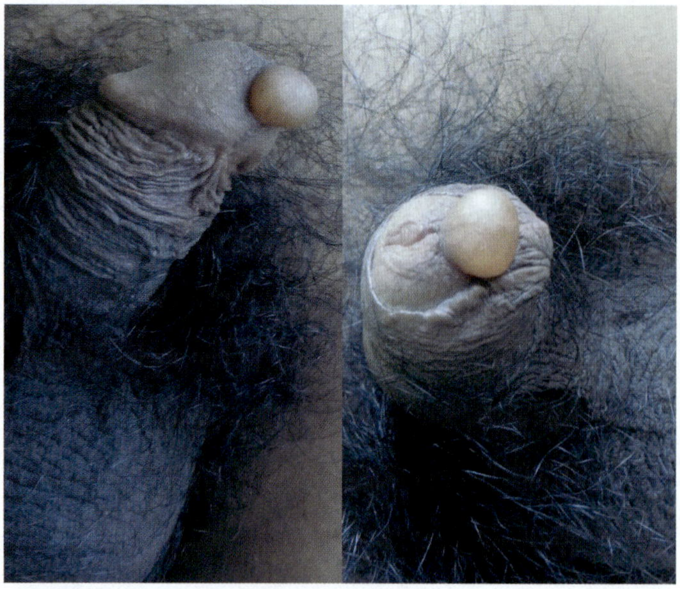

FIGURE 62-1. Median raphe cyst located inferiorly to the urethral meatus. (Reproduced with permission from Syed M, Amatya B, Sitaula S. Median raphe cyst of the penis: a case report and review of the literature. *J Med Case Reports*. 2019;13:214.)

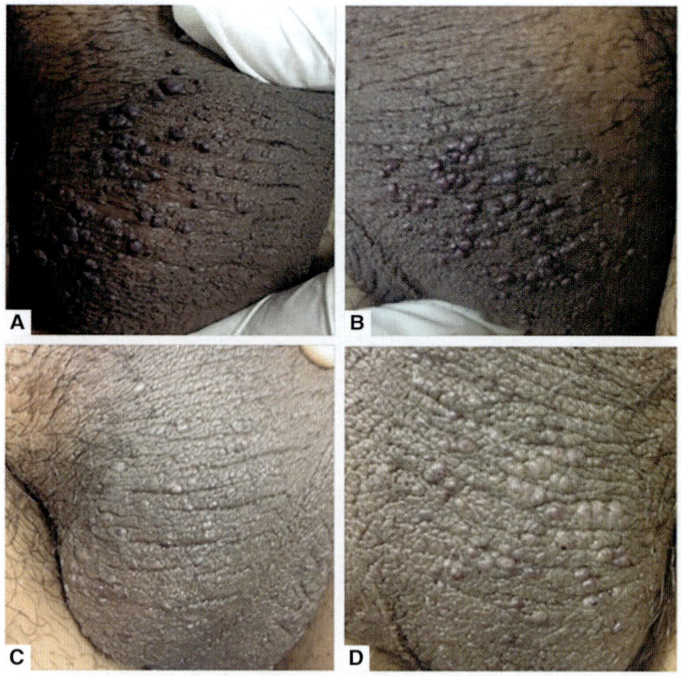

FIGURE 62-3. Angiokeratomas of the scrotum that can be treated with multiple modalities including laser **(A-D)**. (Reproduced with permission from Ibrahim SM. Pulsed dye laser versus long pulsed Nd:YAG laser in the treatment of angiokeratoma of Fordyce: a randomized, comparative, observer-blinded study. *J Dermatolog Treat*. 2016;27(3):270-274.)

INFECTIOUS DISEASES

SEXUALLY TRANSMITTED INFECTIONS

Syphilis

What's New? Rates of syphilis continue to rise, disproportionately impacting marginalized communities. Since 2016, many institutions have implemented the "reverse algorithm" screening method that uses a Treponema-specific test followed by an RPR (rapid plasma reagin) confirmatory titer.[3]

Background Syphilis is a common sexually transmitted infection (STI) caused by the spirochete *Treponema pallidum*, an obligate human pathogen, and its clinical manifestations can mimic other diseases. Syphilis infection can be divided into primary, secondary, latent, and tertiary stages. Transmission usually occurs via direct contact with a primary or secondary lesion. Spirochetes penetrate mucous membranes or broken skin and becomes systemic as the organism travels through the lymphatic system and bloodstream.[3]

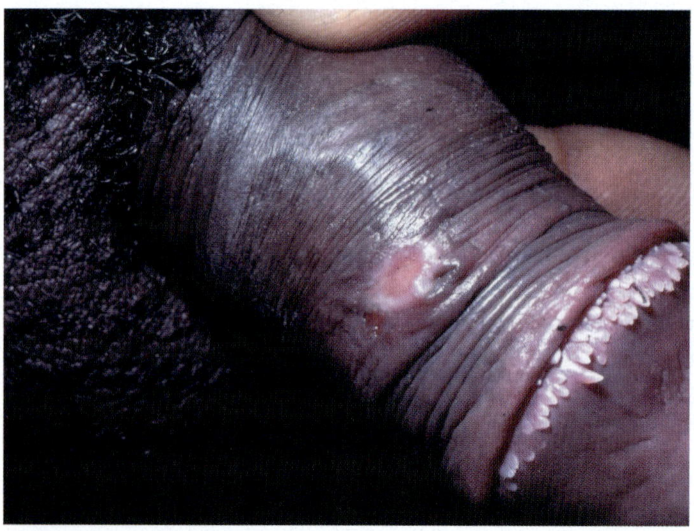

FIGURE 62-2. Punched out, painless ulceration with indurated border of primary syphilis. Incidental pearly penile papules noted on the corona of the penis.

There are 6 million new cases of syphilis each year globally. In the United States, rates of primary and secondary syphilis are higher in Black/African Americans (AA) and Hispanic/Latine populations. Men who have sex with men (MSM), especially Black and Hispanic/Latino males, are disproportionately at risk with rates more than 100-fold higher than heterosexual men. High-risk populations also include female sex workers and their male clients.[3]

Making the Diagnosis Serological testing is the most common assay to screen for and diagnose syphilis including the RPR and a treponemal-specific test (TT). While uncommonly performed, diagnosis can be made via darkfield microscopy, immunochemistry, PCR (polymerase chain reaction), and fluorescent antibody staining. Histologically, staining with Warthin-Starry stain can be performed; however, the stain reacts with melanin, complicating diagnosis in SOC.

What to Look for Clinically? One to 3 weeks after infection, primary syphilis classically manifests with a solitary painless ulcer, also known as a chancre [Figure 62-2]. Multiple lesions on sites involved in sexual contact, and regional lymphadenopathy may also be seen clinically.[3] The chancre generally resolves in 1 week and may be missed by patients. About 6 to 8 weeks later, patients present with secondary syphilis, which is a papulosquamous eruption on the trunk and extremities, and classically involves the palms and soles.[3] Condyloma lata is a form of secondary syphilis that resembles genital warts and can manifest in 6% to 23% of syphilis patients [**Figure 62-4**]. As symptoms subside, an infected individual enters the latent phase but is still considered infectious in the first 1 to 2 years.[3]

Differential Diagnosis Primary syphilis: chancroid, HSV, granuloma inguinale, monkeypox/mpox, Behcet's Disease, squamous cell carcinoma.

What is the Treatment? A single intramuscular injection of 2.4 million units of penicillin G is the standard of care.[3] Partners of persons with syphilis should also be treated. There has never been a report of penicillin-resistant *T. pallidum*. For penicillin-allergic patients, second-line oral antibiotics such as doxycycline or azithromycin are appropriate. Unlike penicillin, there are reports of macrolide-resistant syphilis.

Additional Considerations After treatment, patients should be followed with repeat RPR 6 to 12 months after therapy to confirm clearance.

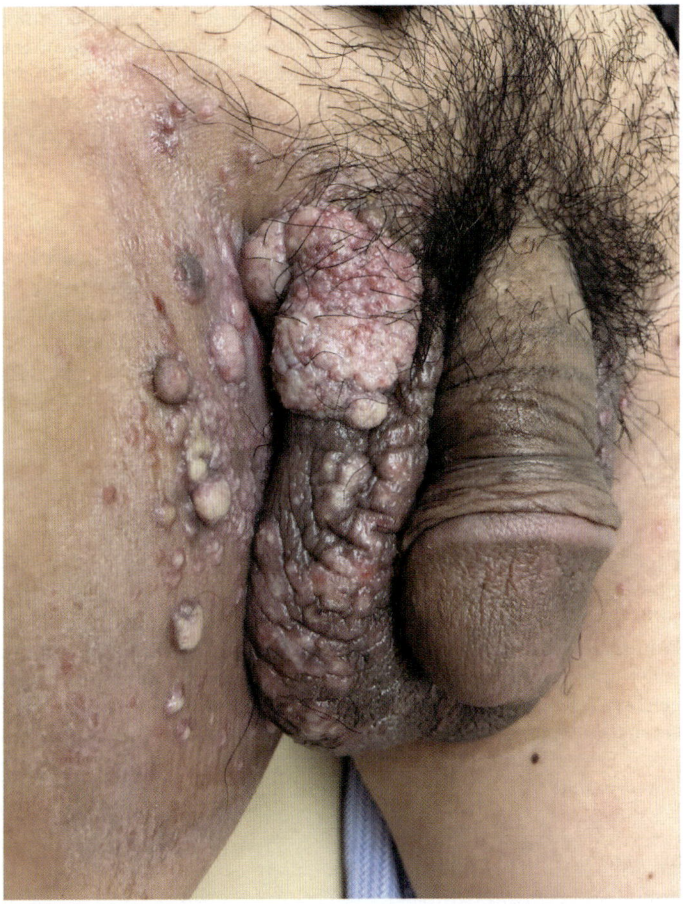

FIGURE 62-4. White, moist-appearing, verrucous papules and nodules that are typical of condyloma lata. (Reproduced with permission from Walkty A, Shute L, Hamza S, Embil JM. Condyloma lata. *IDCases*. 2021;26:e01321.)

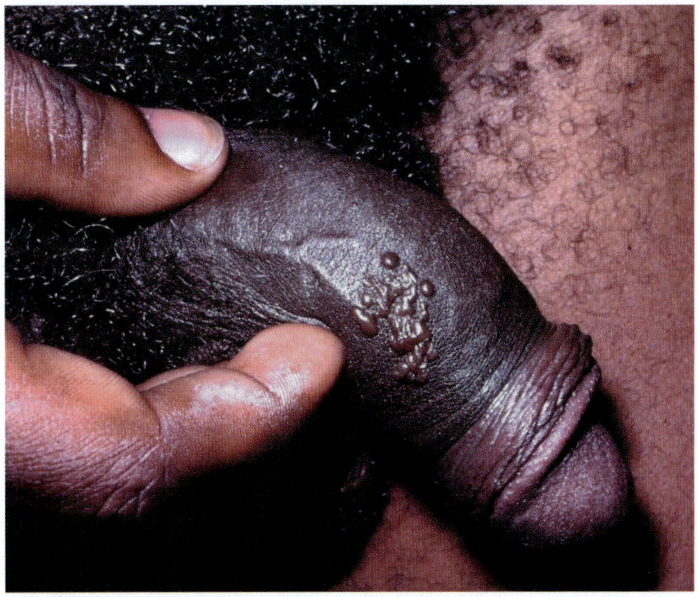

FIGURE 62-5. Genital herpes simplex virus (HSV). Notice the clustered vesicles on the shaft of the penis but background erythematous base is not readily apparent.

In patients who may be reinfected with syphilis, RPR titers may remain elevated. In patients being treated for syphilis, Jarisch-Herxheimer reactions can occur and should not be confused for a penicillin allergy. HIV coinfection rates with syphilis may be as high as 25% among MSM. This should prompt screening for HIV in patients who test positive for syphilis and discussion of preexposure prophylaxis for HIV.

Genital Herpes

What's New? HSV-1 now represents an increasing proportion of genital HSV in the United States.[4]

Background Genital herpes is caused by the herpes simplex virus (HSV), which has two serotypes: HSV-1 and HSV-2, with the former representing one-half of new cases.[4] Black, non-Hispanic, populations have a three- to fourfold increased risk/prevalence of HSV compared to their White counterparts and are more likely to go undiagnosed with HSV-2 infection.

HSV transmission occurs through direct contact with a skin lesion.[4] After infection, primary HSV infection can cause severe mucositis and systemic symptoms including fevers, chills, and myalgias. Subsequent reactivation of HSV leads to the development of genital lesions. In this phase, a person might experience prodrome symptoms, such as tingling or pain at the site of infection. Vesicles that rupture, ulcerate, and reepithelialize commonly occur at the site of inoculation. An outbreak can last 2 weeks with subsequent outbreaks generally being milder and less frequent. HSV persists for life in the latent phase, where it absconds in the peripheral nerves. Upon proper stimulation, HSV is reactivated and travels up neuronal axons, manifesting on the skin or mucosa.[4]

Making the Diagnosis While often a clinical diagnosis, active lesions can be swabbed and diagnosed by PCR testing, which has over 95% sensitivity and specificity.[4] Serologic screening for HSV should be discouraged in most cases as HSV prevalence is very high and the sensitivity and specificity of serologies are low. Importantly, the clinical utility of a positive serologic test is difficult to interpret in the absence of HSV vesicular outbreaks.

What to Look for Clinically? Genital herpes manifests as a cluster of vesicles on an erythematous base in or around the genitals, perineum, buttocks, thighs, or perianal regions.[4] As previously mentioned, erythema may be difficult to appreciate in darker skin [**Figure 62-5**]. Vesicles may erode leaving an ulcer that may demonstrate a scalloped border. Unlike the chancre of primary syphilis, HSV is often painful.

Differential Diagnosis Syphilis, chancroid, herpes zoster, CMV (cytomegalovirus)/EBV (Epstein-Barr virus), Behcet's disease, erosive lichen planus, squamous cell carcinoma, monkeypox/mpox, contact dermatitis.

What is the Treatment? There is no cure for genital herpes, although studies are on-going using CRISPR (clustered regularly interspaced short palindromic repeats) technology to excise latent HSV viral DNA.[5] Nucleoside analogs such as famciclovir, acyclovir, and valacyclovir are approved and well-tolerated antiretroviral therapies.[4] The treatment regimen is based on the frequency of outbreaks and immunosuppression.

Additional Considerations Roughly 65% to 90% of patients are unaware of their genital HSV infection.[4] HSV can spread via asymptomatic shedding, which is more common in the first year of infection and is an important component of counselling patients.

Genital Warts

What's New? Human papillomavirus (HPV) vaccine (Gardasil-9®) is FDA approved for people up to 45 years of age and is protective against 9 strains of HPV. Consider HPV vaccination in patients older than 26 who may be at risk for contracting HPV.

Background Genital warts, also known as condyloma acuminatum, is the most common STI and is caused by HPV.[6] Most infected individuals are between the ages of 15 and 24 years. HPV is ubiquitous with over 180 different strains and is transmitted by skin-to-skin contact. HPV types 6 and 11 are the most common cause of anogenital warts and are considered low-risk strains, although malignant transformation can occur. A history of anogenital warts is associated with penile squamous cell carcinoma, which may be due to coinfection with high-risk HPV strains. Anal HPV and resulting dysplasias are more prevalent among Black men who have sex with men.[7] As with other STIs, the disparity may be a result of poor sexual education programs, which have been shown to impact condom use and highlight the need for reliable sexual health programs for MSM, especially in SOC.[8]

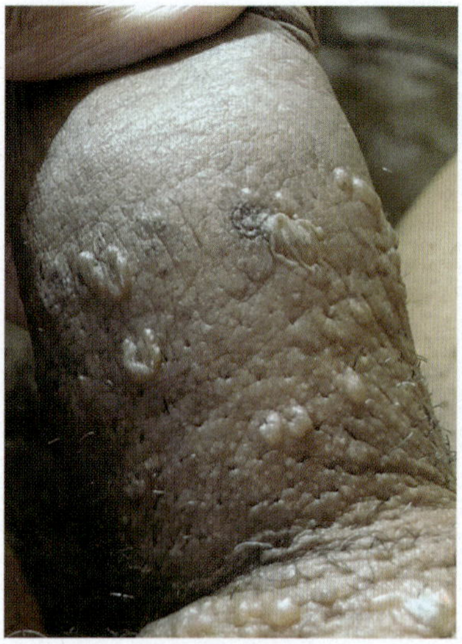

FIGURE 62-6. Condyloma acuminatum, also known as genital warts, are verrucous papules that can present with multiple, clustered lesions on the genitals. (Reproduced with permission from Moore AY, Hurley K, Moore S, Moore L. Topical tirbanibulin resolves recalcitrant condyloma acuminata: Retrospective case series. *JAAD Case Rep.* 2023(4)26;37:58-60.)

Making the Diagnosis Diagnosis of genital warts is clinical; however, a biopsy might be necessary for immunocompromised patients, refractory, or growing lesions.

What to Look for Clinically? Genital warts appear flesh-colored, pink, or hyperpigmented and have a filiform to mammillated texture that range in size and can present after weeks to years after inoculation [**Figure 62-6**].[6] Lesions are typically localized to the anogenital areas.

Differential Diagnosis Condyloma lata, pearly penile papules, skin tag, molluscum contagiosum, Bowenoid papulosis, Bowen disease, squamous cell carcinoma.

What is the Treatment? There is no cure for HPV, and treatment includes immunologic activation with agents such as imiquimod or destructive therapies such as cryotherapy or electrodessication. About 30% of genital warts self-resolve within a few months.[6] Asymptomatic HPV infections are transmissible, and there is conflicting data regarding condoms as infection prevention. Genital warts are likely to recur. Early prevention with HPV vaccination is best done prior to sexual debut.

Additional Considerations Local disfigurement is the most common complication associated with genital warts. In SOC, destructive therapies such as cryotherapy can lead to pigmentary alterations.[6] If patients have periurethral lesions, cystoscopy should be considered. Similarly, anal lesions should prompt anoscopy. Data regarding the utility of anal PAP smears in MSM with HIV have demonstrated a positive effect in treating high-grade lesions.

Bowenoid Papulosis

Background Bowenoid papulosis (BP) is an intraepithelial neoplasia caused by high-risk strains of HPV. It typically effects young, sexually active individuals. The exact prevalence is unknown. BP has been shown to progress to Bowen disease or squamous cell carcinoma in situ in about 1% of cases.

Making the Diagnosis Clinical suspicion of BP must remain high as it often resembles genital warts. Histopathology is diagnostic.

What to Look for Clinically? Look for multiple well-demarcated red to brown, flat to verrucous papules [**Figure 62-7**]. BP is mostly seen on the shaft of the penis but can occur anywhere in the perineal area.

Differential Diagnosis Condyloma lata, melanocytic nevi, mucosal/penile lentigines, skin tag, molluscum contagiosum, condyloma acuminatum, Bowen disease, squamous cell carcinoma.

What is the Treatment? Lesions of BP may regress over the course of a year. However, treatment involves destructive modalities including cryotherapy, electrocoagulation, excision, or carbon dioxide laser. Topical therapies such as imiquimod and 5-fluorouracil have also been used with success.

Additional Considerations Similar to condyloma acuminata, patients with BP who have anal lesions should be evaluated by gastroenterology to assess for internal involvement. Anal pap smears are currently under investigation for clinical utility.

Molluscum Contagiosum

What's New? Berdazimer gel is a novel therapeutic that resulted in 34% clearance of molluscum contagiosum in children at 12 weeks and is an emerging therapeutic option.[9]

Background Molluscum contagiosum (MC) is a self-limited viral infection transmitted by direct or indirect contact.[10] MC infects the epidermis and has an incubation time ranging from 2 to 6 weeks. MC occurs worldwide, but it is more common in warm and humid regions. While mostly seen in children, immunocompromised patients are at risk with prevalence of MC reaching up to 20% in HIV-positive individuals.[10]

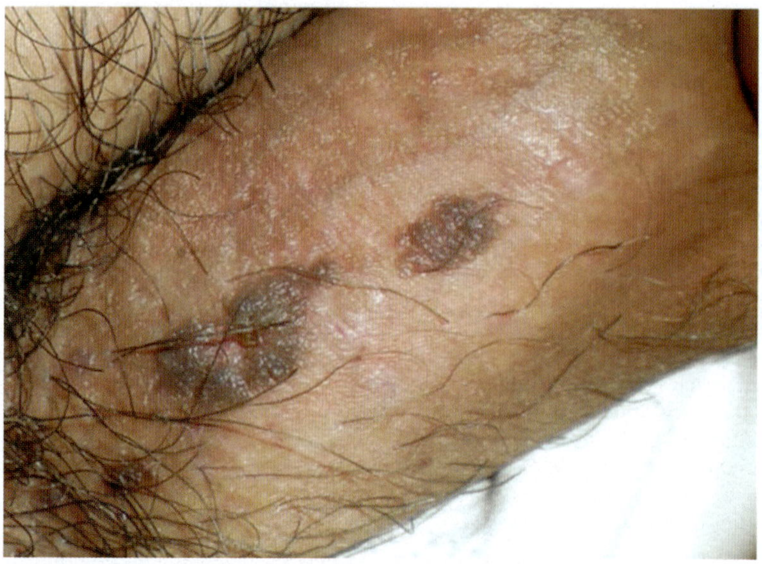

FIGURE 62-7. Bowenoid papulosis. High-risk HPV leading to development of red to brown verrucous papules. (Reproduced with permission from Baykal, C., Yazganoğlu, K.D. Epidermal Precancerous Lesions and In Situ Malignancies. In: Clinical Atlas of Skin Tumors. Springer, Berlin, Heidelberg. (2014). Fig. 2.27.)

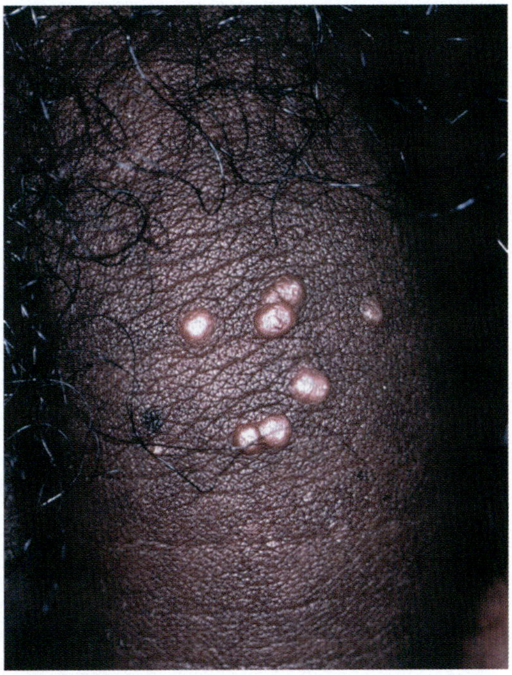

FIGURE 62-8. Molluscum contagiosum. The yellow-pink, umbilicated papules characteristic of MC can be transmitted sexually and seen on the genitals.

Making the Diagnosis Diagnosis is clinical, with or without the aid of dermoscopy. A biopsy is diagnostic.

What to Look for Clinically? MC presents as yellow-pink or flesh-colored, shiny, dome-shaped, umbilicated papules that are generally asymptomatic but can be associated with pruritus [**Figure 62-8**].[10] Dermoscopy may demonstrate central umbilication with round to lobulated white structures centrally that correspond to viral inclusions.

Differential Diagnosis Condyloma acuminatum, condyloma lata, pearly penile papules, epidermal inclusion cysts, median raphe cysts, Fordyce spots/sebaceous glands, syringomas, basal cell carcinoma.

What is the Treatment? MC is self-limited but may last up to 4 years. Treatment is not necessary but may be performed for extensive disease, prevention of autoinoculation or transmission to partners, or aesthetic complaints. Cryotherapy, curettage, or cantharidine are all effective treatments. In a study on children (47% with atopic dermatitis), active treatment does not improve the resolution rate compared to monitoring alone. [10] However, in adults, treatment as outlined above is recommended.

Additional considerations In HIV-positive or other immunocompromised individuals, MC might be extensive, large (giant MC), and refractory to treatment. In patients with atopic dermatitis, eczematous plaques may develop around MC lesions, leading to molluscum dermatitis.

NON-SEXUALLY TRANSMITTED INFECTIONS

Tinea Cruris

Background Tinea cruris, commonly known as "jock itch," is a fungal infection that affects the inguinal and perineal skin. *Trichophyton rubrum* is the most common causative agent of tinea cruris worldwide.[11] Roughly 20% to 25% of the world's population is affected by tinea cruris, with developing and tropical countries having a higher prevalence.

Making the Diagnosis For most cases, diagnosis is clinical, but a potassium hydroxide preparation (KOH) or fungal culture can be diagnostic.[11] Biopsy is rarely needed.

What to Look for Clinically? Tine cruris will appear as an erythematous, scaly, annular plaque with a raised leading edge and central clearing. Patients with darker skin might present with hyperpigmentation instead of erythema and scaling may be absent [**Figure 62-9**]. The eruption is often very pruritic and chronic infection may lead to a lichenified appearance. The penile shaft and scrotum are generally spared.

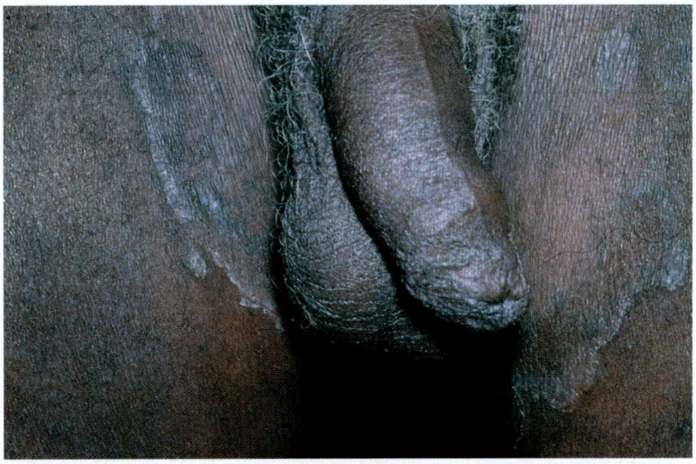

FIGURE 62-9. Tinea cruris demonstrates the classic annular appearance with central clearing. Notice how it typically spares the penis and scrotum.

Differential Diagnosis Inverse psoriasis, candidal intertrigo, irritant/allergic contact dermatitis, acanthosis nigricans, erythema annular centrifugum.

What is the Treatment? Topical antifungal agents such as the azoles applied one to two times daily for 2 weeks are effective in treating tinea cruris. For deep or refractory cases, oral antifungal agents such as fluconazole or itraconazole may be used. Importantly, autoinoculation can occur when dermatophytes spread from the feet to the groin and recurrence is common unless the feet are also treated.

Additional Considerations Misdiagnosis of tinea cruris and application of topical corticosteroid can allow dermatophytes to spread into hair follicles and subcutaneous tissue, causing Majocchi granuloma, a deep inflammatory disease that requires systemic antifungal treatment.[11] Immunosuppression and skin breakdown increases the risk of developing Majocchi granuloma. Emerging tinea infections that may be spread sexually have been described among MSM and may be refractory to topical therapy alone.

Scabies

What's New? Moxidectin, a novel macrolide, is being studied as a single-dose treatment for scabies.[12]

Background Scabies, caused by *Sarcoptes scabiei*, are human parasitic mites that infest the stratum corneum. A single pregnant mite is sufficient to infect another human host, and transmission typically occurs via direct skin-to-skin contact of at least 5 to 10 minutes. Transmission is more likely in communal living or in densely populated areas. Brief contact, such as handshaking, is not usually sufficient to transmit scabies. Mites can survive without a host for 24 to 36 hours making indirect transmission possible. Patients may be unaware of infection for up to 6 weeks.[12]

Making the Diagnosis Diagnosis can be made using physical exam, history, or direct observation. A skin scraping or biopsy may directly observe mites, eggs, or feces (scabala). History of close contact with scabies may also suggest the diagnosis. Dermoscopy can aid diagnosis, but detecting a burrow, mite, eggs, or scabala can be difficult due to secondary changes caused by scratching, crusting, or infection, especially in patients with SOC.[12]

What to Look for Clinically? Manifestations include a characteristic whitish, 3 to 7 mm "J" shaped burrows with an associated papular or papulovesilcular pruritic eruption [**Figure 62-10**].[12] In dark skin, papules may appear brown or hyperpigmented. Regions with thin stratum corneum and low density of sebaceous glands, such as the penis and scrotum, are prone to scabietic infestation.[12] Nodules are more likely to occur on the penis and scrotum, as well as the inguinal and perianal areas [**Figure 62-11**]. Webbed spaces of the digits, axillae, and umbilicus are commonly affected body areas.

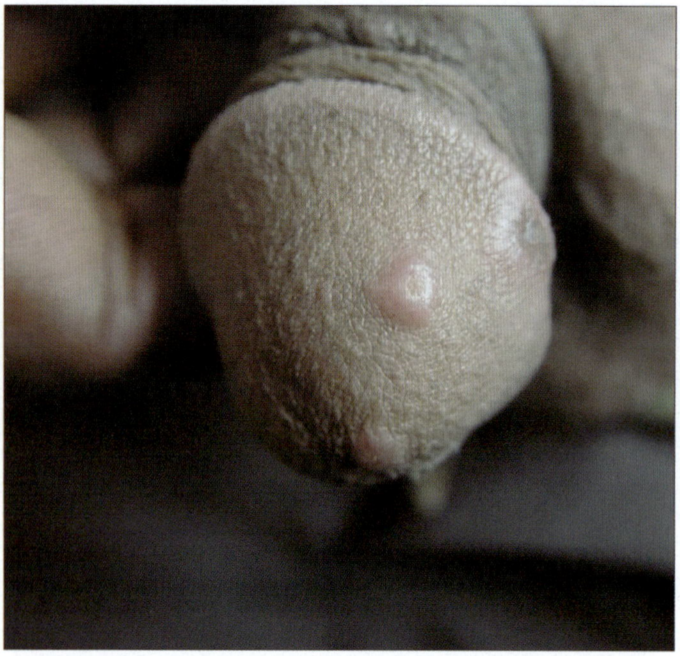

FIGURE 62-10. Pink papules with slight curvature on the head of the penis are signs of scabies. (Reproduced with permission from Mittal A, Garg A, Agarwal N, Gupta L, Khare AK. Treatment of nodular scabies with topical tacrolimus. *Indian Dermatol Online J.* 2013;4(1):52-53.)

Differential Diagnosis Atopic dermatitis, irritant/allergic contact dermatitis, pruritus, papular urticaria, other arthropod assault, prurigo nodularis, folliculitis, delusions of parasitosis, neurotic excoriations, urticarial phase of bullous pemphigoid.

What is the Treatment? Two doses of oral or topical acaricidal or ovicidal medications, such as permethrin 5% cream or ivermectin (200 μg/kg/dose) spaced 1 week apart is typically used. Close contacts should also be treated. In nodular scabies, nodules might persist months after treatment.[12]

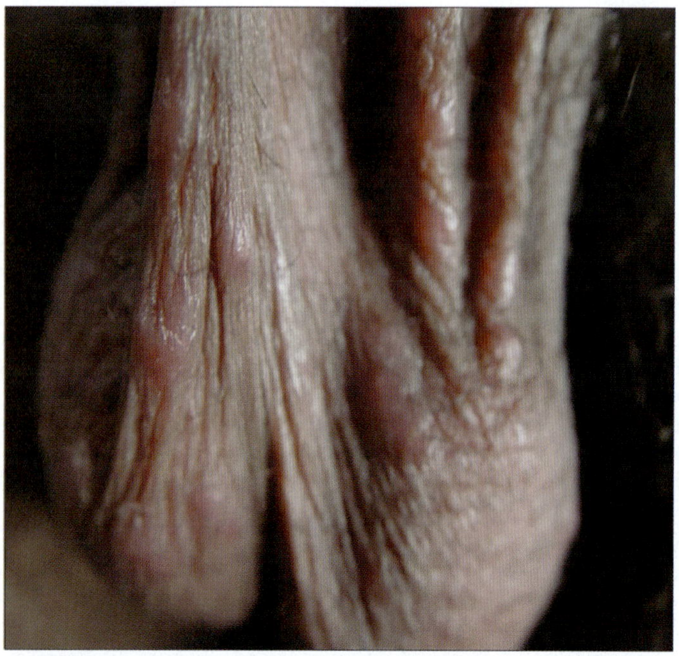

FIGURE 62-11. Papulonodules on the scrotum are a sign of scabies. (Reproduced with permission from Mittal A, Garg A, Agarwal N, Gupta L, Khare AK. Treatment of nodular scabies with topical tacrolimus. *Indian Dermatol Online J.* 2013;4(1):52-53.)

Additional Considerations In immunocompromised persons, the number of scabies present on the skin can reach millions, leading to Norwegian or crusted scabies.[12] In patients with crusted scabies, transmission is more likely to occur after brief contact and indirect transmission is also more likely. Scabies nodules (postscabietic papules) and pruritus (postscabietic itch) can persist for weeks to months after successful treatment and should not be confused for treatment failure.

MULTISYSTEM DISEASES

NONMALIGNANT

Behcet's Disease

What's New? In a double blind controlled study, apremilast was shown to improve the ulcerations caused by Behcet's disease (BD) and may be a forthcoming treatment option.[13] Alemtuzumab, a humanized monoclonal CD52 antibody, is a promising new therapy. [14]

Background BD is a systemic inflammatory disorder of unknown etiology that manifests as recurrent and unpredictable oropharyngeal and genital ulcers.[13] The development of BD involves aspects of the innate, adaptive, and environmental immunity, which leads to an overexpression of proinflammatory cytokines. BD may be hereditary, is more common in male ages 20 to 30 years, and found in those of Japanese and Mediterranean decent. Rates of BD are lower in Japanese and Turkish immigrants living in the United States and Germany, suggesting an environmental component. Herpes simplex and *Streptococcus sanguinis* have been proposed as mediating extrinsic factors.[13] The onset of BD at an early age is typically associated with a worse prognosis.

Making the Diagnosis BD is a diagnosis of exclusion, with varying diagnostic criteria. The International Study Group diagnostic criteria for BD includes recurrent oral ulcerations and two of the following: recurrent genital ulcers, ocular lesions, cutaneous lesions, or positive pathergy test.[15] HLA-B51 haplotype is strongly associated with BD and commercial testing is now available.

What to Look for Clinically? BD manifests as well-defined, painful, genital and/or oropharyngeal ulcers. Lesions are recurrent and typically located on the scrotum but may present on the glans and foreskin. Genital ulcers may scar. Other systemic signs include uveitis, neurological impairment, deep vein thrombosis, arthritis, and gastrointestinal symptoms.[13]

Differential Diagnosis Syphilitic chancre, HSV, chancroid, aphthous stomatitis, pemphigus vulgaris, mucous membrane pemphigoid, systemic lupus erythematosus, lichen planus, lichen sclerosus, monkeypox/mpox.

What is the Treatment? Mucosal hygiene is essential as BD exhibits pathergy. For mild disease, topical low to mid-potency corticosteroids and/or calcineurin inhibitors are first line. Colchicine and dapsone systemic therapy may be added to topical therapy. For severe or refractory disease, systemic corticosteroids, azathioprine, or methotrexate may be used.[13]

Additional Considerations As a diagnosis of exclusion, there is often a significant delay in diagnosis of BD and patients are often frustrated with their disease state. Scarring and dyspigmentation from ulcerations in the genitals can add to patient frustration. A multi-disciplinary team is imperative in patients with BD.

MALIGNANT

Squamous Cell Carcinoma

What's New? Mutations in CASP8 and FBX7 are frequently found in penile squamous cell carcinomas.[16]

Background Although rare, penile squamous cell carcinoma (pSCC) accounts for 95% of malignancies of the penis and has high morbidity and mortality rates. Hispanic/Latino and Black males have the highest incidence of pSCC, present with more advanced disease, and have a mortality of 18%.[17] In the United States, Southern states have high incidence, which corresponds to HPV infection rates. Factors such as income level, employment, and health literacy are significantly associated with HPV vaccination rates, ultimately impacting incidence.[18] Prevalence of pSCC increases with age and is highest in low-income countries in South America and Africa.[16]

pSCC is thought to have two modes of pathogenesis: HPV-associated and inflammatory-mediated.[16] HPV-associated pSCC is more common among younger males who are more likely to have additional risk factors such as smoking and multiple sexual partners.[16] The etiopathogenesis of inflammatory-mediated SCC is less well understood but likely results from chronic inflammation that is present in patients with poor hygiene, trauma, or inflammatory diseases such as lichen sclerosus.[16] Circumcision rates are inversely associated with rates of penile cancer, which may result in decreased inflammatory dermatoses of the penis and limited protection from HPV infection.[17] In addition to higher rates of HPV infection, Black and Latino males have lower rates of circumcision, which may play a role in the disparity of pSCC.

Making the Diagnosis A skin biopsy is diagnostic. Given the rarity of pSCC, a high degree of clinical suspicion must be maintained for nonresolving lesions on the penis. Recent advances in confocal microscopy have shown promise in diagnosing pSCC but is not routinely available.

What to Look for Clinically? pSCC is highly polymorphous and may manifest as an area of erythema, a nonhealing ulceration [**Figure 62-12**], a persistent papule or nodule, or a growing verrucous lesion [**Figure 62-13**]. Associated symptoms can include pruritus, bleeding, discharge, malodor, and tenderness. HPV-associated SCC typically presents with wart-like features.

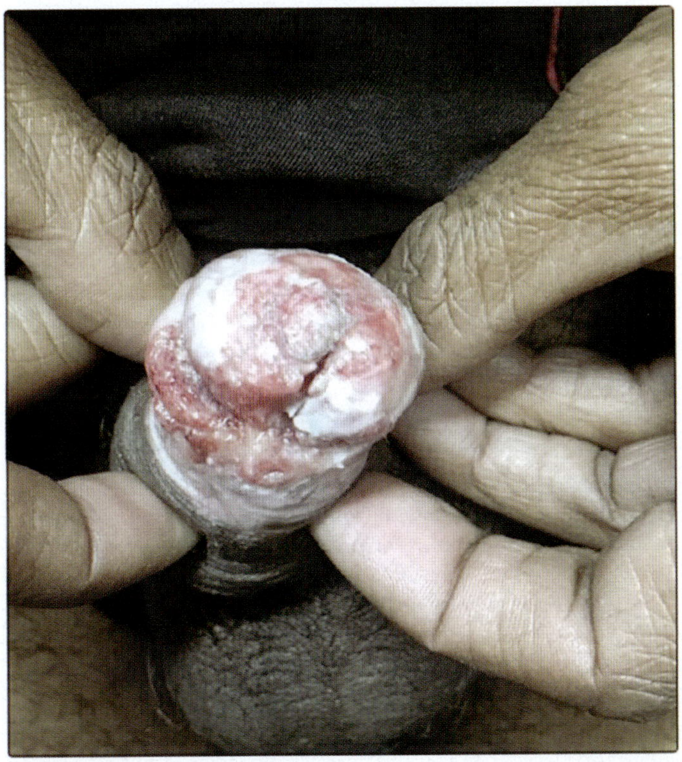

FIGURE 62-12. Penile squamous cell carcinoma may present with many morphologies, including erythema, ulceration, or nonhealing wound. The lower panel demonstrates a higher power of an ulceration in this patient. (Reproduced with permission from Sinha P, Ayub A, Madakshira MG, Praveen L, Bhattacharjee S, Alok K. Donovanosis or Squamous Cell Carcinoma of Penis: Can Dermoscopy Solve this Enigma? *Indian J Dermatol.* 2022 Nov-Dec;67(6):807-810.)

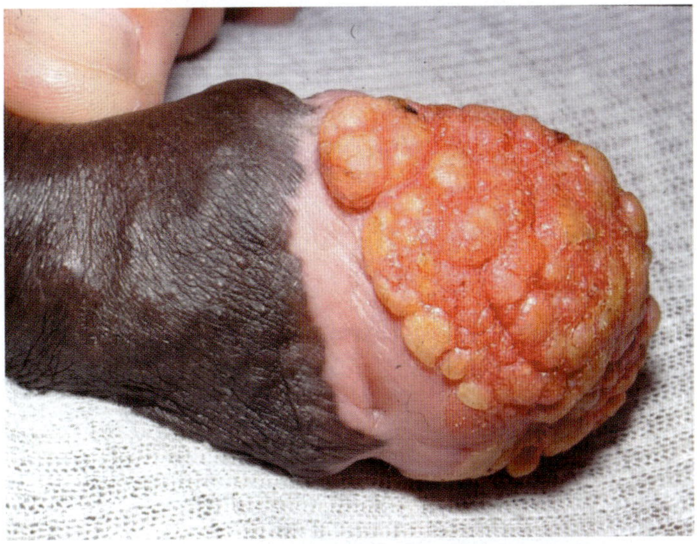

FIGURE 62-13. Verrucous penile squamous cell carcinoma that required a partial penectomy.

Differential Diagnosis Condyloma acuminatum, Bowenoid papulosis, condyloma lata, trauma, lichen sclerosus, lichen planus, psoriasis, contact dermatitis, prurigo nodularis, Behcet disease.

What is the Treatment? Treatment of pSCC involves removal of the lesion while preserving function and cosmesis.[19] Treatment options depend on stage of the tumor. For in situ lesions, treatments include curettage and electrodesiccation, cryosurgery, topical 5-fluorouracil, and photodynamic therapy.[19] For locally invasive lesions, Mohs surgery may be considered versus surgical excision, with cure rates of greater than 90%.[19]

The diagnosis of pSCC is often delayed and many patients present with metastatic disease, which requires systemic therapy. Hispanic/Latino males are more likely to present with high-risk SCC and undergo penectomy rather than Mohs.[20] Black males are less likely to pursue any surgical intervention and therefore tend to have higher mortality rates.[20] Radiation therapy is an alternative for patients who forego surgery but is associated with lower cure rates and a high likelihood of recurrence.[19]

Additional Considerations Immunocompromised individuals such as organ transplant recipients and patients with HIV have a higher risk of developing SCC. In these patient populations, SCC may metastasize to the lymph nodes, lungs, bones, and brain, leading to death.[19] Cemiplimab, an immune checkpoint inhibitor, is approved in the United States for systemic therapy of metastatic SCC. In patients who present with invasive pSCC, imaging of the pelvis should be performed to evaluate for nodal metastasis.

INFLAMMATORY DISEASES

EXOGENOUS

Lichen Simplex Chronicus

Background Lichen simplex chronicus (LSC) is a form of chronic neurodermatitis that is characterized by lichenification due to repeated scratching. Pruritus is a proximal feature, which triggers an itch-scratch cycle. LSC can also be secondary to other dermatoses such as atopic dermatitis, contact dermatitis, and stasis dermatitis. Black patients with HIV may be predisposed to pruritic disease due to skewed Th2-mediated cytokine profiles leading to a higher prevalence of LSC.[21]

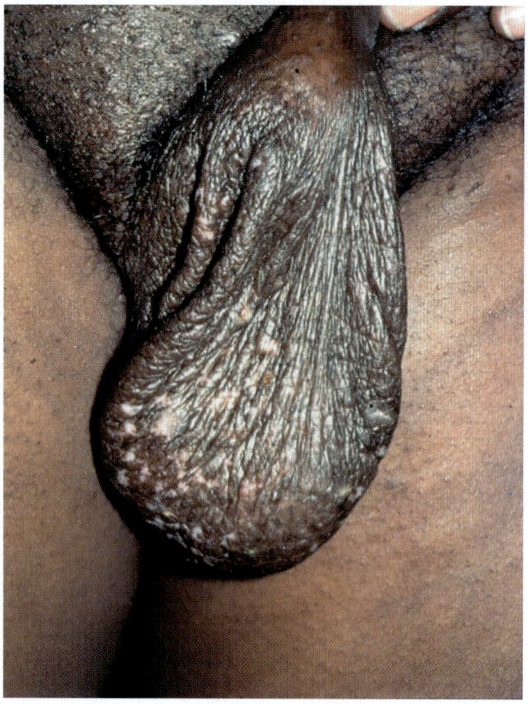

FIGURE 62-14. Lichen simplex chronicus represented as hypertrophic and thickened skin on the scrotum from chronic scratching. Notice hyperpigmentation in this case.

Primary disease can also result from psychological stressors that produce an itch-scratch cycle.

Making the Diagnosis Diagnosis is clinical but steps to evaluate for a primary dermatosis leading to secondary LSC might include patch testing, skin scrapings/KOH prep, and a total body skin exam to evaluate for signs of other dermatoses.

What to Look for Clinically? The epidermis appears hypertrophic with accentuation of the skin lines. Plaques are often scaly and may demonstrate excoriations or prurigo nodules.[22] Color ranges from pink to brown and is often hyperpigmented in darker skin [**Figure 62-14**]. In the groin, LSC is common on the scrotum, where the moist environment may lead to a white and wrinkled rather than thick and scaly appearance.

Differential Diagnosis Allergic/irritant contact dermatitis, inverse psoriasis, prurigo nodularis, tinea cruris, atopic dermatitis, intertrigo, scabies, lichen planus.

What is the Treatment? Scratching cessation is essential with use of barriers and cognitive behavioral therapy being necessary for successful treatment.[22] Other treatments include topical anti-inflammatory medications such as corticosteroids, calcineurin inhibitors, and oral antihistamines. Use of a higher-potency topical corticosteroids, even in the groin, may be necessary to break the itch-scratch cycle. In severe cases, intralesional triamcinolone injection is helpful. For secondary LSC, treatment of the primary dermatitis is needed. Products for sensitive skin are encouraged. New therapies targeting IL-31 and the itch-scratch neurogenic component of this condition may prove useful.

Additional Considerations Super-infection of LSC is common and should be considered in refractory disease. Repeated scratching may also cause scarring and disfigurement.

Contact Dermatitis

Background Contact dermatitis (CD) is a common inflammatory skin disease that is divided into irritant contact dermatitis (ICD) and allergic dermatitis (ACD). ACD is a delayed hypersensitivity reaction due to exposure to allergens, such as poison ivy, which is the most common cause of ACD in the United States and is commonly transferred to genitals from the hands.[23] Other common allergens include nickel, fragrance, and topical neomycin. ICD results from direct damage to the skin barrier, which causes an inflammatory response.

ACD of the genitals can result from exposure to substances such as lubricants, latex, products that delay ejaculation (benzocaine), fragrances, and topical antimicrobials.[24] Rare reports of ACD to seminal fluid have been reported. ICD is common in the groin due to the moist, occlusive environment, and exposure to irritants such as urine, sweat, and stool.[24]

Making the Diagnosis Diagnosis is made clinically with a detailed history. Providers should ascertain exposures and risk factors such as occupation, hobbies, medications, and sexual history. A sexual history should include type of sexual activity (vaginal, anal, oral) and use of protection (latex condoms, spermicidal lubricants, etc). Patch testing can identify causative agents in ACD but a positive patch test can be missed in patients with SOC.[25] Cultural practices and exposures likely result in racial differences in allergen sensitivity. Black patients have been found to have higher rates of ACD to paraphenylenediamine (found in dyes) and imidazolidinyl urea, which is a formaldehyde releaser used in cosmetic products.[25]

What to Look for Clinically? CD manifests with erythema and edema and can be associated with crusting, vesicles, pustules, and tenderness. In SOC, lesions might appear hyperpigmented. Subacute and chronic manifestations are associated with hyperpigmentation and lichenification, respectively. Pruritus is common.[24] Occluded areas are classically spared in CD; however, in adult patients this is not reliable as contactants may be deliberately applied.

Differential Diagnosis Psoriasis, atopic dermatitis, LSC, scabies, lichen sclerosus, lichen planus, fixed drug eruption, lymphedema.

What is the Treatment? Removal of the causative agent is the most important step in treatment, followed by skin barrier protection and optimization. For interval control, treatment with low to mid-potency topical corticosteroids or calcineurin inhibitors is appropriate. Antihistamines may alleviate pruritus. In severe cases, systemic corticosteroids may be necessary.

Additional Considerations Contactants may be spread to the genitals from the hands and review of products applied to areas other than the genitals should be evaluated. In uncircumcised men, CD is more common as the nonkeratinized skin under the prepuce may be less resistant to allergens/irritants. For patients in whom dermatitis correlates to sexual activity, consider postcoital cleansing routines as rinsing the genitals after sexual activity may remove potential irritants such as saliva, vaginal secretions, or feces. Pant zippers or jewelry applied to the genitals may contain nickel and cause ACD.

INFLAMMATORY

Lichen Sclerosus

What's New? Fat grafting, adipose-derived stem cells, and platelet-rich plasma therapies are novel regenerative treatment options.[26]

Background Lichen sclerosis (LS), also known, in men, as balanitis xerotica obliterans (BXO) is chronic inflammatory disease that presents on the anogenital region of unknown etiology. LS is associated with other autoimmune diseases such as alopecia areata and vitiligo. The exact prevalence is unknown, which is likely due to underreporting and misdiagnosis.[27]

Making the Diagnosis Diagnosis is made clinically and may be confirmed with a skin biopsy.

What to Look for Clinically? Hypopigmentation and atrophy are characteristic features of LS. Lesions typically develop as thin, erythematous plaques that develop an ivory to porcelain appearance and can demonstrate a cigarette paper scale.[27] Follicular plugging, fissures, purpura, and ulcerations might also be present. Associated symptoms typically include pruritus, burning, and painful urination and/or bowel movements. In males, LS is commonly found on the foreskin, glans penis, and coronal sulcus penis.[27]

Differential Diagnosis Contact dermatitis, psoriasis, atopic dermatitis, LSC, vitiligo, squamous cell carcinoma, Zoon balanitis.

What is the Treatment? First-line therapy is high-potency topical corticosteroids daily for 4 weeks.[27] Maintenance therapy is often needed and may involve intermittent topical corticosteroids or topical calcineurin inhibitors such as tacrolimus ointment. Phototherapy has been used with success. For refractory cases, use of steroid sparing systemic agents such as methotrexate and azathioprine have been reported. Circumcision is curative and has historically been used to treat LS but is now reserved for only the most severe cases.[27]

Additional Considerations Scarring from LS can lead to anatomical changes and functional impairment including phimosis, which is an emergency.[27] LS has an increased risk of SCCs.

Psoriasis

What's New? Ixekizumab is an IL-17A monoclonal antibody inhibitor approved to treat genital psoriasis.[28]

Background Psoriasis is among the most common dermatoses on the genitalia, with up to 63% of psoriatic patients developing genital lesions during their lifetime.[29] Psoriasis generally presents between the ages of 20 to 30 years and 50 to 60 years. About 3.7% of the U.S. population has psoriasis. Rates are lower in patients of color (2.0% Black and 1.6% Hispanic/Latine); however, SOC patients are more likely to have undiagnosed psoriasis[30]. Black patients with psoriasis may present with more severe psoriasis as measured by total body surface area involvement.[31] Structural barriers including cost, insurance status, lower socioeconomic status, and less education may prevent patients of color from seeking medical care, including seeing a dermatologist leading to more severe disease at diagnosis.[32]

Psoriasis pathophysiology is driven by Th1/Th17 immune activation, resulting in keratinocyte proliferation through TNF-α, IL-17, and IL-23 cytokines. Environmental and genetic factors contribute to psoriasis and can be triggered by medications and trauma, including sexual intercourse.

Making the Diagnosis Psoriasis is often diagnosed clinically with a classic distribution and morphology. Dermoscopy may be used adjunctively with dermoscopic features including dotted vessels and tortuous capillaries. Biopsy may be needed in atypical cases.

What to Look for Clinically? Psoriasis manifests as well-demarcated, erythematous plaques on the genitals and inguinal regions [**Figure 62-15**]. Plaques may lack classic scale given the moist environment. Absence of central clearing may help distinguishing psoriasis from tinea. Evaluation of psoriatic areas (gluteal cleft, scalp, ears, elbows, knees, and nails) can be a clue to the diagnosis. In SOC, erythema may manifest in a violaceous tone with more hyperpigmentation.[1]

Differential Diagnosis Tinea cruris, candida intertrigo, contact dermatitis, Zoon balanitis, squamous cell carcinoma, lichen planus, balanitis circinata.

What is the Treatment? First-line therapy for mild to moderate genital psoriasis include low potency topical corticosteroids, topical vitamin D analogs, and topical calcineurin inhibitors. Psoriasis is chronic and likely requires long-term therapy using a nonsteroidal agent. Tapinarof is a novel aryl hydrocarbon receptor inhibitor that can be used in the groin and may have a remittive effect on psoriasis.[33] For refractory disease, systemic therapies may be considered. Ixekizumab is the only biologic specifically approved for the treatment of genital psoriasis.[28] Other biologic agents targeting IL-17 and/or IL-23 pathways are also effective.

Additional Considerations Comorbidities including cardiovascular disease, dyslipidemia, hypertension, insulin resistance, and obesity are associated with severe psoriasis and disproportionately impact communities of color, especially lower income. Stigmatization of psoriasis can cause significant decreases in quality of life and may also play a role in preventing patients from seeking medical care.

Lichen Planus

What's New? Recent studies have explored additional treatment options for lichen planus (LP) including the use of combination therapy with methotrexate and tofacitinib.[34]

Background LP is a T-cell-mediated, autoimmune disease that may result from cytotoxic T-cells reacting to an unknown antigen in the basement membrane causing destruction of basal keratinocytes.[35] It has an estimated incidence of less than 1% of the population, mostly in middle-aged adults. The prevalence of genital LP is unknown; however, genital involvement occurs in up to 19% of patients with oral LP. LP has genetic and environmental triggers and may be caused by certain medications.[35]

Making the Diagnosis LP may be diagnosed clinically but a biopsy may confirm the diagnosis and rule out SCC in more persistent cases. Evaluation of all mucosal surfaces, particularly in erosive types of LP, is essential.

What to Look for Clinically? LP can have many morphologies in the genitals. Classic LP manifests as small flat-topped, polygonal, violaceous papules. The papules may demonstrate superficial white interlacing lines, known as "Wickham striae." Classic LP is not common on the genitals without involvement of other body surfaces. Annular LP is common on the genitals and demonstrates the classic purple color but with central clearing [**Figure 62-16**]. Genital-only LP most commonly

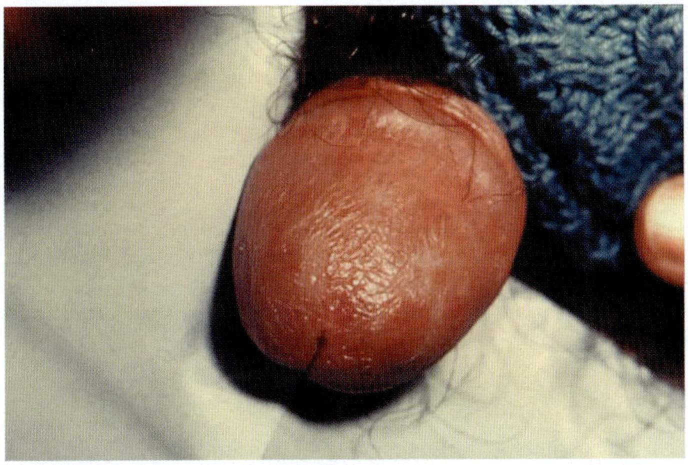

FIGURE 62-15. Psoriasis. Well-circumscribed erythema lacking characteristic scale. (Reproduced with permission from Hill B. Public Health image library. Center for Disease Control and Prevention. 1976. https://phil.cdc.gov/Details.aspx?pid=4052. Accessed August 8, 2023.)

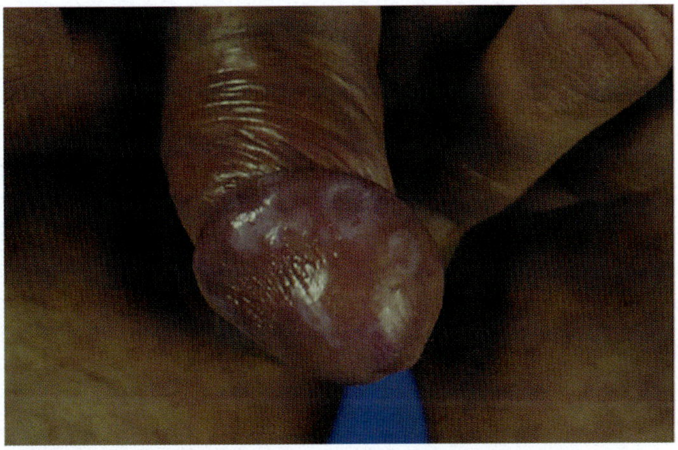

FIGURE 62-16. Annular lichen planus. The purple, flat topped papules in an annular shape suggest a diagnosis of annular lichen planus. (Reproduced with permission from Wagner G, Rose C, Sachse MM. Clinical variants of lichen planus. *J Dtsch Dermatol Ges.* 2013;11(4):309-319.)

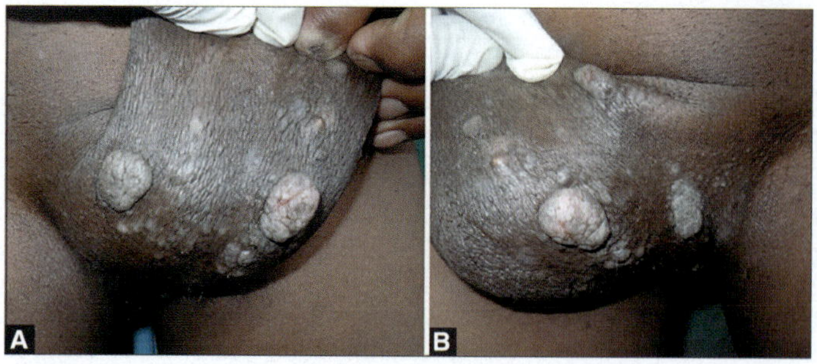

FIGURE 62-17. Hypertrophic lichen planus on **(A)** right side and **(B)** left side of the scrotum can be verrucous and confused for genital warts. (Reproduced with permission from Gayen T, Das A, Shome K, Bandyopadhyay D. Colocalization of lichen planus hypertrophicus and epidermal inclusion cyst: an incident unreported hitherto. *Indian J Dermatol.* 2015;60(5):503-505.)

presents as purple, reticular patches that become white, commonly on the glans penis. Hypertrophic LP may present on the scrotum and can be confused for genital warts or prurigo nodules [**Figure 62-17**]. Erosive LP can occur on the penis, although is much rarer than in female populations. In darker skinned patients, these lesions are highly susceptible to residual pigmentation.

Differential Diagnosis Psoriasis, lichen sclerosus, contact dermatitis, balanitis circinata, Kaposi sarcoma, fixed drug eruption, angiokeratomas.

What is the Treatment? In many cases, LP may remit after several years and treatment is mostly supportive. First-line treatment involves low to mid potency topical corticosteroids. Systemic therapies are rarely needed but include oral corticosteroids (1-2 mg/kg tapered over several weeks), hydroxychloroquine (200-400 mg daily), acitretin (10-30 mg/day), methotrexate (5-25 mg weekly), azathioprine (50-100 mg daily), mycophenolate mofetil (500-1000 mg twice daily), and more recently, JAK inhibitors. In cases of drug-induced LP, cessation of culprit drug will often lead to resolution of the LP.

Additional Considerations LP exhibits the Koebner phenomenon with irritation or friction provoking LP in the groin. There is an association of LP with Hepatitis C, and screening should be considered. Cases of SCC arising within long-standing lesions of LP have been reported.

Zoon's Balanitis

What's New? A recent study suggests that topical cyclosporine 5% cream can be a viable treatment option for Zoon balanitis (ZB) resistant to other treatment modalities.[36]

Background ZB is an underdiagnosed plasma cell-mediated inflammatory process, often associated with middle-aged men who are uncircumcised. The etiology of ZB is unknown. Poor hygiene is thought to relate to its occurrence.[37]

Making the Diagnosis Zoon is diagnosed histologically.

What to Look for Clinically? ZB is a benign inflammatory dermatosis typically found on the glans penis and opposing prepuce.[37] Lesions appear as painless, well-demarcated patches to thin plaques, often appearing red or orange-brown. Ulceration and necrosis may occur in severe cases [**Figure 62-18**].

Differential Diagnosis Psoriasis, contact dermatitis, lichen sclerosus, squamous cell carcinoma, fixed drug eruption.

What is the Treatment? First-line treatment involves low-potency topical corticosteroids. Topical imiquimod and calcineurin inhibitors have also been used.[37] Careful attention to hygienic practices may also lead to improvement in ZB.

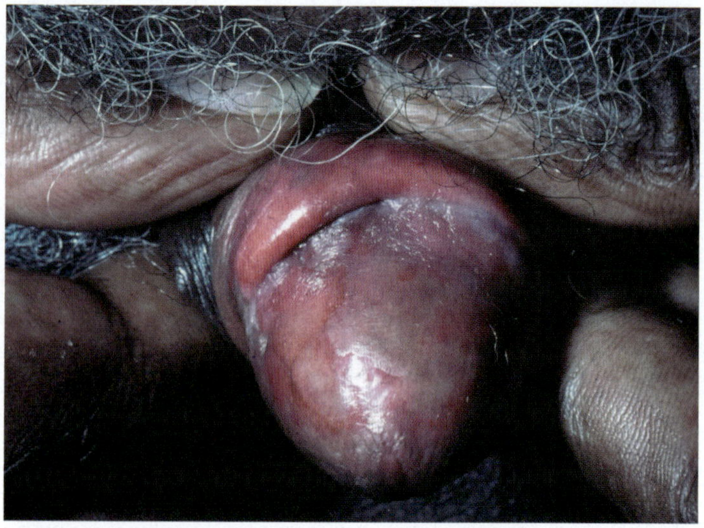

FIGURE 62-18. Zoon's balanitis presents with superficial erosions, often with a pink to orange color.

Additional Considerations There are rare reports of ZB leading to development of SCC.[37]

Intertrigo

What's New? Zinc gluconate-taurine complex containing spray may be a new alternative therapy in intertrigo.[38]

Background Intertrigo is common and affects all races equally. Risk factors include obesity or high BMI (body mass index) and diabetes mellitus, which disproportionately impact historically marginalized communities of color.

Intertrigo results from contact and friction in occluded areas leading to inflammation. Such areas are prone to over colonization by bacteria, fungi, and many *candida species*.[39] Immunocompromised patients are at increased risk of developing intertrigo.

Making the Diagnosis Intertrigo is a clinical diagnosis. Cultures, KOH preparation, and Gram staining can aid in identifying causal organisms. A biopsy may exclude other diagnoses in resistant cases.

What to Look for Clinically? Erythematous to hyperpigmented patches to thin plaques that may have satellite lesions when related to *Candida* infection located in body folds.

Differential Diagnosis Inverse psoriasis, contact dermatitis, tinea cruris.

What is the Treatment? Topical anti-yeast agents such as nystatin powder or azole creams along with skin barrier protection are first-line therapies. Attention to hygiene, nonocclusive clothing, diabetes, and weight management are important for long-term prevention. For very inflamed skin and incidences associated with seborrheic or atopic dermatitis, use of low-potency corticosteroids can help minimize discomfort.[39]

Additional Considerations Intertrigo can be difficult to manage, especially in patients with underlying comorbid conditions and/or pendulous skin. Evaluating patients for hyperhidrosis can be considered. For long-term management, caution should be taken regarding prolonged used of topical corticosteroid leading to skin atrophy.

Hidradenitis Suppurativa

What's New? Recent clinical data indicate that IL-17 modulators may be helpful in hidradenitis suppurativa (HS) treatment.[40]

Background Men have more severe HS and Black Americans have a 2.5 times greater incidence of HS compared to White counterparts.[41,42] There is scarce data regarding prevalence of HS globally but is likely underreported and frequently misdiagnosed. Access to healthcare providers and

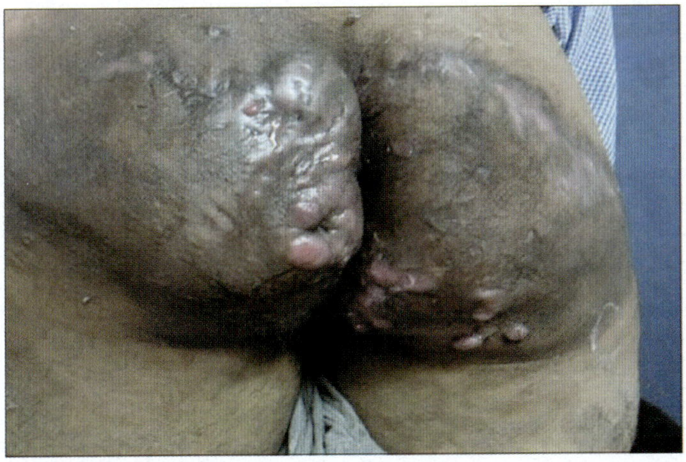

FIGURE 62-19. Hidradenitis suppurativa in skin of color can demonstrate fluctuant nodules, sinus tracts, and significant scarring. (Reproduced with permission from Patil S, Apurwa A, Nadkarni N, Agarwal S, Chaudhari P, Gautam M. Hidradenitis suppurativa: inside and out. *Indian J Dermatol*. 2018;63(2):91-98.)

provider awareness of HS are key components of disparities in HS. HS disease burden negatively impacts quality of life and increases the risk of depression and anxiety.

HS is a disease of follicular occlusion that results in inflammation, abscess formation, and eventual cyst rupture. The inflammatory profile of HS is complex and involves numerous cytokines including IL-1, TNF-α, IL-23, and IL-17.[42]

Making the Diagnosis HS is a chronic disease diagnosed clinically by a relapsing course.[42] The lesions can be staged using the Hurley Staging System.

What to Look for Clinically? Recurrent boil-like lesions that can progress over time to become fistulas and draining sinuses. Scarring can be an important clinical clue to diagnosis and severity of disease [**Figure 62-19**].[42] Lesions can typically be found in intertriginous areas including perineal and inguinal regions. HS in anogenital areas may be associated with a more severe course of the disease, and a higher risk of comorbidities. HS may be seen in association with other diseases of follicular occlusions including dissecting cellulitis, acne conglobata, and pilonidal cyst.[41] In men, lesions generally spare the shaft of the penis, but sinus tracts may develop near the base of the penis and scrotum.

Differential Diagnosis Folliculitis, furuncle/abscess, epidermal inclusion cyst, cutaneous Crohn disease, granuloma inguinale, lymphogranuloma venereum.

What is the Treatment? HS treatment is challenging and requires a multi-modal approach that treats the disease, addresses symptoms, optimizes quality of life, manages expectations, and minimizes progression. Topical antimicrobials such as clindamycin and benzoyl peroxide are first line of treatment. Intralesional corticosteroids are used for isolated lesions. Oral antibiotics such as doxycycline are used for moderate disease. Systemic retinoids may have some benefit, especially in men. In severe cases, immunosuppressants such as corticosteroids and adalimumab can be used. Surgical resection may be appropriate for some patients. Pain management is essential and includes NSAIDs, gabapentin, and topical lidocaine. Lifestyle modifications include weight loss, change in undergarment fabrics, and smoking cessation.

Additional Considerations Patients with long-term HS can develop lymphatic obstruction and scarring from recurrence. Mental health screening and support are recommended in HS patients. Patient and community education may help dispel misconceptions about the disease as well as improve early detection and diagnosis.

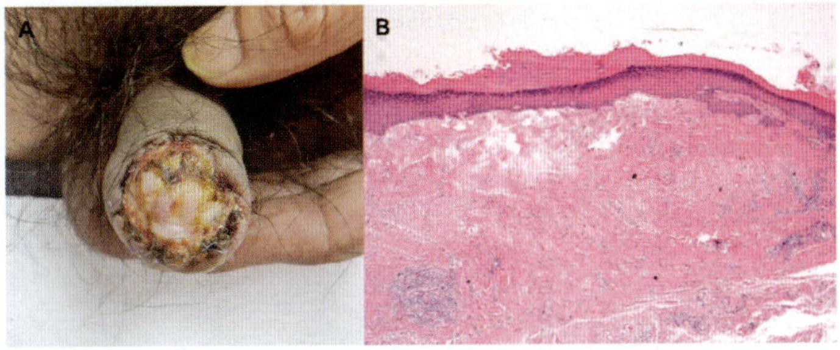

FIGURE 62-20. Vitiligo. Well-demarcated, depigmented patches of vitiligo on the penis. (Reproduced with the permission from Nan Hu, Yongzhen Zou, Xun Deng, Lian Zhang, Zhifang Zhai, Rui Yin, Photodynamic therapy for male genital lichen sclerosus with urethral stricture—Case report, Photodiagnosis and Photodynamic Therapy, Volume 45, 2024, 103947. Figure 1A.)

Vitiligo

What's New? New and emerging treatments for vitiligo include JAK-STAT inhibitors.[43] The FDA has approved topical ruxolitinib cream for the treatment of vitiligo.

Background Vitiligo is an autoimmune disease resulting from the immunologic destruction of melanocytes. Like other autoimmune diseases, genetics plays a role in the development of disease.[44] Vitiligo is associated with other autoimmune diseases, including autoimmune thyroiditis and alopecia areata. Vitiligo may appear at any age, and equally among men and women. The incidence of vitiligo does not differ by race but contrasting color makes lesions more evident in patients with SOC and results in worse quality of life scores in patients with darker skin tones.

Making the Diagnosis Diagnosis is often made clinically. A Wood's lamp may be helpful demonstrating accentuation of depigmented skin. A skin biopsy is rarely needed but may help to distinguish from lichen sclerosus or hypopigmented mycosis fungoides.

What to Look for Clinically? Vitiligo manifests as well-demarcated, depigmented macules and patches in segmental and nonsegmental distributions [**Figure 62-20**]. Vitiligo of the genitals is common, perhaps due to trauma and Koebnerization. Genital vitiligo often appears on the scrotum, pubis, and penile glans and foreskin.[44]

Differential Diagnosis Postinflammatory hypopigmentation, condyloma lata, lichen sclerosus, scars, hypopigmented mycosis fungoides.

What is the Treatment? Treatment is aimed at limiting progression and allowing repigmentation. Topical corticosteroids and calcineurin inhibitors are often first-line therapies. Phototherapy with narrow-band UVB may inhibit inflammatory response and stimulate melanocyte proliferation and pigmentation, though this might not be practical for genital lesions.[43] For severe cases, systemic therapies may be considered including cyclosporine or methotrexate. New studies suggest that inhibition of the JAK-STAT pathway may be effective at treating vitiligo and both topical and oral formulations are currently available.[43]

Additional Considerations Depression and anxiety are commonly associated with vitiligo especially among darker skin types. While there is a paucity of data pertaining to genital vitiligo in patients with SOC, anecdotally patients experience significant reductions in quality of life related to decreased sexual intimacy and fear of stigma.

CONCLUSIONS

This chapter has outlined several of the most common skin diseases of the male genitals. It is important to remember that any skin disease may manifest on the skin in the genital region. A select list of additional diagnoses are presented in **Table 62-2**. Maintaining a broad differential diagnosis [**Table 62-3**] and utilizing appropriate diagnostic algorithms will aid in making accurate diagnoses and providing the best care of patients.

TABLE 62-2 Additional male genital diseases

	Condition	Epidemiology	Morphology	Diagnosis	Treatment
Infectious	Chancroid	STI caused by *Haemophilus ducreyi*. Prevalence has decreased in the United States and worldwide and is now extremely rare.	Painful ulcerations that can be accompanied by regional lymphadenopathy.	Definite diagnosis requires special culture media. There is no FDA-approved PCR.	Azithromycin 1 g orally for one dose; Ceftriaxone 250 mg IM for one dose.
	Granuloma inguinale	STI caused by *Klebsiella granulomatis*. More commonly seen in men in tropical and subtropical climates. Rarely occurs in the United States.	Painless ulcerations that are highly vascular and present without regional lymphadenopathy.	Definitive diagnosis requires visualization of dark-staining Donovan bodies. There is no FDA-approved diagnostic modality.	Azithromycin 1 g orally once weekly for 3 weeks or until lesions have cleared.
	Lymphogranuloma venereum	STI caused by certain strains of *Chlamydia*. Outbreaks are more common among MSM with high rates of HIV coinfection.	Self-limited ulcer or papule at site of inoculation. Clinical manifestations can include lymphadenopathy and proctocolitis.	Definitive diagnosis requires PCR.	Doxycycline 100 mg orally twice daily for 3 weeks.
	Leishmaniasis	Vector-borne disease that afflicts exposed skin and therefore is not common on the genitals.	Ulceration that self-resolves in 3-18 months but can result in scarring and disfigurement.	Definite diagnosis requires visualization of amastigotes.	Liposomal Amphotericin B dosed at 3 mg/kg daily IV on days 1-5, 14 and 21.
Neoplastic	Kaposi sarcoma	Rare tumor that is more prevalent in MSM and immunocompromised populations.	Lesions typically evolve from patch stage to tumor stage. Tumors can ulcerate.	Definite diagnosis requires immunostaining.	Destruction of lesions. Highly active antiretroviral therapy in HIV positive patients.
	Melanoma	Exceedingly rare, representing less than 1.4% of penile cancers and 0.1% of primary melanomas.	Painless pigmented lesion that can ulcerate.	Definite diagnosis requires a biopsy.	Surgical excision.
Inflammatory	Red scrotum syndrome	Uncommon and likely underreported. Etiology is unknown.	Erythema of the scrotum associated with pruritus, hyperalgesia, and burning sensation.	Diagnosis of exclusion.	Avoidance of triggers, topical analgesics, or systemic agents such as gabapentin.
	Sclerosing lymphangitis	Rare and associated with vigorous sexual activity. This disorder can also be associated with underlying STI.	Minimally tender cordlike lesion that typically present circumferentially on the coronal sulcus. [**Figure 62-21**]	Clinical.	Self resolves and typically does not require intervention.
Mechanical	Penile injury	Rare but can result in decreased sexual function and diminished quality of life.	Varies based on type of injury. Injuries include burns, degloving, and blunt trauma.	Clinical.	Self-limited or requires surgical intervention based on extent of injury.

Abbreviations: HIV, human immunodeficiency virus; IM, intramuscular; IV, intravenous; MSM, men who have sex with men; PCR, polymerase chain reaction; STI, sexually transmitted infection.

TABLE 62-3 Differential diagnosis of male genital diseases by morphology

Primary morphology	Color	Differential diagnosis
Macule	Brown	Mucosal lentigines, postinflammatory hyperpigmentation, fixed drug eruption, melanoma
	White	Vitiligo, postinflammatory hypopigmentation, lichen sclerosus
	Pink/red	Psoriasis, squamous cell carcinoma
Papule	Brown/hyperpigmented	Melanoma, nevus, Bowenoid papulosis, condyloma
	White	Condyloma lata, pearly penile papules, milia, scrotal calcinosis, syringomas
	Pink/red	Scabies, Zoon balanitis, SCC (Squamous cell carcinoma), Tyson glands/Fordyce spots, balanitis circinate, chloracne
	Purple	Lichen planus, lichen nitidus
	Flesh color	Median raphe cyst, pearly penile papules, Tyson glands/Fordyce spots, molluscum contagiosum, condyloma acuminatum
Patch	White	Vitiligo, postinflammatory hypopigmentation, lichen sclerosus
	Brown/hyperpigmented	Postinflammatory hyperpigmentation, candida intertrigo, tinea cruris, contact dermatitis, atopic dermatitis
	Purple	Lichen planus, Kaposi sarcoma
	Pink/red	Seborrheic dermatitis, contact dermatitis, SCC, red scrotum syndrome, tinea cruris
Plaque	White	Lichen sclerosus, scars
	Brown/hyperpigmented	Lichen simplex chronicus, tinea cruris
	Pink/red	Psoriasis, balanitis circinata, Zoon balanitis, tinea cruris, lichen simplex chronicus
	Purple	Lichen planus, Kaposi sarcoma, fixed drug eruption
	Flesh color	Sclerosing lymphangitis
Nodule	Pink/red	Scabies, epidermal cyst, squamous cell carcinoma
	White	Scrotal calcinosis
	Flesh color	Epidermal cyst, median raphe cyst, hidradenitis suppurativa
Vesicle		HSV (Herpes simplex virus), contact dermatitis, impetigo, lichen planus
Bulla		Contact dermatitis, lichen planus, fixed drug eruption, autoimmune blistering diseases
Pustule/abscess		Folliculitis, chloracne, hidradenitis suppurativa
Ulcer		Syphilis, chancroid, lymphogranuloma venereum, pyoderma gangrenosum, Behcet disease, penile injury, CMV/EBV

Abbreviations: CMV, cytomegalovirus; EBV, Epstein-Barr virus.

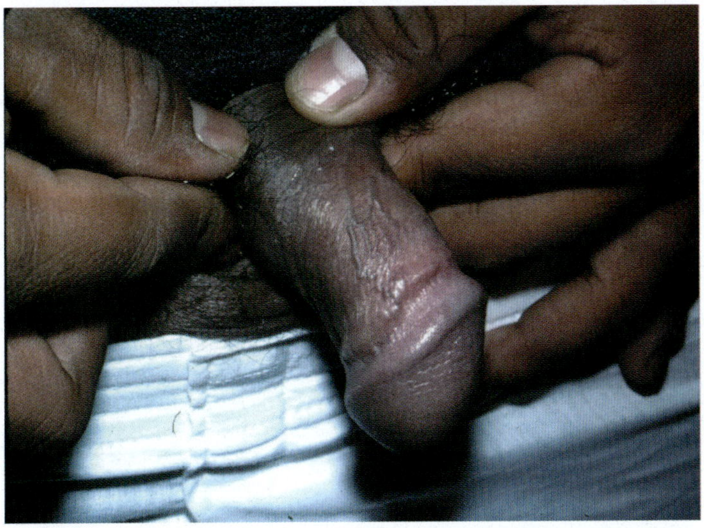

FIGURE 62-21. Sclerosing lymphangitis often presents with a sub-coronal, cordlike plaque.

REFERENCES

1. Alexis AF, Callender VD, Baldwin HE, Desai SR, Rendon MI, Taylor SC. Global epidemiology and clinical spectrum of rosacea, highlighting skin of color: review and clinical practice experience. *J Am Acad Dermatol*. 2019; 80(6):1722-1729.e7.
2. Sloan B. Skin of color images. *J Am Acad Dermatol*. 2021;84(1):35.
3. Peeling RW, Mabey D, Kamb ML, Chen XS, Radolf JD, Benzaken AS. Syphilis. *Nat Rev Dis Primers*. 2017;3:17073.
4. Groves MJ. Genital herpes: a review. *Am Fam Physician*. 2016;93(11):928-934.
5. Yin D, Ling S, Wang D, et al. Targeting herpes simplex virus with CRISPR-Cas9 cures herpetic stromal keratitis in mice. *Nat Biotechnol*. 2021;39(5):567-577.
6. Yanofsky VR, Patel RV, Goldenberg G. Genital warts: a comprehensive review. *J Clin Aesthet Dermatol*. 2012;5(6):25-36.
7. Walsh T, Bertozzi-Villa C, Schneider JA. Systematic review of racial disparities in human papillomavirus-associated anal dysplasia and anal cancer among men who have sex with men. *Am J Public Health*. 2015;105(4):e34-e45.
8. Rasberry CN, Condron DS, Lesesne CA, Adkins SH, Sheremenko G, Kroupa E. Associations between sexual risk-related behaviors and school-based education on HIV and condom use for adolescent sexual minority males and their non-sexual-minority peers. *LGBT Health*. 2018;5(1):69-77.
9. Browning JC, Enloe C, Cartwright M, et al. Efficacy and safety of topical nitric oxide-releasing berdazimer gel in patients with molluscum contagiosum: a phase 3 randomized clinical trial. *JAMA Dermatol*. 2022;e222721.
10. Meza-Romero R, Navarrete-Dechent C, Downey C. Molluscum contagiosum: an update and review of new perspectives in etiology, diagnosis, and treatment. *Clin Cosmet Investig Dermatol*. 2019;12:373-381.
11. Sahoo AK, Mahajan R. Management of tinea corporis, tinea cruris, and tinea pedis: a comprehensive review. *Indian Dermatol Online J*. 2016;7(2):77-86.
12. Sunderkötter C, Wohlrab J, Hamm H. Scabies: epidemiology, diagnosis, and treatment. *Dtsch Arztebl Int*. 2021;118(41):695-704.
13. Scherrer MAR, Rocha VB, Garcia LC. Behçet's disease: review with emphasis on dermatological aspects. *An Bras Dermatol*. 2017;92(4):452-464.
14. Vitale A, Rigante D, Lopalco G, et al. New therapeutic solutions for Behçet's syndrome. *Expert Opin Investig Drugs*. 2016;25(7):827-840.
15. Kiafar M, Faezi ST, Kasaeian A, et al. Diagnosis of Behçet's disease: clinical characteristics, diagnostic criteria, and differential diagnoses. *BMC Rheumatol*. 2021;5(1):2.
16. Ribera-Cortada I, Guerrero-Pineda J, Trias I, et al. Pathogenesis of penile squamous cell carcinoma: molecular update and systematic review. *Int J Mol Sci*. 2021;23(1):251.
17. Goodman MT, Hernandez BY, Shvetsov YB. Demographic and pathologic differences in the incidence of invasive penile cancer in the United States, 1995-2003. *Cancer Epidemiol Biomarkers Prev*. 2007;16(9):1833-1839.
18. Thompson EL, Rosen BL, Maness SB. Social determinants of health and human papillomavirus vaccination among young adults, National Health Interview Survey 2016. *J Community Health*. 2019;44(1):149-158.
19. Fania L, Didona D, Di Pietro FR, et al. Cutaneous squamous cell carcinoma: from pathophysiology to novel therapeutic approaches. *Biomedicines*. 2021;9(2):171.
20. Slopnick EA, Kim SP, Kiechle JE, Gonzalez CM, Zhu H, Abouassaly R. Racial disparities differ for African Americans and Hispanics in the diagnosis and treatment of penile cancer. *Urology*. 2016;96:22-28.
21. Bender AM, Tang O, Khanna R, Ständer S, Kang S, Kwatra SG. Racial differences in dermatologic conditions associated with HIV: a cross-sectional study of 4679 patients in an urban tertiary care center. *J Am Acad Dermatol*. 2020;82(5):1117-1123.
22. Lotti T, Buggiani G, Prignano F. Prurigo nodularis and lichen simplex chronicus. *Dermatol Ther*. 2008;21(1):42-46.
23. Stibich AS, Yagan M, Sharma V, Herndon B, Montgomery C. Cost-effective post-exposure prevention of poison ivy dermatitis. *Int J Dermatol*. 2000;39(7): 515-518.
24. Yale K, Awosika O, Rengifo-Pardo M, Ehrlich A. Genital allergic contact dermatitis. *Dermatitis*. 2018;29(3):112-119.
25. Scott I, Atwater AR, Reeder M. Update on contact dermatitis and patch testing in patients with skin of color. *Cutis*. 2021;108(1):10-12.
26. van der Sluis N, Scheers ECAH, Krenning G, van der Lei B, Oonk MHM, van Dongen JA. Autologous lipoaspirate as a new treatment of vulvar lichen sclerosus: a review on literature. *Exp Dermatol*. 2022;31(5):689-699.
27. Kirtschig G. Lichen sclerosus-presentation, diagnosis and management. *Dtsch Arztebl Int*. 2016;113(19):337-343.
28. Becher G, Burden AD. Ixekizumab in genital psoriasis. *Br J Dermatol*. 2018;179(4):811-812.
29. Kelly A, Ryan C. Genital psoriasis: impact on quality of life and treatment options. *Am J Clin Dermatol*. 2019;20(5):639-646.
30. Kaufman BP, Alexis AF. Psoriasis in skin of color: insights into the epidemiology, clinical presentation, genetics, quality-of-life impact, and treatment of psoriasis in non-white racial/ethnic groups. *Am J Clin Dermatol*. 2018;19:405-423.
31. Alexis AF, Blackcloud P. Psoriasis in skin of color: epidemiology, genetics, clinical presentation, and treatment nuances. *J Clin Aesthet Dermatol*. 2014;7(11):16-24.
32. Bhutani T, Wong JW, Bebo BF, Armstrong AW. Access to health care in patients with psoriasis and psoriatic arthritis: data from National Psoriasis Foundation survey panels. *JAMA Dermatol*. 2013;149(6):717-721.
33. Lé AM, Torres T. New topical therapies for psoriasis. *Am J Clin Dermatol*. 2022;23(1):13-24.
34. Damsky W, Wang A, Olamiju B, Peterson D, Galan A, King B. Treatment of severe lichen planus with the JAK inhibitor tofacitinib. *J Allergy Clin Immunol*. 2020;145(6):1708-1710.
35. Tziotzios C, Lee JYW, Brier T, et al. Lichen planus and lichenoid dermatoses: clinical overview and molecular basis. *J Am Acad Dermatol*. 2018. 79(5):789-804.
36. Giorgio C, Briatico G, Licata G, et al. Topical cyclosporine 5% cream in Zoon's balanitis resistant to other therapies: a case report. *Dermatol Ther*. 2021;34(2). doi:10.1111/dth.14807
37. Fahmy MAB. Zoon's balanitis. In: *Normal and Abnormal Prepuce*. Cham: Springer; 2020.
38. Verzi A, Nasca M, Dall'Oglio F, Cosentino C, Micali F. A novel treatment of intertrigo in athletes and overweight subjects. *J Cosmet Dermatol*. 2021; 20(Suppl 1):23-27.
39. Kalra MG, Higgins KE, Kinney BS. Intertrigo and secondary skin infections. *Am Fam Physician*. 2014;89(7):569-573.
40. Aarts P, Dudink K, Vossen ARJV, et al. Clinical implementation of biologics and small molecules in the treatment of hidradenitis suppurativa. *Drugs*. 2021;81(12):1397-1410.
41. Shih T, Seivright JR, McKenzie SA, et al. Gender differences in hidradenitis suppurativa characteristics: a retrospective cohort analysis. *Int J Womens Dermatol*. 2021;7(5):672-674.
42. Goldburg SR, Strober BE, Payette MJ. Hidradenitis suppurativa: epidemiology, clinical presentation, and pathogenesis. *J Am Acad Dermatol*. 2020;82(5): 1045-1058.
43. Karagaiah P, Valle Y, Sigova J, et al. Emerging drugs for the treatment of vitiligo. *Expert Opin Emerg Drugs*. 2020;25(1):7-24.
44. Pun J, Randhawa A, Kumar A, Williams V. The impact of vitiligo on quality of life and psychosocial well-being in a Nepalese population. *Dermatol Clin*. 2021;39(1):117-127.

CHAPTER 63

Genital Lesions in Women

Melissa Mauskar
Jessica C. Evans
Miriam Pomeranz

KEY POINTS

- Patients, regardless of gender, may delay reporting lesions in the genital area due to a variety of reasons.
- "Normal" vulvar anatomy can vary tremendously among individuals.
- In most cases of vulvar hygiene, less is more. Simply rinsing the vulva with water during a shower is adequate.
- Classic findings of vulvar lesions, such as erythema, may appear differently in individuals with skin of color.

INTRODUCTION

Patients, regardless of gender, may delay reporting lesions in the genital area due to a variety of reasons, ranging from self-consciousness to individual sociocultural beliefs. This can make diagnosing conditions across all skin tones challenging. In addition, patients often try various over-the-counter agents and home remedies before presenting to the doctor's office, and the primary morphology may be obscured by secondary features of irritant or allergic contact dermatitis. Moreover, patients may not examine their genital skin until they notice itch or pain, and normal anatomic variants may be confused for pathologic changes. We will begin this chapter by briefly highlighting normal variants and common cultural beliefs/practices regarding vulvar care before expanding on common genital conditions [**Table 63-1**] seen in women.

VARIATIONS IN NORMAL ANATOMY

The vulva consists of the mons pubis, labia majora (labium majus), labia minora (labium minus), clitoris, urethra, vestibule, Bartholin glands, and vaginal opening [**Figure 63-1**] and can have a myriad of presentations. It is important for providers to convey to their patients that "normal" in terms of size or color of the labia majora, minora, and clitoral hood can vary tremendously among individuals. For instance, regarding size variations, one study of 50 premenopausal women found the average mean width of the labia minora was 21.8 mm with a range from 7 mm to 50 mm.[1] In a separate study of 50 premenopausal and 50 postmenopausal women, the mean labia minora width was significantly smaller in postmenopausal women (15.4 ± 4.7 mm vs 17.9 ± 4.1 mm; $p = 0.01$).[2] In addition to size variation, the vulva may also present with a range of colors from light pink to dark brown-red or black, and the color can vary among different ethnoracial groups. Classically, textbooks show one or only a few representations of how a woman's vulva may appear and fail to include enough images to portray the many possibilities that may still be considered normal architecture. Additionally, the media may highlight certain ideals of normal vulvar anatomy, causing patients to have a negative self-image if their vulva does not resemble those portrayed online, in social media, or even in adult content. Consequently, the number of women pursuing labiaplasty (a surgical procedure to alter the shape or size of the labia minora) has increased over the years.[2]

TABLE 63-1 Differential diagnoses and treatment for common vulvar inflammatory diseases

Lesion/disease	Differential diagnosis	Treatment
Lichen sclerosus	• Lichen planus (chronic) • Morphea • Postinflammatory dyschromia • Squamous cell carcinoma in situ/vulvar intraepithelial neoplasia • Vitiligo	Class I steroids (clobetasol, halobetasol, or betamethasone dipropionate in augmented vehicle ointment) twice daily until the texture normalizes, with follow up every 6-8 weeks; usually requiring about 4 months.
Lichen planus	• Erosive disease • Candidiasis • Cicatricial pemphigoid • Lichen sclerosus • Lupus erythematosus • Pemphigus vulgaris • Bowen disease • Condyloma acuminata (genital warts) • Erythema multiforme • Fixed drug reaction • Lichen simplex chronicus • Psoriasis • Scabies • Secondary syphilis	Class I steroids (clobetasol ointment, etc) twice daily until erosions, white areas heal, and symptoms abate, with follow-up every 6-8 weeks. Taper to least frequent dosing, or lowest potency corticosteroid that maintains control.
Lichen simplex chronicus	• Psoriasis • Contact dermatitis • Hypertrophic lichen planus • Atopic dermatitis • Verruca vulgaris • Acanthosis nigricans	Class I steroids (such as clobetasol or halobetasol ointment) daily, reevaluate monthly. Recommend medication use until the skin is normal, then tapering frequency or potency.
Crohn's disease	• Actinomycosis • Angioedema • Behcet syndrome • Chancroid • Extramammary Paget's disease • Factitious dermatitis • Filariasis • Fixed drug eruption • Granuloma inguinale • Hidradenitis suppurativa	Treatment of vulvar Crohn's disease, in both adults and children, focuses on managing the underlying Crohn's disease, regardless of whether intestinal involvement is present.
Vitiligo	• Discoid lupus erythematosus • Hansen disease (tuberculoid) • Lichen sclerosus (most important) • Postinflammatory dyschromia • Seborrhea • Tinea versicolor (rare on genital skin)	Cosmetic coverup products are camouflage options. Repigmentation therapeutic modalities are available (eg, melanocyte-keratinocyte transplantation or excimer laser treatment), although these are not guaranteed. Corticosteroids are a potential first-line therapy.

CULTURAL BELIEFS/PRACTICES: VULVAR CARE

Intravaginal cleansing (or douching), most often with a mixture of vinegar and water, is the most common intravaginal cleansing method practiced in the United States among reproductive-aged women.[3] Although douching was first adopted for contraception in the 19th century, when it was found to be ineffective, advertisers in the 1920s began marketing douching for cosmetic purposes (under the euphemism of "feminine hygiene").[4] As a result, this practice persists despite adverse health consequences, including reports of increased risk of vaginal and sexually transmitted infections. As well, survey and qualitative research from the United States support that frequent douching is further propagated by advice from other women or family members, and the belief that douching is part of feminine hygiene and protective from sexually transmitted infections. Considering an individual's sociocultural beliefs can help guide discussion regarding both benefits/risks of certain practices

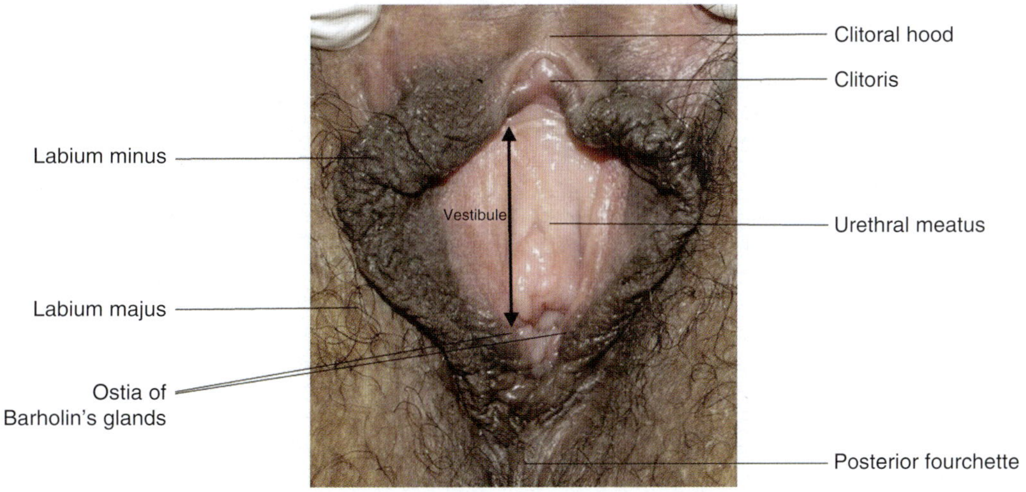

FIGURE 63-1. Vulvar anatomy. (Reproduced with permission from Mauskar MM, Marathe K, Venkatesan A, Schlosser BJ, Edwards L. Vulvar diseases: approach to the patient. *J Am Acad Dermatol.* 2020;82(6):1277-1284, Figure 2.)

(whether related to cleaning/douching or other practices like exfoliation or epilation) so that both the patient and the provider can make better-informed decisions.

RECOMMENDATIONS FOR PROPER VULVAR CARE

It's important for clinicians to take time to review proper cleansing techniques with their patients.[5] In most cases, simply rinsing the vulva with water during a shower is adequate. However, if a patient prefers to use soap, unscented, fragrance-free bar soaps are recommended. Patients should avoid use of soap directly on the vulvar skin; instead, the soap can be lathered in the patient's hands to clean the mons (the hair-bearing skin), then subsequently let the water rinse down. Bland moisturizers are also preferred as one would use on other parts of their body. Often when patients have itching or pain in their vulva, they may believe it is related to their level of cleanliness. As a result, patients may over clean the area by scrubbing with washcloths and using harsh soaps or wet wipes. There is no need to rub and scrub in between the labia or put soap inside of the vagina. This can be very challenging for patients as they have developed habits that can be difficult to break. Additionally, products specifically tailored and marketed toward women for cleaning, douching, or exfoliating are unnecessary. Ultimately, the goal is to keep the vulva dry and free from irritants.

For postmenopausal women who often have dryness or itching related to genitourinary syndrome of menopause or vaginal atrophy, local topical estrogen inserted in the vagina two to three times weekly can help tremendously with restoring moisture and relieving their symptoms.

INFLAMMATORY LESIONS

LICHEN SCLEROSUS

Epidemiology and Pathogenesis Lichen sclerosus (LS) is a chronic inflammatory skin condition in which the exact pathophysiology remains unclear. It is believed to be associated with autoimmunity, genetics, and possible environmental factors or hormonal influences. Autoimmune disorders that have been found to coincide in patients with LS include thyroid disorders, pernicious anemia, psoriasis, and vitiligo. It can occur at any age and in both sexes but is most often seen in prepubertal and postmenopausal women.

Clinical Findings Early LS often presents as fine erythema and texture change, subtle findings that may be missed in patients with skin of color. Other typical skin changes include the development of areas of pallor, ranging from small perifollicular macules to large plaques, as well as atrophic or fragile skin with telangiectasias, purpura, erosions, and tender fissures. Genital lesions with a complete or incomplete "figure of eight" pattern of depigmentation/hypopigmentation around the vulva and anus may also be evident [**Figure 63-2**], with many patients complaining of intractable pruritus and/or soreness of the affected areas. Dysuria, dyspareunia, and pain with defecation are not uncommon. LS is likely an underreported condition and patients often go undiagnosed. Reasons for this are many and may include increased self-consciousness about seeking genital care, sociocultural beliefs surrounding vulvar anatomy/care, issues with access and accessibility to health services and dermatologic care, or possible misdiagnosis from healthcare providers.

Biopsy is not often needed in well-established disease. However, if there is a question of diagnosis or concern for malignancy, biopsy should

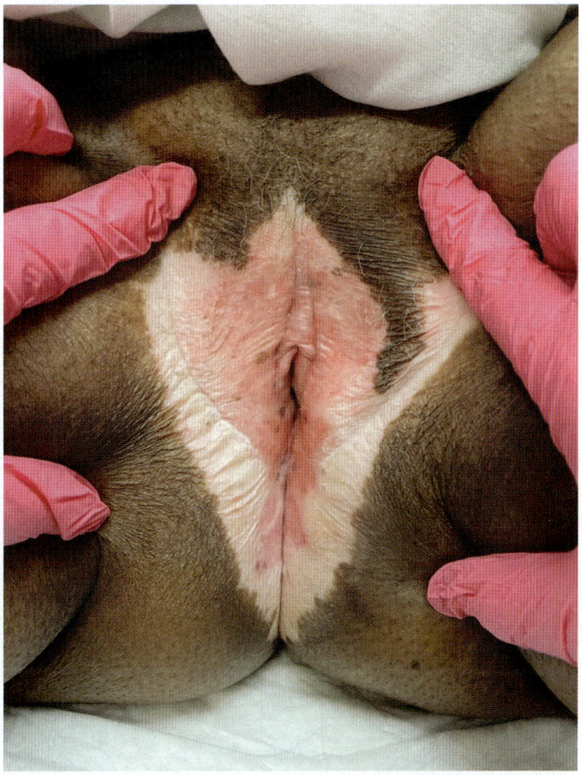

FIGURE 63-2. Lichen sclerosus. Complete "figure of eight" pattern of depigmentation/hypopigmentation around the vulva and anus with retraction of clitoral hood and fusion of the labia majora.

be performed. Classic histologic findings include epidermal atrophy, degeneration of the basal layer, and hyperkeratosis.

Treatment and Clinical Course High-potency topical corticosteroids are the mainstay of treatment. When caught early, scarring may be prevented. Once scarring and obliteration of the architecture have developed, surgery may be required to lyse scars that interfere with normal functioning. Lichen sclerosus is a chronic condition and 5% of women will go on to develop vulvar squamous cell carcinoma (SCC). Therefore, ongoing topical corticosteroid therapy is indicated to maintain control of disease and reduce this risk.[6]

LICHEN PLANUS

Epidemiology and Pathogenesis Lichen planus (LP) is a papulosquamous skin condition thought to be related to T-cell autoimmunity against basilar keratinocytes. LP most commonly affects adults in the third to sixth decade of life. Once thought to be an uncommon occurrence, genital LP is being diagnosed more frequently, especially in women, because more physicians are familiar with the entity and its wide morphologic range. Approximately 1% of the general population has oral LP; of women with oral LP, 20% to 25% also have genital disease.[7]

Clinical Findings Genital LP lesions vary widely in morphology, from papulosquamous to erosive lesions and, rarely, hypertrophic lesions. Erosive disease is the most significant and distressing from of vulvar LP, and commonly involves the posterior vestibule before extending anteriorly to involve the labia minora [**Figure 63-3**]. The erosive form is often associated with inflammatory vaginitis, and patients may experience vaginal discharge, pain, and burning during micturition.[8] Severe longstanding disease can cause loss of normal architecture, including fusion of the labia minora and burying of the clitoris. Vulvar LP, when associated with generalized LP, may resemble the more classic violaceous, polygonal, papular or plaque morphology seen on extragenital skin and involves the labia or mons pubis. In individuals with a darker skin tone, classic lesions are typically deeply pigmented due to the larger amount of melanin displaced from the epidermis. The least common form of vulvar LP is the hypertrophic variant, which presents with extensive white papules/plaques and thickened irregular surface that may or may not have classic-appearing reticulate surface markings. Individuals with genital lesions often experience oral lesions, and oral lesions more commonly may be the presenting symptom. Diagnosis is achieved through biopsy, preferably of a noneroded area. For erosive lesions, a biopsy should be taken at the transition zone between normal and eroded skin. Perilesional samples can be taken for direct immunofluorescence to exclude autoimmune blistering disorders like mucous membrane pemphigoid.

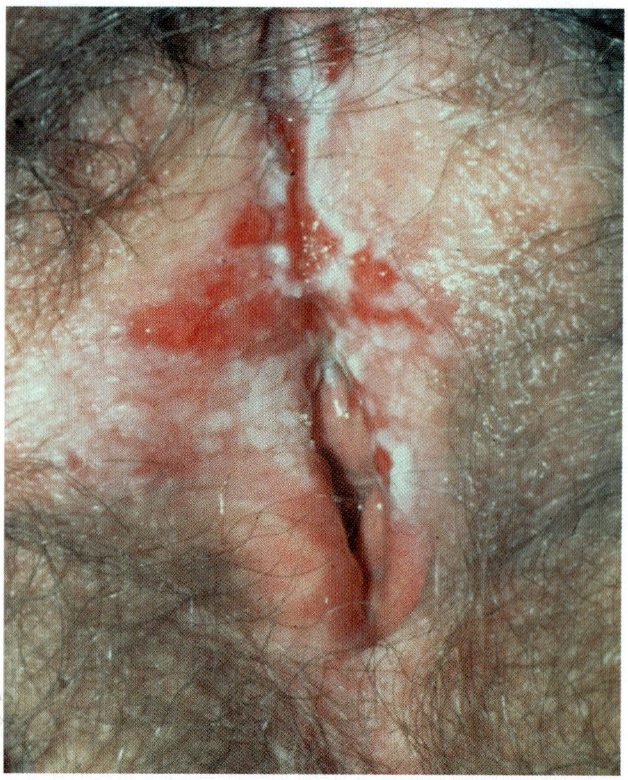

FIGURE 63-3. Lichen planus. Erosive lichen planus resembling genital herpes. (Used with permission from Libby Edwards, MD.)

Treatment and Clinical Course Topical high-potency corticosteroids are first-line therapy for all forms of LP, including genital lesions. Nonerosive lesions may be well controlled with this alone and even fully remit spontaneously. For some patients, systemic immunosuppressive medications may be required for adequate remission. Systemic corticosteroids, methylprednisolone, or prednisone are the most effective treatment modalities in cases of diffuse recalcitrant erosive oral LP or multisite lesions of severe erosive LP. Methotrexate and cyclosporine are also effective systemic therapies. Systemic retinoids, such as acitretin or isotretinoin can additionally be used for treatment. Cyclophosphamide, dapsone, colchicine, and thalidomide may be used as well but should be reserved as third-line options due to less evidence being available for their efficacy compared to other drugs.[9]

Erosive disease tends to be chronic, recalcitrant, and scarring; it can lead to complete vaginal stenosis. The course of erosive LP is one of exacerbations with slow healing, recurrent secondary infections, and slow response to therapy. Patients may develop secondary vulvar pain or pelvic floor dysfunction after their disease is in remission. As erosive LP has been known to have a significant impact on a patient's quality of life, it is important for providers to consider an interdisciplinary approach for severe cases. Management teams may consist of sexual counselors, pelvic floor specialists, psychologists, or psychiatrists.[10]

LICHEN SIMPLEX CHRONICUS

Epidemiology and Pathogenesis Lichen simplex chronicus (LSC) is cutaneous disease characterized by severe and intractable pruritus. Patients may often have an underlying atopic dermatitis but can also develop LSC in preexisting dermatological conditions such as candidiasis, lichen sclerosus, psoriasis, and tinea cruris. The disease manifests as a vicious itch-scratch cycle that leads to its chronic perpetuation. Anogenital LSC is a rather common condition, affecting an estimated 12% of the general population. The condition is more prevalent in middle-aged individuals and affects women more frequently than men, with a 2-to-1 ratio.[11]

Clinical Findings On physical exam, thickening of the genital skin along with associated erythema and/or scaling may be apparent [**Figure 63-4**]. Changes in pigmentation, whether hyper- or hypo-, to the area involved have also been seen. Patients with a darker skin tone may not demonstrate the classic bright pink or red color seen in patients with a lighter skin tone. In addition, the erythema can be masked by postinflammatory hyperpigmentation. Biopsies are rarely done, as the diagnosis can often be made clinically. Not uncommonly, once LSC has been treated, an underlying primary dermatologic condition such as lichen sclerosus or psoriasis may become more apparent. On histological exam, thickening of the epidermis and stratum corneum as a result of chronic trauma due to excessive excoriation is evident.

Treatment and Clinical Course LSC (as the name implies) has a chronic course, though severity may wax and wane. Treatment is aimed at both addressing the underlying condition (if present) and controlling for itch/pruritus. Topical (medium to high potency) corticosteroids are used as first-line therapy to break the itch-scratch cycle. Emollients and barrier cream can also help reduce hyperkeratosis and improve the texture of the skin. Antihistamines, or other agents to control itch, may also be used to deter further scratching. Though the condition itself is considered benign, patients may experience poorer quality of life due to the severe pruritus in an intimate location.

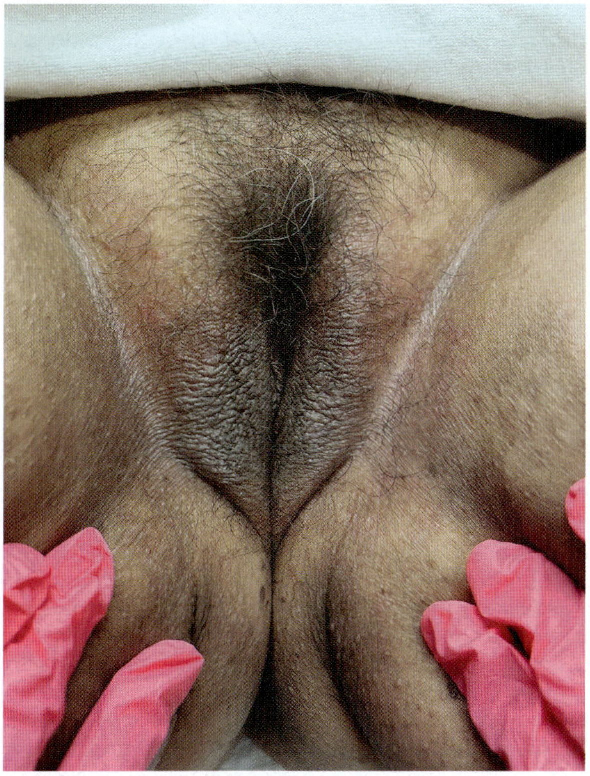

FIGURE 63-4. Lichen simplex chronicus.

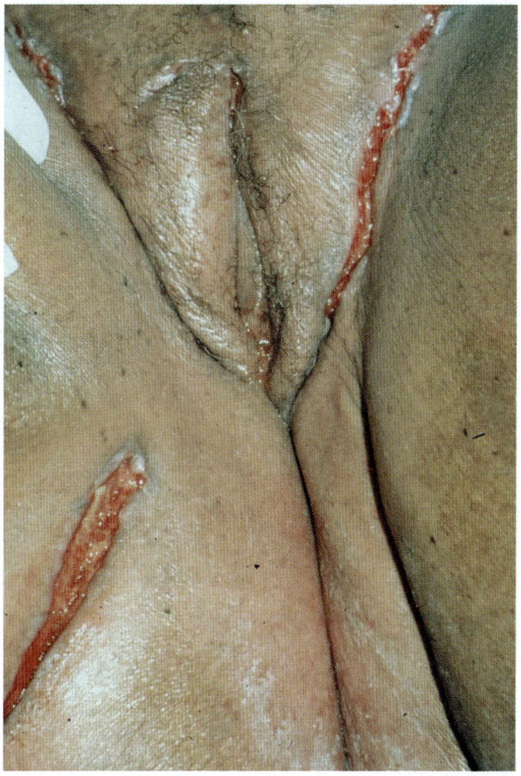

FIGURE 63-5. Cut-like perigenital erosions characteristic of Crohn's disease. (Used with permission from Libby Edwards, MD.)

CROHN'S DISEASE

Epidemiology and Pathogenesis Crohn's disease (CD) is a chronic granulomatous disorder that may involve any portion of the gastrointestinal tract. The disease typically begins between the ages of 15 and 30 years but can persist into the geriatric years. Although commonly thought of as more of a gastrointestinal disease, approximately 40% of all patients affected by CD experience at last one extraintestinal manifestation of disease, with the skin being the most common site of extraintestinal involvement.[12] The skin can be involved by direct extension from the gastrointestinal tract or via involvement away from the gastrointestinal tract, so-called metastatic CD. Genital involvement in CD is less frequent in men than in women. About 2% of women with CD have vulvar involvement.[13] Historically, it was believed that CD predominantly affected White individuals, but growing research suggests increasing incidence among communities of color.[14]

Clinical Findings Patterns of mucocutaneous CD involvement include contiguous, metastatic, and nonspecific/reactive manifestations.[15] Contiguous disease represents direct extension from the involved intestine with the formation of sinuses/fistulas involving perianal/peristomal or orofacial skin. Metastatic disease, albeit rare, consists of plaques, nodules, or ulcers at distant sites from the gastrointestinal tract. Although any body part can be affected, female patients with metastatic CD commonly present with painful swelling and ulceration of the vulvar or perianal area. The classic ulcerations are deemed 'knife cut' linear fissures and are located along the labiocrural fold [**Figure 63-5**]. There are also nonspecific/reactive mucocutaneous lesions, including aphthous ulcers and pyoderma gangrenosum. The diagnosis of cutaneous CD can be made with biopsy that demonstrates granulomatous change 50% of the time. When there is a high index of suspicion, clinicians can check fecal calprotectin, a surrogate marker for gut inflammation.

Treatment and Clinical Course CD may be treated with biologic agents such as tumor necrosis factor (TNF) antagonists, anti-integrin, and anti-interleukin 12 either alone or in addition to immunosuppressants. Although sometimes patients' skin disease will flare with the underlying disease, activity of cutaneous CD is often discordant or independent of gut disease. Dermatologists should discuss with gastrointestinal (GI) physicians but also feel comfortable to aggressively treat skin disease if there is discordance with gut disease. Skin disease may also be the presenting sign of CD, predating diagnosis of gut inflammation.

VITILIGO

Epidemiology and Pathogenesis Vitiligo is a chronic condition characterized by skin depigmentation due to an autoimmune response that destroys the melanocytes. While the etiology is uncertain, it may be related to oxidative stress (triggered by a sunburn, emotional distress, or chemical exposure) and inflammation; a familial predilection is also noted. The disease is very apparent in skin of color, and often extremely psychologically distressing for the patient; this may explain increased rates of vitiligo diagnosis in people of color.[16] The vast majority of cases exhibit onset of the disease before the age of 40 years and there is no gender predilection.

Clinical Findings White/depigmented patches on the skin are the major clinical finding of vitiligo. Frequent sites of involvement tend to be sun-exposed areas, such as the dorsa of the hands and feet and periorificial regions of the face. Other general areas include the armpits, genitals, and navel. In women, involvement of the vulva is common.

Treatment and Clinical Course The clinical course of vitiligo can be highly unpredictable, and it is not possible to calculate if depigmented patches will resolve, spread progressively, or remain stable and persist indefinitely. The speed of the spread of depigmentation also varies. As this is an autoimmune condition, treatment is aimed at suppressing the immune system through use of corticosteroids and calcineurin inhibitors. Recently topical JAK inhibitor have been FDA approved to treat vitiligo.

INFECTIOUS DISEASES

HUMAN PAPILLOMAVIRUS (HPV)

Epidemiology and Pathogenesis Condyloma acuminata, or genital warts, is caused by the human papillomavirus, which is a nonenveloped double-stranded DNA virus. It is quite common in the United States

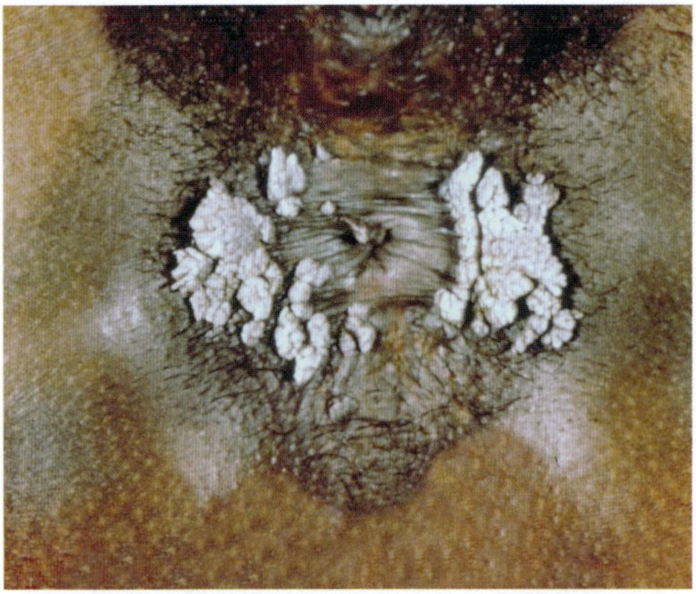

FIGURE 63-6. Condylomata acuminata. Aggregate cauliflower-shaped masses typical of anogenital warts.

with a prevalence of approximately 10% to 20%.[17] There is a reported incidence of 1% in sexually active adults and 3% in sexually active adolescents. Though there are many serotypes, genital warts are typically associated with strains 6 and 11. The virus is transmitted through either skin-to-skin contact or skin-to-mucosa contact.

Clinical Findings The clinical presentation of HPV consists of a distribution of small papules that may develop into skin colored to reddish, filiform, asymptomatic papules [**Figure 63-6**]. These lesions are more commonly referred to as genital warts and develop 2 to 3 months after exposure. The skin around the vaginal introitus and perianal area are most affected, but the cervix may also have lesions. Often, patients will be asymptomatic. Although genital warts are chiefly a clinical diagnosis, confirmation may be achieved through biopsy. Histologically, one may find large dermal papillae lined by hyperplastic squamous epithelium. This leads to the exophytic nature of these lesions.

Treatment and Clinical Course Unfortunately, there is no known cure for HPV, though it may self-resolve. Current treatment modalities consist of both home therapies (imiquimod, podofilox, sinecatechins, topical cidofovir) or office treatment with ablative therapy (cryotherapy, electrodesiccation, laser, scalpel, curettage) or use of topical agents (trichloroacetic acid, dichloroacetic acid, podophyllin) or intralesional therapy. HPV infections tend to have a fluctuating clinical course of visible lesions, latency, and recurrence. The clinical course is approximately 12 months for males and 6 months for females. HPV is responsible for 50% of vulvar cancers.[17] Vaccines have been very effective in reducing the transmission of the virus and thus the progression of squamous cancer. However, individuals living in communities that are underserved are less likely to complete vaccination against the virus for reasons not yet entirely understood, but possibly related to age, income, and education.[18]

SYPHILIS

Epidemiology and Pathogenesis Syphilis is a sexually transmitted infection caused by the spirochete, Treponema pallidum. Inoculation occurs via breaks in the skin or mucosal transmission. After reaching regional lymph nodes, treponemes spread via a hematogenous route to other parts of the body. Recently, there has been a resurgence of syphilis in the United States. Between 2014 and 2018, reported cases of primary and secondary syphilis increased by 71.4% (10.8 vs 6.3 cases per 100,000).[19] While syphilis is more common in men, rates of syphilis are increasing in women (rates increased by just over 30% between 2017 and 2018). Considerable racial and ethnic disparities in syphilis incidence also exist, with Black women and men alike, and particularly Black men who have sex with men, at increased risk. These disparities are likely associated with well-documented structural barriers to quality health access, as well as differences in social determinants of health, which have been shown to influence the incidence of syphilis among marginalized racial and ethnic groups at a local level.[20]

Clinical Findings Primary syphilis is characterized by a solitary ulcerative lesion (or chancre) that is painless and usually regresses on its own. The labia majora and the perineal skin just adjacent to the vaginal orifice are the most frequent sites affected. It is reported that initial symptoms appear as early as 3 weeks after inoculation. Approximately 6 to 8 weeks after primary infection, one will begin to see the secondary manifestation of syphilis, which includes more systemic symptoms such as headache, lymphadenopathy, malaise, and a papulosquamous rash involving the palms and soles. Condyloma lata have been reported to occur in about 6% to 23% of patients with secondary syphilis and can be painful. Moisture, heat, and friction of intertriginous areas are thought to perpetuate the growth and coalescence of syphilitic papules during the secondary stage, leading to plaque-like condylomas.[19] In late-stage tertiary syphilis, destructive gummas may appear, manifesting dermatologically as heavily crusted granulomatous lesions of the skin. Neurologic and cardiovascular structures are vulnerable to gummatous syphilis as well.

In recent years, some laboratories have a adopted a "reverse sequencing" algorithm for diagnosis in which the initial study is an automated treponemal test (usually enzyme immunoassay or chemiluminescent immunoassay) rather than a nontreponemal (RPR or VDRL) test. If the first test has a positive result, a nontreponemal test is then performed for confirmation of an active case.[20] A new diagnosis of syphilis mandates investigation for concomitant human immunodeficiency virus (HIV) infection.

Treatment and Clinical Course First-line therapy for the treatment of syphilis is a one-time dose of penicillin G administered intramuscularly. Patients who have an allergy to penicillin should receive either doxycycline or ceftriaxone. As doxycycline is contraindicated in pregnancy, pregnant people with an allergy to penicillin must first be desensitized and then receive penicillin thereafter. Failure to receive adequate treatment at any stage of syphilis may result in the development of subsequent stages of the disease. However, adequate treatment of primary, secondary, or early latent infectious syphilis should result in disappearance of the clinical manifestations of active disease, although residual postinflammatory pigment alteration is possible in patients with darker skin tones. The titer of RPR or VDRL and the clinical symptoms must be monitored after treatment to verify therapeutic efficacy.

HERPES SIMPLEX VIRUS

Epidemiology and Pathogenesis The herpes simplex virus (HSV) enters the body through the skin or mucous membranes via direct contact with the secretions or mucosal surfaces of an infected individual. After multiplying initially in the epithelial layer, the virus travels in the sensory nerve roots to the dorsal root ganglion, where it becomes latent. Mucocutaneous outbreaks of HSV are triggered by the reactivation of the latent virus, which subsequently travels back down the nerve root. Oral and genital herpes can be caused by either HSV type 2 (HSV-2) or HSV type 1 (HSV-1). Genital herpes is a prevalent infection, with approximately 50 million Americans infected and 500,000 to 700,000 new infections per year.[21] HSV-2 prevalence appears to be highest among historically marginalized groups in the United States and more prevalent among women than among men.[22]

Clinical Findings After an incubation period of 2 to 20 days (average: 7 days), primary lesions develop, consisting of a single or group of painful vesicles that ultimately rupture to become painful ulcers.[23] In women, ulcers may appear on the introitus, urethral meatus, labia, and perineum. Women typically are afflicted with more severe disease, systemic symptoms, and complications than men. Cervical ulcerative lesions are possible, particularly with the initial outbreak. Additionally, women may complain of dysuria and urinary retention secondary to urethral lesions.

Recurrent HSV outbreaks typically are milder than the initial outbreak, and women reportedly have fewer recurrences than men. Although the diagnosis of genital herpes is largely clinical, it may be confirmed using viral culture, a Tzanck smear (showing viral acantholytic giant cells), a polymerase chain reaction (PCR) test for HSV DNA, or characteristic histopathology. PCR testing is preferred.

Treatment and Clinical Course Although there is no known cure for herpes, currently available treatment therapies have been found to reduce disease severity, duration, and frequency of recurrence. HSV is preferably treated with valacyclovir given ease of dosing; however, acyclovir or famciclovir can also be used. Individuals who experience more severe primary infections appear to have recurrent episodes more frequently. Women with HSV who become pregnant are expected to start valacyclovir treatment prophylactically at 36 weeks. Vertical transmission of this disease occurs approximately 50% of the time. Thus, mothers who have active lesions at the time of delivery are recommended to have a cesarean delivery.

ACUTE GENITAL ULCERATION

Epidemiology and Pathogenesis Acute genital ulceration, otherwise known as Lipschutz ulcers, is a nonsexually acquired condition where a small number of ulcers spontaneously appear and then completely resolve. Research studies have shown that the most affected demographic for this condition is women under 20 years of age who have not been sexually active. Very limited data exist that characterize the differences in prevalence based upon race and ethnicity. Some studies have shown that majority of the cases that were included in their study were White women. However, whether this was due to sampling bias or true statistical differences in prevalence remains unclear. The presentation of these ulcers has been associated with a prodrome of flu-like symptoms, sore throat, and fever.[6] There is room for more research to determine the exact pathophysiology of this disease process.

Clinical Findings Patients often start with a clinical prodrome of fever and malaise before these lesions develop. On clinical exam, these ulcers have been described as small (<10 mm), well-demarcated, and painful. On average, there are usually one to three lesions present. They have also been noted to have a necrotic or purulent center and follow a symmetrical distribution. This is often a diagnosis of exclusion; however with the right history, diagnosis is often made clinically without need for microscopic examination (which may show nonspecific changes of mixed inflammatory cell infiltrate in the dermis and sometimes inflammatory vascular reaction).[24] **Table 63-2** includes proposed major and minor diagnostic criteria.

Treatment and Clinical Course The clinical course of these ulcers consists of complete resolution in an average of 21 days. As this disease is self-resolving, treatment consists of local wound care and pain management. Patients may have to be admitted to the hospital for urinary retention due to pain. Ultrapotent topical steroids may be useful. However, most cases require 40 mg to 60 mg per day until lesions start to clinically improve.[6]

TABLE 63-2 Diagnostic criteria for acute genital ulceration (Lipschutz ulcers)[a]

Major diagnostic criteria
Presents with a first flare of acute genital ulcer
Age <20 years
No sexual contact in the past 3 months
No history of immunodeficiency
Acute onset of the genital ulcer and healing within 6 weeks
Minor diagnostic criteria
Single or multiple deeply, painful ulcers, with a necrotic center
Bilateral "kissing" pattern

[a]Reproduced with permission from Govindan B. Lipschütz ulcers: A literature review based on 79 cases *EMJ Reprod Health*. 2016;2(1):73-78.

VULVOVAGINAL CANDIDIASIS

Epidemiology and Pathogenesis Vulvovaginal candidiasis (VVC) is an extremely common yeast infection in women. It has been reported that 70% to 75% of women will experience it at some point in their life. The most common species identified is *Candida albicans*, though other yeast species have been identified, including candida glabrata.[25] *Candida albicans* is a part of the normal microbiome of the vagina and gastrointestinal tract. It becomes pathogenic under certain conditions such as medications, (eg, antibiotics, corticosteroids, or chemotherapy), disease (eg, diabetes or immunodeficiency), and hormones (eg, due to pregnancy or birth control pills). The source of the infection may also be a sexual partner.

Clinical Findings Women may develop candidal vaginitis, vulvitis, or vulvovaginitis, with presenting symptoms being moderate to severe itching or burning. Vaginal discharge varies from thin to a whitish lumpy consistency. In contrast to bacterial vaginosis, the vaginal discharge associated with VVC does not usually have an unpleasant odor. Inflammation with satellite pustules may be seen within the vestibule, in the interlabial crease, and over the labia minora and majora. If the infection is more severe, inflammation may be found in the crural fold and on the upper inner thigh. Vulvar edema, at times severe, may be present. Diagnosis is clinical, with confirmation via culture and/or potassium hydroxide (KOH) wet mount, which will demonstrate pseudohyphae.

Treatment and Clinical Course There are several different options when it comes to the treatment of VVC. These include azoles, polyenes, and ciclopirox olamine. Patients who are asymptomatic should not be started on treatment.[25] Women with vulvovaginitis are susceptible to recurrence because *Candida* is a normal inhabitant of the gastrointestinal tract and vagina. Frequently, recurrent or chronic vaginal candidiasis is a common problem, and there is no simple remedy. In chronic cases, fluconazole may be prescribed for suppression therapy, and patients may need weekly treatment for up to 3 months. It is important that women with recurrent symptoms be evaluated for bacterial vaginosis, *Trichomonas* infection, and infection with a non-*albicans Candida* species, because these conditions will not respond well to conventional treatment. In patients with persistent infection, constant scratching may lead to secondary lichenification, excoriation, and chronic swelling that resembles lichen simplex chronicus or chronic contact dermatitis.[26] In severe infections, particularly those seen in immunocompromised patients, erosions may complicate the disease course.

TINEA CRURIS

Epidemiology and Pathogenesis Tinea cruris, also known as jock itch, is a dermatophyte infection that specifically affects the groin area. This type of infection is more commonly seen in men than women. It is more common in adolescents and adults rather than children. Approximately 10% to 20% of Americans will experience a dermatophyte infection over the course of their life.[25] Tinea cruris (ringworm of the groin) is mostly caused by *Trichophyton rubrum*, the same organism responsible for most cases of tinea corporis. Infection can be spread via sexual contact with infected skin or through autoinoculation from tinea pedis.

Clinical Findings Tinea cruris involves any area from the proximal inner thigh area to the crural crease. It is characterized by a pruritic plaque with an area of central clearing and a peripheral border with overlying scale lending to an annular appearance, though not always present. For some patients, the skin may appear erythematous. However, among individuals with darker skin tones, the lesion may be more consistent with hyperpigmentation. In women, tinea cruris has a propensity to involve the hair-bearing portion of the vulva. Oftentimes the diagnosis of tinea cruris can be made clinically. However, there are several other conditions that may mimic the appearance of tinea (ie, candidiasis), so microscopic examination is commonly performed to confirm the diagnosis. This is done with KOH preparation. One should be able to appreciate hyphae on exam. Species identification is generally not needed, as it usually will not change treatment choice.

Treatment and Clinical Course Topical treatment with clotrimazole or terbinafine are usually sufficient to treat superficial infections.[25] Oral therapy may be required for those who fail topical therapy, have extensive involvement, or are immunocompromised. Affected individuals are at elevated risk for recurrence, although infections may be eradicated temporarily with therapy. Ongoing intermittent therapy with topical antifungals may be indicated to prevent the return of the infection.

NEOPLASTIC VULVAR LESIONS

MALIGNANT

Squamous Cell Carcinoma

Epidemiology and Pathogenesis SCC accounts for 85% to 90% of malignant tumors of the vulva. Historically, this has been classified as HPV dependent and HPV independent. Recent studies show that HPV status may be less of an independent prognostic factor in SCC than it was previously thought to be.[27]

Clinical Findings Approximately half of the affected women complain of pruritus with solitary lesions. Invasive vulvar cancer typically presents often as red glistening tumors, either unifocal or multifocal in nature, that may ulcerate or become nodular morphologically. Lesions appear on the posterior fourchette, labia minora, or interlabial sulcus.[28] Women tend to have larger lesions than men, reaching 2 to 3 cm in diameter.[28] Additionally, women may have significantly more lesions than men. It is important to use a punch biopsy to sample tumors to see if tumors are invasive, as this will change treatment course.

Treatment and Clinical Course Treatment of vulvar SCC is based on TNM staging. For early stages, therapy includes wide local excision with 1 to 2 cm margins or radical vulvectomy. Although Mohs surgery is currently not often performed, use of this technique should be explored further. Stage IB and II warrant a sentinel lymph node biopsy as well. Imaging such as magnetic resonance imaging (MRI) or positron emission tomography (PET) scan may be required to evaluate for total lymph node involvement and direct further treatment. Chemotherapy and external beam radiation are considered in these cases. Routine surveillance for recurrence is crucial.[27]

Melanoma

Epidemiology and Pathogenesis Melanoma is the sixth most common cancer among women. Of the 2.4% of women who will develop a malignant melanoma over their lifetime, 1% will be on the vulva. Melanoma accounts for 5% of vulvar malignancies. The median age at diagnosis is 68. Vulvar melanomas typically affect postmenopausal women, though some cases have occurred in children. It appears that VM is molecularly different from cutaneous melanoma, though the exact pathogenesis of VM is still not fully understood.[29]

Clinical Findings Vulvar melanomas are typically flat or raised pigmented lesions with an average size of 3 cm. Vulvovaginal melanomas are diagnosed at later stages for a variety of reasons. This may be because both patients and providers rarely look in the vulva unless there is a concern, and this condition is often asymptomatic. Late-stage lesions may cause pruritus, bleeding, and pain from ulceration. Vulvar melanomas can physically mimic other vulvar pigmented lesions such as genital nevi, postinflammatory hyperpigmentation, and pigmented seborrheic keratosis; thus, there should be a low threshold to rule out malignancy if one has concerns. Patients with lichen sclerosus often have an activated melanocytic proliferation that can mimic melanoma. Typical ABCDE (asymmetry, border, color, diameter, evolving) assessments are challenging to apply to vulvar melanoma.

Treatment and Clinical Course The first-line treatment for localized disease is surgical excision. Sentinel node biopsy should also be offered. More invasive cases may also require adjuvant therapy such as nivolumab or pembrolizumab. Recent studies have shown that tyrosine kinase inhibitors may have some efficacy against vulvar melanomas specifically if a c-KIT mutation is identified. Even with the recent advancements of immune checkpoint inhibitors and targeted therapy, the prognosis for vulvar melanomas remains very poor. The 5-year survival rate for vulvar melanomas is 47%, compared to 92% in cutaneous melanomas. It was found that vulvar melanomas do not react as well to traditional modalities as cutaneous melanomas.[29] This along with the relative delay in diagnosis makes for a poor prognosis overall.

BENIGN

Cysts

Epidemiology and Pathogenesis Benign genital cysts are very common, with an estimated prevalence of 1 in 200 women affected; this is thought to be an underestimation because most cysts are not reported.[30] Cyst formation appears to increase with age but has no racial predilection.

There are several different types of benign cysts that involve the lower female genitourinary tract. These include Bartholin gland cysts, Skene duct cysts (paraurethral), epidermoid inclusion cyst, and vestibular mucous cyst. Epidermal inclusion cysts are the most common genital cyst in women. They develop from buried epithelial fragments, most commonly following an episiotomy or other surgical procedure, or from a blockage in the pilosebaceous duct. Bartholin duct cysts are due to ductal obstruction within one of the two major vulvar vestibular glands, typically from a previous infection or inspissated mucus. Vestibular mucous cysts are simple cysts of the vulvar vestibule composed of mucus-secreting epithelium. Skene duct cysts (paraurethral duct cysts) are caused by obstruction of the Skene ducts, most commonly secondary to gonorrheal infection.[31]

Clinical Findings Most vaginal cysts are found incidentally on examination. The Bartholin glands are located on both sides of the vulvar vestibule at the 5 and 7 o'clock position. They are typically not palpable unless they are fluid filled. When these glands become obstructed, they may become full of mucus or pus leading to gland enlargement and thus a cyst. They typically are 1 to 3 cm, with some being as large as 5 cm in diameter. Smaller cysts are usually asymptomatic, while larger ones may lead to discomfort, vaginal pressure, or urinary incontinence or retention. Biopsy is usually not needed for diagnosis. However, histologically Bartholin cysts are composed of cuboidal mucin-secreting epithelium. Epidermoid inclusion cysts are typically located on the labia majora and arise from a hair follicle that is obstructed by keratin. These will usually appear as a yellowish papule, though this may be harder to appreciate on darker skin. These cysts tend to be smaller than Bartholin cysts, measuring on average between 1 and 3 mm in diameter but are similar in that they are round, smooth, and mobile. Vestibular mucous cysts range from 0.5 to 1.5 cm in diameter. These are typically located around the introitus and are mobile, nontender, and yellowish or bluish. Vestibular mucous cysts contain mucous-secreting columnar epithelium. Skene duct cysts are located near the edge of the urethral meatus, are mobile, and are skin-colored or translucent.

Treatment and Clinical Course As these cysts are benign and typically asymptomatic, treatment is usually unnecessary. However, if a patient is endorsing more significant pain or urinary symptoms, then excision will be needed as spontaneous remission is unlikely in this case. Patients should be informed that the probability of recurrence may be high.

ACKNOWLEDGMENTS

We would like to acknowledge and thank Dr. Rosen and Dr. Doherty for their excellent work writing the previous chapter on genital lesions in women.

REFERENCES

1. Lloyd J, Crouch NS, Minto CL, Liao LM, Creighton SM. Female genital appearance: "normality" unfolds. *BJOG*. 2005;112(5):643-646.
2. Özer M, Mortimore I, Jansma EP, Mullender MG. Labiaplasty: motivation, techniques, and ethics. *Nat Rev Urol*. 2018;15(3):175-189.

3. Nsereko E, Moreland PJ, Dunlop AL, Nzayirambaho M, Corwin EJ. Consideration of cultural practices when characterizing the vaginal microbiota among African and African American women. *Biol Res Nurs*. 2021;23(1):91-99.
4. Ferranti M. From birth control to that "fresh feeling": a historical perspective on feminine hygiene in medicine and media. *Women Health*. 2009;49(8):592-607.
5. Genital care for women. International society for the study of vulvovaginal disease. Revised 2021. https://www.issvd.org/resources/genital-care-for-women. Accessed June 6, 2023.
6. Mauskar MM, Marathe K, Venkatesan A, Schlosser BJ, Edwards L. Vulvar diseases: conditions in adults and children. *J Am Acad Dermatol*. 2020;82(6):1287-1298.
7. Rosen T. Diseases with unusual features: lichen planus. In: *Clinical Dermatology in Black Patients*. Bari, Italy: PiGreco Press; 1995:36-40.
8. Khurana A, Tandon S, Marfatia YS, Madnani N. Genital lichen planus: an underrecognized entity. *Indian J Sex Transm Dis AIDS*. 2019;40(2):105-112.
9. Solimani F, Forchhammer S, Schloegl A, Ghoreschi K, Meier K. Lichen planus - a clinical guide. *J Dtsch Dermatol Ges*. 2021;19(6):864-882.
10. Mauskar M. Erosive lichen planus. *Obstet Gynecol Clin North Am*. 2017; 44(3): 407-420.
11. Ju T, Vander Does A, Mohsin N, Yosipovitch G. Lichen simplex chronicus itch: an update. *Acta Derm Venereol*. 2022;102:adv00796.
12. Bernett CN, Krishnamurthy K. Cutaneous Crohn disease. In: *StatPearls*. Treasure Island (FL): StatPearls Publishing; January 9, 2023.
13. Das D, Gupta B, Saha M. Metastatic vulvar Crohn's disease-a rare case report and short review of literature. *Indian J Dermatol*. 2016;61(1):70-74.
14. Walker C, Allamneni C, Orr J, et al. Socioeconomic status and race are both independently associated with increased hospitalization rate among Crohn's disease patients. *Sci Rep*. 2018;8(1):4028.
15. Kelly A, Taylor SC, Lim HW, Serrano A. eds. *Taylor and Kelly's Dermatology for Skin of Color*. 2nd ed. New York, NY: McGraw Hill; 2016.
16. Ahmed F, Moseley I, Ragi SD, Ouellette S, Rao B. Vitiligo in underrepresented communities: an all of Us database analysis. *J Am Acad Dermatol*. 2023;88(4):945-948.
17. Leslie SW, Sajjad H, Kumar S. Genital warts. In: *StatPearls*. Treasure Island (FL): StatPearls Publishing; February 14, 2022.
18. Bakir AH, Skarzynski M. Health disparities in the immunoprevention of human papillomavirus infection and associated malignancies. *Front Public Health*. 2015;3:256. Published 2015 Dec 17.
19. Pourang A, Fung MA, Tartar D, Brassard A. Condyloma lata in secondary syphilis. *JAAD Case Rep*. 2021;10:18-21.
20. Amerson EH, Castillo Valladares HB, Leslie KS. Resurgence of syphilis in the US-USPSTF reaffirms screening guidelines. *JAMA Dermatol*. 2022;158(11): 1241-1243.
21. Solomon J, Cannon MJ, Reyes M, et al. Epidemiology of recurrent genital herpes simplex virus types 1 and 2. *Sex Transm Inf*. 2003;79:456-459.
22. Jackson C, Arcelay-Rojas Y. Experiences of African American women living with herpes simplex virus 2. *JSBHS*. 2021;15(1):345-362.
23. Fleming DT, Leone P, Esposito D, et al. Herpes virus type 2 infection and genital symptoms in primary care patients. *SexTransm Dis*. 2006;33:416-421.
24. Sindhuja T, Khaitan BK, Agarwal S, Agarwala S, Bhari N. Lipschutz ulcers in a 4-month-old girl. *Pediatr Dermatol*. 2022;39(5):827-829.
25. Ely JW, Rosenfeld S, Seabury Stone M. Diagnosis and management of tinea infections. *Am Fam Physician*. 2014;90(10):702-710.
26. Fisher BK, Margesson LJ. Infectious diseases of the vulva. In: *Genital Skin Disorders: Diagnosis and Treatment*. St. Louis, MO: Mosby; 1998:128-149.
27. Kolitz E, Lucas E, Hosler GA, et al. Human papillomavirus–positive and –negative vulvar squamous cell carcinoma are biologically but not clinically distinct. *J Invest Dermatol*. 2022;142(5):1280-1290.e7.
28. Fisher BK, Margesson LJ. Tumors and cysts of the vulva. In: *Genital Skin Disorders: Diagnosis and Treatment*. St. Louis, MO: Mosby; 1998:154-176.
29. Wohlmuth C, Wohlmuth-Wieser I. Vulvar melanoma: molecular characteristics, diagnosis, surgical management, and medical treatment. *Am J Clin Dermatol*. 2021;22(5):639-651.
30. Howe HL, Wingo PA, Thun MJ, et al. Annual report to the nation on the status of cancer (1973-1998), featuring cancers with recent increasing trends. *J Natl Cancer Inst*. 2001;93:824-842.
31. Rosen T. Unusual presentation of gonorrhea. *J Am Acad Dermatol*. 1982;6: 369-372.

SECTION 10

Dermatologic Infections

CHAPTER 64

Cutaneous Manifestations of Human Immunodeficiency Virus

Ciara G. Robinson
Henry W. Lim

KEY POINTS

- Human immunodeficiency virus (HIV) infection is associated with a wide range of dermatologic conditions.
- Many HIV-associated skin conditions initially present with deteriorating immunity, particularly when CD4 counts fall less than 200 cells/μL. The extent of skin disease often reflects the patient's immune status.
- Dermatologic conditions in patients with HIV are frequently more robust and refractory to treatment when compared to immunocompetent patients.
- Antiretroviral therapy dramatically reduces morbidity and mortality for patients with HIV and has a profound effect on the appearance and course of many skin conditions such as eosinophilic folliculitis and Kaposi sarcoma.

INTRODUCTION

In 2022, approximately 39 million people were living with human immunodeficiency virus (HIV); 5.5 million of these individuals were unaware that they had HIV.[1] As with many other diseases, Black and Hispanic/Latino communities are disproportionately affected by HIV in the United States.[2] Subpopulations within these racial and ethnic minority groups that are disproportionately affected include gay, bisexual, and other men who have sex with men, Black women, transgender men, and intravenous drug users.[2] HIV diminishes cluster of differentiation (CD) 4 cells, which leads to profound immunodeficiency and subsequent infectious, inflammatory, neoplastic, and metabolic disease. While antiretroviral therapy (ARVT) has revolutionized HIV treatment and reduced the frequency and severity of HIV-related cutaneous disease, 9.2 million people with HIV did not have access to antiretroviral therapy in 2022.[1] This highlights the need for increased access to care to further decrease HIV-specific dermatologic diseases. In this chapter, we will review the cutaneous manifestations of HIV with an emphasis on presentation and treatment in skin of color populations.

NONVIRAL AND NONBACTERIAL DISEASES

EXANTHEM OF ACUTE RETROVIRAL SYNDROME

Acute retroviral syndrome (ARS) occurs in one-half to two-thirds of individuals with HIV; it may present within 2 to 4 weeks and up to 3 months following initial exposure to the virus.[3] Symptoms include fever, malaise, myalgia, pharyngitis, and lymphadenopathy.[3] An estimated 30% to 50% of these patients also have cutaneous findings, which is most commonly erythematous macules and papules scattered on the face, trunk [**Figure 64-1**], and upper extremities. Oral lesions ranging from erythema to ulcers can also be seen. It is important to note that HIV antibody tests are negative in the acute setting and take several months to seroconvert.[3]

SEBORRHEIC DERMATITIS

Seborrheic dermatitis is common in the general population, but prevalence is much higher in patients with HIV. It presents with erythema and greasy, yellow scale in the scalp, nasolabial folds, eyebrows, ears, retroauricular region, and/or beard [**Figure 64-2**]. With poorly controlled HIV and progression to acquired immune deficiency syndrome (AIDS), it becomes more severe, widespread, and refractory to treatment.[4] In skin of color patients, lesions often heal with hyper- or hypopigmentation. Topical antifungals and low-potency topical steroids are typically effective; however, higher potency topical steroids and calcineurin inhibitors are required in some cases.

PSORIASIS

While the prevalence of psoriasis in HIV-infected individuals is similar to that of the general population, psoriasis may be more severe and recalcitrant, and psoriasis arthritis is more prevalent in HIV and AIDS patients.[5] Most patients with both HIV and psoriasis have typical lesions that are characterized by symmetric, well-demarcated erythematous to violaceous papules and plaques with silver scale. It is commonly seen on the scalp, elbows, knees, and intertriginous areas. A distinguishing feature is the presence of more than one type of psoriasis (inverse, classic plaque, annular or polycyclic, and pustular) in the same patient.[3] Improvement in psoriasis is seen as viral load declines with antiretroviral treatment. Treatment options for psoriasis include topical corticosteroids, calcipotriene, tazarotene, phototherapy (narrow-band UVB or psoralen plus UVA), and acitretin.[6] Immunomodulatory drugs should be used with caution. More specifically, methotrexate administration has been related to increased incidence of opportunistic infections and cyclosporine has increased bioavailability when coadministered with protease inhibitors.[6] Biologic agents such as infliximab, ustekinumab, etanercept, and aprelimast are used in patients with HIV and treatment responses are comparable to HIV-negative patients.[7]

DRUG ERUPTIONS

The risk of drug eruptions in patients with HIV is significantly higher than that of the general population.[8-10] Antibiotics and antiretrovirals are common culprits of drug eruptions in HIV patients. Exanthematous eruptions from sulfamethoxazole/trimethoprim have reached rates of 47% when higher than usual doses were used to treat *Pneumocystis jiroveci* pneumonia.[11] Indinavir can cause ingrown toe nails and alopecia, and saquinavir may cause oral ulcerations.[12] Exanthematous eruptions have been reported in 2% to 8% of patients treated with protease inhibitors, including darunavir, lopinavir/ritonavir, fosamprenavir, atazanavir, and tipranavir/ritonavir.[12] Tenofovir can cause pruritus and maculopapular, urticarial, vesiculobullous, or pustular eruptions in 5% to 7% of patients.[12] In the majority of cases, the eruption resolves spontaneously, even if the drug responsible is not discontinued.[12] More serious reactions such as drug reaction with eosinophilia and systemic symptoms/drug-induced hypersensitivity syndrome (DRESS/DIHS) and Stevens-Johnson syndrome/toxic epidermal necrolysis (SJS/TEN) [**Figure 64-3**] occur more frequently in patients with HIV. Abacavir causes DRESS/DIHS in up to 8% of patients and can be fatal. Screening

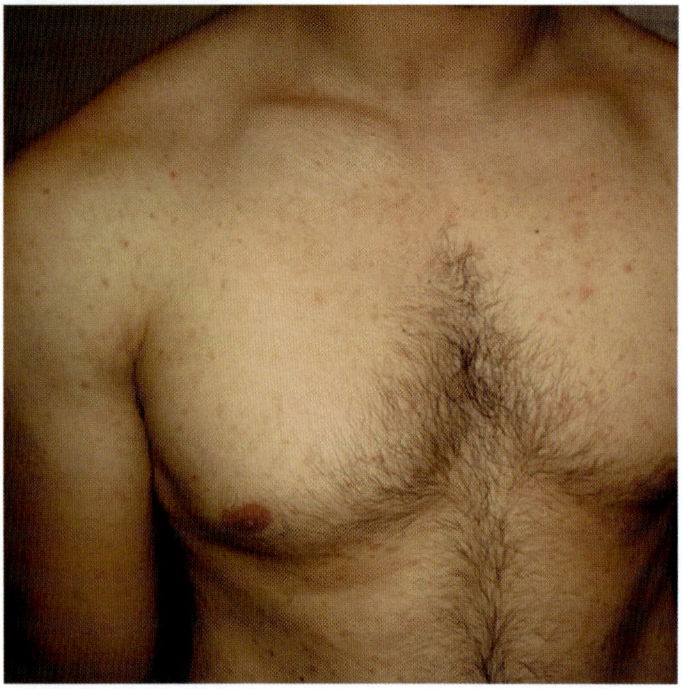

FIGURE 64-1. Poorly defined pink macules on the trunk of a man with acute retroviral syndrome. (Used with permission from the Ronald O. Perelman Department of Dermatology, NYU School of Medicine, NYU Langone Medical Center, NY.)

for HLA-B*5701 is recommended prior to initiation of therapy as it is associated with higher likelihood of developing the reaction. Other causes of DRESS/DIHS in this population include nevirapine, trimethoprim-sulfamethoxazole, and dapsone. Patients with AIDS have a 1000-fold increased risk of developing SJS/TEN. Common culprits include trimethoprim-sulfamethoxazole among other antibiotics, nevirapine, abacavir, efavirenz, etravirine, nonsteroidal anti-inflammatory drugs, and anticonvulsants.[13]

LIPODYSTROPHY

Lipodystrophy is typically seen within 2 years of starting antiretroviral therapy; most notably protease inhibitors and nucleoside reverse transcriptase inhibitors and to lesser extent, nonnucleoside reverse

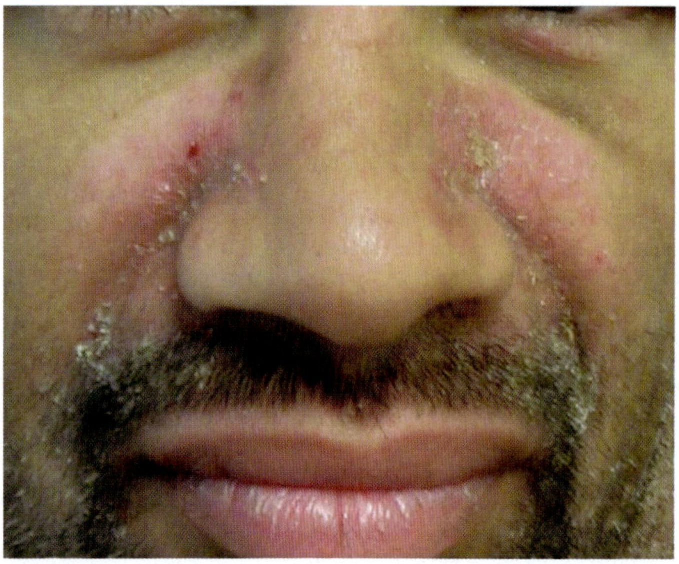

FIGURE 64-2. Severe seborrheic dermatitis with hypopigmented borders on the nasolabial folds of a Hispanic man. (Used with permission from the Ronald O. Perelman Department of Dermatology, NYU School of Medicine, NYU Langone Medical Center, NY.)

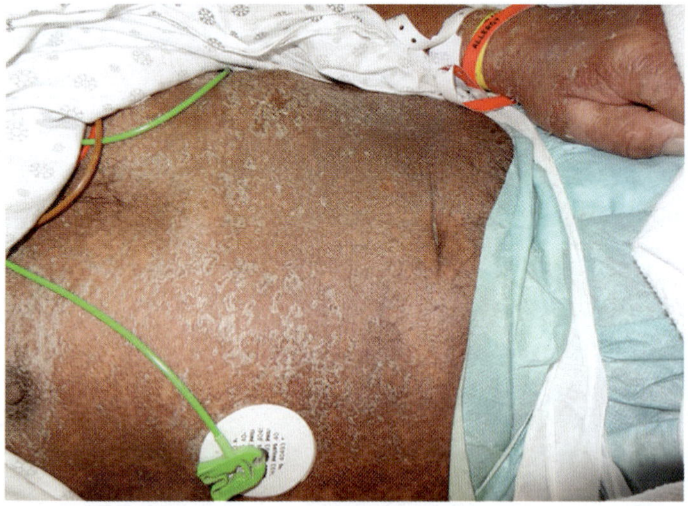

FIGURE 64-3. Toxic epidermal necrolysis due to vancomycin in a patient with human immunodeficiency virus. (Used with permission from the Ronald O. Perelman Department of Dermatology, NYU School of Medicine, NYU Langone Medical Center, NY.)

transcriptase inhibitors. It presents with loss of fat in the face, extremities, and buttocks or accumulation and redistribution of fat to dorsocervical region, neck, or abdomen [**Figure 64-4**]. Lipodystrophy is associated with metabolic disorders (hyperglycemia, hyperlipidemia, and insulin resistance).[14]

IMMUNE RECONSTITUTION INFLAMMATORY SYNDROME

With the recovery of immunity following ARVT, a subset of patients develops clinical deterioration in areas of previous or current infectious (eg, cytomegalovirus, hepatitis B or C, tuberculosis, and Cryptococcus), neoplastic (KS), and autoimmune involvement. Dermatologic manifestations of immune reconstitution inflammatory syndrome (IRIS) include the onset or rapid worsening of molluscum or warts, development of epidermodysplasia verruciformis-like human papillomavirus (HPV) lesions,

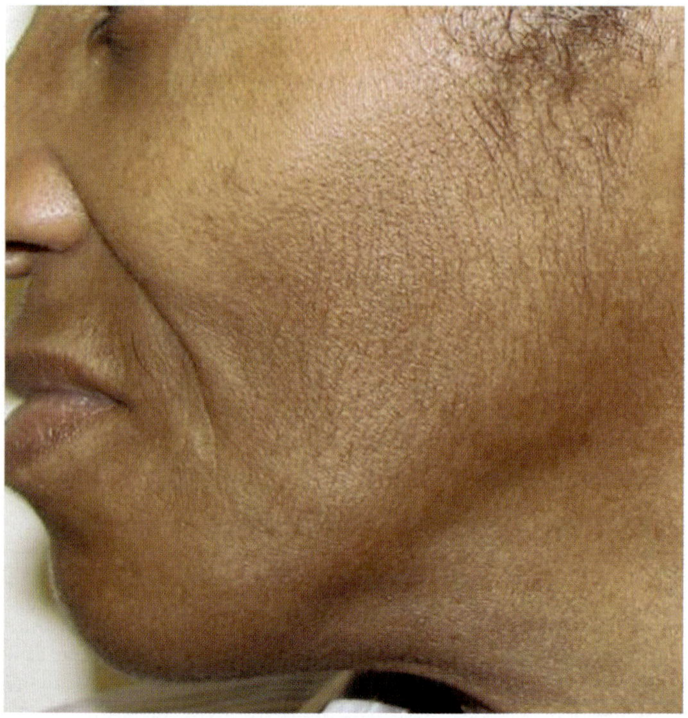

FIGURE 64-4. Human immunodeficiency virus-associated lipodystrophy. (Used with permission from the Ronald O. Perelman Department of Dermatology, NYU School of Medicine, NYU Langone Medical Center, NY.)

reactivation of herpes zoster and ulcerative oral or anogenital herpes, ulcerations from Mycobacterium avium, upgrading of leprosy to the lepromatous spectrum, rapid progression of leishmaniasis, and flare-ups of acne and pruritic papular eruptions (PPEs).[15,16] The etiology involves an exaggerated immune response to antimicrobial or other antigens in the setting of decreasing viral load.[15] This occurs within 2 weeks to 3 months following initiation of ARVT and findings typically improve or resolve within several months. Systemic corticosteroids may be required in some cases to prevent disabling, destructive, or lethal organ damage.[15]

ATOPIC DERMATITIS, PRURITUS, PRURIGO NODULARIS, PRURITIC PAPULAR ERUPTION, AND EOSINOPHILIC FOLLICULITIS

Many individuals with HIV complain of itching, which may be primary HIV-associated pruritus or secondary to skin diseases such as eczema, scabies, drug reactions, pruritic papular eruption, or eosinophilic folliculitis. The prevalence of these conditions is as high as 37.5% in patients with HIV.[17] The degree of dry, pruritic skin reflects the overall burden of immunosuppression and is due to impaired skin barrier. Prurigo nodularis presents as pigmented hyperkeratotic plaques and nodules and is secondary to chronic scratching of the skin. Pruritic papular eruption is an exaggerated immune response to arthropod bites or stings secondary to hyperactive Th-2-driven immune pathways.[17] It manifests as scattered, urticarial papules most commonly on the extremities [**Figure 64-5**]. Eosinophilic folliculitis (EF) is a recurrent, intensely pruritic eruption of pink or pigmented papules and pustules on the face, trunk, and extensor surfaces of upper extremities. Treatment options consist of ARVT, topical steroids, narrow band UVB, systemic steroids, topical calcineurin inhibitors, and tetracyclines.[18]

PHOTODERMATITIS AND PIGMENTARY CHANGES

Photosensitivity to ultraviolet-B and, to a lesser extent, ultraviolet-A, has been reported in patients with HIV. Many of these patients had CD4 counts lesser than 200 cells/μL and most had concomitant eosinophilic folliculitis and/or were on sulfamethoxazole-trimethoprim prophylaxis.[19] Chronic actinic dermatitis [**Figure 64-6**] and porphyria cutanea tarda have been reported in patients with HIV infection.[20,21]

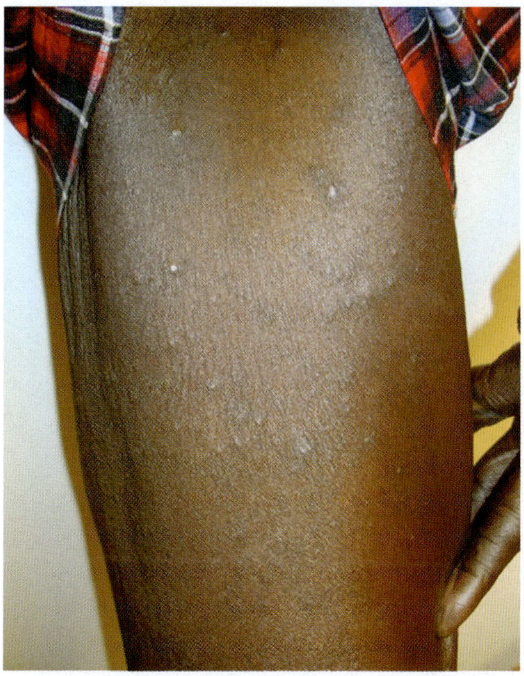

FIGURE 64-5. Discrete excoriated papules in a patient with pruritic papular eruption of human immunodeficiency virus. (Used with permission from the Ronald O. Perelman Department of Dermatology, NYU School of Medicine, NYU Langone Medical Center, NY.)

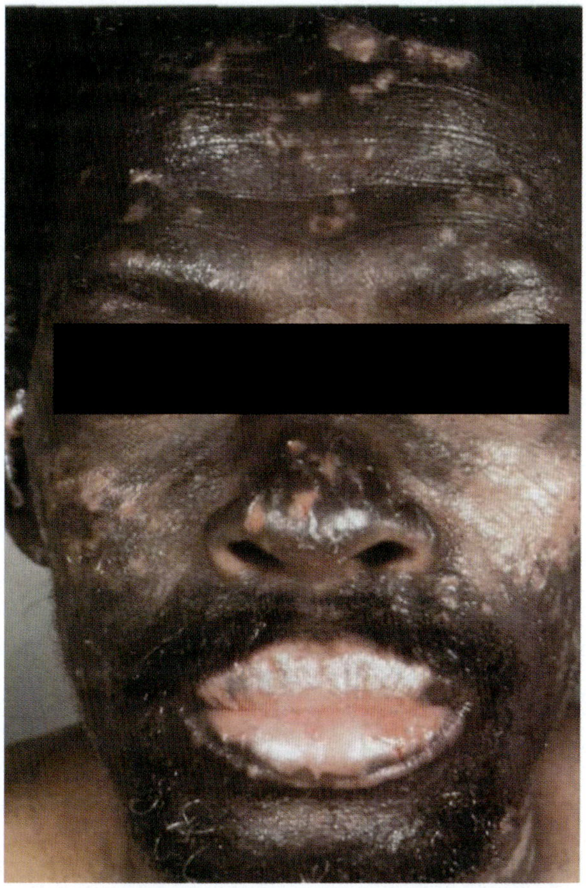

FIGURE 64-6. Hyper- and hypopigmentation with fissures in sun-exposed areas.

Increased photosensitivity in this population can impact the use of phototherapy as a treatment of skin disease. Mucocutaneous pigmentary changes are common in skin of color patients with HIV and are typically drug-induced or secondary to prior cutaneous inflammation. Zidovudine often causes dose-dependent hyperpigmentation of the skin and oral mucosa as well as longitudinal melanonychia.[22] Emtricitabine causes hyperpigmentation of the palms, soles, nails, and oral mucosa, almost exclusively in patients with skin of color.[23]

NONINFECTIOUS HAIR/NAIL DISEASES

Alopecia areata, diffuse alopecia (potentially inflammatory), telogen effluvium, and strikingly elongated eyelashes have been reported in individuals living with AIDS.[24]

SCABIES

With advanced HIV infection, *Sarcoptes scabiei* infestation presents as crusted (Norwegian) scabies with a widespread distribution of hyperkeratotic plaques over the head, dorsa [**Figure 64-7**], trunk, palms, and soles. Diagnosis may be delayed due to absence of typical burrows and pruritus; however, a skin scraping will show numerous mites. Repeated applications of permethrin along with oral ivermectin is usually required.[25]

VIRAL DISEASE

HERPES SIMPLEX VIRUS

Approximately 70% of patients with HIV are infected with herpes simplex virus (HSV)-2 and 95% are infected with either HSV-1 or HSV-2.[26] HSV infection is identical to those of the general population in that it

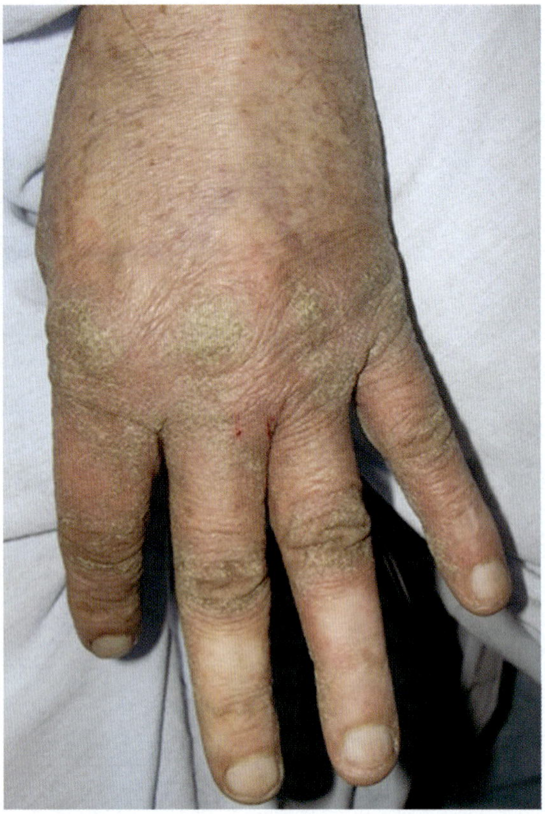

FIGURE 64-7. Hyperkeratotic crusted plaques in a man with crusted (Norwegian) scabies. Similar lesions were present on the trunk, feet, face, and ears. (Used with permission from the Ronald O. Perelman Department of Dermatology, NYU School of Medicine, NYU Langone Medical Center, NY.)

often has prodromal burning, tingling, or pruritus followed by evolution of lesions from papule to vesicle on an erythematous base [**Figure 64-8A** and **B**], to ulcer then crust. In patients with HIV, HSV infections are more likely to be prolonged, severe, and atypical. More specifically, patients with CD4 count of less than 100 cells/μL may develop extensive, nonhealing ulcerations. Gold standard for treatment includes acyclovir, valacyclovir, and famciclovir. Intravenous foscarnet is the treatment of choice of acyclovir-resistant HSV. Other options include topical trifluridine, cidofovir, and imiquimod. Higher doses and prolonged courses may be required for refractory disease.[26]

VARICELLA ZOSTER VIRUS

A person's lifetime risk of herpes zoster is 15% to 20%, with the highest incidence being in elderly and immunocompromised patients. The incidence of herpes zoster is greater than 15-fold higher for patients with HIV compared to age-matched controls.[26] The risk of herpes zoster is less likely to be reduced by ARVT when compared to other opportunistic infections.[26] Herpes zoster can occur in any patient with HIV but there is an increased risk in patients with CD4 count of less than 200 cells/μL. Herpes zoster infection is characterized by a painful eruption of vesicles, pustules, and crusts in a dermatomal distribution [**Figure 64-9A** and **B**]. Similar to HSV infection, it is often preceded by prodromal symptoms such as tingling, pain, or pruritus. Disseminated herpes zoster is almost exclusively seen in immunocompromised patients and is defined as dermatomal disease in addition to greater than 20 lesions outside of dermatome. Visceral involvement can also occur. Acute retinal necrosis may be seen even in patients without trigeminal dermatome involvement.[26] Live attenuated varicella vaccines have been shown to be safe and are recommended for HIV patients with CD4 counts greater than 200 cells/μL.[26] Treatment should be initiated within 1 week of rash onset and continued for 7 to 10 days or longer if the lesions are slow to resolve. Treatment options include oral or IV acyclovir, valacyclovir, or famciclovir.

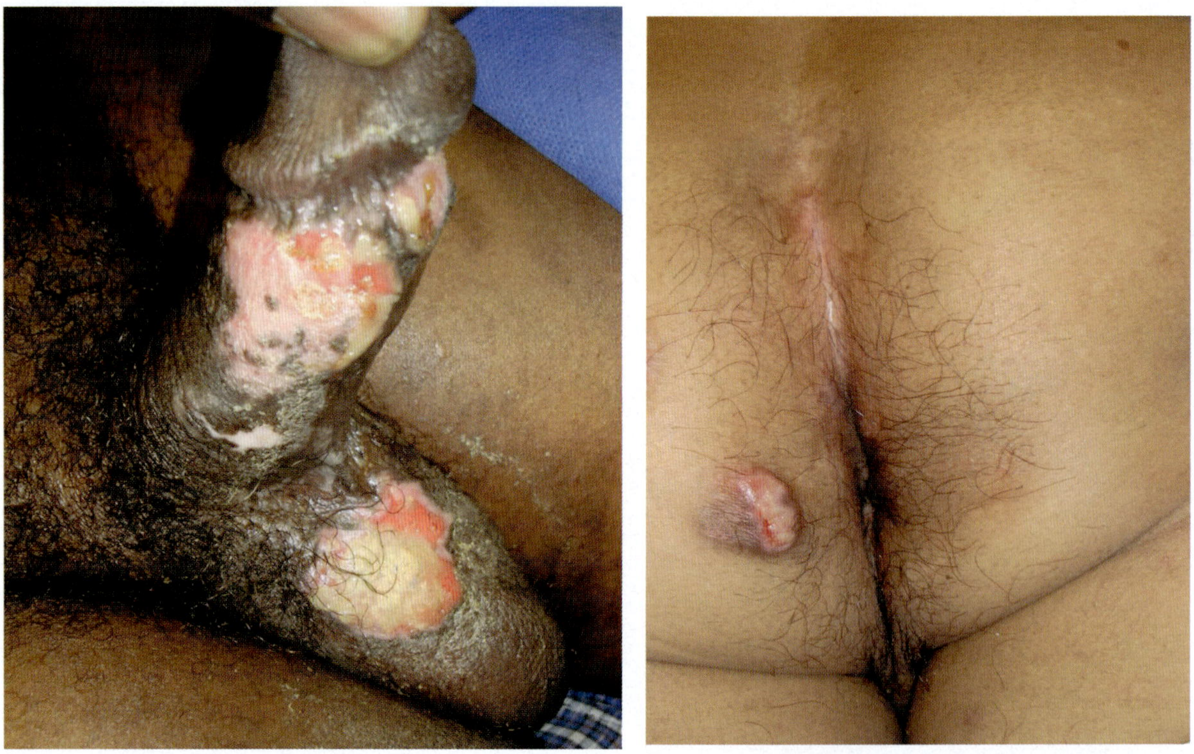

A B

FIGURE 64-8. **(A)** Multiple, large, horizontally expanding, weeping genital ulcers with bright red bases and irregular edges secondary to acyclovir-resistant herpes simplex virus (HSV)-2. **(B)** Chronic, slowly expanding, tumor-like nodule with ulcerated surface caused by HSV-2. (Used with permission from the Ronald O. Perelman Department of Dermatology, NYU School of Medicine, NYU Langone Medical Center, NY.)

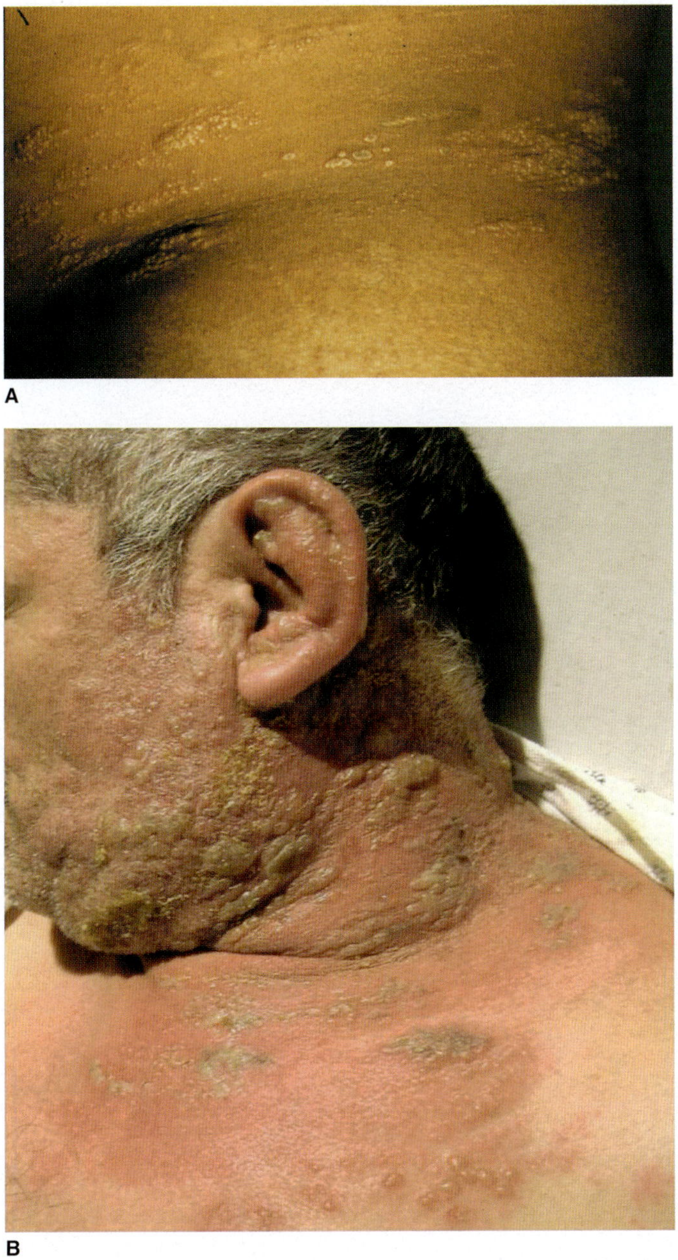

FIGURE 64-9. **(A)** Herpes zoster in the classic dermatomal distribution. **(B)** Severe herpes zoster in a Hispanic man. (Part B used with permission from the Ronald O. Perelman Department of Dermatology, NYU School of Medicine, NYU Langone Medical Center, NY.)

HUMANPAPILLOMA VIRUS

HPV infection rates are high in patients with HIV and clinically manifests as genital, anal, or oral warts. In immunocompromised patients, these lesions spread rapidly, require more aggressive treatment, and are more prone to recur [**Figure 64-10A-C**].[26] Treatment consists of destructive and immunomodulating therapies such as cryotherapy, chemical ablation with trichloroacetic acid, podophyllin/podophyllotoxin or cantharidin, laser or electrocautery, surgical resection, chemoimmunotherapy with imiquimod or sinecatechins, and topical chemotherapy with fluorouracil. Infection with oncogenic HPV subtypes is associated with development of cervical, vaginal, vulvar, anal, and oropharyngeal malignancies; ARVT has limited or no effect on the development of such cancers.[26] Therapeutically recalcitrant warts should be biopsied to exclude squamous cell carcinoma (SCC).

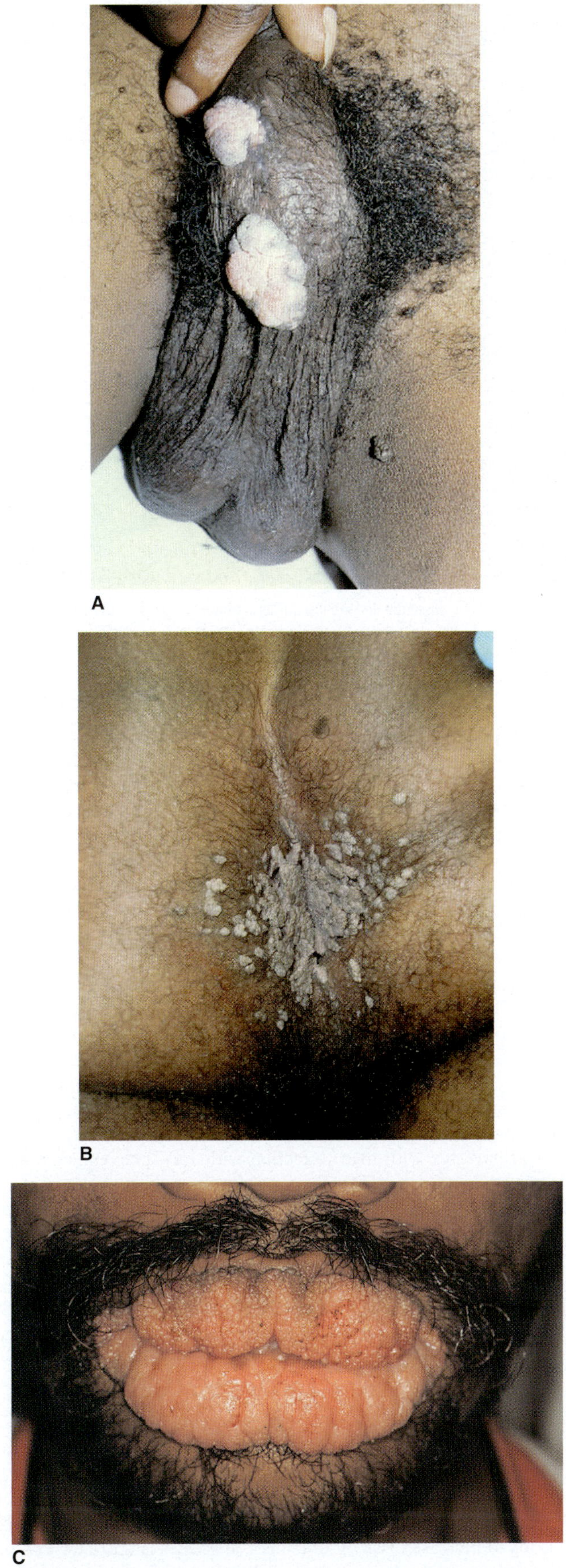

FIGURE 64-10. Condylomata acuminata on **(A)** the shaft of the penis, **(B)** the perianal area, and **(C)** the lips. (Part B used with permission from the Ronald O. Perelman Department of Dermatology, NYU School of Medicine, NYU Langone Medical Center, NY.)

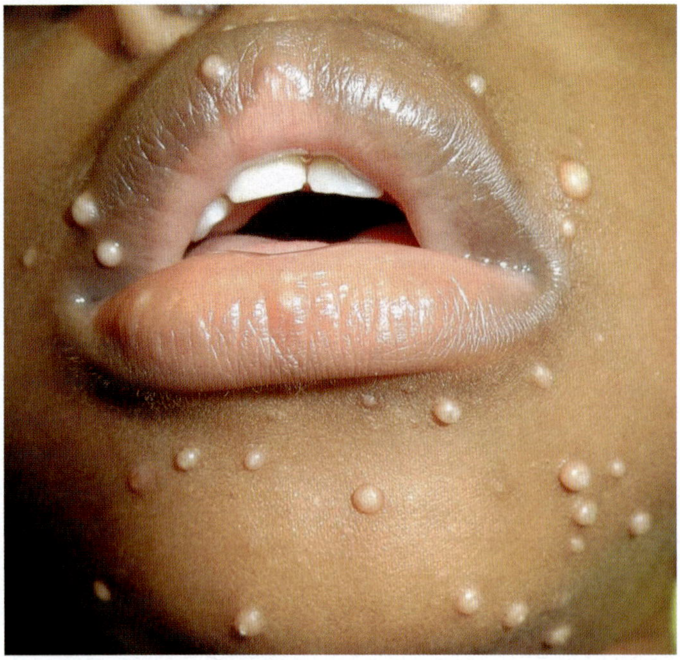

FIGURE 64-11. Disseminated molluscum contagiosum on the face of a child. (Used with permission from the Ronald O. Perelman Department of Dermatology, NYU School of Medicine, NYU Langone Medical Center, NY.)

OTHER VIRAL INFECTIONS

Molluscum contagiosum, caused by poxvirus, is a common infection seen in both immunocompetent patients (especially children) and in patients with HIV. It presents with skin colored, umbilicated papules on the face [**Figure 64-11**], trunk, and flexural surfaces of immunocompetent individuals. When sexually transmitted, lesions are found in the anogenital region and upper thighs. In patients with CD4 count of less than 200 cells/μL, the lesions are numerous, widely disseminated, large (termed "giant molluscum"), and often refractory to conventional treatments.[27]

Epstein-Barr virus causes oral hairy leukoplakia characterized by nonpainful white plaques on the lateral tongue.[28] These lesions resolve with ARVT-induced enhancement of immune function. Polyomavirus results in trichodysplasia spinulosa in immunosuppressed patients; it presents as collections of skin colored to pink spiny papules on the face.[28] Mpox (Monkeypox) disproportionally affects gay and bisexual individuals, and men who have sex with men. Infection with HIV may enhance Mpox virus transmission, as well as vice versa. Moreover, the prevalence of HIV and Mpox coinfection was 40% and the most reported clinical presentation consisted of skin lesions, fever, headache, and lymphadenopathy.[29] Low CD4 count, as seen in patients with HIV, has been associated with clinical severity, dissemination, and mortality from Mpox infection. In patients with HIV and Mpox coinfection, it is recommended that ARVT is continued, and antiviral therapy targeting Mpox is started, if indicated.[29]

BACTERIAL DISEASE

Community acquired bacteria such as *Staphylococcus aureus*, methicillin-resistant *S. aureus* (MRSA), and *Pseudomonas aeruginosa* occur at a higher frequency in patients with HIV.[25] *Staphylococcus aureus* colonization leads to increased risk of folliculitis, abscesses [**Figure 64-12A** and **B**], furuncles, carbuncles, ecthyma, cellulitis pyomyositis, fasciitis, and botryomycosis.[25] When treating these conditions, cultures and sensitivities should guide antibiotic choice. Superficial folliculitis may be treated with topical antibiotics such as clindamycin, benzoyl peroxide, retapamulin, and mupirocin. Treatment of choice for abscesses is incision

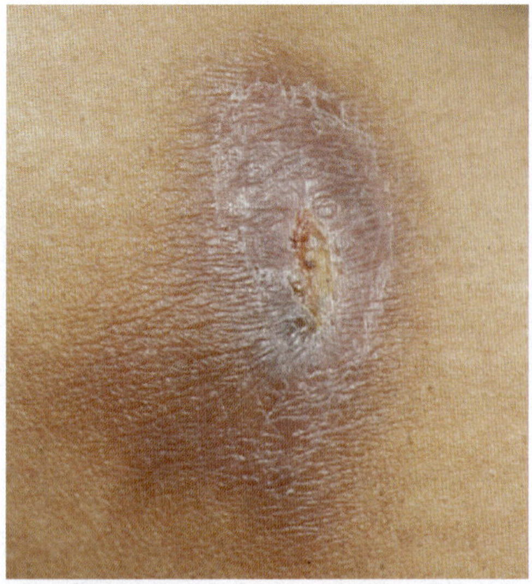

A

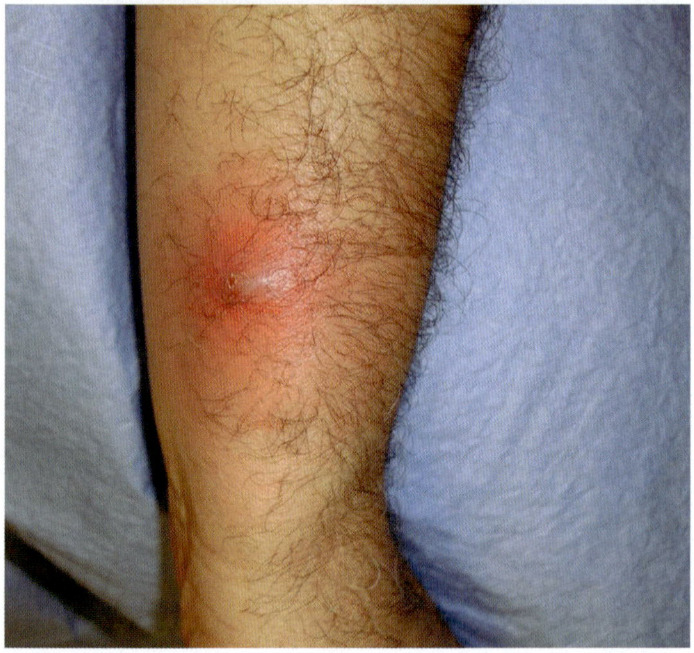

B

FIGURE 64-12. (A) Drained methicillin-resistant *Staphylococcus aureus* (MRSA) abscess. **(B)** Abscess with surrounding cellulitis caused by MRSA on the forearm of a Hispanic man. (Part B used with permission from the Ronald O. Perelman Department of Dermatology, NYU School of Medicine, NYU Langone Medical Center, NY.)

and drainage in addition to antibiotics for immunosuppressed patients. Bacillary angiomatosis, caused by *Bartonella henselae* or *Bartonella quintana*, presents as red, exophytic papules or painful, dusky, subcutaneous nodules.[25] Treatment consists of erythromycin or doxycycline for 2 weeks to 2 months.

SYPHILIS

In the United States and western Europe, the prevalence of syphilis has increased exponentially in the past decade in men who have sex with men, particularly those with HIV infection. According to the Centers for Disease Control and Prevention, approximately 50% of men who have sex with men that are diagnosed with syphilis also have HIV.[30] Primary syphilis presents with a painless, indurated, ulcerated lesion at the site of inoculation. Patients may also have associated lymphadenopathy. Without treatment, these lesions spontaneously resolve in 3 to 6 weeks in comparison to a few days with treatment. Secondary syphilis is more

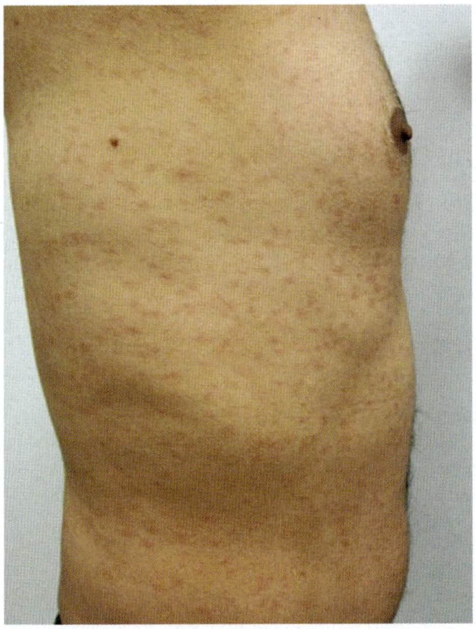

FIGURE 64-13. Typical eruption of secondary syphilis consisting of erythematous, round to oval, barely raised papules following the Langer lines on the trunk of a man. (Used with permission from the Ronald O. Perelman Department of Dermatology, NYU School of Medicine, NYU Langone Medical Center, NY.)

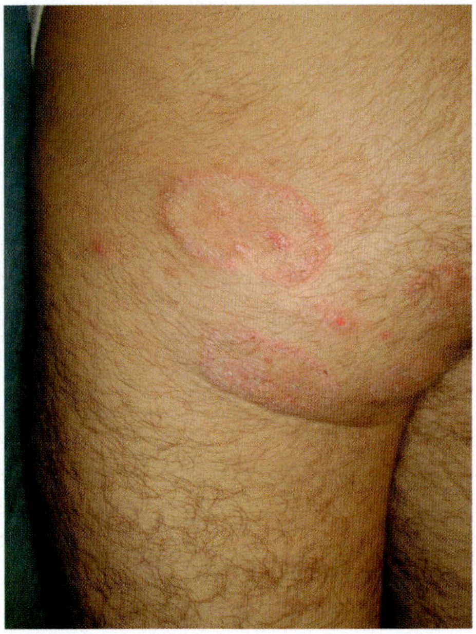

FIGURE 64-15. Widespread tinea corporis on the buttocks of a man infected with human immunodeficiency virus. (Used with permission from the Ronald O. Perelman Department of Dermatology, NYU School of Medicine, NYU Langone Medical Center, NY.)

commonly recognized due to the myriad of clinical symptoms that include a papulosquamous eruption [**Figure 64-13**], copper-colored macules or papules with overlying scale classically on the palms and soles, verrucous lesions on mucosal surfaces called condyloma lata, fever, malaise, headache, and lymphadenopathy.[31] Tertiary syphilis is characterized by gummas, cardiovascular disease, and neurosyphilis. Gummas are locally destructive skin lesions that are prone to recur. Cardiovascular syphilis manifests are aneurysms, coronary artery disease, aortitis, or aortic valve insufficiency.[31] Manifestations of neurosyphilis include pupillary abnormalities, general paresis, and tabes dorsalis. General paresis causes progressive dementia, seizures, and psychiatric symptoms, while tabes dorsalis presents as abrupt lightning pains, ataxia, and loss of proprioception.[31] Accelerated disease course and neurosyphilis are more frequently observed in patients with HIV. Penicillin is the treatment of choice.

FUNGAL DISEASE

Oropharyngeal candidiasis, also known as thrush, is a superficial fungal infection that presents as a painless white exudate that can be easily scraped off in the mouth or pharynx [**Figure 64-14**].[26] It can also present as angular cheilitis or erythematous patches on the anterior or posterior palate or tongue. It is most commonly seen in patients with CD4 count of less than 200 cells/μL. Treatment options include mucoadhesive miconazole, itraconazole or posaconazole, nystatin suspension, or oral antifungals.[26] Patients with HIV are more susceptible to extensive dermatophyte infections including tinea pedis, corporis [**Figure 64-15**], manuum, or capitis, and onychomycosis. Proximal white subungual onychomycosis or superficial white onychomycosis should raise suspicion for HIV infection.[32]

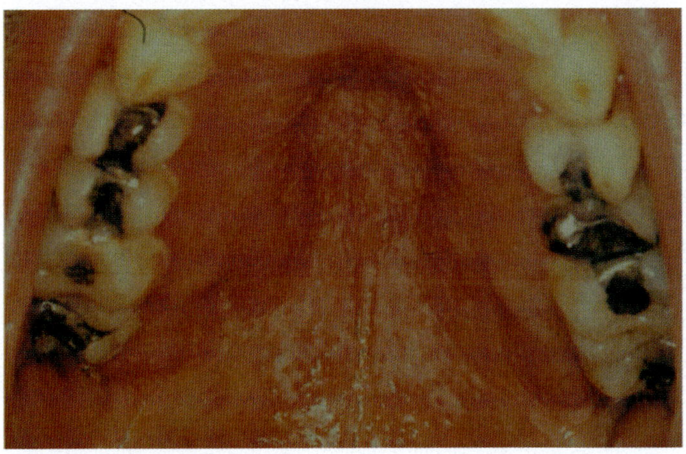

FIGURE 64-14. Oral candidiasis.

Opportunistic deep fungal infections are associated with disseminated disease and high mortality. When dissemination occurs, a variety of cutaneous morphologies can be seen including but not limited to papules, pustules, ulcers, vegetating or granulomatous plaques, nodules, bullae, and vasculitis-like lesions. Histoplasmosis is endemic in Ohio and Mississippi River Valleys and Latin America. It most commonly presents as pulmonary disease; however, skin lesions in disseminated disease appear as reddish, necrotic papules and pustules [**Figure 64-16**]. Patients should be treated with IV amphotericin B followed by oral itraconazole.[26] The incidence of cryptococcal infections among HIV patients has decreased significantly since the development of ARVT. In this population, cryptococcosis most commonly occurs as meningitis. Skin lesions occur with disseminated disease and often mimic molluscum.[26] Treatment of choice is amphotericin B with flucytosine.

MALIGNANCIES

Kaposi sarcoma (KS) is a malignancy of the vascular endothelium caused by human herpesvirus-8. It is characterized by violaceous papules, plaques, or nodules that are often symmetrically distributed on the extremities, trunk, face/neck [**Figure 64-17**], or oral mucosa.[33] The mortality rate of KS has decreased by 90% since ARVT became available and tumors are now more likely to be indolent and spontaneously regress.[33] KS commonly results in vascular obstruction and lymphedema. It can also involve the gastrointestinal tract and lungs; pulmonary disease generally portends a poor prognosis. Treatment options include ARVT, chemotherapy, and locally destructive modalities.[33]

While HIV is associated with an increased risk of keratinocyte skin cancer in both men and women, the exact risk is skin of color patients is uncertain. Patients with HIV have a twofold increased risk of basal cell carcinoma, fivefold increased risk of squamous cell carcinoma (often times

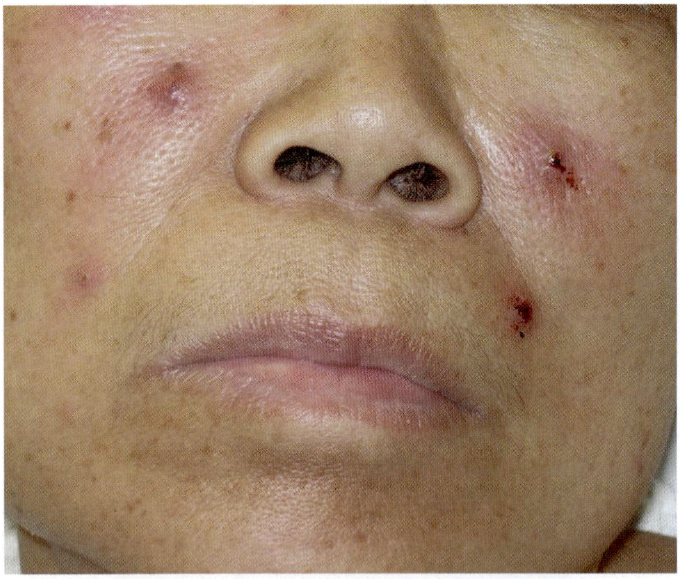

FIGURE 64-16. Case of disseminated histoplasmosis with erythematous pustules that became necrotic and hemorrhagic. (Used with permission from the Ronald O. Perelman Department of Dermatology, NYU School of Medicine, NYU Langone Medical Center, NY.)

anogenital), and twofold increased risk of melanoma compared with their HIV negative counterparts. Viruses, particularly certain subtypes of HPV, are oncogenic and contribute to the development of cutaneous squamous cell carcinoma in this immunosuppressed population.[26]

CONCLUSION

The number of new cases of HIV each year remains high, especially in men who have sex with men, Black women, transgender men, and intravenous drug users. HIV leads to a state of profound immunodeficiency, which increases the likelihood of infection, malignancy, and inflammatory dermatoses associated with the condition. Many cutaneous conditions are indicators of HIV infection, and the extent of disease often reflects the patient's immune status. Cutaneous manifestations remain a common concern for individuals with HIV; even with adequate treatment, patients may still suffer from a wide range of dermatologic conditions, many of which are refractory to standard therapies.

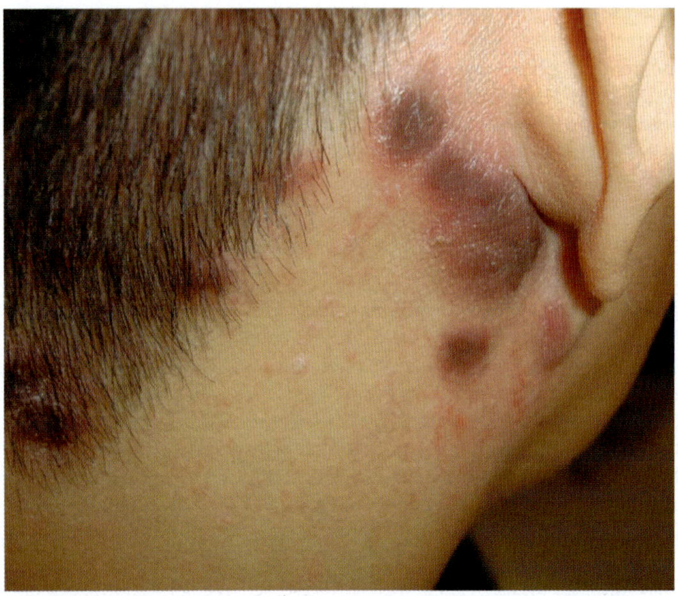

FIGURE 64-17. Violaceous nodular plaques characteristic of epidemic Kaposi sarcoma involving the head and neck. (Used with permission from the Ronald O. Perelman Department of Dermatology, NYU School of Medicine, NYU Langone Medical Center, NY.)

ACKNOWLEDGMENT

We would like to acknowledge Miguel Sanchez, MD for his contributions to Chapter 60: Cutaneous Manifestations of Human Immunodeficiency Virus in *Taylor and Kelly's Dermatology for Skin of Color*, 2nd edition.

REFERENCES

1. Global statistics. Updated November 15, 2023. https://www.hiv.gov/hiv-basics/overview/data-and-trends/global-statistics/. Accessed January 1, 2024.
2. Impact on racial and ethnic minorities. Updated December 18, 2023. https://www.hiv.gov/hiv-basics/overview/data-and-trends/impact-on-racial-and-ethnic-minorities/. Accessed January 1, 2024.
3. Khambaty MM, Hsu SS. Dermatology of the patient with HIV. *Emerg Med Clin North Am*. 2010;28(2):355-368, Table of Contents.
4. Chatzikokkinou P, Sotiropoulos K, Katoulis A, Luzzati R, Trevisan G. Seborrheic dermatitis - an early and common skin manifestation in HIV patients. *Acta Dermatovenerol Croat*. 2008;16(4):226-230.
5. Morar N, Willis-Owen SA, Maurer T, Bunker CB. HIV-associated psoriasis: pathogenesis, clinical features, and management. *Lancet Infect Dis*. 2010;10(7):470-478.
6. Ceccarelli M, Venanzi Rullo E, Vaccaro M, et al. HIV-associated psoriasis: epidemiology, pathogenesis, and management. *Dermatol Ther*. 2019;32(2): e12806.
7. Myers B, Thibodeaux Q, Reddy V, et al. Biologic treatment of 4 HIV-positive patients: a case series and literature review. *J Psoriasis Psoriatic Arthritis*. 2021;6(1):19-26.
8. Coopman SA, Johnson RA, Platt R, Stern RS. Cutaneous disease and drug reactions in HIV infection. *N Engl J Med*. 1993;328(23):1670-1674.
9. Fiszenson-Albala F, Auzerie V, Mahe E, et al. A 6-month prospective survey of cutaneous drug reactions in a hospital setting. *Br J Dermatol*. 2003;149(5):1018-1122.
10. Hoosen K, Mosam A, Dlova NC, Grayson W. An update on adverse cutaneous drug reactions in HIV/AIDS. *Dermatopathology (Basel)*. 2019;6(2):111-125.
11. Caumes E, Roudier C, Rogeaux O, Bricaire F, Gentilini M. Effect of corticosteroids on the incidence of adverse cutaneous reactions to trimethoprim-sulfamethoxazole during treatment of AIDS-associated Pneumocystis carinii pneumonia. *Clin Infect Dis*. 1994;18(3):319-323.
12. Borrás-Blasco J, Navarro-Ruiz A, Borrás C, Casterá E. Adverse cutaneous reactions associated with the newest antiretroviral drugs in patients with human immunodeficiency virus infection. *J Antimicrob Chemother*. 2008;62(5):879-888.
13. Todd G. Adverse cutaneous drug eruptions and HIV: a clinician's global perspective. *Dermatol Clin*. 2006;24(4):459-472, vi.
14. Tanwani LK, Mokshagundam SL. Lipodystrophy, insulin resistance, diabetes mellitus, dyslipidemia, and cardiovascular disease in human immunodeficiency virus infection. *South Med J*. 2003;96(2):180-188; quiz 189.
15. Walker NF, Scriven J, Meintjes G, Wilkinson RJ. Immune reconstitution inflammatory syndrome in HIV-infected patients. *HIV AIDS (Auckl)*. 2015;7:49-64.
16. Novak RM, Richardson JT, Buchacz K, et al. Immune reconstitution inflammatory syndrome: incidence and implications for mortality. *Aids*. 2012;26(6):721-730.
17. Coates SJ, Leslie KS. What's new in HIV dermatology? *F1000Res*. 2019;8: 427-437.
18. Nomura T, Katoh M, Yamamoto Y, Miyachi Y, Kabashima K. Eosinophilic pustular folliculitis: a proposal of diagnostic and therapeutic algorithms. *J Dermatol*. 2016;43(11):1301-1306.
19. Vin-Christian K, Epstein JH, Maurer TA, McCalmont TH, Berger TG. Photosensitivity in HIV-infected individuals. *J Dermatol*. 2000;27(6):361-369.
20. Meola T, Sanchez M, Lim HW, Buchness MR, Soter NA. Chronic actinic dermatitis associated with human immunodeficiency virus infection. *Br J Dermatol*. 1997;137(3):431-436.
21. Franzon VA, Mikilita ES, Camelo FH, Camargo R. Porphyria cutanea tarda in a HIV-positive patient. *An Bras Dermatol*. 2016;91(4):520-523.
22. Radithia D, Subarnbhesaj A, Ayuningtyas NF, et al. Oral hyperpigmentation as an adverse effect of highly active antiretroviral therapy in HIV patients: a systematic review and pooled prevalence. *J Clin Exp Dent*. 2023;15(7):e561-e570.
23. Nelson M, Schiavone M. Emtricitabine (FTC) for the treatment of HIV infection. *Int J Clin Pract*. 2004;58(5):504-510.

24. Jordaan HF. Common skin and mucosal disorders in HIV/AIDS. *South African Family Practice*. 2008;50(6):14-23.
25. Hogan MT. Cutaneous infections associated with HIV/AIDS. *Dermatol Clin*. 2006;24(4):473-495, vi.
26. Kaplan JE, Benson C, Holmes KK, Brooks JT, Pau A, Masur H. Guidelines for prevention and treatment of opportunistic infections in HIV-infected adults and adolescents: recommendations from CDC, the National Institutes of Health, and the HIV Medicine Association of the Infectious Diseases Society of America. *MMWR Recomm Rep*. 2009;58(Rr-4):1-207; quiz CE1-4.
27. Chen X, Anstey AV, Bugert JJ. Molluscum contagiosum virus infection. *Lancet Infect Dis*. 2013;13(10):877-888.
28. Altman K, Vanness E, Westergaard RP. Cutaneous manifestations of human immunodeficiency virus: a clinical update. *Curr Infect Dis Rep*. 2015;17(3):464.
29. Ortiz-Saavedra B, Montes-Madariaga ES, Cabanillas-Ramirez C, et al. Epidemiologic situation of HIV and monkeypox coinfection: a systematic review. *Vaccines (Basel)*. 2023;11(2):246.
30. Syphilis and People with HIV. Updated November 21, 2023. https://www.hiv.gov/hiv-basics/staying-in-hiv-care/other-related-health-issues/syphilis/. Accessed January 12, 2024.
31. Hook EW 3rd. Syphilis. *Lancet*. 2017;389(10078):1550-1557.
32. Daniel CR 3rd, Norton LA, Scher RK. The spectrum of nail disease in patients with human immunodeficiency virus infection. *J Am Acad Dermatol*. 1992;27(1):93-97.
33. Sanchez M. Kaposi's sarcoma. In: Rigel DS, Robinson JK, Ross MI, et al, eds. *Cancer of the Skin*. 2nd ed. Baltimore, MD: Saunders; 2011:168–178.

CHAPTER 65

COVID-19 and Skin of Color

Janet E. Lubov
Esther E. Freeman

KEY POINTS

- The epidemiology of COVID-19 has highlighted existing inequities in our healthcare system.
- Cutaneous manifestations of COVID-19 disease vary by disease severity, and clinical manifestations may have different appearances in different skin tones.
- Cutaneous reactions after SARS-CoV-2 vaccination rarely preclude additional vaccine doses or boosters.
- Dermatologists play a key role in the preparedness, response, and recovery continuum.

INTRODUCTION

Scientists and organizations in both the public and private sectors mobilized during the COVID-19 pandemic to develop and deploy life-saving resources. This unprecedented collaboration had some direct positive outcomes, especially for high-income countries, such as rapid and large-scale vaccination. However, the pandemic simultaneously highlighted systemic issues with the prevention and response in the different phases of the pandemic. This was most apparent in communities with skin of color (SOC) in the United States and globally in low- and middle-income countries. Inequitable vaccine allocation, low uptake in certain communities of vaccination campaigns, and limited buy-in from resource-rich settings to finance measures were issues that curbed the emergence and spread of new and potentially deadlier variants.[1,2] These barriers were layered onto existing inequities in the capacity of national health systems, and widespread problems in healthcare access.[1]

As SARS-CoV-2 variants continue circulating globally, a sustained effort toward understanding how COVID-19 affects different populations will increase our systems' resilience to future waves of this pandemic. These shortcomings are often driven by or exacerbated by complex socioeconomic factors, also seen in the COVID-19 pandemic where Black and Hispanic populations made up 40% of cases of COVID-19 but only received 30% of the vaccines.[3] In COVID-19 dermatology, a scarcity of SOC-focused research has negatively impacted this population's clinical and public health outcomes. Specifically, the skin is a highly immunoreactive organ subject to many genetic and epigenetic factors, which can provide clues to underlying systemic disease processes. These clues are only effective if providers identify these signs in all skin types.

This chapter aims to contribute clinical, preventive, and epidemiologic insight to SOC research on SARS-CoV-2 infection, COVID-19 as a disease, and reactogenicity to COVID-19 vaccines. Additionally, we highlight public health topics such as the equitable distribution of vaccines and access to COVID-19 care in the SOC population from a dermatological perspective.

EPIDEMIOLOGY

The pandemic has lasted more than 2 and a half years as of October 2022 and has claimed millions of lives globally, with over 1,066,000 lives to date in the United States alone.[3] As of October 2022, there has been a promising trajectory toward recovery as the daily average in new cases of COVID-19 and hospitalizations in the United States continue to trend downward.[3] The positive trend in the United States is unfortunately superimposed on a record of high infection, hospitalization, and death rates in SOC populations during the course of this pandemic [**Table 65-1**].[4] For example, from December 2021 to January 2022, weekly cases in non-Hispanic Blacks and Hispanics climbed up to 1124/100,000 people and 1437/100,000, respectively, compared to 731/100,000 in non-Hispanic Whites.[3] Additionally, once infected, death rates among Black non-Hispanics were highest compared to the rest of the population along race and ethnic lines climbing up to 5.82/100,000 population per week in the same time period.[3]

As of October 2022, only 49.9% of non-Hispanic Blacks have received at least one dose of vaccination, and 43.7% have completed a two-dose vaccination series.[3,5] In contrast, 71.0% of Asian Americans have received the first dose of vaccine and 63.7% have completed the primary series in the same time period.[3] Although the U.S. CDC cautions against the generalizability of race/ethnicity stratification data on vaccine uptake due to incomplete race/ethnicity data that may cause significant underestimations,[3,5] we see inequities across different populations.[6] Reasons for poor uptake of vaccination in some racial/ethnic minority communities are multifactorial, including a history of unethical and discriminatory practices in the medical and research system, as well as personal traumatic experiences, that have led to mistrust in the healthcare system.[6-8]

From a dermatologic perspective, there were fewer photos of COVID-19-induced dermatoses in SOC populations. The paucity of pictorial evidence in literature may have contributed to healthcare providers (and possibly patients themselves) underrecognizing and underreporting dermatologic manifestations of COVID-19.[9,10] If an estimated 8% to 10% of patients with active SARS-CoV-2 infection experience

TABLE 65-1 Total COVID-19 cases and deaths/ethnicity (percentages) for all age groups

Race/Ethnicity	Percent of cases	Percent of deaths	Percent of U.S. population
Hispanic/Latino	24.8	17.1	18.45
American Indian/Alaska native non-Hispanic	1	1.1	0.74
Asian non-Hispanic	4.3	3.2	5.76
Black non-Hispanic	12.3	13.1	12.54
Native Hawaiian /other Pacific Islander non-Hispanic	0.3	0.2	0.182
White non-Hispanic	53.3	63.1	60.11
Multiple/other non-Hispanic	3.9	2.2	2.22

Note: CDC's reporting on total cases and deaths by race/ethnicity in all age groups.[3]

skin eruptions,[11-13] and patients with SOC make up about 40% of the total population who has had SARS-CoV-2,[3] then there may be over 3 million people with SOC affected by COVID-19 dermatologic issues—ultimately published literature should reflect this diversity of skin tone. Addressing this gap in the evidence base will require culturally sensitive data-driven approaches to community engagement and education to effectively counter drivers of disparities.

PATHOPHYSIOLOGY

The pathophysiological understanding of COVID-19 dermatoses allows for an avenue to explore SOC-specific differences. While there may be some direct cytopathic effects of the virus on the skin, much of the evidence points to the host immune response to the virus as the major driver in skin manifestations of the virus.[14,15] Factors affecting the host immune response and reaction to the virus include vitamin D levels, expression of angiotensin-converting enzyme 2 (ACE2) receptors, androgen levels, autoimmunity, proinflammatory processes, microthrombi formation, vasculitis development, and even psychological stress.[16,17] Specifically, mild and moderate COVID-19 cases involve humoral-driven immune complex-mediated reactions, while severe cases induce complement-mediated alternative and mannan-binding pathways via cytokine expression.[13,18,19]

Genetic factors associated with COVID-19 immunodermatology include the expression of ACE2 mutations. One hypothesis postulates that the hypo-expression of ACE2 in persons of African descent is believed to induce a passive protective mechanism against SARS-CoV-2 infection.[20] However, in the event of a successful SARS-CoV-2 infection, the same ACE2 hypo-expression exacerbates COVID-19 illness.[20] The SARS-CoV-2 infection triggers a cascade of physiological responses that ultimately can suppress the expression of ACE2, leading to overactivation of the RAAS system and, subsequently, Angiotensin II.[20-22] Clinically, this may translate to an increase in the severity of COVID-19 characterized by the progression of the inflammatory and thrombotic process.[20-22] These factors suggest that the cutaneous manifestation of COVID-19 due to viral spike protein invasion into the dermis (by binding to ACE-2 receptors in keratinocytes) could be altered by the bioavailability of ACE2 in an individual's skin, though this hypothesis is still under investigation.[17]

HISTOPATHOLOGY

The degree of hyperstimulation of the systemic immune system after infection with the SARS-CoV-2 virus also impact the immunogenicity profile of the skin. COVID-19-related skin biopsies reveal varying degrees of spongiosis and epidermal lymphocytic exocytosis, dermal interstitial infiltrates, basal vacuolar changes with interface dermatitis, lymphocytic perivascular infiltrates, and extravasation of red blood cells.[23] Vascular lesions reveal CD4+ T lymphocytes are stimulated by the SARS-CoV-2 virus to produce proinflammatory cytokines (IL-1, IFN-γ, and TNF-α) and recruit eosinophils, CD8+ T lymphocytes, B cells, and natural killer (NK) cells that target keratinocytes.[18] Immunohistochemistry of COVID-19 skin lesions shows perivascular and intraepidermal lymphocytic infiltrates with more CD8+ cells than CD4+ cells, which could serve as a possible modulator of the severity of the associated dermatoses.[24]

DERMATOLOGICAL MANIFESTATIONS OF COVID-19

The COVID-19 registry created by the American Academy of Dermatology (AAD) and the International League of Dermatological Societies (ILDS) contributed to the profiling and cataloging of dermatological manifestations of COVID-19.[14,25] Of the 2000 entries from 52 countries as of September 2022, the provider facing AAD/ILDS registry had recorded over 30 distinct dermatological disorders.[25] The most common dermatological conditions related to COVID-19 include morbilliform (22%), pernio-like (18%), urticarial (16%), macular erythema (13%), vesicular (11%), papulosquamous (9.9%), and retiform purpura (6.4%).[25,26] Less common but severe complications of SARS-CoV-2 infection include multisystem inflammatory syndrome in children (MIS-C).[17]

COVID-19 DERMATOSES

MORBILLIFORM ERUPTION

The association of morbilliform eruption with COVID-19 was reported early in the pandemic.[25,27] Similar to other morbilliform viral eruptions, COVID-19-associated morbilliform is not thought to be a direct cytopathic effect of the virus since there is no detectable viral RNA or protein but rather an immune response to the virus.[17] Another possible cause for morbilliform eruptions in people with COVID-19 may include hypersensitivity to medications given as treatment for COVID-19. Morbilliform eruptions in COVID-19, like morbilliform eruptions from other causes, are pruritic and involve the trunk and extremities.[28] In patients with SOC, erythema may be more subtle; pigmentary changes, violaceous coloration, and warmth should be considered in the assessment for erythema.

PERNIO (CHIBLAIN-LIKE)

COVID-19-associated perniosis, dubbed "COVID toes" in the lay press, is thought to represent a virally triggered exaggerated immune reaction with significant type I interferon signaling,[29] though the relationship with SARS CoV-2 remains controversial.[30] Many patients who develop chilblain-like lesions tend to have mild COVID-19 disease or remain completely asymptomatic, thought to be related to rapid, interferon-mediated viral control.[14,31] Pernio-like eruptions have been noted in the SOC population much less frequently than in White patients.[32,33] This raises questions about disease association, recognition versus nonrecognition in the SOC, where the erythema of pernio may be more subtle, and/or if there could be underlying genetic factors in certain populations or whether it could be a multifactorial combination of all these elements.[34,35] However, the diagnostic assessment in SOC should include a check for swelling of the digits, and detailed history should be elicited, as tingling and burning sensation may be more evident than erythema.[28] Furthermore, heels and subungual region regions should be assessed for hyperpigmented plaques.[28] It is through these approaches that can assist in reduction of missed diagnoses of pernio in darker skin types.

URTICARIA

Urticaria is commonly seen in COVID-19, either as a presenting symptom or after other COVID-19 symptoms. It is unclear if any differences exist in frequency of COVID-19-related urticaria by race. However, it is possible that variations in ACE inhibitors (ACEi) expression in different skin types could, in theory, lead to different cutaneous manifestations of COVID-19 in people with different genetic backgrounds since ACEi-mediated angioedema (ACEi-AE), as seen in urticaria, is reported to be more prevalent in African Americans and Hispanics than in White populations.[36] Urticaria in patients with SOC may present as skin-colored hives or with a violaceous hue, thereby necessitating palpation for changes in skin topography.[28] Also, considering edema of the skin may exist without urticaria, it is important for providers to examine SOC for enlarged follicular openings in order to establish dermal edema.

RETIFORM PURPURA AND LIVEDO RACEMOSA

Retiform purpura stems from vessel obstruction associated with severe COVID-19, leading to cutaneous ischemia, purpura, and necrosis.[14,29]

Patients with retiform purpura and/or cutaneous thrombotic microvascular disease often had moderate to severe COVID-19, some cases necessitating ventilator dependence due to acute respiratory failure.[14] Retiform purpura in COVID-19 has been noted on the acral site and has also been observed in a few cases where the eruption was limited to the buttocks and thighs.[13]

Livedo racemosa is also a thrombotic vasculopathy that stems from partial occlusion of cutaneous vessels and has also been noted in patients with severe COVID-19.[37]

LIVEDO RETICULARIS

Livedo Reticularis is associated with an impairment of blood flow in cutaneous vessels due to vascular stasis or mechanical obstruction of blood flow and has been noted in COVID-19.[28] Livedo reticularis is generally transient and self-resolves within 24 hours; rarely, this may progress to necrosis secondary to small vessel thrombosis.[38] In the SOC context, livedo reticularis may not appear as the classical presentation of a branchable, reticulated vascular pattern with a reddish-blue discoloration and instead may present as an uneven distribution of melanin throughout the skin, causing hyperpigmented patches with a lace-like appearance.[28]

TELOGEN EFFLUVIUM

Telogen effluvium (TE) is the temporary shedding of telogen hair typically noted 3 months after an inciting event, which may include psychosocial and/or physiological stress. Telogen effluvium has been noted in patients with SARS-CoV-2 specifically, and also in the general population during the pandemic due to psychological stress.[39,40] In SARS-CoV-2 specifically, these physiological stressors could include oxidative stress and hypoxemia secondary to SARS-CoV-2-induced lung damage.[41,42] A surge of circulating proinflammatory cytokines during COVID-19 is believed to inhibit the elongation of the hair shaft, impose damage to matrix cells, and encourage catagen development.[41,43] Telogen effluvium after COVID-19 has been noted specifically in the SOC population, specifically in women with an overall mean age of 44 years.[44] A retrospective study by the Henry Ford Health System found that 6 out of 10 patients were Black, one of Middle Eastern heritage experienced hair loss 50 days after the first symptom of COVID-19 infection.[45] This is in line with earlier clinical investigations in Spain and India on COVID-19-associated hair loss, with the average duration from the onset of COVID-19 symptoms to the appearance of acute TE being 74 days.[41]

MIS-C

Multisystem inflammatory syndrome in children (MIS-C) is a rare but severe complication of SARS-CoV-2 infection. In order to diagnose MIS-C, the CDC requires and suspected or confirmed SARS-CoV-2 infection within 4 weeks of presentation, fever greater than 38 degrees Celsius for more than 24 hours, laboratory evidence of inflammation, hospitalization requirement and involvement of two or more organ systems (cardiovascular, respiratory, renal, gastrointestinal, hematological, neurological, and dermatologic).[46] Skin lesions found in children most commonly involve papillitis of the tongue (strawberry tongue), cheilitis, maculopapular eruptions, urticarial lesions, acro-ischemia and dry gangrene.[47,48]

A study analyzed data from the CDC MIS-C database and identified ICU admission was more likely for non-Hispanic Black pediatric patients with shortness of breath, abdominal pain, increased concentrations of inflammatory markers, and other labs.[49] Although some potential age-specific differences among patients with MIS-C could result from differences in nasal expression of receptor used by SARS-CoV-2 for cell entry angiotensin-converting enzyme 2 (ACE2), there are also race and ethnicity disproportionalities.[50] Stierman et al found Black and Hispanic children are more prone to severe outcomes of MIS-C and less frequent in non-Hispanic White children.[51]

COVID-19 PPE-RELATED DERMATOSES

The increased use of personal protective equipment (PPE) during the COVID-19 pandemic has led to a variety of dermatoses. These conditions include associated dermatoses acne, rosacea, "maskne," allergic contact dermatitis (ACD), irritant contact dermatitis (ICD), and seborrheic dermatitis (SD).[52,53] Extensive use of facial masks and the associated contact friction along the chin or jawline may have increased this phenomenon during the pandemic.[54] Many individuals wearing masks noted "maskne" on social media,[52] which is thought to be a subtype of acne mechanica as a result of a warm and humid environment that can increase sebum secretion, occlude pores, and predispose acne flare ups.[53]

Despite their noninflammatory clinical appearance, histologically, SOC patients were found to have striking inflammation with polymorphonuclear leukocyte infiltrates.[55] In SOC, nodulocystic acne (vs comedonal acne) may resolve with hyperpigmented macules, blemishes, scars, spots, discolorations, blotches, or discolorations due to the underlying inflammatory nature that can mask erythema and persist for months to years.[56,57]

COVID-19 VACCINE SKIN REACTIONS

Vaccines currently in wide use for SARS-CoV-2 include modified mRNA in lipid nanoparticles (Pfizer/BioNTech and Moderna), nonreplicating adenoviral vectors (AstraZeneca and Johnson & Johnson), inactivated virus (Sinovac and Sinopharm), protein subunit (NVX-CoV2373/Novavax), DNA plasmid-based (ZyCoV-D), virus-like particles (Covishield, Ad26.COV2.S), self-amplifying RNA, and live attenuated virus.[58,59] The vaccines using mRNA technology, such as Pfizer and Moderna, deliver a laboratory-synthesized mRNA that encodes a protein that is identical to the spike glycoprotein of SARS-CoV-2, allowing the production of immunogenic spike glycoprotein that will then elicit T-cell and B-cell adaptive immune responses.[13]

Vaccine reactogenicity profile, tolerability, and immunogenicity of vaccines in a given individual is influenced by many factors.[60] These different vaccine formulations confer the risk of a range of immunological and autoimmunologic adverse reactions based on factors such as age, gender, race/ethnicity, body mass, general health, and preexisting immunity.[60] The diversity of vaccine reactions, particularly after mRNA vaccination, makes it difficult to categorize these into a single type of hypersensitivity reaction. Some, like the relatively rare anaphylaxis after vaccines, are hypersensitivity type I.[61] Other types of reactions are less clear—for example, delayed large local reactions ("COVID arm") and/or erythema multiforme-like eruptions could be a type IV hypersensitivity reaction.[62]

The AAD/ILDS COVID-19 Dermatology registry found that out of the reactions to mRNA COVID-19 vaccines, delayed large local reactions (66%) were the most frequent morphology, followed by local injection site reactions, urticaria, and morbilliform eruptions.[63]

Less common clinical patterns include subepidermal bullous pemphigoid-like eruptions, dermal hypersensitivity, herpes zoster, lichen planus-like, pernio, other urticarial (acute, exacerbation of preexisting chronic spontaneous urticaria, and chronic spontaneous urticaria), neutrophilic dermatosis, leukocytoclastic vasculitis, erythromelalgia, and other.[15,64-66]

Similarly, a recently published systematic review cataloged 5941 documented SARS-CoV-2 vaccine-related dermatological manifestations cases, representing 75 different types of reactions.[39] The most common vaccine reaction cases involved local injection site reactions (n = 2023/5941), rash/unspecified cutaneous eruption (n = 1954/5941), urticarial rashes (n = 647/5941), angioedema (n = 318/5941), herpes zoster (n = 160/5941), morbilliform/maculopapular/erythematous macular eruption (n = 106/5941), pityriasis rosea and pityriasis rosea-like eruptions (n = 96/5941, and 68 (n = 637/5941) other less common dermatological manifestations.[39] These reactions represented Ad26.COV.S (Johnson & Johnson-Janssen), AZD1222-Vaxzevria (Oxford/AstraZeneca),

BNT162b-Comirnaty (Pfizer/BioNTech), CoronaVac (Sinovac), Covishield (Oxford/AstraZeneca formulation), mRNA-1273 (Moderna), and a minority of unspecified vaccine brands.

Additional work classifying histopathologic reaction patterns characterized skin vaccine reactions into different histopathologic patterns.[15] The most common histopathologic reaction pattern identified was "V-REPP" (vaccine-related eruption of papules and plaques), which was grouped into mild V-REPP, which is eczematous and primarily an interface process, moderate V-REPP, which was pityriasis-rosea like and an overlap of interface and spongiosis, and severe V-REPP, which was vesicular and primarily spongiotic.[15]

LOCAL INJECTION SITE REACTIONS AND DELAYED LARGE LOCAL REACTIONS

It is important to differentiate local injection site reactions occurring within 1 to 2 days of the vaccine, which are frequently noted in other vaccines as well, such as influenza, from delayed large local reactions, which typically occur 7 to 8 days after vaccination.[63] Delayed large local reactions to vaccines were only rarely reported prior to mRNA COVID-19 vaccines and were a novel finding during the pandemic.[62] These reactions, sometimes called "COVID arm" in the lay press, were frequently noted with the first dose of the mRNA-1273 and BNT162b2 vaccines, with less frequent and/or less severe reactions or similar recurrent reactions to the second dose.[39,63,67,68] Avallone et al, a systematic review of SARS-CoV-2 vaccine-related cutaneous manifestations reported in the literature, found that immediate and delayed local injection-site reactions accounted for 2023 of the 5941 cases reported.[39] Of the 2023 reported cases in the literature, Moderna accounted for (1607/2023), followed by Pfizer at (332/2023), AstraZeneca (42/2023), and Johnson & Johnson-Janssen, CoronaVac, and other unspecified vaccines at collectively at (42/2023).[39]

Delayed large local reactions varied in morphology between erythematous targetoid patches and large plaques.[63,67,68] Histologically, these skin lesions are thought to be characteristic of a delayed-type, T-cell–mediated hypersensitivity reaction as evidenced by superficial and deep perivascular lymphocytic infiltrate with rare eosinophils and scattered mast cells.[62,67,68] The trigger of these reactions is not yet clear: whether it is related to the volume of mRNA (with Moderna vaccines having the highest amount) or related to one of the vaccine excipients, such as polyethylene glycol, is still being investigated.[67] Delayed large local reactions to mRNA COVID-19 vaccines in SOC are similar in clinical appearance, may be more subtle, but still have erythema.[69]

URTICARIA

Urticaria after COVID-19 vaccination can occur immediately after vaccination as part of anaphylaxis lesser than 4 hours after vaccination as part of immediate type hypersensitivity, or it can occur with delayed onset greater than 4 hours or several days after the event.[70,71] Delayed type of urticaria, which likely represents a delayed type of hypersensitivity and is not a form of anaphylaxis, typically starts within days of vaccination, and usually lasts 1 to 2 weeks.[63] However, in certain patients can last for more than 6 weeks, becoming chronic. Chronic spontaneous urticaria is characterized by waxing and waning pruritic, erythematous wheals. Omalizumab has shown promise as a treatment for refractory cases.[65] For delayed onset urticaria, patients have successfully been given further doses of the vaccine and boosters, though sometimes with pretreatment with antihistamines.[72]

Patients who experience urticaria after COVID-19 vaccination can still receive further vaccinations. Cases of individuals with a history of immediate reactions (eg, anaphylaxis) should be given future doses in consultation with an allergist. A multicenter, retrospective study showed that 223 of the 265 patients rechallenged the vaccine and tolerated the second dose with minimal symptoms that were self-limited, mild, and/or resolved with antihistamines alone.[73] In the SOC context, it is important to remember that urticarial presentation may not appear erythematous.

ANAPHYLAXIS

Anaphylaxis to the vaccines is thankfully rare, at a rate of approximately 11.1 cases per million doses with the Pfizer-BioNTech BNT162b2 vaccine.[61] A recent study reported 66 cases of anaphylaxis, 47 after the Pfizer-BioNTech vaccine and 19 after the Moderna vaccine, but hospitalizations were rare, and no intensive care unit treatment or deaths were reported.[74]

MORBILLIFORM RASHES

Morbilliform eruptions are also commonly identified reactions to COVID-19 vaccines (106 out of 5941 total reactions).[14,39] Morbilliform eruptions typically occur within 2 to 3 days of vaccination and generally resolve within a week without additional treatment.[67] Histologically, these eruptions feature spongiosis and mild dermal perivascular lymphocytic infiltrates.[67] As mentioned previously, erythema may be more subtle in SOC patients.

VACCINE EQUITY

We may never truly be able to estimate the impact of this pandemic due to the gaps in epidemiological and clinical data. The unquantifiable losses realized from structural inequities (such as racism, segregation, discrimination, and historical trauma), social determinants of health, and healthcare inequities will continue to be felt for decades, not centuries.[7] The historical consignment of Native Americans to reservations with inadequate health resources continues to affect the health in these communities through increased risk factors for the severity and mortality in COVID-19 infection.[7,75,76] The impact of discrimination and scapegoating toward Asian American population during COVID-19 is associated with high vaccine uptake, less testing, lower COVID-19-related healthcare knowledge, and lower telemedicine adoption levels compared to other racial/ethnic groups.[8] The black population experienced historically rooted trauma and mistrusts from experiences born out of unethical biomedical research and medical practices from the Tuskegee syphilis experiments, the legacy of Hela cells from Henrietta Lacks, and many other instances of injustices.[77] This, coupled with the impression that the vaccines were developed very rapidly and only approved based on emergency use authorization, contributed to low uptake. Pervasive misinformation campaigns also had an effect.[1,2,78] What we do know is that in COVID-19 and other diseases, these segregating and isolating acts disproportionately affecting minority groups have been shown to worsen the rates of disease.[7,79,80]

CONCLUSION

Dermatologists are in a position to be part of pandemic readiness, response, and recovery. We can facilitate the vaccination of patients, including those inclined to be vaccine-hesitant due to a medical history of allergic reactions.[81] Furthermore, there is an opportunity to promote and provide high-quality evidence-based services to SOC populations manifesting COVID-19-related dermatoses. These steps can only be effective if dermatologists are comfortable identifying adverse events to vaccines and dermatoses surrounding COVID-19 in all skin types. On the research front, dermatology can extend the reach of vaccination campaigns by developing vaccine delivery technologies, such as skin patches and microneedles, that can reduce the logistical restrictions that come with a heavy reliance on cold-chain supply systems.[59] The need for these innovations can be seen in the lagging global vaccination rates estimated at about 59% coverage of the global population with a single-vaccine dose as of October 2022.[82]

Factors such as access to care and vaccine injustices have exacerbated outcome disparities along socioeconomics, gender, race, ethnicity, immigration status, and geography.[6,7] Bridging the gaps in SOC COVID-19 dermatology knowledge directly influences the intrapersonal and interpersonal attitudes and beliefs toward vaccination willingness and care-seeking. As our world heads toward recovery from the pandemic and prepares for other global health threats, SOC COVID-19 dermatology can be integral in promoting structural drivers for health and vaccine equity.

REFERENCES

1. Griffin S. Covid-19: Commission describes "massive global failures" of pandemic response. *BMJ*. 2022;378:o2237.
2. Sachs JD, Karim SSA, Aknin L, et al. The Lancet Commission on lessons for the future from the COVID-19 pandemic. *Lancet*. 2022;400(10359): 1224-1280.
3. CDC. COVID data tracker. Centers for disease control and prevention. https://covid.cdc.gov/covid-data-tracker. Accessed September 29, 2022.
4. Khanijahani A, Iezadi S, Gholipour K, Azami-Aghdash S, Naghibi D. A systematic review of racial/ethnic and socioeconomic disparities in COVID-19. *Int J Equity Health*. 2021;20(1):248.
5. Troiano G, Nardi A. Vaccine hesitancy in the era of COVID-19. *Public Health*. 2021;194:245-251.
6. Moon S, Alonso Ruiz A, Vieira M. Averting future vaccine injustice. *N Engl J Med*. 2021;385(3):193-196.
7. National Academies of Sciences, Engineering, and Medicine, Health and Medicine Division, Board on Population Health and Public Health Practice, Committee on Community-Based Solutions to Promote Health Equity in the United States. In: Baciu A, Negussie Y, Geller A, Weinstein JN, eds. *Communities in Action: Pathways to Health Equity*. Washington (DC): National Academies Press (US); 2017.
8. Anand S, Cao E, Kimura R, Guo W, Bassi N. Asian American Vaccination, Testing, and Other Healthcare Knowledge & Behaviors during COVID-19, A Systematic Review. *Pathog Glob Health*. 2023;117(2):120-133.
9. Lester JC, Jia JL, Zhang L, Okoye GA, Linos E. Absence of images of skin of colour in publications of COVID-19 skin manifestations. *Br J Dermatol*. 2020;183(3):593-595.
10. Rabin RC. Dermatology has a problem with skin color. *The New York Times*. https://www.nytimes.com/2020/08/30/health/skin-diseases-black-hispanic.html. Accessed October 27, 2022.
11. Visconti A, Bataille V, Rossi N, et al. Diagnostic value of cutaneous manifestation of SARS-CoV-2 infection. *Br J Dermatol*. 2021;184(5):880-887.
12. Mascitti H, Jourdain P, Bleibtreu A, et al. Prognosis of rash and chilblain-like lesions among outpatients with COVID-19: a large cohort study. *Eur J Clin Microbiol Infect Dis*. 2021;40(10):2243-2248.
13. Magro C, Nuovo G, Mulvey JJ, Laurence J, Harp J, Crowson AN. The skin as a critical window in unveiling the pathophysiologic principles of COVID-19. *Clin Dermatol*. 2021;39(6):934-965.
14. Freeman EE, McMahon DE, Lipoff JB, et al. The spectrum of COVID-19-associated dermatologic manifestations: an international registry of 716 patients from 31 countries. *J Am Acad Dermatol*. 2020;83(4): 1118-1129.
15. McMahon DE, Kovarik CL, Damsky W, et al. Clinical and pathologic correlation of cutaneous COVID-19 vaccine reactions including V-REPP: a registry-based study. *J Am Acad Dermatol*. 2022;86(1):113-121.
16. COVID-19 host genetics initiative. Mapping the human genetic architecture of COVID-19. *Nature*. 2021;600(7889):472-477.
17. Pendlebury GA, Oro P, Haynes W, Merideth D, Bartling S, Bongiorno MA. The impact of COVID-19 pandemic on dermatological conditions: a novel, comprehensive review. *Dermatopathology (Basel)*. 2022;9(3):212-243.
18. Birlutiu V, Feiereisz AI, Oprinca G, et al. Cutaneous manifestations associated with anosmia, ageusia and enteritis in SARS-CoV-2 infection - a possible pattern? Observational study and review of the literature. *Int J Infect Dis*. 2021;107:72-77.
19. Lee JSS, Kossard S, McGrath MA. Lymphocytic thrombophilic arteritis: a newly described medium-sized vessel arteritis of the skin. *Arch Dermatol*. 2008;144(9):1175-1182.
20. Vinciguerra M, Greco E. Sars-CoV-2 and black population: ACE2 as shield or blade? *Infect Genet Evol*. 2020;84:104361.
21. Verdecchia P, Cavallini C, Spanevello A, Angeli F. The pivotal link between ACE2 deficiency and SARS-CoV-2 infection. *Eur J Intern Med*. 2020;76:14-20.
22. Guo J, Huang Z, Lin L, Lv J. Coronavirus disease 2019 (COVID-19) and cardiovascular disease: a viewpoint on the potential influence of angiotensin-converting enzyme inhibitors/angiotensin receptor blockers on onset and severity of severe acute respiratory syndrome coronavirus 2 infection. *J Am Heart Assoc*. 2020;9(7):e016219.
23. Fattori A, Cribier B, Chenard MP, Mitcov M, Mayeur S, Weingertner N. Cutaneous manifestations in patients with coronavirus disease 2019: clinical and histological findings. *Hum Pathol*. 2021;107:39-45.
24. Ohsawa R, Sano H, Ikeda M, Sano S. Clinical and histopathological views of morbilliform rash after COVID-19 mRNA vaccination mimic those in SARS-CoV-2 virus infection-associated cutaneous manifestations. *J Dermatol Sci*. 2021;103(2):124-127.
25. Freeman EE, McMahon DE, Fitzgerald ME, et al. The American Academy of Dermatology COVID-19 registry: crowdsourcing dermatology in the age of COVID-19. *J Am Acad Dermatol*. 2020;83(2):509-510.
26. Freeman EE, McMahon DE, Lipoff JB, et al. Pernio-like skin lesions associated with COVID-19: a case series of 318 patients from 8 countries. *J Am Acad Dermatol*. 2020;83(2):486-492.
27. Galván Casas C, Català A, Carretero Hernández G, et al. Classification of the cutaneous manifestations of COVID-19: a rapid prospective nationwide consensus study in Spain with 375 cases. *Br J Dermatol*. 2020;183(1):71-77.
28. Akuffo-Addo E, Nicholas MN, Joseph M. COVID-19 skin manifestations in skin of colour. *J Cutan Med Surg*. 2022;26(2):189-197.
29. Magro CM, Mulvey JJ, Laurence J, et al. The differing pathophysiologies that underlie COVID-19-associated perniosis and thrombotic retiform purpura: a case series. *Br J Dermatol*. 2021;184(1):141-150.
30. Runwal P. Mysterious wave of COVID toes still has scientists stumped. *National Geographic*. March 2022. https://www.nationalgeographic.com/science/article/mysterious-wave-of-covid-toes-still-has-scientists-stumped. Accessed October 25, 2022.
31. Hubiche T, Cardot-Leccia N, Le Duff F, et al. Clinical, laboratory, and interferon-alpha response characteristics of patients with chilblain-like lesions during the COVID-19 pandemic. *JAMA Dermatol*. 2021;157(2):202-206.
32. Cline A, Berk-Krauss J, Keyes Jacobs A, et al. The underrepresentation of "COVID toes" in skin of color: an example of racial bias or evidence of a tenuous disease association? *J Am Acad Dermatol*. 2021;84(2):e91-e92.
33. Daneshjou R, Rana J, Dickman M, Yost JM, Chiou A, Ko J. Pernio-like eruption associated with COVID-19 in skin of color. *JAAD Case Rep*. 2020;6(9): 892-897.
34. Pangti R, Gupta S, Nischal N, Trikha A. Recognizable vascular skin manifestations of SARS-CoV-2 (COVID-19) infection are uncommon in patients with darker skin phototypes. *Clin Exp Dermatol*. 2021;46(1):180-182.
35. Tan SW, Tam YC, Oh CC. Skin manifestations of COVID-19: a worldwide review. *JAAD Int*. 2021;2:119-133.
36. Montinaro V, Cicardi M. ACE inhibitor-mediated angioedema. *Int Immunopharmacol*. 2020;78:106081.
37. Droesch C, Do MH, DeSancho M, Lee EJ, Magro C, Harp J. Livedoid and purpuric skin eruptions associated with coagulopathy in severe COVID-19. *JAMA Dermatol*. 2020;156(9):1-3.
38. Jindal R, Chauhan P. Cutaneous manifestations of coronavirus disease 2019 in 458 confirmed cases: a systematic review. *J Family Med Prim Care*. 2020;9(9):4563-4569.
39. Avallone G, Quaglino P, Cavallo F, et al. SARS-CoV-2 vaccine-related cutaneous manifestations: a systematic review. *Int J Dermatol*. 2022;61(10): 1187-1204.
40. Neera N. How extreme stress causes hair loss. *Forbes Magazine*. June 2020. https://www.forbes.com/sites/neeranathan/2020/06/30/why-extreme-stress-causes-hair-loss/. Accessed October 27, 2022.
41. Gentile P. Hair Loss and Telogen Effluvium Related to COVID-19: The Potential Implication of Adipose-Derived Mesenchymal Stem Cells and Platelet-Rich Plasma as Regenerative Strategies. *Int J Mol Sci*. 2022;23(16):9116.
42. Wambier CG. Reply to: "Comment on 'Androgenetic alopecia present in the majority of patients hospitalized with COVID-19.'" *J Am Acad Dermatol*. 2021;84(1):e53-e54.
43. Aksoy H, Yıldırım UM, Ergen P, Gürel MS. COVID-19 induced telogen effluvium. *Dermatol Ther*. 2021;34(6):e15175.
44. Hussain N, Agarwala P, Iqbal K, et al. A systematic review of acute telogen effluvium, a harrowing post-COVID-19 manifestation. *J Med Virol*. 2022;94(4):1391-1401.

45. Olds H, Liu J, Luk K, Lim HW, Ozog D, Rambhatla PV. Telogen effluvium associated with COVID-19 infection. *Dermatol Ther*. 2021;34(2):e14761.
46. CDC. Information for healthcare providers about multisystem inflammatory syndrome in children (MIS-C). Centers for Disease Control and Prevention. https://www.cdc.gov/mis/mis-c/hcp/index.html. Accessed November 5, 2022.
47. Neale H, Hawryluk EB. COVID-19 pediatric dermatology. *Dermatol Clin*. 2021;39(4):505-519.
48. Singh R, Freeman EE. Viruses, variants, and vaccines: how COVID-19 has changed the way we look at skin. *Curr Dermatol Rep*. 2022;11(4):289-312.
49. Abrams JY, Oster ME, Godfred-Cato SE, et al. Factors linked to severe outcomes in multisystem inflammatory syndrome in children (MIS-C) in the USA: a retrospective surveillance study. *Lancet Child Adolesc Health*. 2021;5(5):323-331.
50. Bunyavanich S, Do A, Vicencio A. Nasal gene expression of angiotensin-converting enzyme 2 in children and adults. *JAMA*. 2020;323(23): 2427-2429.
51. Stierman B, Abrams JY, Godfred-Cato SE, et al. Racial and ethnic disparities in multisystem inflammatory syndrome in children in the United States, March 2020 to February 2021. *Pediatr Infect Dis J*. 2021;40(11): e400-e406.
52. Rubin C. Maskne is the new acne, and here's what is causing it. *The New York Times*. https://www.nytimes.com/article/maskne-acne.html. Accessed October 27, 2022.
53. Abdali S, Yu J. Occupational dermatoses related to personal protective equipment used during the COVID-19 pandemic. *Dermatol Clin*. 2021;39(4): 555-568.
54. Grullon K, Ashi SA, Shea CR, Ruiz de Luzuriaga AM, Stein SL, Rosenblatt AE. Follicular keratosis of the face in pediatric patients of color. *Pediatr Dermatol*. 2022;39(2):231-235.
55. Raju SP, Sachdev M, Khunger N, Madnani N. Mask acne in skin of color: a significant dermatological condition amidst the COVID-19 pandemic. *J Clin Aesthet Dermatol*. 2022;15(4):44-48.
56. Goldsmith L, Katz S, Gilchrest B, Paller A, Leffell D, Wolff K. *Fitzpatrick's Dermatology in General Medicine*. 8th ed. McGraw Hill Professional, New York; 2012.
57. Taylor SC, Paul Kelly A, Lim H, Serrano AMA. *Taylor and Kelly's Dermatology for Skin of Color 2/E*. McGraw Hill Professional, New York; 2016.
58. Prates-Syed WA, Chaves LCS, Crema KP, et al. VLP-Based COVID-19 Vaccines: An Adaptable Technology against the Threat of New Variants. *Vaccines (Basel)*. 2021;9(12):1409.
59. Technologies to advance COVID-19 vaccine equity. *Nat Biotechnol*. 2021;39(12):1477.
60. Hervé C, Laupèze B, Del Giudice G, Didierlaurent AM, Tavares Da Silva F. The how's and what's of vaccine reactogenicity. *NPJ Vaccines*. 2019;4:39.
61. Banerji A, Wickner PG, Saff R, et al. mRNA vaccines to prevent COVID-19 disease and reported allergic reactions: current evidence and suggested approach. *J Allergy Clin Immunol Pract*. 2021;9(4):1423-1437.
62. Blumenthal KG, Freeman EE, Saff RR, et al. Delayed large local reactions to mRNA-1273 vaccine against SARS-CoV-2. *N Engl J Med*. 2021;384(13):1273-1277.
63. McMahon DE, Amerson E, Rosenbach M, et al. Cutaneous reactions reported after Moderna and Pfizer COVID-19 vaccination: a registry-based study of 414 cases. *J Am Acad Dermatol*. 2021;85(1):46-55.
64. Fathy RA, McMahon DE, Lee C, et al. Varicella-zoster and herpes simplex virus reactivation post-COVID-19 vaccination: a review of 40 cases in an international dermatology registry. *J Eur Acad Dermatol Venereol*. 2022;36(1):e6-e9.
65. Strahan A, Ali R, Freeman EE. Chronic spontaneous urticaria after COVID-19 primary vaccine series and boosters. *JAAD Case Rep*. 2022;25:63-66.
66. Tomayko MM, Damsky W, Fathy R, et al. Subepidermal blistering eruptions, including bullous pemphigoid, following COVID-19 vaccination. *J Allergy Clin Immunol*. 2021;148(3):750-751.
67. Sun Q, Fathy R, McMahon DE, Freeman EE. COVID-19 vaccines and the skin: the landscape of cutaneous vaccine reactions worldwide. *Dermatol Clin*. 2021;39(4):653-673.
68. Fernandez-Nieto D, Hammerle J, Fernandez-Escribano M, et al. Skin manifestations of the BNT162b2 mRNA COVID-19 vaccine in healthcare workers. "COVID-arm": a clinical and histological characterization. *J Eur Acad Dermatol Venereol*. 2021;35(7):e425-e427.
69. Samarakoon U, Alvarez-Arango S, Blumenthal KG. Delayed large local reactions to mRNA Covid-19 vaccines in blacks, indigenous persons, and people of color. *N Engl J Med*. 2021;385(7):662-664.
70. Zuberbier T, Abdul Latiff AH, Abuzakouk M, et al. The international EAACI/GA²LEN/EuroGuiDerm/APAAACI guideline for the definition, classification, diagnosis, and management of urticaria. *Allergy*. 2022;77(3):734-766.
71. Anvari S, Samarakoon U, Fu X, et al. Urticaria and/or angioedema secondary to mRNA COVID-19 vaccines: updates from a United States case registry. *Allergy*. 2023;78(1):283-286.
72. Krantz MS, Kwah JH, Stone CA Jr, et al. Safety evaluation of the second dose of messenger RNA COVID-19 vaccines in patients with immediate reactions to the first dose. *JAMA Intern Med*. 2021;181(11):1530-1533.
73. Stone CA Jr, Robinson LB, Li L, et al. Clinical phenotypes of immediate first-dose reactions to mRNA COVID-19: a multicenter latent class analysis. *J Allergy Clin Immunol Pract*. 2023;11(2):458-465.e1.
74. Jaggers J, Samarakoon U, Fu X, et al. Anaphylaxis after COVID-19 vaccination: a registry-based study. *J Allergy Clin Immunol Pract*. 2022;10(11):3020-3023.
75. Heart MYHB, Chase J, Elkins J, Altschul DB. Historical trauma among Indigenous Peoples of the Americas: concepts, research, and clinical considerations. *J Psychoactive Drugs*. 2011;43(4):282-290.
76. Ehrenpreis JE, Ehrenpreis ED. A historical perspective of healthcare disparity and infectious disease in the native American population. *Am J Med Sci*. 2022;363(4):288-294.
77. Wolinetz CD, Collins FS. Recognition of research participants' need for autonomy: remembering the legacy of Henrietta Lacks. *JAMA*. 2020;324(11): 1027-1028.
78. Lee SK, Sun J, Jang S, Connelly S. Misinformation of COVID-19 vaccines and vaccine hesitancy. *Sci Rep*. 2022;12(1):13681.
79. Acevedo-Garcia D. Residential segregation and the epidemiology of infectious diseases. *Soc Sci Med*. 2000;51(8):1143-1161.
80. Wallace R, Wallace D. Socioeconomic determinants of health: community marginalisation and the diffusion of disease and disorder in the United States. *BMJ*. 1997;314(7090):1341-1345.
81. Shavit R, Maoz-Segal R, Iancovici-Kidon M, et al. Prevalence of allergic reactions after Pfizer-BioNTech COVID-19 vaccination among adults with high allergy risk. *JAMA Netw Open*. 2021;4(8):e2122255.
82. WHO COVID-19 Dashboard. Geneva: World Health Organization, 2020. Available online: https://covid19.who.int/ Accessed August 26, 2022.

CHAPTER 66

Mucocutaneous Viral Infections

Susuana T. Adjei
Ashley E. Ojeaga
Stephen K. Tyring

KEY POINTS

- Herpes simplex virus type 1 and type 2 cause primary and recurrent painful vesicular eruptions, with transmission occurring through direct contact with shedding individuals and primarily affects the orolabial and genital mucosa.
- Varicella-zoster virus (VZV) causes varicella (chickenpox) during primary infection, followed by herpes zoster (shingles) upon reactivation, with the virus establishing latency in ganglia.
- Human papillomaviruses (HPVs) are diverse viruses causing various clinical manifestations such as common warts, plane warts, and condyloma acuminata. Transmission occurs through direct skin-to-skin contact.
- Mpox is a DNA virus transmitted via direct contact with infected animals or humans, with a clinical presentation similar to smallpox. It is endemic in Central and West African countries with higher prevalence among men who have sex with men.
- Parvovirus B19, primarily affecting children during winter months, causes erythema infectiosum (fifth disease), characterized by "slapped cheek" rash followed by trunk and extremity involvement, with a lacy pattern resolving spontaneously. This rash is more difficult to recognize in skin of color patients.

- Human Immunodeficiency Virus (HIV) can lead to various mucocutaneous manifestations due to the disease itself, opportunistic infections, or therapy, affecting individuals engaging in high-risk behaviors, men who have sex with men (MSM), and those with low socioeconomic status or IV drug use.
- Polyomaviruses, including Merkel cell polyomavirus (MCPyV) and trichodysplasia spinulosa polyomavirus (TSPyV), can cause mucocutaneous diseases, notably Merkel cell carcinoma (MCC) and Trichodysplasia spinulosa (TS), respectively, primarily affecting immunocompromised individuals.
- MCC is associated with UV exposure and as a result, a lower incidence is seen in darker skin individuals with lower incidence rates.

HERPES SIMPLEX VIRUSES

Herpes simplex virus type 1 (HSV-1) and type 2 (HSV-2) are double-stranded DNA viruses that belong to the alpha-herpesvirus subfamily. They are responsible for primary and chronic, recurrent painful vesicular eruptions, primarily in the orolabial and genital mucosa but infection is most commonly asymptomatic. The prevalence of herpesviruses increases with age and is highest among females, non-Hispanic Blacks, and Mexican Americans.[1]

PATHOGENESIS

HSV transmission occurs through direct contact with mucocutaneous surfaces of infected individuals who are shedding HSV.[2] Approximately 70% of genital HSV-2 is transmitted during periods of asymptomatic shedding.[3] During primary infection, HSV replicates within epithelial cells and subsequently establishes latency in the sacral dorsal root ganglia, remaining noninfectious until reactivation.

CLINICAL PRESENTATION

Primary or recurrent HSV-1 or HSV-2 infection may be asymptomatic or result in prodromal symptoms of localized pain, burning, pruritus, or constitutional symptoms. The lesions initially present as ill-defined erythema with subsequent papulovesicular formation, most commonly on the orolabial area, external genitalia, perianal area, and buttocks [**Figure 66-1**]. The vesicular fluid eventually becomes purulent; the pustule then resolves, leaving a shallow erosion. Primary lesions last between 2 and 6 weeks, while recurrent lesions usually last 1 week.

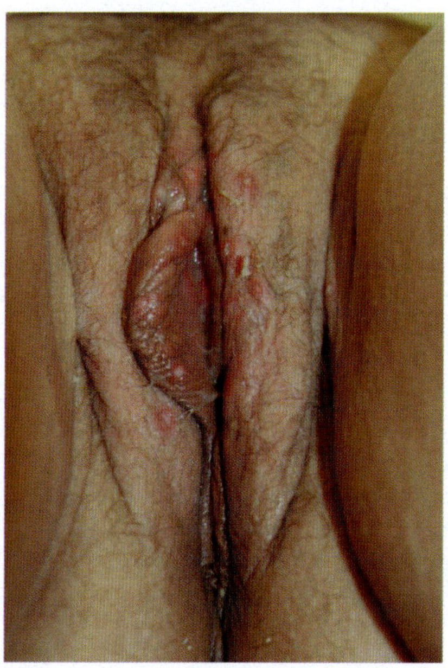

FIGURE 66-1. Herpes simplex virus type 1. Erythematous papulovesicles on female external genitalia.

TABLE 66-1 Genital herpes treatment

Antiviral agent:
Acyclovir
Initial infection: 200 mg five times daily or 400 mg three times daily for 7-10 days
Recurrences: 200 mg five times daily or 400 mg three times daily for 5 days
Suppressive therapy: 400 mg twice daily
Valacyclovir
Initial infection: 1 g twice daily for 7-10 days
Recurrences: 500 mg twice daily for 3-5 days
Suppressive therapy: 1 g daily in patients with more than nine episodes per year; 500 mg daily in patients with fewer outbreaks
Famciclovir
Initial infection: 250 mg three times daily for 7-10 days
Recurrences: 125 mg twice daily for 5 days
Suppressive therapy: 250 mg twice daily

DIAGNOSIS

The gold standard for diagnosis of HSV infection is a viral culture from vesicular lesions. Polymerase chain reaction (PCR) is the most sensitive and specific mechanism. Other diagnostic tests include viral serology, direct fluorescent antibody (DFA) assay, and the Tzanck smear.

TREATMENT

Oral nucleoside analogues, including acyclovir, valacyclovir, and famciclovir, are used to improve symptoms of genital herpes [**Table 66-1**]. They may be used for either episodic treatment or long-term suppressive therapy. Intravenous acyclovir is indicated for disseminated disease.

Episodic therapy is generally indicated for individuals with mild and infrequent recurrences. Chronic suppressive therapy is used for patients with frequent (more than six per year) and severe outbreaks.

VARICELLA-ZOSTER VIRUS

Varicella-zoster virus (VZV) is a human neurotropic alpha-herpesvirus. Primary infection causes varicella (chickenpox, a mild and self-limited disease of childhood). The virus subsequently establishes latency and causes herpes zoster (shingles) with reactivation. Zoster is four times more likely to occur in Caucasians than African Americans.[4]

PATHOGENESIS

VZV is transmitted by aerosolized droplets from the nasopharynx or by direct contact with skin lesions. It is contagious from 1 to 4 days prior to onset of the rash and until all vesicles have crusted.[5] During primary varicella infection, the virus establishes latency in cranial nerve ganglia, dorsal root ganglia, and autonomic ganglia. During reactivation of VZV, the virus travels down peripheral sensory nerves to the skin, resulting in zoster.

CLINICAL MANIFESTATIONS

VZV presents as small, pruritic macules, papules, and vesicles on an erythematous base on the trunk and extremities [**Figure 66-2**]. The lesions then become pustular followed by crust formation and eventual resolution. The rash of zoster is usually localized to a unilateral dermatome, most frequently involving the ophthalmic division of the trigeminal nerve (V_1) and the thoracic nerves [**Figure 66-3**]. A prodrome of dermatomal pain, pruritus, and dysesthesia precedes the rash in most patients and can persist as postherpetic neuralgia (PHN) in over one-third of individuals.[6] Disseminated herpes zoster is a complication primarily in immunocompromised patients.

DIAGNOSIS

VZV is diagnosed clinically and is often morphologically indistinguishable from HSV. Viral culture, serology, direct immunofluorescence,

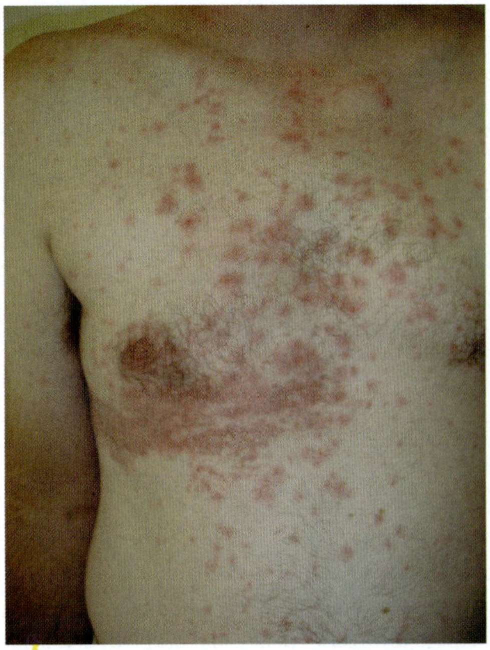

FIGURE 66-2. Disseminated primary varicella-zoster virus. Erythematous macules and papules on the trunk.

dot-blot hybridization, and real-time PCR may be used to differentiate VZV from HSV.

TREATMENT

Children with varicella should receive symptomatic treatment for fever and pruritus. Treatment with acyclovir is most beneficial when initiated within 24 hours of the onset of the rash [**Table 66-2**].[6] Varicella zoster immune globulin is recommended for pregnant, varicella-seronegative women who are exposed to VZV.

There are several antiviral medications available for the treatment of herpes zoster including acyclovir, valacyclovir, and famciclovir [**Table 66-3**]. These medications are most beneficial when initiated within 72 hours of the onset of the rash. Intravenous acyclovir is indicated for immunocompromised individuals, for immunocompetent patients with significant complications, and for those unable to take oral medications.

TABLE 66-2 Varicella treatment

Healthy children: oral acyclovir (20 mg/kg) four times a day for 5 days.
Children who weigh more than 40 kg and immunocompetent adults: oral acyclovir 800 mg four times a day for 5 days; valacyclovir 1 g three times a day and famciclovir 500 mg three times a day for 7 days are also frequently used but not approved by the U.S. Food and Drug Administration for treatment of primary varicella in adults.
Immunocompromised individuals: intravenous acyclovir (10 mg/kg) every 8 hours for 7-10 days.

Symptoms	Treatment
Fever	Antipyretics (acetaminophen): children should not be given aspirin because of its association with Reye syndrome.
Pruritus	Oral antihistamines including diphenhydramine and loratadine, calamine lotion, or tepid baths with baking soda. Fingernails should be clipped to minimize scratching.

There are multiple treatment options to reduce the pain associated with PHN. The duration and severity of PHN are reduced with early initiation of antiviral medications. Additional treatment options include tricyclic antidepressants, anticonvulsants such as gabapentin, and topical medications such as capsaicin cream and lidocaine patches.

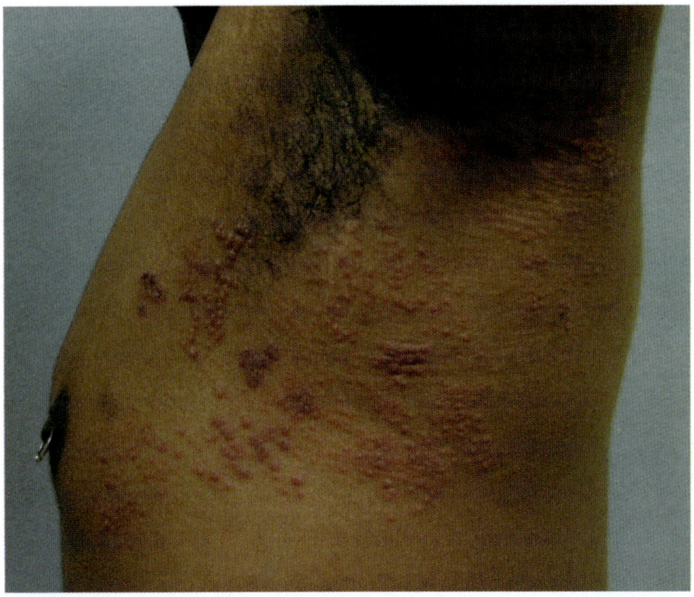

FIGURE 66-3. Herpes zoster. Erythematous papules and vesicles on an erythematous base in a thoracic spinal nerve 4 (T4) distribution.

HUMAN HERPESVIRUS TYPES 4-8

Human herpesvirus 4 (HHV-4), or Epstein-Barr virus (EBV), is most frequently manifested as infectious mononucleosis. Human herpesvirus 5 (HHV-5), or cytomegalovirus (CMV), is the most common congenital infection in the United States and can cause a mononucleosis-like illness in immunocompromised individuals. Human herpesvirus type 8 (HHV-8), or Kaposi sarcoma herpesvirus (KSHV), causes Kaposi sarcoma (KS), a multicentric malignant neoplasm characterized by spindle-shaped tumors of the lymphatic endothelium. HHV-8 is also associated with the development of primary effusion lymphoma (PEL) and multicentric Castleman disease (MCD). HHV-8 is more prevalent in men compared to women and in men who have sex with men. Its seroprevalence is highest in central and southern Africa and lowest in the United States.[7]

PATHOGENESIS

Transmission occurs primarily through saliva but can also be transmitted via sexual contact, pregnancy, breastfeeding, blood transfusions, or stem cell/organ transplantation.[7-11] The infection persists for the life of the host, although the infection predominates in a latent state in most cells.

TABLE 66-3 Zoster treatment

Immunocompetent individuals: oral acyclovir 800 mg five times daily for 7-10 days; oral valacyclovir 1 g three times daily for 7 days, oral famciclovir 500 mg three times daily for 7 days
Immunocompromised individuals: intravenous acyclovir 10 mg/kg every 8 hours for 7 days

Symptoms	Treatment
Pain	Analgesics
Pruritus	Oral antihistamines, calamine lotion

CLINICAL MANIFESTATIONS

While EBV and CMV infections are typically asymptomatic, EBV can cause infectious mononucleosis and CMV can cause a mononucleosis-like illness almost indistinguishable from that of EBV. Cutaneous manifestations are rare but can include morbilliform eruptions, papules/nodules, petechiae/purpura, ulcers, and edema.[8] Furthermore, EBV can manifest as Lipschutz ulcers, painful genital ulcers most commonly in non-sexually active female adolescents.[11] KS typically presents as violaceous lesions on the skin of the lower extremities, most complicated by edema [**Figure 66-4**].[7] Lesions are classified as patches, plaques, and nodules.

DIAGNOSIS

The heterophile test is most used for the diagnosis of infectious mononucleosis and remains positive for 3 to 6 months after primary EBV infection.[9] Other tests include an absolute lymphocytosis and the monospot test, a more sensitive and rapid technique used to measure heterophile antibodies. CMV is commonly diagnosed via serology, PCR, or viral culture. Immunohistochemistry can also be performed on tissue or body fluid samples. Skin biopsy for histopathology is the gold standard of diagnosis of KS.[7]

TREATMENT

Infectious mononucleosis is generally self-limited, and treatment is symptomatic. Antiviral medications such as ganciclovir, valganciclovir, and foscarnet can be used to decrease viral replication. Patients with severe complications are treated with corticosteroids with or without IVIG.[8] KS is incurable but can be electively palliated through various treatments. Localized KS is often treated with surgical excision, cryotherapy, and radiation therapy.[12] In extensive or recurrent KS, treatment is systemic and can include chemotherapy, intralesional injections of vinblastine, surgery, immunotherapy, and radiation.[12]

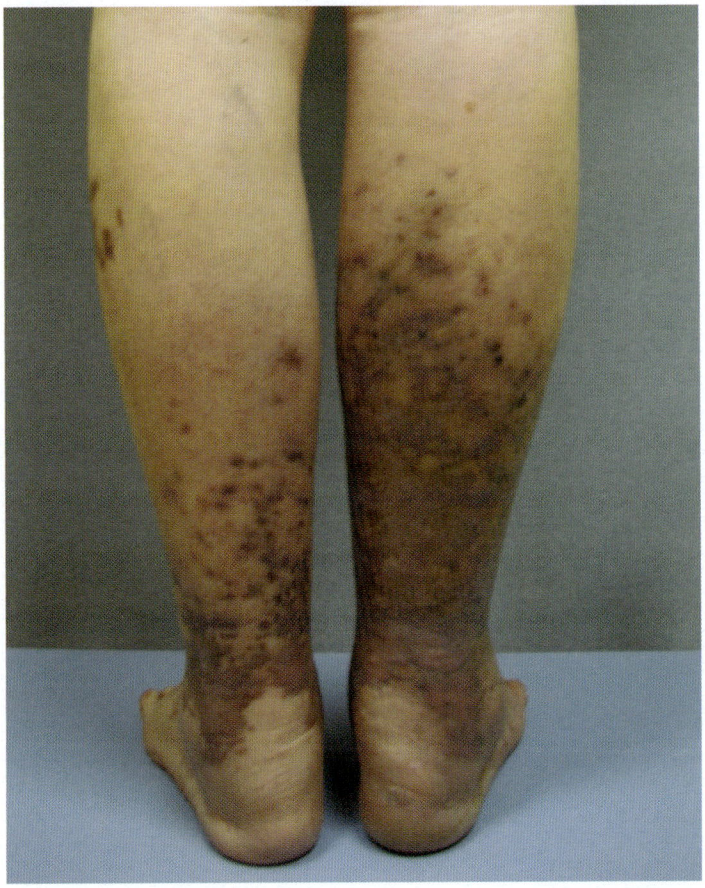

FIGURE 66-4. Kaposi sarcoma. Violaceous plaques and edema on the lower extremities bilaterally.

HUMAN PAPILLOMAVIRUS

Human papillomaviruses (HPVs) are small, nonenveloped, double-stranded DNA viruses classified as members of the Papillomavirus family. There are over 100 types of HPV. Some of the most common nononcogenic or low-risk types include HPV 2, 3, 6, 10, and 11. HPV 2 causes common warts, or verruca vulgaris, while HPV 3 and 10 cause verruca plana, or plane (flat) warts. HPV 6 and 11 are low-risk mucosal types of HPV that cause 90% of all cases of condyloma acuminata (anogenital warts). Within the United States, the prevalence of HPV infection is highest among non-Hispanic Blacks and lowest among Asians.[13]

PATHOGENESIS

HPV transmission occurs through direct skin-to-skin contact with infected skin lesions. HPV invades and replicates in epithelial cells of the skin and mucous membranes.

CLINICAL MANIFESTATIONS

Condyloma acuminata clinically manifest as single or multiple painless papules commonly on the vulva, penis, perineum, perianal area. They can be associated with pruritus, burning, bleeding, and discharge. Common warts typically present as cauliflower-like papules on the dorsa of the hands or fingers but may be palmar, periungual, or plantar.[14] Plane warts are slightly raised, small, skin-colored, flat-topped papules that commonly appear on the palmar and dorsal hands.

DIAGNOSIS

The diagnosis of cutaneous and genital warts is clinical. Biopsy can assist with the diagnosis of atypical lesions or those resistant to treatment.

TREATMENT

The treatment of warts is dependent on the symptoms, the extent and duration of lesions, and the patient's immunologic status. Nonsurgical therapies include salicylic acid, cantharidin, podophyllotoxin, imiquimod, 5-fluorouracil, sinecatechins, and the antiviral cidofovir.[15] Surgical treatments include curettage, cryotherapy, electrosurgery, surgical excision, and laser surgery. Additional therapies include intralesional bleomycin, intralesional recombinant interferon-α, cidofovir, and induction with dinitrochlorobenzene.[15]

MOLLUSCUM CONTAGIOSUM

Molluscum contagiosum (MC) is a cutaneous viral infection that is commonly observed in both healthy and immunocompromised school-age children. The infection is caused by a member of the Poxviridae family, the MC virus (MCV). MC is ubiquitously observed, and several epidemiologic studies conducted on specific racial populations in the United States have similarly concluded that skin color does not appear to impact the prevalence of MCV infection.[16]

PATHOGENESIS

MCV is transmitted by direct contact with infected skin lesions, through fomites, or by autoinoculation. It infects the epidermis and replicates within cells.[17] The estimated incubation period varies from 2 to 6 weeks.

CLINICAL MANIFESTATION

MC presents as asymptomatic 1 mm to 1 cm single or multiple small, pearly white or flesh-colored papules with central umbilication [**Figure 66-5**]. MC usually begins in a localized area of the skin, although the lesions can be transmitted to other areas of the body, such as genital, perineal, pubic, and surrounding skin, through autoinoculation.

DIAGNOSIS

The diagnosis of MC is clinical, but biopsy can aid in the diagnosis. Histopathology demonstrates epidermal hyperplasia producing a crater

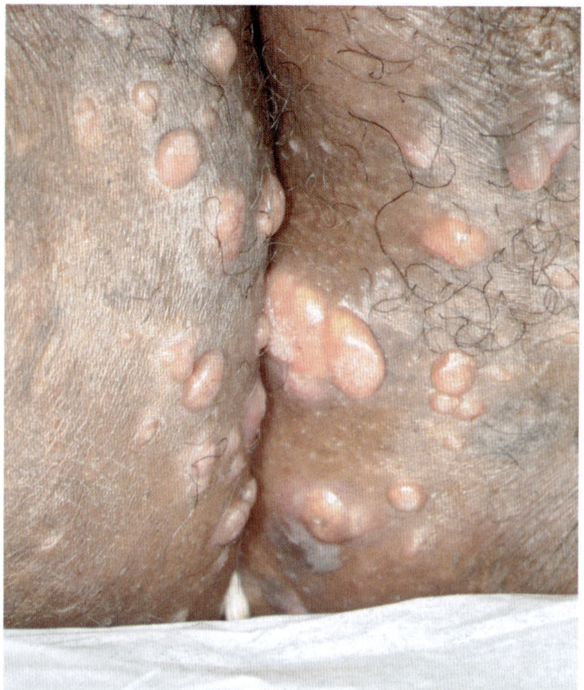

FIGURE 66-5. Molluscum contagiosum. Multiple white and skin-colored papules with central umbilication on the buttocks.

filled with Henderson-Patterson bodies, large eosinophilic cytoplasmic inclusions.

TREATMENT

MC in immunocompetent patients is self-limited; lesions typically resolve without intervention within 6 to 9 months. Current therapeutic intervention in the treatment of MC is intended merely to accelerate the eradication process. Chemical therapies include salicylic acid, cantharidin, potassium hydroxide, podophyllotoxin, trichloroacetic acid, and tretinoin.[17] Immunomodulatory methods include imiquimod, 5-fluorouracil, oral cimetidine, and Candida antigen. Mechanical treatments include curettage, cryotherapy, and pulse dye laser. In immunocompromised patients with extensive or refractory disease, interferon-α and cidofovir can be used.[17]

MPOX

Mpox is a double-stranded DNA virus belonging to the orthopoxvirus genus of the Poxviridae family. It is classically associated with contact with infected prairie dogs, rodents, and primates but human-to-human transmission (ie, sexual transmission) also occurs. It is endemic in Central and West African countries with a higher prevalence among men who have sex with men.[18]

PATHOGENESIS

Mpox is transmitted via direct contact with infected animals or humans via bodily fluids, respiratory droplets, or via fomites.[18] It is currently unknown whether mpox can be sexually transmitted.

CLINICAL MANIFESTATIONS

Mpox has a similar presentation to smallpox. The incubation period ranges from 7 to 21 days. A prodromal phase with fever, lymphadenopathy, and malaise often precedes the characteristic cutaneous widespread eruption. Skin lesions begin as monomorphic erythematous macules, progressing to umbilicated papules, vesicles, then pustules. Within a week, the lesions form an eschar that soon peels off. Patients are considered infectious until resolution of the scabs.[18]

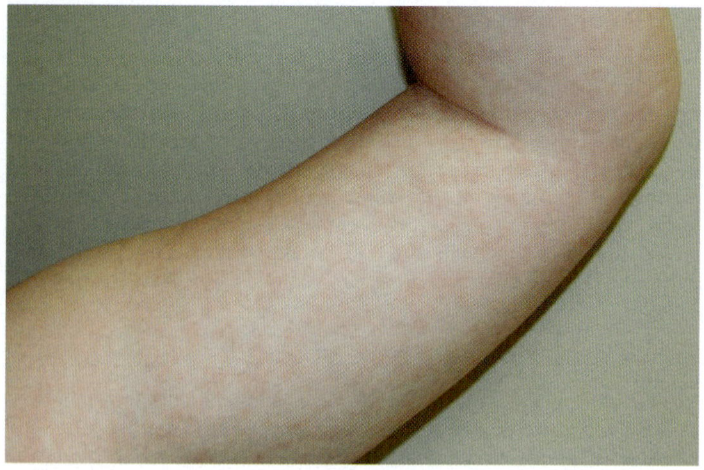

FIGURE 66-6. Parvovirus B19. Pink macules with a lacy, reticular pattern on the arm.

DIAGNOSIS

Diagnosis is made via PCR. Samples should be obtained from vesicular or pustular lesions or eschars.

TREATMENT

The mainstay of treatment of mpox is supportive care. Treatment options for severe cases include the antivirals cidofovir and tecovirimat and brincidofovir, the two FDA-approved treatments for smallpox.[19] Vaccinia immune globulin (VIG), which is FDA approved for treatment of complications due to vaccinia vaccination, is another potential treatment.[19]

PARVOVIRIDAE (PARVOVIRUS B19)

Parvovirus B19 (the only parvovirus that infects humans) is a small ssDNA virus known to cause a myriad of clinical findings, including erythema infectiosum, or fifth disease, in children. Mostly seen in children and mostly in the winter months.[20,21]

PATHOGENESIS

Transmission occurs via aerosol droplets through the respiratory route, blood products, and vertical transmission from mother to fetus. During infection, B19 lyses erythroid precursor cells. The rash subsequently occurs due to immune complex deposition. Individuals are usually not infectious once the rash appears.[21]

CLINICAL MANIFESTATIONS

Erythema infectiosum (fifth disease) is the most common clinical presentation of B19 infection in children. Individuals may experience prodromal symptoms about 7 to 11 days after exposure, leading to "slapped cheek" erythematous edematous plaques on malar eminences.[20] Pink macules and papules then subsequently present on the trunk and extensor surfaces. Adults tend to experience a rash that involves the palms and/or soles. The rash often has a lacy, reticular pattern due to central clearing [**Figure 66-6**] but resolves spontaneously with no permanent sequelae.[20] Erythema is more difficult to decipher in skin of color patients, leading to delayed diagnosis.

DIAGNOSIS

Parvovirus B19 infection is mostly a clinical diagnosis, but in circumstances where clinical diagnosis is unclear, the B19 immunoglobulin M (IgM) can be detected.[21]

TREATMENT

There is no specific treatment for erythema infectiosum. Some patients may benefit from supportive care [**Table 66-4**].

TABLE 66-4 Parvovirus B19 treatment

Symptoms	Treatment
Arthralgias	Nonsteroidal anti-inflammatory medications
Pruritus	Oral antihistamines, starch baths
Fever	Antipyretics
Malaise	Bed rest

ENTEROVIRUSES—HAND, FOOT, AND MOUTH DISEASE (HFMD)

HFMD is a viral illness commonly caused by coxsackievirus A16 (CA16) and enterovirus 71. Enteroviruses are a subgroup of the picornaviridae, a large family of small nonenveloped RNA viruses. Infection rates are higher in young children but can rarely present in adults.[20] While HFMD is a global issue, incidence rates are highest in Asian countries, with cases in China accounting for 87% of all the cases reported to WHO in 2014.[22] Transmission can be primarily through fecal-oral, respiratory routes, or close personal contact with an infected person.[22]

PATHOGENESIS

The viruses infect the gastrointestinal mucosa where they replicate in the lymph tissues. They then cause minor viremia and travel to different anatomical regions to cause disease. These sites are where major viremia occurs and they include the CNS, heart, liver, respiratory tract, skin, mucosal membranes.[20]

CLINICAL MANIFESTATIONS

The exanthem is usually preceded by a prodrome of fever, malaise, sore throat. Macules and papules that evolve into vesicles, typically present on the hands, soles, and oral mucosa [**Figures 66-7** and **66-8**]. Lesions can also be present on other sites such as the buttocks.[20]

DIAGNOSIS

Diagnosis of HFMD is clinical; however, new testing developments can isolate the specific virus, such as RT-PCR.[23] Since the conventional RT-PCR can be time-consuming, real-time RT-PCR has been developed to identify the causal agent within 1 to 2 hours with high sensitivity and specificity.[23]

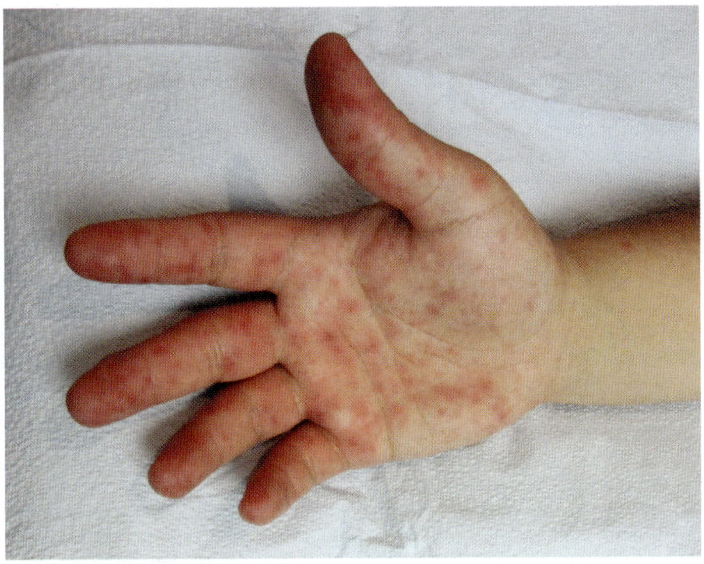

FIGURE 66-7. Hand, foot, and mouth disease. Erythematous papulovesicles on the hands bilaterally.

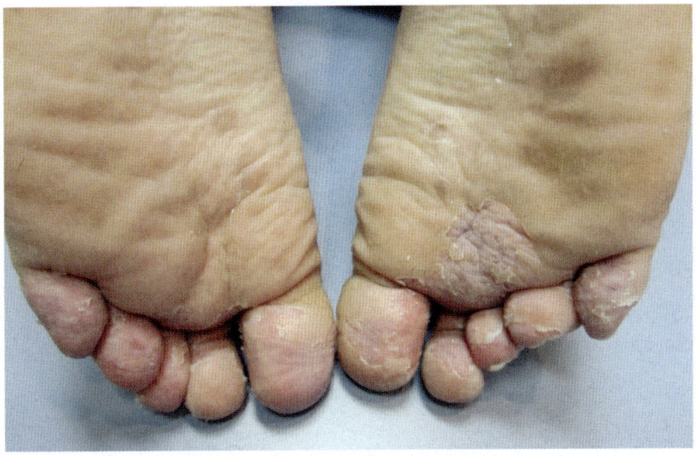

FIGURE 66-8. Hand, foot, and mouth disease. Desquamation of the toes bilaterally.

TREATMENT

The course of disease is frequently self-limited in healthy individuals, requiring only supportive care [**Table 66-5**]. HFMD can cause life-threatening disease in immunocompromised populations so vaccines and antivirals such as ribavirin and acyclovir have been used.[24]

HUMAN IMMUNODEFICIENCY VIRUS

Human Immunodeficiency Virus (HIV) has several associated mucocutaneous manifestations due to the actual disease, opportunistic infections, or due to therapy.[25] HIV affects individuals who engage in high-risk sexual behaviors, men who have sex with men (MSM), individuals with low socioeconomic status, and IV drug users.[25] Currently, sub-Saharan Africa has the highest prevalence of HIV, although the incidence in western countries is still increasing.[25]

PATHOGENESIS

In the acute phase of HIV infection, the virus enters the body through various means (blood, perinatal, breast milk, sexual intercourse) and infects CD4+ T cells, leading to rapid viral replication and a high viral load.[25,26] The viral load then declines after several months to a steady level after the immune system mounts a response by antibodies and CD8+ T cells. Circulating CD4+ T cells eventually steadily decline due to chronic infection, leading to AIDS in most untreated individuals approximately 10 years after initial infection.[25]

CLINICAL PRESENTATION

HIV-related mucocutaneous manifestations are typically due to other opportunistic infections; however, a subset of HIV patients develop a generalized morbilliform rash during the acute phase of the disease.[25] With the waning immunity, opportunistic infections such HSV, MC, EBV, CMV, VZV, and other bacterial, fungal, parasitic infections; neoplasms such as lymphomas, MCC, HPV-induced SCC; inflammatory dermatoses such as psoriasis, seborrheic dermatitis, atopic dermatitis can cause mucocutaneous eruptions.[25] Antiretroviral therapy (ART) is

TABLE 66-5 Hand, foot, and mouth disease treatment

Symptoms	Treatment
Fever	Antipyretics: children should not be given aspirin due its association with Reye syndrome.
Anorexia	Drink water and avoid intake of fruit juices and sodas because they can irritate oral lesions.
Sore throat	Saline water rinses and gargles two or three times daily. Prepare with ½ teaspoon of salt and 1 glass of warm water.

also associated with numerous mucocutaneous manifestations such as DRESS, SJS/TEN, lipodystrophy, hyperpigmentation of skin and nails, and morbilliform rashes.[25]

DIAGNOSIS

The preferred route for diagnosing HIV is currently by obtaining screening (HIV antibodies, p24 antigen) and confirmatory (IgG antibody, nucleic acid testing) laboratory tests.[25]

TREATMENT

Antiretroviral therapy (ART) has completely changed the course of HIV disease where individuals can still lead normal lives.[25]

POLYOMAVIRUS

Polyomaviruses are nonenveloped DNA viruses. Healthy individuals who are infected are typically asymptomatic. Merkel cell polyomaviruses (MCPyV) and trichodysplasia spinulosa polyomaviruses (TSPyV) are typical culprits for mucocutaneous disease in immunocompromised patients.[27] MCC has been associated with UV exposure; thus, SOC individuals have lower incidence than their non-SOC counterparts due to deeper skin pigmentation.[28] Due to the rarity of trichodysplasia spinulosa, there is no solid evidence regarding incidence in SOC patients.[29]

PATHOGENESIS

Merkel cell carcinoma either occurs from the virus integrating its DNA into the tumor genome or due to DNA mutations from ultraviolet (UV) light exposure, where the virus does not contribute.[27] Primary infection of TS is assumed to be during childhood from seroprevalence differences noted across different age groups. The pathogenesis of TS is not clear but presumed to be similar to other polyomaviruses.[30]

CLINICAL MANIFESTATIONS

MCPyV infection can lead to Merkel cell carcinoma (MCC) in some patients that can present as solitary, erythematous nodules or tumors, especially in sun-exposed areas [**Figure 66-9**].[28] Trichodysplasia spinulosa (TS) presents with numerous papules with centralized keratin spines (spicules) that characteristically present around the central part of the face but rarely presents in other areas of the body.[30]

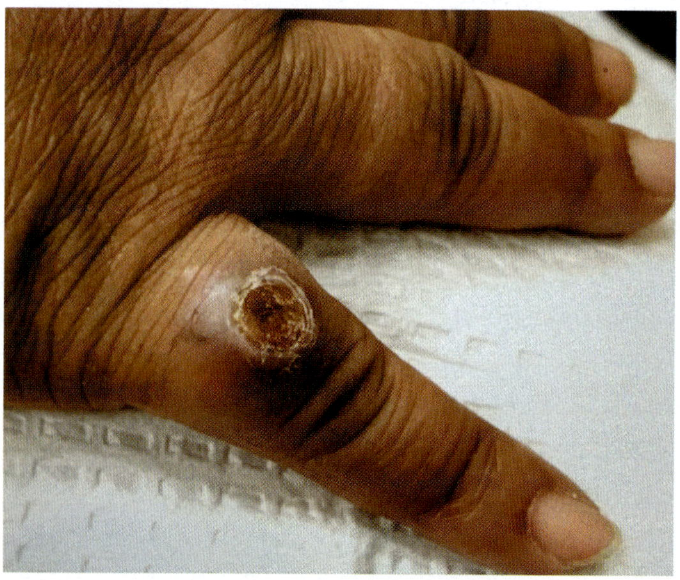

FIGURE 66-9. Merkel cell carcinoma. Ulcerated nodule of the right fifth digit. (Courtesy of Stephen K. Tyring, MD.)

DIAGNOSIS

Diagnosis of MCC can be difficult as the clinical presentation is nonspecific; histopathology assessment is more specific and sentinel lymph node biopsy (SLNB) for staging.[28] TS diagnosis can be confirmed by histopathology and PCR with evidence of high TSPyV burden.[30]

TREATMENT

There is no established treatment for TS; however, antivirals such as 3% topical cidofovir and oral ganciclovir have displayed some degree of efficacy.[30] Standard treatment of MCC is the excision of the primary MCC tumor, with additional excisions, radiotherapy, or systemic therapy for metastases.[28]

REFERENCES

1. McQuillan G, Kruszon-Moran D, Flagg EW, Paulose-Ram R. Prevalence of herpes simplex virus type 1 and type 2 in persons aged 14-49: United States, 2015-2016. *NCHS Data Brief.* 2018;(304):1-8.
2. Gupta R, Warren T, Wald A. Genital herpes. *Lancet.* 2007;370:2127-2137.
3. Azwa A, Barton SE. Aspects of herpes simplex virus: a clinical review. *J Fam Plann Reprod HealthCare.* 2009;35:237-242.
4. Schmader K, George LK, Burchett BM, et al. Racial differences in the occurrence of herpes zoster. *J Infect Dis.* 1995;171:701-704.
5. Patil A, Goldust M, Wollina U. *Herpes zoster*: a review of clinical manifestations and management. *Viruses.* 2022;14(2):192.
6. Creed R, Satyaprakash D, Tyring SK. Varicella-zoster virus. In: Tyring SK, ed. *Mucocutaneous Manifestations of Viral Diseases.* 2nd ed. London: Informa Healthcare; 2010:98-122.
7. Rewane A, Tadi P. Herpes virus type 8. 2022 Jul 19. In: *StatPearls [Internet].* Treasure Island (FL): StatPearls Publishing; 2022 Jan–.
8. Drozd B, Andriescu E, Suárez A, De la Garza Bravo MM. Cutaneous cytomegalovirus manifestations, diagnosis, and treatment: a review. *Dermatol Online J.* 2019;25(1):13030/qt84f936cp.
9. Walling MD, Hudnall SD, A Yen-Moore. Epstein-Barr virus. In: Tyring SK, ed. *Mucocutaneous Manifestations of Viral Diseases.* New York, NY: Marcel Dekker Inc; 2002:145-172.
10. Uldrick TS, Whitby D. Update on KSHV epidemiology, Kaposi Sarcoma pathogenesis, and treatment of Kaposi Sarcoma. *Cancer Lett.* 2011;305(2):150-162.
11. Sangueza-Acosta M, Sandoval-Romero E. Epstein-Barr virus and skin. *An Bras Dermatol.* 2018;93(6):786-799.
12. Antman K, Chang Y. Kaposi's sarcoma. *N Engl J Med.* 2000;342(14):1027-1038.
13. McQuillan G, Kruszon-Moran D, Markowitz LE, Unger ER, Paulose-Ram R. Prevalence of HPV in Adults Aged 18-69: United States, 2011-2014. *NCHS Data Brief.* 2017;(280):1-8.
14. Moore AY, Tyring SK. Cutaneous warts. In: Sterling JC, Tyring SK, eds. *Human Papillomaviruses: Clinical and Scientific Advances.* London, United Kingdom: Arnold; 2001:52-59.
15. Ockenfels HM. Therapeutic management of cutaneous and genital warts. *J Dtsch Dermatol Ges.* 2016;14(9):892-899.
16. Becker TM, Blount JH, Douglas J, Judson FN. Trends in molluscum contagiosum in the United States, 1966-1983. *Sex Transm Dis.* 1986;13(2):88-92.
17. Meza-Romero R, Navarrete-Dechent C, Downey C. Molluscum contagiosum: an update and review of new perspectives in etiology, diagnosis, and treatment. *Clin Cosmet Investig Dermatol.* 2019;12:373-381.
18. Kaler J, Hussain A, Flores G, Kheiri S, Desrosiers D. Monkeypox: a comprehensive review of transmission, pathogenesis, and manifestation. *Cureus.* 2022;14(7):e26531.
19. Titanji BK, Tegomoh B, Nematollahi S, Konomos M, Kulkarni PA. Monkeypox: a contemporary review for healthcare professionals. *Open Forum Infect Dis.* 2022;9(7):ofac310.
20. Mancini AJ, Shani-Adir A, Sidbury R. Other viral diseases. In: Bolognia JL, Schaffer JV, Cerroni L, eds. *Dermatology.* Vol. 2. 4th ed. China: Elsevier; 2018:1425-1446.
21. Gripp AC, Fontenelle E, Wiss K. Parvovirus B19. In: Tyring SK, Yen Moore A, Lupi O, eds. *Mucocutaneous Manifestations of Viral Diseases.* 2nd ed. London: Informa Healthcare; 2010:253-262.
22. Yi Z, Pei S, Suo W, et al. Epidemiological characteristics, routine laboratory diagnosis, clinical signs and risk factors for hand, -foot -and -mouth disease: a systematic review and meta-analysis. *PLoS One.* 2022;17(4):e0267716.
23. Cui A, Xu C, Tan X, et al. The development and application of the two real-time RT-PCR assays to detect the pathogen of HFMD. *PLoS One.* 2013;8(4):e61451.

24. Zhao Y, Sun Y, Alolga RN, Ma G, Wang F. The use of oseltamivir as adjunctive therapy for the treatment of hand-foot-and-mouth disease: a meta-analysis of randomized clinical trials. *Front Pharmacol.* 2021;12:653691.
25. Chan RKW, Chio MTW, Koh HY. Cutaneous manifestations of HIV infection. In: Bolognia JL, Schaffer JV, Cerroni L. *Dermatology*. Vol. 2. 4th ed. China: Elsevier; 2018: 1364-1382.
26. VIRAL DISEASES OF SKIN AND MUCOSA. In: Wolff K, Johnson R, Saavedra AP, Roh EK. eds. *Fitzpatrick's Color Atlas and Synopsis of Clinical Dermatology*, 8e. McGraw-Hill Education; 2017. Accessed May 20, 2025. https://accessmedicine.mhmedical.com/Content.aspx?bookid=2043&sectionid=154894979
27. Prado JCM, Monezi TA, Amorim AT, Lino V, Paladino A, Boccardo E. Human polyomaviruses and cancer: an overview. *Clinics (Sao Paulo)*. 2018;73(suppl 1): e558s.
28. Becker JC, Stang A, DeCaprio JA, et al. Merkel cell carcinoma. *Nat Rev Dis Primers*. 2017;3:17077.
29. Moore MJ, Rampton R. Trichodysplasia Spinulosa. In: *StatPearls*. Treasure Island (FL): StatPearls Publishing; July 5, 2022.
30. Curman P, Näsman A, Brauner H. Trichodysplasia spinulosa: a comprehensive review of the disease and its treatment. *J Eur Acad Dermatol Venereol*. 2021;35(5):1067-1076.

CHAPTER 67

MPox Virus and Skin of Color

Kevin Puerta Durango
Maya Childs
Susan C. Taylor

KEY POINTS

- Populations of color are disproportionately affected by infectious diseases, including Mpox.
- Cutaneous manifestations of the mpox virus can present differently in skin of color.
- Outbreaks were previously endemic to regions of Central and West Africa; however, the 2022 outbreak impacted 117 countries, many of which were nonendemic.
- Vaccines are effective against mpox, but ultimately highlight the inequities experienced by certain marginalized populations in our healthcare system.

INTRODUCTION

Mpox, formerly known as monkeypox (MPXV), is a zoonotic viral infection that was officially renamed by the World Health Organization (WHO) on November 28, 2022.[1,2] Endemic to West and Central Africa, the first documented human case was in 1970, in the Democratic Republic of the Congo (DRC)[3]. Recent outbreaks in numerous nonendemic countries led to a global mpox outbreak in 2022, with more than 90,000 cases diagnosed and sparking worldwide attention.[3] In July 2022, the World Health Organization declared mpox a "public health emergency of international concern."[4] Despite the latest emergence of mpox outbreaks, populations of color have historically been disproportionately affected by this infectious disease, for which the hallmark feature affects the appearance of the skin.[5]

Beyond the dermatologic manifestations of mpox, it is necessary to assess the socioeconomic implications for prevalence, diagnosis, treatment, and prevention in populations of color. By studying and implementing effective prevention measures in demographic regions that are endemic, future populations may be spared. Populations of color are often subject to access inequality with regard to healthcare and regularly experience worse health outcomes.[5,6] In this chapter, mpox will be examined from an epidemiologic, dermatologic, and clinical perspective, specifically highlighting skin of color.

RNA VIRUSES

RNA viruses, including SARS-CoV-2, orthomyxoviruses, Hepatitis C, and Ebola, are single-stranded or double-stranded viruses that express elevated mutation rates.[7] This phenomenon is primarily due to the RNA-dependent polymerases' lack of exonuclease proofreading and replication fidelity, in addition to the occurrence of spontaneous mutations. The resulting genetic variants exhibit distinguishable viral morphogenesis. The lack of proofreading mechanisms provides RNA viruses the ability to avoid pressures from vaccines or antiviral drugs in a manner that DNA viruses are not able to.[8] The fast rate at which RNA viruses replicate results in higher misincorporation of ribonucleotides, but it allows the virus to thrive by rapidly adjusting to varying host environments.[9] Overall, pathogenic RNA viruses are responsible for significant morbidity and mortality in humans, as these viruses mainly represent zoonotic disease transmission and are often involved in global pandemics.[8]

DNA VIRUSES

DNA viruses, such as adenovirus, herpesvirus, and poxvirus, consist of DNA genomes that are replicated by host or virally encoded DNA polymerases. DNA viruses are much larger than RNA viruses, in large part because of the stability of DNA allowing for larger genomes. Like RNA viruses, DNA viruses can be either single-stranded or double-stranded, but these viruses have great variability in their structures and can be linear or circular molecules. Specifics of DNA replication is outside of the scope of this chapter, but it is important to note that different DNA viruses replicate differently depending on size. Smaller DNA viruses rely on host replication machinery, while larger DNA viruses tend to encode their own.[10]

POXVIRIDAE

Mpox is an orthopoxvirus, belonging to the Poxviridae family, Chordopoxvirinae subfamily, and *Orthopoxvirus* genus. Poxviridae consists of large, complex, linear double-stranded DNA viruses that affect numerous species, ranging from mammals, reptiles, birds, and insects, though the natural reservoir remains unknown.[11] Poxviruses contain a large genome that encodes both DNA and RNA polymerases, while replicating and transcribing the genome in the cytoplasm. They also have the ability to encode proteins that are adept at avoiding and inactivating the innate and adaptive immune responses.[12] Mpox is one of four orthopoxvirus species that are pathogenic to humans, including variola major virus (VARV), the causative agent of smallpox, variola minor virus, and cowpox virus (CPXV). Other associated human viruses include camelpox (CMLV), horsepox (HSPV), buffalopox (BPXV).[13] Mpox has such a similar presentation to smallpox that the widespread discontinuation of the smallpox vaccine, due to the eradication of the smallpox virus, has been found to contribute to weakened or nonexistent immunity against mpox.[13]

EPIDEMIOLOGY

The first ever report of mpox was in 1958 when it was observed in two cynomolgus monkeys in a laboratory in Denmark.[14] In 1970, the first recognized case of mpox in a human was identified in a 9-year-old boy in the DRC.[3] Cases of mpox were limited and rarely reported until an outbreak in the DRC in 1996 with 511 patients affected.[15] After this outbreak, 200 cases per year were suspected in the DRC between 1996 and 2004, and greater than 1000 cases per year between 2005 and 2015, after which the number of suspected cases has remained above 2500. The DRC is the endemic region of clade I mpox infections and from January to November 12, 2023, a total of 12,569 cases were suspected, including 581 deaths (case fatality ratio of 4.6%), making it the highest number of cases ever reported in the DRC.[16] Mpox in humans had been limited mostly to Central and West Africa; however, between 2018 and 2021, cases have been reported in Israel (1 case), Singapore (1), United Kingdom (7),

United States (2), all related to travel from Nigeria.[17] Additionally, in 2003, 71 confirmed and suspected cases of mpox were reported in the United States, and connected to contact with prairie dogs who appeared to be infected by Ghanian giant rats.[18] Mpox was relatively contained to the endemic areas until the global mpox clade IIb strain outbreak in 2022. As of November 21, 2023, the mpox 2022 outbreak has reached 117 countries, including 110 (94%) countries that had not historically reported mpox. The case total has surpassed 92,000, and the death total is 167 throughout 25 different countries, with 146 deaths in 19 countries that had not historically reported mpox.[19]

The United States represents the largest number of cases from the clade IIb strain (31,186), and deaths (55).[19] As of November 21, 2023, four Latin American countries, Brazil (10,967 cases), Colombia (4090), Mexico (4066), Peru (3812), one Asian country, China (1531 cases), are also in the top 10 highest number of cases worldwide, accentuating the disproportionate impact mpox has on people of color even outside of Africa. The disparity is further demonstrated by the fact that after the United States, 107 of the 112 clade IIb mpox deaths are from countries in Latin America and Africa.[19] In October of 2023, the number of monthly reported new cases decreased by 22.8% compared to the previous month, and only one country (Oman) reported their first case.[20]

Strikingly, in the 1970s, mpox patients were predominantly young children[3]. Recently, in the United States, patients' age ranges span from approximately 21 to 55 years.[21] People of color, specifically Black or African American men who have sex with men (MSM) have been disproportionately affected by mpox.[22,23] Black people account for approximately 12% of the U.S. population but make up 33% of mpox cases.[24] Further, Hispanic people account for approximately 19% of the U.S. population, but 31% of mpox cases.[25,26] Coinfections in vulnerable populations, such as cisgender MSM and people with HIV (PWH), experienced disproportionately higher clinical manifestations of mpox illness.[27] Mpox research currently focuses on data from White patients. Efforts are needed to accurately capture and reflect the cases of Black or African American patients.[28] Such information would help guide the clinical course and associated outcomes of mpox.

TRANSMISSION

Mpox is known to be transmitted directly from animal-to-human, human-to-human, and indirectly from fomite-to-human.[29] The animal reservoir remains unknown, but mpox has been found in a variety of animal species, including various squirrels, rats, mice and primates, supporting the suspicion that the reservoir is likely a small mammal.[30-33] There is evidence from genomic analyses suggesting that multiple zoonic spillovers have occurred resulting in the infection of humans.[34] The acquisition of mpox is believed to be through percutaneous exposure, direct exposure to mucous membranes, and/or inhalation of infectious particles into the respiratory tract.[29] Animal-to-human transmission was previously the primary method of transmission, as it frequently results from direct contact with an infected animal or due to contact with bodily fluids, such as saliva or respiratory excretions.[35] The recent 2022 outbreak saw human-to-human transmission as the primary method of transmission, with vulnerable populations being at increased risk of infection.[36] Specifically, sexual or intimate contact was seen as the primary method of human-to-human transmission.[37] One European analysis of 41 countries found that as many as 93.9% of cases reported sexual contact as a possible route of transmission.[38]

RECENT OUTBREAKS

Mpox results from two main clades identified in Central (Clade I) and West (Clade IIa/b) Africa, which have caused several outbreaks since the 1970s.[39] These communities of color are often dually impacted by comorbidities, such as parasitic infections, malnutrition, and other major health threats that pose the potential to exacerbate mpox symptoms.[40] Recent mpox outbreaks in Nigeria (2017-2021) and Cameroon (2018) have been documented.[41] Though endemic to Africa, mpox was previously unrecognized and did not garner large-scale international attention until Western countries became infected, with the first reported mpox outbreak outside of Africa being in the United States in 2003.[18] Recent outbreaks since 2018 have been reported in 110 nonendemic countries and territories. Between 2022 and 2023, the Clade IIb strain caused a global outbreak of mpox.[19]

The first reported case in the United States was in Massachusetts on May 17, 2022.[42] By August of 2022, mpox spread to all 50 states, including Washington D.C. and Puerto Rico. The first U.S.-related mpox death was reported on August 30, 2022. The United States had the highest number of mpox cases in the world, representing over one-third of cases and deaths worldwide.[19] The highest recorded number of cases was in the state of California.[43]

On December 7, 2023, the CDC announced a health advisory about the occurrence, geographic spread, and sexual transmission of Clade I mpox in the DRC. At the time of the report, no recent cases had been reported in the United States, but it is important to maintain awareness due to the increased severity and transmissibility of Clade I mpox infections.[44]

DIAGNOSIS

Clinical symptoms of mpox present similarly to smallpox and other infections but are usually less severe.[16] Despite this, mpox can result in fatalities, with a mortality rate of Clade I being as high as 11% to 15%, Clade IIa under 1%, and Clade IIb also having a low mortality in immunocompetent individuals.[45,46] Mpox infections usually have a 5- to 21-day incubation period prior to a 1- to 4-day prodrome of systemic symptoms, which then results in a cutaneous eruption.[47] Due to mpox resembling other conditions, testing is crucial. Chickenpox is the most common differential diagnosis, with secondary syphilis, measles, scabies, and hand, foot, and mouth disease also in the differential.[48,49] The preferred laboratory test for the detection of mpox is reverse transcription polymerase chain reaction (RT-PCR) on lesional skin, fluid, or scab crusts. Alternatively, testing can be completed utilizing oropharyngeal, anal, or rectal swabs.[11]

SIGNS AND SYMPTOMS

The prodromal symptoms of mpox are typically mild and self-limiting, mimicking common influenza symptoms including fever, acute headache, fatigue, asthenia, myalgia, and lymphadenopathy.[11,40,50,51] Lymphadenopathy often occurs with the onset of fever, and is a prominent symptom, presenting in approximately 90% of mpox patients.[51] It is the leading clinical factor distinguishing mpox from smallpox and chickenpox viruses.

Other documented complications of mpox include bronchopneumonia, encephalitis, myocarditis, proctitis, urethritis, sepsis, and gastrointestinal symptoms, including vomiting and diarrhea with dehydration.[40,51,52] Secondary bacterial infections, or superinfections, also occurred, and were found to possibly contribute to dermal scarring.[40] Scarring is likely due to itching, scratching, and ineffective treatments. A relatively uncommon complication of mpox is infection of the cornea, leading to corneal scarring, involvement of the conjunctiva, and subsequent loss of vision or blindness.[40,53]

Mpox is most notable for its characteristic vesiculopustular eruption, which evolves from macules to umbilicated papules to vesicles to pustules to scabs, which then undergo reepithelialization and resolution.[40] Cutaneous eruptions or mucosal lesions are most likely to appear within 1 to 3 days of fever onset, and typically last 2 to 4 weeks.[54,55] The total lesion burden can be low (<25 lesion) or relatively high (>500 lesions).[40]

The pleomorphic skin lesions frequently develop on the face first, but then spread to other parts of the body, often forming on the palms, soles, and near the genitals or anus. It is not uncommon for the eruption to also appear on the chest, mouth, and throat.[11,47] Cutaneous involvement with mpox has been reported as painful and itchy.[47,52] Affected individuals are considered contagious or infectious until all sores have healed, lesions have scabbed, and a new layer of skin has formed.[15] Individuals can be affected with mpox and be asymptomatic.[48,56]

There are notable deviations in skin findings in recent mpox outbreaks compared to previous outbreaks, and across populations.[57] Atypical progression of lesions includes a reduced number of skin or mucocutaneous lesions (<20), and the emergence of skin lesions prior to the onset of systemic illness. The 2022 outbreak also exhibited the involvement of multiple simultaneous morphologies.[58]

Physical manifestations of mpox may present differently in skin of color patients. In one study, the erythema described in traditional mpox was not as distinguishable in the cohort of skin of color patients.[47] For those with skin of color, namely Black and Hispanic populations, the lesions appeared to be a more subtle pink, brown, or gray hyperpigmentation.[47] Scarring following mpox infection was widely reported, and should be evaluated in skin of color, as darker-complected skin can scar differently, resulting in increased negative long-term outcomes.[59]

TREATMENT

Currently, there is no standard for treatment of mpox. Treatment usually involves supportive care and symptom management. Due to similar genetics, research has shown that certain antiviral medications targeting smallpox, namely tecovirimat (TPOXX or ST-246), brincidofovir (oral), and cidofovir (intravenous), may be effective against mpox.[50] Another existing therapeutic is vaccinia immune globulin (VIG); however, further research is needed to prove its efficacy in treating mpox patients. Antiviral treatment is important for individuals who are immunocompromised, pediatric, pregnant, or breastfeeding, have a history of dermatitis, experience skin symptoms of exfoliation, or other lesional complications affecting sensitive areas (eg, eyes, mouth, genitals).[15] Most patients with mpox recover without medical treatment or intervention.[50]

With regard to symptom management, mpox can severely impact multiple organ systems within the host. As the protective barriers of the skin and mucosal surfaces are compromised, an inflammatory response is activated in the lymphatic system and congestion in the lungs.[40] Gastrointestinal complications usually require intravenous or oral rehydration to restore fluid losses. Secondary bacterial infections caused by open lesions are treated with antibiotics. For ocular complications, enhanced lubrication or topical antibiotics are potential treatments.[40]

PREVENTION

To prevent human to human transmission of mpox, it is recommended by the Centers for Disease Control and Transmission (CDC) that individuals avoid skin-to-skin contact with individuals portraying clinical symptoms of the virus (particularly cutaneous involvement), as well as refrain from contact with mpox-contaminated items. It is suggested that using alcohol-containing hand sanitizer and frequent hand washing are used as a routine measure prior to touching the face, eating, and after using the bathroom.[60]

It is also critical to note the needed implementation of strategic infection control and public health measures, and the enhancement of existing systems. Postexposure methods, such as quarantining and other isolation practices, are paramount to prevent the spread of disease. Improved conditions in healthcare environments are also vital, specifically pertaining to practices involving personal protective equipment (PPE), including protective clothing, gloves, and surgical masks.[51] Decisions surrounding protocols for contact and droplet precautions should also be taken into consideration. Immunizations among high-risk sectors of the population could be significantly beneficial, including for healthcare workers.[61] Additionally, increased awareness and education are required to better equip individuals with the ability to identify symptoms and mitigate further spreading. On both a national and international level, systematic surveillance is principal to disease prevention. Notably, vaccine technology has also been effective in preventing infection.

VACCINES

Smallpox vaccination is believed to provide protection against mpox, with a 2022 study showing that serum antibodies from smallpox vaccines were capable of neutralizing the current mpox virus more than 40 years after vaccine administration.[62,63] As of December of 2023, the WHO and CDC agree that mass vaccination for mpox is not required. Rather, vaccination should be reserved for higher-risk individuals who have been or may be exposed to mpox.[61] There are currently three available vaccines in the U.S. Strategic National Stockpile for smallpox: JYNNEOS, a modified vaccinia Ankara (MVA), ACAM2000, and the Aventis Pasteur Smallpox vaccine. The first two are currently approved for mpox.[11] Research shows that Mpox protection levels from smallpox vaccinations are as high as 85%, highlighting why smallpox vaccines have been used for the current mpox outbreak.[64]

The ACAM2000 vaccine is a second-generation smallpox vaccine based on the replication of competent viruses, which causes a cutaneous reaction at the site of inoculation.[50] The ACAM2000 vaccine should be avoided in immunosuppressed persons due to its side effect profile.[65] The JYNNEOS (IMVANEX in Europe) vaccine is a third-generation smallpox vaccine, based on the replication of incompetent vaccine, as such it does not result in any major cutaneous reactions at the inoculation site.[50] The JYNNEOS vaccine has been approved in Europe since 2013 for smallpox, and in the United States for mpox since 2019, for subcutaneous administration. In 2022, it received emergency use authorization for intradermal use in the United States and Europe. The effectiveness of the JYNNEOS vaccine is supported by a U.S. nationwide EPIC-database study, which found that patients with mpox were less likely to have received one or two doses of the vaccine than control patients. Additionally, there was evidence to support that a two-dose series provided better protection against the virus.[66] The second dose is given 4 weeks after the initial dose, and maximum protection is achieved 2 weeks after the second dose.[67] The JYNNEOS vaccine is currently the vaccine of choice recommended by the CDC, due to its more favorable safety profile and its availability among immunosuppressed persons. Vaccination coverage in the United States remains low, as only one in four vaccine-eligible individuals receive the vaccine.[67] Furthermore, it is concerning that vaccine distribution is limited in areas that are more densely populated with MSM and MSM with HIV. Additionally, even in areas where the vaccine is available it is not being equitably distributed. In North Carolina, 70% of cases are Black men, but only 24% of the vaccines are given to Black patients, versus 67% of vaccines being administered to White patients.[68]

CONCLUSION

Further research is needed to better prevent, manage, and treat mpox. Mpox disproportionately affects vulnerable communities, especially people of color, similar to COVID-19.[69] It is necessary to understand the clinical and dermatologic presentations of these groups, to properly distinguish and diagnose their medical conditions accurately, and to improve health outcomes by reducing rates of susceptibility, infection, and mortality.

REFERENCES

1. Gupta PC, Satapathy P, Gupta A, Padhi BK, Sah R. Renaming monkeypox to mpox: correspondence. *Int J Surg*. 2023;109(3):644-645.
2. WHO recommends new name for monkeypox disease. *Neurosciences (Riyadh)*. 2023;28(1):74-75.
3. Ladnyj ID, Ziegler P, Kima E. A human infection caused by monkeypox virus in Basankusu Territory, Democratic Republic of the Congo. *Bull World Health Organ*. 1972;46(5):593-597.
4. WHO director-general declares the ongoing monkeypox outbreak a Public Health Emergency of International Concern. July 23, 2022. https://www.who.int/europe/news/item/23-07-2022-who-director-general-declares-the-ongoing-monkeypox-outbreak-a-public-health-event-of-international-concern.

5. Robertson MM, Shamsunder MG, Brazier E, et al. Racial/ethnic disparities in exposure, disease susceptibility, and clinical outcomes during COVID-19 pandemic in National Cohort of Adults, United States. *Emerg Infect Dis.* 2022;28(11):2171-2180.
6. Javed Z, Haisum Maqsood M, Yahya T, et al. Race, racism, and cardiovascular health: applying a social determinants of health framework to racial/ethnic disparities in cardiovascular disease. *Circ Cardiovasc Qual Outcomes.* 2022;15(1):e007917.
7. Poltronieri P, Sun B, Mallardo M. RNA viruses: RNA roles in pathogenesis, coreplication and viral load. *Curr Genomics.* 2015;16(5):327-335.
8. Villa TG, Abril AG, Sánchez S, de Miguel T, Sánchez-Pérez A. Animal and human RNA viruses: genetic variability and ability to overcome vaccines. *Arch Microbiol.* 2021;203(2):443-464.
9. Fitzsimmons WJ, Woods RJ, McCrone JT, et al. A speed-fidelity trade-off determines the mutation rate and virulence of an RNA virus. *PLoS Biol.* 2018;16(6):e2006459.
10. Payne, S. Introduction to DNA viruses. In: *Viruses: From Understanding to Investigation*. Elsevier; 2023:301-307.
11. Soheili M, Nasseri S, Afraie M, et al. Monkeypox: virology, pathophysiology, clinical characteristics, epidemiology, vaccines, diagnosis, and treatments. *J Pharm Sci.* 2022;25:297-322.
12. Payne, S. Family *Poxviridae*. In: *Viruses: From Understanding to Investigation*. Elsevier; 2023:353-359. Accessed December 11, 2023.
13. Petersen E, Kantele A, Koopmans M, et al. Human monkeypox: epidemiologic and clinical characteristics, diagnosis, and prevention. *Infect Dis Clin North Am.* 2019;33(4):1027-1043.
14. von Magnus P, Andersen EK, Petersen KB, Birch-Andersen A. A pox-like disease in cynomolgus monkeys. *Acta Pathol Microbiol Scand.* 1959;46(2):156-176.
15. Pebody R. Human monkeypox in Kasai oriental, Democratic Republic of Congo, February 1996 – October 1997: preliminary report. Weekly releases (1997–2007). 1997;1(32):1015.
16. World Health Organization (November 23, 2023). Disease Outbreak News; Mpox (monkeypox) in the Democratic Republic of the Congo. Available at: https://www.who.int/emergencies/disease-outbreak-news/item/2023-DON493.
17. McCollum AM, Shelus V, Hill A, et al. Epidemiology of human Mpox - worldwide, 2018-2021. *MMWR Morb Mortal Wkly Rep.* 2023;72(3):68-72.
18. Centers for Disease Control, Prevention. Update: multistate outbreak of monkeypox–Illinois, Indiana, Kansas, Missouri, Ohio, and Wisconsin, 2003. *MMWR Morb Mortal Wkly Rep.* 2003;52(27):642-646.
19. Centers for Disease Control, Prevention. 2022-2023 global map & case count. Updated November 21, 2023. https://www.cdc.gov/poxvirus/mpox/response/2022/world-map.html. Accessed December 11, 2023.
20. 2022-23 Mpox Outbreak: Global Trends. Geneva: World Health Organization, 2023. https://worldhealthorg.shinyapps.io/mpx_global/. Accessed December 11, 2023.
21. Meo SA. Human monkeypox: old virus with new epidemiological and transmission trends. *Pak J Med Sci.* 2022;38(8):2061-2064.
22. Maulsby C, Millett G, Lindsey K, et al. HIV among Black men who have sex with men (MSM) in the United States: a review of the literature. *AIDS Behav.* 2014;18(1):10-25.
23. Ogunbajo A, Euceda A, Smith J, et al. Demographics and health beliefs of black gay, bisexual, and other sexual minority men receiving a mpox vaccination in the United States. *J Urban Health.* 2023;100(1):204-211.
24. Philpott D, Hughes CM, Alroy KA, et al. Epidemiologic and clinical characteristics of monkeypox cases - United States, May 17-July 22, 2022. *MMWR Morb Mortal Wkly Rep.* 2022;71(32):1018-1022.
25. Eustaquio PC, Salmon-Trejo LA, McGuire LC, Ellington SR. Epidemiologic and clinical features of mpox in adults aged >50 years — United States, May 2022–May 2023. *MMWR Morb Mortal Wkly Rep.* 2023;72:893-896.
26. Centers for Disease Control and Prevention. Case demographics. Updated November 28, 2023. https://www.cdc.gov/poxvirus/mpox/response/2022/demographics.html. Accessed December 11, 2023.
27. Karan A, Contag C, Barry M. Health inequities continue to drive the public health threat of mpox. *BMJ.* 2023;381:1391.
28. März JW, Holm S, Biller-Andorno N. Monkeypox, stigma and public health. *Lancet Reg Health Eur.* 2022;23.
29. Beeson A, Styczynski A, Hutson CL, et al. Mpox respiratory transmission: the state of the evidence. *Lancet Microbe.* 2023;4(4):e277-e283.
30. Nolen LD, Osadebe L, Katomba J, et al. Introduction of monkeypox into a community and household: risk factors and zoonotic reservoirs in the Democratic Republic of the Congo. *Am J Trop Med Hyg.* 2015;93(2):410-415.
31. Reynolds MG, Carroll DS, Karem KL. Factors affecting the likelihood of monkeypox's emergence and spread in the post-smallpox era. *Curr Opin Virol.* 2012;2(3):335-343.
32. Arita I, Jezek Z, Khodakevich L, Ruti K. Human monkeypox: a newly emerged orthopoxvirus zoonosis in the tropical rain forests of Africa. *Am J Trop Med Hyg.* 1985;34(4):781-789.
33. Khodakevich L, Jezek Z, Kinzanzka K. Isolation of monkeypox virus from wild squirrel infected in nature. *Lancet.* 1986;1(8472):98-99.
34. Mitja O, Ogoina D, Titanji BK, et al. Monkeypox. *Lancet.* 2023;401(10370):60-74.
35. Kaler J, Hussain A, Flores G, Kheiri S, Desrosiers D. Monkeypox: a comprehensive review of transmission, pathogenesis, and manifestation. *Cureus.* 2022;14(7):e26531.
36. Sharif N, Dey SK. Epidemiology of mpox: focus on men with HIV. *Heliyon.* 2023;9(11):e22129.
37. Pinto P, Costa MA, Goncalves MFM, Rodrigues AG, Lisboa C. Mpox person-to-person transmission-where have we got so far? A systematic review. *Viruses.* 2023;15(5).
38. Vaughan AM, Cenciarelli O, Colombe S, et al. A large multi-country outbreak of monkeypox across 41 countries in the WHO European Region, 7 March to 23 August 2022. *Euro Surveill.* 2022;27(36).
39. Van Dijck C, Hoff NA, Mbala-Kingebeni P, et al. Emergence of mpox in the post-smallpox era-a narrative review on mpox epidemiology. *Clin Microbiol Infect.* 2023;29(12):1487-1492.
40. Reynolds MG, McCollum AM, Nguete B, Shongo Lushima R, Petersen BW. Improving the care and treatment of monkeypox patients in low-resource settings: applying evidence from contemporary biomedical and smallpox biodefense research. *Viruses.* 2017;9(12):380.
41. Saldana CS, Kelley CF, Aldred BM, Cantos VD. Mpox and HIV: a narrative review. *Curr HIV/AIDS Rep.* 2023;20(4):261-269.
42. Centers for Disease Control. Technical report 1: multi-national mpox outbreak, United States, 2022. https://www.cdc.gov/poxvirus/mpox/cases-data/technical-report/report-1.html#:~:text=Domestic%3A%20On%20May%20 17%2C%202022,of%20Columbia%2C%20and%20Puerto%20Rico.
43. 2022 U.S. Map & Case count. Centers for Disease Control and Prevention. Updated November 30, 2023. https://www.cdc.gov/poxvirus/mpox/response/2022/us-map.html. Accessed December 10, 2023.
44. Centers for Disease Control and Prevention. (December 7, 2023). Health Alert Network (HAN) - 00501. Centers for Disease Control and Prevention. https://emergency.cdc.gov/han/2023/han00501.asp#:~:text=The%20Centers%20 for%20Disease%20Control,the%20Democratic%20Republic%20of%20the.
45. Alcamí A. Pathogenesis of the circulating mpox virus and its adaptation to humans. *Proc Natl Acad Sci U S A.* 2023;120(13):e2301662120.
46. Jezek Z, Szczeniowski M, Paluku KM, Mutombo M. Human monkeypox: clinical features of 282 patients. *J Infect Dis.* 1987;156:293-298.
47. Momin ZK, Lee A, Vandergriff TW, et al. A plague passing over: clinical features of the 2022 mpox outbreak in patients of color living with HIV. *HIV Med.* 2023;24(10):1056-1065.
48. Gessain A, Nakoune E, Yazdanpanah Y. Monkeypox. *N Engl J Med.* 2022;387(19):1783-1793.
49. Jezek Z, Szczeniowski M, Paluku KM, Mutombo M, Grab B. Human monkeypox: confusion with chickenpox. *Acta Trop.* 1988;45(4):297-307.
50. Rizk JG, Lippi G, Henry BM, Forthal DN, Rizk Y. Prevention and treatment of monkeypox [published correction appears in Drugs. 2022 Aug;82(12):1343]. *Drugs.* 2022;82(9):957-963.
51. Petersen E, Kantele A, Koopmans M, et al. Human monkeypox: epidemiologic and clinical characteristics, diagnosis, and prevention. *Infect Dis Clin North Am.* 2019;33(4):1027-1043.
52. Thornhill JP, Barkati S, Walmsley S, et al. Monkeypox virus infection in humans across 16 countries - April-June 2022. *N Engl J Med.* 2022;387(8):679-691.
53. Huhn GD, Bauer AM, Yorita K, et al. Clinical characteristics of human monkeypox, and risk factors for severe disease. *Clin Infect Dis.* 2005;41(12):1742-1751.
54. Singhal T, Kabra SK, Lodha R. Monkeypox: a review. *Indian J Pediatr.* 2022;89(10):955-960.
55. Mitjà O, Ogoina D, Titanji BK, et al. Monkeypox [published correction appears in Lancet. 2022;400(10367):1926]. *Lancet.* 2023;401(10370):60-74.
56. Elsayed S, Bondy L, Hanage WP. Monkeypox virus infections in humans. *Clin Microbiol Rev.* 2022;35(4):e0009222.
57. Sale TA, Melski JW, Stratman EJ. Monkeypox: an epidemiologic and clinical comparison of African and US disease. *J Am Acad Dermatol.* 2006;55(3):478-481.
58. Prasad S, Galvan Casas C, Strahan AG, et al. A dermatologic assessment of 101 mpox (monkeypox) cases from 13 countries during the 2022 outbreak: skin lesion morphology, clinical course, and scarring. *J Am Acad Dermatol.* 2023;88(5):1066-1073.
59. Markiewicz E, Karaman-Jurukovska N, Mammone T, Idowu OC. Post-inflammatory hyperpigmentation in dark skin: molecular mechanism and skincare implications. *Clin Cosmet Investig Dermatol.* 2022;15:2555-2565.

60. Huang Y, Mu L, Wang W. Monkeypox: epidemiology, pathogenesis, treatment and prevention. *Signal Transduct Target Ther.* 2022;7(1):373.
61. Centers for Disease Control and Prevention. Mpox vaccine recommendations. Updated August 21, 2023. https://www.cdc.gov/poxvirus/mpox/vaccines/vaccine-recommendations.html. Accessed December 11, 2023.
62. Criscuolo E, Giuliani B, Ferrarese R, et al. Smallpox vaccination-elicited antibodies cross-neutralize 2022-monkeypox virus clade II. *J Med Virol.* 2023;95(3):e28643.
63. Hammarlund E, Lewis MW, Carter SV, et al. Multiple diagnostic techniques identify previously vaccinated individuals with protective immunity against monkeypox. *Nat Med.* 2005;11(9):1005-1011.
64. Fine PE, Jezek Z, Grab B, Dixon H. The transmission potential of monkeypox virus in human populations. *Int J Epidemiol.* 1988;17(3):643-650.
65. Crum-Cianflone NF, Sullivan E. Vaccinations for the HIV-infected adult: a review of the current recommendations, Part II. *Infect Dis Ther.* 2017;6(3):333-361.
66. Deputy NP, Deckert J, Chard AN, et al. Vaccine effectiveness of JYNNEOS against mpox disease in the United States. *N Engl J Med.* 2023;388(26):2434-2443.
67. CDC. Vaccines. Updated August 21, 2023. https://www.cdc.gov/poxvirus/mpox/vaccines/index.html. Accessed December 11, 2023.
68. McNaghten A, Brewer NT, Hung M, et al. COVID-19 vaccination coverage and vaccine confidence by sexual orientation and gender identity — United States, August 29–October 30, 2021. *MMWR Morb Mortal Wkly Rep.* 2022;71.
69. Rodriguez-Diaz CE, Crowley JS, Santiago-Rivera Y, Millett GA. From COVID-19 to monkeypox: unlearned lessons for Black, Latino, and other men with HIV who have sex with men. *Am J Public Health.* 2022;112(11):1567-1571.

CHAPTER 68 Bacterial Infections

Lauren S. Meshkov
Rajiv I. Nijhawan
Jeffrey M. Weinberg

KEY POINTS

- Individuals with skin of color may develop a wide range of cutaneous infections involving either gram-positive or gram-negative organisms.
- In most cases, these infections do not differ significantly from those that occur in the general population.
- *Staphylococcus aureus* and *Streptococcus pyogenes* are the two major Gram-positive organisms that are most often implicated in common skin and soft tissue infections.
- Gram-negative infections of the skin occur more commonly in children, patients with diabetes, and immunocompromised patients.
- Although empirical antibiotic treatment is an important first step in treating bacterial infections, once the diagnosis is established, treatment should then be dictated by the antibiotic sensitivities of the cultured organism.

BACTERIAL BIOFILMS AND THE SKIN

The human body plays host to a diverse world of bacteria, both as single-celled planktonic organisms and in sessile groups. Microbial flora of the skin largely exists within biofilms, sessile bacterial communities encased in an extracellular matrix, with the ability to communicate and regulate its own growth and metabolism.[1] Biofilms exist in both healthy and pathologic skin and may be protective or destructive, influencing host inflammatory cells and host metabolism and conferring antibiotic resistance. Therapeutic approaches to dermatologic disease have shifted recently, as biofilms may require more than traditional culture-based treatment.[2]

Biofilm studies are revealing new information about the skin's bacterial environment. These studies help explain why noninfectious diseases like acne vulgaris, miliaria, and atopic dermatitis respond to antibiotics and why certain lesions have anatomic predilections.[2] More alarming, however, are in vitro studies of biofilms that are 50 to 500 times more resistant to antibiotics than their planktonic counterparts.[3,4] This is due to several mechanisms: a physical barrier that prevents antibiotic diffusion,[5] slowed growth and metabolism of centrally located organisms that escape peripheral antibiotic activity, regulatory genes that change bacterial phenotype in response to environmental stress, spore-like forms that shut down antibiotic targets,[6] and frequent gene transfer through genomic islands of horizontally acquired DNA segments.[7] The complex interaction between biofilms and antibiotic therapy demands attention from the dermatologist, as inappropriate usage with sub-minimum inhibitory concentrations may enhance biofilm formation and confer further resistance.[8,9]

ANTIBIOTIC RESISTANCE

The widespread use of antibiotics for bacterial skin infections contributes to the emergence of resistant organisms and poses a serious threat to public health. Dermatologists wrote approximately 9.5 million prescriptions for oral antibiotics in 2009 alone,[10] and antibiotic resistance is growing among normal skin flora. The first penicillin-resistant *Staphylococcus aureus* was discovered in 1941, shortly after the drug's introduction. Up to 78% of all staphylococcal skin infections are now due to methicillin-resistant *S. aureus* (MRSA).[11] MRSA continues to display resistance to a range of drugs, including mupirocin, erythromycin, clindamycin, tetracycline, sulfonamides, chloramphenicol, cephalosporins, and quinolones.[12]

Propionibacterium acnes, the bacteria involved in acne formation, is just one organism that has shown resistance to oral tetracyclines and topical clindamycin,[13] the most common systemic and topical medications prescribed by dermatologists in 2009.[10] As a result, the recommended treatment now includes topical clindamycin with a benzoyl peroxide agent, retinoids, or clindamycin in a combination product rather than as monotherapy.[14,15] Systemic antibiotics for acne should be limited to the shortest duration possible in order to reduce antibiotic resistance.[16]

Antibiotic resistance is not only the result of overuse but is also caused by infection prophylaxis with topical antibiotics. Seventy-two percent of dermatologists encourage topical antibiotic use after dermatologic procedures, despite the low incidence of postoperative infections[17] and despite allergic contact dermatitis to bacitracin and neomycin.[18] MRSA resistance to mupirocin has grown from 1.6% between 1995 and 1999 to 7% between 2000 and 2004.[19] This is problematic because mupirocin is the cornerstone of treatment for MRSA impetigo infections and nasal carriage.[11]

Clinicians should be aware of local resistance patterns and choose antibiotics based on the target organism, patient profile, and necessity of treatment. Extended courses of antibiotics are not recommended, although in the case of true infections, strict adherence to dosage and duration is imperative.

GRAM-POSITIVE INFECTIONS [TABLE 68-1]

S. aureus and *Streptococcus pyogenes* are the two major gram-positive organisms most often implicated in common skin and soft tissue infections. Infections usually begin and remain contained at the site of

TABLE 68-1 Common Gram-positive bacterial infections
Erythrasma
Impetigo, ecthyma
Infectious folliculitis
Abscess, furuncle, carbuncle
Paronychia
Cellulitis, erysipelas
Blistering distal dactylitis
Cutaneous anthrax
Staphylococcal scalded skin syndrome
Toxic shock syndrome
Scarlet fever

a minor wound or skin abrasion, but once the skin is penetrated, the risk increases for systemic conditions such as sepsis, local necrosis, and endocarditis.

The following infections are typically diagnosed clinically and treated empirically. Gram-positive organisms are treated with an antibiotic, such as a penicillinase-resistant penicillin, a cephalosporin, a macrolide, or a flouroquinolone.[20] Although empiric antibiotic therapy is often important, treatment should be tailored to culture results and antibiotic sensitivities of the offending organisms.

CUTANEOUS MRSA INFECTION

The cost of treating an MRSA infection exceeds that of a methicillin-sensitive *S. aureus* (MSSA) infection by almost $19,000.[21] As the incidence of MRSA increases worldwide, dermatologists must distinguish between community-acquired MRSA (CA-MRSA) and hospital-acquired MRSA (HA-MRSA) strains to best determine treatment.

CA-MRSA most often affects individuals with close infected contacts and those who are exposed to crowded conditions, such as members of athletic teams, prisoners, and military personnel. In identifying those with CA-MRSA, a social history may prove important and should include the following information: intravenous drug use, tobacco use, a recent tattoo, men who have sex with other men, pregnant women, children, newborns, and those with low socioeconomic status. Medical risk factors include recent antibiotic use, chronic skin disease, human immunodeficiency virus, nasal colonization, and history of endocarditis.[22] CA-MRSA carries the *SCCmec* type IV or V gene, which leads to increased interleukin-8, skin necrosis, and leukocytoclasis but not multidrug resistance. HA-MRSA carries the *mecA* gene, which encodes penicillin-binding protein 2a, protects cell wall synthesis, and induces multidrug resistance.[23] HA-MRSA develops in susceptible patients who are hospitalized for over 48 hours. Transmission occurs through skin-to-skin contact, disruption of the skin barrier, or contaminated equipment.[22]

Clinical Description Cutaneous MRSA infections often begin as papules and pustules on the lower extremities that may progress to abscesses with or without necrotic centers. Of those with MRSA skin infections, 58.8% have abscesses, 38.5% have cellulitis, 9.1% have folliculitis/furunculosis, and 2.3% have impetigo.[23] Rare MRSA presentations include acute paronychia, ulcers, necrotizing fasciitis, pyomyositis, bullous erysipelas, staphylococcal scalded skin syndrome, staphylococcal toxic shock syndrome, and purpura fulminans.[23,24]

Treatment Bacterial culture is required to diagnose cutaneous MRSA and to determine appropriate treatment. MRSA colonization is established via a swab and culture of the anterior nasal vestibule. Incision and drainage are required for MRSA abscesses. If an MRSA-confirmed patient suffers systemic symptoms, the Infectious Diseases Society of America recommends blood culture and antibiotic susceptibility testing.[25] Severe MRSA infections warrant an infectious disease consultation and parenteral antibiotics for at least 7 to 10 days.[11] CA-MRSA may be treated with trimethoprim-sulfamethoxazole, doxycycline or minocycline, clindamycin, or rifampin. HA-MRSA may be treated with vancomycin, quinupristin/dalfopristin, or tigecycline. β-Lactam antibiotics cannot be used in either CA-MRSA or HA-MRSA, although it is acceptable to treat a presumed MSSA infection with β-lactam drugs if the patient lacks risk factors for MRSA and there is low MRSA incidence in the geographic region.[22] A thorough epidemiologic history will help distinguish between CA-MRSA and HA-MRSA.

NASAL CARRIAGE AND COLONIZATION OF *S. AUREUS*

The nasal mucosa is a natural habitat for *S. aureus*. Colonization is usually transient, but in those with diabetes, chronic eczema, or atopic diathesis, there is a higher risk of skin disease and wound infection.[11] Between 70% and 90% of atopic patients have *S. aureus* colonization due to an impaired epidermal barrier function and better bacterial adhesion in sites of T-helper 2 cell-mediated inflammation.[26] Reduced antimicrobial sphingosine lipids[27] and less dermcidin in the sweat[28] also contribute to colonization.

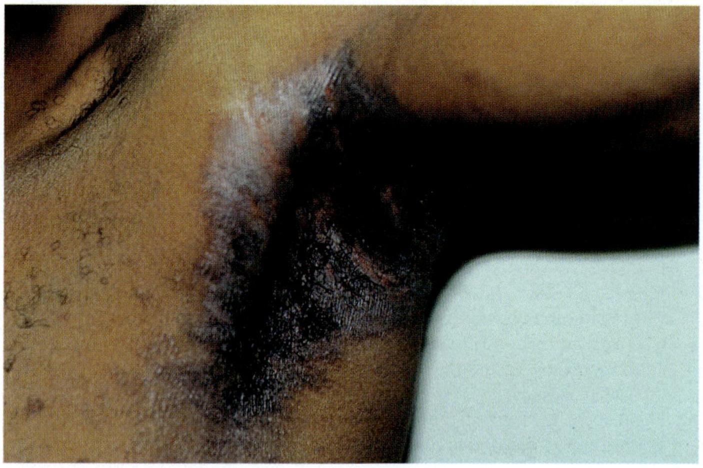

FIGURE 68-1. Skin lesions of erythrasma typically appear in intertriginous areas such as the axillae.

Treatment Colonized atopic patients may be treated with antiseptics, disinfectant baths, silver-threaded clothing or silver-containing therapies, and anti-inflammatory topicals such as tacrolimus or pimecrolimus, or corticosteroids preventatively for previously infected areas.[29] Nasal eradication of laboratory-confirmed MRSA may be accomplished with mupirocin and chlorhexidine soap, but intranasal mupirocin prophylaxis and regular decolonization are not recommended due to increased antibiotic resistance.[11] Frequent hand washing will help prevent spread.

ERYTHRASMA

Erythrasma is a chronic bacterial infection caused by *Corynebacterium minutissimum* that affects the intertriginous areas of the axillae, groin, and toes. Because of these typical locations, it can often mimic a fungal infection.

Clinical Description The skin lesions [**Figure 68-1**] are typically sharply marginated, reddish-brown macules, sometimes with hyperkeratotic white maceration, erosion, or fissures, especially in the webbing of the toes. The condition may be pruritic with resultant secondary excoriation and lichenification.

Treatment As prophylactic measures, looser fitting clothing and the use of an absorbing powder such as Zeasorb AF powder may be useful.[20] The treatment of choice includes a 14-day course of erythromycin 250 mg every other day. Second-line treatments include tetracycline and chloramphenicol. Clarithromycin may also prove to be effective. In interdigital areas, or if erythromycin treatment fails, a combination of topical clindamycin, Whitefield's ointment, sodium fusidate ointment, or antibacterial soaps may be necessary for both treatment and prophylaxis. Whitefield's ointment has shown to have greater efficacy than erythromycin for interdigital areas.[30]

IMPETIGO/ECTHYMA

Impetigo may be bullous or nonbullous in nature, with *S. aureus* being the primary causative agent for bullous impetigo. In industrialized countries, nonbullous impetigo is also primarily caused by staphylococci, whereas in developing nations, nonbullous impetigo can also be caused by *S. pyogenes*, a group A β-hemolytic *Streptococcus*, or both organisms. When both bacteria are found, it is thought to be due to primary infection with *Streptococcus* and secondary infection with *Staphylococcus*. The bacteria initially infect the superficial layer of the epidermis. Although some lesions will resolve spontaneously, others will extend into the dermis, thus causing ecthyma.

Clinical Description Nonbullous impetigo, which accounts for more than 70% of impetigo cases, presents with small superficial pustules that quickly rupture and evolve into a crusted plaque, often of a honey color that appears "stuck on" [**Figure 68-2**]. Surrounding erythema

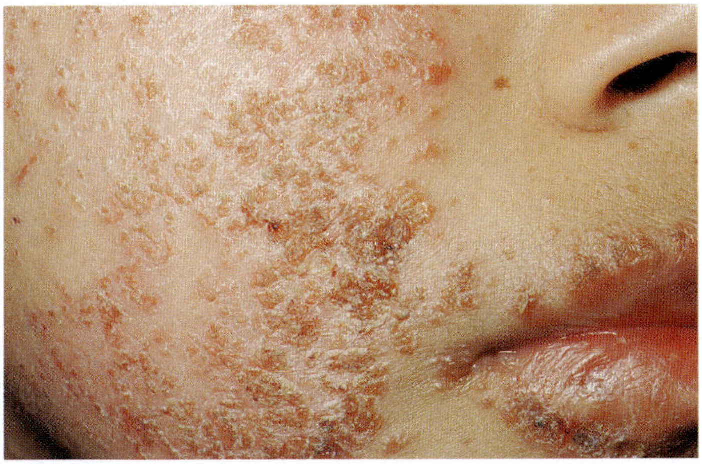

FIGURE 68-2. Nonbullous impetigo.

may be present. Patients lack constitutional symptoms. The most common location for these lesions is the face, but any area may be involved. The lesions are often scattered and discrete, but without treatment will likely coalesce. Autoinoculation may lead to infection at distant sites. Nonbullous impetigo characteristically heals without scarring.

Bullous impetigo is characterized by vesicles containing cloudy-to-yellow fluid arising from skin of normal color, without surrounding erythema [**Figure 68-3**]. Bullous impetigo occurs when staphylococci produce toxins (namely, exfoliative toxins A and B), which causes splitting of the epidermis. Both types of impetigo are most common in, but not limited to, intertriginous areas.

Ecthyma, a deeper form of streptococcal impetigo, presents with punched out ulcerations of the epidermis with a surrounding thick adherent crust [**Figure 68-4**]. Surrounding areas of erythema may occur. Lymphangitis or lymphadenopathy may be associated with ecthyma. Unlike nonbullous impetigo, ecthymas are more commonly found on the extremities and may heal with scarring.

Treatment Pathogen identification in superficial impetigo is unnecessary, because 70% of impetigo infections are caused by *S. aureus*.[31] Topical treatment includes mupirocin applied three times daily to the involved skin and nares, as approximately 25% of people are carriers of *S. aureus*. Although treatment helps reduce autoinoculation and communicable spread, treatment also contributes to the growing resistance of *S. aureus* against mupirocin.[32] Because mupirocin is a cornerstone of MRSA treatment, many authors recommend it to be reserved

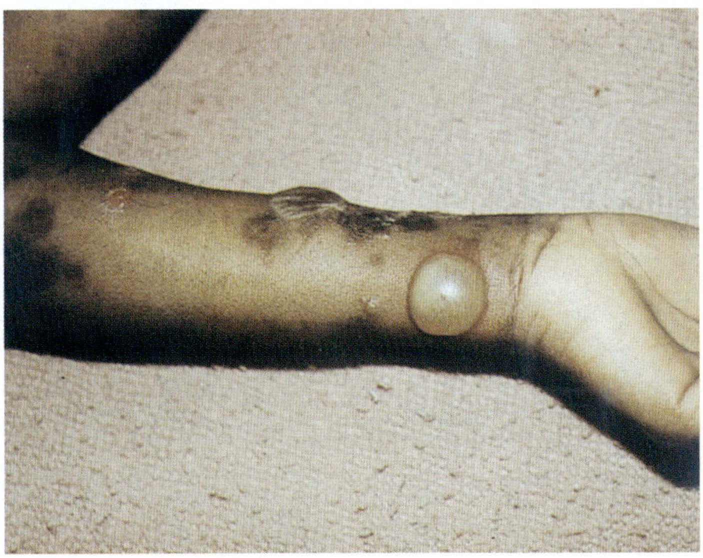

FIGURE 68-3. Bullous impetigo.

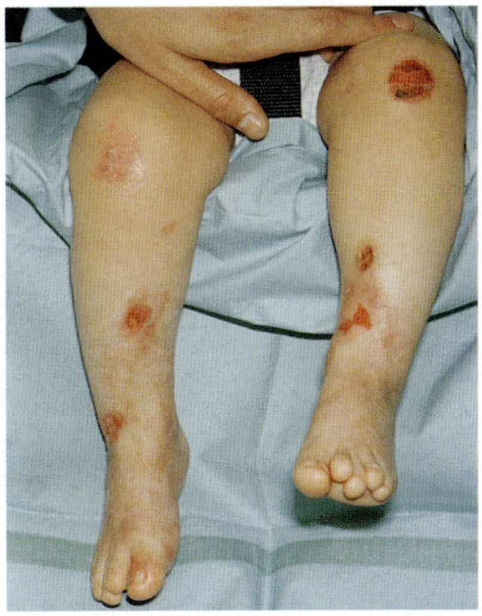

FIGURE 68-4. Ecthyma.

for MRSA carriers with recurrent infections only.[11,23] Although a 1- or 2-week course of mupirocin may not be enough time for the emergence of resistant strains, prolonged treatment with mupirocin is not advised for chronic conditions.[33]

Retapamulin 1% ointment applied twice daily for 5 days is an effective alternative to mupirocin, offering broader coverage of *S. pyogenes* and MSSA.[23] Retapamulin shows no evidence of bacterial resistance due to a threefold mechanism that interferes with the 50s subunit of the bacterial ribosome, blocks p-site interactions, and inhibits peptidyl transfer.[34] A recent study showed that retapamulin inhibited 99% of *S. aureus* isolates in vitro with 4, 16, and 32 times more activity against MSSA, MRSA, and *Streptococcus*, respectively,[31] but there are limited studies on its use in impetigo. Sodium hypochlorite bleach baths and fusidic acid are alternatives.[32]

To eliminate staphylococcal carriage in impetigo patients, rifampin and dicloxacillin are often used, as well as the topical antiseptics polyhexanide, polyvidone, octenidine, and chlorhexidine. For severe infections or impetigo caused by β-hemolytic group A *Streptococcus*, first-line treatment has shifted toward oral cephalexin, dicloxacillin, and amoxicillin/clavulanic acid due to erythromycin and penicillin resistance.[11] Penicillin-allergic patients may take erythromycin. CA-MRSA in impetigo is increasingly common in the pediatric population, and treatment includes clindamycin, trimethoprim-sulfamethoxazole, tetracycline, and flouroquinolones.[12]

INFECTIOUS FOLLICULITIS

Infectious folliculitis affects the upper portion of the hair follicle. When the infection extends to the entire length of the follicle, it is called sycosis. The etiology may include bacterial, fungal, or viral infections. Bacteria include *S. aureus* (seen in both superficial and deep folliculitis), *Pseudomonas aeruginosa* (associated with hot tub folliculitis), and gram-negative folliculitis (associated with acne vulgaris and those who have been treated with oral antibiotics).[35]

Clinical Description Skin lesions typically show a papule or pustule that is confined to the hair follicle but may exhibit surrounding erythema [**Figure 68-5**]. Pustules may rupture, leading to erosions with crusts that can be scattered or more frequently clustered. The superficial infection can progress to an abscess, especially when the causative agent is *S. aureus*.

Although the superficial infection typically heals without scarring, in darkly pigmented people, there can be considerable postinflammatory hypo- and/or hyperpigmentation. Also of note in more darkly pigmented skin is pseudofolliculitis barbae (PFB). PFB is an inflammatory disorder characterized by the formation of papules, pustules, and hyperpigmentation from ingrown hairs often complicated by an *S. aureus* superinfection. Men with skin of color are especially prone to PFB due to

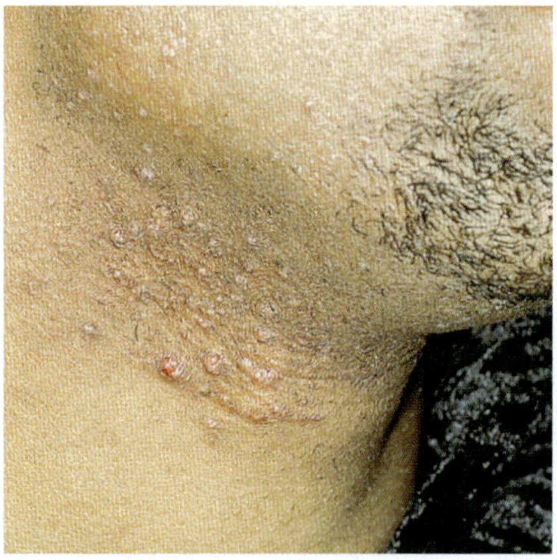

FIGURE 68-5. Infectious folliculitis.

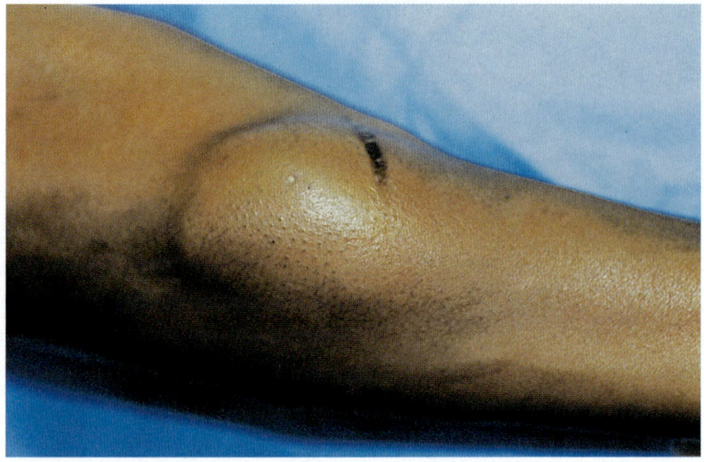

FIGURE 68-6. Abscess.

the curly nature of their hair, which is more prone to becoming ingrown and sometimes infected. It is estimated that PFB affects 45% to 83% of men with darker skin of color who shave regularly. In a recent published study, it was found that twice-daily applications of benzoyl peroxide 5% and clindamycin 1% gel showed reductions in papule and pustule counts ranging from 38.2% at week 2 to 63.9% at week 10.[36] Another type of folliculitis that affects skin of color is keloidal folliculitis. This condition occurs at the nape of the neck with chronically occurring papules and pustules that often lead to extensive hypertrophic scarring and keloid formation. Resulting hair loss may occur in the area. Keloidal folliculitis may also become complicated by bacterial superinfection.

Treatment Affected areas should be cleansed with antibacterial soap or a benzoyl peroxide preparation. Antiseptic or antimicrobial therapy is indicated for widespread folliculitis or immune deregulation. Treatment may include the antiseptics polyhexanide, polyvidone, octenidine, and chlorhexidine, or the oral antibiotics ampicillin or trimethoprim-sulfamthoxazole.[11] Gram-negative folliculitis in acne and rosacea patients is best treated with isotretinoin (0.5-1 mg/kg daily for 4-5 months).[20] For treatment of pseudomonal folliculitis, please see the section on gram-negative infections.

ABSCESS, FURUNCLE, AND CARBUNCLE

Abscesses, furuncles, and carbuncles represent a progression in severity of a process usually caused by a *Staphylococcus* infection.[20] An abscess is a well-circumscribed collection of pus associated with tissue destruction and localized inflammation. A furuncle is acute and deeper than an abscess, is tender and erythematous, and develops around a hair follicle. A carbuncle is a deeper and more extensive lesion and is made up of a confluence of abscesses. The most common cause is *S. aureus*, and these infections occur mostly in individuals who are nasal carriers of this organism.

Clinical Description Cutaneous abscesses present initially as warm, tender, red nodules [**Figure 68-6**] that can occur anywhere on the skin, but typically occur in areas of trauma, burns, or IV catheter insertion. Abscesses will typically enlarge without treatment and form a pus-filled cavity. Furuncles are firmer, tender nodules, larger than abscesses, that occur on hair-bearing skin, such as the beard, neck, scalp, axillae, and buttocks [**Figure 68-7**]. Furuncles may be very painful, develop a surrounding area of cellulitis, and have associated constitutional symptoms. After several days, the nodules will rupture and expel pus and necrotic tissue. Multiple coalescing furuncles comprise a carbuncle, which is typically found on the nape of the neck, back, or thighs. Constitutional symptoms are often present. The involved area is erythematous and indurated and develops a yellow central crater. Carbuncles often resolve with a permanent scar that is very apparent.

Treatment It is advisable for patients susceptible to staphylococcal infections to cleanse daily with an antibacterial soap or a benzoyl peroxide wash. Additionally, mupirocin ointment applied daily to the nares or other known carrier sites is recommended. Application of heat to the lesion can promote consolidation and may even aid in spontaneous drainage if done early in the course of the disease. However, patients must be instructed not to manipulate lesions, particularly on the face, to avoid sinus vein thrombosis.[11] Usually, incision and drainage provide adequate treatment, particularly in otherwise healthy individuals. However, oral antibiotics can hasten resolution and are an absolute requirement for immunosuppressed individuals. Effective oral antibiotics include dicloxacillin, cephalexin, and erythromycin, with clindamycin recommended for penicillin-allergic patients.[11] Intravenous vancomycin is recommended for the most severe cases.

PARONYCHIA

Although the chronic form of paronychia is caused by the yeast *Candida albicans*, the acute form is typically caused by *S. aureus* and is seen in people with hand trauma or those chronically exposed to hand washing or moisture.

Clinical Description In acute paronychia, the proximal and/or lateral nail fold is erythematous, hot, and tender and, if not treated, may evolve into an abscess.

Treatment Treatment includes incision and drainage of an abscess, topical disinfectants, and oral or topical antibiotics.[37] Cephalexin or clindamycin is recommended.[11]

PITTED KERATOLYSIS

Pitted keratolysis, caused by *Micrococcus sedentarius*, is a condition that affects only the feet, specifically the toe web spaces and the soles,

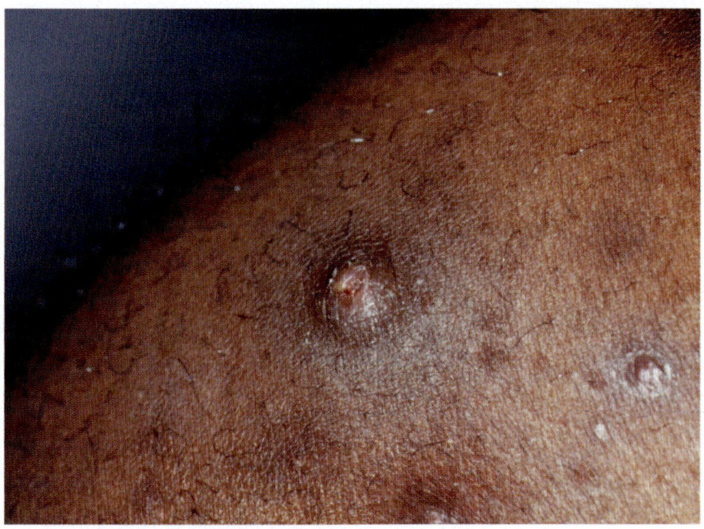

FIGURE 68-7. Furuncle.

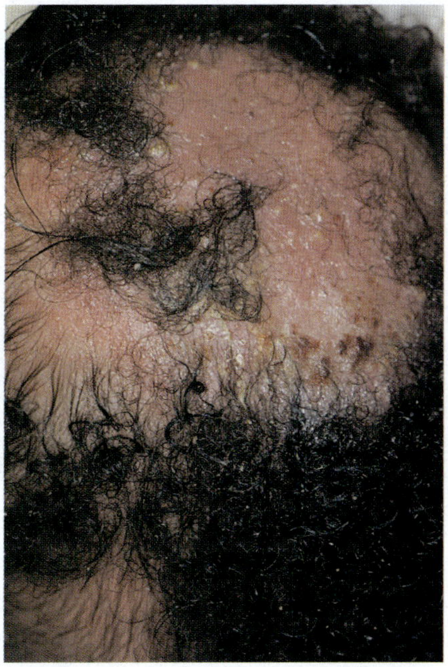

FIGURE 68-8. Cellulitis.

with lesions being most notable on areas of pressure such as the ball or heel of the foot.[38] Predisposing factors include occlusive footwear and hyperhidrosis.

Clinical Description Cutaneous findings show pitting of varying depth within the thickly keratinized skin of one or both soles. The pits range from 1 to 8 mm in diameter and can become confluent.

Treatment Decreasing or minimizing moisture through the selection of less occlusive footwear and the use of an absorbent powder is often a successful treatment modality. Additional treatment may include washing affected areas with a benzoyl peroxide preparation and the daily application of either a topical benzoyl peroxide or an erythromycin gel.

CELLULITIS AND ERYSIPELAS

Cellulitis Cellulitis, although a general term for several types of infections, is, in general, an acute, edematous suppurative inflammation of the dermis and subcutaneous tissues.[39] *S. aureus* and group A *Streptococcus* (GAS) are most commonly identified, but other bacteria may include group B *Streptococcus* in the newborn, pneumococcus, and gram-negative bacilli. It is often associated with systemic symptoms such as fever, malaise, and chills.

Clinical Description Lesions are macular and firm, poorly demarcated from uninvolved skin, and painful upon palpation [**Figure 68-8**]. Necrosis of the overlying epidermis may occur with resulting epidermal sloughing. In some cases, the infection may lead to both dermal and subcutaneous abscess formation and necrotizing fasciitis. Cellulitis is typically found on the extremities and is usually associated with lymphangitis.

Erysipelas Erysipelas is an acute infection of the dermal and subcutaneous tissues that is typically red, hot, and tender. It is most frequently caused by GAS and rarely by *S. aureus*. *Streptococcus* infection is associated with a high morbidity rate. Risk factors for erysipelas include venous insufficiency, toe web intertrigo, lymphedema, and obesity.[40]

Clinical Description Erysipelas differs from cellulitis in that it is a painful, raised, indurated plaque with borders that are markedly distinguishable from the surrounding noninvolved skin. In severe cases, bullous, pustular, or necrotic areas may develop. Patients typically report a prodrome of headache, malaise, and fever. The legs have become the most common areas of infection, with fewer cases affecting the face.[41]

Gangrenous Cellulitis A more severe form of cellulitis is gangrenous cellulitis, or necrotizing fasciitis. In general, gangrenous cellulitis is characterized by the rapid progression of infection with necrosis of both subcutaneous tissue and the overlying skin. The clinical picture, as well as the name of the disease, differs depending on the bacterial organism involved, as well as comorbid conditions and anatomic location of the infection. In general, there is local erythema, heat, and pain in the involved area. Constitutional symptoms are typically present and increase over time. Often there are visible gangrenous changes characterized by a dusky blue hue of the affected area. Vesicles may develop with subsequent rupture of bullae, which is commonly associated with numbness and a black necrotic eschar formation, similar in appearance to a third-degree burn. In some cases, the appearance of the skin may not adequately reflect subcutaneous destruction of small blood vessels and nerve destruction that can produce an anesthetic area.

Treatment is closely aligned with the diagnosis and severity of disease and ranges from incision and drainage to the antibiotics clindamycin and linezolid,[11] and/or surgical debridement of necrotic tissue to life-saving amputations. Of particular concern is necrotizing fasciitis, typically occurring on the leg of an elderly adult with an underlying chronic illness and generally caused by group A β-hemolytic *Streptococcus*. This infection is associated with a high fatality rate and may present with symptoms similar to toxic shock syndrome (discussed later).

Treatment Treatment of cellulitis may be divided into local care, including elevation, immobilization, and the application of cool saline dressings, to systemic antimicrobial therapy that addresses the most frequent isolates, streptococci (groups A, G, and B) and *S. aureus*.[41]

Comorbidities such as diabetes or immunosuppression should also be considered in treatment decisions. The gold standard used to determine the involved organism is a culture obtained from the portal of entry. Often the responsible organism remains elusive and is identified in only about 5% of cases through positive cultures.[41] Empiric treatment for mild cellulitis or erysipelas consists of oral dicloxacillin, which covers both staphylococci and streptococci. Empiric antimicrobial treatment for moderate or severe cellulitis consists of an intravenous cephalosporin (cefazolin or ceftriaxone) or nafcillin (vancomycin in patients with an allergy to penicillin), followed by dicloxacillin or an oral cephalosporin for 7 to 14 days. In patients with recurrent leg cellulitis, identification of interdigital fissures caused by dermatophytes and treatment with topical antifungal agents will likely prevent further recurrences. Daily prophylaxis with oral penicillin G (or amoxicillin) has been suggested for patients who have had more than two episodes of cellulitis at the same site.[41]

BLISTERING DISTAL DACTYLITIS

Blistering distal dactylitis is most often due to GAS, but group B *Streptococcus* may also be a causative agent. Cases of staphylococcal dactylitis have also been reported with an identical clinical picture. Blisters typically occur in children and adolescents.

Clinical Description Blistering distal dactylitis is characterized by a large, purulent, fluid-filled blister on the distal finger or toe pad that often extends distally to the nails. There is often a surrounding erythematous base.

Treatment Blistering distal dactylitis readily responds to incision and drainage, compresses, and oral antibiotics such as penicillin or erythromycin.[42]

CUTANEOUS ANTHRAX

Humans acquire anthrax infections from contact with infected animals or contaminated animal products, such as hides, wool, hair, and ivory tusks. More than 95% of naturally occurring anthrax is the cutaneous form.[43] Cutaneous anthrax is caused by *Bacillus anthracis*.

Clinical Description The primary lesion of anthrax is a painless, pruritic papule occurring at the site of inoculation that appears 1 to 7 days after exposure. One to 2 days after the appearance of the primary lesion, small vesicles surround the papule, or alternatively, a clear or serosanguineous fluid-containing vesicle develops. As the vesicle enlarges, satellite vesicles may develop. A nonpitting, gelatinous edema surrounds the lesion and may become massive, particularly when the primary lesion involves the neck or face. Low-grade fever and malaise are frequent. Necrosis of the vesicle results in the formation of an ulcer covered by a black eschar. The eschar resolves with minimal scarring. Regional lymphadenopathy is present initially. Secondary infection with streptococci or *S. aureus* is uncommon, but fever with lymphangitis, local pain, and purulent drainage is indicative of secondary infection. Bacteremia is a rare complication.[43]

Treatment Without antibiotic treatment, mortality may approach 20%. Incision or debridement of an early-stage lesion should be avoided because it may increase the possibility of bacteremia. For mild cases of cutaneous anthrax in adults, oral treatment with ciprofloxacin 500 mg every 12 hours is recommended. If the strain is susceptible, oral doxycycline at 100 mg every 12 hours or amoxicillin 500 mg every 8 hours is a suitable alternative. Treatment should be continued for 7 to 10 days, unless bioterrorism is suspected, which would necessitate treatment for 60 days. Severe cutaneous anthrax is treated with the same drugs and dosages as inhalation anthrax. The recommended initial therapy for adults with clinically evident inhalation anthrax is 400 mg of ciprofloxacin given intravenously every 12 hours.[43]

STAPHYLOCOCCAL SCALDED SKIN SYNDROME

Staphylococcal scalded skin syndrome (SSSS) is an epidermolytic disease that is caused by two distinct toxins released by a strain of *S. aureus* of phage group II, primarily type 71. The toxins cause erythema with associated detachment of the superficial layers of the epidermis. SSSS occurs in newborns and infants younger than 2 years of age and in immunocompromised adults. There are several different forms of SSSS that range in severity. At one end of the spectrum is the completely localized form, called *bullous impetigo*, and at the other end are more generalized and extensive forms.[44]

Clinical Description The localized form of SSSS is characterized by clusters of intact purulent bullae that rupture and produce erythematous and crusted erosive lesions. The most common sites are the intertriginous areas of the axillae, groin, and neck, as well as periorificial area on the face. The erythema typically deepens in color, and the skin becomes very tender. Lesions become more widespread with time, and there may be accompanying fever. The erythematous eruption can rapidly progress to flaccid bullae that exfoliate, producing a denuded epidermis and a resultant tender and oozing erythematous base.

Treatment Therapy includes baths and compresses for debridement and the use of nonstick dressings.[11] Topical antiseptics include chlorhexidine or polyhexanide solutions and topical antimicrobial agents such as mupirocin, bacitracin, fusidic acid, and sulfadiazine ointment. Successful systemic antimicrobial therapy includes oral cephalexin, clindamycin, or doxycycline for local disease and intravenous nafcillin or cefazolin for generalized disease.[11,13] In known carriers of MRSA, intravenous vancomycin or linezolid is recommended.[11] In severe disease, fluid and electrolyte loss must be replaced.

TOXIC SHOCK SYNDROME

Toxic shock syndrome (TSS) is an acute toxin-mediated febrile illness that is caused by the production and release of exotoxins by *S. aureus*. Systemic symptoms include acute onset of fever, hypotension, generalized skin and mucosal erythema, and multisystem failure. TSS occurs more commonly but not exclusively in women who are using vaginal tampons of high absorbency for extended lengths of time. Nonmenstrual cases, associated with localized infections, surgery, or insect bites, have increased and now account for approximately one-third of all cases. Patients with nonmenstrual TSS have a higher mortality rate than those with menstrual TSS.[45]

Clinical Description The classic cutaneous findings of TSS include a generalized scarlatiniform erythroderma with accompanying fever and hypotension. There is often extensive, generalized, nonpitting, nondependent edema and edema of the feet. One to 2 weeks following resolution of the erythema, there is desquamation of the palms and soles. Intense erythema of the bulbar conjunctivae, mouth, tongue, pharynx, vagina, and tympanic membranes may occur. Often these areas display ulceration. Strawberry tongue and subconjunctival hemorrhages are also typical. Nonspecific gastrointestinal symptoms may also be a manifestation of disease.

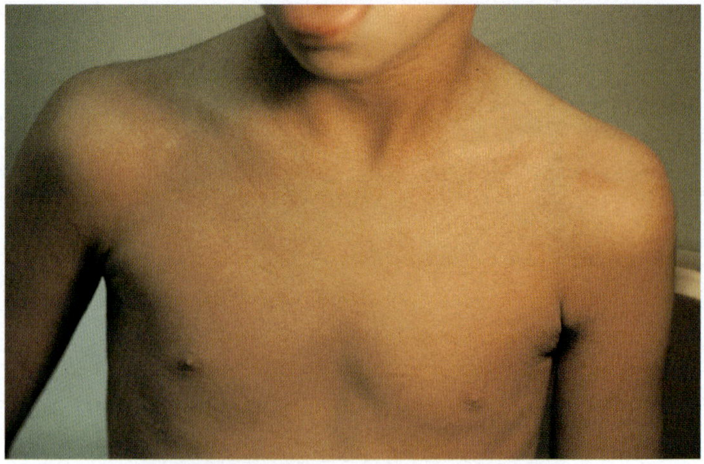

FIGURE 68-9. Scarlet fever exanthem.

Treatment The treatment of TSS is generally supportive.[46] Admission to the intensive care unit for management of fluid replacement for shock, careful organ system monitoring, and intravenous antibiotic therapy for staphylococcal colonization or infection may occur. Commonly prescribed antibiotics include flucloxacillin or cefazolin in combination with clindamycin.[11] In severe cases, methylprednisolone has been given, but benefit is uncertain. In vitro studies have shown that immune globulins may have a future role in the treatment of TTS.

SCARLET FEVER

Scarlet fever is an acute infection of the tonsils and/or skin by an exotoxin-producing strain of GAS. It typically occurs in children.[47]

Clinical Description The initial site of infection is typically the tonsils or pharynx, with resultant pharyngitis or tonsillitis, although a skin lesion or infected wound may be the initiator. The first sign of scarlet fever is finely punctuate erythema on the upper trunk, which may be accentuated in skin folds. The palms and soles are typically spared. The face is flushed with perioral pallor. The initial punctuate lesions become confluent and scarlatiniform. Scattered petechiae and distant lesions may occur [**Figure 68-9**]. The exanthem fades within 4 to 5 days and is followed by truncal and extremity desquamation and exfoliation of the palms and soles. The tongue is characteristically white with scattered hyperkeratotic red papillae (white strawberry tongue). The hyperkeratotic membrane is sloughed and gives way to a strawberry tongue on day 4 or 5. Punctuate erythema and petechiae can also occur in the palate. The patient often appears acutely ill, and there is often appreciable anterior cervical lymphadenitis.

Treatment Treatment includes acetaminophen for fever or discomfort. Penicillin is the drug of choice because of its efficacy in preventing rheumatic fever. Clindamycin can also be used for treatment. Human immune globulin contains toxin-neutralizing antibodies and, if given at an early stage of invasive disease, may have a beneficial effect.[47]

GRAM-NEGATIVE INFECTIONS [TABLE 68-2]

Gram-negative infections of the skin are more common in three groups: children, patients with diabetes, and immunocompromised patients. These infections are typically treated with a second- or third-generation cephalosporin.[20]

TABLE 68-2 Gram-negative infections
Cat scratch disease
Tularemia
Cutaneous *Pseudomonas aeruginosa* infections

CAT SCRATCH DISEASE

Cat scratch disease is usually caused by the gram-negative bacillus *Bartonella henselae*.[48] It is a relatively benign, self-limited disease that typically occurs after being scratched by a cat, but can occur even after contact with a cat without a history of a scratch, bite, or lick.

Clinical Description Following a cat scratch, the area of inoculation develops a small, firm papule or pustule that may be tender. Lesions typically occur on exposed skin. Associated regional lymphadenitis and large tender lymph nodes occur. Alternatively, the site of inoculation of *B. henselae* may be a mucous membrane. In that case, a light yellow granulation on the palpebral conjunctivae, with associated preauricular or cervical lymphadenopathy, occurs. Most patients are afebrile.

Treatment The literature does not definitely report effective antibiotic therapy for cat scratch disease primarily due to the fact that it is a disease in which most patients are not seriously ill and spontaneous resolution is common.[49] The disease is typically self-limiting with a maximum duration of 2 months, although longer disease duration has been reported. Antimicrobial therapy has not been proven to alter the course of the disease. However, ciprofloxacin, doxycycline, and erythromycin are therapeutic suggestions.[50] A small, prospective, comparative study demonstrated that azithromycin may shorten the duration of lymphadenopathy.[51] In a minority of patients (about 15%) with typical cat scratch disease, the affected lymph node undergoes suppuration and becomes exquisitely tender. Drainage with a large-bore needle usually results in the almost immediate relief of pain. However, incision and drainage are seldom necessary and may result in the development of a chronic sinus tract.

TULAREMIA

Tularemia is cause by *Francisella tularensis*, a gram-negative coccobacillus, which is transmitted through direct contact with the flesh of infected animals, typically rabbits and squirrels. Routes of transmission include a puncture or abrasion in the skin, autoinoculation, ingestion, or inhalation. Although accidental exposure can occur through arthropod bites, handling infected animals, or breathing in aerosols, cases are usually isolated and contained. It is important to note that transmission via inhalation is very serious in contrast to cutaneous transmission. The high infectivity of tularemia makes it a major concern to public health officials as a possible biological weapon.[52]

Clinical Description Tularemia has six potential presentations: ulceroglandular, glandular, oculoglandular, oropharyngeal, typhoidal, and pneumonic forms. The ulceroglandular form is the most common and the one that typically presents with skin lesions. If there is an identifiable inoculation site, it is typically an erythematous, tender papule that enlarges with raised, well-demarcated crusted borders surrounded by an area of cellulitis. There is a depressed center that is covered by a black eschar, evidence of rapid necrosis. Mucous membranes involved include the conjunctivae, and typically a purulent, painful, edematous conjunctivitis occurs, with small yellow nodules visible on the conjunctivae. A high fever, chills, headache, and malaise typically accompany the rash, and as bacteremia ensues, painful regional lymphadenopathy develops.

Treatment Management focuses on prevention with complete protective gear when handling wild rabbits. For treatment, streptomycin 1 to 2 g/day until the patient has been afebrile for 7 to 10 days is effective. Gentamicin, tetracycline, and quinolones are also effective.[53]

CUTANEOUS *PSEUDOMONAS AERUGINOSA* INFECTIONS

Pseudomonas aeruginosa produces a host of bacterial infections and is of concern because of its propensity for infecting hospitalized and compromised patients.[54] *Pseudomonas* rarely infects healthy people but instead infects hosts with disruption of the normal flora, with disruption of a normal cutaneous barrier by introduction of a foreign object, or following an injury or trauma. Once local invasion occurs, ecthyma gangrenosum, a necrotizing soft tissue infection, ensues and is associated with blood vessel invasion, sepsis, vascular occlusion, and infarction of tissue throughout the body.

Clinical Description *Pseudomonas* has the potential to colonize many areas on the body and, therefore, can present in a number of manners. *Pseudomonas* colonizes the undersurface of nails in patients with onychomycosis, the hair follicles of healthy individuals exposed to infected hot tubs, and in macerated intertriginous spaces. Outbreaks of *Pseudomonas* may occur in people using hot tubs and whirlpools. Follicular erythematous papules and pustules occur on submerged areas of skin and typically last from 7 to 10 days. *Pseudomonas* hot foot syndrome manifests with tender nodules on the soles of children's feet after using a wading pool.

Treatment Treatment for mild cutaneous cases is usually supportive, with antipruritic agents administered orally or topically. Acetic acid 5% compresses applied for 20 minutes twice daily can also be used for symptomatic relief, as well as sodium hypochlorite solution applied twice daily or topical tobramycin otic or ophthalmic drops under the nail plate.[55] Adequate chlorination and control of the pH level in hot tubs can prevent hot-tub folliculitis.[51] A course of oral ciprofloxacin 500 mg twice daily for 7 days may be warranted if systemic manifestations, including fever, chills, and lymphadenopathy, are present. In patients with immunodeficiencies, granulocytopenia must first be corrected with a colony-stimulating factor. Thereafter, sensitivity-appropriate antimicrobial therapy can be instituted. Antimicrobial therapy for bacteremia is also tailored according to the specific sensitivity of the encountered strain. Antibiotics are given as monotherapy or in combination, as *P. aeruginosa* infections have particularly high mortality rates and the strongest multidrug resistance among all bacteria.[55] Effective agents include aminoglycosides, ciprofloxacin, colistin, and a limited number of β-lactams such as piperacillin, ticarcillin, ureidopenicillins, ceftazidime, carbapenems, aztreonam, and cefepime, which retains the broadest spectrum of activity against *P. aeruginosa*.[55] To prevent further damage to skin and underlying organs, areas of infarction should be surgically debrided once the infection is controlled.[54] For burn victims, topical antimicrobials, such as silver compounds and mafenide acetate, may decrease invasive burn wound sepsis.[55]

In summary, individuals with skin of color may develop a wide range of cutaneous infections involving either gram-positive or gram-negative organisms. In general, most infections do not differ significantly from those that occur in the general population. As expected, *S. aureus* and *S. pyogenes* are gram-positive organisms that are most often implicated in common skin and soft tissue infections. In contrast, gram-negative infections occur more commonly in children, patients with diabetes, and immunocompromised patients. In most cases, treatment is dictated by the antibiotic sensitivities of the cultured organism.

REFERENCES

1. Donlan RM, Costerton JW. Biofilms: survival mechanisms of clinically relevant microorganisms. *Clin Microbiol Rev*. 2002;15:167-193.
2. Vlassova N, Han A, Zenilman JM, James G, Lazarus GS. New horizons for cutaneous microbiology: the role of biofilms in dermatological disease. *Br J Dermatol*. 2011;165:751-759.
3. Prosser BL, Taylor D, Dix BA, Cleeland R. Method of evaluating effects of antibiotics on bacterial biofilm. *Antimicrob Agents Chemother*. 1987;31:1502-1506.
4. Mah TF, O'Toole GA. Mechanisms of biofilm resistance to antimicrobial agents. *Trends Microbiol*. 2001;9:34-39.
5. Anderson GG, O'Toole GA. Innate and induced resistance mechanisms of bacterial biofilms. *Curr Top Microbiol Immunol*. 2008;322:85-105.
6. Lewis K. Persister cells and the riddle of biofilm survival. *Biochemistry (Mosc)*. 2005;70:267-274.
7. Driffield K, Miller K, Bostock JM, et al. Increased mutability of *Pseudomonas aeruginosa* in biofilms. *J Antimicrob Chemother*. 2008;61:1053-1056.
8. Dunne WM. Effects of subinhibitory concentrations of vancomycin or cefamandole on biofilm production by coagulase-negative staphylococci. *Antimicrob Agents Chemother*. 1990;34:390-393.
9. Linares JF, Gustafsson I, Baquero F, Martinez JL. Antibiotics as intermicrobial signaling agents instead of weapons. *Proc Natl Acad Sci U S A*. 2006;103:19484-19489.
10. Leyden JJ, Del Rosso JQ, Webster GF. Clinical considerations in the treatment of acne vulgaris and other inflammatory disorders: focus on antibiotic resistance. *Cutis*. 2007;79(6 Suppl):9-25.

11. Schofer H, Bruns R, Effendy I, et al. Diagnosis and treatment of *Staphylococcus aureus* infections of the skin and mucous membranes. *J Dtsch Dermatol Ges*. 2011;9:953-967.
12. Silverberg N, Block S. Uncomplicated skin and skin structure infections in children: diagnosis and current treatment options in the United States. *Clin Pediatr*. 2008;47:211-219.
13. Del Rosso JQ, Leyden JJ. Status report on antibiotic resistance: implications for the dermatologist. *Dermatol Clin*. 2007;25:127-132.
14. Rosen T. Antibiotic resistance: an editorial review with recommendations. *J Drugs Dermatol*. 2011;10:724-733.
15. Leyden JJ, Del Rosso JQ, Webster GF. Clinical considerations in the treatment of acne vulgaris and other inflammatory disorders: a status report. *Dermatol Clin*. 2009;27:1-15.
16. Toossi P, Farshehian M, Malekzad F, et al. Subantimicrobial-dose doxycycline in the treatment of facial acne. *J Drugs Dermatol*. 2008;7:1149-1152.
17. Neville JA, Housman TS, Letsinger JA, Fleischer AB Jr, Feldman SR, Williford PM. Increase in procedures performed at dermatology office visits from 1995 to 2001. *Dermatol Surg*. 2005;31:160-162.
18. Drucker CR. Update on topical antibiotics in dermatology. *Dermatol Ther*. 2012;25:6-11.
19. Simor AE, Stuart TL, Louie L, et al. Mupirocin-resistant, methicillin-resistant *Staphylococcus aureus* strains in Canadian hospitals. *Antimicrob Agents Chemother*. 2007;51:3880-3886.
20. Stulberg DL, Penrod MA, Blatny RA. Common bacterial skin infections. *Am Fam Physician*. 2002;66:119-124.
21. Filice G, Nyman J, Lexau C, et al. Excess costs and utilization associated with methicillin resistance for patients with *Staphylococcus aureus* infection. *Infect Control Hosp Epidemiol*. 2010;31:365-373.
22. Hansra NK, Shinkai K. Cutaneous community-acquired and hospital-acquired methicillin resistant *Staphylococcus aureus*. *Dermatol Ther*. 2011;24:263-272.
23. Kil E, Heymann W, Weinberg JM. Methicillin-resistant *Staphylococcus aureus*: an update for the dermatologist. Part 2: pathogenesis and cutaneous manifestations. *Cutis*. 2008;81:247-254.
24. Elston D. Community acquired methicillin resistant *Staphylococcus aureus*. *J Am Acad Dermatol*. 2007;56:1-16.
25. Stevens D, Bisno A, Chambers H, et al. Practice guidelines for the diagnosis and management of skin and soft tissue infections. *Clin Infect Dis*. 2005;41:1373-1406.
26. Cho SH, Strickland I, Tomkinson A, et al. Preferential binding of *Staphylococcus aureus* to skin sites of Th2-mediated inflammation in a murine model. *J Invest Dermatol*. 2001;116:658-663.
27. Arikawa J, Ishibashi M, Kawashima M, et al. Decreased levels of sphingosine, a natural antimicrobial agent, may be associated with vulnerability of the stratum corneum from patients with atopic dermatitis to colonization by Staphylococcus aureus. *J Invest Dermatol*. 2002;119:433-439.
28. Rieg S, Steffen H, Seeber S, et al. Deficiency of dermcidin derived antimicrobial peptides in sweat of patients with atopic dermatitis correlates with an impaired innate defense of human skin in vivo. *J Immunol*. 2005;174:8003-8010.
29. Hung SH, Lin YT, Chu CY, et al. *Staphylococcus* colonization in atopic dermatitis treated with fluticasone or tacrolimus with or without antibiotics. *Ann Allergy Asthma Immunol*. 2007;98:51-56.
30. Holdiness MR. Management of cutaneous erythrasma. *Drugs*. 2002;62:1131-1141.
31. Yang LP, Keam SJ. Retapamulin: a review of its use in the management of impetigo and other uncomplicated superficial skin infections. *Drugs*. 2008;68:855-873.
32. Bangert S, Levy M, Hebert AA. Bacterial resistance and impetigo treatment trends: a review. *Pediatr Dermatol*. 2012;29:243-248.
33. Axelsson I. Treatment of impetigo: save mupirocin. *BMJ*. 2004;329:979.
34. Yan K, Madden L, Choudhry AE, et al. Biochemical characterization of the interactions of the novel pleuromutilin derivative retapamulin with bacterial ribosomes. *Antimicrob Agents Chemother*. 2006;50:3875-3881.
35. Boni R, Nehrhoff B. Treatment of gram-negative folliculitis in patients with acne. *Am J Clin Dermatol*. 2003;4:273-276.
36. Cook-Bolden FE, Barba A, Halder R, et al. Twice-daily applications of benzoyl peroxide 5%/clindamycin 1% gel versus vehicle in the treatment of pseudofolliculitis barbae. *Cutis*. 2004;73(6 Suppl):18-24.
37. Scott PM. Drainage for an acute paronychia. *JAAPA*. 2002;15:57-58.
38. Takama H, Tamada Y, Yano K, et al. Pitted keratolysis: clinical manifestations in 53 cases. *Br J Dermatol*. 1997;137:282-285.
39. Hedrick J. Acute bacterial skin infections in pediatric medicine: current issues in presentation and treatment. *Paediatr Drugs*. 2003;5(Suppl 1):35-46.
40. Bonnetblanc JM, Bedane C. Erysipelas: recognition and management. *Am J Clin Dermatol*. 2003;4:157-163.
41. Swartz MN. Clinical practice. Cellulitis. *N Engl J Med*. 2004;350:904-912.
42. McCray MK, Esterly NB. Blistering distal dactylitis. *J Am Acad Dermatol*. 1981;5:592-594.
43. Carucci JA, McGovern TW, Norton SA, et al. Cutaneous anthrax management algorithm. *J Am Acad Dermatol*. 2002;47:766-769.
44. Schenfeld LA. Images in clinical medicine. Staphylococcal scalded skin syndrome. *N Engl J Med*. 2000;342:1178.
45. Manders SM. Infectious disease update. *Dermatol Clin*. 2001;19:749-756.
46. Manders SM. Toxin-mediated streptococcal and staphylococcal disease. *J Am Acad Dermatol*. 1998;39:383-398.
47. Bialecki C, Feder HM Jr, Grant-Kels JM. The six classic childhood exanthems: a review and update. *J Am Acad Dermatol*. 1989;21:891-903.
48. Lamps LW, Scott MA. Cat-scratch disease: historic, clinical, and pathologic perspectives. *Am J Clin Pathol*. 2004;121(Suppl):S71-S80.
49. Adal KA, Cockerell CJ, Petri WA Jr. Cat scratch disease, bacillary angiomatosis, and other infections due to *Rochalimaea*. *N Engl J Med*. 1994;330:1509-1515.
50. Margileth AM. Cat scratch disease. *Adv Pediatr Infect Dis*. 1993;8:1-21.
51. Bass JW, Freitas BC, Freitas AD, et al. Prospective randomized double blind placebo-controlled evaluation of azithromycin for treatment of cat-scratch disease. *Pediatr Infect Dis J*. 1998;17:447-452.
52. Gallagher-Smith M, Kim J, Al-Bawardy R, et al. Francisella tularensis: possible agent in bioterrorism. *Clin Lab Sci*. 2004;17:35-39.
53. Senol M, Ozcan A, Karincaoglu Y, et al. Tularemia: a case transmitted from a sheep. *Cutis*. 1999;63:49-51.
54. Werlinger KD, Moore AY. Therapy of other bacterial infections. *Dermatol Ther*. 2004;17:505-512.
55. Wu DC, Chan WW, Metelitsa AI, et al. *Pseudomonas* skin infection: clinical features, epidemiology, and management. *Am J Clin Dermatol*. 2011;12:157-169.

CHAPTER 69

Fungal and Yeast Infections

Charissa N. Obeng-Nyarko
Aditya K. Gupta
Johnathan J. Ledet
Susan C. Taylor

KEY POINTS

- Susceptibility to fungal infection, which affects people of all races, is influenced by a variety of factors including socioeconomic status, geographic location, and cultural or religious practices.
- Dermatophytes cause most superficial fungal infections.
- In the immunocompromised host, nondermatophyte molds and yeasts may also be cutaneous pathogens.
- Antifungal resistance is an emerging concern

INTRODUCTION

Fungi are ubiquitous and occur worldwide. Cutaneous fungal infections are common among most races.[1] Keratinized tissues including stratum corneum, nails, and hair are an adaptive substrate for the superficial mycoses, such as dermatophytes, which are the primary causative agent of fungal infections. The immune system generally provides adequate defense against fungal invasion. Nondermatophyte molds and yeast occur more common in those with primary or secondary immunodeficiency.

The presence of cutaneous mycoses does not appear to reflect differences in the biologic characteristics of skin color. However, underlying immunologic diseases such as human immunodeficiency virus (HIV) infection and acquired immunodeficiency syndrome (AIDS), which are of epidemic proportions in some low and middle-income countries, have a higher incidence of associated fungal infections.[2] Furthermore, factors such as climate, age, urban environment, health status, socioeconomic level, and cultural habits contribute to the occurrence of cutaneous mycoses.[4] Climatic differences affect the ability of fungi to grow with high ambient temperature and humidity, providing an ideal setting for fungal proliferation. Additional factors such as occlusive clothing and footwear worn in cooler settings may provide suitable microclimates for mycotic activity. Cultural or religious customs, such as communal bathing, may create opportunities for the transmission of fungi. Variation in hygienic practices also may explain increased susceptibility to fungal invasion.

In the last 20 years, there has been an increase in treatment-resistant cutaneous fungal infections and invasive fungal diseases worldwide.[3-4] Antifungal resistance significantly increases disease morbidity, medical complications, negative psychological impact, and cost of medical care.[3] Effective diagnosis and management of superficial fungal infections will lead to better prevention strategies and help to address this global health challenge.[4]

This chapter provides an overview of common superficial fungal infections common to most skin types, including individuals with skin of color. Approaches to addressing antifungal resistance will be discussed. Tinea capitis and seborrheic dermatitis, which are covered in detail in Chapters 25 and 44, are fungal infections found more frequently in people with skin of color.

MYCOLOGIC EXAMINATION

Accurate diagnosis of a fungal infection is necessary before selecting an appropriate treatment regimen. Mycologic methods are similar for most mycoses, the goal being confirmation of the presence of fungi and identification of the pathogenic species.

DIRECT MICROSCOPIC EXAMINATION

Light microscopy and potassium hydroxide (KOH) preparation are used to determine whether fungal organisms are present in the specimen evaluated. Direct examination is performed using 10% to 20% KOH to dissolve the surrounding keratin from skin scrapings or nail clippings. The KOH test can indicate the presence or absence of a fungal element but does not give information as to the type of fungal element detected. The sensitivity of the KOH preparation ranges from 67% to 93%, while the specificity ranges from 38% to 78%.[5] Due to sampling error and nonproliferating fungi that may not be visible on microscopic examination, a negative microscopic result is not necessarily indicative of fungus-free tissue. A KOH result revealing septate hyphae in the setting of clinical suspicion of fungal infection may be sufficient to initiate treatment. In addition, calcofluor white or PAS stain may be added to the KOH preparation to enhance visibility of the fungal organism with high sensitivity of 92%.[6]

FUNGAL CULTURE

Antifungal agents have different spectra of activity necessitating organism identification for disease management.[3,4] Dermatophytes may be identified using culture medium with overall sensitivity ranging from 31% to 59% and specificity from 83% to 100%.[6] Cultures containing cycloheximide and chloramphenicol are used to deter the growth of nonpathogenic molds and bacterial contaminants that may mask proliferation of the dermatophytes.[3] The use of both microscopy and culture as diagnostic tools reduces the rate of false-negative results and aids in accurate diagnosis.

MOLECULAR TECHNIQUES

Polymerase chain reaction (PCR) and other molecular techniques are highly sensitive (95%) and specific (100%) DNA-based methods that allow differentiation of various dermatophyte and nondermatophyte species.[4] Although the high cost, availability, and the use of specialized equipment remain challenges in widespread use, PCR is efficient in fungi identification.[4]

DERMOSCOPY AND WOOD'S LAMP EXAMINATION

Dermoscopy is a noninvasive tool that aids in the diagnosis of tinea capitis, seborrheic dermatitis, and onchomycosis.[4] Dermatoscopic findings can help distinguish between tinea capitis and types of alopecia by revealing comma-shaped hairs, varying lengths of broken hair, and other patterns specific to tinea capitis.[4]

Wood's lamp is a diagnostic aid in discriminating between superficial mycoses and other dermatologic conditions that fluorescence. For example, *Microsporum* species exhibit blue-green fluorescence, while Malassezia species exhibit a yellow-orange fluorescence.[4,7]

Overall, mycologic examination and diagnosis is imperative to appropriately guide treatment options. From KOH prep and light microscopy to PCR, many tools are available to make a precise diagnosis.

TREATMENT

TOPICAL AGENTS

Topical antifungals are first-line therapy for dermatophyte infections in those with uncomplicated, localized infections due to their high efficacy, low systemic side effects, and patient compliance.[8,9] However, topical antifungals may cause irritant and contact dermatitis due to various vehicle components.[8] The main drug classes of topical antifungal agents include imidazoles, triazoles, allylamines, benzylamines, and polyenes.

Azoles Imidazole and triazoles inhibit 14-α-demethylase, preventing synthesis of ergosterol, which is required for fungal cell membrane integrity. Most azoles are fungistatic, but some can be fungicidal at high concentrations. Topical clotrimazole, ketoconazole, miconazole, sertaconazole, fluconazole, and itraconazole have cream, lotion, solution, gel, shampoo, powder, and transdermal patch formulations.[9] Newer topical azoles have associated anti-inflammatory, antiprotozoal, and antipruritic effects, thus broadening the armamentarium against chronic dermatophytoses and nondermatophytoses.[9]

Allylamines and Benzylamines Allylamines and benzylamine inhibit squalene epoxidase, thus interfering with ergosterol synthesis that results in fungicidal levels of intracellular squalene. These topical antifungal agents include terbinafine, naftifine, and butenafine that may possess anti-inflammatory effects and broad antimicrobial activity against *Candida* and *Aspergillus* species.[9]

Polyenes (see Systemics section for more) Polyene antifungal agents bind to the fungi cell membrane and increase permeability; they are fungicidal. With recent advancements in drug delivery, amphotericin B (AmB) is available in a gel formulation that reduces systemic toxicity.[10,11]

Other Antifungal Classes The hydroxypyridinones, ciclopirox and rilopirox, are weak acids that chelate trivalent metal cations causing inhibition of metal-dependent enzymes, thus interfering with the mitochondrial electron transport chain and production of ATP.[9] With its antiprotozoal, antiparasitic, and anti-inflammatory effects, ciclopirox is used for toe fungus and scalp seborrheic dermatitis.[9,12]

Oxaboroles, including tavaborole, act primarily by interrupting protein synthesis via the inhibition of Leucyl-transfer RNA transfer RNA (t-RNA) synthetase confirming both fungicidal and fungistatic activity.[9] This new drug class has activity against some Trichophyton species, *Candida albicans*, and nondermatophyte molds.[9] Other topical agents used for therapy include flucytosine, selenium sulfide, undecylenic acid, and iodoquinol.

SYSTEMIC AGENTS

Systemic antifungal therapy is required for some dermatophyte infections such as onychomycosis, tinea unguium, tinea manuum, tinea capitis, and widespread dermatophytosis. Commonly used systemic antifungals include azoles, polyenes, echinocandins, and griseofulvin.

Azoles Antifungal azoles for systemic therapy include fluconazole, itraconazole, voriconazole, posaconazole, and isavuconazole some of which may have extended-spectrum coverage.[13] These agents are associated with significant drug-drug interactions due to CPY metabolism.[13] Moreover, per the U.S. Food and Drug Administration (FDA) guidelines, oral ketoconazole is no longer considered as a first-line treatment for any fungal infections due to risk of severe liver injury and drug interactions.[14-16]

Polyenes Conventional amphotericin B (AmB) is a systemic therapy in this class that is historically notorious for systemic side effects including electrolyte disturbances, nephrotoxicity, infusion reactions, and hepatoxicity. Since the 1990s, safer lipid-based formulations have been developed that include colloidal dispersion (ABCD), AmB lipid complex (ABLC), and liposomal AmB (LAmB).[13,17] AmB has a broad spectrum of activity against most fungi involved in human pathology including *Cryptococcus neoformans*, most *Candida* species, *Aspergillus* species, and mucormycosis.[13]

Echinocandins Echinocandins interfere with cell wall synthesis and alter permeability by inhibiting synthesis of β-(1,3)-D-glucan. Drugs in this class like caspofungin, anidulafungin, and micafungin have fungicidal activity against *Aspergillus* and the yeast *Candida.*[13] Common side effects of echinocandins include gastrointestinal disturbances (nausea, vomiting, diarrhea), elevated liver enzymes, and cutaneous reactions.[13,18,19]

Griseofulvin Since being approved by the Food and Drug Administration (FDA) in 1959, griseofulvin is one of the most widely used treatments for dermatophytes fungal infections in humans and animals.[20] Griseofulvin inhibits mitosis in dermatophytes by interacting with microtubules. Reported as a safe drug, potential side effects of griseofulvin include elevated serum liver enzymes, hypertriglyceridemia, hyperuricemia, eosinophilia, leukocytosis, and granulocytopenia.[21]

Emerging Antifungals Opelconazole and oteseconazole are synthetic azoles currently being investigated in animal models. Opelconazole has demonstrated in vitro activity against *Aspergillus*, *Cryptococcus*, and many candidial species.[22,23] Oteseconazole was FDA-approved in 2022 for vulvovaginitis.[22,24]

Encochleated amphotericin B is a new vehicle that has emerged as being superior to current formulations of AmB. Encochleated AmB has been shown to have increased chemical stability, safety, and clinical efficacy; higher oral bioavailability, slow drug release, and resistance to enzyme degradation.[22,25] With broad-spectrum activity like conventional AmB, animal studies have shown clinical efficacy in the treatment of systemic candidiasis, cryptococcal meningitis, and invasive pulmonary aspergillosis.[22,25,26]

Rezafungin and ibrexafungerp are new β-glucan inhibitors. Rezafungin's mechanism of action is like currently available echinocandins but with a safer profile and long half-life.[22] In March 2023, it was FDA-approved for candidemia and invasive candidiasis in adults in the United States with no other alternative treatments.[27] Ibrexafungerp is a synthetic derivate of echinocandin with activity against echinocandin-resistant species, fluconazole-resistant species, *Candida*, and *Aspergillus.*[22,28,29] Due to the increased resistance to antifungals, new formulations are being developed for old drugs. Recent milestones in drug delivery have paved the way for safer drug preparations with less side effects, higher bioavailability, and easy applications that could potentially improve patient compliance.

PITYRIASIS VERSICOLOR (TINEA VERSICOLOR)

DEFINITION

Pityriasis (tinea) versicolor (PV) is a noncontagious chronic benign disorder characterized by asymptomatic scaly hypo- or hyperpigmented superficial patches on the trunk and proximal upper extremities caused by the lipophilic fungus *Malassezia.*[30,31] With the exception of children, it seldom occurs on the face and is rare on the lower extremities.

EPIDEMIOLOGY

PV is distributed worldwide geographically with no sex or ethnic predominance; however, it is more common in tropical climates.[30,31] Prevalence of PV reaches up to 50% in tropical climates while it is estimated to be under 5% in moderate and cold climates.[30,31] The disease affects mainly young adults of both sexes due to increased sebum production, although in tropical zones it is also common in infancy and even in neonates.[32] PV is generally rare before puberty and in old age, possibly due to alterations in sebum production. More recently, several studies have investigated the incidence of PV in different Fitzpatrick skin types.[33] A study done by Berry and Khachemoune found that there is no evidence that PV is more prevalent in darker compared to lighter skin, although the presentation may be more visually apparent in individuals with dark skin.[34] A study from the earlier 2000s analyzing National Ambulatory Medical Care data between 1990 and 1999 found that visit rates to physicians for PV were highest among African American patients and American Indians/Eskimos.[35] In addition, an epidemiologic report showed that PV in the United States occurs in 2.2% of patients with darker skin.[36] In southeast London, England, between January and March 1996, a diagnosis of PV was seen in 3.8% of Black patients.[37] Furthermore, in Rwanda on the continent of Africa, PV was one of the most reported cutaneous disease.[38]

ETIOLOGY

The lipophilic yeast *Malassezia* species are the etiologic agents of PV. *Malassezia globosa* and *Malassezia sympodialis* may be the most common etiologic agents, whereas *Malassezia furfur* has been isolated in some lesions.[30,31,39,40] *Malassezia* yeasts are a part of normal skin flora (predominantly *M. sympodialis*); however, in individuals who develop PV, the organisms transform from saprophytic, round-celled, or the yeast phase to the mycelial phase.[30,31] Tropical climates provide the right environment for this conversion due to their high temperature and humidity. Factors such as immunodeficiency, protective face masks, poor nutrition, hyperhidrosis, pregnancy, and use of oral contraceptives and corticosteroids have been implicated in nontropical climates.[30,31] Genetic susceptibility is also likely.[30,31] Though the evidence is limited, some studies suggest that due to the lipophilic nature of the yeast, the frequent use of certain oily emollients and cosmetic products may promote growth of the yeast.[41] These substances contain high concentrations of complex lipids (free acids, free acid esters, and fatty alcohols with a fatty chain length above 12 carbon atoms), some of which have been proven to enhance growth of *M. furfur* in culture media. Dobler and Gonzalez et al found that the presence of saturated acid like palmitic acid or unsaturated acid like oleic acid influenced the compound profile produced by *M. furfur.*[41,42] In addition, substances containing sebum-producing lipids may act to occlude the skin, resulting in increased carbon dioxide concentrations, altered microflora, and altered pH range, leading to subsequent overgrowth of fungi. Frequent application of these products should be avoided in at-risk populations for PV.

CLINICAL PRESENTATION AND DIAGNOSIS

PV is characterized by scaly hypopigmented or hyperpigmented macules and patches in areas rich in sebum production such as the neck, upper arms and trunk, and shoulders.[31] The face is frequently involved in children. Unusual areas of involvement include the areola, pubis, perineum, penile shaft, and vulva.[43-48]

In individuals with skin of color, PV can present as dark brown to gray-black macules and patches in those with dark skin, while lesions are often light brown in lighter skin.[33] PV lesions may present as flaky or mildly pruritic in some, but for most, PV is asymptomatic and mainly a cosmetic concern.

The diagnosis of PV is confirmed by KOH preparations of skin scrapings that demonstrate pseudohyphae and yeast cells. Wood light examination is a useful diagnostic tool for cases of PV in which *M. furfur* is the etiologic agent.[40] The lesions appear coppery-orange, bright yellow, or gold in color. Dermoscopy has emerged as an ancillary tool to confirm the diagnosis of PV.[49,50] Dermatoscopic findings include alteration in the background pigmentation, "contrast halo sign" fine scale on the involved skin, folliculocentricity, and hypopigmentation of the invaded hair follicle.[49-51] Culturing the yeast is not necessary for diagnosis, because the organism is part of normal flora. The differential diagnosis for hypopigmented lesions includes pityriasis alba, vitiligo, hypomelanosis of Ito, and hypopigmented mycosis fungoides.[31,52] For hyperpigmented lesions, the differential diagnosis includes melasma, tinea corporis, pityriasis rotunda, pityriasis rosea, secondary syphilis, acanthosis nigricans, confluent and reticulated papillomatosis, and seborrheic dermatitis.[33,40,53,54] The distinguishing feature of PV is a characteristic "spaghetti and meatballs" appearance under microscopy that results from the transformation of the yeast to a mycelial form.

HISTOPATHOLOGY

Lesional skin samples show that *Malassezia* is present in all layers of the stratum corneum but not in the lower part of the horny layer. The skin cells may swell and split, expelling the cell matrix and organelles, resulting in a "clear zone" around the invading yeast cells. Alternatively, the keratin within the invaded cells may be replaced by lipid-dense material.[40] Generally, histological findings reveal parakeratosis, hyperkeratosis, mild acanthosis in the upper dermis.[30] The classic "spaghetti and meatballs" appearance in the stratum corneum is appreciated on hematoxylin and eosin (H&E), PAS, or Grocott-Gomori methenamine silver stains.[30-31] Hyperpigmented lesions of PV contain more spores and hyphae than either normal or hypopigmented skin. Merkel cells that contain melanosomes and secretory granules may have increased activity, and melanocytes may appear larger, singly distributed, and hypertrophic. Mild perivascular inflammation and lymphocyte infiltration have been reported in both hypopigmented and hyperpigmented skin.[31] In hypopigmented lesions, there may be a decrease in melanosomes in the stratum spinosum, and the horny layer may be hyperkeratotic.[30,40]

TREATMENT

Without treatment, PV is often a chronic disease. After treatment, recurrence of PV is common, up to 80%.[30] Both topical and oral medications have demonstrated efficacy in the treatment of PV. Topical treatments for PV come in various formulations including creams, shampoos, and lotions that are applied once or twice daily that allow for quick improvement of clinical symptoms.[13] Three main drug classes for topical treatment include imidazoles (1% clotrimazole 1%, 2% ketoconazole, econazole, isoconazole, miconazole), allylamines (terbinafine 1%), and 1% ciclopirox olamine.[12,30,31] Nonspecific agents, such as 1% to 2.5% selenium sulfide shampoo or solution, 30% to 50% propylene glycol, and 1% pyrithione zinc shampoo can physically or chemically remove infected stratum corneum.[55,56]

Ketoconazole has been most studied for the treatment of tinea versicolor. As a highly lipophilic antifungal, ketoconazole has been shown to have anti-inflammatory action against all *Malassezia* species and normalize corneocyte proliferation.[30] It can be applied as a cream (twice daily for 2-3 wks), or a shampoo (apply to affected skin, wash off in 5 min daily, for 2-3 wks).

Patients who suffer from severe or widespread involvement of the skin with PV may benefit from oral therapy. Systemic treatment for pityriasis versicolor includes a regimen of 200 mg daily itraconazole for 2 weeks or 300 mg fluconazole once a week for 5 to 7 days.[55-57] Oral terbinafine and ketoconazole are no longer recommended for treatment of PV.[30-31] Treatment selection requires several considerations: extent and location of lesions, risks and benefits of treatment modality, age of patient, likelihood of compliance, and cost. Because relapse commonly occurs, long-term intermittent prophylactic therapy should be considered for patients at-risk for recurrence. Prophylactic administration of topical 2% ketoconazole, 1% clotrimazole 1%, or 2.5 selenium sulfide shampoo applied to the whole body for 10 minutes once a month may lead to decreased relapse rate of tinea versicolor.[30,57,58]

TINEA NIGRA

Tinea nigra is a superficial mycosis that presents as an infection of the stratum corneum affecting the palms, soles, neck, and trunk.[59,60] It is a misnomer since it is not caused by a dermatophyte but has the name *Tinea*. This infection occurs most commonly in tropical and subtropical climates but does occur in the United States, particularly in the southern coastal areas.[61-63] The causative agent, *Hortaea werneckii* (formerly *Exophiala werneckii*), resides in sewage, soil, decaying vegetation, wood, and humid environments.[59,61,62] The most important predisposing factor is hyperhidrosis of the hands and the feet.[64]

Clinical lesions commonly present as slightly scaly, brown to greenish black velvety macules.[59,61-64] Lesions may develop as one or several spots and spread centrifugally, darkening at the border. Heavily pigmented macules may resemble acral melanocytic nevi, benign acral melanocytic lesion, subcorneal hematoma, exogenous pigmentation, syphilis, pinta, and melanoma.[61-63]

On dermoscopy, characteristic brown, fine-dotted, granule-like structure overlapping the light brown amorphous pigmentation are appreciated.[61,65] Diagnosis can be made readily by examination of a KOH preparation and can be confirmed by culture; a skin biopsy will also confirm the diagnosis. Histopathological findings from skin biopsy show hyperkeratosis without dermal inflammation. KOH preparation of scrapings shows dematiaceous hyphae in the upper layers of the stratum corneum that are brownish or olive-colored with branching septate. The therapy of choice for tinea nigra are keratinolytic agents that include urea, salicylic acid, and Whitfield ointment.[65,66]

PIEDRA

Piedra is a superficial asymptomatic infection of the hair shaft. Two varieties of piedra exist: black piedra and white piedra.[63,66,67] Piedras are distinguished by both clinical appearance and microscopic examination. White piedra is characterized by appearance of white or light brown nodules loosely attached to eyelash, facial, axillary, and pubic hair.[66] These nodules lack the organized appearance of black piedra.[63] White piedra is found in the temperate regions of South America, Europe, Asia, and the southern United States. *Trichosporon species, T. beigelii, T. asahii, T. ovoides, T. inkin, T. mucoides, T. asteroides*, and *T. cutaneum* are species that cause white piedra. The infection causes weakening and breaking of the hair by growing through the hair shaft.[63] KOH examination of white piedra shows nondematiaceous hyphae with blastoconidia and arthoconidia. The usual cultures on Sabouraud agar media yield wet, yeast-forming colonies with a brain-shaped appearance.[64]

Black piedra is caused by *Piedraia hortae* and frequently infects scalp and facial hair by forming firm black-colored, irregular nodules in the hair cuticle.[64,67] Black piedra is common in tropical regions of South America, the Far East, and the Pacific Islands and is less frequent in Africa and Asia.[64] KOH preparation of black piedra reveals hard, brown-black nodules on the hair shaft that are cemented together and resemble organized tissue of septate, thick-walled hyphae arthroconidia.[64] Moreover, the fungus grows at room temperature in Sabouraud agar culture media as limited black-greenish acuminate colonies and is identified by its micromorphology.[64] Microscopic examination distinguishes piedra from nits, hair casts, developmental hair defects, and trichomycosis axillaris. Oral terbinafine has been reported to be an effective therapy for black piedra. Treatment for white and black piedra includes imidazoles, ciclopirox olamine, 2% selenium sulfide, 6% precipitated sulfur in petrolatum, chlorhexidine solutions, and zinc pyrithione.[63,64] Clipping of infected hairs is a solution to both black and white piedra.[63,64] Individuals with either black or white piedra are advised to avoid spreading the infection by not sharing combs, hairbrushes, and other hair accessories.[64]

TINEA CORPORIS/CRURIS (RING WORM, JOCK ITCH)

DEFINITION

Tinea corporis (ringworm) includes all superficial dermatophyte infections of the glabrous skin, not including the scalp, beard, face, hands, feet, and groin.[63,68]

Tinea cruris (jock itch) includes infections of the genitalia, pubic area, perineal and perianal skin, and often the upper thigh.[69,70]

ETIOLOGY AND EPIDEMIOLOGY

A variety of dermatophytes may cause tinea corporis; however, *Trichophyton tonsurans, Trichophyton rubrum, Trichophyton mentagrophytes*, and *Microsporum canis* are usually the causative organisms.[63,69] *Trichophyton rubrum* continues to be the most common isolate that causes tinea corporis and cruris.[70]

Tinea corporis is common in children, especially wrestlers and those with family pets with *M. canis*.[8] Tinea cruris is usually caused by *T. rubrum, T. mentagrophytes*, or *Epidermophyton floccosum*.[8,69] A common predisposing factor for these dermatophyte infections in adults is excessive perspiration.[63] Other factors that predispose individuals include occlusive clothing, contact with contaminated clothing or furniture, immunosuppression, diabetes mellitus, and external exposure sites (eg, locker rooms, gymnasiums, wrestlers, outdoor occupations).[14,71] There is a high incidence of tinea corporis/cruris in hot, humid areas of the world, with males being affected by tinea cruris more often than females.

PATHOGENESIS

The responsible dermatophytes generally reside in the stratum corneum and do not penetrate below the epidermis.[14,63] The proteases, produced by dermatophytes, including endopeptidases, exopeptidases, and secreted proteases, are responsible for fungal colonization and keratin degradation during infection.[72] The skin responds to the superficial infection by increasing proliferation, and this results in scale and epidermal thickening.[70]

CLINICAL MANIFESTATIONS

Tinea corporis may take several clinical forms and may be mild to severe. In individuals with skin of color, the lesions may not be erythematous but rather brown or gray in color. Lesions are typically annular with a central clearing but may assume other patterns such as circinate, oval, or arcuate. Likewise, with tinea cruris, the characteristic red scaling plaques may in fact be tan, brown, or gray in color and extend down the sides of the inner thighs, waist area, and buttocks.[65,73]

HISTOPATHOLOGY

Histopathologically, fungal organisms can be seen in the stratum corneum. If compact orthokeratosis is found in a section, there should be a search for fungal hyphae facilitated by staining with PAS.

DIAGNOSIS AND LABORATORY FINDINGS

Diagnosis can be established clinically through review of the patient history and physical examination. However, there is greater diagnostic accuracy if the clinical diagnosis is verified by KOH preparations, skin biopsy with PAS stain, or fungal cultures on Sabouraud agar media.[63,70,74] Generally, the affected area should be disinfected with alcohol or cleansed with water. A 15-blade scalpel or cellophane adhesive tape can be used to obtain a specimen from the active border of the infection.[74]

TREATMENT

Noninflammatory, less severe cases of tinea corporis and cruris infections can be treated with topical antifungals such as imidazoles (eg, bifonazole, clotrimazole, miconazole), triazoles (eg, fluconazole, itraconazole, efinaconazole), allylamines (eg, butenafine, naftifine, terbinafine), and others (eg, amorolfine, ciclopirox, tavaborole).[14] Systemic treatment should be considered when the infection is inflammatory or involves a large surface area of skin, when host immunity is compromised, or when there is poor response to topical therapy, oral antifungal dosing requires a treatment period of 1 to 4 weeks for the following regimens: 250 mg terbinafine once daily, 100 mg itraconazole once daily, 250 to 300 mg fluconazole once weekly for 2 to 4 weeks, and 375 to 1000 mg griseofulvin daily for 2 to 4 weeks.[75] Other factors that determine the choice of therapy include the overall health of the patient, the causative organism, site and extent of the infection, patient preference (oral vs topical treatment), and the cost-effectiveness of therapy.[14] It is important to note that worsening after empiric treatment with a topical steroid should raise the suspicion of a dermatophyte infection. Conversely, if a nonfungal lesion is treated with an antifungal cream, the lesion will likely not improve.[69] While steroids may improve acute inflammation and pruritus, they may also fortify dermatophyte's plasma membranes rendering antifungal medications less effective.[76]

TINEA PEDIS (ATHLETE'S FOOT)

EPIDEMIOLOGY

Tinea pedis is a fungal infection of the foot. It is one of the most common superficial fungal infections, affecting at least 10% of the world population at any given time.[77] In the past, U.S.-based epidemiologic studies have reported the overall prevalence of tinea pedis as between 1.9% and 4.1%.[78,79] Prevalence rates for Europe and Asia are similar, ranging from 3% to 27% and 4% to 20%, respectively.[80-83] In the Middle East, approximately 10% of the population is affected.[84] In general, race does not appear to affect the distribution of this disease. Tinea pedis is more common in men and the elderly.[78,80] Predisposing factors include diabetes, obesity, trauma, immunosuppression, and certain occupations and hobbies.[14,85]

ETIOLOGY

Leading causes of tinea pedis include *T. rubrum, T. interdigitale*, and *E. floccosum*.[14,86] Nondermatophyte pathogens such as *Scytalidium dimidiatum* and *Scytalidium hyalinum* are also associated with this disease.[86]

CLINICAL MANIFESTATIONS

Tinea pedis has three clinical types: interdigital, hyperkeratotic (moccasin), and vesicobullous.[14,77,87] Interdigital (dermatophytosis simplex), the most prevalent and often chronic form, usually affects the toe web space between the fourth and fifth toes, followed by the toe web space between the third and fourth toes. The skin may appear white and macerated with fissures, oozing, and erythematous erosions.[87] The formation of diffuse hyperkeratosis and desquamative erythema on the sole and toes in a chronic and nonseasonal manner is characteristic of hyperkeratotic tinea pedis. This form is often accompanied by *tinea unguium* that is caused by *T. rubrum*.[88] The vesiculobullous form, frequently caused by *T. mentagrophytes*, is characterized by inflammatory vesicles or bullous lesions.[88] It is sometimes associated with a secondary infection (dermatophytosis complex), itching, and maceration.[88] Severe cases are difficult to diagnose because secondary bacterial infections causing inflammation can mask the primary condition.[88]

TREATMENT

Patients should be examined for other fungal infections, especially onychomycosis, because the nails can act as a reservoir of infection.[77,88] Prophylactic measures include wearing nonocclusive footwear, changing socks and shoes regularly, and washing feet with soap and thoroughly drying regularly.[70,77,87] Regular applications of antifungal foot powders may be helpful.[89] Public baths and pools are major sources of infection by dermatophytes, and using these facilities without footwear should be avoided.[90] Topical antifungal agents can be used to treat tinea pedis in most cases. Tinea pedis is usually treated with a topical antifungal cream for 1 month; interdigital tinea pedis may only require 1 week of therapy.[14,70] Various topical antifungals effective against tinea pedis including azoles, allylamines, butenafine, ciclopirox, tolnaftate, and amorolfine are generally curative.[14,75] Dosing for systemic treatment for tinea pedis includes 500 mg twice daily of microsize for griseofulvin for 4 to 8 weeks, 150 mg fluconazole once weekly for 2 to 6 weeks, 200 mg itraconazole twice daily for 1 week, and 250 mg terbinafine once daily for 2 weeks.[75] These regimens have been used in severe cases of tinea pedis or where topical treatment is ineffective and are used off-label in some parts of the world (eg, the United States).[14] Nondermatophyte pathogens are typically recalcitrant to conventional therapy and perhaps best treated with keratolytics.[70,75]

TINEA UNGUIUM (ONCHOMYCOSIS)

DEFINITION

Onychomycosis is a fungal infection involving the nail unit caused by dermatophytes, nondermatophyte moulds, and yeasts.[91]

ETIOLOGY

Approximately 90% of infections are caused by dermatophytes, with *T. rubrum* being the most isolated etiologic agent.[14,87,91,92] Other dermatophyte pathogens include *T. mentagrophytes* and *E. floccosum*.[93] Nondermatophyte molds such as *Scopulariopsis brevicaulis, Acremonium* species, *Aspergillus* species, *Scytalidium* species, *Onychocola canadensis, Alternaria* species, and *Fusarium* species are responsible for 2.1% to 12.5% of onychomycotic infections depending on geographic location.[92,94] *Candida albicans* causes disease in immunocompromised individuals but can also cause primary onycholysis, paronychia, and occasionally nail plate involvement in healthy patients.[92,94]

EPIDEMIOLOGY

In Western countries, onychomycosis accounts for nearly 50% to 75% of all nail disorders.[92,93] North American epidemiologic studies suggest prevalence rates between 8% and 13.8%.[92,93] In Europe, the range is broader and has been reported between 0.5% and 24%.[92] The distribution of onychomycosis does not appear to be directly affected by race, although cultural and socioeconomic factors may play a role.[93] Dermatophytes were isolated from communal bathing areas in several Muslim mosques in a South African study; the incidence of infection reported in males regularly attending these mosques was higher than in non-Muslim males from the same community.[95] Toenails generally are affected more often than fingernails. Predisposing factors include diabetes mellitus, peripheral arterial disease, compromised immune system, smoking, increasing age, and male gender.[91,92,96]

PATHOGENESIS

There are five main routes of entry into the nail unit, each with a corresponding clinical presentation.[87,96] Total dystrophic onychomycosis results from the progression of one or more of the five main presentations or from simultaneous invasion of all nail tissues because of immunosuppression.[87,96]

HISTOPATHOLOGY

Histology is an alternative method that uses PAS or hematoxylin and eosin (H&E) staining to visualize the fungal elements with a high sensitivity of approximately roughly 88%.[96,97] However, this technique has been reported not to identify the causative organism.[96] Histologic examination reveals fungal elements (spores or hyphae) in the stratum corneum, deep portion of the nail plate, or hyponychium depending on the clinical type.[98]

DIAGNOSIS

Clinical suspicion of onychomycosis calls for mycologic examination of the affected nail. Samples should be collected from different sites of the nail unit, including proximal nail clippings, curetted subungual debris, and nail plate shavings from the diseased portion of the nail to maximize positive results.[96,99] Although common techniques used for diagnosis include KOH and microscopy preparations, fungal culture, histopathology, PCR and flow cytometry, microscopy and culture remain the gold standard.[96] Dermoscopy is a recent technique used in the diagnosis of nail disorders. The differential diagnosis of onychomycosis includes psoriasis, chronic onycholysis, lichen planus, yellow nail syndrome, and trauma.[100]

TREATMENT

Treatment options for onychomycosis include oral and topical antifungals but oral antifungal agents are the most effective treatments currently available for onychomycosis [14] Terbinafine, itraconazole, and fluconazole are the main oral antifungal treatments for onychomycosis, having replaced the older antifungal, griseofulvin.[14] Dosing and length of treatment for oral antifungals are largely dependent on the area of nail involvement.[101] For fingernails, 250 mg terbinafine once daily, 200 mg itraconazole once daily for 6 weeks, or 200 to 400 mg once weekly for 6 to 18 months is recommended.[101] Dosing regimens for toenails are the same but require at least 12 weeks of treatment.[101] These drugs are effective in penetrating the nail unit via the nail bed. Systemic agents may be discouraged in polypharmacy patients such as the elderly, immunocompromised, dialysis patients, and organ transplant recipients as drug-drug interactions with antifungal therapies can elicit synergistic and/or antagonistic interactions.[91] Modern topical antifungal nail lacquers and solutions, such as 8% ciclopirox 5% amorolfine, 5% tavaborole, and 10% efinaconazole, are recommended for daily use for 48 weeks.[101] These topical therapies exploit the use of a concentration gradient that promotes penetration of the active compound to the affected portion of the nail.[14,91,92,96] Topical nail lacquers may provide a safe alternative for patients with onychomycosis of mild to moderate disease severity. Removal of the affected portion of the nail by chemical or mechanical means may be used as an adjunct to antifungal therapy to reduce the fungal burden. Nail avulsion or debridement without concomitant antifungal therapy has a high potential for relapse.[91,92,96]

CUTANEOUS CANDIDIASIS

Candidiasis is an acute or subacute fungal infection caused by the fungus of the genus Candida. This infection can affect the mouth, vagina, skin, nails, bronchi, or the lungs, sometimes causing septicemia, endocarditis, or meningitis.[102-104] The most common cause of cutaneous candidiasis *is Candida albicans*. Candida species may become pathogenic when host factors such as immune status are altered. Lesions may affect several body sites, including nails **(see "Onychomycosis (Tinea Unguium)" above)**, with warm, moist intertriginous areas being affected most frequently.

CLINICAL MANIFESTATIONS

There are two types of cutaneous candidiasis: intertriginous and granulomatous. In intertriginous candidiasis, lesions occur on the skin folds of the armpits, groin, intergluteal, breast fold, between fingers or toes, glans penis, and umbilicus in the form of streaks that are demarcated, scaly, wet, and erythematous.[102-104] On the other hand, granulomatous candidiasis is more common in children and presents as reddish papules covered in thick brownish yellow crusts and are firmly attached to the base. This lesion may can often be found on the face, head, nails, body, and legs.[102]

LABORATORY FINDINGS/HISTOPATHOLOGY

For superficial candidal infections, skin scrapings with 10% KOH solution are the easiest and most effective way to diagnose candidiasis though it cannot identify a specific etiology and is less sensitive than culture.[102] Examination of skin scrapings typically shows budding yeasts with hyphae or pseudohyphae in the stratum corneum. Culture results in whitish, mucoid colonies within 2 to 5 days.[102]

TREATMENT

Currently, anticandidal topical therapy includes azoles, polyenes, echinocandins, azoles, ciclopirox, and nystatin. Oral itraconazole or fluconazole is considered if oral therapy is warranted.[102-104]

ANTIFUNGAL RESISTANCE: AN EMERGING CONCERN

The emergence of recalcitrant dermatophytoses, mainly presenting as tinea corporis and cruris, over the past few years has become a global concern.[76,105] Consequently, this emergence has led to renewed research interest in dermatophytoses, the most common fungal infection known to man. More recently, there is limited evidence that factors such as patient nonadherence, widespread availability of topical antifungal-corticosteroid combinations, improper use of antifungal agents, suboptimal drug absorption, and new fungal resistance mechanisms are factors that may contribute to the promotion of antifungal resistance.[4,76,105]

As antifungal resistance increases, newer drugs (third-generation azoles and synthetic echinocandins) have been developed and approved in the United States. For example, Ibrexafungerp (enfumafungin derivative) and oteseconazole (tetrazole) are newer antifungals indicated for vulvovaginal candidiasis.[3] These drugs differ from their respective related drug classes of echinocandins and triazoles by having different structures, which lend these medicines advantage compared to traditional treatment by having a different binding site and more selectivity for fungi respectively.[3]

As more effective antifungal drugs are being developed, antifungal stewardship of existing and newer drugs will be necessary.[4,76,104,105] Concerted efforts at the institutional and individual level should be mobilized to address and limit inappropriate antifungal use.[3] Primary care physicians should be trained in the rational management of dermatophytosis, and patient compliance for prescribed treatments.[105] Patients should be asked about family diseases, and appropriate treatment should be prescribed; prescription sharing should be discouraged.[105] Antifungal drug surveillance systems should be created and promoted globally to create clinical cut off values to guide treatment and monitor drug resistance.[4,76,105]

CONCLUSION

Fungi are ubiquitous, and individuals of all races may be affected. Susceptibility to fungal infection is influenced by a variety of factors including socioeconomic status, geographic location, and cultural or religious practices. Topical antifungals are first-line therapy for dermatophyte infections in those with uncomplicated, localized infections. Systemic antifungal therapy is required for some dermatophyte infections such as onychomycosis, tinea unguium, tinea manuum, tinea capitis, and widespread dermatophytosis. Though fungal infections are generally considered easy to treat, recalcitrant infections, presenting as extensive and difficult to treat tinea corporis and cruris, are on the rise in some parts of the world.[76] This situation demands continued development of newer antifungals, investigation into fungal resistance patterns, and concurrent measures at patient, provider, and institution levels to reduce antifungal resistance.

REFERENCES

1. Taylor SC. Epidemiology of skin diseases in ethnic populations. *Dermatol Clin*. 2003;21:601-607.
2. WHO. Fungal priority pathogens list to guide research, development, and public health action. 2022. https://www.who.int/publications/i/item/9789240060241. Accessed Nov 25, 2023.
3. Koh XQ, Pan JY. Recalcitrant cutaneous fungal infections - a growing problem. *Australas J Dermatol*. 2023;64(3):315-321.
4. Chanyachailert P, Leeyaphan C, Bunyaratavej S. Cutaneous fungal infections caused by dermatophytes and non-dermatophytes: an updated comprehensive review of epidemiology, clinical presentations, and diagnostic testing. *J Fungi (Basel)*. 2023;9(6):669.
5. Ghannoum M, Mukherjee P, Isham N, Markinson B, Rosso JD, Leal L. Examining the importance of laboratory and diagnostic testing when treating and diagnosing onychomycosis. *Int J Dermatol*. 2018;57(2):131-138.
6. Lipner SR, Scher RK. Onychomycosis: clinical overview and diagnosis. *J Am Acad Dermatol*. 2019;80(4):835-851.
7. Dyer JM, Foy VM. Revealing the unseen: a review of wood's lamp in dermatology. *J Clin Aesthet Dermatol*. 2022;15(6):25-30.
8. Garg A, Sharma GS, Goyal AK, Ghosh G, Si SC, Rath G. Recent advances in topical carriers of anti-fungal agents. *Heliyon*. 2020;6(8):e04663.
9. Sahni K, Singh S, Dogra S. Newer topical treatments in skin and nail dermatophyte infections. *Indian Dermatol Online J*. 2018;9(3):149-158.
10. Seify R, Zahednezhad F, Zakeri-Milani P, Valizadeh H. Amphotericin B liposomal formulation: applicable preparation methods, challenges, and tips. *Drug Dev Ind Pharm*. 2023;49(5):367-376.
11. Stone NR, Bicanic T, Salim R, Hope W. Liposomal amphotericin B (AmBisome(®)): a review of the pharmacokinetics, pharmacodynamics, clinical experience and future directions. *Drugs*. 2016;76(4):485-500.
12. Veraldi S, Barbareschi M, Martella A, Milani M. Efficacy and tolerability of 1% ciclopirox shampoo in the treatment of moderate-to-severe scalp seborrheic dermatitis: a multicenter, prospective, assessor-blinded trial. *G Ital Dermatol Venereol*. 2019;154(3):342-346.
13. Nivoix Y, Ledoux MP, Herbrecht R. Antifungal therapy: new and evolving therapies. *Semin Respir Crit Care Med*. 2020;41(1):158-174.
14. Gupta AK, Foley KA, Versteeg SG. New antifungal agents and new formulations against dermatophytes. *Mycopathologia*. 2017;182(1-2):127-141.
15. Gupta AK, Daigle D, Foley KA. Drug safety assessment of oral formulations of ketoconazole. *Expert Opin Drug Saf*. 2015;14(2):325-334.
16. Gupta AK, Lyons DC. The rise and fall of oral ketoconazole. *J Cutan Med Surg*. 2015;19(4):352-357.
17. Hamill RJ. Amphotericin B formulations: a comparative review of efficacy and toxicity. *Drugs*. 2013;73(9):919-934.
18. Aguilar-Zapata D, Petraitiene R, Petraitis V. Echinocandins: the expanding antifungal armamentarium. *Clin Infect Dis*. 2015;61(Suppl 6):S604-S611.
19. Grover ND. Echinocandins: a ray of hope in antifungal drug therapy. *Indian J Pharmacol*. 2010;42(1):9-11.
20. Aris P, Wei Y, Mohamadzadeh M, Xia X. Griseofulvin: an updated overview of old and current knowledge. *Molecules*. 2022;27(20):7034.
21. Chen X, Jiang X, Yang M, et al. Systemic antifungal therapy for tinea capitis in children. *Cochrane Database Syst Rev*. 2016;2016(5):CD004685.
22. Guinea J. New trends in antifungal treatment: what is coming up? *Rev Esp Quimioter*. 2023;36(Suppl 1):59-63.
23. Murray A, Cass L, Ito K, et al. PC945, a Novel inhaled antifungal agent, for the treatment of respiratory fungal infections. *J Fungi (Basel)*. 2020; 6(4):373.
24. Martens MG, Maximos B, Degenhardt T, et al. Phase 3 study evaluating the safety and efficacy of oteseconazole in the treatment of recurrent vulvovaginal candidiasis and acute vulvovaginal candidiasis infections. *Am J Obstet Gynecol*. 2022;227(6):880.e1-880.e11.
25. Aigner M, Lass-Flörl C. Encochleated amphotericin B: is the oral availability of amphotericin B finally reached? *J Fungi (Basel)*. 2020;6(2):66.
26. Faustino C, Pinheiro L. Lipid systems for the delivery of amphotericin B in antifungal therapy. *Pharmaceutics*. 2020;12(1):29.
27. Syed YY. Rezafungin: first approval. *Drugs*. 2023;83(9):833-840.
28. Gamal A, Chu S, McCormick TS, Borroto-Esoda K, Angulo D, Ghannoum MA. Ibrexafungerp, a novel oral triterpenoid antifungal in development: overview of antifungal activity against Candida glabrata. *Front Cell Infect Microbiol*. 2021;11:642358.
29. Sucher AJ, Thai A, Tran C, Mantena N, Noronha A, Chahine EB. Ibrexafungerp: a new triterpenoid antifungal. *Am J Health Syst Pharm*. 2022;79(24):2208-2221.
30. Łabędź N, Navarrete-Dechent C, Kubisiak-Rzepczyk H, Bowszyc-Dmochowska M, Pogorzelska-Antkowiak A, Pietkiewicz P. Pityriasis versicolor-a narrative review on the diagnosis and management. *Life (Basel)*. 2023;13(10):2097.
31. Leung AK, Barankin B, Lam JM, Leong KF, Hon KL. Tinea versicolor: an updated review. *Drugs Context*. 2022;11:2022-9-2.
32. Crespo E, Delgado F. Malassezia species in skin diseases. *Curr Opin Infect Dis*. 2002;15:133.
33. Kallini JR, Riaz F, Khachemoune A. Tinea versicolor in dark-skinned individuals. *Int J Dermatol*. 2014;53(2):137-141.
34. Berry M, Khachemoune A. Extensive tinea versicolor mimicking Pityriasis rubra pilaris. *J Drugs Dermatol*. 2009;8(5):490-491.
35. Mellen LA, Vallee J, Feldman SR, et al. Treatment of pityriasis versicolor in the United States. *J Dermatolog Treat*. 2004;15:18-92.
36. Halder RM, Nootheti PK. Ethnic skin disorders overview. *J Am Acad Dermatol*. 2003;48:S143.
37. Child FJ, Fuller LC, Higgins EM, et al. A study of the spectrum of skin disease occurring in a black population in southeast London. *Br J Dermatol*. 1999;141:512-517.

38. Van Hecke E, Bugingo G. Prevalence of skin disease in Rwanda. *Int J Dermatol.* 1980;19:526-529.
39. Saunte DML, Gaitanis G, Hay RJ. Malassezia-associated skin diseases, the use of diagnostics and treatment. *Front Cell Infect Microbiol.* 2020;10:112.
40. Gupta AK, Bluhm R, Summerbell R. Pityriasis versicolor. *J Eur Acad Dermatol Venereol.* 2002;16:19-33.
41. Dobler D, Schmidts T, Wildenhain S, Seewald I, Merzhäuser M, Runkel F. Impact of selected cosmetic ingredients on common microorganisms of healthy human skin. *Cosmetics.* 2019;6(3):45.
42. Gonzalez M, Celis AM, Guevara-Suarez MI, Molina J, Carazzone C. Yeast smell like what they eat: analysis of volatile organic compounds of *Malassezia furfur* in growth media supplemented with different lipids. *Molecules.* 2019; 24(3):419.
43. Smith BL, Koestenblatt EK, Weinberg JM. Areolar and periareolar pityriasis versicolor. *J Eur Acad Dermatol Venereol.* 2004;18(6):740-741.
44. Romano C, Feci L, Mancianti F, Fimiani M. Perineal and genital pityriasis versicolor due to *Malassezia globosa*. *J Eur Acad Dermatol Venereol.* 2015;29(9):1857-1858.
45. Cinelli E, Vastarella M, Fabbrocini G, Gallo L. Erythrasmoid pityriasis versicolor with exclusive involvement of the pubis and inguinal region. *Ital J Dermatol Venerol.* 2021;156(Suppl. 1 to No. 6):11-12.
46. Day T, Scurry J. Vulvar pityriasis versicolor in an immunocompetent woman. *J Low Genit Tract Dis.* 2014;18(3):e71-e73.
47. Greco V, Megna M, Luciano MA, Fabbrocini G. Pityriasis versicolor with uncommon localizations. *G Ital Dermatol Venereol.* 2020;155(6):786-787.
48. Khaddar RK, Cherif F, Ben Hadid R, Mokni M, Ben Osman A. Penile shaft involvement in pityriasis versicolor. *Acta Dermatovenerol Alp Pannonica Adriat.* 2008;17(2):86-89.
49. Al-Refu K. Dermoscopy is a new diagnostic tool in diagnosis of common hypopigmented macular disease: a descriptive study. *Dermatol Reports.* 2018;11(1):7916.
50. Zhou H, Tang XH, De Han J, Chen MK. Dermoscopy as an ancillary tool for the diagnosis of pityriasis versicolor. *J Am Acad Dermatol.* 2015;73(6): e205-e206.
51. Kapadia F, Kharkar V, Vishwanath T. Dermoscopy to the rescue in an annular enigma: a rare case of annular pityriasis versicolor presenting in an unusual location. *Dermatol Pract Concept.* 2022;12(2):e2022057.
52. Massone C, Cavalchini A, Clapasson A, Nunzi E. Hypopigmented macules: leprosy, atopy or pityriasis versicolor? *G Ital Dermatol Venereol.* 2010;145(6):779-782.
53. Bossini B, Mazzolai M, Berti I, Barbi E. Hyperpigmented pityriasis versicolor misdiagnosed as acanthosis nigricans. *Arch Dis Child.* 2022;107(1):92.
54. Plensdorf S, Livieratos M, Dada N. Pigmentation disorders: diagnosis and management. *Am Fam Physician.* 2017;96(12):797-804.
55. Hu SW, Bigby M. Pityriasis versicolor: a systematic review of interventions. *Arch Dermatol.* 2010;146(10):1132-1140.
56. Gupta AK, Foley KA. Antifungal treatment for pityriasis versicolor. *J Fungi (Basel).* 2015;1(1):13-29.
57. Goldstein BG, Goldstein AO. Tinea versicolor (pityriasis versicolor). In: Dellavalle R, Levy ML, Rosen T (Eds). UpToDate; 2023. Accessed December 16, 2023. https://www.uptodate.com/contents/tinea-versicolor-pityriasis-versicolor.
58. Choi FD, Juhasz MLW, Atanaskova Mesinkovska N. Topical ketoconazole: a systematic review of current dermatological applications and future developments. *J Dermatolog Treat.* 2019;30(8):760-771.
59. Nazzaro G, Ponziani A, Cavicchini S. Tinea nigra: a diagnostic pitfall. *J Am Acad Dermatol.* 2016;75(6):e219-e220.
60. Cappilli S, D'Amore A, Di Stefani A. From direct to confocal microscopy for tinea nigra: time to shift towards in vivo imaging? *J Eur Acad Dermatol Venereol.* 2023;37(7):e850-e851.
61. Lima Dantas M, Serrão Fensterseifer G, Henrique Martins P, Paipilla Hernandez IA, Eibs Cafrune F. Entodermoscopy in the diagnosis of tinea nigra: two case reports. *Dermatol Pract Concept.* 2020;10(3):e2020065.
62. Noguchi H, Hiruma M, Inoue Y, Miyata K, Tanaka M, Ihn H. Tinea nigra showing a parallel ridge pattern on dermoscopy. *J Dermatol.* 2015;42(5): 518-520.
63. Gupta AK, Chaudhry M, Elewski B. Tinea corporis, tinea cruris, tinea nigra, and piedra. *Dermatol Clin.* 2003;21(3):395-400, v.
64. Bonifaz A, Gómez-Daza F, Paredes V, Ponce RM. Tinea versicolor, tinea nigra, white piedra, and black piedra. *Clin Dermatol.* 2010;28(2):140-145.
65. Piliouras P, Allison S, Rosendahl C, Buettner PG, Weedon D. Dermoscopy improves diagnosis of tinea nigra: a study of 50 cases. *Australas J Dermatol.* 2011;52(3):191-194.
66. Dias MF, Quaresma-Santos MV, Bernardes-Filho F, Amorim AG, Schechtman RC, Azulay DR. Update on therapy for superficial mycoses: review article part I. *An Bras Dermatol.* 2013;88(5):764-774.
67. Veasey JV, Avila RB, Miguel BAF, Muramatu LH. White piedra, black piedra, tinea versicolor, and tinea nigra: contribution to the diagnosis of superficial mycosis. *An Bras Dermatol.* 2017;92(3):413-416.
68. El-Gohary M, van Zuuren EJ, Fedorowicz Z, Burgess H, Doney L, Stuart B, Moore M, Little P. Topical antifungal treatments for tinea cruris and tinea corporis. *Cochrane Database Syst Rev.* 2014 Aug 4;2014(8):CD009992. doi: 10.1002/14651858.CD009992.pub2. PMID: 25090020; PMCID: PMC11198340.
69. Ely JW, Rosenfeld S, Seabury Stone M. Diagnosis and management of tinea infections. *Am Fam Physician.* 2014;90(10):702-710.
70. Sahoo AK, Mahajan R. Management of tinea corporis, tinea cruris, and tinea pedis: a comprehensive review. *Indian Dermatol Online J.* 2016;7(2):77-86.
71. Singh S, Verma P, Chandra U, Tiwary NK. Risk factors for chronic and chronic-relapsing tinea corporis, tinea cruris and tinea faciei: results of a case-control study. *Indian J Dermatol Venereol Leprol.* 2019;85(2):197-200.
72. Liu WT, Sun PL, Bramono K, Ezmerli M, Yang CC, Chen W. Annular infectious dermatoses. *Clin Dermatol.* 2022;40(5):427-440.
73. Weinstein A, Berman B. Topical treatment of common superficial tinea infections. *Am Fam Physician.* 2002;65:2095-2102.
74. Drake LA, Dinehart SM, Farmer ER, et al. Guidelines of care for superficial mycotic infections of the skin: tinea corporis, tinea cruris, tinea faciei, tinea manuum, and tinea pedis. Guidelines/Outcomes Committee, American Academy of Dermatology. *J Am Acad Dermatol.* 1996;34:282.
75. Goldstein BG, Goldstein AO. Dermatophyte (tinea) infections. In: UpToDate, Dellavalle R, Levy ML, Rosen T. (Eds), Wolters Kluwer. Accessed on December 16, 2023.
76. Khurana A, Sardana K, Chowdhary A. Antifungal resistance in dermatophytes: recent trends and therapeutic implications. *Fungal Genet Biol.* 2019;132:103255.
77. Gupta AK, Chow M, Daniel CR, et al. Treatments of tinea pedis. *Dermatol Clin.* 2003;21:431-462.
78. Panackal AA, Halpern EF, Watson AJ. Cutaneous fungal infections in the United States: analysis of the National Ambulatory Medical Care Survey (NAMCS) and National Hospital Ambulatory Medical Care Survey (NHAMCS), 1995–2004. *Int J Dermatol.* 2009;48:704-712.
79. Moseley I, Ragi SD, Ouellette S, Rao B. Tinea pedis in underrepresented groups: all of us database analysis. *Mycoses.* 2023;66(1):29-34.
80. Perea S, Ramos MJ, Garau M, et al. Prevalence and risk factors of tinea unguium and tinea pedis in the general population in Spain. *J Clin Microbiol.* 2000;38:3226-3230.
81. Lupa S, Seneczko F, Jeske J, et al. Epidemiology of dermatomycoses of humans in central Poland: III. Tinea pedis. *Mycoses.* 1999;42:563-565.
82. Ungpakorn R, Lohaprathan S, Reangchainam S. Prevalence of foot diseases in outpatients attending the Institute of Dermatology, Bangkok, Thailand. *Clin Exp Dermatol.* 2004;29:87-90.
83. Cheng S, Chong L. A prospective epidemiological study on tinea pedis and onychomycosis in Hong Kong. *Chin Med J (Engl).* 2002;115:860-865.
84. Falahati M, Akhlaghi L, Lari AR, et al. Epidemiology of dermatophytoses in an area south of Tehran, Iran. *Mycopathologia.* 2003;156:279.
85. Ilkit M, Durdu M. Tinea pedis: the etiology and global epidemiology of a common fungal infection. *Crit Rev Microbiol.* 2014;41:374-388.
86. Lopes JO, Alves SH, Mari CR, et al. A ten-year survey of tinea pedis in the central region of the Rio Grande do Sul, Brazil. *Rev Inst Med Trop Sao Paulo.* 1999;41:75-77.
87. Nowicka D, Nawrot U. Tinea pedis-an embarrassing problem for health and beauty - a narrative review. *Mycoses.* 2021;64(10):1140-1150.
88. Masri-Fridling GD. Dermatophytosis of the feet. *Dermatol Clin.* 1996;14:33-40.
89. Pierard G, Wallace R, De Doncker P. Biometrological assessment of the preventive effect of a miconazole spray powder on athlete's foot. *Clin Exp Dermatol.* 1996;21:344.
90. Watanabe K, Taniguchi H, Katoh T. Adhesion of dermatophytes to healthy feet and its simple treatment. *Mycoses.* 2000;43:45-50.
91. Gupta AK, Versteeg SG, Shear NH. Onychomycosis in the 21st century: an update on diagnosis, epidemiology, and treatment. *J Cutan Med Surg.* 2017;21(6):525-539.
92. Gupta AK, Stec N, Summerbell RC, et al. Onychomycosis: a review. *J Eur Acad Dermatol Venereol.* 2020;34(9):1972-1990.
93. Ghannoum MA, Hajjeh RA, Scher R, et al. A large-scale North American study of fungal isolates from nails: the frequency of onychomycosis, fungal distribution, and antifungal susceptibility patterns. *J Am Acad Dermatol.* 2000;43:641-648.
94. Tosti A, Piraccini BM, Lorenzi S, et al. Treatment of nondermatophyte mold and Candida onychomycosis. *Dermatol Clin.* 2003;21:491-497.
95. Raboobee N, Aboobaker J, Peer AK. Tinea pedis et unguium in the Muslim community of Durban, South Africa. *Int J Dermatol.* 1998;37:759-765.

96. Gupta AK, Summerbell RC, Venkataraman M, Quinlan EM. Nondermatophyte mould onychomycosis. *J Eur Acad Dermatol Venereol.* 2021;35(8): 1628-1641.
97. Jung MY, Shim JH, Lee JH, et al. Comparison of diagnostic methods foronychomycosis, and proposal of a diagnostic algorithm. *Clin Exp Dermatol.* 2015;40:479-484.
98. Jerasutus S. Histology and histopathology. In: Scher RK, Daniel CR III, eds. *Nails: Therapy, Diagnosis, Surgery.* 2nd ed. Philadelphia, PA: Saunders; 1997:55-98.
99. Baran R ed. *Baran & Dawber's Diseases of the Nails and their Management.* 5th ed. Hoboken, NJ: Wiley-Blackwell; 2019.
100. Lynde C. Nail disorders that mimic onychomycosis: what to consider. *Cutis.* 2001;68:8-12.
101. Falotico JM, Lipner SR. Updated perspectives on the diagnosis and management of onychomycosis. *Clin Cosmet Investig Dermatol.* 2022;15:1933-1957.
102. Ahronowitz I, Leslie K. Yeast Infections. In: Kang S, Amagai M, Bruckner AL, Enk AH, Margolis DJ, McMichael AJ, Arraigner JS. eds. *Fitzpatrick's Dermatology*, 9e. McGraw-Hill Education (New York?), 2019:2952-2964.
103. Nurdin RSC, Vitayani S, Amin S, Kadir D, Djamaluddin W, Adriani A. Cutaneous candidiasis caused by Candida Kefyr. *Pan Afr Med J.* 2021;38:178.
104. Lu H, Hong T, Jiang Y, Whiteway M, Zhang S. Candidiasis: from cutaneous to systemic, new perspectives of potential targets and therapeutic strategies. *Adv Drug Deliv Rev.* 2023;199:114960.
105. Dogra S, Ramam M. Difficult Dermatophytosis. JAMA Dermatol. 2022;158(11): 1243 -1244.

CHAPTER 70

Deep Fungal Infections

David J. Chandler
Regina Casz Schechtman

KEY POINTS

- Deep fungal infections are chronic infections involving the skin and subcutaneous tissue, caused by a diverse group of fungi and bacteria. They have the potential to invade deeper tissues such as bone, causing significant morbidity, and rarely can disseminate. As a group they are recognized by the WHO as Neglected Tropical Diseases.
- Sporotrichosis is a subacute or chronic infection caused by the fungal genus *Sporothrix* occurring preferably in tropical and subtropical regions, and is considered the most frequent subcutaneous mycosis in Latin America, where it is endemic.
- New species were described based on the phenotypic and molecular characteristics of the Sporothrix complex: *S. globosa*, a globally distributed fungus, *S. brasiliensis*, the species related to the zoonotic epidemic in Brazil, *S. mexicana*, initially limited to Mexico and *S. chilensis* among others.
- There is an advance of human zoonotic sporotrichosis cases in Brazil. Since 1950, sporotrichosis has been well known as subcutaneous mycosis. Around 1998, the number of felines infected by *Sporothrix* sp. has raised significantly, followed by a huge increase in human cases in the poorest areas of Rio de Janeiro state, Brazil. By the year of 2001, Sporotrichosis was considered to be an emergent zoonosis. There are two ways to acquire the cutaneous disease, both by traumatic inoculation of the propagules through the skin.
- The classic clinical presentation known as the "Rose Gardener's disease" is transmitted by plant debris and the atypical "zoonotic disease" is caused by animal transmission.
- Clinical manifestations were divided into a cutaneous (localized and benign form) and extracutaneous disease (usually disseminated). Considering the new pathogenic species described in the last decade and its clinical manifestations, a new classification has been proposed, which also includes the hypersensitivity immune response to the fungus, more frequently seen when there is a zoonotic transmission of the disease.
- Endemic sporotrichosis has been a therapeutic challenge in Brazil. Drug treatments such as azoles, among this group Itraconazole, had shown good therapeutic effects and benefits such as its posology and less side effects than other options.

INTRODUCTION

Deep fungal infections (DFIs) or subcutaneous mycoses are chronic infections of the skin and subcutaneous tissue, in some cases with extension to deeper tissues including bone. They are a heterogeneous group of infections with no logical system of classification; however, they share certain features in common that allow them to be grouped—they are infections of implantation, caused by direct inoculation of environmental organisms into the skin or subcutaneous tissue; they occur predominantly in tropical and subtropical regions where they often affect manual and agricultural workers in rural communities; and they are recognized by the WHO as neglected tropical diseases (NTDs).

OVERVIEW OF DEEP FUNGAL INFECTIONS

The most common DFIs are sporotrichosis, mycetoma, and chromoblastomycosis, although even in endemic settings these infections generally occur infrequently. Rarer infections include phaeohyphomycosis, lobomycosis, rhinosporidiosis, and entomophthoromycosis. These conditions are collectively referred to as deep fungal infections; however, it is important to note that mycetoma can be caused by both fungi (eumycetoma) and filamentous bacteria (actinomycetoma), the latter accounting for the majority of cases in some settings, particularly in Latin America. Rhinosporidiosis is caused by *Rhinosporidium seeberi*, which is now recognized to be a parasitic eukaryote belonging to the class Mesomycetozoea, although it was previously classified as a fungus and continues to be included in discussion of DFIs. In addition to causing subcutaneous infection, both sporotrichosis and phaeohyphomycosis have systemic forms that are often associated with immunosuppression.

Accurate epidemiological data on these conditions are lacking, not least because there are no systems for disease surveillance in endemic countries and many cases will not be reported. Mycetoma is a DFI notable for its progressive course and ability to invade deeper tissues including bone. This leads to deformity and disability, typically in young economically productive individuals, and very rarely can be fatal.

Diagnosis of DFIs often relies on a combination of clinical features, direct examination of clinical material, and analysis of histopathological sections. Culture is usually possible; however, the identification of unusual pathogens and use of special media may require access to a specialist laboratory. Direct examination is particularly useful in patients with chromoblastomycosis and mycetoma, often allowing a diagnosis to be made and in some cases guiding initial treatment. A skin scraping may be adequate for the diagnosis of chromoblastomycosis, whereas for mycetoma a sample of pus containing grains should be collected. Histopathological examination can be performed using hematoxylin and eosin (H&E), although special stains such as Periodic acid-Schiff (PAS) and Grocott-Gomori silver stain are useful particularly when organisms are present in tissue in low numbers. Tissue obtained from skin biopsy can be used for culture but must be stored in a sterile container and is usually placed in sterile saline. Tools for molecular identification are often not available in endemic settings.

The etiological agents of DFI are numerous, with more than 40 causative agents recognized for eumycetoma alone. Conversely, organisms belonging to a single genus can cause more than one disease, such as *Cladophialophora* spp. that are causative agents of phaeohyphomycosis, chromoblastomycosis, and mycetoma. This underscores the importance of close clinicopathological and microbiological correlation; however, this can be challenging especially in the resource-limited settings in which these infections most commonly occur.

Due to their broad geographic distribution, the deep fungal infections occur in a range of skin types. This has implications for the clinical features and sequelae of these infections, although these aspects have received little attention in the literature. For example, features such as scarring and dyspigmentation and their impact on the individual may show a wide variation according to skin type.

SPOROTRICHOSIS

BACKGROUND

Sporotrichosis is a subacute or chronic infection caused by fungi belonging to the Sporothrix Complex: *S. schenckii*, *S. brasiliensis*, *S. mexicana*, *S. globosa*, and *S. albicans*. Sporotrichosis occurs all over the world, mainly in tropical and temperate climes. The infection is normally caused by traumatic inoculation of the fungus into the skin or subcutaneous tissues, and can be either confined to the puncture point or reach the regional lymphatic system. It could even spread through the bloodstream causing systemic infection.[1] Zoonotic transmission has described in isolated cases or in small outbreaks.

REMINISCES

The first report of sporotrichosis was published in the Johns Hopkins Hospital Bulletin in 1898 in Baltimore, Maryland.[2] In 1900, the disease was reported for the second time by Hektoen and Perkins, who classified the etiologic agent as *S. schenckii*, with the pathogen being isolated from a specimen aspirated from the cutaneous lesions of a patient.[3] In 1912, De Beurmann and Gougerot published a complete treatise on the disease.[4,5]

TAXONOMY

S. schenckii is, therefore, a dimorphic pathogenic fungus and the etiologic agent of human and animal sporotrichosis. The fungus belongs to the subdivision Deuteromycotina, class Hyphomycetes.[6] According to Mariat and Taylor, the fungus *Ceratocystis stenoceras* (*Ophiostoma stenoceras*) presents a conidial stage similar to that as *S. schenckii*; however, no conclusions exist regarding the description of the teleomorphic phase of this species.[7] Other investigators have recently postulated that Ophiostoma stenoceras may correspond with the teleomorph of *S. schenckii*.[8] Previous studies based on DNA hybridization experiments, however, provided strong evidence that *O. stenoceras* is not the teleomorph of *S. schenckii*. The degree of hybridization observed among *S. schenckii* and *O. stenoceras* DNAs was as low as 30%, while a high degree of cross-hybridization was observed among *S. schenckii* strains studied.[7]

EPIDEMIOLOGY

S. schenckii is widely distributed in nature and can be found in soil associated with plant organic matter (eg, thorns, dry leaves, and wood), water, and decomposing matter, among others. *S. schenckii* is present in the soil throughout the world. Sporotrichosis is more frequent in tropical and subtropical countries, however, and is endemic in many parts of Latin America. Sporotrichosis has been mainly reported in tropical and temperate zones.[9,10] It is endemic in Mexico, Central America, and South America, as well as other areas such as South Africa. It can also occur in temperate climates such as in southern United States, Japan, and Australia. In the south of the American continent, the disease more frequently occurs in humid autumn or summer seasons.[11,12] Sporotrichosis has been reported from different parts of India.[13,14]

Sporotrichosis can affect persons of all ages,[15] and the number of cases involving men and women varies from region.[9,17] However, typically, the patients are healthy young adults younger than 30 years.

Generally, infection results from inoculation of the fungus through thorns, splinters, scratches, and small traumas during leisure and occupational activities such as floriculture, horticulture, gardening, fishing, hunting, farming and cattle raising, mining, and wood exploration.[11,12,15,16] Laboratory professionals can be accidentally infected while manipulating *S. schenckii* cultures.[17,18] Zoonotic transmission can occur after being scratched or bitten by animals, especially cats, rodents, and armadillos.[5]

Sporotrichosis usually occurs in isolated cases or in small family or professional outbreaks. Epidemics are rare and, if present, have been related to a single source of infection.[19] The largest reported epidemic occurred in South Africa, with about 3000 gold miners infected with the fungus, which occurred in the wood gliders of the mine structure.

Human has been sporadically related to the scratch or bite of animals.[20,21] Since the 1980s, domestic cats have gained importance in the transmission of the mycosis to humans.[22-24] Between animals, the acquired infection is reported in various species. The acquired infection is reported in various species such as horses, rats, dolphins, cows, and fish.[8] Animal to human transmission is rare, however, and there are few reports on animal transmission of sporotrichosis to humans, with the exception of some cases of armadillo transmission in Uruguay[25] and feline transmission in Brazil. Domestic cats can acquire the disease following traumatic injury from infected street cats during fights or from direct inoculation of environmental organisms that inhabit soil and vegetation They transmit the infection to humans in the domestic environment through biting or scratching human skin and consequently inoculating the organisms that are present under the nails. Another way of transmission is through direct contact of human skin with the infected cat skin, mucous membranes, or exudates from open lesions. Domestic dogs have been identified with sporotrichosis, probably transmitted by domestic cats.[26,27]

EPIDEMIOLOGY

Similar to many parts of the developing world, sporotrichosis is also commonly recognized clinically in India; it is endemic in sub-Himalayan West Bengal and Assam in the north-east and Himachal Pradesh in the north-west, however, it has been reported from different parts of India.[13,14,28]

PATHOGENESIS

This subcutaneous mycosis is an infection of implantation. In most cases, it develops following traumatic injury, especially by vegetation such as thorns and wood, and the inoculation of environmental organisms into the host where they affect the subcutaneous tissue, skin, and other adjacent structures. Certain occupational groups such as those who handle plant materials or soil are frequently exposed to the organism and have been known to become infected.

Multiple inoculations may occur simultaneously, not to be confused with spread of a single primary lesion. The presentation and course of sporotrichosis depends on the host immune response as well as the size and virulence of the inoculums. In hosts not previously inoculated, involvement of regional lymphatic ensues. In those with a prior history of exposure to *Sporothrix schenckii*, no lymphatic spread occurs, and a "fixed ulcer" develops at the site of inoculums or granulomatous plaque (particularly on the face).[29]

Extensive cutaneous disease with or without systemic involvement is also possible, especially in an immunocompromised host. Cases of inhaled sporotrichosis have been reported with systemic and cutaneous dissemination, similar to disseminated histoplasmosis and other dimorphic fungal infections.

CLINICAL CONNOTATIONS

Sporotrichosis has diverse clinical manifestations and investigators disagree regarding the clinical classification of the disease.[8] The most frequent clinical form (about 80%) is the lymphocutaneous form. The initial presentation of sporotrichosis is that of a single papule at the precise location of injury, most commonly on the hand appearing several weeks after inoculation. The lesion then becomes eroded or ulcerated

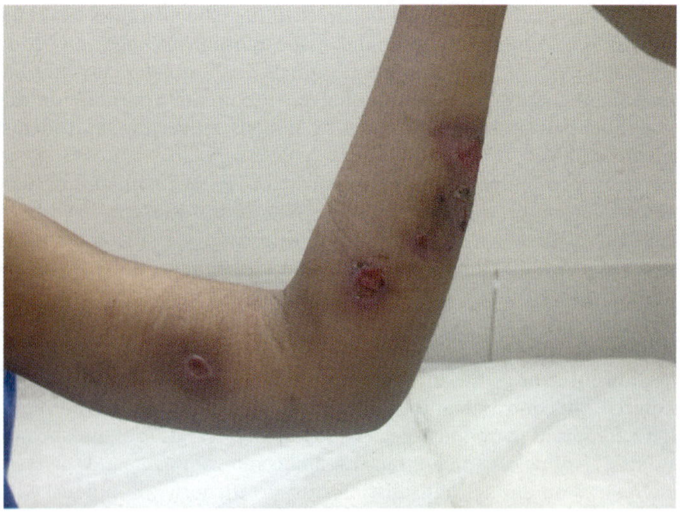

FIGURE 70-1. Lymphocutaneous sporotrichosis in a Brazilian child. (Reproduced with permission from Regina Schechtman, MD, PhD.)

with purulent drainage, and is generally not painful. Weeks after development of the initial lesion, additional lesions appear, typically as dermal and subcutaneous nodules and ulcers along the path of lymphatic drainage (often up the arm). This clinical description led to naming the disease as "ascending nodular lymphangitis."[30] This is the well-known "sporotrichoid" pattern. Usually, lesions located in the deep dermis or subcutaneous tissue result in skin scars [**Figure 70-1**].

In general, the fixed cutaneous form is characterized by infiltrated nodular, ulcerated, or erythmatosquamous lesions located on exposed areas where fungal inoculation occurred [**Figure 70-2**]. The lesions of fixed cutaneous sporotrichosis can appear granulomatous and disseminated lesions typically present as subcutaneous nodules. The disseminated cutaneous forms have mainly been observed among immunosuppressed patients, especially HIV-seropositive individuals.[31,32] Mucosal involvement is not common but may occur, and preferentially affects the ocular mucosa [**Figure 70-3**].[33] Among the extracutaneous forms, osteoarticular and pulmonary involvement are the most common, but there are reports of cases of severe hematogenic dissemination with involvement of multiple organs.

DIAGNOSIS

Sporotrichosis is the only subcutaneous mycosis for which direct examination or histology is of little or no value for diagnosis. The diagnosis rests solely on the isolation of *S. schenckii* in culture. This is best achieved by inoculation of pus on Sabouraud's glucose agar containing chloramphenicol and cycloheximide.[34]

Identification of *S. schenckii*—direct examination/biological samples: aspirate with purulent and seropurulent contents from gummy lesions. Pus need not be collected by painful aspiration from subcutaneous

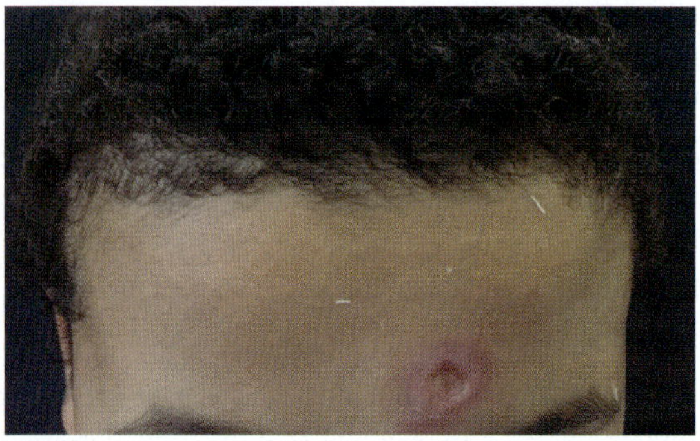

FIGURE 70-2. Fixed cutaneous sporotrichosis in a Brazilian boy. (Reproduced with permission from Regina Schechtman, MD, PhD.)

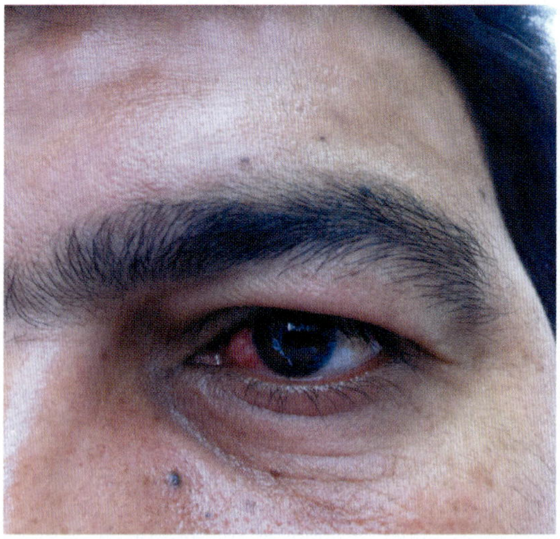

FIGURE 70-3. Hypersensitivity conjunctivitis due to zoonotic sporotrichosis in adult male. (Reproduced with permission from Regina Schechtman, MD, PhD.)

nodules but can be obtained from the ulcerated lesions; after removal of the dry, crusty surface, a small drop of milky pus can readily be recovered. A swab can be used from exudative and/or ulcerated lesions with draining tracts.[34]

Skin biopsy has to be obtained from the border of active lesions and divided into two fragments; one fragment should be fixed in 10% buffered formalin for histopathological examination and stained for hematoxylin and eosin (HE), Wade, Periodic acid-Schiff (PAS), Grocott staining. Another fragment should be kept in sterile saline for mycological examination. Direct microscopic exam is with wet mount preparation with 4% NaOH or 10% KOH. Organisms are rarely seen, except in immunocompromised host. In this case, we could observe, in special colorations like PAS or silver stain, various budding yeasts to cigar-shaped organisms.[34]

In specimen taken from skin biopsy, few organisms are seldom observed and are difficult to be identified. On HE preparations, granulomas with giant body cell are visualized and isolated oval yeast cells surrounded by an eosinophilic substance could be seen. They are called asteroid bodies.[35]

MICROSCOPIC MORPHOLOGY

This fungus is dimorphic with a mycelial phase and a yeast phase. The mycelial saprophytic phase is characterized by slender, hyaline, septated, and branched hyphae containing thin conidiophores whose apex forms a small vesicle with sympodially arranged denticles. Each denticle produces one conidium, each measuring approximately 2 to 4 μm and these conidia are arranged in flower-like groups. The conidia become detached from the conidiophores, sometimes being arranged side by side in a row bilaterally to the hyphae. The yeast parasitic phase is pleomorphic, showing spindle-shaped and/or oval cells measuring 2.5 to 5 μm in diameter and resembling a "cigar."[35]

MACROSCOPIC MORPHOLOGY

As organisms are not typically seen by KOH or histopathology examination, culture (of pus or tissue) is usually required to definitively diagnosis sporotrichosis.

Growth is rapid at 25°C, revealing raised moist colonies with a membranous aspect and a wrinkled or folded surface. In principle, the colonies are white to cream colored, later turning brown to dark gray and black. During subculture, the colonies may irreversibly lose their dark color, becoming creamy white.[35]

PATHOLOGY

Histological, both suppurative and granulomatous inflammation are seen in the dermis and subcutis. The causative organisms are rarely seen;

staining with fluorescent-labeled antibodies may aid in visualizing the cigar-shaped yeasts forms; however, the organisms are still difficult to identify. Asteroid bodies are also seen. When numerous fungi are present, as in the immunocompromised host, budding yeast to cigar-shaped organisms are often identified by PAS or silver stains.[35]

DIFFERENTIAL DIAGNOSIS

Due to the diversity of the clinical forms of sporotrichosis, there is also a vast set of differential diagnosis with other pathological conditions. Examples include leishmaniasis, nocardiosis, chromomycosis, tuberculosis, rosacea, noninfectious granulomatous diseases, and psoriasis, among others.

When there is a sporotrichoid pattern, the major entity to be excluded in endemic areas from Brazil is leishmaniasis. In Europe, Canada, and the United States, the major differential diagnosis is an atypical mycobacterial infection, in particular *Mycobacterium marinum*. Other less common causes are rhinoscleroma, granuloma inguinale, histoplasmosis, leishmaniosis, and *Penicillium marneffei* infection.

The differential diagnosis of fixed plaque sporotrichosis and disseminated lesions is broad and includes other granulomatous disorders, both infectious and inflammatory.

TREATMENT STRATEGIES

Topical therapy is not effective. Saturated solution of potassium iodide (SSKI) has been used with success. Although neither fungistatic nor fungicidal, SSKI is thought to affect the host's immune reaction to the organism. The recommended dose in adults is 250 mg or five drops of SSKI (one drop = 50 mg SSKI), increasing in increments of three drops (150 mg/dose) daily until a maximum dose of 30 to 40 drops (1.5-2.0 g) three times a day is achieved or until the patient experiences side effects. In children, the recommended dose is three drops three times a day, increasing by one drop per kilogram per dose to a maximum of 25 drops three times a day.[36] Its cost is low, but it has a bitter taste as well as potential side effects (eg, iododerma, gastrointestinal upset, and thyroid suppression). SSKI clearly is effective, but this agent have not been subjected to specific treatment trials comparing its efficacy against azoles or allylamine alternatives. Many factors can contribute to the shortage of relevant literature as follows. The duration of therapy in patients taking SSKI will also depend on drug compliance; treatment is limited by side effects; therapeutic dose should be maintained for up to 4 weeks beyond the time of total clinical cure.[5,37,38] Itraconazole, for example, is quite effective against sporotrichosis, compared to ketoconazole, for example, which is ineffective. In a study of 17 patients with lymphangitic and cutaneous sporotrichosis, all had significant clinical improvement and mycological cure when treated with 90 to 180 days of oral itraconazole (100 mg/day).[39] The drug is generally safe and well tolerated, and the relapse rate is low. Amphotericin B may be indicated in severe or disseminated disease.[40] Fluconazole is thought to be effective to fixed cutaneous sporotrichosis and disseminated disease with bone and joints involvement. Terbinafine could be another therapeutic alternative to treat the disease. Some investigators found that patients have demonstrated good response with terbinafine with few adverse reactions.[41] The dosage of terbinafine to treat sporotricosis can range from 250 to 1000 mg/day according to different studies.[42,43]

CONCLUSION

In conclusion, despite effective treatment, sporotrichosis is currently distributed throughout the world. Health professionals need to know control measures that include wearing gloves and long sleeves during high-risk activities such as handling sphagnum moss, wires, rose bushes, hay bales, conifer (pine) seedlings, or other materials that may facilitate the exposure to the fungus. Sporotrichosis in cats requires preventive measures to avoid transmission within the species and from animals to humans. Cats with sporotrichosis should be correctly treated and kept isolated in a proper place. Any physical contact with the animal should be avoided until complete healing of the lesions. When handling the sick cat, during either injury treatment or medication administration, protocols must be adopted to reduce exposure to the fungus, such as using latex gloves. Another important measure is not to abandon the animal, as this facilitates the dissemination of the disease. In the case of cats with extensive lesions and no possibility of treatment, euthanasia and cremation of the body should be standard procedures in a veterinary health centers.

REFERENCES

1. Heidrich D, Senter L, Valente P, Stopiglia CDO, Vetoratto G, Scroferneker ML. Successful treatment of terbinafine in a case of sporotrichosis. *An Bras Dermatol.* 2011;86(4Supl1):S182-S185.
2. Davis BA. Sporotrichosis. *Dermatol Clin.* 1996;14:69-76.
3. Hektoen L, Perkins CF. Refractory subcutaneous abscesses caused by *Sporothrix schenckii.* A new pathogenic fungus. *J Exp Med.* 1900;5:77-89.
4. De Beurmann CL, Gougerot H. *Les Sporotrichoses.* Parise7 Librairie Felix Alcan, Paris; 1912.
5. Ramos-e-Silva M, Vasconcelos C, Carneiro S, Cestari T. Sporotrichosis. *Clin Dermatol.* 2007;25:181-187.
6. Bennett JE. Sporothricosis. In: Kwon-Chung K, Bennet J, eds. *Medical Mycology.* 2nd ed. Philadelphia, PA: Lea & Febiger; 1992:707-729.
7. Travassos LR, Lloyd KO. *Sporothrix schenckii* and related species of ceratocystis. *Microbiol Rev.* 1980;44:683-721.
8. Da Silva Lacaz CS, Porto E, Martins JE, Heins-Vaccari Em, Melo NT, eds. *Tratado de Micologia Médica.* São Paulo, Brazil: Sarvier; 2002:479-497.
9. De Lima Barros MB. Estudo de uma série de casos de esporotricose atendidos no instituto de pesquisa clínica evandro chagas, Rio de Janeiro. Universidade Federal do Rio de Janeiro, Faculdade de Medicina. 2004.
10. Schubach TM, Schubach A, Okamoto T, et al. Evaluation of an epidemic of sporotrichosis in cats: 347 cases (1998-2001). *Jam Vet Med Assoc.* 2004;224:1623-1629.
11. Mackinnon JE, Conti-Diaz IA, Gezuele E, et al. Isolation of *Sporothrix schenckii* from nature and considerations on its pathogenicity and ecology. *Sabouraudia.* 1969;7:38-45.
12. Lopes JO, Alves SH, Mari CR, et al. Epidemiology of sporotrichosis in the central region of Rio Grande do Sul [im Portuguese] . *Rev Soc Bras Med Trop.* 1999;32:541-545.
13. Randhwa HS, Chand R, Mussa AY, Khan ZU, Kowshik T. Sporotrichosis in India: first case in a Delhi resident and an update. *Ind J Med Microbiol.* 2003;21:12-16.
14. Mohan N, Jayaseelan E, Abraham A, Rajendran SC, Stephen J, Sharief S, Macaden R. Cutaneous sporotrichosis in Bangalore, Southern India. *Int J Dermatol.* 2004;43:269-272.
15. Rippon JW. *Medical Mycology: The Pathogenic Fungi and the Pathogenic Actinomycetes.* Philadelphia, PA: WB Saunders; 1988:325-352.
16. De Lima Barros MB, de Oliveira Schubach A, Galhardo MC, et al. Sporotrichosis with widespread cutaneous lesions: report of 24 cases related to transmission by domestic cats in Rio de Janeiro, Brazil. *Int J Dermatol.* 2003;42:677-681.
17. Thompson Dw, Kaplan W. Laboratory-acquired sporotrichosis. *Sabouraudia.* 1977;15:167-170.
18. Cooper Cr, Dixon DM, Salkin IF. Laboratory-acquired sprotrichosis. *J Med Vet Mycol.* 1992;30:169-171.
19. Bustamante B, Campos PE. Endemic sprotrichosis. *Curr Opin Infect Dis.* 2001;14:145-149.
20. Kauffman CA. Sporotrichosis. *Clin Infect Dis.* 1999;29:231-236;quiz 237.
21. Moore JJ, Davis DJ. Sprotrichosis following mouse bite, with certain immunologic data. *J Infect Dis.* 1918;23:252-266.
22. Read SI, Sperling LC. Feline sprotrichosis. Transmission to man. *Arch Dermatol.* 1982;118:429-431.
23. Dunstan RW, Reimann KA, Langham RF. Feline sprotrichosis. *J Am Vet Med Assoc.* 1986;189:880-883.
24. Larsson CE, Goncalves MD, Araujo VC, et al. Feline sprotrichosis: clinical and zoonotic aspects. *Rev Inst Med Trop Sao Paulo.* 1989;31:351-358.
25. Conti Díaz I. Sporotrichosis in Uruguay: epidemiologic and clinical aspects. In: Proceedings of the Fifth International Conference of the Mycoses. Caracas: OPS, 1980: 312-21. (PAHO Scientific Publication, 396).
26. De Lima Barros MB, Schubach TM, Gutierrez-Galhardo MC, et al. Sporotrichosis: an emergent zoonosis in Rio de Janeiro. *Mem Inst Oswaldo Cruz.* 2001;96:777-779.
27. Schubach TMP, Schubach A, Okamoto T, et al. Canine sprotrichosis in Rio de Janeiro, Brazil: clinical presentation, laboratory diagnosis and therapeutic response in 44 cases (1998-20030). *Med Mycol.* 2006;44:87-92.

28. Ghosh A, Chakrabarti A, Sharma VK, Singh K, Singh A. Sporotrichosis in Himachal Pradesh (North India). *Trans Royal Soc Trop Med Hyg.* 1999;93:41-45.
29. Elgart ML. Subcutaneous and miscellaneous mycoses. In: Elewski BE, ed. *Cutaneous Fungal Infections.* Malden, Mass., USA : Blackwell Science, c1998. 1998:155-197.
30. Hoeprich PD. Sporotrichosis. In: Hoeprich PD, Jordan MC, Ronald AR, eds. *Infectious Diseases: A Treatise of Infectious Processes.* 5th ed. JB Lippincott, Philadelphia; 1994:1050-1054.
31. Shaw JC, Levinson W, Montanaro A. Sporotrichosis in the acquired immunodeficiency syndrome. *J Am Acad Dermatol.* 1989;21:1145-1147.
32. Donabedian H, O'Donnell E, Olszewski C, MacArthur RD, Budd N. Disseminated cutaneous and meningeal sporotrichosis in an aids patient. *Diagn Microbiol Infect Dis.* 1994;18:111-115.
33. Vieira-Dias D, Sena CM, Orefice F, Tanure MA, Hamdan JS. Ocular and concomitant cutaneous sporotrichosis. *Mycoses.* 1997;40:197-201.
34. De Vroey C. Identification of agents of subcutaneous mycoses. In: Evans EGV, Richardson MD, eds. *Medical Mycology: A Practical Approach.* IRL Press at Oxford University Press, New York. 1989:134-137.
35. Lacaz CS, Porto E, Heins-Vaccari EM, Melo NT. (1998) Guia para identificação: Fungos, actinomicetos e algas de interesse médico. Sarvier, São Paulo.
36. Bustamante B, Campos PE. Sporotrichosis: a forgotten disease in the drug research agenda. *Expert Rev Anti Infect Ther.* 2004;2:85-94.
37. Kauffman CA, Hajjeh R, Chapman SW. Practice guidelines for the management of patients with sporotrichosis. *Clin Infect Dis.* 2000;30:684-687.
38. Sterling JB, Heymann WR. Potassium iodide in dermatology: a 19th century potassium iodide in dermatology: a 19th century drug for the 21st century—uses, pharmacology, adverse effects, and contraindications. *J Am Acad Dermatol.* 2000;43:691-697.
39. Restrepo A, Robledo J, Gomez I, Tabares AM, Gutierrez R. Itraconazole therapy in lymphangitic and cutaneous sporotrichosis. *Arch Dermatol.* 1986;122:413-417.
40. Elewski BE, Hughey LC, Marchiony Hunt K, Hay RJ. Fungal Diseases. In: Dermatology. Editors: Bolognia JL, Schaffer JV, Cerroni L. 5th Ed. *Elsevier.* 2025. 1343-1376.
41. Hull PR, Vismer HF. Treatment of cutaneous sporotrichosis with terbinafine. *Br J Dermatol.* 1992;126(Suppl 39):51-55.
42. Chapman SW, Pappas P, Kaufman C, et al. Comparative evaluation of the efficacy and safety of two doses of terbinafine (500 and 1000 mg day) in the treatment of cutaneous or lymphocutaneous sporotricosis. *Mycoses.* 2004;47: 62-68.
43. Francesconi G, Valle AC, Passos S, Reis R, Galhardo MC. Terbinafine (250 mg/day): an effective and safe treatment of cutaneous sporotricosis in patients in whom itraconazole use is not possible. *J Eur Acad Dermatol Venereol.* 2009;23:1273-1276.

CHAPTER 71

Parasitic Infections

Shanelle Jackson
Shobita Rajagopalan
Susan C. Taylor

KEY POINTS

- Parasitic infestations and infections are encountered commonly in developing countries, where the environment is ideal for them to thrive. International travel to tropical destinations plays an important part in the acquisition of parasitic diseases.
- Factors such as geography, environment, and low socioeconomic status causing overcrowding and pollution, poor hygiene, food and water contamination, malnutrition, delayed access to medical care, and the presence of appropriate vectors play an important role in transmission of parasitic diseases.
- Skin diseases associated with parasitic infection or infestations, including scabies and cutaneous larva migrans, are encountered in skin of color patients.

INTRODUCTION

Parasites are ubiquitous in nature and associated with a variety of diseases in many different hosts. They are more common in regions of the world where various environmental factors, including climate, population dynamics, food and water sources, and the presence of appropriate vectors, enable them to thrive. In addition, host factors such as nutritional status and immune function play a key role in the transmission and acquisition of parasitic diseases and determine disease severity. Genetic susceptibility to specific parasites may also play a role. Susceptible individuals who travel to destinations where parasites are endemic are at increased risk for acquiring parasitic illnesses.

Racial differences in skin properties, such as including epidermal melanin content, melanosome dispersion, hair structure, and fibroblast and mast cell size and structure may explain differences in disease prevalence and presentation among different groups.[1-4]

Various skin disorders, including those caused by or associated with parasitic infection or infestation, are commonly encountered in people with skin of color, that is, African Americans, Asians, Hispanics/Latinos, and Native Americans. Complex interactions between the host factors, such as genetic makeup, nutritional status, and immune function, and environmental factors, such as geography and climate, play a key role in disease acquisition. Socioeconomic indicators such as poverty, overcrowding, and decreased access to medical care may also contribute to parasitic disease acquisition.[3,4]

This chapter will review some common and important parasitic illnesses that are known to cause significant skin disease in humans and focus on possible race-related variations in disease presentation. Skin manifestations of specific parasitic diseases that will be covered include the ectoparasitic infestations, pediculosis and scabies, the cutaneous migratory endoparasitic phenomenon known as cutaneous larva migrans, and the six plasmodium species of parasites that cause malaria.

SCABIES

BACKGROUND

Scabies is a common and highly contagious ectoparasitic infestation of global and public health significance caused by the arthropod *Sarcoptes scabiei* var. *hominis.* Scabies affects all individuals regardless of age, gender, race/ethnicity, or socioeconomic status. Worldwide, an estimated 300 million cases occur annually.[5,6] Prevalence rates in developing countries are higher than those in developed nations. The estimated prevalence of 0.2% to 71% was identified in a study in diverse global regions, with the highest rates occupying in areas of the Pacific and Latin American areas.[7] Overcrowding, poor hygiene, delayed diagnosis and treatment, and lack of public education are some of the factors that contribute to the prevalence of scabies in both industrial and nonindustrial nations. In developed countries, scabies epidemics occur primarily in institutional settings, such as prisons, long-term care facilities such as nursing homes, and hospitals. Common infestations by nonhuman strains occur and are caused by household animals like dogs and other animals. However, these infections are usually self-limiting.[8] Prevalence rates are observed to be higher in children and sexually active individuals than in other persons. The more severe and crusted variant of scabies, known as *Norwegian scabies* (so named because of its initial description in Norway in the mid-1800s), is common in patients with poor sensory perception due to entities such as leprosy and in immunocompromised persons (after organ or tissue transplantation or with human immunodeficiency virus [HIV] infection) and the aged.[9] These populations typically present with clinically atypical lesions and are frequently misdiagnosed, thus delaying treatment and enhancing the risk of local epidemics. Although scabies is a readily treatable infestation, it remains relatively common primarily because of diagnostic difficulty, inadequate treatment of patients and their contacts, and improper environmental control measures.

PATHOPHYSIOLOGY

The scabies mite is an obligate parasite and completes its entire 30 day life cycle on human skin.[10] Animal scabies mites may cause mild and transient symptoms in humans that generally do not persist. Prolonged direct contact with infected individuals facilitates transmission. Mild, humid environments are conducive to the prolonged survival of mites on the skin, which can endure for up to 3 days after leaving the skin. Due to their attraction to heat and odor, fomites such as infested bedding or clothing may serve as an additional rare transmission source.[11] After copulation, the male mite dies, and the female mite burrows into the superficial skin layers and lays a total of 60 to 90 eggs. The eggs incubate and hatch after 3 to 8 days. About 90% of the hatched mites die, but those that survive go through various stages of molting and reach maturity after approximately 2 weeks. The female adults, who never leave their burrows, die after 1 to 2 months. In classic scabies, 5 to 15 mites (range, 3-50) may live on the host skin. This figure is considerably less than the hundreds that are frequently observed on certain children or the millions that are seen in crusted (Norwegian) scabies.[11,12]

During the initial month of scabies infestation, infested individuals remain relatively asymptomatic. However, approximately 4 weeks of infestation and with subsequent infestations, a delayed-type hypersensitivity reaction develops to the mites, eggs, and scybala (packet of feces). With reinfestation, the sensitized individual may develop a rapid reaction (often within hours). The resulting skin eruption and its associated intense pruritus are the hallmark of classic scabies.

Norwegian Scabies In immunocompromised hosts, frail elderly persons, physically and/or mentally handicapped persons, or individuals with sensory nerve impairment, the fulminant distinctive and highly contagious hyperinfestation due to the crusted or Norwegian form of scabies is relatively common. In this variant of scabies, numerous mites infest the host. Rare cases have been described in immunocompetent patients. Extensive, widespread crusted lesions appear with thick, hyperkeratotic scales over the elbows, knees, palms, and soles. The number of mites in a patient with crusted scabies can exceed 1 million. In these cases, the mite can survive off the host for up to 7 days, feeding on the sloughed skin in the local environment, such as bed sheets, clothing, and chair covers. Failure to implement environmental control measures in this situation may result in relapse and reinfestation after successful treatment of the host. Serum immunoglobulin E (IgE) and immunoglobulin G (IgG) levels are extremely high in these patients, yet the immune reaction does not seem to be protective. Notably, young children are allegedly subjected to recurrent infestations within a brief period in endemic communities.[13] Cell-mediated immune responses in classic scabies demonstrate a predominantly CD4 T-cell infiltrate in the skin, whereas one study suggests CD8 T-cell predominance in crusted scabies. Atypical infestations also can occur in infants and young children.

CLINICAL MANIFESTATIONS

The historical aspects of scabies infestations are quite reliable in suggesting the diagnosis.[14] The incubation period prior to onset of symptoms depends on whether the infestation is an initial exposure or a relapse or reinfestation. Previously sensitized individuals can develop symptoms within hours of reexposure. The hypersensitivity reaction is responsible for the intense pruritus that is the clinical hallmark of the disease.

Lesion distribution, intractable pruritus that is worse at night, and similar symptoms in close contacts should immediately raise a high index of suspicion for scabies. Lesion distribution differs in adults and children. Adults manifest lesions primarily on the flexor aspects of the wrists, the interdigital web spaces of the hands, the dorsal feet, axillae, elbows, waist, buttocks, and genitalia.[15] Children under the age of 6 and older commonly had scalp, neck, and facial lesions as well.[13] Secondary lesions may occur as a result of rubbing and scratching, and they may be the only clinical manifestation of the disease. Pruritic papules and vesicles on the scrotum and penis in men and the areolae in women are highly characteristic. Infants and small children develop lesions predominantly on the face, scalp, neck, palms, and soles, although any site may be involved [**Figure 71-1**]. Widespread pruritic eczematous eruptions in any skin site are common in immunocompromised and elderly patients.

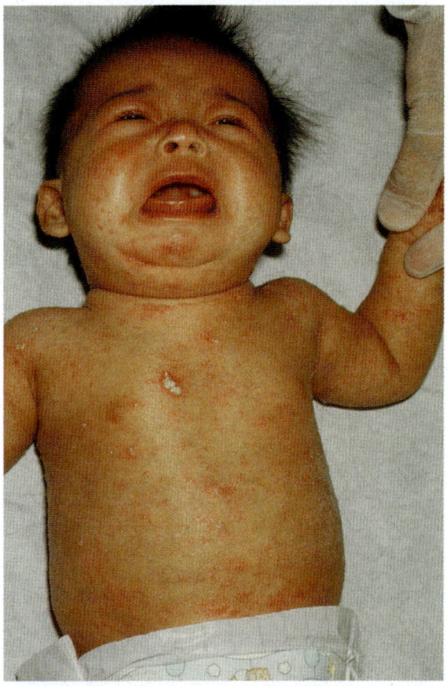

FIGURE 71-1. A Hispanic infant with generalized scabies.

Burrows are a pathognomonic sign of classic scabies and represent the intraepidermal tunnel created by the moving female mite. They appear as inapparent, serpiginous, grayish, threadlike elevations ranging from 2 to 10 mm long [**Figure 71-2**]. Common locations for burrows include the webbed spaces of the fingers; the flexor surfaces of the wrists, elbows, and axillae; the belt line; the feet; the scrotum in men; and the areolae in women. In infants, burrows are commonly located on the palms and soles. The actual mites are not visible to the naked eye and can be visualized only with microscopy. Burrows from the mites may become obscured by scratching the area.[16]

Complications of scabies are rare and generally result from vigorous rubbing and scratching. Disruption of the skin barrier puts the patient at risk for secondary bacterial invasion, primarily by *Streptococcus pyogenes* and *Staphylococcus aureus*. Superinfection with *S. pyogenes* can precipitate acute poststreptococcal glomerulonephritis and even rheumatic fever. More common pyodermas include impetigo and cellulitis, which rarely may result in sepsis. Scabies infestations can exacerbate underlying eczema, psoriasis, and other preexisting dermatoses. Even with appropriate treatment, scabies can leave in its wake the psychosocial burden of residual eczematous dermatitis and postscabietic pruritus, disturbances in sleep, productivity decline, and severe implications for quality of life as seen in 77% of patients in a study. Scabies may be debilitating and recalcitrant.[13,17] Crusted or Norwegian scabies with extensive involvement of the skin carries an increased mortality rate because of the frequency of secondary bacterial infections resulting in sepsis [**Figure 71-3**].

DIAGNOSIS

Dermoscopy Dermoscopy is a valuable diagnostic tool with high sensitivity (98.3%) and specificity (88.5%).[18] When scabies patients are examined using dermoscopy, the delta sign—the mite's mouth and front legs—can be seen. The position of the mite determines whether this indicator is visible; it may be nonexistent, clearly visible, or appear as a

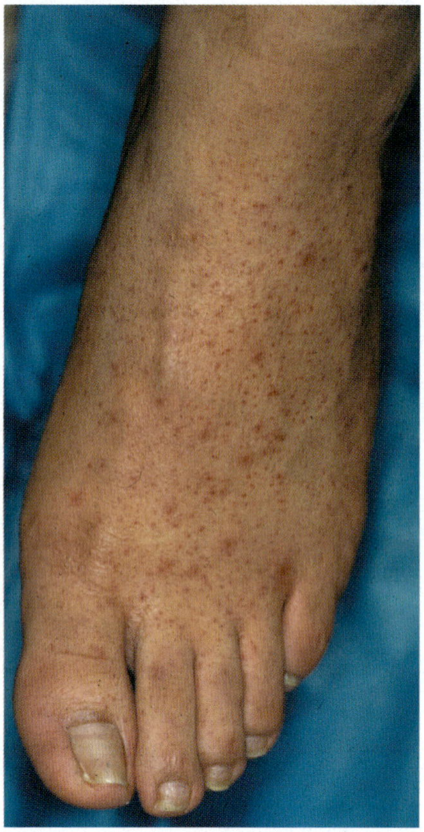

FIGURE 71-2. Classic scabies eruption showing burrows.

brown spot. This is especially true when the mite is deeper in the skin. Using UV dermoscopy equipment that combines UV light characteristics with polarized dermoscopy has been successful for diagnosis. With 365 nm UV light, the UV mode makes the mite and tunnel contents more visible. The UV dermoscope offers a more thorough imaging technique for diagnosis and therapy control because it shows the mite as a whole ball in contrast to polarized dermoscopy. When the mite's polarized mode is unclear, utilizing the mite's response can enhance the clarity of the diagnostic process.[19] Beyond diagnosis, dermoscopy is also helpful in monitoring the resolution of scabies posttreatment.[18]

Light Microcopy The diagnosis may also be confirmed by light microscopic identification of mites, larvae, ova, or scybala in skin scrapings.[20,21] In rare cases, mites are identified in biopsy specimens obtained to rule out other dermatoses. Characteristic histopathology common to a variety

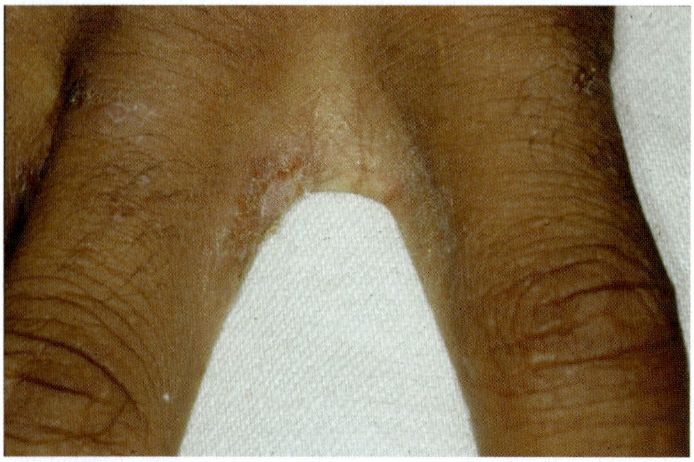

FIGURE 71-3. Scabies infestation of the finger and web spaces.

of arthropod reactions in the absence of actual mites also may suggest the diagnosis. Excision of a burrow may reveal mites, larvae, ova, and feces within the stratum corneum. A superficial and deep dermal infiltrate composed of lymphocytes, histiocytes, mast cells, and eosinophils is characteristic. Spongiosis and vesicle formation with exocytosis of eosinophils and occasional neutrophils is present. Biopsy of older lesions may be nondiagnostic and reveal fibrosis and scale crusts. Crusted scabies demonstrates massive hyperkeratosis of the stratum corneum with numerous mites in all stages of development. Psoriasiform hyperplasia of the underlying epidermis with spongiotic foci and occasional epidermal microabscesses is present. The dermis shows a superficial and deep chronic inflammatory infiltrate with interstitial eosinophils. Nodular variants of scabies reveal a dense, mixed, superficial, and deep dermal inflammatory cell infiltrate. Lymphoid follicles may be present, and the infiltrate occasionally extends into the subcutaneous fat.

Other Tests Elevated IgE titers and eosinophilia may be found in some patients with scabies. Clinically inapparent infection can be detected by amplification of *Sarcoptes* DNA in epidermal scale by polymerase chain reaction.[22]

TREATMENT

The mainstay of scabies treatment is the application of topical scabicidal agents and/or systemic drug treatment.[23,24] The following medications are approved by the U.S. Food and Drug Administration (FDA) for the treatment of scabies.

Permethrin Cream 5% (Brand Name: Elimite) Permethrin, the first-line treatment for scabies, is an FDA-approved synthetic pyrethroid that effectively kills both the mites and their eggs. Two (or more) applications topically, each about a week apart, may be necessary to eliminate all mites, particularly when treating severe crusted (Norwegian) scabies.

Ivermectin Ivermectin is a synthetic macrocyclic lactone belonging to the avermectin group of antibiotics. It is active against a number of human and animal endoparasites and ectoparasites. Ivermectin, although not FDA approved for scabies treatment, is effective in most cases of typical scabies at a dose of 200 to 250 μg/kg given at diagnosis and repeated in 7 to 14 days. Since the medication works by attacking the nerve and muscle function of larvae, nymph, and adult (mobile stages) only, this allows for the medication to treat any newly hatched eggs.[25] Crusted scabies may require three or more doses given at 1- to 2-week intervals. Ivermectin is an ideal agent in patients in whom topical therapy is difficult or impractical, such as in widespread institutional infestations and bedridden patients.[26,27] Ivermectin is contraindicated in patients with allergic sensitization or nervous system disorders and in women who are pregnant or breastfeeding. Children younger than 5 years or weighing less than 15 kg should not be treated with ivermectin.

Patients may experience pruritus for up to 2 weeks after successful treatment. If itching persists beyond this time, the patient must be reevaluated to ensure the correct diagnosis, adequate treatment, and simultaneous treatment of contacts and environment. A second treatment course may be indicated. Rarely, individuals with a history of atopy may require a tapered dose of prednisone for the treatment of severe pruritus. Intranodular injection of dilute corticosteroids may be necessary in patients with nodular scabies. Because of the heavy mite burden, patients with crusted scabies may require repeated applications of topical scabicides or simultaneous treatment with topical permethrin and oral ivermectin.

Symptomatic treatment may require oral antihistamines and topical antipruritics/anesthetics such as menthol and pramoxine. More severe symptoms may require a short course of topical or oral steroids. Secondary infections may require antibiotics, which should be prescribed based on culture and sensitivity.

Detailed verbal and written instructions are critical for compliance and complete eradication and prevention of spread to contacts and are as follows:

- Family members and close contacts must be evaluated and treated, even if they do not have symptoms. Pets do not require treatment.

All carpets and upholstered furniture should be vacuumed and the vacuum bags immediately discarded.

- Patients must be instructed to launder clothing, bed linens, and towels used within the last week in hot water the day after treatment is initiated and again in 1 week. Items that cannot be washed may be professionally dry cleaned or sealed in plastic bags for 1 week.
- Patients with crusted scabies or their caregivers should be instructed to remove excess scale to allow penetration of the topical scabicidal agent and decrease the burden of infestation. This can be achieved with warm-water soaks followed by application of a keratolytic agent such as 5% salicylic acid in petrolatum or Lac-Hydrin cream. (Salicylic acid should be avoided if large body surface areas are involved because of the potential risk of salicylate poisoning.) The scales then are debrided mechanically with a tongue depressor or similar nonsharp device.

Crotamiton 10% Lotion and Cream Crotamiton, although not as effective as topical permethrin, is FDA approved for treating scabies and has shown success when used for at least 28 days.[28] However, frequent treatment failures have been reported with crotamiton.

Lindane Lotion 1% Lindane is an FDA-approved organochloride for the treatment of scabies. Lindane is not recommended as a first-line therapy. Overuse, misuse, or accidentally swallowing lindane can be toxic to the brain and other parts of the nervous system; its use should be restricted to patients who have failed treatment with or cannot tolerate other medications that pose less risk. Because of reported neurotoxicity, lindane should not be used to treat premature infants, persons with a seizure disorder, women who are pregnant or breastfeeding, or infants and children, frail elderly, and persons who weigh less than 110 pounds and have compromised epidermal skin barrier function (marked irritation, erosions, ulcerations).

Antibiotics Topical antibiotic creams like mupirocin or fusidic acid are not advised for instances with widespread lesions; treatment for secondary severe bacterial infections is required. Targeting both *S. aureus* and Group A Streptococcus (GAS), as well as MRSA in some circumstances, is necessary for systemic antibiotics. Trophic endemic areas utilize oral trimethoprim-sulfamethoxazole (cotrimoxazole) or injectable benzathine penicillin G; nontropical sites may use pristinamycin, amoxicillin/clavulanic acid, or cephalexin. The accompanying itching is not advised to be treated in any particular way.

COMPLICATIONS

Treatment failures are uncommon if guidelines are followed. Residual pruritus may require antihistamines or a short course of topical or oral corticosteroids. Secondary bacterial infection usually as a result of *Streptococcus* or *Staphylococcus* species requires administration of an empirical course of antibiotics; although antibiotic susceptibility is usually predictable, culture and sensitivity data should be followed to appropriately tailor the regimen. Scabietic nodules may require intranodular corticosteroid injection for complete resolution. Flaring or reactivation of preexisting eczema or atopic dermatitis requires the use of standard eczema treatments.

PROGNOSIS

Prognosis is usually excellent with proper diagnosis and treatment in otherwise healthy individuals, as well as in immunocompromised or institutionalized hosts.

CUTANEOUS LARVA MIGRANS

BACKGROUND

Cutaneous larva migrans (CLM) is a common dermatology condition caused by the migratory larvae of animal hookworms characteristically encountered in travelers returning from tropical and subtropical destinations.[29] Cases have also been reported from the southwestern United States. CLM is characterized by an erythematous, serpiginous, pruritic cutaneous eruption caused by accidental percutaneous penetration and subsequent migration of larvae of various nematode parasites. The animal hookworm, *Ancylostoma braziliense*, is the species found most frequently in humans.[30,31] These hookworms generally live in the intestines of domestic pets such as dogs and cats who shed their eggs via feces to soil (usually moist soil and sandy areas of beaches or under houses). Humans are incidental hosts and are infected by contact with contaminated soil found in endemic areas of tropical and subtropical regions. The hookworm larvae burrow through intact skin and stay confined to the upper dermis. Migration of larvae through the skin results in an intensely pruritic, linear, or serpiginous track known as a *creeping eruption* [**Figure 71-4**]. Creeping eruptions are not unique to CLM and occur in many other human skin diseases.

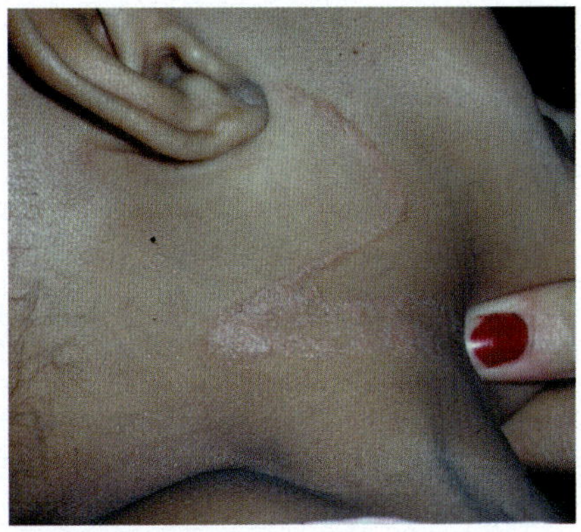

FIGURE 71-4. Cutaneous larva migrans.

In the United States, among helminthic infestations, CLM is rated second to pinworm. The condition is benign and self-limited but can cause a disturbing pruritus. There is neither a specific racial nor gender predilection for CLM; exposure to animal nematode larvae plays the key role in disease acquisition. In addition, CLM can affect persons of all ages, but it tends to be seen more commonly in children than in adults.

ETIOLOGY AND PATHOGENESIS

CLM is caused by several common variables of hookworms that may include the following:

- *Ancylostoma braziliense* (hookworm of wild and domestic dogs and cats) is the most common cause. It can be found in the central and southern United States, Central America, South America, and the Caribbean.
- *Ancylostoma caninum* (dog hookworm) is found in Australia.
- *Uncinaria stenocephala* (dog hookworm) is found in Europe.
- *Bunostomum phlebotomum* (cattle hookworm)
  Rare causes include the following:
- *Ancylostoma ceylonicum*
- *Ancylostoma tubaeforme* (cat hookworm)
- *Necator americanus* (human hookworm)
- *Strongyloides papillosus* (parasite of sheep, goats, and cattle)
- *Strongyloides westeri* (parasite of horses)
- *Ancylostoma duodenale*

The life cycle of the parasites begins when eggs are passed from animal feces into warm, moist soil, where the larvae hatch. The larvae initially feed on soil bacteria and molt twice before the infective third stage. By using proteases, larvae penetrate through follicles, fissures, or intact skin of the new host. After penetrating the stratum corneum, the larvae shed their natural cuticle and begin migration within a few days. In their natural animal hosts, the larvae are able to penetrate through the dermis by secreting hyaluronidase and are transported via the lymphatic and venous systems to the lungs.[32] They break through into the alveoli and migrate to the trachea, where they are swallowed. In the intestine, they mature sexually, and the cycle begins again as their eggs are excreted. Humans are accidental hosts, and the larvae are believed to lack the collagenase enzymes required to penetrate the basement membrane to invade the dermis. Therefore, the disease remains limited to the skin when humans are infected.

CLINICAL FEATURES

Patients complain of tingling or prickling at the site of exposure within 30 minutes of penetration of larvae and then intense pruritus. The affected area can appear as erythematous, linear lesions that traverse the skin. CLM is frequently associated with sunbathing, walking barefoot on the beach, or similar exposure in tropical areas.[20,21] Predispositions include hobbies and occupations that involve contact with warm, moist sandy soil and tropical/subtropical travel. Persons at risk include those who walk barefoot or sunbathe on the beach, children in sandboxes, carpenters, electricians, plumbers, farmers, gardener, and pest exterminators.

Cutaneous signs include pruritic, erythematous, edematous papules and/or vesicles; serpiginous, slightly elevated, erythematous tunnels that are 2- to 3-mm wide and track 3 to 4 cm from the penetration site; nonspecific dermatitis; vesicles with serous fluid; secondary impetiginization; and tract advancement of 1 to 2 cm/day. Systemic signs may include peripheral eosinophilia (Löffler syndrome), migratory pulmonary infiltrates, and increased IgE levels but are rarely seen. Lesions typically are distributed on the distal lower extremities, including the dorsal surfaces of the feet and the interdigital spaces of the toes but also can occur in the anogenital region, the buttocks, the hands, and the knees.

Differential diagnosis includes allergic contact dermatitis, epidermal dermatophytosis, erythema chronicum migrans, migratory myiasis, photoallergic dermatitis, and larva currens caused by *Strongyloides stercoralis*.

DIAGNOSIS

Diagnosis is based primarily on the classic clinical appearance of the eruption.

Dermoscopy has proven to show limitations in diagnosing CLM. A study reported the rate of correct diagnosis being less than 2%.[33] Brown patches on dermoscopy most likely relate to dilated lymphatic pathways rather than the larva's body. The idea that the lymphatic system plays a role in the spread of CLM supports this hypothesis[34]

Ultrasound (US), a noninvasive modality, is helpful for both diagnosing and tracking the course of treatment for CLM, particularly in unusual cases. Under the epidermis, tiny linear hyperechoic and hyperrefringent structures indicate larval fragments. In addition, inflammatory signs unique to the United States and hypoechoic dermal and hypodermal tunnels matching with lymphatic duct dilatation can corroborate the diagnosis. On the other hand, this useful diagnostic tool's restricted availability is a disadvantage.[35]

Serum studies have demonstrated peripheral eosinophilia on a complete blood count and increased IgE levels on total serum immunoglobulin determinations.

Histology from skin biopsy samples from the advancing edge of a tract may show via periodic acid-Schiff larva in a suprabasalar burrow, basal layer tracts, spongiosis with intraepidermal vesicles, necrotic keratinocytes, and an epidermal and upper dermal chronic inflammatory infiltrate with many eosinophils.

TREATMENT

Although the condition is self-limited, the intense pruritus and risk for infection mandate treatment.[36] Topical modalities such as ethyl chloride spray, liquid nitrogen, phenol, piperazine citrate, electrocautery, and radiation have been unsuccessfully because their effectiveness is limited for multiple lesions and the need for daily applications for several days. Topical application of a 10% to 15% thiabendazole solution, ointment, or cream to the affected area has been shown to be effective.[36-40]

Systemic treatment with oral ivermectin or oral albendazole is currently considered the treatment of choice, with ivermectin being preferred. Other effective alternative treatments include albendazole, mebendazole, and ivermectin. The treatment course results in decreased pruritus within 24 to 48 hours, and lesions/tracts resolve in 1 week.

Ivermectin Ivermectin, briefly described in the section on scabies, is also active against *Onchocerca volvulus* and other nematodes, including gastrointestinal helminths. Its mechanism of action is poorly understood.[41,42] A single 12-mg dose for adults and in pediatric patients 150 to 200 ug/kg of ivermectin is recommended for the treatment of patients with CLM. The dose can be repeated if the patient is not cured after the initial dose.[43]

Albendazole Albendazole is a third-generation heterocyclic antihelminthic drug used in the treatment of intestinal helminth infections including ascariasis, enterobiasis, ancylostomiasis, trichuriasis, and strongyloidiasis. Albendazole treatment of CLM with a twice-daily dose of 400 mg for 3 to 7 consecutive days and an 800 mg daily dose for 3 consecutive days has yielded successful results.[43-47] However, other studies suggest that a regimen of 400 to 800 mg/day for 3 to 5 days is appropriate for tourists with CLM.[48] Albendazole is generally well tolerated when used for the treatment of CLM, although gastrointestinal pain and diarrhea from the 800 mg dosage for 3 consecutive days has been reported.[48,49]

Thiabendazole Thiabendazole has been used in the oral treatment of CLM.[40,50-52] Thiabendazole is minimally effective when given as a single dose. The best results have been observed with 50 mg/kg/week of oral thiabendazole for 4 weeks.[36] However, thiabendazole is less well tolerated than either albendazole or ivermectin. Reported adverse effects include nausea, vomiting, dizziness, and headache.[53]

COMPLICATIONS

Complications such as secondary bacterial infection, usually with *S. pyogenes*, may lead to cellulitis and impetigo, or prolonged pruritus.

PROGNOSIS

The prognosis of CLM is excellent. This is a self-limiting disease. Humans are accidental, dead-end hosts, with the larva dying and the lesions resolving within 4 to 8 weeks or as long as a year in rare cases.

PREVENTION

Persons who travel to tropical regions and pet owners should be made aware of CLM. Because tourists are usually infected by walking or lying on tropical sandy beaches contaminated by dog feces, the best way to prevent CLM is to wear shoes when walking in sandy areas. It also may be prudent to lie on sand washed by the tide or to use a mattress; avoid lying on dry sand, even on a towel.

MALARIA

BACKGROUND

Malaria, a parasitic illness, is commonly found in tropical and subtropical regions. The revised WHO estimate places malaria's contribution to the worldwide illness burden at 7.8%, up from the earlier estimate of 4.8%. In 2020 alone, the cases and deaths exceeded 240 million and 600,000, respectively.[54] Malaria is one of the infectious diseases with the most significant mortality with 1.5 to 2.7 million deaths per year. The bulk of these deaths are caused by *Plasmodium falciparum* infections in children under the age of 5.[55]

ETIOLOGY AND PATHOPHYSIOLOGY

The most common vectors of malaria transmission are female *Plasmodium* parasites, which infect red blood cells after being introduced into the bloodstream by an Anopheles mosquito bite, commonly at night. Other modes of transmission include nosocomial transmission, direct inoculation, organ transplantation or blood transfusions, and vertical transfer from the mother.[56-58] The vast range of hosts that are vulnerable to infection by more than 200 species of *Plasmodium*, including mosquitos and animals as well as humans, is primarily defined by host specificity. In comparison to the five species that cause malaria in humans (*P. falciparum, P. vivax, P. malariae, P. ovale, P. knowlesi*), *P. falciparum* causes the most severe presentation.[59]As for this species, the most common geographical location for infectivity is Africa, where coinfection with *P. malariae* or *P. ovale* commonly occurs.[60]

Types of *Plasmodium* species that cause malaria in humans:

The mosquito, anopheles gambiae, is one of the African species that serves as an excellent example of an efficient malaria vector.[61] These mosquitoes are known for their long lifespans, ability to breed readily, ability to live in significant numbers in tropical climates, tendency to rest and bite inside human habitations, and preference for biting humans over other animals.

Since the parasite's life cycle (sporogony) in mosquitoes lasts between 8 and 30 days—from gametocyte consumption to subsequent inoculation—mosquitoes play a critical role in the spread of malaria. When introduced into the bloodstream of a human host by a mosquito bite, sporozoites navigate to the liver, where they can transform into latent hypnozoites (unique to *P. vivax* and *P. ovale*) or asexually reproduce within the hepatocyte. The latter phase leads to the liberation of merozoites back into the circulation, promoting the spread the infection.

After spreading over the surrounding area, the merozoites mature into male and female gametocytes for sexual reproduction, which are then developed into ring-stage trophozoites within another red blood cell (RBC). After maturing, some gametocytes are released into the bloodstream, where another mosquito can consume them. The gametocyte in the mosquito develops into viable gametes, oocytes, and sporozoites in 2 to 3 weeks. The sporozoite migrates to the mosquito's salivary gland so that when it feeds again, it is transferred to the new mammalian host for infection. The type of *Plasmodium* and the temperature of the surroundings affect how long this process takes.[62]

The importance of mosquito lifespans in malaria control efforts is highlighted by the requirement that mosquitoes survive for more than 10 days for sporozoites to mature, which is necessary for successful malaria transmission.

CLINICAL MANIFESTATION

The initial signs and symptoms are nonspecific and can include chills, fever, tachycardia, malaise, and other symptoms. Malaria fever frequently appears at random intervals; in more severe instances, convulsions may accompany the fever. Certain *Plasmodium* species can cause synchronous febrile paroxysms, which happen every other day at regular intervals (*P. vivax, P. ovale*, and *P. falciparum*) or every third day (*P. malariae*) when their infected red blood cells rupture. Physical evidence can include a palpable spleen and symptoms associated with anemia. Results from the laboratory may show minor coagulopathy, anemia, thrombocytopenia, increased transaminases, and parasitemia.[63] Most malaria patients report fever, headaches, and general malaise; however, specific symptoms are rare. Misdiagnosis can sometimes result from digestive problems, jaundice, or respiratory symptoms. Malaria infections are frequently misdiagnosed as influenza, gastroenteritis, hepatitis, or nonspecific viral illnesses.[64]

Children are more likely to appear with general discomfort, tiredness, malaise, and gastrointestinal symptoms.[65,66] Except for the presence of fever, which may not always be apparent and may not display a discernible pattern, physical examination results for patients with uncomplicated malaria are usually normal. Children are more likely than adults to exhibit somnolence, splenomegaly, and hepatomegaly. Patients with severe malaria may exhibit jaundice, disorientation, or seizures if *falciparum* malaria diagnosis is delayed.[67]

LABORATORY DIAGNOSIS

Laboratory diagnosis is essential in preventing overtreatment. Treating patients only based on their symptoms is commonly done in resource-limited areas. Still, it is not encouraged because it raises the possibility of medication resistance, wastes already scarce resources, and adds to the persistent opposition of medical professionals to use the results of diagnostic tests to direct treatment.[68]

Microscopy Giemsa-stained blood smear examination via light microscopy to visualize parasites is standard. This modality should be first line in nonresource-limited endemic settings where experienced and well-trained personnel are available.[69] It is utilized to identify the species and quantify the parasitemia. Blood smears can be classified as thin or thick, depending on whether the erythrocyte shape and integrity are preserved or not, respectively. Both measures can analyze the density, but thin blood smears determine the parasite species, and thick blood smears can determine the absence or presence of parasites. Microscopy should be repeated if the results are initially negative.

Malaria Rapid Diagnostic Tests (MRDT) This technique, which detects antigen or antibody, is ideal in endemic areas that are resource-limited since it does not require a laboratory or electricity and can be performed by personnel with limited training. Results are rapid and are obtained in less than 20 minutes. Immunochromatographic strip (ICS) technology is the foundation of most MRDTs. The device is filled with a liquid sample, often blood, which is then briefly incubated with lysing agents releasing protein from the parasite, buffer solution, and an anti-*Plasmodium* indicator antibody that has been tagged. The solution then migrates down the strip toward capture antibodies that are particular to the indicator antibodies already attached to the parasite antigens or to other epitopes on the antigens. A visible line appears on the immunochromatographic strip, signifying a positive test result.[68]

Rapid diagnostic tests (RDTs) give a practical self-testing alternative when medical professionals are unavailable. A study on malaria self-testing (n = 153) yielded a reported sensitivity of 95% and specificity of 97%; results showed that 84% said it was straightforward to follow the directions, and 75% said it was easy. However, 11% experienced problems that resulted in invalid tests, such as poor blood capture or trouble reading the card. The study highlights that even during a negative test, symptomatic persons should still seek a diagnosis from a healthcare expert. Fixing technical problems with this test to avoid false negatives is crucial. However, this alternative appears appropriate for people who cannot see a medical professional promptly.[70]

Molecular Tests Despite being more sensitive than microscopy, PCR diagnostics can only be used in a lab setting. It is not recommended for critically ill patients due to its lengthy turnaround time for findings and the need for training for optimal performance. Loop-mediated isothermal amplification (LAMP) technology simplifies the process by operating at a single temperature with simple tools like a heating block or water bath. It does away with the need for sophisticated, costly equipment like PCR thermocyclers. [Under isothermal circumstances, the reaction uses a particular set of primers to initiate autocycling strand-displacement DNA synthesis, which produces a highly precise and efficient amplification in under 1 hour. Changes in turbidity or UV fluorescence allow for visual detection, eliminating the need to open reaction tubes after amplification and lowering the possibility of DNA contamination.][71] With specificities and sensitivities higher than 95%, LAMP assays help identify low-level malaria parasites.[72] Although LAMP is not anticipated to displace conventional diagnostic instruments, it does show promise as a sensitive molecular substitute. It helps evaluate returning travelers in nonendemic environments, screening pregnant women for malaria in low-transmission areas, and eliminating malaria.[73]

TREATMENT

Uncomplicated Malaria Artemisinin combination therapy (ACT) is a uniformly successful treatment for chloroquine-resistant and sensitive *P. falciparum* malaria. When ACTs are unavailable, quinine plus clindamycin or atovaquone-proguanil are good alternatives for treating malaria resistant to the chloroquine drug. Where it is sensitive, chloroquine is still an effective treatment when ACTs are unavailable.[54] A more extended ACT therapy or atovaquone-proguanil duration may be required in areas where artemisinin-resistant malaria is prevalent.[74] The World Health Organization (WHO) advises ACT or chloroquine for uncomplicated malaria in cases of *P. vivax*, *P. ovale*, *P. malariae*, and *P. knowlesi*, which are usually chloroquine-sensitive. ACT should be avoided in pregnant women in the first trimester.[54] ACT is advised in place of chloroquine in areas where *P. vivax* resistance to chloroquine is present. When parasites are seen microscopically 48 hours after treatment.[75,76]

Severe Malaria Intravenous administration of at least three dosages of artesunate is the recommended course of treatment. When the parasite density reaches 1% or lower, and the patient can tolerate oral medications, oral artemisinin-based combination therapy (ACT) is initiated in its entirety.[77] It is critical to monitor for hemolysis delayed after artemisinin treatment, as intravenous quinidine is no longer accessible in the United States.[78]

Children In regions where *P. falciparum* is known to cause chloroquine resistance, quinine sulfate oral administration at 25 mg/kg/day in three doses for 3 to 7 days is one option for treating uncomplicated malaria. Another is tetracycline oral intake at 6.25 mg/kg four times daily for 7 days (maximum 1 g/day if over 8 years old), or an alternative is clindamycin oral intake at 7.5 mg/kg four times a day.[66]

PREVENTION

Insecticides Indoor residual spraying (IRS) and long-lasting insecticide-treated netting (ITNs), in addition to many other approaches, constitute the majority of malaria prevention methods that utilize insecticides. IRS uses carbamates, organochlorides, organophosphates, and pyrethroids, as recommended by the WHO. Insecticide resistance develops due to the substantial selection pressure imposed on vector populations by the widespread use of insecticides for agricultural purposes and large-scale malaria control programs.[79] The absence of consistent monitoring in anopheline vector populations across all nations contributes to the ambiguity surrounding the extent of insecticide resistance.

Personal Protective Strategies Reducing exposure to mosquito bites—especially those from Anopheles mosquitoes, which feed primarily at night—is the principal strategy for preventing malaria. Important preventive tactics include taking personal protective precautions including using bed nets impregnated with permethrin and covering exposed skin.[80] Applying permethrin on clothing and applying insect repellent, such as DEET (20-50% diethyltoluamide) or picaridin, on exposed skin are additional examples of personal protection strategies.[81]

Prophylactic Treatment Prophylactic treatment for visitors to malaria-endemic areas taken before departure, while in endemic areas, and continued as predetermined by the provider should be recommended. It is important to note that prophylactic medication does not replace the necessity for personal safety precautions.[80]

Vaccinations To protect children living in endemic areas from *P. falciparum* malaria, the World Health Organization authorized the first widely used malaria vaccine (RTS,S) in 2021. More than a million children have received this vaccination in Ghana, Malawi, and Kenya. The vaccine's approval is good news because it represents a significant advancement in the fight against malaria.[82] Pre-erythrocytic, erythrocytic, transmission-blocking, and multistage are the four primary phases of the parasite lifecycle targeted in developing malaria vaccines. Notably, recent developments have concentrated on prime-boost DNA vaccines. DNA plasmids prime the immunological response, further enhanced by recombinant or viral proteins. Clinical trials are now being conducted on this vaccination method.[55]

PEDICULOSIS HUMANUS CAPITIS

INTRODUCTION

Lice, parasitic insects that live in hairy areas of the body, have long been a cause for concern and have carried a significant social stigma. Current research offers a more complete viewpoint and new research suggests that lice infestations are widespread occurring in all socioeconomic groups. Infections are seldom associated with unsanitary housing circumstances or inadequate personal cleanliness. This revised view alleviates the social disapproval linked to lice infestations in many societies.[83]

EPIDEMIOLOGY

Head lice infestations are more commonly seen in children than adults, impacting millions of school-aged children yearly.[84,85] It is widespread in tropical countries and often affects those with limited access to resources, including people living in rural or low-income locations where proper treatment may be unavailable.[86,87] Head lice, in contrast to *Pediculus humanus corporis*, have significantly smaller bodies and have not been conclusively proven to transmit infectious illnesses.[88] Contrary to prevalent misunderstandings, the frequency of hair brushing or shampooing does not impact the likelihood of head lice infection, and it is not connected to the length of the hair.[89]

LIFE CYCLE

The life cycle of lice consists of three primary phases: eggs or nits, nymphs, and adults. Adult female lice intentionally place nits, which appear as small yellow or white granules, at the base of the hair shaft. Nits may resemble dandruff or residue and they have the potential to alter their color to assimilate with the hair, which presents difficulties in their identification. The incubation period for eggs is 8 to 9 days which is supported by body heat.[89] Nymphs, the early stage in the development of a louse, hatch from eggs and proceed through maturation and become fully grown adults in 9 to 12 days. At this crucial stage, lice reach sexual maturity, which is essential for the ongoing life cycle.[85]

Adult head lice, which resemble sesame seeds, are 3 mm in size and have a brown or gray appearance and six legs.[90] They typically inhabit the human scalp for about 30 days, relying on blood as their primary source of nutrients, eating four times per day. This feeding action causes the host to experience pain and itching. Adult lice rely on the scalp for nourishment as well as essential elements such as warmth, shelter, and moisture, which are vital for their existence. The viability of lice is generally diminished when the eggs are located more than 1 cm away from the scalp. Adult head lice die after 1 to 2 days when removed from a blood supply.[90,91] After a short 2-day period in the adult stage, lice engage in mating once. Following this, a fertilized female can lay 2 to 10 eggs daily for the remainder of the life span.[91]

TRANSMISSION

In addition to the scalp, lice may be detected in the posterior auricular area as well as in the eyebrows and eyelashes. The primary method of transmission is direct contact between people and contact with bedding, caps, and hair care implements.[85,92]

CLINICAL MANIFESTATIONS

Symptoms of head lice infestation include a crawling sensation in the scalp. Pruritus occurs commonly due to an allergic reaction to the saliva left behind by head lice while feeding. Saliva has anticoagulant properties that aid in bloodsucking, and itching sensations usually arise after sensitization, which normally occurs a few weeks after the initial infection.[89] Increased nocturnal lice activity may result in insomnia in certain individuals. Excessive scratching can lead to the formation of sores that may become infected.[83,93]

DIAGNOSIS

To accurately diagnose lice infestation, it is necessary to identify live lice on the scalp. They are usually diagnosed with the naked eye using bright light and magnification. However, finding live lice might be difficult because they tend to avoid light and are fast.[89] For increased diagnostic accuracy, it is advisable to utilize a lice comb to separate the hair and view the lice and nits that become attached to the comb.[94,95]

PEDICULOSIS CORPIS

INTRODUCTION

Pediculus humanus humanus, termed body lice, is a parasite infection that differs from pediculosis capitis or pediculosis pubis. This parasite is found in the seams of clothing and feeds on the human body excluding the pubis and scalp. Body lice infestations are more prevalent in adults than in children.[84]

RISK FACTORS

The unhoused and individuals who sleep in public locations are often found to have body lice infestation. It is particularly prevalent among persons grappling with drug abuse, including alcohol and tobacco addiction, as well as those facing difficulties in maintaining consistent hygienic routines.[96,97] Vulnerable groups encompass those with untreated mental health issues who encounter challenges in adhering to traditional sanitary procedures.[98] These variables contribute to the higher probability of body lice infestations in certain demographic groups, providing insight into the complex nature of this parasitic problem among different vulnerable communities.

LIFE CYCLE

Body lice demonstrate a unique pattern of depositing eggs within the seams, creases and crevices of garments, a vital component of their life cycle and activity. Maintaining humidity levels within the range of 70% to 90% is crucial to establish ideal circumstances for egg hatching. This ensures that newly born lice may quickly migrate to the skin to feed before returning to the clothing. Body lice exhibit optimal physiological activity in the temperature range of 29 to 32°C. While head lice may live a few days when separated from the human body, body lice can exist for up to 60 days when separated. When body temperatures increase during fever or vigorous physical exertion, body lice leave the host, demonstrating their capacity to adjust to external circumstances.[99,100]

CLINICAL MANIFESTATIONS

Symptoms and signs linked to infestation include pruritic papules and vesicles, abrasions, and inflamed skin. The presence of prurigo nodules, lichenification, and hyperpigmentation signals chronic infestation. The cycle of pruritus and scratching predisposes to the secondary bacterial infections, impetigo, ecthyma, or cellulitis. The variety of skin symptoms emphasizes the need for comprehensive treatment approaches to tackle both the infestation and the resulting cutaneous eruptions.[2,101]

DIAGNOSIS

When evaluating individuals for possible body lice infestations, it is essential to conduct a comprehensive evaluation of garments for lice as well as stains that may suggest serum, blood, or louse excrement. Furthermore, a complete blood count is appropriate to evaluate for severe iron deficiency anemia resulting from the loss of blood.[102-104] Eosinophilia may also be observed.[102,104] These evaluations provide insight into the patient's health status and guides the practitioner in determining the appropriate therapeutic intervention.[105-107]

PTHIRUS PUBIS

INTRODUCTION

Pthirus pubis, also termed pubic or crab lice, was initially described in 1892.[108] Although rare, pubic lice have been detected on the scalp and eyelashes.[109] Pubic lice measure 0.8 to 1.2 mm in length and have a width that is about the same as their length. This gives them a less oval form compared to head and body lice. Pubic lice possess caudal legs that are fashioned like claws, even though they have the same number of legs as other types of lice.[110]

LIFE CYCLE

The typical female pubic louse lays three nits daily, with an incubation period of 7 to 8 days before hatching. The duration of adulthood for pubic lice is comparatively briefer than that of head and body lice, lasting 15 days. Data on the life cycle of the pubic louse offer valuable insights into their reproductive activity and lifespan, enhancing our understanding of their biology and potential consequences for persons afflicted by this parasitic infestation.[111]

TRANSMISSION

Transmission is primarily through sexual contact, highlighting the importance of thorough screening for reported concomitant disease. Individuals diagnosed with pubic lice should be screened for HIV, syphilis, gonorrhea, chlamydia, herpes, warts, and trichomonas infections. Knowledge regarding potential associated diseases with pubic lice facilitates the delivery of complete treatment for affected patients.[84,112]

CLINICAL MANIFESTATIONS AND DIAGNOSIS

Pubic lice have been reported to occur the scalp and eyelashes. In the pubic area, clinical manifestations include the presence of blood droplets and crusts and resulting discoloration of undergarments.[84] Pruritus and lesions as a result of excoriation are also prominent manifestations. Deep hemosiderin deposition may lead to the formation of maculae ceruleae, which are blue-gray macules situated in the proximal lower extremities and lower abdomen.[113]

TREATMENT

It is essential to begin treatment for lice infestation only when the diagnosis is verified to prevent the development of treatment resistance. It is important to prioritize the use of prescription pediculicides, as they have demonstrated minimal resistance.[85] When deciding on a treatment strategy, a thorough assessment including the individual's age and body size, as well as the toxicity levels of the pharmaceutical agents is important.[93] Prompt detection, appropriate medical intervention, and efficient control of the environment are central in preventing the spread of lice and reducing their impact on household contacts.

- **Environmental modalities.** Effective management of the environment is a key component to the successful treatment of lice. For treatment of head lice, sanitizing objects that have come into contact with the head include hair care implements, hats, scarves and bedding is essential. For body and pubic lice, washing and drying all garments worn by the impacted individual at temperatures of no less than 50°C (130°F) for a minimum duration of 40 minutes is required. To eradicate unhatched eggs, sealing items that cannot be washed in plastic bags for 2 weeks is recommended.[100,104,114,115] Although home fumigation is not advised, vacuuming furniture, bedding, carpets, vehicle seats, and items that are fabric-covered is recommended. If this is not feasible, abstaining from using upholstered furniture and mattresses for 3 to 5 days will eradicate lice who cannot live without a human host.[89,93,115] Finally, household members and sexual partners of infected individuals must be treated to ensure eradication of lice.[116]
- **Manual Extraction**, a convenient and safe approach for diagnosing and treating head lice, may be used as an alternate or additional therapeutic method to pharmaceuticals. Wet combing or manually removing lice and nits performed meticulously and consistently for a minimum of 5 minutes to many hours has been demonstrated to be effective.[89] The process entails dividing dampened hair into multiple sections, using a lubricating conditioner or substance, and then meticulously combing each segment of hair with a lice comb every 2 days until there are no live lice detected for a continuous period of 10 days.[113] The teeth of the comb should be spaced no more than 0.3 mm apart. Although this approach is affordable and does not require intrusive procedures or pharmaceuticals, it does require a significant amount of time, patience, and careful attention to detail. The process is most effective when conducted after washing and

detangling the hair. It is also recommended for the removal of nits post-pharmaceutical treatment, as pediculicides do not assure complete elimination of ova activity.

- **Permethrin 1% Lotion and Cream**, an FDA-approved nonprescription pediculicidal agent, is a safe and recommended therapy for persons aged 2 months and older. It is classified under pregnancy category B.[89,117] Debuted in the 1980s, its cost-effectiveness renders it a prudent treatment option. Permethrin exerts a neurotoxic effect on hatched lice, leading to their death. Although it does not directly destroy eggs, it leaves a residue that explicitly targets their eradication.[118] If live lice continue to exist after 7 days and to target newly hatched eggs, reapplication is recommended after 7 days.[119] For head lice, to insure efficacy of permethrin treatment, it is advisable to refrain from using conditioning shampoos or conditioners before treatment and apply the permethrin lotion to damp hair with a contact time of 10 minutes, before washing out.[85] For body lice, permethrin is applied to the skin from the neck to the toes including the soles and interdigital spaces, with a contact time of 8 to 14 hours before washing off. For pubic lice, a 20-minute application time to the pubic area is recommended. Adverse events include itching, redness, and swelling, with limited injury to animals.[89] Permethrin resistance is a proven concern in some situations.
- **Pyrethrins and Piperonyl Butoxide** is an FDA-approved over-the-counter options derived from chrysanthemum extract that is recommended for those 2 years old and older. This combination product is offered as mousse, shampoo, or lotion, which is applied to the infested area for 10 minutes before rinsing. For the continued presence of live lice, it is advisable to administer a second treatment after 7 days.[119,120] While pyrethrins have a low impact on mammals, they have neurotoxic effects on lice. Nevertheless, this therapy cannot kill nits due to the absence of a nervous system in nits and reapplication after 7 days when the eggs have hatched is recommended.[118] Reapplication entails following the identical procedure as that for 1% permethrin.[119] The presence of resistance is a significant obstacle, hence diminishing the efficacy of this therapy.[121] Adverse occurrences have been reported as well as a rise in the rate of deaths related to cardiovascular issues.[122]
- **Dimethicone Lotion 4%** is a nonprescription pediculicidal agent that kills head lice and eggs with a single 15-minute application. Research suggests it is more effective than using two applications of 1% permethrin crème rinse when applied for a 15-minute period before shampooing.[123]
- **Malathion 0.5%**, an organophosphate compound that acts as a cholinesterase inhibitor rendering it pediculicidal and ovicidal, is used for the treatment of head or public lice for those ages 6 years and above.[118,124] It is not recommended for children under the age of 2 years. This drug is considered one of the few safe alternatives for usage during pregnancy.[125] Malathion is applied to dry hair for a period of 8 to 12 hours before being washed out. In the United States, the Ovide®, malathion product contains the additional ingredients terpineol, dipentene, and pine needle oil, which also have pediculicidal qualities. These features potentially prevent the development of resistance that is commonly found in European malathion formulation that do not contain these ingredients. Malathion outperforms pyrethrin and permethrin due of its rapid cure rate, and it typically requires only one application. If live lice continue to exist, reapplication is recommended. Because of its elevated alcohol concentration, the treatment is combustible. Ingestion of malathion can decrease respirations that is caused by its ability to block cholinesterase. It is also carcinogenetic for humans.[89,126]
- **Benzyl alcohol 5%**, an FDA-approved prescription medication for head lice in children 6 months and older, eliminates the louse through asphyxiation. It is used by saturating dry hair and scalp for 10 minutes. Since it is not ovicidal, reapplication after 7 days is necessary.[89] Adverse events may include itching, erythema, pyoderma, ocular irritation, and gasping syndrome in neonates.[83]
- **Spinosad Topical Suspension 0.9%**, an FDA-approved prescription medication for head lice, is produced from the bacteria *Saccharopolyspora spinosa*. Both pediculicidal and ovicidal, it interferes with acetylcholine receptors, causing continuous excitation of neurons and resulting in muscular weariness and paralysis.[127] This therapy is suitable pyrethroids demonstrate resistance and has demonstrated superior effectiveness compared to permethrin.[89,128,129] The suspension is applied for 10 minutes prior to washing, and administered again if live lice are still present after a week. Adverse events may include cutaneous and ocular erythema and irritation at the site of application. Safety of this product has not been evaluated in children under the age of 4.[89,129]
- **Ivermectin Lotion 0.5%** is an anthelminthic FDA approved for the treatment of head lice in children ages 6 months or older. It enhances the permeability of chloride ions in muscle cells, resulting in hyperpolarization, paralysis, and death of lice.[130] It is applied to dry hair and scalp for 10 minutes before rinsing. A single application often sufficient. Adverse events include skin or eye irritation, erythema, burning, or dryness.[130,131]
- **Lidane** is a prescription pediculicidal and ovicidal shampoo that is not a first-line treatment for pediculosis. It displays brain and nervous system toxicity and should be avoided in premature infants, individuals with seizure disorders, who weigh less than 110 pounds, are pregnant or breastfeeding, or those allergic to lidane.[132]
- **Abametapir** is a new FDA-approved treatment for head lice in patients 6 months and older, chelates heavy metal cations (iron, copper, and zinc), and inhibits metalloproteinases that are critical for louse ova development, hatching, and nymph and adult survival.[133] It requires a single application and side effects included skin irritation. Due to lack of distribution, this medication is not yet widely available.[134]
- **Crotamiton Lotion 10%**, while lacking FDA approval, is a prescription drug often used for the treatment of scabies and has also been employed for the management of head lice.[135] It is applied to the scalp for 24 hours before washing and it has been demonstrated that application for two consecutive nights is both safe and effective for eliminating lice in adults.[136] Adverse events may include gastrointestinal upset, rash, temporary itching, and an allergic response. [137]
- **Oral Sulfamethoxazole-Trimethoprim,** a sulfa-containing antibiotic, is not FDA approved for treatment of head lice. It eradicates the gut bacteria of lice resulting in direct toxicity.[89] In a small-scale trial, the combination of 1% permethrin with this antibiotic showed efficacy in treating head lice infestation.[137] The potential danger of Steven-Johnson syndrome, a severe hypersensitivity reaction that affects the skin and mucous membranes, renders this treatments as nonpreferred option.
- **Oral Ivermectin,** which is pediculicidal, is not FDA approved for treatment of pediculosis. A single oral dose of 200 mcg/kg repeated in 10 day has been shown to be effective in treating head lice.[138] Furthermore, a single oral dose of 400 mcg/kg repeated in 7 days was demonstrated to be more effective than 0.5% malathion lotion.[139] It is not recommended in children with a body weight below 15 kg. Adverse events include asthenia and fatigue, stomach discomfort, anorexia, and constipation.
- **Natural Remedies** for head lice include essential oils that are not FDA approved. The product, HairClean 1-2-3, which includes essential oils like ylang-ylang oil, has been studied and demonstrated similar effectiveness as permethrin.[101] The adverse events include contact sensitization, which makes its use limited.[89]
- **Occlusive Substances**, such as tea tree or olive oil, mayonnaise, petroleum jelly, or Cetaphil face cleanser are applied to the scalp and left on overnight while wearing a shower cap. They are used to avoid the possible hazards linked to pharmaceutical treatments for lice. It is important to emphasize that although these procedures may decrease the overall number of lice, there is inadequate evidence to verify their efficacy, potential adverse events, or toxicity. Consequently, these alternative remedies are not advised for the treatment of head lice,[114,115,140] but have shown favorable results in the treatment of pubic lice when done at appropriate intervals with retreatment.[141] Occlusive agents have also been useful in treating pubic lice infestation of the eyelashes.[132]

CONCLUSION

Parasitic infestations and infections are encountered in both developing and developed countries. Although they occur in people with skin of color, there does not appear to be a specific predisposition. Other factors such as travel, geography, environment, and socioeconomic and immune status seemingly play important roles in acquiring these disorders.

REFERENCES

1. Bari A, Khan M. Pattern of skin diseases in black Africans of Sierra Leone, West Africa. *J Clin Diagn Res*. 2007:361-368. (Published online.)
2. Shriver MD. Ethnic variation as a key to the biology of human disease. *Ann Intern Med*. 1997;127(5):401.
3. Fitzpatrick TB. The validity and practicality of sun-reactive skin types I through VI. *Arch Dermatol*. 1988;124(6):869.
4. Wesley NO, Maibach HI. Racial (ethnic) differences in skin properties: the objective data. *Am J Clin Dermatol*. 2003;4(12):843-860.
5. Vos T, Allen C, Arora M, et al. Global, regional, and national incidence, prevalence, and years lived with disability for 310 diseases and injuries, 1990–2015: a systematic analysis for the Global Burden of Disease Study 2015. *Lancet*. 2016;388(10053):1545-1602.
6. Burkhart CG, Burkhart CN, Burkhart KM. An epidemiologic and therapeutic reassessment of scabies. *Cutis*. 2000;65(4):233-240.
7. Romani L, Steer AC, Whitfeld MJ, Kaldor JM. Prevalence of scabies and impetigo worldwide: a systematic review. *Lancet Infect Dis*. 2015;15(8): 960-967.
8. Fain A. Epidemiological problems of scabies. *Int J Dermatol*. 1978;17(1):20-30.
9. Guldbakke KK, Khachemoune A. Crusted scabies: a clinical review. *J Drugs Dermatol JDD*. 2006;5(3):221-227.
10. Burgess I. Sarcoptes scabiei and scabies. *Adv Parasitol*. 1994;33:235-292.
11. Heukelbach J, Feldmeier H. Scabies. *Lancet*. 2006;367(9524):1767-1774.
12. Chosidow O. Scabies. *N Engl J Med*. 2006;354(16):1718-1727.
13. Jackson A, Heukelbach J, Filho AF da S, Campelo Júnior E de B, Feldmeier H. Clinical features and associated morbidity of scabies in a rural community in Alagoas, Brazil. *Trop Med Int Health*. 2007;12(4):493-502.
14. Elgart ML. Scabies. *Dermatol Clin*. 1990;8(2):253-263.
15. Fitzpatrick T, Johnson R, Wolff K. Insect bites and infestations. In: Fitzpatrick TJ, Johnson RA, Wolff K, Polano MK, Suurmond R, eds. *Color Atlas and Synopsis of Clinical Dermatology*. 3rd ed. New York, NY: McGraw Hill; 1997:836-861.
16. Thomas C, Coates SJ, Engelman D, Chosidow O, Chang AY. Ectoparasites. *J Am Acad Dermatol*. 2020;82(3):533-548.
17. Worth C, Heukelbach J, Fengler G, Walter B, Liesenfeld O, Feldmeier H. Impaired quality of life in adults and children with scabies from an impoverished community in Brazil. *Int J Dermatol*. 2012;51(3):275-282.
18. Li FZ, Chen S. Diagnostic accuracy of dermoscopy for scabies. *Korean J Parasitol*. 2020;58(6):669-674.
19. Yürekli A. A new sign with UV dermoscope in the diagnosis of scabies: Ball sign. *Skin Res Technol*. 2023;29(5):e13336.
20. Brodell RT, Helms SE. Bedside testing: the diagnostic cornerstone of dermatology. *Compr Ther*. 1997;23(3):211-217.
21. Johnston G, Sladden M. Scabies: diagnosis and treatment. *BMJ*. 2005;331(7517):619-622.
22. Bezold G, Lange M, Schiener R, et al. Hidden scabies: diagnosis by polymerase chain reaction. *Br J Dermatol*. 2001;144(3):614-618.
23. Prevention CC for DC and. CDC - Scabies - resources for health professionals - medications. https://www.cdc.gov/parasites/scabies/health_professionals/meds.html. Accessed December 9, 2023.
24. Elgart GW, Meinking TL. Ivermectin. *Dermatol Clin*. 2003;21(2):277-282.
25. Bernigaud C, Fischer K, Chosidow O. The management of scabies in the 21st century: past, advances and potentials. *Acta Derm Venereol*. 2020;100(9):adv00112.
26. Huffam SE, Currie BJ. Ivermectin for Sarcoptes scabiei hyperinfestation. *Int J Infect Dis*. 1998;2(3):152-154.
27. Aubin F, Humbert P. Ivermectin for crusted (Norwegian) scabies. *N Engl J Med*. 1995;332(9):612-612.
28. Johnstone P, Strong M. Scabies. *BMJ Clin Evid*. 2014;2014:1707.
29. Caumes E, Carrière J, Guermonprez G, Bricaire F, Danis M, Gentilini M. Dermatoses associated with travel to tropical countries: a prospective study of the diagnosis and management of 269 patients presenting to a tropical disease unit. *Clin Infect Dis*. 1995;20(3):542-548.
30. Beaver PC. Larva migrans. *Exp Parasitol*. 1956;5(6):587-621.
31. Chaudhry AZ, Longworth DL. Cutaneous manifestations of intestinal helminthic infections. *Dermatol Clin*. 1989;7(2):275-290.
32. Hotez PJ, Narasimhan S, Haggerty J, et al. Hyaluronidase from infective Ancylostoma hookworm larvae and its possible function as a virulence factor in tissue invasion and in cutaneous larva migrans. *Infect Immun*. 1992;60(3):1018-1023.
33. Veraldi S, Schianchi R, Carrera C. Epiluminescence microscopy in cutaneous larva migrans. *Acta Derm Venereol*. 2000;80(3):233.
34. Hochedez P, Caumes E. Hookworm-related cutaneous larva migrans. *J Travel Med*. 2007;14(5):326-333.
35. Ogueta I, Navajas-Galimany L, Concha-Rogazy M, et al. Very high- and high-frequency ultrasound features of cutaneous larva migrans. *J Ultrasound Med*. 2019;38(12):3349-3358.
36. Caumes E. Treatment of cutaneous larva migrans. *Clin Infect Dis*. 2000;30(5): 811-814.
37. Davies HD, Sakuls P, Keystone JS. Creeping eruption. A review of clinical presentation and management of 60 cases presenting to a tropical disease unit. *Arch Dermatol*. 1993;129(5):588-591.
38. Jelinek T, Maiwald H, Nothdurft HD, Löscher T. Cutaneous larva migrans in travelers: synopsis of histories, symptoms, and treatment of 98 patients. *Clin Infect Dis Off Publ Infect Dis Soc Am*. 1994;19(6):1062-1066.
39. Davis CM, Israel RM. Treatment of creeping eruption with topical thiabendazole. *Arch Dermatol*. 1968;97(3):325-326.
40. Katz R, Ziegler J, Blank H. The natural course of creeping eruption and treatment with thiabendazole. *Arch Dermatol*. 1965;91:420-424.
41. Caumes E, Carriere J, Datry A, Gaxotte P, Danis M, Gentilini M. A randomized trial of ivermectin versus albendazole for the treatment of cutaneous larva migrans. *Am J Trop Med Hyg*. 1993;49(5):641-644.
42. Goa KL, McTavish D, Clissold SP. Ivermectin. A review of its antifilarial activity, pharmacokinetic properties and clinical efficacy in onchocerciasis. *Drugs*. 1991;42(4):640-658.
43. Johanis M, Cheema KS, Young PA, et al. Cutaneous larva migrans in the northeastern US. *Dermatol Online J*. 2023;29(4).
44. Vakil BJ, Bandisode MS, Gaitonde BB, Salunkhe DS, Kulkarni HJ. Clinical trials with a new anthelmintic, thiabendazole. *J Trop Med Hyg*. 1965;68(12): 287-295.
45. Coulaud JP, Binet D, Voyer C, Samson C, Moreau G, Rossignol JF. [Treatment of the cutaneous larva migrans syndrome "Larbish" with albendazole. Apropos of 18 cases]. *Bull Soc Pathol Exot Filiales*. 1982;75(5):534-537.
46. Williams HC, Monk B. Creeping eruption stopped in its tracks by albendazole. *Clin Exp Dermatol*. 1989;14(5):355-356.
47. Orihuela AR, Torres JR. Single dose of albendazole in the treatment of cutaneous larva migrans. *Arch Dermatol*. 1990;126(3):398-399.
48. Sanguigni S, Marangi M, Teggi A, De Rosa F. Albendazole in the therapy of cutaneous larva migrans. *Trans R Soc Trop Med Hyg*. 1990;84(6):831.
49. Pungpak S, Bunnag D, Chindanond D, Radmoyos B. Albendazole in the treatment of strongyloidiasis. *Southeast Asian J Trop Med Public Health*. 1987;18(2):207-210.
50. Katz R, Hood RW. Topical thiabendazole for creeping eruption. *Arch Dermatol*. 1966;94(5):643-645.
51. Katz R, Ziegler J, Blank H. Creeping eruption treated with thiabendazole. *Arch Dermatol*. 1965;91:425-426.
52. Stone OJ, Mullins JF. Thiabendazole effectiveness in creeping eruption. *Arch Dermatol*. 1965;91:427-429.
53. Thomas J, Lugagne J, Rosso AM, et al. Treatment of creeping eruption with thiabendazole (50 cases). *Mars Med*. 1969;106(9):717-721.
54. *WHO Guidelines for Malaria*. World Health Organization; 2022. http://www.ncbi.nlm.nih.gov/books/NBK579022/. Accessed December 8, 2023.
55. Riddell A, Pollard AJ. Tropical disease vaccines. *Expert Rev Vaccines*. 2003;2(1):105-112.
56. Gruell H, Hamacher L, Jennissen V, et al. On taking a different route: an unlikely case of malaria by nosocomial transmission. *Clin Infect Dis*. 2017; 65(8):1404-1406.
57. Mace KE, Lucchi NW, Tan KR. Malaria surveillance - United States, 2017. *MMWR Surveill Summ*. 2021;70(2):1-35.
58. Owusu-Ofori AK, Betson M, Parry CM, Stothard JR, Bates I. Transfusion-transmitted malaria in Ghana. *Clin Infect Dis*. 2013;56(12):1735-1741.
59. Severe malaria. *Trop Med Int Health TM IH*. 2014;19 Suppl 1:7-131.
60. Gnémé A, Guelbéogo WM, Riehle MM, et al. Plasmodium species occurrence, temporal distribution and interaction in a child-aged population in rural Burkina Faso. *Malar J*. 2013;12:67.
61. Naik BR, Tyagi BK, Xue RD. Mosquito-borne diseases in India over the past 50 years and their Global Public Health Implications: a systematic review. *J Am Mosq Control Assoc*. 2023;39(4):258-277.

62. Meibalan E, Marti M. Biology of malaria transmission. *Cold Spring Harb Perspect Med.* 2017;7(3):a025452.
63. Basu S, Sahi PK. Malaria: an update. *Indian J Pediatr.* 2017;84(7):521-528.
64. Jelinek T, Schulte C, Behrens R, et al. Imported Falciparum malaria in Europe: sentinel surveillance data from the European network on surveillance of imported infectious diseases. *Clin Infect Dis.* 2002;34(5): 572-576.
65. Driessen GJ, Pereira RR, Brabin BJ, Hartwig NG. Imported malaria in children: a national surveillance in the Netherlands and a review of European studies. *Eur J Public Health.* 2007;18(2):184-188.
66. Shingadia D, Shulman ST. Recognition and management of imported malaria in children. *Semin Pediatr Infect Dis.* 2000;11(3):172-177.
67. Lalloo DG, Shingadia D, Bell DJ, Beeching NJ, Whitty CJM, Chiodini PL. UK malaria treatment guidelines 2016. *J Infect.* 2016;72(6):635-649.
68. Wilson ML. Malaria rapid diagnostic tests. *Clin Infect Dis.* 2012;54(11): 1637-1641.
69. Kahama-Maro J, D'Acremont V, Mtasiwa D, Genton B, Lengeler C. Low quality of routine microscopy for malaria at different levels of the health system in Dar es Salaam. *Malar J.* 2011;10:332.
70. Whitty CJM null, Armstrong M, Behrens RH. Self-testing for falciparum malaria with antigen-capture cards by travelers with symptoms of malaria. *Am J Trop Med Hyg.* 2000;63(5-6):295-297.
71. Oriero EC, Jacobs J, Van Geertruyden JP, Nwakanma D, D'Alessandro U. Molecular-based isothermal tests for field diagnosis of malaria and their potential contribution to malaria elimination. *J Antimicrob Chemother.* 2015;70(1):2-13.
72. Selvarajah D, Naing C, Htet NH, Mak JW. Loop-mediated isothermal amplification (LAMP) test for diagnosis of uncomplicated malaria in endemic areas: a meta-analysis of diagnostic test accuracy. *Malar J.* 2020;19(1):211.
73. Morris U, Aydin-Schmidt B. Performance and application of commercially available loop-mediated isothermal amplification (LAMP) kits in malaria endemic and non-endemic settings. *Diagnostics.* 2021;11(2):336.
74. Mathieu LC, Cox H, Early AM, et al. Local emergence in Amazonia of *Plasmodium falciparum k13 C580Y* mutants associated with *in vitro* artemisinin resistance. *eLife.* 2020;9:e51015.
75. Chu CS, White NJ. The prevention and treatment of *Plasmodium vivax* malaria. *PLoS Med.* 2021;18(4):e1003561.
76. Price RN, Von Seidlein L, Valecha N, Nosten F, Baird JK, White NJ. Global extent of chloroquine-resistant *Plasmodium vivax*: a systematic review and meta-analysis. *Lancet Infect Dis.* 2014;14(10):982-991.
77. Abanyie F, Acharya SD, Leavy I, Bowe M, Tan KR. Safety and effectiveness of intravenous Artesunate for treatment of severe malaria in the United States-April 2019 through December 2020. *Clin Infect Dis.* 2021;73(11): 1965-1972.
78. Paczkowski MM, Landman KL, Arguin PM, Centers for Disease Control and Prevention (CDC). Update on cases of delayed hemolysis after parenteral artesunate therapy for malaria - United States, 2008 and 2013. *MMWR Morb Mortal Wkly Rep.* 2014;63(34):753-755.
79. Suh PF, Elanga-Ndille E, Tchouakui M, et al. Impact of insecticide resistance on malaria vector competence: a literature review. *Malar J.* 2023;22(1):19.
80. Shahbodaghi SD, Rathjen NA. Malaria: prevention, diagnosis, and treatment. *Am Fam Physician.* 2022;106(3):270-278.
81. Sanford C, McConnell A, Osborn J. The pretravel consultation. *Am Fam Physician.* 2016;94(8):620-627.
82. Nadeem AY, Shehzad A, Islam SU, Al-Suhaimi EA, Lee YS. Mosquirix™ RTS, S/AS01 vaccine development, immunogenicity, and efficacy. *Vaccines.* 2022;10(5):713.
83. Prevention CC for DC and. CDC - lice - head lice - general information - frequently asked questions (FAQs). Published September 17, 2020. https://www.cdc.gov/parasites/lice/head/gen_info/faqs.html. Accessed December 14, 2023.
84. Ko CJ, Elston DM. Pediculosis. *J Am Acad Dermatol.* 2004;50(1):1-12; quiz 13-14.
85. Webber E, McConnell S. Lice update: management and treatment in the home. *Home Healthc Now.* 2018;36(5):289-294.
86. Lesshafft H, Baier A, Guerra H, Terashima A, Feldmeier H. Prevalence and risk factors associated with pediculosis capitis in an impoverished urban community in lima, peru. *J Glob Infect Dis.* 2013;5(4):138-143.
87. Jamani S, Rodríguez C, Rueda MM, et al. Head lice infestations in rural Honduras: the need for an integrated approach to control neglected tropical diseases. *Int J Dermatol.* 2019;58(5):548-556.
88. Coscione S, Kositz C, Marks M. Head lice: an under-recognized tropical problem. *Am J Trop Med Hyg.* 2017;97(6):1636-1637.
89. Devore CD, Schutze GE, Council on School Health and Committee on Infectious Diseases, American Academy of Pediatrics. Head lice. *Pediatrics.* 2015;135(5):e1355-1365.
90. Roberts RJ. Clinical practice. Head lice. *N Engl J Med.* 2002;346(21): 1645-1650.
91. Nash B. Treating head lice. *BMJ.* 2003;326(7401):1256-1257.
92. Cummings C, Finlay JC, MacDonald NE. Head lice infestations: a clinical update. *Paediatr Child Health.* 2018;23(1):e18-e24.
93. Frankowski BL, Bocchini JA, Council on School Health and Committee on Infectious Diseases. Head lice. *Pediatrics.* 2010;126(2):392-403.
94. Jahnke C, Bauer E, Hengge UR, Feldmeier H. Accuracy of diagnosis of pediculosis capitis: visual inspection vs wet combing. *Arch Dermatol.* 2009;145(3):309-313.
95. Mumcuoglu KY, Friger M, Ioffe-Uspensky I, Ben-Ishai F, Miller J. Louse comb versus direct visual examination for the diagnosis of head louse infestations. *Pediatr Dermatol.* 2001;18(1):9-12.
96. Arnaud A, Chosidow O, Détrez MA, et al. Prevalences of scabies and pediculosis corporis among homeless people in the Paris region: results from two randomized cross-sectional surveys (HYTPEAC study). *Br J Dermatol.* 2016;174(1):104-112.
97. Ly TDA, Touré Y, Calloix C, et al. Changing demographics and prevalence of body lice among homeless persons, Marseille, France. *Emerg Infect Dis.* 2017;23(11):1894-1897.
98. Fazel S, Geddes JR, Kushel M. The health of homeless people in high-income countries: descriptive epidemiology, health consequences, and clinical and policy recommendations. *Lancet Lond Engl.* 2014;384(9953):1529-1540.
99. Brouqui P. Arthropod-borne diseases associated with political and social disorder. *Annu Rev Entomol.* 2011;56:357-374.
100. Raoult D, Roux V. The body louse as a vector of reemerging human diseases. *Clin Infect Dis Off Publ Infect Dis Soc Am.* 1999;29(4):888-911.
101. Hansen RC, O'Haver J. Economic considerations associated with Pediculus humanus capitis infestation. *Clin Pediatr (Phila).* 2004;43(6):523-527.
102. Guss DA, Koenig M, Castillo EM. Severe iron deficiency anemia and lice infestation. *J Emerg Med.* 2011;41(4):362-365.
103. Nara A, Nagai H, Yamaguchi R, et al. An unusual autopsy case of lethal hypothermia exacerbated by body lice-induced severe anemia. *Int J Legal Med.* 2016;130(3):765-769.
104. Woodruff CM, Chang AY. More than skin deep: severe iron deficiency anemia and eosinophilia associated with pediculosis capitis and corporis infestation. *JAAD Case Rep.* 2019;5(5):444-447.
105. Takcı Z, Tekin O, Karadağ AS. A pediculid case: autosensitization dermatitis caused by pediculosis capitis. *Turk Parazitolojii Derg.* 2012;36(3): 185-187.
106. Hau V, Muhi-Iddin N. A ghost covered in lice: a case of severe blood loss with long-standing heavy pediculosis capitis infestation. *BMJ Case Rep.* 2014;2014:bcr2014206623.
107. Althomali SA, Alzubaidi LM, Alkhaldi DM. Severe iron deficiency anaemia associated with heavy lice infestation in a young woman. *BMJ Case Rep.* 2015;2015:bcr2015212207.
108. Singh S, Singh N, Ray JC, Roy S, Garg SP. Phthirus pubis infestation of the scalp: report of three cases. *Rev Infect Dis.* 1990;12(3):560.
109. Veraldi S, Pontini P, Nazzaro G. Phthirus pubis Infestation of the scalp: a case report and review of the literature. *Korean J Parasitol.* 2018;56(5): 487-489.
110. Coates SJ, Thomas C, Chosidow O, Engelman D, Chang AY. Ectoparasites: pediculosis and tungiasis. *J Am Acad Dermatol.* 2020;82(3):551-569.
111. Durden LA. Biting and sucking lice. In: Meyerand RP, Madon MB, eds. *Arthropods of Public Health Significance in California.* Mosquito and Vector Control Association of California (MVCAC); 2002:37-44.
112. Pierzchalski JL, Bretl DA, Matson SC. Phthirus pubis as a predictor for chlamydia infections in adolescents. *Sex Transm Dis.* 2002;29(6):331-334.
113. Gunning K, Kiraly B, Pippitt K. Lice and scabies: treatment update. *Am Fam Physician.* 2019;99(10):635-642.
114. Connolly M. Current recommended treatments for head lice and scabies. *Prescriber.* 2011;22(1-2):26-39.
115. Eisenhower C, Farrington EA. Advancements in the treatment of head lice in pediatrics. *J Pediatr Health Care.* 2012;26(6):451-461; quiz 462-464.
116. Salavastru CM, Chosidow O, Boffa MJ, Janier M, Tiplica GS. European guideline for the management of scabies. *J Eur Acad Dermatol Venereol.* 2017;31(8):1248-1253.
117. Chaku A, Lather LA. Pediculosis diagnosis and management: advice for educating about the facts of lice. *Consult 360.* 2015;14(7). https://www.consultant360.com/articles/pediculosis-diagnosis-and-management-advice-educating-about-facts-lice. Accessed December 12, 2023.
118. Meinking TL, Taplin D, Kalter DC, Eberle MW. Comparative efficacy of treatments for pediculosis capitis infestations. *Arch Dermatol.* 1986;122(3): 267-271.
119. Lebwohl M, Clark L, Levitt J. Therapy for head lice based on life cycle, resistance, and safety considerations. *Pediatrics.* 2007;119(5):965-974.
120. Pérez-Gaxiola G, Velásquez-Salazar P, Veroniki AA, et al. Interventions for treating head lice: a network meta-analysis. *Cochrane Database Syst Rev.* 2022;2022(9):CD014735.

121. Burkhart CG. Relationship of treatment-resistant head lice to the safety and efficacy of pediculicides. *Mayo Clin Proc.* 2004;79(5):661-666.
122. Bao W, Liu B, Simonsen DW, Lehmler HJ. Association between exposure to pyrethroid insecticides and risk of all-cause and cause-specific mortality in the general US adult population. *JAMA Intern Med.* 2020;180(3): 367-374.
123. Burgess IF, Brunton ER, Burgess NA. Single application of 4% dimeticone liquid gel versus two applications of 1% permethrin creme rinse for treatment of head louse infestation: a randomised controlled trial. *BMC Dermatol.* 2013;13:5.
124. Meinking TL, Vicaria M, Eyerdam DH, Villar ME, Reyna S, Suarez G. Efficacy of a reduced application time of Ovide lotion (0.5% malathion) compared to Nix creme rinse (1% permethrin) for the treatment of head lice. *Pediatr Dermatol.* 2004;21(6):670-674.
125. Meinking TL, Villar ME, Vicaria M, et al. The clinical trials supporting benzyl alcohol lotion 5% (Ulesfia): a safe and effective topical treatment for head lice (pediculosis humanus capitis). *Pediatr Dermatol.* 2010;27(1):19-24.
126. IARC/WHO. IARC Monographs Volume 112: evaluation of five organophosphate insecticides and herbicides.
127. McCormack PL. Spinosad: in pediculosis capitis. *Am J Clin Dermatol.* 2011; 12(5):349-353.
128. Villegas SC, Breitzka RL. Head lice and the use of spinosad. *Clin Ther.* 2012; 34(1):14-23.
129. Stough D, Shellabarger S, Quiring J, Gabrielsen AA. Efficacy and safety of spinosad and permethrin creme rinses for pediculosis capitis (head lice). *Pediatrics.* 2009;124(3):e389-395.
130. Pariser DM, Meinking TL, Bell M, Ryan WG. Topical 0.5% ivermectin lotion for treatment of head lice. *N Engl J Med.* 2012;367(18):1687-1693.
131. Deeks LS, Naunton M, Currie MJ, Bowden FJ. Topical ivermectin 0.5% lotion for treatment of head lice. *Ann Pharmacother.* 2013;47(9): 1161-1167.
132. Center for Disease Control and Prevention Parasites: Lice. *Cent Dis Control Prev.* https://www.cdc.gov/lice/treatment/pubic-lice.html. Accessed December 12, 2023.
133. Hiel MBV, Breugelmans B, Pagel CN, et al. The ovicidal, larvacidal and adulticidal properties of 5,5′-dimethyl-2,2′-bipyridyl against Drosophila melanogaster. *PLoS One.* 2012;7(11):e49961.
134. Woods AD, Porter CL, Feldman SR. Abametapir for the treatment of head lice: a drug review. *Ann Pharmacother.* 2022;56(3):352-357.
135. Karacic I, Yawalkar SJ. A single application of crotamiton lotion in the treatment of patients with pediculosis capitis. *Int J Dermatol.* 1982;21(10): 611-613.
136. Burkhart CG, Burkhart CN, Burkhart KM. An assessment of topical and oral prescription and over-the-counter treatments for head lice. *J Am Acad Dermatol.* 1998;38(6 Pt 1):979-982.
137. Hipolito RB, Mallorca FG, Zuniga-Macaraig ZO, Apolinario PC, Wheeler-Sherman J. Head lice infestation: single drug versus combination therapy with one percent permethrin and trimethoprim/sulfamethoxazole. *Pediatrics.* 2001;107(3):E30.
138. Dourmishev AL, Dourmishev LA, Schwartz RA. Ivermectin: pharmacology and application in dermatology. *Int J Dermatol.* 2005;44(12):981-988.
139. Chosidow O, Giraudeau B, Cottrell J, et al. Oral ivermectin versus malathion lotion for difficult-to-treat head lice. *N Engl J Med.* 2010;362(10): 896-905.
140. Koch E, Clark JM, Cohen B, et al. Management of Head Louse Infestations in the United States-A Literature Review. *Pediatr Dermatol.* 2016;33(5): 466-472.
141. Burkhart CG, Burkhart CN. Oral ivermectin for Phthirus pubis. *J Am Acad Dermatol.* 2004;51(6):1037; author reply 1037-1038.

CHAPTER 72 Cutaneous Leishmaniasis

Mourad Mokni
Jaime Soto

KEY POINTS

- Cutaneous leishmaniasis (CL) is a parasitic infection caused by a flagellate parasite of the genus Leishmania. It is transmitted by the bite of sandflies. The reservoirs of the disease are most often rodents or canids. More rarely, humans may act as reservoirs.
- The disease is widely distributed across the Americas, Asia, Europe and Africa. Its epidemiology is influenced by environmental, migratory and climatic factors.
- Leishmania are dimorphic parasites, intracellular amastigote in the phagolysosome of the host's immune cells and promastigote, unicellular protozoan flagellate with a kinetoplast in the digestive tract of the vector and in culture.
- The most common clinical form is localized cutaneous leishmaniasis. The other main clinical forms are recurrent, disseminated, diffuse and mucocutaneous leishmaniasis.
- Diagnosis is usually based on the observation of amastigotes on direct smear examination, but molecular biology techniques are becoming increasingly important.
- The natural history of leishmaniasis must also be taken into account in therapeutic strategies. Numerous therapeutic options have been considered in recent decades.
- Antimony derivatives administered intra-lesionally and parenterally remain the standard treatment. Their toxicity requires vigilance and treatment monitoring. Miltefosine, liposomal amphotericin and physical treatments (cryotherapy and thermotherapy) have been added to the therapeutic arsenal.

Leishmaniasis is an infectious disease caused by the parasitization of cells of the mononuclear phagocyte system by flagellate protozoa belonging to the genus of *Leishmania*. It is transmitted by a bite by a dipteran insects belonging to the genus *Phlebotomus* in the Old World and *Lutzomyia* in the New World. In humans, it evolved clinically in three forms: visceral, cutaneous, and mucocutaneous. These diseases have a worldwide distribution. The vast majority of Old World cases are cutaneous, and regress spontaneously within a few weeks to a few years, while in the New World, where subgenus *Viannia* is prevalent, spontaneous healing is only 22% and patients run the major risk of developing a secondary mucosal form.

PARASITOLOGY

Leishmania are flagellate protozoa of the order *Kinetoplastidae* and the family *Trypanosomatidae*. They exist in two different forms in their successive hosts:

- promastigote, flagellated, in the vector's digestive tract or in culture. It has an elongated shape, 20 µm long.
- amastigote, intramacrophagic, nonflagellated, rounded, and immobile, 2 to 6 µm in size, in the vertebrate host.

The most commonly dermotropic *Leishmania* species are represented in the Old World by *L. major*, *L. tropica*, and *L. aethiopica*. Viscerotropic species such as *L. infantum* and *L. donovani* can also be responsible for cutaneous forms. In the New World, they are mainly represented by *L. braziliensis*, *L. guyanensis*, *L. panamensis*, *L. amazonensis*, *L. mexicana*, *L. venezuelensis*, *and L. peruviana*.

EPIDEMIOLOGY

GEOGRAPHIC DISTRIBUTION

The worldwide prevalence of leishmaniasis in humans, including all clinical forms, is estimated at 12 million. It is estimated that 600,000 to 1 million new cases occur worldwide annually but only around 200,000 are reported to the WHO.[1] The geographical distribution of Old World leishmaniasis predominates in the intertropics and temperate regions of Africa, Europe, and Asia. Although it is endemic in 98 countries, roughly 75% of cases of cutaneous leishmaniasis in human beings are reported in only 10 countries: Afghanistan, Algeria, Brazil, Colombia, Costa Rica,

Ethiopia, Iran, Sudan, Peru, and Syria. The disease is underreported and underdiagnosed in most regions, and active detection reveals that the number of cases could increase at least fivefold.

There are cases of tegumentary leishmaniasis from the south of the United States to Argentina, with the exception of Chile and Uruguay. In the period from 2017 to 2022, 253,000 new cases were reported, mainly in the Andean countries and Brazil.[2] These 42,000 annual cases are below the 53,000 annual cases reported in the previous 20 years; this decrease, rather than reflecting a true reduction in infection, shows deficiencies in the surveillance, control, and reporting systems in several countries. Male workers are the most affected but with the colonization of jungle areas, women and children are now one-third of the new cases. Patients with mucosal leishmaniasis (ML) represent 5% of the total in America, but there are countries such as Bolivia, Peru, and Paraguay where ML represents 10% to 25% of cases.

THE VECTOR

The vector is a nematoceran diptera, *Phlebotomus* spp. in the Old World and *Lutzomyia* spp. in the New World, of which only the female is hematophagous. Its activity is crepuscular and nocturnal. The classically painful bite usually goes unnoticed. It is present all year round in intertropical zones, and in summer in temperate regions.

THE RESERVOIRS

Almost 20 to 30 mammalian species, including rodents, carnivores and humans, are incidental hosts.

THE DISEASE TRANSMISSION CYCLE

The female sandfly becomes infected by biting an infected vertebrate during a blood meal. In her digestive tract, the parasites pass from the amastigote to the promastigote form, actively multiplying. The sandfly then bites another vertebrate, transmitting the parasites to it, which are then phagocytosed by macrophages and converted to the amastigote form. The skin is therefore the main entry point.

RISK FACTORS FOR TRANSMISSION

Epidemics of cutaneous leishmaniasis are often associated with migratory movements, armed conflicts, and the introduction of nonimmune people into an endemic area. Poor socio-economic conditions (unplanned, poorly maintained housing, poor waste and water management, overcrowding) encourage the proliferation of sandflies and their access to humans. Urban development work and deforestation can bring naïve populations back to areas with high rodent densities and a very active transmission cycle. Leishmaniasis is thus a disease closely linked to the environment and climatic factors.

CLASSIFICATION

Cutaneous leishmaniasis is considered as a spectrum of parasitic infections with two poles, the high-immune response pole with mucocutaneous leishmaniasis (CML) that corresponds, in its initial phase, to a cutaneous lesion, then a secondary mucosal involvement with cellular hyper-reactivity and a granuloma presenting mixed Th1 and Th2 cytokine profiles. At the opposite pole, diffuse cutaneous leishmaniasis (LCD) represents the severe form, with nodules dissemination over the body, recurrence and resistance to therapy, and associated with a Th2-type cellular response.

Between these two poles, localized cutaneous leishmaniasis (LCL) is consisting of circumscribed lesions, evolving slowly toward spontaneous healing and corresponding to a Th1-type host cellular immune response. Other minor forms of LCL are described in the literature. These include disseminated cutaneous leishmaniasis, and *cutaneous leishmaniasis recidivans*. For localized cutaneous leishmaniasis, a multitude of morphological forms, sometimes with different names for the same clinical appearance, are reported in the literature. This is a major source of confusion. A simpler, practical clinical classification, useful in the therapeutic algorithm, deserves to be proposed.

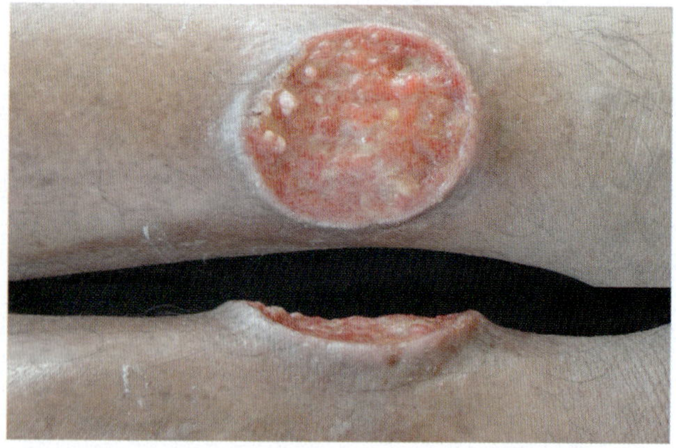

FIGURE 72-1. Semiologic characteristics of cutaneous leishmaniasis ulcer.

CLINICAL MANIFESTATIONS

In all forms of cutaneous leishmaniasis, there is a clinical spectrum.

LOCALIZED CUTANEOUS LEISHMANIASIS

The ulcerative-crust nodule is the most frequently encountered clinical presentation (90%) in Old World cutaneous leishmaniasis, while a clean round ulcer with crateriform edges is seen in 75% of New World patients [**Figure 72-1**]. Following a nocturnal bite by a sandfly, and after an incubation period varying from 1 to 4 months, a small inflammatory raised papule appears rarely pruritic. The papule gradually and steadily increases in size, reaching final nodular lesion size within a few weeks. Subsequently, the nodule will develop a central ulceration that will be covered by a crust of varying thickness [**Figure 72-2**].

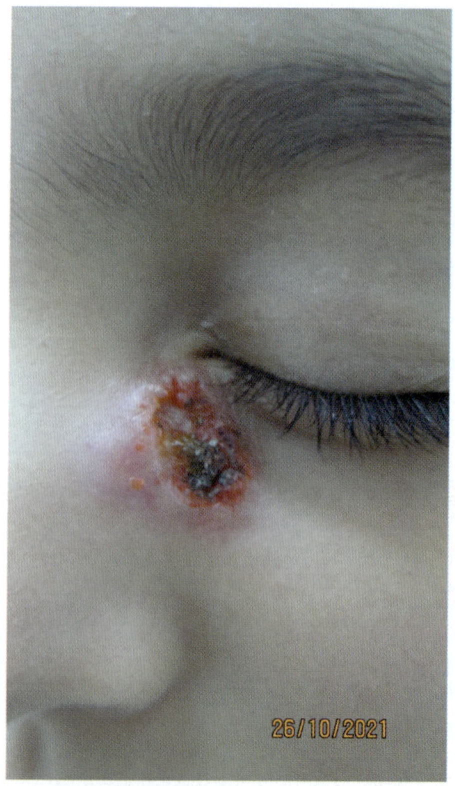

FIGURE 72-2. Ulcero-crusted nodule.

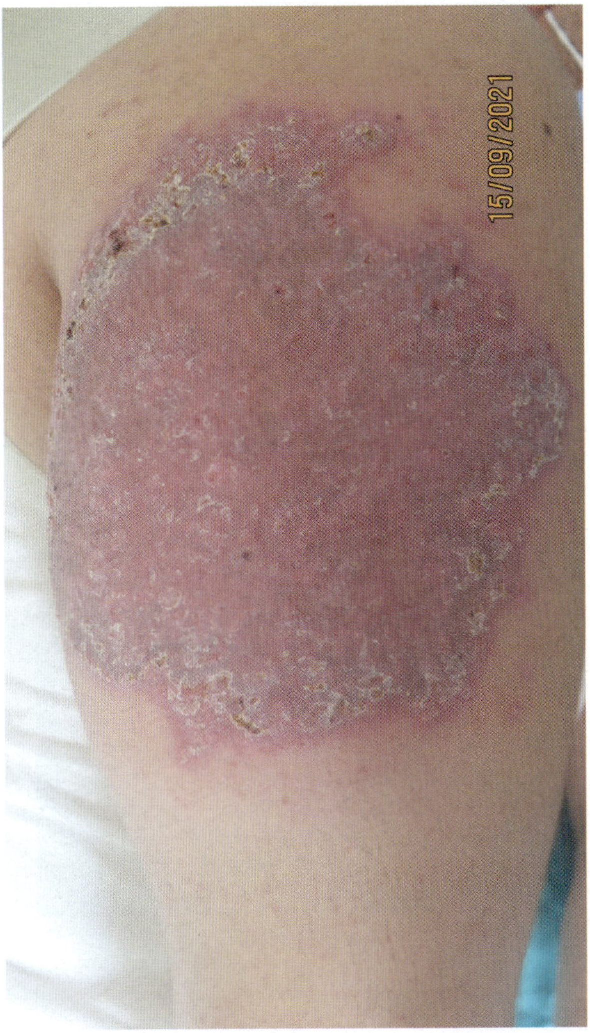

FIGURE 72-3. Infiltrated plaque.

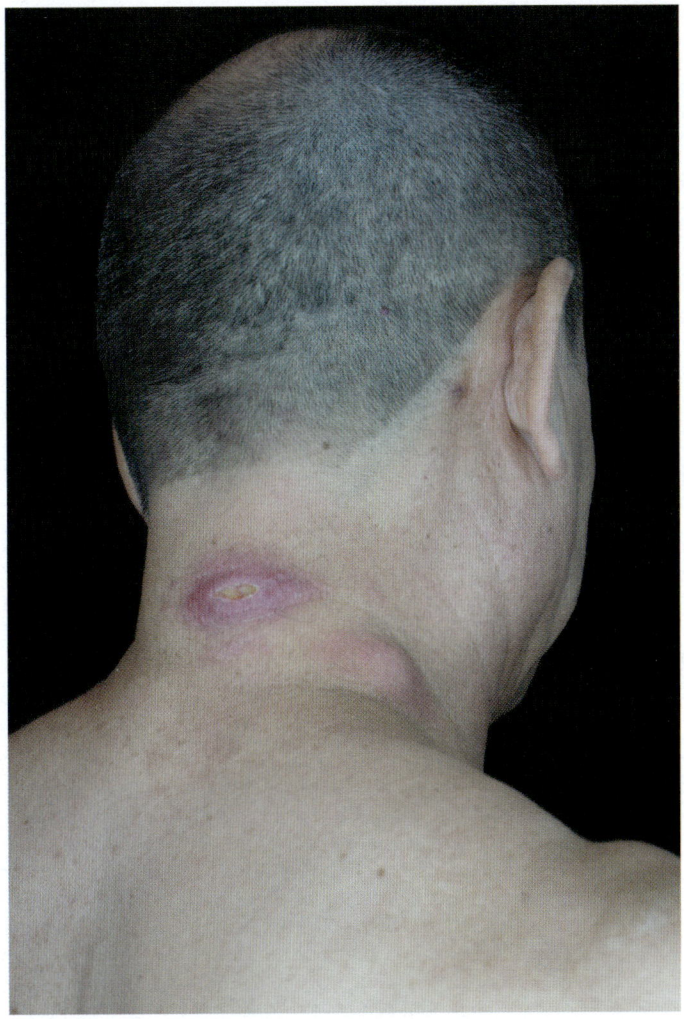

FIGURE 72-5. Regional inflammatory adenopathy.

Less frequently, infiltrated plaque is the other characteristic clinical presentation [**Figure 72-3**]. Satellite papules may emerge around the lesion [**Figure 72-4**]. It is occurring in about 10% of cases. These lesions are generally painless, and eventually heal spontaneously leading to an atrophic scars in at least 50% of cases in the Old World and less than 25% in the New World where swelling adenopathy happens in 25% [**Figure 72-5**] and lymphangitis in 35% of patients [**Figure 72-6**].[3]

Clinical Types

Morphological Types Several morphological forms are described in the literature. Although they reflect a semiological reality, they have little clinical relevance. As a result, there are multiple names describing cutaneous leishmaniasis: erysipelatoid, impetigoid, ulcerative, psoriasiform, echtymatous, eczematiform, verrucous, vegetative, chalazion-like, rhinophyma-like, etc. This is a source of confusion. Size and number of

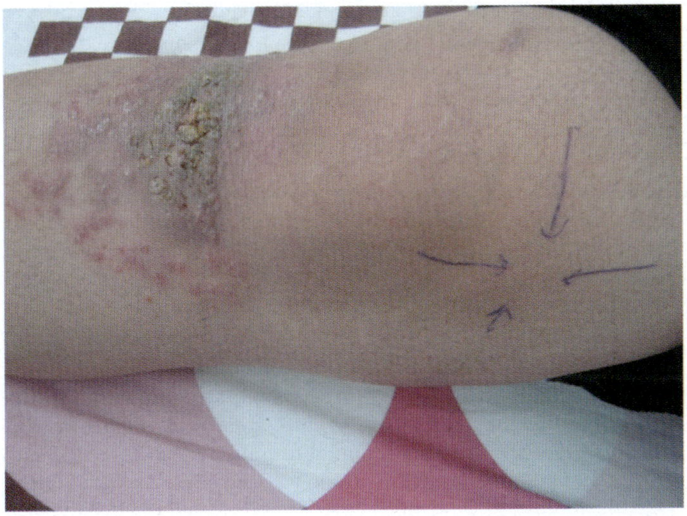

FIGURE 72-4. Satellite papule and nodular lymphangitis with *L. major* cutaneous leishmaniasis.

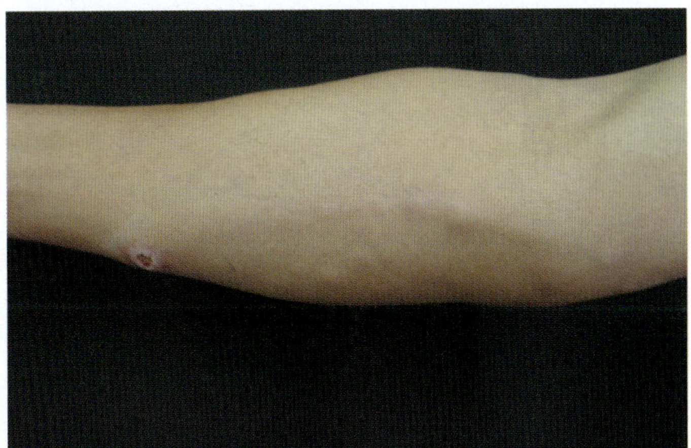

FIGURE 72-6. Local lymphangitis.

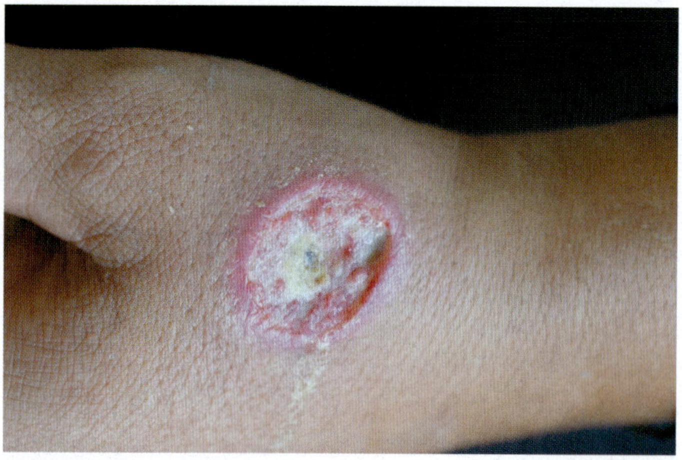

FIGURE 72-7. *L. braziliensis* ulcer.

the lesions are the main criteria for treatment decisions. A simple clinical classification can group all clinical forms together and can aid therapeutic management by only distinguishing between nodules, plaques, or ulcers [Figures 72-1, 72-2, and **72-7**].

Epidemioclinical Types In recent years, it has been possible to individualize certain clinical forms according to their clinical aspects, type of transmission, geographical distribution, and the parasitic species involved.

Sporadic cutaneous leishmaniasis caused by *L. infantum*. Its geographical distribution is based on that of the visceral leishmaniasis. Sporadic cases occur in southern Europe and northern Africa. Cutaneous leishmaniasis is believed to be transmitted by the same vectors as visceral leishmaniasis (*Phlebotomus* spp. of the *Larroussius subgenus*), with the same canine reservoir. Clinically, it affects all ages and both sexes equally. Delay in consultation after sandfly bite varies from 1 month to 2 years, with an average of 3 to 6 months. In the majority of cases, lesions are single and occur on the face in 75% to 90% of cases. Nodules and plaque are usually regular with small or no ulceration [**Figure 72-8**].

Zoonotic cutaneous leishmaniasis caused by *Leishmania major*. It has a widespread distribution in North Africa, Asia Minor and Central Asia, Sub-Saharan Africa, and North-West India.[4] Cutaneous leishmaniasis caused by *L. major* is essentially zoonotic, with epidemic outbreaks. It is transmitted by *Phlebotomus papatasi* or other closely related species, *Ph. duboscqi* and *Ph. salehi*. *Ph. caucasicus* has also been reported as a vector in Iran. The main reservoirs are rodents. *Psammomys obesus* and *Meriones shawi* in North Africa and the Middle East, *Rhombomus opimus* in Central Asia.

In adult populations, a slight male predominance has been reported. This may be linked to the professional activity and clothing habits of these rural regions. *L. major* leishmaniasis is also characterized by a relative clinical polymorphism, with atypical presentation and nodular lymphangitis or sporotrichoid forms [Figure 72-4].

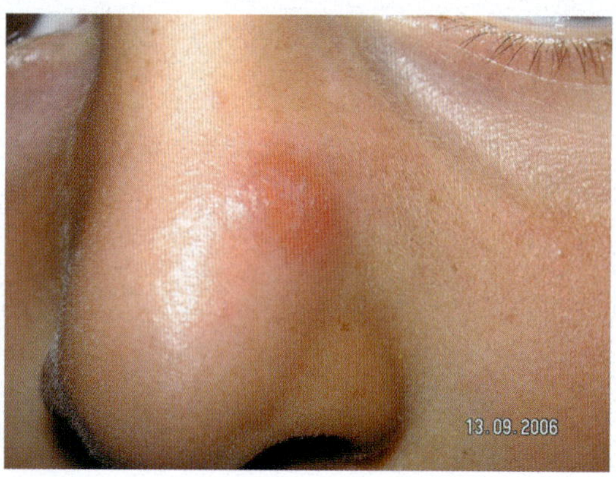

FIGURE 72-8. *L. infantum* cutaneous leishmaniasis.

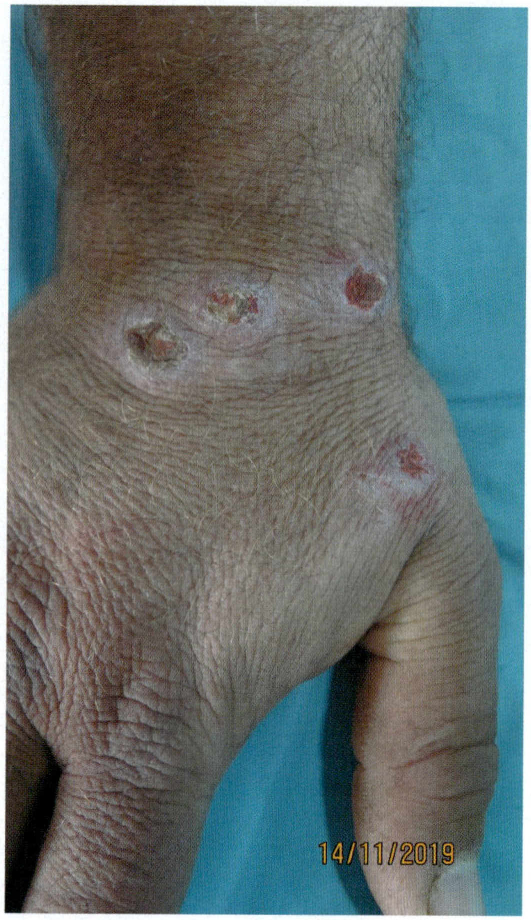

FIGURE 72-9. *L. tropica* cutaneous leishmaniasis.

Cutaneous leishmaniasis caused by *Leishmania tropica*. This parasite is responsible for the "urban dry type"[5] and is distributed in the former USSR, Afghanistan, the Middle East, and Greece. The disease is transmitted by *Ph. Sergenti*. It is anthroponotic and no animal reservoir has been detected to date. However, it could be zoonotic in certain regions of the world.[6] Lesions are unique in 70% of cases. Involvement of the face is observed in 50% of patients. Clinically, the lesions are dominated by dry, ulcerative nodules [**Figure 72-9**]. They are distinguished mainly by their chronicity and recurrence tendency.

Cutaneous leishmaniasis caused by *Leishmania aethiopica*. This form is mainly seen in East Africa. However, most lesions resolve spontaneously in 80% of cases after 2 to 5 years. *Leishmania aethiopica* is mainly responsible for localized chronic nodular forms [**Figure 72-10**], but mucocutaneous and diffuse forms are encountered.

Cutaneous leishmaniasis caused by *Leishmania donovani*. It is distributed mainly in Sudan, Ethiopia, and South Asia. The major reports are from Sri Lanka. Prevalence of the leishmaniasis infections is reported from all the districts of the country, including the endemic areas: north-central, north-western, and southern regions. The disease occurs frequently in young male adults with few and small lesions on the head and neck.

Recurrent cutaneous leishmaniasis (*Leishmania recidivans*)
Recurrent leishmaniasis is a rare, chronic form of cutaneous leishmaniasis caused by *L. tropica*, found in Iran, Iraq, and North Africa. Clinical manifestations begin on the face in 95% of cases, and progress slowly toward centrifugal central scarring, although active papules and nodules continue to appear at the periphery of the lesions [**Figure 72-11**]. Lesions may persist for 20 to 40 years and are often

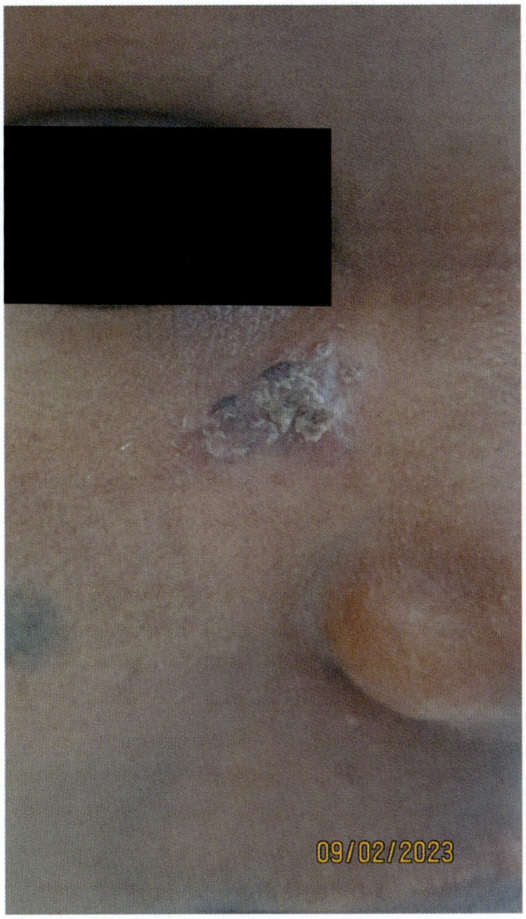

FIGURE 72-10. *L. aethiopica* cutaneous leishmaniasis.

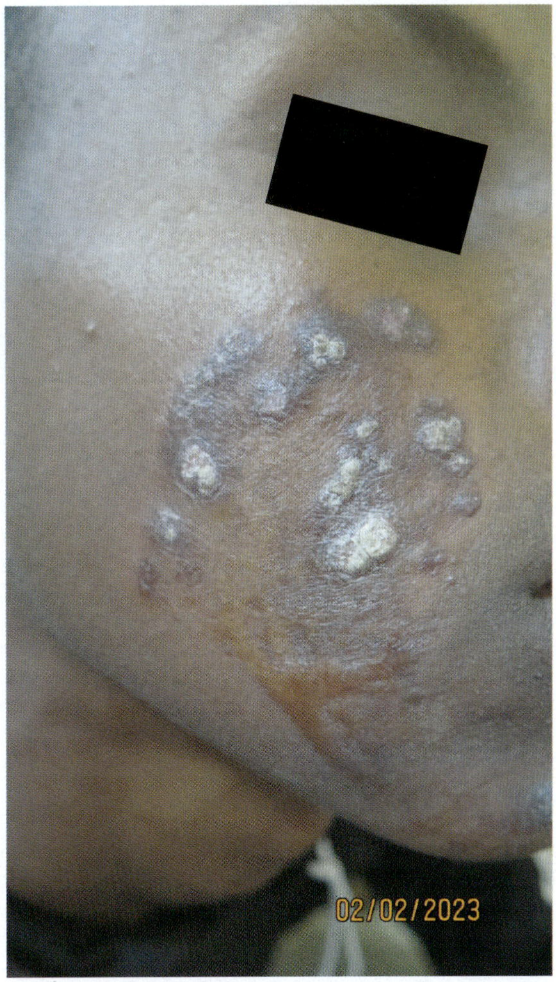

FIGURE 72-11. Leishmania recidivans.

refractory to treatment. This form is sometimes referred to as lupoid or tuberculoid leishmaniasis and could be differentiated from lupus tuberculosis.

In some areas from Brazil and Bolivia where *L. braziliensis* is circulating, there are patients with extensive warty, infiltrative, erosive, and ulcerated cutaneous plaques lasting up to 20 or more years, partially improving with antileishmanial treatments and always relapsing after some months to years [**Figure 72-12**].[7,8]

Disseminated cutaneous leishmaniasis

Often confused in the literature with diffuse cutaneous leishmaniasis, it refers to localized cutaneous leishmaniasis with more than 10 lesions [**Figure 72-13**]. Observations involving several hundred lesions have been described.[9]

MUCOCUTANEOUS LEISHMANIASIS

Months to years after cutaneous leishmaniasis due to *Viannia* subgenus, 5% of patients will develop mucosal lesions in Latin America, but in specific areas such as Bolivia, Paraguay, or Peru, the probability can increase to 10% to 25%.[2] Initial complains of this secondary, severe, and destructive form are nonspecific mild itching or pain and then obstruction, rhinorrhea, and bleeding appear. It affects the nose (95%) [**Figure 72-14**], extends to soft palate (50%) [**Figure 72-15**], hard palate (35%) and can progress to the pharynx (30%), larynx (20%) with mild to severe dysphonia and bronchi (10%) producing respiratory difficulty; there are also difficulties in swallowing which can lead to wasting.[8]

The skin of the nose, cheeks, and upper lip can be affected by extension [**Figure 72-16**]. Involvement of the tongue, gums, and cheeks is extremely rare and should suggest paracoccidioidomycosis, its most common differential diagnosis. ML can be mutilating and destructive [**Figure 72-17**], causing deformities that stigmatize the patient and produce serious physical, psychological, and social consequences. HIV

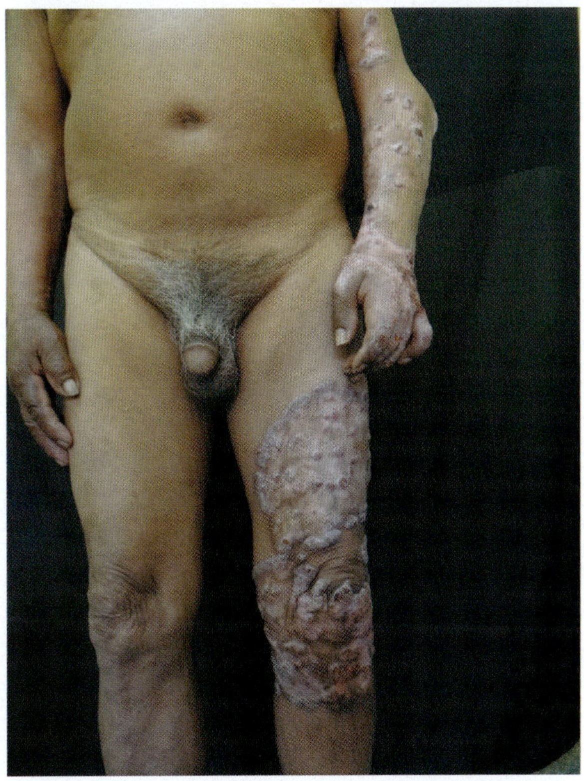

FIGURE 72-12. Chronic recurrents cutaneous leishmaniasis by *L. braziliensis*.

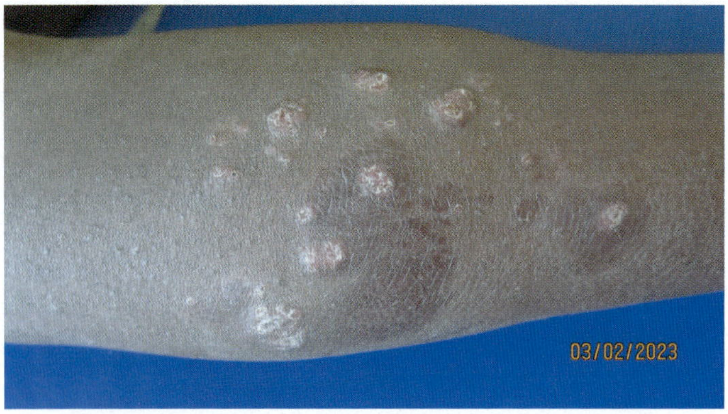

FIGURE 72-13. Disseminated cutaneous leishmaniasis.

infection and cutaneous lesion located above the waist and especially on the face increases the risk of mucosal compromise. A genetic predisposition with association of certain HLA loci and a polymorphism of the TNF-α and β genes has been suspected. Leishmania RNA virus1 (LRV1) has been also mentioned as a possibility. Most mucosal involvement described in Old World leishmaniasis does not represent mucocutaneous leishmaniasis in the classical presentation of the disease. There is no mutilating evolution of the lesions, the transmission is always by direct bite of the sandfly, and mucosal involvement is not preceded by cutaneous lesions. Laryngeal and oral localizations are the most frequent, and the diagnostic smear is generally rich in leishmaniasis.[10]

DIFFUSE CUTANEOUS LEISHMANIASIS

Diffuse cutaneous leishmaniasis is rare. It is caused by *L. aethiopica* in Ethiopia and Kenya for Old World leishmaniasis, and by *L. mexicana* and *L. amazonensis* in Venezuela, Brazil, and Mexico, and more rarely in Colombia, Costa Rica, Dominican Republic, Ecuador, Guatemala, Bolivia, Peru, and the United States. It begins with a single, nonulcerated nodule, most often on the face, followed by the extensive appearance of multiple macules, papules, nodules, plaques, and diffuse infiltration of the skin, especially on the extensor surfaces of the limbs and face, where thickening of the eyebrows and earlobes is reminiscent of lepromatous leprosy. The intradermal leishmanin reaction is consistently negative. Skin smears show numerous amastigotes. Skin histology shows a macrophagic infiltrate containing numerous amastigotes. Such lesions occur mainly in conditions of cellular immunodepression, and when large numbers of parasites are disseminated throughout the integument. The lesions do not ulcerate, the disease does not heal spontaneously, and recurrences are the rule after treatment.

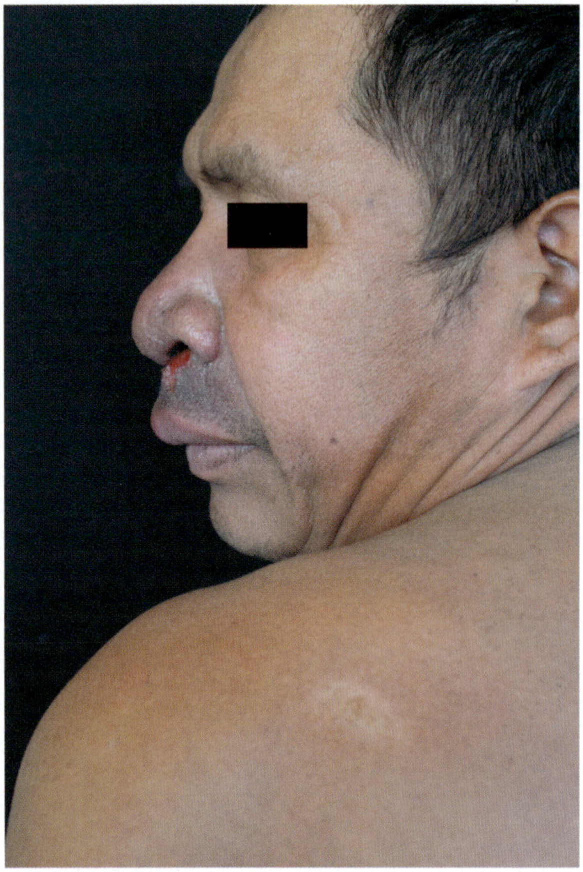

FIGURE 72-14. *L. braziliensis* nasal compromise.

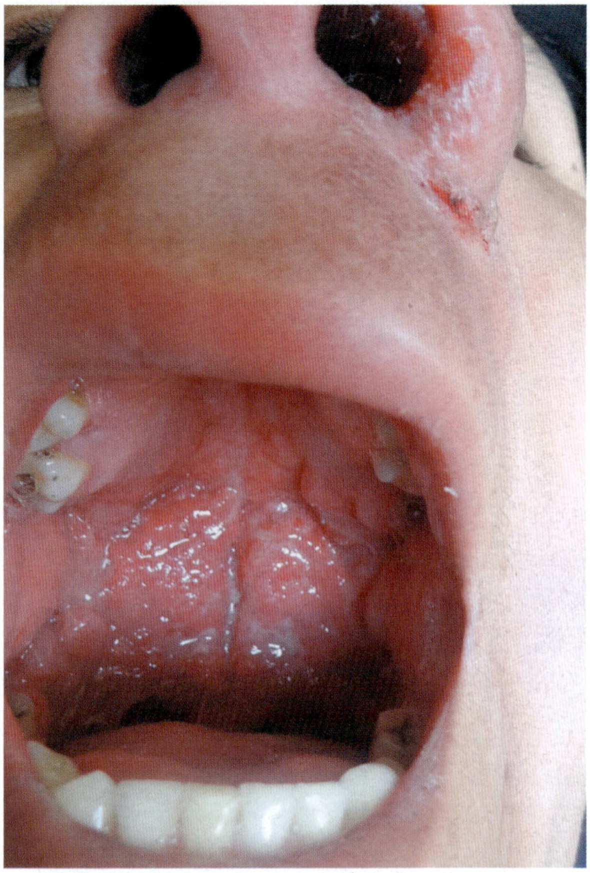

FIGURE 72-15. *L. braziliensis* oral compromise.

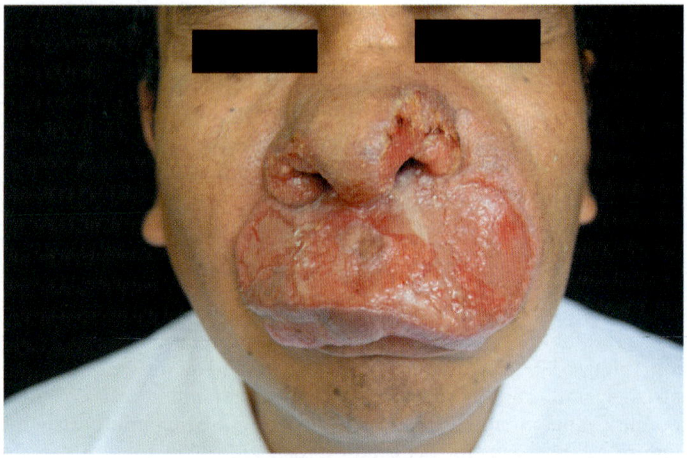

FIGURE 72-16. Extension to facial skin in *L. braziliensis* mucosal leishmaniasis.

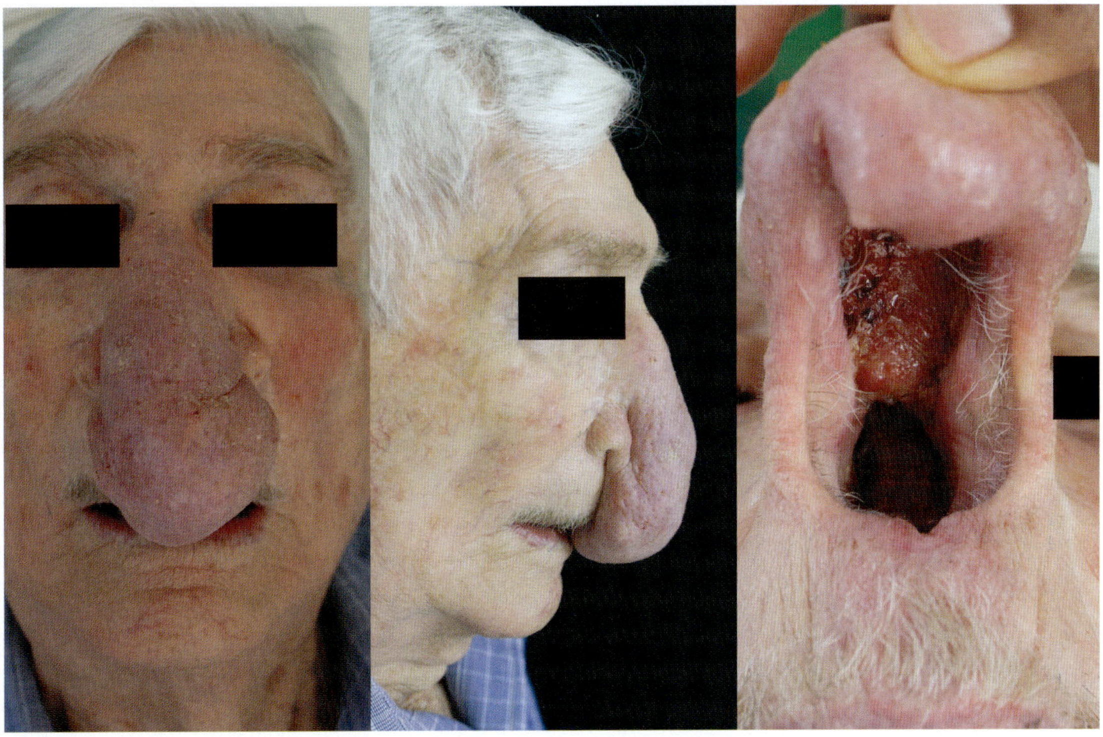

FIGURE 72-17. *L. braziliensis* severe nasal destruction.

POST–KALA-AZAR DERMAL LEISHMANIASIS (PKDL)

Post–kala-azar dermal leishmaniasis (PKDL) is a skin syndrome observed after treatment of visceral leishmaniasis with pentavalent antimony. This complication is more frequent in infants, the malnourished, and in patients who have received incomplete treatment for visceral leishmaniasis. The syndrome is characterized by macules and papules that begin around the mouth. They spread secondarily to the rest of the face and, more rarely, to the extensor surfaces of the limbs and trunk. Initially, they begin as erythematous or hypo-pigmented macules that increase in size and may form nodules resembling those of leprosy.

PKDL occurs in 20% of patients with visceral leishmaniasis in India, with skin lesions appearing 2 to 10 years after successful treatment of visceral leishmaniasis and may persist for several years. PKDL has been reported in over 50% of treated Sudanese patients with visceral leishmaniasis, with lesions appearing some months after treatment. The course of African forms is generally a few months, shorter than that of Asian forms. Histologically, there is a spectrum of cellular response ranging from numerous parasites with few inflammatory cells to a granulomatous reaction with few parasites. Parasites isolated from patients with PKDL are serologically and biochemically identical to *L. donovani* isolated from patients with visceral leishmaniasis. In Asia, as PKDL lesions can persist for up to 20 years, patients can act as a chronic reservoir of infection, and treatment must be instituted.

DIAGNOSIS

Parasitological examination is essential and direct smear is still considered the gold standard specially because its specificity.[11] Its aim is to detect leishmaniasis. Samples should be taken from beneath the adherent crust or from the border of the ulcer or from the bed around the periphery of the lesion, by scraping with a vaccinostyle or curette or surgical blade. We can also aspirate the product of a puncture or make slide smears of a cutaneous biopsy section.

The slide smear, stained with May-Grünwald-Giemsa (MGG), reveals the parasites in amastigote form. Cultures are used to establish the isoenzymatic characteristics of the leishmaniasis, PCR, and to perform in vitro therapeutic sensitivity tests. They are only carried out in specialized laboratories and are not part of routine patient care unless they are included in clinical or research protocols.

Skin histology, with standard hematoxylin and eosin staining or after Giemsa staining, often reveals Leishman bodies in macrophages. In short-stage forms, there is a massive infiltrate of histiocytes and mononuclear cells. In long-standing forms, there is often a nonspecific tuberculoid granuloma appearance.[12]

The leishmanin intradermal reaction (Montenegro test) is of little diagnostic value. It is used to assess the host's cellular immune response.

Gene amplification or polymerase chain reaction (PCR) is today's most widely used technique for detecting parasitic DNA within the sample to be analyzed. It also enables molecular typing of strains without the need for culture. The major advantage of this molecular biology technique is its greater sensitivity than traditional techniques. Serological tests are no useful in cutaneous/mucosal leishmaniasis.

DIFFERENTIAL DIAGNOSIS

As cutaneous leishmaniasis has multiple semiological characteristics (ulcers, plaques, papules, nodules, etc), its differential diagnoses is numerous [**Table 72-1**].

ML located in nasal pyramid and mouth must be differentiated from other infections (such as paracoccidioidomycosis, leprosy, syphilis, and histoplasmosis), proliferative lesions (squamous cell carcinoma, basal cell carcinoma, T-cell lymphoma, and adenocarcinoma) and other septal destructive lesions like perforation by trauma or cocaine abuse, rhinophyma or sarcoidosis.[8]

TREATMENT

A therapeutic regimen that is effective in one region is not necessarily effective in another. It is therefore not possible to recommend a single effective, nontoxic treatment regimen for all forms of the disease in all geographical regions. The therapeutic decision must be considered for each individual patient, taking into account the benefit/risk ratio. As systemic treatment does not always prevent mucosal involvement, use of local treatments in New World forms is now recommended, but it should

TABLE 72-1 Differential diagnosis of cutaneous leishmaniasis[8]

Infections	Inflammatory	Tumors
Pyogenic ulcer	Vascular ulcer	Basal cell carcinoma
Ecthyma	Traumatic ulcer	Squamous cell carcinoma
Sporotrichosis	Diabetic ulcer	Keratoacanthoma
Chromomycosis	Pyoderma gangrenosum	Cutaneous lymphoma
Paracoccidioidomycosis	Insect bites	Lymphocytoma cutis
Cutaneous tuberculosis	Psoriasis	
Atypical mycobacteria	Discoid lupus	
Syphilis	Sickle cell anemia	
Leprosy		
Histoplasmosis		
Boil		

only be considered if close follow-up of the patient can be guaranteed particularly in regions with *L. braziliensis* or *L. panamensis*, with high risk of mucosal leishmaniasis.

LOCAL TREATMENTS

Organic Pentavalent Antimony Salts are still the treatment of choice for all forms of leishmaniasis. There are two widely used presentations: sodium stibogluconate and meglumine antimoniate. Therapeutic indications vary according to the clinical form and species of leishmaniasis involved. For Old World leishmaniasis, local treatment is generally sufficient. In endemic zones, abstention from treatment may be justified for short-course forms (*L. major*), especially for lesions that spare the face, are few in number and uncomplicated. For nodular forms, of low number (<4) and in the absence of lymphatic, cartilaginous, periorificial or periarticular involvement, weekly infiltrations at the three cardinal points of the lesion at a dose of 1 to 3 mL are sufficient.

Thermotherapy is useful for small lesions. After local anesthesia, local heat (50°C for 30 seconds) is applied one or two times with a thermotherapy device. It is as effective as intralesional injections. Bullaes and localized burn reactions may appear.

Cryotherapy involves the application of liquid nitrogen every 3 to 7 days for one to five sessions.

Topical Paromomycin: several formulations have been developed, but their efficacy is controversial. New formulations are in the developing stage.

In New World CL current recommendation in patients with one to four lesions, less than 3 cm not located in face or joints is local therapy with intralesional antimony three to five applications of 1 to 5 mL or thermotherapy (one session of 50°C during 30 seconds).

SYSTEMIC TREATMENTS

Organic Pentavalent Antimony Salts

This treatment is prescribed at a dose of 20 mg pentavalent antimony (Sbv) per kg per day for 2 to 3 weeks. Side effects are frequent, and include hepatic and pancreatic biological disturbances and cardiac toxicity. An ECG should be performed prior to treatment and weekly during administration. In the New World, the schedule is 20 mg per kg per day during 20 days in CL and 20 days in ML.

Pentamidine is administered in two to four intramuscular injections of 4 mg/kg over 4 to 6 days in CL and 7 to 11 doses in ML. These doses are comparable in efficacy and toxicity to pentavalent antimony derivatives. It is mainly reserved for infections caused by *L. guyanensis* and *L. panamensis*. Rhabdomyolysis is frequently observed, usually without renal consequences. Transient diabetes may also be observed.

Amphotericin B Deoxycholate is an effective treatment that has been introduced for visceral leishmaniasis. It may currently be considered in the event of antimony failure in CL or as an alternative in ML when antimonials are contraindicated. It is administered at a dose of 1 mg/kg/day by slow intravenous infusion over 4 to 6 hours, alternating every other day, up to a total dose of 2 to 3 g. Its use is limited due to its toxicity, mainly renal and hematological. Cardiac adverse effects have been reported in patients previously treated with antimony salts. Liposomal Amphotericin B, which is less toxic but more expensive, has been of great help in high-income countries.

Miltefosine was initially developed as an oral anticancer agent. Its antileishmanial effect was shown secondarily. Side effects are mainly digestive: anorexia, nausea, vomiting, and diarrhea. Miltefosine is potentially teratogenic and should not be used in pregnant women. Oral contraception is mandatory in women of childbearing age during treatment and for 6 months after discontinuation. The WHO recommends Miltefosine at a dose of 2.5 mg/kg/day for 28 days for cutaneous leishmaniasis caused by *L. mexicana*, *L. guyanensis*, and *L. panamensis*. Cure rates of 70% to 75% have been observed in *L. braziliensis* cutaneous leishmaniasis in Brazil, Colombia, and Bolivia.[13] Ocular adverse events and male infertility during leishmaniasis treatment with miltefosine were recently reported and WHO established recommendations on the prevention, early detection, and management of eye complications in patients treated with miltefosine.[14]

Other Systemic Treatments are used but are unproven: allopurinol, dapsone, rifampicin, ketoconazole, itraconazole, metronidazole. Controlled studies are needed to assess their effectiveness. The efficacy of fluconazole 200 to 400 mg/day has been demonstrated in *L. major* leishmaniasis.[15] None of these has demonstrated activity in New World CL/ML.

PREVENTION AND CONTROL

VECTOR CONTROL

Reducing the vector population by improving overall sanitary and hygiene conditions could reduce the incidence of cutaneous leishmaniasis. The spraying of dichlorodiphenyl-trichloroethane (DDT) for malaria control has eliminated cutaneous leishmaniasis in several regions, but these actions are now coming to a halt. Individual measures involving the use of DEET-based repellents, permethrin-impregnated clothing, and mosquito nets have shown some effectiveness.

RESERVOIR CONTROL

Ploughing of land containing the burrows of reservoir rodents can reduce the incidence of the disease in some areas. However, these measures are costly for the community, and their effectiveness is short-lived and unsustainable.

VACCINES

Despite the evaluation and development of several candidate vaccines (killed or attenuated promastigotes, recombinant antigens, etc), no effective vaccine has yet seen the light of day.

REFERENCES

1. https://www.who.int/news-room/factsheets/detail/leishmaniasis.
2. "Leishmaniasis: Informe Epidemiológico de Las Américas. Núm. 12 (Diciembre Del 2023)." Washington, D.C.: OPS, -1, 2023. https://iris.paho.org/handle/10665.2/59156.
3. Soto J, Gutiérrez P, Soto P, et al. Treatment of Bolivian leishmania braziliensis cutaneous and mucosal leishmaniasis. *Am J Trop Med Hyg*. 2022;106(4):1182-1190.
4. Postigo JAR, Leishmaniasis in the World Health Organization Eastern Mediterranean Region. *Int J Antimicrob Agents*. 2010;36S:S62-S65.
5. Griffiths WAD: Old World cutaneous Leishmaniasis. In: Peters W, Killick-Kendrick R, eds. *The Leishmaniasis*, Vol. II. Lobdon: Academic Press; 1987:617-636.

6. Bousslimi N, Ben-Ayed S, Ben-Abda I, Aoun K, Bouratbine A. Natural infection of North African gundi (Ctenodactylus gundi) by Leishmania tropica in the focus of cutaneous leishmaniasis, Southeast Tunisia. *Am J Trop Med Hyg.* 2012;86(6):962-965.
7. Guimarães LH, Queiroz A, Silva JA, et al. Atypical manifestations of cutaneous leishmaniasis in a region endemic for Leishmania braziliensis: clinical, immunological and parasitological aspects. *Plos Negl Trop Dis.* 2016;10(12):e0005100.
8. Atlas interactivo de leishmaniasis en las Américas: aspectos clínicos y diagnósticos diferenciales. Washington, D.C.: Organización Panamericana de la Salud; 2020. Licencia: CC BY-NC-SA 3.0 IGO.
9. Couppié P, Clyti E, Sainte-Marie D, Dedet JP, Carme B, Pradinaud R. Disseminated cutaneous leishmaniasis due to Leishmania guyanensis: case of a patient with 425 lesions. *Am J Trop Med Hyg.* 2004;71(5):558-560.
10. Aliaga L, Cobo F, Mediavilla JD, et al. Localized mucosal leishmaniasis due to Leishmania (Leishmania) infantum: clinical and microbiologic findings in 31 patients. *Medicine (Baltimore).* 2003;82:147-158.
11. de Vries HJC, Schallig HD. Cutaneous leishmaniasis: a 2022 updated narrative review into diagnosis and management developments. *Am J Clin Dermatol.* 2022;23(6):823-840.
12. Mokni M, Mebazaa A, Boubaker S. [Histologie de la leishmaniose cutanée]. *Ann Dermatol Venereol.* 2011;138(4):354-356.
13. Soto J, Rea J, Valderrama M, et al. Efficacy of extended (six weeks) treatment with miltefosine for mucosal leishmaniasis in Bolivia. *Am J Trop Med Hyg.* 2009;81:387-389.
14. https://www.who.int/news/item/12-04-2023-acsomp-miltefosine.
15. Alrajhi AA, Ibrahim EA, De Vol EB, et al. Fluconazole for the treatment of cutaneous leishmaniasis caused by *Leishmania major. N Engl J Med.* 2002;346:891-895.

CHAPTER 73 Leprosy

Rochelle Monteiro
Jyoti Jayaraman
Ramesh Bhat M.

KEY POINTS

- Leprosy or Hansen disease caused by the acid-fast bacilli *Mycobacterium leprae* is a neglected tropical disease that continues to be a global health problem.
- The two major structural elements are the capsule and the cell wall, among which phenolic glycolipid 1 (PGL 1) plays an important role in the immunogenicity of the organism.
- The disease is transmitted via the respiratory route and the incubation period greatly varies.
- Macrophages and Schwann cells are the two major host immune cells that interact with *M. Lepra.*
- The Ridley-Jopling classification takes into account the immunological and bacteriological aspects of the disease and classifies it into tuberculoid leprosy (TT), borderline tuberculoid (BT), borderline lepromatous leprosy (BL), mid borderline (BB), and lepromatous leprosy (LL).
- Clinical features in leprosy vary according to the spectrum of the disease and can present as hypopigmented macules, well-defined plaques, or diffuse infiltration of the skin associated with variable loss of sensation and enlarged peripheral nerves.
- The type 1 and 2 lepra reactions are immunologically mediated and occur in the tuberculoid and lepromatous pole of the disease spectrum, respectively.
- Apart from clinical examination, slit skin smear examination and histopathology from skin and or nerve biopsy specimens may aid in the diagnosis and classify the spectrum of disease.
- The standardized treatment of leprosy is based on WHO recommended regimen that comprises the drugs rifampicin, dapsone, and clofazimine available in blister packs and termed as multidrug therapy or MDT.

INTRODUCTION

Leprosy or Hansen disease is a chronic disease that has existed since antiquity. The remains of the earliest human afflicted by leprosy were discovered in an old tomb in the city of Jerusalem and were radiocarbon dated to 1 to 50 AD. The causative organism, *Mycobacterium leprae* was discovered by a Norwegian, Gerard. H. Armauer Hansen in 1873. It is an acid-fast bacillus with a predilection for the skin and peripheral nerves.

GLOBAL EPIDEMIOLOGY

Leprosy or Hansen disease, caused by the acid-fast bacilli *M. leprae*, is a neglected tropical disease that continues to be a global health problem. The average prevalence of cases was 5 million in the 1980s, drastically reducing to 133,802 registered cases in 2021 (number of cases on treatment till December 2021). This is by large attributed to the introduction of MDT in 1981.[1] The current prevalence rate is 16.9 per million population. Region-wise, the distribution is as depicted in **Table 73-1**.

NEW CASES

In 2021, globally, 140,594 new cases were reported, with a case detection rate of 17.93 per million. The global case detection rate increased by 10.2% as compared to the previous year. The South East Asian region (SEAR) reported the maximum number of new cases (66.5%), and the West Pacific Region (WPR) had the fewest new cases (1.8%). India, Brazil, and Indonesia continued to report more than 10,000 cases each.

CASES IN CHILDREN

New case detection in children indicates active and recent transmission. A total of 9052 new cases among children were reported globally in 2021, corresponding to a rate of 4.5 per million population. There was a 4.7% rise in the number of childhood cases in comparison to 2020, and 62.2% of these were in SEAR. In comparison to 2011, there was a decrease of 42% in new adult cases but an increase of 62% in new cases in children.

ETIOLOGY

The etiology of leprosy is the organism *M. leprae*. It is an acid-fast, gram-positive, obligate intracellular bacillus that infects humans, the nine-banded armadillo, and three species of primates. The bacillus has an affinity for the cells of the reticuloendothelial system and the peripheral nervous system, particularly Schwann cells. The organism replicates by binary fission, structurally is slightly curved, and measures 1 to 8 µm in length and 0.3 µm in diameter. The bacilli have been successfully grown in the laboratory in the foot pads of mice. Growth of the organism is optimum between temperatures ranging from 27°C to 30°C. It has a predisposition for infecting the body's colder areas, viz skin, peripheral nerves (superficial), and the nasal mucosa.[2] Though in vitro culture has not been successful, the complete genomic sequencing of the organism has been achieved.

TABLE 73-1 Global leprosy situation[1]

Regions	Registered cases	Prevalence rate (%)
African (AFR)	20,960	18
Americas (AMR)	25,053	24.3
Eastern Mediterranean (EMR)	4206	5.5
South East Asia (SEAR)	81,222	39.4
Western Pacific (WPR)	2360	1.2

AFR, African region; AMR, Americas region; EMR, Eastern Mediterranean region; SEAR, South East Asia region; WPR, Western Pacific region.

STRUCTURE

The two important structural elements of *M. leprae* are the capsule and the cell wall. The capsule is composed of numerous lipids of which most noteworthy are the phenolic glycolipid (PGL-1) and phthiocerol dimycocerosate. PGL 1 is the target of an intense humoral mediated immune response mediated by immunoglobulin M. Lipoarabinomannan is an important component of the cell wall and acts as an antigen for macrophage. Many of the functional genes seen in other mycobacteria have been silenced in *M. leprae*, resulting in pseudogenes. This results in the inactivation of certain functions such as external reproduction. These variations have resulted in the organism having a long reproduction cycle and being an obligate intracellular pathogen.[2]

GENETIC FACTORS

In humans, genetic factors play an important role in the acquisition of infection and the subsequent course of the disease. Single nucleotide polymorphism (SNP) association studies have shown that a major risk factor for the early onset of leprosy was the presence of a low lymphotoxin-producing allele-α (LTA-α). Other SNPs that are associated with disease or development of reactions are vitamin D receptor (VDR), TNF-α, IL-10, IFN-γ, human leukocyte antigen (HLA) genes, and TLR1. Polymorphic risk factors in the promoter region shared by two genes *PARK2*, coding for an E3-ubiquitin ligase designated Parkin, and *PACRG* have been identified by linkage studies. An association between *NOD2* genetic variants and susceptibility to disease and type 1 and 2 reactions has been seen.

DISEASE TRANSMISSION

M. leprae enter the human body mainly through the upper respiratory route. Nasal mucosal secretions have shown bacilli numbers ranging from 10,000 to 10,000,000. As many as 10 million viable bacilli per day can be seen in nasal secretions. In a study, large numbers of bacilli were found in the superficial keratin layer of the skin of lepromatous leprosy patients, suggesting that bacilli could be shed with the sebaceous secretions of the skin.

INCUBATION PERIOD

The average incubation period is between 3 and 10 years. Reports of cases occurring in infants imply that the incubation period could be as little as a few weeks. Conversely, war veterans who were exposed to the disease in endemic areas for short periods went on to develop the disease as long as 30 years later. Thus, the slow onset of the disease and lack of adequate immunological tools make measuring the incubation period difficult.

RISK FACTORS

In regions endemic to leprosy, the common risk factors for acquiring infection are

- Low immunity secondary to other diseases
- Poor and unsanitary living conditions
- Overcrowding
- Prolonged contact

M. LEPRAE AND IMMUNE CELLS

Macrophages and Schwann cells are the two major host immune cells that interact with *M. leprae*. Infection of Schwann cells (which are present in nerves) leads to demyelination of the nerve, neural injury, and subsequent disability. A specific laminin-binding protein of 21KDa and PGL-1 (phenolic glycolipid) aids in the invasion of Schwann cells by *M. leprae*. PGL-1 is a unique glycoconjugate on the surface of *M. leprae*. It has an affinity for laminin-2 on the Schwann cells that explains the predilection of this bacillus for peripheral nerves.[3]

PATHOGENESIS

Once infection occurs, the development of the disease with clinical manifestations depends on the immune status of the patient. Genetic susceptibility, via a locus at chromosome 10p13 near the mannose receptor 1 gene has been described. Class II HLA major histocompatibility complex genes present on chromosome 6, are responsible for the clinical subtype of leprosy a patient develops. Tuberculoid leprosy is linked to *HLA-DR2* and *HLA-DR3* genes, whereas the lepromatous type is linked to *HLA-DQ1*. The clinical phenotype and course of the disease are largely dictated by the immune response of the host. At the tuberculoid pole, there is an intense, organized specific cellular immune response. In contrast, at the lepromatous pole, an absence of immune response is seen. Due to this variable immune response to *M. leprae*, the clinical manifestations can vary spontaneously and may result in type 1 or 2 lepra reactions. Triggers for reactions are related to immune system variations and can be caused by stress, anti-leprosy medications, or pregnancy. The type 1 reaction, also known as the reversal reaction, involves type IV hypersensitivity. It involves activation of the CD4+ T-cells and elevation of interferon-γ and TNF-α. The type 2 reaction, also known as erythema nodosum leprosum, corresponds to the type 3 hypersensitivity reaction. This is seen in dimorphous leprosy or lepromatous leprosy. Immune complex deposition and systemic toxicity are the main features, along with increased TNF levels, complement deposition, and neutrophilic infiltration of the skin.[2]

CLASSIFICATION

Although multiple classification systems have been proposed based on the clinical features and varying degrees of immunity, the most well received and commonly employed was proposed by Ridley and Jopling in 1966. It takes into account immunological and bacteriological aspects of the disease. The spectrum extends from high cell-mediated immunity (CMI) to low CMI and a high humoral immunity and classified as tuberculoid leprosy (TT), borderline tuberculoid (BT), borderline lepromatous leprosy (BL), mid borderline (BB), and lepromatous leprosy (LL).[4] TT and LL represent immunologically stable or polar ends of the spectrum, while borderline groups are associated with variations in the immunity and prone to immunologically mediated *M. leprae* reactions. However, two distinct variants namely pure neuritic leprosy and indeterminate leprosy (I) have not been placed in this classification.

In resource poor settings and for field workers, WHO expert committee on leprosy has classified leprosy into two categories: paucibacillary (PB) and multibacillary (MB).[5]

In India, National Leprosy Eradication Programme (NLEP) classification is currently implemented and it comprises WHO classification with added consideration for pure neuritic leprosy [**Table 73-2**].[5]

CLINICAL FEATURES

Clinical features in leprosy vary according to the spectrum of the disease and cutaneous lesions, nerve involvement gives valuable clue toward diagnosis.

TABLE 73-2 NLEP and WHO classification of leprosy for treatment purpose[5]

Parameters	Pauci bacillary leprosy (PB)	Multi bacillary leprosy (MB)
Number of skin lesions	5 or < 5	>5
Smear status	Negative	Positive
Nerve involvement	Single nerve	Two or more nerves

INDETERMINATE LEPROSY (I)

It presents as hypopigmented macules that often occurs on face, limbs and resembles pityriasis alba or polymorphous light eruption especially when it occurs in children. This stage may last for 5 years or longer before it progresses to TT and due to subtle or no neurological deficits, diagnosis is often missed. Molecular diagnostic techniques such as PCR are of value in such cases.[5,6]

TUBERCULOID LEPROSY (TT)

Well-defined, erythematous plaques or hypopigmented macules usually presenting on extremities and one to three in number are seen [**Figure 73-1**]. Diminished sensation to temperature, touch, or pain is present and due to anhidrosis, the lesions often appear dry in the center.

BORDERLINE TUBERCULOID LEPROSY (BT)

Skin lesions are similar to those in TT but are less well defined and there is an outward sloping noticed in the borders [**Figure 73-2A**]. They may be more numerous than in TT (3-10 in number), some lesions show papules close to the border of larger lesion or plaque that are termed as satellite lesions [**Figure 73-2B**]. Anesthesia over the lesion as well as signs of sensory-motor deficit in area supplied by involved nerve trunk may be present.[6]

MID BORDERLINE LEPROSY (BB)

This group represents an unstable part of the disease spectrum and is characterized by varying morphologies of lesions such as papules, plaques, circinate lesions that have a well-defined punched out inner edge and ill-defined outer edge (inverted saucer appearance) [**Figure 73-3A** and **B**]. Skin within the lesions appears normal and this finding is denoted as Swiss cheese appearance.[5,6] Asymmetrical peripheral nerve enlargement may be also seen.

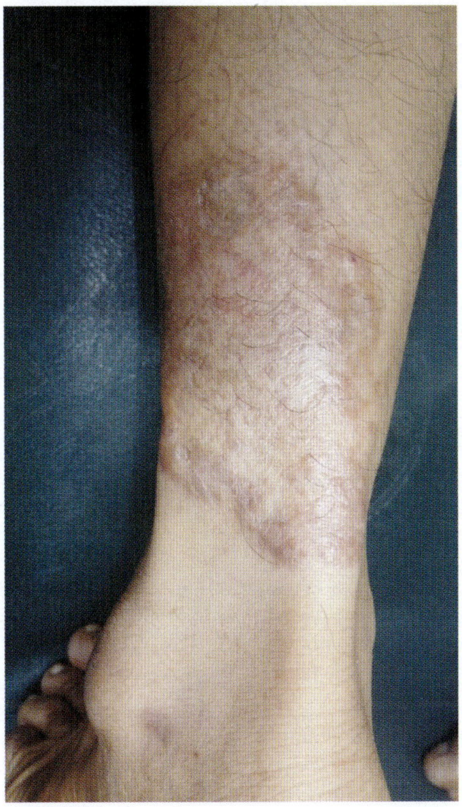

FIGURE 73-1. Well-defined plaque of TT on leg with raised borders and atrophic, hypopigmented center. (Courtesy of the Department of Dermatology, Father Muller Medical College, Mangalore, India.)

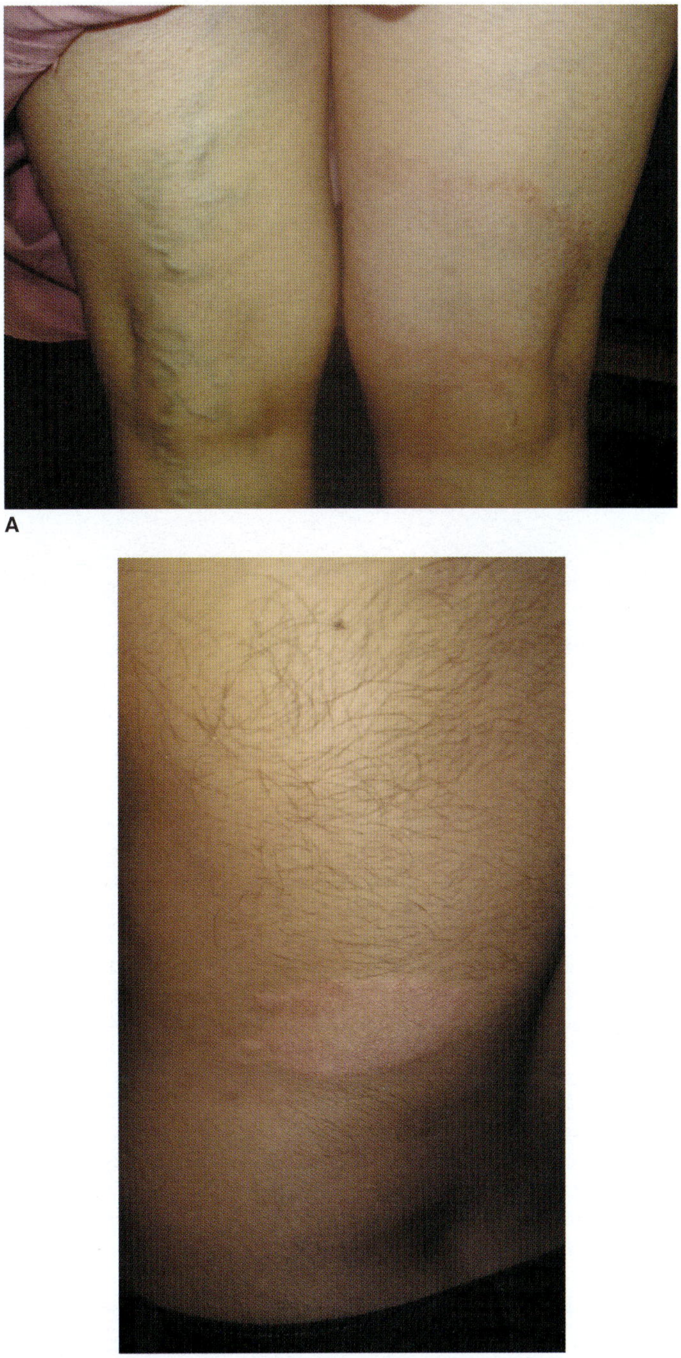

A

B

FIGURE 73-2. **(A)** Patch of borderline tuberculoid (BT) on thigh with partly defined borders and lesion showing xerosis. **(B)** Patch of BT with pseudopod-like extension and satellite lesion. (Courtesy of the Department of Dermatology, Father Muller Medical College, Mangalore, India.)

BORDERLINE LEPROMATOUS LEPROSY (BL)

BL presents as multiple, slightly infiltrated macules and plaques that are asymmetrically distributed over the body with variable loss of sensations, sweating over the area involved [**Figure 73-4**]. Asymmetric peripheral nerve thickening and anesthesia in extremities termed as glove and stocking anesthesia can often be associated with this form of leprosy.[6]

LEPROMATOUS LEPROSY (LL)

This is a multibacillary form and characterized by a myriad of features such as ear lobe infiltration, loss of lateral end of eyebrows (madarosis), diffuse infiltration and thickening of the skin of the face (leonine

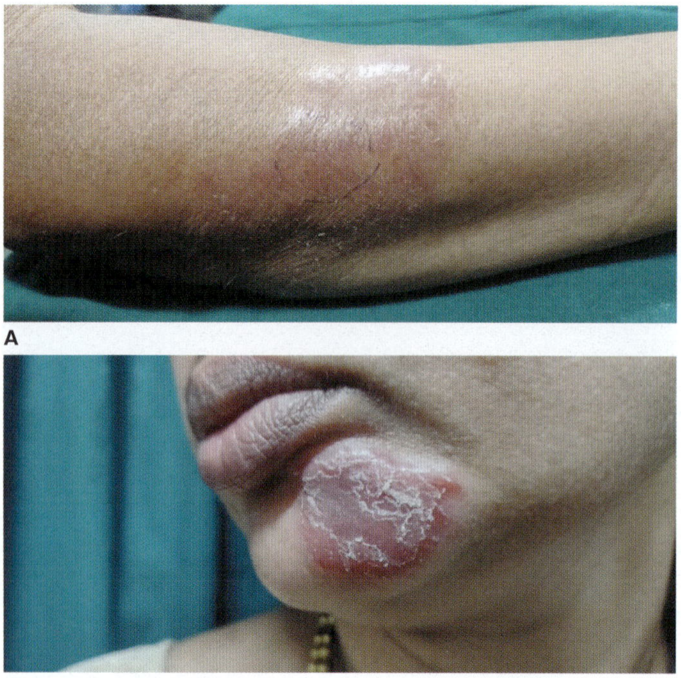

FIGURE 73-3. **(A)** Punched out lesions inner border in mid borderline. **(B)** Inverted saucer appearance. (Courtesy of the Department of Dermatology, Father Muller Medical College, Mangalore, India.)

facies), and diffuse infiltration of skin of the body with red-brown or copper-colored lesions in a symmetrical fashion [**Figure 73-5A** and **B**]. Three distinct forms have been reported: diffuse, nodular, and infiltrated lepromatous leprosy. Systemic involvement of eyes, bones, joints, reticuloendothelial system, and renal system may be seen in cases of lepromatous leprosy. Certain body parts such as scalp, lower back, axilla, groin, sub-umbilical area, and the penile shaft are less commonly involved and are termed as immune zones. Warmth in these areas and a preference of lepra bacilli for cooler body temperature has been attributed to this finding.

Swelling of lower limbs that worsens in the evening, fusiform swelling of digits, symmetrical peripheral nerve thickening, glove, and stocking anesthesia are some of the other clinical features. In up to 80% of cases, nasal mucosal involvement in the form of epistaxis, nasal crusting, and rarely nasal septal perforation leading to a saddle nose deformity is seen.

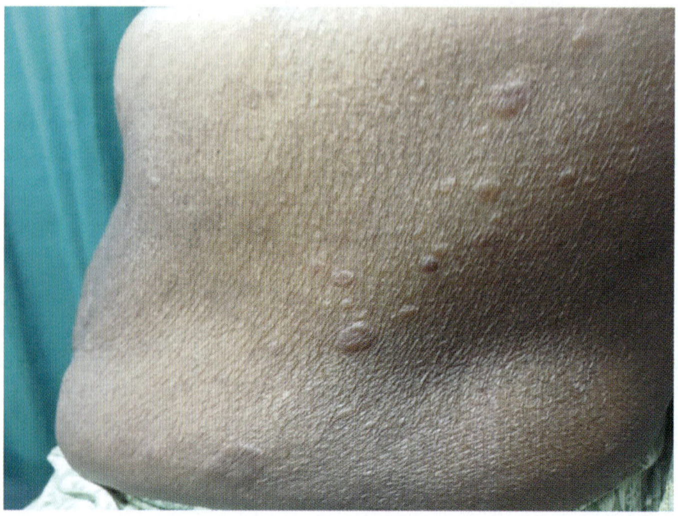

FIGURE 73-4. Multiple skin-colored to brown papules and plaques in borderline lepromatous leprosy. (Courtesy of the Department of Dermatology, Father Muller Medical College, Mangalore, India.)

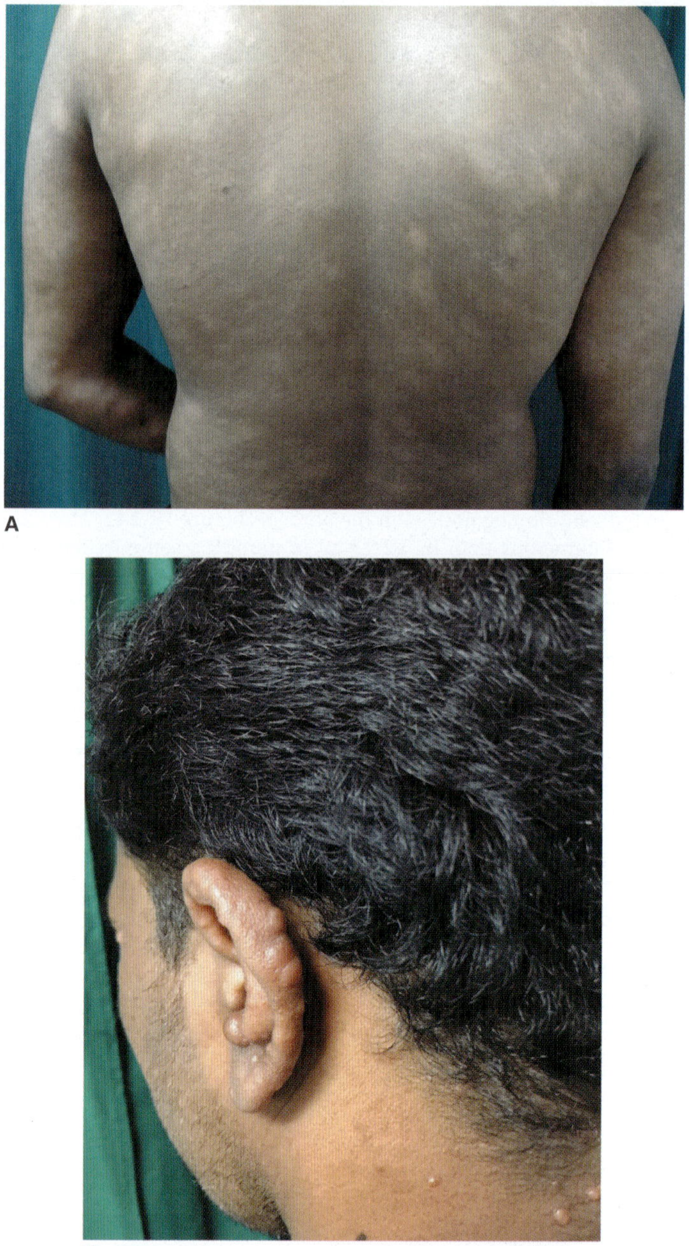

FIGURE 73-5. **(A)** Multiple hypopigmented macules symmetrically distributed over back in LL. **(B)** Ear lobe infiltration. (Courtesy of the Department of Dermatology, Father Muller Medical College, Mangalore, India.)

ADDITIONAL VARIANTS

Histoid Leprosy This is an unusual variant of leprosy first described by Wade. Although cases reported earlier were primarily due to dapsone monotherapy or incomplete therapy, de novo cases are known to occur. It is characterized by shiny, smooth, dome-shaped papules, subcutaneous nodules, and plaques over body [**Figure 73-6**]. It can involve even the immune zones of leprosy and ear lobe infiltration. Madarosis is less common than in lepromatous leprosy. Distinctive histopathology helps in differentiation from the nodular form of lepromatous leprosy.[7,8]

Pure Neuritic Leprosy It is characterized by sensory loss with or without motor involvement along the involved nerve trunk supply without any skin involvement. Nerve conduction studies and nerve biopsy may facilitate the diagnosis and often BT spectrum of disease activity is seen on nerve biopsy.[6]

Lucio Leprosy It is a rare variant of LL reported in Mexico where diffuse and progressive skin infiltration without appearance of any discrete

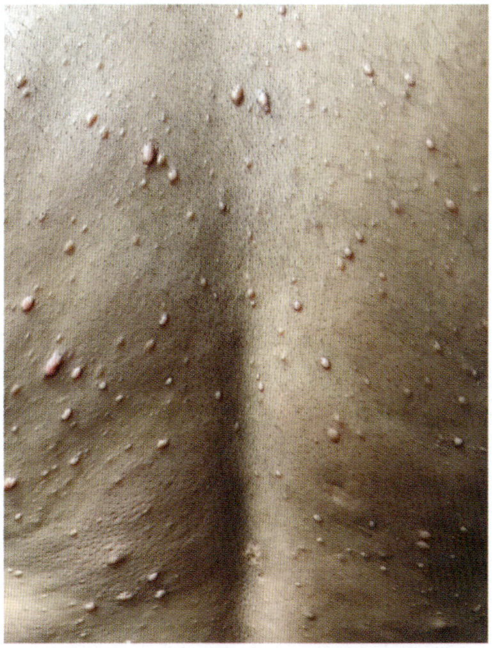

FIGURE 73-6. Multiple skin-colored nodules and papules in histoid leprosy. (Courtesy of the Department of Dermatology, Father Muller Medical College, Mangalore, India.)

skin lesions is seen leading to a smooth, youthful appearance known as lepra bonita or beautiful leprosy.

Lazarine Leprosy This is an uncommon variant of BT in which spontaneous ulcerations have been noticed in the existing skin lesions attributed to a Type 1 hypersensitivity reaction.

Lepra Reactions These are immunologically mediated reactions due to sudden shift in the immunity. Type 1 lepra reaction is commonly seen in tuberculoid pole of leprosy (TT, BT) when it is down grading (due to worsening of immunity) or BB, Bl when it is upgrading (due to improvement in immunity). It is a type 4 hypersensitivity reaction and characterized by a sudden increase in erythema, edema over preexisting skin lesions and neuritis [**Figure 73-7**]. When left untreated, it may lead to sensory motor impairment and deformities.

Type 2 lepra reactions are type 2 or immune complex mediated hypersensitivity reactions that occur commonly in lepromatous pole (BB, BL, LL). It is also known as erythema nodosum leprosum due to the presence of characteristic skin lesions [**Figure 73-8A** and **B**]. In this condition, evanescent, tender, erythematous to violaceous nodules are seen over the body. Systemic complaints such as joint pains, fever, iridocyclitis, glomerulonephritis may be associated.

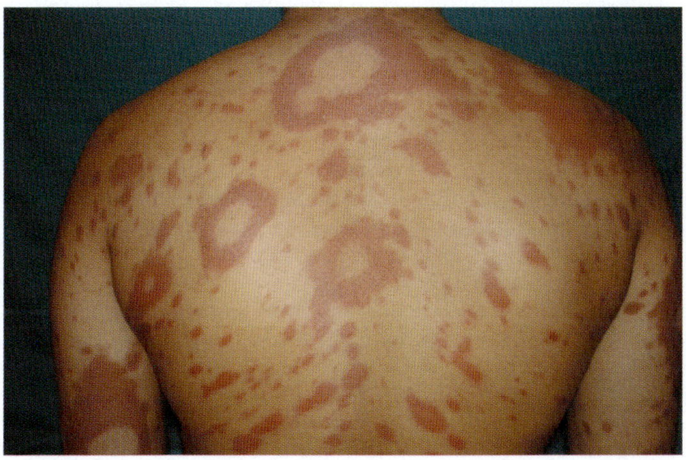

FIGURE 73-7. Borderline tuberculoid patch in type 1 lepra reaction. (Courtesy of the Department of Dermatology, Father Muller Medical College, Mangalore, India.)

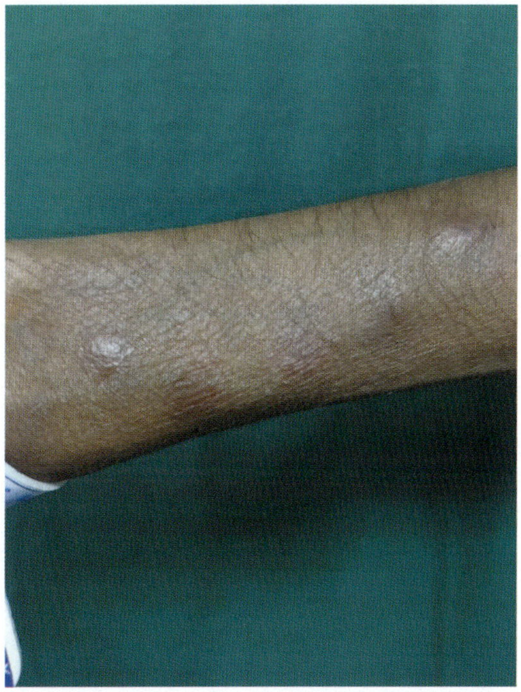

A

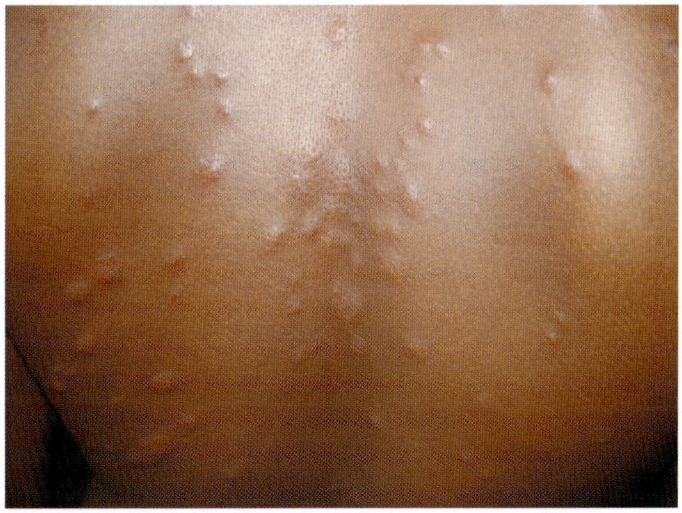

B

FIGURE 73-8. **(A)** and **(B)** Erythema nodosum leprosum. (Courtesy of the Department of Dermatology, Father Muller Medical College, Mangalore, India.)

Type 3 lepra reaction or lucio phenomenon is a lepra reaction occurring in lucio leprosy characterized by painful, purpuric lesions leading to ulcerations with jagged edges due to leukocytoclastic vasculitis and thrombosis of blood vessels.[7,8]

DIAGNOSIS

Cardinal diagnostic signs for leprosy were proposed by WHO Expert Committee on Leprosy in 1997. The sensitivity of the criteria is nearly 97% when all three cardinal features are present. Presence of one or more of these signs in an individual indicates the diagnosis of leprosy.[2]

1. A hypopigmented (or erythematous) anesthetic skin lesion
2. A thickened peripheral nerve
3. A positive skin smear or bacilli observed in a biopsy

Apart from clinical examination, slit skin smear examination and histopathology from skin and or nerve biopsy specimens may aid in the diagnosis and classify the spectrum of disease.

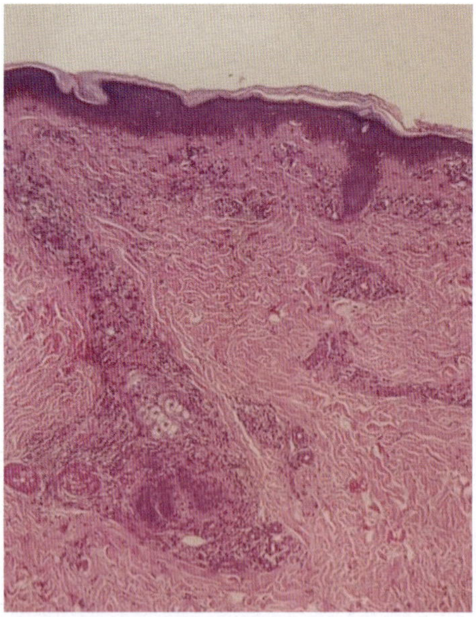

FIGURE 73-9. Hematoxylin and eosin stain showing branching granuloma around pilosebaceous unit in a case of borderline tuberculoid (100× magnification). (Courtesy of the Department of Dermatology, Father Muller Medical College, Mangalore, India.)

Slit Skin Smear test (SSS) involves obtaining a smear from five sites including the ear lobe, forehead, chin, thigh, or buttock. The skin lesions is subjected to modified Ziehl-Neelsen staining and examined for acid-fast bacilli (AFB). Quantification is performed using Ridley logarithmic scale to calculate bacterial load using the bacterial index (BI). High BI suggests presence of multibacillary leprosy.[7,8] In addition, morphological index (MI) may be calculated by studying live bacilli and it has prognostic value in evaluating treatment outcome. The specificity of SSS is 100%, while sensitivity is much less at 50%.

Skin biopsy and histopathology from a representative skin lesion followed by examination with hematoxylin and eosin stain is a useful aid in the diagnosis of leprosy where laboratory facilities are available. The specimen is evaluated for extent, type, and characteristics of cellular infiltrate and Fite Faraco staining is used to detect leprae bacilli.[7] Indeterminate form (I) is a stage of early immunological response and on histopathology, we may find sparse cellular aggregates of lymphocytes and macrophages in periadnexal, perineural or perivascular region. TT is characterized by presence of well-defined, dermal granulomas composed of epithelioid cells, Langhan's giant cells, with a peripheral rim of lymphocytes around neurovascular bundles. In cases of nerve destruction S100 staining may be employed to identify remnants of nerve bundles. Fite Faraco staining of the biopsy specimen usually is negative for AFB. A similar finding is seen in BT but with less well-formed granulomas as compared to TT and AFB may be graded as 1+ to 2+ BI [**Figure 73-9**]. In cases of BB, which is immunologically unstable form, there is a diffuse infiltration of lymphocytes and fewer epithelioid cells as compared to tuberculoid pole. BI is usually 2+ to 3+. In the BL group, aggregates of histiocytes with a foamy cytoplasm (Virchow cells) and lymphocytes are noted. A grenz zone is often present, which is an acellular zone separating epidermis from the dermal cellular infiltrate [**Figure 73-10**]. BI is usually 4+ to 5+. In LL, sheets of foamy macrophages are noticed underneath a well-formed grenz zone and AFB appear in globi giving a 6+BI grading.[4] In histoid leprosy, beneath the grenz zone, numerous spindle-shaped, elongated, histiocytes arranged in a storiform pattern are seen and AFB are long and lie in singles instead of globi formation. This finding is known as histoid habitus.[9] In type 1 lepra reaction, dermal edema, diffuse infiltration by neutrophils and granulomatous destruction of dermal nerves is seen. Type 2 lepra reaction is characterized by evidence of leukocytoclastic vasculitis on histopathology.[8]

In addition, various histopathological indices such as granuloma fraction, bacterial index of granulomna may be used in addition to BI and MI to assess the efficacy of treatment and disease activity following treatment.[8]

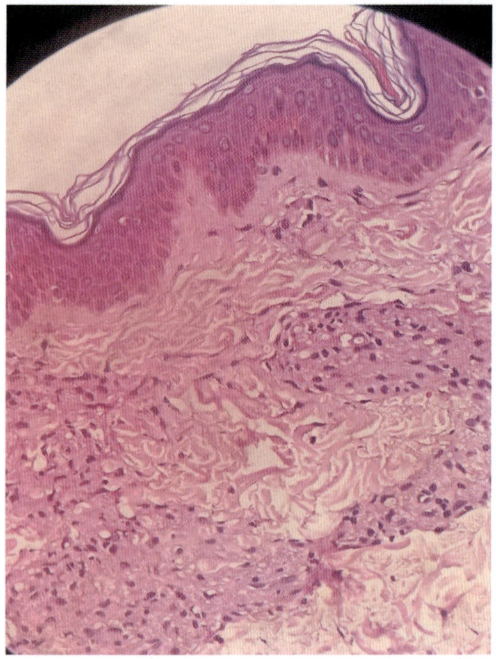

FIGURE 73-10. Hematoxylin and eosin stain showing Grenz zone, aggregates of foamy macrophages in a case of borderline lepromatous leprosy (400× magnification). (Courtesy of the Department of Dermatology, Father Muller Medical College, Mangalore, India.)

Other tests of importance include the lepromin test that assists in the classification of leprosy based on the immunological response noted to an intradermal test utilizing inactivated *M. leprae* extract, bedside tests such as histamine and pilocarpine tests used to test dermal nerve integrity in suspected cases of tuberculoid leprosy.[10]

Serological tests such as detection of antibodies against PG L-1, which is an important antigenic component of *M. leprae*, have been of value to study prevalence and distribution of leprosy in the population as well as gauging the effectiveness of anti-leprosy therapy.[8]

Ultrasonography of peripheral nerves, nerve conduction studies, and needle electromyography is of diagnostic value in cases of pure neuritic leprosy in the absence of skin lesions. These tests also help in the assessment of the severity of nerve damage.[8]

TREATMENT

Standardized treatment of leprosy is based on WHO recommended regimen for diagnosed PB and MB leprosy cases. Drugs are available in a blister pack and composed of rifampicin, dapsone, clofazimine and this is termed as multidrug therapy or MDT that was initiated in 1981.

Dapsone was first introduced as a monotherapy in 1941. It exerts its antibacterial effect by inhibiting folic acid synthesis and has a bacteriostatic effect. Side effects such as headaches, methemoglobinemia, hemolysis, and hepatitis have to be noted while on therapy.[6]

Rifampicin was initially synthesized from a gram-positive bacteria (*Amycolatopsis rifamycinica*) and has a favorable place in MDT due to its potent antibacterial action by inhibition of RNA polymerase enzymes. It renders a person noninfectious within a few days after ingestion. Reddish orange discoloration of body fluids, flu-like symptoms, hepatotoxicity, and skin rashes are some of its side effects.[6]

Clofazimine is a red azo dye first synthesized in Dublin in 1954. It has a mild anti-bacterial effect and an anti-inflammatory effect that renders it useful for type 2 lepra reactions. Brownish hyperpigmentation of skin, xerosis, and gastrointestinal side effects due accumulation of dye crystals in intestinal mucosal surface are some of the side effects noted.[6]

The treatment for PB adult patients includes 28 daily doses of dapsone 100 mg and a monthly dose of rifampicin 600 mg over a 6-month period which is supervised [**Table 73-3A**]. MB adult patients are administered dapsone 100 mg and clofazimine 50 mg once a day for 28 days in addition

TABLE 73-3A Treatment of leprosy with MDT—multibacillary cases MB			
Age	Rifampicin	Dapsone (mg/day)	Clofazimine
Adult > 50 kg	600 mg once a month	100	50 mg/day and 300 mg/month
Children 10-14 years	450 mg once a month	50	50 mg/day and 150 mg/month
Children < 10 years	300 mg once a month	25	50 mg twice a week and 100 mg/month*

TABLE 73-3B Treatment of leprosy with MDT—paucibacillary cases PB		
Age	Rifampicin	Dapsone (mg/day)
Adult > 50 kg	600 mg once a month	100
Children 10-14 years	450 mg once a month	50
Children < 10 years	300 mg once a month	25

to monthly administration of rifampicin 600 mg and clofazimine 300 mg that is supervised for a duration of 12 months [**Table 73-3B**].

A combination of rifampicin, ofloxacin, minocycline ROM treatment regimen was used to treat single-patch PB leprosy and in doubtful cases of indeterminate leprosy with single treatment with rifampicin 600 mg, ofloxacin 400 mg, and minocycline 100 mg.[7,11]

Second-line drugs are minocycline, clarithromycin, ofloxacin that have found utility in case of drug resistance and when alternative drug regimens are required. Rifapentine, which is derivative of rifamycin with superior pharmacokinetic properties and a longer half-life, is yet another useful substitute that has been tried in combination with minocycline and moxifloxacin as a PMM regimen.[11]

Reactions in leprosy pose a significant risk for development of impairment and systemic complications and hence prompt diagnosis and treatment is necessary. In type 1 lepra reactions oral steroids such as prednisolone, immunomodulators such as hydroxychloroquine, or cyclosporine may be used. Steroids, clofazimine, thalidomide, nonsteroidal anti-inflammatory drugs (NSAIDs), azathioprine, methotrexate, pentoxifylline have been tried in the treatment of erythema nodosum leprosum.[11] Ocular care and splinting of limbs in case of neuritis are additional supportive treatments necessary in case of complications associated with reactions.

COMPLICATIONS

Complications in leprosy include (a) infiltration of skin and nerves, and systemic involvement with leprae bacilli (b) nerve damage as a part of disease or during lepra reactions (c) side effects of anti-leprosy drugs. These complications may lead to varying degrees of functional or anatomical impairment and disability [**Figures 73-11** to **73-13**]. Impairment may be primary due to the disease while secondary is as a consequence to primary.[12]

Various impairments have been listed in **Table 73-4**. Deformities often lead to disability and grading of these helps in planning for rehabilitation as well as to assess the efficiency of existing leprosy control programs. In this regard, World Health Organization (WHO) grading (revised in 1988) has been proposed to assess the patients during field surveys. Salient features are tabulated in **Table 73-5**.[12,13]

PREVENTION

Early diagnosis and treatment as well as methods to prevent leprosy are the corner stones of leprosy control measures. Studies of vaccines such as BCG, and more recently *Mycobacterium indicus pranii* (MIP) have shown some efficacy. However, efficacy of BCG vaccine appears to wane with time.

Chemoprophylaxis has been tried since the 1960s in various studies with dapsone, rifampicin, ofloxacin, and minocycline or ROM regimen (as well as a combination of BCG with rifampicin). However, further studies and research are required in this field to validate the use of chemoprophylaxis as a measure to curb this chronic illness.[3]

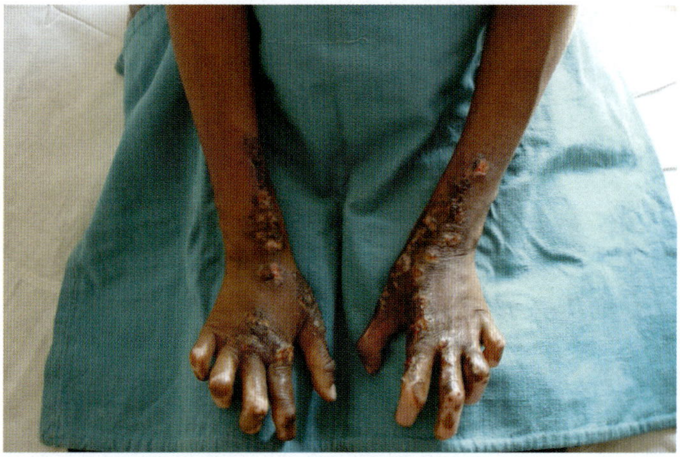

FIGURE 73-11. Claw hands with digital ulcerations. (Courtesy of the Department of Dermatology, Father Muller Medical College, Mangalore, India.)

5-YEAR UPDATE

EPIDEMIOLOGY AND RESERVOIR

Armadillos are a natural host and reservoir for *M. leprae*. A recent study suggested an increased susceptibility to leprosy in individuals in contact with armadillos (living/working in armadillo-inhabited areas, having armadillos as pets, and those who consumed armadillo meat) compared to those having no contact with armadillos. Anti-PGL-1 antibody levels

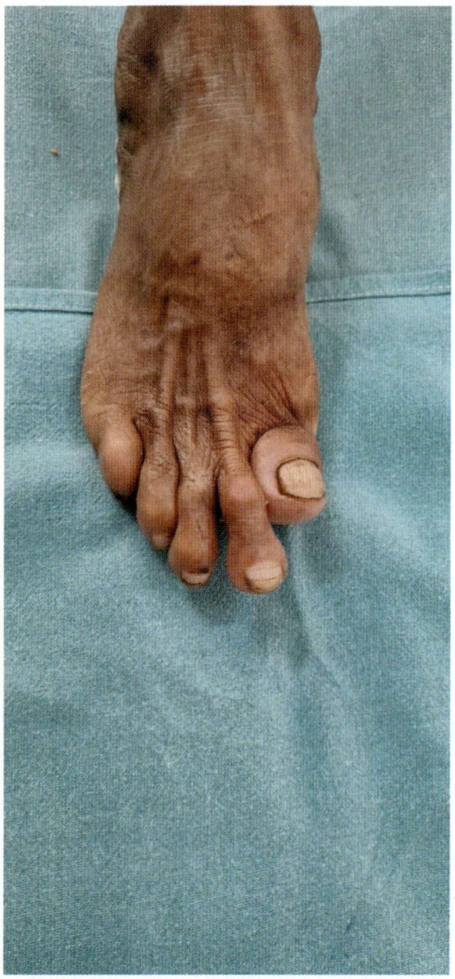

FIGURE 73-12. Claw toe. (Courtesy of the Department of Dermatology, Father Muller Medical College, Mangalore, India.)

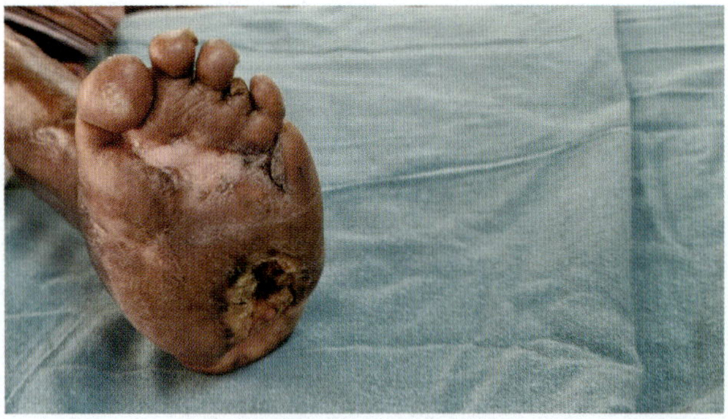

FIGURE 73-13. Amputation of toes with tarsal disorganization. (Courtesy of the Department of Dermatology, Father Muller Medical College, Mangalore, India.)

in the former individuals were seen to be higher than in the latter. Anti–PGL-1 antibodies, although having low sensitivity and predictive value, are a useful biomarker in the exclusion of leprosy.

The Eurasian red squirrels (*Sciurus vulgaris*) found in the British Isles are thought to be a natural reservoir of *M. leprae*. Previously, the only known nonhuman reservoir was the armadillo. *Mycobacterium lepromatosis* isolated from these red squirrels is found to be closely related to *M. leprae*. Although it is found to be a natural reservoir of infection, transmission to humans from squirrels is not so far known. Features of leprosy have also been seen in the sooty mangabey (*Cerocebus atys*) monkey, but transmission to humans has not been described.

GENETICS

A positive association between leprosy and single-nucleotide polymorphisms (SNPs) near HLA genes has been described. SNPs are variations in the DNA between genes. SNPs can aid in predicting the risk of developing the disease or susceptibility to the disease. A novel missense variant in MRPS5 was identified by the genome-wide association study conducted in China.

DISEASE ASSOCIATION

A predisposition to leprosy and type 2 diabetes mellitus that was attributed to the PARK2 gene mutation.

In areas where HTLV-1 coinfection with leprosy was noted, a higher rate of type 1 and 2 reactions and neuritis were seen.

Leprosy coinfection with the SARS-CoV-2 results in uncontrolled cytokine release and inflammatory profile. NET (neutrophil extracellular traps) are associated with severe disease progression and unfavorable outcomes. NETs were seen in patients with ENLs and severe COVID-19. Immunomodulatory drugs have been found useful in this scenario.

DIAGNOSIS

In difficult-to-diagnose cases of leprosy, polymerase chain reaction (PCR) can be performed along with the skin biopsy. 16s RNA and RLEP are the markers used most frequently in PCR testing.

TABLE 73-4 Impairments and deformities in leprosy

Primary impairment	Secondary impairment leading to deformities
Thickening and nodulation of skin and subcutaneous tissue—leonine facies, ear lobe infiltration	"Facies leprosa" that is characterized by (i) atrophy of the anterior nasal spine, (ii) atrophy and recession of the maxillary alveolar processes, and (iii) endonasal inflammatory change
Ocular changes—madarosis, drooping of upper eyelid, punctate keratitis, miliary lepromata, iris pearls	Ocular—iridocyclitis, glaucoma, premature cataract, corneal ulcer, dry eye, lagophthalmos, loss of vision
Sensory loss	Xerosis, anhidrosis, trophic ulcers, banana fingers
Motor paresis	Claw hand (partial or complete), foot drop, wrist drop, frozen hand, claw toes
Testicular atrophy	Gynecomastia, azoospermia, and infertility

TABLE 73-5 WHO grading of disabilities (1988)[13]

Grade	Hands	Feet	Eyes
1	Insensitive hand	Insensitive feet	Redness of conjunctiva
2	Ulcers and injuries and/or mobile claw hand, and/or slight absorption	With trophic ulcer and /or claw toes or foot drop and/ or slight resorption	Lagophthalmos and/or blurring of vision and/or inflammation of globe
3	Wrist drop and/or clawing of fingers with stiff joints and/or severe absorption of fingers	Contracture and/or severe resorption of foot (one-fifth of the sole area is lost)	Severe loss of vision

Source: Reproduced with permission from Kumar B, Kumar HK, IAL Texbook of leprosy. Jaypee Brothers Medical Publishers.

Electroneuromyographic testing is useful in the detection of early cases of leprosy, household contacts, and cases of pure neural leprosy. A reduction or absence in the sensory action potential in the ulnar nerve can precede the development of symptoms in a patient and is thus a useful diagnostic modality. Ultrasonography of the peripheral nerves is another useful diagnostic modality in difficult-to-palpate nerves.

VACCINE

The Bacille Calmette-Guérin (BCG) vaccine and the Indian Cancer Research Centre (ICRC) bacillus vaccine are useful in leprosy; however, simultaneous administration of both vaccines confers double protection when compared to BCG alone. The MIP vaccine can be used to preexposure prophylaxis and also can expedite recovery time from the disease. LepVax is a subunit vaccine, seen to lower bacterial numbers and provide pre- and postexposure prophylaxis. It has also shown a reduction of neuropathy in armadillo studies. In addition, it is cost-effective and safe. LepVax is a hybrid adjuvanted recombinant protein vaccine. It links *M. leprae* antigens ML2531, ML2380, ML2055, and ML2028 (LEP-F1) with a synthetic toll-like receptor

TREATMENT

Fluoroquinolones such as pefloxacin and ofloxacin are useful additives or alternatives to MDT. Minocycline has shown a faster clearance rate of *M. leprae* compared to ofloxacin and pefloxacin. Addition of clarithromycin to rifampicin or fluoroquinolones has an additive effect.

Treatment of *M. lepromatosis* is similar to *M. leprae* although the former shows more similarity to Lucio leprosy.[14]

REFERENCES

1. World population prospects 2019, online edition revision 1. New York City (NY): United Nations, Department of Economic and Social Affairs, Population Division; 2022 revision. https://population.un.org/wpp/Download/Standard/Population/. Accessed July 2022.
2. Eichelmann K, González SE, Salas-Alanis JC, Ocampo-Candiani J. Leprosy. An update: definition, pathogenesis, classification, diagnosis, and treatment. *Actas Dermosifiliogr*. 2013;104(7):554-563.
3. Bhat RM, Prakash C. Leprosy: an overview of pathophysiology. *Interdiscip Perspect Infect Dis*. 2012;2012:181089.
4. Pardillo FE, Fajardo TT, Abalos RM, Scollard D, Gelber RH. Methods for the classification of leprosy for treatment purposes. *Clin Infect Dis*. 2007;44(8):1096-1099.
5. Misra RS, Kataria JK. Classification. In: Kumar B, Kumar HK, eds. *IAL Texbook of Leprosy*. 2nd ed. New Delhi: Jaypee Publishers; 2017;254-262.
6. Fischer M. Leprosy—an overview of clinical features, diagnosis, and treatment. *J Dtsch Dermatol Ges*. 2017;15(8):801-827.
7. Chen KH, Lin CY, Su SB, Chen KT. Leprosy: a review of epidemiology, clinical diagnosis, and management. *J Trop Med*. 2022, 8652062.
8. Chan MMF, Smoller BR. Overview of the histopathology and other laboratory investigations in leprosy. *Curr Trop Med Rep*. 2016;3:131-137.
9. Muthupandian V, Kannan R, Priya BT, Algar K. A retrospective study on histoid Hansen's disease—an insight into aetiopathogenesis and disease pattern. *J Evolution Med Dent Sci*. 2016;5(98):7209-7212.

10. Pande S, Nagar R, Khopkar U. Intradermal tests in dermatology-II: tests for noninfectious diseases. *Indian J Dermatol Venereol Leprol*. 2007;73:57-59.
11. Prasad PV, Kaviarasan PK. Leprosy therapy, past and present: can we hope to eliminate it? *Indian J Dermatol*. 2010;55(4):316-324.
12. Rathod SP, Jagati A, Chowdhary P. Disabilities in leprosy: an open, retrospective analyses of institutional records. *An Bras Dermatol*. 2020;95(1):52-56.
13. Malviya GN. Deformity and disability prevention. In: Kumar B, Kumar HK, eds. *IAL Texbook of Leprosy*. 2nd ed. New Delhi: Jaypee Publishers; 2017:542-560.
14. Randhawa A, Kapila R, Schwartz RA. Leprosy: what is new. *Int J Dermatol*. 2022;61(6):733-738.

CHAPTER 74

Onchocerciasis

Arielle Carolina Mora Hurtado
Chinwe Laura Onyekonwu
Gladys Angela Ozoh
Uche Rowland Ojinmah
Nada Elbuluk
Susan C. Taylor

KEY POINTS

- Onchocerciasis is a chronic, disabling vector-borne disease caused by infection with the filarial nematode worm *Onchocerca volvulus* that can lead to blindness, cutaneous and systemic manifestations, and is also associated with psychosocial sequelae and profound socioeconomic problems.
- An estimated 21 million people are afflicted, the majority residing in Western and Central Africa with the clinical presentation reflecting variations in the host's immune response to the parasite.
- The classic lesion is the onchocercoma, a painless subcutaneous nodule encapsulating female worms and most of the burden of the skin disease occurs as a result of severe, intolerable pruritus.
- Mass treatment with ivermectin and vector control interventions have been highly successful in reducing disease burden and eliminating the transmission of disease in four Latin American countries and in foci in Africa.
- Onchocerciasis is a neglected tropical disease targeted for elimination by the World Health Organization. The elimination of onchocerciasis faces several challenges, especially in areas where *Loa loa* is co-endemic, and in regions experiencing instability and civil conflict.

INTRODUCTION

Onchocerciasis (river blindness) is a vector-borne parasitic disease caused by the filarial nematode worm, *Onchocerca volvulus*. Infection is acquired through the repeated bites of the insect vector, blackflies of the genus *Simulium*, which breed in fast-flowing streams and rivers.[1] Members of the *Simulium damnosum* complex are the major vectors in Africa and the Middle East, whereas *S. neavei* are vectors in parts of East Africa, and numerous other species are vectors of the disease in Latin America.[2,3] People residing in rural areas near fast-flowing rivers and streams have the highest risk of acquiring onchocerciasis.[1] Although the disease occurs in Yemen and in foci in Venezuela and Brazil, 99% of the disease occurs in 31 sub-Saharan African countries, stretching between 15°N and 14°S, from Senegal in the west to Ethiopia in the east, where it causes blindness, cutaneous disease, and systemic manifestations.[4-6]

Onchocerciasis is a neglected tropical disease that is chronic, disabling, and a major public health problem and an even more profound socioeconomic problem that extends beyond the infected individual, affecting families, communities, and countries as a whole.[7] The manifestations of the disease have resulted in abandonment of vast areas of fertile land and an unfavorable attitude with regard to work. The disease has led to the collapse and desertion of families and vast communities and ranks second to trachoma as the leading cause of infectious blindness worldwide.[1]

Onchocerciasis results in significant morbidity, reduction in quality of life, and psychosocial sequelae in those affected.[8] Onchocercal skin disease manifestations have been associated with stigmatization, social rejection, impaired self-esteem, reduced occupational opportunities, and limited marriage prospects for affected women.[6,9,10] The impaired social interaction, low morale, stigmatization, and the socioeconomic impact of the disease must be emphasized.

Estimates indicate there are approximately 21 million individuals infected, mostly residing in Western and Central Africa, and there are 218 million individuals worldwide at risk of contracting onchocerciasis.[11,12] Of those infected, 14.6 million have already had skin disease and 1.15 million have experienced vision loss due to onchocerciasis.[4,11] Nigeria, the Democratic Republic of Congo, South Sudan, and Cameroon are predicted to carry the highest disease burden due to onchocerciasis by the year 2030 due to these countries having the highest numbers of people living in endemic zones or having the blinding savannah parasite strain.[13] O'Neill first reported the presence of filariae in cases of "craw-craw," as onchocerciasis is called in West Africa, in 1875.[14] The term *Onchocerca* is derived from the Greek word *ogkos*, meaning "swelling or mass," and *kerkos*, meaning "tail."[15]

Clinical presentations of onchocerciasis reflect variations in the host's immune response to the parasite, and these range from endemic normal individuals (putatively immune) who are disease free and have a good cellular immune response to the parasite, to individuals with low cellular immunity (with or without generalized onchodermatitis) and significant immune tolerance to millions of microfilariae with tissue damage progressing over many years. Individuals with a strong antibody response and hyperreactive onchodermatitis (*sowda*)[9,16] and human immunodeficiency virus (HIV)-positive patients with a weakened antibody response make up the other groups of susceptible individuals.[17] The severity of complications from onchocerciasis may correspond with the chronicity of infection, continued parasite exposure, and geographic location.[18] Most of the burden of onchocercal skin disease is due to severe intolerable pruritus. The cutaneous manifestations of onchocerciasis are discussed in this chapter.

EPIDEMIOLOGY

The epidemiology of onchocerciasis is determined by several factors including the host's response, parasite and vector competence, the geographic environment (proximity of the home or dwelling to fly breeding sites), and social and demographic influences; even in the same geographic area, onchocerciasis has distinctly variable endemic rates.

Genetic variations in populations exist among the different foci of onchocerciasis worldwide and may affect the biology of the parasites.[19] The parasite and the blackfly vector have reciprocal effects on each other's survival at various stages of the parasite's life cycle.[20]

The disease pattern and severity of onchocerciasis, particularly regarding ocular involvement, varies by geographic areas.[3,5] In the West African savannah (nonforest) areas, ocular involvement is more common.[5] Conversely, onchocercal skin disease predominates in African forest areas where ocular disease is less severe, even among individuals with high parasite load.[5,21] Ocular onchocerciasis can affect the cornea, anterior, and posterior segments of the eye, and in severe cases, lead to blindness.[5,22,23] Lymphatic involvement and dermatologic manifestations (eg, pruritus, chronic papular dermatitis, nodules, depigmentation) are more common in the rainforest than in the savannah.[5,24]

The variation of disease patterns between different geographical zones has been hypothesized to be explained by the existence of two parasite strains, the savannah and the forest strains.[25] This hypothesis postulates the two parasite strains differ in their pathogenicity and distribution in the human body.[25] More recently, following the reanalysis of blindness and transmission data, researchers concluded that evidence for a savannah blinding parasite strain in simple contrast with a nonblinding forest strain is equivocal.[3,26] Researchers have suggested a reappraisal of the two-strain hypothesis to explain ocular disease patterns is necessary to help to advance understanding of onchocerciasis epidemiology and disease burden estimates.[26]

ETIOLOGY AND PATHOGENESIS

O. volvulus is a parasitic filarial nematode worm belonging to the family Filarioidea whose five-stage life cycle occurs in two different hosts: blackflies (the obligate intermediate host) and humans (the definitive host).[27,28] However, infection of nonhuman primates such as the chimpanzee is likely.

Blackflies of the genus *Simulium*, which are tiny ferocious biters, are the only vectors of *O. volvulus*. At least 15 different species of blackflies can transmit onchocerciasis, and they vary by terrain and continent (eg, *S. damnosum* in Africa).[6,27] Their eggs require fast-running rivers for breeding grounds. *Simulium* bites by day and can travel long distances with flights covering several kilometers.[29] Infection occurs when a blackfly introduces an *O. volvulus* stage 3 larva (L_3) into the skin of the human host during a blood meal[30] [Figure 74-1]. These immature larval forms of the parasite create nodules in the subcutaneous tissues of the human host, where the larvae undergo molting to the L_4 stage, and then after reach the adult stage. After the adult worms mate, the female adult worm is capable of producing thousands of microscopic larvae daily.[9] Mature adult worms capable of producing microfilariae develop within 12 to 18 months of infection.[31]

The life span of microfilariae may reach 2 years,[32] in contrast to the adult female worm life span, which is 2 to 15 years.[33,34] The microfilariae migrate throughout the tissues of the body, gathering in the skin, eyes, lymphatics, and lymph nodes,[18] and when they die, they cause a variety of symptoms and signs, including dermatitis, nodular lesions, skin depigmentation, edema, and severe pruritus.[35] Further, the inflammatory response against dying microfilariae over repeated infection causes gradual and eventually blinding sclerosal opacification of the anterior eye by local inflammation and of the posterior eye by autoimmune mechanisms.[30,36] Both the mechanical invasion of microfilariae and deposition of immune complexes appear to be involved in ocular onchocerciasis.[5] While rarely fatal, infection with *Onchocerca* causes debilitating disease, chronic suffering, and lowers the host's immunity and resistance to other diseases, resulting in an estimated 13-year reduction of life expectancy.[3,37]

An intracellular rickettsial bacterium, *Wolbachia* was discovered in the late 1990s to exist in a symbiotic relationship with *O. volvulus*, inhabiting the endodermis of female *O. volvulus* worms and various of its embryonic stages.[30,38] This endosymbiotic bacterium provides essential metabolites to the microfilariae, contributes to reproduction and larval development, and promotes fertility, embryogenesis, and survival of the microfilariae.[3,39] *Wolbachia* also contributes to the clinical presentation of filarial infections, particularly onchocercal eye disease, since bacterial products released from dead worms can activate the host innate immune response, triggering the release of proinflammatory mediators.[21,40,41] The release of *Wolbachia* products from the dead and degenerating worms activates toll-like receptors on corneal epithelial cells and keratinocytes, initiating the immune response in ocular onchocerciasis leading to keratitis.[3,41]

A possible role for *Wolbachia* in immune evasion had previously received little attention,[40] until more recently. A study described the formation of neutrophil extracellular traps (NETosis) induced by *Wolbachia* in human onchocerciasis.[42] The formation of NETs surround the adult worm and function as a physical barrier to the cellular penetration of damaging immune cells toward the parasite.[42-44] In addition, it has been suggested that the formation of NETs may prevent the spread of *Wolbachia*, limiting the collateral inflammatory tissue damage triggered by this bacterium.[9,42-44]

CLINICAL FINDINGS

Onchocerciasis is characterized by dermal, lymphatic, and ocular manifestations. Most of the tissue changes leading to the clinical presentation of this disease appear to be related to the death of microfilariae rather than directly to the presence of adult worms.[6] The clinical manifestations of onchocerciasis can be differentiated across a spectrum, from generalized onchocerciasis on one end of the spectrum to the hyperreactive (*sowda*) form on the other.[45] The more common generalized form presents with a papular dermatitis (acute or chronic),[5] often with intense pruritus. This form of onchodermatitis may progress to alterations in skin pigmentation, atrophy, and loss of elasticity, resulting in disfiguring skin disease.[5] Generalized onchocerciasis is characterized by high parasite burden and immune tolerance to the worms.[5,45-47] At the other end of the spectrum, lichenified dermatitis (*sowda*) presents with pruritic hyperpigmented lichenified plaques that typically localize to one limb and may be accompanied by lymphadenopathy.[9] This clinical manifestation is associated with low parasite burden and stronger immune response.[9,45-47]

Onchocercal depigmentation presents as asymptomatic, depigmented macules and patches located symmetrically on the anterior shins, leading to the "leopard skin appearance."[48,49]

In later stages of onchodermatitis, the host immunologic response encapsulates the adult female worms, which are surrounded by a granulomatous infiltrate, forming an onchocercoma within the subcutaneous tissue.[18] The onchocercoma is a nontender, subcutaneous nodule found over bony prominences, that may be seen anywhere on the body.[6,18] Nodules may vary in size from as small as 0.2 cm in diameter to as large as 6.0 cm and occasionally even larger.[6] Onchocercomas are common on the torso and in African, while in South America, where it is sometimes called *Robles disease*,[50] nodules are favored on the head and shoulders.[30,51,52] Removal of these nodules historically formed the core strategy of control programs in Mexico and Guatemala.[53] However, some studies have suggested that considerable numbers of female worms are hidden in deep-lying, nonvisible nodules, which may be sufficient to maintain a large population of microfilariae in the skin and eyes.[54,55] Angiogenic and lymphangiogenic factors are believed to play a role in the formation of these nodules.[9,56] The number of onchocercomas do not appear to correlate with skin microfilarial load.[6,57] A risk factor for onchocerciasis infection in children in endemic areas, apart from exposure to infected blackflies, may be maternal onchocercal infection during the gestational period.[58,59]

Ocular manifestations of onchocerciasis can include uveitis, punctate keratitis, sclerosing keratitis, uveitis, optic atrophy, onchochorioretinitis, and glaucoma.[5,18] Systemic manifestations of onchocerciasis may also occur and can present as weight loss, general weakness, musculoskeletal pain, and inguinal or femoral hernias.[6,60] There is also evidence that *O. volvulus* may directly or indirectly induce seizures; this is termed onchocerciasis-associated epilepsy (OAE) or "river epilepsy."[61,62] OAE is a type of epilepsy that can present in previously healthy children living in areas where onchocerciasis is endemic.[62,63] Nodding syndrome and Nakalanga syndrome are the most severe and debilitating forms of OAE, and both conditions are irreversible and can progress toward death if not treated.[62,63] OAE is preventable with the elimination of onchocerciasis transmission and improved access to anti-epileptic medications in endemic regions.[63]

CLASSIFICATION

Broadly, cutaneous manifestations of onchocerciasis may be classified into early and late lesions [**Table 74-1**]. Several other classifications for onchocercal dermatitis are in existence, but Murdoch et al[64]

TABLE 74-1 Clinical features of cutaneous onchocerciasis

Symptoms

Pruritus

- Severe pruritus, the most distressing clinical manifestation, interferes with the ability to interact socially, work, farm, or sleep.
- The pruritus may be so intense that patients scratch with twigs, stones, and knives, leading to wounds, sores, and pain.[65]

Psychological sequelae

- Stigmatization, social rejection, impaired self-esteem, reduced occupational opportunities, and limited marriage prospects.[6,9,10]

Signs

- Itching may be mild and intermittent or severe and continuous, leading to superficial excoriation, crusts, secondary infection, and ulceration.
- **Early skin lesions (onchodermatitis)**
  - Urticaria
  - Macules
  - Papules
  - Pustules
  - Subcutaneous edema including swelling of limbs or groin area
  - Scaling
  - Lichenification
  - Lymphadenopathy (particularly in the inguinal and femoral region)
  - Cellulitis, lymphangitis, and lymphadenitis
  - Excoriations
  - Nodules (onchocercomata) found over bony prominences
  - Sowda (intensely itchy localized hyperpigmented papules, pustules, and pachydermia seen in chronic hyperreactive onchodermatitis)
- **Late skin lesions**
  - Atrophy (shiny, fragile skin described as "lizard skin")
  - Dermal scarring and loss of elasticity
  - Loose and hanging skin (face: leonine facies; axilla and groin: hanging groin)
  - Spotty depigmented macules and patches over the anterior shins (leopard skin; see Figure 65-5)
  - Genital elephantiasis
  - Elephantiasis of the limbs (associated with sowda)

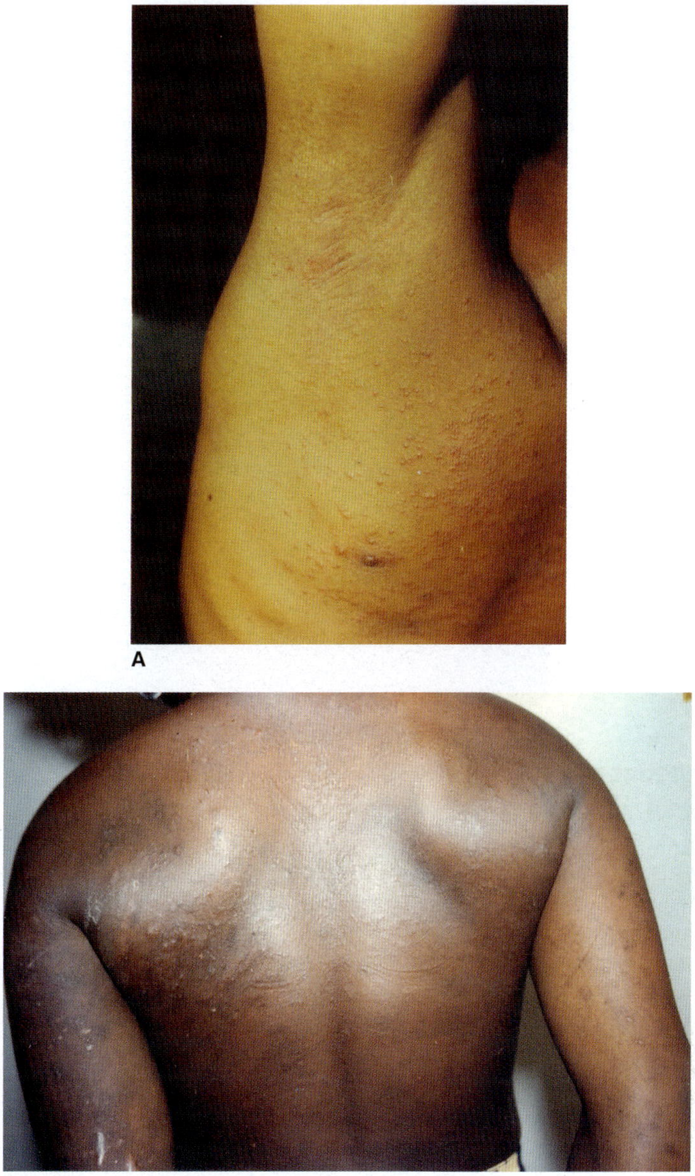

A

B

FIGURE 74-1. (A) Acute papular onchodermatitis. **(B)** Acute papular onchodermatitis on the axilla, neck, and chest.

developed a classification scheme for standardization and comparison of surveys conducted from different parts of the world. This classification describes five main categories of onchocercal dermatitis: (1) acute papular onchodermatitis [**Figure 74-1A and B**], (2) chronic papular onchodermatitis [**Figure 74-2**], (3) lichenified onchodermatitis/sowda [**Figure 74-3**], (4) atrophy, and (5) depigmentation [**Figure 74-4**], with activity, severity (presence of itching or excoriation), and distribution grading as appropriate. Other associated features include lymphadenopathy, lymphedema, onchocercoma [**Figure 74-5**], and hanging groin.

HIV infection may enhance the dermatologic and ocular features of onchocerciasis and may also increase susceptibility to HIV-1 infection among those infected with onchocerciais.[18,66] It has been found that if exposed to HIV, patients with onchocerciasis have a higher possibility of converting to HIV positivity than do those without onchocerciasis, and treatment of onchocerciasis in HIV-infected patients may lower viral replication.[30,66]

DIFFERENTIAL DIAGNOSIS

The differential diagnosis of cutaneous onchocerciasis varies by the clinical manifestations of the disease. **Table 74-2** outlines differential diagnoses by manifestation.

LABORATORY DIAGNOSIS

The gold standard test for the diagnosis of onchocerciasis remains the skin snip microscopy test, which consists of a superficial biopsy to detect microfilariae microscopically.[67] While skin snip microscopy has high specificity, it is invasive and has low sensitivity in early stages of infection and in low intensity infections.[67] In these situations, polymerase chain reaction (PCR) of the skin snip can be performed to increase sensitivity and specificity.[67] An old diagnostic procedure is the diethylcarbamazine (DEC) patch test, which involves applying a DEC-containing transdermal patch to induce the death of skin microfilariae, triggering a reactive urticaria (Mazzotti reaction).[68]

Biochemical methods to detect exposure to *Onchocerca* include enzyme-linked immunosorbent assays (ELISA), enzyme immunoassays, antigen surveys, and antibody-based rapid diagnostic tests.[3,5,30] Recent developments for the detection of parasite in humans include real-time polymerase chain reaction (RT-PCR) [9,69,70] and isothermal loop-mediated amplification (LAMP) assays.[9,71] Other recent developments include assays to detect metabolites produced by adult worms[9,72,73] and parasite microRNA.[9,74,75] The novel development of a urine biomarker

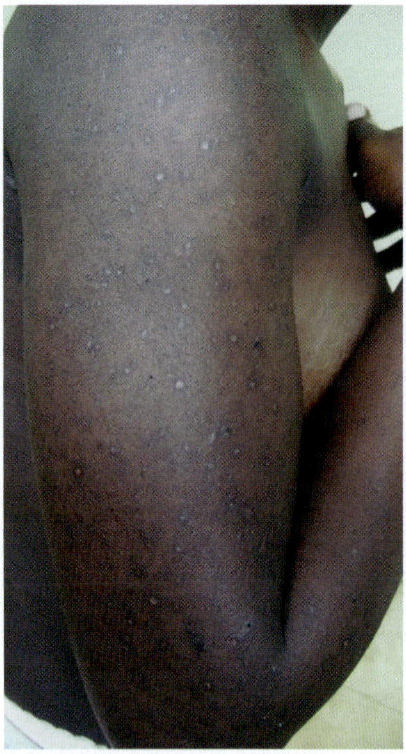

FIGURE 74-2. Chronic papular onchodermatitis on the upper limb.

immunoassay has the potential to serve as a less invasive diagnostic for onchocerciasis.[18,76]

Microfilariae may be seen on slit-lamp examination of the cornea and anterior chamber of the eye. Ultrasonography of subcutaneous nodules may be performed to identify adult worms.[21]

COMPLICATIONS

Complications include secondary bacterial infection, cellulitis, lymphangitis or recurrent lymphangitis, and blindness in the eruptive phase.

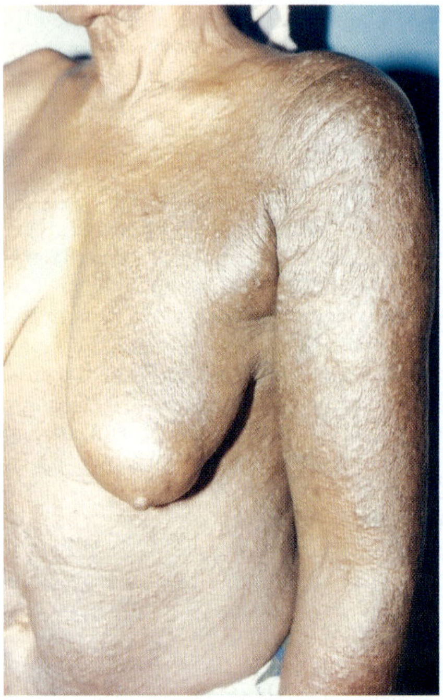

FIGURE 74-3. Lichenified onchodermatitis.

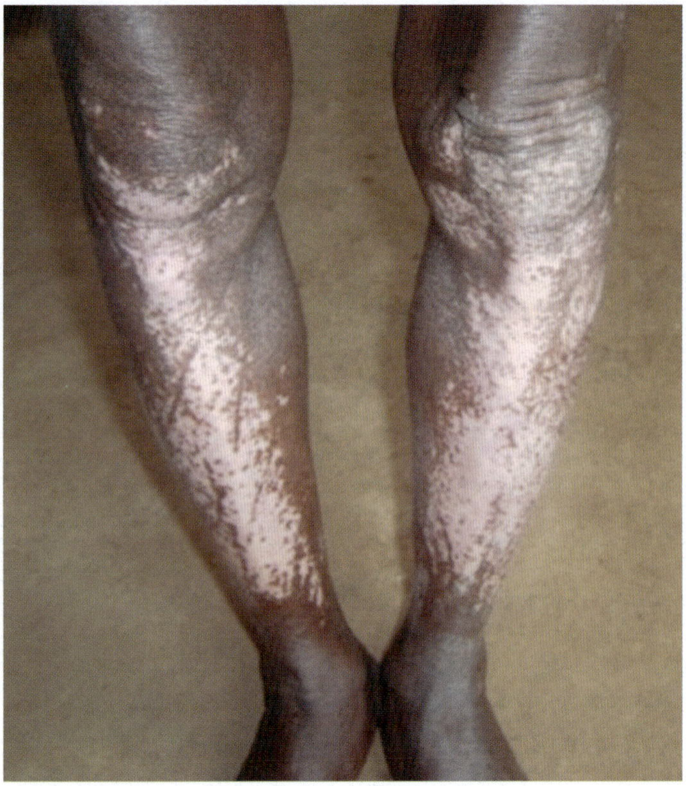

FIGURE 74-4. Bilateral onchocercal depigmentation (leopard skin.)

TREATMENT

Ivermectin is given at a dose of 150 μg/kg administered orally every 3 months, every 6 months, or yearly until the patient is asymptomatic.[21] Repeated treatment may be indicated for as long as the infected individual has symptoms of infection, or until the adult worms die (about 10-15 years). In the treatment of individuals residing in low transmission areas and for those residing in nonendemic areas, experts recommend treatment with one dose of ivermectin, followed by 6 weeks of doxycycline, which targets the *Wolbachia* bacterium.[21,67,77]

In areas where both onchocerciasis and *Loa loa* are endemic, patients must be evaluated for coinfection with *Loa loa* prior to the administration of ivermectin.[21,67] This is due to the risk of a fatal encephalitic reaction to ivermectin in patients infected with *Loa loa*.[5,67]

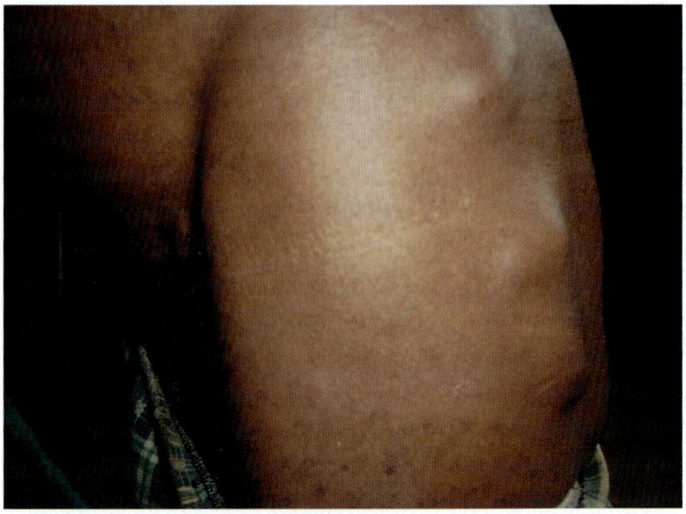

FIGURE 74-5. Multiple onchocercal nodules on the greater trochanter area.

TABLE 74-2 Differential diagnosis of cutaneous onchocerciasis

Manifestation:
Localized nodules
• Epidermoid cyst
• Juxta-articular nodules
• Fibroma
• Lipoma
• Podoconiosis
Generalized eruptive rash
• Pyoderma
• Dermatitis herpetiformis
• Pityriasis lichenoides chronic
• Urticaria
• Lichen planus
• Tinea incognito
• Drug eruption
• Scabies
• Secondary syphilis
• Lichen simplex chronicus
• Chronic idiopathic urticaria
• Atopic dermatitis

DEC, given at a dose of 25 to 50 mg three times a day and increased weekly by 25 mg up to 100 mg, is no longer recommended due to the severe reactions (Mazzotti reaction) that arise as a result of the destruction of microfilariae. An older treatment includes Suramin, a drug that targets adult worms, which is no longer recommended due to multiple systemic toxicities.[67]

An antiparasitic drug, moxidectin, was found to be more effective than ivermectin in reducing skin microfilarial levels in Phase II and III clinical trials.[21,78,79] Moxidectin was approved by the U.S. Food and Drug and Administration in 2018 for the treatment of onchocerciasis in patients 12 years and older.[5,21] Pharmaceuticals in development for the treatment of onchocerciasis include flubentylosin, emodepside, azaquinazolin AWZ1066, oxfendazole, and CC6166.[5]

Furthermore, there are also ongoing efforts in the development of a vaccine for onchocerciasis.[80,81] Nodulectomy may be undertaken for cosmetic purposes, although this procedure alone is not considered curative as worms can be deep lying and undetected. [21]

CONTROL AND PREVENTION

Great progress has been made in the last 50 years in the control of onchocerciasis both in Africa and in the Americas, largely due to international public and private partnerships, sustained funding of regional programs, and new tools and technology.

Until the advent of ivermectin, larvicidal campaigns against the insect vector were the only practical approach for onchocerciasis control. The insecticides used were effective against the vectors but safe for the remainder of the environment because they were biodegradable. They included the organophosphates temephos, chlorphoxin, and pyracolos.[6] Although dichlorodiphenyltrichloroethane (DDT) was relatively cheap, it later fell out of favor because of its persistence in the environment and fears of toxicity. Newer black fly larvicides in use include biolarvicides, which include formulations of insect growth regulators and Bacillus species (*B. thuringiensis israelensis H-14*).[6] This bacterium infects and kills mosquitos and blackfly larvae. Vector control is now recommended as a complementary intervention strategy to mass drug administration in areas that are not progressing toward the elimination of transmission of *Onchocerca*.[6]

In 1987, the manufacturing company, Merck & Co. Inc. committed to donating ivermectin (Mectizan), "as much needed, for as long as needed," to help in the control of onchocerciasis.[82] This unprecedented decision revolutionized the strategy for onchocerciasis control, supporting the mass drug administration of ivermectin to millions of individuals each year.[5,82] Several partnerships such as the Onchocerciasis Control Program (OCP) (1974-2002), the Onchocerciasis Elimination Program for the Americas (OEPA) (1993-present), the African Program for Onchocerciasis Control (APOC) (1995-2015), and the Expanded Special Project for Elimination of Neglected Tropical Diseases (ESPEN) (2016-present), have sustained the mass drug administration of ivermectin.[5,9,83] The transmission of onchocerciasis has been eliminated in four countries including Colombia, Ecuador, Guatemala, and Mexico and in foci in Ethiopia, Nigeria, Sudan, and Uganda.[6]

The Global Onchocerciasis Network for Elimination (GONE) was launched in 2023 by the WHO, with the goal to accelerate progress toward the WHO's 2030 road map targets for onchocerciasis elimination (interruption of transmission). One of these targets includes the elimination of onchocerciasis in 12 endemic countries by the year 2030.[12] In the countries that have achieved the elimination of onchocerciasis, two main strategies have been implemented including mass drug administration of ivermectin, often employed via a community-directed approach, and vector control.[10] While vector control has served as a critical strategy in the fight against onchocerciasis, this strategy is resource intensive, requiring expensive equipment (aircraft) and substantial regional coordination efforts, and thus this strategy may only be cost effective in certain country contexts.[10]

Progress toward the control and elimination of onchocerciasis faces several challenges. In regions where *Loa loa* is co-endemic, mass drug administration with ivermectin is limited.[10,12] This highlights the need for the development of improved screening and treatment approaches in loiasis co-endemic areas.[12] Another limitation of mass drug administration with ivermectin is the lengthy treatment regimen in endemic areas, often spanning 10 to 15 years (the lifespan of the adult worm).[10] Other challenges include the incomplete mapping of transmission zones and concerns for the possible emergence of ivermectin resistance.[84] The elimination of onchocerciasis may be difficult to achieve in countries with nomadic populations as well as in countries experiencing political unrest, civil war, and displacement.[10,84,85] The elimination of onchocerciasis poses many benefits for individuals, communities, and countries, reducing disease burden amongst some of the world's most disadvantaged and impoverished populations.

REFERENCES

1. Centers for Disease Control and Prevention. Parasites—onchocerciasis (also known as river blindness). Updated June 2, 2023. https://www.cdc.gov/parasites/onchocerciasis/. Accessed December 3, 2023.
2. Remme JHF, Feenstra P, Lever PR. et al. Tropical diseases targeted for elimination: chagas disease, lymphatic filariasis, onchocerciasis, and leprosy. In: Jamison DT, Breman JG, Measham AR, et al, eds. *Disease Control Priorities in Developing Countries*. 2nd ed. Washington, DC: The World Bank and Oxford University Press; 2006:433-449.
3. Brattig NW, Cheke RA, Garms R. Onchocerciasis (river blindness)—more than a century of research and control. *Acta Trop*. 2021;218:105677.
4. World Health Organization. Onchocerciasis. Fact sheet. January 12, 2022. https://www.who.int/news-room/fact-sheets/detail/onchocerciasis. Accessed December 3, 2023.
5. Frallonardo L, Di Gennaro F, Panico GG, et al. Onchocerciasis: current knowledge and future goals. *Front Trop Dis*. 2022;3:115.
6. World Health Organization. Entomological manual for onchocerciasis elimination programmes. July 25, 2023. https://www.who.int/publications/i/item/9789240068612. Accessed December 8, 2023.
7. U.S. Agency for International Development. Neglected Tropical Diseases Program. Onchocerciasis. N.d. https://www.neglecteddiseases.gov/about/usaid-targeted-diseases/onchocerciasis/. Accessed December 5, 2023.
8. Alonso LM, Murdoch ME, Jofre-Bonet M. Psycho-social and economical evaluation of onchocerciasis: a literature review. *Soc Med*. 2009;4:8-31.
9. Murdoch ME. Onchodermatitis: where are we now? *Trop Med Infect Dis*. 2018;3(3):94.

10. Dalberg Global Development Advisors. Eliminating onchocerciasis and lymphatic filariasis: reaching the last mile. 2021. https://end.org/report/reaching-the-last-mile-eliminating-onchocerciasis-and-lymphatic-filariasis/. Accessed December 15, 2023.
11. GBD 2017 Disease and Injury Incidence and Prevalence Collaborators. Global, regional, and national incidence, prevalence, and years lived with disability for 354 diseases and injuries for 195 countries and territories, 1990-2017: a systematic analysis for the Global Burden of Disease Study 2017 [published correction appears in Lancet. 2019;393(10190):e44]. *Lancet.* 2018;392(10159):1789-1858.
12. World Health Organization. Ending the neglect to attain the sustainable development goals: a road map for neglected tropical diseases 2021–2030. Geneva: World Health Organization. 2020. https://www.who.int/publications/i/item/9789240010352. Accessed December 15, 2023.
13. Vinkeles Melchers NVS, Stolk WA, van Loon W, et al. The burden of skin disease and eye disease due to onchocerciasis in countries formerly under the African Programme for Onchocerciasis Control mandate for 1990, 2020, and 2030. *PLoS Negl Trop Dis.* 2021;15(7):e0009604.
14. Brown L, Huges AM, Sykes J, et al. eds. *The New Shorter Oxford English Dictionary on Historical Principles.* Oxford: Oxford University Press; 1993.
15. O'Neill J. On the presence of a filaria in "craw craw." *Lancet.* 1875;1:265-266.
16. Ajonina-Ekoti I, Ndjonka D, Tanyi MK, et al. Functional characterization and immune recognition of the extracellular superoxide dismutase from the human pathogenic parasite *Onchocerca volvulus* (OvEC-SOD). *Acta Trop.* 2012;124(1):15-26.
17. Tawill SA, Gallin M, Erttmann KD, Kipp W, Bamuhiiga J, Büttner DW. Impaired antibody responses and loss of reactivity to *Onchocerca volvulus* antigens by HIV-seropositive onchocerciasis patients. *Trans R Soc Trop Med Hyg.* 1996;90(1):85-89.
18. Schwartz RA, Al-Qubati Y, Zieleniewski Ł, Shah R, Kapila R. Onchocerciasis (river blindness): larva-induced eczema (onchodermatitis) from an important oculocutaneous tropical disease spilling over into North America and Europe. *Int J Dermatol.* 2020;59(9):1065-1070.
19. Rodriguez-Perez MA, Unnasch TR, Real-Najarro O. Assessment and monitoring of onchocerciasis. *Adv Parasitol.* 2011;77:175-226.
20. Basáñez MG, Churcher TS, Grillet ME. *Onchocerca-Simulium* interactions and the population and evolutionary biology of *Onchocerca volvulus. Adv Parasitol.* 2009;68:263-313.
21. Murdoch ME. Onchocerciasis. In: *UpToDate,* Post TW (Ed), UpToDate, Waltham, MA. https://www.uptodate.com/contents/onchocerciasis. Accessed December 10, 2023.
22. Remme J, Dadzie KY, Rolland A, Thylefors B. Ocular onchocerciasis and intensity of infection in the community. I. West African Savannah. *Trop Med Parasitol.* 1989;40:340.
23. Otiti-Sengeri J, Omaido BA, Bhwana D, et al. High prevalence of glaucoma among patients in an onchocerciasis endemic area (Mahenge, Tanzania). *Pathogens.* 2022;11(9):1046.
24. Ubachukwu, PO. Socio-economic impact of onchocerciasis with particular reference to females and children: a review. *Anim Res Int.* 2006;3(2):494-504.
25. Duke BO, Lewis DJ, Moore PJ. Onchocerca Simulium complexes. I. Transmission of forest and Sudan-savannah strains of *Onchocerca volvulus,* from Cameroon, by Simulium damnosum from various West African bioclimatic zones. *Ann Trop Med Parasitol.* 1966;60:318-326.
26. Cheke RA, Little KE, Young S, Walker M, Basáñez MG. Taking the strain out of onchocerciasis? A reanalysis of blindness and transmission data does not support the existence of a savannah blinding strain of onchocerciasis in West Africa. *Adv Parasitol.* 2021;112:1-50.
27. Udall DN. Recent updates on onchocerciasis: diagnosis and treatment. *Clin Infect Dis.* 2007;44(1):53-60.
28. Morales-Hojas R, Cheke RA, Post RJ. Molecular systematics of five *Onchocerca* species (Nematoda: Filarioidea) including the human parasite, *O. volvulus,* suggest sympatric speciation. *J Helminthol.* 2006;80(3):281-290.
29. Adler PH, Cheke RA, Post RJ. Evolution, epidemiology, and population genetics of black flies (Diptera: Simuliidae). *Infect Genet Evol.* 2010;10(7):846-865.
30. Wani MG. Onchocerciasis. *Southern Sudan Med J.* 2008;1:14-25.
31. Centers for Disease Control and Prevention. Parasites—onchocerciasis (also known as River Blindness). Onchocerciasis FAQ. Updated September 17, 2020. https://www.cdc.gov/parasites/onchocerciasis/gen_info/faqs.html. Accessed December 8, 2023.
32. Centers for Disease Control and Prevention. DPDx laboratory identification of parasites of public health concern. Onchocerciasis. Updated December 14, 2017. https://www.cdc.gov/dpdx/onchocerciasis/index.html. Accessed December 5, 2023.
33. Somorin AO. Onchocerciasis. *Int J Dermatol.* 1983;22:182-188.
34. Karam M, Schulz-Key H, Remme J. Population dynamics of *Onchocerca volvulus* after 7 to 8 years of vector control in West Africa. *Acta Trop.* 1987;44:445-457.
35. Crump A, Ōmura S. Ivermectin, "wonder drug" from Japan: the human use perspective. *Proc Jpn Acad Ser B Phys Biol Sci.* 2011;87(2):13-28.
36. Hall LR, Pearlman E. Pathogenesis of onchocercal keratitis (river blindness). *Clin Microbiol Rev.* 1999;12:445-453.
37. Otabil KB, Gyasi SF, Awuah E, et al. Prevalence of onchocerciasis and associated clinical manifestations in selected hypoendemic communities in Ghana following long-term administration of ivermectin. *BMC Infect Dis.* 2019;19(1):431.
38. Brattig NW. Pathogenesis and host responses in human onchocerciasis: impact of Onchocerca filariae and Wolbachia endobacteria. *Microbes Infect.* 2004;6(1):113-128.
39. Comandatore F, Cordaux R, Bandi C, et al. Supergroup C Wolbachia, mutualist symbionts of filarial nematodes, have a distinct genome structure. *Open Biol.* 2015;5(12):150099.
40. Hansen RD, Trees AJ, Bah GS, et al. A worm's best friend: recruitment of neutrophils by Wolbachia confounds eosinophil degranulation against the filarial nematode Onchocerca ochengi. *Proc Biol Sci.* 2011;278(1716):2293-2302.
41. Saint André Av, Blackwell NM, Hall LR, et al. The role of endosymbiotic Wolbachia bacteria in the pathogenesis of river blindness. *Science.* 2002;295(5561):1892-1895.
42. Tamarozzi F, Turner JD, Pionnier N, et al. Wolbachia endosymbionts induce neutrophil extracellular trap formation in human onchocerciasis. *Sci Rep.* 2016;6:35559.
43. Schauer C, Janko C, Munoz LE, et al. Aggregated neutrophil extracellular traps limit inflammation by degrading cytokines and chemokines. *Nat Med.* 2014;20(5):511-517.
44. Omar M, Abdelal H. NETosis in parasitic infections: a puzzle that remains unsolved. *Int J Mol Sci.* 2023;24(10):8975.
45. Katawa G, Layland LE, Debrah AY, et al. Hyperreactive onchocerciasis is characterized by a combination of Th17-Th2 immune responses and reduced regulatory T cells. *PLoS Negl Trop Dis.* 2015;9(1):e3414.
46. Hoerauf A, Kruse S, Brattig NW, Heinzmann A, Mueller-Myhsok B, Deichmann KA. The variant Arg110Gln of human IL-13 is associated with an immunologically hyper-reactive form of onchocerciasis (sowda). *Microbes Infect.* 2002;4(1):37-42.
47. Tamarozzi F, Halliday A, Gentil K, Hoerauf A, Pearlman E, Taylor MJ. Onchocerciasis: the role of Wolbachia bacterial endosymbionts in parasite biology, disease pathogenesis, and treatment. *Clin Microbiol Rev.* 2011;24(3):459-468.
48. Hartley M. Onchocerciasis. DermNet NZ. 2010. Updated August 2021. https://dermnetnz.org/topics/onchocerciasis. Accessed December 7, 2023.
49. Le K, Thomas C, Lederman E, Craft N, Burgin S. Onchocerciasis. In: Goldsmith LA, ed. VisualDx. Rochester, NY: VisualDx. Last Updated February 17, 2022. https://www.visualdx.com/visualdx/diagnosis/onchocerciasis?diagnosisId=52070&moduleId=101. Accessed December 10, 2023.
50. Richards F Jr, Rizzo N, Diaz Espinoza CE, et al. One hundred years after its discovery in guatemala by rodolfo robles, *Onchocerca volvulus* transmission has been eliminated from the central endemic zone. *Am J Trop Med Hyg.* 2015;93(6):1295-1304.
51. Wolf R, Orion E, Matz H. Onchocerciasis (river blindness). *Isr Med Assoc J.* 2003;5:522-523.
52. Kapoor U, Sharma V, Chittoria RS. Onchocercoma in a United Nations Peacekeeper. *Med J Armed Forces India.* 2015;71(Suppl 1):S104-S106.
53. Rodriguez-Perez MA, Rivas-Alcala AR. Problems in the investigation of the control of *Onchocerca volvulus* in Mexico. *Salud Publica Mex.* 1991;33:493-503.
54. Schulz-Key H. Observations on the reproductive biology of *Onchocerca volvulus. Acta Leiden.* 1990;59:27-44.
55. Duke BO. Human onchocerciasis: an overview of the disease. *Acta Leiden.* 1990;59:9-24.
56. Attout T, Hoerauf A, Dénécé G, et al. Lymphatic vascularisation and involvement of Lyve-1+ macrophages in the human onchocerca nodule. *PLoS One.* 2009;4(12):e8234.
57. Stingl P. Onchocerciasis: clinical presentation and host parasite interactions in patients of southern Sudan. Int J Dermatol. 1997;36(1):23-28.
58. Kirch AK, Duerr HP, Boatin B, et al. Impact of parental onchocerciasis and intensity of transmission on development and persistence of *Onchocerca volvulus* infection in offspring: an 18 year follow-up study. *Parasitology.* 2003;127:327-335.
59. Colebunders R, Kaiser C, Basáñez MG, Olliaro P, Lakwo T, Siewe Fodjo JN. Reducing onchocerciasis-associated morbidity in onchocerciasis-endemic foci with high ongoing transmission: a focus on the children. *Int J Infect Dis.* 2022;116:302-305.

60. Nelson GS. Hanging groin and hernia complications of onchocerciasis. *Trans R Soc Trop Med Hyg*. 1958;52(3):272-275.
61. Colebunders R, Njamnshi AK, Menon S, et al. *Onchocerca volvulus* and epilepsy: a comprehensive review using the Bradford Hill criteria for causation. *PLoS Negl Trop Dis*. 2021;15(1):e0008965.
62. Hadermann A, Amaral LJ, Van Cutsem G, Siewe Fodjo JN, Colebunders R. Onchocerciasis-associated epilepsy: an update and future perspectives. *Trends Parasitol*. 2023;39(2):126-138.
63. Jada S, Carter J, and Colebunders R. Policy brief: tackling onchocerciasis associated epilepsy: new evidence and recommendations for policymakers. Amref Health Africa; 2022.
64. Murdoch ME, Hay RJ, Mackenzie CD, et al. A clinical classification and grading system of the cutaneous changes in onchocerciasis. *Br J Dermatol*. 1993;129:260-269.
65. Remme JH. Research for control: the onchocerciasis experience. *Trop Med Int Health*. 2004;9(2):243-254.
66. Gopinath R, Ostrowski M, Justement SJ, Fauci AS, Nutman TB. Filarial infections increase susceptibility to human immunodeficiency virus infection in peripheral blood mononuclear cells in vitro. *J Infect Dis*. 2000;182(6):1804-1808.
67. Centers for Disease Control and Prevention. Parasite—onchocerciasis (also known as river blindness). Resources for Health Professionals. Updated November 10, 2021. https://www.cdc.gov/parasites/onchocerciasis/health_professionals/index.html. Accessed December 5, 2023.
68. World Health Organization Neglected Tropical Diseases. Onchocerciasis: diagnostic target product profile to support preventive chemotherapy. 2021. https://www.who.int/publications/i/item/9789240024496. Accessed December 6, 2023.
69. Unnasch TR, Golden A, Cama V, Cantey PT. Diagnostics for onchocerciasis in the era of elimination. *Int Health*. 2018;10(suppl_1):i20-i26.
70. Thiele EA, Cama VA, Lakwo T, et al. Detection of *Onchocerca volvulus* in skin snips by microscopy and real-time polymerase chain reaction: implications for monitoring and evaluation activities. *Am J Trop Med Hyg*. 2016;94(4):906-911.
71. Lagatie O, Merino M, Batsa Debrah L, Debrah AY, Stuyver LJ. An isothermal DNA amplification method for detection of *Onchocerca volvulus* infection in skin biopsies. *Parasit Vectors*. 2016;9(1):624.
72. Globisch D, Moreno AY, Hixon MS, et al. *Onchocerca volvulus*-neurotransmitter tyramine is a biomarker for river blindness. *Proc Natl Acad Sci U S A*. 2013;110(11):4218-4223.
73. Denery JR, Nunes AA, Hixon MS, Dickerson TJ, Janda KD. Metabolomics-based discovery of diagnostic biomarkers for onchocerciasis. *PLoS Negl Trop Dis*. 2010;4(10):e834.
74. Quintana JF, Makepeace BL, Babayan SA, et al. Extracellular Onchocerca-derived small RNAs in host nodules and blood. *Parasit Vectors*. 2015;8:58.1
75. Tritten L, Burkman E, Moorhead A, et al. Detection of circulating parasite-derived microRNAs in filarial infections. *PLoS Negl Trop Dis*. 2014;8(7):e2971.
76. Shirey RJ, Globisch D, Eubanks LM, Hixon MS, Janda KD. Noninvasive urine biomarker lateral flow immunoassay for monitoring active Onchocerciasis. *ACS Infect Dis*. 2018;4(10):1423-1431.
77. Cantey P and Roy S. Onchocerciasis/River Blindness CDC Yellow Book 2024. Centers for Disease Control. Last Updated May 1, 2023. https://wwwnc.cdc.gov/travel/yellowbook/2024/infections-diseases/onchocerciasis-river-blindness. Accessed December 7, 2023.
78. Opoku NO, Bakajika DK, Kanza EM, et al. Single dose moxidectin versus ivermectin for *Onchocerca volvulus* infection in Ghana, Liberia, and the Democratic Republic of the Congo: a randomised, controlled, double-blind phase 3 trial [published correction appears in Lancet. 2018;392(10154):1196]. *Lancet*. 2018;392(10154):1207-1216.
79. Awadzi K, Opoku NO, Attah SK, Lazdins-Helds J, Kuesel AC. A randomized, single-ascending-dose, ivermectin-controlled, double-blind study of moxidectin in *Onchocerca volvulus* infection. *PLoS Negl Trop Dis*. 2014;8(6):e2953.
80. Abraham D, Graham-Brown J, Carter D, et al. Development of a recombinant vaccine against human onchocerciasis. *Expert Rev Vaccines*. 2021;20(11):1459-1470.
81. Ryan NM, Hess JA, de Villena FP, et al. *Onchocerca volvulus* bivalent subunit vaccine induces protective immunity in genetically diverse collaborative cross recombinant inbred intercross mice. *NPJ Vaccines*. 2021;6(1):17.
82. Mectizan Donation Program. History of the Program. N.d. https://mectizan.org/history/. Accessed December 10, 2023.
83. Jesudason T. A new key-player for onchocerciasis elimination. *Lancet Infect Dis*. 2023;23(4):413.
84. Gebrezgabiher G, Mekonnen Z, Yewhalaw D, Hailu A. Reaching the last mile: main challenges relating to and recommendations to accelerate onchocerciasis elimination in Africa. *Infect Dis Poverty*. 2019;8(1):60.
85. Magori K. NTDs, violent conflicts, and the role of military in global health. BioMed Central (BMC) Blog Network. May 4, 2018. https://blogs.biomedcentral.com/bugbitten/2018/05/04/ntds-violent-conflicts-role-military-global-health/. Accessed December 10, 2023.

Cutaneous Manifestations of Systemic Diseases

SECTION 11

CHAPTER 75 Cardiopulmonary

Owen R. Dean
Edward W. Cowen

KEY POINTS

- Coronary artery disease is the leading cause of death globally, with higher morbidity and mortality in Black populations.
- Respiratory diseases, including chronic obstructive pulmonary disease and lower respiratory tract infections, also cause extreme morbidity and mortality and are the third and fourth leading causes of death worldwide, respectively.
- A careful skin examination may suggest the presence of cardiopulmonary disease and/or genodermatoses with cardiopulmonary involvement.
- Inflammatory skin diseases like psoriasis confer an elevated cardiovascular disease risk and affected patients should be referred for appropriate risk stratification.

INTRODUCTION

Cardiovascular disease is the leading cause of death globally, with clear racial and ethnic disparities in care access, morbidity, and mortality.[1] An example is the excess risk of hospitalizations and death from heart failure, the end stage of most heart diseases, in Black men and women in the United States under 50 years old. This risk is driven by the interactions between systemic racism, social determinants of health, delivery of care, and underlying susceptibility.[2] Pulmonary illnesses like chronic obstructive respiratory diseases (COPD), lower respiratory tract infections, lung cancer, interstitial lung diseases, and sarcoidosis also disproportionately affect minority and socioeconomically disadvantaged populations.[3] COPD and lower respiratory tract infections are the third and fourth leading causes of disease-related mortality worldwide.[4] Both children and adults can develop cutaneous findings of cardiopulmonary disease.

CUTANEOUS MANIFESTATIONS OF CARDIOPULMONARY DISEASE

EDEMA

Edema is due to excess interstitial fluid and may be pitting or nonpitting. Pitting edema, when pressure on the skin leaves an indentation for 5 or more seconds, is most often caused by chronic conditions that increase capillary hydrostatic pressure such as heart failure (HF), obstructive sleep apnea, and venous insufficiency. In the United States, chronic, bilateral lower extremity edema and its symptoms such as pain and immobility disproportionately affect older, poorer, and non-White groups.[5] Acute or hyperacute asymmetric pitting edema may be caused by thromboembolic diseases like deep vein thrombosis (erythema, pain, increased limb circumference) and superficial thrombophlebitis (palpable erythema). Medications may also cause soft, symmetric lower extremity edema. Calcium-channel blockers, in particular, are frequently prescribed in the Black population in the United States and may induce peripheral edema.[6]

Nonpitting edema is less common and typically a result of impaired lymphatic flow (lymphedema, **Figure 75-1**), and may result in fibrosis or hyperkeratotic, thickened overlying skin. Nonpitting edema is also seen in chronic thyroid disease (pretibial myxedema).

CYANOSIS

Cyanosis is abnormal coloration of the skin caused by high levels of deoxygenated or abnormal hemoglobin. Cyanosis can appear as shades of blue, purple, gray, white, or green coloration depending on baseline skin color and does not typically blanch with pressure. It is easier to detect where the epidermis is thin, such as the lips, nose, cheeks, ears, and oral mucous membranes, and under bright, fluorescent lighting.[7]

Central cyanosis will be visible on mucous membranes and the extremities will be warm. It often portends serious illness from reduced arterial oxygen saturation (typically less than 85%) due to ventilatory failure or valvular disease. In contrast, in peripheral cyanosis, the extremities will be cold, and the tongue will be pink. Peripheral cyanosis is often the result of increased oxygen extraction in the extremities in the setting of vasoconstriction and can be caused by cold exposure, vasospasm, or be an early sign of shock. Differential cyanosis refers to color change in the lower half of the body and should prompt work-up for pulmonary hypertension and left-to-right anatomic cardiac shunts. Cyanosis may be absent in the setting of severe anemia because the color change is based on the absolute amount of deoxygenated hemoglobin present. Analogously, patients with polycythemia may present with cyanosis at higher arterial oxygen levels. If acute-onset, central cyanosis does not respond to oxygen therapy, hemoglobinopathies like methemoglobinemia should be considered. Mimickers of cyanosis include gold, silver, and amiodarone toxicity (pseudocyanosis).[8]

CLUBBING

Clubbing typically develops with softening of the nail bed followed by an increase in nail convexity. As time goes on, the nail and periungual skin can become shiny, the nail can develop longitudinal ridges, and the depth of the distal phalange may increase [**Figure 75-2**]. A diagnosis of clubbing can be made through the profile sign (nail angle > 180° as it exits the proximal nailfold), a distal phalangeal to interphalangeal ratio of greater than 1, or the loss of the diamond shape when thumbnails are opposed (Schamroth sign).[9]

Clubbing can be primary (pachydermoperiostosis) but is most commonly associated with hypoxic conditions (lung cancer, interstitial lung disease, bronchiectasis), as well as other systemic illnesses such as endocarditis, inflammatory bowel disease, and cirrhosis. In children, acquired clubbing is frequently seen in HIV, hemoglobinopathies, cystic fibrosis, and congenital heart disease. One-sided, acquired clubbing is typically caused by a neurologic insult resulting in hemiplegia, an arteriovenous dialysis fistula, or local trauma resulting in an aneurysm. Primary or secondary clubbing can also be a part of hypertrophic osteoarthropathy (HOA) consisting of bilateral clubbing, joint pain, and long bone periostosis.[10] Notably, COPD does not typically cause digital clubbing, and its presence should prompt consideration for the presence of malignancy or bronchiestasis.[11]

XANTHELASMA

Xanthomas and xanthelasma are characterized by the dermal infiltration of cholesterol containing foam cells. Causes include primary hyperlipidemia syndromes, low high-density lipoprotein (HDL) levels,

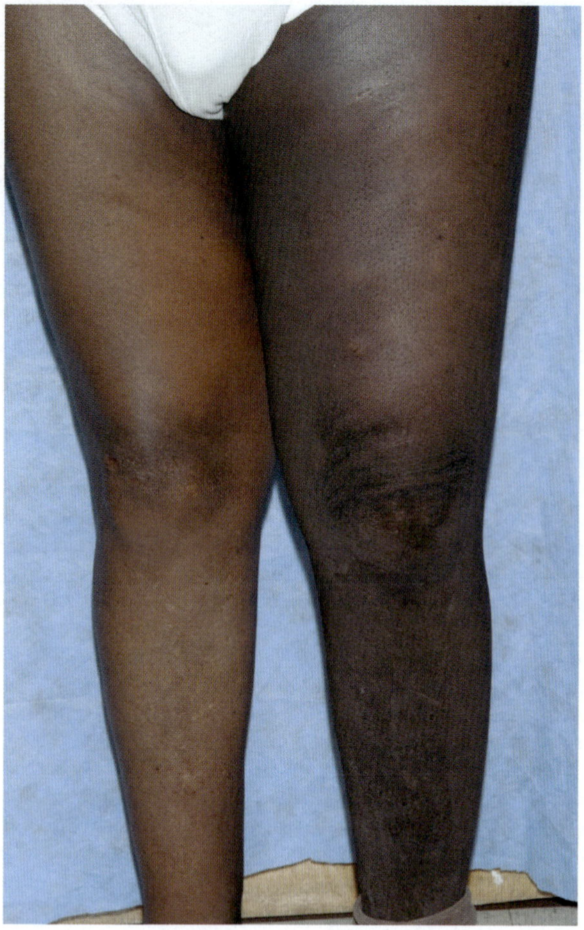

FIGURE 75-1. Lymphedema. Unilateral hyperpigmentation with induration and increased diameter of the left lower extremity in a patient with prostate cancer status-post lymph node dissection. Similar findings can be seen in GATA2 deficiency and deep vein thrombosis. Bilateral disease suggests possible cardiac failure or medication adverse reaction.

hypothyroidism, diabetes mellitus, diets rich in saturated fats and cholesterol, and medications. Xanthelasma palpebrarum (XP) presents as yellow to yellow-white periorbital plaques and is most commonly a marker of underlying atherosclerosis, although it can rarely be seen in other conditions like contact dermatitis and as complications of certain cosmetic procedures.[12] The identification of xanthomata should trigger cardiovascular risk stratification and dyslipidemia evaluation.

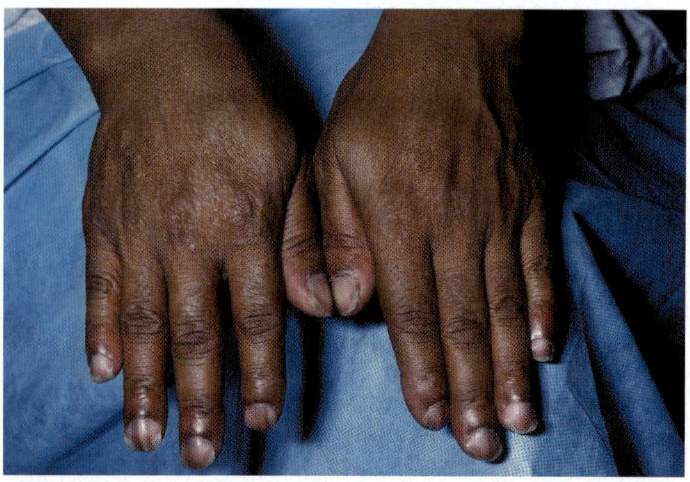

FIGURE 75-2. Digital clubbing. Convexity of the nails is visible, particularly of the first digits in this man with HIV. There is incidental longitudinal melanonychia.

THROMBOEMBOLIC PHENOMENA

INFECTIOUS ENDOCARDITIS (IE)

Infectious endocarditis (IE) is infection of a heart valve (native or prosthetic), endocardium, or a device implanted into the heart, and is most often caused by gram-positive cocci like streptococcus, enterococcus, and staphylococcus. In countries with historically limited financial resources, rheumatic heart disease is the greatest risk factor. In higher income countries, intravenous drug use, diabetes, degenerative and congenital valve disease, and cancer are the most common risk factors. Cutaneous manifestations include petechiae and splinter hemorrhages. Osler nodes (tender, erythematous papules on the digits) and Janeway lesions (painless erythematous macules/hemorrhages on the palms and soles) are other rare findings.[13]

VENOUS THROMBOEMBOLISM (VTE)

Venous thromboembolism (VTE) includes deep vein thrombosis (DVT) and pulmonary embolism (PE). Risk factors include older age, obesity, family history, previous DVT, recent surgery or trauma, hypercoagulable states (eg, malignancy), prolonged immobility, autoimmune disorders, chronic kidney disease, sickle cell disease, and infections like SARS-CoV-2.[14] Cutaneous findings of DVT include warmth, pain, erythema that can be less visible in darker skin, and increased circumference from swelling in the affected limb. PE may present with cyanosis.

CHRONIC VENOUS DISEASE

Chronic venous disease (CVD) is caused by chronic venous hypertension, typically in the setting of obesity, pregnancy, prolonged standing, or a personal or family history of DVT. Skin findings include varicose veins, recurrent leg ulcers, chronic swelling, and pain.[14]

CHOLESTEROL EMBOLIZATION SYNDROME (CES)

Cholesterol embolization syndrome (CES) is caused by cholesterol crystal embolization in the arterial system. It typically occurs after vascular interventional procedures but can also occur after anticoagulation or spontaneously. CES is characterized by livedo reticularis and purple toes, in contrast to arterial thromboembolism, which presents with acute limb ischemia. Skin biopsy demonstrates cholesterol crystal deposits. CES syndrome is often considered rare in dark-skinned populations, but the livedo and purple coloration may be underdiagnosed in heavily pigmented skin.[15]

FAT EMBOLI SYNDROME (FES)

Fat emboli syndrome (FES) occurs when fat globules enter the pulmonary or peripheral circulation, usually in the context of trauma or an orthopedic procedure. It typically presents with respiratory distress around 12 hours after the injury or procedure, followed by global neurologic symptoms. Rarely, petechiae of the head/neck, torso, or subconjunctival and oral mucous membranes may be seen.[16]

COMPRESSIVE SYNDROMES

SUPERIOR VENA CAVA (SVC) SYNDROME

Superior vena cava (SVC) syndrome occurs when the low-pressure SVC is compressed or flow is impeded. Causes include masses, dilation of the aorta, and occlusive thrombi that form on indwelling catheters. Dilated, tortuous cutaneous venules or veins develop above the rib cage. SVC obstruction also causes face, neck, or upper extremity swelling, ruddiness or cyanosis, and respiratory symptoms.[17]

MAY-THURNER SYNDROME

May-Thurner syndrome most commonly occurs when the left common iliac vein is compressed between the spine and the right common iliac artery. It may present as episodic left lower limb swelling that resolves when the limb is elevated. Signs of chronic venous insufficiency, including varicose veins, leg hyperpigmentation, or venous ulcers may occur, as well as deep vein thrombosis. It is most common in women in the second to fourth decades of life.[18]

INFECTIOUS DISEASES

Mycoplasma pneumoniae is a common cause of community-acquired pneumonia that may present with mucocutaneous erosions and crusting, exanthematous skin eruptions, erythema nodosum, urticaria, and erythema multiforme major. Other pulmonary infections, including *Chlamydophila pneumoniae*, Influenza B, enterovirus/rhinovirus, human metapneumovirus, and parainfluenzavirus may lead to similar findings, known as reactive infectious mucocutaneous eruption.[19] Fungal pathogens that can have cutaneous and pulmonary involvement include cryptococcosis, paracoccidiomycosis, coccidioidomycosis, tuberculous, and nontuberculous mycobacteria.

Other infectious diseases with prominent skin findings and cardiac findings include syphilis (painless genital ulcers or chancre in primary syphilis), Lyme disease (annular bulls-eye plaque that in darker skin appears with central clearing and red-purple peripheral rim, also known as erythema migrans), and Chagas disease (unilateral painless swelling at the site of the inoculation or chagoma):

- **Cardiovascular syphilis** occurs 15 to 30 years after primary infection and is typified by ascending aortic aneurysms, aortic insufficiency, coronary artery stenosis, and myocarditis.[20]
- **Lyme carditis** occurs in about 1% of patients with disseminated disease. It classically presents as an atrioventricular block that can fluctuate and progress rapidly. Lyme carditis has an excellent prognosis with appropriate therapy. Myocarditis, valvular disease, and sudden death from Lyme carditis are exceedingly rare.[21]
- Cardiac dysfunction occurs in 14% to 45% of immunocompetent patients with **Chagas disease** and presents with conduction abnormalities, left ventricular dysfunction, dilated cardiomyopathy, cardioembolic stroke, and congestive heart failure.

INFLAMMATORY DISEASES

Patients with immune-mediated inflammatory diseases have increased mortality compared to the general population, and much of this risk is attributed to a greater incidence of cardiovascular disease. **Psoriasis vulgaris,** for instance, has a 50% increased risk of cardiovascular disease, with severe disease conferring a 40% increase in cardiovascular disease mortality.[22]

The first and second leading causes of death from sarcoidosis are complications of pulmonary (eg, progressive lung fibrosis) and cardiac (eg, fatal arrhythmias, pulmonary hypertension) involvement. Recommended evaluation for internal involvement includes chest imaging (x-ray, CT, PET) and 12-lead electrocardiogram.[23] Other inflammatory diseases with cardiopulmonary and cutaneous involvement are shown in **Table 75-1**.

GENODERMATOSES

Genodermatoses with associated cardiopulmonary features are described in **Table 75-2**.

TABLE 75-1 Inflammatory diseases with cutaneous and cardiopulmonary involvement

	Findings			
Disease	**Skin**	**Cardiac**	**Pulmonary**	**Epidemiology**
Amyloidosis	Periorbital purpura, macroglossia, nail dystrophy	Diastolic heart failure with preserved apical systolic function, restrictive cardiomyopathy	Typically asymptomatic but infiltrates can be diffuse or involve tracheobronchial tree	Rare, usually presents in adulthood[24]
Sarcoidosis	Granulomas (often on the face), lupus pernio, erythema nodosum	Conduction abnormalities (high grade AV block), arrhythmia, heart failure, sudden cardiac death	Bilateral hilar lymphadenopathy; may progress to end-stage fibrosis, pulmonary hypertension	Young, middle-aged adults. Black race and female sex are poor prognostic factors[25,26]
Systemic lupus erythematosus	Photosensitivity, acute, subacute, chronic lupus, periungual telangiectasia, Raynaud phenomenon	Increased risk of CAD (lupus activity, antiphospholipid antibodies, homocystinemia, steroid use)	Infectious pneumonias, particularly encapsulated bacteria (*S. pneumoniae*)	Women of child-bearing age, African American women suffer the highest mortality in the United States[27]
Kawasaki disease	Strawberry tongue, cheilitis, conjunctivitis, diffuse polymorphous rash, periungual desquamation	Myocarditis, pericarditis, valvular regurgitation, aortic root enlargement, coronary artery aneurysms	Pulmonary nodules, peribronchial and interstitial infiltrates, pleural effusion, empyema	Children < 5 years, highest incidence in East Asian and Pacific Islander descent[28]
Acute Rheumatic Fever	Erythema marginatum; small, painless subcutaneous nodules on extensor surfaces	Pancarditis, valvulitis (mitral > aortic valve)	Pulmonary edema in setting of severe mitral regurgitation	Incidence is highest children 10-14 years, poverty, social disadvantage; skin findings difficult to discern on dark skin[29]
Systemic Sclerosis (SS)	Skin fibrosis, sclerodactyly, Raynaud phenomenon, telangiectasias, digital ulcer	Asymptomatic perfusion abnormalities, diastolic dysfunction, acute myocarditis, CHF	Pulmonary arterial hypertension, interstitial lung disease (ILD)	SS-ILD is associated with male sex, African American race[30]
Dermatomyositis	Gottron sign/papules, heliotrope rash, poikilodermatous rash, periungual erythema and telangiectasias	Subclinical diastolic dysfunction, myocarditis, myocardial fibrosis, conduction abnormalities, CHF	ILD (rapid progression common in Asian population), pulmonary hypertension, serositis	More common in African Americans and female sex; age onset is bimodal: 4-14, 40-60 y.o.[31]
Granulomatosis with polyangiitis	Saddle nose deformity, oral and nasal ulcers, leukocytoclastic vasculitis, subcutaneous nodules	Myocarditis, pericarditis, endocarditis, pericardial effusion, heart failure (6-20%)	Occurs in most patients (90%), ranges from asymptomatic cavitating granulomas to infiltrates, fulminant alveolar hemorrhage	Onset is usually age 45-65, more common in Caucasian population[32]
Eosinophilic granulomatosis with polyangiitis	Palpable purpura, urticaria, livedo, subcutaneous nodules, ulcers	Myocarditis, pericardial effusion	Asthma, pulmonary infiltrates, alveolar hemorrhage	Rare[33]
Relapsing polychondritis	Erythematous inflammation, swelling of the ear, saddle nose deformity; annular eruptive urticaria	Aortic regurgitation in setting of aortic dilation, mitral regurgitation, pericarditis, aneurysms	Lower respiratory tract infections, laryngeal chondritis, subglottic stenosis, tracheobronchomalacia	Rare

TABLE 75-2 Genodermatoses with cardiopulmonary involvement

	Name	Inheritance pattern	Cutaneous findings	Cardiopulmonary involvement
Heritable connective tissue disorders	Pseudoxanthoma elasticum	PD	Pruritic, yellow papules on the lateral neck w/"gooseflesh" appearance	Peripheral artery disease, valvular disease, cerebrovascular disease[34]
	Ehlers-Danlos Syndrome	AD, AR	Hyperextensibility, fragility, poor scarring	Aneurysmal disease in a minority[35]
	Loeys-Dietz Syndrome	AD	Velvety, thin, and translucent skin with dystrophic scars and striae, eczema	Tortuous arteries and aneurysms, dilation of the aortic root with high risk of rupture[35]
	Marfan Syndrome	AD, de novo mutations in 1/3	Normal skin with striae	Aortic root dilatation that can lead to type A or B dissection, mitral valve prolapse[35]
	Cutis Laxa	AD, AR, X-linked, acquired	Significant skin redundancy, laxity	Emphysema, aortic root dilation[36]
Endocrine, neoplastic, lentiginous syndrome	Carney Complex [**Figure 75-3**]	AD	Spotty lip, conjunctiva, mucosa pigmentation; myxomas	Cardiac myxoma complications: emboli, arrhythmia, cardiomyopathy[37]
Neuro-cardio-facial-cutaneous syndrome	Noonan syndrome	AD, variable penetrance	Pigmented nevi, café au lait macules, keratosis pilaris, thick/curly hair	Congenital heart disease (pulmonary stenosis, hypertrophic cardiomyopathy, atrial defects)[38]
	LEOPARD syndrome	AD	Lentigines on the upper body	Hypertrophic cardiomyopathy, conduction abnormalities[39]
Lysosomal storage disease	Mucopolysaccharidosis types I, II, IV, VI	Varied	Coarse facies, thickened skin, excessive hair growth; melanocytosis (I, II), ivory pebble papules over the scapula (II)	Progressive cardiac valve dysfunction, CAD, endocardial fibroelastosis, conduction abnormalities[40]
Neuro cutaneous syndrome	Tuberous Sclerosis Complex [**Figure 75-4**]	AD	Ash leaf spots, facial angiofibromas, shagreen patches, ungual fibromas	Cardiac rhabdomyomas, LAM[41]
Autoinflammatory syndromes	SAVI	AD	Severe acral vasculopathy, nasal destruction	Recurrent alveolar hemorrhage, ILD, lung fibrosis[42]
	VEXAS	X-linked	Neutrophilic dermatoses, chondritis, subcutaneous edema, LCV	Pulmonary alveolitis, pleural effusions, myocarditis, venous thrombosis[43]
Immunodeficiencies	GATA2 deficiency	AD	Recalcitrant warts/condyloma, panniculitis, neutrophilic dermatosis	Pulmonary alveolar proteinosis, venous thrombosis[44]
	Hyper-IgE syndrome, Autosomal Dominant (Job syndrome)	DN	Prominent forehead, broadened nasal bridge, eczema, recurrent skin abscesses, chronic mucocutaneous candidiasis	Recurrent infectious pneumonia, bronchiectasis, pneumatoceles; coronary artery aneurysms, tortuosity[45]
Other	Hereditary Hemorrhagic Telangiectasia	AD	Telangiectasias on the fingertips, face, lips, tongue, and arms	Pulmonary hypertension and high-output heart failure[46]
	Birt-Hogg-Dube syndrome	AD	Facial fibrofolliculomas, trichodiscomas	Multiple, bilateral pulmonary cysts, pneumothorax[47]
	Alpha 1-antitrypsin deficiency	AC	Neutrophilic panniculitis, vasculitis	Panacinar emphysema, bronchiestasis[48]

Abbreviations: AC, autosomal co-dominant; AD, autosomal dominant; AR, autosomal recessive; DN, dominant negative; E1, enzyme; LAM, lymphangiomyomatosis; LCV, leukocytoclastic vasculitis; PD, pseudodominant; SAVI, STING-associated vasculopathy; VEXAS, vacuoles, X-linked, autoinflammatory, somatic.

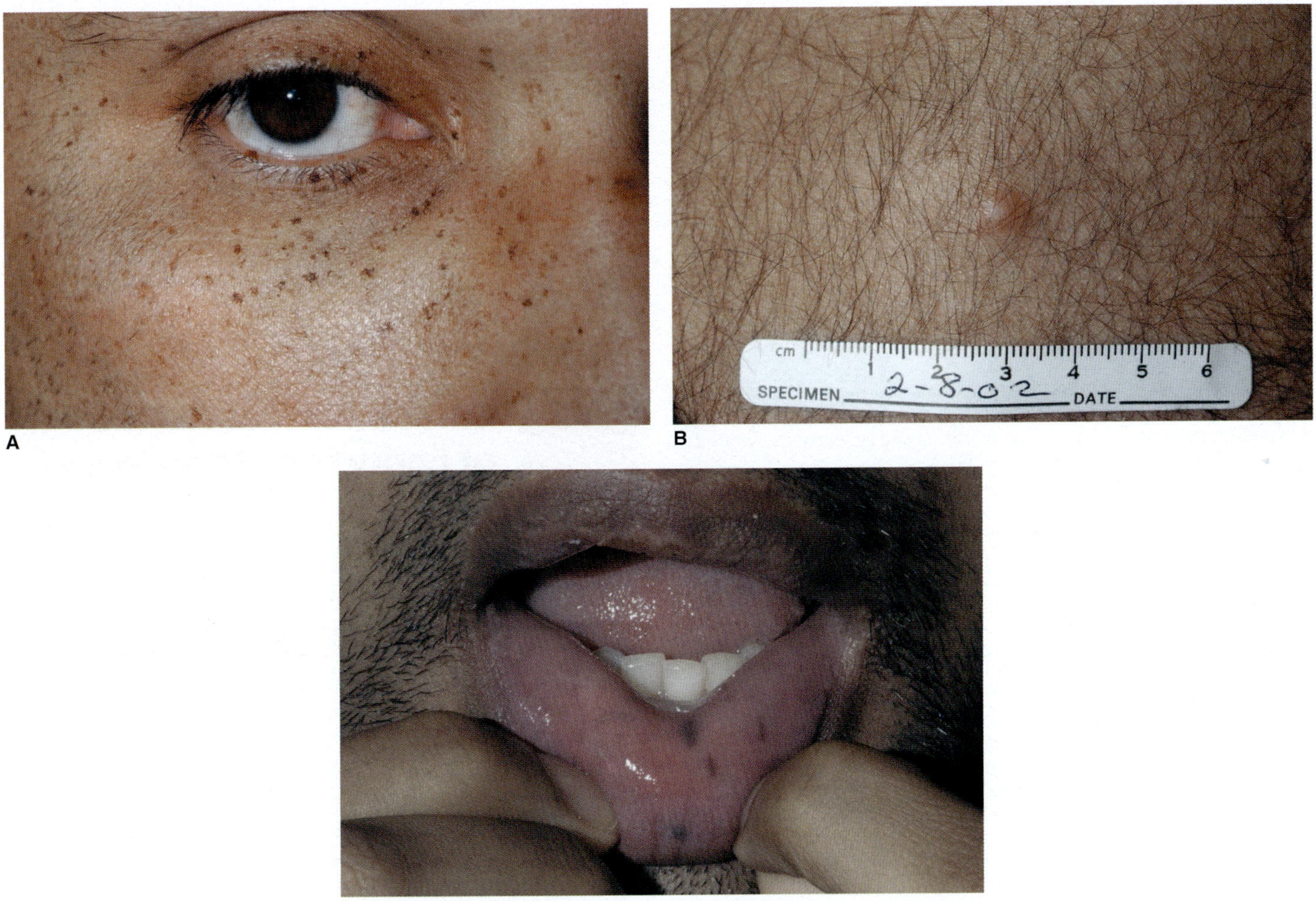

A B C

FIGURE 75-3. Carney complex. Numerous periorificial ink spot lentigines with involvement of lid margin in Hispanic male with Carney complex **(A)**. Cutaneous myxoma on the hip in the same patient **(B)**. Oral mucosal pigmentation in man of Southeast Asian descent **(C)**. Patients with Carney complex are at high risk of one or more cardiac myxomas.

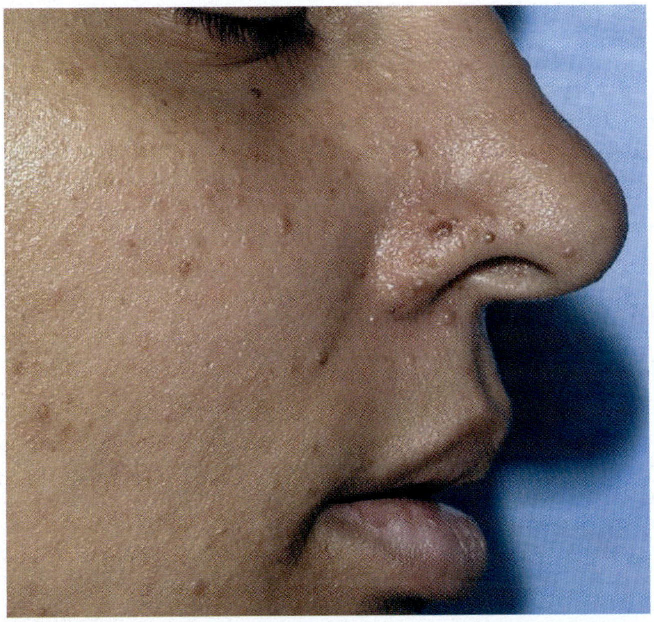

FIGURE 75-4. Pulmonary lymphangioleiomatosis and tuberous sclerosis complex. Perinasal clustering of skin colored and red-brown angiofibromas in African American woman with tuberous sclerosis complex and lymphangioleiomatosis.

CONCLUSION

Cardiopulmonary diseases are responsible for the majority of disease-related deaths worldwide. In addition, recent advances have demonstrated an important contributing role of chronic inflammatory skin diseases in cardiovascular disease risk. Cutaneous findings may provide important clues to previously undetected cardiopulmonary disease. These findings may be more subtle in darker skin and should not be missed given the significant associated morbidity and mortality.

REFERENCES

1. Mazimba S, Peterson PN. Spotlight on racial and ethnic disparities in cardiovascular disease. *J Am Heart Assoc*. 2021;10:e023650.
2. Roger VL. Epidemiology of heart failure: a contemporary perspective. *Circ Res*. 2021;128:1421-1434.
3. Respiratory diseases disproportionately affecting minorities. The NHLBI Working Group. *Chest*. 108: 1380–1392 (1995).
4. World Health Organization. The top 10 causes of death. WHO Newsroom https://www.who.int/news-room/fact-sheets/detail/the-top-10-causes-of-death.
5. Besharat S, et al. Peripheral edema: a common and persistent health problem for older Americans. *PLoS One*. 2021;16:e0260742.
6. Jackson EA, et al. Effect of race and ethnicity on antihypertensive medication utilization among women in the United States: study of Women's Health Across the Nation (SWAN). *J Am Heart Assoc*. 2017;6:e004758.
7. McMullen SM, Patrick W. Cyanosis. *Am J Med*. 2013;126: 210-212.

8. Pahal P, Goyal A. *Central and Peripheral Cyanosis*. St. Petersburg, FL: StatPearls Publishing; 2021.
9. Spicknall KE, Zirwas MJ, English JC 3rd. Clubbing: an update on diagnosis, differential diagnosis, pathophysiology, and clinical relevance. *J Am Acad Dermatol*. 2005;52:1020-1028.
10. Essouma M, Nkeck J R, Agbor VN, Noubiap JJ. Epidemiology of digital clubbing and hypertrophic osteoarthropathy: a systematic review and meta-analysis. *J Clin Rheumatol*. 2022;28:104-110.
11. Myers KA, Farquhar DR. The rational clinical examination. Does this patient have clubbing? *JAMA*. 2001;286:341-347.
12. Rothstein BE, Cohen JL. An updated work-up for patients with xanthelasma palpebrarum. *Dermatol Surg*. 2021;47:1170-1171.
13. Cahill TJ, Prendergast BD. Infective endocarditis. *Lancet*. 2016;387:882-893.
14. Baylis RA, Smith NL, Klarin D, Fukaya E. Epidemiology and genetics of venous thromboembolism and chronic venous disease. *Circ Res*. 2021;128:1988-2002.
15. Ozkok A. Cholesterol-embolization syndrome: current perspectives. *Vasc Health Risk Manag*. 2019;15:209-220.
16. Rothberg DL, Makarewich CA. Fat Embolism and fat embolism syndrome. *J Am Acad Orthop Surg*. 2019;27:e346-e355.
17. Seligson MT, Surowiec SM. Superior vena cava syndrome. St. Petersburg, FL: StatPearls Publishing, 2021.
18. Poyyamoli S. et al. May-Thurner syndrome. *Cardiovasc Diagn Ther*. 2021;11:1104-1111.
19. Ramien ML. Reactive infectious mucocutaneous eruption: mycoplasma pneumoniae-induced rash and mucositis and other parainfectious eruptions. *Clin Exp Dermatol*. 2021;46:420-429.
20. Ghanem KG, Ram S, Rice PA. The modern epidemic of syphilis. *N Engl J Med*. 2020;382:845-854.
21. Radolf JD, Strle K, Lemieux JE, Strle F. Lyme disease in humans. *Curr Issues Mol Biol*. 2021;42:333–384.
22. Weber B, et al. Psoriasis and cardiovascular disease: novel mechanisms and evolving therapeutics. *Curr Atheroscler Rep*. 2021;23:67.
23. Crouser ED, et al. Diagnosis and detection of sarcoidosis. An Official American Thoracic Society clinical practice guideline. *Am J Respir Crit Care Med*. 2020;201:e26-e51.
24. Wechalekar AD, Gillmore JD, Hawkins PN. Systemic amyloidosis. *Lancet*. 2016;387:2641-2654.
25. Drent M, Crouser ED, Grunewald J. Challenges of sarcoidosis and its management. *N Engl J. Med*. 2021;385:1018-1032.
26. Nordenswan H-K, et al. Manifestations and outcome of cardiac sarcoidosis and idiopathic giant cell myocarditis by 25-year nationwide cohorts. *J Am Heart Assoc*. 2021;10:e019415.
27. Fava A, Petri, M. Systemic lupus erythematosus: diagnosis and clinical management. *J Autoimmun*. 2019;96:1-13.
28. Rife E, Gedalia A. Kawasaki disease: an update. *Curr Rheumatol Rep*. 2020;22:75.
29. Karthikeyan G, Guilherme L. Acute rheumatic fever. *Lancet*. 2018;392:161-174.
30. Perelas A, Silver R M, Arrossi AV, Highland KB. Systemic sclerosis-associated interstitial lung disease. *Lancet Respir Med*. 2020;8:304-320.
31. DeWane ME, Waldman R, Lu J. Dermatomyositis: clinical features and pathogenesis. *J Am Acad Dermatol*. 2020;82: 267-281.
32. Guzman-Soto MI, et al. From head to toe: granulomatosis with polyangiitis. *Radiographics*. 2021;41:1973-1991.
33. Fagni F, Bello F, Emmi G. Eosinophilic granulomatosis with polyangiitis: dissecting the pathophysiology. *Front Med*. 2021;8:627776.
34. Brokamp G, Mori M, Faith EF. Pseudoxanthoma elasticum. *JAMA Dermatol*. 2022;158:100.
35. Meester JAN, et al. Differences in manifestations of Marfan syndrome, Ehlers-Danlos syndrome, and Loeys-Dietz syndrome. *Ann Cardiothorac Surg*. 2017;6:582-594.
36. Beyens A, Boel A, Symoens S, Callewaert B. Cutis laxa: a comprehensive overview of clinical characteristics and pathophysiology. *Clin Genet*. 2021;99: 53-66.
37. Shams S, et al. Carney complex syndrome. *Cardiovasc Pathol*. 2020;49:107231.
38. Roberts AE, Allanson JE, Tartaglia M, Gelb BD. Noonan syndrome. *Lancet*. 2013;381.
39. Sarkozy A, Digilio MC, Dallapiccola B. Leopard syndrome. *Orphanet J Rare Dis*. 2008;3:13.
40. Tran MC, Lam JM. Cutaneous manifestations of mucopolysaccharidoses. *Pediatr Dermatol*. 2016;33:594-601.
41. Islam MP. Tuberous sclerosis complex. *Semin Pediatr Neurol*. 2021;37:100875.
42. Frémond M-L, Crow YJ. STING-Mediated lung inflammation and beyond. *J Clin Immunol*. 2021;41:501-514.
43. Grayson PC, Patel BA, Young NS. VEXAS syndrome. *Blood*. 2021;137: 3591-3594.
44. Spinner MA, et al. GATA2 deficiency: a protean disorder of hematopoiesis, lymphatics, and immunity. *Blood*. 2014;123:809-821.
45. Tsilifis C, Freeman AF, Gennery AR. STAT3 Hyper-IgE syndrome-an update and unanswered questions. *J Clin Immunol*. 2021;41:864-880.
46. Kritharis A, Al-Samkari H, Kuter DJ. Hereditary hemorrhagic telangiectasia: diagnosis and management from the hematologist's perspective. *Haematologica*. 2018;103:1433-1443.
47. Daccord C, et al. Birt-Hogg-Dubé syndrome. *Eur Respir Rev*. 2020;29(157): 200042.
48. Strnad P, McElvaney NG, Lomas DA. Alpha-antitrypsin deficiency. *N Engl J Med*. 2020;382:1443-1455.

CHAPTER 76

Cutaneous Manifestations of Endocrine Disorders

Kyla N. Price
Sarah Gonzalez
Nada Elbuluk

KEY POINTS

- Endocrine conditions with dermatologic findings include disorders of the thyroid, parathyroid, ovaries, adrenal glands, hypothalamus, and pituitary glands.
- Some of these conditions occur more commonly in skin of color and have unique presentations in skin of color.
- Endocrine-related genetic syndromes with cutaneous manifestations include multiple endocrine neoplasia, autoimmune polyglandular syndrome, Carney complex, and Cowden syndrome.
- Awareness of the cutaneous manifestations of endocrine disorders in all skin types can allow for earlier diagnosis and treatment of underlying disorders.

INTRODUCTION

Disorders of the endocrine system can demonstrate a variety of cutaneous manifestations. These findings can be the earliest manifestation of an underlying endocrine disorder and can help lead to a more timely diagnosis and earlier therapeutic intervention. This chapter will provide an overview of common dermatologic manifestations of endocrine diseases with an emphasis on unique presentations and considerations in skin of color (SOC).

DISEASES OF THE PANCREAS

DIABETES MELLITUS

Diabetes mellitus (DM) is the most common endocrinopathy in the world affecting around 37.3 million Americans with about 96 million being prediabetic.[1] Type 1 DM often presents in younger patients and is characterized by the autoimmune destruction of the pancreas B-cells. Meanwhile, type 2 DM is more common and occurs because of insulin resistance and impaired insulin secretion. When stratified by racial/ethnic groups, DM is most prevalent in Native Americans (14.5%) and African Americans (12.1%) followed by people of Hispanic origin (11.8%) and Asians (9.5%), and then non-Hispanic Whites (7.4%).[1] The evolving U.S. demographics with a growing SOC population will likely impact the future prevalence of DM.[2] The prevalence of skin disorders among patients with DM has been reported as high as 79.2%.[3] There are a number of cutaneous conditions that are specifically associated with DM including acanthosis nigricans, necrobiosis lipoidica diabeticorum,

TABLE 76-1 Considerations and unique factors of cutaneous conditions associated with diabetes mellitus

Endocrine-associated dermatologic condition	Unique factors and considerations in skin of color
Acanthosis nigricans	• Higher prevalence among African Americans and Latinos • Higher frequency in Fitzpatrick skin type IV compared to types II and II
Necrobiosis lipoidica diabeticorum	• Less often reported in skin of color • Maroon, violaceous, or brown color in darker skin compared to orange-yellow color in lighter skin
Diabetic foot ulcers	• Higher prevalence among African Americans, Hispanics, and Native Americans • Significantly higher risk of amputation among African Americans and Native Americans
Diabetic dermopathy	• Can present as dark brown to violaceous appearing macules and patches in darker skin
Bullous diabeticorum	• Can be associated with scarring and dyspigmentation in darker skin
Granuloma annulare	• Treatment options including steroid injections and cryotherapy; both of which carry a risk of hypopigmentation in skin of color
Scleredema	• Treatment options include steroid injections that carry a risk of hypopigmentation in skin of color

diabetic dermopathy, diabetic foot ulcers, and bullous diabeticorum [**Table 76-1**].

Acanthosis Nigricans Acanthosis nigricans (AN) is a nonspecific cutaneous finding of several endocrinopathies, such as, DM, hyperprolactinemia, acromegaly, Cushing syndrome, excess androgen production, and rarely malignancies, most specifically abdominal adenocarcinomas.[4,5] AN is associated with insulin resistance and hyperinsulinemia, which stimulates keratinocyte proliferation through insulin-like growth factor 1 receptors.[5] In conditions without insulin resistance, AN is thought to be mediated by mutations that activate fibroblast growth receptor 3 also causing keratinocyte proliferation. Rarely, rapidly progressive AN is paraneoplastic and suggestive of underlying malignancy, most commonly gastric adenocarcinoma.[6] AN appears as thick tan to dark brown hyperpigmented velvety plaques often in the axillae, neck, groin, antecubital, popliteal, and periumbilical regions, and rarely on the eyelids and mucosal regions [**Figure 76-1**].[7] In darker skin, AN often appears dark brown to black, whereas in lighter skin colors, the affected skin often appears light to dark brown. The overall prevalence of AN varies based on the population, with rates as low as 7.1% in children and up to 74% among obese adults.[8,9] When stratified based on race and ethnicity, there is often a higher prevalence of AN in African Americans and Latinos compared to other racial groups.[10,11] A cross-sectional study of obese patients also found that patients with Fitzpatrick skin type IV (78.3%) had a higher frequency of AN compared to skin type II (18.8%) and III (52.2%).[7]

Diagnosis of AN is clinical and does not require any tests, although skin biopsy can be diagnostic. Treatment of AN in the setting of insulin resistance involves weight loss and tight glucose control. Anecdotal success has been reported with topical agents such as calcipotriol, salicylic acid, glycolic acid peels, urea, and retinoids. AN associated with malignancy improves with treatment of the underlying malignancy.[12]

Necrobiosis Lipoidica Diabeticorum (NLD) Necrobiosis lipoidica diabeticorum (NLD) is a rare condition and appears in 0.3% to 1.6% of patients with DM, with a predominance in women and insulin-requiring individuals.[13] In addition to DM, NLD is associated with other systemic conditions including sarcoidosis, granuloma annulare, thyroid disorders, inflammatory bowel disease, and rheumatoid arthritis.[14,15] NLD typically arises on the distal legs, as oval indurated, orange yellow plaques, with central atrophy, and occasionally a violaceous margin [**Figure 76-2**].[16] In contrast to patients with lighter skin, erythema in NLD on individuals

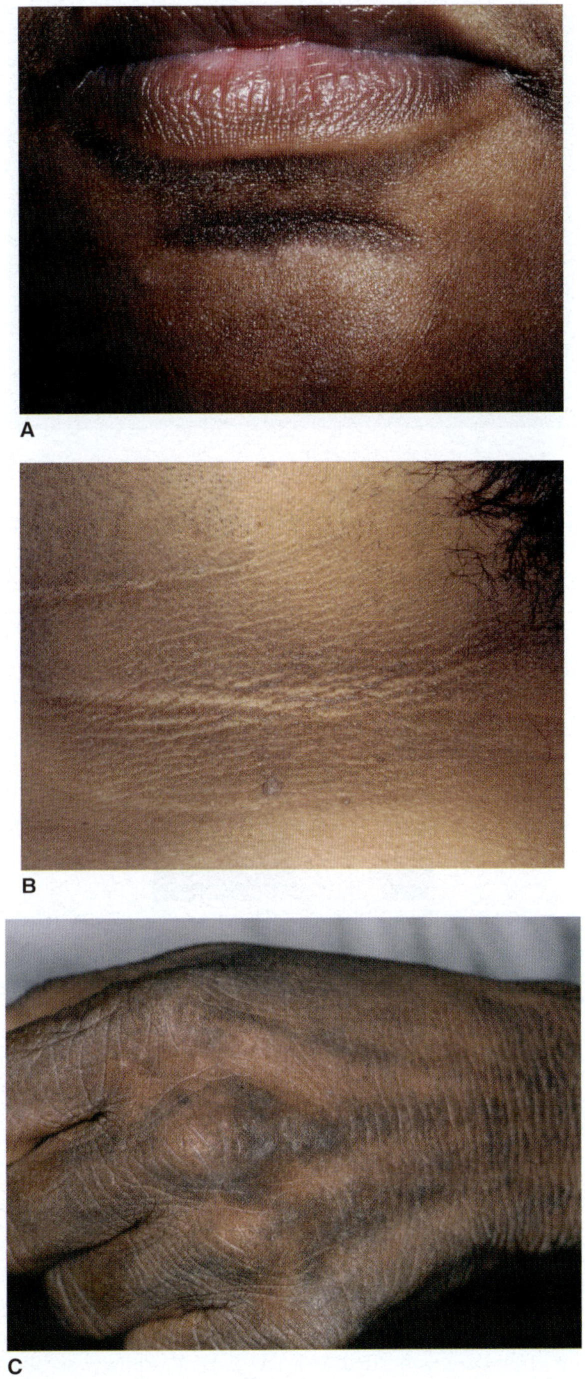

FIGURE 76-1. Acanthosis nigricans of the mouth area **(A)**, neck **(B)**, and hands **(C)**. (Used with permission from the Department of Dermatology, Washington Hospital Center, Washington, DC.)

with darker skin may appear as maroon, violaceous, or brown.[17] Other body sites that may be affected include the scalp, face, dorsal hands, and forearms. NLD is less often reported in SOC individuals.

Skin biopsy is diagnostic for NLD. Histologically, the key features of NLD include pale, acellular degenerated collagen between layers of granulomas. Plasma cells are common in the deep dermis and mucin is often absent. The punch biopsy will often appear rectangular due to sclerosis.

Individuals without a diagnosis of diabetes should have a fasting blood glucose and hemoglobin A1c (HgbA1c). In those with diabetes, severity of NLD does not correlate with glycemic control. The mainstay of treatment for NLD is injury evasion and infection prevention followed by topical and intralesional steroids and topical calcineurin inhibitors.[18] Caution should be taken when using intralesional steroids in SOC

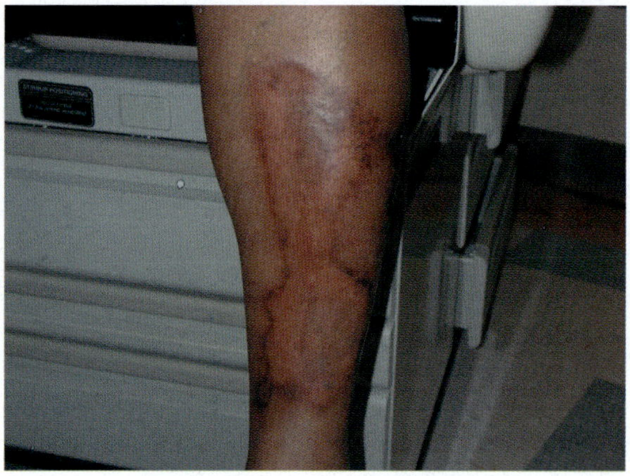

A

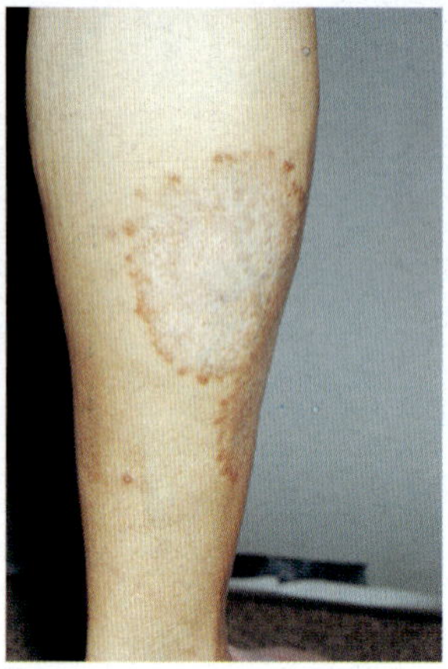

B

FIGURE 76-2. Necrobiosis lipoidica on the anterior shin (**A** and **B**). (Used with permission from the Department of Dermatology, Washington Hospital Center, Washington, DC.)

individuals, due to the risk of hypopigmentation in addition to atrophy. For recalcitrant cases, systemic therapies including pentoxifylline, chloroquine, and fumaric acid esters are considered second line as well as phototherapy.[18] Topical tretinoin may aid with ameliorating discoloration and atrophy in asymptomatic patients.

Diabetic Dermopathy Diabetic dermopathy (DD) is the most common cutaneous manifestation of DM and has been reported in up to half of individuals with diabetes.[19] Despite DD being the most common cutaneous manifestation of DM, incidences as low as 0.2% have been reported among those with darker skin types and has been attributed to difficulty in appreciating DD in SOC.[20,21] Advanced age and longer duration of DM are associated with DD as well as microvascular complications of DM such as retinopathy, neuropathy, and nephropathy.[22] Increased frequency of DD is also reported in those with an increased number of microvascular complications from DM. Some studies have reported a higher frequency in males.[19,22] The condition is asymptomatic and often appear as light, dark brown, or red-brown well-defined macules and/or patches on bilateral anterior shins [**Figure 76-3**]. In darker skin, macules or patches may be dark brown or violaceous. Older areas often appear more atrophic and may have a thin overlying scale. The exact cause of DD remains unclear, but mild trauma, abnormalities in blood flow, thermal disturbances, and subcutaneous nerve degeneration have all been proposed.[19,21,23,24] DD is often self-limited and resolves without treatment. Only variable improvement has been reported with tighter glucose control. Few studies examining the use of low-level laser therapy for the treatment of DD have demonstrated some clinical benefit from laser therapy.[25,26]

Diabetic Foot Ulcers (DFU) Diabetic foot ulcers (DFU) are a commonly recognized complication of diabetes. The cause of DFUs is multifactorial and occurs due to a combination of poor glycemic control, neuropathy, peripheral artery disease, poor foot care, and trauma.[27] DFUs have been reported at rates of up to 34% among those with diabetes. Studies of Medicare beneficiaries have demonstrated that Blacks, Hispanics, and Native Americans have a higher prevalence of DFUs compared to their White counterparts.[28] Among Medicare beneficiaries with DFUs, the risk of amputation was significantly higher among African Americans and Native Americans.[29] Increased risk of amputation among minority groups has been attributed to presentation of a DFU at a more advanced stage, more severe concurrent health conditions, and limited or no access to limb salvage care.[29] Additionally, insurance coverage or lack thereof, an indication of access to healthcare services, is considered one of the major factors contributing to the disparities in lower extremity amputation.[30,31] DFUs commonly present as deep ulcerations surrounded by calluses on the plantar aspect of the foot, tip of the toe, or lateral to the fifth metatarsal [**Figure 76-4**].[32] The treatment of DFUs often requires a multidisciplinary approach often including the primary care provider, endocrinologist, podiatrist, vascular surgeon, and an infectious disease specialist.[33]

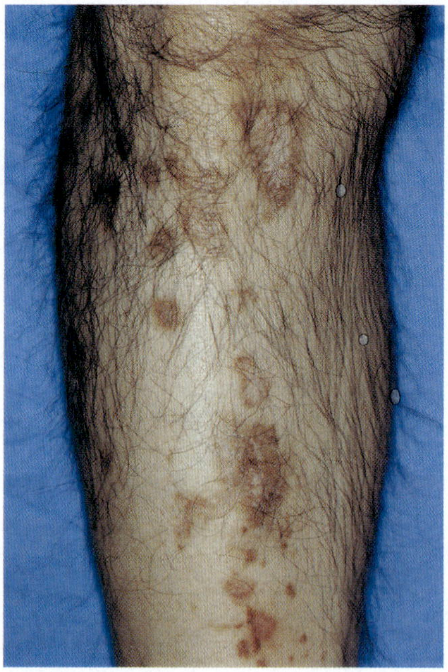

FIGURE 76-3. Diabetic dermopathy on the anterior shin of a male patient. (Used with permission from the Department of Dermatology, Washington Hospital Center, Washington, DC.)

Bullous Diabeticorum (BD) Bullous Diabeticorum (BD) is a rare, spontaneous bullous eruption found in patients with DM with an incidence of about 0.16%.[34,35] BD presents with tense bullae that occur rapidly in as little as 15 minutes and without inciting trauma. The bullae most often involve the extremities, especially the acral feet and present as sterile, fluid containing bullae without underlying erythema or induration [**Figure 76-5**]. Biopsy can be used to differentiate BD from other etiologies but should be used with caution due to the complication risk associated with diabetic neuropathy or a neuroischemic foot. Histology findings are nonspecific with intraepidermal or subepidermal bullae and spongiosis of varying amounts. Direct and indirect immunofluorescence staining is typically negative and can be beneficial in differentiating from other vesiculobullous conditions. When treating BD, some recommend leaving the blister intact while others recommend aspiration or deroofing followed by repeated inspection, application of a nonadherent bandage, regular wound care, foot protection and offloading, and occasionally antibiotics to prevent future complications.[35,36] The reported median healing time is 2.5 months. Although lesions typically heal without scarring, there has been one report of scarring in an African American male.[37]

Granuloma Annulare (GA) Granuloma annulare (GA) is an inflammatory dermatosis that may occur independently but is often associated with a number of systemic diseases including diabetes, hyperlipidemia, and less commonly systemic infections, malignancy, and thyroid

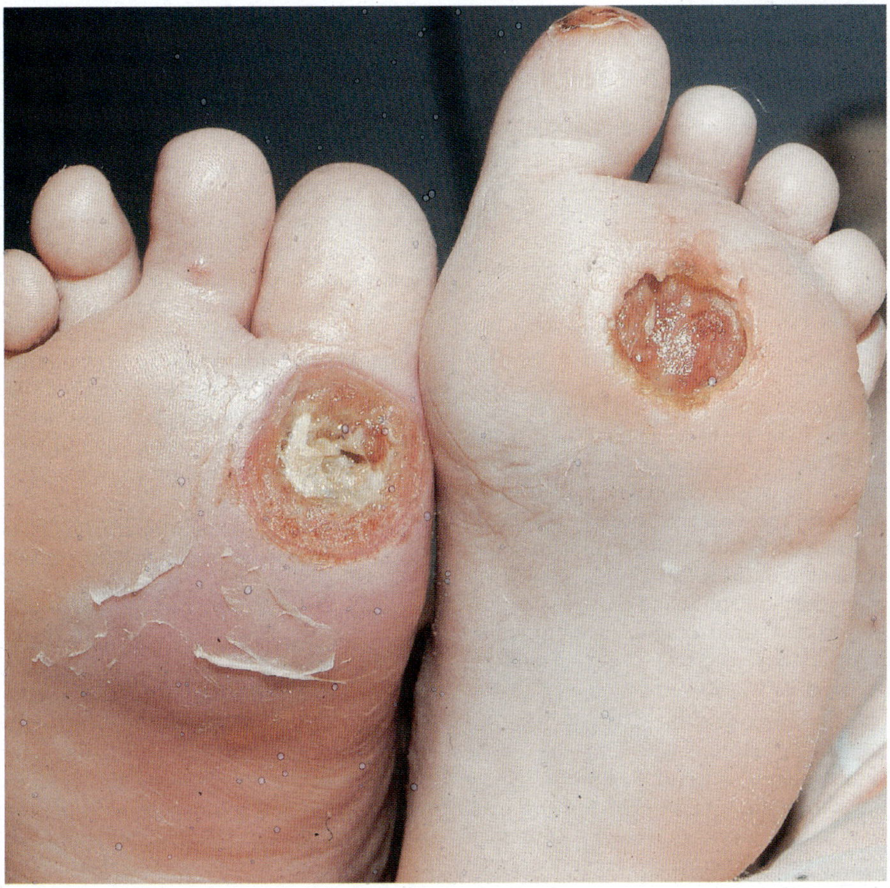

FIGURE 76-4. Diabetic foot ulcers on bilateral plantar feet. (Used with permission from the Department of Dermatology, Washington Hospital Center, Washington, DC.)

disease.[38] The annualized incidence of GA is 0.04%, while the annualized prevalence is 0.06% in the United States.[39] Women are affected at three times the rate as males and there is a predilection for the fifth decade of life. The prevalence of GA among White individuals was higher when compared to Black, Hispanic, or Asian individuals. The pathogenesis of GA remains unknown, but numerous hypotheses have been proposed including potential involvement of a delayed-type hypersensitivity.[38] GA has multiple subtypes and can range in color from flesh-colored to red and red-brown. Localized GA can present with asymptomatic papules in an annular or arciform configuration involving the extremities and rarely the trunk [**Figure 76-6**]. Generalized GA manifests as more extensive

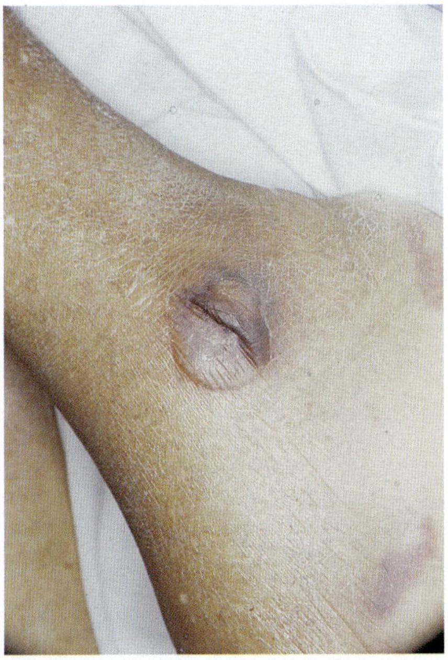

FIGURE 76-5. Diabetic bullae on the ankle. (Used with permission from the Department of Dermatology, Washington Hospital Center, Washington, DC.)

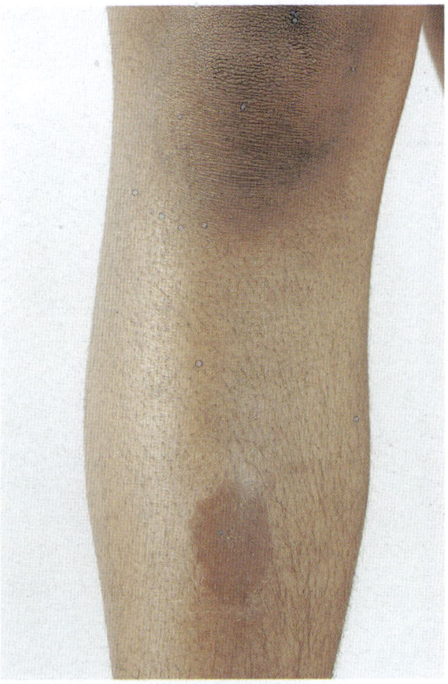

FIGURE 76-6. Granuloma annular on the anterior shin of a patient with darker skin of color. (Used with permission from the Department of Dermatology, Washington Hospital Center, Washington, DC.)

macules, papules, and nodules either discrete or coalescing into reticulate and circinate patches and plaques involving the extremities as well as the trunk. Subcutaneous GA is a subtype of GA seen almost exclusively in children and is characterized by painless, firm subcutaneous nodules on the lower extremities and rarely reported on the forehead and scalp. Perforating GA is rare variant of GA with grouped papules with central scale or an umbilicated plug predominantly involving the extremities. Unlike other forms of GA, perforating GA can ulcerate and thus can result in scarring.

The diagnosis of GA can be achieved clinically or with correlation of clinical presentation with histological findings found on biopsy. Some of the key histological features of GA include necrobiosis, palisading granulomas or interstitial granulomatous infiltration, and an abundance of mucin deposition.

GA is typically self-limited; however, some individuals may be interested in treatment for cosmetic reasons or due to symptoms. The first-line treatment for localized GA is topical corticosteroids or intralesional triamcinolone injections.[40] If unsuccessful, other targeted therapies including calcineurin inhibitors and cryotherapy may beneficial. Special care should be taken with SOC individuals due to the risk of atrophy from steroids and hypopigmentation from both steroids and cryotherapy. For recalcitrant cases or more systemic disease, systemic steroids and phototherapy use have been reported followed by other systemic drug therapies including antibiotics, antimalarials, and fumaric acid esters.[40] Of note, postinflammatory hyperpigmentation can occur particularly in SOC.

Scleredema (Scleredema of Buschke) Scleredema is rare, sclerotic skin disease that is characterized by thickening and tightening of the skin with associated pink to red erythema or tan to dark brown hyperpigmentation [**Figure 76-7**]. Scleredema often begins on the neck and spreads to the upper back and shoulders. Scleredema is divided into three types.[41] Type 1 occurs in patients with a recent bacterial or viral febrile infection, type 2 is often associated with paraproteinemias, while type 3 is associated with diabetes. The pathogenesis of type 3 scleredema is thought to be due to irreversible glycosylation of collagen and disruption of collagenase activity resulting in accumulation of collagen and mucin. Scleredema does not appear to have a racial predilection. Penetration of the dermis causes a woody, *peau d'orange* appearance of the skin. Skin biopsy is diagnostic and often includes extensive fibrosis and thick dermal collagen separated by mucin. Unfortunately, there is no preferred treatment for scleredema and it does not necessarily improve with glycemic control. Numerous treatment modalities for scleredema have been attempted, including topical and intralesional corticosteroids, hyaluronidase injections, methotrexate, systemic glucocorticoids, high-dose intravenous immunoglobulin, antibiotics, factor XIII, cyclosporine, phototherapy, but none have resulted in consistent benefit.[42] Caution must be used in SOC as intralesional steroids may cause hypopigmentation in addition to atrophy.

Acquired Perforating Dermatoses (APD) Acquired perforating disorders (APD) are a collection of disorders classified by transepidermal loss of connective tissue components. The four classic conditions part of APD include Kyrle disease, acquired elastosis perforans serpiginosa, acquired perforating collagenosis (APC), and perforating folliculitis. Most cases of APD occur in association with DM and chronic kidney disease (CKD). Clinically, APD appears as round, skin-colored, erythematous or hypopigmented umbilicated papules and nodules with a central keratin plug involving the extensor surfaces of the extremities and trunk, rarely on the face or scalp. In SOC individuals, erythema is less distinguishable, and papules may take on a brown, violaceous hue compared to those with lighter skin in whom papules range from pink to red. The inner keratin plug is a characteristic clinical finding but is often subject to removal by the individual resulting in an empty cavity. Diagnosis depends on both clinical and histopathologic findings. Histology will demonstrate a crateriform epidermal invagination filled with basophilic cellular debris and a parakeratotic plug.

Treatment of APD revolves around discovery and treatment of the underlying disorder and comorbidities.

While APD may improve with management of the underlying disorder, treatment can be difficult. There are no approved first-line agents for APD. Keratolytics, topical corticosteroids, and topical retinoids have been suggested as first-line topical therapies.[43] Antihistamines and allopurinol have been suggested as first-line systemic therapy. Other potentially helpful medications include phototherapy, systemic retinoids, systemic corticosteroids, and antibiotics.

NECROLYTIC MIGRATORY ERYTHEMA (NME)

Glucagonoma syndrome is secondary to overproduction of glucagon from the alpha cells of pancreas due to a pancreatic neuroendocrine tumor. The associated cutaneous manifestation of glucagonoma syndrome is necrolytic migratory erythema (NME). NME is among the most common (67%) presenting symptoms of glucagonoma, second only to weight loss.[44] Characteristically, NME presents as migratory scaly, annular or centrifugal papules, patches, and plaques classically located in the intertriginous areas, lower abdomen, and distal extremities. In lighter skin, this can be red while in darker skin it can be violaceous to brown. Superficial necrosis of NME can also lead to bullae and subsequently

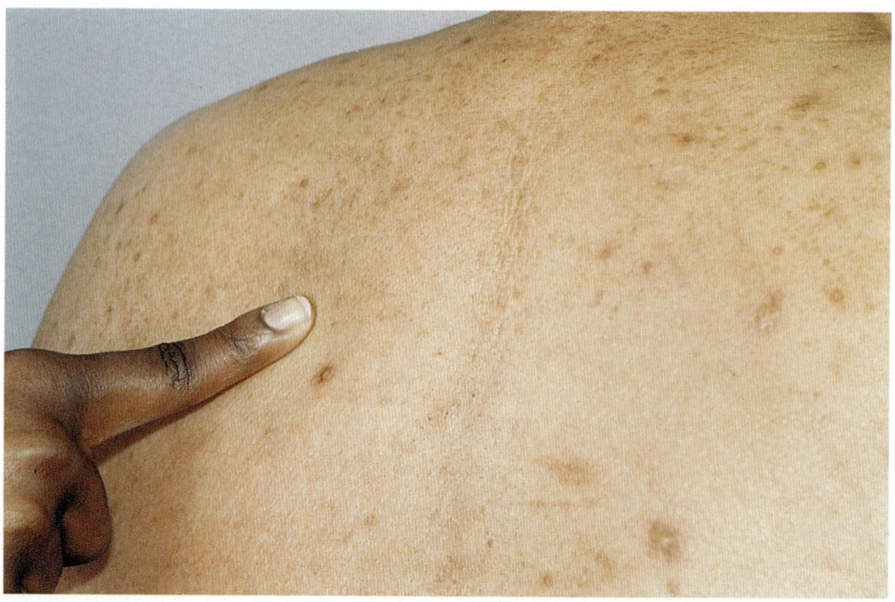

FIGURE 76-7. Scleredema on the upper back. (Used with permission from the Department of Dermatology, Washington Hospital Center, Washington, DC.)

erosions. Additional manifestations of NME include alopecia, angular cheilitis, glossitis, blepharitis, onychoschizia, and other nail changes.[45,46]

Pathogenesis of NME is not understood but excess glucagon and deficiency of zinc, amino acids, and free fatty acids are thought contribute.[47] In some patients, NME exists in the absence of glucagonoma syndrome, associated with other disorders such as malabsorption disorders, inflammatory bowel disease (IBD), liver disease, pancreatitis, and other nonmalignant pancreatic derangements.

Biopsy can be beneficial in narrowing the diagnosis if blood tests or imaging have not been performed. Histological findings of NME include displacement of the stratum spinosum and stratum granulosum with pale, vacuolated keratinocytes.

Resolution of NME often occurs with resection of the glucagonoma when no distal metastases are present. When metastases have occurred, octreotide has also been helpful to treat NME for those with and without glucagonoma syndrome, and streptozocin and 5-fluorouracil have also been shown to be helpful.[48-50] The consequences of NME have not been specifically reported in SOC; however, it is important to know that NME often heals with hyperpigmentation, which can be especially prominent and impactful for SOC individuals.[51]

DISEASES OF THE THYROID

Worldwide thyroid disorders are commonly due to iodine deficiency; however, in the Western world thyroid disease is commonly of autoimmune origin. Autoimmune thyroid disease is associated with other autoimmune disorders such as diabetes mellitus, alopecia, and vitiligo. Due to the many cutaneous manifestations of thyroid disorders and associated conditions, it is not uncommon for dermatologists to be among the first providers to identify signs and symptoms consistent with thyroid disorders and refer patients for further work-up and management.

HYPERTHYROIDISM

Hyperthyroidism is an excess production of thyroid hormone often secondary to autoimmune activation of thyroid stimulating hormone receptors. Graves disease is the most common form of hyperthyroidism and higher rates have been reported among non-Hispanic Blacks and Asian/Pacific Islanders when compared to non-Hispanic Whites.[52,53] The most common skin findings associated with hyperthyroidism include warm and moist skin, palmoplantar hyperhidrosis [**Figure 76-8**], diffuse nonscarring alopecia, onycholysis, Plummers nails, hyperpigmentation, facial flushing, palmar erythema, and pretibial myxedema [**Figure 76-9**].[54] Pigmentary changes may be subtle and thus more difficult to discern in SOC patients.

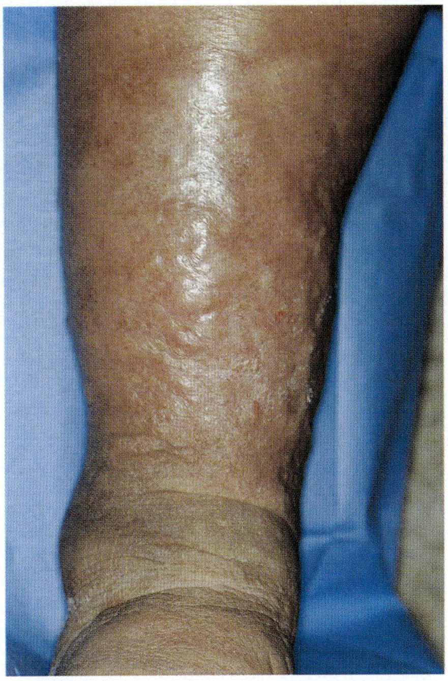

FIGURE 76-9. Pretibial myxedema of the lower extremity. (Used with permission from the Department of Dermatology, Washington Hospital Center, Washington, DC.)

Thyroid Dermopathy Thyroid dermopathy, also referred to as localized myxedema, pretibial myxedema, or infiltrative dermopathy is a skin condition that most commonly manifests in individuals with Graves disease. Thyroid dermopathy is often a late sign of Graves disease that occurs frequently in conjunction with exophthalmos and acropachy [**Figure 76-10**]. Thyroid dermopathy presents as bilateral, painless nonpitting nodules and plaques with a hardened, waxy texture on the bilateral shins; however, it can rarely arise on other regions of the body. The proposed pathogenesis involves autoantibodies binding to the thyroid stimulating hormone receptor (TSHR) on fibroblasts provoking glycosaminoglycan synthesis and subsequent deposition. Biopsy results often demonstrate thickening of the dermis, widened collagen fibrils, and hyaluronic acid in the interstitial space. Topical steroids with occlusion are the mainstay of treatment for thyroid dermopathy and can be helpful for pruritus and cosmesis. Intralesional steroids can also be helpful;

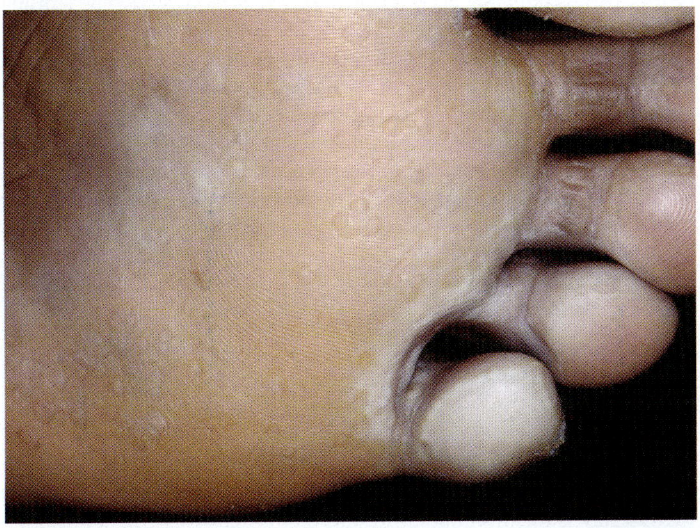

FIGURE 76-8. Plantar hyperhidrosis in a patient with hyperthyroidism. (Used with permission from the Department of Dermatology, Washington Hospital Center, Washington, DC.)

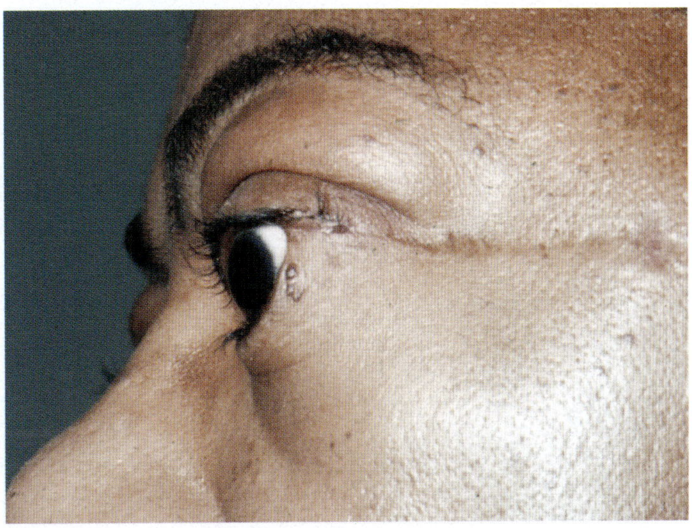

FIGURE 76-10. Exophthalmos in a patient with darker skin of color and Graves disease. (Used with permission from the Department of Dermatology, Washington Hospital Center, Washington, DC.)

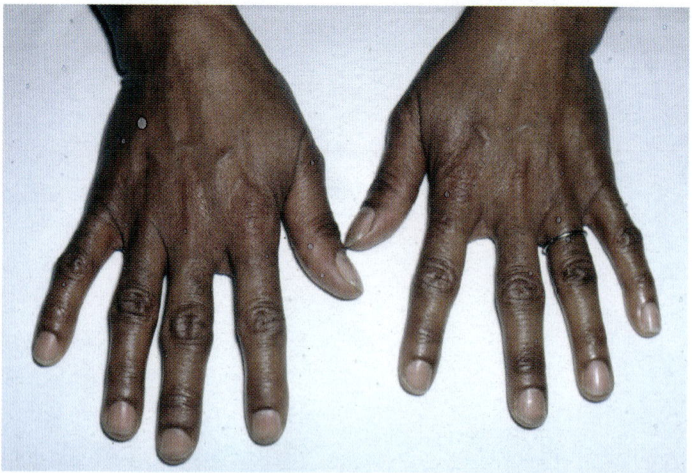

FIGURE 76-11. Thyroid acropachy due to autoimmune thyroid disease in a patient with darker skin of color. (Used with permission from the Department of Dermatology, Washington Hospital Center, Washington, DC.)

however, special attention is warranted prior to use in SOC individuals due to increased risk of postinflammatory hypopigmentation.

Acropachy Thyroid acropachy is a rare manifestation associated with advanced Graves disease that frequently occurs in conjunction with exophthalmos and thyroid dermopathy due to glycosaminoglycan deposition. Acropachy presents with digital clubbing, diaphyseal proliferation, and hypertrophy of the soft tissue [**Figure 76-11**].[55] Treatment of the underlying Graves disease can lead to some improvement in the clinical manifestations of acropachy but often does not result in complete resolution. Use of other treatments such as high-potency steroids, rituximab, radiotherapy, immunosuppressive drugs, and surgery have been reported but often with limited success.

HYPOTHYROIDISM

Hypothyroidism is a deficiency of thyroid hormone with Hashimoto thyroiditis being the most common cause. In contrast to hyperthyroidism, higher rates of hypothyroidism have been reported in non-Hispanic Whites, while the lowest rates have been reported among non-Hispanic Blacks.[53] The most common skin findings in patients with hypothyroidism include coarse, rough, and dry skin, pallor of the skin, nail changes [**Figure 76-12**], diffuse hair loss, carotenoderma, palmoplantar keratoderma, madarosis, and myxedematous facies.[54] Many of the findings associated with hypothyroidism are nonspecific. Pallor of the skin in SOC may have a white or gray appearance and can be subtle and more difficult to appreciate along with carotenoderma.

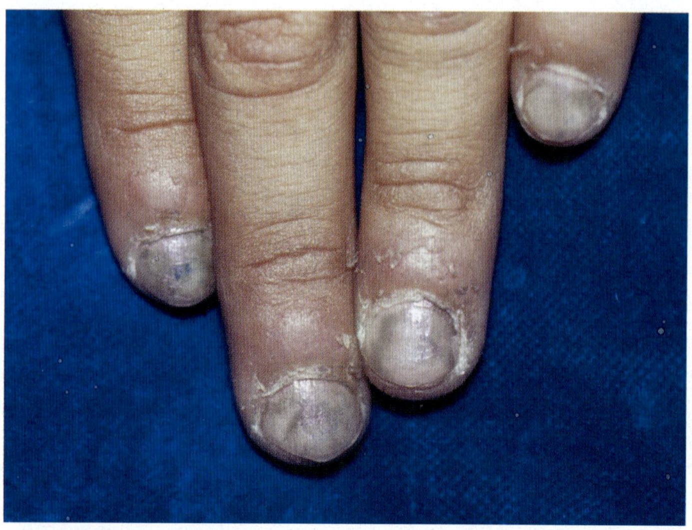

FIGURE 76-12. Nail dystrophy and xerosis in a patient with hypothyroidism. (Used with permission from the Department of Dermatology, Washington Hospital Center, Washington, DC.)

DISEASES OF THE ADRENAL GLANDS

CUSHING SYNDROME

Cushing syndrome is a disorder that occurs because of exposure to excess cortisol hormone. Individuals with Cushing syndrome often present with central obesity of the face, neck, and trunk secondary to excess fat deposition as well as several other cutaneous manifestations including violaceous striae, facial acne, hirsutism, AN, easy bruising, and fungal infections. Increase of ACTH secretion associated with some causes of Cushing syndrome leads to diffuse bronze hyperpigmentation due to stimulation of melanocortin 1 receptor located on the surface of dermal melanocytes. Apart from striae, most skin findings associated with Cushing syndrome will resolve with treatment of the underlying cause.

ADDISON DISEASE

Addison disease, also known as primary adrenal insufficiency or hypoadrenalism, is a rare disease impacting the adrenal glands resulting in a decrease in the hormones cortisol and aldosterone. Like Cushing syndrome, elevated ACTH secretions causes hyperpigmentation due to stimulation of melanocortin 1 receptor on the surface of dermal melanocytes. The bronze hyperpigmentation associated with Addison disease can be diffuse or particularly prominent on the mucous membranes, palmar creases, sun-exposed areas, and areas of trauma.[13] Mucosal involvement presents as streaked or irregular, blue-black to brown macules, papules, patches, and plaques on the tongue, inner surface of the lip as well as the buccal and gingival mucosa. Hyperpigmentation may precede other symptoms of Addison disease by months to years. In darkly pigmented individuals, hyperpigmentation due to Addison disease may frequently be overlooked and can be difficult to distinguish resulting in potential delays in diagnosis.[56,57] Treatment of Addison disease involves hormonal therapy with glucocorticoids and mineralocorticoids, which subsequently results in progressive improvement of the hyperpigmentation.

DISORDERS OF OVARIES

POLYCYSTIC OVARIAN SYNDROME

Polycystic ovarian syndrome (PCOS) is a common endocrine disorder impacting reproductive-aged women. PCOS is characterized by chronic anovulation, hyperandrogenism, and insulin resistance. The cutaneous manifestations of hyperandrogenism include hirsutism, male pattern alopecia, and acne. AN, as discussed previously in this chapter, is a common manifestation of insulin resistance. The prevalence of PCOS is similar across all racial and ethnic groups.[58] However, a 2017 study examined the racial and ethnic differences in phenotype for women with PCOS and found that Hispanic women had a higher prevalence of acne and hirsutism when compared to non-Hispanic Whites and non-Hispanic Blacks.[59] Overall, PCOS treatment is aimed at reducing excess androgens with oral contraceptives and other antiandrogens such as spironolactone.

DISORDERS OF THE HYPOTHALAMUS AND PITUITARY GLAND

ACROMEGALY

Acromegaly is uncommon and results from excessive growth hormone (GH) typically because of a GH-secreting pituitary adenoma. Excess growth hormone leads to both skeletal and soft tissue overgrowth that not only impacts overall physical appearance but can also impact other organ systems including the cardiovascular and respiratory systems.[60] Additionally, excess GH and insulin growth factor-1 act on the skin cells and adnexa.[61] Common skin findings include skin edema, oily skin with large pores, hypertrichosis, excessive sweating, pigmented acrochordons, cutis verticis gyrata, and rarely AN and psoriasis. The mainstay of treatment for acromegaly includes surgical resection of GH-producing tumors and when indicated use of somatostatin analogs, GH receptor antagonists, dopamine agonists, or adjuvant radiotherapy.

GROWTH HORMONE DEFICIENCY

Growth hormone (GH) deficiency is characterized by inadequate or decreased secretion of GH from the anterior pituitary gland. GH deficiency can be further classified into the congenital, acquired, or idiopathic forms. The congenital form of GH deficiency occurs as a result of genetic causes, brain structural defects, or midline facial defects that impact GH synthesis, GH receptors, and overall brain structure.[62] Meanwhile acquired GH deficiency can occur as a result of damage to the CNS system through surgery, trauma, tumors, inflammation, or radiation. However, isolated, sporadic GH deficiency remains the most common form. GH deficiency may be suspected in adults presenting with increased body fat, decreased muscle mass, fatigue, weakness, lethargy, and overall decreased quality of life.[63] GH deficiency in both children and adults can be identified using GH stimulation tests. Skin findings associated with GH deficiency are often nonspecific, but include thin, dry, and pale skin, thin hair, and reduced sweating.[64] The mainstay of treatment for GH deficiency is growth hormone replacement until linear growth has been completed or in adults until symptoms improve.[63]

HYPOPITUITARISM

Hypopituitarism occurs due to disruption of either the pituitary gland or hypothalamus resulting in deficiency of a combination of different pituitary hormones.[16,65] Similar to GH deficiency described above, hypopituitarism can occur due to tumors, radiation, disrupted vascular supply, inflammation, infection granulomatous diseases, or other disorders impacting the pituitary gland or hypothalamus. Pituitary adenomas are among the most common causes of hypopituitarism, and studies have reported higher incidences of pituitary adenomas among both Black males and females.[66,67]

Patients with resulting ACTH deficiency present similar to Addison disease without hyperpigmentation due to the lack of ACTH. Deficiency of TSH results in symptoms consistent with hypothyroidism as described above. Luteinizing hormone and follicle-stimulating hormone and deficiency results in amenorrhea in females and erectile dysfunction with hypogonadism in males. Prolactin secretion under normal pituitary conditions is inhibited, thus with pituitary dysfunction, it becomes elevated causing galactorrhea. Loss of GH can also occur and can lead to nonspecific findings noted above in the previous section. The overall cutaneous manifestations of hypopituitarism are overall similar to the findings of GH deficiency including skin pallor, dryness, thin skin, and thin hair or overall reduction in body hair. Treatment is directed based on the underlying cause of hypopituitarism as wells as supplementation of deficient hormones.

DISORDERS OF THE PARATHYROID GLANDS

HYPERPARATHYROIDISM

Primary hyperparathyroidism occurs from overproduction of parathyroid hormone causing hypercalcemia. Hyperparathyroidism is most commonly caused by a single parathyroid adenoma and less commonly by multiple parathyroid adenomas, hyperplasia of all four parathyroid glands, or parathyroid carcinoma.[68] The incidence of primary hyperparathyroidism has been reported the highest among Blacks, followed by Whites, Asians, Hispanics, and then other races.[69] Unlike hypoparathyroidism, hyperparathyroidism is not commonly associated with specific cutaneous findings. Some case reports have reported chronic urticaria and calcinosis cutis associated with hyperparathyroidism.[70,71] Surgery is the only definitive treatment for hyperparathyroidism and is indicated specifically for those younger than 50, with osteoporosis, fragility fracture, clinically significant hypercalcemia, renal calculi, hypercalciuria, or renal impairment.[68]

HYPOPARATHYROIDISM

Hypoparathyroidism is a disorder that occurs as a result of parathyroid hormone deficiency. Anterior neck surgery is the most common cause of hypoparathyroidism followed by genetic or autoimmune causes.[72] Common presenting symptoms of hypoparathyroidism include paresthesias, muscles cramps, seizures, and laryngospasm, which occur due to hypocalcemia. The most common findings associated with hypoparathyroidism include loss of axillary hair, loss of pubic hair, coarsening of body hair, alopecia areata, brittle nails, nail ridging, and dry skin.[16,73] Less commonly pellagra-like hyperpigmentation, pustular psoriasis, acneiform eruptions, bullous impetigo, and oral candidiasis. In emergent cases such as with life-threatening complications, hypoparathyroidism is treated with IV calcium infusions.[72] In less acute situations, hypoparathyroidism is treated with high-dose vitamin D and calcium supplementation; however, subcutaneous parathyroid hormone therapy has been used for refractory cases.

GENETIC SYNDROMES

MULTIPLE ENDOCRINE NEOPLASIA

Multiple endocrine neoplasia syndromes are a set of rare, autosomal dominant genetic syndromes that are each associated with three or more specific conditions including endocrine tumors.

Multiple endocrine neoplasia type 1 (MEN-1) classically presents with the triad of parathyroid hyperplasia, pancreatic endocrine tumor, and pituitary adenoma. No gender, geographical, racial or ethnic predilections for MEN-1 have been identified.[74] To fit criteria for the diagnosis of MEN-1, a person must have at least two of the previously mentioned tumors and have a first-degree relative that has at least one of the three.[75] In addition, to the three main findings of MEN-1, angiofibromas, especially facial, collagenomas, lipomas, hypopigmented macules, and café au lait macules have all been reported in patients with MEN-1.[76-79] Treatment in MEN-1 is directed at the respective tumor and often requires surgical intervention.[80]

Multiple endocrine neoplasia type 2a (MEN-2a) is characterized by the presence of medullary thyroid carcinoma, unilateral or bilateral pheochromocytoma, and primary hyperparathyroidism most often secondary to parathyroid hyperplasia or adenoma. MEN-2a composes more than 80% of MEN-2 patients.[81] MEN-2a is associated with cutaneous lichen amyloidosis, which manifests as a pruritic, scaly well-demarcated tan to brown plaque on the upper back or intrascapular region.[82,83]

MEN-2b is also associated with specific conditions, which include medullary thyroid carcinoma, pheochromocytoma, multiple neuromas or diffuse ganglioneuromatosis of the gastroenteric mucosa, and marfanoid habitus.[81] Mucosal neuromas appear as flesh-colored to pink to red, papules on the mucosal surface particularly the lips, tongue, and buccal mucosa as well as the eyelids, conjunctivae, and cornea. The marfanoid habitus includes an elongated face and extremities, joint laxity, pectus deformities, and kyphoscoliosis. MEN-2b is the most aggressive MEN-2 variant and on average presents 10 years earlier than in MEN-2a. MEN-2b also has a higher morbidity and mortality than in those with MEN-2a. Surgical interventions for the respective tumors as they arise or even prophylactically is the mainstay of treatment for both MEN-2a and MEN-2b. Regular screening is also important for early detection of new or arising tumors.

AUTOIMMUNE POLYGLANDULAR SYNDROMES (APS)

The autoimmune polyglandular syndromes (APS) are a set of syndromes characterized by distinct patterns of endocrine abnormalities.

Circulating autoantibodies infiltrate tissues and organs resulting in disruption and failure.

In autoimmune polyglandular syndrome 1 (APS-1), also known as autoimmune polyendocrinopathy-candidiasis-ectodermal dystrophy individuals present with chronic mucocutaneous candidiasis and hypoparathyroidism with or without Addison disease.[84] APS-1 occurs as a result of either autosomal dominant or autosomal recessive inheritance of mutations in the autoimmune regular gene. APS-1 has a higher prevalence in Finland, Sardinia, and specifically among Persian Jews living in Israel. APS-1 has a broad number of associations including primary ovarian insufficiency, autoimmune thyroid disease, type 1 diabetes, gastritis, hepatitis, nephritis, enteritis with malabsorption, pancreatitis, retinitis, keratitis, pneumonitis, and enamel hypoplasia.[84,85] The dermatologic conditions associated with APS-1 include vitiligo, alopecia, and nail dystrophy. Treatment for the conditions associated with APS-1 include hormone replacement, antifungal therapy for candidiasis, and immunosuppressants for the conditions caused by underlying autoimmune destruction.[84]

Autoimmune polyglandular syndrome 2 (APS-2) is characterized by at least two of the following: type 1 diabetes, autoimmune thyroid disease, and Addison disease.[84] APS-2 is thought to occur as a result of mutations in a number of different genes as well as environmental factors. APS-2 has been associated with several other conditions including autoimmune gastritis, celiac disease, and primary ovarian insufficiency. In addition to the cutaneous manifestations associated with type 1 diabetes, thyroid disease, and Addison disease that were previously discussed in this chapter, alopecia and vitiligo have also been associated with APS-2. Similar to APS-1, treatment for APS-2 includes hormone replacement.

X-linked immunodysregulation, polyendocrinopathy, and enteropathy (IPEX) is a genetic syndrome that occurs as a result of mutation in the FoxP3 gene that is responsible for producing forkhead box P3 (FoxP3) regulatory T cells that work to inhibit autoreactive cells. Mutations in the FoxP3 leads to lack of inhibition of autoreactive cells. IPEX manifests with autoimmune enteropathy with severe and intractable diarrhea and malabsorption, neonatal type 1 diabetes, and dermatitis that may be eczematous, psoriasiform, or ichthyosiform.[84] IPEX is also associated with autoimmune thyroid disease, hemolytic anemia, and thrombocytopenia. IPEX occurs very early on in life and can be fatal within the first few years of life unless adequately treated with immunosuppressants or bone marrow transplants.

CARNEY COMPLEX

Carney complex is a rare autosomal dominant disorder, characterized by pigmented skin neoplasms, myxomas, and multiple endocrine tumors.[86] The majority of patients with Carney complex have an associated germline inactivation mutation of the *PRKAR1A* gene located on chromosome 17q23-q24.[87] Other associated findings and conditions include growth hormone-producing pituitary adenomas, Cushing syndrome, adrenocortical tumors, thyroid tumors, thyroid cancer (papillary, follicular, or both), testicular tumors, ovarian lesions, cardiac myxomas, breast myxomas, and psammomatous melanotic schwannomas. Common skin findings associated with Carney complex include blue nevi, café au lait macules, lentigines, cutaneous myxomas, and Spitz nevi. Skin findings can be located throughout the body but often have a predilection for the face, lips, genital area, and mucosa. In African Americans, Carney complex may present as slightly raised dark papules.[86]

COWDEN SYNDROME

Cowden syndrome is an autosomal dominant genodermatosis that occurs as a result of germline mutations in the phosphatase and tensin homolog (PTEN) tumor suppressor gene.[88] PTEN is important in downregulating the cell cycle, and thus mutations in PTEN result in increased cell proliferation and survival. Cowden syndrome classically presents with numerous benign mucocutaneous lesions including facial papules, oral papillomas, lipomas, trichilemmomas, and acral and plantar keratoses [**Figure 76-13**]. Other benign tumors associated with Cowden syndrome include benign uterine tumors, hamartomatous polyps, ganglioneuromas, and benign thyroid and breast growths. Patients with Cowden syndrome also have an elevated risk of thyroid, breast, renal, colon, endometrial cancer, and melanoma due to PTEN mutation.

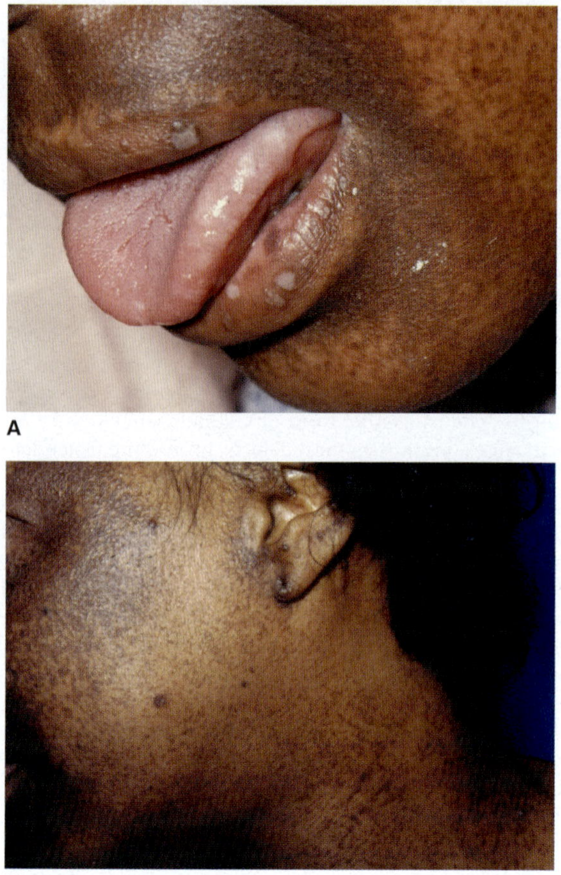

A

B

FIGURE 76-13. Cowden syndrome in a patient with skin of color. (Used with permission from the Department of Dermatology, Washington Hospital Center, Washington, DC.)

CONDITIONS AND SKIN FINDINGS ASSOCIATED WITH ENDOCRINE DISORDERS

ACQUIRED ICHTHYOSIS (AI)

Acquired ichthyosis (AI) is a nonhereditary adult-onset dermatologic disorder manifesting secondary to an underlying disorder or induced by medication. AI is associated with a number of systemic diseases including malignancy, autoimmune/inflammatory diseases, nutritional diseases, infectious disease, and metabolic diseases.[89] Additionally, AI is also associated with medications, including cimetidine, clofazimine, hydroxyurea, cholesterol-lower agents, nicotinic acid, 3-hydroxy-3-methylglutaryl coenzyme A reductase inhibitors, and triparanol. The exact cause of AI remains unknown but is related to abnormal barrier function. Clinically, AI is phenotypically similar to the heritable childhood onset disease ichthyosis vulgaris and has no racial predilection. The skin appears very rough and dry with symmetrical white, brown, or gray scale involving the trunk, limbs, and scalp with sparing of the face and flexural surfaces. Diagnosis is often clinical, but biopsy will demonstrate a noticeably absent or decreased granular layer and orthokeratotic hyperkeratosis. Treatment of the underlying primary condition often results in improvement of AI. Aside from treating the underlying condition, hydration of the skin barrier, preventing water evaporation, and keratolysis are the mainstay treatment.

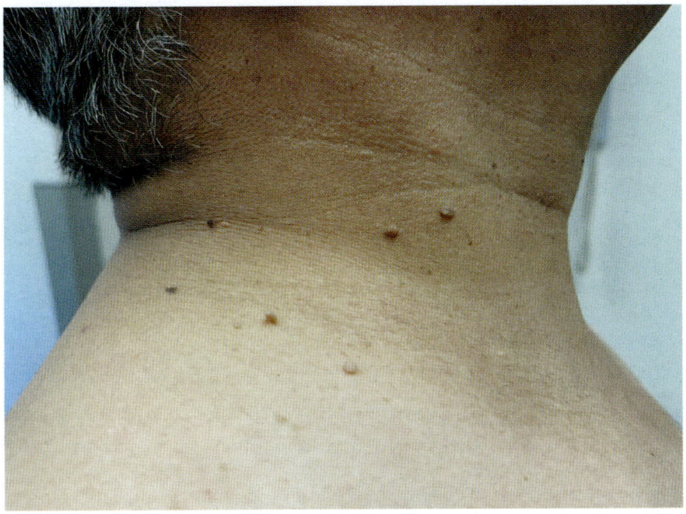

FIGURE 76-14. Acrochordons on the lateral neck. (Used with permission from Dr. Kyla Price.)

ACROCHORDONS

Acrochordons are benign papules most often associated with obesity. Acrochordons are very common with nearly half of the general population having at least one and increasing frequency with age. Acrochordons can also be a finding in the rare autosomal dominant disease, Birt-Hogg-Dubbe Syndrome, as well as acromegaly, acanthosis nigricans, or other disorders with hormone dysregulation. Acrochordons appear as small, skin-colored or brown to black pedunculated papules found on the neck, axilla, eyelids, and inguinal folds and rarely on the oral, anal, or vulvovaginal mucosa [**Figure 76-14**].

Diagnosis is clinical but histology can be helpful in distinguishing acrochordons from other benign neoplasms such as neurofibromas or benign melanocytic nevi. Histology demonstrates a loose array of collagen fibers with abundant dilated lymphatic vessels.

Acrochordons are benign and do not require removal; however, they may become traumatized, inflamed, pruritic, and painful, at which point the individual may desire removal. Removal can be done with scissors, shave excision, electrodessication, or cryotherapy. Special caution must be taken in SOC with use of cryotherapy due to the risk of long-lasting hypopigmentation.

CONCLUSION

Endocrine diseases present with a variety of skin manifestations many of which can look different in darker skin colors. Certain endocrine conditions also have an increased incidence and/or prevalence in SOC populations. Dermatologists and other healthcare providers may be the first to identify the initial dermatologic signs of an underlying endocrine conditions helping to initiate not only timely diagnosis but also early treatment. Once a diagnosis has been made, it is also important for affected individuals to have multidisciplinary care that can involve their primary care provider, endocrinologists, and other specialists for comprehensive care. Early diagnosis and treatment can also help improve health disparities related to many of these endocrine-associated conditions.

REFERENCES

1. *National Diabetes Statistics Report*. Centers for Disease Control and Prevention.
2. Vespa J AD, Medina L. *Demographic Turning Points for the Unitedtates: Population Projections for 2020 to 2060 Population Estimates and Projections Current Population Reports*. U.S. Census Bureau; 2020.
3. Demirseren DD, Emre S, Akoglu G, et al. Relationship between skin diseases and extracutaneous complications of diabetes mellitus: clinical analysis of 750 patients. *Am J Clin Dermatol*. 2014;15(1):65-70.
4. Demirkesen C. Skin Manifestations of endocrine diseases. *Turk Patoloji Derg*. 2015;31(Suppl 1):145-154.
5. Qiu CC, Brown AE, Lobitz GR, Shanker A, Hsu S. The color of skin: black diseases of the skin, nails, and mucosa. *Clin Dermatol*. 2019;37(5):447-467.
6. Arellano J, Iglesias P, Suarez C, Corredoira Y, Schnettler K. Malignant acanthosis nigricans as a paraneoplastic manifestation of metastatic breast cancer. *Int J Womens Dermatol*. 2019;5(3):183-186.
7. Lopez-Alvarenga JC, Garcia-Hidalgo L, Landa-Anell MV, Santos-Gomez R, Gonzalez-Barranco J, Comuzzie A. Influence of skin color on the diagnostic utility of clinical acanthosis nigricans to predict insulin resistance in obese patients. *Arch Med Res*. 2006;37(6):744-748.
8. Stuart CA, Pate CJ, Peters EJ. Prevalence of acanthosis nigricans in an unselected population. *Am J Med*. 1989;87(3):269-272.
9. Hud JA. Prevalence and significance of acanthosis nigricans in an adult obese population. *Arch Dermatol*. 1992;128(7):941.
10. Litonjua P, Piñero-Piloña A, Aviles-Santa L, Raskin P. Prevalence of acanthosis nigricans in newly-diagnosed type 2 diabetes. *Endocr Pract*. 2004;10(2):101-106.
11. Araújo LMB, Porto MV, Netto EM, Ursich MJ. Association of acanthosis nigricans with race and metabolic disturbances in obese women. *Braz J Med Biol Res*. 2002;35(1):59-64.
12. Schachtel A, Kalus A. Diabetes and other endocrine diseases. In: Kang S, Amagai M, Bruckner AL, et al., eds. *Fitzpatrick's Dermatology*. 9th ed. New York, NY: McGraw Hill Education; 2019.
13. Lause M, Kamboj A, Fernandez Faith E. Dermatologic manifestations of endocrine disorders. *Transl Pediatr*. 2017;6(4):300-312.
14. Magro CM, Crowson AN, Regauer S. Granuloma annulare and necrobiosis lipoidica tissue reactions as a manifestation of systemic disease. *Hum Pathol*. 1996;27(1):50-56.
15. Lowitt MH, Dover JS. Necrobiosis lipoidica. *J Am Acad Dermatol*. 1991;25(5 Pt 1): 735-748. doi:10.1016/s0190-9622(08)80961-9.
16. Jabbour SA. Cutaneous manifestations of endocrine disorders: a guide for dermatologists. *Am J Clin Dermatol*. 2003;4(5):315-331.
17. Yahya H. Necrobiosis lipoidica in a Nigerian woman - report of a case. *Niger J Clin Pract*. 2019;22(11):1626-1628.
18. Sibbald C, Reid S, Alavi A. Necrobiosis lipoidica. *Dermatol Clin*. 2015; 33(3):343-360.
19. Melin H. An atrophic circumscribed skin lesion in the lower extremities of diabetics. *Acta Med Scand*. 1964;176(Suppl 423):421-475.
20. Ragunatha S, Anitha B, Inamadar AC, Palit A, Devarmani SS. Cutaneous disorders in 500 diabetic patients attending diabetic clinic. *Indian J Dermatol*. 2011;56(2):160-164.
21. Morgan AJ, Schwartz RA. Diabetic dermopathy: a subtle sign with grave implications. *J Am Acad Dermatol*. 2008;58(3):447-451.
22. Shemer A, Bergman R, Linn S, Drph, Kantor Y, Friedman-Birnbaum R. Diabetic dermopathy and internal complications in diabetes mellitus. *Int J Dermatol*. 1998;37(2):113-115.
23. Wigington G, Ngo B, Rendell M. Skin blood flow in diabetic dermopathy. *Arch Dermatol*. 2004;140(10):1248-1250.
24. Kiziltan ME, Benbir G, Akalin MA. Is diabetic dermopathy a sign for severe neuropathy in patients with diabetes mellitus? Nerve conduction studies and symptom analysis. *Clin Neurophysiol*. 2006;117(8):1862-1869.
25. Hazari A, K. N S, K. Rao K, G. Maiya A. Influence of low-level laser on pain and inflammation in type 2 diabetes mellitus with diabetic dermopathy – a case report. *J Cosmetic Laser Ther*. 2017;19(6):360-363.
26. Abdelhalim NM, Abdelbasset WK, Alqahtani BA, Samhan AF. Low-level laser therapy for diabetic dermopathy in patients with type 2 diabetes: a placebo controlled pilot study. *J Lasers Med Sci*. 2020;11(4):481-485.
27. Armstrong DG, Boulton AJM, Bus SA. Diabetic foot ulcers and their recurrence. *N Engl J Med*. 2017;376(24):2367-2375.
28. Margolis D, Malay D, Hoffstad OJ, et al. Prevalence of diabetes, diabetic foot ulcer, and lower extremity amputation among Medicare beneficiaries, 2006 to 2008: Data Points #1. In: *Data Points Publication Series [Internet]*. Rockville (MD): Agency for Healthcare Research and Quality (US); 2011.
29. Tan T-W, Armstrong DG, Concha-Moore KC, et al. Association between race/ethnicity and the risk of amputation of lower extremities among medicare beneficiaries with diabetic foot ulcers and diabetic foot infections. *BMJ Open Diab Res Care*. 2020;8(1):e001328.
30. Eslami MH, Zayaruzny M, Fitzgerald GA. The adverse effects of race, insurance status, and low income on the rate of amputation in patients presenting with lower extremity ischemia. *J Vasc Surg*. 2007;45(1):55-59.
31. Henry AJ, Hevelone ND, Belkin M, Nguyen LL. Socioeconomic and hospital-related predictors of amputation for critical limb ischemia. *J Vasc Surg*. 2011; 53(2):330-339.e331.
32. Singer AJ, Tassiopoulos A, Kirsner RS. Evaluation and management of lower-extremity ulcers. *N Engl J Med*. 2017;377(16):1559-1567.

33. Oliver TI, Mutluoglu M. Diabetic foot ulcer. In: *StatPearls [Internet]*. Treasure Island (FL): StatPearls Publishing; 2022. https://www.ncbi.nlm.nih.gov/books/NBK537328/. Accessed September 10, 2023.
34. Cantwell AR. Idiopathic bullae in diabetics. *Arch Dermatol*. 1967;96(1):42.
35. Larsen K, Jensen T, Karlsmark T, Holstein PE. Incidence of bullosis diabeticorum - a controversial cause of chronic foot ulceration. *Int Wound J*. 2008;5(4):591-596.
36. Alfaraj DJ, Almuhanna MNA, Alharbi HHB, et al. Bullous disease of diabetes (bullosis diabeticorum). *J Pharma Res Int*. 2021;33:552-557.
37. Vangipuram R, Hinojosa T, Lewis DJ, et al. Bullosis diabeticorum: a neglected bullous dermatosis. *Skinmed*. 2018;16(1):77-79.
38. Piette EW, Rosenbach M. Granuloma annulare: pathogenesis, disease associations and triggers, and therapeutic options. *J Am Acad Dermatol*. 2016;75(3):467-479.
39. Barbieri JS, Rodriguez O, Rosenbach M, Margolis D. Incidence and prevalence of granuloma annulare in the United States. *JAMA Dermatol*. 2021;157(7):824-830.
40. Wang J, Khachemoune A. Granuloma annulare: a focused review of therapeutic options. *Am J Clin Dermatol*. 2018;19(3):333-344.
41. Raboudi A LN. Scleredema. In: *StatPearls*. Treasure Island, FL: StatPearls Publishing; 2022: https://www.ncbi.nlm.nih.gov/books/NBK545159/. Accessed September 10, 2023.
42. Miguel D, Schliemann S, Elsner P. Treatment of scleroedema adultorum buschke: a systematic review. *Acta Dermato Venereologica*. 2018;98(3):305-309.
43. Lukács J, Schliemann S, Elsner P. Treatment of acquired reactive perforating dermatosis – a systematic review. *JDDG: Journal der Deutschen Dermatologischen Gesellschaft. J Dtsch Dermatol Ges*. 2018;16(7):825-842.
44. Wermers RA, Fatourechi V, Wynne AG, Kvols LK, Lloyd RV. The glucagonoma syndrome. Clinical and pathologic features in 21 patients. *Medicine (Baltimore)*. 1996;75(2):53-63.
45. Al-Faouri A, Ajarma K, Alghazawi S, Al-Rawabdeh S, Zayadeen A. Glucagonoma and glucagonoma syndrome: a case report with review of recent advances in management. *Case Rep Surg*. 2016;2016:1-3.
46. Shupack JL, Berczeller PH, Stevens DM. The glucagonoma syndrome. *J Dermatol Surg Oncol*. 1978;4(3):242-247.
47. Tierney EP, Badger J. Etiology and pathogenesis of necrolytic migratory erythema: review of the literature. *MedGenMed*. 2004;6(3):4.
48. Kindmark H, Sundin A, Granberg D, et al. Endocrine pancreatic tumors with glucagon hypersecretion: a retrospective study of 23 cases during 20 years. *Med Oncol*. 2007;24(3):330-337.
49. Virani S, Prajapati V, Devani A, Mahmood MN, Elliott JF. Octreotide-responsive necrolytic migratory erythema in a patient with pseudoglucagonoma syndrome. *J Am Acad Dermatol*. 2013;68(2):e44-e46.
50. Kimbara S, Fujiwara Y, Toyoda M, et al. Rapid improvement of glucagonoma-related necrolytic migratory erythema with octreotide. *Clin J Gastroenterol*. 2014;7(3):255-259.
51. van Beek AP, de Haas ER, van Vloten WA, Lips CJ, Roijers JF, Canninga-van Dijk MR. The glucagonoma syndrome and necrolytic migratory erythema: a clinical review. *Eur J Endocrinol*. 2004;151(5):531-537.
52. Race/ethnicity and the prevalence of thyrotoxicosis in young Americans. *Thyroid*. 2015;25(6):621-628.
53. McLeod DSA, Caturegli P, Cooper DS, Matos PG, Hutfless S. Variation in rates of autoimmune thyroid disease by race/ethnicity in US military personnel. *JAMA*. 2014;311(15):1563.
54. Puri N. A study on cutaneous manifestations of thyroid disease. *Indian J Dermatol*. 2012;57(3):247-248.
55. Perini N, Santos RB, Romaldini JH, Villagelin D. Thyroid acropachy: a rare manifestation of Graves disease in joints. *AACE Clin Case Rep*. 2019;5(6):e36 9-e371.
56. Ross IL, Levitt NS. Addison's disease symptoms–a cross sectional study in urban South Africa. *PLoS One*. 2013;8(1):e53526.
57. Tong CV, Ooi X-Y. Addison's disease presenting with hyperpigmentation. *BMJ Case Rep*. 2021;14(8):e245610.
58. Wolf W, Wattick R, Kinkade O, Olfert M. Geographical prevalence of polycystic ovary syndrome as determined by region and race/ethnicity. *Int J Environ Res Public Health*. 2018;15(11):2589.
59. Engmann L, Jin S, Sun F, et al. Racial and ethnic differences in the polycystic ovary syndrome metabolic phenotype. *Am J Obstet Gynecol*. 2017;216(5):493.e491-493.e413.
60. Capatina C, Wass JAH. 60 Years of neuroendocrinology: acromegaly. *J Endocrinol*. 2015;226(2):T141-T160.
61. Ben-Shlomo A, Melmed S. Skin manifestations in acromegaly. *Clin Dermatol*. 2006;24(4):256-259.
62. Di Iorgi N, Morana G, Allegri AE, et al. Classical and non-classical causes of GH deficiency in the paediatric age. *Best Pract Res Clin Endocrinol Metab*. 2016;30(6):705-736.
63. Kim JH, Chae HW, Chin SO, et al. Diagnosis and treatment of growth hormone deficiency: a position statement from Korean Endocrine Society and Korean Society of Pediatric Endocrinology. *Endocrinol Metab*. 2020;35(2):272-287.
64. Kanaka-Gantenbein C, Kogia C, Abdel-Naser MB, Chrousos GP. Skin manifestations of growth hormone-induced diseases. *Rev Endocr Metab Disord*. 2016;17(3):259-267.
65. Vance ML. Hypopituitarism. *N Engl J Med*. 1994;330(23):1651-1662.
66. McDowell BD, Wallace RB, Carnahan RM, Chrischilles EA, Lynch CF, Schlechte JA. Demographic differences in incidence for pituitary adenoma. *Pituitary*. 2011;14(1):23-30.
67. Heshmat MY, Kovi J, Simpson C, Kennedy J, Fan KJ. Neoplasms of the central nervous system. Incidence and population selectivity in the Washington DC, metropolitan area. *Cancer*. 1976;38(5):2135-2142.
68. Insogna KL. Primary hyperparathyroidism. *N Engl J Med*. 2018;379(11):1050-1059.
69. Yeh MW, Ituarte PH, Zhou HC, et al. Incidence and prevalence of primary hyperparathyroidism in a racially mixed population. *J Clin Endocrinol Metab*. 2013;98(3):1122-1129.
70. Sepriano AR, Pereira Pombo de Araújo FC, Mourão de Almeida Lourenço Dias PM, da Cunha Branco J. Normocalcemic primary hyperparathyroidism presenting as calcinosis cutis. *JCR: J Clin Rheumatol*. 2014;20(6):330-331.
71. Dagher HN, Aboujaoude ZC, Jabbour SA. Chronic urticaria: an unusual initial manifestation of primary hyperparathyroidism. *Endocr Pract*. 2002;8(1):47-49.
72. Gafni RI, Collins MT. Hypoparathyroidism. *N Engl J Med*. 2019;380(18):1738-1747.
73. Sarkar S, Mondal M, Das K, Shrimal A. Mucocutaneous manifestations of acquired hypoparathyroidism: an observational study. *Indian J Endocrinol Metab*. 2012;16(5):819-820.
74. Romei C, Pardi E, Cetani F, Elisei R. Genetic and clinical features of multiple endocrine neoplasia types 1 and 2. *J Oncol*. 2012;2012:1-15.
75. Brandi ML, Gagel RF, Angeli A, et al. CONSENSUS: guidelines for diagnosis and therapy of MEN type 1 and type 2. *J Clin Endocrinol Metab*. 2001;86(12):5658-5671.
76. Darling TN. Multiple facial angiofibromas and collagenomas in patients with multiple endocrine neoplasia type 1. *Arch Dermatol*. 1997;133(7):853.
77. Sakurai A, Matsumoto K, Ikeo Y, et al. Frequency of facial angiofibromas in Japanese patients with multiple endocrine neoplasia type 1. *Endocr J*. 2000;47(5):569-573.
78. Asgharian B, Turner ML, Gibril F, Entsuah LK, Serrano J, Jensen RT. Cutaneous tumors in patients with multiple endocrine neoplasm type 1 (MEN1) and gastrinomas: prospective study of frequency and development of criteria with high sensitivity and specificity for MEN1. *J Clin Endocrinol Metab*. 2004;89(11):5328-5336.
79. Vidal A, Iglesias M, Fernández B, Fonseca E, Cordido F. Cutaneous lesions associated to multiple endocrine neoplasia syndrome type 1. *J Eur Acad Dermatol Venereol*. 2008;22(7):835-838.
80. Piecha G, Chudek J, Wiecek A. Multiple endocrine neoplasia type 1. *Eur J Intern Med*. 2008;19(2):99-103.
81. Marini F, Falchetti A, Del Monte F, et al. Multiple endocrine neoplasia type 2. *Orphanet J Rare Dis*. 2006;1(1):45.
82. Malhotra R, Boro H, Shamim SA, Khadgawat R. Multiple endocrine neoplasia type 2A with cutaneous lichen amyloidosis. *BMJ Case Rep*. 2020;13(8):e238423.
83. Multiple endocrine neoplasia type 2a associated with cutaneous lichen amyloidosis. *Ann Intern Med*. 1989;111(10):802-806.
84. Husebye ES, Anderson MS, Kämpe O. Autoimmune polyendocrine syndromes. *N Engl J Med*. 2018;378(12):1132-1141.
85. Husebye ES, Perheentupa J, Rautemaa R, Kämpe O. Clinical manifestations and management of patients with autoimmune polyendocrine syndrome type I. *J Intern Med*. 2009;265(5):514-529.
86. Correa R, Salpea P, Stratakis CA. Carney complex: an update. *Eur J Endocrinol*. 2015;173(4):M85-M97.
87. Bertherat J, Horvath A, Groussin L, et al. Mutations in regulatory subunit type 1A of cyclic adenosine 5'-monophosphate-dependent protein kinase (PRKAR1A): phenotype analysis in 353 patients and 80 different genotypes. *J Clin Endocrinol Metab*. 2009;94(6):2085-2091.
88. Dragoo DD, Taher A, Wong VK, et al. PTEN Hamartoma tumor syndrome/Cowden syndrome: genomics, oncogenesis, and imaging review for associated lesions and malignancy. *Cancers*. 2021;13(13):3120.
89. Patel N, Spencer LA, English JC 3rd, Zirwas MJ. Acquired ichthyosis. *J Am Acad Dermatol*. 2006;55(4):647-656.

CHAPTER 77

Gastroenterology

Negar Foolad
Jeffery Kwock
Lynn McKinley-Grant
Tarannum Jaleel

KEY POINTS

- Numerous gastrointestinal (GI) conditions, including those of infectious, inflammatory, neoplastic, and metabolic origin, can present with cutaneous manifestations.
- The disease burden and clinical presentation of GI conditions can vary by race/ethnicity and skin color. Conditions such as acanthosis nigricans, gastric cancer, and necrolytic acral erythema are more common in Black individuals.
- Awareness of these cutaneous features can allow earlier detection of underlying GI diseases.

INTRODUCTION

Gastrointestinal (GI) diseases, including infectious, inflammatory, or neoplastic, can present with cutaneous manifestations. Furthermore, the relationship between the gut and skin has been studied through ongoing research on the human microbiome, which is composed of a diverse community of bacteria, fungi, viruses, and multiple other microorganisms.[1] There is evidence that the gut and skin microbiome can modulate immune responses in skin disease and inflammation in certain disease states propagated by gut/skin dysbiosis [**Table 77-1**].[2-5] Increased disease severity in Crohn disease, for example, is associated with a higher degree of gut dysbiosis. Studies are needed to evaluate further the effects of reducing dysbiosis to modulate inflammatory skin conditions.[1] In addition, it is important to note that different GI conditions can present differently in darker skin and/or have racial/ethnic differences in disease morbidity and mortality.

INFECTIOUS

HELICOBACTER PYLORI

In the United States, there is a prevalence of 30% of the population with *Helicobacter pylori* (*H. pylori*), a gram-negative bacterium. Higher rates are reported in African-Americans (50-60%).[20] In one study, the prevalence of *H. pylori* was evaluated in asymptomatic volunteers and found to be significantly more prevalent in Black patients (70%) compared to White patients (34%) ($p < 0.001$).[21] *H. pylori* is one of the most substantial risk factors for gastric cancer. Infections occur as early as childhood in both developed and developing countries.[22] Compared to White patients, the incidence of gastric cancer in African Americans is two times greater.[20]

Chronic Urticaria With an incidence of 0.1% to 3% in the population, chronic urticaria (spontaneous plaques, angioedema, or both for >6 weeks) is a common skin manifestation with various causes.[1] Recent studies have demonstrated that *H. pylori* infection rates were significantly greater in patients with urticaria than in healthy controls.[23] There is an increased prevalence of *H. pylori* among Black patients. If there is a high suspicion of *H. pylori* in chronic urticarial,[21] refer patients to specialists, for example, gastroenterology or primary care, for evaluation. Studies show that *H. pylori* increases gastric mucosal permeability and stimulates immune activation during chronic infection.[1]

TABLE 77-1 The gut microbiome in dermatologic and gastrointestinal conditions

Dermatologic condition	Associated gut microbiota	Additional comments
Acne vulgaris	*Firmicutes* (decrease) *Bacteroides* (increase)	
Alopecia areata	Major differences not reported[2]	Fecal microbiota transplant exhibited beneficial outcomes in hair growth in two patients[6]
Atopic dermatitis	Higher levels: *Faecalibacterium prausnitzii*, *Clostridium*, and *Escherichia* (infants) Lower levels: *Akkermansia*, *Bacteroidetes*, and *Bifidobacterium*	Beneficial impact of probiotics consumption on prevention and severity of atopic dermatitis[7]
Hidradenitis suppurativa	Higher levels: *Ruminococcus gnavus* and *Clostridium ramosum*[8]	Avoidance of food that is made with or contains yeast *S. cerevisiae* may be beneficial[9]
Psoriasis	Higher levels: *Firmicutes* Lower levels: *Bacteroidetes*[10]	Changes in the microbiome after secukinumab use[10]: Increase: *Proteobacteria, Pseudomonadaceae, Enterobacteriaceae, Pseudomonadales* Decrease: *Bacteroidetes, Firmicutes*
Rosacea	Higher levels[11]: *Acidaminococcus, Megasphaera* Lower levels: *Peptococcaceae, Methanobrevibacter*	Increased risk of *Helicobacter pylori* infection[12]
Seborrheic dermatitis	No reports[2]	Consumption of probiotic *Lactobacillus paracasei* associated with symptom improvement in dandruff[13]
Gastrointestinal conditions with skin associations		
Helicobacter pylori	Enhancement of Spirochetes and Proteobacteria phyla[14]	Modification of α-diversity* of gastric microbiome reported among gastric cancer[14] Microorganisms reported frequently in gastric cancer tissue: *Lactobacillus, Shigella, Escherichia, Nitrospirae, fungerum, Burkholderia, Lachospiraceae*
Celiac disease	Increase gram-negative bacteria (*Bacteroides* and *Enterobacteriaceae*) Decrease in gram-positive bacteria (*Bifidobacteria*) *Proteobacteria* more abundant in active celiac disease[15]	Complete restoration of normal microbiome not seen after adherence to gluten-free diet compared to control[16]
Crohn disease	Increased: proteobacteria and fusobacteria Decreased: *Firmicutes* and *Bacteroidetes*[17]	Reduction in diversity of microbiome[17] Gut microbiome may predict disease course when comparing antibiotic use among pediatric population of new-onset CD[18]

α-Diversity: the composition of microbiome in a single sample[19] (including quality and abundance).

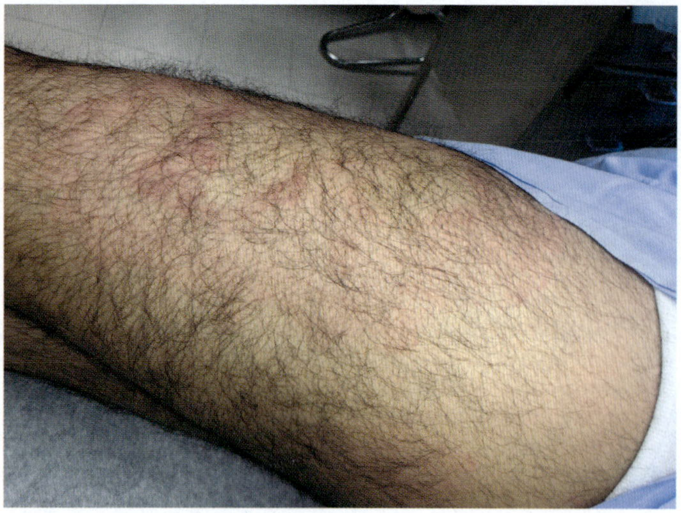

FIGURE 77-1. Chronic urticaria. Chronic urticaria is a symptom of *H. pylori* and can present with serpiginous annular dark pink edematous plaques, shown here on the lower extremity. (Courtesy of Dr. Bahar Bahrani.)

Urticaria is diagnosed as chronic when recurrent edematous, pruritic plaques occur for at least 6 weeks [**Figure 77-1**].[1] By definition, chronic urticaria must last more than 6 weeks, with individual lesions lasting fewer than 24 hours.[1] Pruritus and burning can be associated with urticaria accompanied by angioedema of the face, limbs, or trunk. Angioedema presents as swelling in the lower dermis, subcutis, and edema of mucous membranes. Angioedema can be life-threatening in some cases and has a slower resolution, taking up to 72 hours to resolve.[1]

Triple therapy (amoxicillin, clarithromycin, omeprazole) to treat the underlying *H. pylori* has been found to alleviate urticaria.[1] Second-generation, nonsedating, H1-antagonist antihistamines are commonly used treatments for pruritus. Corticosteroids may be required in some cases of severe urticaria.[1]

NECROLYTIC ACRAL ERYTHEMA

Necrolytic acral erythema (NAE) is common among patients with Hepatitis C Virus (HCV) infection.[1] In the United States, one study reported that all patients with NAE were African American.[24] Equally seen among men and women, NAE has been reported to affect patients of a broad range of ages (11-76 years).[25] The precise pathogenesis has yet to be ascertained. Providers should screen for HCV infection as NAE is highly associated with an underlying infection. HCV is diagnosed for the first time in greater than 75% of patients diagnosed with NAE.[26]

Clinical features of NAE in skin of color include distinct dusky red to violaceous hyperkeratotic plaques with a keratotic border over the dorsum of the feet and toes [**Figure 77-2**].[1] The ankles, legs, and knees may be rarely involved, along with other areas of the body, including the hands, elbows, genitalia, and buttocks [**Figure 77-3**]. NAE presents in three stages: initial, well-developed, and late with a typical progression of spontaneous remission and relapse.[27] Erythematous to violaceous papules and plaques with an overlying scale and a dusky or eroded center can be observed in the initial stage. Smaller papules then combine to form thick, scaly, hyperpigmented plaques. The late stage involves thin, hyperpigmented plaques that are further circumscribed.[27]

Among patients with HCV, treatment with antiviral therapy such as ribavirin and interferon-α has been effective.[27] Zinc therapy has been shown to be an effective treatment option, with reports of clearance after 8 weeks of twice-daily treatment.[27] There have been various responses to other treatment modalities, such as topical and intralesional corticosteroids.

LICHEN PLANUS

In a meta-analysis of 46 studies, the prevalence of lichen planus (LP) in the general population was 0.89%,[28] commonly affecting

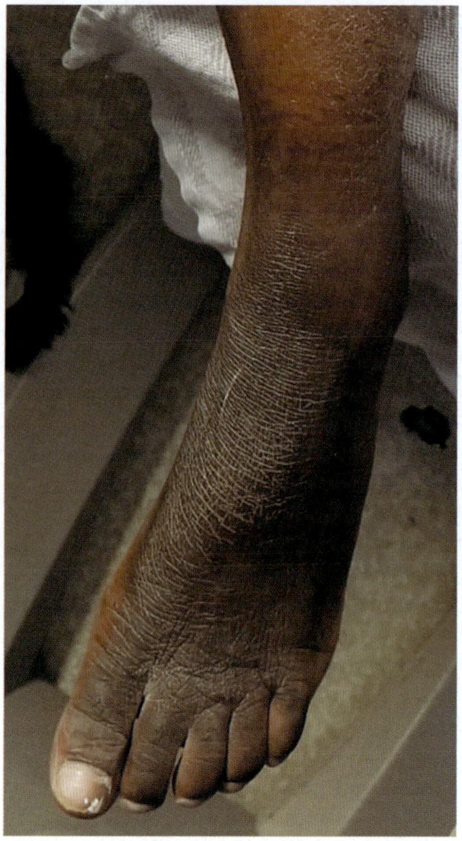

FIGURE 77-2 Necrolytic acral erythema. A hyperpigmented and violaceous to dark brown lichenified plaque on the dorsum of the left foot. (Photo contributed by Dr. Bahar Bahrani.)

middle-aged adults without a particular gender predilection.[28] While patients with HCV had a significantly higher risk of developing LP than noninfected individuals, other viruses (human herpesvirus 6 and 7) and additional environmental factors have also been associated with the development of LP.[27,29] The fundamental pathogenesis of LP involves a T-cell-mediated immune response as well as an upregulation of cytokines such as tumor necrosis factor-α, interferon-γ, and interleukin (IL)-6 and IL-8.[27]

In cutaneous LP, white streaks (Wickham striae) are seen on shiny violaceous firm papules and plaques.[27] In skin of color, LP may appear dark violet or gray with postinflammatory pigmentary changes that just a brown-gray prominence and occasionally have long-term persistent sequelae such as hyperpigmentation. These pruritic papules are typically distributed on the wrists, the lower back, and the ankles [**Figures 77-4** and **77-5**].[27] Mucosal LP generally presents either as painful erosions or peeling of the mucosa with diffuse erythema [**Figure 77-6**]. The two subclasses of mucosal LP include oral and genital LP.[27] In nail LP, there are several alterations to the nails, including thinning of the nail plate, thickening or lifting of the nail bed, shedding or discontinuation of nail growth, destruction of the cuticle, or complete nail disappearance.[27]

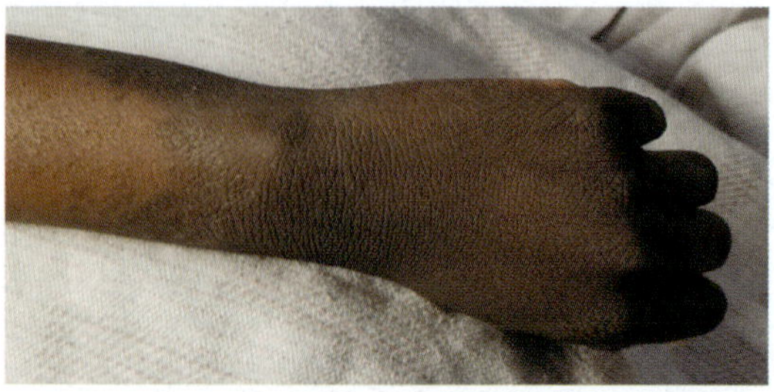

FIGURE 77-3. Necrolytic acral erythema. A hyperpigmented and violaceous lichenified plaque with overlying fine scale on the dorsum of the left hand. (Courtesy of Dr. Bahar Bahrani.)

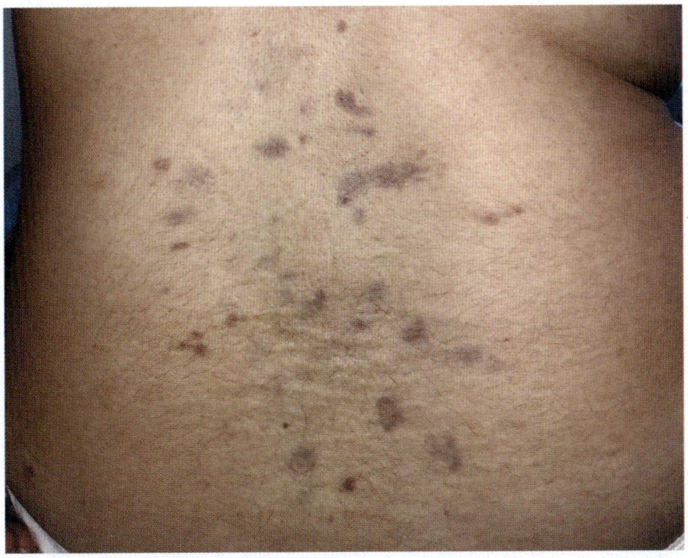

FIGURE 77-4. Lichen planus. Hyperpigmented to violaceous macules and patches seen on the back. (Courtesy of Dr. Bahar Bahrani.)

While spontaneous clearance of cutaneous lesions around 12 to 24 months is observed, there are a variety of treatment modalities that clinicians can utilize in cases of relapse.[27] Topical steroids are the first-line therapy for LP. Other standard options include oral corticosteroids, cyclosporine, and systemic retinoids (acitretin/isotretinoin).[27] Sulfasalazine, narrowband ultraviolet B therapy, ultraviolet A treatment with psoralen, and topical calcineurin inhibitors can be utilized if LP remains unresponsive to the first-line therapies.[27] Hydroxychloroquine, methotrexate, and mycophenolate mofetil are third-line treatment options.

INFLAMMATORY

INFLAMMATORY BOWEL DISEASE

Approximately 1.5 million patients in the United States are affected by inflammatory bowel disease (IBD), specifically, Crohn disease (CD) and ulcerative colitis (UC).[30] There has been an increase in the incidence and prevalence of IBD among African American, Hispanic, and Asian patients in the United States.[30] African American patients are affected by CD at higher rates than UC, while Hispanic Americans have a higher prevalence of UC.[31] With epidemiological studies, the incidence of IBD is increasing worldwide, including in Africa, South America, Asia, and eastern Europe.[32] This has been hypothesized to be related to the increased urbanization and westernization of these countries.[32] With an observed prevalence of up to 50%, extraintestinal manifestations (EIM) involving multiple organ systems have been reported in IBD [**Table 77-2**].[33] Skin findings were reported more often in Hispanic patients, while African American patients experienced ocular and joint involvement.[30] Overall, cutaneous manifestations have been reported to occur more commonly in CD than in patients with UC.[33] With the increased incidence of IBD among various races and ethnic groups, providers need to be cognizant of the range of presentation of EIM. There may be a decrease in the time to diagnosis of IBD if the presence of EIMs prompts a physician to consider underlying IBD.

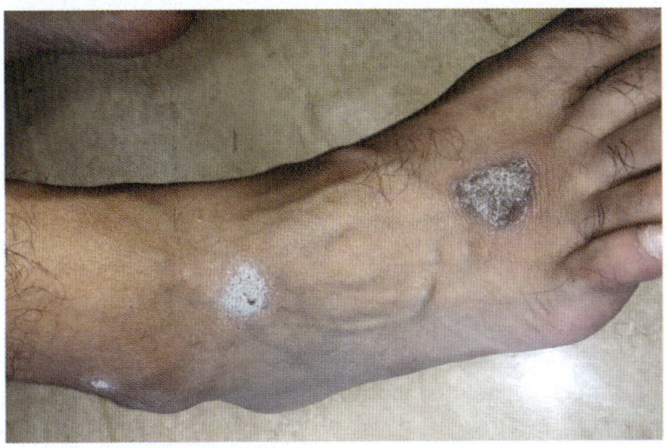

FIGURE 77-5. Hypertrophic lichen planus. Scaly erythematous to violaceous plaques on the dorsal foot. (Courtesy of Dr. Bahar Bahrani.)

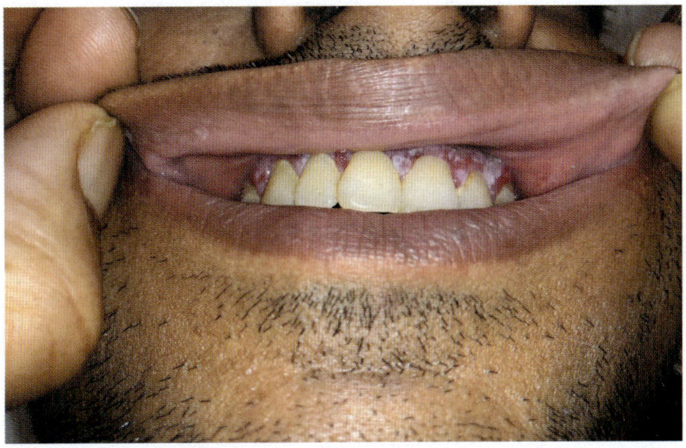

FIGURE 77-6. Erosive lichen planus. Erosions and ulcerations of the upper gingiva. (Courtesy of Dr. Bahar Bahrani.)

IBD patients also have an increased prevalence of immune-mediated inflammatory diseases (IMIDs) involving the skin, such as psoriasis, atopic dermatitis, vitiligo, epidermolysis bullosa acquisita (EBA), cutaneous polyarteritis nodosa, and hidradenitis suppurativa (HS) [Table 77-2].[33] There are a limited number of published studies regarding the prevalence of immune-mediated inflammatory diseases (IMIDs) associated with IBD in skin of color patients.[42-44] Psoriasis has been reported to affect 3.6% of CD patients and 2.8% in UC. Compared to the general population, the incidence rate of HS was ninefold higher in IBD patients.[43] The prevalence of HS is estimated to be 17.3% in CD and 8.5% in UC.[43] Additionally, in a recent study, researchers reported that HS occurs more frequently with a higher incidence of increased severity in African American or Black patients.[44] In Black patients with EBA, the HLA-DRB1*15:03 allele has been significantly associated, suggesting a possible predisposition in patients of African descent.[42] Cutaneous polyarteritis nodosa may present with a violaceous color, requiring the clinician to perform a thorough physical exam as tenderness may also be a helpful clue in diagnosing skin of color patients.

Bowel-associated dermatosis-arthritis syndrome (BADAS), pyoderma gangrenosum (PG), pyodermatitis-pyostomatitis vegetans (PDPSV), and Sweet syndrome are reactive cutaneous manifestations in both UC and CD [Table 77-2].[45] Among patients with CD, PG was reported to be more prevalent in patients of African origin.[35] No racial predilection has been observed in Sweet syndrome.[46] However, the dusky or violaceous plaques and/or nodules seen in Sweet syndrome may result in late and inaccurate diagnosis in skin of color patients [**Figure** 77-7].

Metastatic Crohn disease (MCD) is a rare manifestation of cutaneous Crohn disease characterized by a varied clinical presentation of erythematous and violaceous plaques, nodules, ulcerations, crusts, and linear erosions with a "knife-cut" sign that are disconnected from the gastrointestinal tract.[1,45] An individual may present with MCD before a precise diagnosis of Crohn disease. Although the pathogenesis is not completely clear, a granulomatous response or a type IV hypersensitivity reaction has been thought to contribute to the etiology.[45] A biopsy to aid in diagnosis is imperative.[1] Several treatment options, including topical and systemic steroids, immunomodulators, and tumor necrosis factor-α inhibitors, have been utilized for MCD.[1]

TABLE 77-2 Cutaneous manifestations in inflammatory bowel disease in skin of color[33]

Cutaneous manifestation	Clinical features	Pathogenesis	Treatment	Considerations in skin of color
Erythema nodosum	Dusky red or violaceous subcutaneous nodules on the extensor surface of the lower extremities with postinflammatory hyper- or hypopigmentation Reported in 15% of CD, more common in women	Type IV hypersensitivity reaction (hypothesized)	Mostly self-limiting, supportive measures with lower extremity elevation, analgesics, potassium iodine, and compression stockings Systemic steroids and TNF inhibitors in severe and refractory cases	Erythema nodosum more prevalent among Hispanic patients compared to White patients[34]
Oral diseases *Aphthous stomatitis,* *Periodontitis* *Peristomatitis vegetans*	Aphthous stomatitis: painful oval or round ulcers with yellowish base on buccal or labial mucosa Periodontitis: bleeding, swelling, gingival redness Peristomatitis vegetans: friable pustules with hemorrhagic erosion and ulceration Oral lesions may appear 25% of the time prior to an IBD Seen more commonly in CD compared to UC	Immune complexes hypothesized to be involved in the mechanism	Supplemental therapy with antiseptic mouthwashes and topical corticosteroids Culture for herpes simplex virus (HSV)	
Pyoderma gangrenosum[35]	Single or multiple painful erythematous papules and pustules with necrosis or ulcers along with purulent material commonly on the shins and peristomal area (Figures 77-12 and 77-13) High recurrence rates More prevalent in UC, more common in women	Abnormal function of neutrophil, impairment of cellular immunity	Corticosteroids, tacrolimus, systemic steroids, cyclosporine, or anti-TNF Biopsy and culture (bacterial, viral, fungal) recommended for non-healing lesions	Among patients with CD, PG was more prevalent patients of African origin[35]
Sweet syndrome	Red, brown, or violaceous tender or papulosquamous exanthema or nodules on the face, hands, arms, trunk, and legs with fever (Figure 77-7) More common in women	Type III hypersensitivity reaction and an association with histocompatibility antigens (hypothesized)	Steroids (topical or systemic) and immunomodulators Biopsy recommended to rule out Cutaneous T-Cell Lymphoma or other lymphomas	Differences not observed by race[36] Early and accurate diagnosis in people of color is difficult because of the violaceous color of the erythema
Cutaneous polyarteritis nodosa[37]	Painful pink or violaceous cutaneous and subcutaneous nodules of the lower extremities often in groups along blood vessels Livedo reticularis, cutaneous ulcers, necrosis	Abnormal immune response	Steroid, immunosuppressive agent	Diagnosis in people of color is difficult because of the violaceous color of the erythema. Tenderness may be a helpful clue in diagnosis
Bowel-associated dermatosis arthritis syndrome[38,39]	Erythematous to violaceous papules and plaques with pustules of the upper extremities and trunk Skin symptoms coincide with fever, polyarthralgia, and diagnosis of IBD May be associated with gastric bypass however presents in the absence of bowel surgery	Hypothesized to involve immune-complex formation and deposition in the skin (IBD) Immune-complex formation in the setting of bacterial overgrowth and accumulation of peptidoglycan (gastric bypass)	Steroids Treatment of underlying IBD Antibiotics but may require reversal of bypass in some cases	
Pyostomatitis vegetans[40]	White or yellow pustules of the oral mucosa After rupturing, the pustules have a fissured appearance that may resemble a "snail-track" Only oral manifestation seen more commonly in UC compared to CD; may present as the first sign More common in men	Pathogenesis unknown	Topical steroids for oral lesions Treatment of underlying IBD	
Epidermolysis bullosa acquisita[41]	Vesicle and bullae of the skin, erosions of mucous membranes Mechanobullous and non-mechanobullous Seen more commonly in CD compared to UC	IgG autoantibodies against collagen VII	Avoid trauma Oral steroids, immunosuppressant therapy, anti-neutrophilic agents such as dapsone	Possible predisposition in patients of African descent[42] HLA-DRB1*15:03 allele significantly associated with black patients with EBA
Anti-TNF-induced skin findings	Eczematiform or psoriasiform	Proinflammatory cytokines, and expansion of T-helper cells (Th1 and Th17) (hypothesized)	Discontinuation of anti-TNF and topical corticosteroids	

Abbreviations: CD, Crohn disease; UC, ulcerative colitis.

CELIAC DISEASE

Celiac disease was initially seen most often among patients of European origin but is now recognized with increasing prevalence among patients in North Africa and the Middle East.[47] This is partly due to the more readily available antiendomysial and antigliadin antibodies testing.[47] The global prevalence ranges from 0.7% to 1.4%.[48] When classified by continent, the prevalence was "0.4% in South America, 0.5% in Africa and North America, 0.6% in Asia, and 0.8% in Europe and Oceania." Interestingly, among a diverse cohort of patients that included African (56.4%), Asian Indian (31.7%), White (4.5%), and multiracial (7.4%) with type 1 diabetes mellitus in South Africa, no differences by ethnicity were found in prevalence when screened for celiac disease. In addition, while one-third of patients had positive celiac antibodies and approximately 6% had histologic evidence of celiac disease, none of the patients had classic clinical symptoms of celiac disease, which include chronic diarrhea, weight loss, and abdominal discomfort.[49]

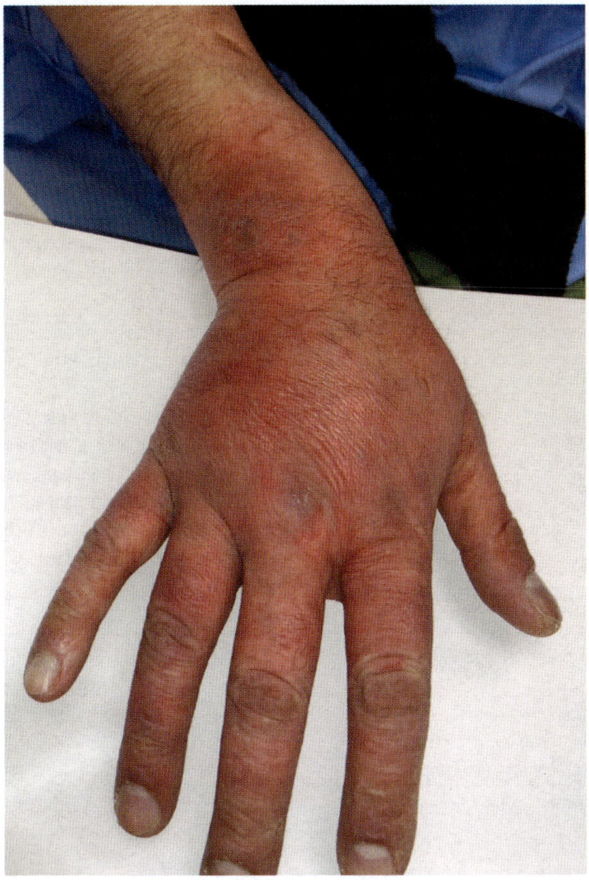

FIGURE 77-7. Sweet syndrome. A violaceous and edematous hand. (Courtesy of Dr. Bahar Bahrani.)

Dermatitis Herpetiformis Dermatitis herpetiformis (DH) is the most common skin manifestation of celiac disease.[1] The prevalence of DH is more common among untreated patients, with a higher prevalence among men than women (1.5-2:1).[50] The mean age at diagnosis is around 43 years. The pathogenesis of DH has been hypothesized to involve IgA antitransglutaminase (TG) antibodies, specifically the elevation of TG2 and TG3.[48] When individuals with CD consume gluten, it is transported across the gastrointestinal mucosa to the lamina propria and is deaminated to form a covalent bond with tissue transglutaminase-2 (TTG-2).[48] IgA antibodies recognize the TG2-gliadin complex and epitope spreading leads to generating IgA autoantibodies against epidermal TTG3. Circulating anti-TTG3 IGA binds to TTG-3 within the dermal papilla leading to subepidermal blisters.[48]

Clinical manifestations of DH in skin of color individuals include small pruritic grouped vesicles and violaceous papules on the elbows, knees, and buttocks with postinflammatory macules.[1] Excoriations can obscure the primary lesions. The scalp, face, neck, shoulders, and sacral region may be involved.[1] Direct immunofluorescence (DIF) of perilesional skin is the gold standard for diagnosing DH.[1]

Once a patient has been placed on a strict gluten-free diet, DH tends to improve over months to years.[1] Persistent disease may necessitate a course of topical and oral dapsone for its anti-inflammatory properties.[50]

NEOPLASTIC

CARCINOID SYNDROME

Carcinoid syndrome occurs secondary to the metastasis of neuroendocrine tumors to the liver, resulting in excess serotonin production and leading to increased gut motility and flushing.[51] Although most neuroendocrine tumors responsible for causing carcinoid syndrome arise initially from the midgut, tumors of the foregut, hindgut, respiratory tract, ovaries, testicles, and kidneys have also been reported. In 2004, the incidence of neuroendocrine tumors within the United States, Netherlands, and the United Kingdom was 5.25/100,000, with Black patients having a higher incidence (6.82/100,000) compared to White patients (4.92/100,000) [**Table 77-3**].[51] The most common location for neuroendocrine tumors in White patients was the lung (30%). Jejunal/ileal neuroendocrine tumors were seen more commonly in Black (15%) and White (17%) patients compared to Asian/Pacific Islanders and Native Americans. Skin of color patients had a higher much higher rate of rectal neuroendocrine tumors, with Asian/Pacific Islanders (41%) having the highest rate, followed by Native Americans (32%) and Black patients (26%), all of whom had a higher rate compared to White patients (12%).[51]

Most patients (85%) with carcinoid syndrome present with intermittent flushing, erythema, and warmth that is short-lived from 30 seconds to 30 minutes and occurs most commonly in conjunction with a midgut neuroendocrine tumor.[1] In darker skin types, warmth may be a helpful adjunct in identifying skin erythema that can present with varying shades of red. Chronic diarrhea is also a common symptom in 80% of patients with carcinoid syndrome resulting in nutritional deficiencies [Table 77-3].[1] There is cardiac involvement in 60% to 70% of patients with carcinoid syndrome.[1] Less common manifestations include bronchospasm (10-20%), pellagra, muscle wasting, and ureteral obstruction.[1]

In carcinoid syndrome, complete surgical resection of all tumors is curative.[1] Surgical debulking can significantly alleviate symptoms and reduce mortality even in patients with a high metastatic tumor burden. Symptom relief can be achieved using somatostatin analogs such as octreotide and lanreotide.[1]

CRONKHITE-CANADA SYNDROME

Cronkhite-Canada syndrome is not associated with a familial inheritance pattern and appears sporadically. Despite that, 75% of known cases have been documented in Japanese individuals [Table 77-3].[54] There is a peak incidence within the age group of 50 to 70 years old with a 3:2 male predominance.[54] The underlying pathophysiology of Cronkhite-Canada syndrome is not well elucidated.

Individuals with Cronkhite-Canada syndrome present with GI hamartomatous polyps that often result in protein-losing enteropathy and chronic diarrhea. These polyps have a relatively low risk of progressing to malignancy, although gastric and colorectal cancers have been documented.[1] Alopecia, nail dystrophy, and lentigines of the hands, feet, and buccal mucosa represent the most common cutaneous findings in Cronkhite-Canada syndrome.[1]

Given the malabsorption seen in this syndrome, repletion of crucial nutrients such as electrolytes, vitamins, and minerals, in conjunction with prednisone, have been shown in some cases to provide symptomatic improvement and occasionally remission.[1]

NECROLYTIC MIGRATORY ERYTHEMA

Necrolytic migratory erythema (NME) has an incidence of 1 in 20 million, and onset peaks between 50 and 60 years.[57] Most NME cases are associated with an underlying glucagonoma, a specific type of pancreatic islet cell tumor. A population-based epidemiological study from 1973 to 2003 included 1310 patients and examined the incidence and prevalence of all pancreatic islet cell tumors (including glucagonomas).[57] Although they found that pancreatic islet cell tumors are not seen more frequently in one demographic versus another, this study did demonstrate that the median age of diagnosis of pancreatic islet cell tumors was significantly younger ($p = 0.02$) in Black patients at age 55 (mean 54.5, SD 16.5) and in other non-White racial groups at age 55.5 (mean 57, SD 16.5) compared to the age of presentation in White patients at age 60 (mean 58, SD 14.9) [Table 77-3].[57]

The exact mechanism underlying necrolytic migratory erythema is unknown but appears to be associated with hyperglucagonemia. The catabolic state associated with elevated glucagon levels leads to derangement of zinc metabolism, hypoalbuminemia, hypoproteinemia, and essential fatty acid dysfunction, all of which contribute to cutaneous inflammation.[1] NME often appears as part of glucagonoma syndrome,

TABLE 77-3 Cutaneous paraneoplastic manifestations associated with GI malignancy

Paraneoplastic disorder	Dermatologic manifestations	Underlying GI malignancy	Considerations in skin of color
Acanthosis nigricans	Velvety brown to dark brown hyperpigmented patches in the face, posterior neck, hands, axilla, groin	Gastric and colorectal cancer	Acanthosis nigricans is more common in Hispanics, Native Americans, and African Americans[52]
Acquired hypertrichosis lanuginosa	Fine, lanugo hairs most commonly seen on the face	Colorectal cancer (most common), followed by lung and breast cancer	
Acrokeratosis paraneoplastica (Bazex syndrome)	Hyperkeratotic erythematous papules and plaques on fingers, toes, ears, lip, elbows, and knees and nail dystrophy	Squamous cell carcinoma of the esophagus, oropharynx, and larynx	Vital to distinguish Bazex from occupational/contact dermatitis or manual laborers
Carcinoid syndrome	Flushing of the face, neck, and upper trunk with increased warmth, and skin signs of pellagra (red, brown, violaceous flaky skin with thick crusts and scale on the chest, tender gums, tongue, and lips)[51]	Neuroendocrine tumors with liver metastases	Higher incidence of neuroendocrine tumors in African Americans compared to White patients. Jejunal/ileal neuroendocrine tumors more common in all skin of color patients. Rectal neuroendocrine tumors more common in African American and White patients.[51] Nutritional deficiencies[53]: Niacin (B3), B12, 25-OH vitamin D
Cronkhite-Canada syndrome	Lentigo-like hyperpigmentation, alopecia, nail dystrophy	Colon and gastric cancer, GI hamartomatous polyps	Japanese individuals comprise 75% of all documented cases[54]
Leser-Trelat syndrome	Numerous eruptive seborrheic keratoses	Esophageal, gastric, pancreatic, and colorectal cancer[55]	
Muir-Torre syndrome (MTS)	Sebaceous adenoma, sebaceoma, sebaceous carcinomas, multiple keratoacanthomas[56]	Colon cancer (most common), GU cancer (second most common), gastric, ovarian, endometrial cancers, and lymphoma	Few cases of MTS reported by ethnicity[56]
Necrolytic migratory erythema	Arcuate erythematous, scaly papules and plaques with overlying blisters[27]	Glucagonoma	Occurs at an earlier age (55 yo) in African American patients compared to White patients (60 yo)[57]
Peutz-Jeghers syndrome	Pigmented macules on mucosal and acral surfaces[27]	GI hamartomatous polyps	
Tripe palms	Thick, wrinkled palms and soles	Gastric and pulmonary carcinomas, although other cancers have been reported[56]	

characterized by a classic triad of diabetes mellitus, weight loss, and necrolytic migratory erythema.[1]

Lighter skin colors presenting with necrolytic migratory erythema will often initially present with erythematous papules and plaques on areas such as the genitals, buttocks, lower abdomen, and lower legs.[1] Those with darker skin may present with more violaceous to dark brown papules and plaques. These papules and plaques then develop central bullae that rupture and resolve with hyperpigmentation and residual crust. Patchy hypopigmentation and persistent erythema can also be appreciated in darker skin.[1] As the lesions enlarge, the central portion may start to heal. The erythema and hyperpigmentation often expand centrifugally, developing blisters in new areas of activity that can coalesce. These lesions are often exacerbated by trauma and can wax and wane in severity. Superimposed infection by Staphylococcus aureus or Candida albicans can be seen in NME and is indicated by the formation of overlying pustules.[1] Additional mucocutaneous findings seen in NME include glossitis, stomatitis, and angular cheilitis, which are present in about 30% of patients with NME.[1] Nail findings such as onychoschizia (horizontal nail splitting) and other nail changes have also been reported.

Excision of the underlying glucagonoma is curative in patients with localized disease. Unfortunately, greater than 50% of patients present with metastatic disease at initial diagnosis, with the most common sites of metastases being the liver, followed by the peripancreatic lymph nodes.[1] Metastatic glucagonoma is typically resistant to chemotherapy and not amenable to surgical resection. Despite that, resection of the primary tumor in metastatic glucagonoma has been shown to improve survival and should be performed when possible. Medical therapy can be beneficial in patients with metastatic disease or who are poor surgical candidates. Palliative treatment with somatostatin analogs such as octreotide or lanreotide and interferon alpha antagonize glucagon effects and increase the progression-free survival rate.[1] Topical corticosteroid may help treat the cutaneous findings of necrolytic migratory erythema. As nutritional deficiency appears to play an essential role in the pathogenesis of NME, the repletion of zinc, fatty acids, and amino acids has led to improvement in several cases of NME.[1]

PEUTZ-JEGHERS SYNDROME

Peutz-Jeghers syndrome (PJS) has an incidence of approximately 1 in 25,000 to 300,000 births. The syndrome affects males and females equally and does not have a predilection for any ethnic group (PMID: 34893571). Serine/threonine kinase 11 (STK11) is responsible for regulating the cell cycle, and mutations in STK11 can lead to abnormal cell proliferation. Mutations in STK11 (LKB1), a gene that can be found on chromosome 19b13.3, have been shown to lead to the development of Peutz-Jeghers syndrome.[1] Mutations in STK11 are seen in an autosomal-dominant, inherited familial pattern in ~70% of patients, while the remaining patients acquire the mutation de novo.

Patients with PJS classically present with mucocutaneous brown macules and GI hamartomatous polyps.[1] These hyperpigmented brown macules are seen on the lips, buccal mucosa, perioral areas, eyes, nostrils, fingertips, palms, soles, and perianal areas [**Figure 77-8**]. Most macules are not present at birth but appear before age 5. Brown macules that are present on cutaneous surfaces may fade during adolescence, but macules on the buccal mucosa persist through adulthood [**Figure 77-9**]. Melanocytic macules seen in PJS do not undergo malignant transformation.

GI hamartomatous polyps are present within the first decade of life and can be found anywhere along the GI tract but may also be present in the bronchus, renal pelvis, and urinary bladder. These polyps can lead to intussusception of the small intestine in 69% of patients; the first episode typically occurs between 6 and 18 years of age.[58] GI polyps can also lead

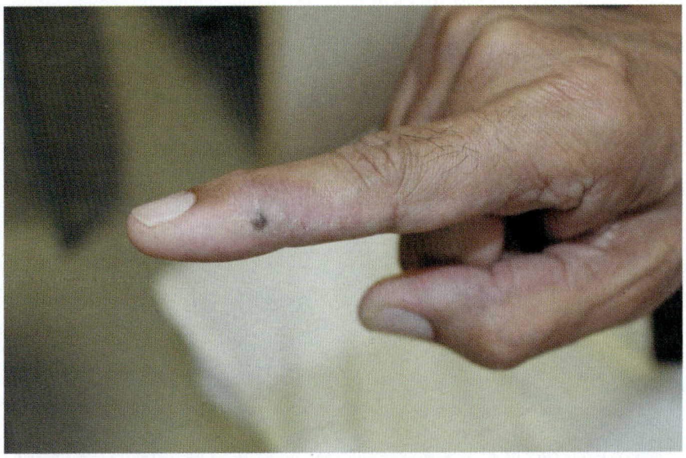

FIGURE 77-8. Peutz-Jeghers syndrome. A dark brown to black hyperpigmented round macule with slightly irregular borders surrounded by erythema and light scale on the index finger. (Courtesy of Dr. Bahar Bahrani.)

to bleeding and chronic anemia. Ninety-three percent of patients with Peutz-Jeghers syndrome develop cancer before age 65, with GI cancer (small intestine, colon, stomach, esophagus) being the most common, followed by lung and breast cancer.[58]

Surveillance, prevention of disease manifestation, and treatment of complications are three critical components of managing patients with PJS. Given that patients may develop GI polyposis as early as 10 years old, early surveillance is key.[59] Screening of the small intestine, the most common site of intestinal polyposis, should begin at age 12.[59] Endoscopy screening should take place every 2 to 3 years, and colonoscopy screening should take place every 1 to 3 years unless a polyp is found in which case these tests should be repeated annually.[59] Screening for pancreatic, breast, gynecologic, and testicular cancer should also be pursued in these patients.[59]

ACANTHOSIS NIGRICANS

In the United States, the prevalence of acanthosis nigricans is higher in skin of color individuals, such as Hispanics, Native Americans, and African Americans, compared to Caucasian or Asian individuals [Table 77-3].[52] African Americans have been estimated to be 25 times more likely to develop acanthosis nigricans compared to Americans of European descent.[60] Acanthosis nigricans is also highly prevalent amongst Native Americans, although the prevalence varies depending on the tribe.[61] The incidence of malignant acanthosis nigricans is overall rare. Most cases of acanthosis nigricans are associated with underlying insulin resistance. However, malignant acanthosis nigricans can occur as a paraneoplastic phenomenon with GI and other cancers.

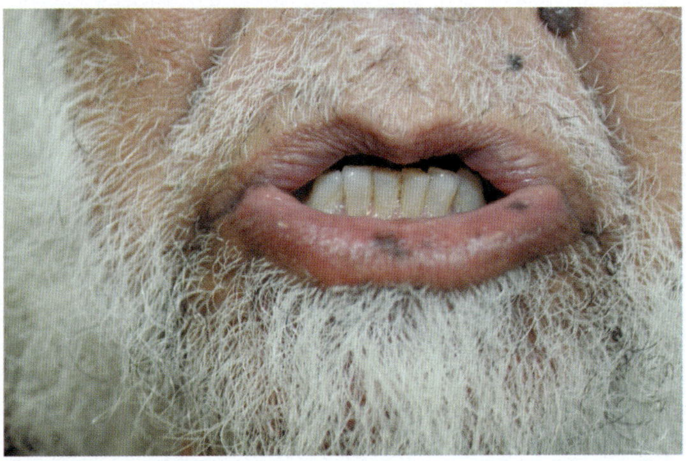

FIGURE 77-9. Peutz-Jeghers syndrome. Several dark red to black hyperpigmented macules and papules on the mucosal lip. (Courtesy of Dr. Bahar Bahrani.)

Type 2 diabetes mellitus is twice as common in patients with acanthosis nigricans compared to those without acanthosis nigricans.[52] In patients with benign acanthosis nigricans, elevated levels of insulin-like growth factor appear to stimulate keratinocytes and fibroblasts, leading to the proliferation of fibroblasts and enhanced stimulation of epidermal keratinocytes. High insulin levels can generate proliferative effects by binding to IGF-1 receptors, a phenomenon observed in a metabolic syndrome that leads to faster cell differentiation and growth.[52] Given the rarity of malignant acanthosis nigricans, the pathogenesis behind the development of malignant acanthosis nigricans has not yet been fully elucidated. It is often seen as a paraneoplastic phenomenon associated with gastrointestinal adenocarcinomas, genitourinary cancers, and others such as prostate, breast, and ovarian cancer. There have also been reports of malignant acanthosis nigricans arising in lung cancer and lymphoma settings.[52] In malignant acanthosis nigricans, one-third of patients will present with skin changes that precede a diagnosis of cancer, one-third of patients will present with skin changes concurrent with their cancer diagnosis, and the final one-third will present with skin findings after being diagnosed with cancer.[52]

Acanthosis nigricans presents as velvety, hyperpigmented brown to dark brown patches and plaques most commonly seen in the groin, axilla, or posterior neck [**Figure 77-10 A** and **B**].[1] Other areas of involvement include the nipple in women and, less frequently, the mucous

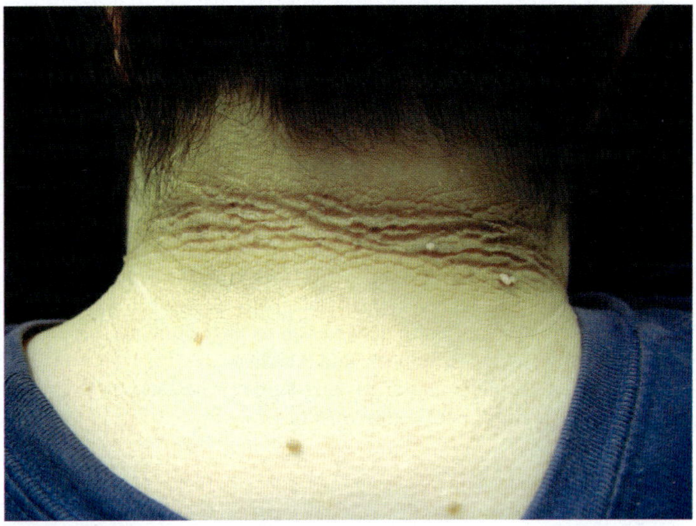

A

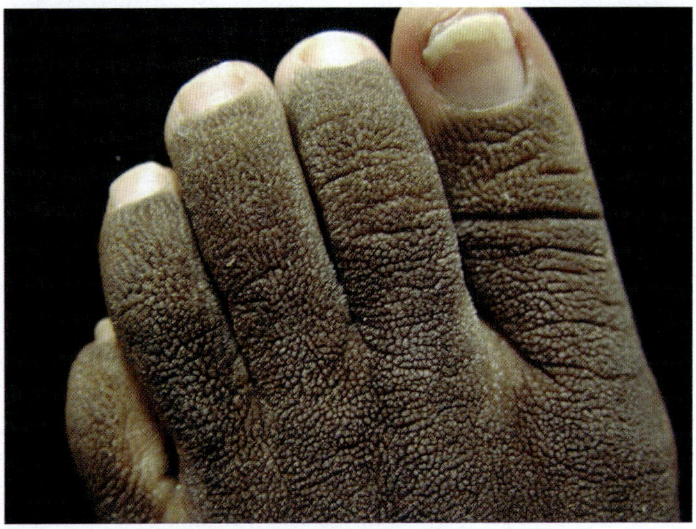

B

FIGURE 77-10 **(A)** Acanthosis nigricans. Hyperpigmented, velvety plaques on the neck. **(B)** Diffuse acanthosis nigricans with involvement of the dorsal foot.

membranes of the nose, oral cavity, esophagus, and larynx. In patients with malignant acanthosis nigricans, velvety, hyperpigmented plaques may be accompanied by additional skin findings such as acrochordons, multiple seborrheic keratoses (ie, Leser-Trelat), or tripe palms [Table 77-3].[1]

Treatment for acanthosis nigricans revolves around addressing the underlying cause. In benign acanthosis nigricans, treating insulin resistance through exercise, diet, and better blood glucose control can often improve symptoms. In malignant acanthosis nigricans, it is crucial to treat the underlying malignancy.[1] Topical treatment for acanthosis nigricans has been used with varying effects. Keratolytics, such as topical tretinoin 0.1% or 12% ammonium lactate, have been used, as well as topical vitamin D analogs, such as calcipotriol (calcipotriene 0.005%).[1] Metformin, etretinate, octreotide, and melatonin have been tried with variable degrees of success.[1] Procedural treatments such as alexandrite laser, fractional ablative CO_2 laser, dermabrasion, and chemical peels have all been reported in the literature.[59]

METABOLIC AND NUTRITIONAL

ACRODERMATITIS ENTEROPATHICA

Acrodermatitis enteropathica results from a mutation in *SLC39A4* on Chromosome 8.[1] *SLC39A4* encodes for a zinc-ligand binding protein, ZIP4, known to play a key role in epidermal differentiation and development within the skin.[62] In a large study examining over 100 worldwide populations, it was found that there was a nearly complete selective sweep in favor of the single nucleotide polymorphism Leu-372Val in ZIP4 within the Sub-Saharan African population.[63] Although more studies are needed, one hypothesis is that reduced zinc uptake may have been beneficial within Sub-Saharan Africa by depriving specific pathogens of zinc.

Infants with lighter skin color who develop acrodermatitis enteropathica most commonly present with erythematous scaly plaques on the perioral, anogenital, and acral surfaces.[1] In infants with darker skin color, these scaly plaques can appear violaceous to dark brown. Nail and hair changes are also common. In addition to the cutaneous symptoms, patients may present with alopecia and diarrhea.

Lifelong zinc supplementation of 3 mg/kg/day is necessary for patients with inherited acrodermatitis enteropathica.[1]

PELLAGRA

Pellagra is the term used to describe the cutaneous and systemic manifestations associated with niacin (vitamin B_3) deficiency.[1] Although uncommon in most industrialized nations, persons from low socioeconomic backgrounds or with specific diets, such as a vegetarian diet without fortified grains, can be susceptible to niacin deficiency, as well as those from certain parts of Africa, India, and China.[64] Patients with pellagra present with a classic triad of diarrhea, dermatitis, and dementia, with cutaneous findings manifesting as brown to violaceous scaly plaques on sun-exposed surfaces such as the face, neck, upper chest, arms, and legs.[1]

Treatment of pellagra entails supplementation with oral nicotinamide 250 to 500 mg/day.[1] Additionally, sun and alcohol avoidance is recommended to limit the cutaneous exacerbations of this condition.

PORPHYRIA CUTANEA TARDA

Porphyria cutanea tarda has been reported worldwide with a similar presence among all ethnicities.[65] Although this is the most common porphyria, the exact incidence of this hepatic porphyria remains unclear.[65] Commonly seen among patients ages 40 to 50, this has been noted to occur more often in men. There are three types of PCT (Types I-III). Type I is the most frequent, constituting 75% to 80% of cases without the hepatic enzyme uroporphyrinogen decarboxylase (UROD) mutation.[65] In the United States, approximately 70% to 80% of patients with PCT have HCV. In southern Europe, a strong association was found between HCV and acquired PCT, with almost 80% of patients with type I PCT coinfected with HCV.[66] PCT is caused by decreased hepatic UROD activity.[1] Various factors make patients susceptible to PCT, including hepatitis C virus infection, HIV infection, alcohol abuse, and cigarette smoking.[65]

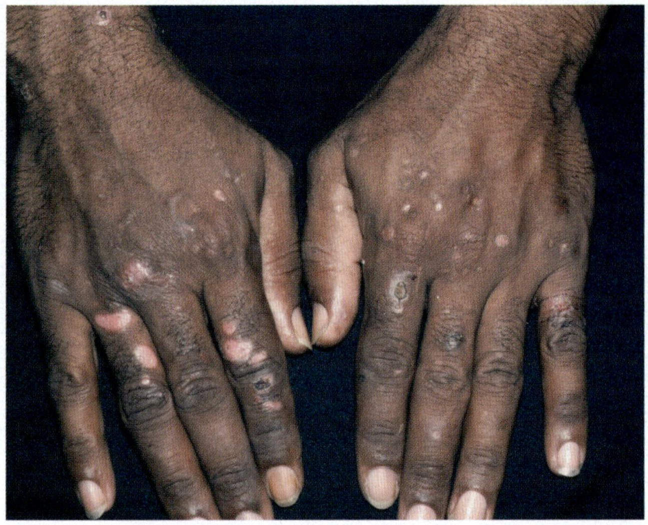

FIGURE 77-11. Porphyria cutanea tarda presenting with postinflammatory hypopigmentation and milia on the hands. (*Source:* Image appears with permission from VisualDx.)

Photosensitivity is a classic symptom of PCT due to the excess circulating porphyrins.[67] The dorsal hands and other photo-exposed areas present with chronic bullae that may result in prominent dyspigmentation upon resolution in skin of color individuals [**Figure 77-11**].[65] Other areas of involvement include the face, ears, neck, and forearms.[1] Patients have also experienced skin fragility after minor trauma and delayed wound healing.

This treatable condition involves phlebotomy as first-line and hydroxychloroquine when contraindications to phlebotomy are present.[1] Treatment of the underlying infection (HCV, HIV) is also pertinent. Additionally, photoprotection, alcohol avoidance, and smoking cessation should be encouraged. Following successful treatment, relapses may present.[65]

MEDICATIONS USED FOR DERMATOLOGIC CONDITIONS WITH GI SIDE EFFECTS

Several medications used to treat dermatologic conditions are associated with significant GI side effects. For instance, the rate of a ruptured colon with prednisone is dose-dependent, with the highest risk in patients on prolonged periods of high-dose prednisone (>20 mg/day). One hundred percent mortality was seen in patients who experienced bowel perforation.[68] Additionally, methotrexate, colchicine biologics, and tetracycline antibiotics commonly prescribed for skin diseases are notable for the frequency and severity of their GI side effects, detailed in **Table 77-4**.

TABLE 77-4 Selected dermatologic medications and their GI side effects

Medication	GI side effects
Prednisone	GI rupture at high doses (>20 mg/day)
Colchicine	Diarrhea (23%), vomiting (17%), nausea (4-17%)
Methotrexate	Liver fibrosis (at cumulative doses >1.5-4 g), nausea, vomiting, diarrhea
Biologics	Increased risk of Hepatitis B reactivation (particularly in TNF-α inhibitors, rituximab, and ustekinumab)
Doxycycline	Nausea, vomiting, epigastric pain
Clindamycin	Increased risk for *C. diff* colitis
Nonsteroidal Anti-inflammatory drugs	GI ulceration or bleeding, nausea, vomiting, diarrhea

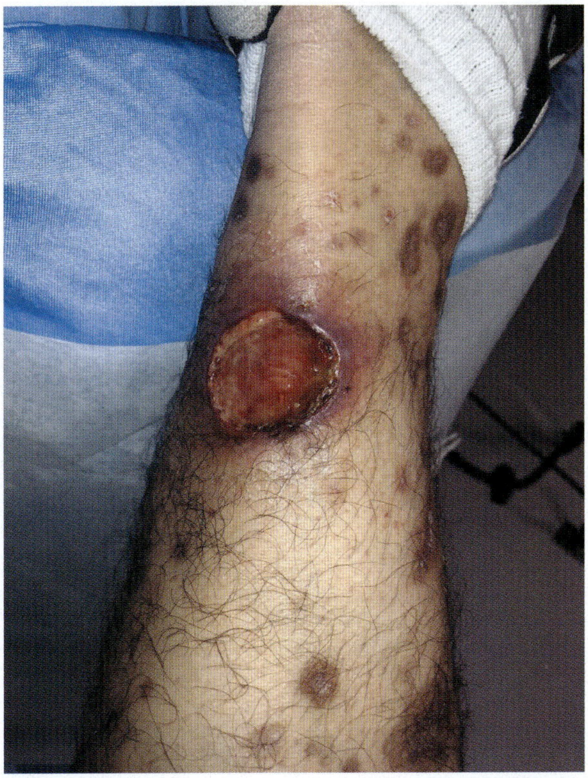

FIGURE 77-12. Pyoderma gangrenosum. A large annular ulcer with violaceous rolled borders on the leg. Scattered hyperpigmented, atrophic macules and patches with erosions are concerning for trauma. Consider injection drug use in the differential. (Courtesy of Dr. Bahar Bahrani.)

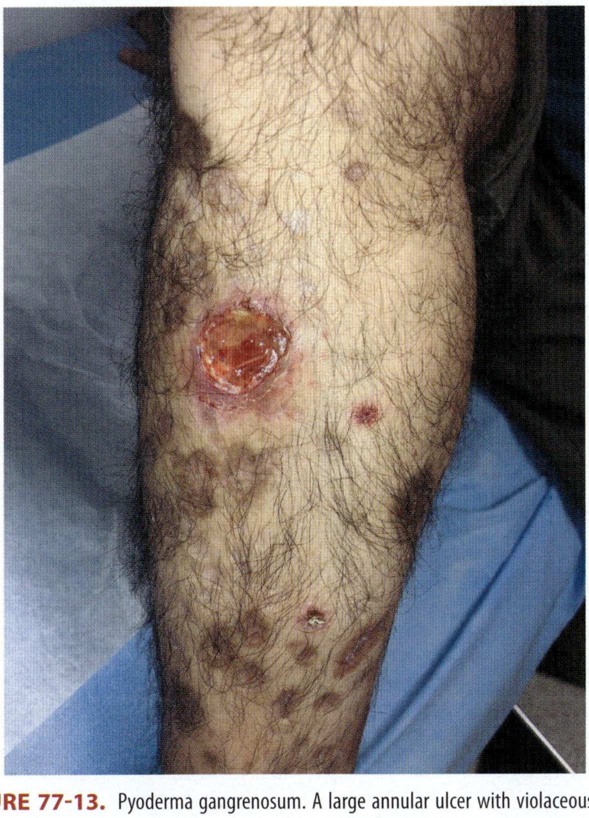

FIGURE 77-13. Pyoderma gangrenosum. A large annular ulcer with violaceous rolled borders on the leg. Scattered hyperpigmented, atrophic plaques, some with erosions are also evident. (Courtesy of Dr. Bahar Bahrani.)

SUMMARY

Epidemiological studies of many cutaneous diseases associated with underlying gastrointestinal conditions have demonstrated an increased incidence within skin of color individuals. Acanthosis nigricans, necrolytic acral erythema, acrodermatitis enteropathica, and Cronkhite-Canada syndrome are all notable examples. The cause of this increased incidence is heterogeneous, with diseases such as acrodermatitis enteropathica linked to a genetic sweep of single nucleotide polymorphism within the ZIP4 and other diseases such as acanthosis nigricans being associated with differences in the rate of underlying insulin resistance. Despite the increased incidence of GI-related skin disease within skin of color populations, disease-specific morbidity and mortality do not vary between skin of color and nonskin of color populations. Notably, skin erythema in skin of color patients may not be readily perceptible, as skin erythema may appear as more violaceous to dark brown compared to its presentation in White skin, where similar conditions may present as red to pink. Alterations in the gut microbiome have also been associated with numerous skin conditions, including acne vulgaris, atopic dermatitis, psoriasis, and others. Currently, differences in microbial flora between skin of color and nonskin of color patients with dermatologic disease have yet to be elucidated. Awareness of cutaneous disease presentation of gastrointestinal conditions in all skin types is important for improving health equity. Additional research is needed to better understand the increased incidence of certain conditions in skin of color populations as well as the role of the gut microbiome in cutaneous diseases.

REFERENCES

1. Bolognia J, Schaffer JV, Cerroni L. *Dermatology*. 4th ed. Amsterdam: Elsevier; 2018: 2 volumes: chaps 11, 12, 18, 19, 31, 49, 51, 53, 106, 112.
2. De Pessemier B, Grine L, Debaere M, Maes A, Paetzold B, Callewaert C. Gut-skin axis: current knowledge of the interrelationship between microbial dysbiosis and skin conditions. *Microorganisms*. 2021;9(2):353.
3. Benyacoub J, Bosco N, Blanchard C, et al. Immune modulation property of Lactobacillus paracasei NCC2461 (ST11) strain and impact on skin defences. *Benef Microbes*. 2014;5(2):129-136.
4. Chapat L, Chemin K, Dubois B, Bourdet-Sicard R, Kaiserlian D. Lactobacillus casei reduces CD8+ T cell-mediated skin inflammation. *Eur J Immunol*. 2004;34(9):2520-2528.
5. Gueniche A, Benyacoub J, Buetler TM, Smola H, Blum S. Supplementation with oral probiotic bacteria maintains cutaneous immune homeostasis after UV exposure. *Eur J Dermatol*. 2006;16(5):511-517.
6. Rebello D, Wang E, Yen E, Lio PA, Kelly CR. Hair growth in two alopecia patients after fecal microbiota transplant. *ACG Case Rep J*. 2017;4:e107.
7. Foolad N, Brezinski EA, Chase EP, Armstrong AW. Effect of nutrient supplementation on atopic dermatitis in children: a systematic review of probiotics, prebiotics, formula, and fatty acids. *JAMA Dermatol*. Mar 2013;149(3):350-355.
8. McCarthy S, Barrett M, Kirthi S, et al. Altered skin and gut microbiome in Hidradenitis Suppurativa. *J Invest Dermatol*. 2022;142(2):459-468 e15.
9. Aboud C, Zamaria N, Cannistra C. Treatment of hidradenitis suppurativa: surgery and yeast (Saccharomyces cerevisiae)-exclusion diet. Results after 6 years. *Surgery*. 2020;167(6):1012-1015.
10. Yeh NL, Hsu CY, Tsai TF, Chiu HY. Gut microbiome in psoriasis is perturbed differently during secukinumab and ustekinumab therapy and associated with response to treatment. *Clin Drug Investig*. 2019;39(12):1195-1203.
11. Nam JH, Yun Y, Kim HS, et al. Rosacea and its association with enteral microbiota in Korean females. *Exp Dermatol*. 2018;27(1):37-42.
12. Rebora A, Drago F, Parodi A. May Helicobacter pylori be important for dermatologists? *Dermatology*. 1995;191(1):6-8.
13. Reygagne P, Bastien P, Couavoux MP, et al. The positive benefit of Lactobacillus paracasei NCC2461 ST11 in healthy volunteers with moderate to severe dandruff. *Benef Microbes*. Oct 13 2017;8(5):671-680.
14. Fakharian F, Asgari B, Nabavi-Rad A, et al. The interplay between Helicobacter pylori and the gut microbiota: an emerging driver influencing the immune system homeostasis and gastric carcinogenesis. *Front Cell Infect Microbiol*. 2022;12:953718.
15. Gorkiewicz G, Moschen A. Gut microbiome: a new player in gastrointestinal disease. *Virchows Arch*. 2018;472(1):159-172.

16. Sanchez E, Donat E, Ribes-Koninckx C, Fernandez-Murga ML, Sanz Y. Duodenal-mucosal bacteria associated with celiac disease in children. *Appl Environ Microbiol.* 2013;79(18):5472-5479.
17. Hu J, Cheng S, Yao J, et al. Correlation between altered gut microbiota and elevated inflammation markers in patients with Crohn's disease. *Front Immunol.* 2022;13:947313.
18. Gevers D, Kugathasan S, Denson LA, et al. The treatment-naive microbiome in new-onset Crohn's disease. *Cell Host Microbe.* 2014;15(3):382-392.
19. Olejniczak-Staruch I, Ciazynska M, Sobolewska-Sztychny D, Narbutt J, Skibinska M, Lesiak A. Alterations of the skin and gut microbiome in psoriasis and psoriatic arthritis. *Int J Mol Sci.* 2021;22(8).
20. Epplein M, Signorello LB, Zheng W, et al. Race, African ancestry, and Helicobacter pylori infection in a low-income United States population. *Cancer Epidemiol Biomarkers Prev.* 2011;20(5):826-834.
21. Cardenas VM, Graham DY. Smoking and Helicobacter pylori infection in a sample of U.S. adults. *Epidemiology.* 2005;16(4):586-590.
22. Everhart JE. Recent developments in the epidemiology of Helicobacter pylori. *Gastroenterol Clin North Am.* 2000;29(3):559-578.
23. Cui YL, Zhou BY, Gao GC. A systematic review and meta-analysis of the correlation between Helicobacter pylori infection and chronic urticaria. *Ann Palliat Med.* 2021;10(10):10584-10590.
24. Raphael BA, Dorey-Stein ZL, Lott J, Amorosa V, Lo Re V 3rd, Kovarik C. Low prevalence of necrolytic acral erythema in patients with chronic hepatitis C virus infection. *J Am Acad Dermatol.* 2012;67(5):962-968.
25. Inamadar AC, Shivanna R, Ankad BS. Necrolytic acral erythema: current insights. *Clin Cosmet Investig Dermatol.* 2020;13:275-281.
26. el Darouti M, Abu el Ela M. Necrolytic acral erythema: a cutaneous marker of viral hepatitis C. *Int J Dermatol.* 1996;35(4):252-256.
27. Bolognia J, Schaffer JV, Cerroni L. *Dermatology.* 4th ed. Amsterdam: Elsevier; 2018: 2 volumes.
28. Li C, Tang X, Zheng X, et al. Global prevalence and incidence estimates of oral lichen planus: a systematic review and meta-analysis. *JAMA Dermatol.* 2020;156(2):172-181.
29. Ma SH, Tai YH, Dai YX, Chang YT, Chen TJ, Chen MH. Association between hepatitis C virus infection and subsequent chronic inflammatory skin disease. *J Dermatol.* 2021;48(12):1884-1891.
30. Afzali A, Cross RK. Racial and ethnic minorities with inflammatory bowel disease in the United States: a systematic review of disease characteristics and differences. *Inflamm Bowel Dis.* 2016;22(8):2023-2040.
31. Basu D, Lopez I, Kulkarni A, Sellin JH. Impact of race and ethnicity on inflammatory bowel disease. *Am J Gastroenterol.* 2005;100(10):2254-2261.
32. Ng SC, Shi HY, Hamidi N, et al. Worldwide incidence and prevalence of inflammatory bowel disease in the 21st century: a systematic review of population-based studies. *Lancet.* 2017;390(10114):2769-2778.
33. Greuter T, Navarini A, Vavricka SR. Skin manifestations of inflammatory bowel disease. *Clin Rev Allergy Immunol.* 2017;53(3):413-427.
34. Nguyen GC, Torres EA, Regueiro M, et al. Inflammatory bowel disease characteristics among African Americans, Hispanics, and non-Hispanic Whites: characterization of a large North American cohort. *Am J Gastroenterol.* 2006;101(5):1012-1023.
35. Farhi D, Cosnes J, Zizi N, et al. Significance of erythema nodosum and pyoderma gangrenosum in inflammatory bowel diseases: a cohort study of 2402 patients. *Medicine (Baltimore).* 2008;87(5):281-293.
36. Vashisht P, Goyal A, Hearth Holmes MP. Sweet syndrome. *StatPearls.* 2022.
37. Komatsuda A, Kinoshita K, Togashi M, et al. Cutaneous polyarteritis nodosa in a patient with Crohn's disease. *Mod Rheumatol.* 2008;18(6):639-642.
38. Johns HR, Shetty N, Cash J, Patel T, Pourciau C. Bowel-Associated-dermatosis-arthritis syndrome (BADAS) as early presentation of ulcerative colitis in an adolescent girl. *Pediatr Dermatol.* 2022;39(4):643-645.
39. Jorizzo JL, Schmalstieg FC, Dinehart SM, et al. Bowel-associated dermatosis-arthritis syndrome. Immune complex-mediated vessel damage and increased neutrophil migration. *Arch Intern Med.* 1984;144(4):738-740.
40. Atarbashi-Moghadam S, Lotfi A, Atarbashi-Moghadam F. Pyostomatitis vegetans: a clue for diagnosis of silent Crohn's Disease. *J Clin Diagn Res.* 2016;10(12):ZD12-ZD13.
41. Reddy H, Shipman AR, Wojnarowska F. Epidermolysis bullosa acquisita and inflammatory bowel disease: a review of the literature. *Clin Exp Dermatol.* 2013;38(3):225-229; quiz 229-230.
42. Zumelzu C, Le Roux-Villet C, Loiseau P, et al. Black patients of African descent and HLA-DRB1*15:03 frequency overrepresented in epidermolysis bullosa acquisita. *J Invest Dermatol.* 2011;131(12):2386-2393.
43. Principi M, Cassano N, Contaldo A, et al. Hydradenitis suppurativa and inflammatory bowel disease: an unusual, but existing association. *World J Gastroenterol.* 2016;22(20):4802-4811.
44. Vlassova N, Kuhn D, Okoye GA. Hidradenitis suppurativa disproportionately affects African Americans: a single-center retrospective analysis. *Acta Derm Venereol.* 2015;95(8):990-991.
45. Alvarez-Payares JC, Ramirez-Urrea S, Correa-Parra L, Salazar-Uribe D, Velasquez-Lopez M. mucocutaneous manifestations of inflammatory bowel disease. *Cureus.* 2021;13(8):e17191.
46. Joshi TP, Friske SK, Hsiou DA, Duvic M. New practical aspects of Sweet syndrome. *Am J Clin Dermatol.* 2022;23(3):301-318.
47. Catassi C, Gatti S, Lionetti E. World perspective and celiac disease epidemiology. *Dig Dis.* 2015;33(2):141-146.
48. Singh P, Arora A, Strand TA, et al. Global prevalence of celiac disease: systematic review and meta-analysis. *Clin Gastroenterol Hepatol.* 2018;16(6):823-836 e2.
49. Paruk IM, Naidoo VG, Pirie FJ, et al. Prevalence and characteristics of celiac disease in South African patients with type 1 diabetes mellitus: results from the Durban Diabetes and Celiac Disease Study. *J Gastroenterol Hepatol.* 2019;34(4):673-678.
50. Graziano M, Rossi M. An update on the cutaneous manifestations of coeliac disease and non-coeliac gluten sensitivity. *Int Rev Immunol.* 2018; 37(6):291-300.
51. Yao JC, Hassan M, Phan A, et al. One hundred years after "carcinoid": epidemiology of and prognostic factors for neuroendocrine tumors in 35,825 cases in the United States. *J Clin Oncol.* 2008;26(18):3063-3072.
52. Kong AS, Williams RL, Rhyne R, et al. Acanthosis nigricans: high prevalence and association with diabetes in a practice-based research network consortium–a PRImary care Multi-Ethnic network (PRIME Net) study. *J Am Board Fam Med.* 2010;23(4):476-485.
53. Clement DS, Tesselaar ME, van Leerdam ME, Srirajaskanthan R, Ramage JK. Nutritional and vitamin status in patients with neuroendocrine neoplasms. *World J Gastroenterol.* 2019;25(10):1171-1184.
54. Goto A. Cronkhite-Canada syndrome: epidemiological study of 110 cases reported in Japan. *Nihon Geka Hokan.* 1995;64(1):3-14.
55. Ozlu E, Uzuncakmak TK, Takir M, Akdeniz N, Karadag AS. Comparison of cutaneous manifestations in diabetic and nondiabetic obese patients: a prospective, controlled study. *North Clin Istanb.* 2018;5(2):114-119.
56. Wargo JJ, Plaza JA, Carr D. Sebaceous neoplasia leading to the diagnosis of Muir-Torre syndrome in an African American man. *JAAD Case Rep.* 2021;11:72-73.
57. Yao JC, Eisner MP, Leary C, et al. Population-based study of islet cell carcinoma. *Ann Surg Oncol.* 2007;14(12):3492-3500.
58. Wu M, Krishnamurthy K. Peutz-Jeghers syndrome. *StatPearls.* 2022.
59. Signoretti M, Bruno MJ, Zerboni G, Poley JW, Delle Fave G, Capurso G. Results of surveillance in individuals at high-risk of pancreatic cancer: a systematic review and meta-analysis. *United European Gastroenterol J.* May 2018;6(4):489-499.
60. Stuart CA, Gilkison CR, Smith MM, Bosma AM, Keenan BS, Nagamani M. Acanthosis nigricans as a risk factor for non-insulin dependent diabetes mellitus. *Clin Pediatr (Phila).* 1998;37(2):73-79.
61. Stuart CA, Smith MM, Gilkison CR, Shaheb S, Stahn RM. Acanthosis nigricans among Native Americans: an indicator of high diabetes risk. *Am J Public Health.* 1994;84(11):1839-1842.
62. Bin BH, Hojyo S, Seo J, et al. The role of the Slc39a family of zinc transporters in zinc homeostasis in skin. *Nutrients.* 2018;10(2):219.
63. Engelken J, Carnero-Montoro E, Pybus M, et al. Extreme population differences in the human zinc transporter ZIP4 (SLC39A4) are explained by positive selection in Sub-Saharan Africa. *PLoS Genet.* 2014;10(2):e1004128.
64. Dietary Reference Intakes for Thiamin, Riboflavin, Niacin, Vitamin B(6), Folate, Vitamin B(12), Pantothenic Acid, Biotin, and Choline. 1998. The National Academies Collection: Reports funded by National Institutes of Health.
65. Singal AK. Porphyria cutanea tarda: recent update. *Mol Genet Metab.* 2019;128(3):271-281.
66. To-Figueras J. Association between hepatitis C virus and porphyria cutanea tarda. *Mol Genet Metab.* 2019;128(3):282-287.
67. Heymans B, Meersseman W. Porphyria: awareness is the key to diagnosis! *Acta Clin Belg.* 2022;77(3):703-709.
68. ReMine SG, McIlrath DC. Bowel perforation in steroid-treated patients. *Ann Surg.* 1980;192(4):581-586.

CHAPTER 78

Hematology

Cheri Frey
Jewell Dinkins
Becky Li
Lynn McKinley-Grant

KEY POINTS

- Hematologic diseases are a diverse range of conditions affecting the constituents of blood. This includes disorders of red blood cells, white blood cells, and platelets.
- Red blood cell disorders are conditions that affect the number or function of red blood cells. Pallor, a common manifestation of anemia, is especially difficult to detect in skin of color.
- White blood cell disorders can be the result of cell overproduction, underproduction, or dysfunction. While benign diseases may exist, leukemias, lymphomas, and plasma cell disorders are the main categories of malignant diseases.
- Coagulation disorders can result in either uncontrolled blood clotting or uncontrolled bleeding. Antiphospholipid syndrome and disseminated intravascular coagulation are both coagulopathies that may result in nonspecific retiform purpura.
- Drugs that are used in the treatment of specific hematological conditions can have toxicities that manifest on the skin. This includes hydroxyurea-induced skin changes, warfarin-induced skin necrosis, and heparin-induced skin necrosis.

INTRODUCTION

Hematologic disorders such as anemia, lymphomas, and leukemias can have cutaneous manifestations on the skin. Physicians and healthcare providers play a vital role in assessing these manifestations and should be aware of their presentation in different skin colors. This chapter will provide an overview of the cutaneous manifestations of hematologic diseases and unique differences in epidemiology and presentation in skin of color.

DISORDERS OF RED BLOOD CELLS

According to the World Health Organization, anemia is defined as hemoglobin less than 13 g/dL in adult men and less than 12 g/dL in adult nonpregnant women. A mean corpuscular volume (MCV) between 80 and 100 femtoliters (fl) is considered normocytic. Anemias are classified into microcytic, normocytic, and macrocytic. An MCV less than 80 fl results in microcytic anemias and an MCV greater than 100 fl is considered macrocytic. Iron deficiency anemia, a microcytic anemia, is the most common type of anemia.[1]

SICKLE CELL ANEMIA

Introduction Sickle cell anemia (SCA) is caused by a mutation in the hemoglobin β gene on chromosome 11, which replaces glutamic acid with valine and results in a rigid and sickle-shaped erythrocyte. Sickling of erythrocytes leads to vaso-occlusion, ischemia, hemolysis, and anemia. This condition typically affects individuals who are of African, Asian, Caribbean, and Mediterranean descent. Africa has the highest prevalence of SCA by far. Nearly 90% of the world's sickle cell disease population lives in Nigeria, India, and the Democratic Republic of Congo, where the disease affects approximately 2% of the population, and the carrier prevalence is as high as 10% to 30%.[2] According to the Centers for Disease Control and Prevention, it is estimated that SCA occurs in 1 out of every 365 Black or African American births and one out of every 16,300 Hispanic American births. Additionally, about 1 in 13 Black or African American babies is born with the sickle cell trait.[3] Cutaneous presentations include leg ulcers and skin infections; however, the first manifestation of SCA is often hand-foot syndrome, which typically presents in early childhood.[4]

Cutaneous Manifestations Pallor and jaundice are the most common cutaneous manifestations in patients with SCA. Pallor can be difficult to detect in darker skin colors and may present as ashen, gray, or yellow. Conjunctival pallor may be a more accurate indicator of anemia in skin of color. Alternatively, the palmar surfaces of the hand can also appear paler.[5] Jaundice in an infant can be one of the earliest signs of sickle cell anemia. In skin of color, yellowing of the sclera may be the most noticeable sign of jaundice.

Patients with SCA can also develop nonhealing wounds and indolent leg ulcers. The exact pathogenesis is unclear, but it is thought to be related to repeated injury of small vessels by sickled cells, a decrease in oxygen delivery to the distal blood vessels, venous incompetence, and persistent inflammation. Ulcers usually occur in areas of the leg with less subcutaneous fat and decreased blood flow, with the skin overlying the medial and lateral malleoli being the most frequent site of formation. The ulcerations are round and punched out with a raised border and deep necrotic base associated with tenderness on palpation. These ulcers are often slow to heal, resistant to treatment, and recurrent. Frequently, there is evidence of postinflammatory pigment alteration in areas of healed ulcers.[4]

Dactylitis is another common finding in patients with SCA. It presents as swelling of the hands and feet in infants and young children. The overlying skin appears to be tense and shiny, and there is effacement of the skin folds. Children typically have limited mobility in the affected extremities. In more severe cases, areas of necrosis may result in shortening of the digits, leaving these children with a permanent deformity.[4]

Diagnosis and Treatment Laboratory findings include anemia and reticulocytosis on complete blood counts, and sickled cells can be observed on peripheral blood smears. Confirmatory tests include hemoglobin electrophoresis and high-performance liquid chromatography. The overall management of SCA is aimed at addressing the increased risk for infection, bone marrow aplasia, and painful crises. Individuals are typically given prophylactic penicillin until the age of five, as well as the appropriate vaccinations to prevent an infection from encapsulated organisms. Patients may later require blood transfusion or exchange transfusions to treat symptomatic anemia or to support severe life-threatening complications, such as acute stroke or acute chest syndrome. Several treatments have been proposed to manage leg ulcers and interventions include systemic antibiotics, vasodilators, reconstructive surgery, skin or cell transplant, and laser treatments. Despite the variety of options available, a single effective modality of treatment has not yet emerged. Standard treatments typically include bed rest, hygienic maintenance, and dressings, such as Unna boots. On the contrary, hand-foot syndrome is a self-limited phenomenon. Therefore, the care offered by physicians is usually largely supportive, including hydration, analgesics, antibiotics in the presence of fever and leukocytosis, and reassurance for the patient's parents and family. Folic acid is often given as a daily regimen to reduce the risk of bone marrow aplasia in patients with chronic hemolysis. Effective pain management is extremely important for improving the quality of life of these individuals. Physicians usually prescribe a variety of analgesics and encourage patients to maintain an appropriate level of hydration. Patients can also receive hydroxyurea as a disease-modifying drug, which also increases their hemoglobin F levels. Bone marrow transplant offers curative therapy.[4]

IRON DEFICIENCY ANEMIA

Introduction Iron deficiency anemia (IDA) is the most common nutritional deficiency in the world, with 30% of the population being affected with this condition. Low-income families, women of child-bearing age, and women of color are particularly at risk.[6] Iron deficiency may result from insufficient iron intake, decreased absorption, or blood loss. In older patients, IDA is most often from blood loss, but it may also be seen with low dietary intake, increased systemic requirements for iron, and decreased iron absorption. Studies have shown that anemia is three times more common in African Americans than in Whites.[7]

Cutaneous Manifestations The cutaneous manifestations of IDA may appear on the oral mucosa, nails, and hair. Oral mucosa findings can include angular stomatitis and alterations in tongue papillae. Nail manifestations include koilonychia, or spoon-shaped nails.[8] Diffuse hair thinning as well as changes in hair quality, such as increased splitting, dryness, and dullness, can also be observed. Curlier hair types are often dryer than straighter hair types at baseline, thus it may be more difficult to assess dullness and dryness in such patients.

Diagnosis and Treatment Diagnosis requires laboratory-confirmed evidence of anemia, as well as evidence of low iron stores. Serum ferritin is currently the most efficient and cost-effective diagnostic method.[9] Once IDA is confirmed, oral iron supplementation or infusions may be warranted for treatment. Patients with an underlying condition that causes IDA should be treated or referred to a subspecialist (eg, gynecologist, gastroenterologist) for definitive treatment.[10]

ANEMIA OF CHRONIC DISEASE

Anemia of chronic disease is the second most common cause of anemia after iron deficiency anemia (IDA). It is seen in several disease states, such as malignancies, chronic infections, and auto-immune diseases.[11] Increased iron uptake as well as iron retention within cells leads to reduced iron available for hemoglobin production. Cutaneous manifestations present similarly to IDA; however, symptoms of the associated disease typically take precedence over mild or moderate anemia symptoms. Treatment depends on the underlying disease.[12]

POLYCYTHEMIA VERA

Introduction Polycythemia vera (PCV) is a rare myeloproliferative disorder caused by uncontrolled amplification of hematopoietic progenitor cells. A mutation in Janus-Kinase-2 (JAK2) is present in 90% of PCV cases, leading to clonal proliferation of red blood cells, with an associated increase in leukocytes and megakaryocytes. This increased cellularity of the blood leads to hyperviscosity, which accounts for most of the disease sequelae. In the United States, the prevalence of polycythemia vera ranges from 0.6 to 1.6 per million persons. PCV is slightly more common in men than in women and the median age of diagnosis is 60 years.[13] It is more prevalent among Jews of Eastern European descent than other Europeans or Asians.[14] Although PCV is more common in Whites, the REVEAL study showed that non-White patients, including African Americans, Asians, and Pacific Islanders, had worse symptom burdens, lower functional scores, and greater disability.[15]

Cutaneous Manifestations Polycythemia vera is frequently associated with ruddy cyanosis or facial redness. Skin color is especially important in assessing cyanosis. In patients with lighter skin, cyanosis presents with a dark blue tint to the skin and mucous membranes that reflects the blue color of unoxygenated hemoglobin. In darker skin, however, cyanosis may present as gray or gray-white skin periorally, and the conjunctivae may appear gray or blue. In patients with yellow skin undertones, cyanosis may cause a gray-green skin discoloration.[16] Another striking feature of PCV is pruritus, specifically aquagenic pruritus (AP), characterized by itching, stinging, or burning sensation following contact with water, without visible skin findings. In a German study of 441 PCV patients, 64.8% reported a history of aquagenic pruritus. Although aquagenic pruritus preceded the diagnosis of PCV by an average of 2.9 years, AP led to the diagnosis of PCV in only 15.4%.[17] The etiology of AP in patients with PCV is poorly understood; however, increased basophil and mast cell degranulation in addition to iron deficiency are proposed mechanisms. Acrocyanosis, a blue-purple hue of the distal extremities, and erythromelalgia, redness, and burning of the distal extremities, may occasionally be observed.[18] Other cutaneous manifestations such as livedo reticularis and ulcerations have been reported but occur less frequently in patients with PCV when compared to other myeloproliferative disorders such as essential thrombocytosis. In darker skin, the erythema in livedo reticularis may be subtle or appear deep red, maroon, or violaceous. In the darkest skin tones, it may be masked completely.[19]

TABLE 78-1 Major and minor criteria for polycythemia vera

Criteria
Major criteria:
• Hemoglobin (Hgb) > 16.5 g/dL (male), 16g/dL (female) (6g/dL in women) **OR** Hematocrit (Hct) > 49% in men (48% in women) **OR** red blood cell mass > 25% above mean normal predicted
• Bone marrow biopsy demonstrating hypercellularity for age with pan proliferation of erythroid, granulocytic, and megakaryocytic cell lines with pleomorphic, mature megakaryocytes
• JAK2 V617For JAK2 exon 12 mutation
Minor criteria:
• Serum erythropoietin level below the reference range for normal

Diagnosis In 2016, the World Health Organization revised the criteria for diagnosis of PCV [**Table 78-1**]. Patients suspected of having PCV must meet all three major criteria or two major criteria plus one minor criterion.

Treatment Cutaneous manifestations of PCV, such as cyanosis, should first be addressed with the treatment of the underlying condition. Treatment of PCV is aimed at reducing the risks associated with thrombosis. Patients are stratified based on age and history of thrombotic events. Low-risk patients (age 60 or younger without a history of thrombosis) are treated with phlebotomy and low-dose aspirin. High-risk patients (age 60 years and older or patients with a history of thrombosis) are treated with hydroxyurea in addition to phlebotomy and low-dose aspirin. Ruxolitinib and pegylated interferon may be considered if patients are unresponsive to hydroxyurea.[13] Antihistamines and phototherapy may also benefit patients with AP. Other AP-specific treatment options include topical capsaicin and topical anesthetics. Serotonin-reuptake inhibitors and pregabalin may be considered as second- and third-line treatments, respectively.[18]

DISORDERS OF WHITE BLOOD CELLS

White blood cell disorders can be the result of cell overproduction, underproduction, or dysfunction. While benign diseases may exist, leukemias, lymphomas, and plasma cell disorders are the main categories of malignant diseases. Leukemia cutis occurs in the setting of leukemia. Lymphomas can be further subdivided into Hodgkin and non-Hodgkin lymphomas. The non-Hodgkin lymphomas that will be discussed in this chapter include cutaneous T- and B-cell lymphoma.

CUTANEOUS T-CELL LYMPHOMA

Cutaneous T-cell lymphoma (CTCL) refers to a group of non-Hodgkin lymphomas characterized by infiltration of malignant monoclonal T lymphocytes in the skin.[20] Initially, CTCL was categorized into two broad categories: mycosis fungoides (MF) and Sézary syndrome (SS). However, this schematic has since been replaced by the World Health European Organization for Research and Treatment of Cancer (WHO-EORTC) classification, which stratifies disease into indolent, intermediate, or aggressive behavior and combines clinical presentation with histologic features and immunophenotype. This classification provides valuable information on staging, the preferred mode of treatment, clinical behavior, and prognosis, and serves as a useful guide to optimize management.

Epidemiology MF is a rare condition with an incidence of 6.4 persons per million annually, while SS is even more uncommon. It is suggested that Agent Orange may be a causative factor for the development of MF. MF typically affects older adults (55-60 years), though it may occur in children and adolescents as well. There is a 1.5 times greater incidence in Black individuals than White individuals. Black patients also tend to present with earlier and more aggressive disease with increased BSA involvement compared to White patients. Unfortunately, MF in skin of color (SOC) portends a worse prognosis and overall survival. It has been suggested that these differences in presentation and survival may be attributed to genetic and immunological/molecular differences in the pathogenesis of CTCL in SOC.[21]

Pathogenesis The development and pathogenesis of malignant monoclonal T lymphocytes in the skin require further elucidation; however, genetic, environmental, and immunologic factors have all been considered. A single-institutional study showed that Black patients with MF and SS had increased blood eosinophil count when compared to White patients.[21] IL-6 levels were also shown to be higher in Black patients. Besides these differences in immunologic factors, other factors, such as access to care leading to delayed diagnoses, missed diagnoses, social inequities, and disparities in risk factors (eg, exposure to pollution) likely contributes to prognostic differences seen in SOC.

Cutaneous Manifestations MF classically presents as erythematous, brown annular or arcuate, atrophic patches or plaques on photoprotected areas, though there are other forms of the disease, including plaque, tumor, and erythrodermic. In SOC, the erythematous patches and plaques may have a red, purple, or gray hue. Patch and plaque stage MF presents as patches or thin plaques with fine scale that measure 2 to 20 cm and favor the photo-protected areas of the body, including buttocks and posterior axillary folds. A classic feature of patches is a wrinkled surface that resembles "cigarette paper." A poikilodermatous variant of patch stage MF comprises atrophy, telangiectasias, and hyper- and hypopigmentation. Annular, serpiginous, horseshoe-shaped, and bizarrely shaped plaques are frequently seen in plaque-stage disease. Tumor stage MF presents with violaceous, exophytic tumors that predominantly affect the face and body folds. Tumors often undergo ulceration or necrosis and secondary infection.[22] SOC patients are likely to present with areas of hypopigmentation as well as hyperpigmentation. (**Figures 78-1** through **78-5**).[21] There can also be secondary lichenification and overlying scale, further challenging diagnosis as it can resemble atopic dermatitis. Overall, SOC patients present with an increased incidence of disease, earlier onset, greater body surface area (BSA) involvement, and worse survival.[21] Recently, a single-institutional exploratory study found a substantial impact on quality of life in the setting of having CTCL, with certain aspects being more affected among patients with

FIGURE 78-1. Mycosis fungoides. Mycosis fungoides can present in skin of color as hypopigmented patches, seen here on the ventral upper extremity. (Reproduced with permission from Dr. Ginette Okoye, Howard University Department of Dermatology.)

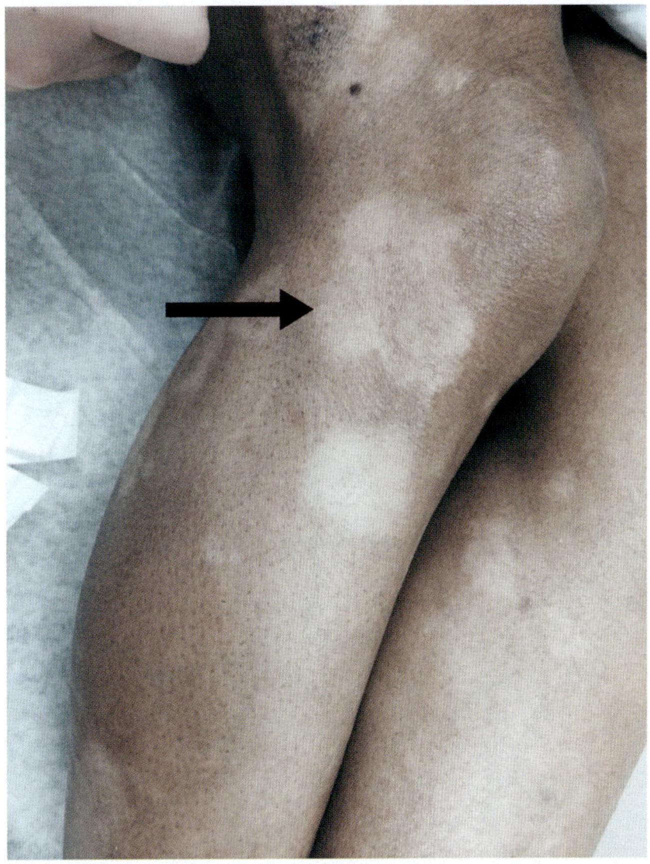

FIGURE 78-2. Hypo- to depigmented atrophic patches with some areas of central repigmentation. Note the accentuation of vasculature in the larger plaque inferior to the right knee.

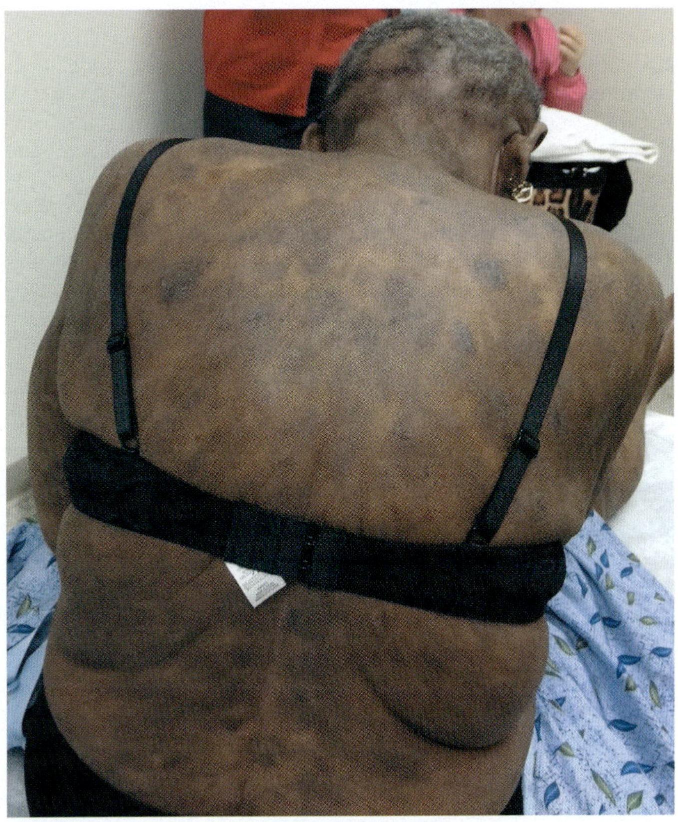

FIGURE 78-3. Coalescing hyperpigmented patches and plaques, some with overlying scale on the back.

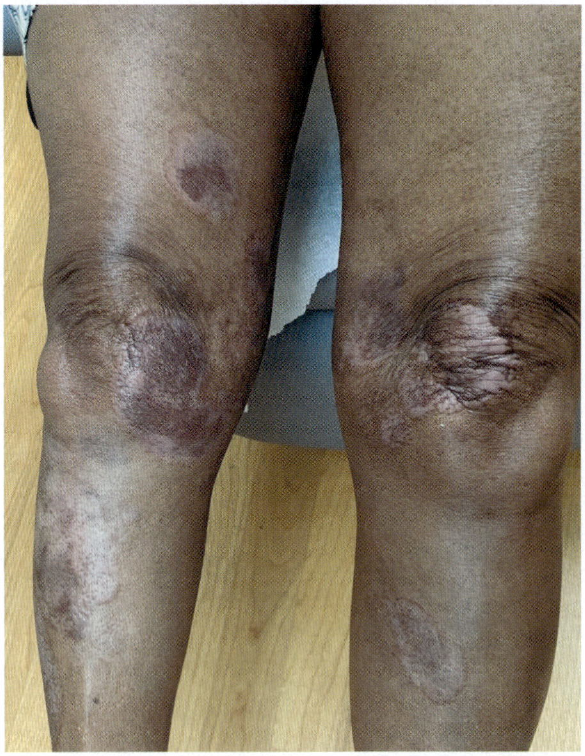

FIGURE 78-4. Multiple red-brown nummular scaly plaques on the lower legs.

SOC.[23] This included pruritus being reported with greater severity, and affected individuals being more self-conscious and uncomfortable with themselves from before-to-after diagnosis.

On the other hand, SS is the leukemic form of MF, characterized by generalized erythroderma, lymphadenopathy, and atypical T-cells located in the peripheral blood.

Diagnosis The single most important diagnostic tool for CTCL is a skin biopsy. TNM staging, as well as WHO-EORTC classification, is pertinent to determine the preferred mode of treatment, clinical behavior, prognosis, and overall survival. The early diagnosis of MF is important because the appropriate management of early disease portends a prognosis similar to individuals without MF.[20]

In order to diagnose SS, there must be a T-cell clone in the peripheral blood (preferably the same T-cell clone as in the skin), in combination with an absolute Sézary cell count greater than or equal to 1000 cells/mcl or immunophenotypical abnormalities (an expanded CD4+ T-cell population resulting in a CD4/CD8 ratio >10 and/or aberrant expression of pan-T-cell antigens).

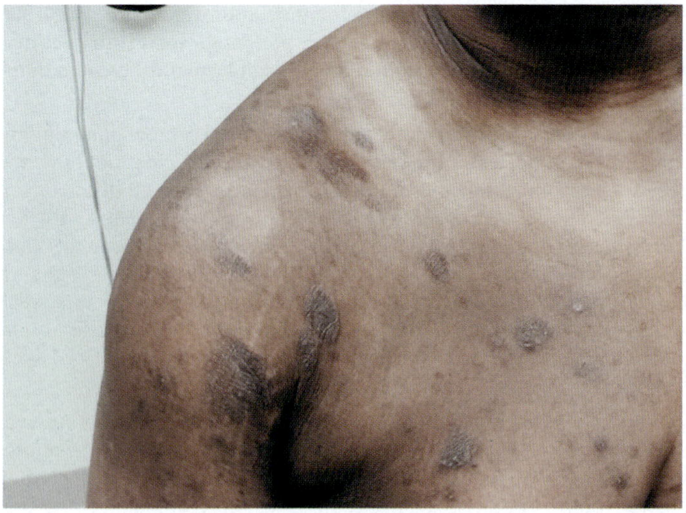

FIGURE 78-5. Well-demarcated brown scaly plaques on right chest extending onto right upper extremity.

Pathology On pathology of MF, there is a vacuolar interface dermatitis. Atypical lymphocytes are present in the epidermis (epidermotropism) and dermis, with epidermal lymphocytes being larger, darker, and more angulated than lymphocytes in the dermis. Dermal lymphocytes can appear on the epidermal side of the superficial vascular plexus, producing the "bare underbelly sign." Spongiosis is usually not seen in most cases, unlike atopic dermatitis.

Treatment Treatment of CTCL includes utilizing skin-directed therapies and systemic therapies.[20] Skin direct therapies include topical corticosteroids, topical nitrogen mustard, topical bexarotene, phototherapy, and total skin electron beam. Phototherapy is optimal for patients with hypopigmented MF. When selecting treatment modalities for patients, especially for SOC patients, it is imperative to counsel on drug adverse effects (eg, hyperpigmentation after total skin electron beam) and to consider these adverse effects in the context of patient medical comorbidities (eg, dyslipidemia in the setting of oral bexarotene use).

CUTANEOUS B-CELL LYMPHOMA

B-cell lymphomas are non-Hodgkin lymphomas and represent approximately a quarter of all primary cutaneous lymphomas. According to the World Health Organization, primary cutaneous B-cell lymphomas (PCBCLs) are classified into three groups: primary cutaneous marginal zone lymphoma (PCMZL), primary cutaneous follicle-center cell lymphoma (PCFCL), and diffuse large B-cell lymphoma, leg type (PCDLBCL, LT) [**Figure 78-6**].[24]

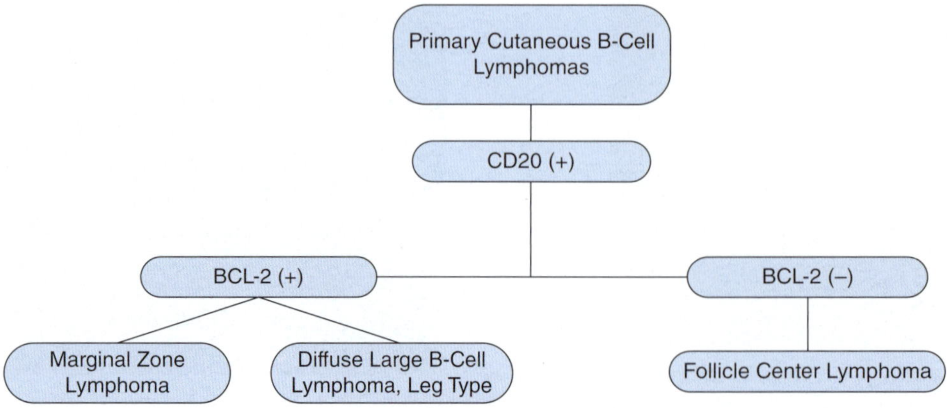

FIGURE 78-6. Classifications of primary B-cell lymphomas.

Epidemiology PCBCLs seem to occur more frequently in specific regions of the world with U.S. cases only representing about 4% of all primary cutaneous lymphomas. In contrast, PCBCLs represented 22.5% of all primary cutaneous lymphomas in Europe. PCDLBCL, LT does appear to have a gender predilection, affecting mostly elderly women in the seventh decade of life.[25] Compared to White patients, Black patients with PCBCL are diagnosed at younger ages and are more likely to present with head and neck involvement, as well as regional or generalized distributions.[26] Data suggest that African American patients with diffuse large B-Cell Lymphoma present at a younger age, more advanced stage, and have lower survival rates.[27]

Pathogenesis The pathogenesis of PCBCLs is unknown, though infectious etiologies such as *Borrelia burgdorferi* and *Helicobacter pylori* have been implicated.[25] Immune dysregulation may also play a role in the development of disease, as PCBCLs have been described in immunosuppressed patients (eg, patients with AIDS and solid organ transplant recipients), as well as those receiving methotrexate for rheumatoid arthritis.

Cutaneous Manifestations Each type of PCBL presents with unique characteristics. PCFCLs commonly present as solitary or localized red to purple papules or nodules, plaques, or tumors in all skin colors. Affected areas may be on an erythematous background and are typically on the trunk. Acneiform papules on the face and scalp have also been described [**Figures 78-7** and **78-8**]. PCMZLs manifest as red, purple, and brown papules or nodules and plaques on the arms, legs, and trunk. PCDLBCL, LT presents as solitary or localized red to brown ulcerated papules or nodules on the distal leg. Some cases may occur elsewhere on the skin surface. Diagnosis requires histological examination with immunohistochemical staining, as well as a further workup for systemic disease. PCMZL and PCFCL are considered indolent lymphomas associated with good prognosis. PCFCL tends to present on the head and neck, whereas PCMZL prefers the upper extremities and trunk. Of note, PCFCL may be confused for acneiform scars. Both confer a good prognostic outcome and rarely present with systemic symptoms (eg, fever, night sweats, weight loss). In contrast, PCDLBCL, LT is considered an aggressive lymphoma with a poor prognosis. Ulceration is more common, as well as B symptoms. Treatment includes observation, and local or systemic therapy.[28]

Diagnosis Diagnosis relies heavily on skin biopsy and immunohistochemical staining. For PCDLBCL, LT, further laboratory and imaging workup is needed, as well as frequent follow-up consisting of a complete cutaneous and nodal clinical examination and annual restaging.[27] Serum lactate dehydrogenase, if elevated, is suggestive of a more aggressive disease and poor prognosis.

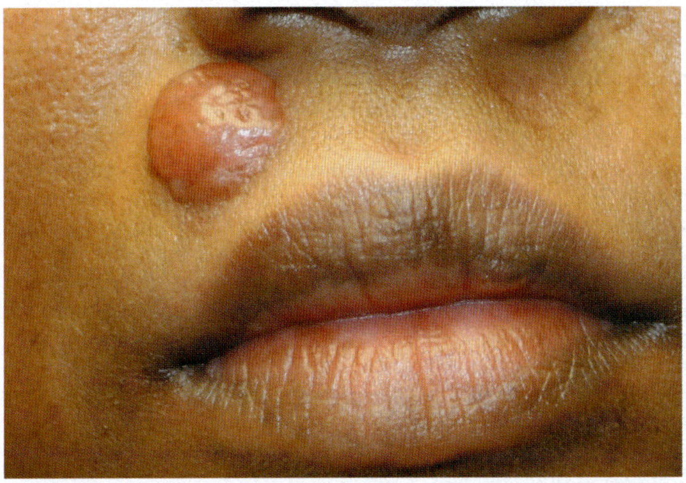

FIGURE 78-7. Primary cutaneous B-cell lymphoma presenting as solitary pink nodule on the upper cutaneous lip of a woman of color. (Reproduced with permission from Dr. Ginette Okoye, Howard University Department of Dermatology.)

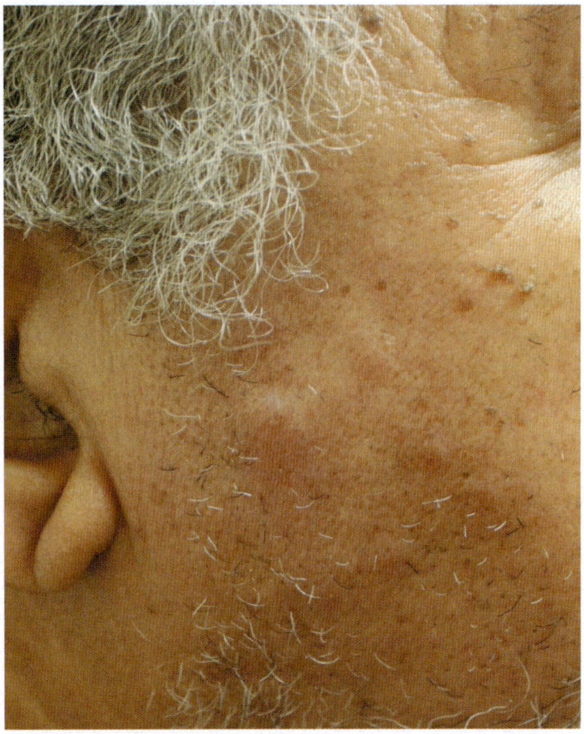

FIGURE 78-8. Primary cutaneous follicle-center lymphoma presenting as faint erythematous papules on the right cheek. (Reproduced with permission from Dr. Ginette Okoye, Howard University Department of Dermatology.)

Pathology On histology, nodular or diffuse lymphocytic infiltrates within the entire dermis is alarming for cutaneous lymphomas. CD20 staining can confirm the presence of lymphocytes, and Bcl-2, Bcl-6, and MUM-1 can help differentiate PCFCL, PCMZL, and PCDLBCL, LT.

Treatment As PCFCL and PCMZL are associated with excellent prognosis, it is not uncommon to simply observe these conditions. However, if lesions are bothersome to patients, surgical excision may be considered. For PCDLBCL, LT, a combination of local radiation with an immunochemotherapy regimen (eg, R-CHOP) may be utilized for treatment.[29]

LEUKEMIA CUTIS

Leukemia cutis is a rare complication of leukemia, and different types of leukemia exist in different demographics of patients. Acute lymphoblastic leukemia (ALL) typically occurs in childhood, while acute myelogenous leukemia (AML) and chronic myelogenous leukemia (CML) occur primarily in adults. Chronic lymphocytic leukemia (CLL) is most common in elderly patients. Studies suggest that in patients with AML, African Americans have worse overall survival than Whites when given similar initial therapies.[30]

Leukemia cutis happens when malignant leukocytes or their precursors invade the skin and presents similarly to PCBCLs with discrete or multiple firm pink to red-brown or purple papules and nodules on the head, neck, and trunk. Overlying ulceration and/or bleeding often occur. Currently, there is no treatment for leukemia cutis. Management of underlying leukemia typically results in the resolution of cutaneous manifestations.

GRAFT-VERSUS-HOST DISEASE

Introduction Graft-versus-host disease (GVHD) is a well-known complication of allogeneic hematopoietic stem cell transplantation (HSCT). GVHD occurs when immunocompetent donor T-cells recognize foreign antigens present in recipient cells. Many studies have shown an increased risk of acute GVHD in African Americans.[31] When the immunocompromised recipient is unable to mount a response against donor lymphocytes, GVHD results. While unmatched recipients are at a higher risk of developing graft-versus-host disease, up to 50% of HLA-matched allogeneic bone marrow transplant recipients will develop acute GVHD. Acute GVHD is a life-threatening complication with a guarded prognosis typically presenting 1 to 3 weeks following the transplant. Chronic GVHD, while classically presenting more than 100 days following transplant, may occur at any time posttransplant. Therefore, the distinction between acute and chronic GVHD is sometimes made based on clinical features as opposed to the time of onset. Acute GVHD commonly presents with a coalescent morbilliform eruption, elevated bilirubin, and/or diarrhea. Chronic GVHD is characterized by mucocutaneous findings (eyes, mouth, genitalia), as well as liver, gastrointestinal, and lung involvement.[32]

Cutaneous Manifestations The skin is the most common organ involved in GVHD; however, cutaneous manifestations are often nonspecific. Acute GVHD may present initially as a morbilliform eruption localized to acral skin. Erythroderma, bullae formation, or full-thickness skin necrosis resembling toxic epidermal necrolysis are found in more severe diseases. While erythroderma may be easily identified in patients with lighter skin tones, it may be subtle in darker skin. The staging of acute GVHD includes an evaluation of the extent of skin involvement. The long-term survival rate for severe acute GVHD is 5%, therefore the extent of skin involvement is an important prognostic factor.[32]

Chronic GVHD skin findings include red to purple scaly papules and plaques resembling lichen planus, perifollicular erythema, and poikiloderma. Atrophic, white plaques resembling lichen sclerosis, and fibrotic skin changes may also develop. Mucosal plaques and ulcerations of the mouth, eyes, and genitalia are other common findings of chronic GVHD [**Figure 78-9**].[32]

Pathology Lichenoid and sclerodermoid features are the most common histopathologic patterns observed on biopsy. Lichenoid patterns of acute GVHD reveal a mildly spongiotic epidermis with interface vacuolar changes, necrotic keratinocytes, and a dermal perivascular lymphocytic infiltrate. Satellite cell necrosis and scattered eosinophils may also be present. Early biopsies of acute GVHD, like the skin findings, may be indistinguishable from other acute processes such as drug hypersensitivity reactions. Sclerodermoid patterns resemble scleroderma with fibrosis or thickened collagen within the papillary and reticular dermis, as well as the subcutaneous fat.[32]

Treatment Up to 15% of patients with acute GVHD will have limited skin disease without systemic involvement. For these patients, topical steroids are the first-line treatment.[33] Symptoms of internal involvement are treated more aggressively with high-dose oral corticosteroids, such as prednisone. Patients are often at an increased risk of infection; therefore, appropriate prophylaxis is recommended. In 2019, ruxolitinib was approved for the treatment of acute GVHD. Second-line treatments such as etanercept, mycophenolate mofetil, and extracorporeal photopheresis have been used for patients not responsive to steroids. In all cases, optimizing immunosuppressive regimens is imperative.[34]

Mild chronic GVHD can be managed with mid- to high-potency topical steroids or phototherapy. The benefits of phototherapy with UVB or UVA must be weighed against the risk of skin cancer. Moderate to severe cases will need systemic therapy with corticosteroids. In 2017, Ibrutinib, an inhibitor of Bruton tyrosine kinase, was approved by the U.S. Food and Drug Administration (FDA) as second-line treatment for chronic GVHD.[35]

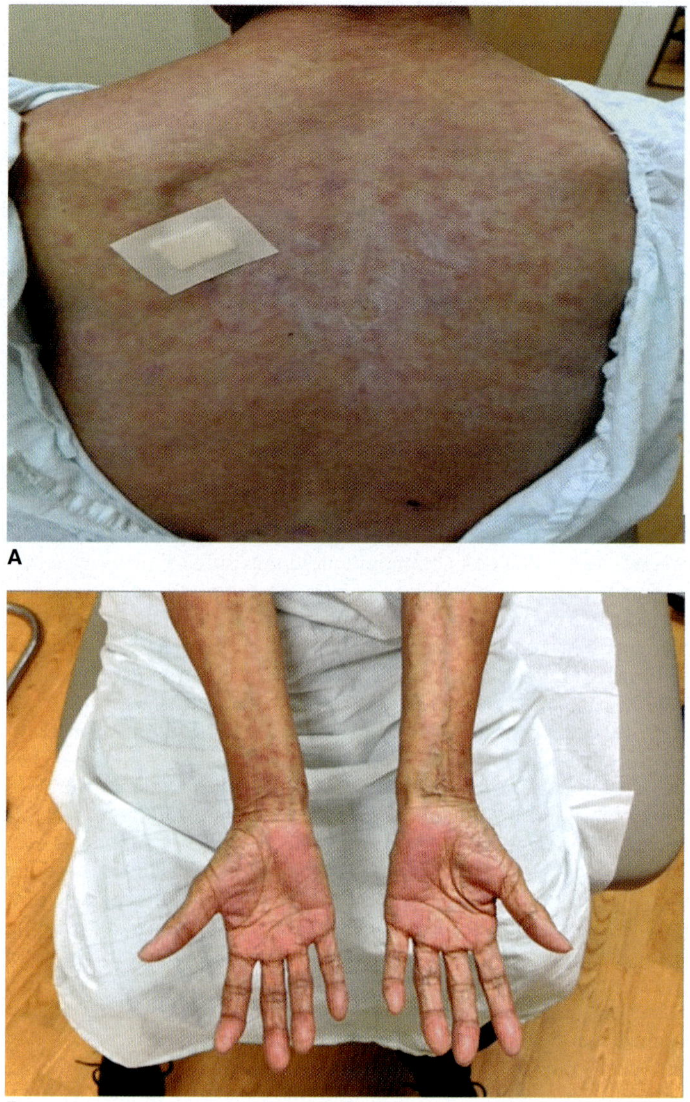

A

B

FIGURES 78-9. Graft-versus-host disease presents as numerous erythematous, dusky, and edematous annular macules and papules on the trunk **(A)** and palmar hand **(B)**. (Reproduced with permission from Dr. Cheri Frey.)

MASTOCYTOSIS

Mastocytosis is a rare neoplasm resulting from an abnormal proliferation of mast cells in various organs including the skin, liver, bone marrow, gastrointestinal tract, and spleen. Nearly 80% of cases of mastocytosis have been linked to a gain of function mutation of the proto-oncogene, c-kit at the 816 codons. The two forms of mastocytosis are systemic mastocytosis (SM) and cutaneous mastocytosis (CM), with CM being the more predominant form. Cutaneous mastocytosis (CM) includes maculopapular cutaneous mastocytosis (MPCM), also known as urticaria pigmentosa (UP), diffuse cutaneous mastocytosis (DCM), and cutaneous mastocytoma.[36] C-kit mutations are more common in pediatric cases of CM than in adults. Uncontrolled activation of mast cells and release of inflammatory mediators have also been discovered in cases of long-COVID, or postacute sequelae of COVID-19.[37] Mastocytosis can be indolent or aggressive, with the most aggressive forms including mast cell leukemia. The incidence of mastocytosis is estimated to be 1 in 10,000 and approximately 65% of all cases occur in children, although it can present at any stage in life from the neonatal period to adulthood.[38]

Cutaneous Manifestations The most common cutaneous presentation is UP. In UP, 0.5 to 1 cm red-brown round to oval macules and papules appear in early childhood with a predilection for the trunk and proximal extremities [**Figure 78-10**]. Areas such as the face, scalp, and acral surfaces are typically spared. UP may take on a monomorphic or polymorphic appearance. Telangiectasia macularis eruptiva perstans is a subset of UP where erythema and telangiectatic vessels appear, in addition to the more classic red-brown macules and papules. Mastocytomas are isolated tan-brown nodules or plaques that may present at birth or shortly thereafter. They are commonly located on the extremities and more than one mastocytoma may occur in a single patient. Furthermore, more than four mastocytomas should be classified as UP.[38]

Diffuse cutaneous mastocytosis (DCM) presents as a generalized redness and thickening of the skin at, or near the time of birth. Erythema may take on a brown or dusky purple hue in darker skin tones.

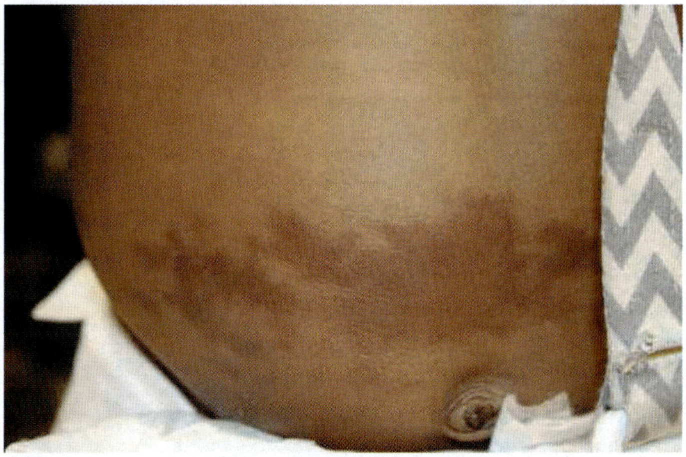

FIGURE 78-10. Mastocytosis presenting as a red-brown urticarial plaque on the trunk. (Reproduced with permission from Dr. A. Yasmine Kirkorian.)

Dermatographism is commonly associated with DCM in infancy. DCM in childhood and adulthood is marked by bulla formation, and in some cases, desquamation. A hallmark feature of cutaneous mastocytosis is the Darier sign, where swelling can be elicited by gentle stroking. Darier sign should not be performed on patients suspected of having DCM to avoid massive release of histamine resulting in systemic symptoms such as hypotension.[38]

Pathology Histopathologic features of cutaneous mastocytosis reveal a dense infiltration of mast cells in the superficial dermis and dilated vessels. The neoplastic mast cells show strong positivity for the CD117 stain.[39]

Treatment Patients with less aggressive forms of mastocytosis, such as CM, have an excellent prognosis. Cutaneous mastocytosis in children often follows a self-limited course. Only a few cases will persist into adulthood. Antihistamines are first-line treatments for CM. Solitary mastocytomas can be treated with intralesional steroids or removed with surgical excision.[39]

DISORDERS OF PLATELETS

ESSENTIAL THROMBOCYTOSIS

Essential Thrombocytosis (ET) is the most common myeloproliferative neoplasm, characterized by a platelet count greater than 45,000 in the presence of a mutation in one of the following genes: Janus Kinase (JAK2), Calreticulin (CALR), or myeloproliferative leukemia virus oncogene (MPL). ET presents more commonly in the sixth and seventh decades of life and has a female predominance.[40] Prior studies have indicated there are similar incidences and survival rates across different races for patients with myeloproliferative disorders including ET.[41] However, a more recent study conducted at the University of Illinois demonstrated non-Whites, particularly African Americans, were at significant risk for hemorrhagic complications of ET.[42]

The most common cutaneous manifestation in ET is pruritus. Erythromelalgia, painful redness, and swelling of the distal extremities have also been reported. Livedo reticularis, minor bleeding, acrocyanosis, and Raynaud phenomenon can occur in a minority of patients.[33] Patients are stratified into low-risk and high-risk categories based on age (<60 vs >60) and history of thrombosis. Low-risk patients are often treated with aspirin, while hydroxyurea is the first-line treatment for high-risk patients.[43]

PURPURA

Purpura is the name given to the discoloration of the skin or mucous membranes due to hemorrhage from blood vessels. Petechiae are pinpoint purpuric macules, while ecchymoses are larger extravasations of blood. Palpable purpura is due to inflammation of the blood vessels and is seen in vasculitis. Petechiae usually presents in the setting of thrombocytopenia, and coagulation defects usually present with large ecchymoses. Purpura can occur in the setting of thrombocytopenia including thrombotic thrombocytopenic purpura (TTP) as well as solar (actinic) purpura. The latter is a common benign disorder of dermal connective tissues due to skin damage from chronic sun exposure. It is characterized by dark purple macules or patches on sun-exposed areas, especially the dorsal hands and the extensor forearms of elderly patients. These findings may spontaneously resolve without intervention. The best treatment for solar purpura is preventive and involves protection from excessive sun exposure through the application of sunscreen and wearing long-sleeved shirts.[44]

PLASMA CELL DISORDERS

CRYOGLOBULINEMIA

Cryoglobulinemia is a rare condition that presents as retiform purpura at acral sites. It affects about 1 in 100,000 individuals.[45] Cryoglobulins are immunoglobulins in the blood that reversibly precipitate with cold exposure. In the cold, cryoglobulins change their configuration and become water-insoluble, resulting in increased blood viscosity and possible occlusion. Cryoglobulins cause disease via two mechanisms: occlusion (type I) or immune complex-mediated vasculitis (types II, III). Type I cryoglobulinemia commonly occurs in the setting of an underlying plasma cell dyscrasia or lymphoproliferative disorder, while types II and III often present with chronic inflammatory disorders, for example, HCV infection.

Cryoglobulinemia presents as purpuric or necrotic plaques, often retiform, at acral sites of cold exposure. Other findings include acral cyanosis, livedo reticularis, Raynaud phenomenon, arthralgia, and myalgia. Of note, it is imperative to treat acral skin lesions before the development of digital gangrene. Skin biopsy in the setting of cryoglobulinemia does not provide as definitive of a diagnosis as other skin conditions, as histology may show nonspecific findings seen in other vasculitides and vasculopathy (eg, leukocytoclastic vasculitis, vessel occlusion). Instead, laboratory tests are helpful. The presence of cryoglobulin coupled with a low C4 complement level is highly suggestive of cryoglobulinemia. Management includes cold avoidance and treatment of any underlying disorder. Plasmapheresis or plasma exchange provides short-term improvement. However, for more severe cases, oral corticosteroids in combination with rituximab may be utilized.[45]

DISORDERS OF COAGULATION

ANTIPHOSPHOLIPID SYNDROME

Antiphospholipid syndrome (APS) is an acquired autoimmune disorder characterized by hypercoagulability, resulting in recurrent thrombotic events, pregnancy loss, thrombocytopenia, valvular heart disease, and/or nephropathy. APS may develop as a primary disease or secondary to other medical conditions such as systemic lupus erythematosus, malignancy, or infection.[46]

Epidemiology To date, the only population-based study of newly diagnosed APS in the United States was performed in Olmsted County, Minnesota, with a predominantly White cohort (97%). Based on limited data, the estimated incidence of APS is 1 to 2 cases per 100,000 persons per year and the estimated prevalence is 40 to 50 cases per 100,000 persons. The mean age of diagnosis is 50 years. Worldwide, there is a slight female predominance, but the female-to-male ratio approaches 1:1 after the exclusion of patients with lupus.[47] The risk of thrombotic events is elevated in patients with systemic lupus erythematosus (SLE) and has been attributed to both systemic inflammations and to the presence of antiphospholipid antibodies.[47]

Pathogenesis The pathogenesis of APS is multifactorial. Antiphospholipid syndrome can occur in otherwise healthy persons without an underlying systemic autoimmune disease (primary APS) or with other systemic autoimmune diseases, particularly SLE. Compared with SLE patients without antiphospholipid antibodies (aPL), those with aPL have a higher prevalence of thrombosis, pregnancy morbidity, valve disease, pulmonary hypertension, livedo reticularis, thrombocytopenia, hemolytic anemia, acute/chronic renal vascular lesions, and moderate/severe cognitive impairment; worse quality of life; and higher risk of organ damage.[48] The presence of aPL, specifically antibeta2-GPI, is crucial to clot formation. While thrombotic events are the hallmark of APS, platelet activation, complement activation, disruption of innate anticoagulants (proteins C and S), and fibrinolysis are also important mediators of disease. A "second hit" theory has been proposed whereby innate immune responses trigger clot formation in APS.[49] In a study of 97 patients with a history of venous thromboembolic events meeting criteria for SLE, African American patients were less likely to have a clinically significant aPL profile. Thus, the authors concluded that a negative aPL profile in African American patients did not decrease VTE risk.[50]

Cutaneous Manifestations Cutaneous manifestations are common in APS, with a significant number of patients reporting skin findings as the initial presenting sign of disease. These cutaneous manifestations include livedo reticularis, livedo racemosa, necrotizing vasculitis, skin ulcerations, superficial thrombophlebitis, and gangrene. As such, dermatologists may play a key role in identifying patients at risk for APS based on cutaneous evidence of thrombotic disease.[51] In livedo racemosa, the reticular configuration is discontinuous. There are asymmetric patchy areas on the lower extremities, and the trunk and upper extremities may also be involved. Erythema may be subtle in darker skin or it may appear violaceous. Livedo reticularis and livedo racemosa may appear deep red, maroon, violaceous, or brown in darker skin colors. They may be masked completely in the darkest skin colors. In superficial thrombophlebitis, the superficial vein is often palpable as a tender cord with erythema and edema of the overlying skin and soft tissues. Induration, pain, and erythema are often present along the course of the vein. In darker skin, erythema may appear gray, dark brown, or violaceous.

Diagnosis APS classification is based on the Sydney criteria where at least one clinical criterion and one laboratory criterion must be present for the diagnosis. Clinical criteria include venous or arterial thrombosis or fetal loss. Laboratory criteria can be met by the presence of medium to high levels of IgG or IgM anticardiolipin, lupus anticoagulant, or anti–beta-2 glycoprotein I, on at least two occasions at least 12 weeks apart.[52]

Treatment Treatment of APS is only indicated once a thrombotic event has occurred. Once treatment is initiated, lifelong use of anticoagulation or antiplatelet therapy is necessary. In pregnancy, heparin with or without low-dose aspirin is utilized. Other treatments include systemic therapy for associated autoimmune disorders and the elimination of other risk factors (eg, oral contraceptives, smoking, hypertension, and/or hyperlipidemia). Vitamin D may be useful as prophylaxis against thrombosis in patients with SLE due to the effects of vitamin D on tissue factors.[53]

DISSEMINATED INTRAVASCULAR COAGULATION

Disseminated intravascular coagulation (DIC) is a life-threatening syndrome characterized by disseminated and uncontrolled activation of coagulation. This leads to intravascular thrombosis and progressive consumption coagulopathy, which results in an increased bleeding risk. A breadth of pathological conditions may trigger DIC, including sepsis, cancer, trauma, and obstetric complications.[54] DIC, like other coagulopathies, presents with nonspecific retiform purpura. A skin biopsy may not be as helpful as a thorough history and physical exam, along with a laboratory workup. A coagulation panel can confirm the disease, while D-dimer is an inexpensive, rapid test that screens for thrombosis (though not specific for DIC). Early diagnosis and treatment are of critical importance to favorable patient outcomes.

Treatment of the underlying disorder is of paramount importance in all cases of DIC. Suppression of coagulation activation is also important, though the benefit of anticoagulation therapy must be weighed against the risk of increased bleeding. If bleeding is observed due to a significant decrease in platelets and coagulation factors (consumption coagulopathy), replacement therapy is warranted. Fresh frozen plasma may be utilized.[55]

DRUGS

HYDROXYUREA-INDUCED SKIN CHANGES

Hydroxyurea (HU) is an antimetabolite used in the treatment of myeloproliferative disorders. Hydroxyurea interferes with DNA synthesis and repair through noncompetitive inhibition of ribonucleotide reductase. Cutaneous side effects of HU include leg ulcers, commonly localized to the perimalleolar region. Although the underlying myeloproliferative disorders may induce vascular occlusion, leg ulcers have been reported after long-term HU use in patients with stable disease. HU-induced cytotoxicity of basal cell keratinocytes and HU-induced macrocytosis are thought to be underlying causes. Other cutaneous side effects of HU include nonmelanoma skin cancer, hyperpigmentation of the skin and nails, and alopecia.[56]

WARFARIN-INDUCED SKIN NECROSIS

Warfarin is an anticoagulant used frequently in the treatment of thrombotic disorders. Warfarin necrosis occurs in approximately 1 in 10,000 patients receiving this therapy. It occurs more commonly in females and in those with an underlying history of thrombophilic disease, such as protein C deficiency. African Americans are at an increased risk of bleeding induced by warfarin.[57]

Painful purpuric plaques progressing to necrotic ulcerations occur 2 to 5 days after warfarin initiation with a predilection for fatty areas such as the breast, thighs, and buttocks. In darker skin colors, erythema may appear violaceous, gray, or black. The suspected etiology of warfarin necrosis involves a transient hypercoagulable state induced by the initial rapid reduction in protein C without a corresponding reduction in clotting factors. Treatment consists of warfarin discontinuation, heparin administration, intravenous vitamin K, FFP or 4-factor prothrombin complex concentrate, and wound care.[58]

HEPARIN-INDUCED SKIN NECROSIS

Heparin-induced thrombocytopenia is a rare, antibody-mediated side effect of anticoagulation therapy. Antibodies form to the heparin/platelet-factor-4 complex leading to platelet aggregation, consumption, and occasionally, thrombosis. It typically develops around day 5 of heparin administration. It is important to note that patients with thrombosis do not always have thrombocytopenia. Cutaneous necrosis presents with painful purpuric plaques with or without marginal retiform purpura. Treatment requires the discontinuation of heparin. Finding a suitable alternative for anticoagulation may be challenging as the use of warfarin during an acute episode of HIT can lead to the progression of thrombosis due to its early effects on protein C.[59]

CONCLUSION

Hematologic disorders include disorders of red blood cells, white blood cells, platelets, and plasma cells. Several of these conditions disproportionately affect populations of color and have increased disease morbidity and mortality in these populations. Common skin manifestations of these disorders include cyanosis, erythema, hyperpigmentation, and purpura that present vastly different in darker skin tones. Dermatologists can play an important role in the detection of underlying hematologic conditions through awareness of these cutaneous manifestations and their appearance across skin colors.

REFERENCES

1. *Hematology glossary*. Hematology Glossary - Hematology.org. (n.d.). https://www.hematology.org/education/patients/blood-basics. Accessed 1 Dec. 2023.
2. Piel FB, Hay SI, Gupta S, Weatherall DJ, Williams TN. Global burden of sickle cell anaemia in children under five, 2010-2050: modelling based on demographics, excess mortality, and interventions. PLoS Med. 2013;10(7):e1001484.
3. Centers for Disease Control and Prevention. *Data & statistics on Sickle Cell Disease*. Centers for Disease Control and Prevention. https://www.cdc.gov/ncbddd/sicklecell/data.html. Accessed 1 Dec. 2023.
4. *Identifying AEFI in diverse skin colour*. The Melbourne Vaccine Education Centre(MVEC).https://mvec.mcri.edu.au/references/identifying-aefi-in-diverse-skin-colour/. Accessed 1 Dec. 2023.
5. Wawer AA, Jennings A, Fairweather-Tait SJ. Iron status in the elderly: a review of recent evidence. *Mech Ageing Dev*. 2018;175:55-73.
6. Zakai NA, McClure LA, Prineas R, et al. Correlates of anemia in American blacks and whites: the REGARDS Renal Ancillary Study. *Am J Epidemiol*. 2009;169(3):355-364.
7. Le CH. The Prevalence of Anemia and Moderate-Severe Anemia in the US Population (NHANES 2003-2012). PLoS One. 2016;11(11):e0166635. Published 2016 Nov 15. doi:10.1371/journal.pone.0166635.
8. DeLoughery TG. Iron deficiency anemia. *Med Clin North Am*. 2017;101(2):319-332.
9. Johnson-Wimbley TD, Graham DY. Diagnosis and management of iron deficiency anemia in the 21st century. *Therap Adv Gastroenterol*. 2011;4(3):177-184.
10. Weiss G. Pathogenesis and treatment of anaemia of chronic disease. *Blood Rev*. 2002;16:87-96.
11. Weiss G, Goodnough LT. Anemia of chronic disease. *N Engl J Med*. 2005;352:1011-1023.
12. Lu X, Chang R (2022). *Polycythemia Vera*. Treasure Island, FL: StatPearls Publishing; 2022.
13. Chaiter Y, Brenner B, Aghai E, Tatarsky I. High incidence of myeloproliferative disorders in Ashkenazi Jews in northern Israel. *Leuk Lymphoma*. 1992;7(3):251-255.
14. Altomare I, Colucci P, Parasuraman S, Paranagama DC, Al-Janadi A. Disease characteristics of minority patient populations with polycythemia vera: an analysis from the reveal study. *Blood*. 2018;132(Supplement 1):4735.
15. *Color awareness: A must for patient assessment*. American Nurse. https://www.myamericannurse.com/color-awareness-a-must-for-patient-assessment/. Accessed 1 Dec 2023.
16. Siegel FP, Tauscher J, Petrides PE. Aquagenic pruritus in polycythemia vera: characteristics and influence on quality of life in 441 patients. *Am J Hematol*. 2013;88(10):925.
17. Nguyen HT, Nguyen CTH. Cutaneous manifestations indicate an underlying polycythemia vera. *J Clin Rheumatol*. 2021;27(3):e109-e110.
18. Pincelli MS, Echavarria AMJ, Criado PR, et al. Livedo racemosa: clinical, laboratory, and histopathological findings in 33 patients. *Int J Low Extrem Wounds*. 2021;20(1):22-28.
19. Hinds GA, Heald P. Cutaneous T-cell lymphoma in skin of color. *J Am Acad Dermatol*. 2009;60(3):359-378.
20. Brown-Korsah JB, McKenzie S, Omar D, Syder NC, Elbuluk N, Taylor SC. variations in genetics, biology, and phenotype of cutaneous disorders in skin of color. Part I: genetic, biological, and structural differences in skin of color. *J Am Acad Dermatol*. 2022;S0190-9622(22)02243-5.
21. Pulitzer M. Cutaneous T-cell lymphoma. *Clin Lab Med*. 2017;37(3):527-546.
22. Abraham J, Wei G, Desai SR, Seminario-Vidal L. A cross-sectional analysis of quality of life in skin of color patients with cutaneous T-cell lymphoma: an exploratory study. *J Am Acad Dermatol*. 2022;S0190-9622(22)00100-1.
23. McKenzie S, Brown-Korsah JB, Syder NC, Omar D, Taylor SC, Elbuluk N. Variations in genetics, biology, and phenotype of cutaneous disorders in skin of color. Part II: differences in clinical presentation and disparities in cutaneous disorders in skin of color. *J Am Acad Dermatol*. 2022;S0190-9622(22)02242-3.
24. Vitiello P, Sica A, Ronchi A, Caccavale S, Franco R, Argenziano G. Primary cutaneous B-cell lymphomas: an update. *Front Oncol*. 2020;10:651.
25. Geller S, Pulitzer M, Myskowski P, Kheterpal M. Low-grade cutaneous b-cell lymphoma in African American patients. *J Drugs Dermatol*. 2018;17(12):1334-1337.
26. Cerroni L. *Skin Lymphoma: The Illustrated Guide*. Hoboken, NJ: John Wiley & Sons; 2020.
27. Chen ST, Barnes J, Duncan L. Primary cutaneous B-cell lymphomas-clinical and histopathologic features, differential diagnosis, and treatment. *Semin Cutan Med Surg*. 2018;37(1):49-55.
28. Shenoy PJ, Malik N, Nooka A, et al. Racial differences in the presentation and outcomes of diffuse large B-cell lymphoma in the United States. *Cancer*. 2011;117(11):2530-2540.
29. Sekeres MA, Peterson B, Dodge RK, et al. Cancer and Leukemia Group B. Differences in prognostic factors and outcomes in African Americans and whites with acute myeloid leukemia. *Blood*. 2004;103(11):4036-4042.
30. Morishima Y, Kawase T, Malkki M, et al. Significance of ethnicity in the risk of acute graft-versus-host disease and leukemia relapse after unrelated donor hematopoietic stem cell transplantation. *Biol Blood Marrow Transplant*. 2013;19(8):1197-1203.
31. Justiz Vaillant AA, Modi P, Mohammadi O. Graft versus host disease. Treasure Island, FL: StatPearls Publishing; 2022.
32. Sharma N, Efebera Y. Acute graft-versus-host disease, prophylaxis and therapy. *OBM Transplant*. 2021;5(1):1.
33. Johnston R. *SD–Weedon's Skin Pathology Essentials E-Book*. London: Churchill Livingstone; 2011.
34. Jaglowski SM, Blazar BR. How ibrutinib, a B-cell malignancy drug, became an FDA-approved second-line therapy for steroid-resistant chronic GVHD. *Blood Adv*. 2018;2(15):2012-2019.
35. Hartmann K, Escribano L, Grattan C, et al. Cutaneous manifestations in patients with mastocytosis: Consensus report of the European Competence Network on Mastocytosis; the American Academy of Allergy, Asthma & Immunology; and the European Academy of Allergology and Clinical Immunology. *J Allergy Clin Immunol*. 2016;137(1):35-45.
36. Arun S, Storan A, Myers B. Mast cell activation syndrome and the link with long COVID. *Br J Hosp Med (Lond)*. 2022;83(7):1-10.
37. Di Raimondo C, Del Duca E, Silvaggio D, et al. Cutaneous mastocytosis: a dermatological perspective. *Australas J Dermatol*. 2021;62(1):e1-e7.
38. Matito A, Azaña JM, Torrelo A, Alvarez-Twose I. Cutaneous mastocytosis in adults and children: new classification and prognostic factors. *Immunol Allergy Clin North Am*. 2018;38(3):351-363.
39. Ashorobi D, Gohari P. (2022). *Essential Thrombocytosis*. Treasure Island, FL: StatPearls Publishing; 2022.
40. Saraf S, Shergill A, Patel PR, et al. Role of ethnicity in clinical outcomes of patients with ph-negative myeloproliferative neoplasms. *Blood* 2012;120 (21):2076.
41. Khan I, Shergill A, Saraf SL, et al. Outcome disparities in Caucasian and non-Caucasian patients with myeloproliferative neoplasms. *Clin Lymphoma Myeloma Leuk*. 2016;16(6):350-357.
42. Cozzani E, Iurlo A, Merlo G, Cattaneo D, Burlando M, Pierri I, Gugliotta L, Parodi A. Essential thrombocythemia: the dermatologic point of view. *Clin Lymphoma Myeloma Leuk*. 2015;15(12):739-747.
43. Hafsi W, Masood S, Badri T. *Actinic Purpura*. Treasure Island, FL: StatPearls Publishing; 2021.
44. Bhandari J, Awais M, Aeddula NR. *Cryoglobulinemia*. Treasure Island, FL: StatPearls Publishing; 2022.
45. Caporuscio S, Sorgi M, Nisticò S, et al. Cutaneous manifestations in antiphospholipid syndrome. *Int J Immunopathol Pharmacol*. 2015:270-273.
46. Bustamante JG, Goyal A, Rout P, Singhal M. Antiphospholipid Syndrome. In: StatPearls. Treasure Island (FL): StatPearls Publishing; May 6, 2024.
47. Ünlü O, Zuily S, Erkan D. The clinical significance of antiphospholipid antibodies in systemic lupus erythematosus. *Eur J Rheumatol*. 2016;3(2): 75-84.
48. Duarte-García A, Pham MM, Crowson CS, et al. The epidemiology of antiphospholipid syndrome: a population-based study. *Arthritis Rheum*. 2019;71(9):1545-1552.
49. Dieudonné Y, Guffroy A, Poindron V, et al. B cells in primary antiphospholipid syndrome: Review and remaining challenges. *Autoimmun Rev*. 2021;20(5):102798.
50. Gkrouzman E, Peng M, Davis-Porada J, Kirou KA. Venous thromboembolic events in African American lupus patients in association with antiphospholipid antibodies compared to White patients. *Arthritis Care Res* (Hoboken). 2022;74(4):656-664.
51. Meroni PL, Borghi MO, Raschi E, Tedesco F. Pathogenesis of antiphospholipid syndrome: understanding the antibodies. *Nat Rev Rheumatol*. 2011;7(6):330-339.
52. Rahman, A. Management of antiphospholipid syndrome. *Clin Rheumatol*. 2020;39:2111-2114.
53. Petri M. Antiphospholipid syndrome. *Transl Res*. 2020;225:70-81.
54. Papageorgiou C, Jourdi G, Adjambri E, et al. Disseminated intravascular coagulation: an update on pathogenesis, diagnosis, and therapeutic strategies. *Clin Appl Thromb Hemost*. 2018;24(9_suppl):8S-28S.

55. De T, Alarcon C, Hernandez, W, et al. Association of genetic variants with warfarin-associated bleeding among patients of African descent. *JAMA* 2018;320:1670-1677.
56. Malato A, Rossi E, Palumbo GA, Guglielmelli P, Pugliese N. Drug-related cutaneous adverse events in Philadelphia chromosome-negative myeloproliferative neoplasms: a literature review. *Int J Mol Sci.* 2020;21(11):3900.
57. Pourdeyhimi N, Bullard Z. Warfarin-induced skin necrosis. *Hosp Pharm.* 2014;49(11):1044-1048.
58. Handschin AE, Trentz O, Kock HJ, Wanner GA. Low molecular weight heparin-induced skin necrosis – a systematic review. *Langenbecks Arch Surg.* 2005;390:249-225.
59. Sator P, Kiprov A, Feldmann R, Breier F, Steiner A. Heparin-induced skin necrosis. *J Eur Acad Dermatol Venereol.* 2016;30(1):161-163.

CHAPTER 79

Cutaneous Manifestations of Renal Disease

Courtney Squirewell
Sebastian Cruz
Scott Worswick

KEY POINTS

- Racial and ethnic minority populations are at the greatest risk of chronic kidney disease, with diabetes mellitus, hypertension, and obesity being the major contributing factors.
- Prominent cutaneous manifestations of renal failure include pruritus, nail changes, and pigmentary alterations.
- Common treatments for end-stage renal disease, such as dialysis, can also lead to cutaneous side effects.
- While renal transplantation may help treat dialysis-induced cutaneous conditions, patients are still at risk for posttransplant cutaneous diseases.
- Cutaneous manifestations of renal disease can disrupt quality of life, so early detection particularly in SOC where conditions may have varied presentation and proper management are vital.

INTRODUCTION

Chronic kidney disease (CKD) affects between 8% and 16% of the world population, with minority populations being at greater risk. Diabetes, hypertension, and obesity constitute the major causes. In the United States, the prevalence of CKD in 2015-2016 was 13% in non-Hispanic Whites, 15.3% in Mexican Americans, and 16.5% in non-Hispanic Blacks.[1] With increasing loss of kidney function and decreasing ability to properly filter the blood, excess toxins and waste products accumulate and lead to uremia.

There are a variety of cutaneous manifestations of CKD, including uremic pruritus, ichthyosis, xerosis, pallor, and nail changes. These conditions may alter a patient's quality of life, causing severe complications such as sleep deprivation and depression.[2] These changes continue to worsen as the disease progresses to end-stage renal disease (ESRD), which is fatal without treatment. Similar to their most common predisposing conditions, both CKD and ESRD are 1.5 to 4.0 times more common in minority adults.[3] The major cause of ESRD in all racial and ethnic groups is diabetes mellitus, which occurs at a higher rate in African Americans, Hispanics, and Native Americans.[4] African Americans also have the highest rate of hypertension-related ESRD.[4] Studies have shown that African Americans are most likely to progress to ESRD and require renal replacement therapy.[3] The incidence rate of pediatric ESRD is also increasing across the globe.[5] Despite the available therapies, such as renal transplantation or dialysis, ESRD remains a leading cause of death worldwide.

RENAL DYSFUNCTION LEADING TO NONSPECIFIC CUTANEOUS MANIFESTATIONS

XEROSIS AND ICHTHYOSIS

Xerosis is the most common skin change seen in CKD patients, occurring in about 50% to 85% of patients. It is most noticeable on the extremities.[6] Atrophy of the eccrine sweat glands and pilosebaceous follicles has been documented as a possible driver of its pathogenesis. The decrease in lipid levels in the skin surface causes decreased water content in the stratum corneum and a loss of its integrity. Impairment of the skin barrier, metabolic imbalances, and depletion of volume due to diuretics have also been postulated to be contributing factors.[6] Thus, use of emollients, avoiding irritants, and topical corticosteroids can help provide relief. With ESRD, transplantation can provide permanent resolution.

Uremia that results in xerosis may also lead to acquired ichthyosis, which appears clinically as white, gray, or dark brown "fish scales." Notably, like xerosis, ichthyosis can also occur in association with many other diseases and is not specific to patients with renal disease.[1]

UREMIC PRURITUS

About 15% to 49% of patients with chronic renal failure are affected by pruritus.[7] Pruritus is known to worsen after starting hemodialysis treatment, and about 90% of patients receiving hemodialysis suffer from pruritus.[2] Pruritus is often severe and can be localized or generalized, although the back is most commonly affected.[7,8] There is no associated primary dermatitis, but chronic scratching and rubbing can lead to excoriations, lichen simplex chronicus, and prurigo nodularis on examination.[2,7] The pathophysiology of uremic pruritus is multifactorial. There are many hypotheses described, including the chronic inflammatory state of CKD, increased μ-opioid receptor activity and κ-opioid receptor blockade,[9] and elevated levels of neurotrophin-4.[2,10] Xerosis, decreased ability to sweat, deposition of uremic toxins, calcium and phosphate dysregulation, hyperparathyroidism, and vitamin excess and deficiencies are other potential contributing factors.[2,7] Pruritus can lead to significantly decreased quality of life, interfering with daily activities and sleep. Potential treatments are numerous and include topical agents (emollients, capsaicin, corticosteroids, and calcineurin inhibitors), phototherapy, oral agents (antihistamines, gabapentin, naltrexone, rifaximin, dronabinol, and montelukast), or intravenous treatments (naloxone).[2,7] In severe renal disease, renal transplantation is the best therapeutic option.[7,11]

NAIL CHANGES

Nail changes occur in about one in five patients with renal failure, with Mees lines (transverse bands of leukonychia) and half-and-half nails being most common.[6,7,11] Half-and-half nails (also known as Lindsay nails) can be seen in association with several conditions, but they are most characteristic of renal failure and are particularly common in dialysis patients. Both fingernails and toenails demonstrate proximal white discoloration and distal red to brown color, neither of which are blanchable.[7] Although the pathogenesis is not well understood, it has been attributed to hyperpigmentation and increased levels of β-melanin-secreted hormone (β-MSH). The nail bed is believed to be the primary pathologic site since the bands do not move with nail growth. Renal transplantation may lead to resolution. Leukonychia, koilonychia, and splinter hemorrhages have also been noted in association with ESRD patients.[8]

PIGMENTARY CHANGES

There are multiple pigmentary changes that have been described in the skin of renal failure patients: pallor, hyperpigmentation, and yellow discoloration are the most common. Pallor occurs in 8% of uremic patients, hyperpigmentation in an estimated 22%, and yellow discoloration in 40%.[12] Pallor is commonly attributed to erythropoietin deficiency and anemia of chronic disease. While pallor in skin of color may be difficult to appreciate, patients have also been noted to have distinct pallor of the mucosal surfaces.[13] Hyperpigmentation is due to increasing melanin production, a result of the poor metabolism of β-melanocyte-stimulating hormone (β-MSH) by the kidneys.[1] Pigmented macules are slightly more common in patients with CKD than in those without. While hyperpigmentation may be subtle in skin of color, it may be more appreciable on acral surfaces.[13] Yellow discoloration has been attributed to dermal and subcutaneous deposition of pigment (lipochromes and carotenoids) and may present more subtly in skin of color. Brown or gray discoloration is caused by hemosiderin deposition in the skin, especially on the lower legs.[1,12] Patients may also notice easier bruising or purpura as a result of hematologic abnormalities.[11]

UREMIC FROST

Uremic frost is a rare manifestation of chronic renal failure associated with serum urea levels greater than 200 mg/dL. Urea deposits in the skin as a result of urea accumulation in sweat glands.[8,11] It only occurs in about 3% of patients with CKD and responds well to hemodialysis.[6] With dialysis, this finding has become rare in the United States. The skin may appear grayish with a metallic hue and have underlying hyperpigmentation and/or pallor. It is a finding that can look different in patients with skin of color.[11]

ACQUIRED PERFORATING DERMATOSIS

The acquired perforating disorders include perforating folliculitis, Kyrle disease, elastosis perforans serpiginosa (EPS), and reactive perforating collagenosis (RPC). They are commonly associated with CKD and diabetes mellitus.[11] There is a predominance of this disorder in African American patients.[11] It is characterized by a disruption in the transepidermal elimination of dermal connective tissue components, a process through which structurally altered connective tissue components (such as collagen or elastic fibers) are eliminated through the epidermis without damage to the surrounding tissue.[11,12] It is hypothesized that fibronectin deposition in the dermal matrix and diabetic vasculopathy-mediated epidermal abnormalities may play a role in the disease process.[12] Scratching-induced trauma, calcium deposition, and defects in the metabolism of vitamins A or D are also thought to contribute.

Lesions are typically dome-shaped papulonodules with a centrally crusted crater.[7,8] In Kyrle disease, the trunk and extremities are affected before the scalp and face. Kyrle lesions are verrucous, folliculocentric papules that may be hyperpigmented and dark brown to black in darker skin types [**Figure 79-1**]. The lesions of EPS are commonly found on the face and neck and typically are characterized by umbilicated red to red brown papules, often in a serpiginous configuration and sometimes with overlying keratosis.

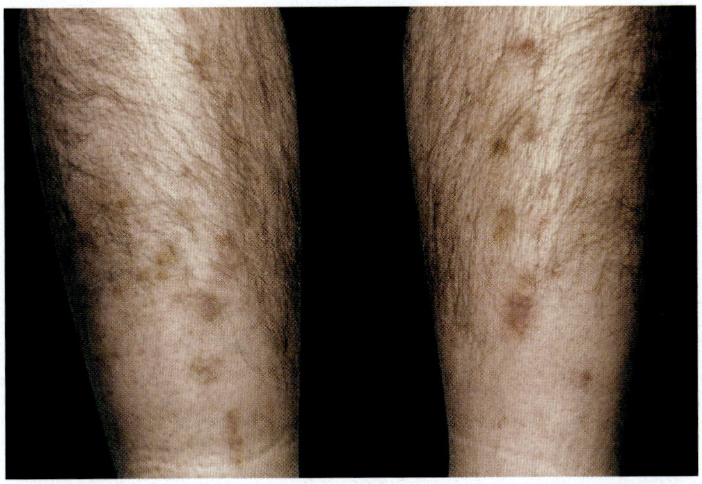

FIGURE 79-1. Kyrle disease is a perforating skin condition characterized by the presence of large keratotic papules distributed widely throughout the body, as seen on this patient. (Used with permission from the Department of Dermatology, Washington Hospital Center, Washington, DC.)

Perforating lesions may spontaneously resolve as newer lesions develop.[11] Spontaneous and complete resolution of lesions is common, but when symptomatic or progressive there are some treatment options available. These treatments aim to provide symptomatic relief and include narrowband ultraviolet B (UVB) phototherapy, topical steroids, oral retinoids, cryotherapy, and ablative lasers.[11,12]

ACUTE INTERSTITIAL NEPHRITIS SECONDARY TO DRUG

Acute interstitial nephritis (AIN) is characterized by inflammation in the renal interstitium. When affecting the skin, drug-induced AIN is characterized by a triad of dermatitis, fever, and eosinophilia. Dermatitis occurs in fact in only 20% to 30% of patients and is often symmetric and morbilliform morphologically.[14] Manifestations occur within a few days to weeks after drug initiation.

AIN is in some cases associated with drug reaction with eosinophilia and systemic symptoms (DRESS), which is characterized by internal organ involvement, fever, lymphadenopathy, facial edema, and rash. Also known as drug-induced hypersensitivity syndrome (DIHS), DRESS is rare but can be fatal if left untreated. The dermatitis is often morbilliform, pruritic, and starts on the face and upper body. It can progress or evolve to bullous, erythrodermic, purpuric, or other rarer presentations. Renal involvement is particularly common when allopurinol is the causative agent, whereas vancomycin is a more recently implicated common trigger for DRESS syndrome with renal involvement.[14,15] Cessation of the offending medication is of paramount importance, and systemic immunosuppressive medications are often used to treat this eruption, most notably corticosteroids and cyclosporine.

BULLOUS DERMATOSES

The two bullous dermatoses that patients with chronic renal failure most commonly develop are porphyria cutanea tarda (PCT) and pseudoporphyria. Prevalence of PCT in hemodialysis patients ranges from 1.2% to 18%.[8] PCT is an autosomal dominant disorder caused by a defect in heme biosynthesis due to a deficiency in uroporphyrinogen decarboxylase.[8,9] Like pseudoporphyria, PCT presents with photodistributed vesiculobullous lesions, particularly on the forearms and dorsal hands. The face, chest, feet, and legs may also be involved. Lesions may heal with scarring, milia, or hyperpigmentation.[7,9,12] Hypertrichosis and sclerodermoid plaques can be seen in PCT but are not usually found in patients with pseudoporphyria. First-line treatments of PCT include serial phlebotomy in conjunction with hematology and oral antimalarials.[9,12]

In addition to chronic renal failure and hemodialysis, pseudoporphyria can be associated with medications and ultraviolet A (UVA) exposure. Although it resembles PCT clinicopathologically, psuedoporphyria does not result from abnormal porphyrin metabolism. Photodistributed vesiculobullous lesions are the characteristic cutaneous finding. Commonly located on dorsal hands and face, blisters may burst early and resolve with scarring, milia, and crusting over a few weeks.[7,8] Scarring in skin of color individuals can include dyspigmentation of the skin. Sun protection and discontinuation of any triggering medications are the mainstays of treatment.

CALCIPHYLAXIS AND CALCINOSIS CUTIS

Calciphylaxis is life-threatening and commonly develops in association with chronic renal failure and hemodialysis; hepatic disease, medications, solid organ malignancies, and connective tissue diseases are lesser associations. It is characterized by widespread calcification of tissues and blood vessels, resulting in livedo reticularis, retiform purpura, and eventual progression to necrotic plaques[8] [**Figure 79-2A** and **B**]. Lesions are commonly found in fat-bearing areas such as the thighs, abdomen, buttocks, and upper extremities.[7,8] Pain is often excruciating, and the prognosis is poor with a 5-year mortality rate of greater than 50% often attributable to superinfection and resultant sepsis.[1] Treatments including bisphosphonates, cinacalcet, phosphate binders, sodium thiosulfate (intravenous, intralesional, and/or topical), low calcium dialysates, tissue plasminogen activator (tPA), and anticoagulants have been tried with varying levels of success.[11] There is no standard of care, though current practice is to treat patients with sodium thiosulfate during dialysis.

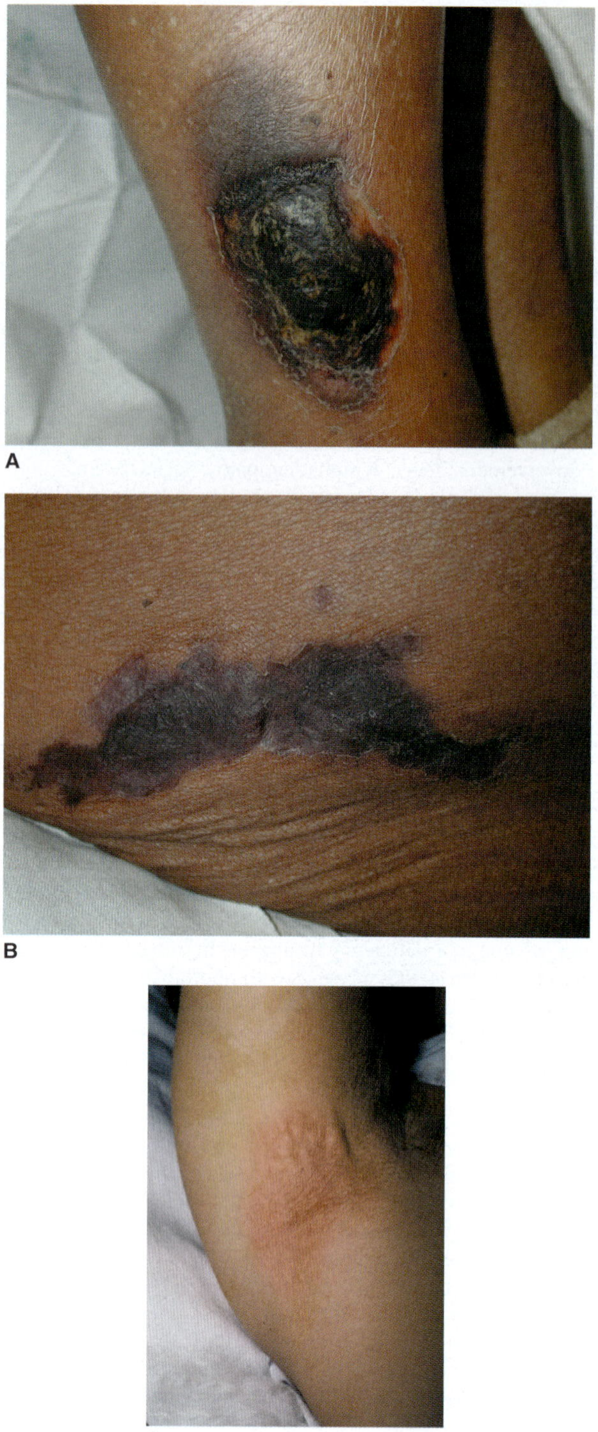

A

B

C

FIGURE 79-2. (A) Calciphylaxis with necrotic plaque on an edematous erythematous base appearing on the lower extremity of an African American patient on dialysis. **(B)** Calciphylaxis can be seen on the proximal lower extremity of a patient on dialysis; the acute onset of this condition manifested with painful burgundy, necrotic, depressed plaques. **(C)** A case of calcinosis cutis axilla in a Hispanic female patient. (Used with permission from the Department of Dermatology, Washington Hospital Center, Washington, DC.)

Calcinosis cutis develops due to calcium salt deposits in the skin and subcutaneous tissues. Calcium deposition can be seen with both normal (as in dystrophic calcinosis cutis) or imbalanced calcium and/or phosphate levels (as in metastatic calcinosis cutis). Dystrophic calcinosis cutis is commonly associated with underlying connective tissue diseases, whereas the most common cause of metastatic disease is chronic renal failure with or without hemodialysis. This condition manifests clinically as firm, white to skin-colored papules, plaques, and nodules commonly located on the fingertips[9] [Figure 79-2C]. A chalky white discharge may also be noticed. Lesions are normally painless but may cause discomfort if the deposits lead to joint dysfunction.[11] Treatment of the underlying process is crucial, and adjunctive therapies with some reported success include diltiazem, bisphosphonates, intravenous immunoglobulin (IVIg), rituximab, and intralesional or topical sodium thiosulfate.[9]

CUTANEOUS MANIFESTATIONS OF DIALYSIS AND RENAL TRANSPLANTATION

DIALYSIS

Dialysis treatment, while necessary in many patients who have a loss of kidney function, may also lead to adverse cutaneous effects. Dialysis-induced pruritus is episodic, mild, and localized. Peritoneal dialysis has a lower severity of pruritus than hemodialysis.[9] Calciphylaxis can occur in association with either type of dialysis. Dialysis-associated amyloidosis occurs in almost all patients who have been on dialysis for 15 or more years and develops due to the deposition of β-2-microglobulin amyloid fibrils in soft tissue, joints, and bone. It presents with musculoskeletal symptoms, carpal tunnel syndrome, pedunculated sacral masses, lichenoid papules, and localized hyperpigmentation.[9]

RENAL TRANSPLANTATION

Immunosuppressive agents used to prevent organ failure after renal transplantation can lead to cutaneous effects in the skin, including an increased susceptibility to infection. *Staphylococcus aureus* and group A *Streptococcus* are the two most common culprits of bacterial infections, leading to impetigo, cellulitis, and erysipelas.[9] Patients in an immunosuppressed state are more susceptible to reactivation of viruses such as herpes simplex virus and varicella zoster virus. Common fungal infections such as pityriasis versicolor, candidiasis, and onychomycosis have been reported in higher numbers in renal transplant patients, and angioinvasive and deep fungal infections are also more prevalent.[9] Specific transplant medications can have unique adverse mucocutaneous effects, such as hypertrichosis, sebaceous hyperplasia, and gingival hyperplasia from cyclosporine. The skin is also the most common site of posttransplant malignancies. The skin also accounts for close to 40% of all posttransplant malignancies, with squamous cell carcinoma and basal cell carcinoma accounting for more than 90% of cases.[9] Children with renal disease are noted to have a higher incidence of warts, hypertrichosis, and gingival hypertrophy.[5] The incidence of hypertrichosis approximates 70% in children with renal transplantation, whereas the incidence of gingival hypertrophy is between 19% and 81%.[5] Children of color with renal transplantation have been found to develop more warts and fewer fungal infections compared to White children.[5] Cutaneous effects of transplantation can also impact children psychologically, leading to appearance-related distress and depression, and must be carefully managed.[5]

DISEASES AFFECTING THE KIDNEYS WITH SPECIFIC CUTANEOUS MANIFESTATIONS

SYSTEMIC SARCOIDOSIS

Sarcoidosis is characterized by granulomatous inflammation throughout the body, most often of the lungs, lymph nodes, skin, and eyes. It is most common in women ages 30 to 50 and in patients with northern European and African ancestry. Cutaneous signs predate other organ involvement and symptoms in approximately 30% of initial cases.[16] Red-brown to violaceous macules, papules, infiltrated plaques, and nodules have been reported. Treatment depends on the severity of the disease and includes systemic, intralesional or topical corticosteroids, steroid-sparing immunosuppressive agents, and biologics.

IgA VASCULITIS (HENOCH-SCHONLEIN PURPURA) AND OTHER VASCULITIDES

Cutaneous manifestations are often the first presenting sign of systemic vasculitides. Most commonly found in children, IgA vasculitis involves IgA deposition in blood vessels and the renal mesangium. It classically presents with the tetrad of palpable purpura, abdominal pain, hematuria, and arthralgias. Bullous lesions and necrotic ulcers may be present, particularly in adults. While most children will improve with supportive care, prolonged disease is more common in adults and can be managed with dapsone, colchicine, systemic corticosteroids, other immunosuppressive agents, rituximab, and IVIg. Of note, dapsone has been shown to be effective in treating chronic cutaneous involvement.[17]

Cryoglobulinemia is defined by the presence of circulating immunoglobulins that precipitate in the blood at colder temperatures. It is most strongly associated with underlying gammopathy, infection (particularly with hepatitis C virus), and connective tissue diseases. Cutaneous findings include palpable purpura, livedo reticularis, acrocyanosis, and Raynaud's phenomenon.[14] Systemic symptoms are common, including arthralgias and peripheral neuropathy.

Other common systemic vasculitides that commonly involve the kidneys include granulomatosis with polyangiitis (GPA) and microscopic polyangiitis (MPA). The latter is a small- and medium-vessel nongranulomatous vasculitis associated with p-ANCA positivity and rapidly progressive glomerulonephritis. The former is associated with c-ANCA positivity and presents with upper and lower respiratory disease, renal involvement, and cutaneous signs. Cutaneous clues of systemic vasculitis include palpable purpura, necrotic ulcers, livedo reticularis, nodules, and sometimes urticarial lesions.[14] Therapy includes systemic immunosuppression with corticosteroids, rituximab, cyclophosphamide, or steroid-sparing agents.

FABRY DISEASE

Fabry disease (FD) is an X-linked lysosomal storage disorder due to deficient or absent lysosomal α-galactosidase A activity. Although most patients are asymptomatic during the first stages of life, the deposition of glycosphingolipids within lysosomes leads to organ failure as the disease progresses.[18] The skin, kidneys, heart, and brain are most often affected. Angiokeratomas, a presenting feature for FD, are dark red to violaceous and are found in a swimsuit distribution on the buttocks, upper thighs, umbilicus, and groin. Hypohidrosis, anhidrosis, corneal changes, tinnitus, fatigue, and weight gain are other common symptoms. Renal involvement increases in severity as the patient ages. Untreated FD leads to end-stage renal failure, uremia, and death.[18] Treatment involves enzyme replacement therapy where available, supportive care, and electrodessication or laser therapy for angiokeratomas.

TUBEROUS SCLEROSIS

Tuberous sclerosis complex (TSC) is a multisystem genetic disorder that affects the skin, brain, retina, heart, kidneys, and lungs. It is caused by inactivating mutations of *TSC1* or *TSC2*, which encode hamartin and tuberin, respectively.[19] Note that 48% to 80% of patients have renal involvement, most commonly cysts and angiomyolipomas.[19] Cutaneous manifestations include facial angiofibromas, subungual or periungual fibromas, hypomelanotic macules ("ash-leaf spots"), connective tissue nevi ("Shagreen patches"), fibrous forehead papules, and confetti-like macules. Both systemic and topical mTOR inhibitors may help improve cutaneous findings.[19]

BIRT-HOGG-DUBE SYNDROME

Birt-Hogg-Dube syndrome (BHD) is a rare autosomal dominant disorder caused by a mutation in the *FLCN* gene that encodes folliculin. Clinically, it presents with multiple pulmonary cysts, bullous emphysema, recurrent spontaneous pneumothoraces, cutaneous findings, and various renal tumors. Skin lesions normally present during the third decade of life as white to skin-colored, dome-shaped papules around the nose, cheeks, neck, and trunk known as fibrofolliculomas and trichodiscomas.[20] Acrochordons are also common.[20,21] Cutaneous findings can be treated with laser therapy, curettage, and electrocautery.

FAMILIAL LEIOMYOMATOSIS CUTIS ET UTERI (REED SYNDROME)

Reed syndrome is an autosomal-dominant condition associated with an increased predisposition to developing benign smooth muscle tumors as well as cutaneous leiomyosarcomas. Resulting from a mutation of fumarate hydratase, a tumor suppressor protein, it is characterized by the association of multiple cutaneous and uterine leiomyomas (fibroids) with an increased risk of renal cell carcinoma (RCC) in a subset of patients.[22] Cutaneous leiomyomas are skin-colored or red-brown papulonodules.[23] The skin findings can remain asymptomatic, but there have been reported cases where the lesions have exhibited severe pain on cold exposure.[23] Treatment of cutaneous leiomyomas involves surgical excision (although recurrence is common), laser therapy, and other procedural interventions including botulinum toxin for associated pain.

SYSTEMIC LUPUS ERYTHEMATOSUS

Systemic lupus erythematosus (SLE) is a chronic autoinflammatory disease that affects multiple organ systems, including the skin and kidneys (the latter in about 50% of cases). Glomerulonephritis is the most characteristic form of renal involvement. There are three recognized subtypes of cutaneous lupus erythematosus: acute (ACLE), subacute (SCLE), and chronic (CCLE).[24] ACLE classically presents with an erythematous malar dermatitis involving the cheeks and nasal bridge with sparing of the nasolabial folds. SCLE often manifests as photodistributed annular, polycyclic and scaly erythematous papules and plaques. CCLE most commonly presents with scaly erythematous to violaceous plaques on the scalp or sun-exposed areas that can scar and result in patches with depigmented centers and surrounding peripheral hyperpigmentation. First-line cutaneous treatments include topical corticosteroids, photoprotection, and antimalarials.

SCLERODERMA

Scleroderma is characterized by inflammation and fibrosis in the skin and internal organs due to excess deposition of collagen and microvascular damage. Specific subtypes of systemic sclerosis include limited systemic sclerosis (CREST syndrome) and diffuse cutaneous systemic sclerosis (SSc), which is more common in African-Americans.[25] Patients with SSc have a higher prevalence of and more rapid progression of renal and pulmonary involvement, with renal crisis occurring in 5% to 10% of patients.

In CREST syndrome, the most common cutaneous manifestations are sclerosis of the distal extremities, matted telangiectasias, and tightening of the face and mouth. These patients also carry a high risk of developing calcinosis cutis, Raynaud phenomenon, and esophageal dysmotility.[25] In SSc, there exists diffuse sclerosis of the skin including not only the distal but also the proximal extremities. Raynaud phenomenon is present in 75% of SSc patients.

Treatment of SSc involves systemic corticosteroids and steroid-sparing immunosuppressive agents.[26] Calcium channel blockers and phosphodiesterase inhibitors may be helpful for Raynaud phenomenon. Patients with severe disease may require stem cell transplant.

NAIL-PATELLA SYNDROME

Nail-patella syndrome (NPS) is a rare autosomal dominant pleiotropic disorder characterized by dysplasia or absence of the nails, aplasia or hypoplasia of the patella, glaucoma, and progressive nephropathy.[27] Nails may be dystrophic, ridged, pitted, discolored, or separated by a longitudinal cleft of skin. Triangular lunulae may also be observed and are pathognomonic. The kidneys are affected in 40% of patients, with severity ranging from mild proteinuria to ESRD (the latter seen in about 5% of cases).[28]

CONCLUSION

Affecting nearly 843.6 million people worldwide as of 2017 (and 25% of the United States population), CKD and ESRD have become prominent causes of morbidity and mortality throughout the world. These conditions as well as their predisposing medical and socioeconomic factors are more common in African American, Hispanic, and other minority patients. African Americans, Native Americans, Asian Americans, and Hispanic Americans are 3.9, 2.7, 1.6, and 1.5 times more likely than white Americans to develop ESRD, respectively.[1,4] The cutaneous manifestations of renal disease in the skin are many. Pruritus, xerosis, nail changes, and pigmentary alterations are most common and can be non-specific. While such findings may be more subtle in skin of color, it is nevertheless crucial for clinicians to identify them and treat patients appropriately to prevent quality of life disruption and further complications. There are also a myriad of specific cutaneous findings including the triangular lunulae seen in nail-patella syndrome, the matted telangiectasias found in scleroderma, or the numerous leiomyomas seen in Reed syndrome. Skin and nails are often viewed as a window into internal disease: this is certainly the case for the aforementioned renal diseases. In promptly recognizing these conditions, clinicians can make a life-altering diagnosis and promote timely initiation of appropriate treatment.

REFERENCES

1. Kovesdy CP. Epidemiology of chronic kidney disease: an update 2022. *Kidney Int Supp*. 2022;12(1):7-11.
2. Trachtenberg A, Collister D, Rigatto C. Recent advances in the treatment of uremic pruritus. *Curr Opin Nephrol Hypertens*. 2020;29(5):465-470.
3. Norris KC, Williams SF, Rhee CM, et al. Hemodialysis disparities in African Americans: the deeply integrated concept of race in the social fabric of our society. *Semin Dial*. 2017;30(3):213-223.
4. T. Palmer Alves and J. Lewis. Racial differences in chronic kidney disease (CKD) and end-stage renal disease (ESRD) in the United States: a social and economic dilemma. *Clin Nephrol*. 2010;74:72-77.
5. Silverberg NB, Singh A, Laude TA. Cutaneous manifestations of chronic renal failure in children of color. *Pediatr Dermatol*. 2001;18(3):199-204.
6. Lupi O, Rezende L, Zangrando M, et al. Manifestações cutâneas na doença renal terminal. *An Bras Dermatol*. 2011;86(2):319.
7. Kurban MS, Boueiz A, Kibbi AG. Cutaneous manifestations of chronic kidney disease. *Clin Dermatol*. 2008;26(3):255-264.
8. Robles-Mendez JC, Vazquez-Martinez O, Ocampo-Candiani J. Skin manifestations of chronic kidney disease. *Actas dermo-sifiliográficas*. 2015;106(8):609-622.
9. Goel V, Sil A, Das A. Cutaneous manifestations of chronic kidney disease, dialysis and post-renal transplant: a review. *Indian J Dermatol*. 2021;66(1):3-11.
10. Thomas EA, Pawar B, Thomas A. A prospective study of cutaneous abnormalities in patients with chronic kidney disease. *Indian J Nephrol*. 2012;22(2):116-120.
11. Taylor SC, Kelly AP, Lim HW, Anido Serrano AM, eds. *Taylor and Kelly's Dermatology for Skin of Color*. 2nd ed. New York, NY: McGraw Hill; 2016.
12. Abdelbaqi-Salhab M, Shalhub S, Morgan MB. A current review of the cutaneous manifestations of renal disease. *J Cutan Pathol*. 2003;30(9):527-538.
13. Falodun O, Ogunbiyi A, Salako B, George AK. Skin changes in patients with chronic renal failure. *Saudi J Kidney Dis Transpl* 2011; 22:268-272.
14. Esson GA, Hussain AB, Meggitt SJ, Reynolds NJ, Sayer JA. Cutaneous manifestations of acute kidney injury. *Clin Kidney J*. 2022;15(5):855-864.
15. Madigan LM, Fox LP. Vancomycin-associated drug-induced hypersensitivity syndrome. *J Am Acad Dermatol*. 2019;81(1):123-128.
16. Noe M, Rosenbach M. Cutaneous sarcoidosis. *Curr Opin Pulm Med*. 2017;23(5):482-486.
17. Roman C, Dima B, Muyshont L, Schurmans T, Gilliaux O. Indications and efficiency of dapsone in IgA vasculitis (Henoch-Schonlein purpura): case series and a review of the literature. *Eur J Pediatr*. 2019;178(8):1275-1281.
18. Germain DP. Fabry disease. *Orphanet J Rare Dis*. 2010;5:30-30.
19. Rakowski SK, Winterkorn EB, Paul E, Steele DJ, Halpern EF, Thiele EA. Renal manifestations of tuberous sclerosis complex: incidence, prognosis, and predictive factors. *Kidney Int*. 2006;70(10):1777-1782.
20. Menko FH, van Steensel MA, Giraud S, et al. Birt-Hogg-Dube syndrome: diagnosis and management. *Lancet Oncol*. 2009;10(12):1199-1206.
21. Daccord C, Good JM, Morren MA, Bonny O, Hohl D, Lazor R. Birt-Hogg-Dube syndrome. *Eur Respir Rev*. 2020;29(157):200042.
22. Emer JJ, Solomon S, Mercer SE. Reed's syndrome: a case of multiple cutaneous and uterine leiomyomas. *J Clin Aesthet Dermatol*. 2011;4(12):37-42.
23. Basendwh MA, Fatani M, Baltow B. Reed's syndrome: a case of multiple cutaneous leiomyomas treated with liquid nitrogen cryotherapy. *Case Rep Dermatol*. 2016;8(1):65-70.
24. Walling HW, Sontheimer RD. Cutaneous lupus erythematosus: issues in diagnosis and treatment. *Am J Clin Dermatol*. 2009;10(6):365-381.
25. Ferreli C, Gasparini G, Parodi A, Cozzani E, Rongioletti F, Atzori L. Cutaneous manifestations of scleroderma and scleroderma-like disorders: a comprehensive review. *Clinic Rev Allerg Immunol*. 2017;53(3):306-336.
26. Denton CP, Lapadula G, Mouthon L, Muller-Ladner U. Renal complications and scleroderma renal crisis. *Rheumatology (Oxford)*. 2009;48 Suppl 3:iii32-5.
27. Hoyer JR, Michael AF, Vernier RL, Sisson S. Renal disease in nail-patella syndrome: clinical and morphologic studies. *Kidney Int*. 1972;2(4):231-238.
28. Virani ZA, Rajput P, Vora H, Shah BV. Retrospective diagnosis of nail-patella syndrome. *Indian J Nephrol*. 2021;31(5):485-487.

CHAPTER 80 Paraneoplastic Dermatology

Christina Topham
Abraham M. Korman
Lauren M. Madigan

KEY POINTS

- Cutaneous eruptions may serve as the presenting feature of an underlying malignancy or signal recurrence.
- Early recognition of paraneoplastic eruptions presenting within the skin may lead to improved outcomes.
- A lack of familiarity with how paraneoplastic disorders present in skin of color may further compound the disparities that exist in outcomes among racial and ethnic minority groups.

INTERNAL MALIGNANCY AND THE SKIN

The skin serves an important role as an indicator of systemic disease and may be the presenting feature of an underlying malignancy—or herald recurrence. While many paraneoplastic eruptions are nonspecific, others are morphologically distinct and can be identified by a trained observer. These may occur due to metabolic products of the neoplasm itself, represent secondary epidermal proliferation, or present as a recognizable inflammatory disorder with a known malignancy association. As such, dermatologists are vital to the early recognition of these disorders as—in some instances—identification can lead to improved outcomes. Conversely, a lack of familiarity with how these disorders present in skin of color may lead to a poor prognosis and further compound the disparities that exist in cancer diagnosis, treatment, and outcomes among racial and ethnic minority groups.[1]

EPIDEMIOLOGY

The American Cancer Society's 2022 Cancer Statistics, which compiled and analyzed population-based cancer occurrence and outcome data, highlights significant and distressing differences between racial and ethnic groups in the United States.[2] Alarmingly, Black individuals have lower survival rates for nearly every cancer type, with a cancer-related mortality rate among Black women that is 12% higher compared to White women despite a lower overall incidence.[2] When stratified by sex, Black men have the highest incidence of malignancy.[2] American Indian/

Alaska Natives have the second highest cancer mortality rate and, notably, this population has the highest incidence and mortality related to renal cancers. Compared to non-Hispanic Whites, Hispanics/Latinos have higher cancer incidence and mortality rates related to stomach, liver/intrahepatic biliary duct, and uterine/cervical malignancies.[2] Asian/Pacific Islanders have lower incidences for all cancer types but have a predilection toward infection-associated malignancies (hepatocellular and gastric) and a higher mortality related to these when compared to White individuals.[2] Numerous additional racial/ethnic disparities exist and the roots of these inequities are complex, including socioeconomic, environmental, institutional, behavioral, and biological factors. Later presentation and decreased access to healthcare likely play large roles in the disproportionately poor prognoses in these populations. This chapter describes the morphology of paraneoplastic eruptions with a focus on presentation in skin of color in an effort to improve early identification and consequently improve clinical outcomes.

DISORDERS ASSOCIATED WITH THE METABOLIC PRODUCTS OF MALIGNANCY

NECROLYTIC MIGRATORY ERYTHEMA

Necrolytic migratory erythema (NME) is a presenting sign of disease in up to 70% of patients with glucagonoma syndrome.[3] It is characterized by erythematous to brown, hyperpigmented macules and papules that expand centrifugally to form arcuate and circinate plaques with associated vesiculation, pustules, and scale. These plaques demonstrate a predilection for the perioral and intertriginous areas and distal extremities. A similar eruption can present in the setting of liver dysfunction, celiac disease, nutritional deficiency, inflammatory bowel disease, pancreatitis, and other malignancies.[4]

Glucagonomas are malignant, neuroendocrine tumors originating from pancreatic α-islet cells. These glucagon-secreting neoplasms are rare, with islet tumors comprising only 1.3% of all pancreatic malignancies.[5] The average age of onset is the fifth to sixth decades and cases are evenly distributed among sexes, with an unknown prevalence among different racial groups.[6] The most common presenting sign is weight loss, affecting 70% to 90% of patients, with most developing diabetes mellitus and diarrhea.[3,6] Neuropsychiatric symptoms and thrombosis may be present and laboratory features (in addition to an elevated fasting glucagon level) often include normocytic anemia, hyperglycemia, and a reduction in amino acids.[6] Cutaneous manifestations include NME—with a prominence of hyperpigmentation in skin of color—but also stomatitis, nail dystrophy, and glossitis. Following assessment of serum glucagon levels, the diagnosis is often confirmed via imaging as tumors are frequently large (>3 cm) in size with most found within the tail of the pancreas. Unfortunately, metastatic disease is common at the time of diagnosis.[6]

HYPERPIGMENTATION SECONDARY TO ECTOPIC ADRENOCORTICOTROPIC HORMONE (ACTH)

While less specific cutaneous features of hypercortisolism—such as striae, acne, hirsutism, and bruising—may be present in patients with Cushing syndrome of any etiology, diffuse hyperpigmentation is only present in the setting of excess adrenocorticotropic hormone (ACTH).[7] In addition to pituitary hypersecretion, ectopic production has been associated with a variety of neoplasms but is most often derived from neuroendocrine tumors or small-cell carcinomas of the lung. When present in association with the latter, it is a poor prognostic feature.[7,8] Hyperpigmentation is frequently generalized but most prominent in sun-exposed sites and those with repetitive friction. These features may be overlooked in patients of color as pigmentation may appear subtly and be incorrectly attributed to ethnicity. As such, mucosal, nail, and periungual involvement can serve as an important clue to diagnosis when presenting with additional features such as obesity, hypertension, osteopenia, and glucose intolerance.[9] Pigmentation in these patients likely occurs as ACTH, a precursor to α-melanocyte-stimulating hormone (α-MSH), is also able to activate the melanocortin-1 receptor in the skin leading to an increase in melanin synthesis.[10] This differs from the abnormal deposition of melanin present in diffuse cutaneous melanosis, a distinct paraneoplastic disorder presenting in the setting of advanced melanoma.

TABLE 80-1 Additional disorders associated with the metabolic products of malignancy

Disorder	Cutaneous presentation	Malignancy association
Carcinoid syndrome	Episodic flushing/erythema of the face and upper trunk. Telangiectasia, pellagra-like dermatitis, and sclerodermoid changes may be present when advanced.	Associated with mid-gut tumors (with requisite liver metastasis) as well as type III gastric and bronchial tumors (without liver metastasis necessary)
Eruptive hemangiomatosis	Abrupt appearance of multiple, benign vascular growths/cherry angiomas [Figure 72-1].	Secondary to elevated IL-6 and VEGF, associated with multicentric Castleman disease ± POEMS, lymphoproliferative disorders[15]

PANCREATIC PANNICULITIS

Pancreatic panniculitis is an uncommon disorder associated with both benign and malignant pancreatic disorders.[11] Morphologically, pancreatic panniculitis presents with scattered erythematous, red-brown or violaceous subcutaneous nodules. These are commonly bilateral and observed on the distal extremities—though cases in association with malignancy can be more widespread.[12,13] These lesions are associated with ulceration and drainage of an oily, yellow-brown fluid resulting from direct liquefactive destruction of the fat.[12,14] Elevation in pancreatic enzymes is typically observed, and favored to be pathologic. Polyarthralgias are also common in both malignant and benign cases—though the triad of polyarthritis, panniculitis, and eosinophilia in the setting of pancreatic cancer (known as Schmid triad) is particularly associated with a poor prognosis.[12,13] While metastatic disease is common at the time of diagnosis, prompt recognition of this paraneoplastic presentation remains vital for cases in which intervention is possible.

ADDITIONAL DISORDERS [TABLE 80-1]

BAZEX SYNDROME (ACROKERATOSIS PARANEOPLASTICA)

Bazex syndrome, or acrokeratosis paraneoplastica, is a rare manifestation of occult malignancy presenting with psoriasiform plaques on acral surfaces such as the hands, feet, nose, and ears. The plaques are associated with a distinctive, powdery scale and may range in color from erythematous to violaceous or hyperpigmented, the latter being more common in darker skin phenotypes.[16-18] Nail changes often precede the development of the aforementioned skin findings and include subungual hyperkeratosis, onycholysis, longitudinal streaks, and yellow discoloration.[16] Associated pruritus or pain is frequently described.[16] Bazex syndrome is classically associated with squamous cell carcinoma of the upper aerodigestive tract (pharynx, esophagus, and larynx) and precedes symptoms secondary to the underlying malignancy in most cases.[16] As such, early recognition of these distinct cutaneous findings is important and should prompt a broad investigation for malignancy with emphasis on the upper aerodigestive tract. Treatment of the underlying malignancy results in improvement of the skin and relapse of cutaneous manifestations is associated with disease progression.

ACQUIRED HYPERTRICHOSIS LANUGINOSA

Acquired hypertrichosis lanuginose (AHL), also known as hypertrichosis lanuginosa acquisita or malignant down, classically manifests as the rapid onset of diffuse lanugo hairs—long, fine hairs with little to no pigment—and often progresses in a craniocaudal fashion.[19] Strikingly, AHL affects cutaneous sites that typically lack hair growth and

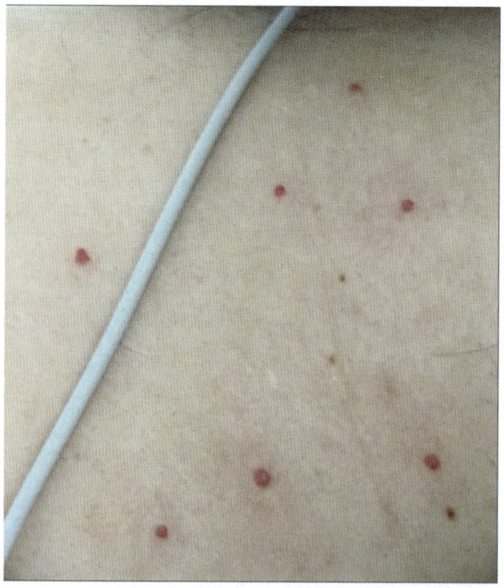

FIGURE 80–1. Eruptive hemangiomatosis. Multiple, eruptive angiomas presenting in a Japanese man with TAFRO syndrome, a variant of multicentric Castleman disease.

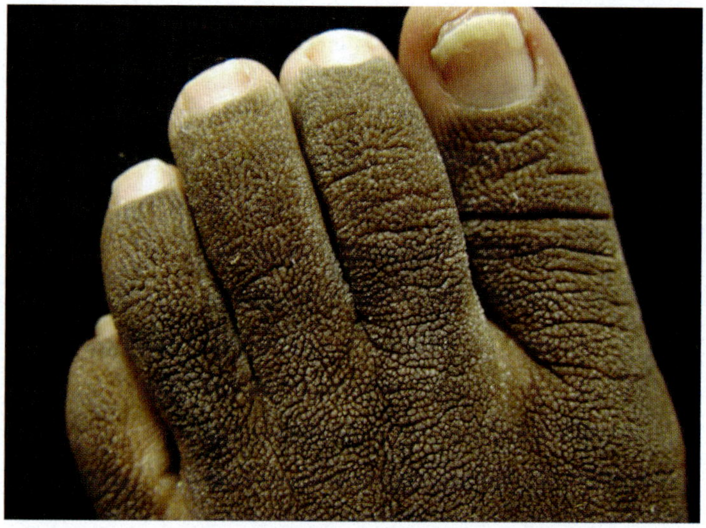

FIGURE 80–2. Tripe palms/malignant acanthosis nigricans. Velvety, rugose thickening of the skin on the dorsal foot.

previously perceived by patients as "hairless," such as the glabrous skin of the face. Notably, in skin of color populations, lanugo hairs may be pigmented so differentiating from terminal hairs—which are thicker and more deeply pigmented—is necessary to recognize AHL in these patients. Additionally, detection can prove difficult in patients with a higher density of background thicker hairs or those who utilize various hair removal techniques. Concurrent acanthosis nigricans, glossitis, and lingual papillary hypertrophy may also be present.[20] AHL is classically associated with breast, lung, and colorectal carcinomas.[19] Comprehensive evaluation for an underlying malignancy should be pursued, including age-appropriate screenings (colonoscopy, mammography) and chest imaging.

TRIPE PALMS

Tripe palms, also known as acanthosis palmaris, is a form of acquired palmoplantar keratoderma associated with underlying malignancy, especially carcinomas of the lung and stomach. Tripe palms characteristically present as velvety, rugose thickening of the skin resulting in marked accentuation or distortion of the dermatoglyphic ridges and sulci [**Figure 80-2**]. In individuals with darker skin phenotypes, cutaneous findings can be densely pigmented appearing brown to black in color as opposed to white, yellow, or tan in those with lighter skin phenotypes.[21,22] Findings are most pronounced over pressure-bearing areas, such as the fingertips and thenar and hypothenar eminences.[23] Concurrent malignant acanthosis nigricans is common.[23] In most reported cases, the skin changes of tripe palms precede the diagnosis of a new or recurrent malignancy but may present at any point during the course.[24] As more than 90% of cases are associated with malignancy, thorough screening should be pursued including both upper endoscopy and pulmonary imaging.[25]

ADDITIONAL DISORDERS [TABLE 80-2]

NEUTROPHILIC DERMATOSES

Sweet Syndrome Sweet syndrome (SS) is characterized by rapidly developing, tender, edematous erythematous to violaceous papules and plaques predominantly on acral-facial locations or at sites of trauma [**Figures 80-4** and **80-5**].[27] The presence of neutrophils imparts a deep erythema, which is perceived as duskiness in skin of color. Extracutaneous symptoms are common, and include fever, malaise, and ocular disturbances. Leukocytosis with neutrophilia is often present. SS can be associated with a variety of triggers, though when associated with malignancy often occurs in the setting of acute myelogenous leukemia and other myeloproliferative disorders. The diagnosis is clinicopathologic and is supported histologically by marked papillary dermal edema and a brisk neutrophilic infiltrate.[28] Cultures by necessity remain sterile, as infection must be ruled out to render this diagnosis. Treatment of paraneoplastic SS consists of treating the underlying malignancy and using systemic corticosteroids and neutrophil-targeting agents (dapsone, colchicine) to control inflammation. In patients presenting with SS without a known trigger, evaluation for malignancy should include a complete blood count, peripheral smear, and serum immunofixation and free light chains.

Pyoderma Gangrenosum Pyoderma gangrenosum (PG) in the classic ulcerative subtype commonly presents on the lower extremities as a pustule or tender nodule that rapidly ulcerates [**Figure 80-6**]. The

TABLE 80-2 Additional proliferative disorders (disorders with associated hyperkeratosis or epidermal proliferation) occurring secondary to malignancy

Disorder	Cutaneous presentation	Associated malignancies	Screening
Malignant acanthosis nigricans	Rapid onset of velvety hyperpigmentation on both typical and atypical (perioral and mucosal) locations	Gastric adenocarcinoma	Upper endoscopy, symptom-directed malignancy screening
Hypertrophic osteoarthropathy	Digital clubbing, periostitis of long tubular bones, large joint arthritis/effusion [**Figure 80-3**]	When paraneoplastic, associated with lung cancer, other thoracic malignancies	Pulmonary imaging
Eruptive disseminated porokeratosis	Rapid onset (<2 months) of disseminated monomorphic papules/plaques with fine peripheral scale on multiple regions, ± pruritus	When paraneoplastic, associated with hepatocellular and ovarian carcinomas, cholangiocarcinoma, lymphoma	Abdominal imaging, transvaginal ultrasound or CA-125[26]
Sign of Leser-Trélat (controversial)	Rapid increase in number and/or size of seborrheic keratoses, ± inflamed keratoses	Gastrointestinal adenocarcinoma, lymphoid malignancies	Colorectal and/or gastric endoscopic exams

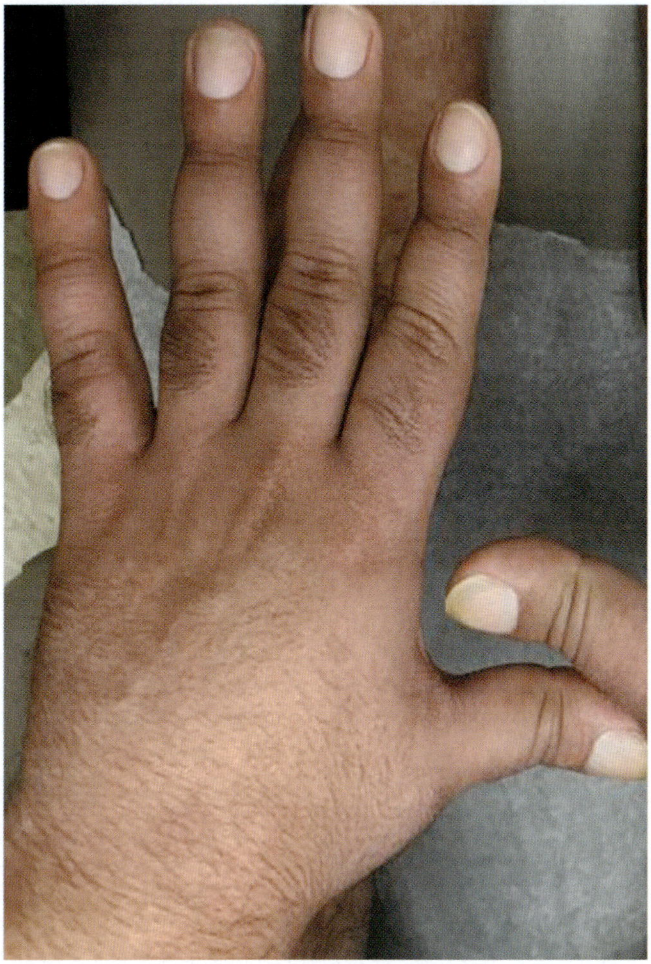

FIGURE 80–3. Neutrophilic dermatosis of the dorsal hands. An ulcer on the dorsal thumb with surrounding dusky, violaceous edema.

ulcer has a peripheral, violaceous border that is often undermined.[29] In skin of color, the border can appear as brown hyperpigmentation rather than violaceous and when healed classically results in cribriform scarring. PG is associated with many conditions, though when paraneoplastic is most commonly observed in association with malignant hematologic neoplasms including acute myelogenous leukemia as well as myelodysplastic syndrome. The diagnosis is rendered after competing etiologies are excluded. Histopathology demonstrates an ulcer with an undermined neutrophilic infiltrate and serves to exclude competing diagnoses of infection, malignancy, vasculitis, and vasculopathy. Treatment of paraneoplastic PG aims to treat the underlying neoplasm,

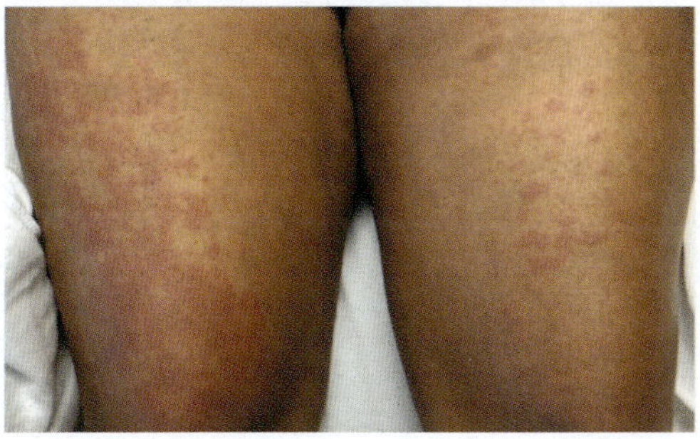

FIGURE 80–4. Neutrophilic Sweet syndrome. Edematous, erythematous plaques on the thighs.

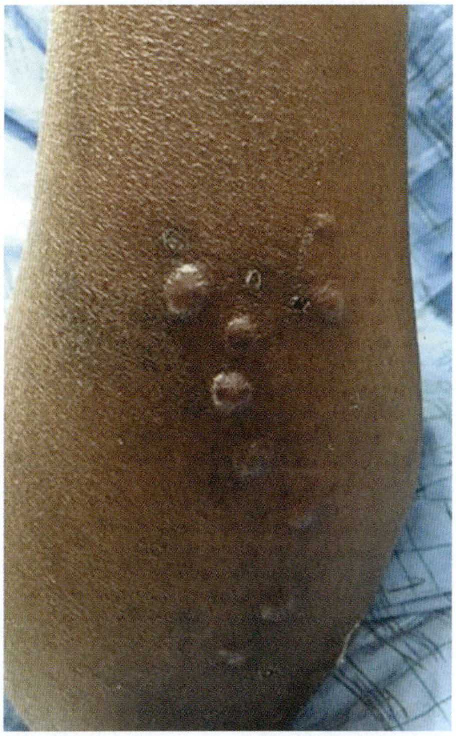

FIGURE 80–5. Sweet syndrome. Pink-brown edematous plaques and pustules on the extremities.

eliminate the neutrophilic infiltrate from the skin, and obtain adequate wound healing.

Neutrophilic dermatosis of the dorsal hands is a localized variant of neutrophilic dermatosis occurring on the spectrum of SS and PG [**Figure 80-7**].[30] While principles of evaluation and management are the same, when ulceration and inflammation occur overlying a joint,

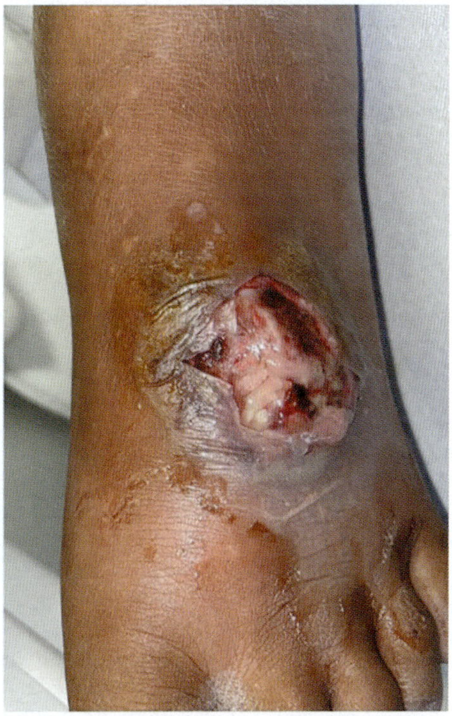

FIGURE 80–6. Pyoderma gangrenosum. Ulceration of the dorsal foot with associated violaceous erythema, surrounding hyperpigmentation, and an undermined edge.

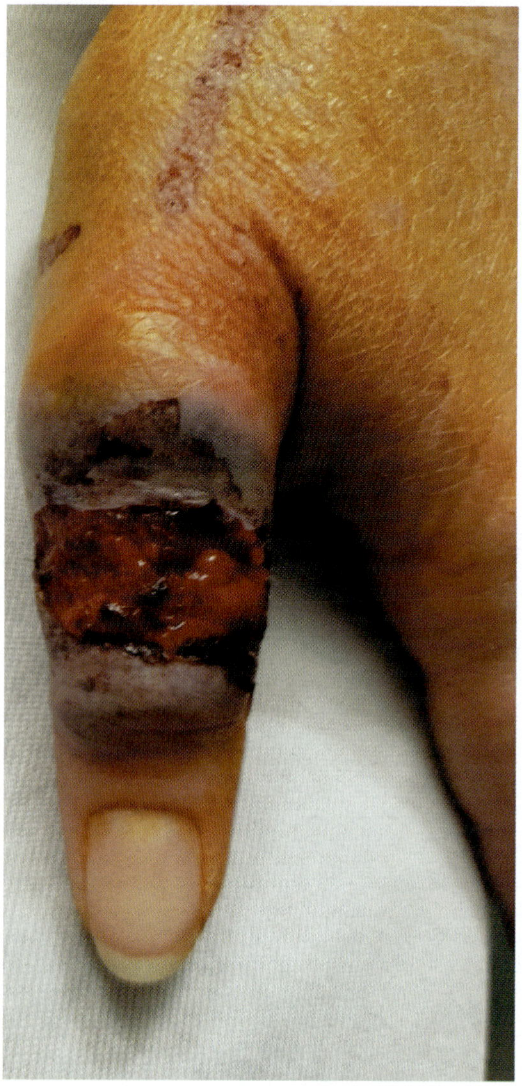

FIGURE 80–7. Neutrophilic dermatosis presenting as an ulcer on the dorsal thumb with surrounding dusky, violaceous edema.

measures to prevent joint contractures and/or permanent deformity are necessary.

VEXAS SYNDROME

VEXAS (vacuoles, E1 enzyme, X-linked, autoinflammatory, somatic) syndrome is an acquired autoinflammatory disorder characterized by bone marrow abnormalities (vacuolated precursors), cytopenias, elevated inflammatory markers, fevers, and cutaneous findings. The cutaneous features of VEXAS syndrome include neutrophilic dermatitis, cutaneous vasculitis, periorbital edema, and chondritis.[31] Patients with VEXAS are also predisposed to progressive marrow dysplasia with up to 55% meeting criteria for myelodysplastic syndrome as well as other clonal disorders, including myeloma, monoclonal gammopathy of uncertain significance, and monoclonal B-cell lymphocytosis. This diagnosis should be considered in any adult patient—particularly male—who presents with the aforementioned skin findings in conjunction with cytopenias and signs of autoinflammation.

DERMATOMYOSITIS (ADULT)

Dermatomyositis (DM) is an inflammatory disease that predominantly affects the skin, muscles, and lungs, and carries an increased risk of malignancy. Cutaneous manifestations are protean but include the pathognomonic Gottron papules and sign as well as heliotrope rash [**Figure 80-8**].[32] Photodistributed erythema, which appears dusky

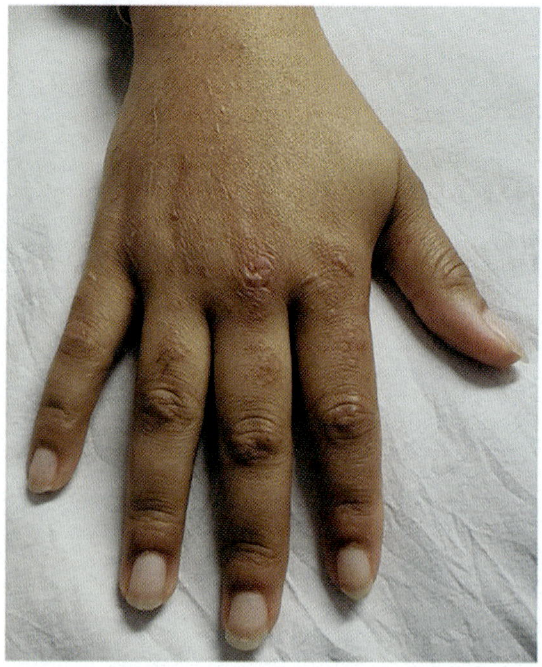

FIGURE 80–8. Dermatomyositis. Pink-brown to skin-colored Gottron papules overlying the metacarpophylangeal, proximal interphalangeal, and distal interphalangeal joints.

to violaceous in skin of color, and poikiloderma occurring on the chest and back as the V-sign and shawl sign, respectively, is often seen [**Figure 80-9**]. Muscle disease presents as symmetric, proximal muscle weakness; elevated laboratory markers including creatine kinase are often observed. The most common pulmonary presentation is interstitial lung disease. Diagnosis is rendered clinically, with supportive biopsy findings showing vacuolar interface dermatitis with epidermal

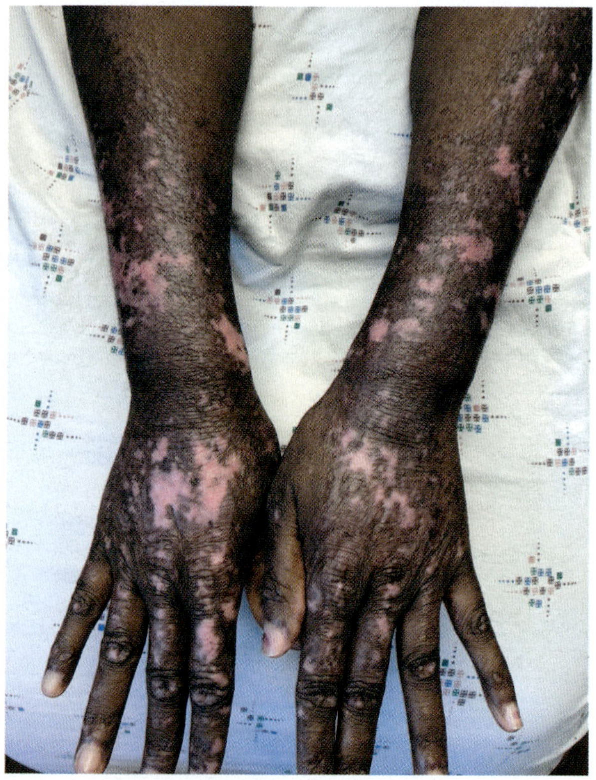

FIGURE 80–9. Dermatomyositis. Pink macules and patches on the bilateral dorsal forearms and hands.

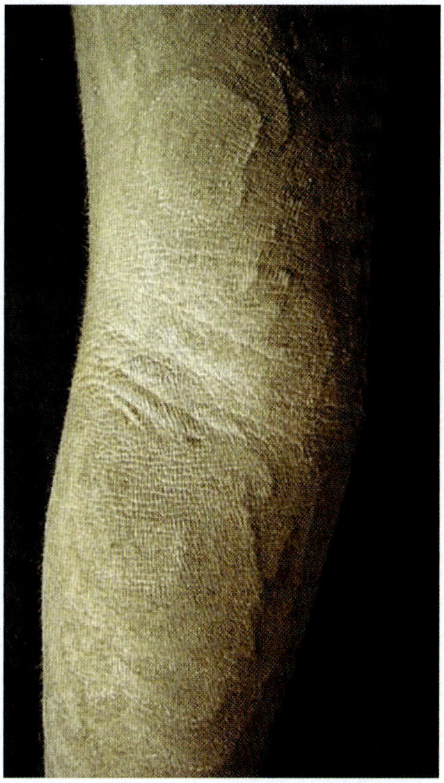

FIGURE 80–10. Erythema gyratum repens. Polycentric, skin-colored to gray scaly plaques with a wood-grain appearance on the volar upper extremity.

atrophy and increased dermal mucin.[33] Myositis-specific antibodies can be drawn to further classify the type of DM and associated risks (eg, lung disease, malignancy risk).

Treatment is aimed at halting disease activity and screening for malignancy is vital. Age-appropriate cancer screening is recommended along with pelvic ultrasound and CT imaging of the chest/abdomen/pelvis, particularly for those with high-risk antibody phenotypes (eg, TIF-1-gamma or NXP-2 positivity). Individualized risk-based screening should also be considered (such as nasopharyngeal imaging in patients from high-risk areas).

ERYTHEMA GYRATUM REPENS

Erythema gyratum repens (EGR) is a paraneoplastic skin condition with a striking presentation characterized by polycentric, pink, scaly plaques with a wood-grain appearance rapidly migrating over the skin surface.[34] The skin lesions can appear violaceous or hyperpigmented in skin of color [**Figure 80-10**]. EGR is classically associated with lung cancer but can be associated with any solid organ malignancy. A thorough workup for underlying malignancies including pulmonary imaging is warranted.[35] The lesions of EGR remit with successful treatment of the underlying associated disorder.

TABLE 80-3 Blistering disorders associated with malignancy

Disorder	Mucocutaneous presentation	Malignancy association
Paraneoplastic pemphigus[36]	Severe hemorrhagic stomatitis, with or without flaccid bullae on the skin. In skin of color the classic erythema of bullae may be absent, instead presenting with hyperpigmentation or a purplish hue, mimicking interface dermatitides	Non-Hodgkin lymphoma, chronic lymphocytic leukemia, Castleman disease
Antilaminin 332 mucous membrane pemphigoid[37]	Erosions and scarring of mucous membranes (most commonly oral) [**Figure 80-11**]	Solid organ malignancies

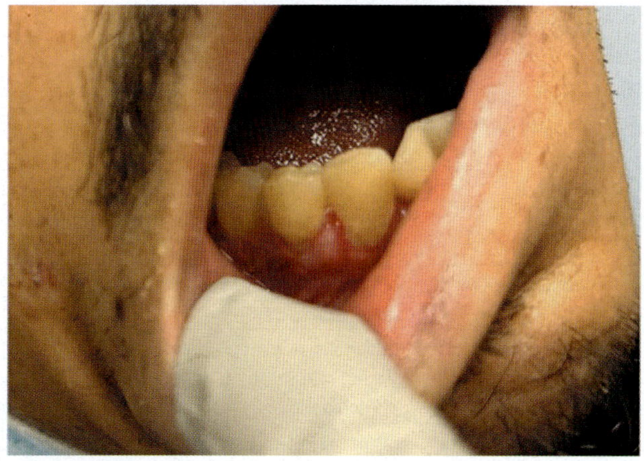

FIGURE 80–11. Antilaminin 332 mucous membrane pemphigoid. Ulceration on the inferior gingival mucosa.

BLISTERING DISORDERS ASSOCIATED WITH MALIGNANCY [TABLE 80-3]

MULTICENTRIC RETICULOHISTIOCYTOSIS

Multicentric reticulohistiocytosis (MRH) is a rare, inflammatory, dermatosis that is associated with inflammatory and erosive arthritis, autoimmune diseases, and malignancy (usually solid organ cancers). The presentation is that of numerous, firm, reddish brown papules on the bilateral dorsal hands, elbows, and ears.[38] In skin of color, the contrast between the brown lesions and background skin can be more subtle [**Figure 80-12**]. Histopathology confirms the diagnosis, demonstrating dermal histiocytes with a characteristic "ground-glass" cytoplasm.

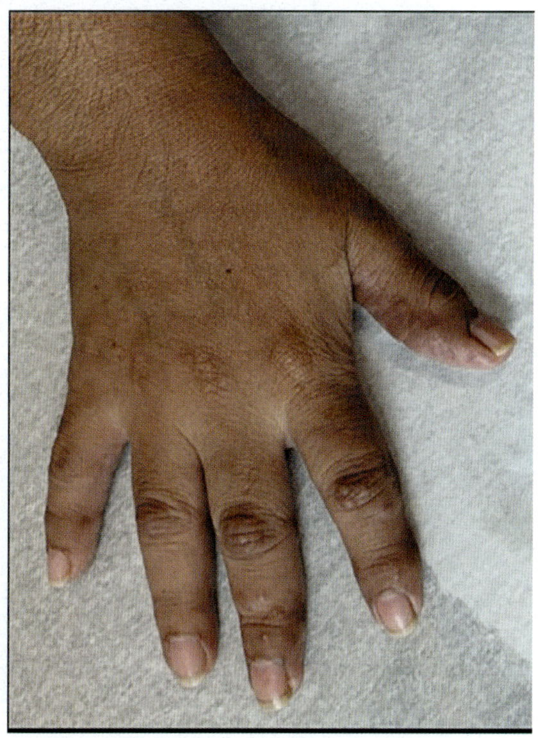

FIGURE 80–12. Multicentric reticulohistiocytosis. Firm, reddish-brown papules on the metacarpophylangeal and distal interphalangeal joints of the dorsal hand.

TABLE 80-4 Disorders associated with monoclonal gammopathy

Disorder	Cutaneous presentation	Malignancy association
AESOP (adenopathy, and extensive skin patch overlying a plasmacytoma)	Large, slowly expanding erythematous to violet-brown patch or thin plaque	The underlying plasmacytoma may be solitary or associated with POEMS/monoclonal gammopathy, Castleman disease, or (in one reported case) a blue-cell sarcoma.[41]
Systemic amyloidosis	Waxy, yellow papules, noninflammatory petechia and macular purpura (often in areas of minor trauma, eg, periorbitally), bullous hemorrhagic lesions, macroglossia [**Figure 80-13**]	May occur in the setting of multiple myeloma or, less commonly, Waldenström macroglobulinemia
Type I cryoglobulinemia	Retiform purpura, cyanosis, and ischemia/necrosis favoring acral sites, livedo reticularis	Clinical lesions result from monoclonal immunoglobulins produced in the setting of monoclonal gammopathy, multiple myeloma, Waldenström macroglobulinemia, CLL
Necrobiotic xanthogranuloma	Yellow-orange, red-brown, or violaceous, infiltrative papules and plaques with atrophy, telangiectasia, and ulceration. Classically in a periorbital location though may present at other sites	Associated with paraproteinemia, most often IgG with kappa light chain, less commonly a malignant disorder (of which multiple myeloma is most common)[42]
Normolipemic plane xanthoma	Patches and thin, yellow plaques favoring the periocular region/face, upper trunk, and intertriginous sites	Associated with a monoclonal gammopathy and, less commonly, multiple myeloma and other lymphoproliferative disorders
POEMS (polyneuropathy, organomegaly, endocrinopathy, M-protein and skin changes) syndrome	Hyperpigmentation, angiomas (including classic glomeruloid hemangiomas), sclerodermatous thickening, acrocyanosis, hyperhidrosis, digital clubbing, nail changes, plethora	Associated with a lambda light chain monoclonal gammopathy. Cases of Castleman disease, solitary plasmacytoma, and osteosclerotic myeloma reported
Schnitzler syndrome	Persistent urticarial plaques (with a neutrophil-rich infiltrate) in the setting of bone/joint pain and fever	Associated with an IgM, typically kappa light chain, paraproteinemia. Approximately 15% of patients will develop a lymphoplasmacytic malignancy
Scleredema (type II)	Slowly progressive, firm induration of the skin on the posterior neck and upper back which may develop secondary hyperpigmentation or a "peau d'orange" appearance	Associated with monoclonal gammopathy and, less commonly, multiple myeloma
Scleromyxedema	Firm, monomorphic waxy, papules diffusely, often in a linear assortment. Leonine facies may develop	Associated with IgG, typically lambda light chain, monoclonal gammopathy. Less than 10% develop overt multiple myeloma

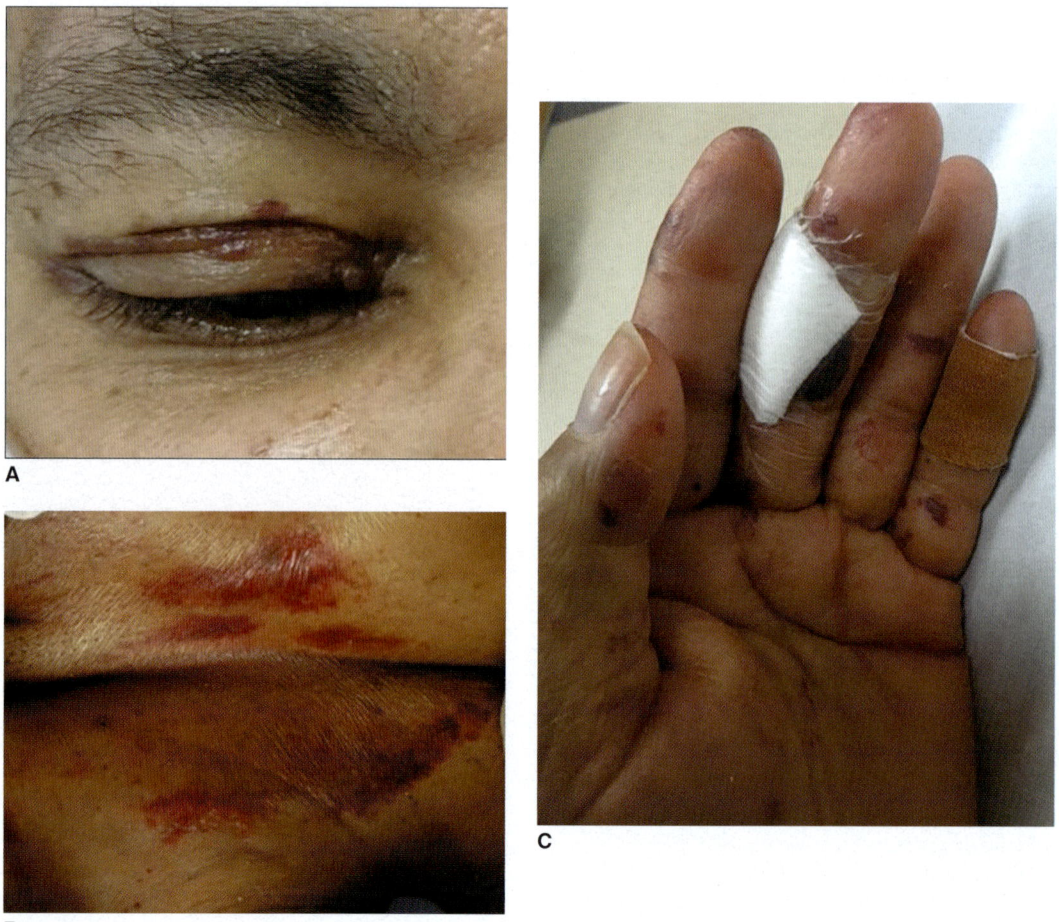

FIGURE 80–13. Systemic amyloidosis. Waxy red-purple papules, purpura, and hemorrhagic bullae involving the superior eyelids **(A)**, intertriginous folds **(B)**, and palmar hand **(C)**.

PITYRIASIS ROTUNDA

Pityriasis rotunda is a rare dermatosis that is associated with solid organ cancers, most characteristically liver. It presents with strikingly circular, well-demarcated, scaly pink to brown patches on the trunk and extremities.[39] Histopathology is nonspecific, and the diagnosis is rendered clinically. Treatment of any underlying diseases can improve the condition, and topical corticosteroids can be employed for symptomatic treatment.

EOSINOPHILIC DERMATOSIS OF HEMATOLOGIC MALIGNANCY

Eosinophilic dermatosis of hematologic malignancy is an inflammatory dermatosis that occurs most commonly in response to underlying chronic lymphocytic leukemia.[40] It presents with pruritic, pink papules to nodules on the trunk and extremities that may appear darker in skin of color. Histopathology confirms diagnosis, demonstrating a superficial and deep perivascular lymphocytic infiltrate with many eosinophils.

DISORDERS ASSOCIATED WITH MONOCLONAL GAMMOPATHY

Cutaneous features may also herald the presence of clinically meaningful paraproteinemias as well as overt multiple myeloma and other lymphoproliferative disorders [**Table 80-4**].

CONCLUSION

This chapter covered many paraneoplastic presentations with distinct morphologies; however, paraneoplastic eruptions can also be less specific manifesting as dermal hypersensitivity, acquired ichthyosis, exfoliative erythroderma, and small vessel vasculitis among others. Of course, malignancy can also present directly as metastatic disease within the skin. Finally, there are numerous familial cancer syndromes with cutaneous features that may, at times, be the most prominent or identifiable presentation.

The ability to recognize the ways in which the skin can herald a systemic malignancy in all skin types is essential to providing equitable care and a skill that dermatologists uniquely offer to patients both in the ambulatory and hospital settings.

REFERENCES

1. Zavala VA, Bracci PM, Carethers JM, et al. Cancer health disparities in racial/ethnic minorities in the United States. *Br J Cancer*. 2021;124(2):315-332.
2. Siegel RL, Miller KD, Fuchs HE, Jemal A. Cancer statistics, 2022. *Cancer J Clin*. 2022;72(1):7-33.
3. Remes-Troche JM, García-de-Acevedo B, Zuñiga-Varga J, Avila-Funes A, Orozco-Topete R. Necrolytic migratory erythema: a cutaneous clue to glucagonoma syndrome. *J Eur Acad Dermatol Venereol*. 2004;18(5):591-595.
4. Tierney EP, Badger J. Etiology and pathogenesis of necrolytic migratory erythema: review of the literature. *MedGenMed*. 2004;6(3):4.
5. Yao JC, Eisner MP, Leary C, et al. Population-based study of islet cell carcinoma. *Ann Surg Oncol*. 2007;14(12):3492-3500.
6. Wermers RA, Fatourechi V, Wynne AG, Kvols LK, Lloyd RV. The glucagonoma syndrome. Clinical and pathologic features in 21 patients. *Medicine (Baltimore)*. 1996;75(2):53-63.
7. Young J, Haissaguerre M, Viera-Pinto O, Chabre O, Baudin E, Tabarin A. Management of endocrine disease: Cushing's syndrome due to ectopic ACTH secretion: an expert operational opinion. *Eur J Endocrinol*. 2020;182(4):R29-R58.
8. Nagy-Mignotte H, Shestaeva O, Vignoud L, et al. Prognostic impact of paraneoplastic Cushing's syndrome in small-cell lung cancer. *J Thorac Oncol*. 2014;9(4):497-505.
9. Sandoval MAS, Bruno RG. Nail hyperpigmentation in ACTH-secreting pituitary adenoma (Cushing's disease) and its resolution after successful transsphenoidal excision. *BMJ Case Rep*. 2020;13(4):e234905.
10. Wakamatsu K, Graham A, Cook D, Thody AJ. Characterisation of ACTH peptides in human skin and their activation of the melanocortin-1 receptor. *Pigment Cell Res*. 1997;10:288-297.
11. Requena L, Yus ES. Panniculitis. Part II. Mostly lobular panniculitis. *J Am Acad Dermatol*. 2001;45(3):325-364.
12. Dahl PR, Su WP, Cullimore KC, Dicken CH. Pancreatic panniculitis. *J Am Acad Dermatol*. 1995;33(3):413-417.
13. García-Romero D, Vanaclocha F. Pancreatic panniculitis. *Dermatol Clin*. 2008;26(4):465-470, vi.
14. Anand NC, Takaichi M, Johnson EF, Wetter DA, Davis MDP, Alavi A. Suggestions for a new clinical classification approach to panniculitis based on a mayo clinic experience of 207 cases. *Am J Clin Dermatol*. 2022;23(5):739-746.
15. Fajgenbaum D, Rosenbach M, van Rhee F, Nasir A, Reutter J. Eruptive cherry hemangiomatosis associated with multicentric Castleman disease: a case report and diagnostic clue. *JAMA Dermatol*. 2013;149(2):204.
16. Räßler F, Goetze S, Elsner P. Acrokeratosis paraneoplastica (Bazex syndrome) - a systematic review on risk factors, diagnosis, prognosis and management. *J Eur Acad Dermatol Venereol*. 2017;31(7):1119-1136.
17. Zarzour JG, Singh S, Andea A, Cafardi JA. Acrokeratosis paraneoplastica (Bazex syndrome): report of a case associated with small cell lung carcinoma and review of the literature. *J Radiol Case Rep*. 2011;5(7):1-6.
18. Poligone B, Christensen SR, Lazova R, Heald PW. Bazex syndrome (acrokeratosis paraneoplastica). *Lancet*. 2007;369(9560):530.
19. Slee PH, van der Waal RI, Schagen van Leeuwen JH, et al. Paraneoplastic hypertrichosis lanuginosa acquisita: uncommon or overlooked? *Br J Dermatol*. 2007;157(6):1087-1092.
20. Wendelin DS, Pope DN, Mallory SB. Hypertrichosis. *J Am Acad Dermatol*. 2003;48(2):161-179.
21. Chakraborty PP, Datta S, Mandal SK, Kumar M. Tripe palm: a cutaneous manifestation of gastric carcinoma. *BMJ Case Rep*. 2014;2014:bcr2014206004.
22. Boyce M, Flower C. Tripe palms. *N Engl J Med*. 2022 Jul 28;387(4):355.
23. Lo WL, Wong CK. Tripe palms: a significant cutaneous sign of internal malignancy. *Dermatology*. 1992;185(2):151-153.
24. Cohen PR, Grossman ME, Silvers DN, Kurzrock R. Tripe palms and cancer. *Clin Dermatol*. 1993;11(1):165-173.
25. Clarke J. Malignant acanthosis nigricans. *Clin Exp Dermatol*. 1977;2(2):167-170.
26. Shoimer I, Robertson LH, Storwick G, Haber RM. Eruptive disseminated porokeratosis: a new classification system. *J Am Acad Dermatol*. 2014;71:398-400.
27. Weiss EH, Ko CJ, Leung TH, et al. Neutrophilic dermatoses: a clinical update. *Curr Dermatol Rep*. 2022;11(2):89-102.
28. Su WP, Liu HN. Diagnostic criteria for Sweet's syndrome. *Cutis*. 1986;37(3):167-174.
29. Ashchyan HJ, Nelson CA, Stephen S, James WD, Micheletti RG, Rosenbach M. Neutrophilic dermatoses: pyoderma gangrenosum and other bowel- and arthritis-associated neutrophilic dermatoses. *J Am Acad Dermatol*. 2018;79(6):1009-1022.
30. Micallef D, Bonnici M, Pisani D, Boffa MJ. Neutrophilic dermatosis of the dorsal hands: a review of 123 cases. *J Am Acad Dermatol*. 2023;88(6):1338-1344.
31. Beck DB, Ferrada MA, Sikora KA, et al. Somatic mutations in UBA1 and severe adult-onset autoinflammatory disease. *N Engl J Med*. 2020;383(27):2628-2638.
32. DeWane ME, Waldman R, Lu J. Dermatomyositis: clinical features and pathogenesis. *J Am Acad Dermatol*. 2020;82(2):267-281.
33. Waldman R, DeWane ME, Lu J. Dermatomyositis: diagnosis and treatment. *J Am Acad Dermatol*. 2020;82(2):283-296.
34. Liau MM, Long V, Yang SS. Erythema gyratum repens: a paraneoplastic eruption. *Case Rep*. 2016;2016:bcr2016214665.
35. Gore M, Winters ME. Erythema gyratum repens: a rare paraneoplastic rash. *West J Emerg Med*. 2011;12(4):556-558.
36. Ouedraogo E, Gottlieb J, de Masson A, et al. Risk factors for death and survival in paraneoplastic pemphigus associated with hematologic malignancies in adults. *J Am Acad Dermatol*. 2019;80(6):1544-1549.
37. Bernard P, Antonicelli F, Bedane C, et al. Prevalence and clinical significance of anti-laminin 332 autoantibodies detected by a novel enzyme-linked immunosorbent assay in mucous membrane pemphigoid. *JAMA Dermatol*. 2013;149(5):533-540.
38. Selmi C, Greenspan A, Huntley A, Gershwin ME. Multicentric reticulohistiocytosis: a critical review. *Curr Rheumatol Rep*. 2015;17(6):511.
39. Batra P, Cheung W, Meehan SA, Pomeranz M. Pityriasis rotunda. *Dermatol Online J*. 2009;15(8):14.
40. Farber MJ, La Forgia S, Sahu J, Lee JB. Eosinophilic dermatosis of hematologic malignancy. *J Cutan Pathol*. 2012;39(7):690-695.
41. Sanchez EG, Ramos C, Ratnarajah K, et al. Adenopathy and extensive skin patch overlying plasmacytoma syndrome-the clue to early diagnosis of polyneuropathy, organomegaly, endocrinopathy, monoclonal gammopathy, and skin changes: a case series and literature review. *SAGE Open Med Case Rep*. 2022;10:2050313X221091602.
42. Nelson CA, Zhong CS, Hashemi DA, et al. A multicenter cross-sectional study and systematic review of necrobiotic xanthogranuloma with proposed diagnostic criteria. *JAMA Dermatol*. 2020;156(3):270.

SECTION 12

Inpatient Dermatology

CHAPTER 81 Severe Cutaneous Adverse Reactions*

Brenda Umenita Imo
Benjamin Eduardo Swaby
Helena Pasieka

KEY POINTS

- Erythema may be less noticeable in patients with deeply pigmented skin, and different ethnic groups may exhibit variations in facial proportions, such as lip fullness, nasolabial fold angle, and eyelid anatomy. When assessing facial, periocular, or lip swelling, it is best to compare the patient to their own baseline. Knowing common offending agents is crucial for identifying and discontinuing the correct medication in drug reactions.
- The timeline of tolerance and a thorough drug history, including drugs started 6 or more weeks ago, help diagnose severe cutaneous adverse reactions (SCARs).
- Some SCARs are not medication related; in cases of erythema multiforme and reactive infectious mucocutaneous eruption, the etiology is thought to be an infection or idiopathic.
- Physicians and other care team members must maintain a high index of suspicion for drug reactions in patients with skin of color. Even when signs and symptoms are subtle, it is crucial to avoid any dismissive tendencies. Delaying the cessation of the offending agent can lead to a later stage of presentation and increased severity of illness.

INTRODUCTION

Severe cutaneous adverse reactions (SCARs) are a group of rare but potentially life-threatening dermatological conditions that involve a severe immune-mediated reaction to drugs or infections. SCARs are characterized by the development of widespread skin lesions, mucosal involvement, and systemic symptoms that can affect multiple organs. In cases of drug-induced SCARs, it is essential to identify the causative drug as soon as possible and discontinue it immediately. Delayed discontinuation of the offending drug can lead to more severe or prolonged reactions and may increase the risk of complications such as infections or multiorgan involvement.

Early diagnosis of SCARs in patients with deeply pigmented skin can be more challenging than in lighter skin tones due to differences in the clinical presentation. Patients with skin of color may present with subtle skin findings, which can be easily missed or misdiagnosed. This can lead to delayed recognition and treatment of SCARs, resulting in increased morbidity and mortality.

ACUTE GENERALIZED EXANTHEMATOUS PUSTULOSIS

Acute generalized exanthematous pustulosis (AGEP) is a severe rash with a reported incidence of one to five cases per million per year and an overall estimated mortality of less than 5%.[1,2] There is a slight predilection for women with most cases occurring in patients 27 to 74 years of age, and a mean age of 56 years.[1] Approximately 90% of cases are attributed to drugs, most commonly β-lactam antibiotics; however, a minority of cases with triggers attributed to acute infections, spider bites, and iodine-based intravenous contrast media have also been reported.[1-5]

The pathogenic mechanism of AGEP is thought to involve a T-cell-mediated delayed type IV hypersensitivity response in which drug-specific T-cells use granzyme B and perforin to induce apoptosis of epidermal keratinocytes.[1-4] This reaction results in the formation of vesicles containing CD4+ T-cells and keratinocytes that release CXCL8/IL-8 for neutrophil recruitment, leading to tissue destruction.[1]

The histopathologic findings demonstrate sterile intracorneal, subcorneal, and/or intraepidermal pustules with papillary edema consisting mainly of neutrophils. Necrotic keratinocytes, epidermal spongiosis with exocytosis of neutrophils and eosinophils, and perivascular lymphocytic infiltrates with a predominance of CD4+ cells can also be observed.[1-3]

Clinically, AGEP is characterized by disseminated erythematous plaques and papules with superimposed nonfollicular pinpoint pustules [**Figure 81-1**].[1-4] These lesions initially manifest in the intertriginous areas or face and spread rapidly to the trunk and extremities within hours.[1] Skin findings may present with signs of systemic manifestations, including fever, neutrophilia, mildly elevated hepatic enzymes, creatinine, and C-reactive protein.[1-3,5] Symptoms typically appear within 2 to 5 days after exposure to the offending agent(s); however, time to onset is not routinely included in the diagnostic criteria.[1-3]

Most AGEP cases have a favorable prognosis with spontaneous resolution of signs and symptoms within 2 weeks following removal of the causative agent(s).[1-6] Rare complicated cases with multiorgan involvement or superimposed infections can be fatal.[1,3] Such severe cases may require management in an intensive care setting and supportive care with antibiotics, systemic corticosteroids, or immunosuppressants.[1,3,4,6]

DRUG REACTION WITH EOSINOPHILIA AND SYSTEMIC SYMPTOMS/DRUG-INDUCED HYPERSENSITIVITY SYNDROME

Drug reaction with eosinophilia and systemic symptoms (DRESS), also known as drug-induced hypersensitivity syndrome (DiHS), is characterized by a morbilliform skin rash, hematologic alterations,

*The opinions and assertions expressed herein are those of the author(s) and do not reflect the official policy or position of the Uniformed Services University of the Health Sciences or the Department of Defense.

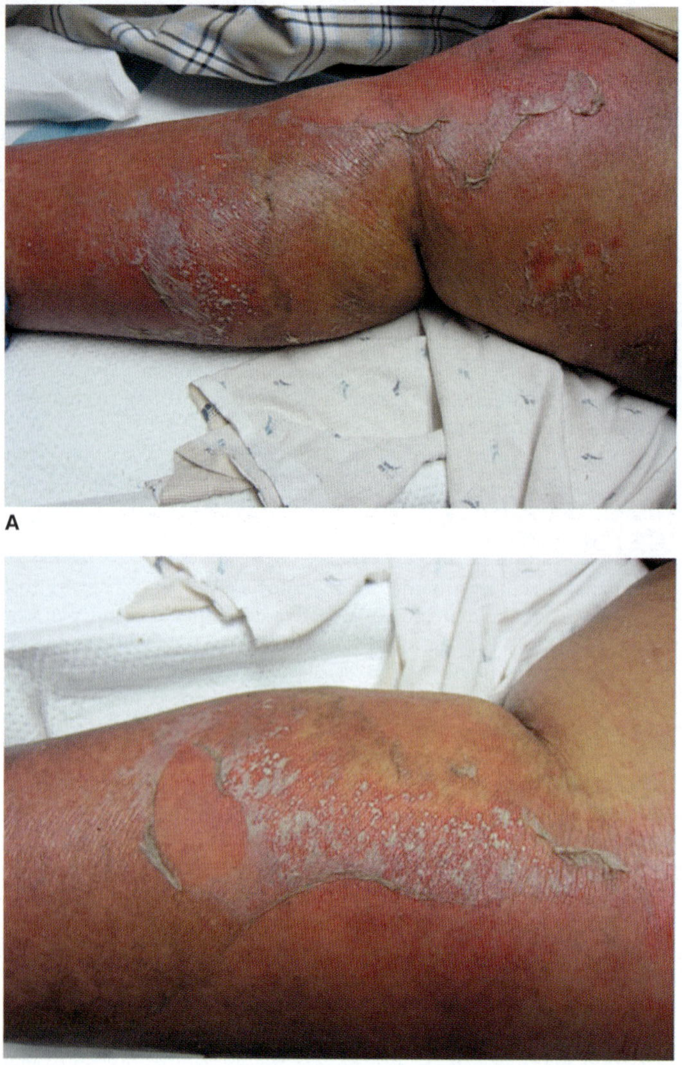

A

B

FIGURE 81-1 (A and B) Acute generalized exanthematous pustulosis (AGEP). Lower legs with erythema and multiple, nonfollicular, sterile pustules with desquamation in patient with skin of color.

lymphadenopathy, and internal organ involvement in response to medication.[1,2,5] Drug causality has been reported in approximately 80% of cases[5]; namely antiepileptics, sulfonamides, antibiotics, and uricosurics.[1] The exact incidence of DRESS/DiHS is difficult to calculate due to its variable presentation[5]; nonetheless, a recent U.S.-based study estimated the population risk as 0.9 to 2 per 100,000 patients per year with no gender predilection and average age of 47.8 years.[1]

DRESS/DiHS manifests as a delayed hypersensitivity reaction to an offending drug in susceptible individuals.[2] Several mechanisms have been proposed including reduced activity of certain drug detoxification enzymes leading to the accumulation of drug or reactive metabolites that go on to bind to endogenous proteins or directly to major histocompatibility complex (MHC) proteins or T-cell receptors to illicit an immune response, agents that induce cytochrome P450 (CYP450) activity resulting in decreased glutathione levels, and immunosuppression.[1,2] Various HLA-I genotypes have been linked to the development of DRESS/DiHS after ingestion of specific medications (eg, abacavir, allopurinol, carbamazepine, dapsone, phenytoin, and vancomycin).[1]

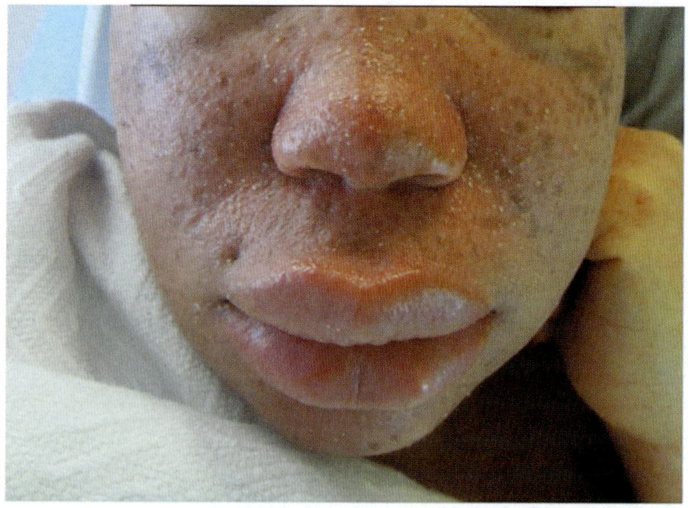

FIGURE 81-2. Drug reaction with eosinophilia and systemic symptoms (DRESS) as it appears in pigmented skin. Notice the prominent facial edema (including swollen lips and effacement of the nasolabial folds) with modest erythema.

Skin biopsy of DRESS/DiHS lesions is not typically required, as immunohistopathologic features are heterogenous.[1] Findings may include dermal-epidermal infiltrates with lymphocytic exocytosis, dermal edema, and superficial perivascular infiltrates of mostly lymphocytes with or without eosinophils.[2]

Clinical manifestations present on average 2 to 8 weeks after drug exposure. The first sign is typically a high fever that may precede a pruritic polymorphous rash by up to 2 weeks.[1,2] The rash classically affects more than 50% body surface area and often demonstrates follicular accentuation.[1] Facial edema is seen in most cases and can present with facial erythema that spares the periorbital region[1,2] and effaces the nasolabial folds [**Figure 81-2**]. Mucosal involvement is present in more than half of cases, usually affecting the oral cavity with oral erosions or tonsillitis and the keratinized lips with cheilitis.[1] Lymphadenopathy and liver injury are common, and kidney injury is often seen. Lung involvement and cardiac involvement occur rarely but are associated with increased mortality when noted.[1,2] Almost all cases of DRESS/DiHS have hematologic abnormalities [**Table 81-1**].[2]

The mainstay management of DRESS/DiHS requires withdrawing the suspected inciting drug and close monitoring, along with the evaluation of hepatic and renal function.[5] Mild cases may be managed with potent topical steroids; however, severe cases with significant internal organ involvement typically require systemic corticosteroids with gradual tapering over 6 to 8 weeks.[1,2] Mortality is estimated between 2% and 10%, typically due to fulminant hepatitis, requiring organ transplantation for effective treatment.[1] Other causes of mortality are associated with the reactivation of HHV-6/7, Epstein-Barr virus, or provocation of autoimmune sequelae.[1,2] The sequelae of DRESS/DiHS include autoimmune derangements such as thyroiditis, type 1 diabetes mellitus, and autoimmune hemolytic anemia, vitiligo, systemic lupus

TABLE 81-1 Hematological abnormalities in DRESS/DiHS[2]

Eosinophilia	95% of cases
Leukocytosis with atypical lymphocytes	75% of cases
Lymphopenia	25% of cases
Thrombocytopenia	25% of cases

Abbreviation: DRESS/DiHS, drug reaction with eosinophilia and systemic symptoms/drug-induced hypersensitivity syndrome.

erythematosus, which can develop several months to years after the resolution.[1,7]

STEVENS-JOHNSON SYNDROME AND TOXIC EPIDERMAL NECROLYSIS

Stevens-Johnson syndrome (SJS) and toxic epidermal necrolysis (TEN) are rare, life-threatening severity variants of the same clinical condition, characterized by extensive bullae formation and sloughing of skin and mucosal surfaces, mimicking burned skin.[1,5] SJS and TEN are differentiated by the percentage of body surface area (BSA) that is detachable or denuded,[1] where SJS represents less than 10% BSA involvement, SJS-TEN overlap represents between 20% and 30% BSA involvement, and TEN represents greater than 30% BSA involvement. The incidence of SJS is reported to be eight to nine cases per million per year, while TEN occurs less frequently, with between one and two cases per million per year.[1] A longitudinal study conducted among United Kingdom inpatients found no gender predilection; however, patients who identified as Black and Asian were found to have a higher incidence than White patients.[2]

The most common inciting drugs in SJS/TEN are antibiotics, antiepileptic drugs (with aromatic antiepileptics constituting 35% of cases), nonsteroidal anti-inflammatory drugs (NSAIDs), and allopurinol (identified in 20% of cases).[1,2] The principal mechanism is most consistent with a delayed hypersensitivity reaction resulting in full-thickness necrosis of all epidermal layers with dermoepidermal detachment.[2,5] Certain HLA genotypes have been associated with the development of SJS/TEN among racial and ethnic groups [**Table 81-2**].[2,5]

Histologic features of early SJS/TEN demonstrate scattered necrotic keratinocytes in the lower layer of the epidermis with vacuolization at the epidermal-dermal junction.[1,2] Established SJS/TEN shows extensive full-thickness keratinocyte necrosis and subepidermal bullae.[2]

Most cases of SJS/TEN present less than 4 weeks after initiation of the inciting medication.[2] The acute phase manifests as unspecific symptoms of fever, malaise, sore throat, and cough that typically precede cutaneous manifestations by a few days.[8] Subsequent cutaneous and mucosal involvement typically appear as erythematous macules or atypical target lesions on the trunk that progress to become confluent areas of erythema with dusky centers and flaccid blisters with a positive Nikolsky sign [**Figures 81-3** and **81-4**].[1,2,8] The mucosal lesions are most frequently oral (80% of cases), ocular, and sometimes genital.[2]

In addition to the identification and cessation of the causative agent, supportive care is the mainstay treatment of SJS/TEN, ideally in an intensive care unit, with the goal of maintaining a urinary output of 0.5 to 1.0 mL/kg per hour.[1,2,8] Adjunctive therapies include systemic corticosteroids and intravenous immunoglobulins (IVIG) although these methods have shown varying degrees of success.[2,8] Combination of corticosteroids and IVIG has been associated with a better prognosis in some cases than corticosteroids alone.[2] Cyclosporine and etanercept have also been used in the treatment of SJS/TEN.

Morbidity and mortality vary widely in SJS/TEN patients and are much higher in patient with TEN.[2,8] On the spectrum of disease, as the extent of BSA involvement increases, so does mortality: 5% for SJS, 30% for SJS/TEN overlap, and up to 50% for TEN.[1] Mortality can be predicted by using one of two scoring systems, the severity-of-illness score for TEN (SCORTEN) or ABCD10 [**Table 81-3**].[9]

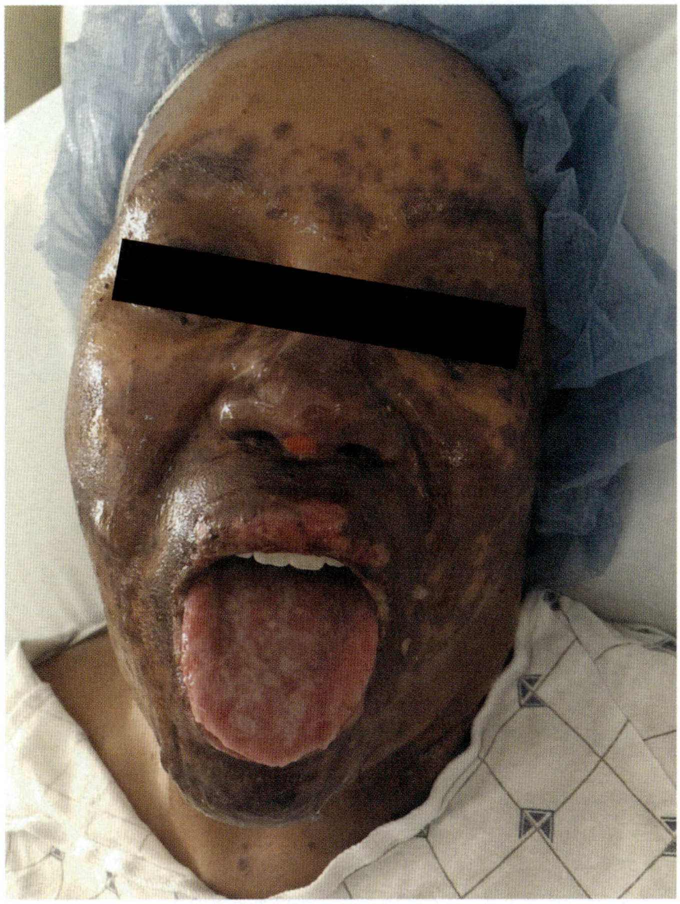

FIGURE 81-3. Stevens-Johnson syndrome (SJS). Early lesions in SJS may appear more violaceous or hyperpigmented in deeply pigmented skin as shown in this image.

TABLE 81-2 HLA genotypes associated with the development of SJS /TEN among ethno-racialized groups[2,5]

Asians (SJS/TEN)	HLA-A*0206 HLA-B*15:02 HLA-B*58:01
Europeans (TEN)	HLA-B*12

Abbreviations: HLA, human leukocyte antigen; SJS-Stevens-Johnson syndrome; TEN, toxic epidermal necrolysis.

ERYTHEMA MULTIFORME

Erythema multiforme (EM) is a cytotoxic dermatosis characterized by round, erythematous papules with concentric color changes, typically seen on the limbs.[10] Erythema multiforme is classified into minor and major types based on the involvement of mucosal tissues. Generally, EM is a self-limiting condition that subsides within 1 to 2 weeks of symptom onset, but there are instances of recurring or persistent forms of the disease.[11]

Historically, erythema multiforme (EM) was considered part of the spectrum of SJS and TEN. These conditions were believed to represent different severities of the same disease process, with EM being the mildest form, SJS being more severe, and TEN being the most severe. Over time, researchers and clinicians have come to recognize that EM, SJS, and TEN are distinct entities with different etiologies, clinical features, and prognoses [see Table 81-4]. Although the exact incidence of EM is unclear, it has been estimated to exist between 0.01% and 1%.[12] EM occurs most commonly in young adults with a slight female preponderance and no racial or ethnic predilection.[12]

Numerous exposures, including drugs, cancers, autoimmune disease, radiation, and immunization, have been linked to erythema multiforme, but infectious agents—most frequently the herpes simplex virus (HSV) in adults and *Mycoplasma pneumonia* in

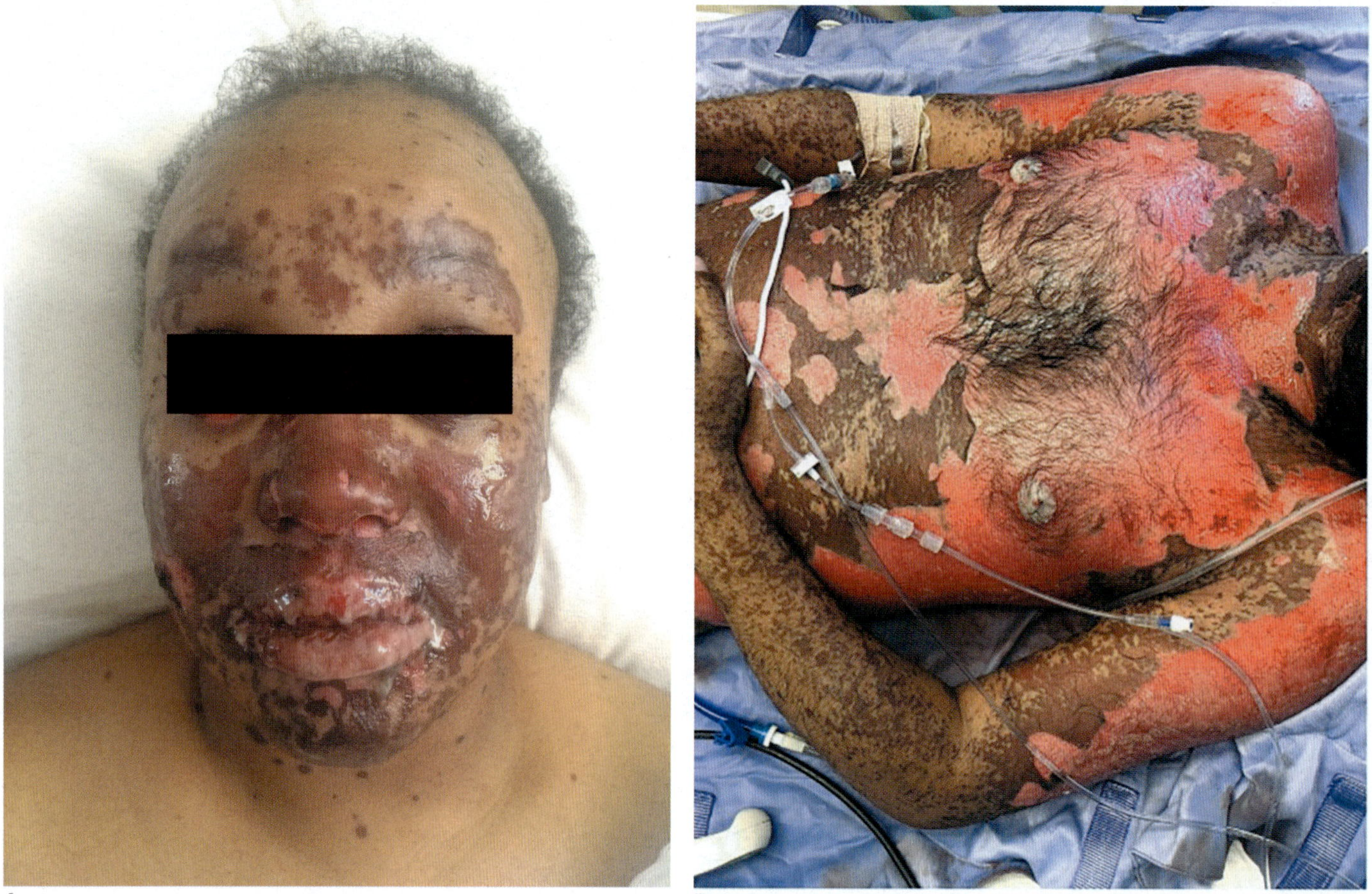

A B

FIGURE 81-4. Toxic epidermal necrolysis (TEN) as it appears in two patients with skin of color. Extensive cutaneous sloughing of the face **(A)** and body **(B)** resulting in exposure of the dermis.

children—are responsible for roughly 90% of cases.[11,12] Some EM patients may be predisposed due to genetic susceptibility. HSV-associated EM has been correlated with the HLA-DQB1*0301 allele. HLA-B35, HLA-B62, 15, and HLA DR-53 alleles have all been associated with recurrent EM.[12]

Histopathologic features in EM depend on both timing and depth of biopsy. Findings may include necrotic keratinocytes, lymphocyte exocytosis, basal epidermal cell liquefactive necrosis, and vacuolar degeneration that result in subepidermal clefts and vesiculation. The dermo-epidermal junction can be obscured by a lichenoid pattern of mild to moderate lymphohistiocytic infiltrate and dermal layers typically reveal lymphohistiocytic infiltrate along superficial and mid-dermal vessels. Cutaneous and mucous membrane EM generally share similar microscopic characteristics.[12]

TABLE 81-3 Mortality prognostication tools for SJS/TEN

SCORTEN		ABCD-10	
Parameter	Weight	Parameter	Weight
Age ≥ 40 years	1	Age ≥ 50 years	1
Malignancy—Yes	1	Serum Bicarbonate < 20 mmol/L	1
BSA detached > 10%	1	Active Cancer—Yes	2
Serum bicarbonate < 20 mmol/L	1	Dialysis prior to admission—Yes	3
Serum glucose > 252 mg/dL	1	BSA involvement > 10%	1
Maximum score possible	7		8

Abbreviations: BSA, body surface area; SCORTEN, severity-of-illness score for toxic epidermal necrolysis; SJS, Stevens-Johnson syndrome; TEN, toxic epidermal necrolysis.

EM lesions typically display a time-dependent morphology. Typically, the first EM lesions are round, erythematous, edematous papules surrounded by regions of blanching that may mimic insect bites or papular urticaria. These papules can expand and undergo concentric changes in their morphology and color, evolving to become the familiar targetoid

TABLE 81-4 Erythema multiforme vs SJS/TEN

	Erythema Multiforme (EM)	SJS/TEN
Classic distribution	Face, extremities, acral surfaces	Face, trunk
Hallmark lesion	Papular, typical target lesions	Macular, ill-defined borders that may progress to bullae and vesicles and sloughing of skin. Atypical targetoid lesions
Mucosal involvement	Less commonly	> 80%, usually two or more sites
Constitutional symptoms	Uncommon	Common
Typical age	All ages; commonly third to fifth decades	All ages; commonly fifth to eight decades
Precipitating factors	More commonly: infectious (HSV-1 in adults; mycoplasma in children) Less commonly: drugs	More commonly: drugs (aromatic antiepileptics, NSAIDs, allopurinol, antibiotics) Less commonly: infections
Duration of symptoms	1-2 weeks	Acute phase: 8-12 days Reepithelialization: 2-4 weeks

Abbreviations: HSV, herpes simplex virus; NSAIDS, nonsteroidal anti-inflammatory drugs; SJS, Stevens-Johnson syndrome; TEN, toxic epidermal necrolysis.

lesions of EM. Target lesions are circular, less than 3 cm in diameter, and feature three zones: an outer ring with a well-defined boundary, a middle zone of paler edema, and a core region of dusky erythema or purpura [**Figure 81-5**].[12]

The differential diagnosis for EM is broad and includes papular urticaria, SJS, fixed drug eruption (FDE), bullous pemphigoid, paraneoplastic pemphigus, Sweet syndrome, Rowell syndrome, polymorphous light eruption, cutaneous small vessel vasculitis, lupus erythematosus as well as other bullous autoimmune dermatoses.[12]

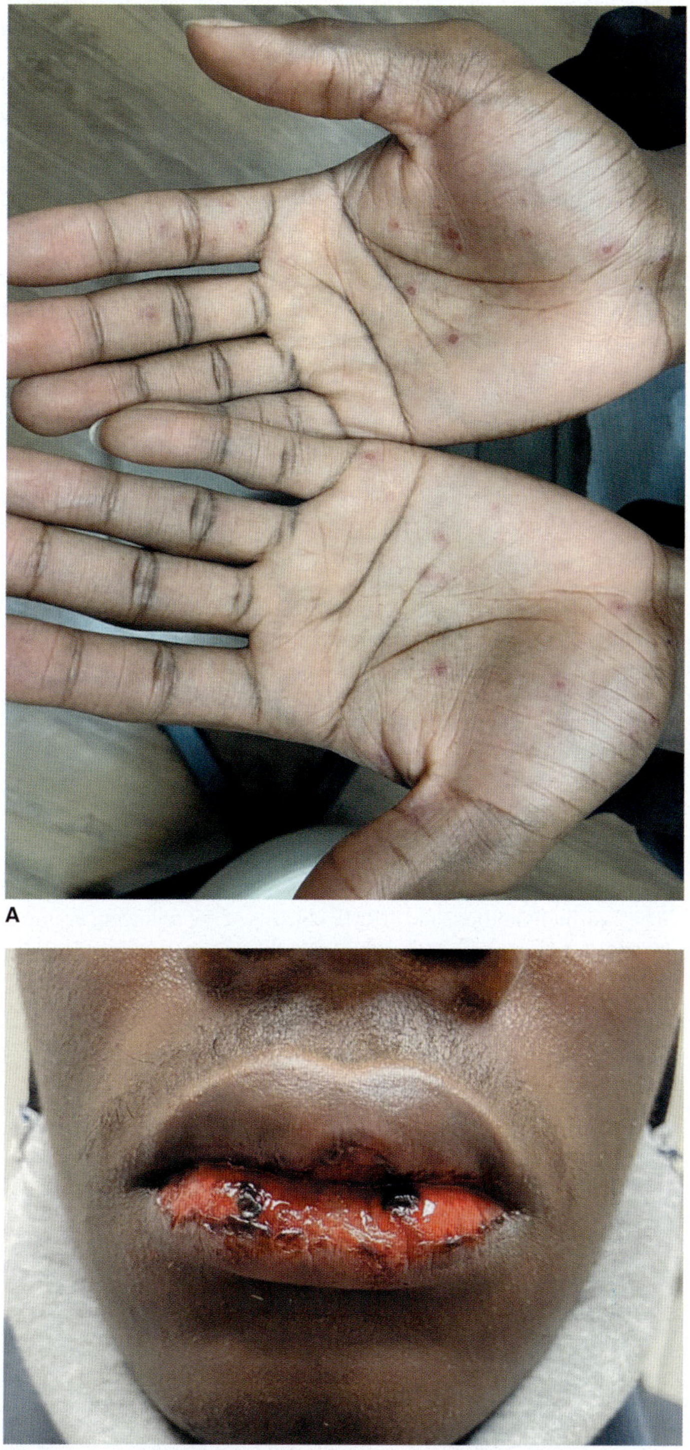

A

B

FIGURE 81-5. Erythema multiforme (EM). **(A)** Palmar cutaneous skin with typical target lesions. **(B)** Lips (especially lower lip) with erosions complicated by hemorrhagic exudate and crusts.

There is a lack of evidence-based guidance for EM treatment.[10] For drug-induced EM, discontinuation of inciting medications is critically important. Due to the highly variable presentation and disease severity of EM, individualized treatment strategies should be employed. Supportive therapies for acute EM flares range from antihistamines and topical corticosteroids for mild symptomatic treatment to inpatient hospitalization for more severe cases. Many interventional regimens have been trialed for prophylactic treatment of EM.[10] Limited evidence supports continuous acyclovir therapy for recurrent, HSV-associated EM. Alternative prophylactic regimens such as thalidomide, corticosteroids, antibiotics, and immunosuppressive regimens have been tried but lack evidence to be codified for the prevention of recurrent EM.[10,12]

GENERALIZED BULLOUS FIXED DRUG ERUPTION

FDE is a severe cutaneous adverse drug hypersensitivity reaction characterized by sharply defined erythematous patches or plaques that develop at the same spot on the body every time a specific drug is administered.[13,14] Repeated exposure to the causative medication in individuals with a prior history of FDE can precipitate a rare, more severe variant of FDE known as generalized bullous FDE (GBFDE). GBFDE is described as conventional FDE lesions as well as blisters and erosions affecting at least 10% of body surface area across three of six distinct anatomic regions (namely, the head and neck, anterior trunk, back, upper extremities, lower extremities, and genitalia).[13] The risk of a GBFDE increases with repeated exposure to the causative drug.

FDE has been reported in all age groups but most commonly occurs in young to middle-aged adults with no gender, racial, or ethnic predilection. The overall incidence of FDE is geographically highly variable and dependent upon the frequency of use of any particular medication.[13]

The pathogenesis of FDE and GBFDE alike is unclear but is thought to be caused by intraepidermal CD8+ T-cell activation. Activation of basal CD8+ T-cells by the causative agent causes upward epidermal migration of T-cells, the release of cytokines such as interferon-γ and TNF-α, and T-cell expression of CD56, perforin, and granzyme B, which directly cytolyze adjacent keratinocytes promoting the further release of numerous proinflammatory cytokines into the surrounding tissue.[14] Despite the geographic-dependent variability, common causative medications include NSAIDs, acetaminophen, amoxicillin, levofloxacin, doxycycline, trimethoprim/sulfamethoxazole, phenytoin, carbamazepine, phenobarbital, intravenous contrast, and the influenza vaccine.[14]

GBFDE is characterized by vacuolar changes at the dermoepidermal junction, a subepidermal blister or denuded epidermis, and a variable amount of necrotic keratinocytes within the epidermis. There is often a rapid, fairly dense perivascular infiltration of lymphocytes and interstitial eosinophils despite the varied infiltrate of inflammatory cells. Neutrophils may also be present in response to the necrosis of the epidermis.[14]

The majority of individuals with GBFDE mention a history of previous comparable lesions at the time of presentation. GBFDE invariably manifests 1 to 2 weeks (but most typically 48 hours) after administration of the offending agent. Local sensations like pruritus or burning may sometimes accompany the eruption of the lesions, which might appear as blisters, vesicles, or bullae that burst readily and leave erosions or shallow ulcers. GBFDE bullae and patches often have clearly defined borders and broad areas of healthy skin in between lesions [**Figure 81-6**].[14]

Invariably, SJS and TEN are part of the differential diagnosis for GBFDE due to the generalized nature of the reaction and considerable overlap in morphology.[13]

Management of GBFDE most critically requires identification and cessation of the offending drug. Other treatments described in the literature include supportive care, topical and/or systemic corticosteroids, and cyclosporine. The utilization of antibiotics has also been documented to promote healing and reduce the risk of infection.[13,14]

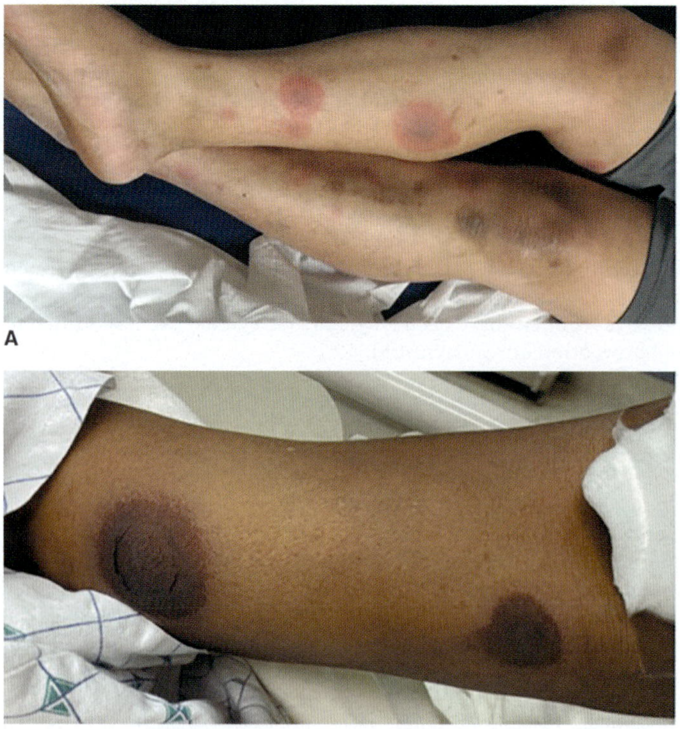

FIGURE 81-6. Multiple bullous fixed drug eruptions among different skin tones. Compared to individuals with lighter skin tones, individuals with darker skin tones may project less erythema and more hyperpigmentation. **(A)** Notice characteristic round morphology, dusky centers, and large swaths of intervening normal skin. **(B)** Multiple bullous fixed drug eruption with well-developed central bulla distally.

REACTIVE INFECTIOUS MUCOCUTANEOUS ERUPTION (RIME)/ MYCOPLASMA PNEUMONIAE RASH AND MUCOSITIS (MIRM)

Reactive infection mucocutaneous eruption (RIME) is a postinfectious mucocutaneous eruption characterized by mucositis with sparse yet prominent vesiculobullous and/or target-like eruptions. The term RIME refers to all postinfectious mucocutaneous eruptions, including the rash and mucositis caused by *Mycoplasma pneumoniae*, also known as *Mycoplasma pneumoniae* rash and mucositis (MIRM).[15]

The exact incidence of RIME is largely unknown though one study reported an incidence rate of 5.34/10,000 among children hospitalized with *Mycoplasma pneumoniae* infection. *Mycoplasma*-associated cases of RIME are more commonly observed in children with a slight predilection for young male populations, although cases in adults have been reported.[16,17]

Although the pathophysiology of RIME is unknown, it is hypothesized to be associated with the proliferation of polyclonal B cells, the development of particular antibodies, and the formation of immunological complexes that are then deposited in the skin, causing activation of cytotoxic T-cells via molecular mimicry and subsequent skin damage.[17] Serologic analysis of patients with recurring episodes of *Mycoplasma*-associated RIME have been shown to reveal consistently high *Mycoplasma pneumoniae* IgG levels, which may contribute to its pathogenesis.[16] Additionally, reports of RIME family aggregation and recurrence are hypothesized to be influenced by genetic predisposition.[15] Classically, MIRM has been associated with recent *Mycoplasma pneumoniae* infection. Given that other organisms, such as *Chlamydophila pneumoniae* and viral infections, such as influenza B, may cause a similar constellation of symptoms, the name "reactive infectious mucocutaneous eruption" (RIME) better represents MIRM.[16]

There is minimal documented evidence of histopathologic analysis of mucocutaneous manifestations of RIME. Documented histopathologic analysis of mucosal lesions reveal epidermal necrosis, whereas documented microscopic analysis of skin lesions has revealed interface dermatitis with sub-basilar microvesicle formation and significant keratinocyte apoptosis with minimal dermal change demonstrating considerable overlap with SJS/TEN.[15,18]

The diagnosis of RIME is difficult due to significant clinical and histopathologic overlap with SJS/TEN. RIME presents clinically with a prominent mucositis and cutaneous involvement that demonstrates a distinctive, sparse vesiculobullous and/or targetoid eruption.[17] The suggested diagnostic criteria for classic MIRM includes the following: clinical and laboratory evidence of atypical pneumonia caused by *Mycoplasma pneumoniae* with at least two involved mucosal sites, less than 10% of skin surface area involved, few vesiculobullous lesions or atypical scattered targets with or without targetoid lesions.[18]

The differential diagnosis for RIME/MIRM is broad and includes SJS/TEN and other pathogenic causes of mucocutaneous lesions including herpes simplex (HSV), cytomegalovirus, *chlamydia* species, coxsackie virus, influenza B, *Staphylococcus aureus*, Varicella-Zoster as well as an array of autoimmune processes due to the coexistence of mucositis and skin eruption. Due to the considerable overlap in clinical presentation, a combination of detailed medical history taking and pathogenic identification is required in order to distinguish RIME/MIRM from SJS/TEN and HSV.[17] Notably, the mucositis and skin involvement of MIRM/RIME tends to be sparse and can occur independently of one another, which can help distinguish it from SJS/TEN and HSV.[17]

Despite the lack of defined treatment guidelines for patients with MIRM, supportive therapy, which includes pain control, intravenous hydration, and mucosal care, is the cornerstone of treatment.[18]

PROGRESSIVE IMMUNOTHERAPY-RELATED MUCOCUTANEOUS ERUPTION (PIRME)

Progressive immunotherapy-related mucocutaneous eruption (PIRME) is a newly characterized immunotherapy-related generalized bullous dermatosis characterized initially by a mild rash that progresses to generalized, Nikolsky-positive bullous dermatoses that can present with or without mucosal involvement.[19] The epidemiology of PIRME has not been characterized.[19]

The pathogenesis and etiology of PIRME have not been fully elucidated but appear to be associated with a "two-hit mechanism" whereby patients on immune checkpoint inhibitors develop an SJS-like rash within 2 months of starting a concomitant medication classically associated with SJS.[19]

The two-hit hypothesis for PIRME consists of the following events:

1. The first hit: The immunotherapy treatment, such as a checkpoint inhibitor, activates the patient's immune system, enhancing its ability

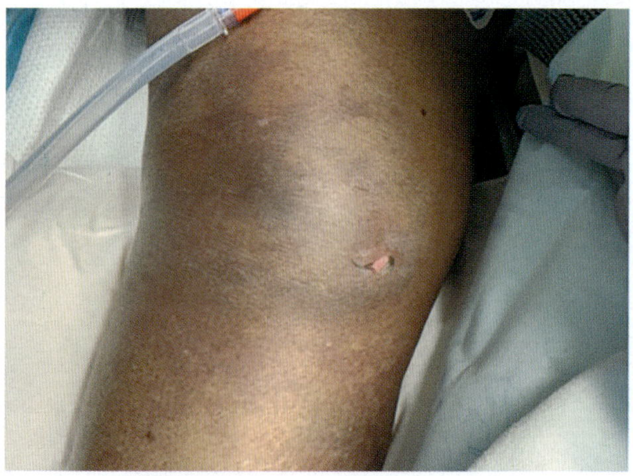

FIGURE 81-7. PD-1 induced rash and mucositis. Note the violaceous to purpuric patches along the medial knee that formed a bullae to frictional provocation (Nikolsky sign +).

Example of Drug Chart																		
	Symptoms						*cellulitis of leg*						*fever, malaise*	*mouth pain, nausea*	*rash, with oral pain*	*bullae,to ED*	*transfer to hospital*	
Drug	**Date**	**Daily in June**	**1-Jul**	**2-Jul**	**3-Jul**	**4-Jul**	**5-Jul**	**6-Jul**	**7-Jul**	**8-Jul**	**9-Jul**	**10-Jul**	**11-Jul**	**12-Jul**	**13-Jul**	**14-Jul**	**15-Jul**	**16-Jul**
ASA		x	x	x	x	x	x	x	x	x	x	x	x	x	x	x	x	x
Lisinopril		x	x	x	x	x	x	x	x	x	x	x	x	x	x	x	x	x
Metformin		x	x	x	x	x	x	x	x	x	x	x	x	x	x	x	x	x
Atorvastatin		x	x	x	x	x	x	x	x	x	x	x	x	x	x	x	x	x
Polyethylene glycol eye drops		x	x	x	x	x	x	x	x	x	x	x	x	x	x	x	x	x
Trimethoprim-Sulfamethoxazole								x	x	x	x	x	x	x	x	x		
Acetaminophen with dextromethorphan HBr														x	x	x	x	
Ibuprofen				x	x	x	x	x					x	x				
Piperacillin/tazobactam																x	x	

* Here you can identfy TMP-SMX as having been started 5 days prior to the onset of systemic symptoms, making it the most likely offending agent on this chart

FIGURE 81-8. Example of a drug timeline chart. The chart identifies trimethoprim-sulfamethoxazole (TMP-SMX) as having been started 5 days prior to the onset of the systemic symptoms, making it the most likely offending agent.

to identify and target cancer cells. During this phase, patients generally tolerate the checkpoint inhibitor without experiencing mucocutaneous eruptions.

2. The second hit: An additional trigger, such as drug exposure, further stimulates the immune system. This trigger exacerbates the autoimmune response, causing immune cells, such as T-cells, to target and attack healthy mucocutaneous tissues in the body. This immune-mediated attack on the skin and mucosal cells lead to the development of mucocutaneous eruptions seen in PIRME.

In most cases, the rash has mild initial presentation with lichenoid, urticarial, and morbilliform morphologies. From its initial benign presentation, PIRME progresses to a generalized, Nikolsky-positive bullous dermatosis with occasional mucosal involvement [**Figure 81-7**].[19] The histopathologic presentation of PIRME closely resembles that of SJS/TEN such as full-thickness epidermal necrosis, subepidermal clefting.[19] However, although SJS/TEN tends to be pauci-inflammatory, PIRME tends to exhibit either lichenoid or interface dermatitis.

The differential for PIRME most notably includes SJS/TEN. Despite their similarities, obtaining a detailed medical history, including a comprehensive medication list and known drug allergies can be utilized to distinguish PIRME from SJS/TEN. Unlike SJS/TEN, PIRME has a delayed onset and mild initial morphologic presentation and is rarely associated with ocular involvement.[19]

Cessation of the offending, concomitant medication is the mainstay of treatment for PIRME. Initiation of systemic therapy, such as IV corticosteroids and cyclosporine has been documented; however, cessation of the offending agent alone has shown to be effective for achieving complete and rapid resolution of PIRME.[19]

TIPS AND PEARLS FOR CLINICAL EVALUATION

1. Utilize patients' baseline photograph to detect early central facial, lip, and eyelid swelling. This can be facilitated by using their identification card or a photo on their phone.
2. Creating a "drug timeline chart" can be helpful in identifying the correct offending agent, as it visually highlights the timeline and may prompt the care team and the patient not to omit any of the medication history [**Figure 81-8**]. Mark the dates of constitutional symptoms and the development of a rash on the chart, and consider drugs ingested before that date when appropriate.
3. For MIRM/RIME and EM, assessment of recent symptoms of infectious diseases such as oral or genital ulcers seen in HSV or cough associated with mycoplasma may help to determine which infectious disease evaluation to undertake.
4. Always perform a comprehensive review of systems and assess all the mucosal sites for patients whom you suspect may be having a drug reaction.
5. Good lighting is paramount. A handheld LED flashlight or an illuminated magnifying glass are inexpensive and will improve the clinician's ability to discern early erythema or mucositis.

REFERENCES

1. Owen CE, Jones JM. Recognition and management of severe cutaneous adverse drug reactions (including drug reaction with eosinophilia and systemic symptoms, Stevens-Johnson syndrome, and toxic epidermal necrolysis). *Med Clin North Am.* 2021;105:577-597.
2. Alvarado SA, Munoz-Mendoza D, Bahna SL. High-risk drug rashes. *Ann Allergy Asthma Immunol.* 2018;121:552-560.
3. Reap LE, Rodd C, Larios J, Marshall M. Hydrochlorothizide-induced acute generalised exanthematous pustulosis presenting with bilateral periorbital impetigo. *BMJ Case Rep.* 2019;12(2):e223528.
4. Svoboda SA, Bisbee EL, Bender N, Motaparthi K. Acute generalized exanthematous pustulosis sine pustules: a case series. *JAAD Case Rep* 2022;23:24-26.
5. Bellon T. Mechanisms of severe cutaneous adverse reactions: recent advances. *Drug Saf.* 2019;42:973-992.
6. Yanes D, Nguyen E, Imadojemu S, Kroshinsky D. Cyclosporine for treatment of acute generalized exanthematous pustulosis: a retrospective analysis. *J Am Acad Dermatol.* 2020;83:263-265.
7. Miyagawa F, Asada H. Current perspective regarding the immunopathogenesis of drug-induced hypersensitivity syndrome/drug reaction with eosinophilia and systemic symptoms (DiHS/DRESS). *Int J Mol Sci.* 2021;22(4):2147.
8. Frantz R, Huang S, Are A, Motaparthi K. Stevens-Johnson syndrome and toxic epidermal necrolysis: a review of diagnosis and management. *Medicina (Kaunas).* 2021;57(9):895.
9. Koh HK, Fook-Chong S, Lee HY. Assessment and comparison of performance of ABCD-10 and SCORTEN in prognostication of epidermal necrolysis. *JAMA Dermatol.* 2020;156:1294-1299.
10. de Risi-Pugliese T, Sbidian E, Ingen-Housz-Oro S, Le Cleach L. Interventions for erythema multiforme: a systematic review. *J Eur Acad Dermatol Venereol.* 2019;33:842-849.
11. Paulino L, Hamblin DJ, Osondu N, Amini R. Variants of erythema multiforme: a case report and literature review. *Cureus.* 2018;10:e3459.
12. Sokumbi O, Wetter DA. Clinical features, diagnosis, and treatment of erythema multiforme: a review for the practicing dermatologist. *Int J Dermatol.* 2012;51:889-902.
13. Mitre V, Applebaum DS, Albahrani Y, Hsu S. Generalized bullous fixed drug eruption imitating toxic epidermal necrolysis: a case report and literature review. *Dermatol Online J.* 2017;23(7):13030/qt25v009gs.
14. Anderson HJ, Lee JB. A review of fixed drug eruption with a special focus on generalized bullous fixed drug eruption. *Medicina (Kaunas).* 2021;57(9):925.
15. Song A, Nicholson C, Maguiness S. Recurrent reactive infectious mucocutaneous eruption (RIME) in two adolescents triggered by several distinct pathogens including SARS-CoV-2 and influenza A. *Pediatr Dermatol.* 2021;38:1222-1225.
16. Gandelman JS, Kim EY, Grzegorczyk AM, Zejnullahu K, Edson RS. Mycoplasma pneumoniae-induced rash and mucositis in a previously healthy man: a case report and brief review of the literature. *Open Forum Infect Dis.* 2020;7:ofaa437.
17. Chen N, Li M. Case report and literature review: clinical characteristics of 10 children with mycoplasma pneumoniae-induced rash and mucositis. *Front Pediatr.* 2022;10:823376.
18. Lofgren D, Lenkeit C. Mycoplasma pneumoniae-induced rash and mucositis: a systematic review of the literature. *Spartan Med Res J* 2021;6:25284.
19. Molina GE, Yu Z, Foreman RK, Reynolds KL, Chen ST. Generalized bullous mucocutaneous eruption mimicking Stevens-Johnson syndrome in the setting of immune checkpoint inhibition: a multicenter case series. *J Am Acad Dermatol.* 2020;83:1475-1477.

CHAPTER 82

Neutrophilic Dermatoses in Skin of Color

Hadir Shakshouk
Shannon Kody
Alex G. Ortega-Loayza

KEY POINTS

- The pathogenesis of neutrophilic dermatoses is complex and incompletely understood.
- Underlying inflammatory and autoimmune comorbidities are commonly associated with neutrophilic dermatoses and some of these diseases may also have extracutaneous manifestations.
- Some neutrophilic dermatoses are associated with higher rates of hospitalization or more severe disease in patients with skin of color.
- Diagnostic criteria have been developed for many of these conditions but lesions classically characterized as erythematous may appear grayish, black, or violaceous in skin of color.
- Insufficient research data exist on neutrophilic dermatoses in skin of color.

INTRODUCTION

Neutrophilic dermatoses (ND) encompass a heterogeneous group of inflammatory skin diseases. All share sterile neutrophil infiltration on skin biopsy and underlying systemic diseases or associated comorbidities. Cutaneous manifestations are variable and may include pustules, papules, plaques, nodules, or ulcers. Additionally, pathergy is a common feature among most neutrophilic dermatoses. The characteristic histopathological finding is a marked neutrophilic infiltrate with no detectable infection or true vasculitis. This infiltrate may be epidermal, dermal, and/or hypodermal.

The precise pathogenesis of neutrophilic dermatoses is not fully understood. An interplay between neutrophil dysfunction, aberrant expression of inflammatory effector molecules, and genetic predisposition is implicated. Emerging evidence supports the role of proinflammatory cytokines, namely, interleukin (IL)-1-β, IL-17, and tumor necrosis factor-α (TNF-α). Ongoing research continues to unravel the intricate pathogenesis.

ND can be classified according to the predominant location of neutrophilic infiltrate [**Figure 82-1**] into hypodermal including pyoderma gangrenosum, hidradenitis suppurativa, and Behçet disease; dermal such as Sweet syndrome, erythema elevatum diutinum, and neutrophilic eccrine hidradenitis; or epidermal such as amicrobial pustulosis of the folds, subcorneal pustular dermatosis, and IgA pemphigus.[1]

Extracutaneous involvement can be detected in some cases, hence the use of the term "neutrophilic disease" that was initially coined by French colleagues. Dermatologists should be aware of the possibility of neutrophilic infiltrates in other organs and the immune-mediated diseases associated with each type of ND to guide a thorough work-up, screening, and management.[2]

NEUTROPHILIC DERMATOSES IN SKIN OF COLOR PATIENTS

The literature lacks adequate studies about ND in patients with skin of color. The majority of ND do not exhibit any racial predilections. Few exceptions exist; Behçet disease occurs more frequently in patients from the Mediterranean and eastern Asia, and hidradenitis suppurativa disproportionately affects patients from historically marginalized groups, including Black/African American and possibly Latine/Hispanic patient populations although there is conflicting evidence.[3,4] Outcomes may also differ in patients with skin of color. For instance, the rate of hospitalization due to pyoderma gangrenosum is higher in Black patients.[5] Similarly, hidradenitis suppurativa may be more severe in patients with skin of color.[6] Skin lesions may vary clinically with darker skin.[7] In particular, inflammatory dermatoses characterized by erythematous lesions can create diagnostic confusion in darker skin as lesions typically described as erythematous may appear more grayish, black, or even violaceous.[8] Insufficient data exist regarding the clinical presentations of ND in skin of color. Recognition of important clinical features in skin of color and careful consideration of social determinants of health is important for effective management of patients with ND (refer to Chapter 11).

In this chapter, we will discuss the most representative neutrophilic dermatoses such as Sweet syndrome and pyoderma gangrenosum in detail. We will briefly discuss Behçet disease, neutrophilic eccrine hidradenitis, amicrobial pustulosis of the fold, IgA pemphigus, and neutrophilic panniculitis as they are less prevalent in a general dermatology practice. Hidradenitis suppurativa, acute generalized exanthematous pustulosis, and pustular psoriasis will be discussed in other chapters.

SWEET SYNDROME

EPIDEMIOLOGY

Sweet syndrome (SS), also known as acute febrile ND, is regarded as the prototype of ND. It can occur at any age; however, it usually affects middle-aged women (30-60 years old) without racial predilection. SS can be classified as classic, malignancy-associated or drug-induced.

Classic or idiopathic SS can be triggered by upper respiratory tract or gastrointestinal infection, vaccination, inflammatory bowel disease, or pregnancy. Malignancy-associated SS is frequently reported with hematologic malignancies and myeloproliferative or myelodysplastic disorders (MDS), most commonly acute myeloid leukemia (AML) followed by MDS. It can also occur in the setting of solid-organ tumors. SS may precede or follow a diagnosis of malignancy and can be a marker of recurrence.[9]

Common drugs incriminated in drug-induced SS are granulocyte colony stimulating factor and all-trans retinoic acid. A temporal relationship between drug exposure and clinical presentations of SS is required for the diagnosis.[10]

CLINICAL FEATURES

Clinically, SS is typified by the abrupt onset of tender, elevated, erythematous papules, or coalescent plaques, variable in size from one to several centimeters [**Figures 82-2** and **82-3**]. Lesions are often asymmetrical and favor the upper extremities, head, and neck. Lesions may have central yellowish discoloration, creating a target-like appearance, or marked edema producing pseudo-vesiculations. True pustulation and blistering may occur. Plaques are characteristically tender and not pruritic. Patients also have fever, peripheral neutrophilia, arthralgia, and generalized malaise. Lesions usually resolve spontaneously within 5 to 12 weeks; however, recurrence occurs in a third of the patients. Other less frequent clinical variants of SS include pustular, bullous, necrotizing, and subcutaneous.

Features typical of malignancy-associated SS are older patient age, vesiculobullous lesions, leukopenia, anemia, thrombocytopenia, elevated erythrocyte sedimentation rate (ESR), and absence of arthralgia.[11-14]

Extracutaneous involvement can occur in muscles, bones, the central nervous system, ears, eyes, mouth, kidneys, intestines, liver, spleen, heart, and lung. A wide variety of ocular manifestations are possible and may be the presenting symptom of SS.

HISTOPATHOLOGICAL FEATURES

Skin biopsy reveals marked dermal edema and diffuse infiltrates of mature neutrophils in the superficial dermis. Neutrophilic infiltrates can extend deeper into the subcutaneous tissue. Lesions typically lack features of leukocytoclastic vasculitis. Pathologic variants of SS are cryptococcoid, histiocytoid, lymphocytic, subcutaneous, and xanthomatized. Histiocytoid Sweet syndrome exhibits histiocytoid immature mononuclear myeloid cells. This variant may have a higher risk of associated hematologic malignancy.

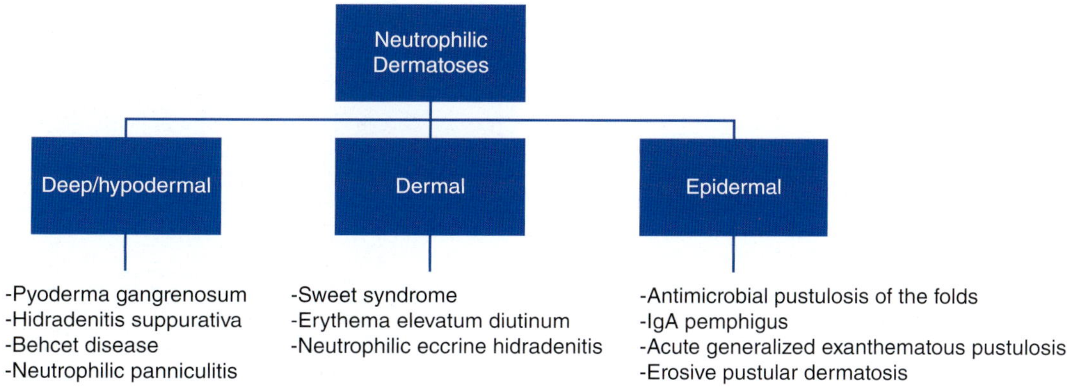

FIGURE 82-1. Histopathological classification of neutrophilic dermatoses.

DIAGNOSIS

Major diagnostic criteria rely on the abrupt onset of characteristic skin lesions and typical histopathologic features as illustrated in **Table 82-1**.[15] Criteria for diagnosing drug-induced SS are outlined in **Table 82-2**. Laboratory investigations required for diagnosis include complete blood count (CBC) with differential, C-reactive protein (CRP), and ESR. Tissue culture for bacterial, fungal, and mycobacterial organisms may be helpful to exclude infection. Appropriate work-up to detect underlying conditions should be based on clinical suspicion. Screening for hematological malignancies is recommended.

MANAGEMENT

Treatment relies on systemic corticosteroids. Prednisone is used at a dose of 0.5 to 1 mg/kg/day with subsequent slow tapering over 4 to 6 weeks. Topical and intralesional steroids can be used as well. Marked improvement on systemic steroids confirms the diagnosis. If recurrence while tapering systemic corticosteroids or lack of improvement is noted, underlying malignancy should be considered.

Potassium iodide (900 mg/day) and colchicine (1.5 mg/day) are other effective treatment options. Dapsone (100–200 mg/day), indomethacin, and cyclosporine have also been used.[16,17] Biologics (tumor necrosis factor-α (TNF-α) inhibitors and ustekinumab) and small molecules (eg, baricitinib) can be used with good efficacy.

PYODERMA GANGRENOSUM

EPIDEMIOLOGY

Pyoderma gangrenosum (PG) is primarily an ulcerative ND with an estimated prevalence of 5.8 cases per 100,000 adults in the United States. Prevalence is comparable in White and Black/African American patients.[18] PG was the most common reason for inpatient dermatology consultation involving ulcers in a multi-center study.[19] It is more common in females than males. The burden of hospitalization in PG has been linked to female sex, Black race, and accompanying comorbidities.[5] About half of patients with PG have associated comorbidities, mainly inflammatory bowel diseases, inflammatory arthritis, and hematological disorders. Rheumatoid arthritis is the most common arthritis and often precedes the diagnosis of PG.[20] PG might also occur in association with solid organ malignancies.[21] Neutrophilic infiltrates have been detected in other organs, especially the lungs, reinforcing the concept of the use of the term "neutrophilic disease" over neutrophilic dermatosis.[22] Given its chronic nature, prolonged wound healing, and associated comorbidities, PG profoundly impairs patients' quality of life.[23] There is also an estimated threefold increase in the mortality rate for patients with PG.[24]

CLINICAL FEATURES

PG usually starts as an erythematous papule, pustule, or vesicle that rapidly ulcerates and expands centrifugally. Some cases also start as an inflammatory nodule. Ulcers characteristically exhibit violaceous undermined border and are consistently painful [**Figure 82-4**]. When healing occurs, projections of epithelium extends from the wound edge toward the center, known as Gulliver sign. After healing, cribriform scarring can be seen [**Figure 82-5**]. The lower extremities are the most common site of disease.[25] Other less common subtypes of PG include bullous, vegetative, pustular, verrucous [**Figure 82-6**], peristomal, and postoperative.

Unlike ulcerative PG, bullous PG favors the face and upper extremities and is more frequently associated with malignancy. Vegetative PG, also known as the superficial granulomatous subtype, manifests with superficial ulcers with a verrucous surface. It lacks the classic violaceous, undermined border of ulcerative PG. Pustular PG appears as multiple painful pustules surrounded with erythematous halos.

Peristomal PG represents 15% of all PG cases and develops around a stoma as a painful papule or plaque that rapidly evolves into a classic PG

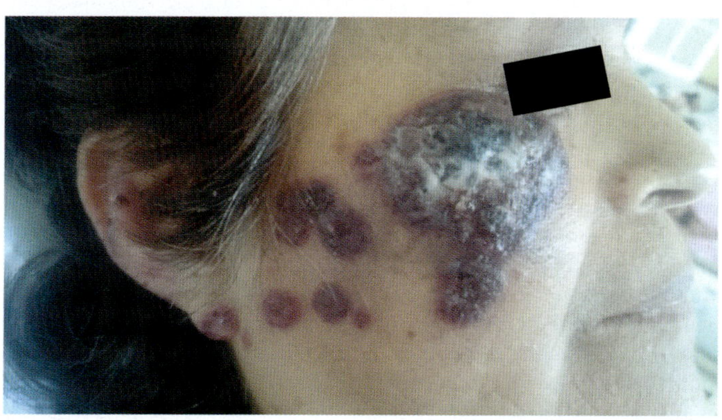

FIGURE 82-2. Sweet syndrome—edematous and violaceous plaques with some hyperpigmentation on the face.

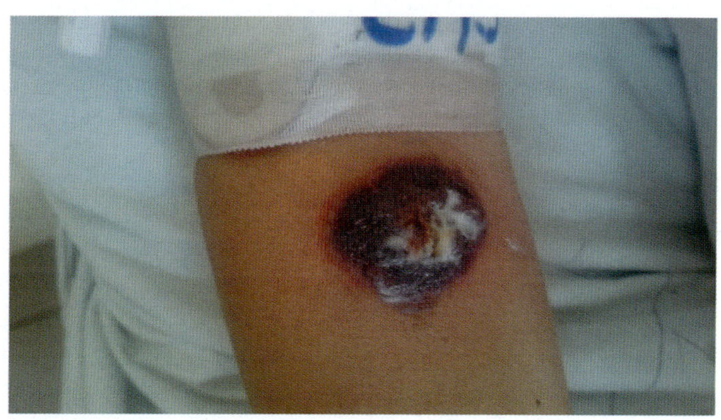

FIGURE 82-3. Sweet syndrome—plaque on arm started after venipuncture representing pathergy; a clue for diagnosis of neutrophilic dermatoses.

TABLE 82-1 Diagnostic criteria for Sweet syndrome[15]*

Major criteria
1. Abrupt onset of typical cutaneous lesions
2. Typical histopathologic features of Sweet syndrome
Minor criteria
1. Preceded by infections or vaccinations; associated with malignancies or inflammatory disorders; drug exposure or pregnancy
2. Presence of fever and constitutional signs and symptoms
3. Leukocytosis
4. Excellent response to systemic corticosteroids

*Both major and two minor criteria are required for diagnosis.

ulcer. Postoperative PG is frequently misdiagnosed as a wound infection. Within 11 days of the procedure, it starts as erythema around suture lines or the incision, then foci of punctate ulcerations with discharge develop with subsequently larger areas of wound dehiscence.[26] This is explained by the pathergy phenomenon, in which PG lesions appear at the site of trauma. Delayed diagnosis of PG can lead to unnecessary surgical debridement or even limb amputations.[27]

HISTOPATHOLOGICAL FEATURES

Classically, biopsy shows dense diffuse infiltrates of neutrophils occupying the dermis without vasculitis. The bullous type shows epidermal necrosis, whereas the superficial granulomatous type demonstrates marked pseudo-epitheliomatous hyperplasia and may have dermal suppurative granulomata with plasma cells and eosinophils. In many cases (between 30% and 89% cases depending on the publication), biopsy findings are nonspecific and definitive diagnosis depends on the clinical assessment in conjunction with a neutrophilic infiltrate without evidence of leukocytoclastic vasculitis and negative tissue cultures for fungi, bacteria, and mycobacteria.[28]

DIAGNOSIS

The diagnosis of PG is challenging due to overlap with other ulcerative diseases, and lack of specific markers and nonspecific histopatholoic features. Also, lack of awareness and provider specialty may impact the ability to diagnose PG. PG used to be considered a diagnosis of exclusion. However, diagnostic criteria for ulcerative PG have been suggested as outlined in **Table 82-3**. More recent studies have shown that the PARACELSUS score has higher sensitivity in identifying PG than the Su and Delphi criteria.[32,33] PARACELSUS is also the criteria preferred by PG experts.[34]

Proper diagnosis entails exclusion of other differential diagnosis and evaluation for underlying comorbities as summarized in **Table 82-4**. Adequate skin biopsy from the ulcer edge is recommended but not necessary. Tissue culture is required if there is suspicion for superimposed infection or infectious etiology. Given the frequent associated comorbidities in PG, further work up should be considered. A thorough history, CBC, age-appropriate screening for malignancy (eg, colonoscopy), and fecal calprotectin are recommended. A panel of laboratory tests including tests such as rheumatoid factor, anti-cyclic citrullinated peptide (CCP), anti-nuclear antibody (ANA), and antineutrophil cystoplasmic antibody (ANCA) may be needed to detect underlying comorbidities or

TABLE 82-2 Diagnostic criteria for drug-induced Sweet syndrome.[10] All criteria are required for diagnosis

1. Abrupt onset of typical cutaneous lesions
2. Typical histopathologic features of Sweet syndrome
3. Presence of fever and constitutional signs and symptoms
4. Temporal relationship between drug ingestion and clinical presentation or temporally related recurrence after oral rechallenge
5. Temporally related resolution of lesions after drug withdrawal or treatment with systemic corticosteroids

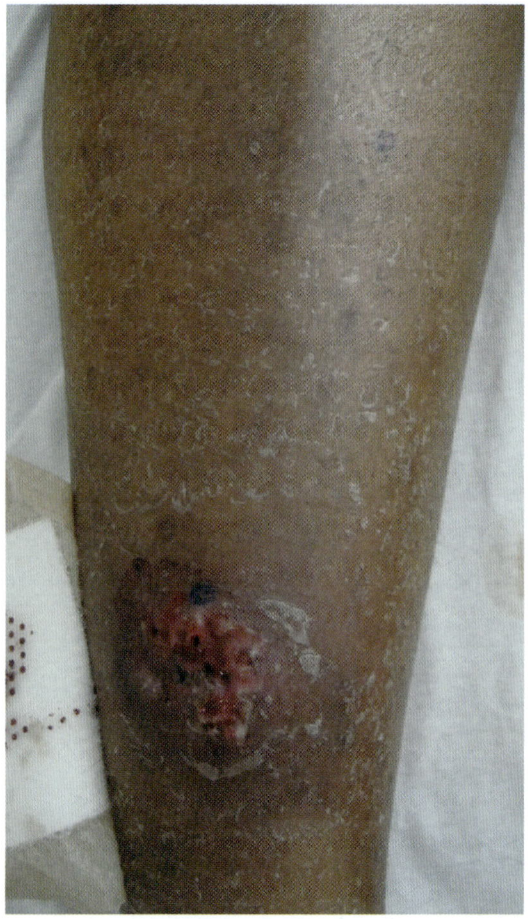

FIGURE 82-4. Ulcerative pyoderma gangrenosum—classic ulcer with some violaceous erythema and hyperpigmentation around ulcer with early necrotic tissue in the center.

mimickers.[35] Duplex ultrasonography and ankle-brachial index are helpful in evaluating for primary or superimposed vascular disease in ulcers of the lower limbs.

MANAGEMENT

Initial treatment relies on classic immunosuppression with systemic corticosteroids and/or cyclosporine. Management aims to halt neutrophil infiltration and promote wound healing. Newer biologic and small-molecules drugs show promising results and combination therapy with classic immunosuppression while waiting for these drugs to exert their effects has become the standard of care in clinical practice.[36,37] As concluded by a systematic review in 2018, the most effective options with the highest level of evidence are systemic corticosteroids, cyclosporine, infliximab, and canakinumab; however, no treatment is FDA-approved for use in PG.[38] If biologics cannot be used, mycophenolate mofetil and dapsone may be considered as they have the highest evidence among older immunosuppressants.[39]

Prednisone with a dose of 0.5 to 2.0 mg/kg/day yields rapid improvement of the ulcers with a significant decrease in the ulcer size. Cyclosporine 4 mg/kg/day proved to have similar healing time, rate of recurrence, and frequency of side effects compared to oral prednisolone 0.75 mg/kg/day.[40] TNF-α inhibitors, particularly infliximab, have shown efficacy.[41] Adalimumab is now officially approved to treat PG in Japan.[42] One study showed less side effects and shorter time to remission with TNF inhibitors. In this study, systemic corticosteroids were linked to higher mortality, prompting recognitions of the need for safer treatment options.[43] Ustekinumab and new IL-23 inhibitors also seem to be effective.[44-46] JAK inhibitors may be another alternative for PG treatment; however, randomized controlled trials are warranted to test their efficacy.[39]

For patients with a few (<3) and/or small (<3 cm in diameter) ulcers, topical therapy with a corticosteroid and/or calcineurin

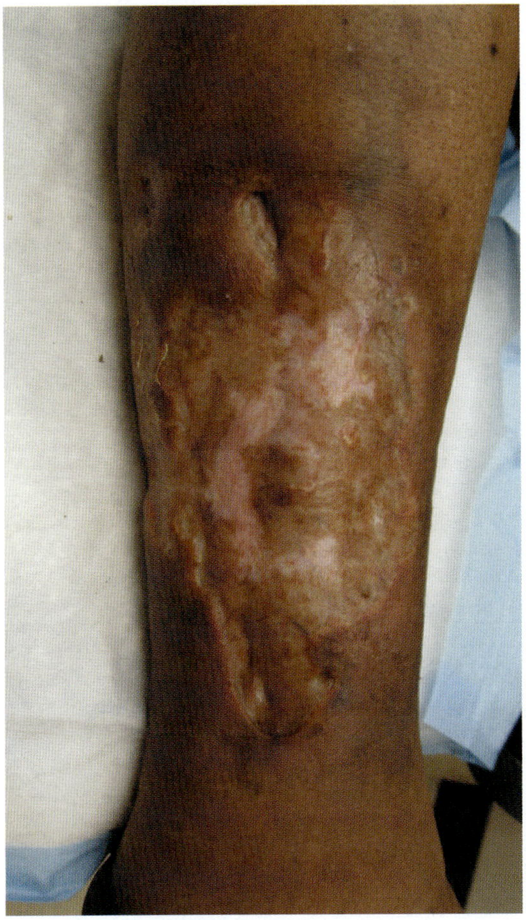

FIGURE 82-5. Healed pyoderma gangrenosum—note the early cribriform appearance close to the borders as well as postinflammatory changes.

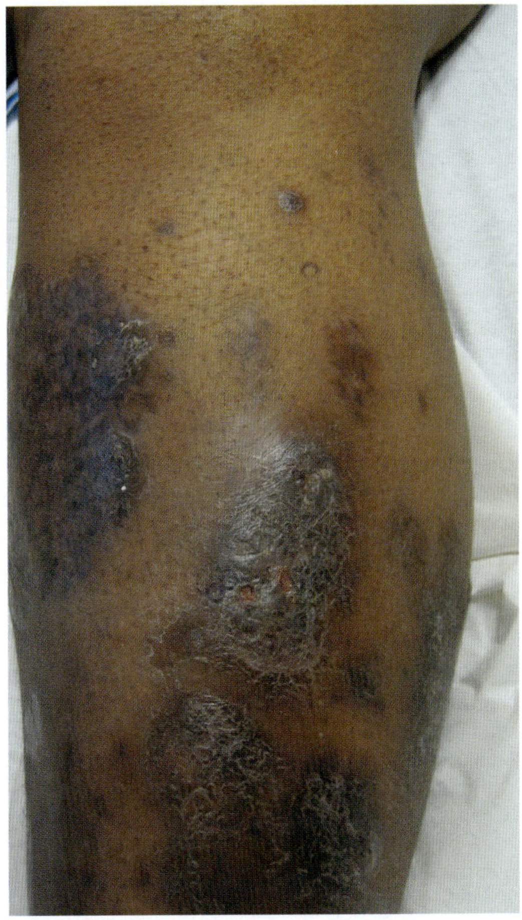

FIGURE 82-6. Verrucous pyoderma gangrenosum—rare form of pyoderma gangrenosum with verrucous plaques. Cribriform scar present in this photo was a clue for diagnosis.

inhibitor may be used.[39] Adequate wound care (dressings and compression) is crucial to optimize the healing process of PG ulcers.[47] Pain control is another challenge in the management of PG. Short courses of opioids should be considered on an individual basis. Other alternatives for pain control include topical anesthetics (eg, lidocaine) and systemic medications such as gabapentin, pregabalin, or duloxetine.

BEHÇET DISEASE

EPIDEMIOLOGY

Behçet disease (BD) is a chronic inflammatory condition with multiple organ involvement. Its predilection for patients from the Mediterranean and eastern Asia has been linked to HLA-B51. Patients are usually in their third to fourth decades and are at increased risk for malignancy.[48]

TABLE 82-3 Three diagnostic frameworks for the diagnosis of ulcerative pyoderma gangrenosum

	Su criteria (2004)[29]	Delphi consensus criteria (2018)[30]	PARACELSUS score (2019)[31]
Criteria met for diagnosis	Both major criteria and ≥2 minor criteria	Major criteria and ≥4 minor criteria	Score ≥ 10 Major criteria = 3 points Minor criteria = 2 points Additional criteria = 1 point
Major criteria	• Rapid progression of a painful, necrotic cutaneous ulcer with an irregular, violaceous, and undermined border • Other causes of cutaneous ulceration have been excluded	• Biopsy with neutrophilic infiltrate	• Progressive course of disease • Absence of relevant differential diagnoses • Reddish-violaceous border of the ulcer
Minor criteria	• History suggestive of pathergy or clinical finding of cribriform scarring • Systemic disease associated with PG (IBD, rheumatoid arthritis) • Histopathologic findings of sterile dermal neutrophilia ± mixed inflammation ± lymphocytic vasculitis • Rapid response to systemic corticosteriods	• Exclusion of infection on histology • Pathergy • Associated IBD or inflammatory arthritis • Papule, pustule, vesicle that rapidly ulcerates • Peripheral erythema, undermined border, and tenderness • Cribriform or wrinkled paper scars at healed ulcer sites • Decrease in ulcer size after immunosuppressives • Multiple ulcerations (at least one on anterior lower leg)	• Amelioration due to immunosuppressant • Characteristically bizarre ulcer shape • Extreme pain > 4 (Visual analog score) • Localized pathergy phenomenon
Additional criteria	None	None	• Suppurative inflammation on histopathology • Undermined wound margin • Associated systemic disease

TABLE 82-4 Proposed diagnostic work-up for pyoderma gangrenosum

Aim	Investigation
To confirm diagnosis	Clinical assessment (there is no specific marker)
To exclude other differential diagnoses	
Infection (including atypical etiologies)	Tissue culture
Venous insufficiency	Duplex ultrasound and venous reflux studies
Peripheral arterial disease	Ankle-brachial index
Vasculitis or connective tissue disease	ANA, ANCA
Vasculopathies	Hypercoagulable panel
To detect underlying comorbidities	
Hematological malignancy	CBC with differential, SPEP, UPEP, blood smear
Solid organ malignancy	Age-appropriate cancer screening
Arthritis	RF, anti-CCP
Inflammatory bowel disease	Endoscopy or colonoscopy (if suspicious)

Abbreviations: ANA, anti-nuclear antibody; ANCA, antineutrophil cytoplasmic antibody; CBC, complete blood count; CCP, cyclic citrullinated peptide; RF, rheumatoid factor; SPEP, serum protein electrophoresis; UPEP, urine protein electrophoresis.

TABLE 82-5 Diagnostic criteria for Behçet's disease

International Study Group for Behçet's Disease criteria[49]	International Criteria for Behçet's Disease[51]	
One major and two minor criteria are required for diagnosis	Score ≥ 4 is required for diagnosis	
Major criteria	Ocular lesions	2 points
Recurrent oral ulceration: minor aphthous, major aphthous, or herpetiform ulceration recurred at least three times in one 12-month period	Genital aphthosis	2 points
Minor criteria	Oral aphthosis	2 points
1. Recurrent genital ulceration or scarring	Skin lesions	2 points
2. Eye lesions: anterior uveitis, posterior uveitis, or cells in vitreous on slit lamp examination; or retinal vasculitis	Neurological manifestations	1 point
3. Skin lesions: erythema nodosum observed by physician or patient, pseudofolliculitis, or papulopustular lesions; or acneiform nodules observed by physician in post adolescent patients not on corticosteroid treatment	Vascular manifestations	1 point
4. A positive pathergy test		

CLINICAL FEATURES

BD is characterized by recurrent mucocutaneous ulcers involving the oral cavity and genitalia. Oral ulcers are the most common manifestations and often precede other symptoms. Ulcers are typically painful and recurrent, ranging in size from a few millimeters to centimeters, most commonly on the lips, buccal mucosa, tongue, and soft palate. Initially, erythematous papules or pinpoint pustules appear, which then progress to round-to-oval ulcers with rolled borders and a white-yellow necrotic base with surrounding erythema. Oral ulcers heal spontaneously within 1 to 3 weeks and do not scar.

Genital ulcerations are the most specific feature of BD. They arise on the vulva in women or scrotum and penis in men. Unlike oral ulcers, genital ulcers tend to be larger with irregular margins, more painful and heal with scarring.[49]

Other less frequent cutaneous manifestations include papulopustular eruptions, erythema nodosum-like lesions, superficial thrombophlebitis, and PG-like lesions. Similar to PG, pathergy may be observed.

Extracutaneous involvement results from systemic vasculitis, which can affect both the arterial and venous circulation including vessels of all sizes. Ocular involvement in the form of uveitis and retinal vasculitis is commonly seen. Involvement of joints, central nervous system, cardiopulmonary, and renal systems can occur. When the gastrointestinal tract is affected, bowel perforation can occur. Vascular involvement can lead to substantial morbidity and mortality. For example, aneurysm of the large proximal pulmonary artery branches is relatively specific to BD and carries a mortality of 25%.[50]

HISTOPATHOLOGICAL FEATURES

Various degrees of vasculopathy and/or vasculitis can be seen. Angiocentric, neutrophilic infiltrates with leukocytoclasia and erythrocyte extravasation are frequent, as well as leukocytoclastic vasculitis with or without mural thrombosis and necrosis. It is controversial whether vasculitis is primary or secondary to intense inflammation.

DIAGNOSIS

Diagnosis hinges upon the constellation of clinical manifestations. Diagnostic criteria are summarized in **Table 82-5**. Ophthalmology consultation is needed.

MANAGEMENT

Therapy is chiefly symptomatic and directed toward the clinical manifestations. Dermatologists are usually consulted to manage the mucocutaneous aspects of Behcet. Topicals are typically sufficient for the oral and genital ulcers; this includes topical corticosteroids and supportive care with lidocaine gel, chlorhexidine, and sucralfate suspension.[52] Papulopustular or acne-like lesions are treated with topical or systemic measures as used in acne vulgaris.[53]

For severe disease, systemic therapy, of which colchicine is the first line, is indicated. Colchicine or dapsone can be used for the prevention of recurrent mucocutaneous lesions particularly when the dominant lesion is erythema nodosum or a genital ulcer. Apremilast has been FDA approved for adult patients with mucocutaneous Behcet.[54] Ustekinumab is also considered an effective treatment for patients with BD with recurrent oral ulcers refractory to colchicine.[55] Other systemic agents include azathioprine, minocycline, thalidomide, interferon, and TNF-α inhibitors. Referrals to rheumatology, gastroenterology and ophthalmology are appropriate based on the systemic manifestations.

NEUTROPHILIC ECCRINE HIDRADENITIS

EPIDEMIOLOGY

In neutrophilic eccrine hidradenitis (NEH), neutrophil infiltration is centered around eccrine glands. It typically occurs in patients with acute myeloid leukemia receiving chemotherapy, most commonly cytarabine followed by daunorubicin. Numerous chemotherapeutic agents as well as other drugs have been incriminated in NEH.[56] Another subtype of NEH occurs in children as a benign self-limited eruption during summer.

CLINICAL FEATURES

The clinical picture is variable and ranges from single to multiple asymptomatic or painful erythematous papules or plaques. The eruption usually occurs on the trunk but the extremities and face can also be involved [**Figure 82-7**]. Pathergy and fever can also occur in NEH. If chemotherapy is the inciting factor, lesions develop approximately 10 days after initiation.[56]

In pediatric patients, NEH appear as urticarial erythematous nodules and plaques on the limbs, trunk, or scalp.[57] Idiopathic plantar hidradenitis is a variant of NEH reported in healthy children with lesions occurring on the planter surface of the feet.[58]

HISTOPATHOLOGICAL FEATURES

The main pathology lies in the eccrine glands, which exhibit degenerative vacuolar changes in the secretory coils and ducts, sparing the acrosyringium. Dense neutrophilic infiltrates around the eccrine glands is a characteristic feature. Eccrine squamous syringometaplasia may be noted.[59]

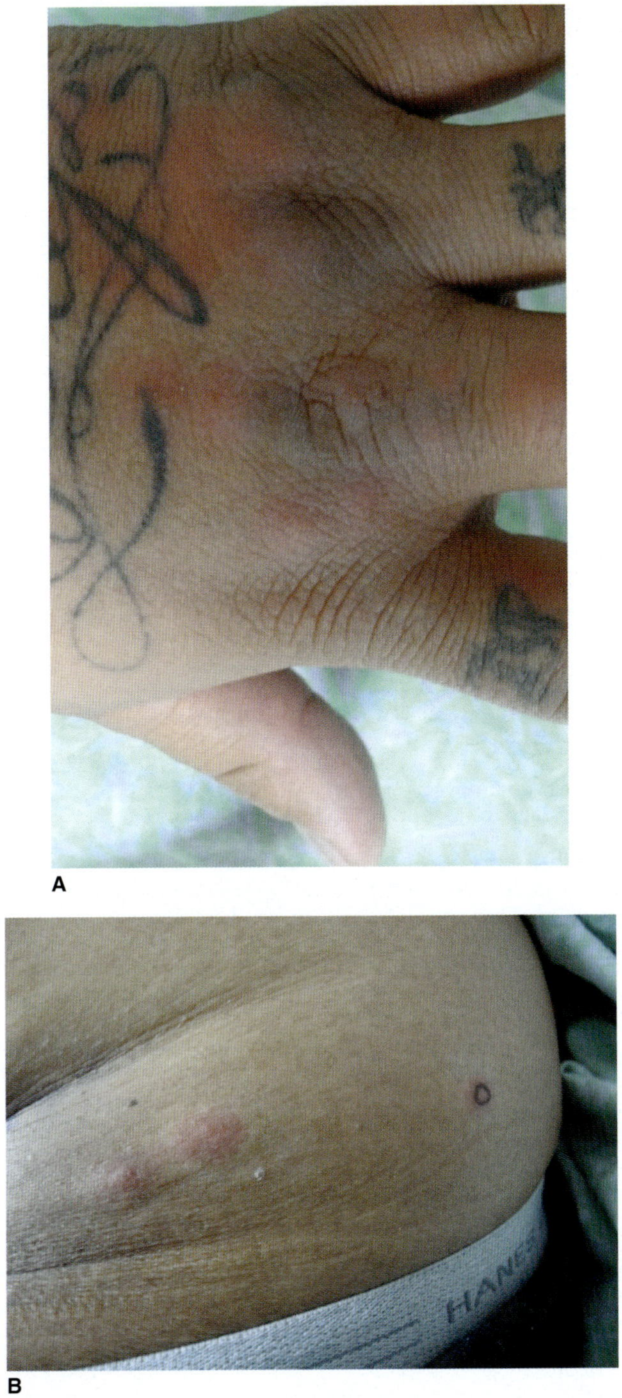

FIGURE 82-7. Neutrophilic eccrine hidradenitis—dorsal hand (A) and trunk (B) with erythematous papules and plaques. (Courtesy of Dr. Arturo Dominguez.)

DIAGNOSIS

Diagnosis is based on the characteristic histopathology of the skin lesions. Tissue culture is an important step in diagnosis as patients with hematologic malignancies and patients undergoing treatment with chemotherapeutics are often granulocytopenic and at risk for infection.[56]

MANAGEMENT

Lesions tend to spontaneously resolve within days to weeks after discontinuation of chemotherapy; however, they may recur in subsequent cycles. Systemic corticosteroids and nonsteroidal anti-inflammatory drugs are effective in reducing pain or fever. The depth of inflammation around the eccrine glands renders topical treatment ineffective.[56] Dapsone can be beneficial to prevent recurrences.[60]

AMICROBIAL PUSTULOSIS OF THE FOLDS

EPIDEMIOLOGY

Amicrobial pustulosis of the skin folds (APF) is a rare neutrophilic dermatosis that exclusively occurs in the skin folds of young women with underlying autoimmune diseases.[61]

CLINICAL FEATURES

Follicular and nonfollicular sterile pustules suddenly appear and favor cutaneous folds, particularly the anogenital region and scalp, with a symmetrical distribution. The nostrils, retroauricular regions, and external auditory canals may also be involved. Generalized forms of this pustulosis rarely occur. The pustules are erythematous and eczematous with macerated skin surfaces. Lesions may coalesce forming oozing, crusted or eroded areas associated with burning or pain. Onychodystrophy with suppurative vegetating paronychia is a common finding. The disease has a relapsing course, particularly after tapering or discontinuing treatment.[62]

HISTOPATHOLOGICAL FEATURES

Lesions display spongiform pustulation in the upper layer of the epidermis and a predominately neutrophilic infiltrate in the dermis.

DIAGNOSIS

APF can be challenging to diagnose owing to wide variety of differential diagnoses such as bacterial infections, subcorneal pustular dermatosis, and acute generalized exanthematous pustulosis. Diagnosis relies on histopathologic findings along with negative microbiological cultures. Diagnostic criteria are outlined in **Table 82-6**.

MANAGEMENT

Systemic corticosteroids remain the most effective therapy. Emerging drugs such as anakinra and anti-TNF-α inhibitors have shown promising results.[61]

IgA PEMPHIGUS

EPIDEMIOLOGY

IgA pemphigus, a rare autoimmune blistering disease, is characterized by the presence of IgA autoantibodies that target the keratinocyte cell surface. These antibodies can be detected by direct immunofluorescence

TABLE 82-6 Diagnostic criteria for amicrobial pustulosis of the folds. All major criteria and at least one minor criterion are required to establish diagnosis[62]

Major criteria	Minor criteria
• Pustulosis involving one or more major folds*, one or more minor folds⁺ and the anogenital area • Histological pattern consisting of intraepidermal spongiform pustules with predominantly neutrophilic dermal infiltrate • Negative culture from intact pustule	• Association with one or more autoimmune or autoinflammatory disorders • Positive ANA at a titer of 1/160 or higher • Presence of one or more serum autoantibodies (notably anti-ENA, anti-dsDNA, antiphospholipid, antihistone, antismooth muscle, antimitochondrial, antigastric parietal cell, antiendomysial)

*Major folds = groin and axilla.

⁺Minor folds = pedal interdigital spaces, retroauricular folds, external auditory canal.

Abbreviations: ANA, antinuclear antibody; dsDNA, double-stranded deoxyribonucleic acid; ENA, extractable nuclear antigen.

Source: Reproduced with permission from Marzano AV, Ramoni S , Caputo R. Amicrobial Pustulosis of the Folds: Report of 6 Cases and a Literature Review. Dermatology. 2008;216(4):305-11.Copyright © 2012 Karger Publishers, Basel, Switzerland

(DIF) and indirect immunofluorescence (IIF) microscopy. IgA pemphigus can be divided into two types: subcorneal pustular dermatosis (SPD) and intraepidermal neutrophilic dermatosis (IEN). It is agreed that the target antigen in SPD is desmocollin 1 (Dsc1), whereas in IEN, the antigen remains controversial with various reports suggesting desmoglein 1-3 and desmocollin 1-3.[63] A 2020 systematic review revealed an average age of 51 years and a slight female predominance with a female-to male ratio of 1.1:1.[64]

CLINICAL FEATURES

Patients present with pruritic vesicles and pustules, which characteristically exhibit a circinate pattern showing central crusts and peripheral vesiculation. Sometimes, the pus localizes to the lower half of the blister resulting in the "hypopyon sign." Lesions commonly involve the trunk and proximal extremities but can also affect the flexures and scalp.[65] Approximately 13% of patients show mucosal involvement, and 18% of patients are found to have concomitant malignancies. IgA monoclonal gammopathy is the most common.[64]

HISTOPATHOLOGICAL FEATURES

Intraepidermal separation and acantholysis with a predominantly neutrophilic infiltrate are typical features on biopsy. A mixed neutrophilic and eosinophilic infiltrate is also common. The subtype names correspond with the level of separation and subcorneal separation is seen in the SPD type, whereas lower epidermal separation is seen in the IEN type.[66]

Intercellular deposition of IgA is characteristically detected on DIF of perilesional skin biopsy specimens. Less commonly, a mixture of IgA, IgG, and complement C3 can be observed. IIF is positive for IgA intercellular antibodies in patient sera in two-thirds of the cases.[64]

DIAGNOSIS

In addition to clinical and histopathological features, DIF is essential for confirming a diagnosis of IgA pemphigus.[64]

MANAGEMENT

Common treatments used in IgA pemphigus include dapsone and systemic corticosteroids. Treatments such as colchicine, acitretin and adalimumab have been reported too. Of these treatments, complete resolution appears to be most frequently seen with adalimumab, systemic corticosteroids and dapsone. Recurrences are not uncommon.[67]

NEUTROPHILIC PANNICULITIS

EPIDEMIOLOGY

Neutrophilic panniculitis is a very rare disease that tends to be underdiagnosed and is often confused with other causes of panniculitis.[68] Females appear to be more frequently affected.[69]

CLINICAL FEATURES

Lesions appear as painful, erythematous, subcutaneous nodules, mainly involving the extremities. Patients usually have constitutional symptoms as fever, arthralgias, and malaise.[69] Nodules and plaques last 15 days or more and usually heal with transient hyperpigmentation and atrophy. Neutrophilic panniculitis can be associated with myelodysplasia.[70]

HISTOPATHOLOGICAL FEATURES

Skin biopsy specimens show a lobular neutrophilic infiltrate without vasculitis.[69] Distinction from other neutrophilic panniculitides such as pancreatic, erythema nodosum, infectious, and subcutaneous SS can be challenging.

DIAGNOSIS

Diagnosis can be made with the presence of five positive criteria and absence of three negative criteria as illustrated in **Table 82-7**.[68]

TABLE 82-7 Criteria for diagnosis of neutrophilic panniculitis[69]

Positive criteria	Clinical	Lesions in the form of nodule or plaque
		Constitutional symptoms (fever, arthralgias, malaise)
	Histopathology	Lobular infiltrate of neutrophils
	Association	Myelodysplasia
	Treatment	Excellent response to oral steroids
Negative criteria	Histopathology	Lack of septal involvement with neutrophilic infiltrate
		Lack of vasculitis
	Association	No other cause of panniculitis

MANAGEMENT

Systemic corticosteroids provide a good response and work within days.[69] Other therapeutic options include dapsone, TNF antagonists, and anakinra (IL-1 receptor antagonist).[71]

REFERENCES

1. Marzano AV, Borghi A, Wallach D, et al. A comprehensive review of neutrophilic diseases. *Clin Rev Allergy Immunol*. 2018;54:114-130.
2. Prat L, Bouaziz JD, Wallach D, et al. Neutrophilic dermatoses as systemic diseases. *Clin Dermatol*. 2014;32:376-388.
3. Lee DE, Clark AK, Shi VY. Hidradenitis suppurativa: disease burden and etiology in skin of color. *Dermatology*. 2017;233:456-461.
4. Sachdeva M, Shah M, Alavi A. Race-specific prevalence of hidradenitis suppurativa. *J Cutan Med Surg*. 2021;25(2):177-187.
5. Narla S, Silverberg JI. The inpatient burden and comorbidities of pyoderma gangrenosum in adults in the United States. *Arch Dermatol Res*. 2021;313:245-253.
6. Kilgour JM, Li S, Sarin KY. Hidradenitis suppurativa in patients of color is associated with increased disease severity and healthcare utilization: A retrospective analysis of 2 U.S. cohorts. *JAAD Int*. 2021;3:42-52.
7. Alexis AF, Callender VD, Baldwin HE, et al. Global epidemiology and clinical spectrum of rosacea, highlighting skin of color: review and clinical practice experience. *J Am Acad Dermatol*. 2019;80:1722-1729.e7.
8. Abdel-Naser MB, Verma SB, Abdallah MA. Common dermatoses in moderately pigmented skin: uncommon presentations. *Clin Dermatol*. 2005;23:446-456.
9. Cohen PR. Sweet's syndrome – a comprehensive review of an acute febrile neutrophilic dermatosis. *Orphanet J Rare Dis*. 2007;2:34.
10. Walker DC, Cohen PR. Trimethoprim-sulfamethoxazole-associated acute febrile neutrophilic dermatosis: case report and review of drug-induced Sweet's syndrome. *J Am Acad Dermatol*. 1996;34:918-923.
11. Nelson CA, Noe MH, McMahon CM, et al. Sweet syndrome in patients with and without malignancy: a retrospective analysis of 83 patients from a tertiary academic referral center. *J Am Acad Dermatol*. 2018;78:303-309.e4.
12. Rochet NM, Chavan RN, Cappel MA, et al. Sweet syndrome: clinical presentation, associations, and response to treatment in 77 patients. *J Am Acad Dermatol*. 2013;69:557-564.
13. Zheng S, Li S, Tang S, et al. Insights into the characteristics of sweet syndrome in patients with and without hematologic malignancy. *Front Med*. 2020;7.
14. Marcoval J, Martín-Callizo C, Valentí-Medina F, et al. Sweet syndrome: long-term follow-up of 138 patients. *Clin Exp Dermatol*. 2016;41:741-746.
15. Su WP, Liu HN. Diagnostic criteria for Sweet's syndrome. *Cutis*. 1986;37:167-174.
16. Amouri M, Masmoudi A, Ammar M, et al. Sweet's syndrome: a retrospective study of 90 cases from a tertiary care center. *Int J Dermatol*. 2016;55:1033-1039.
17. Cohen PR, Kurzrock R. Sweet's syndrome: a review of current treatment options. *Am J Clin Dermatol*. 2002;3:117-131.
18. Xu A, Balgobind A, Strunk A, et al. Prevalence estimates for pyoderma gangrenosum in the United States: an age- and sex-adjusted population analysis. *J Am Acad Dermatol*. 2020;83:425-429.
19. Haynes D, Hammer P, Malachowski SJ, et al. Characterisation and diagnosis of ulcers in inpatient dermatology consultation services: a multi-centre study. *Int Wound J*. 2019;16:1440-1444.
20. Sawka E, Zhou A, Latour E, et al. Inflammatory arthritis-associated pyoderma gangrenosum: a systematic review. *Clin Rheumatol*. 2021;40:3963-3969.
21. Gupta AS, Ortega-Loayza AG. Pyoderma gangrenosum: a too often overlooked facultative paraneoplastic disease. *Ann Hematol*. 2019;98:2247-2248.

22. Borda LJ, Wong LL, Marzano AV, et al. Extracutaneous involvement of pyoderma gangrenosum. *Arch Dermatol Res*. 2019;311:425-434.
23. Ighani A, Al-Mutairi D, Rahmani A, et al. Pyoderma gangrenosum and its impact on quality of life: a multicentre, prospective study. *Br J Dermatol*. 2019;180:672-673.
24. Langan SM, Groves RW, Card TR, et al. Incidence, mortality, and disease associations of pyoderma gangrenosum in the United Kingdom: a retrospective cohort study. *J Invest Dermatol*. 2012;132:2166-2170.
25. Alavi A, French LE, Davis MD, et al. Pyoderma gangrenosum: an update on pathophysiology, diagnosis and treatment. *Am J Clin Dermatol*. 2017;18:355-372.
26. Tolkachjov SN, Fahy AS, Cerci FB, et al. Postoperative pyoderma gangrenosum: a clinical review of published cases. *Mayo Clin Proc*. 2016;91:1267-1279.
27. Haag CK, Nutan F, Cyrus JW, et al. Pyoderma gangrenosum misdiagnosis resulting in amputation: a review. *J Trauma Acute Care Surg*. 2019;86:307-313.
28. Crowson AN, Mihm MC, Jr., Magro C. Pyoderma gangrenosum: a review. *J Cutan Pathol*. 2003;30:97-107.
29. Su WP, Davis MD, Weenig RH, et al. Pyoderma gangrenosum: clinicopathologic correlation and proposed diagnostic criteria. *Int J Dermatol*. 2004;43:790-800.
30. Maverakis E, Ma C, Shinkai K, et al. Diagnostic criteria of ulcerative pyoderma gangrenosum: a Delphi consensus of international experts. *JAMA Dermatol*. 2018;154:461-466.
31. Jockenhöfer F, Wollina U, Salva KA, et al. The PARACELSUS score: a novel diagnostic tool for pyoderma gangrenosum. *Br J Dermatol*. 2019;180:615-620.
32. Haag C, Hansen T, Hajar T, et al. Comparison of three diagnostic frameworks for pyoderma gangrenosum. *J Invest Dermatol*. 2021;141:59-63.
33. Min MS, Kus K, Wei N, et al. Evaluating the role of histopathology in diagnosing pyoderma gangrenosum using Delphi and PARACELSUS criteria: a multicentre, retrospective cohort study. *Br J Dermatol*. 2022.
34. Kohn AH, Alavi A, Armstrong AW, et al. International dermatology outcome measures (IDEOM): report from the 2020 Annual Meeting. *Dermatology*. 2022;238:430-437.
35. Shakshouk H, Gibson LE. Pyoderma gangrenosum-like skin ulceration in antineutrophil cytoplasmic antibody-associated vasculitis: a retrospective case series. *Clin Exp Dermatol*. 2022;47:1716-1719.
36. Goldust M, Hagstrom EL, Rathod D, et al. Diagnosis and novel clinical treatment strategies for pyoderma gangrenosum. *Expert Rev Clin Pharmacol*. 2020;13:157-161.
37. Afifi L, Ortega-Loayza AG, Shinkai K. Management of classic ulcerative pyoderma gangrenosum. *Cutis*. 2020;106:119-23;e2;e3.
38. Partridge ACR, Bai JW, Rosen CF, et al. Effectiveness of systemic treatments for pyoderma gangrenosum: a systematic review of observational studies and clinical trials. *Br J Dermatol*. 2018;179:290-295.
39. Maronese CA, Pimentel MA, Li MM, et al. Pyoderma gangrenosum: an updated literature review on established and emerging pharmacological treatments. *Am J Clin Dermatol*. 2022;23(5):615-634.
40. Ormerod AD, Thomas KS, Craig FE, et al. Comparison of the two most commonly used treatments for pyoderma gangrenosum: results of the STOP GAP randomised controlled trial. *BMJ*. 2015;350:h2958.
41. Brooklyn TN, Dunnill MG, Shetty A, et al. Infliximab for the treatment of pyoderma gangrenosum: a randomised, double blind, placebo controlled trial. *Gut*. 2006;55:505-509.
42. Yamasaki K, Yamanaka K, Zhao Y, et al. Adalimumab in Japanese patients with active ulcers of pyoderma gangrenosum: twenty-six-week phase 3 open-label study. *J Dermatol*. 2020;47:1383-1390.
43. Schøsler L, Fogh K, Bech R. Pyoderma gangrenosum: a retrospective study of clinical characteristics, comorbidities, response to treatment and mortality related to prednisone dose. *Acta Derm Venereol*. 2021;101:adv00431.
44. Ben Abdallah H, Fogh K, Vestergaard C, et al. Pyoderma gangrenosum and interleukin inhibitors: a semi-systematic review. *Dermatology*. 2022;238:785-792.
45. Westerdahl JS, Nusbaum KB, Chung CG, et al. Ustekinumab as adjuvant treatment for all pyoderma gangrenosum subtypes. *J Dermatolog Treat*. 2022;33:2386-2390.
46. Reese AM, Erickson K, Reed KB, et al. Modified dose of guselkumab for treatment of pyoderma gangrenosum. *JAAD Case Rep*. 2022;21:38-42.
47. Strunck JL, Cutler B, Latour E, et al. Wound care dressings for pyoderma gangrenosum. J *Am Acad Dermatol*. 2022;86:458-460.
48. Wang X, Peng Y, Gao J, et al. Risk of malignancy in Behcet disease: a meta-analysis with systematic review. *Medicine (Baltimore)*. 2019;98:e17735.
49. Criteria for diagnosis of Behçet's disease. International Study Group for Behçet's Disease. *Lancet*. 1990;335:1078-1080.
50. Hamuryudan V, Er T, Seyahi E, et al. Pulmonary artery aneurysms in Behçet syndrome. *Am J Med*. 2004;117:867-870.
51. The International Criteria for Behçet's Disease (ICBD): a collaborative study of 27 countries on the sensitivity and specificity of the new criteria. *J Eur Acad Dermatol Venereol*. 2014;28:338-347.
52. Nakamura K, Iwata Y, Asai J, et al. Guidelines for the treatment of skin and mucosal lesions in Behçet's disease: a secondary publication. *J Dermatol*. 2020;47:223-235.
53. Hatemi G, Christensen R, Bang D, et al. 2018 update of the EULAR recommendations for the management of Behçet's syndrome. *Ann Rheum Dis*. 2018;77:808-818.
54. Hatemi G, Mahr A, Ishigatsubo Y, et al. Trial of apremilast for oral ulcers in Behçet's syndrome. *N Engl J Med*. 2019;381:1918-1928.
55. London J, Régent A, Dion J, et al. Efficacy and safety of ustekinumab in Behçet disease: results from the prospective phase 2 STELABEC trial. *J Am Acad Dermatol*. 2022;87:681-684.
56. Bachmeyer C, Aractingi S. Neutrophilic eccrine hidradenitis. *Clin Dermatol*. 2000;18:319-330.
57. Shih IH, Huang YH, Yang CH, et al. Childhood neutrophilic eccrine hidradenitis: a clinicopathologic and immunohistochemical study of 10 patients. *J Am Acad Dermatol*. 2005;52:963-966.
58. Stahr BJ, Cooper PH, Caputo RV. Idiopathic plantar hidradenitis: a neutrophilic eccrine hidradenitis occurring primarily in children. *J Cutan Pathol*. 1994;21:289-296.
59. Shakshouk H, Johnson EF, Peters MS, et al. Cutaneous eccrine inflammation and necrosis: review of inflammatory disorders affecting the eccrine apparatus including new associations. Hum Pathol. 2021;118:71-85.
60. Shear NH, Knowles SR, Shapiro L, et al. Dapsone in prevention of recurrent neutrophilic eccrine hidradenitis. *J Am Acad Dermatol*. 1996;35:819-822.
61. Schissler C, Velter C, Lipsker D. Amicrobial pustulosis of the folds: where have we gone 25 years after its original description? *Ann Dermatol Venereol*. 2017;144:169-175.
62. Marzano AV, Ramoni S, Caputo R. Amicrobial pustulosis of the folds. *Dermatology*. 2008;216:305-311.
63. Hashimoto T, Yasumoto S, Nagata Y, et al. Clinical, histopathological and immunological distinction in two cases of IgA pemphigus. *Clin Exp Dermatol*. 2002;27:636-640.
64. Kridin K, Patel PM, Jones VA, et al. IgA pemphigus: a systematic review. *J Am Acad Dermatol*. 2020;82:1386-1392.
65. Tsuruta D, Ishii N, Hamada T, et al. IgA pemphigus. *Clin Dermatol*. 2011;29:437-442.
66. Tekin B, Johnson EF, Wieland CN, et al. Histopathology of autoimmune bullous dermatoses: what's new? Hum Pathol. 2022;128:69-89.
67. Geng RSQ, Sood S, Bestavros S, Waked J, Towheed S, et al. Treatment Outcomes in IgA Pemphigus: A Systematic Review. J Cutan Med Surg. 2025 Jul-Aug;29(4):420-421. doi: 10.1177/12034754251316289. Epub 2025 Jan 29. PMID: 39881552.
68. Filosa A, Filosa G. Neutrophilic dermatoses: a broad spectrum of disease. *G Ital Dermatol Venereol*. 2018;153:265-272.
69. Sutra-Loubet C, Carlotti A, Guillemette J, et al. Neutrophilic panniculitis. *J Am Acad Dermatol*. 2004;50:280-285.
70. Qian L, Shen J, Cen J, et al. Myelodysplastic syndrome with neutrophilic panniculitis: a report of two cases and a literature review. *Oncol Lett*. 2015;9:1954-1956.
71. Lipsker D, Perrigouard C, Foubert A, et al. Anakinra for difficult-to-treat neutrophilic panniculitis: IL-1 blockade as a promising treatment option for neutrophil-mediated inflammatory skin disease. *Dermatology*. 2010;220:264-267.

CHAPTER 83

Purpuric Eruptions

Megan Zhao
Robert G. Micheletti

KEY POINTS

- Purpuric eruptions can be difficult to diagnose due to their low prevalence and broad differential diagnosis; timely diagnosis may also be more challenging in patients with skin of color.
- Careful clinical-pathologic correlation is necessary to confirm the diagnosis of purpuric eruptions and identify potential systemic complications.

- Vasculitis is classified according to the size of the affected blood vessels; evaluation for systemic manifestations of vasculitis and potential underlying disease states should follow a systematic and stepwise approach.
- Other conditions mimicking vasculitis include coagulopathy, depositional diseases, and infections; skin biopsy and evaluation for underlying hypercoagulable states is essential.

PURPURIC ERUPTIONS

The differential diagnosis of a patient presenting with a purpuric eruption—livedo reticularis, petechiae, purpura, cutaneous infarct, or ulceration—is broad, encompassing a range of disorders of bleeding, clotting, and vascular inflammation. Careful evaluation and clinical-pathologic correlation is necessary to differentiate these entities and identify potential systemic complications.

PURPURIC ERUPTIONS IN PATIENTS WITH SKIN OF COLOR

Accurate and timely diagnosis of purpuric eruptions can be difficult due to their low prevalence and potential to mimic one another. This task may be harder in those with darker skin tones. In such patients, purple hues may be less prominent and less clearly purpuric (vs hyperpigmented, **Figure 83-1**) compared to those with lighter skin tones. Because the conditions are uncommon, images available in most dermatology textbooks are few and largely limited to individuals with lighter skin. Subtler clinical presentations and decreased provider awareness may contribute to delayed diagnosis of purpuric skin conditions in those with darker skin, but unfortunately little is known about this topic.

Knowledge regarding the prevalence and diagnosis of various types of vasculitis and vasculopathy in different ethnic groups is also incomplete. Available data suggest certain conditions, like antineutrophil cytoplasmic antibodies (ANCA) associated vasculitis and polyarteritis nodosa, may be more common in those of European compared to non-European descent, while IgA vasculitis may be more common in White and Asian populations.[1,2] Environmental as well as genetic factors are thought to play a role. Likely, missing data and underdiagnosis contribute to an incomplete picture of the epidemiology of this group of diseases.

This chapter presents a framework to conceptualize and diagnose purpuric eruptions, complemented by clinical images, to improve recognition of purpuric eruptions in patients with skin of color.

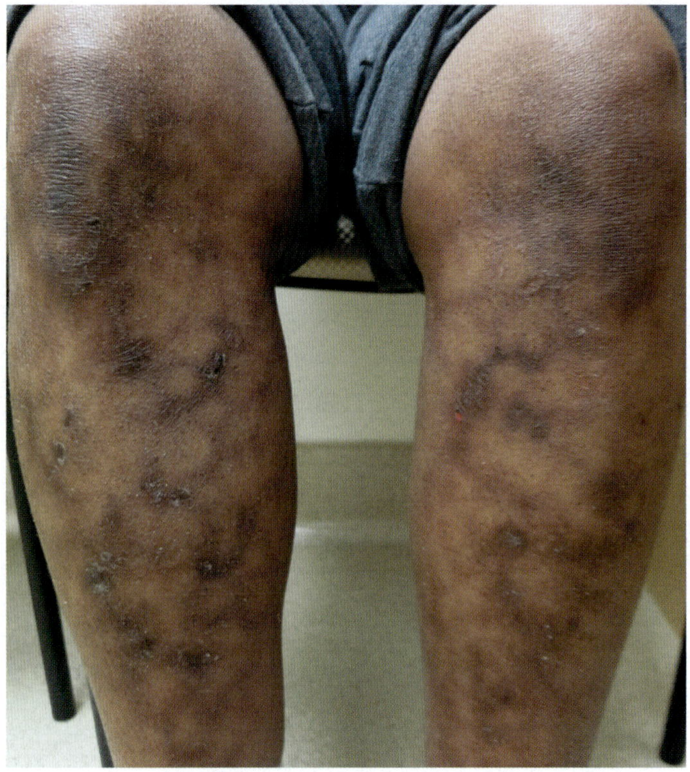

FIGURE 83-1. Erythema ab igne characterized by hyperpigmented livedoid patches, in contrast to the violaceous hue of true livedo reticularis or racemosa.

VASCULITIS

Vasculitis results from inflammation and destruction of blood vessels, leading to downstream ischemic tissue damage. Vasculitis can be, and often is, limited to the skin. However, cutaneous lesions of vasculitis may also be a feature or presenting sign of systemic disease. Vasculitis is classified according to the size of the affected blood vessels.[3,4] Generally speaking, small vessel vasculitis results in purpuric macules and papules, petechiae, urticarial papules, and/or vesicles; medium vessel vasculitis is characterized by livedo reticularis, retiform purpura, subcutaneous nodules, ulceration, and/or digital necrosis. A size-based classification of vasculitis is shown in **Table 83-1**.

SMALL VESSEL VASCULITIS

Most vasculitis encountered by dermatologists involves small-sized vessels and is mediated by immune complex deposition. Patients typically present with purpuric macules and papules on the lower extremities and other dependent areas (ie, "palpable purpura") [**Figure 83-2**]. Petechiae, hemorrhagic vesicles, urticarial papules, targetoid lesions, and rounded small ulcerations also occur. Lesions may itch, burn, or sting, or they may be asymptomatic.

TABLE 83-1 Vasculitis classification and treatment[a]

Vessel size	Classification/subclassification	Clinical features	First- and second-line therapies
Small	Cutaneous small vessel vasculitis (CSVV), IgM/IgG immune complex vasculitis, IgA vasculitis, urticarial vasculitis, erythema elevatum diutinum, acute hemorrhagic edema of infancy	Palpable purpura (most common), petechiae, macular purpura, urticarial papules, vesicles, pustules, targetoid lesions, rounded ulcers	Address potential triggers Rest, elevation, compression Colchicine,[5] dapsone,[6,7] azathioprine[8] Corticosteroids[9]
Small and Medium	Cryoglobulinemic vasculitis	Petechiae, palpable purpura, livedo racemosa, retiform purpura, ulcers, digital necrosis	Treatment of underlying disease (eg, hepatitis C), if present[10] Corticosteroids, rituximab[11]
	ANCA-associated vasculitis (granulomatosis with polyangiitis (GPA); microscopic polyangiitis (MPA); eosinophilic granulomatosis with polyangiitis (EGPA))	Petechiae, purpura, urticaria, livedo racemosa, retiform purpura, ulcers, subcutaneous nodules, digital necrosis	Corticosteroids, rituximab[12] Methotrexate, mepolizumab (EGPA),[13] avacopan (GPA and MPA),[14] cyclophosphamide
Medium	Polyarteritis nodosum (systemic) Cutaneous polyarteritis nodosum	Livedo racemosa, retiform purpura, ulcers, subcutaneous nodules, digital necrosis	Corticosteroids, azathioprine, methotrexate, cyclophosphamide (systemic) Colchicine, dapsone, azathioprine, corticosteroids (cutaneous)[15]

[a]For additional information on evidence-based management of cutaneous vasculitis, refer to the referenced manuscripts.[16,17]

Abbreviation: ANCA, antineutrophil cytoplasmic antibodies.

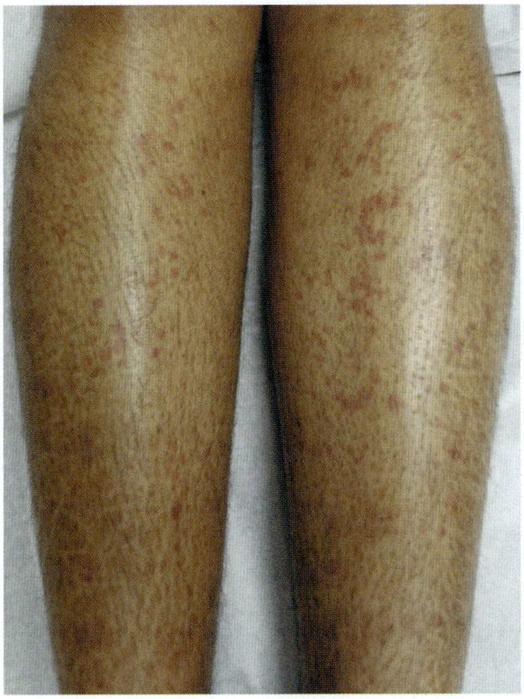

FIGURE 83-2. Immune complex-mediated small vessel vasculitis demonstrating purpuric macules and papules.

Terms used in clinical practice to describe the most common type of small vessel vasculitis of the skin include leukocytoclastic vasculitis (LCV) and cutaneous small vessel vasculitis (CSVV). It should be noted, however, that the former is a histologic descriptor seen in other types of vasculitis (and is therefore not specific), while CSVV is an umbrella term encompassing a number of types of small vessel vasculitis occurring in the skin (eg, erythema elevatum diutinum). In the dermatologic addendum to the Chapel Hill Consensus Conference Nomenclature,[4] **IgM/IgG vasculitis** is the preferred term, defined as a skin-limited type of immune complex-mediated small vessel vasculitis mediated by IgM or IgG and not belonging to one of the other defined categories.

IgA vasculitis (also called Henoch-Schonlein) is a special category of immune complex-mediated small vessel vasculitis which presents with palpable purpura resulting from IgA deposition in postcapillary venules. This disease most commonly affects children and may follow a preceding viral illness or Streptococcal pharyngitis. The key histologic feature is the presence of IgA on direct immunofluorescence study. Because IgA vasculitis carries an increased risk of gastrointestinal, joint, and renal involvement, a thorough review of systems is necessary. Patients should be screened regularly for glomerulonephritis with a urinalysis and blood pressure monitoring, especially within the first 1 to 6 months of diagnosis, when the risk is highest.[18]

Urticarial vasculitis presents with erythematous and edematous papules that resemble hives but that persist greater than 24 hours and frequently result in non-blanching purpura [**Figure 83-3**]. Patients may have systemic symptoms, such as fever and arthritis. Those with normal C3 and C4 levels (so-called normocomplementemic urticarial vasculitis) are best thought of as a subset of skin-limited small vessel vasculitis presenting with hive-like lesions. Those with low complement levels (hypocomplementemic urticarial vasculitis) are much more likely to meet criteria for systemic lupus erythematosus (about 50%) and to have systemic manifestations, including arthritis, nephritis, and obstructive lung disease.[19]

Additional types of small vessel vasculitis presenting in the skin include **erythema elevatum diutinum**, characterized by symmetric violaceous, red-brown, or yellowish papules, plaques, or nodules favoring extensor surfaces. Histologic findings include leukocytoclastic vasculitis

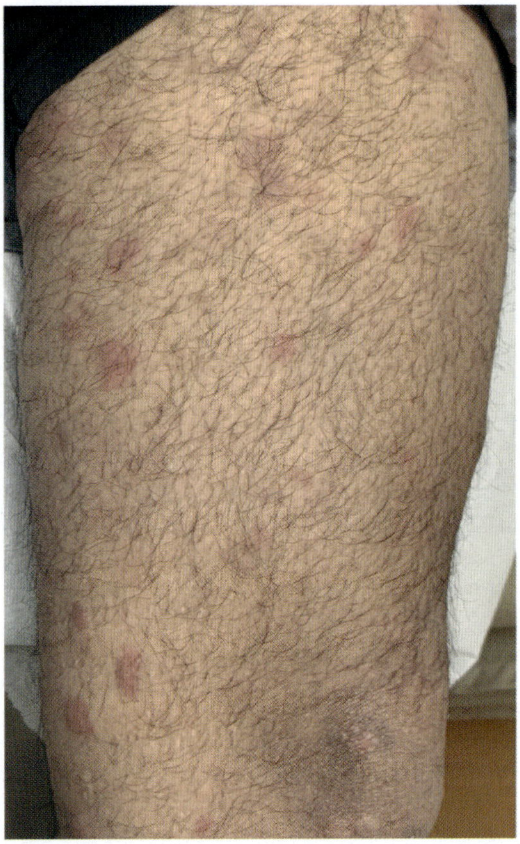

FIGURE 83-3. Hypocomplementemic urticarial vasculitis; note the purpuric urticarial papules on the leg.

and angiocentric fibrosis. The disease has a relapsing-remitting course and is considered skin-limited.

Acute hemorrhagic edema of infancy is an uncommon small vessel vasculitis affecting children 4 to 24 months of age that manifests abruptly with large erythematosus patches or urticarial lesion on the face and extremities. These lesions evolve into annular or targetoid purpuric plaques. Fever is common, but otherwise the condition has a benign clinical course.

SMALL AND MEDIUM VESSEL VASCULITIS

Cryoglobulinemic vasculitis is a type of immune complex-mediated vasculitis that results from the presence of IgM autoantibodies that bind IgG antibodies to form immune complexes that precipitate in cold temperatures (so-called mixed cryoglobulins). This process occurs secondary to B-cell stimulation and expansion in the setting of a chronic inflammatory state, most commonly hepatitis C infection.[20] As in other types of small vessel vasculitis, cryoglobulinemic vasculitis most commonly presents with palpable purpura of the lower extremities. However, livedo reticularis, retiform purpura, necrosis, and ulceration—manifestations more often associated with medium vessel disease—are also seen. Common extracutaneous findings include weakness, arthritis, peripheral neuropathy, and glomerulonephritis.

The ANCA-associated vasculitides (AAV)—including **granulomatosis with polyangiitis (GPA)**, **microscopic polyangiitis (MPA)**, and **eosinophilic granulomatosis with polyangiitis (EGPA)**—are characterized by vasculitis involving small to medium-sized vessels. Cutaneous manifestations of AAV occur in one-third to one-half of patients at the time of presentation.[21] Common findings include purpuric macules and papules, livedo reticularis, retiform purpura, and splinter hemorrhages [**Figure 83-4**]. Patients with EGPA frequently present with nonspecific or "allergic" findings, such as hives, itching, and eczematous eruption. Potential systemic manifestations of AAV include sinusitis

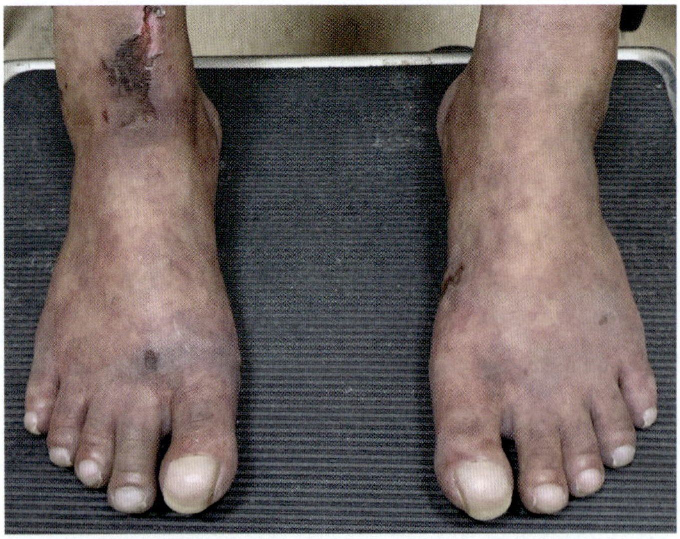

FIGURE 83-4. Retiform purpura and livedo racemosa in a patient presenting with MPO+ microscopic polyangiitis. MPO: myeloperoxidase.

and epistaxis (GPA), asthma and allergic rhinitis (EGPA), glomerulonephritis, mononeuritis, pulmonary nodules, diffuse alveolar hemorrhage, and others. When present, cutaneous manifestations of AAV portend a more severe systemic course.[21] Positive ANCA and antiproteinase 3 (PR3) or antimyeloperoxidase (MPO) ELISA are suggestive of a diagnosis of AAV in the appropriate clinical context. Drugs associated with ANCA-associated vasculitis include levamisole-tainted cocaine [**Figure 83-5**] and medications such as propylthiouracil, minocycline, and hydralazine.

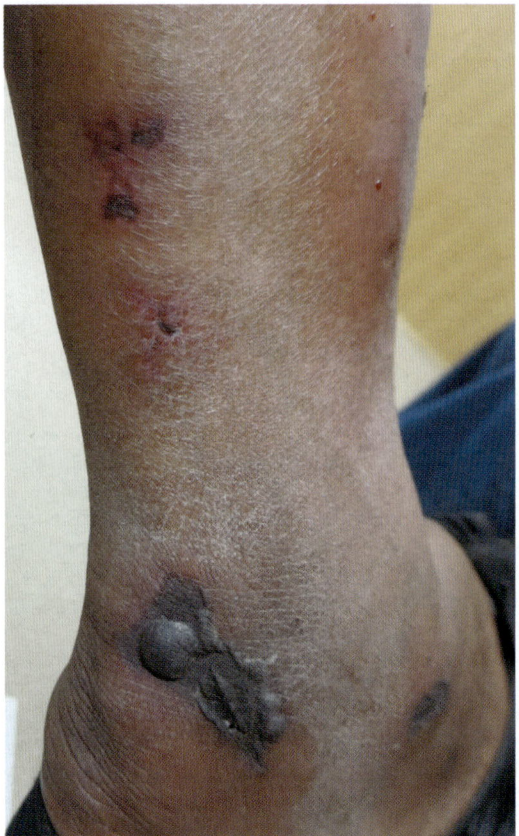

FIGURE 83-5. Levamisole-induced vasculitis/vasculopathy from contaminated cocaine, resulting in retiform purpura and bullous necrosis.

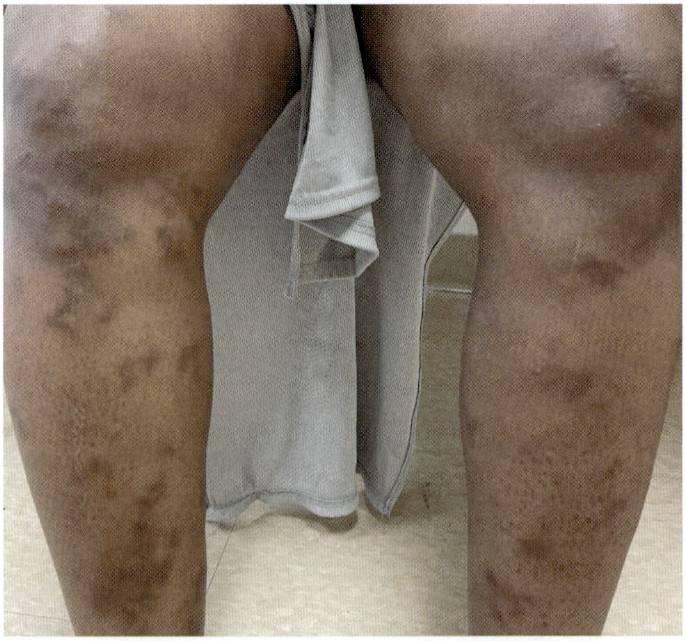

FIGURE 83-6. Cutaneous polyarteritis nodosa characterized by subcutaneous nodules and broken rings of "starburst" livedo reticularis.

MEDIUM VESSEL VASCULITIS

Polyarteritis nodosa (PAN) affects medium-sized vessels. Cutaneous manifestations include fixed livedo reticularis or livedo racemosa [**Figure 83-6**], subcutaneous nodules, retiform purpura, ulceration, and digital necrosis. PAN may be skin-limited (cutaneous PAN) or systemic. Potential systemic manifestations include fever, weight loss, arthritis, peripheral neuritis, renovascular hypertension, and intestinal infarction.

EVALUATION OF THE PATIENT WITH SUSPECTED VASCULITIS

When a patient presents with purpura or other skin lesions suspicious for vasculitis, the clinician must determine (1) whether the lesions are, in fact, due to vasculitis (or a vasculitis mimic); (2) whether other organ systems are involved; and (3) whether there are findings that help establish a particular diagnosis.[16]

A skin biopsy demonstrating leukocytoclasis and fibrinoid necrosis of vessel walls helps confirm the diagnosis of vasculitis. However, careful clinical-pathologic correlation is essential to distinguishing true cases of vasculitis from those entities in which vasculitis can be seen as a secondary finding (eg, arthropod bite or ulceration). Appropriate site selection and sufficient tissue sampling enhance biopsy utility. In general, a well-established but not old lesion should be chosen. Clinically, such a lesion may exhibit both erythema and purpura. Palpable purpura, retiform purpura, and subcutaneous nodules are generally more likely to exhibit diagnostic histologic findings when biopsied than livedo reticularis or ulceration. In cases of suspected small vessel vasculitis, biopsy of a new lesion for direct immunofluorescence studies should be performed. Specifically, the presence of perivascular IgA, as seen in IgA vasculitis, is prognostically important, as such patients are more likely to develop gastrointestinal, joint, and renal complications.

Evaluation for systemic manifestations of vasculitis and potential underlying disease states should follow a systematic and stepwise approach, as outlined in **Figure 83-7**, beginning with a thorough review of systems, history, and examination. The presence of constitutional symptoms, arthritis, abdominal pain, hematuria or proteinuria, neuropathy, sinusitis, epistaxis, or other symptoms is a potential "red flag" for systemic disease. Initial work-up should include a complete blood count, basic metabolic panel, and urinalysis with microscopy. Second-level tests—including serologies for hepatitis B and C, HIV, antistreptolysin-O,

History, examination, and review of systems

- Evaluate signs and symptoms of extracutaneous disease
  - Fever, weight loss, fatigue
  - Arthralgias / arthritis, myalgias
  - Hematuria, frothy urine
  - Abdominal pain, bloody stools
  - Paresthesias, numbness, weakness
  - Cough, shortness of breath, chest pain, hemoptysis
  - Nasal crusting, sinusitis, epistaxis
- Review medications, evidence of infection
- Consider associated inflammatory disorders or malignancy

Skin Biopsy

- If suspecting small vessel vasculitis, perform punch biopsies for routine histology (1-2 day old lesion) and direct immunofluorescence (early lesion, < 1 day old)
- If suspecting medium vessel vasculitis, perform deep punch or incisional biopsy to include subcutaneous fat (nodule > retiform purpura > livedo reticularis or ulcer edge)
- Exercise rigorous clinical-pathologic correlation

Initial laboratory evaluation (may be repeated during flares)

- CBC with differential, basic metabolic panel, creatinine, urinalysis with microscopic

Additional evaluation (dictated by systemic symptoms or chronic / recurring skin lesions)

Infectious	▪ Antistreptolysin-O; Hepatitis B/C and HIV serologies ▪ Cultures, if indicated
Autoimmune	▪ ANA, Rheumatoid factor; anti-SSA/SSB ▪ C3/C4 if suspecting urticarial vasculitis
Inflammatory	▪ Cryoglobulins ▪ ANCAs (including MPO/PR3 ELISA)
Neoplastic	▪ SPEP / immunofixation; peripheral blood smear ▪ Age-appropriate cancer screening; lung cancer screening (IgA vasculitis, especially if older, male)
Other	▪ Any other organ-specific, targeted work-up dictated by signs and symptoms

Evaluation for extracutaneous involvement in systemic vasculitis:

- Chest X-ray, CT of chest and sinuses (especially ANCA-associated vasculitis)
- Mesenteric/renal CT or MR angiogram (especially polyarteritis nodosa)
- Electromyogram/nerve conduction studies if sensory or motor neuropathy
- Echocardiogram/electrocardiogram if concern for cardiac involvement
- Biopsy of affected tissues (eg, kidney, nerve, respiratory tract), if indicated

FIGURE 83-7. Stepwise approach to the evaluation of cutaneous vasculitis. ANA, antinuclear antibody; ANCA, antineutrophil cytoplasmic antibodies; CBC, complete blood count; CT, computed tomography; MPO, myeloperoxidase; MR, magnetic resonance; PR3, proteinase-3; SPEP, serum protein electrophoresis. (Reproduced with permission from Micheletti RG. Cutaneous Small Vessel Vasculitis: A Practical Guide to Diagnosis and Management. *Am J Clin Dermatol.* 2023;24(1):89-95.)

antinuclear antibody, rheumatoid factor, serum protein electrophoresis, C3 and C4 complement levels, antineutrophil cycoplasmic antibodies, cryoglobulins, and diagnostic imaging—should be guided by the patient's presenting signs and symptoms [Figure 83-7].[16]

VASCULOPATHY, COAGULOPATHY, AND OTHER PURPURIC ERUPTIONS

Besides vasculitis, the differential for purpuric eruptions remains broad. The presence of retiform purpura suggests a pathology of medium-sized vessels in the deep dermis or subcutis. In addition to medium and small-to-medium vessel vasculitis (eg, PAN, cryoglobulinemic, ANCA-associated vasculitis), vasculopathic or hypercoagulable conditions like antiphospholipid antibody syndrome, depositional diseases like calciphylaxis, and angiodestructive infectious processes like gram-negative bacterial or angioinvasive fungal infections should be considered.

In such cases, a skin biopsy is typically necessary to investigate the presence of fibrin thrombi, medial calcification, cholesterol emboli, infection, or other processes. Laboratory evaluations vary depending on the clinical and histologic appearance.

VASCULOPATHY AND HYPERCOAGULABLE STATES

Evaluation for the following entities should be considered in those presenting with suspected vasculopathy/hypercoagulability: **antiphospholipid antibody syndrome** (APS), **protein C or S deficiency**, **factor V Leiden deficiency**, **prothrombin gene mutation**, **methylenetetrahydrofolate reductase (MTHFR) mutation**, **hyperhomocysteinemia**, **antithrombin III deficiency**, connective tissue disease, and malignancy. Initial testing may include a complete blood count, activated partial thromboplastin time (aPTT), prothrombin time (PT), fibrinogen level, anti-cardiolipin and anti-β-2 glycoprotein assays, protein C and S levels, activated protein C resistance assay, total homocysteine concentration, plasma antithrombin activity assay, and genetic testing [**Table 83-2**].[22]

Depending on the clinical context, other considerations include **thrombotic thrombocytopenic purpura** (TTP), **disseminated intravascular coagulation** (DIC), **heparin-induced thrombocytopenia**, and **coumadin necrosis**. **Purpura fulminans** is the sudden appearance of diffuse retiform purpura rapidly progressing to hemorrhagic skin necrosis, particularly of acral sites [**Figure 83-8**]. Usually occurring secondary to bacterial septicemia or viral infection, purpura fulminans is accompanied by fever, shock, and DIC. All these conditions can present initially

TABLE 83-2 Hypercoagulable work-up[a]

Condition	Testing
Antiphospholipid syndrome	IgG and IgM antibodies to cardiolipin and β-2-glycoprotein; functional assay for lupus anticoagulant
Protein C/S deficiency	Functional protein C assay and free protein S antigen assay; ~50% of normal is considered low
Factor V leiden	Functional (activated Protein C resistance assay) or Genetic testing
Prothrombin gene mutation	Prothrombin G20210A point mutation testing
Antithrombin III deficiency	Antithrombin-heparin (AT) cofactor assay using factor Xa or thrombin
MTHFR deficiency	Total homocysteine concentration, genetic testing permissible in symptomatic individuals
Malignancy	Age-appropriate cancer screening, basic laboratory testing, thorough physical exam and review of systems (ROS), chest radiograph; other testing dependent upon suspicion
Connective tissue disease	Thorough exam and ROS, basic laboratory testing; autoimmune serologies dependent upon suspicion

[a]Refer to published guidelines for additional information on when and how to test for hereditary and acquired thrombophilia.[22]

with retiform purpura or other purpuric eruption in the skin and can result in systemic thrombosis, morbidity, and mortality.

DEPOSITIONAL DISORDERS

Calciphylaxis is a rare condition in which calcium-phosphate dyshomeostasis results in calcium deposition and subsequent clotting of small-to-medium sized vessels (also see Chapter 86). Cutaneous findings include painful subcutaneous nodules and retiform purpura leading to necrosis and ulceration [**Figure 83-9**]. The condition most often occurs in the setting of end-stage renal disease. With a mortality rate of 50% at 1 year, treatment is multimodal, including sodium thiosulfate, bisphosphonates, cinacalcet, noncalcium phosphate binders, pentoxifylline, vitamin K, wound management, and pain control.[23]

In those with severe atherosclerosis, intravascular instrumentation can dislodge lipid plaques, resulting in **cholesterol emboli**. Prominent livedo reticularis, cyanosis, purpura, ulceration, and gangrene are clinical manifestations, along with peripheral eosinophilia, pain, acute renal failure, and bowel ischemia. Potential treatments include fluid resuscitation and pain management, as well as systemic corticosteroids.

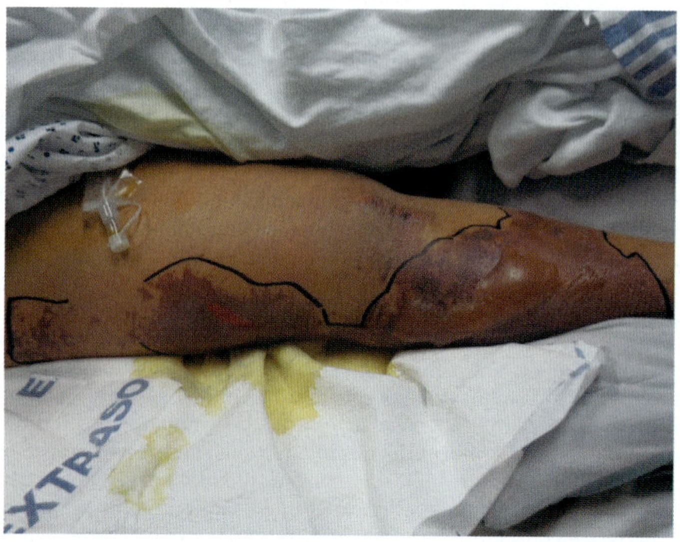

FIGURE 83-8. Purpura fulminans with diffuse retiform purpura and hemorrhagic necrosis.

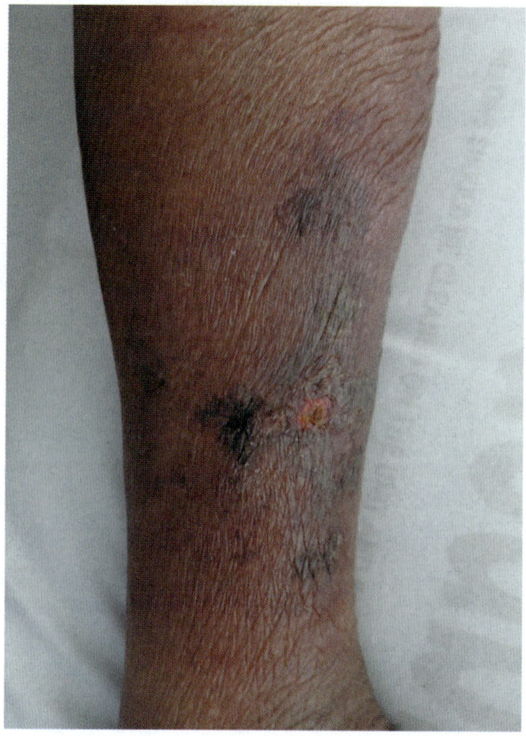

FIGURE 83-9. Calciphylaxis of the lower leg characterized by firm, painful retiform purpura with ulceration.

INFECTIOUS ETIOLOGY

Infectious organisms that directly destroy blood vessels or compromise blood flow should also be considered in this category of purpuric eruptions. **Ecthyma gangrenosum** secondary to *Pseudomonas* or mucormycosis a rare but serious fungal infection manifests with an infarcted appearance, as vascular destruction leads to ischemic necrosis. Biopsy and tissue culture are essential for diagnosis and for determining appropriate antibiotic coverage.

PETECHIAE AND PURPURIC MACULES

The clinical differential diagnosis for petechiae and purpuric macules includes thrombocytopenia, capillaritis, golfer vasculitis, and livedoid vasculopathy. **Thrombocytopenia** has many potential causes, including immune-mediated and drug-induced. **Capillaritis**, or pigmented purpuric dermatosis (PPD), can mimic small vessel vasculitis. A chronic and benign condition, PPD affects primarily the lower extremities and may either be asymptomatic or pruritic/burning. Golfer vasculitis, also called exercise-induced vasculitis, results from vascular damage secondary to physical activity, warmth, or humidity. Areas of exposed skin (eg, above the sock line) are typically affected, resulting in purpuric patches, swelling, itching, and stinging. These conditions lack systemic involvement/disease associations.

Livedoid vasculopathy results from occlusion of small-sized vessels by fibrin thrombi and is therefore a cutaneous sign of an underlying hypercoagulable state. Livedoid vasculopathy mimics small vessel vasculitis by presenting with painful purpuric macules and ulcerations [**Figure 83-10**]. Upon healing, lesions appear porcelain-white in color, with atrophic scarring and peripheral telangiectasis, termed "atrophie blanche." Successful management involves anticoagulant and vasodilatory agents, often in combination, for example, the so-called CHAP regimen, which includes a calcium channel blockers (nifedipine or amlodipine), hydroxychloroquine, aspirin, and pentoxifylline.[24] A systematic hypercoagulable work-up [Table 83-2] is an essential part of evaluation and management.

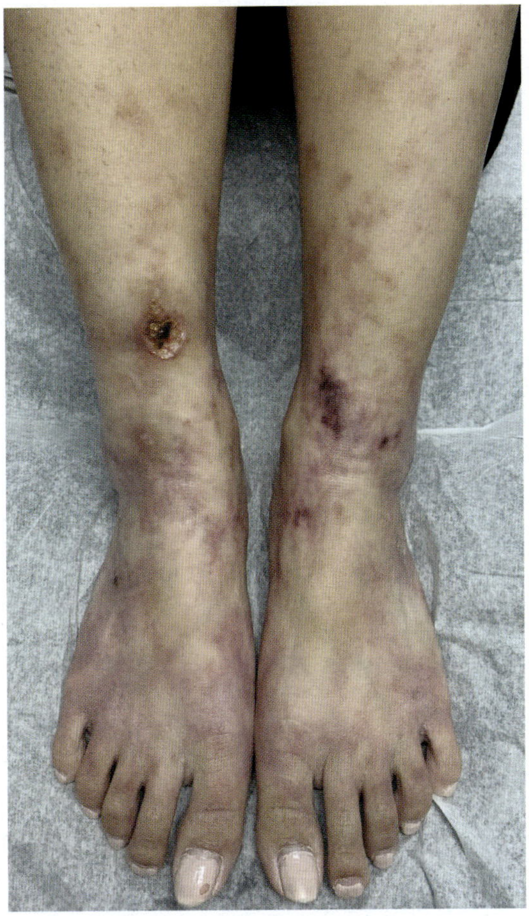

FIGURE 83-10. Livedoid vasculopathy with prominent livedo reticularis, painful purpuric macules, and ulceration on the lower legs and dorsal feet.

OTHER PURPURIC ERUPTIONS

Other rare but important purpuric eruptions include Degos disease, Buerger disease, diffuse dermal angiomatosis, and generalized essential telangiectasia.

Degos disease, also known as malignant atrophic papulosis, is a rare occlusive vasculopathy that presents with pathognomonic white atrophic skin lesions with telangiectatic rim. Degos can either be skin-limited or systemic, with potentially fatal gastrointestinal and central nervous system infarction. Workup should include a laparoscopy for evaluation of gastrointestinal involvement.[25] Though speculative, eculizumab and treprostinil may hold promise as treatments for Degos.

Buerger disease, or thromboangiitis obliterans, results from segmental inflammation and occlusion of small- and medium-sized vessels of the extremities. It typically affects male tobacco smokers less than 45 years of age, with a related condition secondary to marijuana smoking (cannabis arteritis) also described. Cold sensitivity, superficial thrombophlebitis, and ultimately digital ischemia and necrosis characterize the condition.

Diffuse dermal angiomatosis is a rare condition most commonly affecting the lower extremities or breasts of patients with severe peripheral vascular disease. Lesions result from a proliferation of capillaries in the dermis secondary to tissue hypoxia. These present as violaceous, indurated plaques that ulcerate and are associated with ischemic pain [**Figure 83-11**].

Generalized essential telangiectasia is characterized by diffuse, innumerable telangiectasias with preference for the feet and lower legs. Lesions tend to be lacy or branch-like and blanch with diascopy. The condition is usually asymptomatic and is not thought to be associated with systemic disease.

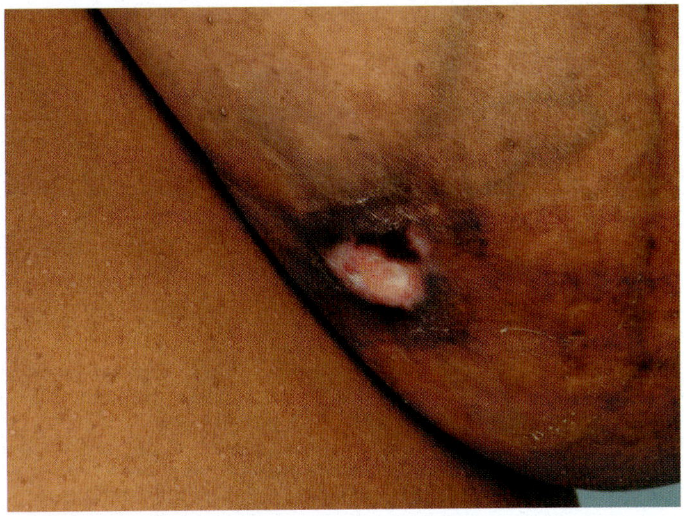

FIGURE 83-11. Diffuse dermal angiomatosis characterized by a firm, violaceous, livedoid plaque with ulceration.

REFERENCES

1. Leung AKC, Barankin B, Leong KF. Henoch-Schönlein purpura in children: an updated review. *Curr Pediatr Rev*. 2020;16(4):265-276.
2. Mahr A, Guillevin L, Poissonnet M, Aymé S. Prevalences of polyarteritis nodosa, microscopic polyangiitis, Wegener's granulomatosis, and Churg-Strauss syndrome in a French urban multiethnic population in 2000: a capture-recapture estimate. *Arthritis Rheum*. 2004;51(1):92-99.
3. Jennette JC, Falk RJ, Bacon PA, et al. 2012 revised International Chapel Hill Consensus Conference Nomenclature of Vasculitides. *Arthritis Rheum*. 2013;65(1):1-11.
4. Sunderkötter CH, Zelger B, Chen KR, et al. Nomenclature of cutaneous vasculitis: dermatologic addendum to the 2012 revised International Chapel Hill Consensus Conference Nomenclature of Vasculitides. *Arthritis Rheumatol*. 2018;70(2):171-184.
5. Sais G, Vidaller A, Jucglà A, Gallardo F, Peyrí J. Colchicine in the treatment of cutaneous leukocytoclastic vasculitis. Results of a prospective, randomized controlled trial. *Arch Dermatol*. 1995;131(12):1399-1402.
6. Fredenberg MF, Malkinson FD. Sulfone therapy in the treatment of leukocytoclastic vasculitis. Report of three cases. *J Am Acad Dermatol*. 1987;16(4):772-778.
7. Iqbal H, Evans A. Dapsone therapy for Henoch-Schönlein purpura: a case series. *Arch Dis Child*. 2005;90(9):985-986.
8. Callen JP, Spencer LV, Burruss JB, Holtman J. Azathioprine. An effective, corticosteroid-sparing therapy for patients with recalcitrant cutaneous lupus erythematosus or with recalcitrant cutaneous leukocytoclastic vasculitis. *Arch Dermatol*. 1991;127(4):515-522.
9. Kolkhir P, Grakhova M, Bonnekoh H, Krause K, Maurer M. Treatment of urticarial vasculitis: a systematic review. *J Allergy Clin Immunol*. 2019;143(2):458-466.
10. Cacoub P, Si Ahmed SN, Ferfar Y, et al. Long-term efficacy of interferon-free antiviral treatment regimens in patients with hepatitis C virus-associated cryoglobulinemia vasculitis. *Clin Gastroenterol Hepatol*. 2019;17(3):518-526.
11. De Vita S, Quartuccio L, Isola M, et al. A randomized controlled trial of rituximab for the treatment of severe cryoglobulinemic vasculitis. *Arthritis Rheum*. 2012;64(3):843-853.
12. Jones RB, Furuta S, Tervaert JW, et al. Rituximab versus cyclophosphamide in ANCA-associated renal vasculitis: 2-year results of a randomised trial. *Ann Rheum Dis*. 2015;74(6):1178-1182.
13. Wechsler ME, Akuthota P, Jayne D, et al. Mepolizumab or placebo for eosinophilic granulomatosis with polyangiitis. *N Engl J Med*. 2017;376(20):1921-1932.
14. Jayne DRW, Merkel PA, Schall TJ, Bekker P; ADVOCATE Study Group. Avacopan for the treatment of ANCA-associated vasculitis. *N Engl J Med*. 2021;384(7):599-609.
15. Bettuzzi T, Jachiet M, Sbidian E, et al. Efficacy and safety of treatments in cutaneous polyarteritis nodosa: a French observational retrospective study. *J Am Acad Dermatol*. 2022;86(5):1035-1041.
16. Micheletti RG. Cutaneous small vessel vasculitis: a practical guide to diagnosis and management. *Am J Clin Dermatol*. 2023;24(1):89-95.

17. Micheletti RG. Treatment of cutaneous vasculitis. *Front Med (Lausanne).* 2022;9:1059612.
18. Narchi H. Risk of long term renal impairment and duration of follow up recommended for Henoch-Schonlein purpura with normal or minimal urinary findings: a systematic review. *Arch Dis Child.* 2005;90(9):916-920.
19. Jachiet M, Flageul B, Deroux A, et al. The clinical spectrum and therapeutic management of hypocomplementemic urticarial vasculitis: data from a French nationwide study of fifty-seven patients. *Arthritis Rheumatol.* 2015;67(2):527-534.
20. Kolopp-Sarda MN, Miossec P. Cryoglobulinemic vasculitis: pathophysiological mechanisms and diagnosis. *Curr Opin Rheumatol.* 2021;33(1):1-7.
21. Micheletti RG, Chiesa Fuxench Z, Craven A, et al. Cutaneous manifestations of antineutrophil cytoplasmic antibody-associated vasculitis. *Arthritis Rheumatol.* 2020;72(10):1741-1747.
22. Middeldorp S, Nieuwlaat R, Baumann Kreuziger L, et al. American Society of Hematology 2023 guidelines for management of venous thromboembolism: thrombophilia testing. *Blood Adv.* 2023;7(22):7101-7138.
23. Rick J, Rrapi R, Chand S, et al. Calciphylaxis: treatment and outlook-CME part II. *J Am Acad Dermatol.* 2022;86(5):985-992.
24. Coromilas AJ, Micheletti RG. A novel combination ("CHAP") regimen for management of livedoid vasculopathy in 12 patients. *J Am Acad Dermatol.* 2023;88(3):672-674.
25. Toledo AE, Shapiro LS, Farrell JF, Magro CM, Polito J. Laparoscopy shows superiority over endoscopy for early detection of malignant atrophic papulosis gastrointestinal complications: a case report and review of literature. *BMC Gastroenterol.* 2015;15:156.

CHAPTER 84

Severe and Inpatient Presentations of Common Dermatoses

Joyce XiaAlice Tan
Daniela Kroshinsky

KEY POINTS

- Severe infection, development of erythroderma, systemic involvement, and disease refractory to treatment may indicate reasons for inpatient admission in patients with common dermatoses such as eczema and psoriasis.
- Immediate identification and cessation of causative drugs is critical in the management of AGEP, SJS/TEN, and DRESS, with certain ethnicities demonstrating greater risk profiles for drug reactions.
- Patients with skin of color may present with specific subtypes of dermatologic disease, more advanced disease, and/or greater number of hospitalizations with longer length of stay, reflecting disparities in care.
- Early dermatologic consultation as well as coordinated multidisciplinary care is paramount in managing sequelae of skin barrier disruption and organ involvement.

INTRODUCTION

Atopic dermatitis, psoriasis, and other dermatoses are typically managed in the outpatient setting. In some cases, common dermatoses complicated by infection, widespread erythema and scaling, or continued severe symptomatology despite therapy may benefit from hospitalization.[1] In this chapter, we review common dermatoses in addition to erythroderma, drug eruptions, neutrophilic dermatoses, and calciphylaxis that may require inpatient management and consider nuances in patients with skin of color.

ATOPIC DERMATITIS

INTRODUCTION

Atopic dermatitis (AD) is a chronic disorder characterized by pruritus, eczematous lesions, and lichenification. Prevalence and disease burden of AD varies across racialized groups, with Black Americans having a higher prevalence of AD and higher burden of moderate to severe disease presumably driven by intrinsic (ie, hereditary predisposition, skin barrier dysfunction, immune disruption) and extrinsic factors (including socioeconomic status, race, and environment).[2] While AD is typically managed in the outpatient setting, hospitalization may be necessary in severe disease complicated by erythroderma (see Erythroderma section) or infection.[1]

ECZEMA HERPETICUM

Presentation Eczema herpeticum (EH) occurs due to secondary infection of AD by herpes simplex virus (HSV). EH is characterized by rapid onset of numerous, painful, vesicular to pustular lesions progressing into punched-out crusted ulcers [**Figures 84-1** and **84-2**]. New lesions appear over the course of 7 to 10 days and resolve within 2 to 6 weeks.[1] Associated symptoms include fever, lymphadenopathy, and malaise.

Differential Impetigo, eczema coxsackium, primary varicella zoster virus (VZV), herpes zoster (localized or disseminated, see **Figure 84-3**), molluscum contagiosum, dermatitis herpetiformis.

Diagnosis Diagnosis can be made clinically but may be reinforced with testing including direct fluorescent antibody (DFA) stain, polymerase chain reaction (PCR), or viral culture. Of these, PCR is the most sensitive and specific.[3] Biopsy may demonstrate multinucleated giant cells with intranuclear inclusions. Tzanck smear is quick to result but reliability and sensitivity is user dependent, and it does not distinguish between HSV1, HSV2, and VZV.[3]

Management Limited disease may be treated orally with acyclovir, famciclovir, or valacyclovir. Immunocompromised patients and severe cases with extensive skin involvement should receive intravenous antivirals.[1] Topical steroids are not associated with longer hospital length of stay and may be resumed within 72 hours of starting acyclovir.[4] Other

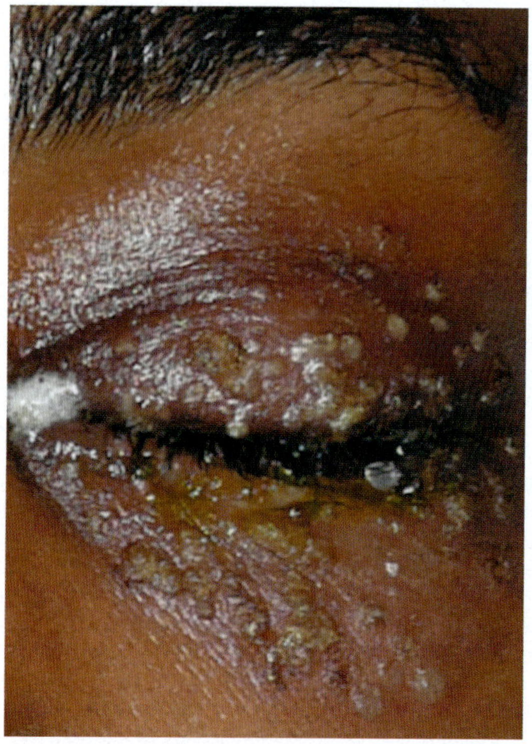

FIGURE 84-1. Periocular eczema herpeticum.

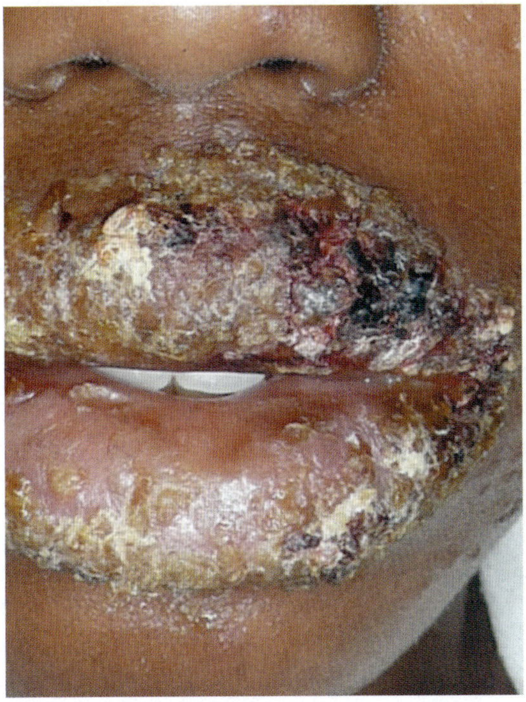

FIGURE 84-2. Herpetic gingivostomatitis.

cornerstones of management include pain and itch control, and cultures/antibiotics for secondary infection. Ophthalmologic consultation and evaluation for herpetic keratitis is recommended for rash with periocular involvement.[1] For recurrent cases of EH, consider a chronic daily oral suppressive antiviral regimen.

Complications Disseminated viremia, multiorgan involvement (eg, hepatitis, encephalitis, meningitis), loss of vision, keratoconjunctivitis, secondary bacterial infection.

Prognosis May be fatal in the absence of antiviral therapy, but in recent years mortality rates have been found to be as low as 0.1%.[5]

BACTERIAL INFECTION

Presentation Bacterial superinfection of AD is common and can result in impetigo, cellulitis, erysipelas, skin abscesses, or bacteremia. Up to 90% of AD patients are colonized with *Staphylococcus aureus*, the most common infectious agent.[1] In impetigo, patients may develop pustules or honey crusted papules on an erythematous base [**Figure 84-4**]. Bullous impetigo may present as fluid filled blisters or crusted tender erosions. Erysipelas and cellulitis can be identified by focal erythema, edema, warmth, tenderness, fever, bacteremia, or worsening dermatitis with failure to respond to therapy. Abscess may present as fluctuant or nonfluctuant nodules and pustules. Patients with bacteremia may be febrile or present with other instability of vital signs indicating progression to sepsis.

Differential Eczema herpeticum, eczema coxsackium, thrombophlebitis, contact dermatitis, drug reactions, scabies.

Diagnosis Typically clinical, with cultures recommended for guidance of antibiotic therapy.

Management Minor cases of impetigo may be treated with topical antibiotics such as bacitracin, neomycin, or mupirocin only. **Table 84-1** includes management of more extensive skin infection.[6] Prevention of future infection necessitates control of pruritus with treatments such as topical anti-inflammatories, antihistamines, phototherapy, cyclosporine, dupilumab, and skin moisturization to address scratching and further barrier breakdown. Efficacy of bleach baths is equivocal, but they remain an inexpensive and well-tolerated adjunctive measure.[7]

Complications Sepsis, endocarditis, septic arthritis, osteomyelitis, bursitis, staphylococcal scalded skin syndrome.

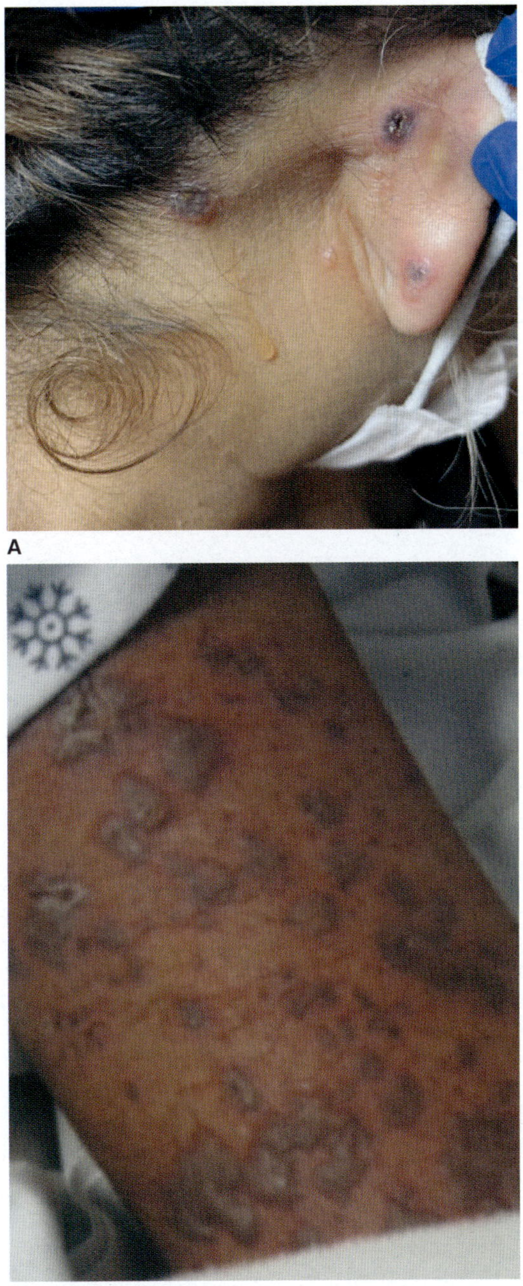

A

B

FIGURE 84-3. (A) Localized herpes zoster. **(B)** Disseminated zoster.

Prognosis Favorable with prompt treatment. In general, recurrence of cellulitis is relatively common, with up to 49% of patients reporting a history of the disease.[6]

PSORIASIS

INTRODUCTION

Psoriasis is a chronic, inflammatory, immune-mediated disease affecting the skin and joints. There are five major subtypes: plaque psoriasis (psoriasis vulgaris), guttate (eruptive) psoriasis, inverse/intertriginous/flexural psoriasis, pustular psoriasis, and erythrodermic psoriasis. Patients with pustular psoriasis or erythrodermic psoriasis (see Erythroderma section) more often require hospitalization due to systemic complications. Whether partly explained by population-specific effects of HLA variants or inequities in the social determinants of health, erythrodermic and pustular psoriasis are more likely to be seen in patients with skin of color.[8]

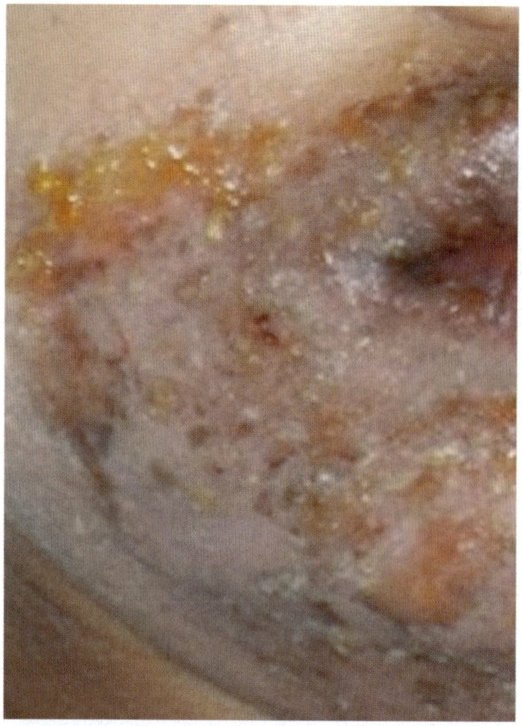

FIGURE 84-4. Impetiginized eczema.

GENERALIZED PUSTULAR PSORIASIS

Presentation Pustular psoriasis can be present as localized or generalized forms. Local disease includes the palmoplantar and acrodermatitis continua of Hallopeau variants. Generalized pustular psoriasis (GPP), which is more likely to require inpatient admission, can be further subcategorized (see **Table 84-2**).[9-11] Patients present with sterile pustules on an erythematous base, though psoriasis on darker skin types may additionally appear gray to violaceous. Median age of onset is in the fifties, though familial subtypes may have an earlier age of onset.[9] In the most severe and common von Zumbusch subtype, progression of the lesions can be rapid and life-threatening. Patients may present with fever, malaise, neutrophilic leukocytosis, elevated c-reactive protein (CRP), and peripheral eosinophilia. For a list of triggering factors, see **Table 84-3**.[9,10]

TABLE 84-1 Treatment of Cellulitis[6]

Uncomplicated Cellulitis*	Severe Cellulitis** and Immunocompromised Patients
Empiric treatment should cover both *S. aureus* and β-hemolytic streptococci Nonpurulent, uncomplicated cellulitis • Trial oral non-MRSA antibiotics such as amoxicillin-clavulanate, cephalexin, or dicloxacillin • If patient does not improve consider intravenous antibiotics covering MSSA such as cefazolin, ceftriaxone, or penicillin G Purulent, uncomplicated cellulitis • Consider risk of MRSA infection • If low, proceed with oral non-MRSA antibiotics as detailed above • If high, proceed with oral MRSA antibiotics such as clindamycin, tetracyclines, or trimethoprim-sulfamethoxazole If patient does not improve, consider intravenous MRSA antibiotics such as clindamycin, daptomycin, vancomycin	Treat empirically for MSSA and MRSA with broad-spectrum IV coverage. • Consider intravenous vancomycin PLUS piperacillin/tazobactam or meropenem Later changes to antibiotic regimen should be targeted based on culture results.

*Cellulitis in patients without comorbidities or systemic symptoms such as fever, diabetes, or immunosuppressive disorders.

**Cellulitis in patients demonstrating ≥2 SIRS criteria, hypotension, or rapid disease progression.

Rrapi R, Chand S, Kroshinsky D. Cellulitis: a review of pathogenesis, diagnosis, and management. *Med Clin North Am.* 2021;105(4):723–735.

TABLE 84-2 Subtypes of GPP[9-11]

Generalized pustular psoriasis	
von Zumbusch subtype	**Annular subtype**
• Diffuse pustular eruption that may coalesce to form lakes of pus • Base of painful dark or erythematous patches • Rapid onset (7 days or fewer) • Up to 90% of GPP • Most severe presentation • Associated systemic symptoms and laboratory abnormalities (fevers, arthralgias, malaise, neutrophilic leukocytosis, elevated CRP, and peripheral eosinophilia) • Referred to as impetigo herpetiformis during pregnancy	• Annular lesions with pustules along the advancing edge • Develops between 7 days and 3 months • Relatively mild symptoms

Differential Acute generalized exanthematous pustulosis (AGEP), annular pustular psoriasis, palmoplantar pustular psoriasis, disseminated tinea corporis, dermatitis herpetiformis, IgA pemphigus, pustular miliaria, pustular erythema multiforme, dermatitis with secondary infection, pemphigus foliaceus.

Diagnosis Diagnostic criteria, including skin biopsy, are listed in **Table 84-4**.[9] In patients with early onset GPP, consideration may be given to screening for known associated mutations including IL36RN, CARD14, and AP1S3, though this is not routinely indicated.[10]

Management In adults, first-line treatment options include retinoids, cyclosporine, methotrexate, and infliximab. Cyclosporine has a relatively quick onset of action as compared to methotrexate, with improvements noted as soon as 2 weeks after initiation.[9] Infliximab is also considered a first-line treatment for severe cases given its rapid onset of action.[9] Retinoids have been historically used with high efficacy but have also been shown to have a greater incidence of side effects and complications. In children, retinoids may lead to premature epiphyseal closure and so cyclosporine is the first-line treatment.[9] Methotrexate is not approved for use in children under age 2. Second-line options include adalimumab, etanercept, topical agents such as calcipotriene and tacrolimus, and PUVA phototherapy. Pregnant patients may be treated with systemic

TABLE 84-3 GPP triggers[9,10]

Factors associated with pustular eruption
• Sudden withdrawal of systemic steroids*
• Infection
• Medications (lithium, iodine, penicillin, interferon-α, terbinafine, ramipril, rituximab, clopidogrel, amoxicillin, calcipotriol, NSAIDs, aspirin, sulfonamides, morphine, coal tar, potassium iodide, progestins, hydroxychloroquine)
• Pregnancy
• Phototherapy
• Vaccinations (BCG and H1N1)
• Emotional stress

*Notably, the occurrence of severe psoriatic flares following systemic steroid administration remains a controversial topic. Systemic prednisone remains in common use for psoriatic control in Europe and by nondermatologists. Preliminary studies have found that only about 1.5% of patients receiving systemic corticosteroids developed a subsequent flare; of these, most cases involved worsening plaque psoriasis rather than GPP or erythroderma. While post steroid flares are a possible phenomenon, the true incidence of severe flare may be less widespread than commonly taught.[12]

TABLE 84-4 Diagnosis of GPP[9]

Suggested diagnostic criteria for GPP by Umezawa et al[a]
• Multiple sterile pustules overlying erythematous or gray to violaceous skin*
• Fever, malaise, and other systemic symptoms
• Kogoj spongiform pustules on histopathology
• Laboratory abnormalities including left shift leukocytosis, elevated ESR or CRP, elevated anti-streptolysin O antibody levels, elevated IgG or IgA levels, hypoproteinemia, hypocalcemia
• Recurrence of these clinical and histological findings

*Psoriasis on darker skin tones/types may additionally appear gray to violaceous.

[a]Reproduced with permission from Hoegler KM, John AM, Handler MZ, Schwartz RA. Generalized pustular psoriasis: a review and update on treatment. *J Eur Acad Dermatol Venereol*. 2018;32(10):1645-1651.

corticosteroids, cyclosporine, and infliximab. Risks of steroid treatment include premature labor, macrosomia, and gestational diabetes.[9] GPP typically resolves after delivery, and early induction of labor may be required as part of treatment. Adjunctive measures for comfort include wet wraps, oatmeal baths, emollient use, pain control, and antihistamines and topical corticosteroids for itch control. Supportive care should also include prevention and treatment of secondary infection.

Complications Cholestasis/cholangitis, osteoarthritis, uveitis, interstitial pneumonitis/ARDS, cardiovascular shock, renal failure, otitis media, polymicrobial infection.

Prognosis Given the rarity of GPP, prognostic data are limited and variable. It is common for the condition to recur or flare in response to triggers.

ERYTHRODERMA

INTRODUCTION

Erythroderma, also known as exfoliative dermatitis, is a rare and potentially life-threatening condition characterized by erythematous skin and scaling affecting greater than or equal to 90% of body surface area. Erythroderma can occur at any age, but average onset is 41 to 61 years with a male predominance.[13] Acute erythroderma typically presents as widespread erythema followed by exfoliative scaling 2 to 6 days later, with associated symptoms of skin pain and pruritus.[13,14] Onset and duration of erythroderma are highly variable and dependent on the underlying cause.

Presentation Erythroderma presents with erythematous and warm skin affecting greater than or equal to 90% of body surface area [**Figure 84-5**]. Severe skin pain or pruritus is common, the latter particularly in patients with atopic dermatitis or Sezary syndrome.[13] Clinical features that may help differentiate diagnoses include palmoplantar hyperkeratosis in pityriasis rubra pilaris, nail dystrophy in psoriasis, unexplained weight loss and lymphadenopathy in Sezary syndrome, and mucocutaneous blisters or erosions in immunobullous diseases.[14,15] Associated extracutaneous symptoms include chills/shivering, hypothermia, malaise, fatigue, lymphadenopathy, and in extreme cases, signs of high-output cardiac failure (tachycardia, peripheral edema).[12-15] Lab abnormalities are nonspecific and may include leukocytosis, anemia, and elevated erythrocyte sedimentation rate.[15] Eosinophilia may be associated with drug eruptions, atopic dermatitis, or bullous pemphigoid.[13]

Differential Erythroderma can represent a wide range of cutaneous and systemic diseases, most commonly from exacerbation of preexisting inflammatory dermatoses (atopic dermatitis, psoriasis, lichen planus, pityriasis rubra pilaris). Other etiologies include infection (scabies, staphylococcal scalded skin syndrome (SSSS), toxic shock syndrome, dermatophytoses, leprosy), infiltration (Sezary syndrome, mycosis fungoides, diffuse cutaneous mastocytosis, internal malignancy), ingestion (drug hypersensitivity reaction, systemic contact dermatitis), immunologic (graft-vs-host disease, dermatomyositis, systemic lupus erythematosus, sarcoidosis), immunobullous (pemphigus foliaceus, bullous pemphigoid), or idiopathic.[15,16] Erythroderma may also result from sudden withdrawal of systemic or potent topical steroids.[14]

Diagnosis Diagnosis is made clinically in patients with diffuse erythema and scaling involving greater than or equal to 90% body surface area. Examination should be performed in a well-lit environment as darker skin tones may make identification of erythema difficult. Palpation to assess blanching may also be a helpful clinical clue to assess degree of erythema relative to patient's baseline unaffected skin. The rate of disease progression and morphology of the rash can vary significantly depending on the underlying cause. Age at onset, initial site of involvement, types of lesions, predisposing factors, and family history are also crucial in determining the etiology.[15] Erythroderma due to drug hypersensitivity, contact allergy, cutaneous T-cell lymphoma, leukemia, and SSSS are characterized by rapid progression, whereas primary cutaneous disease, such as atopic dermatitis and psoriasis, develops more gradually.[13,15] The utility of a biopsy is low as diagnostic features may be masked by nonspecific histopathological changes of erythroderma, such as hyperorthokeratosis, acanthosis, and chronic perivascular inflammatory infiltrate with or without eosinophilia.[13] A biopsy can be repeated when clinical signs begin to improve, and multiple biopsies may increase histopathologic accuracy.[13]

Complications Complications include thermoregulatory disturbances, reactive lymphadenopathy, fluid and electrolyte disturbances, acute respiratory distress syndrome, and anemia. Monitoring for high-output cardiac failure is important especially in older or compromised patients.[13] Superimposed bacterial infections may occur and lead to sepsis from *S. aureus*, particularly in HIV positive patients or widespread herpes simplex virus (HSV) infection.[13-15]

Management Early diagnosis when possible and supportive therapy are critical in reducing morbidity and mortality. Management is focused on treatment of the underlying etiology. Patients who are unstable may require hospital admission for initial evaluation. Inpatient management includes replacement of fluid and electrolytes, nutritional support, a warm and humid room to prevent hypothermia, and treatment of any superinfections such as methicillin-resistant *S. aureus* or HSV.[13,17]

Symptomatic treatment with low- to mid-potency topical steroids and oral antihistamines can help reduce pruritus and inflammation. Other topical measures include wet dressings and emollients. The oral mucosa, eyes, and genitourinary tract should be evaluated for involvement. Treatment will ultimately be based on cause and may take 4 to 6 weeks; however, for rapid improvement, cyclosporine or infliximab can be considered.[17] Other immunosuppressive therapies including mycophenolate mofetil, dupilumab, methotrexate, azathioprine, and ruxolitinib may also be considered. Tumor necrosis factor-α (TNF-α) inhibitors (adalimumab, etanercept) and biologics targeting interleukin-12 (IL-12) and/or 23 (ustekinumab, guselkumab, risankizumab) and IL-17 (secukinumab, ixekizumab, brodalumab) receptors have also proved beneficial in erythrodermic psoriasis.

Prognosis A cross-sectional analysis of the National Inpatient Sample found Black and Asian ethnicity to be associated with increased hospital costs and longer length of stay in patients admitted for erythroderma.[18] Although recent advances in diagnosis and treatment have resulted in lower mortality, mortality rates range from 3.73% to 64%.[13] Prevention of relapses of erythroderma involves treatment of the underlying cause.

DRUG ERUPTION RASHES

INTRODUCTION

Most adverse drug reactions are cutaneous and benign, consisting of maculopapular eruptions or urticaria, with only 2% considered truly life-threatening.[19] These are AGEP, Stevens-Johnson syndrome (SJS), toxic epidermal necrolysis (TEN), and drug reaction with eosinophilia and systemic symptoms (DRESS). Ethnicity has been observed to influence risk profiles for specific drug reactions such as SJS and TEN due to the relative prevalence of predisposing HLA alleles, with many of these alleles found at greater frequencies in Asian populations.[20] Belonging to

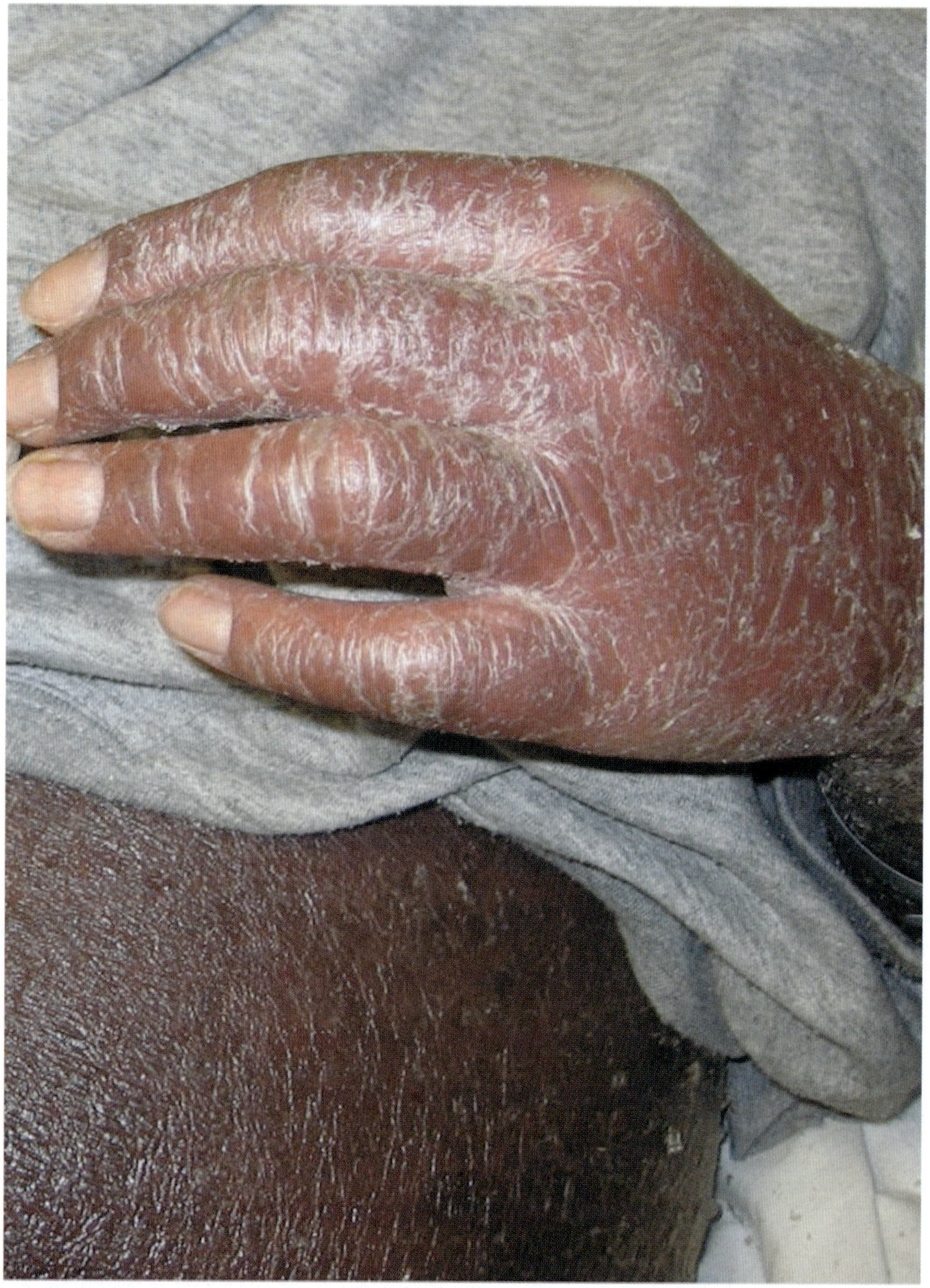

FIGURE 84-5. Erythrodermic psoriasis.

a racial or ethnic minority has not been observed to be associated with risk of developing DRESS.[21]

ACUTE GENERALIZED EXANTHEMATOUS PUSTULOSIS (AGEP)

AGEP affects patients of all ages, with a slight female predominance. Certain genetic mutations may predispose toward development of AGEP, with higher levels of IL-36 receptor antagonist gene mutations found in AGEP patients as compared to control.[22]

Presentation AGEP presents rapidly after exposure to a causative drug (90% of cases), with onset typically occurring within 48 hours [**Table 84-5**].[22,23] AGEP appears as many small nonfollicular pustules on an erythematous base [**Figure 84-6A**], usually involving the trunk and intertriginous regions, frequently progressing to confluence [**Figure 84-6B**]. There tends to be minimal to no mucous membrane involvement.[23] AGEP is typically pruritic and sometimes painful. During the resolution phase of the rash, superficial collarette-shaped desquamation may also be observed. Presenting symptoms include leukocytosis with elevated neutrophil counts ($\geq 7.5 \times 10^9$/L) and fever (≥38C).[23]

Differential GPP, pustular vasculitis, subcorneal pustular dermatosis (Sneddon-Wilkinson), DRESS, SJS/TEN, Sweet syndrome, bullous impetigo.

TABLE 84-5 Precipitating AGEP medications, infections, and exposures[23]

Medications	Infections and exposures
• Antibiotics: pristinamycin, aminopenicillins, sulfonamides	• Parvovirus B19
• Antifungals: terbinafine, ketoconazole, and fluconazole	• Cytomegalovirus (CMV)
• Antimalarials: quinolones, hydroxychloroquine	• Chlamydia pneumoniae
• Diltiazem	• Spider bites
	• Mercury
	• Iodine contrast

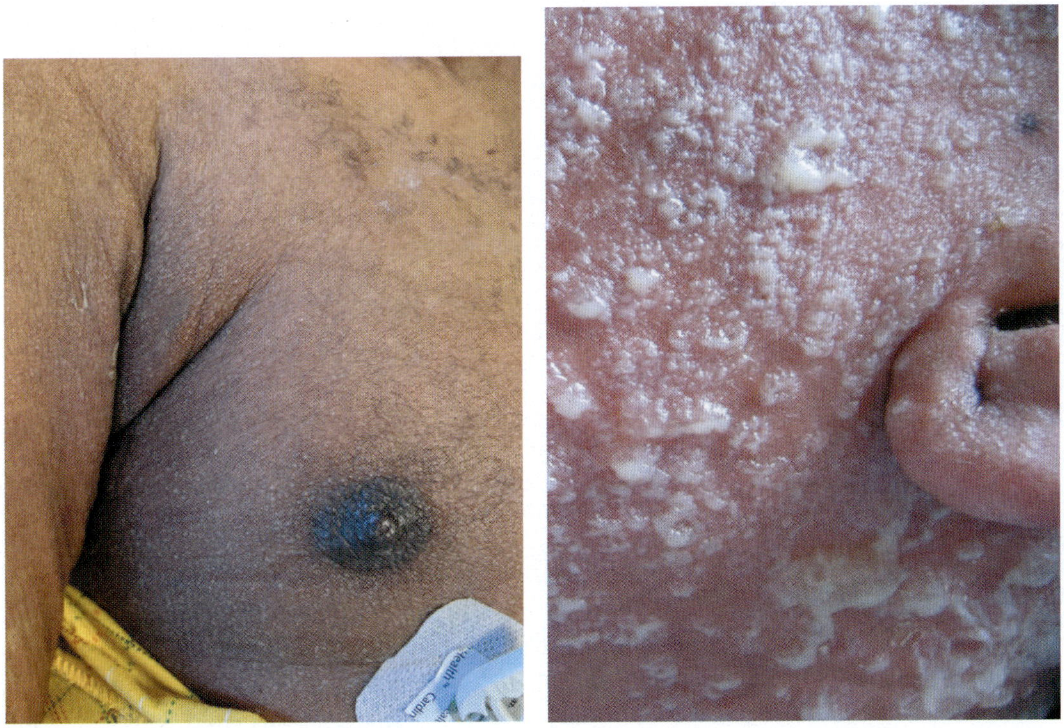

A B

FIGURE 84-6. **(A)** Acute generalized exanthematous pustulosis (AGEP) appears as many small nonfollicular pustules on an erythematous base. **(B)** AGEP with confluence of erythema and subcorneal pustules.

Diagnosis In addition to a thorough medical history, identifying possible causative exposures, and timing of exposure, skin biopsy is necessary to confirm AGEP. Histology should reveal spongiform intracorneal, subcorneal, and/or intraepidermal pustules with papillary dermal edema, and neutrophilic and eosinophilic infiltrates. Epidermal changes seen may include spongiosis with exocytosis of neutrophils and necrotic keratinocytes.[23] The EuroSCAR validation score may be used to classify patients by likelihood of having AGEP. Finally, patch testing 4 to 6 weeks after disease resolution may be useful in identifying the causative exposure.[22] A positive patch test is confirmatory, but a negative test is not exclusionary.

Management AGEP is self-limiting, though patients are usually hospitalized for monitoring and treatment. Suspected causative drugs should be discontinued immediately. Patients must be monitored for evidence of systemic involvement and bacterial superinfection of lesions. Itch and inflammation can be symptomatically managed with medium to high-dose topical or systemic steroids. Cyclosporine, infliximab, or IVIG may be attempted in recalcitrant cases.[22] Topical emollients may also be used during the desquamating phase of healing to help restore the skin barrier. Patients should avoid causative drugs in the long term, as reexposure can prompt another reaction.

Complications Systemic involvement with hepatic, renal, or pulmonary insufficiency occurs in 20% of cases.

Prognosis Prognosis is generally favorable, with mortality rates of under 5% reported.[24] Once the causative drug is discontinued, the rash resolves spontaneously in days.

STEVENS-JOHNSON SYNDROME/TOXIC EPIDERMAL NECROLYSIS (SJS/TEN)

SJS and TEN lie along a spectrum of delayed-type hypersensitivity reactions characterized by epidermal necrosis and detachment. SJS involves less than 10% of total body surface area, whereas TEN involves greater than 30% of the skin. Between 10% and 30% detachment is referred to as SJS/TEN overlap. The incidence of disease in the United States is approximately 8.61 to 9.69 per million for SJS, 1.46 to 1.84 per million for SJS/TEN, and 1.58 to 2.26 per million for TEN.[25] For Asian and Black populations, national data indicate substantially higher risk of SJS/TEN in the context of urate-lowering drug adverse effects (ie, allopurinol) compared to White or Hispanic populations, correlating well with corresponding frequencies of HLA-B*5801 among each group in the United States.[26]

Presentation Onset of SJS/TEN is usually within 4 to 8 weeks after exposure to an inciting medication [**Table 84-6**].[25] Symptoms begin with a prodrome of malaise, fever, myalgias, and arthralgias, followed by the development of painful cutaneous and mucous membrane (90% of cases) lesions. Lesions typically begin on the face or torso before spreading symmetrically and appear as coalescing erythematous macules with dusky centers [**Figure 84-7**]. The scalp, palms, and soles are usually spared. Atypical target lesions, vesicles, bullae, and positive Nikolsky sign may be seen. This acute phase lasts 1 to 2 weeks, with healing and reepithelialization occurring by 2 to 4 weeks.

TABLE 84-6 Commonly implicated drugs in SJS/TEN[25]

Medications
Allopurinol
Aminopenicillins
Carbamazepine
Cephalosporins
Lamotrigine
Levetiracetam
Macrolides
Nevirapine
Oxicam-NSAIDs
Pantoprazole, omeprazole
Phenobarbital
Phenytoin
Quinolones
Rifampin
Sertraline
Sulfonamide antibiotics (sulfasalazine)
Terbinafine
Tetracyclines

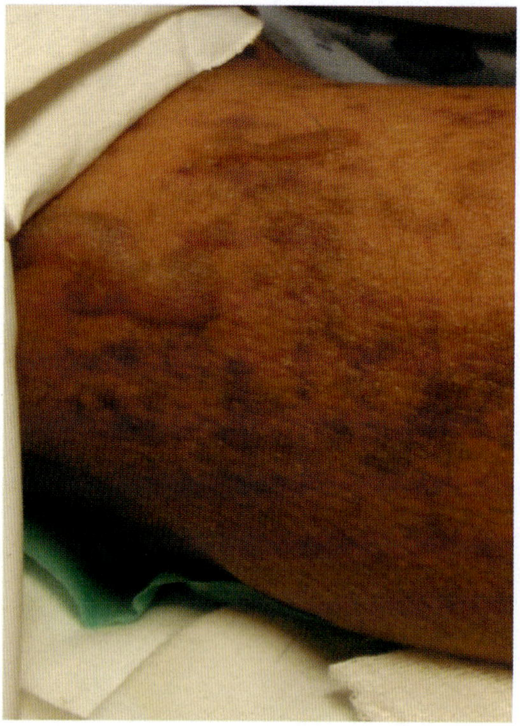

FIGURE 84-7. Early Stevens-Johnson syndrome/toxic epidermal necrolysis.

Differential AGEP, bullous lupus erythematosus, epidermolysis bullosa acquisita, erythema exsudativum multiforme majus, generalized fixed bullous drug eruption, graft versus host disease, linear IgA dermatosis, staphylococcal scalded skin syndrome (SSSS).

Diagnosis Diagnosis is clinical, with a careful history of drug exposures and timelines, prodromal symptoms, and characteristic skin findings. Histology is nonspecific, but skin biopsy may be used to rule out similar conditions. Pathology may show subepidermal blisters with necrosis, apoptotic keratinocytes, and minimal lymphocytic inflammatory infiltrate.[25] Direct immunofluorescence is negative. ALDEN (algorithm of drug causality for epidermal necrolysis) score may be used to determine probable culprit drugs. Otherwise, after the acute phase has resolved, patch testing, in vitro drug tests (eg, lymphocyte transformation test, CD69, IFN-γ), and HLA variant testing may be used with variable reliability to determine the cause of the reaction.[25]

Management Management includes immediate identification and removal of potential causative drugs. Prognosis improves in patients promptly transferred to burn centers, intensive care units, or specialized dermatology units.[25] Acute phase of treatment includes supportive care due to barrier disruption (eg, fluid and electrolyte management, wound care, nutritional support, pain control, infection prevention). Support in the event of organ dysfunction is also required. Skin shearing is minimized with silver dressings and air fluidized beds. Debridement is not recommended, and outcomes are similar to that of a conservative approach.[25] Otherwise, isolation and barrier methods should be employed to reduce risk of infection. There are no clinically proven standard treatments for SJS/TEN. However, commonly utilized interventions that may have benefit include systemic corticosteroids, IVIG, cyclosporine, and etanercept.[25] If trialed, these agents should be administered during the acute phase (up to 8 days from onset of symptoms).

Complications Adverse sequelae include acute and chronic ocular complications (possibly more severe in darker skin phototypes),[27] bacterial infection, disseminated intravascular coagulation, encephalopathy, esophageal ulceration, perforated diverticulitis, hepatitis, myocarditis, pneumonia, bronchiolitis obliterans, long-term pulmonary dysfunction, renal failure, septicemia, urogenital strictures/adhesions/stenosis, and psychiatric disorders (eg, post-traumatic stress disorder, depression, anxiety).

Prognosis Multiple illness severity scores are available to calculate mortality. Of these, SCORTEN and ABCD-10 are similar in reliability and widely used. Mortality of SJS, SJS/TEN, and TEN are estimated at 4.8%, 19.4%, and 14.8%, respectively.[25]

DRUG REACTION WITH EOSINOPHILIA AND SYSTEMIC SYMPTOMS (DRESS)

DRESS and drug-induced hypersensitivity syndrome (DIHS) are used interchangeably to refer to a severe cutaneous drug reaction characterized by fever, lymphadenopathy, hematologic abnormalities, and multiorgan involvement. It is considered a T-cell-mediated hypersensitivity reaction to a causative drug. Viral reactivation (eg, HHV6, EBV, CMV) may also contribute to the pathophysiology of the disease, due to T-cell cross-reactivity leading to autoimmune attack on tissues. Several HLA variants and genetic polymorphisms may contribute to increased susceptibility. Incidence has been reported at approximately 10 per million, with all ages affected.[28]

Presentation Symptoms of DRESS typically occur 2 to 3 weeks following exposure to a causative drug, though may range up to 3 months or longer[28,29] [**Table 84-7**]. Patients may present with a symmetric polymorphous maculopapular eruption to the trunk and extremities, erythema, and facial edema. The eruption may appear as pustules, purpura, plaques, blisters, target lesions, urticarial lesions, or exfoliative dermatitis.[28] Other symptoms include fever, lymphadenopathy, hematologic abnormalities (eg, eosinophilia, leukocytosis, neutrophilia, lymphocytosis, monocytosis, atypical lymphocytes), and organ involvement (see Complications).[28]

Differential Acute cutaneous lupus erythematosus, AGEP, angioimmunoblastic T-cell lymphoma, hypereosinophilic syndrome, infection (eg, measles, rubella, parvovirus, meningococcemia, mononucleosis), morbilliform drug eruption, Sezary syndrome, SJS/TEN.

Diagnosis In addition to drug exposure in the preceding 2 to 12 weeks and characteristic rash, other presenting features like fever, lymphadenopathy, hematologic and multisystem abnormalities should be assessed. Laboratory testing including CBC with differential, peripheral blood smear, liver function tests, kidney function tests, cardiac enzymes, amylase, lipase, viral serology, and viral hepatitis panels should be evaluated. Biopsy may rule out alternative causes, but histology seen in DRESS is frequently nonspecific. Among the most widely used criteria for diagnosis is the RegiSCAR (European Registry of Severe Cutaneous Adverse Reactions to Drugs and Collection of Biological Samples) scoring system[28] [**Table 84-8**]. Patch testing may have utility following resolution of symptoms to evaluate drug causality.[28]

Management The principal treatment for DRESS is to discontinue the causative drug. Isolating the offending drug may prove difficult given

TABLE 84-7 Inciting medications in DRESS[28,29]

Commonly implicated medications in DRESS
Abacavir
Allopurinol
Antibiotics: amoxicillin, ampicillin, piperacillin
Anticonvulsants: carbamazepine, phenytoin, lamotrigine, oxcarbazepine, phenobarbital
Fluoxetine
Mexiletine
Minocycline
Nevirapine
NSAIDs
Olanzapine
Sulfonamides: sulfasalazine, dapsone, TMP-SMX, sulfadiazine
Tuberculosis medications: rifampicin, ethambutol, isoniazid, pyrazinamide
Vancomycin

TABLE 84-8 RegiSCAR for diagnosis of DRESS[28]

RegiSCAR criteria
• Acute skin reaction (Body surface area >50%, biopsy, rash suggestive of DRESS)
• Fever (>38C)
• Lymphadenopathy to at least two sites
• Involvement of at least one internal organ
• Atypical lymphocytes
• Eosinophilia
• Thrombocytopenia

the variable latency in onset of symptoms; therefore, all high-risk medications should be held. Hospitalization is considered depending on the extent of rash and involvement of other organs. Patients may be provided supportive care with antihistamines and topical corticosteroids for control of pruritus and inflammation, antipyretics for fever, and fluid, electrolyte, and nutritional management. Emollients and warm baths or wet dressings may be applied. In severe disease with multiple organ involvement, systemic glucocorticoids are considered first-line therapy despite a lack of randomized controlled trials.[28] For steroid refractory disease, cyclosporine, plasmapheresis, cyclophosphamide, mycophenolate mofetil, rituximab, and tofacitinib have been used with reported success.[28] Antivirals are atypical, but evidence for viral reactivation causing severe consequences may be addressed with ganciclovir or valganciclovir. Patients should avoid the causative drug as well as potentially cross-reactive drugs in the future.

Complications Arthralgia/arthritis, colitis, encephalitis, hepatic failure, myocarditis, pneumonitis/ARDS, renal failure, acute interstitial nephritis, venous thrombosis, long-term autoimmune sequelae (eg, autoimmune thyroiditis, vitiligo, diabetes mellitus, hemolytic anemia, systemic lupus erythematosus).

Prognosis The estimated mortality of DRESS ranges between 5% and 10%.[28] Viral reactivation is associated with increased severity of outcome. Relapses and flares are common, with up to 25% of patients suffering recurrence.[28]

NEUTROPHILIC DERMATOSIS: PYODERMA GANGRENOSUM & SWEET SYNDROME

INTRODUCTION

Neutrophilic dermatoses are conditions characterized histopathologically by neutrophilic inflammatory cell infiltrates with frequent systemic manifestations and associations (please also see Chapter 82). This section will focus on the most common neutrophilic dermatoses: pyoderma gangrenosum and Sweet syndrome.

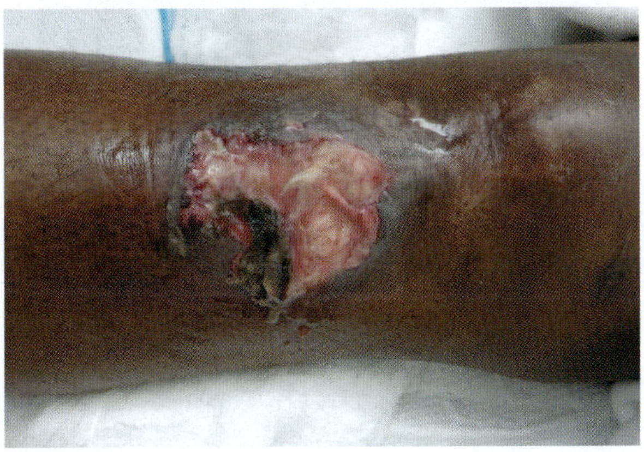

FIGURE 84-8. Pyoderma gangrenosum. (Courtesy of Dr. Arturo Dominguez.)

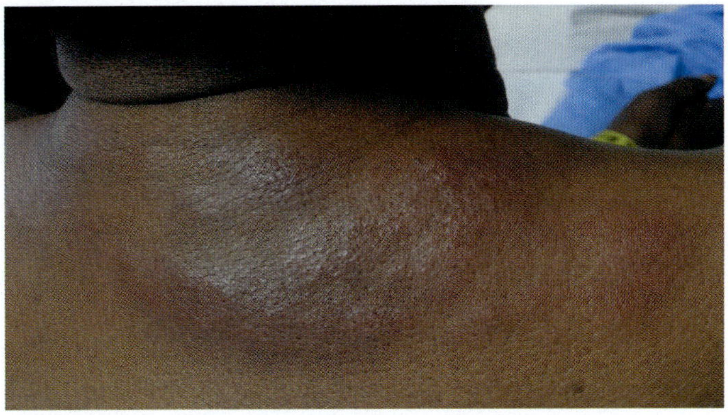

FIGURE 84-9. Sweet syndrome. (Courtesy of Dr. Arturo Dominguez.)

Pyoderma gangrenosum (PG) is a condition commonly associated with trauma or systemic diseases and characterized by severely painful necrotic ulcers with violaceous or gray undermined borders [**Figure 84-8**] and peripheral erythema that heals with cribriform scarring.[30]

Sweet syndrome (SS), also known as acute febrile neutrophilic dermatosis, is characterized by the abrupt onset of painful edematous erythematous papules, plaques, or nodules accompanied by pyrexia and leukocytosis [**Figure 84-9**].[31,32] Individuals aged 30 to 60 years old and predominantly females are affected.[31] There are three subtypes: classical, malignancy-associated, and drug-induced.[31,32] Classical SS is associated with infection (particularly upper respiratory tract and gastrointestinal), inflammatory bowel disease, and pregnancy. Malignancy-associated SS is most commonly secondary to acute myelogenous leukemia (AML) and rarely solid tumors. Finally, the most frequent inciting therapy in drug-induced SS is granulocyte-colony stimulating factor; however, checkpoint inhibitor immunotherapy, nonsteroidal anti-inflammatory drugs, antivirals, and antibacterial medications have also been implicated. Lesions typically develop 2 weeks after drug exposure.[31]

Presentation Patients with PG typically present with rapid progression of an inflammatory papule or pustule to necrotic ulceration with a violaceous border and purulent base, pain out of proportion, and/or history of preceding trauma. The lower extremity is most commonly affected, but other sites such as the face, upper extremities, peristomal area, genital region, and extracutaneous locations can also be involved.

SS cutaneous lesions are characteristically tender and inflamed, distribution is often asymmetrical, and the head and upper extremities are most commonly affected. Systemic symptoms include fever, arthralgias, malaise, headache, and myalgias.[31] Anemia and/or platelet abnormalities may also be present in malignancy-associated or drug-induced SS.

Differentials PG: Cellulitis, venous stasis ulcer, malignancy, ulcerative necrobiosis lipoidica, cutaneous Crohn, antiphospholipid antibody syndrome, granulomatosis with polyangiitis, polyarteritis nodosa, livedoid vasculopathy, cryoglobulinemia, exogenous injury.

SS: erythematous plaques (cellulitis, urticaria, PG, neutrophilic eccrine hidradenitis, Behcet syndrome, cutaneous Crohn, drug eruption), nodules (deep fungal infection, Majocchi granuloma, atypical mycobacterial infection, leukemia cutis, metastatic carcinoma, sarcoidosis, vasculitis, erythema nodosum), bullous (bullous PG, bullous leukocytoclastic vasculitis, bullous pemphigoid, bullous systemic lupus, inflammatory epidermolysis bullosa acquisita, linear IgA bullous dermatosis, bullous cellulitis, aspergillosis, ecthyma gangrenosum)

Diagnosis See **Table 84-9** for diagnostic criteria of PG and SS.[30,33]

TABLE 84-9 Sweet syndrome diagnostic criteria[33]

Major (2)	Minor (2+)
1. Abrupt onset of painful edematous erythematous plaques or nodules 2. Histopathologic evidence of dense neutrophilic infiltrate without evidence of leukocytoclastic vasculitis	1. Pyrexia >38C 2. Association with underlying hematologic or visceral malignancy, inflammatory disease, or pregnancy OR preceded by upper respiratory or gastrointestinal infection / vaccination 3. Excellent response to treatment with systemic steroids or potassium iodide 4. Abnormal lab values at presentation (3/4: ESR >20, positive CRP, >8000 WBC, >70% neutrophils)

Both major findings and two minor criteria are required for the diagnosis.

Complications Complications from PG include pathergy, infection, and immobility.

Complications from SS include pathergy and extracutaneous involvement (most commonly ocular). Neuro-Sweet syndrome, characterized by central nervous involvement following skin lesion development, has been reported to be more common in patients of Asian descent than White patients.[34]

Management The mainstays of treatment for PG are wound and pain management, immunosuppression, and treatment of underlying disorders. In cases of limited disease consisting of few superficial ulcers or a solitary plaque, topical steroids are attempted for 2 to 3 weeks, and if no improvement, tacrolimus ointment can be added. More extensive disease necessitates systemic therapy consisting of systemic glucocorticoids or cyclosporine. Systemic prednisone often results in rapid improvement and can be initiated in the inpatient setting but is typically tapered over 4 to 10 weeks with a bridging glucocorticoid-sparing agent (mycophenolate mofetil, cyclosporine, azathioprine, infliximab).[31] Strict avoidance of wound debridement is critical in preventing complications from pathergy.[32]

SS with involvement limited to the skin frequently resolves spontaneously and without scarring. First-line therapy consists of systemic glucocorticoids and typically results in dramatic clinical improvement. Alternative first-line agents include colchicine, dapsone, and potassium iodide.[31] Similar to PG, the inpatient setting warrants close monitoring of iatrogenic causes of pathergy, including skin biopsies and intravenous catheter placements. Age-appropriate cancer screening can be considered in cases where malignancy is suspected.[31]

Prognosis Greater than 50% of patients with PG achieve complete wound healing within 1 year, although disease recurrence and scarring are common. Primary admission for PG has been associated with female sex, Black race/ethnicity, lower household income, and public or no insurance, highlighting potential disparities in outpatient management of PG and barriers to high-value dermatologic care.[35]

Cutaneous lesions from SS typically heal without scarring although postinflammatory hyperpigmentation can take months to years to resolve. Death from SS is rare. Relapse is more likely in malignancy-associated disease, particularly in patients with hematologic disorders.

CALCIPHYLAXIS

INTRODUCTION

Calciphylaxis is a rare condition characterized by severely painful necrotic skin lesions with high morbidity and mortality most commonly seen in patients with end-stage renal disease (ESRD) on dialysis. Calciphylaxis primarily affects females with a mean age of 50 to 70 years old.[36,37] In a U.S. study involving 1030 patients with calciphylaxis who were dependent on hemodialysis, 49% were White and 28% were Black individuals, a racial distribution approximating that of patients undergoing hemodialysis in the United States.[36,38] No differences in misdiagnosis rate or delay in diagnosis were observed among racialized or ethnic groups in a single site, retrospective study.[39] Please refer to Chapter 86 for more information.

Presentation Clinical features of calciphylaxis include dusky violaceous discoloration, induration, nodules, plaques, and/or retiform purpura followed by necrosis and painful ulcer formation with black eschars [**Figure 84-10**]. Ninety percent of cases affect the lower extremities, while the buttocks and breasts are also commonly affected. Acral and penile lesions have also been reported.[37]

Diagnosis Diagnosis is frequently by clinical exam, features include painful subcutaneous nodules or plaques, nonhealing ulcers, and/or cutaneous necrosis particularly on the legs. The utility of skin biopsy is limited given the high rate of false negative and false positive results, and clinical correlation is necessary.

Differential Cellulitis, cholesterol embolization, venous stasis ulcer, warfarin necrosis, atherosclerotic vascular disease, endarteritis obliterans, vasculitis, purpura fulminans, oxalate vasculopathy, antiphospholipid antibody syndrome, nephrogenic systemic fibrosis, PG, and Martorell ulcer.

Complications Chronic and extensive ulceration, secondary infection with sepsis, death.

Management Calciphylaxis management involves a multidisciplinary team consisting of nephrology, dermatology, dermatopathology, pain management, wound or burn center, and nutrition. First-line therapy is intravenous sodium thiosulfate (STS), an inorganic compound with vasodilatory, antioxidant, and anticalcific properties.[37,40] The ideal dosing and duration is not standardized, and there have been no randomized control trials to date. Resistant disease, defined by severe pain, progression, or lack of recovery for 3+ months, warrants second-line therapy, including hyperbaric oxygen therapy and bisphosphonates.[40] Wound management involves nonstick dressings, chemical debridement, negative pressure wound therapy, and avoidance of local trauma to the skin. Surgical wound debridement should be reserved for actively infected lesions given the risk of calciphylaxis and propagation with skin trauma.[37,40] Early involvement of a pain specialist is imperative.

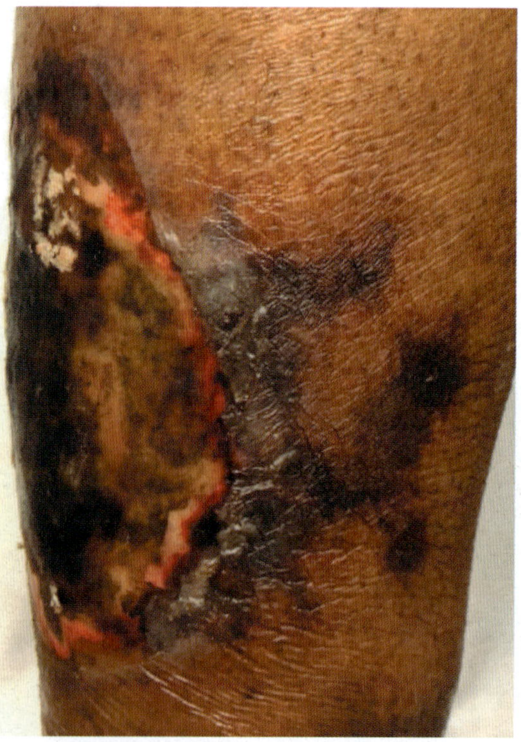

FIGURE 84-10. Calciphylaxis.

A high index of clinical suspicion should be maintained for infected wounds. Calcium, phosphorus, and parathyroid hormone abnormalities should be corrected. Medications that may contribute to calciphylaxis such as vitamin D, calcium supplements, warfarin, and iron should be discontinued.[37]

Prognosis Calciphylaxis has high morbidity and mortality rates, with mortality up to 40% at 6 months and up to 44% at 1 year in patients with ESRD.[36,37] Mortality is significantly lower in patients without ESRD and is reduced with early diagnosis and intervention.[36] Infection, such as sepsis from an ulcer, is the primary cause of mortality.[36] Features that worsen prognosis include more advanced disease at time of therapy, proximal ischemic necrotic lesions in the skin and soft tissue, presence of cardiovascular disease, and use of warfarin.

REFERENCES

1. Cathcart SD, Theos A. Inpatient management of atopic dermatitis. *Dermatol Ther*. 2011;24(2):249-255.
2. Tackett KJ, Jenkins F, Morrell DS, McShane DB, Burkhart CN. Structural racism and its influence on the severity of atopic dermatitis in African American children. *Pediatr Dermatol*. 2020;37(1):142-146.
3. Traidl S, Roesner L, Zeitvogel J, Werfel T. Eczema herpeticum in atopic dermatitis. *Allergy*. 2021;76(10):3017-3027.
4. Aronson PL, Shah SS, Mohamad Z, Yan AC. Topical corticosteroids and hospital length of stay in children with eczema herpeticum. *Pediatr Dermatol*. 2013;30(2):215-221.
5. Hsu DY, Shinkai K, Silverberg JI. Epidemiology of eczema herpeticum in hospitalized U.S. children: analysis of a nationwide cohort. *J Invest Dermatol*. 2018;138(2):265-272.
6. Raff AB, Kroshinsky D. Cellulitis: a review. *JAMA*. 2016;316(3):325-337.
7. Wang V, Boguniewicz J, Boguniewicz M, Ong PY. The infectious complications of atopic dermatitis. *Ann Allergy Asthma Immunol*. 2021;126(1):3-12.
8. Yan D, Afifi L, Jeon C, Cordoro KM, Liao W. A cross-sectional study of the distribution of psoriasis subtypes in different ethno-racial groups. *Dermatol Online J*. 2018;24(7).
9. Hoegler KM, John AM, Handler MZ, Schwartz RA. Generalized pustular psoriasis: a review and update on treatment. *J Eur Acad Dermatol Venereol*. 2018;32(10):1645-1651.
10. Ly K, Beck KM, Smith MP, Thibodeaux Q, Bhutani T. Diagnosis and screening of patients with generalized pustular psoriasis. *Psoriasis (Auckl)*. 2019;9:37-42.
11. Zheng M, Jullien D, Eyerich K. The prevalence and disease characteristics of generalized pustular psoriasis. *Am J Clin Dermatol*. 2022;23(Suppl 1):5-12.
12. Gregoire ARF, DeRuyter BK, Stratman EJ. Psoriasis flares following systemic glucocorticoid exposure in patients with a history of psoriasis. *JAMA Dermatol*. 2021;157(2):198-201.
13. Mistry N, Gupta A, Alavi A, Sibbald RG. A review of the diagnosis and management of erythroderma (generalized red skin). *Adv Skin Wound Care*. 2015;28(5):228-236; quiz 237-228.
14. Tso S, Satchwell F, Moiz H, et al. Erythroderma (exfoliative dermatitis). Part 1: underlying causes, clinical presentation and pathogenesis. *Clin Exp Dermatol*. 2021;46(6):1001-1010.
15. Inamadar AC, Ragunatha S. The rash that becomes an erythroderma. *Clin Dermatol*. 2019;37(2):88-98.
16. Miyashiro D, Sanches JA. Erythroderma: a prospective study of 309 patients followed for 12 years in a tertiary center. *Sci Rep*. 2020;10(1):9774.
17. Rosenbach M, Hsu S, Korman NJ, et al. Treatment of erythrodermic psoriasis: from the medical board of the National Psoriasis Foundation. *J Am Acad Dermatol*. 2010;62(4):655-662.
18. Kim YH, Bhandarkar AR, Adeleye O, Zhu A, Bydon M, Vidal NY. Socioeconomic predictors of cost and length of stay for erythroderma: a cross-sectional analysis of the national inpatient sample. *Arch Dermatol Res*. 2022.
19. Hoetzenecker W, Nägeli M, Mehra ET, et al. Adverse cutaneous drug eruptions: current understanding. *Semin Immunopathol*. 2016;38(1):75-86.
20. Ghattaoraya GS, Middleton D, Santos EJ, Dickson R, Jones AR, Alfirevic A. Human leucocyte antigen-adverse drug reaction associations: from a perspective of ethnicity. *Int J Immunogenet*. 2017;44(1):7-26.
21. Blumenthal KG, Alvarez-Arango S, Fu X, et al. Risk Factors for vancomycin drug reaction with eosinophilia and systemic symptoms syndrome. *JAMA Dermatol*. 2022;158(12):1449-1453.
22. Hadavand MA, Kaffenberger B, Cartron AM, Trinidad JCL. Clinical presentation and management of atypical and recalcitrant acute generalized exanthematous pustulosis. *J Am Acad Dermatol*. 2022;87(3):632-639.
23. Szatkowski J, Schwartz RA. Acute generalized exanthematous pustulosis (AGEP): a review and update. *J Am Acad Dermatol*. 2015;73(5):843-848.
24. Creadore A, Desai S, Alloo A, et al. Clinical characteristics, disease course, and outcomes of patients with acute generalized exanthematous pustulosis in the US. *JAMA Dermatol*. 2022;158(2):176-183.
25. Lerch M, Mainetti C, Terziroli Beretta-Piccoli B, Harr T. Current perspectives on Stevens-Johnson syndrome and toxic epidermal necrolysis. *Clin Rev Allergy Immunol*. 2018;54(1):147-176.
26. Lu N, Rai SK, Terkeltaub R, Kim SC, Menendez ME, Choi HK. Racial disparities in the risk of Stevens-Johnson syndrome and toxic epidermal necrolysis as urate-lowering drug adverse events in the United States. *Semin Arthritis Rheum*. 2016;46(2):253-258.
27. Thorel D, Delcampe A, Ingen-Housz-Oro S, et al. Dark skin phototype is associated with more severe ocular complications of Stevens-Johnson syndrome and toxic epidermal necrolysis. *Br J Dermatol*. 2019;181(1):212-213.
28. Cardones AR. Drug reaction with eosinophilia and systemic symptoms (DRESS) syndrome. *Clin Dermatol*. 2020;38(6):702-711.
29. Mukit W, Cooper R, Moudgil H, Ahmad N. DRESS syndrome: an important differential for eosinophilia with systemic organ dysfunction. *BMJ Case Rep*. 2020;13(5).
30. Maverakis E, Ma C, Shinkai K, et al. Diagnostic criteria of ulcerative pyoderma gangrenosum: a Delphi consensus of international experts. *JAMA Dermatol*. 2018;154(4):461-466.
31. Shah N, Asdourian MS, Jacoby TV, Chen ST. Neutrophilic dermatosis and management strategies for the inpatient dermatologist. *Curr Dermatol Rep*. 2022;11(3):146-157.
32. Biesbroeck LK, Shinohara MM. Inpatient consultative dermatology. *Med Clin North Am*. 2015;99(6):1349-1364.
33. Su WP, Liu HN. Diagnostic criteria for Sweet's syndrome. *Cutis*. 1986;37(3):167-174.
34. Drago F, Ciccarese G, Agnoletti AF, Sarocchi F, Parodi A. Neuro sweet syndrome: a systematic review. A rare complication of Sweet syndrome. *Acta Neurol Belg*. 2017;117(1):33-42.
35. Narla S, Silverberg JI. The inpatient burden and comorbidities of pyoderma gangrenosum in adults in the United States. *Arch Dermatol Res*. 2021;313(4):245-253.
36. Nigwekar SU, Thadhani R, Brandenburg VM. Calciphylaxis. *N Engl J Med*. 2018;378(18):1704-1714.
37. Nigwekar SU, Kroshinsky D, Nazarian RM, et al. Calciphylaxis: risk factors, diagnosis, and treatment. *Am J Kidney Dis*. 2015;66(1):133-146.
38. Nigwekar SU, Zhao S, Wenger J, et al. A Nationally representative study of calcific uremic arteriolopathy risk factors. *J Am Soc Nephrol*. 2016;27(11):3421-3429.
39. Gabel CK, Blum AE, François J, et al. Clinical mimickers of calciphylaxis: a retrospective study. *J Am Acad Dermatol*. 2021;85(6):1520-1527.
40. Udomkarnjananun S, Kongnatthasate K, Praditpornsilpa K, Eiam-Ong S, Jaber BL, Susantitaphong P. Treatment of calciphylaxis in CKD: a systematic review and meta-analysis. *Kidney Int Rep*. 2019;4(2):231-244.

CHAPTER 85

Nutritional Deficiencies

Nivedita Sriram
Cristina Thomas

KEY POINTS

- Dermatologic manifestations of nutritional deficiencies may be the first sign of a deficiency.
- Features of multiple deficiencies may exist concomitantly in the setting of food insecurity, unbalanced diets, increased metabolic demands, and malabsorptive conditions.
- Low- and middle-income countries carry a large burden of nutritional deficiencies, including nutrient deficiencies and protein-energy malnutrition, which can lead to long-term health sequelae.

- Certain cutaneous manifestations of nutritional deficiencies may appear skin-colored to violaceous rather than erythematous in patients with skin of color. Some manifestations, such as hemorrhage in scurvy, may be more subtle in patients with skin of color.

INTRODUCTION

Nutritional deficiencies can be associated with serious and potentially life-threatening sequelae, and mucocutaneous findings may be the initial manifestation of the underlying deficiency. It is crucial for dermatologists to be able to identify and treat nutritional deficiencies based on their dermatologic manifestations. The dermatological manifestations of nutritional deficiencies often overlap, due to similar metabolic pathways and presence of concomitant multiple deficiencies with poorly balanced diets and/or conditions causing malabsorption. Thus, testing should include an evaluation of the suspected deficiency and related deficiencies. **Table 85-1** demonstrates the dermatologic manifestations, diagnostic testing, and treatment of several nutritional deficiencies.

PROTEIN ENERGY MALNUTRITION

MARASMUS, KWASHIORKOR, AND MARASMIC KWASHIORKOR

Introduction Marasmus, kwashiorkor, and marasmic kwashiorkor are illnesses of protein-energy malnutrition (PEM) that primarily affect pediatric populations. Marasmus is due to caloric and protein deficiency, which results in loss of muscle and subcutaneous fat to meet the body's energy requirements. Kwashiorkor is due to protein deficiency but with sufficient calorie intake. As the name suggests, marasmic kwashiorkor has characteristics of both diseases.

Dermatologic Manifestations Marasmus presents with xerotic, wrinkled, and loose skin due to loss of subcutaneous fat [**Figure 85-1**]. Temporal wasting and loss of the buccal fat pad can lead to a characteristic hollow-faced appearance in patients with marasmus. In patients with kwashiorkor, dark hair can become lighter and take on a yellow-red or gray-white hue [**Figure 85-2**]. Hair and nails can also demonstrate the "flag sign," which is an alternating pattern of hypopigmented horizontal

TABLE 85-1 Dermatologic manifestations, diagnostic testing, and management recommendations for protein energy malnutrition and vitamin deficiencies.

Vitamin deficiency	Dermatologic manifestations	Diagnosis	Management
Marasmus	• Xerotic, wrinkled, and loose skin • Temporal wasting and hollow-faced appearance	• Low serum protein, prealbumin and serum amino acid levels • Mid-upper arm circumference and weight-for-height *Z*-scores	• Fluid and electrolyte resuscitation • Nutritional supplementation via oral or enteral feeding • Liberal emollient use and topical corticosteroids
Kwashiorkor	• "Flag sign" • "Flaky paint" dermatosis		
Vitamin A	• Generalized xerosis • Phrynoderma	• Serum retinol levels < 20 µg/dL	• 50,000 IU/day for acute cases • 5000 IU/day for maintenance • Topical keratolytics
Vitamin B_1 (Thiamine)	• Glossitis, glossodynia, and cheilitis • Edema and overlying waxy skin with wet beriberi	• Erythrocyte transketolase activity <120 nmol/L	• Mild: oral 3-10 mg/day for 6 weeks • Critical illness: 5-30 mg intravenous or intramuscular (IM) followed by oral 5-30 mg daily for 1 month
Vitamin B_2 (Riboflavin)	• Cheilitis and glossitis • Magenta, pebbled tongue • Oral-ocular–genital syndrome • Seborrheic-like dermatitis	• Erythrocyte glutathione reductase activity coefficient of 1.30 or higher	• Oral 5 mg/day • Circumcision may be necessary for male patient with genital symptoms
Vitamin B_3 (Niacin)	• Photodistributed hyperpigmented plaques with shellac-like scale • "Casal necklace" • "Gauntlet of pellagra"	• Whole blood niacin number < 130	• Nicotinamide 300 mg daily or 100 mg every 6 hours when symptomatic • 50-100 mg daily for maintenance
Vitamin B_7 (Biotin)	• Intertriginous and periorificial exfoliative dermatitis • Candidal superinfection • Glossitis • Alopecia • Conjunctivitis	• Plasma levels are not reflective of deficiency	• Oral 200 mcg every day for 2-5 days for adults • Oral 1 mg daily for pediatric cases
Vitamin B_9 (folate) Vitamin B_{12} (cobalamin)	• Glossitis, cheilitis and aphthous ulcers • Hyperpigmentation in photodistribution, palmar creases, and flexural regions • Vitiligo	• Serum folate < 4 ng/mL and serum cobalamin <200 pg/mL	• Oral 1-5 mg/day folic acid for 1-4 months • Vitamin B_{12} deficiency w/ neurologic involvement: IM cyanocobalamin • Vitamin B_{12} deficiency w/o neurologic involvement: IM or oral cyanocobalamin
Vitamin C	• Petechiae, ecchymoses • Perifollicular hemorrhage • Bleeding gums • Follicular hyperkeratosis • Corkscrew hairs	• Serum ascorbic acid < 0.4 mg/dL	• 800-1000 mg/day
Zinc	• Acrodermatitis enteropathica • Necrolytic erythema-like eruption • Blepharitis • Glossitis, angular cheilitis • Alopecia	• AM plasma zinc < 70 microgram/dL • Normal levels do not rule out zinc deficiency	• 3 mg/kg/day of elemental zinc

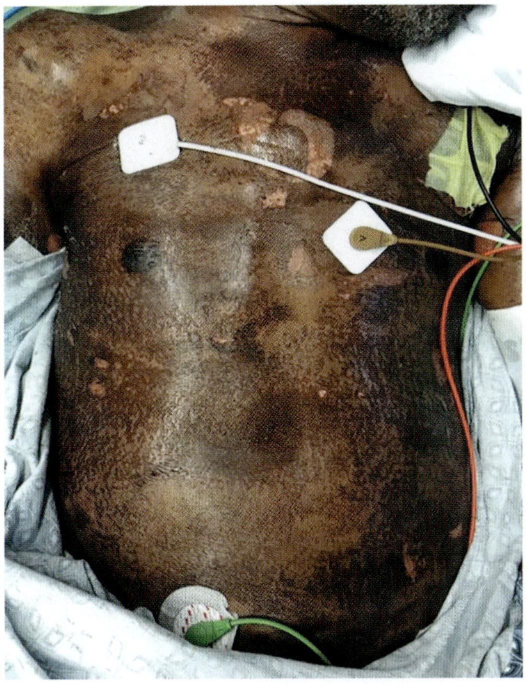

FIGURE 85-1. Protein-energy malnutrition. An adult with flaky paint dermatosis on the trunk due to poor diet in the setting of alcohol use disorder. The patient also had full-thickness epidermal detachment in areas of trauma.

bands marking periods of insufficient nutrition. In chronic kwashiorkor, the characteristic "flaky paint" dermatosis may be seen, in which shiny hyperpigmented scale and superficial desquamation is present overlying anasarca or edema [**Figures 85-1** and **85-2**]. Edema is a helpful clue to the diagnosis and is due to third-spacing in the setting of hypoalbuminemia. Marasmic kwashiorkor presents with overlapping symptoms in between.

Risk Factors PEM is primarily seen in low- or middle-income countries but can also be present in more economically developed countries in patients with restrictive diets or chronic disease. Marasmus can be seen in anorexia nervosa, bulimia nervosa, and other psychiatric diseases that cause patients to restrict calories. Since kwashiorkor presents in calorie-sufficient but protein deficient states, it can be seen in chronic illness or inflammatory states such as cystic fibrosis. Other risk factors include dietary restriction, specifically in the absence of breastfeeding or dietary restriction due to milk or other protein allergy.

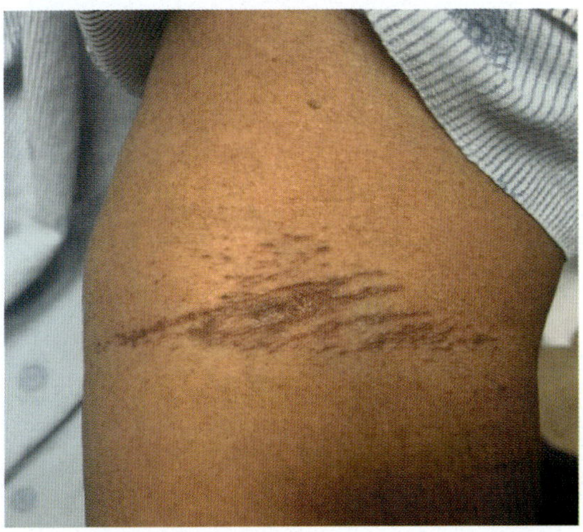

FIGURE 85-2. Protein-energy malnutrition. An adult with flaky pain dermatosis on the antecubital fossa due to poor diet.

Diagnosis Serum protein, prealbumin, and serum amino acid levels can be a marker for PEM; however, they can be affected by states of inflammation. The World Health Organization (WHO) recommends using mid-upper arm circumference, weight-for-height *Z*-score, and the presence or absence of symmetrical pitting edema in the diagnosis of malnutrition.[1] Skin biopsy can also aid in the diagnosis although findings are like those seen in many nutritional deficiencies, including parakeratosis, epidermal pallor, and psoriasiform hyperplasia.[2]

Management Management begins with correcting the underlying malnutrition through fluid and electrolyte resuscitation and nutritional supplementation via oral or tube feeding. Liberal emollient use and topical corticosteroids can be helpful.[2]

VITAMIN A DEFICIENCY

Introduction Vitamin A is a fat-soluble vitamin that is required for cell proliferation and keratinization. Dietary vitamin A is found in animal sources such as fish, fish oil, green and yellow vegetables, and eggs.

Dermatologic Manifestations Because vitamin A is necessary for normal keratinization, deficiency manifests as generalized xerosis, alopecia, and phrynoderma. Phrynoderma is defined as asymptomatic follicular-based hyperkeratotic papules often distributed symmetrically on the extensor surfaces, including the elbows, knees, buttocks, and shoulders. These papules may have a central keratotic plug and broken hair. Particularly in patients with darker skin tones, papules can be hyperpigmented rather than skin colored.

Risk Factors Vitamin A deficiency is rare in economically developed countries, and when seen, is often associated with conditions that cause fat malabsorption, such as bowel resection or pancreatic disease. Chronic alcohol abuse also predisposes patients to several micronutrient deficiencies including vitamin A deficiency, and cutaneous findings are often the first sign of deficiency in these cases. In low- or middle-income countries, vitamin A deficiency is much more common especially among children and is often associated with malnutrition.

Diagnosis The diagnosis of vitamin A deficiency is made when serum retinol levels are less than 20 μg/dL. It is important to note that acute inflammation will lower serum retinol levels because of decreased retinol-binding protein.[3] A diagnosis based on dermatological findings alone is difficult, because while phrynoderma is found in vitamin A deficiency, similar findings can be seen in other disorders, including pityriasis rubra pilaris and perforating disorders. Vitamin C deficiency, or scurvy, may present with similar follicular hyperkeratosis but is also associated with bleeding and gingival disease. Assessing for ophthalmologic findings associated with vitamin A deficiency, such as light sensitivity, night blindness, and xerophthalmia, can assist in the diagnosis when classic cutaneous findings are present.[4]

Management Oral, intramuscular, and intravenous vitamin A treatment are all viable methods to treat acute deficiency.[5] Dosage and frequency of supplementation are dependent on age and clinical severity, but 50,000 IU/day followed by a taper to 5000 IU/day for maintenance is a standard recommendation.[4] High-dose treatment can increase the risk of hepatotoxicity and thus, patients with liver dysfunction should be monitored.[6] Phrynoderma can be treated with topical keratolytic such as salicylic acid alongside the above regimen.[5]

VITAMIN B DEFICIENCY

All B vitamins are water-soluble and as such are not sufficiently stored in the body. In the United States, B vitamins are fortified in most foods. Therefore, deficiency is primarily associated with inadequate consumption or malabsorptive states, such as restrictive diets, inflammatory bowel disease, bariatric surgery, among others. Since several B vitamins have metabolic similarities, many of the cutaneous findings overlap. In these cases, laboratory testing and characteristic noncutaneous findings are often helpful in diagnosis.

VITAMIN B_1

Introduction Vitamin B_1 (thiamine) is responsible for energy metabolism by acting as an enzyme cofactor. Thiamine is found in unprocessed rice, juices, meat, nuts, and seeds.

Dermatologic Manifestations Vitamin B_1 deficiency is associated with symptoms of glossitis, glossodynia, and cheilitis. Wet beriberi is a manifestation of thiamine deficiency characterized by high-output heart failure and dependent edema with overlying waxy skin.

Risk Factors Alcohol use reduces thiamine phosphorylation, impacts thiamine storage in the liver, and limits intestinal absorption. Other risk factors include anorexia nervosa, hyperemesis of pregnancy, cystic fibrosis, loop diuretics, and chemotherapeutic agents such as 5-fluorouracil that increase thiamine metabolism.

Diagnosis Noncutaneous signs of thiamine deficiency can be useful in making the diagnosis. In dry beriberi, a symmetric sensory or motor peripheral neuropathy may be noted. In wet beriberi, high-output heart failure characterized by dyspnea and peripheral edema can be seen. Wernicke encephalopathy is an acute state of thiamine deficiency characterized by altered mental status, oculomotor abnormalities, and ataxic gait while Korsakoff syndrome is associated with confabulation and memory loss seen in more chronic states of thiamine deficiency. Laboratory testing, including plasma thiamine or thiamine metabolite levels, may not reflect true systemic thiamine levels. Whole blood or erythrocyte levels of thiamine diphosphate are better tests, but clear cutoffs have not been defined. Erythrocyte transketolase activity in erythrocyte hemolysates is a sensitive functional assay but is not widely available. Some suggest a threshold of less than 120 nmol/L to indicate deficiency with this test.[7]

Management According to the WHO, mild thiamine deficiency can be treated with oral supplementation of 10 mg daily for 1 week, then 3 to 5 mg daily for at least 6 weeks. In those who are critically ill, 5 to 30 mg intravenously or intramuscularly per day followed by 5 to 30 mg orally daily for 1 month is recommended.[8]

VITAMIN B_2

Introduction Vitamin B_2 (riboflavin) is found in sufficiently absorbable quantities in meat and dairy products. It is required for hormone production, collagen production, and as a coenzyme for oxidation-reduction reactions through its biologically active forms flavin mononucleotide and flavin adenine dinucleotide.

Dermatological Manifestations The characteristic dermatologic manifestation of riboflavin deficiency is oral-ocular–genital syndrome. In this syndrome, oral findings include angular cheilitis and glossitis with the tongue initially having a pebbled appearance and appearing magenta in color followed by atrophy. Photophobia and conjunctivitis may occur. Genital involvement of the syndrome affects men more than women. Red papules and scaly plaques occur over the scrotum and thighs but classically spare the midline. Balanitis and phimosis can also occur. Additionally, a seborrheic-like dermatitis can be seen.

Risk Factors Riboflavin deficiency can be caused by acute borate ingestion/poisoning and phototherapy due to degradation of riboflavin. Medication-induced riboflavin deficiency has been attributed to oral contraceptives, probenecid, and several antiepileptics.

Diagnosis An erythrocyte glutathione reductase activity coefficient value of 1.30 or higher before and after addition of flavin adenine dinucleotide is considered diagnostic of deficiency.[9] Serum and urine riboflavin levels are less sensitive but more readily available.[10] Riboflavin deficiency should be distinguished from thiamine deficiency as both present with angular cheilitis, cheilosis, and glossitis. The ocular involvement associated with riboflavin deficiency including photophobia, blepharitis angularis, conjunctivitis, and cataracts can help distinguish the two.

Management Treatment of riboflavin deficiency consists of 5 mg per day of oral supplementation.[10] In male patients with associated oral-ocular–genital syndrome, circumcision may be necessary to treat balanitis or phimosis.

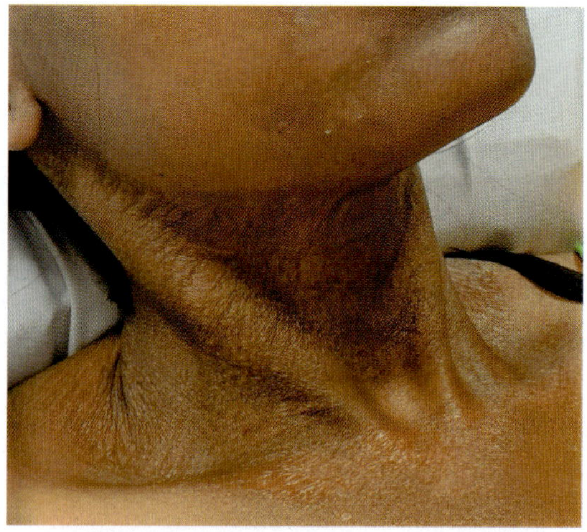

FIGURE 85-3. Pellagra. An adult with "Casal necklace" on the anterior neck.

VITAMIN B_3

Introduction Vitamin B_3 (niacin, nicotinic acid, or nicotinamide) is found in meat products, fortified grains, cereals, nuts, and seeds. The active forms of niacin are nicotinamide adenine dinucleotide (NAD) and NAD phosphate (NADP), both of which are cofactors involved in ATP production and cellular metabolism. Thus, niacin is critical for keratinocyte turnover.

Dermatologic Manifestations Niacin deficiency, caused either directly by niacin insufficiency or lack of its precursor tryptophan, is called pellagra. Pellagra is characterized by a photo-distributed eruption initially presenting with painful or pruritic erythema, edema, and at times vesiculobullous lesions ("wet pellagra"), which then progress to well-demarcated hyperpigmented plaques with an overlying shellac-like scale. "Casal necklace" refers to involvement over the neck and upper chest [**Figures 85-3** and **85-4**], while involvement in a glove distribution on the dorsal hands is called the "gauntlet of pellagra." Lesions may also involve the ankles and dorsal feet in a boot distribution. Chronic cases develop papery-thin, atrophic skin with a yellow hue, although this

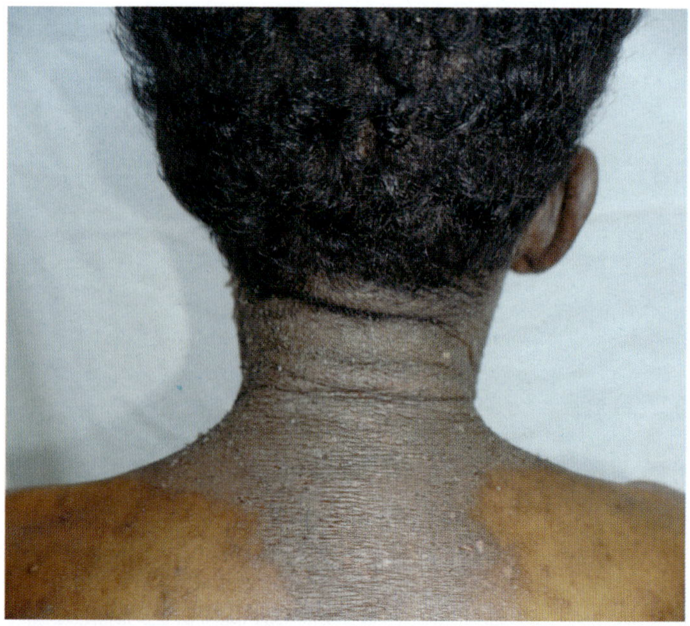

FIGURE 85-4. Pellagra. An adult with "Casal's necklace" on the posterior neck.

may be more subtle in darker skin types. Nail changes can include "half and half nails" in which the distal nail bed appears red-brown while the proximal portion appears white.

Risk Factors Apart from dietary and absorption issues, another risk factor for pellagra is carcinoid syndrome, in which tryptophan is converted to serotonin rather than niacin. In Hartnup disease, tryptophan absorption is impaired due to an inherited defect in kidney and intestinal tryptophan transportation resulting in niacin deficiency. Medications such as isoniazid and antiretroviral medications can also cause niacin deficiency.

Diagnosis A whole blood niacin number can be calculated as the ratio of NAD to NADP multiplied by 100, and a value less than 130 suggests pellagra.[11] While this test is easily performed and accessible, it can be altered by dietary niacin consumption prior to testing. As such, pellagra is often diagnosed clinically by recognition of its characteristic cutaneous manifestations, neurologic involvement (dementia, anxiety, encephalopathy), and diarrhea.

Management Supplementation with nicotinamide is preferred to niacin as the latter can cause undesirable cutaneous flushing.[12] The recommended treatment regimen is nicotinamide orally 300 mg daily or 100 mg every 6 hours. This can be reduced to a maintenance dose of 50 to 100 mg daily as symptoms improve.[13] Skin symptoms can take up to a month to resolve and reduced exposure to sunlight may aid recovery.[12]

VITAMIN B_7

Introduction Vitamin B_7, or biotin, is a cofactor for certain carboxylase enzymes. While it is present in meat, fish, and egg yolks, it is also produced by human gut flora.

Dermatologic Manifestations Biotin deficiency causes a red exfoliative dermatitis on the face, concentrated around the eyes and mouth, but can also involve the intertriginous areas. Candida superinfection is common. Additional findings include conjunctivitis, glossitis, and alopecia.

Risk Factors Risk factors for biotin deficiency include, short-gut syndrome, use of parenteral alimentation, genetic biotin metabolism defects including holocarboxylase synthetase and biotinidase deficiencies, pregnancy, breastfeeding mothers, antiepileptic medications, and excessive egg white consumption that lowers biotin absorption.

Diagnosis Direct measurement of biotin levels is not reflective of deficiency. If there is concern for holocarboxylase synthetase of biotinidase deficiency, genetic testing can be performed.

Management For adults, 200 mcg of biotin daily for 2 to 5 days can be used for treatment of biotin deficiency.[14] For neonates and children, oral treatment of 1 mg a day is recommended.[15] While the cutaneous symptoms of biotin deficiency will resolve rapidly with supplementation, hair changes may take longer to improve.

VITAMIN B_9 AND B_{12}

Introduction Vitamin B_9 (folate or folic acid) and vitamin B_{12} (cobalamin) are critical for DNA synthesis. Additionally, vitamin B_{12} is a cofactor for methylmalonyl-CoA mutase and methionine synthase. Vitamin B_9 is found in leafy greens, meat, dairy, and yeast, and vitamin B_{12} is found in meat, dairy, and seafood.

Dermatologic Manifestations Cutaneous findings of folic acid and cobalamin deficiency include glossitis, cheilitis, and aphthous ulcers. In vitamin B_{12} deficiency, the tongue can be red, painful, and the lingual papillae may be atrophic, termed Hunter glossitis. Hyperpigmentation occurs in both deficiencies over sun-exposed areas, palmar creases, and flexural surfaces. Longitudinal melanonychia has also been reported.

Risk Factors Risk for both deficiencies can be increased by achlorhydria, as in the case of *Helicobacter pylori* infection. Severe vegetarianism, alcoholism, and certain medications including methotrexate and metformin can predispose to both deficiencies. Vitamin B_{12} deficiency can also occur in the setting of pernicious anemia, in which autoantibodies exist against intrinsic factor preventing absorption of vitamin B_{12}.

Diagnosis Plasma folate and cobalamin levels are used in the diagnosis of folate and cobalamin deficiency. Additional signs suggesting a diagnosis of folate or cobalamin deficiency are megaloblastic anemia and specifically in cobalamin deficiency, neuropsychiatric abnormalities including mood changes, ataxia, and paresthesia.[16,17]

Management Folate deficiency is treated with 1 to 5 mg/day of oral folic acid for 1 to 4 months. For patients with neurologic involvement, intramuscular supplementation is recommended.[18]

VITAMIN C DEFICIENCY

Introduction Vitamin C, or ascorbic acid, is a water-soluble vitamin, and deficiency causes scurvy. Vitamin C has a role in collagen production through hydroxyproline and hydroxylysine formation and plays a role as an antioxidant. Body stores last around 2 months, after which severe deficiency can occur with poor consumption or absorption of vitamin C. Vitamin C is found in citrus fruits and green vegetables; however, oxidation of foods can decrease active vitamin C levels.

Dermatologic Manifestations Due to altered collagen production, scurvy is characterized by hemorrhagic cutaneous findings, including petechiae, ecchymoses, and perifollicular hemorrhage. In darker skin, hemorrhage may be subtle. Other findings of subcutaneous or intramuscular hemorrhage include aching subcutaneous nodules and bone pain or tenderness as a manifestation of subperiosteal bleeding. Periungual and retinal hemorrhage can occur, but bleeding gums are more commonly seen. Gingivitis may present initially with gingival swelling that can progress to ulceration and bleeding. Follicular hyperkeratosis of the trunk and extremities and corkscrew hairs are also common manifestations of scurvy [**Figure 85-5**].

Risk Factors Vitamin C deficiency is more commonly seen in lower-income populations that have limited access to fresh fruits and vegetables. Strict diets and malabsorption are also associated with scurvy. Iatrogenic scurvy can occur with dialysis and tyrosine kinase inhibitors.

Diagnosis Resolution of symptoms with vitamin C treatment is diagnostic of scurvy. Serum ascorbic acid can corroborate vitamin C deficiency if less than 0.4 mg/dL but often clinical history in conjunction with physical examination is sufficient.[19] Biopsy of follicular papules may demonstrate perifollicular hemorrhage, follicular plugging, and follicular hyperkeratosis.[20] Additional symptoms suggestive of scurvy include fatigue, arthralgias, poor wound healing, and diarrhea.

Management Oral ascorbic acid 800 to 1000 mg/day is recommended for patients with vitamin C deficiency and rapid improvement is expected with initiation of supplementation.[19,21] Any reversible underlying risk factors should be addressed. Some patients may require a maintenance dose of 100 to 200 mg daily if underlying cause for deficiency cannot be reversed.[22]

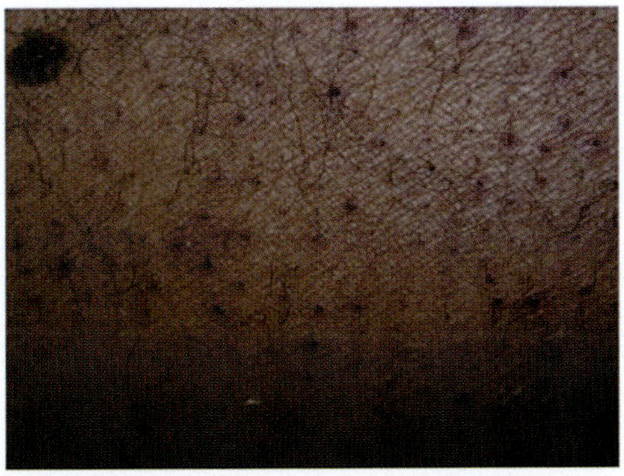

FIGURE 85-5. Perifollicular hemorrhage and corkscrew hairs in a patient with scurvy. (Reproduced with permission from Goldberg LJ, Lenzy Y. Nutrition and hair. *Clin Dermatol.* 2010;28(4):412-419, Figure 1.)

ELEMENT DEFICIENCY

ZINC

Introduction Zinc is a trace element that serves as an important coenzyme with regulatory, structural, and catalytic roles. It is found in red meat, shellfish, breastmilk, cereals, and legumes. Cereals and legumes have lower zinc bioavailability because of high phytate content that prevents zinc absorption.

Dermatologic Manifestations Because zinc is required for keratinocyte proliferation, the skin is commonly affected in zinc deficiency. The most recognized cutaneous manifestation of zinc deficiency is acrodermatitis enteropathica (AE). AE presents with symmetric well-demarcated pink scaly and psoriasiform plaques that can become vesiculobullous, pustular, or erosive [**Figures 85-6** and **85-7**]. In skin of color, lesions tend to be hyperpigmented. Lesions generally affect the perioral region in a U-shaped configuration, anogenital region, and acral sites. Because zinc plays a key role in immune system regulation, lesions can be secondarily impetiginized or superinfected with candida. Zinc deficiency has been implicated in a necrolytic migratory erythema-like eruption, characterized by well-demarcated pink to violaceous annular plaques with peripheral scaling and crusting.

Risk Factors AE can be acquired or inherited in an autosomal recessive pattern. The inherited form is due to a mutation in SLC39A4, resulting in altered zinc absorption in the intestine. Because breastmilk contains zinc, deficiency is most often seen in infants soon after breastfeeding weaning. Infants fed with formula or those with transient neonatal zinc deficiency, wherein breastmilk is deficient of zinc, may present with acrodermatitis enteropathica soon after birth. Acquired AE can be due to altered zinc absorption and transport, as in Crohn disease, inflammatory bowel disease, celiac disease, cirrhosis, hypoalbuminemia, nephrotic syndrome, and cystic fibrosis. Other risk factors include nutritionally deficient parenteral nutrition, anorexia nervosa, and some antiepileptic drugs.

Diagnosis Normal plasma zinc levels are between 70 and 100 μg/dL.[23] Definitive diagnosis of zinc deficiency relies on plasma zinc levels, although normal zinc levels do not rule out zinc deficiency.[24] Low levels of zinc-dependent enzymes such as alkaline phosphatase in serum can suggest zinc deficiency. Histopathology of AE lesions demonstrate parakeratosis, epidermal pallor, loss of the granular cell layer, and psoriasiform hyperplasia. Associated symptoms that can suggest AE include diarrhea and neurologic issues.[24]

Management In cases of AE, 3 mg/kg/day of elemental zinc is recommended with dose adjustments based on subsequent plasma zinc levels.[24] If deficiency is due to decreased zinc intake, oral supplementation with 1 to 2 mg/kg/day is generally sufficient. Cutaneous symptoms usually resolve within days, sometimes before serum levels return to normal.[23]

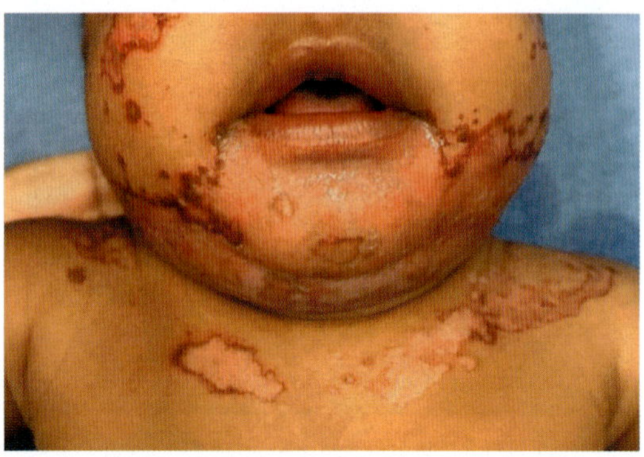

FIGURE 85-6. Acrodermatitis enteropathica. An infant with desquamating plaques in a U-shaped configuration in the perioral region. (Courtesy of Dr. Smridhi Mahajan.)

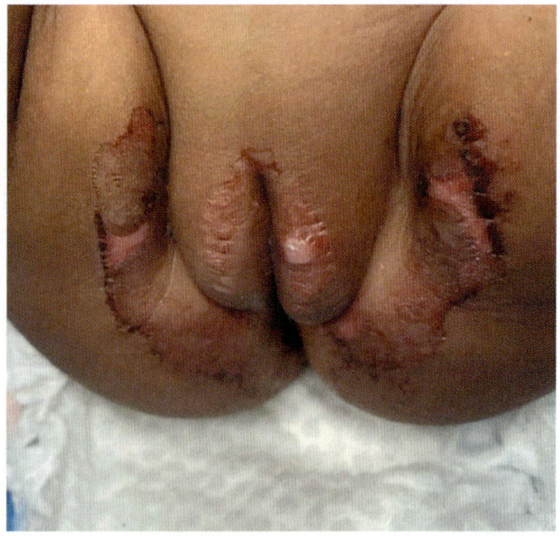

FIGURE 85-7. Acrodermatitis enteropathica. An infant with desquamating plaques in a U-shaped configuration in the genital region. (Courtesy of Dr. Smridhi Mahajan.)

REFERENCES

1. WHO. WHO child growth standards and the identification of severe acute malnutrition in infants and children. A Joint Statement by the World Health Organization and the United Nations Children's Fund; 2009.
2. Kuhl J, Davis MDP, Kalaaji AN, Kamath PS, Hand JL, Peine CJ. Skin signs as the presenting manifestation of severe nutritional deficiency: report of 2 cases. *Arch Dermatol.* 2004;140(5):521-524.
3. de Pee S, Dary O. Biochemical indicators of vitamin A deficiency: serum retinol and serum retinol binding protein. *J Nutr.* 2002;132(9):2895S-2901S.
4. Di Stefani A, Orlandi A, Chimenti S, Bianchi L. Phrynoderma: a cutaneous sign of an inadequate diet. *Can Med Assoc J.* 2007;177(8):855-856.
5. Ragunatha S, Kumar VJ, Murugesh SB. Therapeutic response of vitamin A, vitamin B complex, essential fatty acids (EFA) and vitamin E in the treatment of phrynoderma: a randomized controlled study. *J Clin Diagn Res.* 2014;8(1):116-118.
6. Kowalski TE, Falestiny M, Furth E, Malet PF. Vitamin A hepatotoxicity: a cautionary note regarding 25,000 IU supplements. *Am J Med.* 1994;97(6):523-528.
7. Praharaj SK, Munoli RN, Shenoy S, Udupa ST, Thomas LS. High-dose thiamine strategy in Wernicke–Korsakoff syndrome and related thiamine deficiency conditions associated with alcohol use disorder. *Indian J Psychiatry.* 2021;63(2):121-126.
8. WHO. Thiamine deficiency and its prevention and control in major emergencies. World Health Organization Micronutrient series.
9. Hill MHE, Bradley A, Mushtaq S, Williams EA, Powers HJ. Effects of methodological variation on assessment of riboflavin status using the erythrocyte glutathione reductase activation coefficient assay. *Br J Nutr.* 2008;102(2):273-278.
10. Ajayi OA, James OA. Effect of riboflavin supplementationon riboflavin nutriture of a secondary school population in Nigeria. *Am J Clin Nutr.* 1984;39(5):787-791.
11. Shah GM, Shah RG, Veillette H, Kirkland JB, Pasieka JL, Warner RR. Biochemical assessment of niacin deficiency among carcinoid cancer patients. *Am J Gastroenterol.* 2005;100(10):2307-2314.
12. Arif T, Adil M. Pellagra: an uncommon disease in the modern era-A case report. *J Pak Assoc Dermatol.* 2018;28:360-363.
13. WHO. Pellagra and its evention and control in major emergencies. World Health Organization, Micronutrient Series; 2000.
14. Baugh CM, Malone JH, Butterworth CE, Jr. Human biotin deficiency: a case history of biotin deficiency induced by raw egg consumption in a cirrhotic patient. *Am J Clin Nutr.* 1968;21(2):173-182.
15. Fujimoto W, Inaoki M, Fukui T, Inoue Y, Kuhara T. Biotin deficiency in an infant fed with amino acid formula. *J Dermatol.* 2005;32(4):256-261.
16. Kuroki Y, Okamoto Y, Ishibashi S, Kawada K, Ishikawa Y. Clinical study of vitamin B12 therapy to Hunter glossitis. *Oral Ther Pharmacol.* 2015;34:9-15.
17. Stoopler ET, Kuperstein AS. Glossitis secondary to vitamin B12 deficiency anemia. *Can Med Assoc J.* 2013;185(12):E582.
18. Devalia V, Hamilton MS, Molloy AM. Guidelines for the diagnosis and treatment of cobalamin and folate disorders. *Br J Haematol.* 2014;166(4):496-513.
19. Li R, Byers K, Walvekar RR. Gingival hypertrophy: a solitary manifestation of scurvy. *Am J Otolaryngol.* 2008;29(6):426-428.

20. Moya-Martínez C, Haya-Martínez L, Fuertes-Vega L, Santonja C, Requena L. Co-occurring features of scurvy and phrynoderma in the same patient. *JAAD Case Rep.* 2022;19:14-17.
21. Walters RW, Vinson EN, Soler AP, Burton CS. Scurvy with manifestations limited to a previously injured extremity. *J Am Acad Dermatol.* 2007;57(2 Suppl):S48-49.
22. Singer R, Rhodes HC, Chin G, Kulkarni H, Ferrari P. High prevalence of ascorbate deficiency in an Australian peritoneal dialysis population. *Nephrology (Carlton).* 2008;13(1):17-22.
23. Kelly S, Stelzer JW, Esplin N, Farooq A, Karasik O. Acquired acrodermatitis enteropathica: a case study. *Cureus.* 2017;9(9):e1667.
24. Nistor N, Ciontu L, Frasinariu O-E, Lupu VV, Ignat A, Streanga V. Acrodermatitis enteropathica: a case report. *Medicine.* 2016;95(20):e3553.

CHAPTER 86 Calciphylaxis

Arturo R. Dominguez
Jessica C. Evans
Melissa M. Mauskar

KEY POINTS

- Calciphylaxis is a cutaneous small vessel vasculopathy that can present with severe pain, noninflammatory retiform purpura, skin necrosis, and ulceration in primarily adipose-rich areas.
- Calciphylaxis predominantly affects patients with advanced chronic kidney disease (CKD), but other common risk factors include malignancy, alcohol-related liver disease, obesity, connective tissue disorders, diabetes mellitus, chronic corticosteroid, and long-term warfarin use.
- Diagnosis of calciphylaxis relies on identifying individual risk factors, lesion morphology, and location. Skin biopsy could be a valuable diagnostic tool in atypical cases or in situations where confirmation is necessary to guide therapy.
- Delays in diagnosis in patients of skin of color may occur due to challenges in early recognition of early dermatological signs of calciphylaxis, such as livedo, inflammation, and retiform purpura.
- Despite improved patient survival in recent years, calciphylaxis remains a life-threatening condition (with mortality rates approximately 44-50% within 1 year of diagnosis). A multimodal therapy approach and multidisciplinary care involving various specialists such as dermatology, renal/endocrine, cardiology, hepatology, wound care, pain management, general surgery, and the patient's primary care provider is recommended for optimal treatment.

INTRODUCTION

Calciphylaxis, a cutaneous small vessel vasculopathy, is characterized by progressive calcification and thrombosis of dermal and subcutaneous arterioles and capillaries. The condition typically presents with intractable pain, noninflammatory retiform purpura, skin necrosis, and ulceration, primarily affecting adipose-rich tissue areas. Mortality rates are approximately 44% to 50% within 1 year of diagnosis, making calciphylaxis a life-threatening disease.[1] In addition to the morbidity of poor wound healing, infection, and hospitalization, the high mortality rate underscores the urgent need for appropriate diagnosis and management.

While the mortality rate associated with calciphylaxis in patients of skin of color (SOC) is currently unknown, the increased prevalence of comorbidities and health disparities in these marginalized communities may potentially affect outcomes. Moreover, delays in diagnosis in patients of SOC may occur due to challenges in early recognition of early dermatological signs of calciphylaxis, such as livedo, inflammation, and retiform purpura, which may be obscured by darker skin types. Furthermore, pain, which is often a key early symptom of calciphylaxis, may be discounted in patients of SOC, as previous studies have indicated that pain is frequently under-addressed in this population.[2]

In this chapter, we will review the clinical features of patients suspected of having calciphylaxis with the goals of improving diagnosis, treatment outcomes and recognizing health disparities that may exist in patients of SOC.

INCIDENCE

Once regarded as a rare disease, greater awareness and improved recognition of calciphylaxis have contributed to rising incidence. A recent study[3] reported a rise in cases from 3.7 to 5.7 per 10,000 patients on chronic hemodialysis (HD) between 2007 and 2011 in the United States. Nevertheless, the incidence and prevalence of calciphylaxis specifically among individuals of SOC is understudied, apart from one cross-sectional study conducted in an urban hospital that reported a prevalence rate of 4%, with 90% of cases occurring in individuals of SOC.[4]

PATHOPHYSIOLOGY

Calciphylaxis is believed to progress in a stepwise manner, beginning with calcification in the tunica media of dermal arteries (<0.6 mm in diameter), arterioles, and subcutaneous capillaries followed by extravascular calcification and intimal thrombosis.[5] Numerous molecular pathways—nuclear factor kappa B (NF-κB), tumor necrosis factor (TNF), Wnt/β-catenin, and phosphoinositide 3-kinase (PI3K)—are thought to drive the epithelial-mesenchymal transition (EMT), which transforms medial vascular smooth muscle cells into cells displaying an osteoblastic phenotype.[6] Other factors likely contributing to calciphylaxis include disturbances in calcium and phosphorus metabolism, reduced activity of inhibitors of vascular calcification like vitamin K-dependent Matrix Gla protein (MGP), and hypercoagulable states.[7] Recent studies challenge the theory that stepwise progression is necessary in calciphylaxis, as biopsy samples of early calciphylaxis lesions demonstrate thromboses in subcutaneous capillaries, both with and without calcification.[8] Furthermore, the presence of medial calcification and even thrombosis in biopsy samples cannot be considered specific to calciphylaxis, as similar changes have been observed in biopsy samples from patients with chronic kidney disease (CKD) who do not have calciphylaxis.[9-11] Finally, the role of genetic susceptibility in the development of calciphylaxis among patients with shared risk factors has been proposed as a potential contributing factor.

RISK FACTORS

Calciphylaxis primarily affects patients with advanced CKD, particularly those with end-stage renal disease (ESRD). Nevertheless, in recent years, there has been an increased recognition of calciphylaxis in patients with normal renal function, which has been termed nonuremic/non-nephrogenic calciphylaxis. Among patients with ESRD, common risk factors include hyperphosphatemia, calcium-based phosphate binders, vitamin D analogs, and hypoalbuminemia. Other risk factors associated with both nephrogenic and non-nephrogenic calciphylaxis include female sex, and comorbid conditions such as primary hyperparathyroidism, malignancy, alcohol-related liver disease, obesity, connective tissue disorders, diabetes mellitus, chronic corticosteroid, and long-term warfarin use.[12]

Current literature suggests that calciphylaxis may occur more frequently in individuals of White race. However, many calciphylaxis studies are limited by their small sample sizes and single-center experiences.[7] In reality, the relationship between race (a social construct) and calciphylaxis is complex. Risk factors associated with calciphylaxis are likely influenced both by the social determinants of health (also see Chapter 11) and ancestry. As a result, while certain risk factors may be more common among racial and ethnic minoritized groups [**Table 86-1**], data on incidence or prevalence may be underestimated due to access issues or misdiagnoses affecting these groups. For example, Black patients have

TABLE 86-1 Risk factors for calciphylaxis among ethnoracial groups[a]

Risk factor	Mechanism	Ethnoracial groups disproportionately affected
ESRD and HD	↑ RANkL, Hemodialysis ↓fetuin-A, high levels of inactive MGP	Black/African American (AA) are more likely to have ESRD and be placed on HD.[14]
Alcoholic liver disease	IL-1 and TNF-α ↑ RANkL, ↓ active MGP, ↓ Protein C&S, ↓ Fetuin-A	Though studies have found that White individuals have the highest prevalence of current alcohol consumption, Black and Native Americans were found to be the most vulnerable to alcohol-related health consequences.[15]
Hyperphosphatemia and hypercalcemia	↑metastatic calcification and precipitation, ↑ NFkB	Black CKD patients are significantly more likely to have hyperphosphatemia than non-Black patients.[16]
Glucocorticoids	↑ RANkL, ↓ OPG	Chronic glucocorticoid use 5× more likely in Black patients with systemic lupus erythematosus.[17]
Warfarin\dietary Vitamin K deficiency (gastric bypass)	↓ of Vitamin K-dependent MGP	Black patients are more likely to have erratic warfarin levels and less likely to be prescribed DOACs.[18]
Aluminum	↑ calpain, an inhibitor of NFkB inhibitory protein	Studies suggest that White patients undergoing HD may have greater serum aluminum levels than Black patients.[19]
Autoimmune disease (AID) and inflammation	IL-1 and TNF-α ↑ RANkL upregulation, ↓ fetuin-A	Of the 22 AIDs analyzed in one study, prevalence rates were higher in the multiracial group compared to White patients. For 8 of 22 of the AIDs, prevalence rates were higher in the Black/AA group.[20]
Obesity	Chronic tension on septae and arterioles promotes dystrophic calcification. Increased adipose tissue leads to increased expression of TNF.[13]	Data from the National Health and Nutrition Examination Survey (NHANES) demonstrate that obesity rates have increased overtime for all racialized groups, but increases were markedly greater in non-Hispanic Black and Mexican Americans.[21]
Female sex, age > 50 (menopause)	Estrogen: ↑OPG expression	Race/ethnicity did not particularly moderate the association between traditional CVD risk factors measured across the menopause transition and late midlife subclinical vascular disease.[13]
Vitamin D analogues	↑ RANkL	Black patients have a 15-20-fold higher prevalence of severe vitamin D deficiency, consequently making them more likely to be placed on Vitamin D analogues.[22]

[a]For a more in-depth discussion on the pathophysiology of calciphylaxis, please see Nigwekar SU, Thadhani R, Brandenburg VM. Calciphylaxis. *N Engl J Med.* 2018;378(18):1704-1714.

Abbreviations: AID, autoimmune disease; CKD, chronic kidney disease; CVD, cardiovascular disease; DOACs, direct-acting oral anticoagulants; ESRD, end-stage renal disease; HD, hemodialysis; IL-1, interleukin-1; MGP, matrix Gla protein; NF-κB, nuclear factor kappa B; TNF, tumor necrosis factor; OPG, Osteoprotegerin; RANKL, receptor activator of nuclear kappa beta ligand.

increased rates of ESRD compared with Whites, despite having similar rates of CKD.[23] Recently, studies have suggested that the use of a race coefficient in race-based estimations of Glomerular Filtration Rate (GFR) leads to an overestimation of GFR in these populations and has contributed to these disparities.[24]

Moreover, studies have demonstrated that Black patients, despite experiencing more suboptimal anticoagulation control with warfarin, are more frequently prescribed warfarin over direct oral anticoagulants (DOACs) in comparison to White patients.[18] As a result, Black patients are more likely to remain on warfarin, which as mentioned earlier, is a direct risk factor for calciphylaxis.

DIAGNOSIS

HISTORY

Calciphylaxis is primarily a clinical diagnosis that relies on identifying individual risk factors, lesion morphology, and location, as there are no universally accepted diagnostic criteria. However, for patients with ESRD and other identifiable risk factors that present with painfully indurated subcutaneous nodules and plaques with overlying livedoid skin changes in adipose-rich areas, the diagnosis of calciphylaxis should be considered until proven otherwise.

Obtaining a thorough patient history is crucial for identifying risk factors, acute triggers, and excluding conditions that could mimic calciphylaxis. The differential diagnosis also varies depending on the stage of the disease. Considering the patient's history and physical exam is helpful for excluding common alternative etiologies, which according to a recent study include cellulitis (31%), skin infection (8%), and peripheral vascular disease (6.9%) (also see **Table 86-2**).[25] In this same study, while the misdiagnosis rates did not differ among racial groups, the study was limited by a small number (18/101 [14.3%]) of non-White patients. Notably, there was a trend toward patients of SOC experiencing a greater delay in obtaining a correct diagnosis of calciphylaxis following an initial misdiagnosis compared to White patients (57.5 vs 32 days, $p = 0.62$).

Although calciphylaxis primarily affects the skin, involvement of other organ systems has been reported. However, apart from cases of peripheral neuropathy and myopathy in patients with typical skin lesions, it is unclear whether other reported cases of extra-cutaneous "calciphylaxis" represent the same thrombotic pathophysiological process.[26]

PHYSICAL EXAM AND LOCATION

When evaluating a patient with suspected calciphylaxis, it is important to inquire about pain in commonly affected sites, which include adipose-rich areas such as the medial and lateral thighs, calves, buttocks, abdominal pannus, lower back, and breasts. A comprehensive skin examination should be performed, including palpation of all commonly affected areas while taking care not to cause further discomfort. Additionally, as acral calciphylaxis can result in genital and digital necrosis, a thorough examination of all digits in the upper and lower extremities, as well as the genitalia should be performed.

MORPHOLOGY

Lesion morphology is dependent on the stage of the disease. Patients with early disease may present with pain out of proportion to exam with nondescript subcutaneous papules and nodules on adipose-rich areas. No livedoid skin changes may be present in this stage. As the disease progresses, patients may develop livedo racemosa and noninflammatory retiform purpura over exquisitely painful indurated subcutaneous nodules or plaques [**Figure 86-1A-C**]. In patients of SOC, noninflammatory retiform purpura may appear hyperpigmented rather than violaceous or purple when compared to lighter skin tones [**Figure 86-2**]. Erythema, which is secondary to ischemic injury, may not be as readily apparent when there is overlying xerosis and powdery scale [**Figure 86-3A**]. Dampening the dry skin with an alcohol pad or moist towel can make the underlying purpura or inflammation more visible in these patients

TABLE 86-2 Differential diagnosis for calciphylaxis

Condition	Distinguishing characteristic(s) of alternative diagnosis	Distinguishing characteristic(s) of calciphylaxis
Cellulitis	Ill-defined erythema, warmth, painful but not exquisite pain	Severe pain out of proportion to exam, deeper more indurated component; livedoid changes
Warfarin skin necrosis	History: Recent initiation of warfarin use; also involves adipose-rich body areas.	History: Associated with long-term warfarin use
Acute lipodermatosclerosis	Distribution: bilateral lower legs Morphology: painful subcutaneous nodules without livedo, purpura, ulceration; stasis change	Distribution: localized Morphology: typically overlying livedo (but it may be lacking in very early disease)
Livedoid vasculopathy	Location: medial malleolus, dorsal feet Morphology: stasis change; small punched out purpuric papules without underlying induration; atrophie blanche	Location: adipose rich areas; typically calves on lower legs Morphology: indurated deep component
Septic vasculitis	History: Bacteremia Location: digits, acral Morphology: typically lacks indurated component of calciphylaxis	Location: adipose-rich areas Morphology: indurated nodules
ANCA-associated and other medium vessel vasculitides	Morphology: inflammatory retiform purpura (although inflammation may not be presented in late lesions); dermal to subcutaneous nodules. Ear and nose involvement, and agranulocytosis could suggest drug-induced ANCA vasculitis.	Morphology: noninflammatory retiform purpura
antiphospholipid syndrome (APLS)	Serum antiphospholipid antibodies. Cutaneous lesions are more common during multisystem catastrophic APLS. Morphology: noninflammatory retiform purpura without the subcutaneous component of calciphylaxis	Morphology: indurated nodules
Heparin-induced thrombocytopenia and thrombosis	History of heparin use; thrombocytopenia Location: near site of injection	Labs: not antibody-mediated Location: not localized to site of injection
Cryoglobulinemia	History: history of hepatitis C, plasma cell dyscrasias Labs: positive cryoglobulins Distribution: distal, acral	Labs: not antibody-mediated Distribution: adipose-rich areas
Peripheral vascular disease	History: symptoms of claudication Abnormal ABI. Distribution: distal extremities, digits, anterior tibia of lower leg Exam: lack of peripheral pulses, hairless, shiny skin	Distribution: can be proximal or distal distribution; severe pain Skin biopsy: dermal arteriolar calcification
Necrotizing cellulitis	History: signs of sepsis (including SIRS) Morphology: ill-defined erythema, retiform purpura could be present	History: no signs of systemic infection
Venous stasis ulcer	Morphology: irregular shaped ulcers; excessive fibrinous exudate; surrounding stasis change. Location: Ulcers typically near medial malleolus	Morphology/Location: stellate shaped ulcers on adipose-rich areas
Hematoma	History of trauma. Morphology: ill-defined ecchymosis. Rarely, large hematomas can compromise blood flow to the skin and cause retiform purpura	Morphology: typically, retiform purpura; ulceration and necrosis
Steal syndrome	Distribution: digital ischemia on ipsilateral side of AV fistula or graft (symptoms may mimic acral calciphylaxis) Changes noted on arterial doppler studies.	No change seen on arterial doppler studies with compression of HD access device.

Abbreviations: ABI=Ankle Brachial Index, ANCA= Antineutrophil cytoplasmic antibodies, APLS=Antiphospholipid syndrome, AV=arteriovenous, HD=Hemodialysis, SIRS=Systemic inflammatory response syndrome.

[**Figure 86-3B**]. Other techniques that may be helpful include taking pictures both with and without flash [**Figure 86-4A** and **B**]. Eventually, the skin demonstrates signs of epidermal ischemic injury such as duskiness, pallor, and hemorrhagic bullae, which when ruptured exposes dermis [**Figure 86-5**]. Depending on the degree of ischemia, the dermis may initially appear shiny and pink but eventually becomes dull and devitalized. Ultimately, stellate-shaped ulcers with black eschar or yellow fibrinous exudate [**Figure 86-6**] will develop, sometimes accompanied by the presence of pale and devitalized necrotic fat in the ulcer bed [**Figure 86-7**].

Patients whose ulcers heal may develop stellate-shaped atrophic scars with surrounding dyschromia [**Figure 86-8**], and occasionally calcinosis cutis at the previously involved area. Individuals of SOC are prone to keloid development[27] and pigmentary alteration, which can impact their quality of life even after ulcer healing.

Patients with acral calciphylaxis may present with pain, tenderness, and a burning sensation or numbness in the affected digits. Initially, the skin over the affected area may show subtle livedoid changes, but eventually, a mottled appearance characterized by purple or black discoloration, splinter hemorrhages, and pallor in the nail beds with reduced capillary refill may develop. As the ischemia worsens and progresses to digital necrosis, ulceration and eschar may form [**Figure 86-9**]. Over time, the digit will develop dry gangrene and may autoamputate. Similar changes occur in penile calciphylaxis with the glans being the most commonly area affected [**Figure 86-10**].

HISTOPATHOLOGY AND ROLE OF SKIN BIOPSY

Biopsy samples from suspected calciphylaxis cases typically demonstrate medial calcification and thrombosis of dermal small arteries, arterioles, and subcutaneous capillaries.[8] Other findings include lobular and septal panniculitis, fat necrosis, and extravascular soft-tissue calcification. Von Kossa and Alizarin red stains are useful for highlighting subtle intravascular and extravascular calcifications, especially perieccrine stippled calcification. However, the specificity of these classic histopathological findings has recently been called into question, as a retrospective review found that only 18% of samples exhibited these features. Furthermore, other studies have shown that many

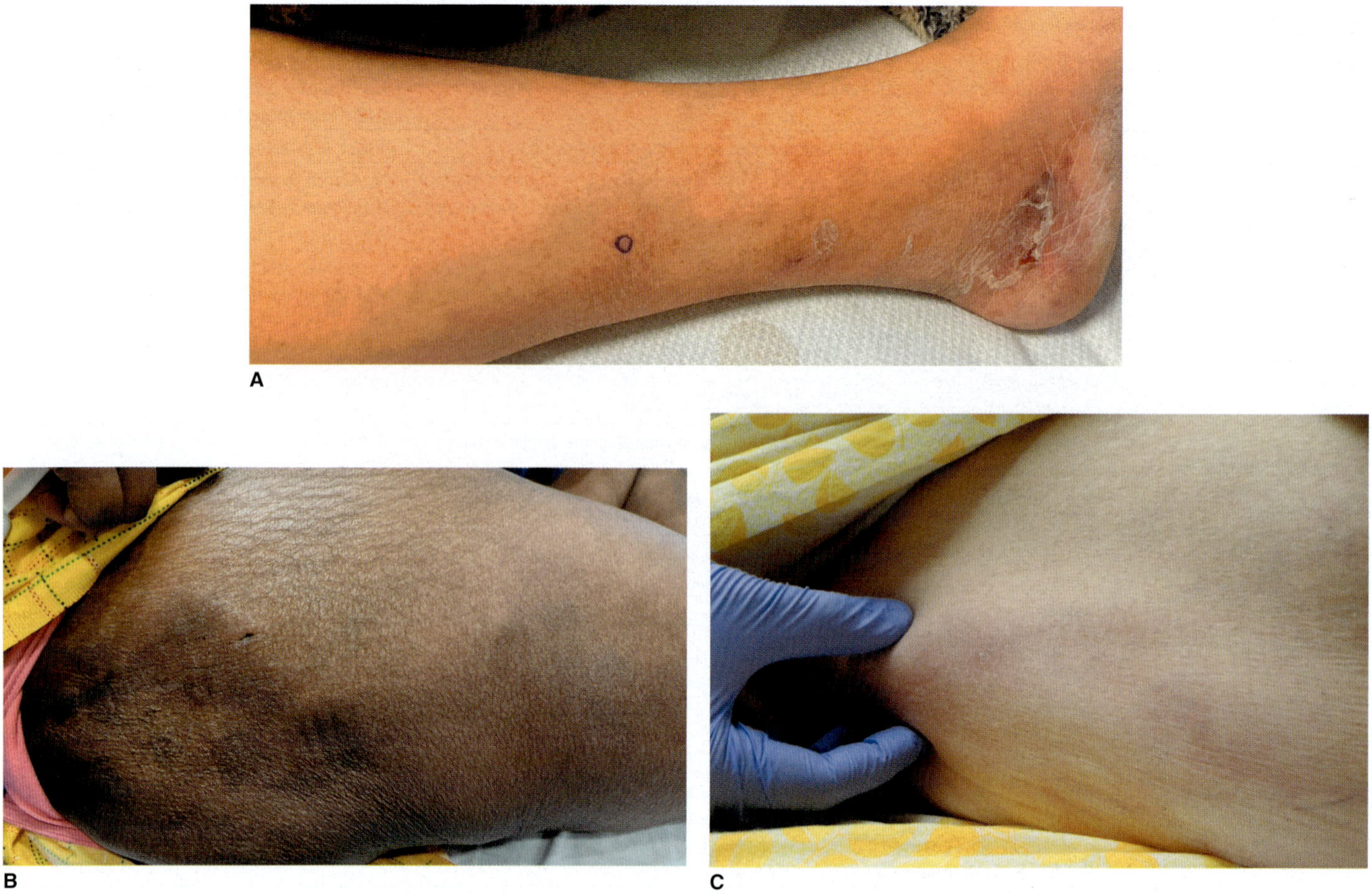

FIGURE 86-1 (A-C) These three images show subtle livedoid changes over deeper, nodular involvement across several different skin types.

histopathological findings previously considered pathognomonic to calciphylaxis can also be seen in biopsy samples from patients with CKD who do not have calciphylaxis.[9-11]

For acral calciphylaxis, the histopathology has not been well described, and it is unclear whether it represents the same disease as microvascular peripheral arterial disease (PAD) or if there is any overlap between the two.

Performing a skin biopsy requires careful consideration of various factors, such as the risk of complications, which include pathergy, ulceration, slow healing, and infection.[28] Furthermore, as mentioned above, the biopsy findings may lack specificity, and the sensitivity may vary depending on the lesion's location, stage, and technique used (eg, punch vs excisional biopsy). Recent studies suggest that image-guided core needle biopsy may be associated with fewer complications

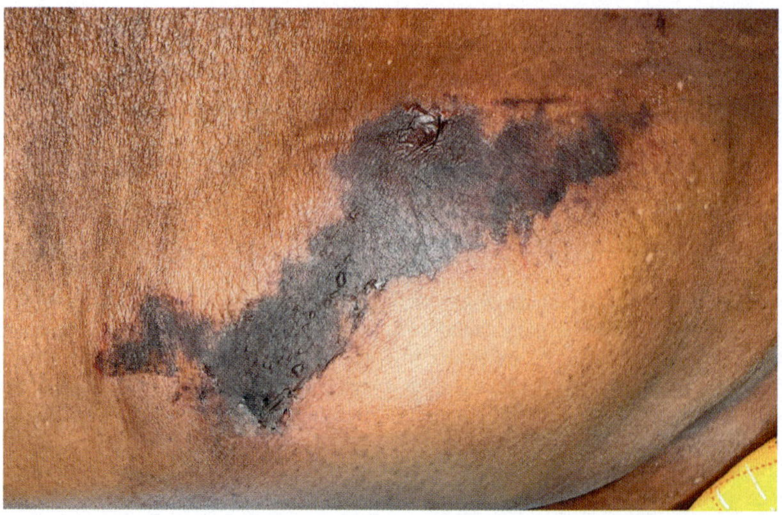

FIGURE 86-2. Noninflammatory retiform purpura with overlying necrotic epidermis. This may appear hyperpigmented in individuals with darker skin rather than purple in individuals with lighter skin.

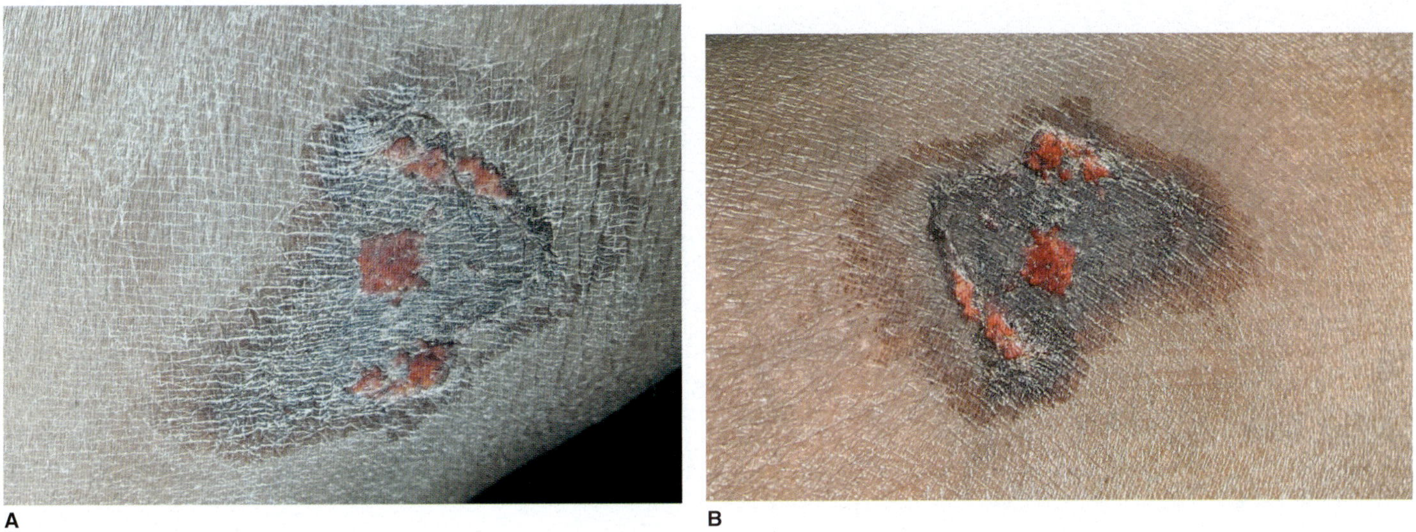

FIGURE 86-3. (A) Overlying xerosis can mask underlying purpura and inflammation. (B) Dampening dry skin with an alcohol pad or moist towel can make underlying purpura and inflammation more visible.

than a punch biopsy and more likely to demonstrate thrombosis on histopathology.[29,30]

Overall, skin biopsy may be a valuable diagnostic tool in atypical cases or in situations where confirmation is necessary to guide complex management decisions in calciphylaxis [**Table 86-3**]. However, it should be used judiciously and in combination with clinical and laboratory findings, as it may not provide additional diagnostic information.

LAB EVALUATION

Lab testing for patients with suspected calciphylaxis has two major goals: identifying potential risk factors and ruling out other potential causes of the patient's thrombotic vasculopathy. It is important to note that there are no specific laboratory findings that are indicative of calciphylaxis. Previously, an elevated calcium-phosphorus product was believed to be more prevalent in patients with calciphylaxis, but recent studies have disproven this association.[7] Additionally, because studies have

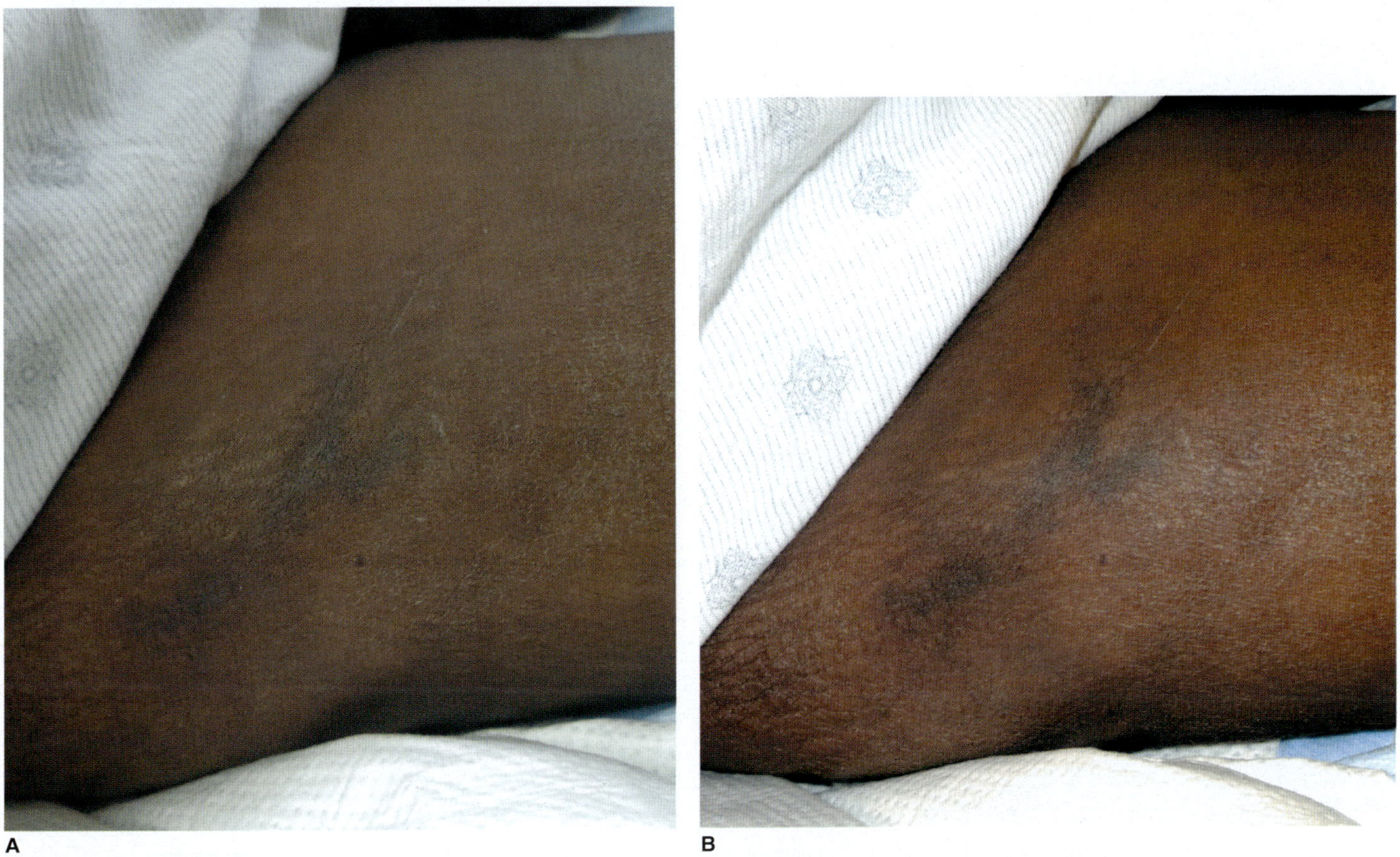

FIGURE 86-4. (A) Retiform purpura without flash photography and (B) with flash photography. Using flash photography is helpful for visualizing erythema in darker skin tones.

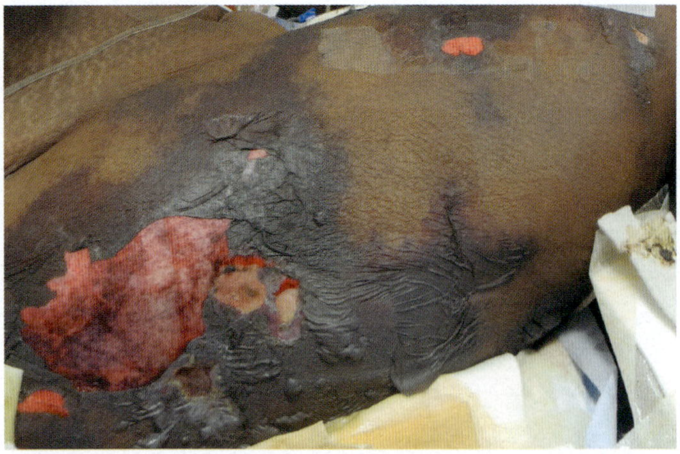

FIGURE 86-5. Extensive epidermal ischemic injury due to underlying thrombosis. This image demonstrates retiform purpura, hemorrhagic bullae, and ruptured bullae with exposed dermis and ulceration.

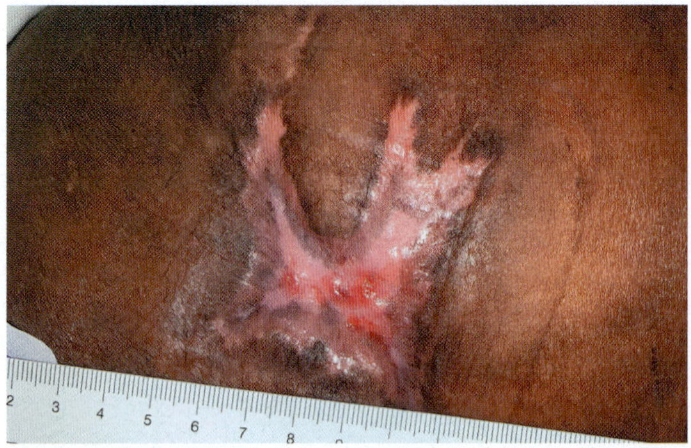

FIGURE 86-8. As the wounds heal, the stellate-shaped atrophic scars often have surrounding dyschromia.

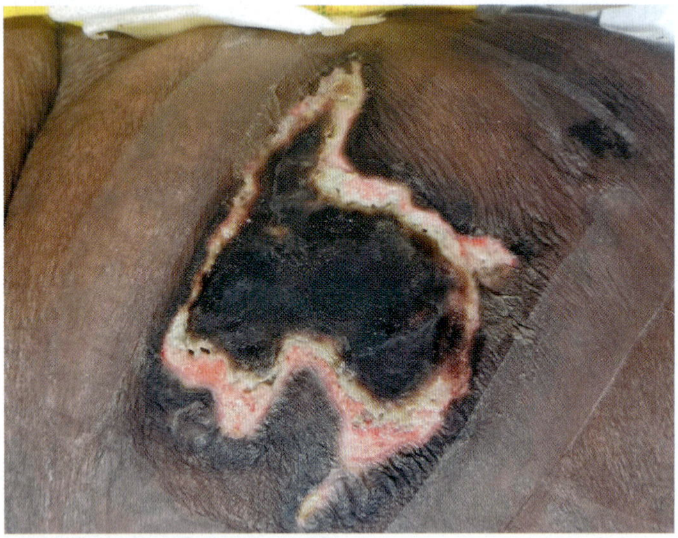

FIGURE 86-6. End stage stellate-shaped ulcers with yellow fibrinous exudate and overlying black eschar.

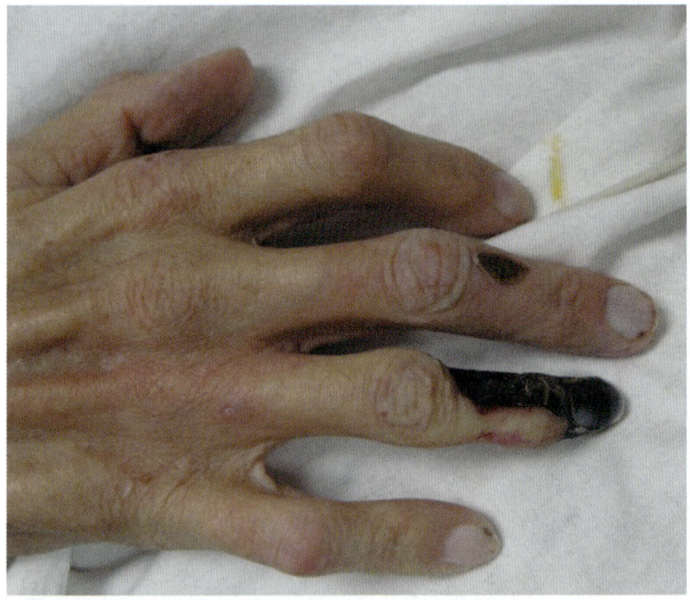

FIGURE 86-9. Acral calciphylaxis, often confused for peripheral artery disease.

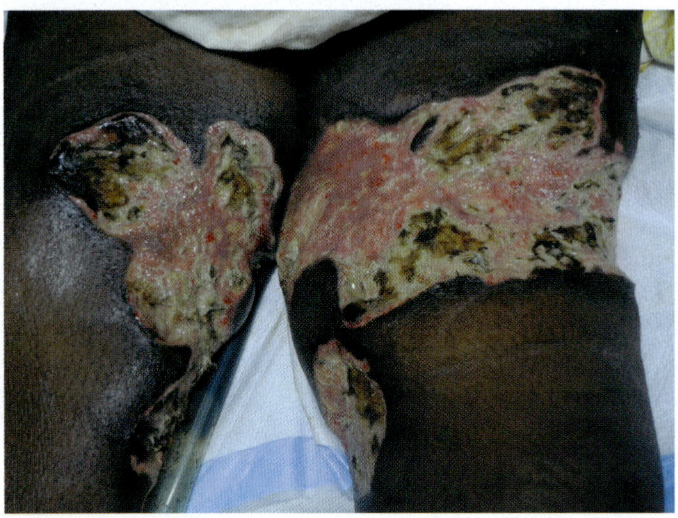

FIGURE 86-7. Bilateral thighs with stellate-shaped ulcers, overlying fibrin, and devitalized necrotic fat in the ulcer bed.

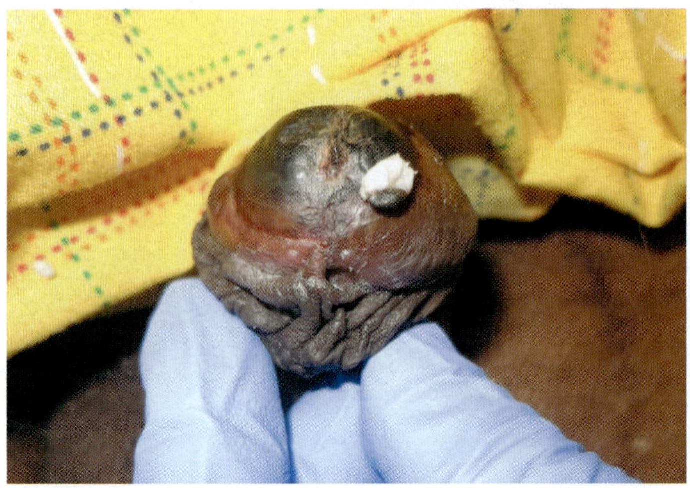

FIGURE 86-10. Necrotic eschar of the glans. Penile calciphylaxis has a high mortality rate.

TABLE 86-3 Potential indications for biopsy to confirm calciphylaxis

Scenario
Nonuremic calciphylaxis
Atypical location
Morphology: "early disease" subcutaneous nodules without overlying livedoid change
Immunosuppressed patient
Septic or bacteremic patient
Concern for malignancy: lymphomas, cutaneous metastases
Insurance company refusal to pay for STS or other treatment
Changing from PD to HD in patient with recalcitrant calciphylaxis
Renal transplantation candidacy
Determining goals of care
Stopping warfarin in difficult scenarios such as valvular disease (DOAC contraindicated)

Abbreviations: DOAC, direct-acting oral anticoagulant; HD, hemodialysis; PD, peritoneal dialysis; STS, sodium thiosulfate.

demonstrated that a significant percentage of patients with calciphylaxis have an underlying thrombophilia, a hypercoagulable workup can be considered [**Table 86-4**].[31,32]

IMAGING

Various radiological imaging modalities, including x-ray, ultrasound, and nuclear imaging, have been utilized for the diagnosis of calciphylaxis.[33] Possible benefits of radiological imaging include the ability to monitor response to treatment as well as avoid the need for a skin biopsy, which as mentioned above, is associated with a significant risk of complications. However, the specificity of these radiological findings is not well-established due to the lack of controlled studies. Therefore, radiological imaging should be considered in conjunction with clinical, laboratory, and histopathological data to ensure an accurate diagnosis.

Imaging plays an important role in the evaluation of patients with suspected acral calciphylaxis. If clinically indicated, a transthoracic or transesophageal echocardiogram should be performed to exclude embolic disease. Ankle-brachial index (ABI), arterial duplex ultrasound, and run-off computed tomography angiography (CTA) are useful tools for evaluating peripheral vascular disease, a condition that can mimic calciphylaxis and complicate wound healing. For suspected penile calciphylaxis, penile Doppler ultrasound should be performed to assess large vessel patency. Finally, for patients with ESRD that have an arteriovenous (AV) fistula for hemodialysis and present with acral ischemia, it is important to rule out steal syndrome in the ipsilateral limb. This can be done using arterial Doppler studies, performed both with and without compression of the fistula.

TABLE 86-4 Recommended hypercoagulable workup in patient with calciphylaxis.

PTT, PT/INR, D-dimer, Fibrinogen, LDH
Antiphospholipid antibodies
• Lupus anticoagulant
• Anticardiolipin (IgM and IgG)
• Anti-β-2-glycoprotein (IgM and IgG)
Serum protein electrophoresis
Cryoglobulins and cryofibrinogens
Rheumatoid factor
Protein C&S
Anti-thrombin III
Factor V Leiden mutation
Prothrombin mutation
HITT antibody (if clinically indicated)

Abbreviations: LDH, lactate dehydrogenase; PT/INR, prothrombin time/international normalized ratio; PTT, partial thromboplastin time.

TREATMENT

The management of calciphylaxis is primarily based on retrospective observational studies and expert opinion. A multimodal therapy approach and multidisciplinary care involving various specialists such as dermatology, renal/endocrine, cardiology, hepatology, wound care, pain management, general surgery, and the patient's primary care provider is recommended for optimal treatment. Initial therapies may vary depending on the patient's comorbidities and whether they have chronic kidney disease and are on HD. Treatment goals include halting ischemic injury, minimizing risk factors for comorbid conditions, managing pain, promoting tissue healing, and treating complications such as infection. Recognition of early disease and initiation of multimodal treatment are vital steps to reduce the morbidity and mortality associated with calciphylaxis.

MAXIMIZATION OF CKD PARAMETERS

In patients with calciphylaxis who have ESRD, collaboration with nephrology to optimize HD according to the National Kidney Foundation-Kidney Disease Outcomes Quality Initiative (KDOQI) guidelines is recommended.[7] Interventions may include increasing the frequency or duration of dialysis sessions to improve calcium-phosphate balance and prevent further calcification. Additionally, the nephrologist may adjust the patient's medication regimen, including phosphate binders (sevelamer), discontinuing vitamin D supplements, and calcimimetics to help manage the underlying metabolic abnormalities that contribute to calciphylaxis.[7]

In some cases, renal transplantation may be considered as a treatment option for calciphylaxis as healing following transplantation has been reported.[34] Currently, controversy exists as some solid organ transplant centers consider calciphylaxis to be a contraindication to renal transplant, due to infection risk and reports of worsening disease following transplantation.[35]

As mentioned previously, ESRD is a particularly difficult condition for patients of SOC with CKD as they are more likely to progress to it and experience worse outcomes.[36] Moreover, HD can also pose challenges for patients of SOC due to higher rates of complications with vascular access such as infection and bleeding.[14] Patients of SOC also encounter barriers accessing renal transplantation as they are less likely to be referred for transplant evaluation due to inadequate health care access. Additionally, they experience delays in transplant referral partially due to race-based estimations of GFR, resulting in an overestimation of GFR above the ≤ 20 mL/min/1.73 m^2 cutoff for kidney transplant priority.[37] Furthermore, patients of SOC who undergo transplant evaluation are less likely to be placed on the waitlist or receive an organ.[38]

SODIUM THIOSULFATE (STS)

Intravenous sodium thiosulfate (IVSTS) is commonly utilized as the primary treatment for most patients with calciphylaxis undergoing hemodialysis (HD). The recommended dosage ranges from 12.5 to 25 g, administered three to five times per week. IVSTS is thought to enhance the solubility of calcium and form a dialyzable salt, although its precise mechanism of action remains incompletely understood. Reported side effects include metabolic acidosis, QT interval prolongation, headache, nausea, and vomiting. Moreover, the medication can be expensive, and obtaining insurance approval for patients without renal disease may pose challenges. The duration of treatment varies among providers, with some continuing until complete healing of ulcers, while others suggest a shorter duration of about 3 months or until signs of ischemia (livedo and induration) have resolved. This shorter duration is recommended due to potential risks of STS, including osteoporosis and bone fractures. Notably, a meta-analysis did not show significant differences in mortality, wound progression, or amputation rates between calciphylaxis patients treated with IVSTS and those who were not.[39] Additional prospective studies are needed.

In cases of localized and limited disease or in patients who cannot tolerate IVSTS, intralesional sodium thiosulfate (ILSTS) may be used as an alternative. Moreover, a recent study reported no mortality differences between patients treated with a combination of IVSTS and ILSTS versus ILSTS alone.[40]

VITAMIN K

Like other treatments, there is limited evidence for vitamin K supplementation in the treatment of calciphylaxis. Nevertheless, vitamin K1 (phylloquinone) 30 mg weekly (divided 10 mg three times per week) can be considered based on studies demonstrating an improvement in serum levels of active matrix Gla protein (MGP), a potent vitamin-K-dependent inhibitor of vascular calcification, following supplementation. A recent phase II randomized control trial demonstrated a reduction in mortality compared to placebo in patients with calciphylaxis.[41] However, safety remains a concern due to one patient developing portal vein thrombosis in this study.

BISPHOSPHONATES

Bisphosphonates can be useful in the treatment of calciphylaxis, specifically for those with non-nephrogenic calciphylaxis. Although typically contraindicated in advanced CKD, it can be considered in recalcitrant cases in patients with ESRD. Numerous case reports using various dosing regimens have reported efficacy in patients with nonnephrogenic calciphylaxis.[42]

ANTICOAGULATION

Although studies have shown that a significant percentage of patients presenting with calciphylaxis have hypercoagulable states,[31,32] patients without another indication are not usually fully anticoagulated. Nevertheless, it is crucial to acknowledge that calciphylaxis is primarily a thrombotic process that may benefit from anticoagulation, especially during early stages of the disease. Indeed, antiplatelet agents such as aspirin, clopidogrel, and pentoxifylline are often prescribed. In cases where calciphylaxis develops in patients receiving warfarin for other indications such as stroke prevention in atrial fibrillation or chronic thromboembolic disease, discontinuation of warfarin and initiation of an alternative agent such as low molecular weight heparin or apixaban is advised.[43] Vitamin K supplementation in patients previously on warfarin should also be considered. In patients with CKD and ESRD on HD, apixaban 5.0 mg bid can be utilized and dose-adjusted to 2.5 mg po bid in patients aged greater than 80 years or with body weight less than 60 kg. However, there may be instances where apixaban and other direct oral anticoagulants (DOACs) are contraindicated and no alternative available, such as in patients with mechanical heart valves or left ventricular assist devices where warfarin is the only approved option.

WOUND CARE

Effective wound care is a critical component in the treatment of calciphylaxis, as chronic ulcers are highly susceptible to infection, which is the leading cause of mortality in this condition. Therefore, prompt and specialized wound care management is essential to minimize the risk of infection and other complications. Referral to a wound care clinic can be considered as well.

During the active ischemic phase, it is generally recommended to avoid trauma and surgical debridement, unless there are signs of active infection. In this stage, prevention of skin breakdown and ulceration is the goal. For inactive wounds without livedo or surrounding induration that need debridement due to necrotic tissue and eschar, gentle autolytic or chemical debridement using hydrocolloid dressings, water jet irrigation, sterile *Leptospermum* honey, and collagenase can be used.

Foam dressings can help minimize trauma and pain by reducing the frequency of dressing changes. In cases where conservative debridement is ineffective or if there is severe infection, surgical removal of eschar may be considered. It is essential to tailor wound care strategies to each patient's unique needs, such as wound size, location, comorbidities, and overall health status.

PAIN MANAGEMENT

As previously discussed, managing pain is crucial to address the significant discomfort experienced by patients with calciphylaxis. For optimal pain control, it is recommended to involve a pain specialist or palliative care provider, but limited access to these resources and lack of training in dermatologists may contribute to inadequate pain management. Effective pain control typically involves a combination of long-acting and breakthrough medications. Long-acting agents include fentanyl transdermal patches as well as methadone. Hydromorphone is the preferred choice for treating breakthrough pain and dressing changes, as it is not renally cleared. However, due to concerns regarding the effectiveness of opiates in controlling calciphylaxis-related pain, other adjuncts such as ketamine, gabapentin, pregabalin, and lidocaine gel may be used.

Patients of SOC often encounter challenges in obtaining sufficient pain management due to systemic biases that exist within our healthcare system.[2] By being aware of potential biases and addressing them proactively, healthcare providers can improve the quality of care provided to patients with calciphylaxis, particularly those from marginalized communities.

PROGNOSIS AND PALLIATIVE CARE

Despite recent studies demonstrating improved patient survival in recent years, calciphylaxis remains a life-threatening condition with high mortality rates. The 6-month survival rate for nephrogenic calciphylaxis ranges from approximately 50% to 62%, with a median survival time of approximately 6.2 months.[1,44] Several risk factors are associated with poor outcomes, including the use of vitamin K antagonists such as warfarin, high levels of C-reactive protein, low albumin and hemoglobin, ulceration, proximal disease, and penile involvement.[45,46] While some studies suggest differences in outcomes according to race and ethnicity (with poorer prognosis reported for White individuals), larger studies are limited by small sample sizes and single-center experiences. Additionally, racial disparities in access to healthcare and the higher prevalence of comorbidities among marginalized communities (including Black and Latin American/Hispanic patients) could contribute to uncertain outcomes. Further research is needed to fully understand the relationship between racialized groups and prognosis in calciphylaxis, as well as to identify strategies for reducing disparities and improving outcomes for all patients.

To provide optimal care for patients with calciphylaxis- a rare condition with a poor prognosis, questionable treatment efficacy, and a significant impact on quality of life- early involvement of palliative care is critical. Palliative care can help manage pain, address symptom burden, and provide support for patients and their families as they navigate the challenges of this complex illness. In addition, palliative care providers can facilitate discussions about goals of care, advanced directives, and end-of-life planning. By involving palliative care early in the disease course, patients can receive the necessary support and guidance to ensure that their care aligns with their values and preferences.

Patients of SOC, especially Latin American/Hispanic and Black patients, often face challenges and disparities when it comes to palliative care, defining goals of care, and end-of-life planning. These disparities are due to a variety of factors, including a lack of cultural sensitivity and understanding among healthcare providers, historical mistrust of the healthcare system, and systemic barriers to accessing healthcare. Additionally, there may be differences in cultural beliefs and practices related to death and dying that can impact end-of-life care for patients of SOC. To address these disparities, it is important for healthcare providers to engage in culturally responsive care that considers the patient's values, beliefs, and cultural background.

ACKNOWLEDGMENTS

The authors would like to thank Dr. Daniela Kroshinsky for her scientific contributions to our understanding of calciphylaxis as well as her content review of this chapter. We would like to also thank Dr. Cristina Thomas for her review as well.

REFERENCES

1. Gabel CK, Nguyen ED, Chakrala T, et al. Assessment of outcomes of calciphylaxis. *J Am Acad Dermatol.* 2021;85(4):1057-1064.
2. Goree JH, Jackson J. Do racial and ethnic disparities lead to the undertreatment of pain? Are there solutions? *Curr Opin Anaesthesiol.* 2022;35(3):273-277.
3. Nigwekar SU, Solid CA, Ankers E, et al. Quantifying a rare disease in administrative data: the example of calciphylaxis. *J Gen Intern Med.* 2014;29(Suppl 3): S724-S731.
4. Angelis M, Wong LL, Myers SA, Wong LM. Calciphylaxis in patients on hemodialysis: a prevalence study. *Surgery.* 1997;122(6):1083-1090.
5. Karwowski W, Naumnik B, Szczepański M, Myśliwiec M. The mechanism of vascular calcification - a systematic review. *Med Sci Monit.* 2012;18(1):RA1-RA11.
6. Nigwekar SU, Thadhani R, Brandenburg VM. Calciphylaxis. *N Engl J Med.* 2018;378(18):1704-1714.
7. Nigwekar SU, Kroshinsky D, Nazarian RM, et al. Calciphylaxis: risk factors, diagnosis, and treatment. *Am J Kidney Dis.* 2015;66(1):133-146.
8. Mochel MC, Arakaki RY, Wang G, Kroshinsky D, Hoang MP. Cutaneous calciphylaxis: a retrospective histopathologic evaluation. *Am J Dermatopathol.* 2013;35(5):582-586.
9. Ellis CL, O'Neill WC. Questionable specificity of histologic findings in calcific uremic arteriolopathy. *Kidney Int.* 2018;94(2):390-395.
10. Chen TY, Lehman JS, Gibson LE, Lohse CM, El-Azhary RA. Histopathology of calciphylaxis: cohort study with clinical correlations. *Am J Dermatopathol.* 2017;39(11):795-802.
11. Chaudet KM, Dutta P, Nigwekar SU, Nazarian RM. Calciphylaxis-associated cutaneous vascular calcification in noncalciphylaxis patients. *Am J Dermatopathol.* 2020;42(8):557-563.
12. Jeong HS, Dominguez AR. Calciphylaxis: controversies in pathogenesis, diagnosis and treatment. *Am J Med Sci.* 2016;351(2):217-227.
13. Barinas-Mitchell E, Duan C, Brooks M, et al. Cardiovascular disease risk factor burden during the menopause transition and late midlife subclinical vascular disease: does race/ethnicity matter? *J Am Heart Assoc.* 2020;9(4):e013876.
14. Woo K, Yao J, Selevan D, Hye RJ. Influence of vascular access type on sex and ethnicity-related mortality in hemodialysis-dependent patients. *Perm J.* 2012;16(2):4-9.
15. Delker E, Brown Q, Hasin DS. Alcohol consumption in demographic subpopulations: an epidemiologic overview. *Alcohol Res.* 2016;38(1):7-15.
16. Gutiérrez OM, Isakova T, Andress DL, Levin A, Wolf M. Prevalence and severity of disordered mineral metabolism in Blacks with chronic kidney disease. *Kidney Int.* 2008;73(8):956-962.
17. Sullivan JK, Littlejohn EA. Utilization of glucocorticoids among White and Black patients with systemic lupus erythematosus: observations from the enrollment visit of a prospective registry. *Lupus.* 2021;30(14):2298-2303.
18. Essien UR, Holmes DN, Jackson LR 2nd, et al. Association of race/ethnicity with oral anticoagulant use in patients with atrial fibrillation: findings from the outcomes registry for better informed treatment of atrial fibrillation II. *JAMA Cardiol.* 2018;3(12):1174-1182.
19. Salahudeen AK, Deogaygay B, Fleischmann E, Bower JD. Race-dependent survival disparity on hemodialysis: higher serum aluminum as an independent risk factor for higher mortality in whites. *Am J Kidney Dis.* 2000;36(6): 1147-1154.
20. Roberts MH, Erdei E. Comparative United States autoimmune disease rates for 2010-2016 by sex, geographic region, and race. *Autoimmun Rev.* 2020;19(1):102423.
21. Cossrow N, Falkner B. Race/ethnic issues in obesity and obesity-related comorbidities. *J Clin Endocrinol Metab.* 2004;89(6):2590-2594.
22. Ames BN, Grant WB, Willett WC. Does the high prevalence of vitamin D deficiency in African Americans contribute to health disparities? *Nutrients.* 2021;13(2):499.
23. Albertus P, Morgenstern H, Robinson B, Saran R. Risk of ESRD in the United States. *Am J Kidney Dis.* 2016;68(6):862-872.
24. Hsu CY, Yang W, Parikh RV, et al. Race, genetic ancestry, and estimating kidney function in CKD. *N Engl J Med.* 2021;385(19):1750-1760.
25. Gabel CK, Blum AE, François J, et al. Clinical mimickers of calciphylaxis: a retrospective study. *J Am Acad Dermatol.* 2021;85(6):1520-1527.
26. Aouizerate J, Valleyrie-Allanore L, Limal N, et al. Ischemic myopathy revealing systemic calciphylaxis. *Muscle Nerve.* 2017;56(3):529-533.
27. Limmer EE, Glass DA 2nd. A review of current keloid management: mainstay monotherapies and emerging approaches. *Dermatol Ther (Heidelb).* 2020;10(5):931-948.
28. Dobry AS, Nguyen ED, Shah R, Mihm MC, Kroshinsky D. The role of skin biopsy in diagnosis and management of calciphylaxis: a retrospective analysis. *J Am Acad Dermatol.* 2021;85(3):765-767.
29. Pyle HJ, Shedd CM, Begovic J, et al. Complications and histopathological findings of image-guided core needle biopsy in diagnosis of cutaneous calciphylaxis. *Am J Dermatopathol.* 2023;45(6):414-417.
30. Mask-Bull L, Lee MP, Wang A. Image-guided core-needle biopsy for the diagnosis of cutaneous calciphylaxis. *JAMA Dermatol.* 2019;155(7):856-857.
31. El-Azhary RA, Patzelt MT, McBane RD, et al. Calciphylaxis: a disease of pannicular thrombosis. *Mayo Clin Proc.* 2016;91(10):1395-1402.
32. Dobry AS, Ko LN, St John J, Sloan JM, Nigwekar S, Kroshinsky D. Association between hypercoagulable conditions and calciphylaxis in patients with renal disease: a case-control study. *JAMA Dermatol.* 2018;154(2):182-187.
33. Bonchak JG, Park KK, Vethanayagamony T, Sheikh MM, Winterfield LS. Calciphylaxis: a case series and the role of radiology in diagnosis. *Int J Dermatol.* 2016;55(5):e275-e279.
34. Nordheim E, Dahle DO, Syse IM, Åsberg A, Reisæter AV, Hartmann A. Resolution of calciphylaxis after urgent kidney transplantation in 3 patients with end-stage kidney failure. *Transplant Direct.* 2016;2(11):e113.
35. Guillén-Olmos E, Torregrosa JV, Garcia-Herrera A, Ganau S, Diekmann F, Cucchiari D. Development of calciphylaxis in kidney transplant recipients with a functioning graft. *Clin Kidney J.* 2021;15(4):663-671.
36. Lopes AA. Relationships of race and ethnicity to progression of kidney dysfunction and clinical outcomes in patients with chronic kidney failure. *Adv Ren Replace Ther.* 2004;11(1):14-23.
37. Ahmed S, Nutt CT, Eneanya ND, et al. Examining the potential impact of race multiplier utilization in estimated glomerular filtration rate calculation on African-American care outcomes. *J Gen Intern Med.* 2021;36(2): 464-471.
38. Wesselman H, Ford CG, Leyva Y, et al. Social determinants of health and race disparities in kidney transplant. *Clin J Am Soc Nephrol.* 2021;16(2): 262-274.
39. Wen W, Portales-Castillo I, Seethapathy R, et al. Intravenous sodium thiosulphate for calciphylaxis of chronic kidney disease: a systematic review and meta-analysis. *JAMA Netw Open.* 2023;6(4):e2310068.
40. Gabel CK, Nguyen ED, Dobry AS, et al. Assessment of outcomes of calciphylaxis lesions treated with intralesional sodium thiosulfate. *J Am Acad Dermatol.* 2021;85(3):770-773.
41. Nigwekar SU, Krinsky S, Thadani RI, et al. Phase 2 trial of phytonadione in calciphylaxis. Presented at the American Society of Nephrology's Kidney Week 2019 meeting held Nov. 5 to 10 in Washington, DC. Poster TH-PO1188.
42. Truong DH, Riedhammer MM, Zinszer K. Non-uraemic calciphylaxis successfully treated with pamidronate infusion. *Int Wound J.* 2019;16(1): 250-255.
43. Garza-Mayers AC, Shah R, Sykes DB, Nigwekar SU, Kroshinsky D. The successful use of apixaban in dialysis patients with calciphylaxis who require anticoagulation: a retrospective analysis. *Am J Nephrol.* 2018;48(3):168-171.
44. Weenig RH, Sewell LD, Davis MD, McCarthy JT, Pittelkow MR. Calciphylaxis: natural history, risk factor analysis, and outcome. *J Am Acad Dermatol.* 2007;56(4):569-579.
45. Chinnadurai R, Huckle A, Hegarty J, Kalra PA, Sinha S. Calciphylaxis in end-stage kidney disease: outcome data from the United Kingdom calciphylaxis study. *J Nephrol.* 2021;34(5):1537-1545.
46. Gabel C, Chakrala T, Shah R, et al. Penile calciphylaxis: a retrospective case-control study. *J Am Acad Dermatol.* 2021;85(5):1209-1217.

CHAPTER 87

Blistering Disorders

Chia-Chun Ang
Victoria Werth

KEY POINTS

- The causes of cutaneous blistering diseases are multiple and can be broadly differentiated based on the age of onset and the chronicity of the disease. The clinical context provides further clues for diagnosing cutaneous blistering diseases.
- Potential issues that affect the management of autoimmune blistering diseases in patients with skin of color include a difference in prevalence of specific autoimmune bullous diseases, disease presentation, postinflammatory/posttreatment dyspigmentation, and access to care.
- A difficulty in the clinical assessment of autoimmune blistering disease activity can be the difficulty in discerning erythema in inflamed skin lesions.
- Large multicenter controlled trials are needed to determine whether treatment responses vary among patients with autoimmune bullous diseases across diverse skin tones.

INTRODUCTION

Cutaneous blisters appear because of disruption of the desmosome or hemidesmosome cell junctions or due to cytolysis of keratinocytes. The differential diagnoses are diverse, and their epidemiology and presentation can be different in patients with darker skin. In the following sections, we will present an approach to the diagnosis of blistering diseases. We will highlight some of the diagnostic and management issues specific to individuals with skin of color. We will then focus on the epidemiology, clinical presentation, and treatment of common autoimmune blistering disease, and highlight the recent literature involving Black/African American, Hispanic/Latine and Asian patient populations.

APPROACH TO DIAGNOSING BLISTERING DISEASES

An approach to the differential diagnoses of blistering diseases is to consider the age of the patient and the tempo of the clinical presentation [**Figures 87-1** and **87-2**]. Blistering from the effects of exogenous agents is mostly episodic and the triggers can be identified by a careful history and physical examination. Blistering dermatoses from autoimmune, inflammatory, inherited, and neoplastic causes are usually chronic, relapsing, and progressive. Although genodermatoses should always be considered when evaluating a child with blistering diseases,

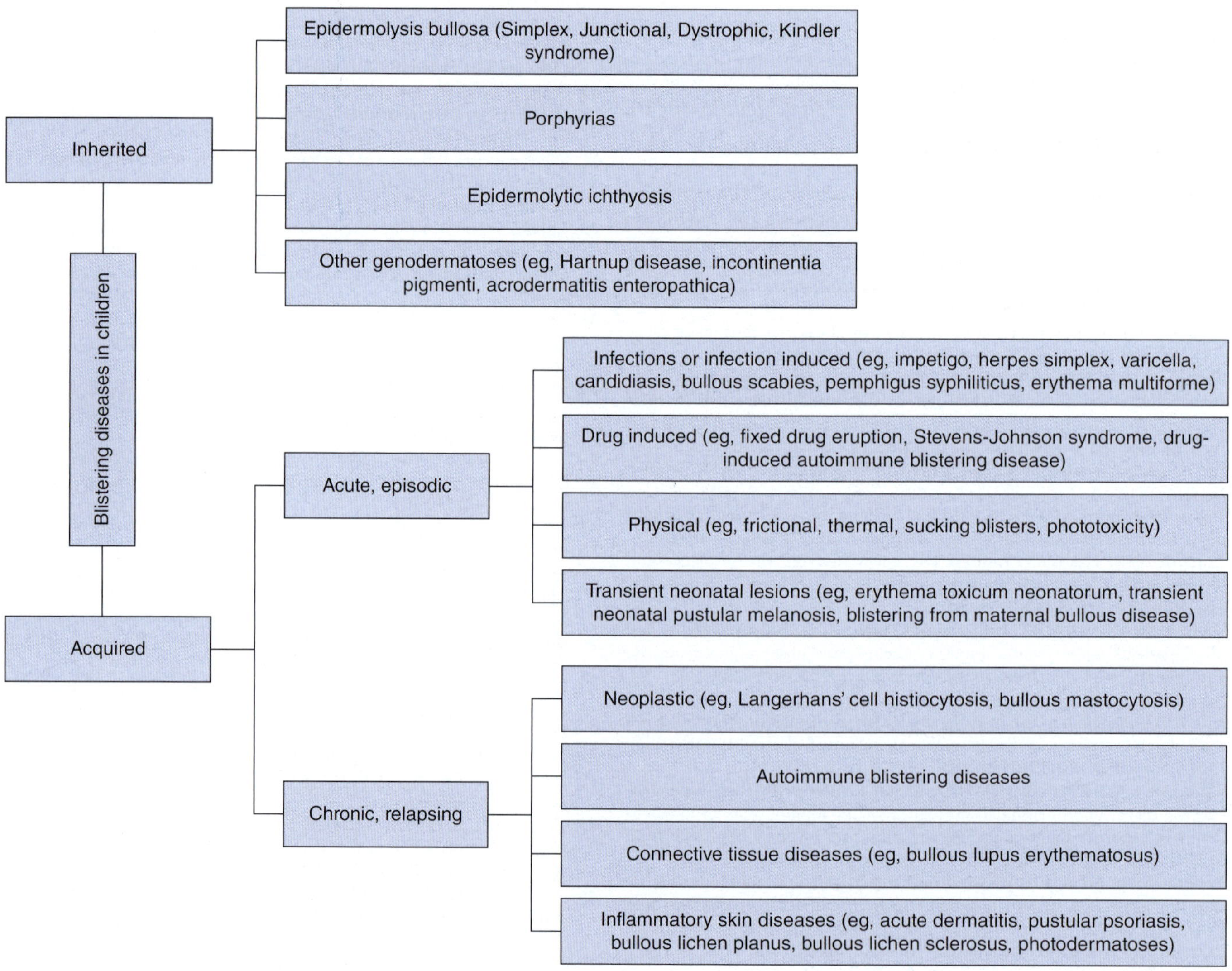

FIGURE 87-1. Approach to diagnosing blistering diseases in children.

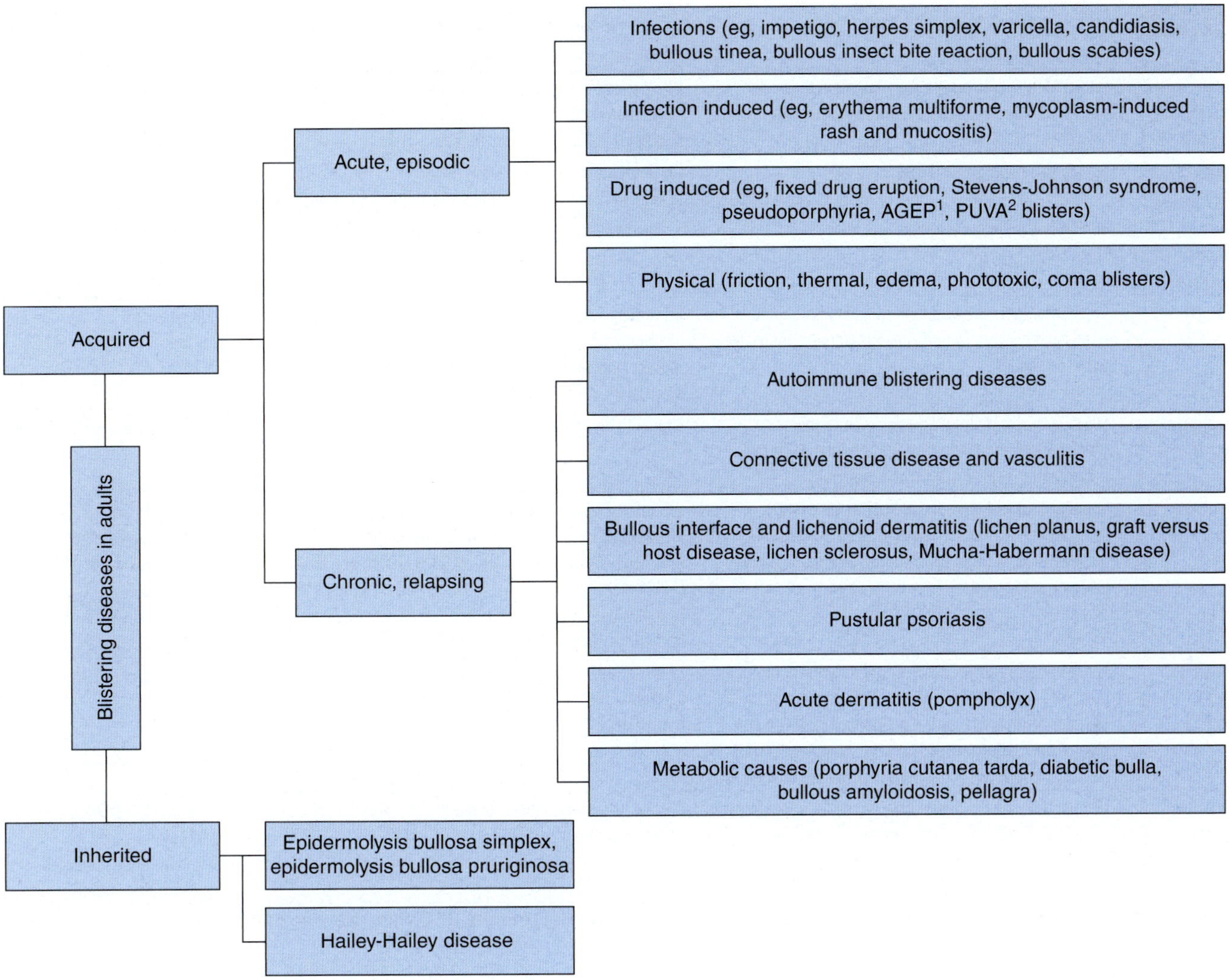

FIGURE 87-2. Approach to diagnosing blistering diseases in adults.
[1]Acute generalized exanthematous pustulosis (AGEP); [2]Psoralen and ultraviolet light A (PUVA)

some genodermatoses can manifest in adolescence and adulthood. These include localized epidermolysis bullosa simplex with palmoplantar bulla, late onset junctional epidermolysis bullosa, epidermolysis bullosa pruriginosa, and Hailey-Hailey disease.

The presence of specific desmosome or hemidesmosome targeting autoantibodies is central to the diagnosis of an autoimmune blistering disease.[1,2] Direct immunofluorescence (DIF) of perilesional skin and indirect immunofluorescence (IIF) test using patient's sera are good screening tests that demonstrate tissue bound or circulating autoantibodies, respectively. False negative DIF can arise from technical issues (eg, biopsy of inflamed skin or blister where the epidermis then separates), while false positive DIF can occur from nonspecific epidermal binding of antibodies in inflammatory and infectious cutaneous diseases.[3] Successful IIF testing depends on the titers of circulating autoantibodies and the use of an appropriate substrate that is enriched with the antigen of interest. False positive detection of intercellular autoantibodies on monkey esophagus (IIF) in nonpemphigus patients has been described, and these patients subsequently developed subepidermal autoimmune blistering diseases or inflammatory dermatoses.[4] Commercial enzyme-linked immunosorbent assay (ELISA) systems detect and quantify circulating autoantibodies targeting specific epitopes in common autoimmune blistering diseases and are used to monitor disease activity. Immunoblot and immunoprecipitation tests detect circulating autoantibodies targeting uncommon desmosome and hemidesmosome antigens. They are highly sensitive and specific but are only available in specialized laboratories. Proper diagnosis of an autoimmune blistering disease requires good clinic-pathological correlation [**Tables 87-1** and **87-2**].

CONSIDERATIONS IN THE DIAGNOSIS AND MANAGEMENT OF AUTOIMMUNE BLISTERING DISEASES IN SKIN OF COLOR PATIENTS

The incidence, presentation, complications, and treatment outcomes of autoimmune blistering diseases in skin of color patients are influenced by skin tone, genotype, and the social determinants of health (SDOH) affecting these patients. Erythema can be difficult to discern in darker skin tones, while dyspigmented and hypertrophic scarring are more common and affect the quality of life.[5] Some autoimmune blistering diseases are more commonly seen in darker skin tones (eg, lichen planus pemphigoides reported in epidemiologic studies from India[6] and Kuwait[7] compared to other published epidemiologic studies[8]).

Darker skin tones and cultural practices are associated with lower vitamin D levels.[9] Assessing and replacing vitamin D should be done when initiating long-term systemic steroid therapy. Pharmacogenomic differences in different ethnic populations can affect the selection and dosing of immunomodulatory and immunosuppressive agents. Patients treated with dapsone should be screened for glucose-6-phosphate dehydrogenase (G6PD) deficiency, which is more prevalent in patients from Africa, the Middle East, and Asia, compared to the Americas and Europe.[10] HLA-B*13:01 is associated with dapsone-induced cutaneous

TABLE 87-1 Histological and immunofluorescence features of intraepidermal autoimmune blistering diseases

	Histological findings	Immunofluorescence findings	Main target antigen(s)
Pemphigus foliaceus (PF)	Intraepidermal blister with acantholysis in the upper epidermis, dermal mixed inflammatory cell infiltrate.	DIF: Intercellular IgG, may be more intense in the upper epidermis. IIF (human skin): Intercellular IgG Anti Dsg 1 ELISA+, anti Dsg 3 ELISA -	Desmoglein 1
• Pemphigus erythematosus	Similar to pemphigus foliaceus	DIF: Intercellular IgG with lupus band IIF human skin: Intercellular IgG and antinuclear antibodies.	Desmoglein 1
• Endemic pemphigus (fogo Selvagem)	Similar to pemphigus foliaceus	Similar to pemphigus foliaceus	Desmoglein 1
Pemphigus vulgaris (PV)	Suprabasal cleft with acantholysis and tomb-stoning of basal keratinocytes. Dermal inflammatory cell infiltrate with eosinophils.	DIF: Intercellular IgG, may be more intense in the lower epidermis. IIF (monkey esophagus): Intercellular IgG Mucocutaneous PV: anti-Dsg 1 ELISA+, anti-Dsg 3 ELISA+ Mucosal PV: Anti Dsg 1 ELISA−, anti Dsg 3 ELISA+	Desmoglein 3 ± Desmoglein 1
• Pemphigus vegetans	Suprabasal acantholysis, acanthosis and papillomatosis, intraepidermal micro-abscesses, intense dermal inflammatory cell infiltrate with eosinophils	Similar to pemphigus vulgaris	Desmoglein 3 ± Desmoglein 1
Paraneoplastic pemphigus	Suprabasal acantholysis, necrotic and dyskeratotic keratinocytes, lymphocytic exocytosis, basal vacuolar degeneration, or lichenoid lymphocytic inflammatory infiltrate in the dermis	DIF: Intercellular and BMZ IgG, can be negative IIF (rat bladder): Intercellular IgG can be negative. Anti-Dsg1, anti-Dsg3, and anti-BP230 ELISA can be positive. ELISA for antibodies against the N-terminal fragment of Envoplakin+ Immunoprecipitation or Western blotting	Envoplakin, periplakin, bullous pemphigoid antigen 1 (BP230), desmoplakin I, desmoplakin II, plectin, α-2-macroglobulin-like-1, desmoglein 1, desmoglein 3, plakophilin 3 and desmocollins 1-3
IgA pemphigus (also see Chapter 82)	Epidermal acantholytic clefts. Intraepidermal neutrophilic pustules localized to the subcorneal region in subcorneal pustular dermatosis type IgA pemphigus (SPD-IgA pemphigus) and to the mid epidermis in the intraepidermal neutrophils type IgA pemphigus (IEN-IgA pemphigus)	DIF: Intercellular IgA > IgG or C3 IIF (human skin or monkey esophagus): Intercellular IgA, may be negative.	Desmocollin 1-3; desmoglein 1 and 3.
Drug-induced pemphigus	Histologically similar to pemphigus vulgaris or pemphigus foliaceous. Eosinophils are present in some cases	DIF and IIF findings follows either PF (66%) or PV (33%) or are negative (rarely)	Desmoglein 1 (66%), Desmoglein 3 (33%) Non immune mediated acantholysis (rarely)

Abbreviations: BMZ, basement membrane zone; BP230, bullous pemphigoid antigen 1; DIF, direct immunofluorescence; Dsg, Desmoglein; ELISA, enzyme-linked immunosorbent assay; IIF, indirect immunofluorescence.

adverse drug reactions in patients of Asian descent.[11] While screening of thiopurine S-methyltransferase (TPMT) genetic polymorphisms can predict azathioprine-induced myelotoxicity in populations of European descent, screening for Nudix hydrolase 15 (NUDT-15) genetic polymorphisms predicts azathioprine-induced myelotoxicity in populations of Asian descent more accurately.[12]

Disparate social determinants of health (also see Chapter 11) influence access to dermatologic care as well as increase the risk of acquiring infectious diseases. Worsening of existing infection (such as COVID-19), acquiring uncommon infections (such as pneumocystis jiroveci pneumonia), or reactivation of latent infections (such as hepatitis B, hepatitis C, human immunodeficiency virus, tuberculosis, strongyloidiasis, JC virus, and herpes zoster) can occur with immunosuppression. Prior to the initiation of immunosuppressive therapy, patients with autoimmune blistering diseases should be screened for latent or chronic infections and receive anticipatory vaccinations or prophylactic treatment where available.[13-15] The patient should be referred to the infectious disease physician for further management if any of these infections are detected.

PEMPHIGUS FOLIACEUS AND PEMPHIGUS VULGARIS

Pemphigus is an intraepidermal autoimmune blistering disease.[16] The three main forms of pemphigus are pemphigus foliaceus, pemphigus vulgaris, and paraneoplastic pemphigus. Patients with pemphigus foliaceus (PF) and its variants (pemphigus erythematosus and fogo selvagem/endemic pemphigus foliaceus) harbor antibodies against desmoglein 1. Patients with mucosal pemphigus vulgaris (PV) and pemphigus vegetans harbor antibodies against desmoglein 3, while patients with mucocutaneous pemphigus carry anti-desmoglein 1 and 3 antibodies. Upon binding of the anti-desmoglein antibody to its target antigen, steric hindrance of desmosome adhesion and disruption of normal desmoglein homeostasis through p38-MAPK signaling occurs, leading to acantholysis and subsequent blistering and erosions. The distribution of mucocutaneous lesions depends on the differential expression of desmoglein 1 and 3 in the skin and mucosa, and their compensatory effects in the presence of anti-desmoglein 1 and 3 autoantibodies.[17] Pemphigus patients can occasionally harbor nondesmoglein autoantibodies that targets other antigens (α-catenin, desmocollin-1/3, α-acetylcholine receptor, pemphaxin, ATP2C1, E-cadherin, periplakin, and desmoplakin).[18] The pathogenic role of these autoantibodies remains to be defined.

Nonendemic pemphigus predominately affects adults and is slightly more frequent in females than males. Pemphigus vulgaris is more common compared to sporadic pemphigus foliaceus in most populations studied. In comparison, endemic pemphigus foliaceus is the predominant phenotype in rural South America and Tunisia. The risk of pemphigus vulgaris is higher in those with Jewish and Mediterranean ethnicity. Certain HLA haplotypes, medications, vaccines, and environmental triggers such as drugs and Lutzomyia sand fly exposure in endemic pemphigus foliaceus have been associated with an increased risk of pemphigus.[19] De novo and aggravation of pemphigus has been noted in patient receiving different forms of SARS-CoV-2 vaccines.[20] The mortality associated with untreated pemphigus has improved tremendously since the use of systemic steroids, steroid-sparing immunosuppressants, and anti-CD20 therapy. Infections, cardiovascular diseases, peptic ulcer diseases, and malignancies were the main causes of death in various epidemiological studies.[19]

Patients with PV commonly present with oral mucosal erosions [**Figure 87-3**] and desquamative gingivitis [**Figure 87-4**]. Involvement

TABLE 87-2 Histological and immunofluorescence features of subepidermal autoimmune blistering diseases

	Histological findings	Immunofluorescence findings	Main target antigens
Bullous pemphigoid (BP)	Pre-bullous phase: eosinophilic spongiotic dermatitis Bullous phase: subepidermal blister, dermal inflammatory cell infiltrate with eosinophils	DIF: Linear IgG and C3 or C3 alone at BMZ, n-serrated IIF (salt split skin): epidermal (roof) binding IgG BMZ antibodies Anti BP180 NC16a ELISA+ in 75-90% of patients, titers can be used to monitor disease activity. Anti BP230 ELISA + in 50-70% of patients, useful in diagnosis of BP in patients with + DIF and negative anti BP180 ELISA.	BP 180 NC16a domain, BP 230.
Pemphigoid gestationis (PG)	Similar to bullous pemphigoid	DIF: Linear C3 +/- IgG at BMZ IIF (salt split skin): Epidermal (roof) binding C3>>IgG. Complement fixing IgG demonstrable with modified IIF technique. Anti BP180 NC16a ELISA+ in 90% of patients	BP180 NC16a domain
Mucous membrane pemphigoid (MMP)	Subepidermal blister with a lympho-histiocytic infiltrate and plasma cells. Dermal fibrosis is seen in advanced lesions	DIF: Linear deposits of IgG, IgA and C3 at BMZ, n- or u-serrated. DIF may be negative. IIF (salt split skin): Anti-BP 180 and anti-BP 230 IgG or IgA antibodies bind the epidermal side. Anti-laminin-332 and anti Col VII IgG or IgA antibodies binds the dermal side. IIF may be negative. Anti BP180 NC16a ELISA, BP230 ELISA and Col VII ELISA may be +	BP180, BP 230, Laminin 332, Collagen VII.
Linear IgA bullous dermatosis (LABD)	Subepidermal blister with neutrophilic or eosinophilic dermal inflammatory infiltrate	DIF: Linear deposits of IgA at BMZ, n-serrated in lamina lucida type, u-serrated in sublamina densa type. Weak linear IgG and C3 is rarely seen on DIF IIF (salt split skin): Epidermal (more common) or dermal (less common) binding, or combined epidermal-dermal staining with IgA BMZ autoantibodies Anti BP180 NC16a ELISA may be +	Shed ectodomains of BP180 (LAD-1/120kDa, 97kDa), BP180 NC16-A domain, type VII collagen, laminin γ1
Dermatitis herpetiformis (DH)	Subepidermal blister with neutrophilic micro-abscesses at the dermal papilla	DIF: Granular or fibrillar IgA deposits at dermal papillae. Rarely continuous BMZ IgA staining. IIF (monkey esophagus): Endomysium binding IgA. IIF (normal human skin) is negative. ELISA for IgA anti-tissue (TG2) or epidermal (TG3) transglutaminase. Level of autoantibodies reduces with a gluten free diet. IgG anti TG2 or TG 3 antibodies should be screen if patients have IgA deficiency.	Epidermal (TG3) transglutaminase is the main antigen in DH and is more specific for DH. Tissue (TG2) transglutaminase is the main antigen in celiac disease and is less specific for DH.
Epidermolysis bullosa acquisita (EBA)	Basal vacuolar alteration or frank subepidermal blister. Dermal inflammatory infiltrate may be present (neutrophil rich) or minimal. Milia and fibrosis can be seen in biopsies of older lesions.	DIF: Linear homogenous IgG ± C3, occasionally IgM or IgA at BMZ, u-serrated. IIF (salt split skin): Dermal (floor) binding IgG BMZ antibodies. May be negative. Advanced tests to confirm EBA: Serology-based assays (Immunoblot, ELISA for type VII collagen, Biochip™ IIF, IIF on skin deficient in type VII collagen or indirect immunoelectron microscopy) or tissue-based assays (electron microscopy or direct immunoelectron microscopy, fluorescent overlay antigen mapping) where available	Type VII collagen
Bullous systemic lupus erythematosus (BSLE)	Subepidermal blister with neutrophils in the papillary dermis (DH or LABD like). Histological features of cutaneous lupus are occasionally present.	DIF: Linear or granular IgG and C3, IgM or IgA at BMZ. u-serrated. IIF (salt split skin): Negative or dermal (floor) binding IgG BMZ autoantibodies.	Type VII collagen is the most common target.
Anti-p200 pemphigoid	Subepidermal blister with neutrophilic or eosinophilic dermal inflammatory infiltrate.	DIF: Linear IgG and C3 at BMZ, n-serrated. IIF (salt split skin): Dermal (floor) binding IgG BMZ antibodies. Immunoblotting or ELISA for laminin β4 and/or Laminin γ1 antibody where available	Laminin β4, Laminin γ1 subunit

Abbreviations: BMZ, basement membrane zone; BP180, type XVII collagen/bullous pemphigoid antigen 2; BP180 NC16a domain, type XVII collagen noncollagenous 16a domain; BP230, bullous pemphigoid antigen 1; DIF, direct immunofluorescence; Dsg, desmoglein; ELISA, enzyme-linked immunosorbent assay; IIF, indirect immunofluorescence; LAD-1, linear IgA bullous dermatosis antigen I; TG2, tissue transglutaminase 2; TG3, tissue transglutaminase 3/epidermal transglutaminase.

of other mucosal surfaces can occur as an initial or concurrent presentation in PV, leading to considerable morbidity. The typical skin lesions of mucocutaneous PV are flaccid blisters or erosions that heal with hyperpigmentation in skin of color [**Figure 87-5**]. The scalp and nail unit can be affected by pemphigus vulgaris, leading to alopecia, paronychia, and onychomadesis. Pemphigus vegetans presents with pustules and vegetative plaques involving the scalp, face, and intertriginous areas.

Pemphigus foliaceus is characterized by erosions with overlying cornflake like scales [**Figure 87-6**] in the face, scalp, and trunk [**Figure 87-7**] with no mucosal involvement. Erythroderma can occur in severe cases of PF. Senear-Usher syndrome (pemphigus erythematosus) presents with erythematous scaly plaques on the malar cheeks reminiscent of the malar rash of acute cutaneous lupus. Endemic pemphigus foliaceus is clinically identical to pemphigus foliaceus and less commonly presents with annular exfoliative plaques, erythroderma, diffuse hyperpigmentation (involving lesional and nonlesional skin), or keratotic lesions. Drug-induced pemphigus can present as pemphigus foliaceus or pemphigus vulgaris. Patients can go into remission if the offending drug is identified and stopped. The Pemphigus Disease Area Index (PDAI) can be used to grade the severity of pemphigus and to guide therapeutic decisions[21].

The goal of treatment is to achieve and maintain disease remission with the least treatment-related side effects.[22-25] Rituximab is the only drug with a U.S. Food and Drug Administration-approved indication for treating adult patients with moderate to severe pemphigus vulgaris in combination with oral glucocorticoids.[26,27] Many other systemic medications for the treatment of pemphigus are used off-label. For milder forms of pemphigus (mild: PDAI score ≤ 15), a tapering course of oral prednisone 0.5 to 1 mg/kg/day with anti-inflammatory immunomodulating therapy (dapsone, tetracycline antibiotics) or steroid-sparing immunosuppressive agents (mycophenolate mofetil, azathioprine), or early use of intravenous rituximab can be considered. The treatment of choice for moderate to severe pemphigus foliaceus and pemphigus vulgaris (moderate: PDAI score >15 to ≤ 45, severe: PDAI score > 45) is intravenous rituximab and a tapering course of oral prednisone 0.5 to 1 mg/kg/day. Patients with recalcitrant pemphigus can be treated with intravenous immunoglobulins, immunoadsorption, intravenous pulsed corticosteroid, cyclophosphamide, or novel agents in a clinical trial. Pretreatment

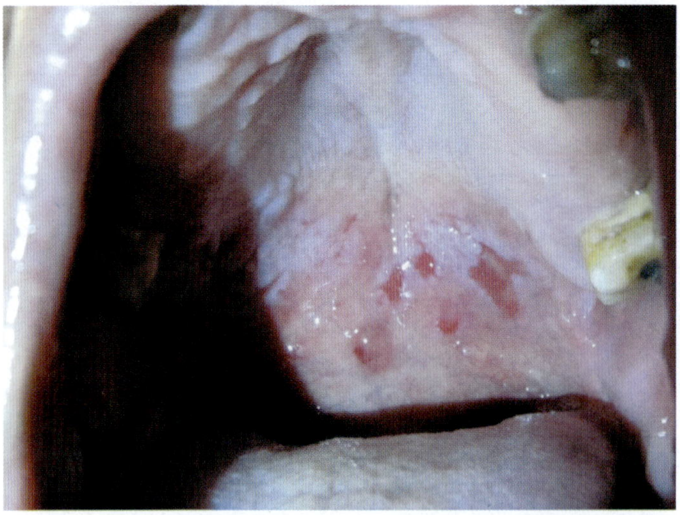

FIGURE 87-3. Erosions on the palatal mucosa in a patient with pemphigus vulgaris.

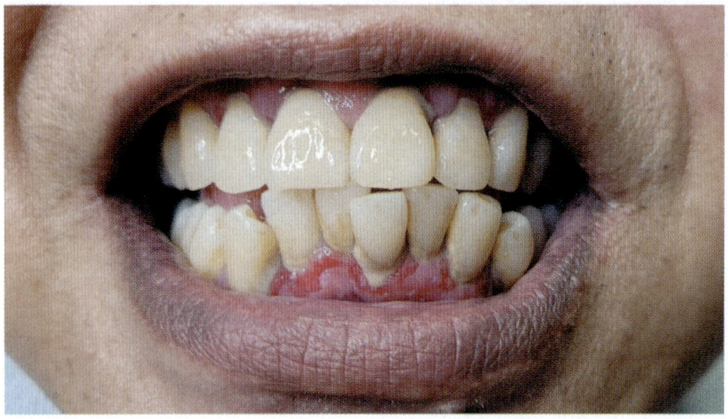

FIGURE 87-4. Desquamative gingivitis in a patient with pemphigus vulgaris.

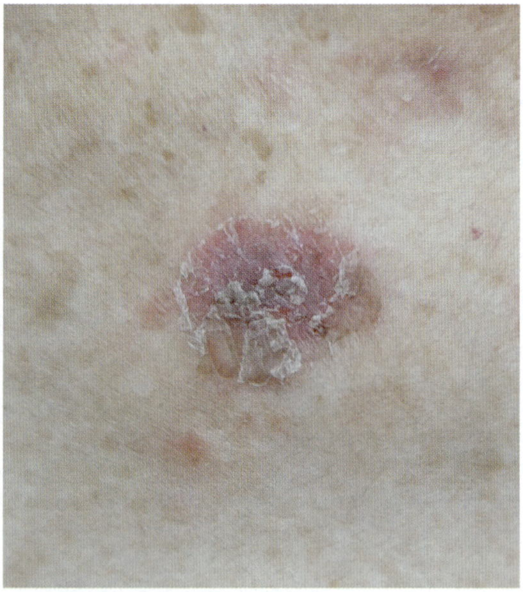

FIGURE 87-6. Single macular lesion of pemphigus foliaceus demonstrating superficial thin corn-flake-like peeling scale and underlying erythema.

assessment of disease severity, comorbidities, active or chronic infections, and malignancies will determine the chosen treatment modality and timing of treatment initiation. The therapeutic pipeline for pemphigus appears promising with several agents targeting B cells and immunoglobulins in preclinical and phase 2 to 3 trials.[17,22]

Local therapy with topical glucocorticoids or topical calcineurin inhibitors, wound care, and pain relief contribute to the patient's recovery. Concurrent impetigo or herpes simplex infections should be screened for and treated appropriately when faced with slow healing skin or mucosal erosions. Patients with oral erosions benefit from a diet with a soft consistency and maintenance of oral hygiene with antiseptic or antibacterial/anticandida mouth wash. Referral to an oral medicine specialist, otorhinolaryngologist, or gastroenterologist may be necessary if other mucosal surfaces are involved.

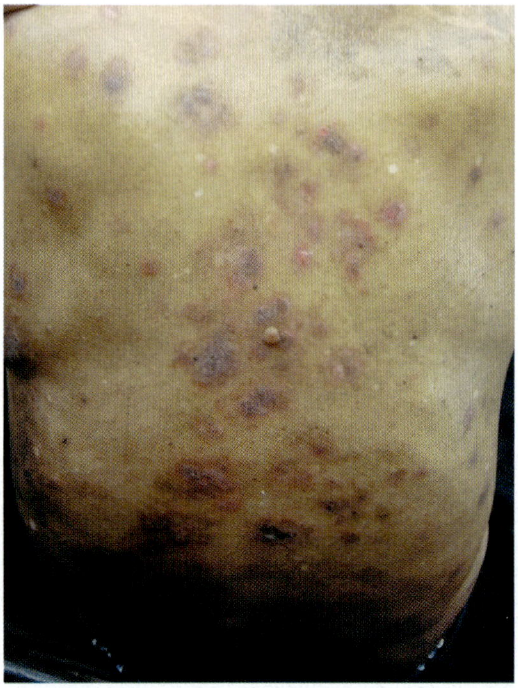

FIGURE 87-5. Resolving pemphigus vulgaris plaques on the back of an Asian patient demonstrating erythema and postinflammatory hyperpigmentation.

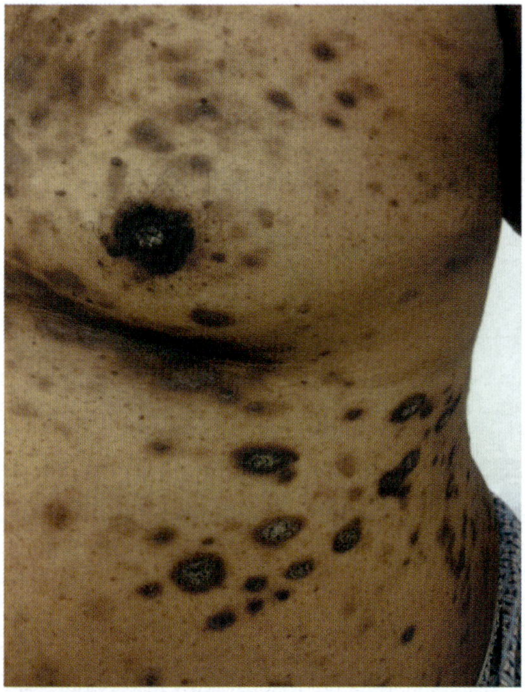

FIGURE 87-7. Hyperpigmented macules with overlying hyperkeratotic scale on the trunk of an African patient with pemphigus foliaceus.

PARANEOPLASTIC PEMPHIGUS

Paraneoplastic pemphigus (PNP) is also known as paraneoplastic autoimmune multiorgan syndrome (PAMS).[28] It is a distinct neoplasia-associated multiorgan inflammatory reaction mediated by both the humoral and cellular immune responses to epithelial cell junction proteins. Autoantibodies against the plakin family of cell junction proteins (envoplakin, periplakin, bullous pemphigoid antigen 1 (BP230), desmoplakin I, desmoplakin II, plectin), α-2-macroglobulin-like-1, desmoglein 1, desmoglein 3, plakophilin 3, and desmocollins 1 to 3 have been described.[29] The mean age of presentation is 51 years with near equal female-to-male ratio.[19] Twenty-two percent of patients with PNP/PAMS presented at the age of 30 years or less.[19] The commonest associated neoplasm in childhood, Chinese, and South Korean patients is Castleman disease. Lymphoproliferative malignancies accounts for the majority of malignancies described with adult PNP/PAMS in the western literature, while thymoma, Castleman disease, carcinomas, and sarcomas are less common.[19] In a case series of Chinese patients, myasthenia gravis was found to coexist with PNP/PAMS in 35% of their cohort, and was mostly seen in patients with PNP/PAMS due to thymoma and Castleman disease.[30]

Mucosal involvement is present in the majority of patients with PNP/PAMS and may be the sole manifestation. Recalcitrant extensive stomatitis that extends to the vermillion lip is the commonest presentation. The bronchial, conjunctival, anogenital, oropharyngeal, and esophageal mucosa can be affected. Skin involvement can range from pemphigoid-like tense blisters, pemphigus-like erosions, erythema multiforme-like lesions, lichenoid plaques [**Figure 87-8**], graft versus host disease-like lesions, erythroderma, and toxic epidermal necrolysis-like presentation. The mortality rate of PNP/PAMS is high. Infections, progression of underlying neoplasia, or respiratory failure from bronchiolitis obliterans are the main causes of death. Erythema multiforme-like skin lesions with extensive mucocutaneous involvement predicted a worse outcome in a French case series.[31]

The histology of PNP/PAMS depends on the clinical presentation and predominant underlying immune response. Tissue bound and circulating disease-specific autoantibodies can be demonstrated through various immunologic tests[29] [Table 87-1]. These autoantibodies may be difficult to detect in patients after receiving rituximab or other immunosuppressive therapy for the underlying malignancy. A combination of clinical, histopathological, and immunological features is required to diagnose PNP/PAMS.[28] Treatment of PNP/PAMS is difficult. The disease may progress despite treatment of the underlying neoplasm. High-dose systemic steroids, steroid-sparing immunosuppressive agents, rituximab, and intravenous immunoglobulin have been reported to be useful but should be initiated in consultation with the oncologist.[22,28]

BULLOUS PEMPHIGOID

Bullous pemphigoid (BP) is caused by autoantibodies targeting the hemidesmosome proteins type XVII collagen (BP180/BPAG2) and bullous pemphigoid antigen 1 (BP230/BPAG1). Binding of the autoreactive IgG1, IgG4, and IgE autoantibodies to the target antigens leads to a downstream cascade that include FcγR- and FcεR-mediated complement activation, infiltration and activation of neutrophils, eosinophils, and mast cells; as well as IgG4-induced BP180 and BP230 internalization via macropinocytosis and secretion of IL-6 and IL-8 by basal keratinocytes. The end result is cutaneous inflammation and subepidermal blister formation.[17] Medications, isomorphic responses to cutaneous trauma (radiotherapy, phototherapy, stoma sites, and burns) and neuropsychiatric conditions were found to be associated with a higher risk of developing BP.[32] The high-risk medications include furosemide, spironolactone, phenothiazine, penicillamine, terbinafine, rivaroxaban, angiotensin-converting enzyme inhibitors, SARS-CoV-2 vaccination,[20] dipeptidyl peptidase IV inhibitors,[33] and immune checkpoint inhibitors.[34] Bullous pemphigoid can occur in patients with concurrent chronic inflammatory dermatoses such as lichen planus, atopic dermatitis, and psoriasis. Acquired hemophilia A is an uncommon bleeding disorder that has a strong association with bullous pemphigoid.[35] It is due to autoantibodies to Factor VIII and presents with a prolonged activated partial thromboplastin time and increased risk of life-threatening bleeding.

Bullous pemphigoid is very common, with an estimated incidence of 10 to 43 per million persons per year.[32] It is typically seen in elderly patients who are also frail and have multiple comorbidities.[36] Adolescent and childhood bullous pemphigoid cases are rare.[37,38] The 1-year standardized mortality ratio was 2.93 from a meta-analysis of the world-wide published literature with no significant difference in standardized mortality ratio between the United States, Europe, and Asia.[39] The main causes of death were infectious and cardiovascular diseases.[39]

Early or prebullous BP appears as intensely pruritic eczematous or urticated papules and plaques. It can be mistaken for other inflammatory skin diseases. Large tense blisters arising on normal or inflamed skin develop subsequently [**Figure 87-9**] and heal with significant dyschromia and occasionally milia formation [**Figure 87-10**]. The blisters can be localized at particular sites (pretibial, peristomal, periumbilical,

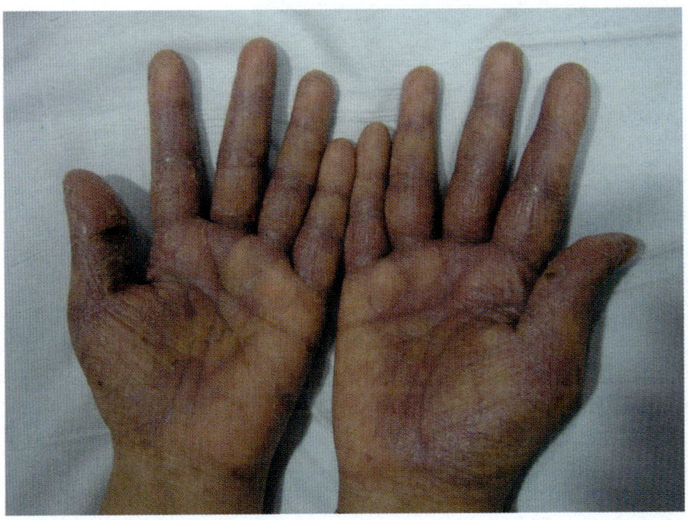

FIGURE 87-8. Violaceous scaly plaques on the palms of an Asian patient with paraneoplastic pemphigus.

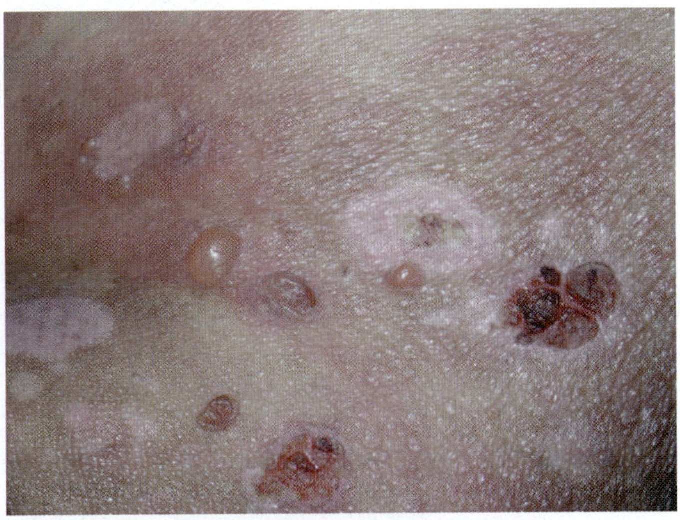

FIGURE 87-9. Tense blisters arising on an erythematous plaque, crusted erosions, and postinflammatory hypopigmented macules on the trunk of an Asian patient with bullous pemphigoid. (Used with permission from Dr. Shan-Xian Lee, Changi General Hospital, Singapore.)

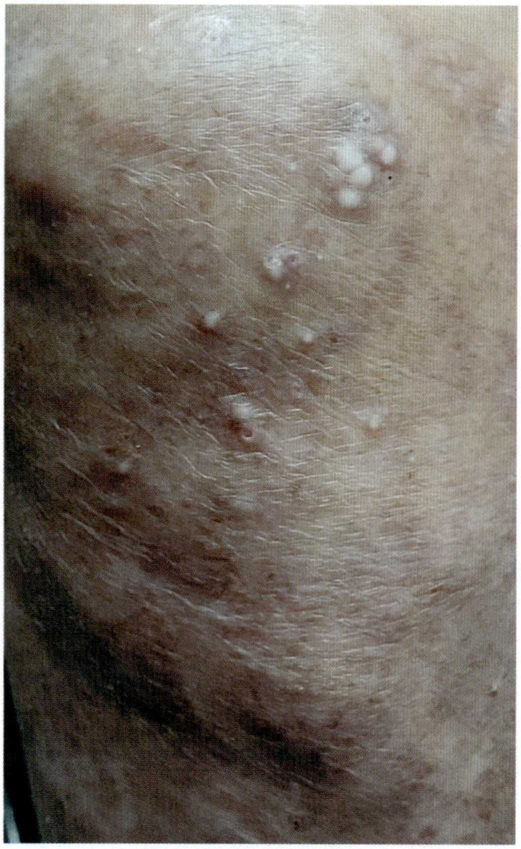

FIGURE 87-10. Cluster of milia and multiple postinflammatory hypopigmented macules on the right knee of an Asian patient with bullous pemphigoid.

genital, extremities) or in a zosteriform distribution [**Figure 87-11**]. The blisters can be distributed predominantly on acral skin [**Figure 87-12**], mimicking severe pompholyx or bullous scabies. Prurigo-like lesions is the predominant feature in pemphigoid nodularis [**Figure 87-13**]. Predominant flexural involvement, generalized erythrodermic or toxic epidermal necrolysis-like pemphigoid are not commonly seen. Oral mucosal involvement occurs in about 10% to 30% of patients. Nail involvement is occasionally seen. Childhood BP has a predilection for acral skin and genitalia. The Bullous Pemphigoid Disease Area Index (BPDAI) can be used to grade the severity of bullous pemphigoid.[40,41]

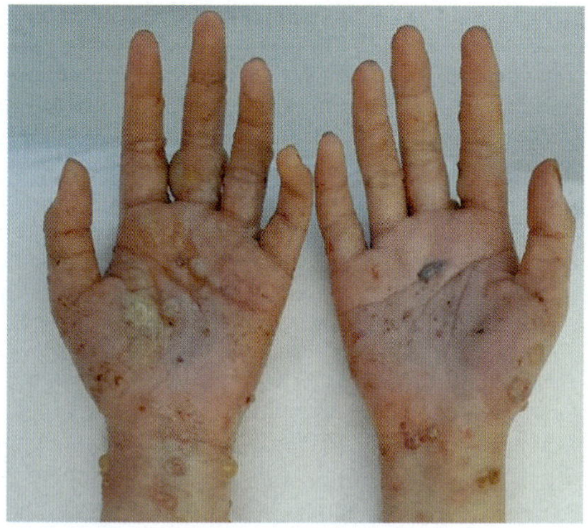

FIGURE 87-12. Clusters of pompholyx-like pseudovesicles and tense bulla on the palms of a patient with acral dyshidrosiform bullous pemphigoid.

Clinical, pathological, and immunofluorescence correlation is required to confirm the diagnosis of bullous pemphigoid [Table 87-2]. The goals of treatment in BP are to achieve clinical remission with the least treatment-related side effects. In frail elderly pemphigoid patients, this should take into account the comorbid conditions, presence of chronic infections, potential drug interactions, compliance, and the presence of a reliable caregiver to administer topical and systemic therapy. In patients with localized pemphigoid lesions, topical steroid therapy, wound care, and treatment of secondary skin infection are often sufficient. Patients who have mild to moderate disease (mild: BPDAI score < 20, moderate: BPDAI score between 20 and <57) not responding to topical therapy or have moderate to severe bullous pemphigoid (severe: BPDAI score ≥ 57) can be treated with whole body (excluding face) application of potent topical steroid (eg, clobetasol propionate 0.05% cream) in a tapering regimen[42] or oral prednisone taper at a starting dose of 0.5 to 0.75 mg/kg/day.[41,43] Adjunctive therapy with doxycycline, dapsone, methotrexate, azathioprine, or mycophenolate can be considered for their steroid sparing effect.[41,43] Patients with severe and steroid resistant disease can be treated with IV rituximab, intravenous immunoglobulins, cyclophosphamide, immunoadsorption, or plasma exchange.[41,43] Omalizumab and dupilumab have been used to treat bullous pemphigoid off-label, and a trial of dupilumab is ongoing.[41,43] Therapies targeting complements, leukotriene B4, Ig E, Eotaxin-1, and interleukins 4, 5, 12, and 23 are currently being investigated for bullous pemphigoid.[17]

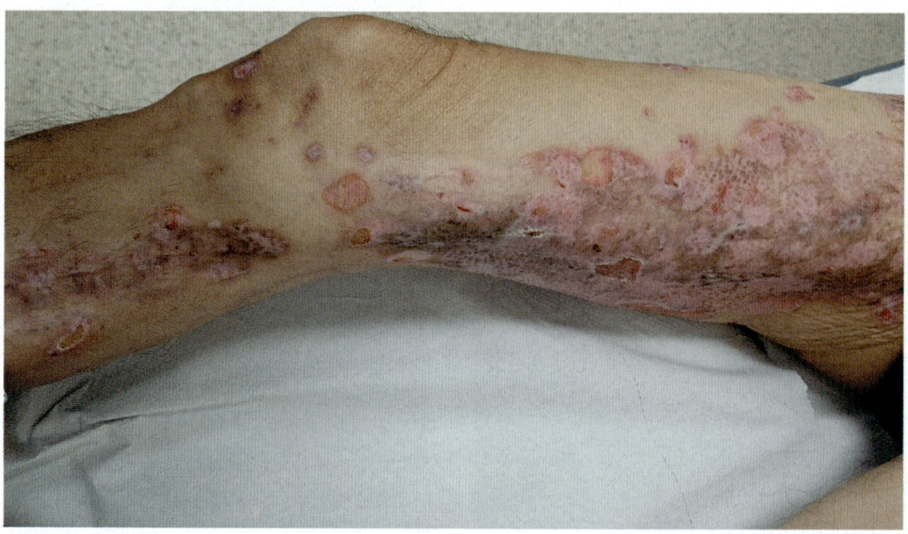

FIGURE 87-11. Zosteriform bullous pemphigoid on the right inner thigh and right medial calf of an Asian patient, demonstrating intact blisters, healing erosions, and multiple postinflammatory depigmented patches with follicular repigmentation.

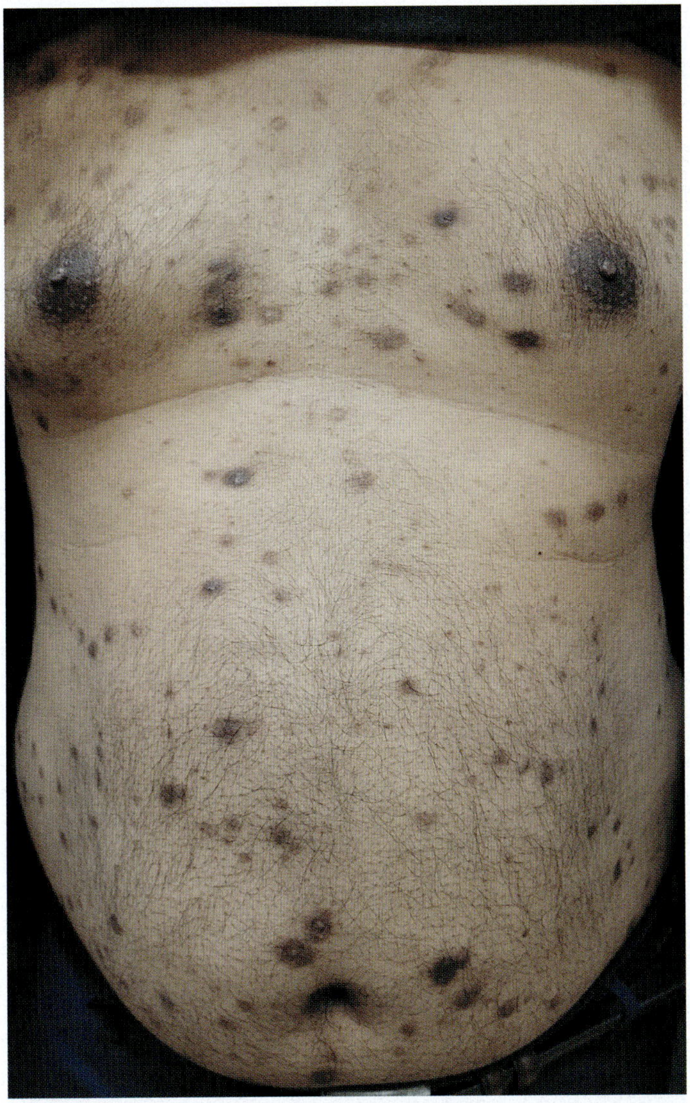

FIGURE 87-13. An Asian patient with pemphigoid nodularis demonstrating multiple prurigo-like papules and nodules and postinflammatory hyperpigmented macules on the anterior trunk.

LINEAR IgA BULLOUS DERMATOSIS

Linear IgA bullous dermatosis (LABD) is a rare subepidermal autoimmune blistering disease that is defined by a mucocutaneous blistering eruption in the presence of linear IgA autoantibody deposits at the basement membrane zone on direct immunofluorescence.[32] The IgA autoantibodies target various proteins in the hemidesmosome and can be classified into the lamina lucida type (targeting the 97-kDa and 120-kDa cleaved ectodomains or NC16a domain of type XVII collagen/BP180) and sublamina densa type (targeting type VII collagen or laminin γ-1).[44] LABD has been associated with various genes (*HLA Cw7*, *B8*, *DR3*, and the *TNF-2* gene), medications (mostly antibiotics and especially vancomycin[45]), vaccines (including the SARS-CoV-2 vaccine[20]), malignancies, inflammatory bowel diseases, autoimmune conditions, and infections by various organisms.[46]

The incidence of LABD was estimated to be 1 per million people per year in Germany, while the incidence was estimated to be higher in African countries (Uganda, Mali, and South Africa), probably due to its younger population.[47] It can be seen in both adults and children and is rarely reported in neonates. Disease remission in childhood LABD was seen in 64% of cases within 2 years of disease while neonatal cases have a poor prognosis from respiratory mucosal involvement.[46] Elderly idiopathic LABD patients above 70 years old without mucosal involvement have a better chance of disease remission compared to younger adult LABD patients.[48] Cessation of the culprit drug can lead to disease remission in drug-induced LABD.[45]

Urticated annular plaques with central healing and peripheral tense blisters ("string of pearls" sign) are classically found in LABD [**Figure 87-14**]. These lesions are commonly located on the abdomen, perioral, and perineal region in childhood LABD.[32,46] Adult LABD presents with scattered vesicles or bulla, while "string of pearls" or herpetiform lesions are less commonly seen. LABD can affect mucosal sites and cause scarring and morbidity.[46,48] Drug-induced LABD can present with typical lesions or atypically with less frequent mucosal involvement (erythema multiforme-like, toxic epidermal necrolysis-like, morbilliform and localized forms).[45]

Histologic and immunofluorescence features are highlighted in Table 87-2. Most patients respond to dapsone treatment. Systemic corticosteroids can be added if the patient does not respond fully to dapsone or in more extensive disease. Other immunomodulatory (nicotinamide, colchicine, sulfapyridine, antibiotics, and IVIG) or immunosuppressive (azathioprine, cyclosporine, mycophenolate mofetil, rituximab, and tumor necrosis factor-α (TNF-α) inhibitors) agents can be used if

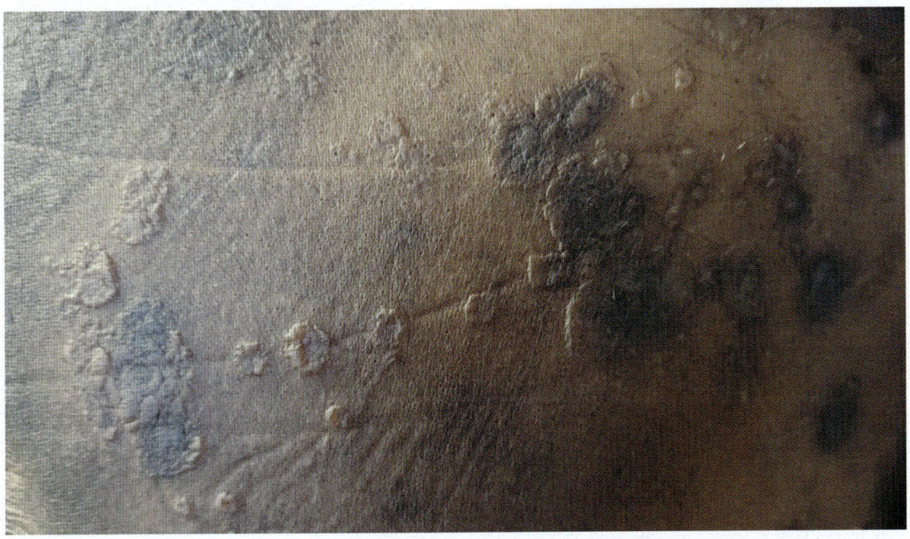

FIGURE 87-14. Annular "string of pearls" blisters with central patches of postinflammatory hyperpigmentation in a south Asian male (Fitzpatrick type V skin) with vancomycin-induced linear IgA bullous dermatosis. Note the difficulty in discerning erythema on the affected skin.

dapsone and prednisone are contraindicated or are ineffective, although this is based on data from case reports and case series.[41,46,48]

DERMATITIS HERPETIFORMIS

Dermatitis herpetiformis (DH) is a unique autoimmune blistering disease arising from gluten (found in wheat, barley, rye, and oat) hypersensitivity. It is seen in patients of Northern European descent and is rare in Asians and African Americans. In genetically predisposed individuals with HLA-DQ2 or DQ8 haplotypes, intestinal tissue transglutaminase 2 modify gliadin in gluten into an autoantigen that binds strongly to HLA-DQ2 or DQ8 on antigen presenting cells. This results in T- and B-cell stimulation and an inflammatory response against gliadin and tissue transglutaminase 2-gliadin complexes in the intestinal mucosa, leading to celiac disease. High-affinity IgA autoantibodies against epidermal transglutaminase 3 are produced by epitope spread. These form immune complexes with keratinocyte derived epidermal transglutaminase 3 in the dermal papillae, leading to a neutrophilic inflammatory response with subepidermal blister formation in DH.[32,49,50]

Patients present with itchy urticated plaques and excoriated papulovesicles predominantly distributed on the extensor surfaces (scalp, shoulders, back, buttocks, elbows, and knees). Acral purpura [**Figure 87-15**] is characteristically seen in DH. Mucosal involvement is rare. Patients with DH have concurrent celiac disease that can range from asymptomatic to severely symptomatic. All patients with DH should receive gastroenterological evaluation. Associations with other organ specific autoimmune diseases (such as autoimmune thyroid disease, type 1 diabetes mellitus, Addison disease, vitiligo, alopecia areata), non-Hodgkin lymphomas (mucosa-associated lymphoid tissue and B-cell lymphoma), splenic atrophy, partial IgA deficiency, neurologic involvement, and iodine sensitivity have been reported. Patients should be monitored accordingly.[32,49,50]

The diagnosis of DH requires consistent findings from histology and direct immunofluorescence studies [Table 87-2]. Indirect immunofluorescence microscopy and ELISA can detect circulating IgA autoantibodies against the endomysium and tissue transglutaminases accordingly. ELISA testing for IgG antitransglutaminase antibodies can be used if patients have concurrent IgA deficiency.[32,49,50]

Patients with symptomatic DH respond rapidly to dapsone. However, clinical remission of dermatitis herpetiformis and celiac disease and a reduced risk of lymphoma is possible only with a lifelong gluten-free diet. Patients who are unable to tolerate dapsone can be treated with sulfasalazine. Other immunosuppressive or immunomodulatory agents that have shown efficacy in case reports include tetracycline antibiotics, nicotinamide, colchicine, methotrexate, mycophenolate, azathioprine and rituximab.[41,49,50]

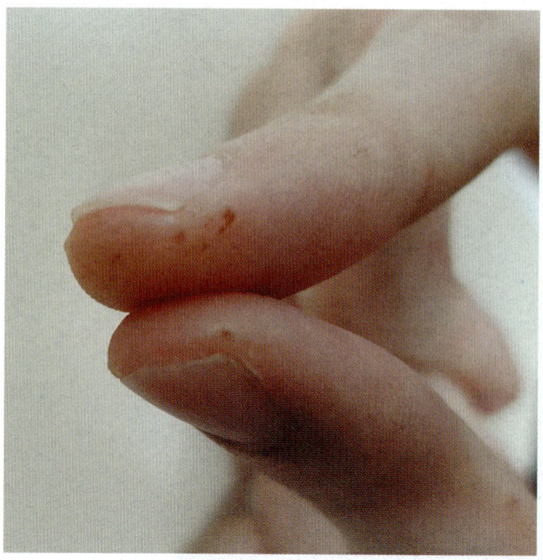

FIGURE 87-15. Acral petechiae in an Asian patient with dermatitis herpetiformis. Biopsy of the petechial lesion revealed typical histological findings of dermatitis herpetiformis (not shown).

MUCOUS MEMBRANE PEMPHIGOID

Mucous membrane pemphigoid (MMP)[51-53] refers to a group of autoimmune subepithelial blistering disease with different immunoglobulin class specificity and/or hemidesmosome antigen targets that shares the common phenotype of predominant mucosal involvement. In the latest 2021 European guidelines on MMP,[51,52] entities such as linear IgA disease and epidermolysis bullosa acquisita with predominant mucosal involvement were subsumed under the diagnosis of MMP. MMP is seen mainly in the elderly. Its incidence was 1 per million per year in France[54] to 2 per million persons per year in Germany,[47] and was reported to be rare among autoimmune blistering diseases in Turkey,[55] Sudan,[56] and Iran.[57] BP180 is more frequently targeted compared to BP230, laminin 332, α6β4 integrin, and collagen VII.[51] Dipeptidyl peptidase-4 inhibitors and immune checkpoint inhibitor-associated MMP has been described.[51] Patients with anti-laminin 332 MMP may benefit from screening for an associated solid organ malignancy.[51]

Multiple mucosal surfaces can be involved either singly or in combination in MMP. Skin involvement tends to be mild and uncommon except for the Brunsting-Perry mucosal pemphigoid variant where the skin of the scalp, head, and neck is predominantly affected. The oral mucosa [**Figure 87-16**] is more frequently involved compared to the other mucosal surfaces (ocular [**Figure 87-17**], laryngeal, esophageal, tracheal, and genitourinary mucosa). Inflammation and scarring of mucosal surfaces other than the oral mucosa can lead to significant morbidity (eg, blindness) or mortality (eg, from airway impairment). The Oral Disease

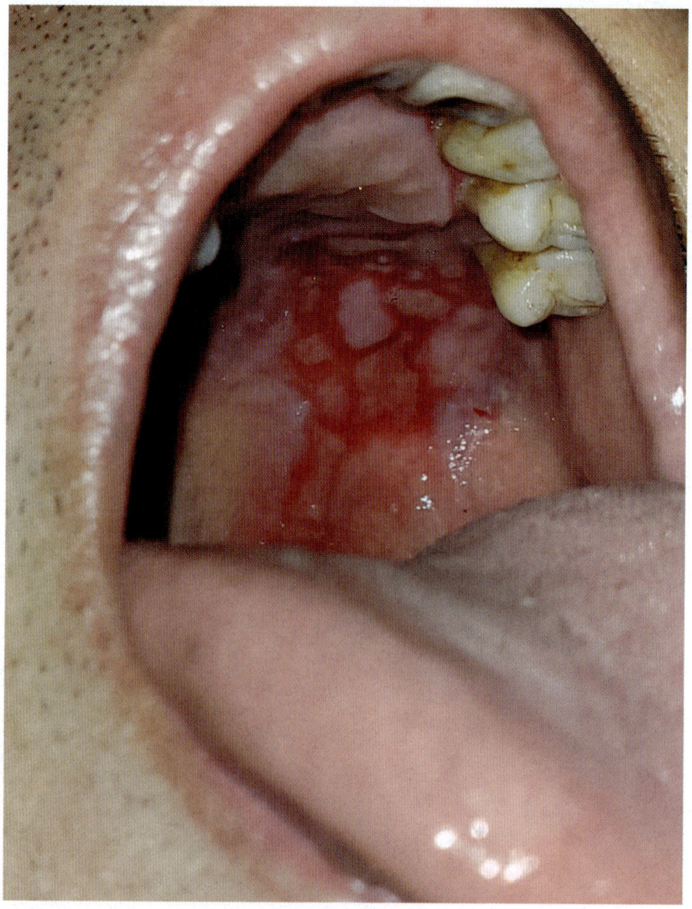

FIGURE 87-16. Erosions on the left palate in an Asian patient with mucous membrane pemphigoid.

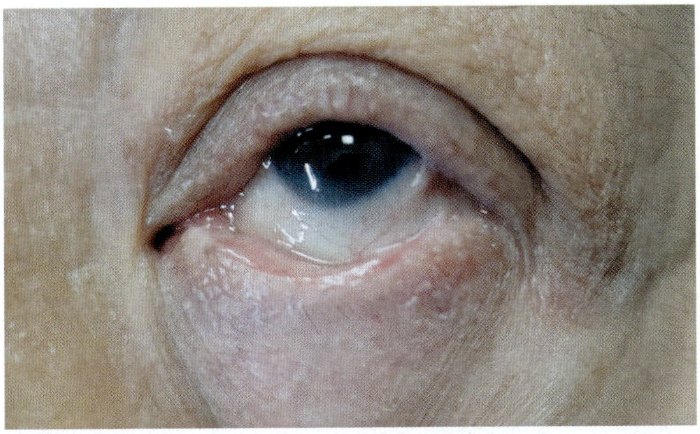

FIGURE 87-17. Symblepharon, entropion, and upper and lower eyelid trichiasis affecting the left eye of an Asian patient with mucous membrane pemphigoid.

Severity Score (ODSS) is a validated scoring system to assess the severity of oral MMP.[58] The Mucosal Membrane Pemphigoid Disease Activity Index (MMPDAI) can be used to grade the severity of milder forms of MMP although it has not been validated formally.[59]

It is more difficult to confirm the diagnosis of MMP because the site of involvement may not be amenable to a biopsy, and the yield of direct and indirect immunofluorescence studies is lower, especially for ocular MMP[51,53] [Table 87-2]. Treatment is tailored to the site(s) of disease and degree of activity and scarring, and requires a multidisciplinary approach. Oral MMP is usually mild to moderately severe and can be managed with anti-inflammatory agents (dapsone, methotrexate, tetracycline antibiotics, topical corticosteroids) initially. Patients with extra-oral mucosal involvement is deemed to have severe MMP and require aggressive systemic immunosuppressive therapy (steroids, cyclophosphamide, rituximab, IV immunoglobulins, or anti-TNF-α biologic) to prevent scarring.[52]

EPIDERMOLYSIS BULLOSA ACQUISITA

Epidermolysis bullosa acquisita (EBA) is a subepidermal blistering disease characterized by autoantibodies against type VII collagen (predominantly the NC1 domain) on the anchoring fibrils of the dermoepidermal junction.[60] It was reported to be rare in Germany (0.5 per million per year)[47] and France (0.17-0.26 per million per year).[54] In comparison, EBA was more common in skin of color populations,[61-64] and was found to be associated with HLA-DRB1*15:03 in French cohort of African Black patients,[62] HLA-DR2 in an American cohort,[63] and HLA- DRB1*13 in a Korean cohort.[64] EBA affects all age groups with a median age of 50 years and a slight female preponderance.[65]

Affected patients manifest either a noninflammatory mechanobullous phenotype [**Figure 87-18**] or mimic the presentation of other subepidermal autoimmune blistering diseases (bullous pemphigoid, mucous membrane pemphigoid, Brunsting Perry pemphigoid, or linear IgA bullous dermatosis).[66] Occasionally, a patient can have both inflammatory and noninflammatory mechanobullous lesions simultaneously.[65,66] Inflammatory bowel diseases (predominantly Crohn disease),[67] rheumatoid arthritis, and thyroiditis were more commonly associated with EBA.[62] The histologic and immunofluorescence findings[66] are summarized in Table 87-2. EBA can be chronic and refractory to treatment. Patients should actively protect the skin from trauma. Because of its rarity, there are no randomized controlled therapeutic trials to date. Milder forms of EBA can respond to anti-inflammatory agents (such as dapsone and colchicine).[41] Systemic corticosteroids and steroid-sparing immunosuppressive medications (such as azathioprine, mycophenolate mofetil, cyclosporine, methotrexate, cyclophosphamide, IVIG, and rituximab) can be used in more severe disease, although patients are often less steroid responsive and require a longer course of systemic steroids.[41,65]

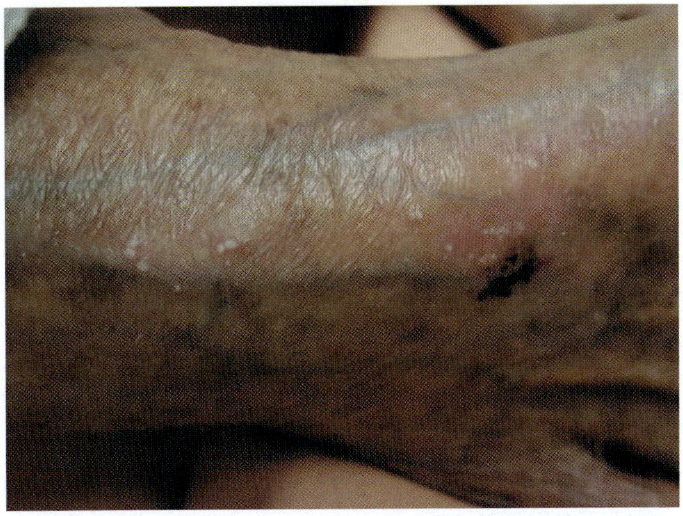

FIGURE 87-18. Two clusters of milia on the dorsum of the right foot in an Asian patient with epidermolysis bullosa acquisita.

REFERENCES

1. Witte M, Zillikens D, Schmidt E. Diagnosis of autoimmune blistering diseases. *Front Med (Lausanne)*. 2018;5:296.
2. Mutasim DF, Adams BB. Immunofluorescence in dermatology. *J Am Acad Dermatol*. 2001;45:803-822.
3. Miller DD, Bhawan J. Bullous tinea pedis with direct immunofluorescence positivity: when is a positive result not autoimmune bullous disease. *Am J Dermatopathol*. 2013;35:587-594.
4. Kridin K, Bergman R. The usefulness of indirect immunofluorescence in pemphigus and the natural history of patients with initial false-positive results: a retrospective cohort study. *Front Med (Lausanne)*. 2018;5:266.
5. P Shah, K Svigos, L Yin, et al. Differences in the clinical presentation of bullous pemphigoid in patients with skin of colour and patients with white skin. *Br J Dermatol*. 2021;185:430-432.
6. De D, Khullar G, Handa S, et al. Clinical, demographic and immunopathological spectrum of subepidermal autoimmune bullous diseases at a tertiary center: a 1-year audit. *Indian J Dermatol Venereol Leprol*. 2016;82:358.
7. Nanda A, Dvorak R, Al-Saeed K, et al. Spectrum of autoimmune bullous diseases in Kuwait. *Int J Dermatol*. 2004;43:876-881.
8. Hübner F, Langan EA, Recke A. Lichen planus pemphigoides: from lichenoid inflammation to autoantibody-mediated blistering. *Front Immunol*. 2019;10:1389.
9. Webb AR, Kazantzidis A, Kift RC, et al. Colour counts: sunlight and skin type as drivers of vitamin D deficiency at UK latitudes. *Nutrients*. 2018;10:457.
10. Nkhoma ET, Poole C, Vannappagari V, et al. The global prevalence of glucose-6-phosphate dehydrogenase deficiency: a systematic review and meta-analysis. *Blood Cells Mol Dis*. 2009;42:267-278.
11. Tangamornsuksan W, Lohitnavy M. Association between HLA-B*1301 and dapsone-induced cutaneous adverse drug reactions: a systematic review and meta-analysis. *JAMA Dermatol*. 2018;154:441-446.
12. Shipman KE, Shipman AR, Marinaki AM. Genotyping before azathioprine administration in dermatology. *Clin Exp Dermatol*. 2022;47:503-504.
13. Laniosz V, Lehman JS, Poland GA, et al. Literature-based immunization recommendations for patients requiring immunosuppressive medications for autoimmune bullous dermatoses. *Int J Dermatol*. 2016;55:599-607.
14. Li TF, Tang-Lin L, Ang CC. A retrospective cohort study of hepatitis B reactivation in patients with autoimmune bullous diseases on immunosuppressive therapy in Singapore. *J Am Acad Dermatol*. 2021;85:1017-1020.
15. Keith PJ, Wetter DA, Wilson JW, et al. Evidence-based guidelines for laboratory screening for infectious diseases before initiation of systemic immunosuppressive agents in patients with autoimmune bullous dermatoses. *Br J Dermatol*. 2014;171:1307-1317.
16. Montagnon CM, Tolkachjov SN, Murrell DF, et al. Intraepithelial autoimmune blistering dermatoses: clinical features and diagnosis. *J Am Acad Dermatol*. 2021;84:1507-1519.
17. Ellebrecht CT, Maseda D, Payne AS. Pemphigus and pemphigoid: from disease mechanisms to druggable pathways. *J Invest Dermatol*. 2022;142(3 Pt B): 907-914.

18. Di Lullo G, Calabresi V, Mariotti F, et al. Identification of a novel non-desmoglein autoantigen in pemphigus vulgaris. *Front Immunol.* 2019;10:1391.
19. Kridin K, Schmidt E. Epidemiology of pemphigus. *JID Innov.* 2021;1:100004.
20. Calabria E, Canfora F, Mascolo M, et al. Autoimmune mucocutaneous blistering diseases after SARS-Cov-2 vaccination: a case report of pemphigus vulgaris and a literature review. *Pathol Res Pract.* 2022;232:153834.
21. Boulard C, Duvert Lehembre S, Picard-Dahan C, et al. Calculation of cut-off values based on the autoimmune bullous skin disorder intensity score (ABSIS) and Pemphigus Disease Area Index (PDAI) pemphigus scoring systems for defining moderate, significant and extensive types of pemphigus. *Br J Dermatol.* 2016;175:142-149.
22. Montagnon CM, Lehman JS, Murrell DF, et al. Intraepithelial autoimmune bullous dermatoses disease activity assessment and therapy. *J Am Acad Dermatol.* 2021;84:1523-1537.
23. Joly P, Horvath B, Patsatsi A, et al. Updated S2K guidelines on the management of pemphigus vulgaris and foliaceus initiated by the European academy of dermatology and venereology (EADV). *J Eur Acad Dermatol Venereol.* 2020;34:1900-1913.
24. Harman KE, Brown D, Exton LS, et al. British Association of Dermatologists' guidelines for the management of pemphigus vulgaris 2017. *Br J Dermatol.* 2017;177:1170-1201.
25. Murrell DF, Peña S, Joly P, et al. Diagnosis and management of pemphigus: Recommendations of an international panel of experts. *J Am Acad Dermatol.* 2020;82:575-585.e1.
26. Joly P, Maho-Vaillant M, Prost-Squarcioni C, et al. First-line rituximab combined with short-term prednisone versus prednisone alone for the treatment of pemphigus (Ritux 3): a prospective, multicentre, parallel-group, open-label randomised trial. *Lancet.* 2017; 389:2031-2040.
27. Werth VP, Joly P, Mimouni D, et al. Rituximab versus mycophenolate mofetil in patients with pemphigus vulgaris. *N Engl J Med.* 2021;384:2295-2305.
28. Didona D, DI Zenzo G, Joly P. Paraneoplastic autoimmune multiorgan syndrome. *Ital J Dermatol Venerol.* 2021;156:174-183.
29. Poot AM, Diercks GF, Kramer D, et al. Laboratory diagnosis of paraneoplastic pemphigus. *Br J Dermatol.* 2013;169:1016-1024.
30. Wang R, Li J, Wang M, et al. Prevalence of myasthenia gravis and associated autoantibodies in paraneoplastic pemphigus and their correlations with symptoms and prognosis. *Br J Dermatol.* 2015;172:968e75.
31. Leger S, Picard D, Ingen-Housz-Oro S, et al. Prognostic factors of paraneoplastic pemphigus. *Arch Dermatol.* 2012;148:1165e72.
32. Montagnon CM, Tolkachjov SN, Murrell DF, et al. Subepithelial autoimmune blistering dermatoses: clinical features and diagnosis. *J Am Acad Dermatol.* 2021;85:1-14.
33. Kridin K, Avni O, Damiani G, et al. Dipeptidyl-peptidase IV inhibitor (DPP4i) confers increased odds of bullous pemphigoid even years after drug initiation. *Arch Dermatol Res.* 2023;315(1):33-39.
34. Asdourian MS, Shah N, Jacoby TV, et al. Association of bullous pemphigoid with immune checkpoint inhibitor therapy in patients with cancer: a systematic review. *JAMA Dermatol.* 2022;158(8):933-941.
35. Abdul-Halim NA, Ng HJ. Bullous pemphigoid is a common associated disorder with acquired haemophilia A. *Int J Hematol.* 2021;113:58-62.
36. Sim B, Fook-Chong S, Phoon YW, et al. Multimorbidity in bullous pemphigoid: a case–control analysis of bullous pemphigoid patients with age- and gender-matched controls. *J Eur Acad Dermatol Venereol.* 2017;31:1709-1714.
37. Patsatsi A, Kyriakou A, Werth VP. Bullous pemphigoid in adolescence. *Pediatr Dermatol.* 2019;36:184-188.
38. Fisler RE, Saeb M, Liang MG, et al. Childhood bullous pemphigoid: a clinicopathologic study and review of the literature. *Am J Dermatopathol.* 2003;25:183-189.
39. Tedbirt B, Gillibert A, Andrieu E, et al. Mixed individual-aggregate data on all-cause mortality in bullous pemphigoid: a meta-analysis. *JAMA Dermatol.* 2021;157:421-430.
40. Murrell DF, Daniel BS, Joly P, et al. Definitions and outcome measures for bullous pemphigoid: recommendations by an international panel of experts. *J Am Acad Dermatol.* 2012;66:479-485.
41. Montagnon CM, Lehman JS, Murrell DF, et al. Subepithelial autoimmune bullous dermatoses disease activity assessment and therapy. *J Am Acad Dermatol.* 2021;85:18-27.
42. Joly P, Roujeau JC, Benichou J, et al. A comparison of two regimens of topical corticosteroids in the treatment of patients with bullous pemphigoid: a multicenter randomized study. *J Invest Dermatol.* 2009;129:1681-1687.
43. Borradori L, Van Beek N, Feliciani C, et al. Updated S2 K guidelines for the management of bullous pemphigoid initiated by the European Academy of Dermatology and Venereology (EADV). *J Eur Acad Dermatol Venereol.* 2022;36(10):1689-1704.
44. Hashimoto T, Yamagami J, Zone JJ. History, diagnosis, pathogenesis, and nomenclature in sublamina densa-type linear IgA disease. *JAMA Dermatol.* 2021;157:907-909.
45. Garel B, Ingen-Housz-Oro S, Afriat D, et al. Drug-induced linear immunoglobulin A bullous dermatosis: a French retrospective pharmacovigilance study of 69 cases. *Br J Clin Pharmacol.* 2019;85:570-579.
46. Mori F, Saretta F, Liotti L, et al. Linear immunoglobulin A bullous dermatosis in children. *Front Pediatr.* 2022;10:937528.
47. Bertram F, Bröcker EB, Zillikens D, et al. Prospective analysis of the incidence of autoimmune bullous disorders in Lower Franconia, Germany. *J Dtsch Dermatol Ges.* 2009;7:434-440.
48. Gottlieb J, Ingen-Housz-Oro S, Alexandre M, et al. Idiopathic linear IgA bullous dermatosis: prognostic factors based on a case series of 72 adults. *Br J Dermatol.* 2017;177:212-222.
49. Görög A, Antiga E, Caproni M, et al. S2k guidelines (consensus statement) for diagnosis and therapy of dermatitis herpetiformis initiated by the European Academy of Dermatology and Venereology (EADV). *J Eur Acad Dermatol Venereol.* 2021;35:1251-1277.
50. Nguyen CN, Kim SJ. Dermatitis herpetiformis: an update on diagnosis, disease monitoring, and management. *Medicina (Kaunas).* 2021;57:843.
51. Rashid H, Lamberts A, Borradori L, et al. European guidelines (S3) on diagnosis and management of mucous membrane pemphigoid, initiated by the European Academy of Dermatology and Venereology - Part I. *J Eur Acad Dermatol Venereol.* 2021;35:1750-1764.
52. Schmidt E, Rashid H, Marzano AV, et al. European Guidelines (S3) on diagnosis and management of mucous membrane pemphigoid, initiated by the European Academy of Dermatology and Venereology - Part II. *J Eur Acad Dermatol Venereol.* 2021;35:1926-1948.
53. Du G, Patzelt S, van Beek N, Schmidt E. Mucous membrane pemphigoid. *Autoimmun Rev.* 2022; 21:103036.
54. Bernard P, Vaillant L, Labeille B, et al. Incidence and distribution of subepidermal autoimmune bullous skin diseases in three French regions. Bullous Diseases French Study Group. *Arch Dermatol.*1995;131:48-52.
55. Durdu M, Bozca BC, Enli S, et al. A multicentre prospective analysis of the incidence of pemphigoid diseases in Turkey. *Australas J Dermatol.* 2021;62:e496-e503.
56. Siddig O, Mustafa MB, Kordofani Y, et al. The epidemiology of autoimmune bullous diseases in Sudan between 2000 and 2016. *PLoS One.* 2021;16:e0254634.
57. Ghiasi M, Daneshpazhooh M, Ismonov M, et al. Evaluation of autoimmune bullous diseases in elderly patients in Iran: a 10-year retrospective study. *Skinmed.* 2017;15:175-180.
58. Ormond M, McParland H, Thakrar P, et al. Validation of an Oral Disease Severity Score (ODSS) tool for use in oral mucous membrane pemphigoid. *Br J Dermatol.* 2020;183:78-85.
59. Murrell DF, Marinovic B, Caux F, et al. Definitions and outcome measures for mucous membrane pemphigoid: recommendations of an international panel of experts. *J Am Acad Dermatol.* 2015;72:168-174.
60. Chen M, Kim GH, Prakash L, et al. Epidermolysis bullosa acquisita: autoimmunity to anchoring fibril collagen. *Autoimmunity.* 2012;45:91-101.
61. Daneshpazhooh M, Fazlolahi S, Mahmoudi H, et al. Epidermolysis bullosa acquisita: the most frequent pemphigoid disease in patients with dermal binding autoantibodies by indirect immunofluorescence microscopy on human salt-split skin in Tehran, Iran. *J Eur Acad Dermatol Venereol.* 2021;35:e370-e372.
62. Zumelzu C, Le Roux-Villet C, Loiseau P, et al. Black patients of African descent and HLA-DRB1*15:03 frequency overrepresented in epidermolysis bullosa acquisita. *J Invest Dermatol.* 2011;131:2386-2393.
63. Gammon WR, Heise ER, Burke WA, et al. Increased frequency of HLA-DR2 in patients with autoantibodies to epidermolysis bullosa acquisita antigen: evidence that the expression of autoimmunity to type VII collagen is HLA class II allele associated. *J Invest Dermatol.* 1988;91:228-232.
64. Lee CW, Kim SC, Han H. Distribution of HLA class II alleles in Korean patients with epidermolysis bullosa acquisita. *Dermatology.* 1996;193:328-329.
65. Iwata H, Vorobyev A, Koga H, et al. Meta-analysis of the clinical and immunopathological characteristics and treatment outcomes in epidermolysis bullosa acquisita patients. *Orphanet J Rare Dis.* 2018;13:153.
66. Prost-Squarcioni C, Caux F, Schmidt E, et al. International Bullous Diseases Group: consensus on diagnostic criteria for epidermolysis bullosa acquisita. *Br J Dermatol.* 2018;179:30-41.
67. Reddy H, Shipman AR, Wojnarowska F. Epidermolysis bullosa acquisita and inflammatory bowel disease: a review of the literature. *Clin Exp Dermatol.* 2013;38:225-229.

CHAPTER 88 Oncodermatology

Arturo P. Saavedra
Ellen K. Roh
Richard H. Flowers

KEY POINTS

- Inequities in care disproportionally affect historically marginalized communities and patients with skin of color.
- Untimely identification and improper treatment of cutaneous side effects of cytotoxic drugs and checkpoint inhibitors contribute to disparities in care.
- Radiation dermatitis and ensuing postinflammatory hyperpigmentation are more commonly seen in patients with skin of color for treatment of specific but common malignancies such as breast cancer.
- In patients with graft-versus-host disease, dyspigmentation contributes to decreased patient satisfaction when compared to the development of sclerodermoid induration.
- Dyspigmentation often impacts patients with skin of color more significantly than physicians recognize. Often, these concerns are judged by patients to be more impactful in measures of quality of life than other concerns that physicians may have.
- Understanding cutaneous side effects in patients with skin of color may improve compliance, morbidity, and mortality during the treatment of malignant disorders.

ONCODERMATOLOGY

According to the National Cancer Institute, nearly 1.8 million cases of cancer were diagnosed at the turn of the decade with an estimated cost of care of about $21 billion dollars. Through the development of improved screening and novel therapies, improvements in morbidity and mortality have been noted in some populations. Yet, inequities still exist and disproportionately impact historically marginalized communities (including Black/African American, Hispanic/Latine, and American Indian/Alaskan Native). The dermatologist must be equipped to narrow such gaps by recognizing important clinical features in skin of color and understanding the systemic inequities that drive the social determinants of health in the care of patients with cancer (also see Chapter 11). This chapter describes important dermatologic features in patients treated for cancer with cytotoxic, targeted, immune checkpoint inhibitors, and radiation therapies. In addition, the role of bone marrow transplantation and the most common cause of nonrelapse mortality, graft-versus-host disease (GVHD), are also discussed.

DRUG EFFECTS

CYTOTOXIC CHEMOTHERAPIES

Cytotoxic chemotherapies inhibit cell division. Their goal is to target cancer's more rapidly proliferative cells. Because of skin's fast turnover, it is also often affected. **Table 88-1** lists common side effects seen with these medications including alopecia, hand-foot syndrome, nail changes, hyperpigmentation, and mucositis.[1] Other reported complications include photosensitivity, radiation recall, localized scleroderma, Raynaud, hypersensitivity reaction, and capillary leak reaction.[1]

TARGETED CHEMOTHERAPIES

Targeted chemotherapies target specific genes and proteins that promote cancer growth. They are thought to have less systemic toxicity but still frequently produce cutaneous adverse reactions. Dermatologic issues have been reported in 65% to 90% of patients on epidermal growth factor receptor (EGFR) inhibitor therapy.[3] **Table 88-2** shows dermatologic side effects from targeted chemotherapies. Both cytotoxic and targeted chemotherapies can affect hands and feet; however, they differ in

TABLE 88-1 Cytotoxic chemotherapy and dermatologic side effects

Chemotherapy type	Mechanism	Indications	Dermatology side effects
Antimetabolites 5-Fluorouracil (5FU), gemcitabine, pemetrexed, cytarabine, methotrexate	Interfere with deoxyribonucleic acid (DNA) and ribonucleic acid (RNA) synthesis	Leukemia Breast, ovarian, gastrointestinal cancer	Hand-foot syndrome Alopecia Nail changes (Beau lines, melanonychia) Hyperpigmentation [**Figure 88-1**] Mucositis Radiation recall
Antitumor antibiotics Anthracyclines (doxorubicin, daunorubicin) Bleomycin	Change DNA in cancer cells Isolated from Streptomyces	Leukemia, lymphoma Breast, stomach, lung, uterine, ovarian cancers Hodgkin, head/neck cancers, testicular	Hand-foot syndrome Extravasation Radiation recall Flagellate hyperpigmentation Localized scleroderma Raynaud phenomenon
Platinum agents Cisplatin, carboplatin, oxaliplatin	Cross link DNA	Testicular, bladder, ovarian cancers	Hyperpigmentation Type 1 hypersensitivity reaction Alopecia
Taxanes Docetaxel, paclitaxel	Disruption of microtubule function	Breast cancer, non-small cell lung cancer (NSCLC)	Hand-foot syndrome Nail changes (hemorrhagic onycholysis) [**Figure 88-2**] Dermatitis (flexural)[2] Alopecia Radiation recall Edema[2]
Topoisomerase inhibitors Irinotecan, etoposide	Block topoisomerase function	Colorectal, small cell lung, hematologic cancers	Alopecia Hand-foot syndrome Nail changes (hyperpigmentation) Hypersensitivity reaction
Vinca alkaloids Vincristine, vinblastine	Prevent tubulin polymerization (arrest in metaphase)	Acute lymphoblastic leukemia (ALL), Hodgkin and non-Hodgkin lymphoma, rhabdomyosarcoma, neuroblastoma, Wilms	Hand-foot syndrome Alopecia Hypersensitivity reaction

TABLE 88-2 Targeted chemotherapies and dermatologic side effects

Chemotherapy Type	Mechanism	Indications	Dermatology Side Effects
Epidermal growth factor receptor (EGFR) inhibitors Erlotinib, gefitinib, cetuximab, panitumumab, lapatinib, canertinib	Block EGFR to prevent unregulated cell division	Non-small cell lung cancer (NSCLC), colorectal cancer, pancreatic cancer, head/neck cancer	P—papulopustules, paronychia R—regulatory hair abnormalities I—itch D—dryness due to EGFR inhibitors
KIT and BCR-ABL inhibitors Imatinib, nilotinib, dasatinib	Inhibits c-Kit, which is essential for normal hematopoiesis, and BCR-ABL tyrosine kinase, which is important in the pathogenesis of chronic myelogenous leukemia (CML)	Hematologic cancers, gastrointestinal stromal tumor (GIST)	Edema Morbilliform eruption Pigmentary changes
Mammalian target of rapamacyin (mTOR) inhibitors Sirolimus, everolimus, temsirolimus	Mammalian target of rapamycin (mTOR) inhibitors stops rapamycin that regulates cell growth and angiogenesis	Renal cell cancer	Impaired wound healing Mucositis Lymphedema
Vascular endothelial growth factor receptor (VEGFR) inhibitors Selective inhibitors: bevacizumab, ranibizumab Nonselective inhibitors: sorafenib, sunitinib, pazopanib	Impairs angiogenesis	Kidney, colon, lung, liver, breast cancers, glioblastoma	Mucocutaneous hemorrhage Disturbed wound healing Hand-foot skin reaction [**Figure 88-3**] Inflammatory eruptions Hair changes (alopecia, curling, depigmentation)
BRAF inhibitors vemurafenib, dabrafenib, encorafenib	Interferes with the mitogen-activated protein kinase (MAPK) pathway that regulates the proliferation and survival of melanoma cells	BRAF-mutant melanoma	Keratinocytic lesions Pruritus Hand foot skin reaction Photosensitivity Alopecia, curly hair
Mitogen-activated protein kinase kinase (MEK) inhibitors Trametinib, binimetinib, selumetinib, cobimetinib	Targets Ras/Raf/MEK/ERK signaling *pathway*, inhibiting cell proliferation	Melanoma, NSCLC, thyroid cancer, neurofibroma	Xerosis Papulopustular rash Photosensitivity

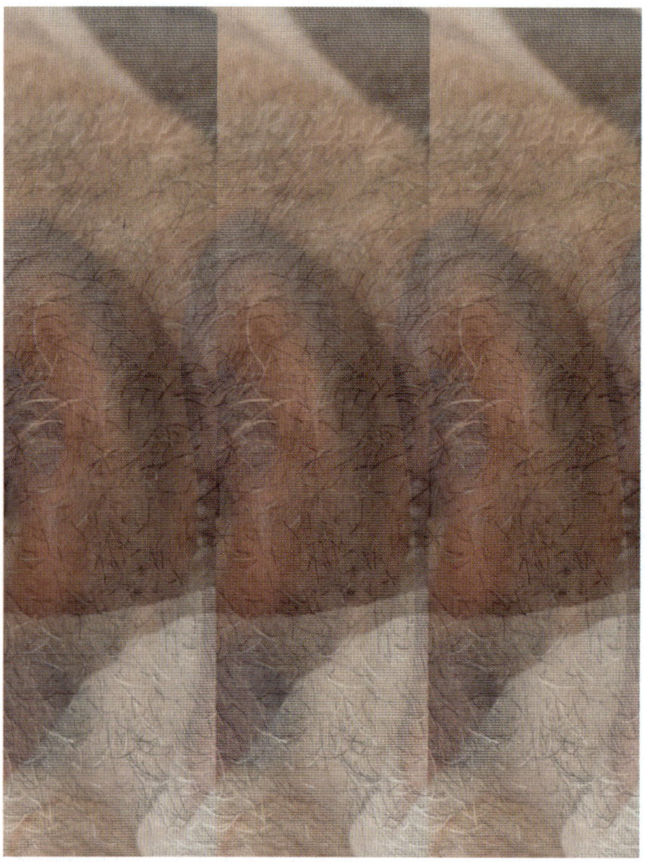

FIGURE 88-1. Mucosal hyperpigmentation in a patient treated with antimetabolite chemotherapy. Note irregular borders of hyperpigmentation on the tongue. The patient was otherwise asymptomatic.

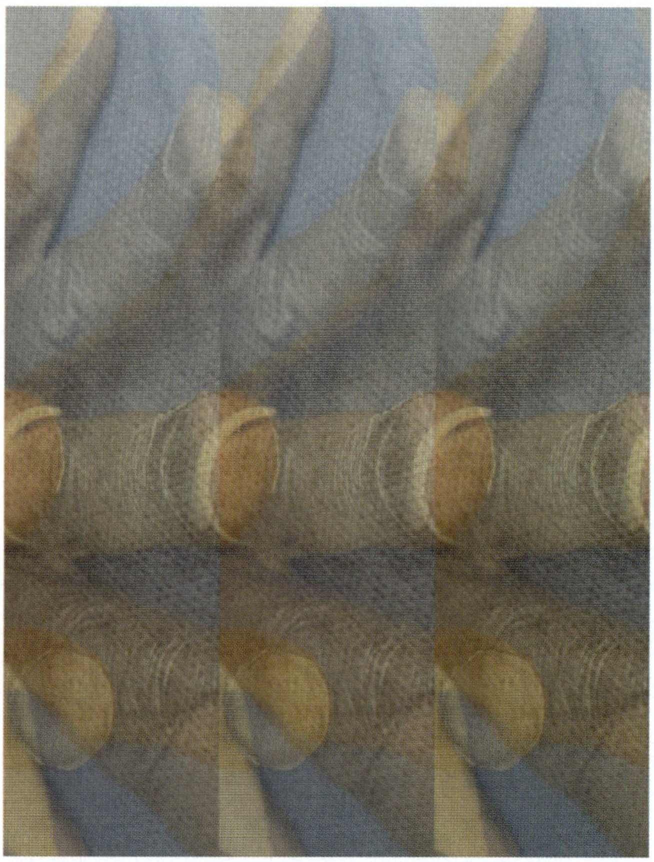

FIGURE 88-2. Hemorrhagic onycholysis in a patient treated with docetaxel. The patient experienced significant discomfort. It is common for only a few digits to be involved.

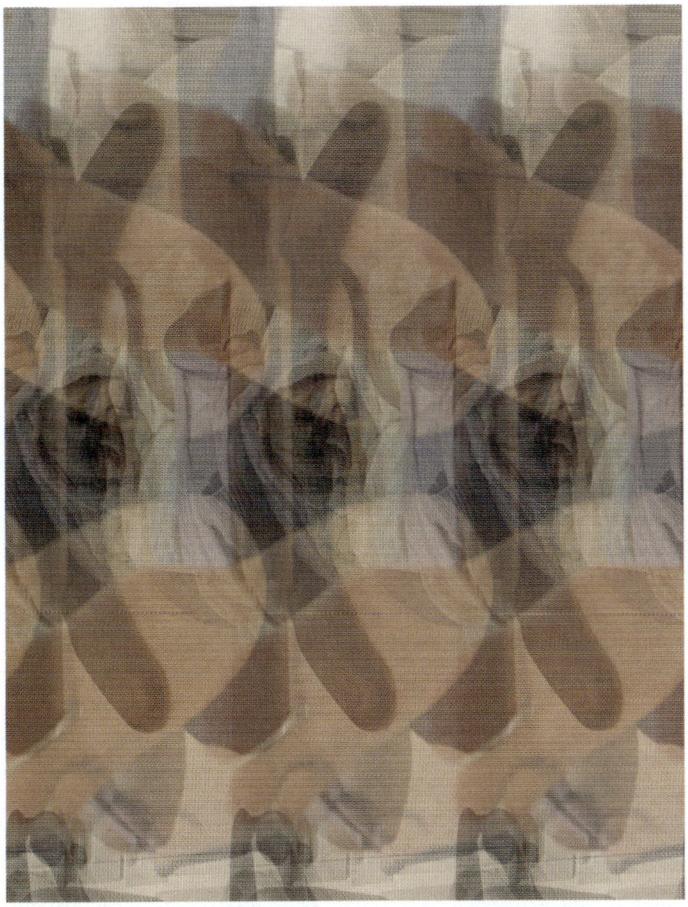

FIGURE 88-3. Hand-foot skin reaction in a patient treated with VEGFR inhibitors. Note focal hyperkeratotic papules and desquamation.

presentation. Hand-foot syndrome occurs with cytotoxic chemotherapy and is also referred to as acral erythema, palmar-plantar erythrodysesthesia, and toxic erythema of chemotherapy. Diffuse erythema, edema, and pain appear on the palms and soles within the first few months of treatment and may develop scale and blisters. Hand-foot skin reaction is a dose-dependent and common side effect of multikinase inhibitors that presents within the first month of treatment with painful focal hyperkeratotic lesions and blisters.

Because many of these adverse reactions are inflammatory, postinflammatory hyperpigmentation is a concern in skin of color. Patients should be treated quickly and counseled on sun protection when appropriate.

IMMUNE-CHECKPOINT INHIBITORS

Immune checkpoint inhibitors (ICIs) have revolutionized cancer treatment since the approval of ipilimumab (a cytotoxic T-lymphocyte-associated protein 4 or CTLA-4 inhibitor) in 2011 for the treatment of melanoma. Indications for the use of programmed death-1 (PD-1) inhibitors (pembrolizumab, nivolumab, cemiplimab) and programmed death-ligand 1 (PD-L1) inhibitors (atezolizumab, durvalumab, avelumab) have accelerated. Indications include non-small and small cell lung cancer, urothelial carcinoma, Hodgkin lymphoma, Merkel cell carcinoma, squamous cell carcinoma, and hepatocellular carcinoma. Dermatologists play a crucial role in ICI therapy, as the skin is the most common site for immune-related adverse events (irAEs).

Immune checkpoint inhibitors are monoclonal antibodies that increase anti-tumor response by blocking downregulation of immune surveillance. Specifically, CTLA-4 inhibition increases T-cell CD28 binding to B7 on antigen-presenting cells, promoting T-cell activation. PD-1 or PD-L1 inhibition impairs the normal decrease in T-cell proliferation, cytokine production, and survival associated with this receptor-ligand interaction.

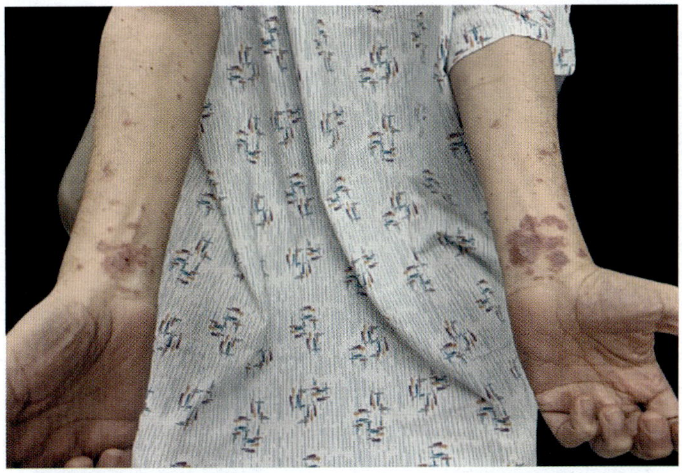

FIGURE 88-4. Lichenoid eruption due to nivolumab. Violaceous papules and thin plaques in a symmetric distribution. (Courtesy of Dr. Cristina Thomas.)

While increased T-cell activity is desirable for anti-tumor response, widespread and nonspecific activation results in a range of off-target effects. Overall, irAEs occur in up to 90% of patients on CTLA-4 inhibitors and 70% of patients treated with PD-1 or PD-L1 inhibitors.[4] These include autoimmune arthritis, colitis, pneumonitis, hepatitis, thyroid dysfunction, hypophysitis, and myocarditis, in addition to cutaneous irAEs.

Cutaneous irAEs occur in up to half of patients, may limit use, and can have a significant impact on patient quality of life.[5] Morbilliform exanthems are most common and occur in approximately one quarter of patients receiving ipilimumab or combination therapy, and less commonly in patients on anti-PD-1 monotherapy. Other common cutaneous irAEs include generalized pruritus, lichenoid dermatoses, and psoriasiform and eczematous eruptions [**Figures 88-4** and **88-5**]. Vitiligo-like depigmentation occurs in up to a quarter of patients treated for melanoma (and rarely in the setting of other malignancies) and is associated with improved overall and melanoma-specific survival[6] [**Figure 88-6**]. ICI-induced alopecia can be particularly distressing to patients. Bullous pemphigoid is a rare but well-described reaction and is often delayed. Severe cutaneous adverse reactions like Stevens-Johnson syndrome/toxic epidermal necrosis and drug reaction with eosinophilia and systemic symptoms are also rare but generally necessitate therapy discontinuation [**Figures 88-7** through **88-9**]. Treatment for mild irAEs typically consists

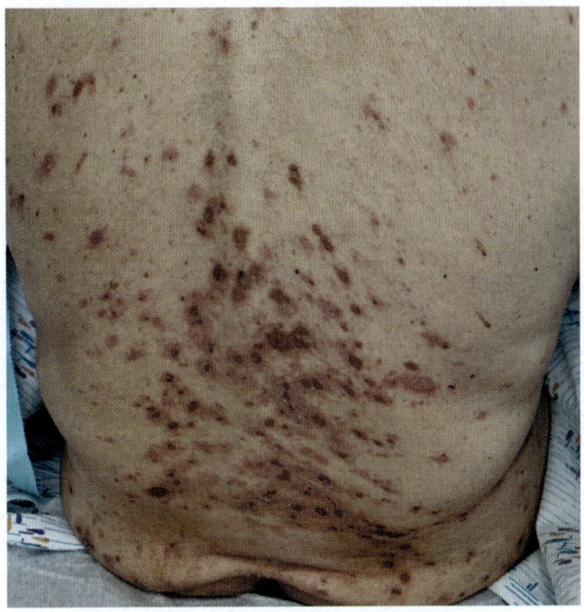

FIGURE 88-5. Lichenoid eruption due to nivolumab. Violaceous plaques on the lower back. Note erosive component in this patient. (Courtesy of Dr. Cristina Thomas.)

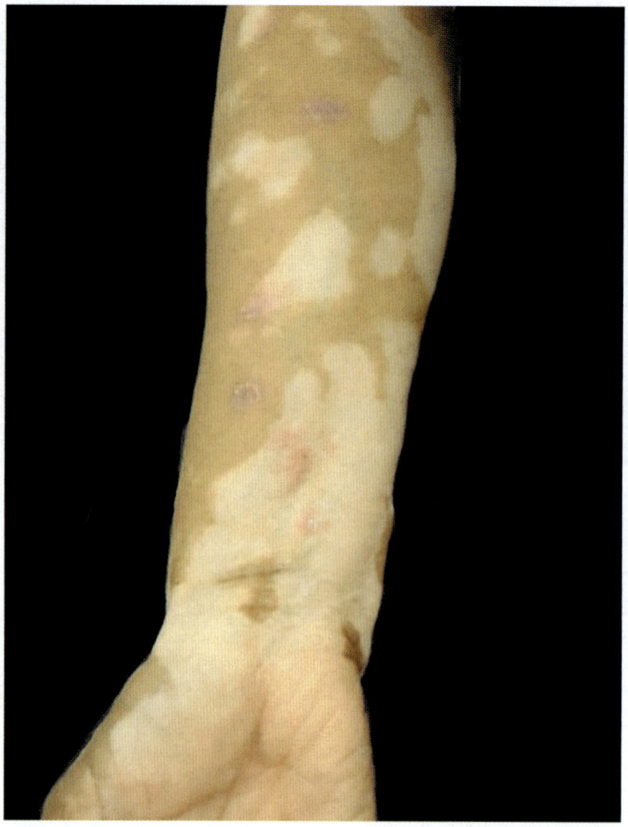

FIGURE 88-6. Vitiligo-like depigmentation due immune checkpoint inhibitor therapy. Note the admixed lichenoid eruption. (Courtesy of Dr. Jennifer Gill.)

of topical emollients and topical corticosteroids. More severe, extensive, or persistent reactions may require oral corticosteroids, other immunomodulators, or cessation of ICI.

Overall, the distribution/type, severity or grade of cutaneous irAE do not significantly differ between White patients and patients with skin of color (SOC).[7] More patients with SOC required a skin biopsy compared to White patients, perhaps reflective of difficulties in diagnosing cutaneous adverse effects in darker skin tones.[7] Non-White patients are also less likely than White patients to be diagnosed with an irAE and more likely to be referred to a dermatologist.[8] Disparities in use of ICI therapy do exist. Black or African Americans as well as lower income patients are less likely to receive immunotherapy for melanoma and experience longer delays prior to ICI initiation.[9,10] Ongoing underrepresentation of historically marginalized patients in clinical trials may contribute to this disparity. Acral melanoma, which is overrepresented in SOC patients, responds poorly to PD-1 therapy as compared to nonacral melanoma. This difference may be secondary to lower mutational burden of acral melanoma and highlights the need to advance research in this melanoma subtype.[11] As the use of ICIs continues to expand, equitable use and ongoing research into specific impact on populations of SOC are critical.

RADIATION

Radiation dermatitis occurs in about 95% of patients receiving radiation treatment for malignancy overall.[12] Toxicities are traditionally defined as acute (transient erythema, epilation, dry or moist desquamation, or ulceration) and late (fibrosis, alopecia, atrophy, telangiectasia, or necrosis) [**Figure 88-10**]. The presence and severity of radiation dermatitis depends on the energy of radiation used, the dose and fractionation schedule, the size of the area exposed, the presence of radiosensitizing chemotherapy, and the proximity of the radiation target to the skin. Radiation dermatitis can have a significant negative impact on patients' quality of life both during and after therapy. Treatment of radiation dermatitis is generally supportive, including washing with mild soap and

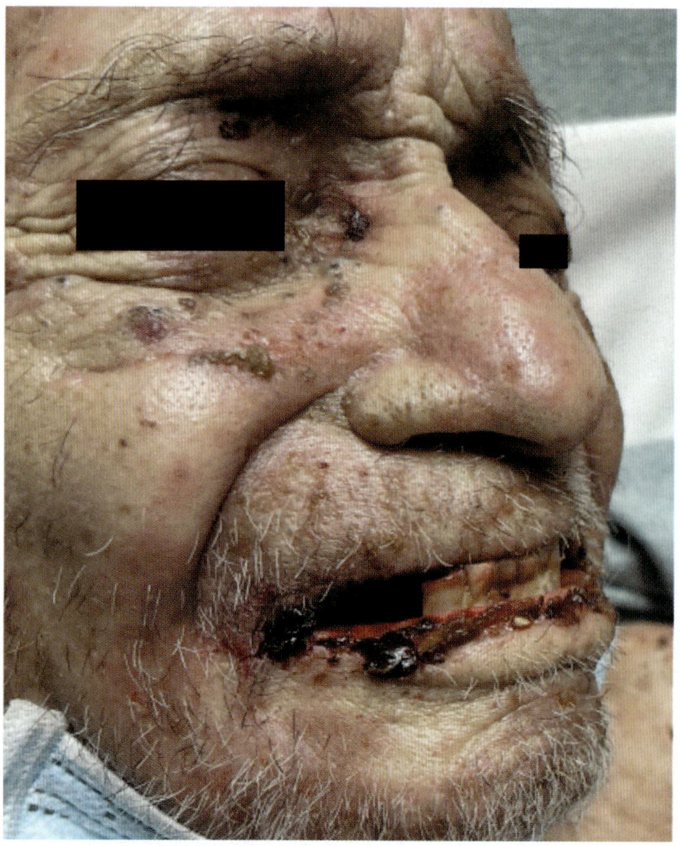

FIGURE 88-7. Stevens-Johnson syndrome secondary to nivolumab. Hemorrhagic mucositis and focal facial erosions. (Courtesy of Dr. Cristina Thomas.)

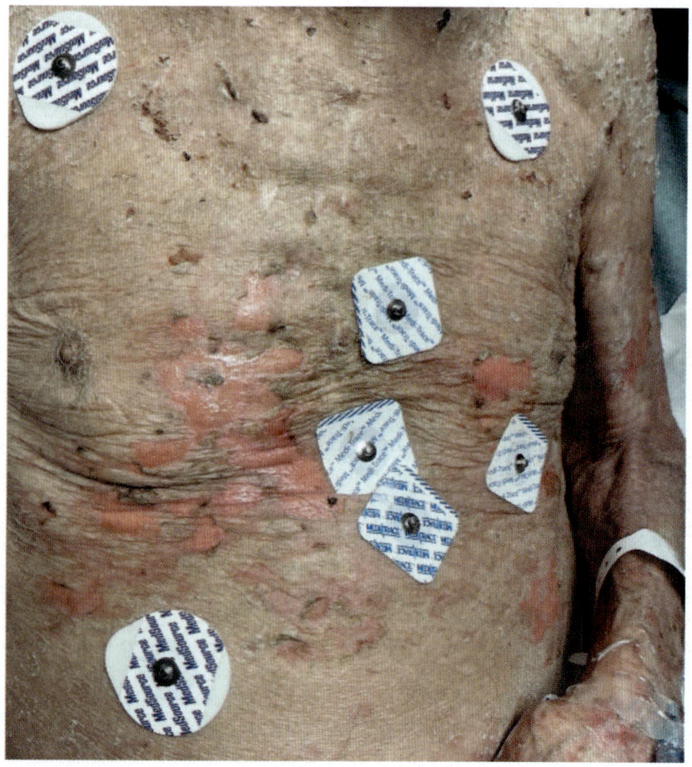

FIGURE 88-8. Stevens-Johnson syndrome secondary to nivolumab. Extensive erosions on the chest overlying broad patches of dusky erythema. (Courtesy of Dr. Cristina Thomas.)

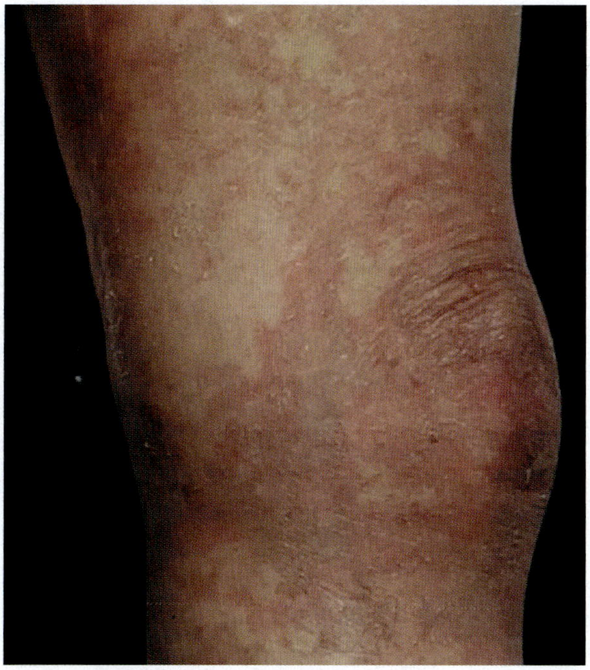

FIGURE 88-9. Stevens-Johnson syndrome secondary to nivolumab. Dusky red patches on the lower leg. (Courtesy of Dr. Cristina Thomas.)

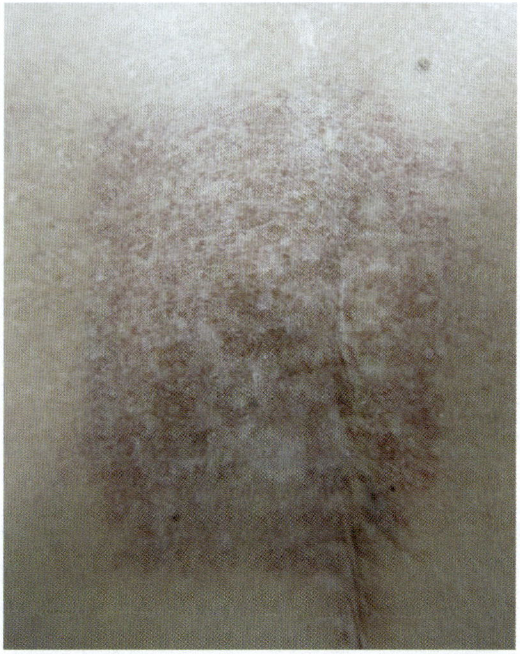

FIGURE 88-10. Poikiloderma occurring after radiation therapy. Hyperpigmentation, hypopigmentation and cutaneous atrophy with visible telangiectasias in this patient. (Reproduced with permission from Burgin S, ed. *Guidebook to Dermatologic Diagnosis*. New York, NY: McGraw Hill; 2021, Figure 3.6.)

using bland emollients. Topical steroids may provide benefit. Modification of radiation therapy intensity may be required as well.

Several special considerations for radiation therapy in patients with skin of color deserve mention. In a large prospective study of a diverse population of breast cancer patients undergoing radiation, Black or African American were more likely to experience radiation dermatitis.[13] This was attributed to increased risk factors for skin toxicity including higher body mass index, higher disease stage, and larger breast volume. Overall, Black patients receiving radiation therapy for cancer reported more severe posttreatment skin problems than White patients.[14] Published scoring systems for radiation dermatitis define grade 1 and 2 reactions by the degree of erythema, which may be more difficult to appreciate in patients with darker skin tones.[15] Skin phototype may predict radiation outcomes in some populations: a study in Japan of radiation recipients for breast cancer predicted significant radiation-induced skin pigmentation in self-reported "suntan" ability, whereas "sunburn" phenotype did not predict radiation-induced erythema.[16]

GRAFT-VERSUS-HOST DISEASE

Hematopoietic stem cell transplantation (HSCT) has offered potential cure for many malignant and immunologic diseases. As approaches to HSCT and its complications have improved, so have patient morbidity and mortality. GVHD, both acute and chronic, can present with cutaneous manifestations. In addition to understanding differences in the evaluation of the clinical exam in skin of color, it is also important to consider social determinants of health in an effort to improve disparities in all aspects of care following HSCT. GVHD, particularly the chronic variant, is the most common cause of non-relapse mortality following HSCT. Therefore, understanding pathophysiological mechanisms, the clinical exam, and the goals of therapy is of utmost importance.

Pathophysiology Acute GHVD is caused by inflammation due to tissue injury often following radiation or chemotherapy. In addition, release of inflammatory cytokines leads to activation of donor T-cells that attack recipient tissue. The most common risk factors include mismatch in donor and recipient human leukocyte antigen (HLA) types, the use of peripheral blood stem cell graft, advanced age, and previous pregnancy status of a female donor. In addition to tissue injury and activated donor T-cell proliferation, chronic GVHD is thought to result from dysregulation of both T- and B-cell subtypes as well as tissue repair and subsequent fibrosis.[17] Risk factors are similar to the acute variant, such as donor and recipient HLA mismatch and advanced age. Prior history of acute GVHD also imparts a higher risk for the development of chronic disease.

Clinical Features Acute GVHD is generally seen in the early post-transplant period. Traditionally defined as occurring in the first 100 days following transplantation, clinical features are now more important in distinguishing acute versus chronic disease. Chronic GVHD is seen months after transplantation. Importantly, overlap syndromes have also been described making it increasingly important to discern important clinical features in the evaluation of skin, hair, nails, and mucosal surfaces.

Involvement of skin, gut, and liver are typical in acute GVHD. Cutaneous features are generally the most common, and oncologists rely on dermatologist to make this diagnosis while they pursue abnormalities in liver function enzymes and the evaluation of diarrhea. Elevated bilirubin and alkaline phosphatase are generally seen. The skin may present with a pruritic exanthem covering various degrees of the skin surface. Erythroderma and bullae portend a worse prognosis and patients can present almost identically to patients with toxic epidermal necrolysis [**Figure 88-11**]. **Table 88-3** shows clinical stages of acute cutaneous GVHD.

The clinical exam in chronic disease is particularly important in patients with skin of color. Common features of chronic disease include lichen planus-like lesions [**Figure 88-12**], sclerodermoid induration [**Figure 88-13**], and dyspigmentation [**Figure 88-14**]. Xerosis, icthyosis, panniculitis-like changes, keratosis pilaris and bullae can also be noted. Nail changes include longitudinal ridging, Beau lines, onychomadesis, paronychia, trachyonychia, onycholysis, leukonychia, and pterigyum [**Figure 88-15**]. A recent report showed nail matrix changes are more common than nail bed changes and that these findings are not correlated to the extent of cutaneous disease.[18] Alopecia is common and may be scarring or nonscarring [**Figure 88-16**]. Other features include premature graying, thinning, brittleness, rash with follicular accentuation as well as comedone formation.[19] About half of the time, patchy nonscarring alopecia is noted. Other variants in order of prevalence include diffuse nonscarring alopecia, diffuse sclerotic disease, and patchy sclerotic changes.[20] **Figure 88-17** shows the National Institutes of Health skin severity scoring for patients with chronic GVHD.

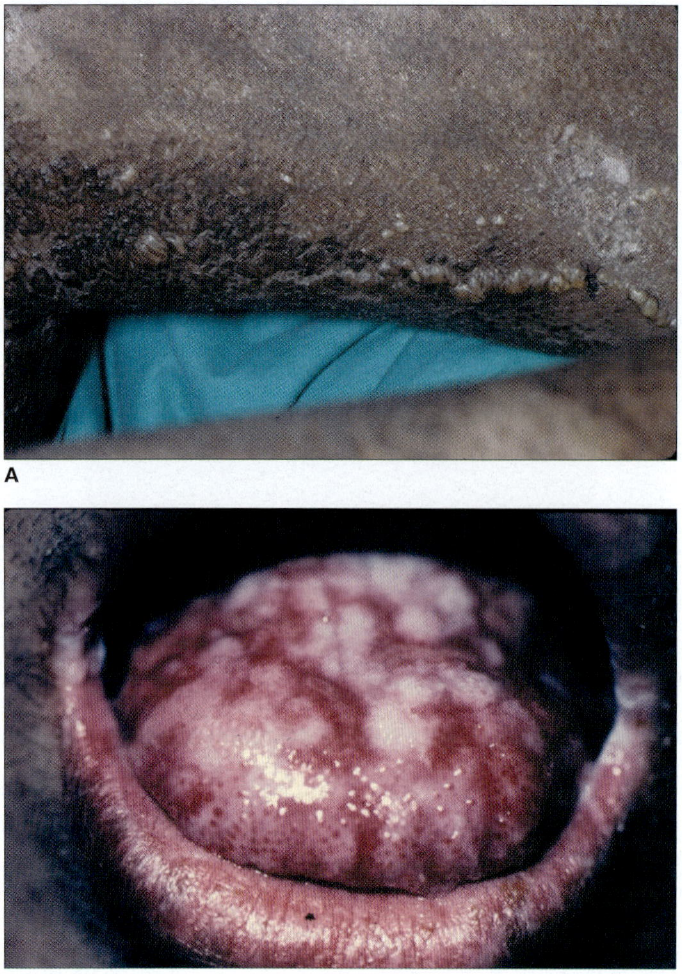

A

B

FIGURE 88-11. Blistering acute GVHD. Evolution of these clinical findings often resemble toxic epidermal necrolysis in the skin **(A)** and in the mouth **(B)**. (Courtesy of Dr. Kenneth Greer.)

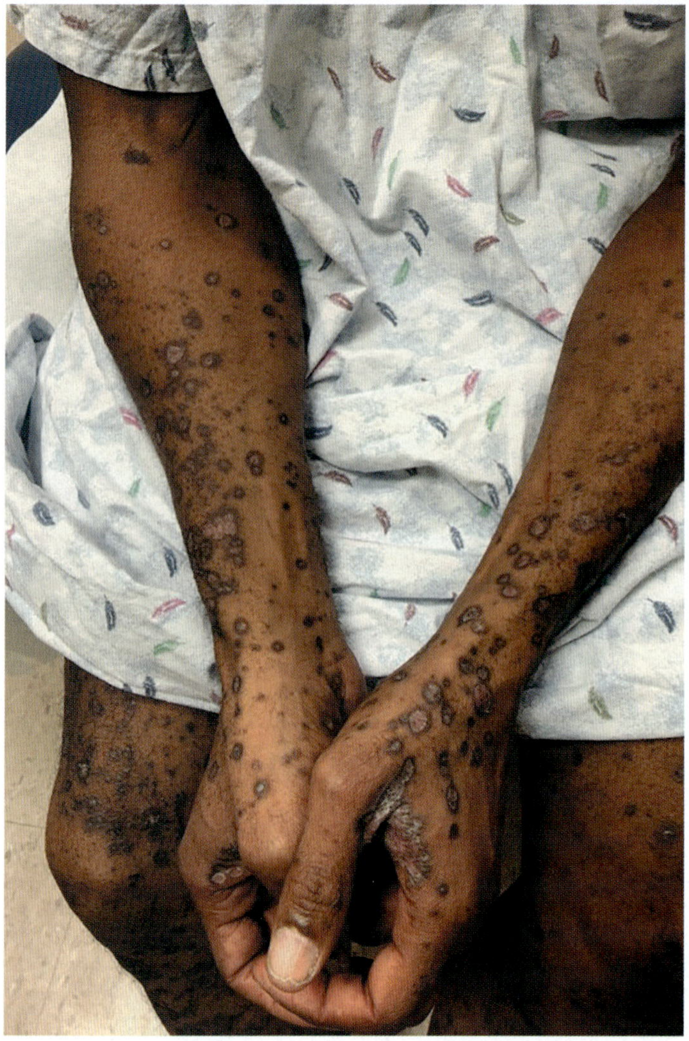

FIGURE 88-12. Lichen-planus like GVHD. Note that these lesions may reach confluence. Follicular prominence, xerosis, and scaling are also important features to distinguish. (Courtesy of Dr. Kenneth Greer.)

Dyspigmentation has a particularly profound influence on quality of life in skin of color. Patients with skin type III to VI and both epidermal and sclerotic changes report higher clinical severity than patients with either subtype alone. Importantly, patients with inactive GVHD but with significant dyspigmentation reported higher clinical severity when compared to physician assessment of those with active sclerotic disease. Furthermore, patients with active disease involving epidermal changes such as color change, dermatitis, erosions, ulceration, and pruritus reported increased dissatisfaction compared to patients with sclerotic disease.[21] Because sclerotic disease is considered to be more aggressive by clinicians and is more likely to be steroid-refractory, equal attention must be placed on the evaluation of pigmentation and its impact as relayed by patients.

Histopathology Vacuolar dermatitis, dyskeratosis, satellitosis, and subepidermal cleft formation are features of acute disease. Orthokeratosis, parakeratosis, epidermal growth disarray, lichenoid dermatitis, dermal sclerosis, scant perivascular, and interstitial infiltrates and vacuolization can be seen alone or in combination in patients with chronic disease.[22] Nevertheless, histopathologic changes can often be insufficient to make a definitive diagnosis. Because GVHD continues to be a clinical diagnosis, the development of novel serologic and molecular markers may improve diagnostic accuracy in the future.

Treatment First and foremost, approach to treatment requires evaluation for multi-system disease. Localized acute cutaneous GVHD is

TABLE 88-3	Clinical staging of acute GVHD
Stage 1	Maculopapular rash < 25% of total body surface area
Stage 2	Maculopapular rash over 25 but under 50% of total body surface area
Stage 3	Generalized erythroderma
Stage 4	Generalized erythroderma with bullous formation

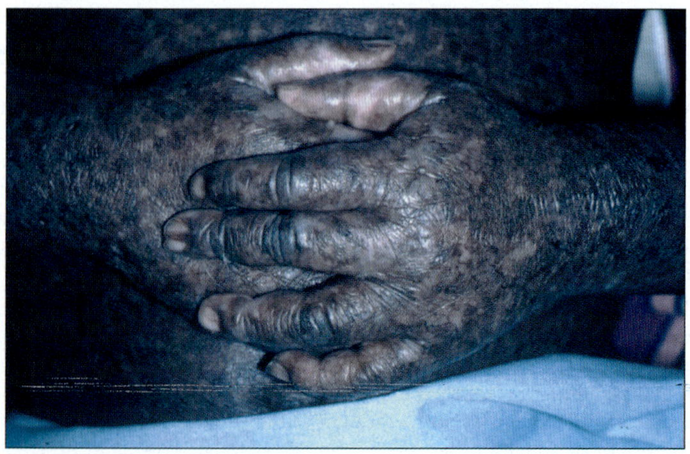

FIGURE 88-13. Sclerodermatous induration and dyspigmenation in a patient with chronic GVHD. Note the ivory-colored areas in the thumbs and nail plate dyspigmentation. (Courtesy of Dr. Kenneth Greer.)

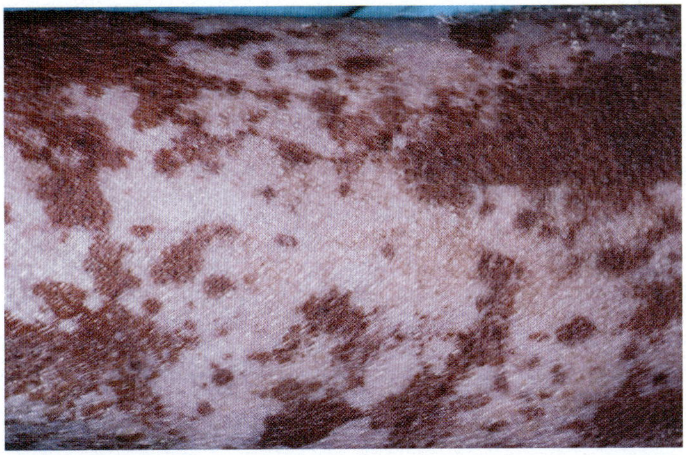

FIGURE 88-14. Residual dyspigmentation in patients with inactive chronic GHVD. These clinical features have been shown to be of greater concern to patients than to physicians, even when compared to other findings such as sclerodermoid induration. (Courtesy of Dr. Kenneth Greer.)

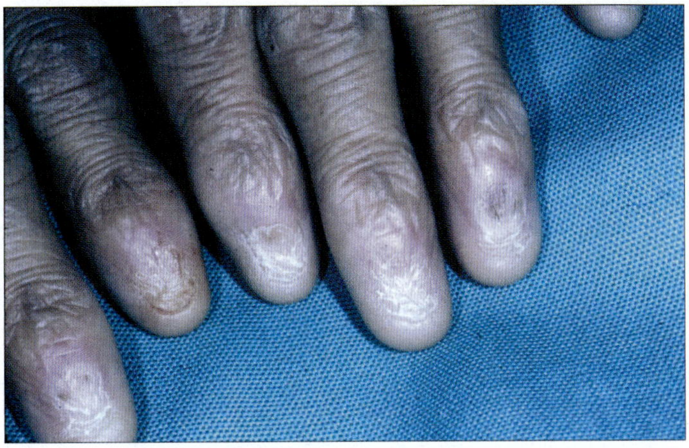

FIGURE 88-15. Features of GVHD in nails. Features resemble lichen planus with prominent periungual erythema. (Courtesy of Dr. Kenneth Greer.)

treated with topical corticosteroids and calcineurin inhibitors. Recalcitrant disease or that involving greater than 25% body surface area will require systemic corticosteroids at doses between 1 and 2 mg/kg/day. Steroids are tapered according to treatment response. Additional treatments reported in the literature include phototherapy, mycophenolate mofetil, calcineurin inhibitors, sirolimus, pentostatin, denileukin diftitox, extracorporeal phototherapy, and various monoclonal antibodies

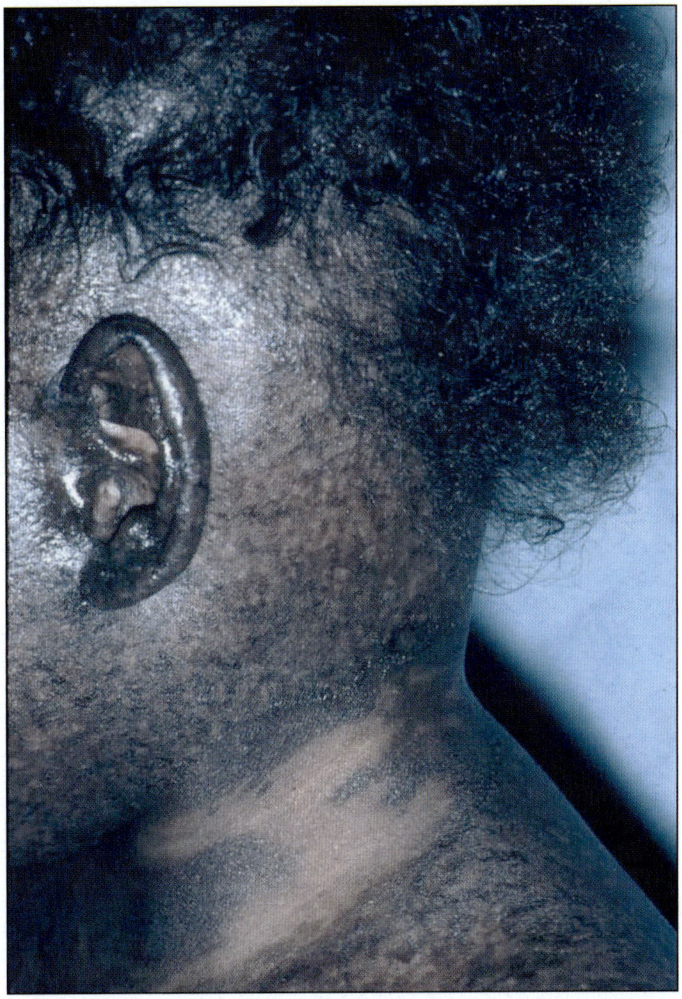

FIGURE 88-16. Features of alopecia in GVHD. Both patchy and diffuse hair loss is noted. In addition, poikilodermatous skin changes can also be appreciated. (Courtesy of Dr. Kenneth Greer.)

such as anti CD-25 and anti-CD52 agents. Recently, the U.S. Food and Drug Administration has approved the use of ruxolitinib, a JAK1/2 inhibitor, for use in steroid-refractory acute GVHD.[17]

Patients with chronic disease will generally undergo long-term therapy often requiring 2 to 3 years of treatment. Therapy requires 0.5 to 1 mg/kg/day of systemic corticosteroids. Steroids are tapered based on clinical response. Treatment of steroid-refractory or steroid-dependent disease is complicated and often requires a multi-specialty approach that considers patient clinical status, co-morbidities, social and economic factors as

	0	1	2	3
Score %BSA ____ *GVHD features to be scored by BSA:*	No BSA involved	1-18% BSA	19-50% BSA	>50% BSA
Check all that apply: ☐ Maculopapular rash/ erythema ☐ Lichen planus-like features ☐ Sclerotic features ☐ Papulosquamous lesions or ichthyosis ☐ keratosis pilaris-like	No sclerotic features		Superficial sclerotic features "not hidebound" (able to pinch)	**Check all that apply:** ☐ Deep sclerotic features ☐ "Hidebound" (unable to pinch) ☐ Impaired mobility ☐ Ulceration
☐ Abnormality present but explained entirely by non-GVHD documented cause (specify) ____				

FIGURE 88-17. National Institutes of Health skin severity score in chronic GVHD.

well as the availability of clinical trials in the treating facility. Evidenced-based guidance on second-line agents is scarce. Steroid-sparing agents such as mycophenolate mofetil, azathioprine, and calcineurin inhibitors are generally used first. Additionally, treatment responses targeting B-cells have also been published. Single courses of rituximab have been shown to improve clinical features in some patients.

The role of immunomodulatory agents to prevent relapse and to decrease treatment-related morbidities has increased. Interleukin-2 and extracorporeal therapy have been previously reported to be helpful by exerting immunomodulatory activity. Three important recent treatments should be highlighted. Tyrosine kinase inhibitors, most notably ibrutinib, have shown benefit. Ruxolitinib as well as belumosudil, a rho-associated coiled-coil kinase (ROC) inhibitor, have also been approved for patients 12 years and older who have tried at least two other systemic therapies.[23,24]

Special mention should be made of treatment for dyspigmentation in patients with skin of color given its significant impact on quality of life. Early control of cutaneous inflammation with topical and systemic therapy may prevent some of these changes. Depigmentary agents should also be considered in the treatment course as long as they do not cause irritation, pruritus, or active inflammation of the skin that may lead to further dyspigmentation. Hydroquinone can be helpful but patients must be followed closely for any secondary depigmentation or exogenous ochronosis. Tretinoin may also be of use in those who do not develop retinoid dermatitis. Triple combination agents that add a topical steroid to hydroquinone and tretinoin could be considered but their significant costs can preclude their potential benefit. Azelaic acid can also be used but could lead to mild irritation. Peels and laser treatment should be performed by those with expertise in skin of color to avoid exacerbation of pigmentary changes. The use of sunscreen and protective garments should be discussed with all patients particularly those on any photosensitizing systemic medications.

REFERENCES

1. Guillot B, Bessis D, Dereure O. Mucocutaneous side effects of antineoplastic chemotherapy. *Expert Opin Drug Saf.* 2004;3(6):579-587.
2. Sibaud V, Lebœuf NR, Roche H, et al. Dermatological adverse events with taxane chemotherapy. *Eur J Dermatol.* 2016;26(5):427-443.
3. Fabbrocini G, Panariello L, Caro G, Cacciapuoti S. Acneiform rash induced by EGFR inhibitors: review of the literature and new insights. *Skin Appendage Disord.* 2015;1(1):31-37.
4. Puzanov I, Diab A, Abdallah K, et al. Managing toxicities associated with immune checkpoint inhibitors: consensus recommendations from the Society for Immunotherapy of Cancer (SITC) Toxicity Management Working Group. *J Immunother Cancer.* 2017;5(1):1-28.
5. Villadolid J, Amin A. Immune checkpoint inhibitors in clinical practice: update on management of immune-related toxicities. *Trans Lung Cancer Res.* 2015;4(5):560.
6. Teulings HE, Limpens J, Jansen SN, et al. Vitiligo-like depigmentation in patients with stage III-IV melanoma receiving immunotherapy and its association with survival: a systematic review and meta-analysis. *J Clin Oncol.* 2015;33(7):773-781.
7. Ngo T, Hossain C, Guzman AK, et al. Spectrum of PD-1 and PD-L1 inhibitor cutaneous adverse events in skin of color: a retrospective, single-institutional study in an urban community. *Acta Oncologica.* 2021;60(4):559-563.
8. Thompson LL, Pan CX, Chang MS, et al. Impact of ethnicity on the diagnosis and management of cutaneous toxicities from immune checkpoint inhibitors. *JAAD.* 2021;84(3):851-854.
9. Haque W, Verma V, Butler EB, et al. Racial and socioeconomic disparities in the delivery of immunotherapy for metastatic melanoma in the United States. *J Immunother.* 2019;42(6):228-235.
10. Tripathi R, Archibald LK, Mazmudar RS, et al. Racial differences in time to treatment for melanoma. *JAAD.* 2020;83(3):854-859.
11. Ogata D, Haydu LE, Glitza IC, et al. The efficacy of anti-programmed cell death protein 1 therapy among patients with metastatic acral and metastatic mucosal melanoma. *Cancer Med.* 2021;10(7):2293-2299.
12. Ryan JL. Ionizing radiation: the good, the bad, and the ugly. *J Invest Derm.* 2012;132(3):985-993.
13. Wright JL, Takita C, Reis IM, et al. Prospective evaluation of radiation-induced skin toxicity in a race/ethnically diverse breast cancer population. *Cancer med.* 2016;5(3):454-464.
14. Ryan JL, Bole C, Hickok JT, et al. Post-treatment skin reactions reported by cancer patients differ by race, not by treatment or expectations. *Br J Cancer.* 2007;97(1):14-21.
15. Dzul S, Ninia J, Jang H, et al. Predictors of acute radiation dermatitis and esophagitis in African American patients receiving whole-breast radiation therapy. *Pract Radiat Oncol.* 2022;12(1):52-59.
16. Yamazaki H, Yoshida K, Nishimura T, et al. Association between skin phototype and radiation dermatitis in patients with breast cancer treated with breast-conserving therapy: suntan reaction could be a good predictor for radiation pigmentation. *J Rad Res.* 2011;52(4):496-501.
17. Hamilton BK. Updates in chronic graft-versus-host disease. *Hem Am Soc Hematol Educ Program.* 2021;1:648-654.
18. Lee YK, Kim HS, Lee JY, et al. Nail changes in patients with graft-versus-host disease. *J Am Acad Dermatol.* 2011;64:AB91.
19. Silveira L, eSouza MN, Sternberg F. Graft-versus-host disease with acute hair loss: A distinctive manifestation of chronic graft-versus-host disease. *J Am Acad Dermatol.* 2016;74:AB135.
20. Marks DH, Naftulin JS, Penzi LR, et al. Chronic hair loss in patients with cutaneous chronic graft-versus-host disease. *J Am Acad Dermatol.* 2019:81(5):1134-1141.
21. Smith ZI, Rosenstein RK, Banerjee S. et al. Quality of life in patients with skin of color and chronic graft-versus-host disease. *JAMA Dermatol.* 2020;156:589-590.
22. Shulman HM, Kleiner D, Lee SJ, et al. Histopathologic diagnosis of chronic graft-versus-host disease: national institutes of health consensus development project on criteria for clinical trials in chronic graft-versus-host disease. *Biol Blood Marrow Transplan.* 2006;12:31-47.
23. Zeiser R, Polverelli N, Ram R, et al. Ruxolitinib for glucocorticoid-refractory chronic graft-versus-host disease. *N Engl J Med.* 2021;385:228-238.
24. Cutler C, Lee SJ, Arai S, et al. Belumosudil for chronic graft-versus-host disease after 2 or more prior lines of therapy: the ROCKstar study. *Blood.* 2021;138:2278-2289.

SECTION 13

Cosmetic and Procedural Dermatology

CHAPTER 89 Cultural Beauty Around the World

Chidubem A. V. Okeke
Cheryl M. Burgess

KEY POINTS

- It is essential to challenge and broaden the understanding of beauty by embracing diverse representations across various cultures and ethnicities.
- Emphasizing inclusivity and promoting the celebration of beauty in all its forms.
- Attractiveness is subjective. Beauty is influenced by cultural, societal, and individual preferences.

INTRODUCTION

Beauty perceptions and standards vary significantly around the world. They can be shaped by various factors, including historical, social, economic, and cultural influences. Although there are a few dominant beauty ideals that are universally agreed upon, many are largely impacted by historical, geographic, and cultural practices.

Beauty ideals often reflect historical and traditional values. For example, in many East Asian cultures, pale skin has been historically associated with wealth and nobility, while in some African cultures, beauty may be associated with fuller figures or specific hairstyles. Different geographic regions can also impact beauty standards as in societies with limited exposure to sunlight, lighter skin tones may be preferred; however, in sunnier regions, tanned or darker skin may be considered more attractive.[1] Beauty ideals can also be influenced by cultural practices and symbolism. Body modification, such as scarification or elongated necks with the use of neck rings, is considered beautiful in certain African and Southeast Asian cultures.

Beauty is a complex phenomenon influenced by various factors, including societal norms, historical contexts, and individual preferences.[2] While beauty standards have been prevalent across different cultures, women, in particular, often find themselves grappling with the expectations imposed by these standards. This chapter aims to explore the dynamic nature of cultural beauty worldwide, focusing on female beauty standards. It will delve into the universal attractiveness variables, discuss beauty standards in various countries, and examine the Western world's adoption of beauty standards from other cultures.

BEAUTY DEFINED

Beauty, whether in nature or art, is often tied to uniqueness, awe-inspiring elements, or intricate design. However, when it comes to the female form, we tend to seek a standardized ideal, overlooking diversity. Beauty is culturally defined, evolving with time, yet certain attractiveness traits are deemed universal across cultures [see **Table 89-1**].

CULTURAL DIFFERENCES OF BEAUTY

Throughout history, there have been political, cultural, and social, regional, religious, and Western factors impacting the perception of beauty. However, culture plays a critical part in influencing our ideas about what is beautiful. For example, in the Western world, beauty is often associated with clear skin, facial symmetry, and low waist to hip ratios. In contrast, outside the western world, many cultures place a higher value on inner beauty and factors such asymmetry, high waist to hip ratio, and imperfect teeth are deemed beautiful.

When considering the impact of regional differences on beauty standards, we can look at the varying Asian regions. The ideal woman in these cultures tend to appear youthful and fair-skinned as a symbol of luxury and success in Asian cultures.

One of the most prominent beauty features in East Asia (eg, China, Korea, Japan, Hong Kong, Taiwan) is the size of an individual's eyes.[11] Larger eyes are viewed as more attractive because it makes females seem cuter and almost baby-like. Therefore, double eyelid surgery remains one of the most popular aesthetic surgeries, especially among East Asian populations. A study by Hwang and Spiegel[12] assessed how attractiveness is interpreted by Chinese and non-Chinese observers in terms of eyelid structure. Findings demonstrated that a statistically significant number of participants considered the medium-height upper eyelid crease most attractive and absent upper eyelid crease less attractive. Another beauty ideal strongly held by East Asians is having pale, clear skin. This trait is associated with femininity, youth, and power. Therefore, many women from these regions try skin lightening products, limit sun exposure, and have attitudes of excessive sun protection.[13] Similarly, Southeast Asian countries (eg, Thailand, Singapore, Indonesia, Philippines) value features such as fair skin, a small nose, V-shaped facial structure, and large eyes.

In South Asia (eg, Pakistan, Maldives, Bangladesh, Afghanistan), beauty standards are influenced by the intersection of culture and religion. Given the region's status as home to the world's largest Muslim population, religious factors play a significant role. In many Muslim cultures, the hijab is a symbol of sexual modesty and religious devotion, emphasizing a woman's adherence to religious values over her appearance.

When considering Middle Eastern beauty standards, such as those in Iran, we can see features like large, expressive eyes, long and thick eyelashes, and a slender yet curvaceous figure prioritized. The example of Iran brings us into a discussion regarding Western influences on beauty standards. Because the hijab only allows the face to be exposed, this can lead to body dysmorphia and a fixation on the nose, resulting in a desire to surgically modify a dorsal hump or drooping tip to emulate Western media; thus, rhinoplasty is the most popular plastic procedure in Iran.[14] Now, a surgical bandage from rhinoplasty has become a part of a fashion trend, and signifies social status and financial power.

African countries also see different beauty standards based on region. In West Africa, beauty is often associated with fuller figures, including curvaceous hips and a rounder buttock region. In Northwestern countries such as Mauritania,[15] larger body sizes are considered a symbol of beauty and prosperity, leading to practices like force-feeding young girls to enhance their weight, sometimes to the point of morbid obesity. Here we can see an example of body image greatly impacting a woman's place in society and politics, as the focus on gaining and maintaining the weight limits their ability to engage with the community and politics.

TABLE 89-1 Universal attractiveness variables

Reproductive fitness	Evolutionarily, traits that indicate reproductive fitness, such as youthfulness and health, are universally valued as attractive.
Symmetry	Symmetrical features, whether in the face or body, are generally perceived as more attractive due to their association with good health and genetic fitness in many cultures.[3,4]
Waist-to-hip ratio	A waist-to-hip ratio of 0.7 in Western women, 0.6 in Latinx in women, and 0.9 in northern Asian women are often considered attractive, as it signifies fertility and reproductive capability.[5]
High-pitched female voice	A high-pitched voice is culturally associated with femininity and is considered more attractive in many societies.[6]
Healthy hair	Shiny, lustrous, and well-maintained hair is considered attractive, as it indicates good health and grooming habits.[7]
Smile	A genuine, confident smile is universally perceived as attractive, as it signals warmth, approachability, and happiness. White teeth are favored in most cultures; however, crooked teeth are acceptable in most Asian cultures.[8]
Natural appearance with little to no makeup	The preference for a natural appearance varies across cultures, with many societies valuing minimal makeup or an effortless look over heavy cosmetics.[9]
The color red	The color red has cultural significance in various contexts, including beauty. It is associated with attractiveness, passion, and desirability in many cultures. Evolutionary factors have linked red to aspects of health, vitality, and fertility. The cultural significance is associated with love, passion, and romance but can symbolize power and energy. The visual impact of red is highly noticeable, stimulating, and attention-grabbing thus creating a sense of excitement or attraction.[10]

Eastern European beauty ideals prioritize slender body types. Due to an earlier onset of photoaging in this population,[16] there's an emphasis on skincare early in age.

Latine beauty standards encompass a rich tapestry of diverse cultural influences, yet they often reflect certain commonalities. Traditionally, these standards have celebrated features such as dark, expressive eyes, lush hair, and varying shades of skin tones that span a spectrum from fair to deep. However, it's important to acknowledge that Eurocentric ideals have also influenced perceptions of beauty within Latinx communities. This influence has sometimes placed a greater emphasis on lighter skin tones and more European facial features. Moreover, there exists a significant emphasis on achieving a specific physique, with an average weight range of 110 to 125 lbs being often aspired to. A noteworthy trend is the pursuit of aesthetic enhancements. Brazil, in particular, ranks second only to the United States in plastic surgery procedures, with a particular emphasis on augmentations for the buttocks and breasts.[17] This cultural emphasis on physical appearance is further exemplified by the substantial investment individuals make, allocating nearly half of their income toward various beauty treatments.

In New Zealand, 7.4% of the population identifies with Pacific ethnic groups.[18] However, there are limited studies on beauty standards among Pasifika Island women.[19] These women are often portrayed "tropical" and "exotic" through a Western lens in magazines, tourist materials, and postcards.[20] In a study of 121 Samoan adults,[21] larger body sizes were considered attractive in Samoa, representing power and wealth. However, among Samoan adults in New Zealand, bigger frames were perceived as unhealthy, signifying low self-confidence. In the Māori community of New Zealand, Tāmoko (tattoos) are symbols of an individual's beauty and ancestry. For example, Tāmoko placement on the chin area represents prestige and authority.

North American beauty reflects a spectrum of diversity. Blonde hair and blue eyes were once the benchmark of beauty, but since 2008, the preference has shifted. A study surveying 130 men and 112 women demonstrated that light skin tones and brunette hair were perceived more attractive.[1] In the past decade, women such as Ashley Graham, a plus-sized model of German and Russian decent, have redefined attractiveness by challenging conventional beauty standards. As America continues to blend cultures, the National Geographic predicts that by 2050, the average American will have a multiracial appearance.

LACK OF DIVERSITY IN MEDIA

Beauty is an abstract and subjective concept; it encompasses characteristics that are aesthetically pleasing to the senses or possesses qualities that evoke admiration and satisfaction. It also goes beyond physical appearance and includes elements such as personality, charisma, and inner qualities. It is crucial to recognize that beauty standards are not inherently defined solely through the lens of Eurocentric or Western beauty standards. This perception or attractiveness is a result of historical power dynamics, colonialism, and the global influence of Western culture. Beauty ideals should instead be understood within a broader context of cultural diversity and influences and should not be universally attributed to a single racial or ethnic group.

The influence of media, particularly through globalization, has led to the spread of certain Western beauty standards across the world. Eurocentric features, such as fair skin, slim figures, and special facial characteristics, have disproportionally been highlighted and promoted in mainstream media, contributing to a perceived dominance of white-centric beauty standards. This is why proper representation matters in the beauty industry, television, and social media. In the beauty industry, fashion, modeling, and makeup brands have been forced to place a greater emphasis on representing different body and skin types. This is done to reject the idea that those with darker skin tones and a plus-size figure should not have access to products that can increase their confidence. However, a more continuous effort is needed as approximately 25% of GenZ consumers do not feel represented by current beauty advertisements. The lack of inclusivity in some aspects of media can make some demographics feel ignored by certain brands; the constant usage of filters and models with surgical enhancements heightens insecurities and takes a negative toll on consumers' mental health.

EMPHASIZING INCLUSIVITY

Female beauty standards, in particular, have long been a subject of criticism and concern. In many societies, women face immense pressure to conform to narrow and often unattainable beauty ideals. These standards can contribute to body image issues, low self-esteem, and a sense of inadequacy among women.[22] The emphasis on physical appearance often overshadows other important aspects of a woman's identity, reinforcing harmful stereotypes and objectification.

It is important to emphasize inclusivity and promote beauty in all its forms as not doing so catalyzes low self-esteem, confidence, and body dysmorphia. For example, historically, darker skin types have been seen as less desirable than their counterparts with lighter skin tones. As a result, movements such as "Black is Beautiful" was created to promote black women's self-esteem as challenge colorist beauty standards. Social standards regarding featurism and hair texturism are also unfairly placed on minority communities. Preferred features uphold the Eurocentric standards of beauty; characteristics such as full lips and broad noses result in discrimination due to unfair beauty standards. Preferred hair textures include hair with a smoother or looser texture, with criticism against those with "kinky" coarse hair, afros, locks, or even braids. As a result, numerous states across the United States have passed the CROWN Act ("Creating a Respectful and Open World for Natural Hair")[23] to prohibit hair-based discrimination in workplaces and schools. While this marks significant progress, there remains work to be done, particularly in states where the Act has not yet been implemented. Black women, in particular, continue to face the risk of discrimination in those areas without the Act's protections. It is imperative that we continue to advocate for inclusivity and educate communities about the significance of this issue.

When we discuss cultural beauty standards, we must also discuss the exploitation of minority aesthetics on racially ambiguous White women.

With the rise of social media, there is a history of racially ambiguous women adopting beauty standards seen in other cultures—such as a darker complexion, more plump lips, and curvaceous figure—to be seen as "exotic" and "interesting." These women are now able to benefit socially and financially from features their minority counterparts have been fetishized and admonished for. This supports an industry that profits off those changing their natural features to fit unattainable social standards.

CONCLUSION

Cultural beauty around the world is a multifaceted and ever-evolving concept. While beauty is culturally defined, certain universal attractiveness variables transcend cultural boundaries. However, the problem of female beauty standards persists, often leading to unrealistic expectations and negative consequences for women. Recognizing and appreciating diverse beauty standards across cultures can foster inclusivity and promote a healthier and more accepting environment for women. The Western world's adoption of beauty practices from other cultures demonstrates the global influence and ongoing evolution of beauty standards. Embracing cultural diversity without appropriation can enrich our understanding of beauty and pave the way for more inclusive beauty standards worldwide.

ACKNOWLEDGMENT

We would like to thank Nina C. Nwade, Howard University College of Medicine, for her contributions to this chapter.

REFERENCES

1. Swami V, Furnham A, Joshi K. The influence of skin tone, hair length, and hair colour on ratings of women's physical attractiveness, health and fertility. *Scand J Psychol.* 2008;49(5):429-437.
2. Lorenzo GL, Biesanz JC, Human LJ. What is beautiful is good and more accurately understood. Physical attractiveness and accuracy in first impressions of personality. *Psychol Sci.* 2010;21(12):1777-1782.
3. Little AC, Apicella CL, Marlowe FW. Preferences for symmetry in human faces in two cultures: data from the UK and the Hadza, an isolated group of hunter-gatherers. *Proc Biol Sci.* 2007;274(1629):3113-3117.
4. Wade TJ. The relationships between symmetry and attractiveness and mating relevant decisions and behavior: a review. *Symmetry.* 2010;2(2):1081-1098.
5. Brooks RC, Shelly JP, Jordan LA, Dixson BJW. The multivariate evolution of female body shape in an artificial digital ecosystem. *Evol Hum Behav.* 2015;36(5):351-358.
6. Feinberg DR, DeBruine LM, Jones BC, Perrett DI. The role of femininity and averageness of voice pitch in aesthetic judgments of women's voices. *Perception.* 2008;37(4):615-623.
7. Fink B, Hufschmidt C, Hirn T, Will S, McKelvey G, Lankhof J. Age, health and attractiveness perception of virtual (rendered) human hair. *Front Psychol.* 2016;7:1893.
8. Tracy JL, Beall AT. Happy guys finish last: the impact of emotion expressions on sexual attraction. *Emotion.* 2011;11 6:1379-1387.
9. Jones AL, Kramer RS, Ward R. Miscalibrations in judgements of attractiveness with cosmetics. *Q J Exp Psychol (Hove).* 2014;67(10):2060-2068.
10. Elliot AJ, Niesta D. Romantic red: red enhances men's attraction to women. *J Pers Soc Psychol.* 2008;95(5):1150-1164.
11. Chen T, Lian K, Lorenzana DI, Shahzad N, Wong R. (2020). Occidentalisation of Beauty Standards: Eurocentrism in Asia. Across the Spectrum of Socioeconomics 1 issue 2. https://doi.org/10.5281/zenodo.4325856.
12. Hwang HS, Spiegel JH. The effect of "single" vs "double" eyelids on the perceived attractiveness of Chinese women. *Aesthet Surg J.* 2014;34(3):374-382.
13. Jang H, Koo FK, Ke L, et al. Culture and sun exposure in immigrant East Asian women living in Australia. *Women Health.* 2013;53(5):504-518.
14. Kalantar Motamedi MH, Ebrahimi A, Shams A, Nejadsarvari N. Health and social problems of rhinoplasty in Iran. *World J Plast Surg.* 2016;5(1):75-76.
15. Thompson CS. Body image in Mauritania: bigger is better. *Utah Hist Rev.* 2014;VI:171-177.
16. Vashi NA, de Castro Maymone MB, Kundu RV. Aging differences in ethnic skin. *J Clin Aesthet Dermatol.* 2016;9(1):31-38.
17. Batista BN. State of plastic surgery in Brazil. *Plast Reconstr Surg Glob Open.* 2017;5(12):e1627.
18. *The profile of Pacific peoples in New Zealand.* Pasefika Proud, Ministry of Social Development; 2016.
19. Latu M. *Pacific Women, Beauty and Race: The Communication of Beauty Ideals and the Experiences of Pacific Women in Contemporary Society.* Auckland: Auckland University of Technology; 2020.
20. Sua'ali'i-Sauni T. Deconstructing the 'exotic' female beauty of the Pacific Islands and 'white' male desire. *Women's Stud J.* 1997;13(2):75.
21. Brewis AA, McGarvey ST, Jones J, Swinburn BA. Perceptions of body size in Pacific Islanders. *Int J Obes Relat Metab Disord.* 1998;22(2):185-189.
22. Cash, T. F., & Smolak, L. (Eds.) Cognitive-behavioral perspectives on body image. *Body Image: A Handbook of Science, Practice, and Prevention.* 2nd ed. New York, NY: The Guilford Press; 2011:39-47.
23. Lee MS, Nambudiri VE. The CROWN act and dermatology: taking a stand against race-based hair discrimination. *J Am Acad Dermatol.* 2021;84(4):1181-1182.

CHAPTER 90 Photoaging in Skin of Color

Yemisi Dina
Chee Leok Goh
Angeline Anning Yong
Anna Chien
Sewon Kang

KEY POINTS

- Race, cultural behavior, nature of occupation, hobbies, and smoking habit can affect the photoaging process.
- The skin varies considerably in its response to sun exposure and the process of photoaging, influenced by the wide range of skin phototypes.
- The melanin in darker skin types appears to confer protection against photoaging from ultraviolet B and A radiation.
- Fairer-skinned individuals tend to develop earlier onset of photoaging and develop more prominent wrinkles than those with skin of color.
- People with skin of color tend to have less coarse wrinkles, telangiectasia, actinic keratoses, and skin cancers but tend to manifest with more pigmentary disorders (eg, lentigo and melasma) and uneven skin tones. In addition, as a result of the reduced extrinsic aging changes, signs of intrinsic aging, such as volume loss, can appear accentuated.

INTRODUCTION

Skin aging in all skin types can be divided into two basic processes: intrinsic aging and extrinsic aging.[1] Photoaging, a term first coined in 1986, is a form of extrinsic aging that refers to the complex process of skin changes caused by chronic exposure to solar radiation.[1,2] While intrinsic aging is a natural process that occurs with time and manifests as skin thinning, laxity, fine wrinkles, and xerosis, photoaging results in premature skin aging on chronically photodamaged skin and is thought to be the major determinant in skin aging. [3,4] Photoaging is characterized by deep wrinkles, senile purpura, pigmentary disorders (eg, solar lentigines and seborrheic keratoses), telangiectasais, skin sagging, actinic keratoses, and skin cancers.[3] Race, cultural behavior, nature of occupation, hobbies, and smoking habit can affect the photoaging process.[5] In this chapter, we will discuss the differences in photoaging between people with skin of color and Caucasians.

OVERVIEW OF PHOTOAGING

Intrinsic aging occurs in all skin types and is determined by genetics while extrinsic aging or photoaging is secondary to mostly cumulative sun exposure.[5] Photoaging is thought to account for 90% of visible skin aging. Risk factors for photoaging include fairer skin, older age, male sex, residence in a location with high sun irradiation and high occupational or recreational sun exposure.[6] Intrinsic aging is characterized by soft tissue volume loss and redistribution due to gravity as well as a decrease in skin elasticity.[7] Photoaging is superimposed upon intrinsic aging and is characterized by decreased skin elasticity, rhytides, solar lentigines, textural roughness, and irregular pigmentation.[7,8]

Histologically, aged skin shows epidermal atrophy and flattening of the rete ridges. In addition to these findings, in photoaged skin, there is also an accumulation of disorganized elastin in the upper dermis and fragmentation of collagen.[7,9] The loss of integrity in elastic fibers and effacement of the dermal-epidermal junction (DEJ) leads to a decline in skin elasticity and therefore manifests as deep coarse wrinkles and skin laxity.[10]

Chronic ultraviolet radiation exposure (290-400 nm) is thought to be the primary driving factor leading to the appearance of photoaged skin.[11] While UVC (200-290 nm) is filtered out by the ozone layer, both ultraviolet A (UVA, 320-400 nm) and ultraviolet B (UVB, 290-320 nm) are contributors to the photoaging process.[7,12] Seventy percent of UVB that reaches the skin is absorbed by the stratum corneum, 20% reaches the epidermis and only about 10% penetrates to the level of the superficial dermis.[13] Twenty to thirty percent of UVA on the other hand reaches the deep dermis.[13]

UVB is directly absorbed by cellular DNA in the epidermis and causes direct damage via the formation of cyclobutane pyrimidine dimers and pyrimidine-pyrimidone (6-4) photoproducts.[14] Due to its shorter wavelengths, UVB penetrates the skin less than UVA. However, because of that wavelength property, UVB is a lot more energetic than UVA and is responsible for erythema, sunburns, inflammation, and the development of skin cancers.[7,14] Given that UVA is far more prevalent than UVB and is able to penetrate deeper into the dermis, UVA is thought to play the larger role in photodamage.[13,15] UVA causes indirect DNA damage through the formation of reactive oxygen species (ROS).[16] These ROS activate cell surface receptors such as epidermal growth factor (EGF) and tumor necrosis factor-α (TNF-α).[16,17] ROS also induce transcription factors such as activator protein-1 (AP-1) and NF-κB.[17]

Matrix metalloproteinases (MMPs) serve an important role in the aging process.[7] Consisting of several members, MMPs collectively act to degrade dermal matrix macromolecules. The collagenases, for example, working in concert with other MMPs (gelatinases and stromelysins), break down collagen and therefore lead to the accumulation of fragmented collagen associated with aging skin.[7] AP-1 is the important transcription factor that upregulates MMPs-1, -3, and -9, leading to the degradation of dermal collagen I and III.[17] AP-1 also inhibits transforming growth factor-β (TGF-β) signaling that is necessary for the production of procollagen.[18] Additionally, UV radiation also depletes endogenous antioxidants including glutathione, tocopherol, and ubiquinone[7], thereby promoting further signaling through AP-1 transcription factor.

Visible light (400-760nm) has more recently been implicated in photoaging. VL makes up about 40% of solar irradiation and penetrates deeper into the skin than UV radiation.[7,16] Similar to UVA, VL causes indirect DNA damage, leading to the production of reactive oxygen species, proinflammatory cytokines, and MMPs in the dermis.[7,16]

DEFINING SKIN OF COLOR

Most of the world's population are individuals with skin of color, including Asians, Hispanics, and Africans. Asians can be subdivided into East Asians (Chinese, Koreans, Japanese), Southeast Asians (Indonesians, Malaysians, Singaporeans, Thais, Cambodians, Vietnamese, Filipinos), and South Asians (Bangladeshis, Pakistanis, Sri Lankans, Indians). Both East Asians and Southeast Asians are of Mongoloid background. Those from East Asia have lighter skin color, whereas Southeast Asians have darker brownish skin color. South Asians, on the other hand, are of Caucasian origin but have brown to dark brown skin.[19]

Hispanics are a large group with varied skin color. A large number of Hispanics worldwide are brown-skinned, but European Hispanics who are of Caucasian origin are lighter in skin color. There are also Hispanics who are of mixed ancestry, with Caucasian and African American or Native American heritage. The geographic areas for brown-skinned Hispanics include North America, Mexico, Central and South America, and the Caribbean.[19]

Thus, the term skin of color includes an extremely heterogeneous group of people. Patients with skin of color generally have Fitzpatrick skin phototypes III to VI. With this wide range of skin colors, their skin varies considerably in its response to sun exposure and the process of photoaging.[19]

PHOTOAGING IN SKIN OF COLOR

Skin of color has varying properties from Caucasian skin that help to determine the response to cumulative photodamage. While skin of color has a thicker stratum corneum, greater lipid content and greater intercellular cohesion, it also has an increased rate of desquamation and decreased ceramide content that is correlated with increased transepidermal water loss and manifests as dry skin.[20,21]

Skin pigmentation is determined by the amount of melanin an individual possesses. Melanin is produced by melanocytes, and while the number of melanocytes is similar across ethnicities, individuals with skin of color have larger and more numerous melanosomes, the organelles within which melanogenesis occurs.[22] Melanocytes transfer melanin to keratinocytes where it is arranged in a supranuclear cap and protects cellular DNA from external insult. There is therefore a direct correlation between the amount of melanin present and the amount of photoprotection DNA receives.[13] The increased melanin in skin of color leads to greater photoprotection through absorption, reflection, and scatter, with UV filtration being five times more effective in skin of color.[23] Additionally, while Caucasian skin possesses more pheomelanin, skin of color possesses more eumelanin. Pheomelanin is prooxidative and releases more ROS than eumelanin upon UV exposure.

In a 1979 study, Kaidbey et al compared the transmission of UV radiation between Caucasian and dark skin of color cadaver skin. They found that the mean protective factor for UVB in the epidermis of dark skin of color was 13.4 compared with 3.4 in the lighter-skinned epidermis, and the mean UVB transmission into the dermis was 5.7% in the epidermis of dark skin of color versus 29.4% in the epidermis of lighter-colored skin.[23] For UVA, the mean protective factor of dark skin of color epidermis was 5.7 compared to 1.8 in lighter-colored epidermis, and the mean UVA transmission into dark skin of color epidermis was 17.5% compared with 55.5% for lighter-colored epidermis.[23] Therefore, three to four times more UVA reaches the upper dermis of fairer-skinned individuals than that of people with dark skin of color. The main site of UV filtration in the former was the stratum corneum, whereas the Malpighian layers removed twice as much UVB radiation as the overlying stratum corneum in the latter.[23]

Studies have also demonstrated differences in the damaging effects of chronic sun exposure in skin of color. Yamaguchi et al[24] reported that the incidence of UV-induced apoptosis was greater in darker skin compared to lighter skin, suggesting that photodamaged cells may be more efficiently removed in darker skin. Del Bino et al[25] reported the relationship between skin color and response to UV exposure using ex vivo light and dark skin samples. A biologically efficient UV dose was determined for each sample by quantifying sunburn cells. The biologic markers include DNA damage, apoptosis, and p53 accumulation. A statistically significant correlation was reported between the biologically efficient dose and DNA damage. In light, intermediate, and tanned skin samples, DNA-damaged lesions were distributed throughout the epidermis and the uppermost dermal cells. In brown and dark skin samples, DNA-damaged lesions were confined to the suprabasal epidermal layers. These results demonstrate a progressive decrease in sensitivity to UV exposure with increasing skin pigmentation. This inverse relationship between skin color and UV damage allowed prediction on individual's propensity for skin cancer development and photoaging and confirmed that skin pigmentation can have a natural protective role against photodamage.[25]

On a histological level, skin of color has more undulations at the DEJ with an increased number of dermal papillae that are more evenly distributed than Caucasian skin.[7] These histologic findings are characteristically seen in more youthful skin and allow for a greater area of contact between the dermis and epidermis, facilitating a more efficient transfer of essential nutrients.[7,26] The elastic fibers in skin of color are thicker and more numerous in the reticular dermis.[7] Additionally, skin of color is able to maintain skin elasticity in both photo-exposed and photoprotected sites, while lighter skin loses elasticity in photo-exposed sites making it more prone to photoaging.[21]

Fibrillin-rich microfibrils (FRMs) are an integral component of the elastic fiber network, the primary effector of skin elasticity.[10,27] The loss of FRMs at the DEJ along with the deposition of disorganized elastotic material in the reticular dermis are signs of photoaging and affect skin elasticity.[10,27] While patients with darker skin of color have an increased number of FRMs that are less susceptible to the remodeling effects of chronic UV radiation, it is unclear whether the ultrastructure of FRMs themselves are influenced by ethnicity.[28] FRMs have a characteristic "beads on a string" ultrastructural appearance.[28] Langton et al demonstrated that while there were no significant differences in the ultrastructure of FRMs between European and African participants in the reticular dermis of a photoprotected site, in the more superficial papillary dermis, there is a larger inter-bead periodicity in FRMs extracted from European participants than that of African participants.[28] Given that there were no significant FRM ultrastructure differences in neonates, there are likely changes that are acquired over time that lead to these differences.[28] The significance of these changes warrants further investigation.

Despite the additional photoprotection that increased melanin grants to persons with skin of color, studies have shown that there is significant impairment of biomechanical function with flattening of rete ridges and marked depletion of elastic fibers and fibrillar collagens.[10] Using a Cutometer and a ballistometer, Langton et al were able to evaluate the biomechanical properties of skin of color. This study showed that in young buttock and forearm skin, there is high resilience and elasticity that decreased with intrinsic aging. In chronically photoexposed skin, there was a decline in both resiliency and elasticity.[10]

In Fitzpatrick skin types IV to VI, visible light has been shown to contribute to clinical manifestations of photoaging such as increased pigmentation. In a study utilizing a light source emitting 98.3% visible light, Mahmoud et al showed that although both UVA-1 and visible light can induce pigmentation in darker skin types, the pigmentation induced by visible light was darker and more sustained.[29] In this study, no pigmentation was induced in light-skinned participants. Increased pigmentation induced by visible light in skin of color has been attributed to shorter wavelengths of visible light. Regazzetti et al demonstrated that OPN3 is the key sensor in melanocytes responsible for this hyperpigmentation[30] Blue light-induced pigmentation results from activation of opsin 3 that then activates extracellular signal regulated kinase and p38 pathways.[30] This leads to the phosphorylation of micropthlamia-associated transcription factor (MITF), resulting in increased tyrosinase and dopachrome tautomerase activity and therefore melanin production in melanocytes.[30]

SPECIFIC PHOTOAGING CHANGES IN SKIN OF COLOR

PHOTOAGING IN DARK SKIN OF COLOR

Photoaging does occur in individuals with dark skin of color but is less common or mild because the epidermis and upper dermis are protected against photodamage by the increased number of melanosomes and melanin in the keratinocytes. Photoaging is seen more frequently in African Americans than in Africans or Afro-Caribbeans. This may be because African Americans consist of a heterogeneous mix of African, Caucasian, and Native American ancestry.[19] Published reports on photoaging in individuals with dark skin have been limited to African Americans.

Histologic preservation of epidermal and dermal components has been demonstrated in sun-exposed African American skin in contrast to sun-exposed Caucasian skin. Montagna and Carlisle[31] compared 19 dark-skinned women of African descent and 19 lighter-skinned women and found that long-term sun exposure resulted in only minor changes in the former compared to profound alterations in the latter. The majority of the lighter-skinned women aged between 45 and 50 years had wrinkles beside the lateral canthi of the eyes and at the corners of the mouth, whereas none of the dark skin of color women showed any obvious wrinkles. In their study, punch biopsies obtained from the malar eminences showed that in fair sun-exposed skin, the stratum lucidum was usually distorted, swollen, and distinctly cellular, whereas darker sun-exposed skin remained compact and rarely showed any evidence of alteration in the stratum lucidum regardless of age. A greater amount of solar elastosis was also found in fairer skin compared to darker skin.[31] This presence of elastotic material in fairer skin is an important factor in dermal photodamage.[32] The deposition of elastotic material occurs less precipitously in the facial skin of young and middle-aged women with dark skin of color.[31] Consequently, a naturally youthful appearance can be maintained well into later life, with photoaging appearing usually late in the fifth or sixth decades of life in this group.[33]

Clinical features of photoaging in African Americans include fine wrinkling and laxity with aging, particularly in the deeper muscular layers of the face, with sagging of malar fat pads toward the nasolabial fold.[34] Hyperpigmentation and uneven skin tone have also been reported to be a greater concern in African American skin compared to Caucasian skin.[35] Although melanin has photoprotective effects as discussed previously, the increased melanin in darker skin of color places these individuals at a higher risk of dyspigmentation. In this patient population, overall pigmentation decreases with age as was demonstrated by Chien et al who analyzed sun-protected buttock skin and sun-exposed forearm skin of 40 Caucasian and 43 African American participants using colorimetry readings.[36] In Caucasians, sun-exposed skin darkens with age and is darker than sun-protected skin, while in African Americans, sun-exposed skin lightens with age and is lighter than sun-protected skin.[36]

Mottled pigmentation and dermatosis papulosa nigra (DPN) are other common manifestations of photoaging in individuals with dark skin of color [**Figure 90-1**]. Although the pathogenesis for the formation of DPN is not completely understood, Niang et al[37] proposed that UV radiation is a potential pathogenic factor because lesions were found to be limited to sun-exposed areas in the African population of Senegal.

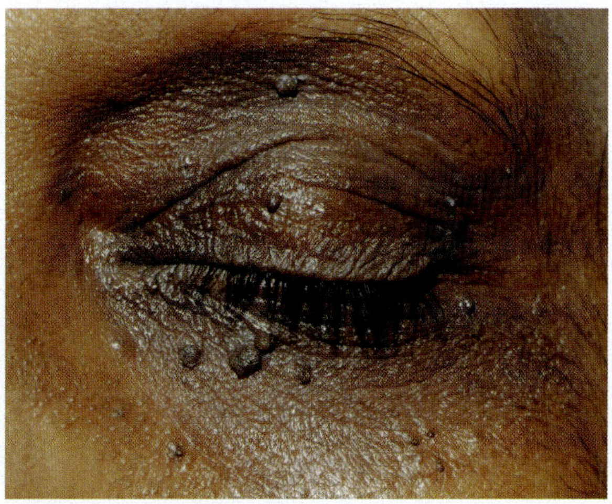

FIGURE 90-1. Clinical features of photoaging in individuals with dark skin of color include mottled pigmentation and dermatosis papulosa nigra, as seen in this patient. (Courtesy of National Skin Centre, Singapore.)

Given that there is a variability in the clinical features of photoaging in darker skin types compared to lighter skinned individuals, a 9-point photonumeric scale has been created to assess the severity of photoaging in the African-American population. Similar scales have been developed for Caucasian and Asian skin types, and are necessary for an objective assessment of photoaging in darker skin types. Using this photonumeric scale, Chien et al assessed photographs of 75 African-American participants and found age and BMI to be significant contributing factors to intrinsic skin aging phenotype in this population.[38]

PHOTOAGING IN HISPANICS

The Hispanic population in the United States includes persons of Puerto Rican, Dominican, Cuban, Venezuelan, Mexican, and other Latin American or mixed populations. This contributes to the wide variation of skin complexions in this population. Sanchez[39] showed that photoaging was the third most common dermatologic diagnosis in 1000 Hispanic patients treated in a dermatology practice in the United States, accounting for 16.8% of visits. Major concerns in this population included a yellow tone and dullness of their skin. Because the Hispanic population comprises individuals with varying skin phototypes, the lighter-pigmented Hispanics tend to exhibit photoaging signs similar to Caucasians individuals, whereas the darker-skin Hispanics tend to show photoaging signs similar to African Americans and other populations of African descent.[40]

Photoaging in European and lighter-skin Hispanics occurs in the same frequency and degree as in Caucasians. As such, the clinical manifestation is primarily wrinkling rather than pigmentary alterations. Coarse wrinkling also appears at roughly the same age at which it would appear in Caucasians. Darker-skin Hispanics who have skin phototypes IV and V and who live in sunny tropical climates such as Mexico, Central America, or South America tend to have clinical photoaging manifestations similar to those of South Asians and African Americans. These manifestations include fine wrinkling and mottled pigmentation. Melasma is a common pigmentary disorder [**Figure 90-2**] that occurs in the late fourth through sixth decades of life.[19] Hernández-Pérez and Ibiett[41] listed photoaging effects in Salvadorans, including fine wrinkles, dilated pores, thick skin, oily skin, telangiectasias, lentigines, and laxity of the skin, which responded well to intense pulsed light treatment.

PHOTOAGING IN ASIANS

Much attention has been directed toward the effects, prevention, and treatment of photoaging, in particular skin discoloration, in Asians in recent years. Many studies on photoaging have been carried out recently in East and Southeast Asians. In that region, photoaging is common because of the geographic proximity to the equator where sunlight exposure is continuous throughout the year. In addition, the traditional desire of Asians to have fair and flawless facial skin, uniform in color and texture, has led to individuals seeking treatment of pigmentary disorders that are associated with photoaging. Thus, the pigmentary changes associated with photoaging in Asians are significant cosmetic problems for these patients.[42]

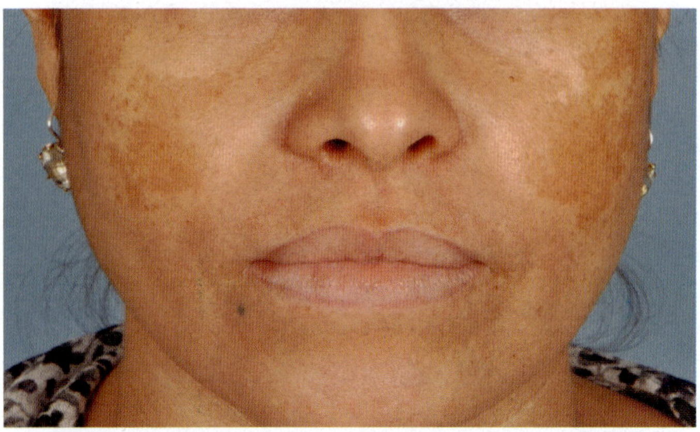

FIGURE 90-2. Darker-skinned Hispanics who have skin phototypes IV and V tend to have photoaging changes that are similar to South Asians and African Americans. This patient has melasma over her cheeks.

Characteristic features of photoaging in the Asian population have been well described. The effects are attributed not only to inherent genetic differences in the biologic defenses of the skin but may also be augmented by the different cultural practices related to sun exposure. Unlike Caucasians, Asians, such as Koreans, Japanese, and Chinese, traditionally avoid direct sunlight by wearing long-sleeved clothes, carrying umbrellas, or seeking shade. Asians have natural photoaging protection, including a thicker stratum corneum, and increased epidermal melanin. The primary difference between Caucasian and Asian skin, however, is attributed to melanocytic function. Because Asian skin is more pigmented, its acute and chronic cutaneous responses to UV radiation differ from Caucasian skin.[43]

In an evaluation of 1500 Asian patients with skin phototypes III and IV from Singapore, Indonesia, and Malaysia, Goh[44] reported that the main features of photoaging included hyperpigmentation, tactile roughness, and coarse and fine wrinkling. However, skin wrinkling was not readily apparent in these populations until about 50 years of age, and even then, the extent of wrinkling was less marked than in Caucasian skin. In another study conducted on Chinese and Japanese patients by Griffiths et al,[45] pigmentary changes seemed to be a more important feature in photoaged skin than wrinkling. Histologic diagnoses of photoaging in this group include seborrheic keratoses, solar lentigines, and solar elastosis.[45]

A later study by Chung,[43] however, showed that rhytide formation could also be a major feature of photoaging in Koreans. This study showed that Asians have thicker, coarser, and deeper rhytides concentrated on the forehead as well as the periocular and perioral areas, whereas Caucasians have relatively fine wrinkles on their cheeks and the crow feet area.[43] These differences in the pattern of skin wrinkling suggest the possibility that there may be wrinkle-associated genes or single-nucleotide polymorphisms in certain genes, such as those for collagen, elastin, or matrix metalloproteinase.[43] However, no scientific evidence has been established to date. In Koreans, patterns of pigmentary change related to aging have been shown to be dependent on gender. The most common pigmented lesions in sun-exposed skin include ephelides (freckling), melasma, lentigo, mottled pigmentation, and pigmented seborrheic keratoses. The appearance of solar lentigines increases with age and is more common in women, whereas the incidence of seborrheic keratosis also increases with age but is more common in men.[46]

Nonetheless, the primary clinical feature of photoaging in East and Southeast Asians is that of discrete pigmentary changes and growths, which predominate over acquired rhytides. These include solar lentigines, pigmented seborrheic keratoses, and mottled hyperpigmentation [**Figure 90-3A–C**], with very little manifestation of skin wrinkling. Sun-induced facial melasma is also more common in this group than in Caucasians and should be considered a form of actinic dyspigmentation and a contributor to photoaging in this instance.[19,42,47] It is not uncommon for photoaging in these individuals to present as a combination of multiple skin pigmentary disorders (eg, lentigines, melasma, acquired dermal melanocytosis) [**Figure 90-4**].

There are few studies describing photoaging changes in South Asians with skin of color. Sun-related hyperpigmentation, seborrheic keratoses, and DPN have been reported with increasing age, but fine wrinkling is not as apparent.[42] Durai et al[3] reported 500 consecutive elderly individuals with skin phototypes IV and V attending the dermatology outpatient department in Puducherry, India, and found that the majority (83%) of the cases were found to have chronologic aging without photoaging. In addition, only a minority (17%) of cases had photoaging along with chronologic aging.[3] Cutaneous changes suggestive of photoaging such as dyspigmentation (13%), freckles (4.8%), thick skin (3.2%), deep wrinkles (2.4%), melasma (2.4%), citrine skin (1%), senile purpura (1%), pseudostellate scars (0.4%), acrokeratoelastoidosis marginalis (0.4%), and lentigines (0.2%) were less frequently observed in this study than other reports. In contrast, Beauregard and Gilchrest[27] observed elastosis in 95.6%, lentigines in 70.6%, senile purpura in 11.9%, and stellate pseudoscars in 5.9% of their Caucasian patients in the United States.

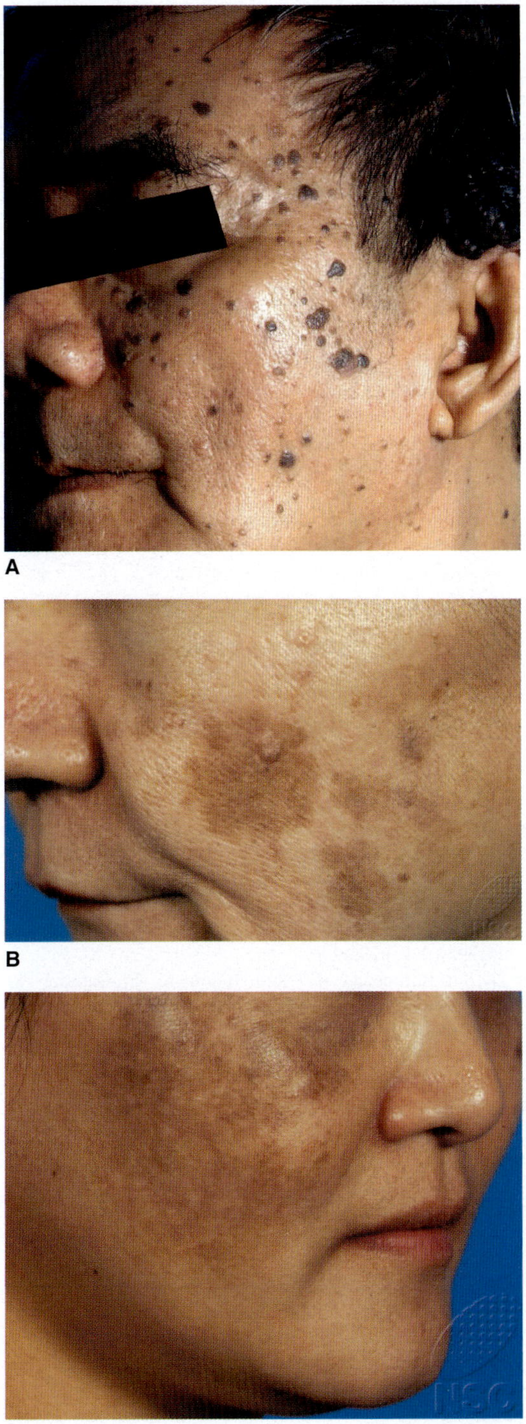

FIGURE 90-3. (A–C) Photoaging in Chinese is characterized by solar lentigines, flat pigmented seborrheic keratoses, mottled hyperpigmentation, and fine wrinkles. (Courtesy of National Skin Centre, Singapore.)

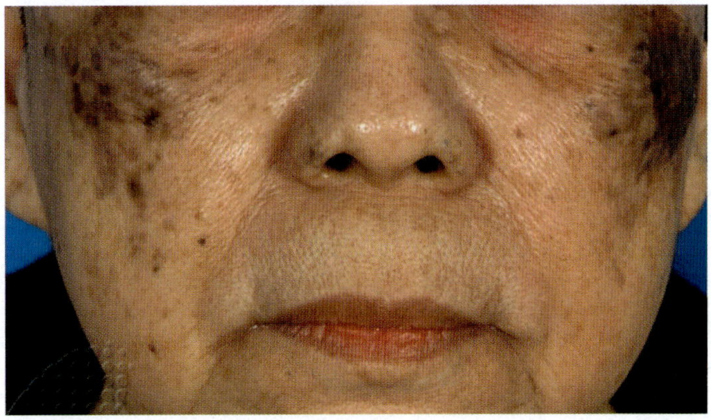

FIGURE 90-4. Typical photoaging changes in a Chinese woman include combination pigmentary disorders (eg, melasma, lentigines, acquired dermal melanocytosis) on sun-exposed areas with little fine wrinkling. Coarse wrinkling is generally absent. (Courtesy of National Skin Centre, Singapore.)

OTHER CONTRIBUTORY FACTORS TO PHOTOAGING IN SKIN OF COLOR

Smoking has been associated with an increased risk of premature photoaging and rhytide formation. This has been found predominantly in fairer skin and less often in skin of color.[48] In Caucasians, premature wrinkling was found to increase with the number of smoking pack-years. Kadunce et al[49] found that individuals who smoked more than 50 pack-years were 2.3 to 4.7 times more likely to develop facial wrinkles than nonsmokers. When excessive sun exposure and smoking coexisted, their effects on wrinkling on skin were synergistic. In the brown skin of Koreans, the odds ratios of wrinkling associated with 30 and 50 pack-years of smoking were 2.8 and 5.5, respectively, after controlling for age, gender, and sun exposure.[46] The effects of sun exposure and smoking were synergistic with an 11-fold increased risk for wrinkling compared to nonsmokers in a less sun-exposed group.[46] Yin et al[50] also reported a 22-fold increase in more severe skin wrinkling in Japanese participants who smoked more than 30 pack-years and were exposed to the sun for more than 2 hours per day, compared to those of the same age who never smoked and had sun exposure levels of less than 2 hours per day.[50] These studies suggest that cigarette smoking is an independent risk factor for the development of rhytides in Asians, as in the Caucasians. Similar studies have not been performed in other skin of color populations.

Pollutants have also been implicated as contributors in skin aging. Air pollutants can be classified into two main categories, particulate matter (PM) that can be fine or coarse and gases (O_3, CO_2, CO, SO_2, NO_2), also known as volatile organic compounds.[51] NO_2 is a primary air pollutant that results from the burning of fuel, contributing to traffic related air pollution. Utilizing data from the Chinese Taizhou cohort, Huls et al found that in Chinese women older than 50 years of age, after adjusting for age, BMI, smoking history, socioeconomic status, and sun-exposure history, an increase of 10 μg/m^3 in NO_2 was associated with the development of 24% more lentigines on the cheeks.[52] These findings were consistent with a similar study that showed increased pigmentation on the cheeks of German women secondary to NO_2.[52,53] Indoor pollution from the cooking with solid fuels such as coal have also been implicated in skin aging in the Chinese population. These individuals were found to have a 5% to 8% more severe wrinkle appearance on the face and a 74% increased risk of having fine wrinkles on the dorsal hands.[54]

PHOTOPROTECTION IN SKIN OF COLOR

Photoprotection includes seeking shade, avoiding sunlight during peak hours, wearing sun protective clothing, and applying sunscreen. Many people with skin of color do not protect themselves with sunscreen when exposed to the sun, and studies have shown that sunscreen use is less prevalent in the African American and Hispanic populations than among Caucasians, even among those who have experienced severe sunburns.[55-57] Note that 10.9% of Black individuals and 24.7% of Hispanic individuals reported using sunscreen with an SPF of 15 or higher for sun protection, compared with 40.4% of non-Hispanic Whites.[18] When sunscreens are applied in Black and Hispanic individuals, they are often applied insufficiently and with inadequate reapplication.[57] This behavior is slowly changing now with improved public education.

Broad-spectrum sunscreens in the United States provide protection against wavelengths shorter than 370 nm and are typically considered the mainstay of photoprotection. These products, however, do not protect against VL and UVA-1, which as discussed earlier in this chapter, are significant contributors to hyperpigmentation in skin of color patients. Grimes et al[58] demonstrated that the daily utilization of sunscreen that offers both broad-spectrum and UVA protection for 12 months in Hispanic females with skin types IV and V improved signs of photoaging including hyperpigmentation, fine lines, skin texture, and overall skin quality. Inorganic sunscreens containing iron oxide, titanium dioxide, and zinc oxide can absorb, reflect, and scatter solar radiation, thus making them effective in the prevention and treatment of dyspigmentation induced by UVA and VL.[59] Individuals with skin of color should therefore be counseled to incorporate sunscreens that offer broad-spectrum, UVA, and VL protection. It is important to note that physical sunscreens that offer protection again UV radiation and visible light often leave a white hue on darker-skinned individuals and thus, may be less accepted in this population. Alternative options include tinted sunscreens that can be matched to an individual's skin type and offer similar or potentially even better protection.[60] Individuals with skin of color should also be encouraged to utilize other modalities of photoprotection including seeking shade and wearing sun protective clothing.

TREATMENT OF PHOTOAGING IN SKIN OF COLOR

The treatment of photoaging is particularly challenging in patients with skin of color due to the innate increased risk of postinflammatory pigmentary changes and scarring in darker skin types. Topical retinoids are the cornerstone of medical management of photoaging. Tretinoin and tazarotene are both FDA approved for this indication, and they have been found to significantly improve dyspigmentation, skin texture, fine wrinkles, lentigines, and elastosis.[61] In patients with skin of color, there is an increased risk of irritant contact dermatitis with a potential for ensuing post inflammatory hyperpigmentation (PIH). However, the benefit of topical retinoids for the treatment of photoaging likely outweighs the risk of PIH in these patients. Utilizing lower strengths of topical retinoids and decreasing frequency of use may be helpful in preventing irritant contact dermatitis.

Photorejuvenation utilizes nonablative visible or infrared light energy to improve the manifestations of photoaging such as fine wrinkles, dyspigmentation, and coarse texture[62] When utilized in skin of color patients, it is imperative to not only limit the fluence of visible wavelengths to prevent excessive absorption by melanin but to also ensure adequate epidermal cooling to prevent conversion of light absorbed by melanin to heat, which can lead to thermal injury.[62] Photorejuvenation has been studied extensively in Asian skin, demonstrating that intense pulse light (IPL) therapy is safe and effective in improving pigmentation, skin texture and tone, telangiectasias, and elasticity.[63]

Other therapies have the potential to reverse evidence of existing photoaging but have not been well studied in patients with skin of color include photodynamic therapy (PDT), platelet-rich plasma (PRP), oral isotretinoin, chemical peels, 5-fluorouracil cream, and antioxidants such as vitamin C, vitamin E, coenzyme Q and lipoic acid, soy, ginseng, and gingko biloba among others.[61]

CONCLUSION

Aging is a global issue, and the desire to halt, retard, or reverse this process is observed in all patient population. Although Caucasian skin is more prone to UV light injury while those with skin of color are more protected against its effect, the latter also exhibit their own characteristic photoaging changes.

The cutaneous manifestations of photoaging can differ significantly between Caucasians and those with skin of color. Pigmentation disorders are more commonly observed with photoaging in individuals with skin of color, whereas wrinkles and telangiectasia are more common in Caucasians. As in light-skinned individuals, adequate photoprotection is important in preventing the detrimental effects of solar radiation in individuals with skin of color.

REFERENCES

1. Gilchrest BA. Skin aging and photoaging: an overview. *J Am Acad Dermatol.* 1989;21(3, Part 2):610-613.
2. Han A, Chien AL, Kang S. Photoaging. *Dermatol Clin.* 2014;32(3):291-299.
3. Durai PC, Thappa DM, Kumari R, Malathi M. Aging in elderly: chronological versus photoaging. *Indian J Dermatol.* 2012;57(5):343-352.
4. Themes UFO. Evaluation of Beauty and the Aging Face. 2019. https://plasticsurgerykey.com/evaluation-of-beauty-and-the-aging-face/. Accessed October 3, 2022.
5. Farage MA, Miller KW, Elsner P, Maibach HI. Intrinsic and extrinsic factors in skin ageing: a review. *Int J Cosmet Sci.* 2008;30(2):87-95.
6. Green AC, Hughes MCB, McBride P, Fourtanier A. Factors associated with premature skin aging (photoaging) before the age of 55: a population-based study. *Dermatology.* 2011;222(1):74-80.
7. Lim H, Kang S, Chien AL. Photodamage in skin of color. In: Watson REB, Griffiths CEM, eds. *Cutaneous Photoaging.* London: Royal Society of Chemistry; 2019:31-58.
8. Krutmann J, Berneburg M. Photoaging of the skin: What's new? *Dermatologist.* 2020;72(2):2-5.
9. Khavkin J, Ellis DAF. Aging skin: histology, physiology, and pathology. *Facial Plast Surg Clin North Am.* 2011;19(2):229-234.
10. Langton AK, Alessi S, Hann M, et al. Aging in skin of color: disruption to elastic fiber organization is detrimental to skin's biomechanical function. *J Invest Dermatol.* 2019;139(4):779-788.
11. Talwar HS, Griffiths CEM, Fisher GJ, Hamilton TA, Voorhees JJ. Reduced type I and type III procollagens in photodamaged adult human skin. *J Invest Dermatol.* 1995;105(2):285-290.
12. Panich U, Sittithumcharee G, Rathviboon N, Jirawatnotai S. Ultraviolet radiation-induced skin aging: the role of DNA damage and oxidative stress in epidermal stem cell damage mediated skin aging. *Stem Cells Int.* 2016;2016:7370642.
13. Battie C, Jitsukawa S, Bernerd F, Bino SD, Marionnet C, Verschoore M. New insights in photoaging, UVA induced damage and skin types. *Exp Dermatol.* 2014;23(s1):7-12.
14. Benjamin CL, Ullrich SE, Kripke ML, Ananthaswamy HN. p53 tumor suppressor gene: a critical molecular target for UV induction and prevention of skin cancer. *Photochem Photobiol.* 2008;84(1):55-62.
15. Yaar M, Gilchrest BA. Photoageing: mechanism, prevention and therapy. *Br J Dermatol.* 2007;157(5):874-887.
16. Liebel F, Kaur S, Ruvolo E, Kollias N, Southall MD. Irradiation of skin with visible light induces reactive oxygen species and matrix-degrading enzymes. *J Invest Dermatol.* 2012;132(7):1901-1907.
17. Fisher GJ, Kang S, Varani J, et al. Mechanisms of photoaging and chronological skin aging. *Arch Dermatol.* 2002;138(11):1462-1470.
18. Tsai J, Chien AL. Photoprotection for skin of color. *Am J Clin Dermatol.* 2022;23(2):195-205.
19. Halder R, Richards G. *Photoaging.* 1st ed. Boca Raton, FL: CRC Press; 2004.
20. Rawlings AV. Ethnic skin types: are there differences in skin structure and function? *Int J Cosmet Sci.* 2006;28(2):79-93.
21. Berardesca E, Maibach H. Racial differences in skin pathophysiology. *J Am Acad Dermatol.* 1996;34(4):667-672.
22. Videira IFdS, Moura DFL, Magina S. Mechanisms regulating melanogenesis. *An Bras Dermatol.* 2013;88(1):76-83.
23. Kaidbey KH, Agin PP, Sayre RM, Kligman AM. Photoprotection by melanin—a comparison of black and Caucasian skin. *J Am Acad Dermatol.* 1979;1(3):249-260.
24. Yamaguchi Y, Takahashi K, Zmudzka BZ, et al. Human skin responses to UV radiation: pigment in the upper epidermis protects against DNA damage in the lower epidermis and facilitates apoptosis. *FASEB J.* 2006;20(9): 1486-1488.
25. Del Bino S, Sok J, Bessac E, Bernerd F. Relationship between skin response to ultraviolet exposure and skin color type. *Pigment Cell Res.* 2006;19(6): 606-614.

26. Girardeau-Hubert S, Pageon H, Asselineau D. In vivo and in vitro approaches in understanding the differences between Caucasian and African skin types: specific involvement of the papillary dermis. *Int J Dermatol.* 2012;51 Suppl 1:1-4.
27. Watson RE, Griffiths CE, Craven NM, Shuttleworth CA, Kielty CM. Fibrillin-rich microfibrils are reduced in photoaged skin. Distribution at the dermal-epidermal junction. *J Invest Dermatol.* 1999;112(5):782-787.
28. Langton AK, Hann M, Costello P, et al. Heterogeneity of fibrillin-rich microfibrils extracted from human skin of diverse ethnicity. *J Anat.* 2020;237(3):478-486.
29. Mahmoud BH, Ruvolo E, Hexsel CL, et al. Impact of long-wavelength UVA and visible light on melanocompetent skin. *J Invest Dermatol.* 2010;130(8):2092-2097.
30. Regazzetti C, Sormani L, Debayle D, et al. Melanocytes sense blue light and regulate pigmentation through Opsin-3. *J Invest Dermatol.* 2018;138(1):171-178.
31. Montagna W, Carlisle K. The architecture of black and white facial skin. *J Am Acad Dermatol.* 1991;24(6 Pt 1):929-937.
32. Montagna W, Kirchner S, Carlisle K. Histology of sun-damaged human skin. *J Am Acad Dermatol.* 1989;21(5 Pt 1):907-918.
33. Halder RM. The role of retinoids in the management of cutaneous conditions in blacks. *J Am Acad Dermatol.* 1998;39(2 Pt 3):98.
34. Courtiss E. Ethnic considerations in facial aesthetic surgery. *Plast Reconst Surg.* 1998;102(5):1755.
35. Grimes P, Edison BL, Green BA, Wildnauer RH. Evaluation of inherent differences between African American and white skin surface properties using subjective and objective measures. *Cutis.* 2004;73(6):392-396.
36. Chien AL, Suh J, Cesar SSA, et al. Pigmentation in African American skin decreases with skin aging. *J Am Acad Dermatol.* 2016;75(4):782-787.
37. Niang SO, Kane A, Diallo M, Choutah F, Dieng MT, Ndiaye B. Dermatosis papulosa nigra in Dakar, Senegal. *Int J Dermatol.* 2007;46 Suppl 1:45-47.
38. Chien AL, Qi J, Grandhi R, et al. Chronological aging in African-American Skin: a reliable photonumeric scale demonstrates age and body mass index as contributing factors. *J Natl Med Assoc.* 2018;110(6):534-539.
39. Sanchez MR. Cutaneous diseases in Latinos. *Dermatol Clin.* 2003;21(4):689-697.
40. Taylor SC. Skin of color: biology, structure, function, and implications for dermatologic disease. *J Am Acad Dermatol.* 2002;46(2 Suppl Understanding):41.
41. Hernández-Pérez E, Ibiett EV. Gross and microscopic findings in patients submitted to nonablative full-face resurfacing using intense pulsed light: a preliminary study. *Dermatol Surg.* 2002;28(8):651-655.
42. Munavalli GS, Weiss RA, Halder RM. Photoaging and nonablative photorejuvenation in ethnic skin. *Dermatol Surg.* 2005;31(9 Pt 2):1250-1260; discussion 1261.
43. Chung JH. Photoaging in Asians. *Photodermatol Photoimmunol Photomed.* 2003;19(3):109-121.
44. Goh SH. The treatment of visible signs of senescence: the Asian experience. *Br J Dermatol.* 1990;122 Suppl 35:105-109.
45. Griffiths CE, Goldfarb MT, Finkel LJ, et al. Topical tretinoin (retinoic acid) treatment of hyperpigmented lesions associated with photoaging in Chinese and Japanese patients: a vehicle-controlled trial. *J Am Acad Dermatol.* 1994;30(1):76-84.
46. Chung JH, Lee SH, Youn CS, et al. Cutaneous photodamage in Koreans: influence of sex, sun exposure, smoking, and skin color. *Arch Dermatol.* 2001;137(8):1043-1051.
47. Alexis A, Rossi A. Photoaging in skin of color. *Cosmetic Dermatology.* 2011;24(8):367-370.
48. Allen HB, Johnson BL, Diamond SM. Smoker's wrinkles? *JAMA.* 1973;225(9):1067-1069.
49. Kadunce DP, Burr R, Gress R, Kanner R, Lyon JL, Zone JJ. Cigarette smoking: risk factor for premature facial wrinkling. *Ann Intern Med.* 1991;114(10):840-844.
50. Yin L, Morita A, Tsuji T. Skin aging induced by ultraviolet exposure and tobacco smoking: evidence from epidemiological and molecular studies. *Photodermatol Photoimmunol Photomed.* 2001;17(4):178-183.
51. Krutmann J, Bouloc A, Sore G, Bernard BA, Passeron T. The skin aging exposome. *J Dermatol Sci.* 2017;85(3):152-161.
52. Hüls A, Vierkötter A, Gao W, et al. Traffic-related air pollution contributes to development of facial lentigines: further epidemiological evidence from Caucasians and Asians. *J Invest Dermatol.* 2016;136(5):1053-1056.
53. Vierkötter A, Schikowski T, Ranft U, et al. Airborne particle exposure and extrinsic skin aging. *J Invest Dermatol.* 2010;130(12):2719-2726.
54. Li M, Vierkötter A, Schikowski T, et al. Epidemiological evidence that indoor air pollution from cooking with solid fuels accelerates skin aging in Chinese women. *J Dermatol Sci.* 2015;79(2):148-154.
55. Hall HI, Jones SE, Saraiya M. Prevalence and correlates of sunscreen use among US high school students. *J Sch Health.* 2001;71(9):453-457.
56. Holman DM, Berkowitz Z, Guy GP, Hawkins NA, Saraiya M, Watson M. Patterns of sunscreen use on the face and other exposed skin among US adults. *J Am Acad Dermatol.* 2015;73(1):83-92.e1.
57. Summers P, Bena J, Arrigain S, Alexis AF, Cooper K, Bordeaux JS. Sunscreen use: non-Hispanic Blacks compared with other racial and/or ethnic groups. *Arch Dermatol.* 2011;147(7):863-864.
58. Grimes P, Halder R, Verschoore M, et al. Long-term benefits of daily Photo-Protection with a broad-spectrum sunscreen in United States Hispanic female population. *J Drugs Dermatol.* 2020;19(3):236-242
59. Taylor SC, Alexis AF, Armstrong AW, Chiesa Fuxench ZC, Lim HW. Misconceptions of photoprotection in skin of color. *J Am Acad Dermatol.* 2022;86(3S):S9-S17.
60. Lyons AB, Trullas C, Kohli I, Hamzavi IH, Lim HW. Photoprotection beyond ultraviolet radiation: a review of tinted sunscreens. *J Am Acad Dermatol.* 2021;84(5):1393-1397.
61. Poon F, Kang S, Chien AL. Mechanisms and treatments of photoaging. *Photodermatol Photoimmunol Photomed.* 2015;31(2):65-74.
62. Munavalli GS, Weiss RA, Halder RM. Photoaging and nonablative photorejuvenation in ethnic skin. *Dermatol Surg.* 2005;31(9 Pt 2):1250-1260; discussion 1261.
63. Shin J-, Lee D-, Choi S-, et al. Objective and non-invasive evaluation of photorejuvenation effect with intense pulsed light treatment in Asian skin. *J Eur Acad Dermatol Venereol.* 2011;25(5):516-522.

CHAPTER 91

Photoprotection

Mustufa A. Jafry
Joseph W. Fakhoury
Henry W. Lim

KEY POINTS

- Both UV radiation (UVR) and visible light (VL) contribute to photodamage and dyspigmentation in people with skin of color (SOC)
- Sunscreens containing organic and/or inorganic UV filters provide protection against UVA and UVB while the addition of tints (iron oxides or pigmentary titanium dioxide) and antioxidants provide additional protection against UVA1 and VL.
- Recent controversies surrounding sunscreens include concerns about systemic absorption of organic filters, association with frontal fibrosing alopecia (FFA), and environmental impacts of organic filters
- SOC patients would benefit most from sunscreen with SPF 30+ and UVA-protection combined with either a tint or antioxidants.

INTRODUCTION

On the spectrum of electromagnetic radiation emitted by the sun, only a small percentage of wavelengths ultimately reach the surface of the Earth, which includes ultraviolet radiation (UVR; 290-400 nm), visible light (VL; 400-700 nm), and infrared (IR; 700 nm to 1mm).[1] Within UVR, UVA (320-400 nm) and UVB (290-320 nm) reach the Earth's surface, while UVC (100-290 nm) does not as it is absorbed by the ozone layer.[1] The vast majority of currently available nontinted sunscreens mitigate the effects of UVR, but they do not protect against VL, which contributes to dyspigmentation in people with skin of color (SOC).[2] This chapter reviews effects of UVR and VL on SOC, followed by a review of sunscreens, including various UV filters, tinted sunscreens, U.S. Food and Drug Administration's (FDA) most recent regulations and health controversies of UV filters, and concludes with recommendations for effective photoprotection in SOC. The term "sunscreen" refers to the final product on the shelves, while "UV filters" are the active ingredients of sunscreens.

EFFECTS OF UV AND VL

Sun damage from UV and VL exposure can occur in all skin types, although with varying clinical presentation. In SOC, photodamage most commonly presents with pigmentary changes.[2]

EFFECTS OF UV

A common effect of UV radiation in SOC is skin pigmentation, also known as tanning. Skin pigmentation has three phases: immediate pigment darkening (IPD), persistent pigment darkening (PPD), and delayed tanning (DT).[3] IPD occurs within minutes of irradiation and resolves in 2 hours; it is followed by PPD, occurring within hours after irradiation and lasting up to about 24 hours. Both IPD and PPD are predominantly induced by UVA and VL; they are due to photooxidation of preformed melanin and redistribution of melanosomes within keratinocytes.[3] DT occurs within about 3 to 5 days following UVA and/or UVB irradiation; in contrast to IPD and PPD, DT is caused by neogenesis of melanin.[3]

EFFECTS OF VL

As VL has longer wavelength range than UV, VL has greater penetration depth. The most significant effects of VL on skin are from violet-blue light (400-500 nm) compared to lower energy VL such as red light.[4] VL has been shown to induce erythema in light- and dark-skinned subjects, and intense and long lasting dyspigmentation in SOC.[4-6] VL induces production of free radicals and reactive oxygen species (ROS), which results in DNA damage, inflammation, and melanogenesis.[4]

OVERVIEW OF SUNSCREENS

Since the first commercial sunscreen became available about a century ago, there has been a vast expansion of UV filters. Active ingredients of sunscreens, ie, UV filters, can be classified as organic filters and inorganic filters. In the United States, UV filters are considered to be over-the-counter drugs, and need to be approved by the FDA. Currently, there are 14 organic UV filters listed in FDA sunscreen monograph, 2 inorganic filters, and another organic filter (ecamsule) approved through New Drug Application process [**Table 91-1**].[7]

In a FDA Proposed Administrative Order released in September 24, 2021, the inorganic filters (titanium dioxide and zinc oxide) were considered GRASE (generally recognized as safe and effective), two organic filters (aminobenzoid acid and trolamine salicylate) were considered not GRASE, while the remaining 12 filters were considered not GRASE because additional safety data are needed.[7] However, until a Final Administrative Order is issued, FDA does NOT require the removal of these filters from the market.

While UV filters have been studied for many decades, the importance of photoprotection from VL has only recently been recognized.[4] In SOC patients, effective sunscreens must provide protection from both UVR and VL in order to prevent the photobiologic effects previously discussed.

TABLE 91-1 UV Filters listed in the FDA monograph

Inorganic filters	
	Zinc oxide
	Titanium dioxide
Organic filters	
	Avobenzone
	Ensulizole
	Homosalate
	Meradimate
	Octinoxate
	Octisalate
	Octocrylene
	Oxybenzone
	Padimate O
	Sulisobenzone

ORGANIC FILTERS

Organic UV filters, also known as chemical filters, are aromatic compounds conjugated to a carbonyl group. The conjugated structure of organic filters allows them to absorb high-energy UVR and convert it into a lower energy state that is then released.[1]

Current U.S. FDA-approved organic UV filters only provide protection against shorter wavelength UVA1 (340-370 nm), with no protection against longer UVA1 wavelengths (370-400 nm).[1] UVA1 represents about 80% of UVR reaching the surface of the earth, and is known to induce pigmentary changes and accentuate the pigmentary effects of VL in SOC.[4] Likewise, no FDA-approved filters have absorption in the VL range, which as stated earlier, has significant biologic effects in SOC. In the European Unions, there are two novel filters that have been approved and marketed: methoxypropylamino cyclohexenylidene ethoxyethylcyanoacetate (MCE; also known as Mexoryl 400), with absorption to 400 nm,[8] and phenylene bis-diphenyltriazine (TriAsorB), has an absorption to 450 nm.[9] These represent a welcome development for photoprotection, especially for those with SOC.

INORGANIC FILTERS

Inorganic filters, also known as mineral or physical filters, are metal oxides: zinc oxide (ZnO) and titanium dioxide (TiO_2). TiO_2 occurs naturally in three crystalline structures: rutile, brokite, and anatase. Rutile is the most stable form, with a higher refractory index and density, and the most common form used in mineral sunscreen.[11] ZnO exists in two forms, zinc blend and wurtzite. Wurtzite is commonly used in mineral sunscreen as it has high refractory index and density with thermodynamic stability at ambient temperatures.[11]

ZnO and TiO_2 are available in different particle sizes, from micronized (>1000 nm) to submicronized (100-1000 nm) to nanosized (<100 nm).[10] Submicronized ZnO (200-400 nm) and TiO_2 (150-300 nm) can reflect and absorb both UVR and VL,[10] but their application can result in white chalky appearance on the skin so they are not cosmetically appealing, especially for individuals with SOC. Therefore, in sunscreens, nanosized particles are commonly used to improve the cosmesis and acceptability of the final product. Photoprotective property of TiO_2 are influenced by its size: reduction in particle size decreases its UVA absorption, shifting its effectiveness further into the UVB spectrum.[11] In contrast, the UV absorption of ZnO is not significantly affected by its size, with a uniform absorption curve across the UVB and UVA spectrum.[11]

TINTED SUNSCREENS

Tinted sunscreens combine color-based coverage with UV filters. The tint is a blend of iron oxides and, in some products, pigmentary non-nanosized titanium dioxide, which are broader-spectrum filters across the UV and VL range.[10] Both iron oxides and pigmentary titanium dioxide can provide opacity and coverage. Iron oxide is a transition metal oxide that can appear as yellow, red, or black. A desired shade of tint can be synthesized by mixing the three colors of iron oxide, with or without pigmentary titanium dioxide.[10]

In addition to protection against UV rays, tinted sunscreens provide the additional benefit of protection against VL. Kaye et al showed that tinted sunscreens (iron oxides combined with ZnO) were more effective than nontinted inorganic or organic sunscreens at protecting against VL.[12] Other studies have shown a tinted sunscreen formulation with 4.5% yellow iron oxide minimized the development of pigmentation induced by VL,[13] and that sunscreens with higher concentration of iron oxides with mineral filter afforded superior protection against blue light sensitivity caused by topical aminolaevulinic acid.[14] Another study showed that while the attenuation of VL by darker shades products was slightly higher than lighter shades, different shades of the same sunscreen brand did not result in a significant difference in the degree of photoprotection against VL.[15,16] Moreover, Dumbuya et al showed that iron-oxide containing sunscreen formulations, when compared to SPF 50+ nonmineral sunscreens, both masked against current pigmentation and reduce prevention of further pigmentation after sun exposure.[16]

ANTIOXIDANTS INCORPORATED INTO SUNSCREENS

VL combined with UVA1 can induce erythema and hyperpigmentation in people with SOC. Hyperpigmentation from VL combined with UVA1 has previously been shown to be induced, at least in part, by oxidative stressors.[17,18] Thus, antioxidants (AO) hold a potential therapeutic potential in mitigating the combined effects of VL and UVA1.

Ruvolo et al studied the effects of AO on combined VL and UVA1 irradiation in skin types IV to VI patients.[17] Four sunscreen products (organic sunscreen with no AO, organic sunscreen with three AO, organic sunscreen with five AO, and tinted mineral sunscreen with one AO) and control were tested. The nontinted five AO sunscreen (with vitamin E, vitamin C, diethylhexyl syringylidenemalonate, licochalcone A, and glycyrrhetinic acid) provided comparable photoprotection against the VL and UVA1 induced erythema and pigmentation to the tinted sunscreen. In another study, Lyons et al showed that an topical antioxidant blend containing a variable concentration of diethylhexyl syringylidenemalonate (singlet oxygen quencher; at 1% and 2%) and fixed concentrations of vitamin E (0.25%) and vitamin C (0.01%) reduced pigmentation in SPT IV to VI caused by VL and UVA.[18]

CONTROVERSIES OF SUNSCREENS

These include systemic absorption and potential effects on health, frontal fibrosing alopecia (FFA), and environmental impacts of UV filters.

SYSTEMIC ABSORPTION

Scientists at FDA has conducted two studies to investigate systemic absorption of organic sunscreens.[18,19] The FDA has previously recommended that topical agents with systemic absorption resulting in plasma levels of greater than 0.5 ng/mL should be subject to nonclinical toxicology assessment including developmental and reproductive studies as well as systemic carcinogenicity.[19] The first trial included 24 healthy participants and application of 2 mg/cm^2 of four commercial sunscreens (containing avobenzone, oxybenzone, octocrylene, and ecamsule) applied to 75% of body surface area (BSA) four times per day for 4 days, with blood samples collected over 1 week from each participant.[19] Systemic concentrations reached greater than 0.5 ng/mL for all four products after four applications on the first day.[19] In a follow-up randomized control trial, 48 healthy participants were randomized to one of four sunscreen products (lotion, aerosol spray, nonaerosol spray, and pump spray), and 2 mg/cm^2 of sunscreen was applied to 75% of BSA once on day 1 and then four times on days 2 through 4, with blood samples collected over 21 days from each participant.[20] All six organic sunscreen active ingredients tested (avobenzone, oxybenzone, octocrylene, homosalate, octisalate, and octinoxate) resulted in plasma levels above 0.5 ng/mL, and were reached after one application on the first day.[20] The FDA has stated that while the clinical relevance of these studies is unclear, future studies need to be performed to better understand the effects of these systemic absorptions.[20] Finally, based on a recent systemic review examining 29 studies, current evidence is not sufficient to support the causal relationship between the elevated systemic level of oxybenzone or octinoxate and adverse health outcomes.[21]

In contrast to organic UV filters, inorganic filters are not readily absorbed beyond the stratum corneum and pilosebceous unit and are thus considered to be systemically safe.[22] However, there are concerns regarding inhalation of mineral nanoparticles as the lung is unable to clear them, resulting in potential increased alveolar concentration and subsequent systemic absorption.[22] While human studies have not shown acute systemic effects from inhalation of ZnO nanoparticles, TiO_2 remains classified by the International Agency for Research on Cancer (IARC) as a possible carcinogen when inhaled in large doses due to an increased risk of cancer in animal models.[22] Thus, the Environmental Working Group (EWG) recommends against powdered products or spray sunscreens containing ZnO or TiO_2.[22]

FRONTAL FIBROSING ALOPECIA (FFA)

FFA is a cicatricial alopecia of unclear pathogenesis, although recent reports have described a potential association between skin care products and this condition.[23] A recent systematic review, examining nine studies with 1248 patients with FFA and 1459 controls, found a significantly increased risk of FFA with the use of facial moisturizer or sunscreen.[23] However, while an association does exist, there is insufficient evidence to suggest a direct causal relationship.[23]

ENVIRONMENTAL IMPACT

Prior work has identified certain organic UV filters (octocrylene, oxybenzone, ethylhexyl salicylate, and octinoxate) in nearly all water sources of the world.[22,24] Notably, these filters are difficult to remove with common wastewater treatment plant techniques. Other organic UV filters (octinoxate, 4-methylbenzylidene camphor, octocrylene, and oxybenzone) have been identified in various fish species worldwide, which can affect fertility and various systemic organs. Moreover, these chemicals are not broken down by lower-order organisms on the food chain and have the potential to increase in concentration as other animals or humans ingest these organisms. Additionally, in vitro studies, using concentrations higher than those detected in sea water, have implicated oxybenzone as a possible contributor to coral reef bleaching. In general, inorganic filters do not negatively impact the environment as they tend to form sediments at ocean floor. In fact, the report from National Academies, released on August 9, 2022, recommended that the U.S. Environmental Protection Agency should conduct an ecological risk assessment study on UV filters.[24]

PHOTOPROTECTION RECOMMENDATIONS

There are many benefits of outdoor activities, therefore, the general public should continue to be encouraged to participate. However, for skin health, proper photoprotection should be practiced. This includes staying in the shade when outdoors, wearing photoprotective clothing, wide brimmed hat and sunglasses, and applying sunscreen on otherwise exposed area.

Many individuals with SOC believe that their natural pigmentation serves as effective protection and thus they do not need to practice photoprotection. Studies have shown that SOC individuals having experienced a severe sunburn were over seven times less likely to wear sunscreen than White patients who had experienced a severe sunburn.[2] However, public education has been shown to be beneficial. Studies examining photoprotection education in elementary school students found a 30% increase in use of photoprotection after educational interventions were implemented.[2]

SPF, BROAD SPECTRUM PROTECTION, AND TINTED SUNSCREENS

Broad spectrum sunscreens currently available in the United States protect against 90% of wavelengths under 370 nm and do not protect against VL and UVA1.[2] A majority of U.S. dermatologists and consumers have been shown to use SPF as their primary measure for selection of sunscreen.[25] However, SPF serves as a measure of protection against erythema, which is predominantly the effect of UVB, and to a lesser extent, short-wave UVA [UVA2 (320-340 nm)].[25] Long-wave UVA and VL, which are highly relevant to SOC, are not taken into consideration with SPF. Long-wave UVA and VL have been shown to contribute to pigmentary disorders such as melasma and PIH.[2] As such, public education regarding broad-spectrum sunscreens with UVA1 and VL protection is important for reduction of photoaging and improvement in dyspigmentation.

The biologic effects of sunlight differ based on skin phototypes. Light-skinned individuals are more prone to UV erythema, and with chronic exposure, photoaging and photocarcinogenesis. In contrast, dark-skinned individuals are less likely to develop sunburn, photoaging, and photocarcinogenesis but are more prone to develop UV-induced hyperpigmentation, which could be persistent. As such, in the past few years, individualized advice for the type of sunscreen used has been developed [**Figure 91-1**].

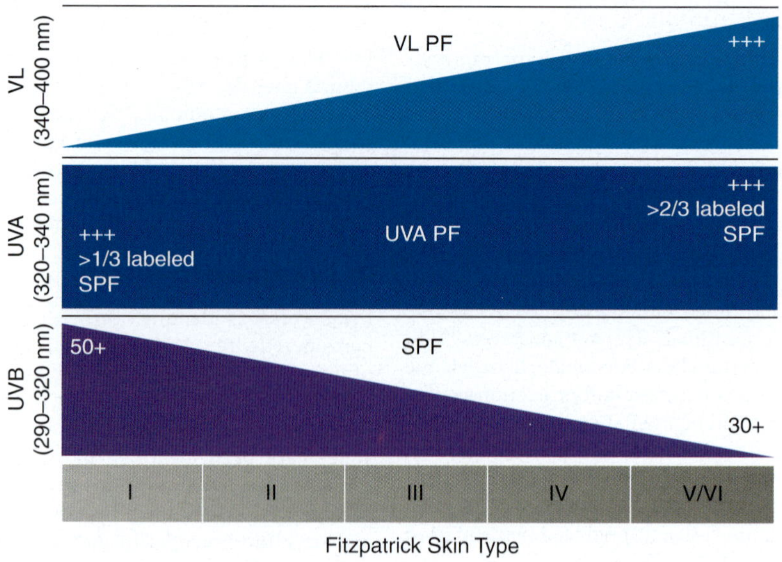

FIGURE 91-1. UV and VL protection factors according to skin phototype. (Reproduced with permission from Rigel DS, Lim HW, Drealos ZD, Weber TM, Taylor Sc. Photoprotection for all: current gaps and opportunities. *J Am Acad Dermatol.* 2022;86(3S): S18-S26.)

Individuals with SOC should be encouraged to use sunscreen with SPF 30+ and an UVA-protection factor (UVA-PF)/SFP ratio of greater than two-thirds (eg, UVA-PF should be at least 30 for an SPF45 sunscreen). Light-skinned subjects should be encouraged to use SPF50+, and an UVA-PF/SPF ratio of >1/3 (ie, UVA-PF of at least 15 for an SPF 45 sunscreen).[25,26]

Tinted sunscreens are beneficial for individuals with SOC. They should be advised to try different formulations of tinted sunscreen to best match their skin-tone.[26] If the individual uses topical medication, sunscreen should be applied after the application of medication, with make-up (if desired) as the last step. Moreover, patients should be encouraged to rub the product thoroughly into their skin in order to decrease the cast caused by the sunscreen. Tinted sunscreens do stain clothing; however, the stain can easily be washed off.

SUNSCREENS WITH ANTIOXIDANTS, AND ORAL PHOTOPROTECTIVE AGENTS

Although tinted sunscreens have been shown to reliably protection from VL and UVA1, studies are underway to find additional compounds that may also provide similar protection. Antioxidants scavenge ROS and have been shown to provide protection from VL and UVA1.[17,18] While not as extensively studied as tinted sunscreens, sunscreens with antioxidants may provide a future alternative to tinted sunscreens for patients who would prefer to use nontinted products.

Oral photoprotection has also been shown to provide photoprotection from VL in SOC.[25] *Polypodium leucotomos* is a fern native to South America that has anti-inflammatory, photoprotective, and antioxidant effects. *P. leucotomos* has been previously shown to decrease persistent pigmentation in SOC, highlighting the VL photoprotective effects of *P. leucotomos*.[25] Other oral agents that have been studied to show photoprotective effects include carotenoids, green tea, pomegranate, resveratrol (grape seed, grape peel, and red wine), curcumin (Turmeric), and silymarin (milk thistle).[27]

CONCLUSION

Photoprotection is critically important in all skin types, including in SOC. Both UVR and VL contribute to dyspigmentation in SOC. Sunscreens containing organic and/or inorganic UV filters provide protection against UVB and UVA. The addition of iron oxides, pigmentary titanium dioxide, as well as antioxidants provide additional protection against UVA1 and VL. Studies on oral agents also show potential additional benefits. Individuals with SOC would most benefit from sunscreen with SPF 30+ and an UVA-PF/SPF ratio of greater than two-thirds, combined with either a tint or antioxidants. Continued public education on photoprotection needs to be done.

REFERENCES

1. Austin E, Geisler AN, Nguyen J, Kohli I, Hamzavi I, Lim HW, Jagdeo J. Visible light. Part I: Properties and cutaneous effects of visible light. *J Am Acad Dermatol.* 2021;84(5):1219-1231.
2. Taylor SC, Alexis AF, Armstrong AW, Chiesa Fuxench ZC, Lim HW. Misconceptions of photoprotection in skin of color. *J Am Acad Dermatol.* 2022;86(3S):9-17.
3. Maddodi N, Jayanthy A, Setaluri V. Shining light on skin pigmentation: the darker and the brighter side of effects of UV radiation. *Photochem Photobiol.* 2012;88(5):1075-1082.
4. Lim HW, Kohli I, Ruvolo E, Kolbe L, Hamzavi IH. Impact of visible light on skin health: The role of antioxidants and free radical quenchers in skin protection. *J Am Acad Dermatol.* 2022;86(3S):27-37.
5. Randhawa M, Seo I, Liebel F, Southall MD, Kollias N, Ruvolo E. Visible light induces melanogenesis in human skin through a photoadaptive response. *PloS One.* 2015;10(6):e0130949.
6. Ramasubramaniam R, Roy A, Sharma B, Nagalakshmi S. Are there mechanistic differences between ultraviolet and visible radiation induced skin pigmentation? *Photochem Photobiol Sci.* 2011;10(12):1887-1893.
7. Geisler AN, Austin E, Nguyen J, Hamzavi I, Jagdeo J, Lim HW. Visible light. Part II: Photoprotection against visible and ultraviolet light. *J Am Acad Dermatol.* 2021;84(5):1233-1244.
8. Marionnet C, Tran C, Bastien P. A broader filtration of UVA1 wavelengths improves skin photoprotection. *J Dermatol Sci.* 2018;91(3):337-340.
9. Bacqueville D, Jacques-Jamin C, Dromigny H. Phenylene bis-diphenyltriazine (TriAsorB), a new sunfilter protecting the skin against both UVB + UVA and blue light radiations. *Photochem Photobiol Sci.* 2021;20:1475-1486.
10. Lyons AB, Trullas C, Kohli I, Hamzavi IH, Lim HW. Photoprotection beyond ultraviolet radiation: a review of tinted sunscreens. *J Am Acad Dermatol.* 2021;84(5):1393-1397.
11. Smijs TG, Pavel S. Titanium dioxide and zinc oxide nanoparticles in sunscreens: focus on their safety and effectiveness. *Nanotechnol Sci Appl.* 2011;13(4):95-112.
12. Kaye ET, Levin JA, Blank IH, Arndt KA, Anderson RR. Efficiency of opaque photoprotective agents in the visible light range. *Arch Dermatol.* 1991;127(3):351-355.
13. Ruvolo E, Fair M, Hutson A, Liebel F. Photoprotection against visible light-induced pigmentation. *Int J Cosmet Sci.* 2018;40(6):589-595.
14. Bissonnette R, Nigen S, Bolduc C, Méry S, Nocera T. Protection afforded by sunscreens containing inorganic sunscreening agents against blue light sensitivity induced by aminolevulinic acid. *Dermatol Surg.* 2008;34(11):1469-1476.

15. Bernstein EF, Sarkas HW, Boland P, Bouche D. Beyond sun protection factor: an approach to environmental protection with novel mineral coatings in a vehicle containing a blend of skincare ingredients. *J Cosmet Dermatol.* 2020;19(2):407-415.
16. Grimes PE. Impact of iron-oxide containing formulations against visible light-induced skin pigmentation in skin of color individuals. *J Drugs Dermatol.* 2020;19(7):712-717.
17. Ruvolo E, Boothby-Shoemaker W, Kumar N, Hamzavi IH, Lim HW, Kohli I. Evaluation of efficacy of antioxidant-enriched sunscreen products against long wavelength ultraviolet A1 and visible light. *Int J Cosmet Sci.* 2022;44: 394-402.
18. Lyons AB, Zubair R, Kohli I, et al. mitigating visible light and long wavelength UVA1-induced effects with topical antioxidants. *Photochem Photobiol.* 2022;98(2):455-460.
19. Matta MK, Zusterzeel R, Pilli NR. Effect of sunscreen application under maximal use conditions on plasma concentration of sunscreen active ingredients: a randomized clinical trial. *JAMA.* 2019;321(21):2082-2091.
20. Matta MK, Florian J, Zusterzeel R. Effect of sunscreen application on plasma concentration of sunscreen active ingredients: a randomized clinical trial. *JAMA.* 2020;323(3):256-267.
21. Suh S, Pham C skin-lightening and cleansing, Smith J, Mesinkovska NA. The banned sunscreen ingredients and their impact on human health: a systematic review. *Int J Dermatol.* 2020;59(9):1033-1042.
22. Schneider SL, Lim HW. Review of environmental effects of oxybenzone and other sunscreen active ingredients. *J Am Acad Dermatol.* 2019;80(1): 266-271.
23. Maghfour J, Ceresnie M, Olson J, Lim HW. The association between frontal fibrosing alopecia, sunscreen, and moisturizers: a systematic review and meta-analysis. *J Am Acad Dermatol.* 2022;87(2):395-396.
24. Council NR. *Review of Fate, Exposure, and Effects of Sunscreens in Aquatic Environments and Implications for Sunscreen Usage and Human Health [Internet].* Washington, DC: The National Academies Press; 2022.
25. Rigel DS, Lim HW, Draelos ZD, Weber TM, Taylor SC. Photoprotection for all: current gaps and opportunities. *J Am Acad Dermatol.* 2022;86(3S): S18-S26.
26. Torres AE, Awosika O, Maghfour J, Taylor S, Lim HW. Practical guide to tinted sunscreens. J Am Acad Dermatol. 2022;87(3):656-657.
27. Torres AE, Luk KM, Lim HW. Botanicals for photoprotection. *Plast Aesthetic Res.* 2020;7:57.

CHAPTER 92

Cosmeceuticals in Skin of Color

Cheryl M. Burgess
Porcia B. Love
Jennifer David
Chloe Walker

KEY POINTS

- Cosmeceuticals have become one of the largest profitable market-segments of the beauty industry with products widely available from diverse marketers.
- First- and second-generation cosmeceuticals contain bioactive ingredients that impact the skin's biological function by penetrating the stratum corneum barrier more deeply for enhanced health benefits.
- Cosmeceuticals are designed with multifunctionality for the treatment of common ethnic skin concerns including sensitive skin, dyschromia, skin laxity, rhytids, and sun-induced aging.
- Cosmoleculars™ or designer molecules for cosmetics will mark the introduction of new skin care technology for the 21st Century.
- The cosmetic industry continues to hold promise in providing novel agents for maintaining healthy skin with an uptrend in clinical efficacy and safety data provided over time.

INTRODUCTION TO COSMECEUTICALS

WHAT ARE COSMECEUTICALS?

The term "cosmeceuticals" describes a rapidly expanding product category hybrid between cosmetics and pharmaceuticals, designed with multifunctionality and less side effects. Cosmeceuticals have been referred to as functional cosmetics in their ability to enhance functioning when applied topically. Cosmeceuticals contain bioactive ingredients that may penetrate the stratum corneum barrier more deeply to enhance the skin's biological function.[1]

COMMON USE OF COSMECEUTICALS

There is a wide variety for the clinical use of cosmeceutical formulations promoting optimal skin health. Cleansing cosmeceutical technologies including toners, cleansing cloths, exfoliating scrubs, mechanized and unmechanized beauty devices, and medicated cleansers are important for treating oily and acne-prone skin.[2] Moisturizing cosmeceuticals with barrier repair agents including ceramides, fatty acids, and cholesterol are crucial for the management of dermatologic conditions that cause excessively dry skin. Anti-inflammatory cosmeceutical agents aid in the treatment of sensitive skin; skin-lightening cosmeceutical agents aid in the treatment of dyschromia, anti-aging cosmeceutical agents aid in the treatment of skin laxity and wrinkle-prone skin, and photoprotective cosmeceutical agents prevent photodamage contributing to sun-induced aging skin **[Figure 92-1]**.[3] Botanicals are an important source of bioactive ingredients that are often formulated in combination with other cosmeceuticals for improved effectiveness. **Table 92-1** lists a variety of botanical agents that may be utilized for anti-inflammation, anti-aging, skin-lightening, moisturizing, and cleansing in patients of all skin types.[4]

COSMECEUTICAL MULTI-FUNCTIONALITY

An advantage of cosmeceuticals like many pharmaceuticals is that there is multi-functionality of use that can be recommended for a variety of skin conditions. For example, topical vitamins like niacinamide is known for its exfoliative effects in treating acne inflammation while it is also beneficial for skin-lightening and cleansing.[5,6] Vitamin A has cleansing, anti-inflammatory, and anti-aging properties.

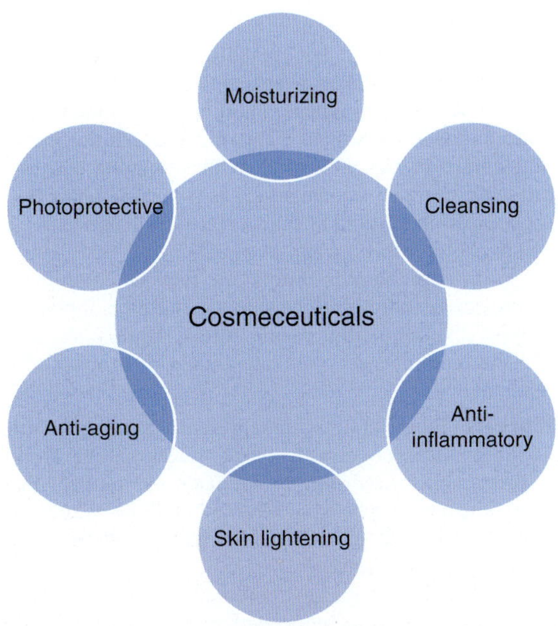

FIGURE 92-1. Cosmeceuticals include a diverse group of hybrid products containing both cosmetic and medicinal properties for cleansing, moisturizing, anti-aging, skin-lightening, anti-inflammatory, and photoprotective management.

TABLE 92-1 Plant derivatives for cosmetic use[4]

Botanical agent (active component)	Skin care properties
Soy (isoflavones, saponins, essential amino acids, phytosterols, calcium, potassium, iron, STI, BBI)	Antioxidant, antiproliferative, anticarcinogenic, depigmentation, increased skin elasticity, oil production control, moisturizing, delayed facial/body hair regrowth
Green/Black/White Tea extracts/polyphenols (epigallocatechin-3-gallate [EGCG])	Antioxidant, anti-inflammatory, anticarcinogenic, photoprotective, wound healing
Chamomile (terpenoids, flavonoids, hydroxycoumarins, mono-/oligosaccharide, mucilages)	Antimicrobial, antiallergic, anti-inflammatory, antioxidant, analgesic
Caffeine	Anticarcinogenic, antioxidant
Coffeeberry extract	Antioxidant, skin rejuvenation

Abbreviations: BBI: Bowman-Birk inhibitor; STI: soybean trypsin inhibitor.

Vitamins C and E as well as α-lipoic acids have skin-lightening and anti-aging properties. α-Hydroxy acids (AHA) may be used for anti-inflammatory and skin-lightening properties.[7] Taking individual preferences into consideration with the formulation of cosmeceuticals may improve compliance of use.[1]

DEVELOPMENT OF COSMECEUTICAL INDUSTRY

HISTORY OF COSMECEUTICALS

The term cosmeceuticals was first introduced in 1961 by Raymond Reed, founding member of the U.S. Society of Cosmetic Chemists. Cosmeceuticals were further popularized in the 1970s by dermatologist Dr. Albert Kligman through his significant contributions in the anti-acne and anti-aging effects of topical retinoid.[1]

MARKETING OF COSMECEUTICALS

Cosmeceuticals are considered the largest growth segment of the personal care industry, representing approximately 80% of the combined U.S. and European cosmeceutical market in skincare.[1] Market growth is encouraged by consumer demand, competition between doctor brands and major manufacturers, accessibility of new ingredients, financial incentive, and increased knowledge in skin physiology.[8] Cosmeceuticals are widely available through mass, direct, and prestige retailers.[1]

The Consumer Consumer demographics and demand continues to shift and become more complex over time with the rapid growth of the cosmeceutical industry. Aging baby boomers have traditionally driven cosmeceutical sales in the United States and Western Europe, accounting for an upward of U.S. $150 million in anti-aging cosmeceuticals. Nontraditional consumer segments such as young men have become an important population targeted by the cosmeceutical market in cleansing, moisturizing, photoprotection, and shaving.[9,10]

Today's knowledgeable consumers are seeking credible scientific backing to their skin care products and alternative noninvasive treatment options. Consequently, cosmeceutical companies have partnered with dermatologists to validate claims of product efficacy to consumers.[1]

Ethnic Markets Ethnic groups also represent a growing consumer segment in cosmeceuticals targeting hyperpigmentation, uneven skin tone, and acne-prone skin.[9] According to equitable market predictions, the U.S. beauty industry is expected to reach $73 billion by 2025 at a compound annual growth rate (CAGR) of 5% with a potential $9.2 billion revenue from ethnic consumers.[11]

Cofounder, Dr. Cheryl Burgess, and representatives of U.S. Black Opal note the success of distributors with operations in the UK, including destinations in the Caribbean, Botswana, Brazil, and Zaire. Another indicator of the success of products targeting ethnic populations is the acquisition of cosmetic companies in non-Western countries: For example, L'Oréal's purchase of Yue-Sai Kan cosmetics and Carson, Inc.[12,13]

REGULATION OF COSMECEUTICALS

The hybrid function of cosmeceuticals presents unique challenges for classification and regulation. The Federal Food, Drug, and Cosmetic Act of 1906 within which the Food and Drug Administration (FDA) operates does not recognize the term cosmeceuticals.[1,2] In some cases, regulators have attempted to distinguish drugs from cosmetics based on the concentration of an active ingredient. This poses a challenge for active ingredients such as AHA in which their efficacy on the skin is more vehicle versus concentration dependent.[14]

MOISTURIZING COSMECEUTICALS

OVERVIEW AND THERAPEUTIC SIGNIFICANCE IN SKIN OF COLOR

Individuals with darker skin types are known to have an increased propensity to dry, cracked skin that often precipitates chronic pruritus, atopic eczema, nummular eczema, and asteatotic eczema in this patient population.[15,16] Reduced ceramides, an important stratum corneum lipid for skin barrier function, contribute to the development of these common conditions. Moisturizers are the conventional treatment for dermatologic conditions driven by skin barrier dysfunction through creating a suitable environment for skin repair and healing. Moisturizer ingredients can be classified into four basic categories: (1) occlusive agents, (2) humectants, (3) emollients, and (4) rejuvenators [**Table 92-2**].[17,18]

Occlusive Agents Occlusive agents are the most popular formulation ingredient due to their ability to prevent water loss by forming a hydrophobic layer on the skin surface promoting barrier repair. Occlusives

TABLE 92-2 Moisturizer ingredients[17–19]

Category (Function)	Moisturizer ingredients
Occlusive agents (Create a water impermeable barrier over the stratum corneum preventing epidermal water loss)	• Hydrocarbons: petrolatum, mineral oil, paraffin, squalene • Silicones: dimethicone, cyclomethicone, amodimethicone • Animal and vegetable fats: lanolin, shea butter, grape seed oil, avocado oil, hemp oil, jojoba oil, sesame seed oil, nut oil • Fatty acids: lanolin acid, stearic acid • Fatty alcohols: lanolin alcohol, cetyl alcohol • Polyhydric alcohols: propylene glycol, butylene glycol • Wax esters: lanolin, beeswax, stearyl stearate • Vegetable waxes: carnauba, candelilla • Phospholipids: lecithin • Sterols: cholesterol
Humectants (Draw water to the stratum corneum)	Alpha-hydroxy acids, amino acids, collagen, elastin, glycerin, gelatin glycogen, glycosphingolipids, glycosaminoglycans, hyaluronic acid, honey, lecithin, phospholipids, polysaccharides, proteins, pyrrolidone carboxylic acid (sodium PCA), propylene glycol, sodium lactate, sorbitol, sugars, urea
Emollients (Smooth and soften skin by filling spaces between corneocytes)	• Protective/smooth film: diisopropyl dilinoleate, isopropyl isostearate • Fatting/greasy film: castor oil, propylene glycol, jojoba oil, isostearyl isostearate, octyl stearate • Dry/nongreasy: isopropyl palmitate, decyl oleate, and isostearyl alcohol • Astringent/minimal greasy: dimethicones, cyclomethicones, isopropyl myristate, octyl octanoate
Rejuvenators (Smooth skin by restoring essential proteins)	Collagen, keratin, elastin

work most effectively when applied to dampened skin. Examples include petrolatum, lanolin, silicones, and mineral oils. Despite its greasy feel, petrolatum is the prototypic occlusive, known for its hypoallergenic, noncomedogenic, and nonacnegenic qualities, as well as its ability to reduce transepidermal water loss (TEWL) by 99%. Dimethicone is the second most common silicone-based active agent in moisturizers. Although dimethicone has comparable qualities to petrolatum, petrolatum is superior in reducing facial dehydration lines and in skin healing [Table 92-2].[17,18]

Humectant Agents Humectants promote skin hydration by attracting water from the deeper dermal layer to the epidermis. The efficacy of humectants are optimized when used in conjunction with occlusive agents to prevent further TEWL. Examples of common humectants include hyaluronic acid, glycerin, hydroxy acids, propylene glycol, and urea [Table 92-2].[17-19]

Emollient Agents Emollients promote soft, smooth skin by depositing in the spaces between desquamating corneocytes. The proper selection of emollient use in skin care products is influenced by their unique aesthetic properties including greasiness and spreadability. Examples of common emollients found in moisturizers include essential fatty acids such as linoleic acid [Table 92-2].[17-19]

Rejuvenator Agents Similar to emollients, rejuvenator agents may improve skin smoothness and function to restore essential proteins including collagen, keratin, and elastin. Successful penetration of large essential proteins into the skin is a noted limitation.[17]

Skin Care Regimens for Dry Skin Skin care regimens for dry skin should preserve essential skin lipids from the protective bilayer membrane with a hydrating nonfoaming cleanser free of detergents and surfactants used both morning and evening. Cleansers should be followed by a barrier repair moisturizer that restores ceramides, cholesterol, and fatty acids in the morning and evening. A hydrating mineral sunscreen should be applied in the morning as a final step.[3]

CLEANSING COSMECEUTICALS

OVERVIEW AND THERAPEUTIC SIGNIFICANCE IN SKIN OF COLOR

Oily skin is another common concern of patients with skin of color. While there is no direct association between darker skin subtypes and increased sebum production, enhanced light reflection from a darker skin surface may produce a more oily appearance. Cleansing cosmeceuticals are essential to remove excess sebum, bacteria, and other debris from the skin surface for optimal skin health, preventing acne and other inflammatory skin conditions.[3]

Cleansers are generally characterized as soaps or synthetic detergents. Soaps have higher alkaline pH properties that often result in excess stripping of important intercellular lipids. Soaps include traditional fatty acid salts and modern blends of tallow and nut oil. Synthetic detergents or syndets have comparatively more natural alkalinity resulting in less lipid removal. Combars are cleansers composed of both modern soaps and synthetic detergents such as antibacterial bars.[20]

Cleansers may be further classified by chemical or physical cleansing properties. Surfactants and solvents are two classes of chemicals for cleansing. Cationic, anionic, amphoteric, and nonionic surfactants aid to emulsify skin surface oils to facilitate removal. Polar and nonpolar solvent-based cleansers aid by homogenous dissolution of skin surface oils. Physical cleansing requires friction through the use of cleansing cloths, mechanical devices, etc. Furthermore, there are various forms of cleansing technologies including foaming/emollient cleansers, milks, scrubs, toners, and cleansing cloths/mechanical devices with cosmeceutical components. The cleanser category recommended is contingent upon specific skin care needs by skin type. It is important to avoid certain additives in cleansers, especially if there is a history of sensitive skin.[21] **Table 92-3** lists several types of cleansers and their main attributes.

TABLE 92-3 Cleansers[20]

Cleanser type	Composition	pH	Skin issues	Examples
Traditional soaps	Animal fat interacting with an alkali, such as lye, resulting in a fatty acid salt	9-10, strongly alkaline	Excessive removal of intercellular lipids, stratum corneum swelling	Homemade soaps
Modern soaps	Blend of tallow and nut oil, or the fatty acids derived from these products	9-10, strongly alkaline	Removes intercellular lipid, less stratum corneum swelling	Ivory (P&G)
Syndets	Synthetic detergents: sodium lauryl sulfate, sodium laurate, and sodium cocyl isethionate	5.5-7, neutral to slightly alkaline	Less alkaline pH reducing protein denaturation	Dove (Unilever)
Combars	Combine modern soap and synthetic detergents	7, slightly alkaline	Intermediate skin damage between soap and syndet, includes most antibacterial bars	Dial (Henkel)

Source: Reproduced with permission from Zoe Diana Draelos. The science behind skin care: Cleansers. J Cosmet Dermatol. 2018;17(1):8-14.

EXFOLIANT AGENTS

α-hydroxy Acids AHAs are organic carbolic acids that are naturally derived from fruit, sour milk, sugar cane, and molasses. As opposed to true keratolytic agents, AHAs reduce corneocyte cohesion at newly formed deeper stratum corneal layers leading to increased flexibility for reduced fissuring. AHAs can be used as peeling agents as they further promote the exfoliation of dead skin cells and removal of excess skin oil.[22,23] As two of the most common AHA agents, glycolic acid and lactic acid have been shown to significantly improve clinical signs of photodamage including hyperpigmentation and roughness.[23,24] While prescription and over-the-counter (OTC) AHAs vary in Ph and concentration, AHA preparations with higher acidity have increased efficacy in absorption independent of concentration level.[22]

Polyethylene Beads Polyethylene beads or microbeads are synthetic scrub particles often combined with surfactants for use as a mild exfoliant. Polyethylene beads utilize van der Waals forces to absorb oil when rolled over the skin surface. However, microbead use has raised environmental disposal concerns challenging there continued use in several states.[1]

TOPICAL VITAMIN AGENTS

Topical vitamins are popular active micronutrients in the cosmeceutical industry. Vitamins carry diverse therapeutic benefits for the skin including antioxidant protection from UV-induced free radicals.[25]

Niacinamide Niacinamide or biologically active vitamin B_3 (niacin) is important for its sebostatic effect in oil-reducing moisturizers. Niacinamide also plays a key role in the NADPH anabolic pathway, resulting in diverse cutaneous properties including the disruption of melanogenesis through inhibition of melanosome transfer.[5,26]

Vitamin A Vitamin A is a fat-soluble natural compound that is well-known for its role in cellular proliferation and differentiation.[27,28] Cosmeceutical-grade retinoids, available OTC (retinyl esters, retinol, and retinaldehyde), undergo conversion to the biologically active metabolite, retinoic acid, leading to diminished potency. Prescription-grade retinoids (tretinoin, tazarotene) directly bind and activate retinoic acid receptors for enhanced efficacy and consequently more potential side effects (dryness, irritation).[8,28] Innovative drug delivery systems (solid lipid nanoparticles, microemulsions, liposomes) may improve retinoid response and tolerability.[25] Retinoids are invaluable for daily maintenance as they promote prevention and repair of photodamaged skin by stimulating collagen synthesis.[29]

BOTANICAL TONER AND ASTRINGENT AGENTS

Toners or astringents are liquid formulations that are often used following cleansing technologies to enhance sebum removal. Toners vary in alcohol to humectant concentrations depending on the targeted skin type, with higher alcohol concentrations found in oily skin astringents.[3] See Table 92-1 for a list of botanical toners and astringent agents beneficial for oily skin.

SKIN CARE REGIMENS FOR OILY SKIN

Skin care regimens for oily skin should include a foaming, detergent-containing facial cleanser to remove sebum from the skin both morning and evening. Cleansing may be followed by the optional use of a toner in the T-zone area for additional sebum removal both morning and evening. Regimens for oily skin may avoid application of a facial moisturizer. However, if use of a moisturizer is preferred after cleansing, use of a niacinamide (morning and/or evening) or retinoid moisturizer (evening) is recommended.[2] Finally, an oil-free mineral broad-spectrum sunscreen containing zinc oxide and titanium dioxide with a sun protection factor (SPF) of 30 or higher should be applied in the morning. Tinted mineral sunscreen may be a more elegant option for patients with skin of color to reduce an opaque appearance.[3] Regimens may be supplemented with the use of polymer bead oil-absorbing creams and oil-absorbing facial powders/tissue papers.[2,30] Regimens should avoid the use of comedogenic products.[3]

ANTI-INFLAMMATORY COSMECEUTICALS

OVERVIEW AND THERAPEUTIC SIGNIFICANCE IN SKIN OF COLOR

Underlying erythema is often masked in individuals with darker skin tones and therefore may be challenging to appreciate in skin of color.[3] Hyperpigmentation is often more notable on presentation in skin of color that may occur secondary to prior inflammatory disease including acne, rosacea, and allergic or irritant dermatitis known as postinflammatory hyperpigmentation (PIH).[31] Burning and stinging of the skin may be present in the absence of underlying erythema as primary cutaneous symptoms pointing to sensitive skin and inflammation. Cosmeceuticals for these conditions are aimed at reducing inflammation in conjunction with avoidance of irritating triggers that further exacerbate the skin.[3]

COSMECEUTICALS FOR ACNE-PRONE SKIN

Salicylic Acid Salicylic acid (SA) is a lipophilic β-hydroxy acid commonly used as an active ingredient in the treatment of acne, PIH, and melasma due to its strong comedolytic and low-level anti-inflammatory effects.[6,32] SA may be incorporated into many vehicles including lower concentration (2% or less) cleansers, moisturizers, and facial foundations. SA is often used at higher concentrations (20% to 30%) as a chemical peeling agent with routinely safe and effective use in skin of color.[32,33] Beta-lipohydroxy acid (LHA) is an SA derivative with an additional fatty chain resulting in enhanced lipophilic properties with more uniform cutaneous exfoliation for a smooth skin appearance.[32]

Glycolic Acid Glycolic acid is a common hydrophilic AHA with similar clinical use as SA active ingredients but with less comedolytic potency.[6]

Lactobionic Acid Lactobionic acid is an important polyhydroxy acid for acne-prone sensitive skin types with humectant and antioxidant properties and comparatively less comedolytic potency.[6]

SKIN CARE REGIMENS FOR SENSITIVE SKIN

Skin care regimens for acne-prone sensitive skin should use combination therapy that will vary between oily/dry/combination skin types. A hydroxy acid gentle exfoliating cleanser to clear pores may be used both morning and evening. Morning cleansing may be followed by a combination benzoyl peroxide/antibiotic topical to kill bacteria and reduced resistance and finally a barrier repair moisturizer with a broad-spectrum sunscreen. Evening cleansing may be followed by a moisturizer then a topical retinoid to prevent irritation. Regimens may be further supplemented with hormonal agents, oral antibiotics, and other adjunctive treatments.[34]

Skin care regimens for rosacea-prone sensitive skin may include a soothing cleanser to calm the skin morning and evening, followed by a broad-spectrum sunscreen in the morning. Regimens may be supplemented with the use of anti-inflammatory botanicals in combination with a vasoconstrictive agent including caffeine, oxymetazoline, and brimonidine.

Skin care regimens for allergic/irritant dermatitis should generally include the use of fragrance-free products with a nonfoaming gentle cleanser followed by a barrier repair moisturizer morning and evening.[3]

SKIN LIGHTENING COSMECEUTICALS

OVERVIEW AND THERAPEUTIC SIGNIFICANCE IN SKIN OF COLOR

Acquired skin disorders of hyperpigmentation including melasma, PIH, freckles, and lentigines, are a common concern in skin of color and can be very challenging to treat. Skin-lightening cosmeceuticals are important for targeting hyperactive melanocytes causing dyschromia through inhibition of tyrosinase, inhibition of melanosome transfer, and/or removal of epidermal pigment.[35] The most common approach by skin-lightening agents is through tyrosinase inhibition as the key rate-limiting enzyme of melanin biosynthesis. Hydroquinone and triple combination therapies for a synergistic effect are considered first line for the management of dyschromia.[36,37]

QUINONE-RELATED COMPOUNDS

Hydroquinone and Arbutin Hydroquinone (HQ) or 1,4-dihydroxybenzene is a naturally occurring phenolic compound found in plants, coffee, tea, beer, and wine. Hydroquinone is the gold-standard of depigmenting agents as one of the most effective melanocyte cytotoxic agents for the treatment of hyperpigmentary disorders.[36,38] HQ gradually suppresses melanin synthesis through reduced tyrosinase activity and impact on DNA and RNA synthesis leading to the reversible-inhibition of cellular metabolism.[38,39] Available prescription HQ formulations often include tretinoin, glycolic acid, microsponges, and/or sunscreen ingredients to increase the skin-lightening potency.[40] The risk of dermatological side effects of HQ including skin irritation, contact dermatitis, and rarely exogenous ochronosis increase with higher concentration and extended use of HQ especially with Fitzpatrick skin types IV to VI.[38,39] An HQ-free holiday for 4 to 12 weeks is recommended generally after 2 to 3 months of use for individuals that do not respond well to treatment or require extended treatment during which an alternative lightening agent may be used for maintenance including arbutin, kojic acid, licorice extract, azelaic acid, and tretinoin.[39]

Liposomal conductive systems are microscopic vesicles made of phospholipid bilayers used to introduce water and lipid soluble medications leading to reduced side effects. While liposomal HQ has demonstrated significant therapeutic effects for dyschromia, there is minimal added benefit for its use compared to conventional HQ. A double-blind randomized controlled trial (RCT) demonstrated no superiority of 4% liposomal hydroquinone once daily treatment compared to standard formulations of 4% HQ for 12 weeks.[41]

Arbutin (hydroquinone-O-beta-D-glucopyranoside) is a naturally occurring derivative of hydroquinone that also functions to inhibit tyrosinase activity and thereby reduces melanin synthesis.[35] Further research is warranted for the recommendation of use of arbutin for melasma therapy.[37]

FLAVONOID-LIKE AGENTS

Licorice Extract Licorice extract is a skin-lightening agent that originates from the root *Glycyrrhiza Glabra Linneva*. Glycyrrhizic acid and flavonoids are the primary bioactive components of licorice extract. Specific isolated flavonoids, including licuraside, isoliquiritin, and licochalcone A, have demonstrated competitive inhibition for monophenolase activity of tyrosinase with no significant inhibition of diphenolase activity with an L-DOPA substrate.[42,43] Glabridin, a major ingredient in the hydrophobic fraction of licroice extract, also demonstrates melanocyte tyrosinase inhibition. Additional isoflavene and chalcone derivatives from licorice extract including glabrene and isoliquiritigenin (2′,4′,4-trihydroxychalcone), respectively, have demonstrated both mono- and diphenolase tyrosinase activities.[43]

Hydroxystilbenes Hydroxystilbene derivatives including resveratrol, oxyresveratrol, and gnetol all function to reversibly inhibit tyrosinase, with the latter two isomer derivatives demonstrating increased efficiency. Resveratrol structure analog, 4,4′-dihydroxybiphenyl, is a potent tyrosinase inhibitor in B16 mouse melanoma cells. 4,4′-dihydroxybiphenyl has demonstrated diverse inhibitory mechanisms for melanin synthesis including glutathione synthesis activation, reduced activity of the cAMP-dependent PKA signaling pathway, and reduced Mift gene expression.[36]

NATURALLY OCCURRING ORGANISMS

Kojic Acid Kojic acid or 5-hydroxy-4-pyran-4-one-2-methyl is a natural metabolite extracted from Aspergillus, Acetobacter, and Penicillium fungal species.[44] Kojic acid is a mixed tyrosinase inhibitor that acts through copper ion chelation.[38] Kojic acid treats hyperpigmentation in 1% to 4% strength formulations often combined with topical corticosteroids and penetration enhancers (glycolic acid) for increased efficacy.[35] Kojic acid has minimal side effects including contact dermatitis, stinging, and erythema.[44,45] A review of existing RCTs gave a weak recommendation for kojic acid in combination with other agents such as 2% HQ, 0.1% betamethasone, and 2.5% ascorbic acid with insufficient evidence to support use as monotherapy agent for melasma.[37]

Azelaic Acid A natural occurring dicarboxylic acid derived from pityrosporum ovale and commonly found in wheat, rye, and barley.[35,38] Azelaic acid is both a competitive and reversible inhibitor of tyrosinase that appears to function selectively on highly active melanocytes.[38,46] Azelaic acid was given a weak recommendation for melasma due to lack of well-designed existing RCTs for up to 20% azelaic acid formulations with use twice daily.[37]

PEPTIDE AGENTS

Tetrapeptide-30 and Undecylenoyl phenylalanine Tetrapeptide-30, a natural skin-derived tetrapeptide, and undecylenoyl phenylalanine, an amino acid and lipid residue containing compound, both function to treat dyschromia through reduction in melanocyte activation. Studies have demonstrated a statistically significant clinical improvement in as few as 4 weeks of both skin-lightening peptides, PKEK, and 2% undecylenoyl phenylalanine, respectively.[35,47,48]

THIOL COMPOUNDS

Cysteamine Cysteamine is a tyrosinase inhibitor with a beneficial safety profile. In two double-blind RCTs, including up to 50 patients with melasma receiving 4 months daily treatment with 5% cysteamine or placebo, cysteamine significantly reduced Melasma Area and Severity Index (MASI) scores.[49,50] Another double-blind single-center RCT, including 20 participants with melasma treated with hydroquinone or cysteamine for 16 weeks, demonstrated no statistically significant difference in modified MASI (mMASI) scores between groups ($p = 0.3$) suggesting comparable efficacy.[51]

SYSTEMIC AGENTS

Polypodium Leucotomos Extract Oral polypodium leucotomos extract (PLE) is a natural substance derived from tropical fern leaves with many dermatologic applications consistent with its notable antioxidant, photoprotective, and anti-inflammatory properties. PLE promotes a reduction in UV-induced phototoxicity including increased cyclobutene pyrimidine dimers as well as improved cell membrane integrity and elastin expression.[52]

Tranexamic acid Oral tranexamic acid (TXA) is a procoagulant that functions through inhibition of the plasminogen activation pathway.[35] In a systematic review of RCTs involving TXA, TXA demonstrated strong recommendation for the treatment of melasma with comparable efficacy to HQ and favorable side effect profile. TXA is prescribed with caution due to theoretical risk for thrombosis; however, there is little to no evidence for increased clotting among low-risk patients.[37]

BOTANICAL AGENTS FOR SKIN LIGHTENING

Soy Soybean-derived protein proteinase inhibitors including soybean trypsin inhibitor (STI) and the Bowman-Birk protease inhibitor (BBI) are known natural skin-lightening agents. Soybean extracts have demonstrated in vivo and in vitro reduced pigmentation by blocking melanosome transfer through the protease-activated receptor 2 (PAR-2) pathway.[52,53] Soymilk and STI have also demonstrated prevention of UVB-induced pigmentation.[52]

Soybeans are rich in isoflavones including genistein and daidzein with noted anti-inflammatory, anticarcinogenic, and antioxidant properties.[54] Through tyrosine kinase inhibition and upregulation of alpha 2 (I) collagen (COL1A2) gene expression, genistein may additionally demonstrate collagen stimulating properties.[54,55] Robust soy-mediated skin care properties support its safety and efficacy in postmenopausal women and pigmentary disorders excluding melasma with a noted hormonal estrogen component [Table 92-1].[4]

SKIN CARE REGIMENS FOR SKIN LIGHTENING

A morning regimen may include a gentle hydroxy acid exfoliating cleanser followed by vitamin C and a broad-spectrum sunscreen. In the evening, gentle cleansing may be followed by a triple combination product (hydroquinone, retinoid, and a steroid). A moisturizer may be applied before or after triple combination therapy for sensitive or dry skin types.[3]

ANTI-AGING COSMECEUTICALS

OVERVIEW AND THERAPEUTIC SIGNIFICANCE IN SKIN OF COLOR

Aging is a complex process that is driven by genetic influences (chronological aging) as well as various environmental stressors including UV damage (epigenetic aging).[56]

Unique ethnic characteristics in facial anatomy and skin biology impact the signs and onset of aging.[57,58] Generally African Americans (Fitzpatrick skin type [FST] III to VI) have an upward 20-year delayed onset of visible aging followed by Latino and Hispanics compared to patients with lighter skin.[59] While increased melanin, melanosome dispersion and intrinsic skin features of increased elasticity provide a natural skin protective factor against UV damage, skin of color is still at risk for UV-induced damage commonly leading to sagging skin.[3,57] Classic signs of aging in skin of color are attributed to volume loss and decline of thick, heavy soft tissue as opposed to fine lines and wrinkles attributed to decreased skin laxity in lighter-skinned individuals.[57]

ANTIOXIDANT AGENTS

Coenzyme Q10 Coenzyme Q10 (ubiquinone, Q10) facilitates mitochondrial energy production as part of the mitochondrial respiratory chain. The endogenously reduced form, ubiquinol, has cutaneous antioxidant properties that preserve cellular energy metabolism. The degree to which the aging process may impact Q10 biosynthesis and plasma levels is unclear; however, reduced Q10 levels in the skin have been demonstrated with increasing age and external stress.[60,61]

Topical Q10-containing formulas have shown promising results. A randomized controlled study showed a significant increase in both superficial and deeper layer skin quinone levels following 2 weeks treatment with twice-daily application of Q10-containing formulas. Increased oxygen consumption rate as a measure of energy metabolism, a significant decrease in free radicals, and increased antioxidant capacity were also demonstrated in stressed skin.[60]

Furfuryladenine N6-Furfuryladenine (Kinetin) is classified as a cytokinin plant-derived hormone with anti-aging effects in plants, cultured human fibroblast cells, and fruit flies. While its exact antioxidant mechanism is still unclear, kinetin has demonstrated protective properties against DNA oxidative damage. Compared to other anti-aging compounds, kinetin may delay aging onset without impacting proliferative capacity.[62,63]

COSMECEUTICALS FOR ANTI-AGING SKIN

Alpha-Lipoic Acid Alpha-lipoic acid (LA) is a natural dithiol compound that facilitates mitochondrial energy production as a key cofactor. LA's unique structural properties are influenced by its enantiomer activity (R-LA vs S-LA) and cellular concentration.[56]

LA is well-known for its robust antioxidant properties. LA has demonstrated increased cellular glutathione levels promoting antioxidant potential. LA also functions as a free radical scavenger preventing lipid peroxidation.[56]

Low concentrations of up to 100 μM are adequate to achieve favorable results with minimal side effects.[64] Topical and oral treatments containing LA have shown positive anti-aging outcomes in reducing UV-induced skin damage; however, topical vehicles advantageously target application of a controlled concentration.[56,65,66] LA has also demonstrated a therapeutic role in the management of chronic disease such as diabetic neuropathy. One such study showed intravenous LA diminished neuropathic pain, paresthesia, and numbness.[67]

Idebenone Idebenone is classified as a benzoquinone and Q10 analogue initially synthesized for cerebral ischemic lesions.[68] Idebenone has become a popular active agent in anti-aging cosmeceuticals known for its potent antioxidant properties. Compared to other topical antioxidants, including tocopherol, kinetin, ubiquinone, ascorbic acid, and lipoic acid, idebenone has surpassed in antioxidant capacity.[69] Idebenone has specifically demonstrated a role in protection from endogenous oxidative stress in Friedreich Ataxia-patient-derived fibroblasts.[68]

In a double-blinded study, topical idebenone in 0.5% and 1% formulations demonstrated comparable efficacy in improving UV-induced roughness, dyschromia, fine lines, and wrinkles with no reported adverse events. These positive outcomes were further supported on immunofluorescent staining with decreased matrix metalloproteinase (MMP), interleukin (IL)-6, and IL-1b expression and increased collagen 1.[70]

VITAMIN AGENTS

Vitamin C (L-ascorbic acid) Vitamin C or its active form, L-ascorbic acid, is a natural water-soluble antioxidant sourced through diet. Optimal skin levels of vitamin C are maintained through direct topical application as absorption and delivery to the skin through dietary supplementation is limited biologically.[54] Topical formulations with L-ascorbic acid derivatives including magnesium ascorbyl phosphate and ascorbyl-6-palmitate increase stability but do not effectively optimize vitamin C levels in the skin.[54]

Vitamin C functions as a potent antioxidant by donating electrons to neutralizing free radicals. Topical vitamin C has demonstrated photoprotective effects in porcine and human skin.[71] A 6-month, double-blinded, randomized trial demonstrated improvement in photodamaged skin among the vitamin C-treated group including significant reappearance of small furrows (<20 μm) and reduction in deep furrows.[72] Multi-functionality of vitamin C, in addition to its antioxidant properties for photoprotection, include collagen production and preservation, improved hyperpigmentation via tyrosinase inhibition, and anti-inflammatory effects via downregulation of transcription factor nuclear factor kappa B (NF-κB).[54,72]

Vitamin E Vitamin E is a physiologic, fat-soluble antioxidant that exists as eight molecular forms including tocopherols and tocotrienols. Vitamin E is also sourced by diet with free D-alpha-tocopherol being the most biologically active form.[54,73] The biologic inactivity of vitamin E acetate, in the absence of a free phenolic hydroxyl group, favors this provitamin in topical formulations. Vitamin E acetate exerts its antioxidant effect in the skin by hydrolysis to active α-tocopherol.[74] In fact, α-tocopherol has significantly demonstrated protection against UVB-induced lipid peroxidation, sun-burn, and DNA damage in cultured skin.[75]

Many studies have explored the controversial role of vitamin E in skin cancer protection and wound healing. Vitamin E also demonstrates anti-inflammatory and immunomodulatory properties contributing to its therapeutic potential in diverse dermatologic conditions including granuloma annulare, discoid lupus erythematosus, and psoriasis.[73,76] Antioxidant effect of vitamin E is synergistic with vitamin C as it replenishes its oxidized form as well as with vitamin A for optimal levels.[73,77]

PEPTIDE AGENTS

Short amino acid chains or peptides are increasingly popular cosmeceutical agents that may be classified as signal, neurotransmitter, and carrier peptides.

Carrier Peptides Carrier peptides that transport copper into cells have demonstrated a vital role in wound-healing properties in acute, chronic, and ischemic open wounds.[78] The tripeptide-copper complex (TCC), glycyl-histidyl-lysine-Cu2+ (GHK-Cu), promotes extracellular matrix remodeling by regulating the expression of MMPs and tissue inhibitors of metalloproteinases (TIMPs).[78,79] GHK-Cu was found to directly stimulate dermal fibroblast proMMP-2 synthesis with simultaneous increase in TIMP-1 and TIMP-2 synthesis that may facilitate regulation of MMP proteolytic activity.[79] Topical TCC was found to also decrease wound concentrations of cytokines and proteinases, which in excess may contribute to chronicity. TCC-treated ischemic wounds demonstrated significantly lower concentrations of active/pro-MMP-2, pro-MMP-9, and TNF-α compared to controls by day 6.[78]

Copper's direct role in angiogenesis for wound healing is well-established. Copper sulfate was found to target human keratinocyte expression of vascular endothelial growth factor (VEGF), a potent angiogenic stimulator.[80] TCC also promotes wound repair through synthesis of collagen and glycosaminoglycans and proteoglycans by dermal fibroblasts.[81,82] TCC injections increased wound production of type I collagen, decorin mRNA, chondroitin sulfate, dermatan sulfate,[82] and heparan sulfate.[81]

Signal Peptides (Pentapeptide Pal-KTTKS) Signal peptides promote collagen preservation through stimulating collagen synthesis or preventing collagen degradation. Palmitoyl pentapeptide palmitoyl-lysine-threonine-threonine-lysine-serine (pal-KTTKS) is well-known signal peptide for its ability to improve photoaged skin.[83,84] A double-blind randomized controlled study demonstrated tolerability (no irritation) and significant reduction of fine lines/wrinkles with topical pal-KTTKS at weeks 8 and 12.[84]

Neurotransmitter-Affecting Peptides Neurotransmitter-affecting peptides are cosmeceuticals marketed as noninvasive replicates to botulinum neurotoxins. Neuropeptides reportedly increase the signal threshold for facial muscle contraction leading to reduced fine lines and wrinkles.[83] Synthetic neuropeptide, acetyl hexapeptide-3 (AC-gly glu-met-gln-argarg-NH2) or Argireline, targets the soluble N-ethylmaleimide-sensitive factor attachment protein receptors (SNARE) complex preventing acetylcholine vesicle docking and release. While Argireline demonstrated reduced efficacy in blocking neurotransmitter release compared to botulinum neurotoxin type A (BTX-A), argireline is advantageous in reduced acute toxicity as a biosafe alternative.[83,85]

GROWTH FACTOR-CONTAINING PREPARATIONS

Growth factors, important in wound healing, are present in a number of cosmeceuticals. Among the growth factors found in new cosmeceutical products, TGF-β is an important collagen-stimulating growth factor.[86] Fetal fibroblasts have been used to develop skin contracts with horse collagen and have been clinically shown to produce complete closure of burn wounds in pediatric patients without traditional grafting.[87] Fetal fibroblasts express transient and lower amounts of TGF-β 1 than adult fibroblasts, which may be resulting in scarless healing of skin during the first trimester of pregnancy.[88]

A novel skin cream containing processed skin-cell proteins (PSP), a proprietary growth factor and cytokines extracted from cultured first trimester fetal human dermal fibroblasts, has shown to be effective for skin rejuvenation. In a clinical study, 18 patients with Fitzpatrick class II or greater facial photodamage applied this growth factor and cytokine skin cream twice daily for 60 days. The patients were evaluated for clinical grading of photodamage on a five-point scale and facial photography. The results showed an statistically significant improvement in average wrinkle score in periorbital and perioral areas extending to day 74 after a 2-week wash-out period.[89]

An additional novel skin cream shown to be effective for skin rejuvenation contains liposome-encapsulated TGF-β 1, L-ascorbic acid, and black cohosh (*Cimicifuga racemosa*) extract in a silicone base. In a clinical study, 12 patients with facial wrinkling applied TGF-β 1 containing cream on one-half of the face and a skin cream without TGF-β 1 on the other half of the face twice daily for 3 months. The patients were evaluated for clinical grading of photodamage on a five-point scale and facial photography. The results showed a statistically significant ($p < 0.05$) improvement in wrinkle score for TGF-β 1 containing cream as compared to cream with only L-ascorbic acid and black cohosh extract.[90]

BOTANICAL ANTI-AGING AGENTS

Green Tea Green Tea contains polyphenols known to have superior antioxidant activity when taken orally or topically applied. In cosmetic science, the term *Green Tea* does not refer to common herbal tea. Instead, Green Tea refers to the product of a careful process in which the leaves of the plant, *Camellia sinensis*, are processed taking care to prevent the oxidation and polymerization breakdown of polyphenolic compounds. In Green Tea, the most powerful of these polyphenols is (−)-epigallocatechin-3-gallate (EGCG), contributing to its anti-inflammatory and anticarcinogenic properties.[91]

Preclinical studies in mouse models have provided evidence that Green Tea polyphenols provide protection against UV-B radiation-induced immunosuppression, generation of reactive oxygen species, and biochemical markers of chemical carcinogenesis. Inhibition of UV-induced leukocyte infiltration and inhibition of cyclobutane pyrimidine dimer formation in DNA are mechanisms through which Green Tea may reduce the development of oxidative stress-driven skin disease in humans and mice.[91]

Liao and Hiipakka have shown that Green Tea polyphenols are potent inhibitors of type 1,5-α-reductase, suggesting the potential use of Green Tea polyphenols in the treatment of androgen-mediated skin disorders, such as androgenetic alopecia.[92]

Presently, numerous products are supplemented with Green Tea, even though the concentration of active polyphenols in these products is inconsistent and few controlled clinical trials have been conducted.[91,93]

Grape Seed Extract Grape seed extract contains polyphenols, mainly flavonoids, including oligomeric proanthocyanidins (OPC), which have antioxidant capabilities 20 times greater than vitamin E, and 50 times greater than vitamin C.[94] An in vitro model demonstrated up to 81% inhibition of free radicals with a 100 mg/L concentration of IH636 grape seed proanthocyanidin extract (GSPE). GSPE inhibition was superior to both Vitamin C at 12% to 19% and Vitamin E at 36% to 44% free radical inhibition.[95]

Studies suggest that grape seed extract binds to collagen, where its antioxidant effects enhance young, healthy skin, elasticity, and flexibility.[94] Studies also support OPCs protection against several age-related diseases, including cardiovascular disease and cancer.[94]

GSPE is known for its wound healing properties.[96,97] Topical GSPE demonstrated upregulation of VEGF transcription and tenascin expression and promoted tissue oxidation for facilitating dermal wound healing in human keratinocytes.[96] Increased tissue oxidation may be attributed to inadequate capacity to regenerate oxidized antioxidants at the wound site.[96,97]

SKIN CARE REGIMENS FOR ANTI-AGING SKIN

An anti-aging skin regimen may include gentle cleansing followed by an antioxidant such as ascorbic acid and a moisturizer with broad SPF in the morning. In the evening following cleansing, a moisturizer may be applied followed by a retinoid to promote collagen production. Retinoids should be slowly up-titrated based on patient tolerability and skin type.[46]

SUN PROTECTION

BROAD-SPECTRUM SUNSCREEN

Ultraviolet (UV) B (280 to 320 nm), UVA (320 to 400 nm), visible light (400 to 800 nm), and infrared radiation (800 nm and above) are all components of terrestrial sunlight. To protect human skin from free radical generation, skin has a sophisticated antioxidant system that includes superoxide dismutase, glutathione reductase, and glutathione peroxidase. However, UV light damages skin throughout life because the cutaneous antioxidant system is less than 100% effective. In addition, these cutaneous antioxidant systems, themselves, experience continuous damage from the sun, compromising their effectiveness.[99] All skin types and ethnic groups are advised to use sun protection.[3]

While UVB light is known to be major contributor to the development of sunburn and skin cancer, there is growing evidence to support UVA light as another contributor to oxidative damage that may lead to skin cancer as it penetrates more deeply into the skin.[98] Therefore, use of broad-spectrum sunscreen is recommended that includes UVA light protection with a minimum critical wavelength of 370 nm.[100]

Sunscreens may contain chemical filters, physical filters, or a combination of both to optimize UV protection [**Table 92-4**].[100,101] Chemical sunscreen ingredients are composed of organic aromatic compounds that function to absorb high-energy UV light and convert to thermal energy.[100,102] Avobenzone is an organic UVA filter limited by its photoinstability requiring a photostabilizer such as octocrylene, a UVB filter, to preserve efficacy.[99,101] Mexoryl SX is a broad-spectrum UVA absorber that has demonstrated increased efficacy of sunscreen formulations against

TABLE 92-4 Sunscreen filters currently approved under the 2011 FDA monograph[101]

Sunscreen filter	Maximum concentration	Peak absorption λ (nm)	UV action spectrum
Inorganic filters			
Titanium dioxide Zinc oxide	25%		UVB, UVA[b]
Organic UVA filters			
Oxybenzone (benzophenone-3)	6%	288, 325	UVB, UVA II
Sulisobenzone (benzophenone-4)	10%	366	
Dioxybenzone (benzophenone-8)	3%	352	
Avobenzone (butyl methoxydibenzoyl-methane (Parsol 1789)	3%	360	UVA I
Meradimate (menthyl anthranilate)	5%	340	UVA II
Ecamsule[a] (terephthalylidene dicamphor sulfonic acid, Mexoryl SX)	10%	345	UVB, UVA
Organic UVB filters			
PABA (para-aminobenzoic acid)	15%	283	UVB
Padimate-O (octyl dimethyl PABA)	8%	311	UVB
Cinoxate (2-ethoxyethyl p-methoxycinnamate)	3%	289	UVB
Octinoxate (octyl methoxycinnamates (OMC))	7.5%	311	UVB
Octisalate (octyl salicylate)	5%	307	UVB
Homosalate (homomenthyl salicylate)	15%	306	UVB
Trolamine salicylate (triethanolamine salicylate)	12%		UVB
Octocrylene	10%	303	UVB, UVA II
Ensulizole (phenylbenzimidazole sulfonic acid)	4%	310	UVB

Modified with permission from Burnett ME, Hu JY, Wang SQ. Sunscreens: Obtaining adequate photoprotection. *Dermatol Ther.* 2012;25(3):244-251.

[a]Only allowed as a component of certain sunscreen formulations approved under a new drug application.

[b]UV absorption spectrum varies by particle size.

UV-induced damage since FDA approval in 2006.[99] In a clinical study on Fitzpatrick type III skin, Mexoryl SX-containing formulations demonstrated protection against pigmentation at concentration-dependent levels.[99,103] Mexoryl SX has also demonstrated significant protection against DNA damage through reduced pyrimidine dimer and p53 expression. Furthermore, Mexoryl SX-containing formulations also promote immunoprotection against suppression of delayed-type hypersensitivity reactions to recall antigens.[99]

Physical sunscreen ingredients are inorganic compounds that function to reflect UV light.[100,102] Titanium dioxide and zinc oxide are inorganic filters available in nanosized formulations for more cosmetically elegant application minimizing the undesirable white film among traditional sunscreens.[101,104] In an article addressing the safety of nanosized particles, current findings suggest no evidence of significant penetration into the stratum corneum contributing to potential toxicity; however, further real-world studies evaluating safety in human models are recommended.[104]

SPF is a traditional measure of sunscreen efficacy that is defined as "the ration of the dose of UVR (290-400nm) required to produce 1 minimal erythema dose (MED) on sunscreen-protected skin (after application of 2 mg/cm^2 of product) over the dose to produce 1 MED on unprotected skin."[105] An SPF of 30 or higher applied to all exposed skin with reapplication every 2 hours with sweating, swimming, or outdoor activities is recommended by the American Academy of Dermatology (AAD).[106] The amount and frequency of sunscreen application are two important factors that may impact the sunscreen efficacy.[105] Sunscreen use with higher SPF may help to counteract these factors.[100]

NATURAL PHOTOPROTECTIVE AGENTS

There is a growing interest in botanicals for sun protection and research has found that plants contain active metabolites including polyphenols, carotenoids, terpenoids, alkaloids, and glucosides with many constituting natural photoprotective properties [Table 92-1].[107] For example, topical and oral cocoa-derived polyphenols especially flavanol-rich concentrations have demonstrated effective protection against UV radiation-induced damage.[108]

Evidence is growing that the addition of antioxidants to sunscreen formulations can protect human skin against UVB, UVA, and IR irradiation. A study including 30 patients demonstrated significant protection from a cocktail of antioxidants (5% vitamin E linoleate, 0.03% butylated hydroxytoluene, 0.01% nordihydroguaradinic acid, and 1% magnesium-ascorbyl phosphate). Results indicated protection from UVB (163% protection against erythema), UVA (76% protection against immediate pigment darkening or IPD), and IR irradiation (52% and 43% protection against erythema and blood flow, respectively).[98]

THE FUTURE OF COSMECEUTICALS

Anti-aging skin is one market area for growth and development of future cosmeceuticals. While stem cells in aging skin are present in youthful concentration with functional potential, stem cells no longer receive and respond to key signals driving differentiative processes. The Wnt signaling pathway is one fundamental mediator of cell division triggered by coactivators cAMP response element binding protein (CREB)-binding protein (CBP) and p300 binding beta-catenin, respectively. These Wnt signaling networks may be utilized to increase recruitment of stem cells in aging skin for normal proliferation directed toward youth-promoting processes including wound healing, tissue repair, and collagen synthesis for reinvigorated growth of skin, hair, nails, and mucous membranes.[109]

One of latest technologies with great promise in development is the novel therapeutic use of nitrones or "spin traps" in dermatology. These synthetic antioxidant compounds function to stabilize or trap free radical intermediates preventing oxidative damage. Spin traps were initially utilized in the late 1960s within analytical chemistry systems progressing into biochemical systems. Phenyl butyl nitrone (PBN) and PBN-related nitrones are well-known spin traps for their potent activity of which mechanism is still being further explored.[110,111]

Draelos discusses nanoparticles as a revolutionizing frontier in cosmetic dermatology.[112] The high surface area to volume ratio of nanoparticles increases penetrability of active ingredients into the stratum corneum. The invisibility of nanoparticles, less than the wavelength of light, improve application of mineral-based sunscreen as well as promote reduced wrinkles and dyspigmentation.[112]

CONCLUSION

The cosmetic industry is an ever-changing, ever-growing market that promises to continue providing novel agents for maintaining healthy skin. The true clinical efficacy of some of these products remains to be proven. However, many products are known to provide clinically relevant results. In time, clinical efficacy and safety data will be supplied.

The development and tremendous growth in cosmeceutical sales is a response to consumer demands for more scientific and sophisticated cosmetic products. The first generation of cosmeceuticals provided supplements and antioxidants. The second generation of cosmeceuticals focused on growth factors to help stimulate repair of photoaged skin. While the 20th century brought the development of cosmeceuticals, the 21st century will mark the introduction of new skin care technology in the form of cosmoleculars™—designer molecules for cosmetics.

REFERENCES

1. Bellad K, Nanjwade B, Kamble M, Srichana T, Idris N. Development of Cosmeceuticals. *World J Pharm Pharm Sci.* 2017;6(4):643-691.
2. Draelos ZD. Cosmeceuticals: What's Real, What's Not. *Dermatol Clin.* 2019;37(1):107-115. doi:10.1016/j.det.2018.07.001
3. Baumann L. Cosmeceuticals in skin of color. *Semin Cutan Med Surg.* 2016;35(4):233-237. doi:10.12788/j.sder.2016.056
4. Stallings AF, Lupo MP. Practical Uses of Botanicals in Skin Care. *J Clin Aesthetic Dermatol.* 2009;2(1):36-40.
5. Wohlrab J, Kreft D. Niacinamide - Mechanisms of Action and Its Topical Use in Dermatology. *Skin Pharmacol Physiol.* 2014;27(6):311-315. doi:10.1159/000359974
6. Draelos ZK, Dover JS, Alam M, Hitchen M, Bajor J. *Cosmeceuticals.* 3rd ed. Elsevier; 2016.
7. Crous C, Pretorius J, Petzer A. Overview of popular cosmeceuticals in dermatology. *Skin Health Dis.* 2024;4(2):e340. doi:10.1002/ski2.340
8. Draelos ZD. The cosmeceutical realm. *Clin Dermatol.* 2008;26(6):627-632. doi:10.1016/j.clindermatol.2007.09.005
9. Kumar S. Exploratory analysis of global cosmetic industry: major players, technology and market trends. *Technovation.* 2005;25(11):1263-1272. doi:10.1016/j.technovation.2004.07.003
10. Draelos ZD. Cosmeceuticals for Male Skin. *Dermatol Clin.* 2018;36(1):17-20. doi:10.1016/j.det.2017.09.003
11. Black representation in the beauty industry | McKinsey. Accessed June 20, 2023. https://www.mckinsey.com/industries/consumer-packaged-goods/our-insights/black-representation-in-the-beauty-industry
12. Tenerelli MJ. Ethnic Skin-Care: —Special Products for a Special Sector. *Glob Cosmet Ind.* 2000;167(4):32-32.
13. Another Breakthrough For The Group In China: After Mininurse, L'Oreal Acquires Yue-Sai. L'Oréal. Accessed November 21, 2024. https://www.loreal.com/en/press-release/group/another-breakthrough-for-the-group-in-china-after-mininurse-loreal-acquires-yuesai/
14. Vermeer BJ, Gilchrest BA. Cosmeceuticals. A proposal for rational definition, evaluation, and regulation. *Arch Dermatol.* 1996;132(3):337-340. doi:10.1001/archderm.132.3.337
15. Cole P, Hatef D, Taylor S, Bullocks J. Skin Care in Ethnic Populations. *Semin Plast Surg.* 2009;23(03):168-172. doi:10.1055/s-0029-1224795
16. Anthony V Rawlings, James J Leyden. *Skin Moisturization.*; 2002.
17. Nolan K, Marmur E. Moisturizers: reality and the skin benefits. *Dermatol Ther.* 2012;25(3):229-233. doi:10.1111/j.1529-8019.2012.01504.x

18. Draelos ZD. The science behind skin care: Moisturizers. *J Cosmet Dermatol.* 2018;17(2):138-144. doi:10.1111/jocd.12490
19. Diana Draelos Z. THERAPEUTIC MOISTURIZERS. *Dermatol Clin.* 2000;18(4):597-607. doi:10.1016/S0733-8635(05)70210-2
20. Draelos ZD. The science behind skin care: Cleansers. *J Cosmet Dermatol.* 2018;17(1):8-14. doi:10.1111/jocd.12469
21. Draelos ZD. Facial Cleansers and Cleansing Cloths. In: *Cosmetic Dermatology: Products and Procedures.* John Wiley & Sons, Incorporated; 2015. Accessed November 24, 2022. http://ebookcentral.proquest.com/lib/bu/detail.action?docID=4443318
22. Vidt DG, Bergfeld WF. Cosmetic use of alpha-hydroxy acids. *Cleve Clin J Med.* 1997;64(6):327-329. doi:10.3949/ccjm.64.6.327
23. Van Scott EJ, Yu RJ. Hyperkeratinization, corneocyte cohesion, and alpha hydroxy acids. *J Am Acad Dermatol.* 1984;11(5 Pt 1):867-879. doi:10.1016/s0190-9622(84)80466-1
24. Stiller MJ, Bartolone J, Stern R, et al. Topical 8% Glycolic Acid and 8% L-Lactic Acid Creams for the Treatment of Photodamaged Skin: A Double-blind Vehicle-Controlled Clinical Trial. *Arch Dermatol.* 1996;132(6):631-636. doi:10.1001/archderm.1996.03890300047009
25. Desai J, Mallya R. A Review on Novel Topical Formulations of Vitamins. *J Rep Pharm Sci.* 2021;10(2):159. doi:10.4103/jrptps.JRPTPS_91_20
26. Burgess C. Topical vitamins. *J Drugs Dermatol JDD.* 2008;7(7 Suppl):s2-6.
27. Hakozaki T, Minwalla L, Zhuang J, et al. The effect of niacinamide on reducing cutaneous pigmentation and suppression of melanosome transfer. *Br J Dermatol.* 2002;147(1):20-31. doi:10.1046/j.1365-2133.2002.04834.x
28. Griffiths CEM. The role of retinoids in the prevention and repair of aged and photoaged skin. *Clin Exp Dermatol.* 2001;26(7):613-618. doi:10.1046/j.1365-2230.2001.00892.x
29. Motamedi M, Chehade A, Sanghera R, Grewal P. A Clinician's Guide to Topical Retinoids. *J Cutan Med Surg.* 2022;26(1):71-78. doi:10.1177/12034754211035091
30. Draelos ZD. The science behind skin care: Cleansers. *J Cosmet Dermatol.* 2018;17(1):8-14. doi:10.1111/jocd.12469
31. Draelos ZK, Dover JS, Alam M, Hitchen M, Bajor J. Oily Skin. In: *Cosmeceuticals.* 3rd ed. Procedures in cosmetic dermatology. Elsevier; 2016:173-174.
32. Candrice R. Heath; Raechele Cochran Gathers; Susan C. Taylor. Postinflammatory Hyperpigmentation/Periorbital Hyperpigmentation. In: *Taylor and Kelly's Dermatology for Skin of Color, 2e | AccessMedicine | McGraw Hill Medical.* Accessed November 24, 2022. https://accessmedicine-mhmedical-com.ezproxy.bu.edu/Book.aspx?bookid=2585
33. Cheng J, Vashi NA. Chemical Peels in Ethnic Skin. In: Vashi NA, Maibach HI, eds. *Dermatoanthropology of Ethnic Skin and Hair.* Springer International Publishing; 2017:437-448. doi:10.1007/978-3-319-53961-4_24
34. Love PB, Kundu RV, eds. *Clinical Cases in Skin of Color: Adnexal, Inflammation, Infections, and Pigmentary Disorders.* Springer International Publishing; 2016. doi:10.1007/978-3-319-22392-6
35. Callender VD. Acne in ethnic skin: special considerations for therapy. *Dermatol Ther.* 2004;17(2):184-195. doi:10.1111/j.1396-0296.2004.04019.x
36. Burgess, Cheryl, David, Jennifer. Specific Use: Cosmeceuticals for Skin Brightening and Lightening. In: *Aesthetic Dermatology.* Vol 5. S.Karger AG; 2021. doi:10.1159/000491849
37. Solano F, Briganti S, Picardo M, Ghanem G. Hypopigmenting agents: an updated review on biological, chemical and clinical aspects. *Pigment Cell Res.* 2006;19(6):550-571. doi:10.1111/j.1600-0749.2006.00334.x
38. Topical Treatments for Melasma: A Systematic Review of Randomized Controlled Trials. *JDDonline - J Drugs Dermatol.* 2019;18(11). Accessed December 1, 2024. https://jddonline.com/articles/topical-treatments-for-melasma-a-systematic-review-of-randomized-controlled-trials-S1545961619P1156X/
39. Parvez S, Kang M, Chung HS, et al. Survey and mechanism of skin depigmenting and lightening agents. *Phytother Res.* 2006;20(11):921-934. doi:10.1002/ptr.1954
40. Tse TW. Hydroquinone for skin lightening: Safety profile, duration of use and when should we stop? *J Dermatol Treat.* 2010;21(5):272-275. doi:10.3109/09546630903341945
41. Draelos ZD. Skin lightening preparations and the hydroquinone controversy. *Dermatol Ther.* 2007;20(5):308-313. doi:10.1111/j.1529-8019.2007.00144.x
42. Taghavi F, Banihashemi M, Zabolinejad N, et al. Comparison of therapeutic effects of conventional and liposomal form of 4% topical hydroquinone in patients with melasma. *J Cosmet Dermatol.* 2019;18(3):870-873. doi:10.1111/jocd.12744
43. Fu B, Li H, Wang X, Lee FSC, Cui S. Isolation and Identification of Flavonoids in Licorice and a Study of Their Inhibitory Effects on Tyrosinase. *J Agric Food Chem.* 2005;53(19):7408-7414. doi:10.1021/jf051258h
44. Nerya O, Vaya J, Musa R, Izrael S, Ben-Arie R, Tamir S. Glabrene and Isoliquiritigenin as Tyrosinase Inhibitors from Licorice Roots. *J Agric Food Chem.* 2003;51(5):1201-1207. doi:10.1021/jf020935u
45. Searle T, Al-Niaimi F, Ali FR. The top 10 cosmeceuticals for facial hyperpigmentation. *Dermatol Ther.* 2020;33(6):e14095. doi:10.1111/dth.14095
46. Lim JTE, Frcpi, Fams. Treatment of Melasma Using Kojic Acid in a Gel Containing Hydroquinone and Glycolic Acid. *Dermatol Surg.* 1999;25(4):282-284. doi:10.1046/j.1524-4725.1999.08236.x
47. Breathnach AS. Melanin hyperpigmentation of skin: melasma, topical treatment with azelaic acid, and other therapies. *Cutis.* 1996;57(1 Suppl):36-45.
48. Katoulis A, Alevizou A, Soura E, et al. A double-blind vehicle-controlled study of a preparation containing undecylenoyl phenylalanine 2% in the treatment of melasma in females. *J Cosmet Dermatol.* 2014;13(2):86-90. doi:10.1111/jocd.12089
49. Farwick M, Maczkiewitz U, Lersch P, Summers B, Rawlings AV. Facial skin-lightening benefits of the tetrapeptide Pro-Lys-Glu-Lys on subjects with skin types V–VI living in South Africa. *J Cosmet Dermatol.* 2011;10(3):217-223. doi:10.1111/j.1473-2165.2011.00569.x
50. Mansouri P, Farshi S, Hashemi Z, Kasraee B. Evaluation of the efficacy of cysteamine 5% cream in the treatment of epidermal melasma: a randomized double-blind placebo-controlled trial. *Br J Dermatol.* 2015;173(1):209-217. doi:10.1111/bjd.13424
51. Farshi S, Mansouri P, Kasraee B. Efficacy of cysteamine cream in the treatment of epidermal melasma, evaluating by Dermacatch as a new measurement method: a randomized double blind placebo controlled study. *J Dermatol Treat.* 2018;29(2):182-189. doi:10.1080/09546634.2017.1351608
52. Segars K, McCarver V, Miller RA. Dermatologic Applications of Polypodium leucotomos: A Literature Review. *J Clin Aesthetic Dermatol.* 2021;14(2):50-60.
53. Paine C, Sharlow E, Liebel F, Eisinger M, Shapiro S, Seiberg M. An Alternative Approach to Depigmentation by Soybean Extracts via Inhibition of the PAR-2 Pathway. *J Invest Dermatol.* 2001;116(4):587-595. doi:10.1046/j.1523-1747.2001.01291.x
54. Seiberg M, Paine C, Sharlow E, et al. The protease-activated receptor 2 regulates pigmentation via keratinocyte-melanocyte interactions. *Exp Cell Res.* 2000;254(1):25-32. doi:10.1006/excr.1999.4692
55. Pinnell SR. Cutaneous photodamage, oxidative stress, and topical antioxidant protection. *J Am Acad Dermatol.* 2003;48(1):1-22. doi:10.1067/mjd.2003.16
56. Greenwel P, Hu W, Kohanski RA, Ramirez F. Tyrosine dephosphorylation of nuclear proteins mimics transforming growth factor beta 1 stimulation of alpha 2(I) collagen gene expression. *Mol Cell Biol.* 1995;15(12):6813-6819.
57. Matsugo S, Bito T, Konishi T. Photochemical stability of lipoic acid and its impact on skin ageing. *Free Radic Res.* 2011;45(8):918-924. doi:10.3109/10715762.2011.587420
58. Fabi SG, Burgess C, Edwards CD, Kanaris NP, Dayan S. Aesthetic considerations when treating patients of African descent: Thriving in diversity international roundtable series. *J Cosmet Dermatol.* 2023;22(6):1870-1878. doi:10.1111/jocd.15688
59. Fabi SG, Park JY, Ho WWS, Vachiramon V, Dayan S. Aesthetic considerations for treating the Asian patient: Thriving in diversity international roundtable series. *J Cosmet Dermatol.* 2023;22(6):1805-1813. doi:10.1111/jocd.15787
60. Fabi SG, Callender VD, Lee WW, Dayan S. Aesthetic considerations for treating the North American MULTI-ETHNIC patient: Thriving in diversity international roundtable series. *J Cosmet Dermatol.* 2022;21(12):6976-6984. doi:10.1111/jocd.15422
61. Knott A, Achterberg V, Smuda C, et al. Topical treatment with coenzyme Q10-containing formulas improves skin's Q10 level and provides antioxidative effects. *BioFactors.* 2015;41(6):383-390. doi:10.1002/biof.1239
62. Lenaz G, Bovina C, D'Aurelio M, et al. Role of mitochondria in oxidative stress and aging. *Ann N Y Acad Sci.* 2002;959:199-213. doi:10.1111/j.1749-6632.2002.tb02094.x
63. Rattan SI, Clark BF. Kinetin delays the onset of ageing characteristics in human fibroblasts. *Biochem Biophys Res Commun.* 1994;201(2):665-672. doi:10.1006/bbrc.1994.1752
64. Olsen A, Siboska GE, Clark BF, Rattan SI. N(6)-Furfuryladenine, kinetin, protects against Fenton reaction-mediated oxidative damage to DNA. *Biochem Biophys Res Commun.* 1999;265(2):499-502. doi:10.1006/bbrc.1999.1669
65. Sen CK, Roy S, Han D, Packer L. Regulation of Cellular Thiols in Human Lymphocytes by α-Lipoic Acid: A Flow Cytometric Analysis. *Free Radic Biol Med.* 1997;22(7):1241-1257. doi:10.1016/S0891-5849(96)00552-7
66. E Thom. A Randomized, Double-blind, Placebo-controlled Study on the Clinical Efficacy of Oral Treatment with DermaVite™ on Ageing Symptoms of the Skin. *J Int Med Res.* 2005;33:267-272. doi:10.1177/147323000503300301
67. Beitner H. Randomized, placebo-controlled, double blind study on the clinical efficacy of a cream containing 5%α-lipoic acid related to photoageing of facial skin. *Br J Dermatol.* 2003;149(4):841-849. doi:10.1046/j.1365-2133.2003.05597.x

68. Jin HY, Joung SJ, Park JH, Baek HS, Park TS. The effect of α-lipoic acid on symptoms and skin blood flow in diabetic neuropathy. *Diabet Med.* 2007;24(9):1034-1038. doi:10.1111/j.1464-5491.2007.02179.x
69. Jauslin ML, Wirth T, Meier T, Schoumacher F. A cellular model for Friedreich Ataxia reveals small-molecule glutathione peroxidase mimetics as novel treatment strategy. *Hum Mol Genet.* 2002;11(24):3055-3063. doi:10.1093/hmg/11.24.3055
70. Farris P. Idebenone, green tea, and Coffeeberry® extract: new and innovative antioxidants. *Dermatol Ther.* 2007;20(5):322-329. doi:10.1111/j.1529-8019.2007.00146.x
71. McDaniel D, Neudecker B, DiNardo J, Lewis II J, Maibach H. Clinical efficacy assessment in photodamaged skin of 0.5% and 1.0% idebenone. *J Cosmet Dermatol.* 2005;4(3):167-173. doi:10.1111/j.1473-2165.2005.00305.x
72. Farris PK. Topical Vitamin C: A Useful Agent for Treating Photoaging and Other Dermatologic Conditions. *Dermatol Surg.* 2005;31(s1):814-818. doi:10.1111/j.1524-4725.2005.31725
73. Humbert PG, Haftek M, Creidi P, et al. Topical ascorbic acid on photoaged skin. Clinical, topographical and ultrastructural evaluation: double-blind study vs. placebo. *Exp Dermatol.* 2003;12(3):237-244. doi:10.1034/j.1600-0625.2003.00008.x
74. Keller KL, Fenske NA. Uses of vitamins A, C, and E and related compounds in dermatology: a review. *J Am Acad Dermatol.* 1998;39(4 Pt 1):611-625. doi:10.1016/s0190-9622(98)70011-8
75. Beijersbergen van Henegouwen GM, Junginger HE, de Vries H. Hydrolysis of RRR-alpha-tocopheryl acetate (vitamin E acetate) in the skin and its UV protecting activity (an in vivo study with the rat). *J Photochem Photobiol B.* 1995;29(1):45-51. doi:10.1016/1011-1344(95)90251-1
76. Nakayama S, Katoh EM, Tsuzuki T, Kobayashi S. Protective effect of alpha-tocopherol-6-O-phosphate against ultraviolet B-induced damage in cultured mouse skin. *J Invest Dermatol.* 2003;121(2):406-411. doi:10.1046/j.1523-1747.2003.12351.x
77. Katsimbri P, Korakas E, Kountouri A, et al. The Effect of Antioxidant and Anti-Inflammatory Capacity of Diet on Psoriasis and Psoriatic Arthritis Phenotype: Nutrition as Therapeutic Tool? *Antioxidants.* 2021;10(2):157. doi:10.3390/antiox10020157
78. Burke KE. Interaction of vitamins C and E as better cosmeceuticals. *Dermatol Ther.* 2007;20(5):314-321. doi:10.1111/j.1529-8019.2007.00145.x
79. Canapp SO, Farese JP, Schultz GS, et al. The effect of topical tripeptide-copper complex on healing of ischemic open wounds. *Vet Surg VS.* 2003;32(6):515-523. doi:10.1111/j.1532-950x.2003.00515.x
80. Siméon A, Emonard H, Hornebeck W, Maquart FX. The tripeptide-copper complex glycyl-L-histidyl-L-lysine-Cu2+ stimulates matrix metalloproteinase-2 expression by fibroblast cultures. *Life Sci.* 2000;67(18):2257-2265. doi:10.1016/s0024-3205(00)00803-1
81. Sen CK, Khanna S, Venojarvi M, et al. Copper-induced vascular endothelial growth factor expression and wound healing. *Am J Physiol Heart Circ Physiol.* 2002;282(5):H1821-1827. doi:10.1152/ajpheart.01015.2001
82. Wegrowski Y, Maquart FX, Borel JP. Stimulation of sulfated glycosaminoglycan synthesis by the tripeptide-copper complex glycyl-L-histidyl-L-lysine-Cu2+. *Life Sci.* 1992;51(13):1049-1056. doi:10.1016/0024-3205(92)90504-i
83. Siméon A, Wegrowski Y, Bontemps Y, Maquart FX. Expression of glycosaminoglycans and small proteoglycans in wounds: modulation by the tripeptide-copper complex glycyl-L-histidyl-L-lysine-Cu(2+). *J Invest Dermatol.* 2000;115(6):962-968. doi:10.1046/j.1523-1747.2000.00166.x
84. Lupo MP, Cole AL. Cosmeceutical peptides. *Dermatol Ther.* 2007;20(5):343-349. doi:10.1111/j.1529-8019.2007.00148.x
85. Robinson LR, Fitzgerald NC, Doughty DG, Dawes NC, Berge CA, Bissett DL. Topical palmitoyl pentapeptide provides improvement in photoaged human facial skin. *Int J Cosmet Sci.* 2005;27(3):155-160. doi:10.1111/j.1467-2494.2005.00261.x
86. Blanes-Mira C, Clemente J, Jodas G, et al. A synthetic hexapeptide (Argireline) with antiwrinkle activity. *Int J Cosmet Sci.* 2002;24(5):303-310. doi:10.1046/j.1467-2494.2002.00153.x
87. Ehrlich M, Rao J, Pabby A, Goldman MP. Improvement in the appearance of wrinkles with topical transforming growth factor beta(1) and l-ascorbic acid. *Dermatol Surg.* 2006;32(5):618-625. doi:10.1111/j.1524-4725.2006.32132.x
88. Hohlfeld J, de Buys Roessingh A, Hirt-Burri N, et al. Tissue engineered fetal skin constructs for paediatric burns. *Lancet Lond Engl.* 2005;366(9488):840-842. doi:10.1016/S0140-6736(05)67107-3
89. Cass DL, Meuli M, Adzick NS. Scar wars: implications of fetal wound healing for the pediatric burn patient. *Pediatr Surg Int.* 1997;12(7):484-489. doi:10.1007/BF01258707
90. Gold MH, Goldman MP, Biron J. Efficacy of novel skin cream containing mixture of human growth factors and cytokines for skin rejuvenation. *J Drugs Dermatol JDD.* 2007;6(2):197-201.
91. Katiyar Sk, Ahmad N, Mukhtar H. Green tea and skin. *Arch Dermatol.* 2000;136(8). doi:10.1001/archderm.136.8.989
92. Liao S, Hiipakka RA. Selective inhibition of steroid 5 alpha-reductase isozymes by tea epicatechin-3-gallate and epigallocatechin-3-gallate. *Biochem Biophys Res Commun.* 1995;214(3):833-838. doi:10.1006/bbrc.1995.2362
93. Liao R, Parker T, Bellerose K, Vollmer D, Han X. A Green Tea Containing Skincare System Improves Skin Health and Beauty in Adults: An Exploratory Controlled Clinical Study. *Cosmetics.* 2022;9(5):NA-NA. doi:10.3390/cosmetics9050096
94. Shi J, Yu J, Pohorly JE, Kakuda Y. Polyphenolics in Grape Seeds—Biochemistry and Functionality. *J Med Food.* 2003;6(4):291-299. doi:10.1089/109662003772519831
95. Bagchi D, Bagchi M, Stohs SJ, Ray SD, Sen CK, Preuss HG. Cellular Protection with Proanthocyanidins Derived from Grape Seeds. *Ann N Y Acad Sci.* 2002;957(1):260-270. doi:10.1111/j.1749-6632.2002.tb02922.x
96. Bagchi D, Sen CK, Ray SD, et al. Molecular mechanisms of cardioprotection by a novel grape seed proanthocyanidin extract. *Mutat Res.* 2003; 523-524:87-97. doi:10.1016/s0027-5107(02)00324-x
97. Khanna S, Venojarvi M, Roy S, et al. Dermal wound healing properties of redox-active grape seed proanthocyanidins. *Free Radic Biol Med.* 2002;33(8):1089-1096. doi:10.1016/S0891-5849(02)00999-1
98. Muizzuddin N, Shakoori AR, Marenus KD. Effect of antioxidants and free radical scavengers on protection of human skin against UVB, UVA and IR irradiation. *Skin Res Technol.* 1999;5(4):260. doi:10.1111/j.1600-0846.1999.tb00139.x
99. Fourtanier A, Moyal D, Seité S. Sunscreens containing the broad-spectrum UVA absorber, Mexoryl SX, prevent the cutaneous detrimental effects of UV exposure: a review of clinical study results. *Photodermatol Photoimmunol Photomed.* 2008;24(4):164-174. doi:10.1111/j.1600-0781.2008.00365.x
100. McDonald KA, Lytvyn Y, Mufti A, Chan AW, Rosen CF. Review on photoprotection: a clinician's guide to the ingredients, characteristics, adverse effects, and disease-specific benefits of chemical and physical sunscreen compounds. *Arch Dermatol Res.* 2023;315(4):735-749. doi:10.1007/s00403-022-02483-4
101. BurnettME,HuJY,WangSQ.Sunscreens:Obtainingadequatephotoprotection. *Dermatol Ther.* 2012;25(3):244-251. doi:10.1111/j.1529-8019.2012.01503.x
102. Sabzevari N, Qiblawi S, Norton SA, Fivenson D. Sunscreens: UV filters to protect us: Part 1: Changing regulations and choices for optimal sun protection. *Int J Womens Dermatol.* 2021;7(1):28-44. doi:10.1016/j.ijwd.2020.05.017
103. Moyal D. Prevention of ultraviolet-induced skin pigmentation. *Photodermatol Photoimmunol Photomed.* 2004;20(5):243-247. doi:10.1111/j.1600-0781.2004.00111.x
104. Newman MD, Stotland M, Ellis JI. The safety of nanosized particles in titanium dioxide– and zinc oxide–based sunscreens. *J Am Acad Dermatol.* 2009;61(4):685-692. doi:10.1016/j.jaad.2009.02.051
105. Kullavanijaya P, Lim HW. Photoprotection. *J Am Acad Dermatol.* 2005;52(6):937-958. doi:10.1016/j.jaad.2004.07.063
106. American Academy of Dermatology. What to wear to protect your skin from the sun. Accessed November 14, 2024. https://www.aad.org/public/everyday-care/sun-protection/shade-clothing-sunscreen/what-to-wear-protect-skin-from-sun
107. Kathuria D. Cosmeceutical applications of natural oils and fats. In: *Specialized Plant Metabolites As Cosmeceuticals.* 1st ed. Elsevier; 2024.
108. Scapagnini G, Davinelli S, Renzo LD, et al. Cocoa Bioactive Compounds: Significance and Potential for the Maintenance of Skin Health. *Nutrients.* 2014;6(8):3202. doi:10.3390/nu6083202
109. Dahl MV. Stem cells and the skin. *J Cosmet Dermatol.* 2012;11(4):297-306. doi:10.1111/jocd.12008
110. Deletraz A, Tuccio B, Roussel J, et al. Para-Substituted α-Phenyl-N-tert-butyl Nitrones: Spin-Trapping, Redox and Neuroprotective Properties. *ACS Omega.* 2020;5(48):30989-30999. doi:10.1021/acsomega.0c03907
111. Floyd RA, Kopke RD, Choi CH, Foster SB, Doblas S, Towner RA. Nitrones as therapeutics. *Free Radic Biol Med.* 2008;45(10):1361-1374. doi:10.1016/j.freeradbiomed.2008.08.017
112. Draelos ZD. Cosmetics, diet, and the future. *Dermatol Ther.* 2012;25(3):267-272. doi:10.1111/j.1529-8019.2012.01500.x.

CHAPTER 93

Skin and Lip Typology

Diane Baras
Laurence Caisey

KEY POINTS

- Diversity of skin color covers a large and continuous color space where different racial groups overlap each other.
- Racial or ethnic origins and cultural backgrounds play a major role in self-perception of skin tone, undoubtedly influencing makeup strategy.
- Four main makeup strategies have been identified.
- The lip color space is as large as the skin color space.

INTRODUCTION

The ideal makeup is a tailor-made product that respects a woman's individuality. Individual uniqueness can be characterized by biophysical as well as psychological features. A thorough understanding of a woman based on her own characteristics entails these two dimensions.

The diversity of women comes from the various types of skin tone, lips, and eyelashes, all of which could be enhanced, corrected, or transformed by makeup according to the user's expectations.

These expectations are linked to self-perception of the biophysical properties of the face. A woman's features and concerns about skin tone, lips, and lashes strongly depend on racial or ethnic origin, as well as on the cultural and geographic environment. There may be a discrepancy between self-perception and objective assessment.

Objective assessments are provided by instrumental measurements of physical and biophysical properties of the face. Several characteristics are recorded, such as color and unevenness of skin tone and morphologic and biomechanical hydration properties of the lips. Such measurements emphasize the diversity among different population groups as well as within each individual group.

This chapter expands on the main results of our dual approach, combining qualitative assessments and quantitative measurements in women with different skin of color and cultural background. It focuses on the two main cosmetic supports of the facial appearance: skin complexion and lips through their colorimetric features.

THE COLOR OF THE SKIN

For most women, applying a "colored" makeup to the skin is the first step, or foundation, of the makeup routine. A woman enhances her face by matching or changing the color of her skin.

A qualitative and quantitative study was conducted on a large panel of diverse women to better understand how individual women think about their makeup strategy and how it is influenced by skin color, race, ethnicity, and geographic location. The study consisted of (1) an examination of various skin colors or hues to define skin color worldwide, to highlight the differences between racial groups, and to observe the diversity within each group; (2) an exploration of how women self-perceive facial skin complexion, what their ideal skin tone is, how they managed to achieve it, specifically what they did, and how much they were satisfied with their makeup results; and (3) a colorimetric assessment of makeup results and comparison between that data and a woman's feelings.

Our investigations involved two studies, the first of which began in 1999 and now includes 3721 women living in nine countries, that determined the skin color of women. In 2003, colorimetric measurements were performed on 507 women from different racial groups before and after applying foundation. Measurements were followed by an in-depth interview to record the subject's self-description of her face as well as her satisfaction level. Data were tabulated in a way to assess the needs of women.

SKIN TONES: A HIGH DIVERSITY

A number of studies have explored the differences in skin color among different population groups. However, they often do not provide adequate information about the diversity and intermixing of the involved populations. The scale of most of these studies was small, and the places where measurements were performed were too limited to reflect the large range of skin tones within each racial group or to reveal the overlapping of skin color range between groups.[1-7] In our study, which began in 1999, we measured skin tones and classified them independent of racial origin in order to emphasize their diversity and overlap.

Panel A total of 3721 female volunteers from six different racial origins living in nine different geographic locations have been included. They range in age from 18 to 65 years and include 1993 Asians, 160 Indians, 1120 Caucasians, 219 Hispanics, 127 French Africans, and 102 African Americans [**Table 93-1**]. None suffer from disease that might impair or change color or facial skin condition.

Methods Forehead and cheek color is measured using a spectroradiometer inside a Chromasphere. The Chromasphere, developed and patented by L'Oreal Research,[8] is a stable, reliable, and diffuse lighting system that faithfully mimics natural daylight (CIE illuminant D65). This device does not involve contact measurements that have the potential to alter blood flow when pressure is applied to the skin, thus altering skin color. The volunteer places her face into the Chromasphere, and standardized cameras are used to obtain pictures of the face.[9] The unevenness of skin color is then assessed through image analysis.

A spectroradiometer that measures the reflectance of forehead and cheek in the visible light range (400-700 nm) was used. The recorded spectrum is expressed in the CIE 1976 standard colorimetric space L^*C^*hD65/10°, where each color is described through three coordinates that reflect perception by human eye: h for hue angle (angular coordinate), C^* for chroma (radius coordinate), and L^* for lightness (z axis) [**Figure 93-1**]. The hue h is the approximate psychosensorial translation of the dominant wavelength. This is why the hue is that aspect of a color described with names such as *red* and *yellow*. The chroma C^*, or saturation, refers to the pureness or vividness. Highly colorful skin is vivid and intense, whereas less colorful skin appears more muted, even close to gray. The lightness L^*, or brightness coordinate, grades skin color (more or less light, more or less dark) using a gray scale.

Statistics Significant differences between racial groups were demonstrated using univariate analysis on L^*, C^*, and h data on both forehead and cheeks. The diversity of skin tones was described using principal component analysis (PCA) from L^*, C^*, and h data on forehead and cheeks of subjects. PCA allowed us to classify skin tones from different population groups on a hierarchical ascending classification.

Results From measurements performed on 3721 volunteers, a large color space has been defined [**Figure 93-2**]. The darkest skin tones were found in African American, French African, and Indian women. At the opposite end of the spectrum, Caucasians had the lightest complexions and the reddest cheeks. Asian and Indian women had the yellowest skin [**Figure 93-3**]. Interestingly, Caucasian, Asian, and Hispanic women covered the same lightness range, Caucasian and Hispanic women the same chroma (saturation) range, and African American and Caucasian women the same hue range [Figure 93-3]. These are the first data that highlight this type of diversity between groups. However, such analyses

TABLE 93-1 Population and place of residence of the 3721 female volunteers involved in the study

Population	Place of residence	Frequency
African American	United States	102
Asian	China, Japan, Korea, Thailand	1993
Caucasian	France, Russia, United States	1120
French African	France	127
Hispanic	Brazil, United States	219
Indian	India	160

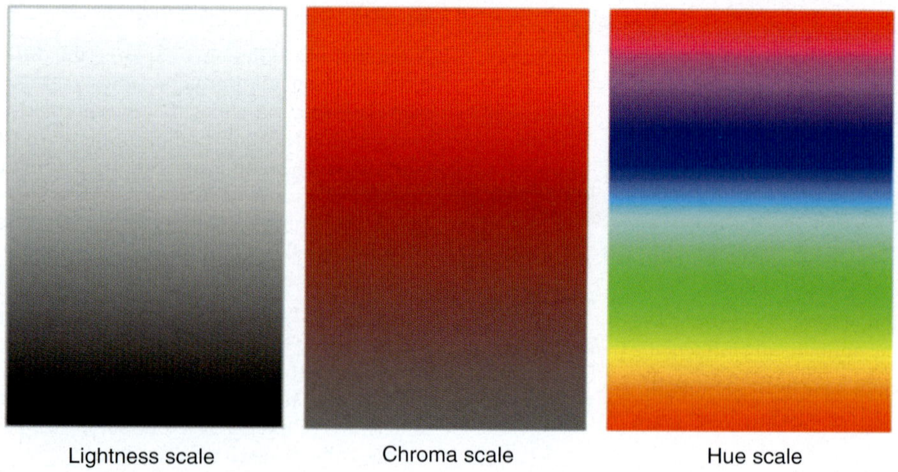

FIGURE 93-1. Scales of lightness, chroma, and hue. When the chroma/saturation is low, the color appears gray.

do not evaluate the diversity within each population group, which motivated us to investigate differences within the skin color space.

Our classification emphasizes six groups of skin tones [Figures 93-2 and **93-4**].

Group 1 encompasses the darkest and the less saturated skin tones (L^* = 42.0; C^* = 19.4 on the forehead; Figure 93-3), including African American, French African, Brazilian, and Indian women.

Group 2 is composed of women with significantly lighter skin than group 1 but still significantly darker skin than in the other groups (L^* = 54.4 on forehead; Figure 93-3). It includes not only some African American, French African, and Indian women but also some Asian (living in Thailand) and Hispanic (living in Brazil and the United States) women. Even among dark skin, there is a high level of diversity.

Group 3 has significantly lighter and the most saturated skin (L^* = 61.2 and C^* = 26.5 on the forehead; Figure 93-3). These skin tones could be termed *tanned skin*. This group is the meeting point where many racial or ethnic groups (eg, Caucasian, Asian, Hispanic, and French African) overlap one other.

Group 4, primarily composed of Caucasian women but also some Asian and Hispanic women who also show such "pink" skin tones, displays significant redness (h = 51.4 and 46.3 on forehead and cheeks, respectively; Figure 93-3).

Group 5 has the lightest skin tones, with a good balance between red and yellow components and a low saturation level that reinforces the white visual appearance of the skin (L^* = 66.2, C^* = 22.1, and h = 55.9 on the forehead; Figure 93-3). With the exception of French Africans, African Americans, and Indians, all the racial or ethnic groups are found in Group 5. Group 6, which includes not only Asian but also Caucasian and Hispanic women, has skin that is significantly yellow (h = 59.9 on forehead; Figure 93-3). Contrary to prejudgment, group 6 is not insignificant in proportion.

It is essential to note that these results show a tremendous diversity of skin color covering a large and continuous color space where different racial or ethnic groups overlap one another.

SELF-PERCEPTION AND SATISFACTION LEVEL OF SKIN COLOR BEFORE AND AFTER APPLYING FOUNDATION MAKEUP

In 2006, we reported a study[10] on self-perception of facial skin by women from different population groups, showing how it was influenced by skin color, origin, and living place.

Panel The study involved 507 healthy women from distinct population groups using foundation on a daily basis and living in different geographic locations (112 French Caucasians in Paris, 107 American Caucasians in New York, 118 Japanese in Tokyo, and 75 African Americans and 95 Hispanic Americans in New York). The volunteers were 25 to 65 years old, including 170 women aged 25 to 35 years, 174 women aged 36 to 45 years, and 163 women aged 46 to 65 years.

Methods Fourteen women selected from each group were involved in semidirected, in-depth interviews based on a specific guideline to establish self-perception about their skin complexion. The interviewer belonged to the same specific population group in each case. The interviews were designed to explore self-perceptions and description of skin complexion and skin tone by the volunteers and their expectations from liquid foundation.

Results For the African American women, skin color was an important part of their identity. They described themselves as "people of color." In general, dark skin complexion was well regarded by the African American community. It was reflected in the use of positive expressions to describe their skin tone, such as "dark chocolate" and "mahogany" to depict dark skin and "toast" or "pecan" for lighter hues. None of the women used negative words about color itself. While women appeared to be fairly satisfied

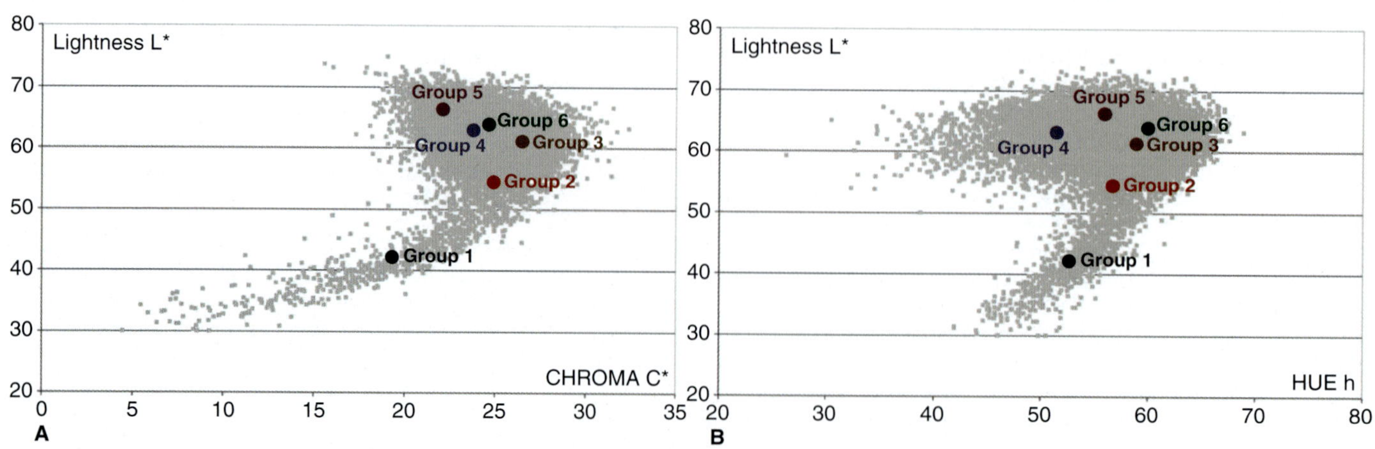

FIGURE 93-2. The worldwide skin color space depicted in two dimensions: **(A)** C^*, L^* and **(B)** h, L^*.

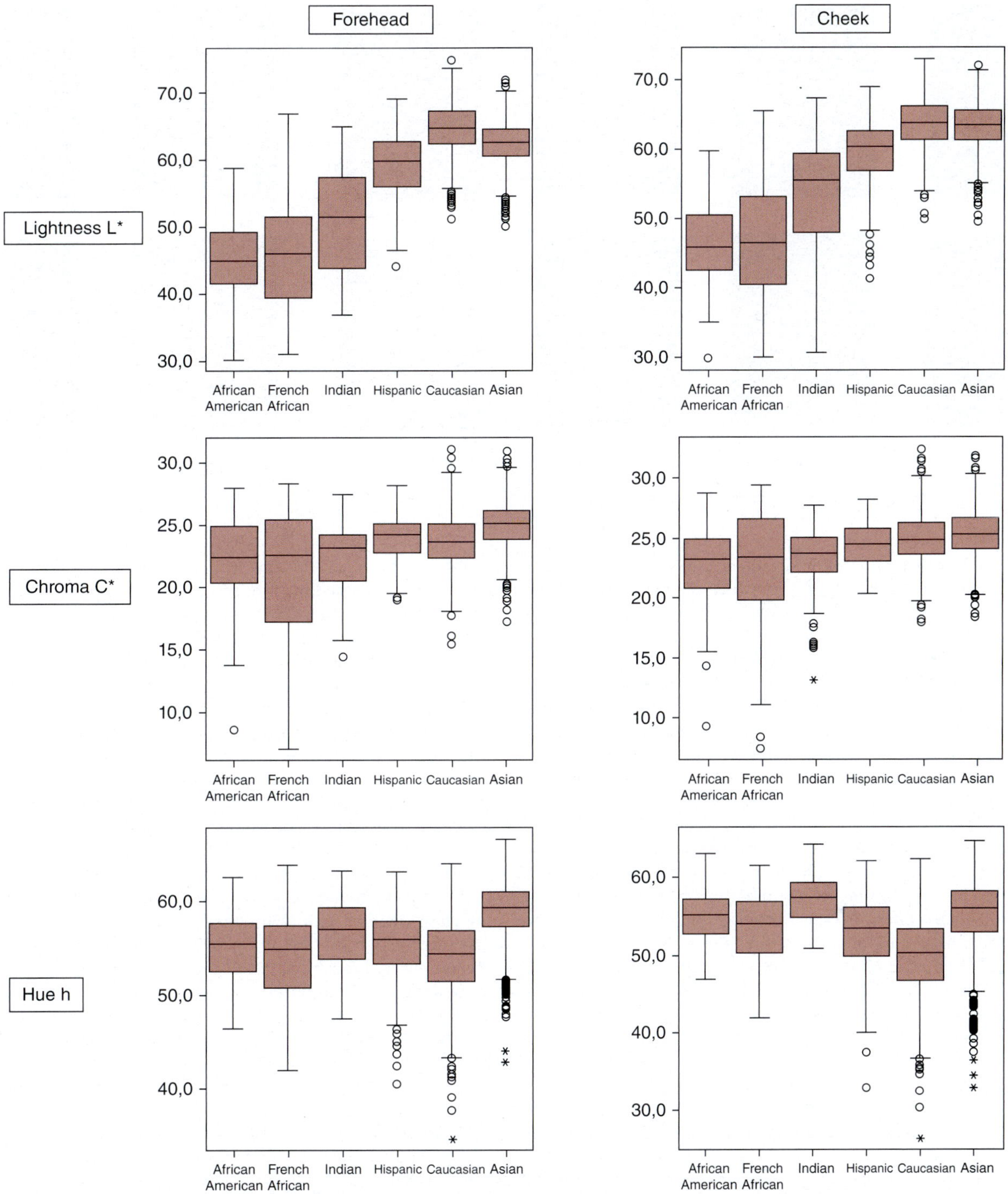

FIGURE 93-3. Boxplots bringing out the ranges of lightness, chroma, and hue of the different population groups on the forehead and cheek. It is interesting to note that Caucasian and Asian women practically cover the same lightness range, Caucasian and Hispanic women the same chroma range, and French African and African American women the same hue range.

with their skin tone, they were concerned about color and texture unevenness. Subjects frequently complained about light/dark color variations, visible texture irregularities such as dark marks or scars, and skin blemishes such as pimples, wrinkles, rough skin, large pores, and facial hair.

The major issue addressed when applying foundation was to provide evenness by covering up blemishes. Makeup application resulted in shades darker than the natural skin tone. Women in this group chose shades at least as dark as their darkest skin area to even face color. They also expected shades that brought glow and clarity from dullness. They used "vibrant" shades that were dark but not dull, such as "ebony," or with a slightly reddish undertone, such as "mahogany." A few individuals chose to lighten darker areas with a light foundation.

These interviews show that African American women have a positive self-perception of their own color. Although they declared themselves not satisfied with their usual foundation product because appropriate foundation shades were not available in stores, they managed to improve evenness by mixing several products.

Two independent groups of Caucasian women were also involved in the study; one included women in Paris, France, and the other one was made up of American women living in New York. We noticed a clear similarity between the results obtained from these two groups. The range of color used to depict skin included descriptors such as "beige," "medium beige," and "bronze-like." Skin defects most commonly mentioned included pimples, acne, blackheads, and wrinkles. They were often described as "redness" by the French subjects and as "dark blotches" by the American group. However, as a general observation from the in-depth interviews, we noted that Caucasian women were the least concerned group about skin unevenness. Ideal facial skin complexion was depicted

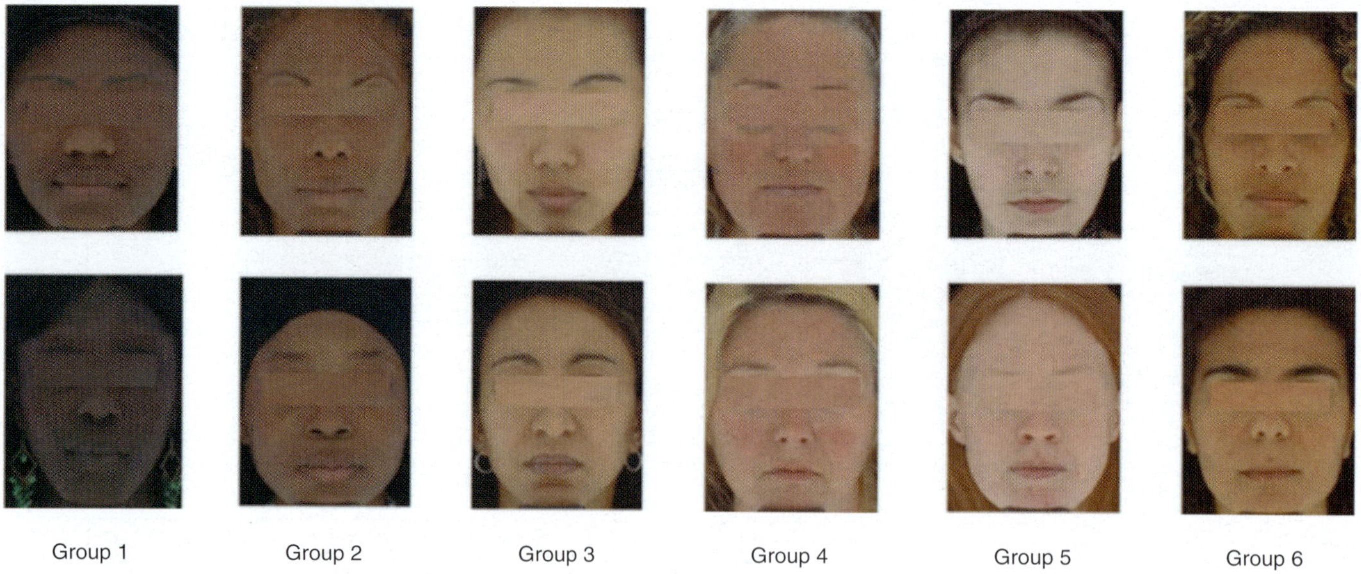

FIGURE 93-4. The six groups of skin tones reflecting the diversity in skin color.

as a healthy look with even color and radiance. Most women chose a shade slightly darker than their skin tone, which they felt allowed them to look "healthy" (*bonne mine*), provided a better coverage by covering the darkest areas or skin imperfections, and thereby helped them obtain evenness of color. They selected colors that impart a "healthy" look, such as "tan" or "bronze-like" colors—"sun tan," "gold," "sand on the beach." Otherwise, they selected "rosy-orangy" (the French group) and "blush pink" (the American group) to enhance a glowing look.

In this study, Asian skin was represented by Japanese women. It is worth noting that Japanese women described their skin complexion using a skin tone scale: pink, ocher, and beige. Some of them described themselves as "yellow." Japanese women did not describe their yellow skin color as a source of dissatisfaction but seemed to be more concerned by unevenness of their skin color because of the presence of pigment spots. Makeup strategies in this group consistently focused on improving skin evenness, irrespective of age or skin tone subgroup. Interestingly, the Japanese women were the only group that expected a "lightly tinted," "white," lucid, and bright skin color. They chose "white peach," "boiled egg," and "chinaware" shades or a color not different from the bare skin of the neck. To achieve this, they "played with color" by blending different foundation shades and by balancing powder and foundation shades.

Unlike the preceding groups, Hispanic Americans originated from a wide range of geographic areas that may have resulted in specific cultural characteristics. The Hispanic group included women from Puerto Rico, Dominica, Cuba, Venezuela, and Mexico, and many were recent immigrants. In contrast to the African American group, we found that some Hispanic American women tended not to enhance their own skin color by using descriptors such as "olive" and "dull." They complained about the "yellow tone" of their skin, which had a negative association with conditions such as jaundice and other types of sickness. Furthermore, they commented on uneven color, notably beneath the eyes, and reddish marks. The perception of skin color influenced makeup strategy. They expected color evenness with "one color all over the face" and a "healthy" skin color. This meant enhancing the yellow skin using shades that bring radiance, such as "golden bronze," "sun kissed," and "honey." Their approach to cosmetics undoubtedly also was influenced by the fact that the Hispanic American group included women from a wide range of cultural backgrounds, which likely contributed to a certain discrepancy between skin makeup result and declared cosmetic approach. Even when subjects verbally described a consistent desire to seek darker skin tones with a view to achieve a "sun kissed" skin color and to resolve perceived unevenness, the result was either lightened or darkened or reddened skin.

To clarify our conclusions from the previous study, a new qualitative study was carried out more recently on self-perception and makeup expectations of women according to their native countries. The in-depth interviews took place in Los Angeles, Miami, and New York. Women involved in the study in Los Angeles originated from Mexico, Honduras, Guatemala, and Nicaragua, with an equal number of light, medium, and dark complexions according to their self-perceptions to get a wide range of skin tones. Women involved in Miami originated from Cuba, Colombia, Venezuela, and Argentina with the same distribution over the lightness scale. Women involved in New York were natives of Puerto Rico and the Dominican Republic, with an equal number of light, medium, and dark complexions too. The women were aged 25 to 65 years.

This study confirmed that the self-perception and approach of Hispanic Americans to cosmetics is undoubtedly influenced by lightness of skin complexion and native country. Those with the lightest skin were the least satisfied with skin complexion, except for women of Cuban and Mexican origin. A too light skin tone was referred to as "pale," "yellowish," "illness," and "sickly." A medium complexion was much more appreciated, especially in women from the Dominican Republic, Puerto Rico, and South America. Although not unsatisfied with medium complexions, Cuban and Mexican women expressed preference for lighter complexions. The darkest skin tones were very well appreciated, and women referred to tanned skin as robust to the sun and not sickly.

However, the level of satisfaction with skin tone depended on social background and native country. The darkest complexions were hard to come to terms with for Mexican and Central American women, whereas the lightest skin tones were reported to be "less discriminating," "more elegant," and "cleaner." Women from Puerto Rico and the Dominican Republic were much more satisfied with their dark complexions, particularly because they were living in New York, where the high level of mixing between people of different backgrounds and origins makes complexion less of a source of concern.

Cuban women living in Miami belonged to a large community, which could explain why they generally accepted dark complexions very well. They did, however, express appeal for "rosy" tones. Women from South America living in Miami often came from favored social backgrounds and so assumed a dark skin tone. All in all, the ideal color this group identified was a "tanned," "bronze" skin tone that brings radiance to the face. To achieve such a complexion, women with fair skin tones chose darker shades, especially those native of the Dominican Republic. Those originating from Mexico and Cuba preferred to slightly lighten the skin with "rosy" or "bronze" shades that corrected the disliked "yellow" component. Most of those with medium complexions looked for a

TABLE 93-2 Percentage of each makeup strategy in different population groups

	Makeup strategies			
	"Golden look"	"Matching"	"Glow Look"	"Whitening"
French Caucasian	**54%**	20%	20%	6%
Russian Caucasian	**32%**	**54%**	14%	0%
American Caucasian	**33%**	**31%**	**28%**	8%
African American	**35%**	14%	**46%**	5%
French African	**36%**	20%	**38%**	6%
American Hispanic	**32%**	19%	**41%**	8%
Chinese	2%	14%	**48%**	**37%**
Japanese	6%	22%	**46%**	**26%**

Note: The percentages higher than 25% are highlighted in boldface.

matching foundation. However, they preferred to slightly darken the face if they could not get the appropriate shade, except for Cuban, Mexican, and some Puerto Rican women, who sought to slightly lighten the skin. Those with the darkest skin tones liked to match their own skin tones, but because of uneven skin color, they finally decided to darken the face and achieve a homogeneous result.

Regarding the colorimetric overlap of the different groups, it is obvious that racial origin and cultural background play a major role in self-perception of skin tone and undoubtedly influence makeup strategy.

THE COLOR OF THE SKIN AFTER APPLYING MAKEUP: MAIN STRATEGIES, SPECIFICITIES, AND COMMON STRATEGIES

The second stage of the 1999 study was to colorimetrically assess and classify women's makeup strategies. Women were asked to apply their usual and most preferred foundation with their own makeup routine. Measurements were done before (see the first part of the study) and after making up. The difference was computed for each color coordinate L^*, C^*, and h on both forehead and cheek to evaluate makeup strategy.

Panel The trial involved 2047 women aged 18 to 65 years from five different origins who lived in five different geographic locations: 1319 Asians (living in China and Japan), 432 Caucasians (living in France, Russia, and the United States), 98 Hispanics living in the United States, 112 French Africans, and 86 African Americans.

Statistics Makeup strategies were investigated from the differences in L^*, C^*, and h coordinates (ΔL^*, ΔC^*, and Δh, respectively) on the forehead and cheek using PCA. PCA brought out the significant components on which a hierarchical ascending classification was carried out to classify the strategies.

Results There emerged four main strategies involving the three attributes: lightness L^*, saturation C^*, and hue h [**Table 93-2** and **Figure 93-5**]. The first strategy made the skin darker, with most of the women making the skin more saturated and/or redder at the same time ($\Delta L^* = -1.6$, $\Delta C^* = +1.3$, $\Delta h = -2.1$ on forehead and $\Delta L^* = -1.9$, $\Delta C^* = -1.3$, $\Delta h = -1.6$ on cheek). We named it the "golden look." The second main strategy did not change the color, thus matching the skin tone. We named it "matching." The third main strategy made the skin redder and slightly less saturated ($\Delta h = -2.0$, $\Delta C^* = -1.1$ on forehead; $\Delta h = -1.6$, $\Delta C^* = -1.0$ on

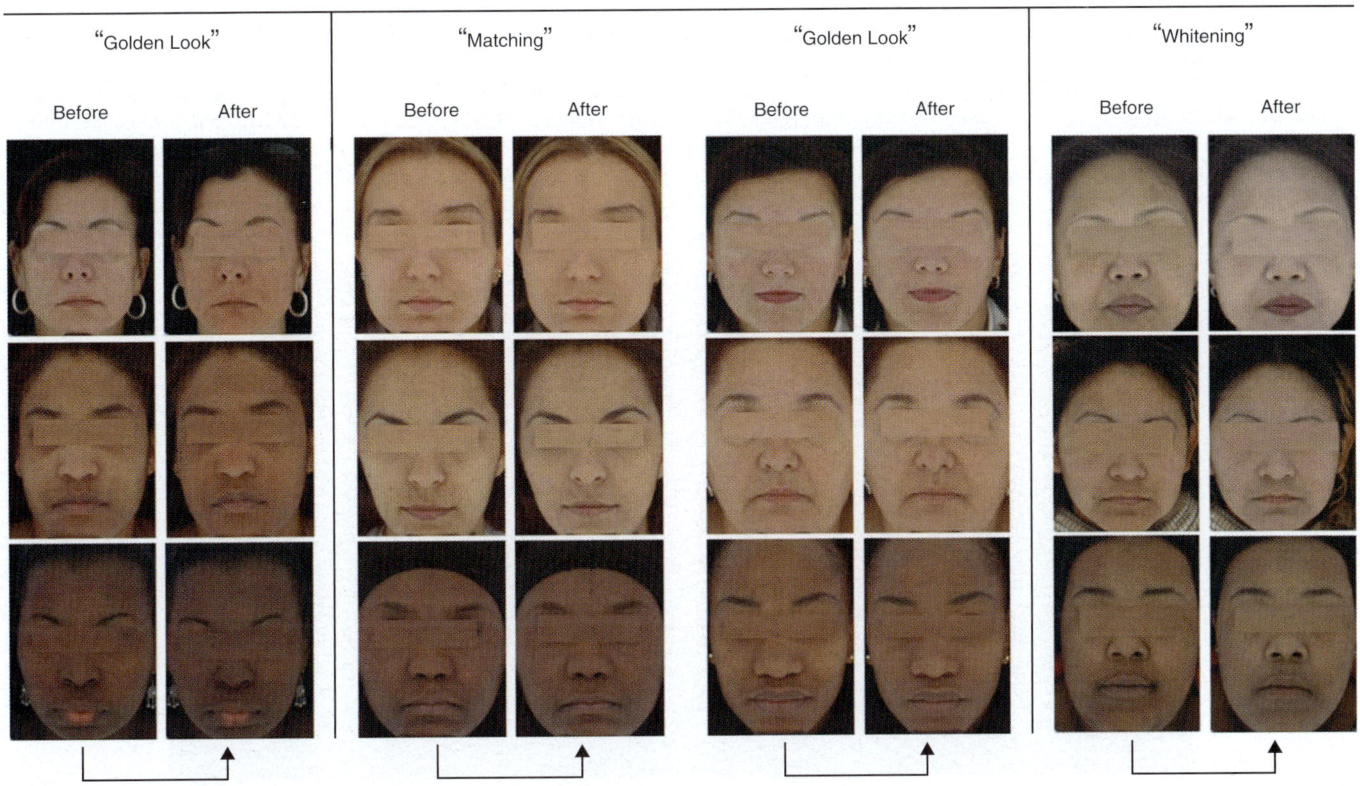

FIGURE 93-5. The four main strategies of women from different skin color groups.

cheek). We named it the "glow look." The last strategy made the skin highly less saturated to mute the color, with most of the women making the skin redder and lighter at the same time ($\Delta C^* = -3.0$, $\Delta h = -3.2$, $\Delta L^* = +1.4$ on forehead and $\Delta C^* = -2.7$, $\Delta h = -2.5$, $\Delta L^* = +1.3$ on cheek). We named it "whitening."

A sizeable portion of the African American women (35%; Table 93-2 and Figure 93-5) made their skin darker, which shows good consistency with the qualitative study. Many of the women explained that a darkening strategy was the easiest way to homogenize and/or the way to get a vibrant dark complexion. However, 46% preferred the "glow look," which does not alter the lightness, and 14% made up the skin without changing skin tone. We found that only 5% of African American women made the skin strongly less saturated and at the same time lighter and redder. This extreme strategy could be considered as a "whitening" strategy. The weak percentage confirms that most of the African American women are not willing to lighten their skin tone.

Most of the Chinese and Japanese women (85% and 72%, respectively) [Table 93-2 and Figure 93-5] made their skin less saturated. More detailed analysis showed that 37% and 26%, respectively, obtained a visible "white" appearance by strongly unsaturating the skin and making it lighter and redder. Only 14% of the Chinese and 22% of the Japanese women decided not to change their skin tone. It is worth noting that skin complexion in Asia strongly influences makeup strategy. Women who decide to strongly unsaturate skin have a bare skin tone significantly darker and more saturated, and women who decide to match their skin tone have significantly less saturated and redder skin, which means a pinkish complexion. Cross-correlating all data, we may suggest that the ideal Asian skin tone is a fair, not too saturated, and pink-ochre skin complexion.

In good agreement with their expectations, most Caucasian women made the skin darker (54% of French, 32% of Russian, and 33% of American Caucasians, respectively) [Table 93-2 and Figure 93-5]. Twenty percent and 31% of the French and American women, respectively, preferred to match their skin tone. The percentage increased to 54% in Russian Caucasians. Still consistent with the in-depth interview, 20% and 28% of the French and American women, respectively, brought a glow look to their faces. Few of these women decided to lighten their skin. Six percent of the French and 8% of the American women made the skin highly less saturated principally to mute a too vivid color.

As detailed in the qualitative study, the makeup strategies are much more varied in Hispanic women depending on native country and skin complexion. Nevertheless, 41% preferred to get a "glow look," and 32% darkened the skin to get a "tanned," "bronze" complexion [Table 93-2 and Figure 93-5], whereas 19% chose to match their skin tone. When looking deeper, only 8% strongly unsaturated the skin to get an apparent whitening/lightening effect.

There is a real diversity of makeup strategies. The matching strategy is transversal across different population groups. It is the way to enhance a well-appreciated skin color by hiding unevenness. The darkening strategy is either a way to homogenize the face or a way to make the skin more "tanned" and "radiant." The brightening strategy that goes through the unsaturation of color is either a way to mute a too vivid color or a cultural routine to get brightened fair skin.

CONCLUSION

A woman's uniqueness is striking with regard to the diversity of skin tones and various perceptions, expectations, and makeup strategies. Taking into account this diversity is of prime importance when formulating a makeup foundation range. It also means that proper advice should be provided to women to help them in selecting the most appropriate shades of makeup, which entails using their own words to meet their expectations.

THE LIPS

Lip makeup has a special place in the makeup routine. It could be the overall finish of the makeup routine or a way to enlighten skin tone. Unlike skin tone makeup, lip makeup is highly diversified in terms of color ranges and optical effects from matte to extreme shiny. Anatomically, lips are composed of the upper and lower vermilion borders and the perilabial skin that includes the area from the nose to the chin.

LIP COLOR

Our approach consisted in defining the color space of the vermilion border, juxtaposing it to the skin color space, enlightening various contrasts, and determining the differences between different populations.

Panel The colorimetric study included 1940 subjects—166 French Caucasian, 169 Russian Caucasian, 292 Chinese, 315 Japanese, 409 American Caucasian, 416 African American, and 160 Indian women.

Methods Colorimetrical measurements were done inside the Chromasphere using a spectroradiometer as described earlier.

Statistics The significant differences between population groups were demonstrated using univariate analysis on L^*, C^*, and h data. The limit for significance was $p < 0.05$.

Results Surprisingly, the lip color space is as large as skin color space [**Figure 93-6**]. Some differences between groups were brought out. Indian and African American women have the darkest and least saturated lips ($L^* = 42.9$ and 43.1, $C^* = 17.7$ and 18.5, respectively) [**Figure 93-7**], whereas Asian and Caucasian women showed the lightest

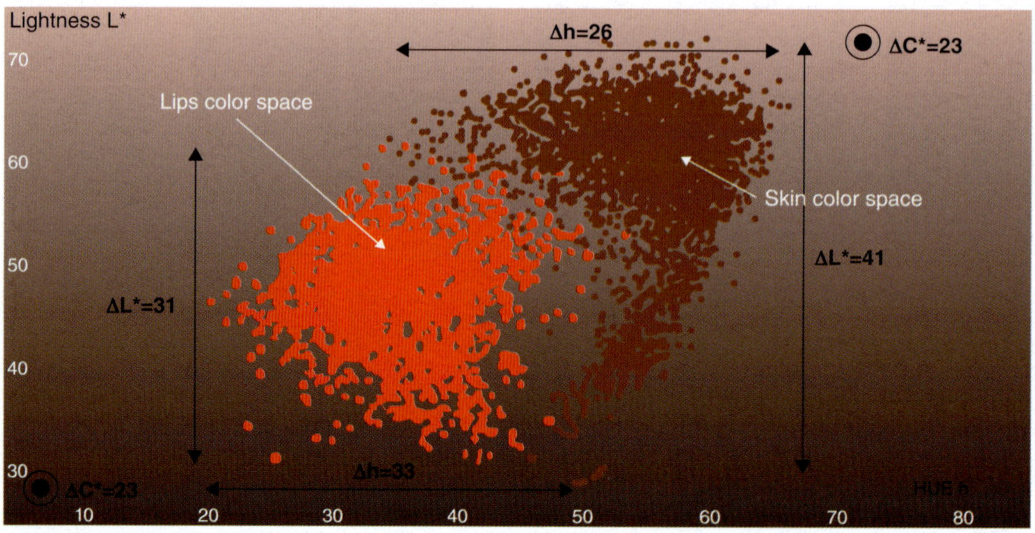

FIGURE 93-6. The lip and skin color spaces.

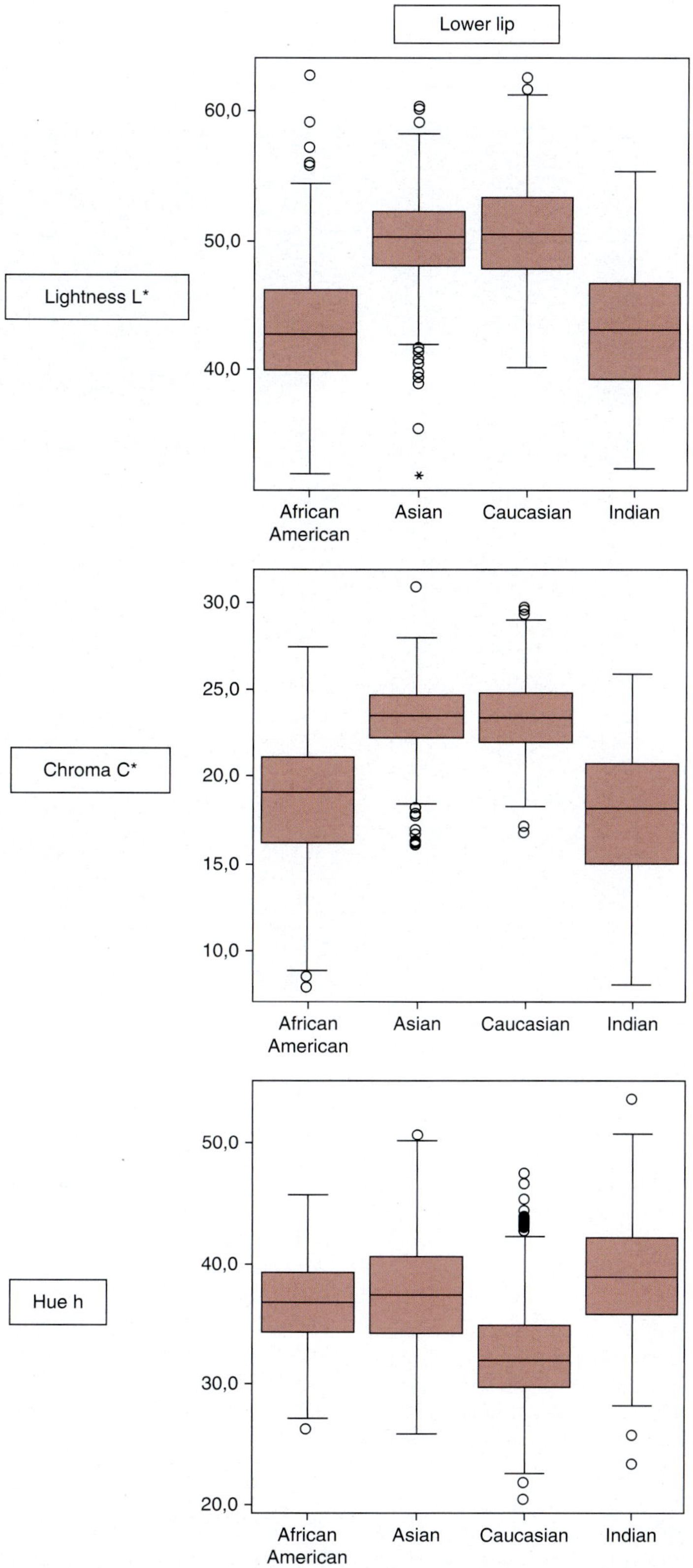

FIGURE 93-7. Boxplots bringing out the ranges of lightness, chroma, and hue of the different population groups on the lower lip. It is interesting to note that Caucasian and Asian women practically cover the same lightness and chroma ranges but are distinguished by the hue. African American and Indian women also have the same lightness and chroma ranges, but Indian lips are significantly more yellowish.

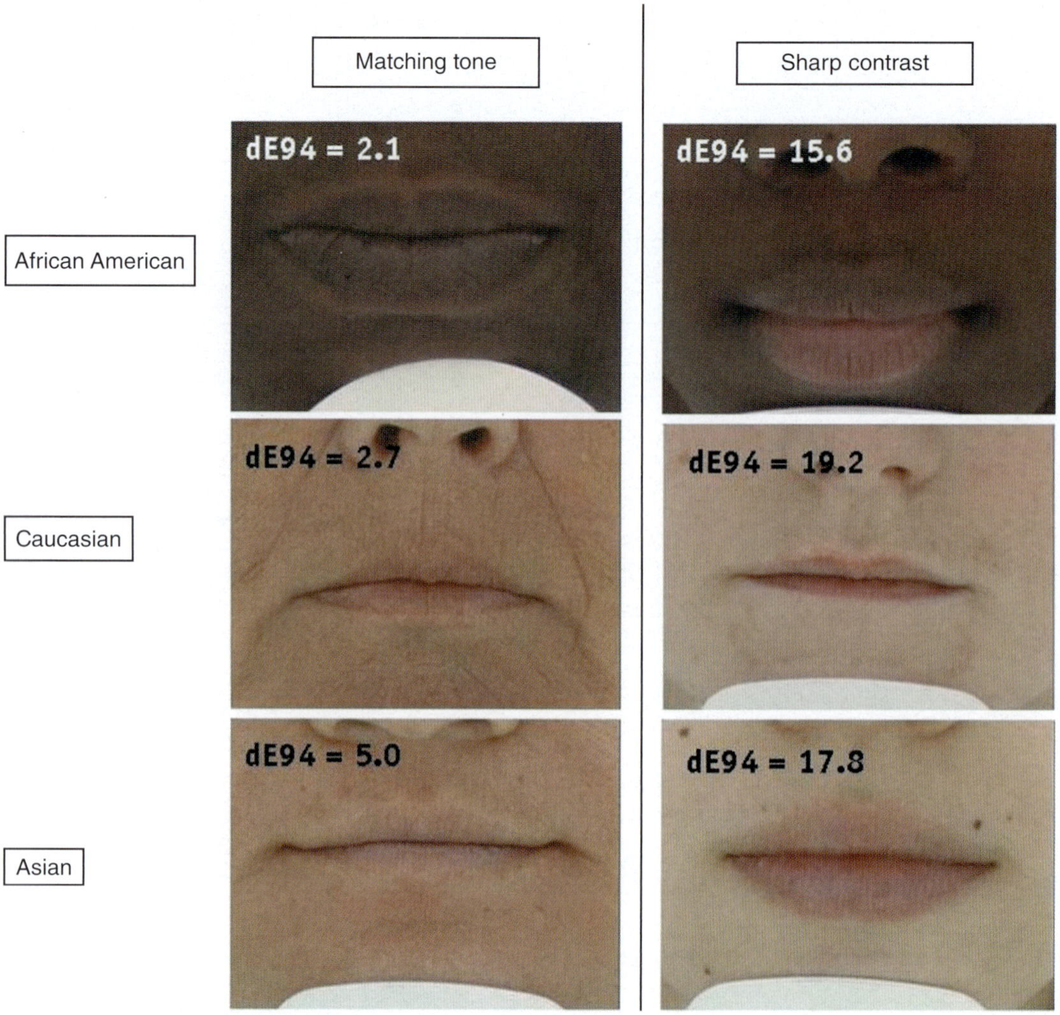

FIGURE 93-8. Various contrasts between the vermilion border and the perilabial skin expressed by the dE94 value.

and most saturated lip complexions (L^* = 50.0 and 50.6, C^* = 23.3 and 23.4, respectively) [Figure 93-7]. However, the hue distinguished Caucasian and Asian women. Caucasian women have redder lips than Asian women, and Indian women have the most yellowish lips (h = 32.4, 37.5, and 39.1, respectively) [Figure 93-7].

LIP COLOR CONTRAST

Comparison of the vermilion border and perilabial skin color refers to colorimetric contrasts. Indeed, lips can be likened to a colored object placed on a colored background (ie, the skin tone). The resulting contrast effect may change our visual perception of the color of the lips in relation to the color of skin tone. This issue was documented by the following study.

Panel A total of 914 women were involved in a colorimetric study using the same devices as described earlier to characterize the contrast between vermilion border and perilabial skin—238 African American, 238 American Caucasian, 225 French Caucasian, and 213 Japanese women equally distributed in the three age ranges of 18 to 35, 36 to 50, and 51 to 65 years.

Statistics A comparison between the vermilion border and the perilabial skin was carried out using the Student t test in cases of normal distribution, and the nonparametric Wilcoxon test was used if this was not the case. The difference was significant if $p < 0.05$.

Results Measurements show widely varying contrasts between the vermilion border and the perilabial skin from sharp differences to matching tones [**Figure 93-8**]. In all population groups except African American women, lips were made up to appear significantly darker than the perilabial skin [**Figure 93-9**]. In African American women, the vermilion border was lighter or darker, impacting the contrast [**Figure 93-10**]. Not surprisingly, the lips of women are significantly redder than the perilabial skin. However, some women show matching tones between lips and skin that decrease lip highlighting visually. In each group, there was no significant difference in saturation between the lips and perilabial skin. Consequently, lips could be either more saturated or less saturated than the skin.

CONCLUSION

The great number of contrasts between skin and lips offers a new perspective to enhance skin tone, lip color, or both. New studies should be conducted to explore the most appreciated contrasts for women. Other lip characteristics, such as morphologic, biomechanical, and hydration properties, could be investigated. Women express various concerns about these characteristics that also strongly depend on their racial origin, as well as on cultural and geographic environment.

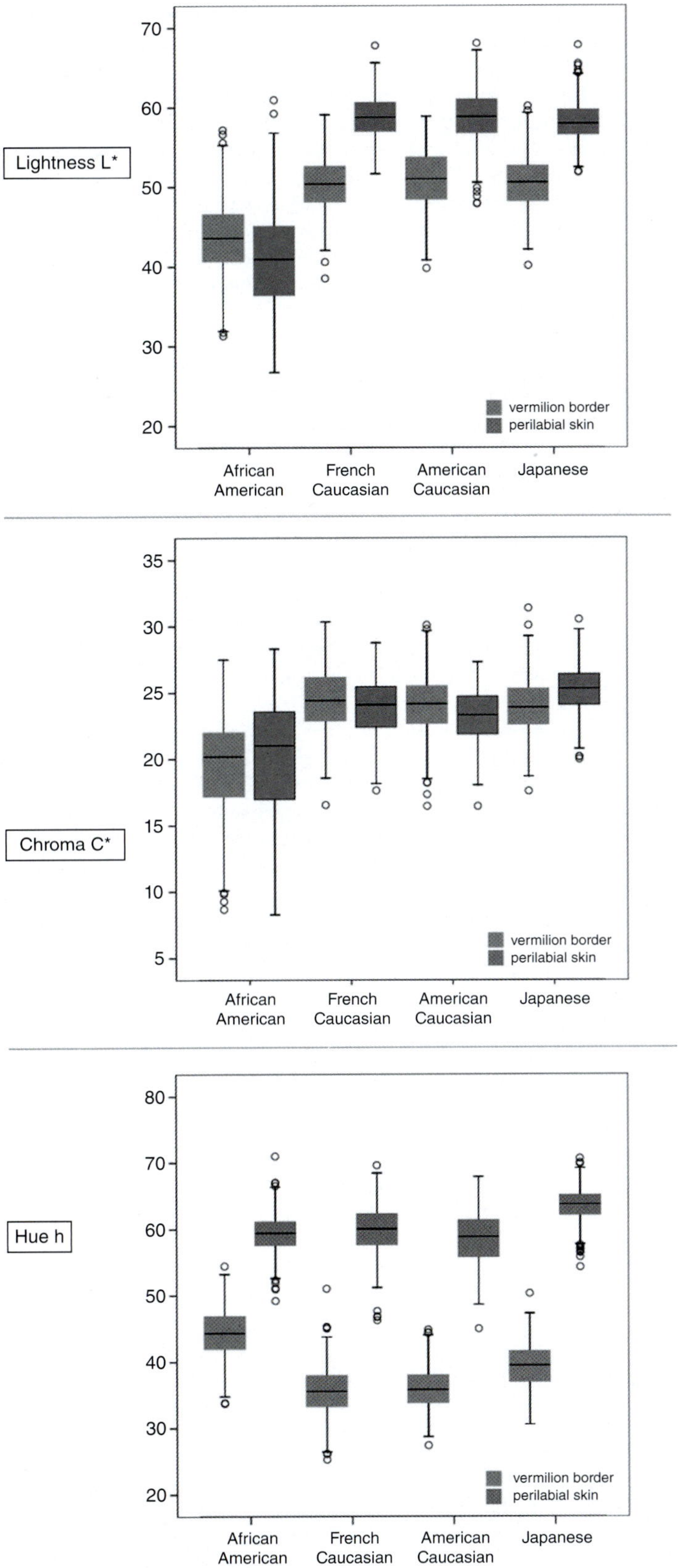

FIGURE 93-9. Boxplots bringing out the differences of lightness, chroma, and hue between the vermilion border and the perilabial skin.

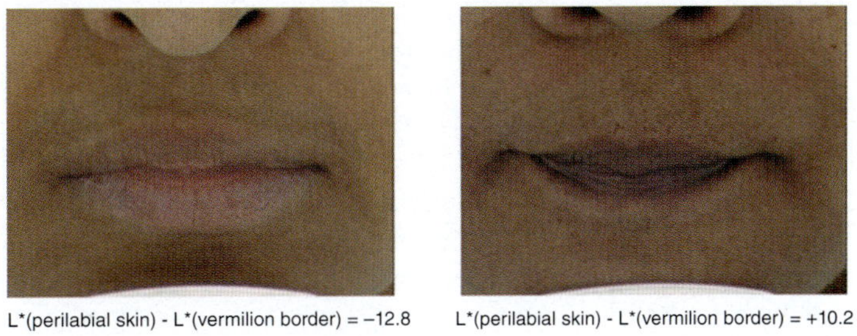

FIGURE 93-10. Two extreme contrasts.

REFERENCES

1. Sonoda I, Hirai Y, Okabe N, et al. On the preference of the color of makeup products related to the skin color in Japanese women. *J Soc Cosmet Chem.* 1987;21:219-224.
2. Lee KY, Shimagami K, Sato M, et al. Measurement of the color for bare skin and foundation-applied skin in women in their 20s: comparison of Japanese and Korean. *J Physiol Anthropol Appl Hum.* 2001;20:301.
3. Richards GM, Oresajo CO, Halder RM. Structure and function of ethnic skin and hair. *Dermatol Clin.* 2003;21:595-600.
4. Morizot F, Jdid R, Dheurle S, et al. Features related to skin pigmentation: differences between Japanese and French women. *Skin Res Technol.* 2005;11:76-77.
5. Minami J, Minami T. Designing the color of cosmetic foundations: Analysis on consumers' opinions about changing face color and measurement of colorimetric properties of foundation layers. *FRAGR J.* 1999;27:21-26.
6. Chardon A, Cretois I, Hourseau C. Skin colour typology and sun tanning pathways. *Int J Cosmet Sci.* 1991;13:191-208.
7. Liu W, Wang XM, Lai W. Skin color measurement in the Chinese female population: analysis of 407 cases from four cities of China. *Int J Dermatol.* 2007;46:835-839.
8. Giron F. Dispositif d'acquisition d'au moins une image d'au moins une partie du visage ou de la chevelure d'une personne. French patent 0111215. Paris, France: L'Oréal; 2001.
9. Caisey Bluteau L, Aubert J. Procédé et dispositif de mesure de la couleur. French patent 9606425. Paris, France, L'Oréal, 1996.
10. Caisey L, Grangeat F, Lemasson A, et al. Skin color and makeup strategies of women from different racial or ethnic groups. *Int J Cosmet Sci.* 2006;28:427-437.

CHAPTER 94

Skin Resurfacing—Lasers, Chemical Exfoliation, and Devices

Alicia Edwards
Janeth R. Campbell
Camille Robinson
Chesahna Kindred
Valerie Callender
Cheryl Burgess

KEY POINTS

- The use of lasers in people of color requires an understanding of laser physics and laser tissue interactions. Epidermal melanin in people of color acts as a competing chromophore; this not only decreases the effect of laser treatment but is also likely to cause nonselective thermal injury to the epidermis.
- With the proper selection of device, wavelength, and parameters, cutaneous dermatologic lasers can be used safely on people of color. To minimize unwanted side effects, the use of aggressive parameters is discouraged.

- With the ideal candidate and the proper clinical setting, intense pulsed light (IPL) often treats numerous dermatologic conditions. However, IPL must be used with caution in patients with Fitzpatrick Skin Phototypes IV and is not the desired treatment for those with phototypes V or VI.
- Fractional lasers show promise in the treatment of melasma, acne scarring, and skin rejuvenation in patients with darker phototypes.
- Test spots are highly encouraged when treating people with darker skin phototypes.
- Skin cooling and postoperative skin care are highly recommended for people of color.

INTRODUCTION TO LASERS IN PEOPLE OF COLOR

In 1983, the use of brief pulses of selectively absorbed optical radiation was reported to cause selective damage to pigmented structures, cells, and organelles in vivo. This description of target thermal energy delivery set in motion the advancement of cutaneous laser surgery.[1] Decades later, laser technology has been refined, allowing clinicians to successfully treat a wide variety of skin conditions, including vascular and pigmented lesions, tattoos, scars, and unwanted hair.[2] The Aesthetic Plastic Surgery National Databank reported 431,485 cutaneous laser procedures for the year of 2021.[3] Non-Hispanic Whites will no longer be the majority of the United States populations as early as 2045.[4] The demographics of the United States is changing, as racial minority populations are steadily growing. From 2000 to 2010, the African American population increased by 12%, and the Hispanic and Asian populations both increased by 43%.[5] With the United States becoming more racially and ethnically diverse, it is imperative that clinicians have a thorough understanding of laser use in people of color (POC). This section will discuss laser types, safety and efficacy, adverse events, and techniques associated with their use for resurfacing in POC patients.

POC patients have larger and more heavily concentrated melanosomes throughout the epidermal layer compared to their White counterparts.[6] To treat dermal chromophores, laser light must pass through this heavily melanized epidermis. The light that is emitted from the laser beam is monochromatic, coherent, collimated, and of high energy. Once the laser light reaches the skin, it can be reflected, scattered, transmitted, or absorbed. Laser light is absorbed by chromophores, which are "light-loving" substances within the skin. There are three main endogenous chromophores in the skin: melanin, hemoglobin (oxyhemoglobin), and water [**Figure 94-1**]. Given the increased concentration and increased wavelength absorption (240-1200 nm) of melanin, laser light in POC is often absorbed into the pigmented epidermis rather than the dermis. Thus, the efficacy of older laser technology may be reduced in POC. Additionally, side effects of blistering, dyspigmentation, and scarring can occur as this absorbed light is converted into epidermal heat. Newer technology in lasers utilizes longer wavelengths for the penetration of deeper, dermal chromophores to improve efficacy and reduce epidermal injury in POC patients.[7] Generally, POC typically seek laser therapy for the treatment of scars and pigmentation changes and less often for the treatment of rhytids.

LASER AND LIGHT-BASED TREATMENTS FOR COMMON SKIN DISORDERS

VASCULAR DISORDERS

Port-Wine Stains Port-wine stains (PWS) affect 0.3% to 0.5% of newborns.[8,9] Occurring less often in African Americans, there is an equal frequency in males and females [**Figure 94-2**]. PWS are thought to be related to the varying depth of the ectatic vessels, which are typically 30 to 300 μm in diameter, in the papillary and reticular dermis. There is a deficiency of nerves in the papillary plexus of the affected skin. Interestingly, with PWS, the adjacent bone and soft tissue can become hyperplastic.

The most common location of a PWS is on the face, with only one-third of stains occurring on nonfacial areas.[10] In general, PWS get darker and worsen over time. Approximately two-thirds of all patients develop nodularity by the fifth decade of life.[10] Negative prognostic variables for laser treatment are lesions with a "cobblestone" texture, patients over 50 years old, those with Fitzpatrick skin phototypes V and VI, and those with larger lesions or nonfacial PWS.[11,12]

The pulsed dye laser (PDL), with a wavelength of 585 or 595 nm, is traditionally the laser of choice in the treatment of PWS for all individuals. Specifically, the variable PDL, with a 595-nm wavelength and equipped with cooling, is the ideal laser for treating PWS in skin phototypes IV to VI. The slightly longer wavelength of the 595-nm PDL allows for deeper penetration into the dermis and the ectatic vasculature of the PWS, and is thus a better choice for darker-skinned individuals.[13-15]

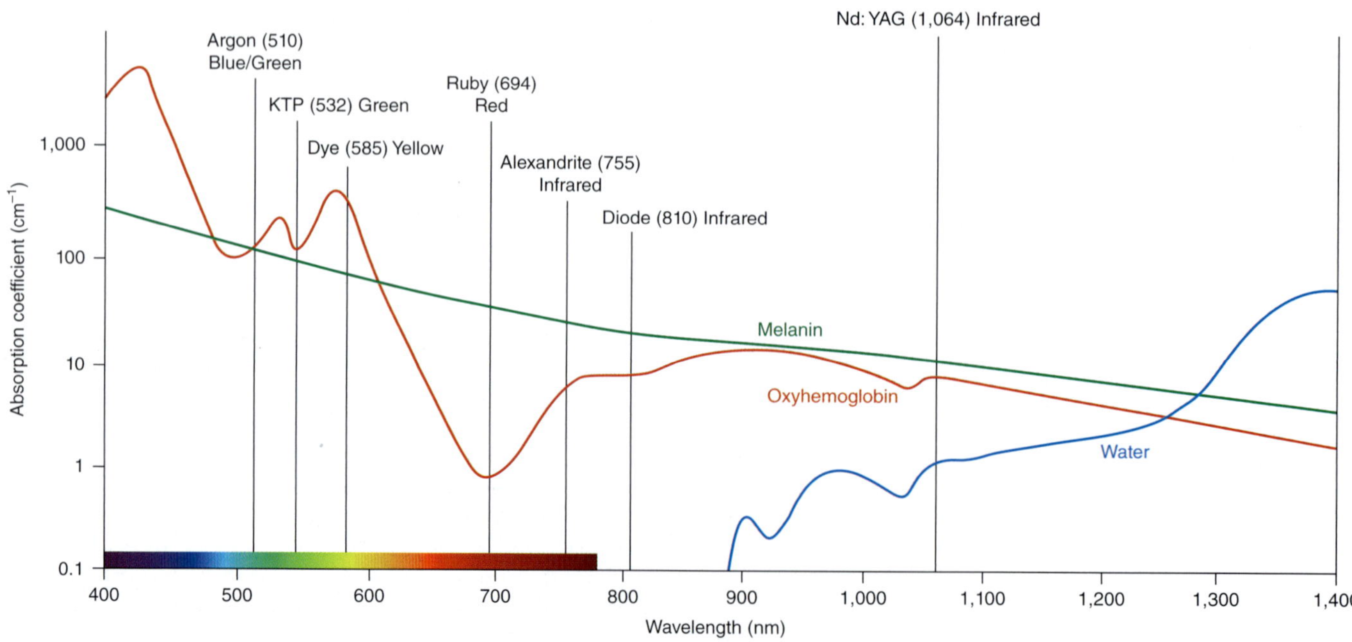

FIGURE 94-1. Endogenous chromophore. (Reproduced with permission from Allemann IB, Kaufman J. Laser principles. *Curr Probl Dermatol.* 2011:42:7-23.)

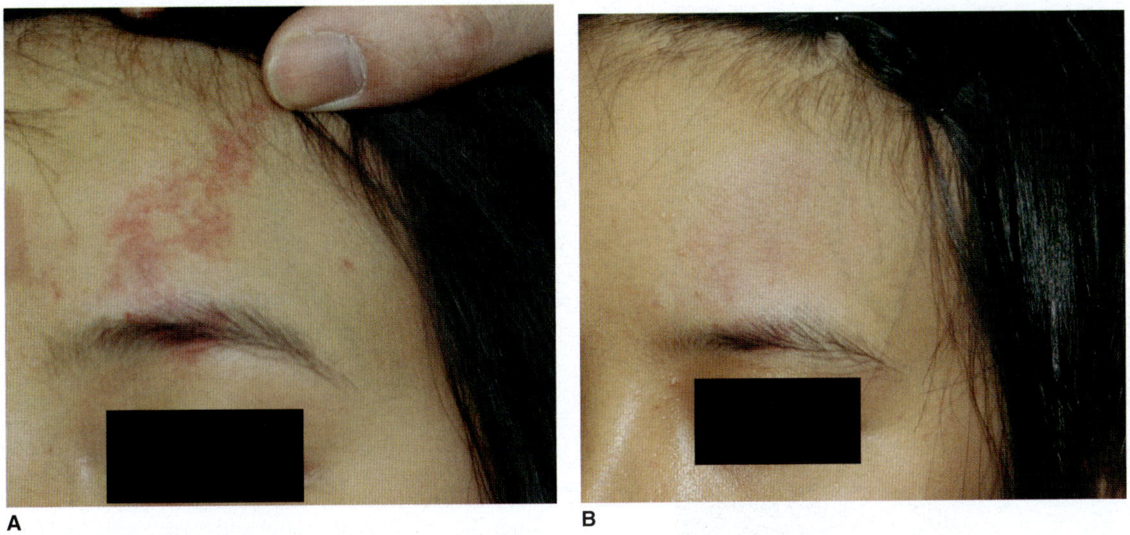

FIGURE 94-2. **(A)** Port-wine stain on the forehead of a young female patient before treatment. **(B)** Significant improvement was observed after three pulsed dye laser treatments at 595 nm. (Used with permission from Dr. Zhong Lu, Dermatology Department, Huashan Hospital, Fudan University, Shanghai, China.)

The TRT of different blood vessels is important in determining the appropriate pulse duration. For smaller vessels (of ≤20 μm in diameter), a pulse duration of 450 μs is adequate; vessels with a larger diameter (30 to 150 μm) should have a pulse duration of approximately 1 to 10 ms.[16] Longer pulse durations are generally indicated for darker skin types (V and VI), which require pulse durations of 10 ms or longer in most clinical situations.

It is crucial that test spots are performed on patients before they undergo laser treatment of the entire lesion. These test spots allow determination of the appropriate fluence and should be performed by delivering several juxtaposed pulses onto the PWS lesion. Varying fluences should be used to determine the best clinical outcome. Stacked or double pulsing is not recommended for patients with POC. The patient should return after 1 month so the dermatologist can check the clinical outcome of the test spot. The treatment should then be performed at a setting that provokes a clinical subpurpuric tissue response. With the PDL, transient violaceous discoloration of the treated area is normal. Limited exposure to sun, heat, and exercise is an important postlaser care measure to prevent the recanalization of the blood vessels.

Conventionally, 4-week treatment intervals are the most common. Decreasing the treatment intervals and initiating treatment early can result in better treatment outcomes and responses, as was seen in a study of 24 infants with PWS by Anolik et al.[17] The reason for this may be twofold: infant skin is commonly subjected to less sun exposure and is also thinner than adult skin. In POC, intervals between treatments should allow sufficient time for the skin to heal.

As the PWS lightens with subsequent laser treatments, due to the decreasing number of chromophores, higher fluences are necessary. The exact number of treatments necessary to improve the color and texture of PWS in POC is unknown. The side effects of treating PWS with lasers are minimal, although transient hyperpigmentation has been reported in 44% to 46% of patients.[18] Transient hypopigmentation, permanent hypopigmentation, and scarring are rarely encountered.[19]

Unfortunately, the results of treating PWS with laser therapy remain disappointing. It is reported that only 10% to 20% of patients obtain a complete resolution of their PWS.[20,21] Hence, the majority of treated patients either experience lighter PWS or no change at all. For POC, the rate of any significant degree of improvement is thought to be significantly less than that of the general population.

There are new therapies that may help address difficult-to-treat PWS and thus may benefit darker-skinned individuals. Emerging light-based technology includes the use of longer wavelength devices—such as the 755-nm alexandrite laser, 810-nm diode laser, or the 1064-nm neodymium-doped yttrium-aluminum-garnet (Nd:YAG) laser—either simultaneously with PDL or alone.[22,23] Although there is deeper penetration with these adjunct lasers, there is decreased absorption by the hemoglobin, which thus requires the use of higher fluences for sufficient photocoagulation. This can result in the nonselective bulk-like heating of the surrounding tissue, thus increasing the risk of scarring.[22] Interestingly, the PDL/Nd:YAG dual laser is a system that works by first using the 595-nm PDL to cause a conversion of the oxyhemoglobin to methemoglobin, which has an absorption peak near 1064 nm. The subsequent synergistic use of the 1064-nm Nd:YAG then decreases the amount of fluence necessary for the photocoagulation of the blood vessels.[23] Unfortunately, there are no published reports of this laser on POC, so it is not known if this combination is successful on their skin types.

Combining PDL with the prescription of posttreatment imiquimod has shown promise; this combination was seen to improve PWS in a recent small study.[24] The proposed mechanism of action of imiquimod is the inhibition of angiogenesis. However, more clinical trials are needed to establish its true efficacy and safety. Likewise, the immunosuppressant sirolimus, a macrolide antibiotic, has antiangiogenic properties that appear to help reduce PWS when used in combination with PDL therapy.[25]

Intense pulsed light (IPL) is a broadband light source that emits noncoherent light in wavelengths of between 500 and 1200 nm. IPL provides an option for the treatment of PWS in individuals with lighter complexions and has been used to treat patients with skin phototype IV. Ho et al were able to achieve a 25% to 50% clearance in a group of patients with skin phototype IV undergoing five to seven treatments every 3 to 4 weeks.[26] However, IPL is not recommended for the treatment of PWS in patients with darker phototypes. POC are more likely to experience hyperpigmentation, vesiculation, hypopigmentation, scarring, and permanent hair reduction.

Finally, another vascular laser device used in the treatment of PWS is the frequency-doubled 532-nm Nd:YAG laser. It is best suited for patients with lighter skin types of phototype IV or fairer.

Hemangiomas Infantile hemangiomas occur in 10% of children.[27] There is a greater predilection in Caucasians compared with African Americans and in females compared with males [**Figure 94-3**].[27,28] Hemangiomas are benign vascular tumors of the skin. There is a rapid intermittent growth phase within the first year of life; the tumors usually reach their maximum size by the time the patient is 9 months old. It is during this proliferation phase that there is the highest risk of complications, which can include bleeding, ulceration, infection, or the obstruction of vital organs.[29,30] Regression is approximately 90% complete by the time the patient reaches the age of 9 years.[31] Generally, laser treatment

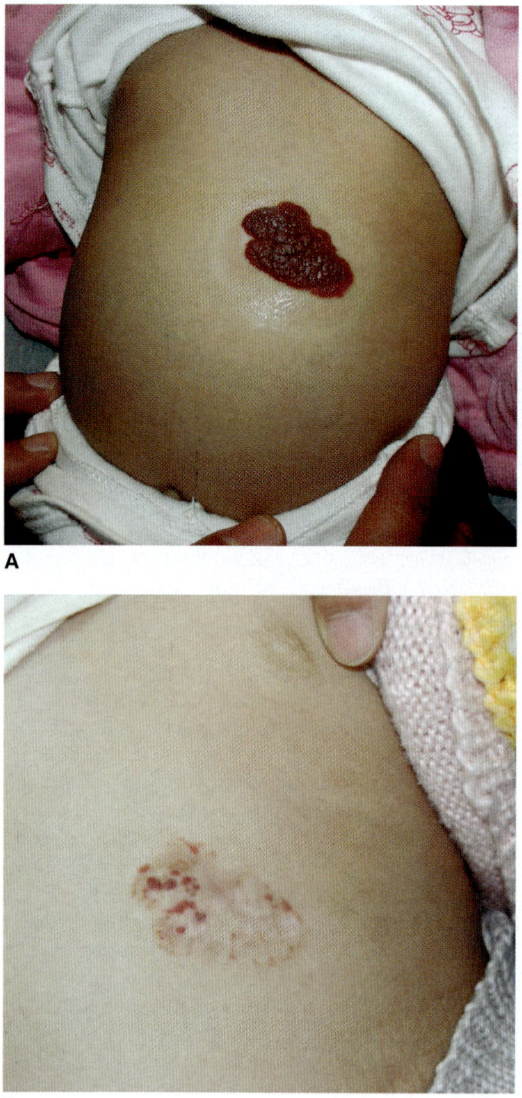

A

B

FIGURE 94-3. (A) Hemangioma on the stomach of an infant before treatment. **(B)** Significant improvement was observed after four long-pulsed neodymium-doped yttrium-aluminum-garnet laser treatment at 1064 nm. (Used with permission from Dr. Zhong Lu, Dermatology Department, Huashan Hospital, Fudan University, Shanghai, China.)

for hemangiomas is not necessary because the majority involute or resolve spontaneously, and thus a "wait and see" philosophy is commonly adopted. However, new ideologies are slowly emerging advocating the early intervention and treatment of hemangiomas, especially complicated ones.

Approximately 10% of hemangiomas will require active medical treatment to avoid the advent of life-threatening complications.[32] Treatment modalities range from topical and oral β-adrenergic blockers, such as propranolol, to topical corticosteroids, oral glucocorticoids, intralesional steroid injections, lasers, and surgical excision.[33]

Treatments aim to halt any further growth of the hemangioma, accelerate regression, and prevent loss of function. When using lasers as an early adjunctive treatment modality for uncomplicated hemangiomas in darker-skinned patients, it is important that the benefits clearly outweigh the risks.

The laser of choice for the treatment of hemangiomas is PDL. The 595-nm PDL reaches a depth of 1.5 mm, and thus superficial hemangiomas respond better to PDL than others.[34-36] Propranolol can help to reduce the size of thicker hemangiomas. For patients receiving propranolol, laser treatments are sometimes performed during or just prior to the weaning of propranolol to counteract any potential rebound growth effects. With the 595-nm PDL, the number of treatments varies depending on the patient—therapy is usually continued until involution is achieved. Pre- and postcooling are beneficial. As with PWS lesions, initial treatments for hemangiomas should be performed at pulse durations that result in a clinical subpurpuric change in the skin. It is best to maintain a conservative fluence during the initial treatment. In subsequent visits, the parameters can be adjusted according to clinical outcome and tissue response. Some experts advocate treating patients more frequently, for example, every 2 weeks instead of every 4 to 6 weeks. However, there should be enough time between treatments for the patient and/or doctor to notice any adverse cutaneous changes.

Similar to PWS therapies, adjunctive therapies seem promising for the treatment of hemangiomas in the future—particularly the use of imiquimod and sirolimus combined with PDL treatment and the single use of long-pulsed Nd:YAG lasers.

Leg Veins Sclerotherapy remains the gold standard for the treatment of leg veins. However, laser therapy may be considered for patients who have an allergy to the sclerosing agent, a fear of needles, small vessels that cannot be cannulated, postsclerotherapy matted telangiectasias, vessels in areas that are prone to ulceration, for instance the ankle, or superficial vasculature.

The following light sources are typically used to treat leg veins: 595-nm PDL; 800-, 810-, 940-, and 980-nm diode lasers; 1064-nm Nd:YAG; and 515- to 1200-nm IPL.[37] Wavelengths of between 700 and 1200 nm penetrate into the skin to a depth of approximately 3 mm, thereby targeting the superficial vessels. High fluences are required to achieve photocoagulation of the blood vessels. Pulse durations of 40 to 60 ms are adequate for leg veins measuring 0.2 to 0.8 mm in diameter, based on a TRT of 20 to 300 ms.[38] Clinically there is usually evidence of immediate vessel clearance, intravascular thrombosis, and rupture of the vessel resulting in purpura. With all factors taken into consideration, blue and larger vessels respond better to the 1064-nm Nd:YAG laser in comparison to the smaller red vessels. The fluence for larger vessels (1.5-3 mm in diameter) is generally lower and ranges from 100 to 200 J/cm^2 with longer pulse durations. For smaller vessels, the fluence is typically higher, in the range of 250 to 400 J/cm^2 with shorter pulse durations. Spot sizes of 2 to 3 mm are typical. With laser-assisted leg vein therapy, multiple treatments are necessary. Unlike sclerotherapy, compression stockings are not necessary.

It should be stated that treatment for patients with skin phototype V should be approached cautiously; cosmetic laser treatment of leg veins is not recommended for those with phototype VI. Moreover, IPL in particular is not the best treatment for POC, especially those with phototypes IV to VI.

For optimal results, it is best that individuals undergoing laser leg vein treatment are not tanned. Additionally, it is prudent to first treat conditions like venous insufficiency, feeder vessels, and larger varicosities. Pre- and postlaser cooling are necessary to protect the skin from thermal damage and altered pigmentation. Postinflammatory hyperpigmentation or hemosiderin are common side effect, often lasting several months. However, cutaneous ulceration is rare.

SCLEROTHERAPY

Varicose veins are a very common cosmetic complaint and are observed in a large majority of the population. In fact, 41% of women in the fifth decade of life have varicose veins, whereas 72% have varicosities in the seventh decade.[39] Sclerotherapy for varicose and spider veins is a common procedure performed in dermatologic practices and has been used by dermatologists since the 1980s.[40,41] It is a first-line therapy for treatment of small varicose veins.

Patient Selection A detailed history and physical examination should be performed on all patients with varicose veins considering sclerotherapy. Based on an individual's history and physical examination, a noninvasive diagnostic test of the venous system may be necessary.[42] The "gold standard" of this testing is duplex ultrasound, which assesses for blood clots within the veins. After the patient has been deemed a good candidate, informed consent is obtained.

Contraindications

- Reflux at the saphenofemoral junction
- Patients confined to bed
- Severely restricted arterial flow to legs
- History of deep venous thrombosis
- Allergy to sclerosing agents
- Obesity
- Pregnancy

Types of Sclerosing Agents Numerous classes of sclerosing agents are available [**Table 94-1**]. The selection of an agent depends on factors such as the size and location of the vessel undergoing treatment. There are three major classes of sclerosing agents, and they include osmotic, detergent, and corrosive agents. Osmotic solutions are milder and less capable of initiating a cascade of inflammation, which could result in PIH, a common side effect of sclerotherapy in patients with skin of color.

Sclerosing agents are effective in treatment by causing endothelial damage of the vein, which induces fibrosis of the veins, followed by eventual resorption of the vessel.[43]

Hypertonic saline is used in different concentrations ranging from 10% to 30%. Although allergenicity is low with this solution, it may cause skin necrosis if extravasation occurs at the injection site. Ulcerations after injection of hypertonic saline are the leading cause of malpractice cases associated with sclerotherapy in the United States.[44] Pain associated with hypertonic saline injections is due to irritation of the nerves in the adventitia and muscular tissue.[45] Other potential side effects with the use of hypertonic saline are exacerbation of hypertension, necrosis of the cortex of the kidneys, hemolysis, hematuria, central nervous system disorders,[44] hypernatremia,[45] and membranous fat necrosis.[43]

The hypertonic saline and dextrose solution contains a mixture of dextrose, sodium chloride, propylene glycol, and phenethyl alcohol. It is predominantly marketed in Canada and used for treatment of smaller vessels. It is used off label in the United States for the treatment of telangiectasias.

Polidocanol is a detergent-based sclerosing agent that contains hydroxypolyethoxydodecane dissolved in distilled water with 5% ethanol. It was approved by the U.S. Food and Drug Administration (FDA) as a sclerosing agent in the United States in June 2010 for the treatment of lower extremity veins, with the 0.5% concentration being used for telangiectasias and the 1% concentration being used for small reticular veins.[43] The recommended volume of injection is less than 10 mL for patients weighing 50 kg or more or a dose of 2 mg/kg.[45] Injection with this agent is relatively painless, and it has a low incidence of cutaneous necrosis. In a study of 285 Chinese patients, polidocanol 0.5%, 1%, and 3% (dose used was dependent on the type of varicose vein being treated) was found to be efficacious, with all response rates greater than 85%, superior to placebo, and safe.[46]

Sodium tetradecyl sulfate is considered a detergent and is a very effective sclerosing agent. It is also FDA approved for the treatment of lower extremity veins. In high doses, this agent has been reported to cause an increased incidence of posttreatment pigmentation.

Sodium morrhuate consists of a 5% solution of salts of saturated and unsaturated fatty acids in cod liver oil. This agent has an increased potential for cutaneous necrosis and is used rarely for treatment of varicose veins due to its side effects. Fatalities due to anaphylaxis from this agent have been reported.[47]

Chromated glycerin is considered a chemical irritant and is not approved by the FDA. It is a weak sclerosing agent but does have the ability to destroy the endothelium.

Polyiodinated iodine is also a chemical irritant and a strong sclerosing agent. It has a very toxic effect on the endothelium and is not approved by the FDA.

Technique Sclerotherapy is performed beginning with treatment of the largest proximal varicosities and extending to the smaller distal vessels. Injection is performed using a 30-gauge needle that is inserted at a 10° to 30° angle with the bevel up. Initial treatment of telangiectatic webs begins with the lowest concentration of sclerosing agents. The agents used most commonly are 0.1% sodium tetradecyl sulfate or 0.2% polidocanol. Sclerosing usually occurs 1 to 6 months after the procedure is done, and if it is not successful, the concentration is increased during subsequent treatments.

Foam sclerotherapy is a technique that consists of a detergent sclerosing agent that is combined with air and is found to be more potent than liquid sclerosing agents.[48]

Complications Hyperpigmentation following sclerotherapy [**Figure 94-4**] occurs at a rate of 0.3% to 10%, with rates as high as 30% in some studies.[49] The cause of this complication appears to be multifactorial and includes

TABLE 94-1 Comparison of commonly used sclerosing agents

Sclerosing solution	Category	Advantages	Disadvantages	Vessels treated	Concentrations
Sodium tetradecyl sulfate (Sotradecol)	Detergent	FDA approved Painless unless injected extravascularly	May cause breakdown rarely found to be equivalent to polidocanol in clinical studies	All sizes	0.1-0.2% telangiectasias 0.-0.5% reticular 0.5-1.0% varicose 1.0-3.0% axial varicose
Polidocanol	Detergent	Painless Low ulceration risk at low concentrations		Small to medium	0.2-0.5% telangiectasias 0.5-1.0% reticular 1.0-3.0% varicose
Hypertonic saline	Hyperosmolar	Low risk of allergic reactions	Ulcerogenic Painful to inject	Small	23-11.7% telangiectasias 23.4% reticular
Hypertonic saline + dextrose (Sclerodex)	Hyperosmolar	Low risk of allergic reaction Mild stinging Low ulcerogenic potential	Not FDA approved Relatively weak sclerosant	Small	Undiluted—telangiectasias Undiluted—reticular
Sodium morrhuate (Scleromate)	Detergent	FDA approved	Allergic reactions highest	Small	Undiluted—telangiectasias Undiluted—reticular
Chromated glycerin (glycerin with 6% chromium salt; Scleremo)	Chemical irritant	Low skin ulcer potential	Not FDA approved Very weak sclerosant	Smallest	Undiluted to one-half strength—telangiectasias
Glycerin—plain	Chemical irritant	Painless, low risk of allergic reaction, decreased risks of pigmentation and matting	FDA approved for reduction of cerebral edema	Smallest	50-72%
Polyiodinated iodine (Varigloban)	Chemical irritant	Highly corrosive allows treatment of largest veins	Not FDA approved Avoid in iodine-allergic patients	Largest	1-2% for up to 5-mm veins 2-6% for the largest veins

Abbreviation: FDA, U.S. Food and Drug Administration.

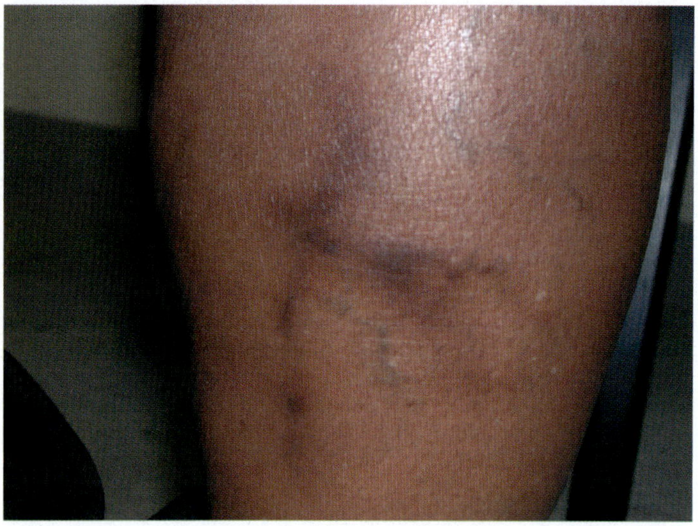

FIGURE 94-4. Hyperpigmentation following sclerotherapy.

type and concentration of the sclerosing agent [**Table 94-2**], technique used, intravascular pressures, and postsclerotherapy care.[50] Initially, this pigmentation is due to deposition of hemosiderin, and eventually the hemosiderin is replaced by melanin. Within 6 months, the hyperpigmentation clears in 70% of patients.[50] For more persistent cases of hyperpigmentation, various treatments, including hypopigmenting agents, chemical peeling, and lasers,[51] which have demonstrated limited success, have been used.

Other complications of sclerotherapy include erythema, edema, pruritus, pain, urticaria, localized hypertrichosis, telangiectatic matting, cutaneous necrosis and ulceration, superficial thrombophlebitis, and pulmonary embolism.

Patient Instructions and Follow Up Four to 8 weeks are usually allowed between subsequent treatments if needed. Patients are instructed to wear compression stockings for at least 2 weeks following treatment with sclerotherapy. Graduated 20 to 30 or 30 to 40 mm Hg support hose are recommended after treatment of larger veins, and over-the-counter 15 mm Hg compression stockings are recommended for smaller veins. In a study that evaluated postsclerotherapy compression with class II (30-40 mm Hg) stockings in 37 women who underwent sclerotherapy for leg telangiectasia, hyperpigmentation decreased from 40.5% to 28.5%.[52] Edema in the ankle and calf also was reduced.

HYPERTROPHIC SCARS AND KELOIDS

While both hypertrophic scars and keloids are forms of scarring, hypertrophic scars are confined to the borders of the skin injury, whereas keloids extend beyond this boundary. African Americans have the highest incidence of keloids, reported to be as high as 16%.[53]

PDL is effective in remodeling scar tissue and reducing the appearance of scars, although the mechanism of this effect is not yet fully understood. Young scars fare better with PDL. Nouri et al[54] found decreased formation of scar tissue when treating postsurgical scars with the 585-nm PDL on the day of suture removal. Additionally, adjunctive therapy with compression stockings was found to improve the height and erythema of burn scars.[55] The use of intralesional triamcinolone and the antimetabolite 5-fluorouracil immediately after PDL treatment showed more improvement than with PDL alone.[56]

TABLE 94-2 Sclerosing agents associated with hyperpigmentation

Chromated glycerin (glycerin with 6% chromium salt)
Hypertonic saline
Hypertonic saline + dextrose
Polidocanol
Polyiodinated iodine
Sodium tetradecyl sulfate

The 595-nm PDL is a better choice in treating POC.[57] It has been observed that purpuric pulse durations with conservative fluences improve erythematous hypertrophic scars and keloidal scars. For POC, longer pulse durations are recommended, and multiple treatments are necessary.

Fractional laser technology and the long-pulsed Nd:YAG are efficacious in reducing scars and pigmentary alterations. These are discussed in subsequent sections of this chapter.

PSORIASIS

Psoriasis is a chronic inflammatory skin disorder that is characterized by silvery scaly erythematous papules and plaques. It affects males and females equally and is estimated to occur in 2.6% of individuals in the United States.[58]

The PDL and ultraviolet B 308 nm excimer laser are used in the control of psoriasis vulgaris, with the latter being the most commonly used one. Hacker and Rasmussen[59] initially used PDL to treat psoriasis vulgaris in 1992. It is thought that the PDL targets the altered microvasculature in the psoriatic lesion. Generally, the parameters used for psoriasis vulgaris are mild to moderate fluence with a purpuric or short pulse duration on a spot size of 5 to 10 mm. PDL treatments can be used in conjunction with topical, oral, and injectable treatments. There was a 71% improvement, with a remission period of 10.7 months, seen in hand and feet psoriasis after treatment with PDL and either salicylic acid or calcipotriol.[60] There seems to be no difference between short PDL systems (0.450 ms) and long PDL systems (1.5 ms).[28]

For nail psoriasis, Oram et al[61] used the 595-nm PDL in five patients; although subungual hyperkeratosis and onycholysis responded well, nail pitting did not. Treewittayapoom et al[62] treated one hand (40 nails) with the 595-nm PDL on a 7-mm spot at 9 J/cm^2 for 6 ms, with 20 ms of cryogen and a 10-ms delay. The other hand (39 nails) was treated with the 595-nm PDL at 6 J/cm^2 for 0.45 ms, with 20 ms of cryogen and 10-ms delay, again on a 7-mm spot. The lateral and proximal nail folds were treated, including the lunula. Two passes were performed with a 10% overlap on a monthly basis for a total of 6 months. The fingernails on both hands improved from their baseline, independent of pulse duration.[62] Huang et al[63] used tazarotene 0.1% cream on all nails. A 7-mm spot on one hand was treated with the 595-nm PDL at 9 J/cm^2, for a pulse duration of 1.5 ms, with 30 ms of cryogen and a 30-ms delay. The treatment included one pass of pulses with a 10% overlap to the proximal and lateral nail folds. Investigators found a statistically significant decrease in the Nail Psoriasis Severity Index score in the PDL treatment group versus the non-PDL treatment group.[63]

The treatment of psoriasis in POC with the PDL has not shown consistent results. To enhance treatment with the PDL, it is best to remove scale prior to treatment. Conservative fluences and multiple treatments every 2 to 4 weeks are necessary. A more reliable and reproducible laser to help control psoriasis is the excimer laser. The 308-nm excimer laser has been approved by the U.S. FDA to treat mild, moderate, and severe psoriasis.[64] The xenon chloride laser produces a 308-nm monochromatic band of ultraviolet (UV) B radiation. Unlike traditional narrowband UVB (NB-UVB), the excimer laser only targets the affected psoriatic papules and plaques, sparing uninvolved skin. This allows for higher dosimetry to be used on the involved skin. The initial starting dose is dependent on the minimal erythema dose, which is then adjusted on subsequent treatments as per the clinical response. The mechanism of action is through T-cell cytotoxicity.

With their initial left-right comparison study of traditional NB-UVB versus the excimer laser, Bónis et al[64] demonstrated that there was less cumulative dosing, fewer treatments, and shorter treatment duration with the latter. Other studies have confirmed longer periods of remission with fewer treatments when using the excimer laser compared to traditional phototherapy. Therefore, there is a lower cumulative dose of UV light with a lower risk for carcinogenicity. The side effects are localized to the treated site and include crusting, erythema, burning, and superficial erosion.

It appears that the excimer laser works best for truncal psoriasis. However, the excimer laser can be used in the treatment of scalp psoriasis and palmoplantar psoriasis. In addition, the excimer laser can be used in combination with other treatments, or as a monotherapy.

VERRUCA VULGARIS

Warts can prove very difficult to treat, and the PDL and CO_2 laser are the most common laser devices known to be effective. However, the CO_2 ablative laser is not recommended in POC. The PDL is a therapeutic option. In POC, it is recommended for the initial treatment to either keep the pulse duration short while decreasing the fluence or to keep the fluence moderate with a longer pulse duration. Subsequent treatments can be altered depending on the clinical response. During the pulse delivery onto the skin, the patient should not experience any graying, vesiculation, or extreme discomfort. The PDL can be used alone or in combination with other forms of treatment. Clearance rates are reportedly as high as 62.7% after an average of 3.4 treatments.[65,66]

PIGMENTED LESIONS

Q-switched lasers are well suited to treat POC for a variety of pigmented dermatologic disorders. The three major Q-switched laser systems are the Q-switched ruby (694 nm), alexandrite (755 nm), and Nd:YAG (1064 nm) lasers. The Q-switched ruby laser is best suited for patients with phototype IV or lighter, whereas the Q-switched alexandrite laser is best for phototype V or lighter. The Q-switched Nd:YAG laser can be used for all skin types. The frequency-doubled Nd:YAG (532 nm) is another Q-switched laser system but is not used commonly for patients with darker phototypes.

Additionally, the fractional laser is used on all skin types and has gained acceptance for improving a variety of pigmentary disorders. IPL has gained popularity not only in medical offices, but medical spas. Nevertheless, it should be stated that although patients with skin phototype IV can use these treatments with caution, IPL is not suitable for patients with phototypes V or VI.

LENTIGINES

Often appearing as signs of aging and sun damage, lentigines are considered cosmetically undesirable by most patients. For fair-complexioned individuals, the Q-switched ruby laser is efficacious. In addition, the frequency-doubled 532-nm Q-switched Nd:YAG laser is an alternative if it is used at the lowest possible fluence. Usually, only one or two treatment sessions are needed. Postinflammatory hyperpigmentation is common in patients with skin phototype IV and darker; it is more common with the use of lower-wavelength Q-switched lasers. Typically, frostlike whitening is observed as an after effect. It is important that the patient avoids excessive sun exposure when healing from the laser treatment [**Figure 94-5**].

The IPL system has been used to treat lentigines. Kawada et al[67] treated 66 Japanese patients with facial lentigines and ephelides using three to five IPL treatments. Approximately 48% of patients showed more than 50% improvement, with 20% of patients experiencing over 75% clearing of the lentigines. The expected mild crusting with pigmented lesions was experienced by over half of the patients, and one patient was burned. The authors postulated that this was due to the darker lesion and darker skin tone.[67] Wang et al[68] found a preference for the IPL for lentigines and the Q-switched alexandrite laser for ephelides, when comparing the two treatments in a group of Asian women.

NEVI OF ITO AND OTA

These dermomelanocytic lesions are best treated with Q-switched laser systems. Multiple treatments are necessary to achieve a clinically acceptable outcome. On average, treatments range from four to eight sessions and can be performed every 1 to 2 months. It is believed that 2-month intervals between treatments may reduce the overall number of treatments required over time. Watanabe and Takahashi[69] found good results after three or more treatments with the Q-switched ruby laser on 114

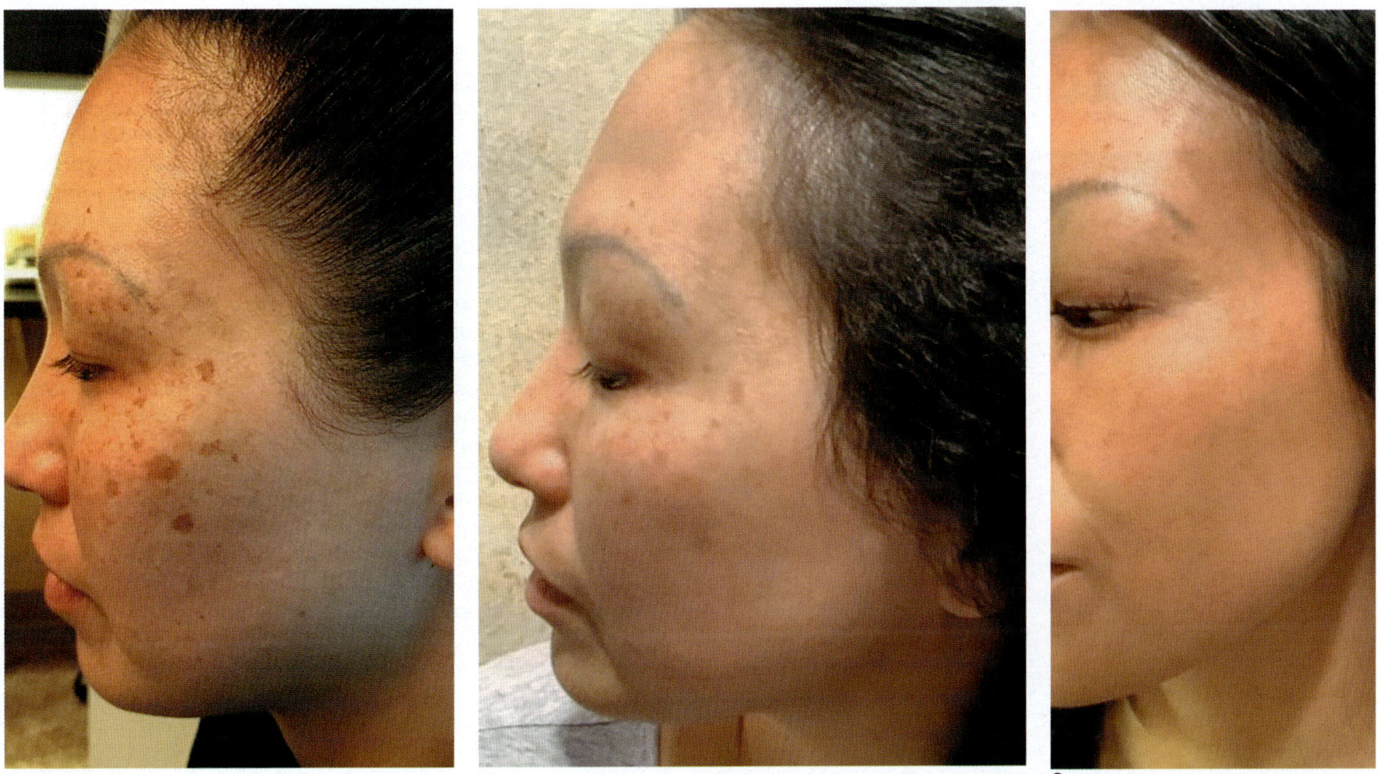

A B C

FIGURE 94-5. Lentigo treatment with IPL in Asian woman FST IV: **(A)** pretreatment, **(B)** 6 weeks posttreatment, **(C)** 6 months posttreatment. (Courtesy of Cheryl Burgess, MD, FAAD.)

Asian patients with a nevus of Ota. As previously stated, the choice of device should be based on the individual patient's phototype, with the Q-switched ruby laser most suitable for type IV, the Q-switched alexandrite laser for types IV and V, and the Q-switched Nd:YAG laser for all types.

In addition, depending on the clinical response and the depth of the dermal melanocytes, laser systems may need to be interchanged. The longer-wavelength lasers are better suited for the more deeply situated dermal melanocytic cells. Chan et al[70] found that the Q-switched Nd:YAG laser was clinically more effective than the Q-switched alexandrite laser after three or more treatments. The most common side effect was transient postinflammatory altered pigmentation [**Figure 94-6**].

MELASMA

Melasma is a common disorder of hyperpigmentation that is most commonly found in women with skin phototypes III through VI who live in areas of intense sunlight exposure. Other factors that are thought to play a role in the pathogenesis of melasma include hormonal factors, phototoxic drug effects, ovarian dysfunction, and underlying thyroid disease. However, recent studies have shown that melasma may also have a vascular component in its pathogenesis,[71] as well as a genetic predisposition.[72]

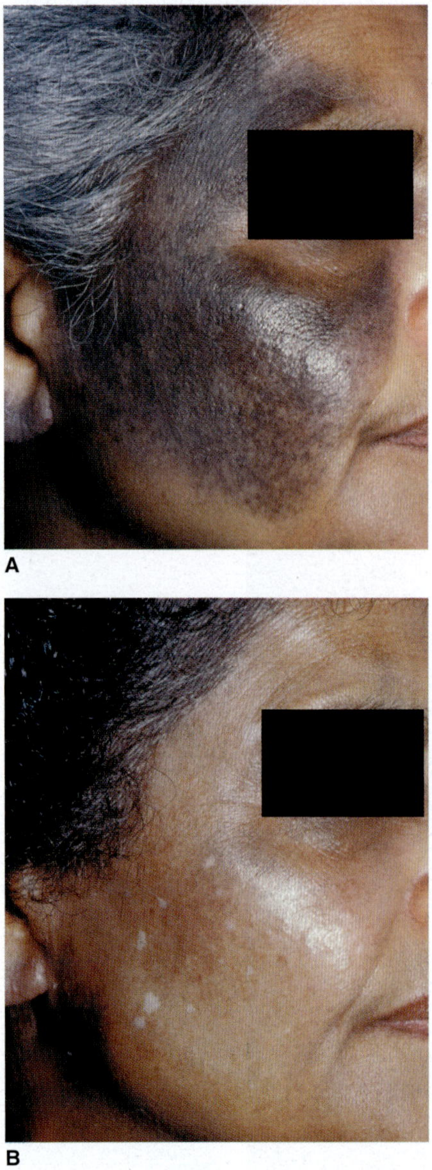

FIGURE 94-6. Nevus of Ota before **(A)** and after **(B)** several Q-switched ruby laser treatments. Note the mild transient hypopigmentation but excellent clearance. (Used with permission from H. Lui, MD.)

Although still not reported in the U.S. literature, there are reports of success abroad and the increased popularity of treating melasma with the Q-switched laser using a technique referred to as "laser toning" or "laser facial." It is widely used in Asian countries for skin rejuvenation and melasma.[73] In Thailand, Wattanakrai et al[74] treated 22 Asian patients in a split-face study. The combination of the Q-switched laser and 2% hydroquinone topical therapy was compared to treatment with the 1064-nm Q-switched Nd:YAG on a 6-mm spot size, with a fluence of 3 to 3.8 J/cm^2 for five sessions at 1-week intervals. The monotherapy laser showed improvement in relative lightness and in the melasma area and severity. However, mottled hypopigmentation developed in three patients. In addition, the improvement in hyperpigmentation proved temporary in four of the 22 patients; these patients developed rebound hyperpigmentation. All patients had recurrence of the melasma.[74] To avoid serious side effects, it is recommended that too many (eg, >6 to 10 sessions) or overly frequent (eg, every week) sessions with the Q-switched Nd:YAG laser be avoided. Hypopigmentation should be investigated after every session, and further treatments should be stopped if evidence of this side effect is found.[75] To summarize, the use of the Q-switched laser in the treatment of melasma needs greater study and analysis to determine its efficacy and safety.

Overall, the IPL system appears to modestly improve melasma in the Asian population when used as an adjunctive therapy in cases of melasma refractory to topical therapy alone.[76] It is not recommended in Fitzpatrick Skin Type IV to VI. In one study, 89 Asian females who were unresponsive to topical therapy and chemical peels were treated with IPL every 3 weeks for a total of four sessions.[77] Melanin and erythema measurements showed improvement. Interestingly, the IPL system has been reported in the literature to exacerbate subclinical melasma when aggressive fluences are used. Negishi et al[78] postulated that patients with latent melasma detected by UV photography should be treated with mild IPL parameters to avoid erythema. It is important to note that IPL-induced erythema should only last a few minutes and not hours. Nonablative lasers are helpful in improving melasma in patients with skin phototypes IV to VI. The nonablative long pulse 1064-nm laser has also been noted, in unpublished reports, to improve melasma as well as postinflammatory pigmentation changes. The exact mechanism of this improvement is unclear. However, there appears to be dermal remodeling with the release of cytokines, which enhances the quality of the skin. Multiple treatments every 3 to 6 weeks are necessary, but the treatment is a safe option for all phototypes with limited risk for patients with tanned skin. Adjunctive treatments with topical retinoids, sunscreens, and hydroquinone, as well as the use of chemical or mechanical peels, are helpful to improve the condition. The laser parameters with the long-pulsed 1064-nm laser should use a 5-mm spot size for 0.3 ms and 5 Hz, with a fluence range of 11 to 14 J/cm^2 depending on skin tone.

Another nonablative laser technique that is helpful in controlling melasma is fractional photothermolysis. After treatment with fractional laser resurfacing, patients with melasma showed a decrease in the number of melanocytes as well as the amount of melanin granules within the keratinocytes on light and electron microscopy.[78] Lee et al[79] studied 25 Asian patients with melasma who received four monthly treatments; early improvement was found overall, but a decline in improvement was noted at 24 weeks, and a loss of efficacy was seen at 6 months. No change in elasticity was noted in the group, and hyperpigmentation was observed in 13% of the patients.[80] When treating melasma in POC, low density and low depth of penetration are recommended. The recommended density for the 1550-nm erbium-doped fractional nonablative laser is 11% to 14% (level 4 or 5) with an energy level of 6 to 8 mJ/cm^2. To avoid a rebound effect, it is best not to perform continued treatments in an effort to achieve 100% clearance. Strict sun avoidance and pre- and posttreatment hydroquinone are imperative [**Figure 94-7**].

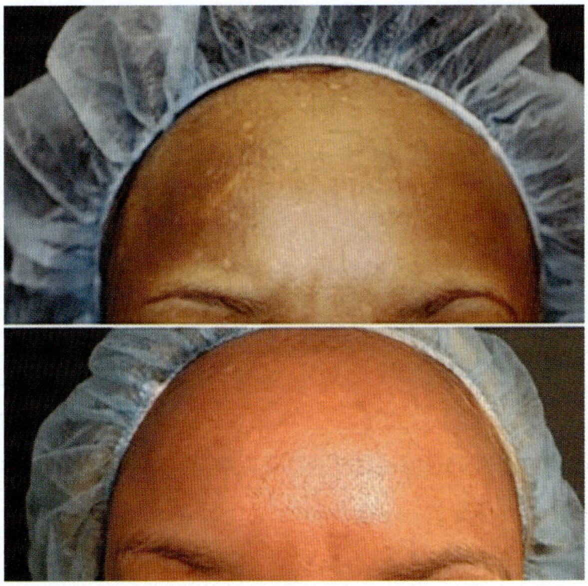

FIGURE 94-7. Sun avoidance and HQ (melasma and ochronosis treated with 650 microsecond 1064 nm Nd:YAG laser). (Courtesy of Cheryl Burgess, MD, FAAD.)

Overall, the complex pathogenesis and the recurrent and refractory nature of melasma make it difficult to treat.

LASER AND LIGHT-BASED COSMETIC TREATMENTS

SKIN REJUVENATION

There is evidence that PDL has thermal effects on perivascular tissue to induce neocollagenesis. This concept is well established in the literature. The earliest studies were done by Zelickson et al[67] in patients with perioral and periorbital wrinkling; 10 patients were considered to have mild rhytides, and 10 patients had moderate rhytides. A 585-nm PDL was used, with a fluence of 3 to 6.5 J/cm^2 and pulse duration of 450 μs on spots of 7 to 10 mm in diameter. Approximately 14 months after the initial treatment, there was a 90% clinical improvement for those with mild rhytides and a 40% improvement for those with moderate rhytides. Histologically, there was increased staining of the elastin and collagen fibrils in the papillary dermis and increased mucin.[81] In a split-face study, Hsu et al[82] found a statistically significant improvement in periorbital rhytides following one to two sessions of the 585-nm PDL. Histologically, there was an increase in type III procollagen, type I collagen mRNA, and chondroitin sulfate.[82] Furthermore, after one PDL treatment to treat facial rhytides, an increase in dermal collagen was observed using ultrasonography.[83] These findings suggest that the PDL promotes new collagen production through the release of certain mediators within the skin. Neocollagenesis is seen after as little as one to two treatments with PDL. However, PDL skin rejuvenation is best used in patients with lighter phototypes.

The IPL system has been used to improve skin texture. In a cohort of 97 Asian patients with skin phototypes IV and V, Negishi et al[84] observed improvement in pigmentation, telangiectasias, and skin texture in 90%, 83%, and 65% of patients, respectively. Cut-off filters for shorter wavelengths were used, and the patients underwent multiple treatments. There were no reports of scarring or changes in pigmentation.[70] However, transient erythema and blistering have been noted with the use of IPL in Chinese patients.[85] Hernandez-Perez and Ibiett[86] treated five Hispanic women using five IPL sessions. Moderate to very good improvements were noted in their patients' skin, including for conditions like mild rhytides and dilated pores. Histologically, there was a statistically significant difference in epidermal thickness, suggesting not only a dermal improvement but also an epidermal textural improvement.[86] However, it is the authors' opinion that the IPL should not under any circumstance be used on patients with skin phototypes V or VI.

Fractional laser therapy is now considered a fundamental device for treatment for skin rejuvenation. The remodeling of collagen within the treatment zones facilitates skin rejuvenation. In addition to long-pulse 1064 nm devices, new technology has led to the use of fractional, nonablative Q-switched 1064-nm Nd:YAG laser systems for treating acne scarring as well as performing skin rejuvenation.

TATTOO REMOVAL

It is estimated that 21% of adults in the United States have at least one tattoo.[87] Tattoos can be exogenous (eg, decorative or amateur) or traumatic (eg, asphalt, gravel). Laser-assisted tattoo removal is considered the gold-standard treatment. With laser-assisted tattoo removal, there is decreased risk of scarring and pigmentary alteration. Professional tattoos generally require more treatments than amateur tattoos. Traumatic tattoos can often be cleared after only a few treatments.

Depending on the absorption spectrum of the ink, a particular wavelength can be chosen. Red inks are best treated with a 532-nm laser, whereas green or teal inks are best treated with a 755-nm laser, and black ink can be treated with 694-, 755-, or 1064-nm lasers. However, the 1064-nm laser has been used most frequently to remove black tattoo ink and is the wavelength of choice when treating pigmented skin.[88]

There are few precautions and contraindications to be aware of concerning laser tattoo removal. The most severe reaction, and hence contraindication, is an allergy to the tattoo ink. In this case, the tattoo should either be surgically removed or vaporized with an ablative laser. Second, cosmetic tattoos that use flesh tones or white inks may undergo immediate pigment darkening with Q-switched lasers. This occurs when the ferric oxide in the ink is reduced to ferrous oxide by the laser. This pigment-darkening reaction cannot always be removed successfully.[89] Therefore, a test spot is highly recommended before treatment begins. Third, although not a contraindication, patients who are known to form keloids should be treated with caution. Although somewhat controversial, it is prudent to wait a minimum of 6 months after using isotretinoin, a medication primarily used for cystic acne, before most laser procedures to reduce the risk of scarring and keloid formation.[90,91] Tattoos resulting from combustible substances, for example, gunpowder or fireworks, can cause ignition when treated with Q-switched lasers.[92] Finally, those who are taking gold salts have been known to develop chrysiasis with the Q-switched lasers.[93]

The majority of tattoos are never completely removed. For the most part, faint to imperceptible remnants of color remain; this signifies an excellent outcome. Shorter-wavelength lasers often cause hypopigmentation, although this is transient in most cases and rarely permanent. Patients who "do-over" or "cover-up" their original tattoo with a second one are at risk for further side effects. Negative prognostic variables include smoking, older tattoos, short treatment intervals, brightly colored tattoos, tattoos with white ink, and tattoos located on the legs and feet; these were noted by Bencini et al[94] in their prospective study of 397 patients.

New on the market is the ultra-short Q-switched laser system. This technology provides a faster and more precise deposit of light energy to the target, causing the target to heat and expand more rapidly, resulting in the more precise and efficient dissolution of the ink or pigment. This means that there is less disruption of the surrounding tissue. The benefits of using ultra-short Q-switched devices (measured in ps) include lower fluences, faster clearance of the tattoo or pigment target, and fewer side effects.[95-97] In particular, the 1064-nm ultra-short Q-switched laser shows promise in pigmented skin, although studies are pending.

HAIR REMOVAL

Laser-assisted hair removal is used to ensure the permanent reduction of hair. Multiple treatments are necessary. Thick black hairs show the best response to treatment, with gray, blonde, white, red, and light brown hairs showing either no or little response to laser-assisted hair removal. Side effects are rare; one uncommon side effect is the aberrant induction of hair growth, which mostly occurs in persons of Mediterranean descent. Anecdotally, it has been observed that those with fine to intermediate hairs located in the temple area or the lateral forehead are at greater risk. The increased hair growth is often difficult to treat and requires multiple treatments, sometimes with alternative laser-assisted hair removal devices

ERBIUM:YTTRIUM-ALUMINUM-GARNET (ER:YAG) LASER

Ablative laser treatments, which include carbon dioxide (CO_2) and Er:YAG lasers, are highly effective in skin resurfacing. However, CO_2 lasers are not typically used in POC as they may cause hyperpigmentation, hypopigmentation, and burns. The short-pulsed Er:YAG is an ablative laser that can be used in POC for skin resurfacing. This laser emits a wavelength of 2900 nm, ablating approximately 2 to 5 μm per pass with equally narrow zones of thermal necrosis.[98,99] Compared to its CO_2 counterpart, the Er:YAG laser is absorbed 12 to 18 time more efficiently by the superficial dermis. These mechanisms result in decreased rates of hyperpigmentation and posttreatment erythema, and the shorter duration of healing after treatment compared to CO_2 lasers.[98,99] The Er:YAG laser has shown efficacy in the treatment of mild-moderate rhytids, photodamage, and atrophic scars through implementing multiple passes and sessions and high fluences.[99-103] One study of 50 Asian patients examined the efficacy of the Er:YAG laser in the treatment of rhytids, scars, pigmentary alteration, and a variety of cutaneous growths. All of the subjects had Fitzpatrick skin phototypes (FST) III to V. The Er:YAG laser used had a wavelength of 2940 nm, pulse duration of 250 microseconds, output energy of 1 Joule per pulse, and a spot size of 2 to 5 mm with a repetition rate of 1 to 10 Hz. The fluences used ranged between 5 and 15 J/cm^2. Objective improvement of rhinophyma (90%), chicken pox scars (90%), wrinkles (80%), photoaged skin (70%), melasma (60%), and acne scars (50-60%) was reported. Postinflammatory hyperpigmentation (PIH) occurred in 30% of the subjects, which resolved after an average of 1 to 2 months. Transient hypopigmentation was observed in 2% of the patients, resolving at 2 months. Scarring was not observed in any of the treated subjects. This group concluded that the Er:YAG laser is a safe and effective treatment for wrinkles, photoaged skin, scarring, and various skin lesions in Asian skin.[104] Chathra et al conducted a retrospective study of 80 patients with FTS IV and V to determine efficacy and safety of the variable squared pulse Er:YAG laser for the treatment of acne scars. Each patient underwent a minimum of four treatment sessions. Statistically significant improvement of acne scars was noted using the Qualitative Global Acne Scarring System. Adverse events were limited but included prolonged erythema in two patients, prolonged crusting in one patient and proinflammatory hyperpigmentation in another patient.[105] Studies suggest the safety and efficacy of Er:YAG laser use in POC for skin resurfacing.

1064 NM NEODYMIUM-DOPED YTTRIUM ALUMINUM GARNET (ND:YAG) LASER

Nonablative lasers have a better safety profile than ablative lasers. The 1064 nm Nd:YAG is a 650 microsecond laser that delivers energy in a collimated beam. This laser penetrates deeper and delivers higher energy than q-switched lasers. The combination of short pulse and high energy allows for efficacy, comfort, and a greater margin of safety, therefore decreasing the risks of burns or pigmentation changes.[106] The 1064 nm Nd:YAG laser has the capability to remove the dermal and epidermal melanosis in patients of all skin types.[107] A pilot study of nine patients demonstrated a low risk of adverse events with the use of 1064 nm Nd:YAG in FST V to VI treated for acne scarring. Acne scarring improved in all the subjects.[108] Another study looked retrospectively at 22 patients with FST III to VI that were treated with the 1064 nm Nd:YAG for atrophic scarring. An average of six treatments was performed on each patient approximately 3 weeks apart. Fluence of 14 to 16 J/cm^2 was used with a pulse duration of 300 to 500 microseconds and repetition rate of 5 to 7 Hz. Statistically significant improvement of scarring, texture, and pigment was observed, and pigment complications were minimal.[109] Greywal et al treated 10 FST II to V patients with melasma with the 1064 nm Nd:YAG laser. This group reported the lightening of pigmentation as early as 3 weeks post treatment. All 10 subjects required several treatments to achieve adequate resolution of their melasma. Advantages of this laser for the treatment of melasma included no pain or down-time, lower risk of rebound, and the safety in use of all skin types.[110] Overall, in POC, the successful treatment of melasma, acne, PIH, pseudofolliculitis barbae, hair removal, acne keloidalis nuchae, and aging in POC.[93] The combination of the 1064-nm Nd:YAG with chemical peel and topical medications may help clinicians in skin resurfacing.[111]

1550 NM ERBIUM-DOPED FRACTIONAL LASER

The 1550-nm erbium-doped fractional laser may be used in POC for skin resurfacing at lower treatment densities (microthermal zones (MTZ cm^{-2}), as higher treatment densities were associated with a higher frequency of PIH among Chinese patients. [112,113] Alexis provides recommendations for treatment when using this laser in POC depending on the skin condition, stating 40 to 70 mJ and 200 to 392 MTZ cm^{-2}, and 15 mJ and 125 MTZ per pass with eight passes for melasma. In addition, there may be a role of hydroquinone 4% beginning 2 to 4 weeks prior to the first laser treatment for melasma and continued for 4 weeks after each treatment. Finally, allowing time for skin cooling lowers the risk PIH in higher FST.[113,114] The most common complications with the use of the 1550-nm erbium-doped fractional laser in all skin types are acneiform eruptions (1.87%), outbreaks of herpes simplex virus (1.77%), and erosions (1.35%). Similar rates of complications are seen in POC, except PIH, which is seen more in POC with this laser use.[115,116]

1927 NM THULIUM LASER

A prospective, multi-center study of FST I-IV enrolled 40 subjects to investigate the safety and efficacy of the fractionated 1927 nonablative thulium laser for photo-induced pigmentation. An energy level of 10 mJ was used with a coverage of 40% and four to six passes. Results showed that two treatments with this laser type produce moderate to marked improvement in overall appearance of pigmentation. The response to treatment was maintained at 1 and 3 months. Treatment was well tolerated, and no serious adverse events related to treatment were observed or reported.[117] In nine patients with FST IV, PIH was treated using the 1927-nm thulium laser followed by topical hydroquinone 4% cream for 6 weeks. This pilot interventional study reported 37.5% of patients with excellent response, 50% of patients with satisfactory response, and 12.5% of patients with nonsatisfactory response. None of the subjects in this study had pigmentation changes after treatment.[118] More studies are needed on this laser in FST IV to VI.

PEARLS FOR LASER USE IN PEOPLE OF COLOR

Clinicians should have a thorough discussion with POC to determine patient expectations and engage in shared decision-making regarding laser treatment. Risks and side effects associated with skin resurfacing must be reviewed. Ablative CO_2 and intense pulsed light source lasers are not used in skin resurfacing for POC as they can lead to PIH, hypopigmentation, and burns. Cooling devices can help decrease unwanted side effects when using lasers in POC. A test patch may be of utility in observing how a patient's skin reacts to the desired treatment. Prompt follow up after treatment allows for early intervention if adverse events occur. Appropriate laser selection and application allows for the safe, effective use of lasers in POC patients for skin resurfacing.

INTRODUCTION TO SKIN RESURFACING IN PEOPLE OF COLOR

Chemical and mechanical skin resurfacing were developed to improve the overall appearance and well-being of skin. The first chemical peels were utilized by Egyptians. They used sour milk baths (lactic acid), various chemicals (eg, alabaster and salt), and sandpaper in order to attain a smoother skin surface.[119] In 1882, a German dermatologist named P.G. Unna pronounced the properties of salicylic acid, resorcinol, phenol, and trichloroacetic acid (TCA) and used these chemicals as peeling agents.[120] In 1976, Resnik et al explained the functionality of TCA peels in various skin conditions.[121] In the late 1980s, early 1990s, α-hydroxy acids (AHAs) became available for superficial peeling agents. For nearly 20 years, microdermabrasion has become a key player in the field of noninvasive antiaging medicine. Over the last several decades, the science behind resurfacing procedures has expanded. The expansion and newer techniques has the public's increasing demand for cosmetic surgery and skin rejuvenation. Today, chemical peeling and microdermabrasion are among the most common procedures performed in dermatologic offices and often require modifications and special considerations when performed on darker skin tones.

CHEMICAL EXFOLIATION

Chemical resurfacing has a long and well-documented history.[119] Since the late 1800s, physicians have been investigating various procedures and techniques involving both chemical and mechanical skin resurfacing. Chemical exfoliation procedures involve the application of a chemical agent to the skin, which then produces a controlled, partial-thickness injury. The controlled partial-thickness injury will promote the growth of new skin with improved surface characteristics. The wound-healing response is dependent on the depth of injury. The process involves (1) removal of actinic keratoses (AK) and lentigines, (2) epidermal regeneration by epithelial migration from adnexal structures, (3) decrease in solar elastosis, and (4) replacement of new dermal connective tissue.[122]

SUPERFICIAL EXFOLIATION PEELING

There are three types of exfoliation: superficial, medium-depth, and deep [**Table 94-3**]. In this section, we will focus on superficial peels with a target depth penetration to the superficial papillary dermis (0.06 mm). Superficial exfoliation peels are divided into two subgroups: very light and light. Very light superficial exfoliation peels include low-potency concentrations (20-60%) of glycolic acid, α-hydroxy acids, 10% to 20% TCA, tretinoin, Jessner solution, and salicylic acid. Light superficial exfoliation peels such as 70% glycolic acid, 25% to 30% TCA, and dry ice slush target depth penetration includes the entire epidermis extending down to the basal cell layer or upper papillary dermis, stimulating the regeneration of a new epithelium.[132]

INDICATIONS

Superficial exfoliation peeling is indicated for mild rhytids, photoaging, actinic and seborrheic keratoses, acne, dyspigmentation in the form of melasma and postinflammatory hyperpigmentation (PIH), and to improve the overall texture of the skin. There are many different exfoliation agents classified under superficial peels. In this section, we will discuss glycolic acid (20-70%), salicylic acid, Jessner solution, solid CO_2 and TCA (10-35%).

CONTRAINDICATIONS

There are several contraindications to superficial, medium-depth, and deep chemical peeling. These contraindications are listed in **Table 94-4**.

PATIENT SELECTION

There are several factors that must be considered to determine if the patient is a suitable candidate for skin resurfacing. A thorough history and physical examination needs to be taken during the initial evaluation. The patient's skin type should be evaluated using Fitzpatrick's classification measuring pigmentary responsiveness of the skin to ultraviolet (UV) light. Ethnic FST skin types IV to VI can be peeled, but the risk of unwanted pigmentary change in the form of hypopigmentation and hyperpigmentation is greater when compared to skin types I to III.[132] Skin types IV to VI are recommended to avoid deep peels in order to reduce the risk for potential damaging side effects like ochronosis.[133]

TABLE 94-3 Types of chemical peeling agents

Type of agent	Key facts

Glycolic acid	• Most readily available peeling agent
	• Commonly used for melasma, PIH, photodamage, and acne
	• How it works:
	  • Thins the stratum corneum, diminishes intercellular bonding, promotes epidermolysis, disperses basal layer melanin, and increases collagen synthesis within the dermis.[123,124]
	• Skin test should always occur prior to using on skin of color
	• Concentration levels: 30-70%
	• 70% gel formulation delivers a high concentration of GA to the skin with a reduced risk of scarring[125]
	• Important considerations:
	  • Asian and darker skin shows benefits with GA peels, especially skin that is sensitive or dry[126,127]

Lactic acid	• Inexpensive • Safe and effective for melasma and acne scarring in darker skin
Phytic acid	• Does not require neutralization • Excessive peeling and burning is avoided • Applied and left on the face overnight once a week • Five to six sessions typically yield results • Used for melasma
Pyruvic acid	• Stimulates the formation of new collagen and elastin fibers[13] • Side effect of intense burning has limited use • No studies regarding efficacy in ethnic skin
Salicylic acid	• Effective keratolytic agent • Improves penetration of other peeling agents when use in 3-5% concentrations • Anti-inflammatory properties • Useful for acne, melasma, and PIH
Lipohydroxy Acid	• Modifies the stratum corneum, making it thinner, flexible, and resistant to wrinkling and cracking[128] • Greater keratolytic effect than the traditional SA[128,129] • Similar PH to normal skin, making it safe for darker skin • Effective for treatment of acne
Salicylic-mandelic acid peel	• No studies regarding efficacy in ethnic skin • Slow and uniform quick penetration • Ideal for sensitive skin, beneficial for PIH[130]
Trichloroacetic acid	• Used alone or in combination with GA or SA • Useful for acne scarring in ethnic skin • Typically used in 10-30% solutions; however, the risks of PIH and scarring increase with the use of higher concentrations in skin of color
Jessner's solution	• Well tolerated in Fitzpatrick skin types IV to VI • Contains the phenolic skin-lightening agent resorcinol (can cause depigmentation if not used correctly) • A combination of Jessner's solution followed by a 35% concentration of TCA have been found to be safe and effective in treating acne scars in patients with dark skin.[131]

TABLE 94-4 Contraindications

Contraindications of chemical peeling
• Active herpes simplex infection, or verrucae
• Atopic dermatitis
• Wounded, sunburned, or excessively sensitive skin
• Inflammatory rosacea
• Isotretinoin use within a year
• Salicylate allergy (for SA peels)
• Pregnancy or active breast-feeding

ADVERSE EFFECTS

Superficial peels are generally well tolerated in all skin types. The majority of patients will experience mild stinging and burning during the application of the chemical agent, which is an expected side effect and is not considered a procedural complication. Pigmentary changes in the form of both hypopigmentation and hyperpigmentation are possible complications. The risk of hyperpigmentation is greater in patients with darker skin types. Typically, hypopigmentation resolves within months after the peel. Hyperpigmentation can be treated effectively with hydroquinone regimens.[132] Prolonged erythema, milia, pustulocystic acne, reactivation of latent herpes simplex infection, and superficial bacterial infection are all potential complications.[133] Prolonged erythema may be treated with a low-dose topical steroid such as hydrocortisone or with desonide 0.05% lotion twice daily for 2 to 3 days. Milia or acne that occurs post peel may be irritated by thick ointments applied to the treated area. The risk of hypertrophic scarring is less than 1% with superficial peels.[134]

OUTCOME

Patients who complete a series of treatments with superficial exfoliation peels experience regeneration of new skin and improvement in their overall complexion, texture, and appearance.[132] Superficial exfoliation peels are beneficial to patients because there are minimal risks as well as no downtime post procedure. Of note, superficial peels, especially glycolic acid and salicylic acid, are well tolerated in patients with darker complexions with minimal side effects since these peels only affect the epidermis and do not penetrate into the dermis.[132]

ETHNIC SKIN CONSIDERATIONS

When considering applying chemical peels in ethnic skin, it is critical to identify the patient's Fitzpatrick skin type, as well as determine the patient's ethnicity prior to selecting the peeling agent. Indications for chemical peeling in darker skin include acne vulgaris, PIH, melasma, scarring, photodamage, and pseudofolliculitis barbae. However, the primary indication for chemical peeling in skin types III to VI is for pigmentation dyschromias.[132]

Dermatologists treating richly pigmented patients should consider the different properties and the effects of superficial chemical peeling agents in order to choose the most appropriate agent to address the patient's dermatological needs. For example, glycolic acid and salicylic acid peels are excellent tools to treat acne in POC. Additionally, salicylic acid in ethanol solutions is a great peeling agent for richly pigmented patients with melasma and PIH. Glycolic acid is a less favorable agent compared to salicylic acid to treat melasma and PIH because of its potential to induce PIH in skin types V and VI. At low concentrations of 10% to 25%, Trichloroacetic acid efficiently treats acne scarring in POC. When Trichloroacetic acid is used in combination with 70% glycolic gel, it also rejuvenates uneven blotchy facial pigmentation. Jessner solution may create depigmentation in patients with skin types V and VI but may be a practical treatment in spot-peeling for PIH in ethnic skin. In addition, TCA 25% and salicylic acid are effective tools for spot-peeling for PIH.[132]

Asian and Asian Americans seeking treatment for melasma respond well to serial glycolic peels maintained at the same concentration. Africans and darker African Americans (skin types V and VI) have better results with salicylic acid peels compared to glycolic acid peels. Glycolic acid peels have a higher risk for PIH, thus salicylic acid peels are used instead.[132] Serial glycolic acid peels and salicylic acid peels have been successful in improving the skin texture in patients with pseudofolliculitis barbae, which has a higher prevalence in African Americans.[135]

When choosing a superficial agent in ethnic/dark skin, it is critical to start a prepeel regimen that includes a morning regimen of sunscreen with UVA/UVB SPF 30 and an evening regimen of moisturizer containing α-hydroxy acid, a combination of retinoid, hydroquinone, kojic acid, or azelaic acid and possibly at low-potency steroid. The duration of this pre- and postpeel regimen is comparative in all skin types. [132]

GLYCOLIC ACID PEELS

Glycolic acid is an AHA. It belongs to a class of naturally occurring compounds derived from food sources such as sugar cane.[133] Glycolic acid peels range in concentration from 20% to 70% glycolic acid. This particular peel is generally performed every 3 to 4 weeks for a total of four to six treatments per month.[132] Glycolic acid peels are indicated in the treatment of melasma, postinflammatory hyperpigmentation, mild photoaging (Glogau I and II), and acne. Glycolic acid peels are generally well tolerated by all skin types I to VI. Several studies have shown glycolic acid peels with a concentration up to 70% is well tolerated with minimal adverse effects. They have shown to improve melasma and postinflammatory hyperpigmentation.[137,138] Glycolic acid peels may be used as monotherapy, combined with a topical preprocedure rejuvenation regimen consisting of tretinoin and hydroquinone, or even combined with 5-fluorouracil (5-FU) for the treatment of actinic keratosis with an improved overall cosmesis.[139]

A previous study by Moy et al revealed that glycolic acid has a stimulatory effect on collagen production in fibroblasts. This proposed mechanism may account for the decrease in fine wrinkling, leading to improvement of fine rhytids.[140]

SALICYLIC ACID PEELS

Salicylic acid (SA) is a β-hydroxy acid that is naturally found in the bark of the willow tree. Salicylic acid peels range in concentration from 20% to 30%, and are performed a total of three to five times every 3 to 4 weeks. Salicylic acid peels are indicated in the treatment of acne vulgaris, melasma, postinflammatory hyperpigmentation, rough/oily skin with enlarged pores, and mild to moderate photodamaged skin.[132] Salicylic acid peels are safe and efficacious in skin types I to VI.[141] Salicylic acid is a lipophilic agent that induces desquamation of the upper lipophilic layers of the stratum corneum.[141] Because it is a lipid-soluble comedolytic, salicylic acid acts by decreasing corneocyte cohesion at the follicular opening and assists in comedone plug extrusion.[123] In order to expedite the clearing of hyperpigmented lesions and significantly decrease the occurrence of post peel hyperpigmentation seen more commonly in skin types V and VI, the salicylic acid peel can be combined with hydroquinone 4%.[141]

The majority of patients tolerate this procedure without side effects. Some side effects seen are transient dryness and hyperpigmentation. The side effects typically resolve within 1 to 2 weeks. Additional side effects include temporary superficial crusting and edema, which usually clear in a week. This agent causes significantly more desquamation than glycolic acid peels.[142]

JESSNER PEEL

Jessner peel is a solution that combines resorcinol (14 g), salicylic acid (14 g), 85% lactic acid (14 g), and 95% ethanol (q.s.a.d. 100 mL).[132] Jessner peels are indicated in the treatment of inflammatory and comedonal acne, melasma, and hyperkeratotic skin disorders.

Jessner solution has intense keratolytic activity, initially causing loss of corneocyte cohesion within the stratum corneum and subsequently creating intercellular and intracellular edema within the upper epidermis if application is continued.[143]

TRICHLOROACETIC ACID 10% TO 30%

TCA produces superficial peeling when used in strengths from 10% to 30%.[144] At these strengths, TCA is indicated for the treatment of fine rhytids, actinic damage, mild epidermal dyschromia, reduction of superficial keratoses, scars, and comedone formation.[132] TCA precipitates epidermal proteins and induces necrosis and exfoliation of normal and actinically damaged cells. Partial epidermal exfoliation occurs with 20% TCA; therefore, a series of peels may be necessary in order to optimize the rejuvenating effects of papillary dermal remodeling.[145] Complete reepithelialization takes place within 7 to 10 days. Depending on the desired appearance, the patient may undergo a second treatment within a week or two.[146] Superficial TCA peels are well tolerated by most patients and thus do not require sedation.[132]

SOLID CARBON DIOXIDE

Solid CO_2, (dry ice)/solid GO, slush is the final superficial peel discussed in this section. Solid CO_2 is not a true chemical peeling agent but a physical modality for peeling. It is applied by a small hand towel dipped in a solution of approximately 3:1 acetone and alcohol.[134] CO_2 ice causes mechanical injury to the epidermis, which results in microvesiculation and disruption of the stratum corneum barrier. It may be used alone (superficial peel) or to amplify TCA as a medium-depth peel.[127]

MEDIUM-DEPTH CHEMICAL PEELING

Medium-depth peels are chemical peeling agents used to exert a controlled injury extending to the papillary dermis.[148] The prototypical medium-depth peeling agent, composed of 50% TCA, is no longer the gold standard because of its high risk of complications. Scarring and postpeel dyschromias are possible consequences of higher concentrations of TCA. The higher levels of concentration may lead to an unpredictable pattern of absorption and resultant "hot spots." Many clinicians have replaced the higher-level TCA peels for combination peels using 35% TCA with Jessner solution, 70% glycolic acid, or solid CO_2.[136] Pyruvic acid is a new addition to the medium-depth chemical peel armamentarium showing many of the same clinical benefits as the traditional medium-depth peeling agents.[146] The combination peels can achieve the same depth of penetration as the solitary 50% TCA but without the associated risks.[132]

SCIENTIFIC BACKGROUND

TCA is widely accepted as the gold standard of chemical peeling agents. It is appealing because of its stabilizing properties that help establish a shelf life greater than 6 months. It is also not light sensitive and requires no refrigeration. By priming the skin with 70% glycolic acid, Jessner solution, or solid CO_2, the cosmetic surgeon can allow for penetration of a lower and safer concentration of TCA (35%) that is deeper and more evenly distributed. The evenly distributed controlled injury leads to uniform peeling with fewer complications. Glycolic acid at a concentration of 70% penetrates the epidermal barrier by breaking up the individual keratinocytes.[132] Jessner solution destroys the epidermis in a manner similar to that of 70% glycolic acid; however, solid CO_2 with acetone creates epidermal necrosis. Both Jessner and CO_2 enhance the penetration of the less potent 35% TCA.[132]

Following the chemical peel, the process of wound healing is responsible for the smoothening and tightening outcome of the skin. In the following 2 weeks, reepithelization is completed, as revealed by the appearance of an erythematous fresh epidermal layer. Within the next 3 to 4 months, collagen remodeling will take place.[148] Less popular medium-depth peels include pyruvic acid, a potent peeling agent at concentrations of 40% to 70%.[149] Pyruvic acid converts to lactic acid, a small molecule capable of penetrating down to the upper papillary dermis.[150] Its effects result in increased production of collagen, elastin, and glycoproteins.[151]

INDICATIONS

Medium-depth chemical peels are best suited for the treatment of superficial epidermal lesions, lentigines, actinic keratosis, pigmentary dyschromias, textural irregularities due to acne scarring, and mild to moderate rhytids associated with photoaging.[152] This level chemical peel is also used in combination with laser resurfacing or deep chemical peels, to blend the lines of demarcation between treated and untreated skin. Chun et al utilized the focal application of TCA at concentrations of 10% to 65% to safely remove or improve benign pigmented lesions, including seborrheic keratoses, lentigines, freckles, and melasma in richly pigmented patients.[153]

PATIENT SELECTION

Patients with mild to moderate facial rhytids and minimal pigmentary disturbances achieve the best outcomes with medium-depth peels.[149] Mild atrophic acne scarring and diffuse AK have shown consistent improvement with peels of this depth.[132] Medium-depth peels are traditionally avoided in richly pigmented patients but are now being safely and successfully performed in these patients with some pre- and post-treatment precautions. Although there has been successful application to isolated lesions in richly pigmented skin types, full-face medium-depth chemical peels are best avoided in very dark skin types (Fitzpatrick VI) because of the possibility of postpeel hyper- or hypopigmentation.

ADVERSE EFFECTS

Side effects of medium-depth peel are fewer with the development of the combination peel but are not negligible. The most common complication following a TCA peel is hyperpigmentation, and the most common factor responsible is early sun exposure.[149] Patients are routinely instructed to avoid sun exposure in the weeks leading up to and following a medium-depth peel.[132] A sunscreen with a UVA/UVB block is to be worn regularly, and some doctors even recommend the cessation of oral contraceptives, 2 months prior and after the peeling because their use may stimulate pigmentary changes.[133,149] The pretreatment and posttreatment precautions include retinoic acid and hydroquinone, which can reduce the risk of postoperative hyperpigmentation. Patients with darker skin types and or those being treated for pigment problems are at even greater risks of postoperative hyperpigmentation. If hyperpigmentation is noted, it can be managed with retinoic acid, hydroquinone products, mid-potency topical steroids, and follow-up peels (approximately 3-6 months later) until a lightening effect is achieved.[133,149] Although previously thought only to be a complication of deep peels, hypopigmentation has been reported following application with 20% TCA and 35% TCA chemical peels.[133] In richly pigmented patients, this potentially permanent side effect can be devastating.[132]

Other complications reported after medium-depth chemical peels include milia, acne flares, and cyst formation, hypertrophic scars,[154] and keratoacanthomas[155] following chemical peeling.

OUTCOME

In most cases of actinic damage, the medium-depth peel has been effective, as evidenced by a reduction of AK and softening of fine lines and wrinkles. Ise et al compared two medium-depth combination peels, 70% glycolic acid/35% TCA versus Jessner solution/35% TCA, with respect to clinical and histological effects on facial skin.[156] Clinically, both peeling agent combinations were effective at treating solar lentigines and AK, yet the glycolic acid/TCA combination revealed an advantage in eliminating AK. Neither peel was significantly effective at treating fine wrinkles. Recovery time for both agents was comparable at 7 to 10 days, but the Jessner/TCA combination created more postoperative erythema.

Pigmentary dyschromias, including postinflammatory hyperpigmentation, and melasma have both been successfully treated with medium-depth peels. The epidermal component of these pigmentary aberrations is more responsive to medium-depth chemical peels compared to the dermal component. In addition to removing the epidermis, medium-depth peels also affect the melanocytes in the pilar apparatus during the process of reepithelization.[152] This mechanism, adjunct with pre/post-treatment regimens with retinoic acid and hydroquinone, allows for a reduction in the risk of rebound hyperpigmentation, an unwanted pigmentary problem most often seen in POC.[132] By focally applying TCA at concentrations ranging from 10% to 65%, Chun et al safely treated a host of benign pigmented lesions in 106 richly pigmented patients. The results revealed that 42 of 49 (86%) patients with solar lentigines, 19 or 23 (83%) patients with seborrheic keratosis, 8 of 14 (58%) patients with freckles, and 11 of 20 (55%) patient with melasma experienced a good clinical response without significant complications.[153]

ETHNIC SKIN CONSIDERATIONS

The chemical percentage of medium-depth peeling agents, combinations, and even the vehicle selected may vary based on skin tone. Roberts describes a technique of using glycolic acid 70% gel in place of solution before applying TCA 25% solution for the treatment of acne scars in darker skin.[132] Although the glycolic acid enhances the effect of the TCA, the gel vehicle limits the harshness of this second product, allowing for more control of the peeling process.[125] This author also emphasized that the TCA should not be allowed to frost completely but, rather, be neutralized with 10% sodium bicarbonate after 2 to 4 min, depending on the type of lesion being treated. For areas of postinflammatory hyperpigmentation, Roberts recommended "spot peel" using TCA 25% salicylic acid or Jessner solution on discrete areas in combination with or without full-face peeling.[132] Treating dermal pigment in POC should be avoided because of the inherent risk of permanent depigmentation and hypertrophic scarring. Strict control of peel depth is critical to achieving a successful outcome in skin types IV to VI. Treatment of pigmentary and scarring disorders via medium-depth peeling agents can lead to outcomes worse than the original chief complaint.[132]

DEEP EXFOLIATION PEELING

SCIENTIFIC BACKGROUND

Deep exfoliation peels create a controlled injury through the papillary dermis into the upper reticular dermis and may even extend into the mid-reticular dermis, approximately 0.6 mm. Deep peeling agents include phenol-containing preparation, or TCA in concentrations above 50%. Due to the risks associated with 50% TCA, such as scarring, TCA at these concentrations is not recommended for deep exfoliation peeling.[132] Instead, solutions containing phenol are substituted for deep exfoliation peels.[157]

INDICATIONS

Deep peels involve the use of chemexfoliants that penetrate to the mid-reticular dermis.[158]

Indications for the use of deep peeling agents include deep rhytids secondary to photoaging, treatment of severe or extensive AK, and solar lentigines.[132]

PATIENT SELECTION

There are many relative contraindications to deep chemical peels, which depend on the patient's Fitzpatrick skin type and medical history. Therefore, patient selection is critical in deep chemical peeling. Patients with Fitzpatrick skin type IV to VI are not candidates for deep chemical peels secondary to the increased risk of pigmentary changes, especially hypopigmentation and scarring.[133]

ADVERSE EFFECTS

The most notable side effects include hypertrophic scarring, textural changes, and pigmentary disturbances.[132] Permanent pigmentary changes may occur as a complication of phenol peels. Hypopigmentation occurs when susceptible Fitzpatrick skin types III to VI undergo deep peeling and thus are advised against this treatment. Deep phenol peels may lead to irreversible hypopigmentation, hyperpigmentation, scarring, or keloid formation, especially in richly pigmented patients with Fitzpatrick skin types IV to VI.[159] Temporary hypopigmentation is common and expected; the final skin color cannot be determined until all the postpeel erythema has resolved. Once the erythema resolves, if the hypopigmentation is still present, the pigmentary change is irreversible. Hyperpigmentation is a common postoperative side effect in richly pigmented patients but usually resolves spontaneously with time, topical tretinoin, and hydroquinone therapy.[160]

TECHNIQUES AND PATIENT INSTRUCTIONS FOR CHEMICAL EXFOLIATION

Prior to treating a patient with a chemical peel, a careful history should be obtained and a thorough skin examination performed. Patients should avoid the following procedures 1 week prior to chemical peeling: electrolysis, waxing, use of depilatory creams, and laser hair removal. Two to 5 days prior to the procedure, patients should discontinue use of topical retinoids and products that contain retinol, AHA, β-hydroxy acid, or benzoyl peroxide. Prophylactic antiviral therapy should be given to patients with a history of herpes simplex infection. Prior to applying chemical peeling agents to the skin, all makeup should be removed, the eyes should be protected with moistened cotton pads or eye shields, and petrolatum should be applied to sensitive areas, such as the corners of the nose and lips. The peel is applied with sponges or brushes for approximately 3 to 5 minutes, neutralized when appropriate, and then rinsed off. For the treatment of pigmentary disorders, pre- and posttreatment hyperpigmentation therapy is often essential and consists of treating the affected areas for 1 month prior to and after peeling with a combination skin-lightening agent containing hydroquinone, azelaic acid, or other cosmeceuticals with skin-lightening properties.[161] For specific technique on certain agents, please see **Table 94-5**.

Following the peel, patients are instructed to wash the skin with gentle cleansers, apply emollients twice daily, and use daily sun protection (SPF > 30). When treating disorders of pigmentation, an effective interval between superficial peels is 3 to 6 weeks. Following the last peel of the series, the patient is maintained on daily ultraviolet (UV) protection sunscreen and often receives nightly application of a hydroquinone-based skin-lightening agent for a 4- to 8-week period. Chronic melanocyte suppression can be accomplished by rotating the skin-lightening agents to avoid any of the adverse side effects of any one agent.[162]

TABLE 94-5 Technique for specific agents

Type of agent	Technique
Glycolic acid	• For skin of color, a partially buffered solution of 30-50% may be used.[6] • Contacts the skin for 2-4 minutes and then is rinsed off with cool water. • Comedone extractor after peeling is suggested for maximum benefit and results.
Salicylic acid	• A 20-30% solution is applied to the skin with a sponge applicator and to individual papules and pustules with a cotton-tipped swab. • Typically, 4-5 minutes of a tingling or burning sensation occur before a white frost appears, signaling the end of the peel.

Trichloroacetic acid	• After application, a white frost usually marks the end point of the peel.
	• In skin types V to VI, proceed with caution regarding the frost as it is associated with higher risks of adverse effects.
	• A combination of 70% GA gel and 25% TCA is a viable option as the gel formulation limits the harshness of TCA.
	  • First, GA gel is applied generously; then TCA is applied over it.
	  • The peel remains on the face for 2-4 minutes before removal.
	  • The procedure is usually repeated in 4-6 weeks, and if tolerated well, the peel may be left on 1 or 2 minutes longer with subsequent treatments.

Topical retinoids, azelaic acid, or other cosmeceutical skin-lightening agents as maintenance therapy also can be used as an alternative to hydroquinone therapy.

MICRODERMABRASION

Microdermabrasion has gained much popularity since its development in Italy in 1985.[132] The various machine types can be divided into the higher power physician's model and the lower power aesthetician's model. The physician's model is capable of creating pressures up to 70 mm Hg, affecting deeper layers of skin, and requires the supervision of a physician.[163] The technique of microdermabrasion relies on two basic functions: (1) superficially abrading the skin with fine, sharp crystals aluminum oxide, salt, or sodium bicarbonate) via positive- or negative-flowing pressure, and (2) a vacuum closed-loop suction device to remove the crystals, along with dead skin, oil, and surface debris.[163,164]

SCIENTIFIC BACKGROUND

Aluminum oxide crystal particles (corundum crystals) are composed of white-fused alumina and bauxite. These particles are inert, water insoluble, and approximately 100 μm in diameter.

The abrasive effect of these crystals results from their sharp edges, coupled with the flow generated by the positive stream of crystals flowing via a hand piece with vacuum suction.[163] The depth of penetration is controlled by the level of suction, the duration of time the suction handpiece is held in contact with the skin, and the number of passes.[110] Microdermabrasion treatments directly impact the stratum corneum and epidermis. The exfoliating effect is responsible for the improvement seen in clogged pores. Improved skin texture is a direct outcome of removing superficial skin layers.[163] It has also been theorized that microdermabrasion stimulates dermal collagen deposition.[165]

INDICATIONS

Microdermabrasion is indicated for similar skin issues treated by laser resurfacing, exfoliation peels, and dermabrasion but with the limitation of having relatively superficial results. It is an excellent option for the patient who is unable to tolerate peels or for whom extensive recovery time is not an option. Microdermabrasion is used to treat atrophic acne scars, mild facial rhytids, clogged pores, traumatic scars (Bi), enlarged pores, brown spots, stretch marks,[166] melasma, keratosis pilaris, and to improve skin texture.[163] It has also been used as a preprocedure before superficial exfoliation peels by stripping the stratum corneum to ensure more even absorption of the peeling agent.[163] The combination treatment of microdermabrasion and traditional superficial exfoliation peeling agents can help achieve medium-depth exfoliation peel results with fewer adverse side effects.[163]

PATIENT SELECTION

With predictably superficial results, microdermabrasion has been safely done on all skin types. The concerns of hyperpigmentation limiting many patients from elective resurfacing procedures are greatly reduced in microdermabrasion. People whose expectations for dramatic change are high, or photodamage and/or acne scars are too extreme, would not be appropriate for microdermabrasion as a sole therapy.[167] Other poor candidates include those with cutaneous malignancies, active skin infections (eg, herpes simplex, verruca vulgaris, impetigo), acute skin inflammation (eg, rosacea, atopic dermatitis, pustular acne, sunburn, heat rash, bruises), Koebnerizing skin conditions (eg, psoriasis, lichen planus, vitiligo), isotretinoin use within 1 year, broken skin (eg, cuts, abrasions) on the treatment area, unstable diabetes, and autoimmune disorders.[163]

ADVERSE EFFECTS

Unlike traditional dermabrasion, the risk for scarring, hyperpigmentation, and postoperative wound infections is quite low.[168] Following treatment, the most common complications patients can experience is tenderness, swelling, and erythema. Less common complications include petechiae, purpura, or skin wounding if the vacuum suction power is increased, which result in PIH.[169]

Although a very well-tolerated procedure, the noncutaneous complications of microdermabrasion warrant precautions. The risk of eye irritation and corneal abrasion[151,164] from the crystals has many technicians and patients using protective eye wear during the procedure. Pulmonary fibrosis and tracheal and laryngeal papillomas have been linked to aluminum oxide dust exposure.[170] The presence of aluminum in the brain senile plaques of Alzheimer patients has raised the question of the risk of chronic exposure to aerosolized aluminum oxide, but the larger particles used in microdermabrasion are inert and too heavy to become aerosolized and are not likely to pose a risk to the respiratory or cognitive systems.[164] Finally, patients with a history of herpes simplex should be treated with antiviral prophylaxis prior to the procedure as reactivation of the virus is a possibility.[171]

TECHNIQUES

There are a variety of microdermabrasion systems. Most systems being used in practice operate with aluminum oxide crystals. Other options include less abrasive sodium chloride and sodium bicarbonate crystals, or diamond wands that are crystal-free. Crystal-based systems are normally propelled at a predetermined rate. Prior to starting the procedure, the area of desired treatment should be cleaned with a cleanser and protective eye coverings should be applied. To start, the device uses negative pressure to pull the skin into the handpiece. Thus, the device superficially abrades the skin with either a diamond chip or crystals, which are simultaneously removes surface debris from the stratum corneum layer. The number of passes in a session varies with the patient's tolerance and desired effect, but most patients require at least three passes. Depth of ablation depends on the amount of force used to spray the crystals onto the skin, the flow rate of the crystals, the crystal size, and the angle at which the crystals are applied to the skin.[172]

Three levels of microdermabrasion may be used in the treatment of the skin[172]:

- Level one produces a superficial abrasion of the epidermis for gentle exfoliation.
- Level two is more aggressive, extends to the papillary dermis, and is used to treat superficial scars, striae, and fine wrinkles.
- Level three is most aggressive, extends to the level of the papillary and upper reticular dermis, and is used to treat striae.

It is important to note that levels two and three must be used with caution in POC due to an increased risk of hyperpigmentation.

FOLLOW UP AND PATIENT INSTRUCTIONS

Following a treatment with microdermabrasion, patients are instructed to use mild cleansers, emollients, and sun protection (SPF 30). For maximal results, microdermabrasion is recommended 2 to 4 weeks apart for four to six treatments until desired results have been achieved.

OUTCOME

Reepithelialization is usually complete within 1 week, but erythema may persist just beyond 2 weeks. The benefits of microdermabrasion have been proven for the treatment of acne and acne scarring. Investigators demonstrated the efficacy of the procedure in 25 patients with grade II or III acne.[173] The patients received eight treatments at weekly intervals. Overall, 96% of the patients were pleased with their results and reportedly would recommend this procedure to others. The efficacy of microdermabrasion was also accessed in 28 patients ranging in age from 40 to 75 with Fitzpatrick skin types I to IV by Shim et al.[174] Of those enrolled, there were 14 patients with photoaging, 11 with comedonal acne or milia, and 3 with severe acne scarring. Following 12 to 14 weeks of treatment, microdermabrasion produced statistically significant improvement in skin roughness, mottled pigmentation, and overall skin appearance, but not in rhytides. Some acne scarring improved, but most patients required deeper ablation. Adverse events, namely, PIH, did not occur.[174]

Microdermabrasion is also useful for other types of facial scarring. A study evaluated 41 Asian patients with scars (16 acne scars, 18 traumatic scars, 3 surgical scars, 2 chickenpox scars, 1 burn scar, and 1 other scar) that were treated with microdermabrasion over a 2-year period in a Taiwan hospital. All patients reported good to excellent clinical results. [175] Mean frequencies of treatment were 19 treatments for acne scars, 4 for traumatic scars, 4 for surgical scars, and 5.5 for chickenpox scars.

It has been found that microdermabrasion has benefit for patients with vitiligo. A study was performed demonstrating the efficacy of pimecrolimus 1% cream combined with microdermabrasion in the treatment of nonsegmental childhood vitiligo. This was a 3-month, randomized, placebo-controlled study in which three vitiliginous patches were treated in each subject.[176] One lesion was treated with pimecrolimus 1% cream alone, another lesion was treated with microdermabrasion on day 1 followed by the application of pimecrolimus 1% cream and the third lesion was treated with placebo. The treatment course was for 10 days, and microdermabrasion was performed on day 1 until erythema was observed on the skin. Pimecrolimus 1% cream was applied to the affected areas daily for the duration of the treatment course. Sixty-five children were enrolled and 60 completed the study. Significant clinical response was noted as greater than 50% repigmentation of the treated lesions. A total of 60.4% of the patches treated with combination treatment showed a significant clinical response at the 3-month follow-up, compared with 32.1% and 1.7% of those treated with pimecrolimus alone and placebo, respectively. The only side effect noted was a mild burning sensation in 30% of the patients treated with microdermabrasion.[176] Another study demonstrated the efficacy of vitiligo treated with microdermabrasion in combination with 5-fluorouracil cream. The response rate with this combination treatment was 73.3%.[177]

Alam et al treated 10 female patients (mean age 43) split face with six consecutive weekly 20% glycolic acid peels and mild-setting microdermabrasion to investigate comparative reviews of patient ratings and investigator ratings.[132] The skin features under review included redness, brown spots, smoothness, softness, and wrinkles. The comparative reviews results described skin color improvement more by glycolic acid peels in four patients, by microdermabrasion in one patient, equally in three patients but not at all in two patients. An overall preference for glycolic acid peels was stated by 7 of the 10 patients while, of the remaining three, one preferred microdermabrasion and two revealed no preference.[178] Chemical peels and microdermabrasion will likely remain among the most popular "cosmetic procedures" of younger generations whose early intervention may afford them the luxury of preventive rather than therapeutic practices.[132]

MICRONEEDLING

Microneedling (MN) has been used for various cosmetic improvements, skin rejuvenation, skin tightening including treatment of striae, scar remodeling of the face and body, and hair growth.[179] It stands out from other resurfacing modalities such as chemical peels and lasers, because there is no full thickness destruction of the epidermis. This proves to be advantageous to POC (Fitzpatrick IV through VI) because it lowers the possibility of complications such as postinflammatory hyperpigmentation.[180]

In the United States, MN devices exist as both rollers, stampers, and pens (electrically powered or otherwise). When those devices are combined with radiofrequency (RF)—known as fractional radiofrequency microneedling (FRF-MN)—they can deliver energy below the epidermal surface. A common trend among aesthetic procedures is that they lack a standardized protocol. MN and FRF-MN require further clinical studies to determine optimal number of passes, number of treatment sessions, intertreatment duration intervals, and maintenance therapy.[179]

SCIENTIFIC BACKGROUND

MN is effective by creating microchannels and microwounds at the level of the dermis breaking down compact, thickened collagen and inducing the wound healing process. The creation of microchannels is safe to use in darker skin tones because they cause little epidermal damage. Gene expression profiling before and after MN treatment demonstrates an upregulation in type I collagen expression, as well as glycosaminoglycans, vascular endothelial growth factor (VEGF), fibroblast growth factor (FGF)-7, epidermal growth factor (EGF), and transforming growth factor-β (TGF-β).[179] All of these signaling molecules play an important role in collagen production, as well as neovascularization. Furthermore, tissue histology after MN shows thickened epidermis and an increase in dermal collagen and elastic fiber deposition. MN effect of skin tightening and the improvement of scars or rhytides appearance continues over a period of weeks to months as newly formed type III collagen becomes mature type I collagen.[181]

INDICATIONS

MN has shown to be effective and safe for the treatment of acne, postacne scarring, melasma/melanosis, and hyperhidrosis in POC.[180] MN has also been used to treat hypertrophic or keloid scars, and those resulting from surgery, trauma, varicella, or smallpox.[179] MN may also be used for transdermal drug delivery of tranexamic acid and depigmenting serums by the process of forming evenly spaced micropores in the stratum corneum. Furthermore, Microneedling in conjunction with subcision has been successful in treating POC with postacne scarring.[182] Although there are a limited number of studies examining microneedling in the use of hair loss, some studies have shown follicle stimulation when MN is paired with other hair growth promoting therapies, such as minoxidil, platelet-rich plasma, and topical steroids. It is hypothesized that microneedling efficacy lies in its ability to facilitate penetration of first-line medications.[183]

ADVERSE EFFECTS

Overall, MN is a minimally invasive, well-tolerated procedure with minimal downtime in POC.[184] Adverse events (AEs) due to MN or FRF-MN were mostly of minimal severity; no serious AEs were reported. Some of the most common AEs reported were pain and bleeding during the procedure; postprocedure AEs included transient postprocedure pain/discomfort/burning, erythema, and/or swelling.[179] Although less frequently reported, there have been cases of postinflammatory hyperpigmentation, herpes simplex reactivation that was successfully treated with oral valacyclovir, and an allergic reaction to the nickel contents in the MN devices needles, which was subsequently treated with oral prednisolone and topical steroids.[185] One of the most severe AE of MN treatment is the "railroad" or "tram track" scarring that can occur with overly aggressive treatment.[181] MN and FRF-MN were reportedly tolerated better by patients than their laser resurfacing counterparts, namely the CO_2, Er:glass, and diode lasers, with less reported downtime.[179]

CONCLUSION

This chapter reviews key information regarding the use of lasers, chemical peels, microdermabrasion, and microneedling in POC. The cosmetic procedures reviewed are being performed more than ever and as noted, they are safe and effective in this population when performed with skill and caution.

REFERENCES

1. Maiman T. Stimulated optical radiation in ruby. *Nature*. 1960;187:4.
2. Tanzi EL, Lupton JR, Alster TS. Review of lasers in dermatology: four decades of progress. *Am Acad Dermatol*. 2003;4:1-31.
3. Aesthetic Plastic Surgery National Databank Statistics 2020-2021. Procedural Statistics, The Aesthetic Society. https://Cdn.theaestheticsociety.org/media/statistics/2021-TheAestheticSocietyStatistics.pdf
4. Vespa J, Medina L, Armstrong DM, "Demographic turning points for the united states: Population projections for 2020 to 2060," current population reports, P25-1144. Washington, DC: U.S. Census Bureau; 2020.
5. U.S. Census Bureau. Overview of race and Hispanic origin: 2010; 2010 Census Briefs. http://www.census.gov/prod/cen2010/briefs/c2010br-02.pdf. Accessed February 10, 2012.

6. Montagna W, Carlisle K. The architecture of black and white facial skin. *J Am Acad Dermatol.* 1991;24(6 pt 1):929-937.
7. Battle EF Jr, Hobbs LM. Laser therapy on darker ethnic skin. *Dermatologic Clin.* 2003;21(4): 713-723.
8. Jacobs HA, Walton RG. The incidence of birth marks in the neonate. *Pediatrics.* 1976;58:218-222.
9. Alper JC, Holmes LB. The incidence and significance of birthmarks in a cohort of 4641 newborns. *Pediatr Dermatol.* 1983;1:58-68.
10. Geronemus R, Ashinoff R. The medical necessity of evaluation and treatment of port-wine stains. *J Dermatol Surg Oncol.* 1991;17:76-79.
11. Morelli JG, Weston WL, Huff JC, et al. Initial lesion size as a predictive factor in determining the response of port-wine stains in children treated with pulsed dye laser. *Arch Pediatr Adolesc Med.* 1995;149:1142-1144.
12. Ho WS, Chan HH, Ying SY, et al. Laser treatment of congenital facial port wine stains: long term efficacy and complication in Chinese patients. *Lasers Surg Med.* 2002;30:44-47.
13. Tong AK, Tan OT, Eng JB, et al. Ultrastructure: effects of melanin pigment on target specificity using a pulsed dye laser (577 nm). *J Invest Dermatol.* 1987;6:747-752.
14. Van Kampen EJ, Zijlstra WG. Determination of hemoglobin and its derivatives. In: Sobotka H, Stewart CP, eds. *Advances in Clinical Chemistry.* Vol 8. New York, NY: Academic Press; 1965:158-187.
15. Scherer K, Lorenz S, Wimmershoff M, et al. Both the flashlamp-pumped dye laser and the long pulsed tunable dye laser can improve results in port-wine stain therapy. *Br J Dermatol.* 2001;145:79-84.
16. Anderson RR. Laser-tissue interactions in dermatology. In: Arndt KA, Dover JS, Olbricht SM, eds. *Lasers in Cutaneous and Aesthetic Surgery.* Philadelphia, PA: Lippincott-Raven; 1977:25-51.
17. Anolik R, Newlove T, Weiss ET, et al. Investigation into optimal treatment intervals of facial port-wine stains using the pulsed dye laser. *J Am Acad Dermatol.* 2012;67:985-990.
18. Sommer S, Sheehan-Dare RA. Pulsed dye laser treatment of port-wine stains in pigmented skin. *J Am Acad Dermatol.* 2000;42:667-671.
19. Chang CJ, Kelly KM, van Gemert MJ, et al. Comparing the effectiveness of 585 nm vs 595 nm wavelength pulsed dye laser treatment of port wine stains in conjunction with cryogen spray cooling. *Lasers Surg Med.* 2002;31:352-358.
20. Huikeshoven M, Koster PH, de Borgie CA, et al. Redarkening of port-wine stains 10 years after pulsed-dye-laser treatment. *N Engl J Med.* 2007;356: 2745-2746.
21. Kelly KM, Choi B, Mc Farlane S, et al. Description and analysis of treatments for port-wine stain birthmarks. *Arch Facial Plast Surg.* 2005;7:287-294.
22. Chen JK, Ghasri P, Guillermo A, et al. An overview of clinical and experimental treatment modalities for port wine stains. *J Am Acad Dermatol.* 2012;67:389-304.
23. Alster TS, Ranzi EL. Combined 595-nm and 1064-nm laser irradiation of recalcitrant and hypertrophic port-wine stains in children and adults. *Dermatol Surg.* 2009;35:914-919.
24. Tremaine AM, Armstrong JA, Yu-Chin H, et al. Enhanced port-wine stain lightening achieved with combined treatment of selective photothermolysis and imiquimod. *J Am Acad Dermatol.* 2011;66:634-641.
25. Jia W, Sun V, Tran N, et al. Long-term blood vessel removal with combined laser and topical rapamycin antiangiogenic therapy: implications for effective port-wine stain treatment. *Lasers Surg Med.* 2010;42:105-112.
26. Ho WS, Ying SY, Chan PK, et al. Treatment of port wine stains with intense pulsed light: a prospective study. *Dermatol Surg.* 2004;30:887-891.
27. Kilcline C, Frieden IJ. Infantile hemangiomas: how common are they? A systematic review of the medical literature. *Pediatr Dermatol.* 2008;25:168-173.
28. Kanada K, Reyes-Merin M, Munden A, et al. A prospective study of cutaneous findings in newborns in the United States: correlation with race, ethnicities, and gestational status using up dated classification and nomenclature. *J Pediatr.* 2012;161:240-245.
29. Drolet BA, Esterly NB, Frieden IJ. Hemangioma in children. *N Engl J Med.* 1999;341:173-181.
30. Kim HJ, Colombo M, Frieden IJ. Ulcerated hemangiomas: clinical characteristics and response to therapy. *J Am Acad Dermatol.* 2001;44:962-972.
31. Bowers RE, Graham EA, Tomlinson KM. The natural history of the strawberry nevus. *Arch Dermatol.* 1960;82:667-680.
32. Li J, Chen X, Zhao S, et al. Demographic and clinical characteristics and risk factors for infantile hemangioma. *Arch Dermatol.* 2011;9:1049-1056.
33. Maguiness SM, Frieden IJ. Current management of infantile hemangiomas. *Semin Cutan Med Surg.* 2010;29:106-114.
34. Kono T, Hiroyuki S, William FG. Comparison study of traditional pulsed dye laser versus a long-pulsed dye laser in the treatment of early childhood hemangiomas. *Lasers Surg Med.* 2005;38:112-115.
35. Rizzo C, Brightman L, Chapas AM, et al. Outcomes of childhood hemangiomas treated with the pulsed-dye laser with dynamic cooling: a retrospective chart analysis. *Dermatol Surg.* 2009;35:1947-1954.
36. Hunzeker C, Geroneumus R. Treatment of superficial infantile hemangiomas of the eyelid using the 595-nm pulsed dye laser. *Dermatol Surg.* 2010; 36:590-597.
37. McCoppin HH, Hovenic WW, Wheeland RG. Laser treatment of superficial leg veins: a review. *Dermatol Surg.* 2011;37:729-741.
38. Parlette EC, Groff WF, Kinshella MJ, et al. Optimal pulse durations for the treatment of leg telangiectasias with a neodymium YAG laser. *Lasers Surg Med.* 2006;38:98-105.
39. Engel A, Johnson ML, Haynes SG. Health effects of sunlight exposure in the Unites States: results from the first national health and nutrition examination survey 1971-1974. *Arch Dermatol.* 1988;124:72.
40. Weiss RA, Weiss MA. Sclerotherapeutic agents used for treatment of spider and varicose veins: update 2002. *J Drugs Dermatol.* 2002;1:53-59.
41. Duffy DM. Small vessel sclerotherapy: an overview. *Adv Dermatol.* 1988;3:221.
42. Weiss RA. Vascular studies of the legs for venous or arterial disease (review). *Dermatol Clin.* 1994;12:175.
43. Peterson JD, Goldman MP, Weiss RA, et al. Treatment of reticular and telangiectatic leg veins: double-blind, prospective comparative trial of polidocanol and hypertonic saline. *Dermatol Surg.* 2012;38:1322-1330.
44. Duffy DM. Sclerosants: a comparative review. *Dermatol Surg.* 2010;36: 1010-1025.
45. Goldman MP, Guex JJ, Weiss RA. *Sclerotherapy: Treatment of Varicose and Telangiectatic Veins.* 5th ed. Philadelphia, PA: Saunders Elsevier; 2011.
46. Zhang J, Jing Z, Schliephake DE, et al. Efficacy and safety of Aethoxysklerol (polidocanol) 0.5%, 1% and 3% in comparison with placebo solution for the treatment of varicose veins of the lower extremities in Chinese patients (ESA-China Study). *Phlebology.* 2012;27:184-190.
47. van Haarst EP, Liasis N, Van Ramshorst B, et al. The development of valvular incompetence after deep vein thrombosis: a 7-year follow-up study with duplex scanning. *Eur J Vasc Endovasc Surg.* 1996;12:295.
48. Rao J, Goldman MP. Stability of foam in sclerotherapy: differences between sodium tetradecyl sulfate and polidocanol and the type of connector used in the double system technique. *Dermatol Surg.* 2005;31:19-22.
49. Goldman MP. Sclerotherapy treatment for varicose and telangiectatic leg veins. In: Coleman WP, Hanke WK, Alt TH, Asken S, eds. *Cosmetic Surgery of the Skin.* Philadelphia, PA: BC Decker; 1991:197.
50. Weiss RA, Weiss MA. Resolution of pain associated with varicose and telangiectatic leg veins after compression sclerotherapy. *J Dermatol Surg Oncol.* 1990;16:333.
51. Tafazzoli A, Rostan E, Goldman MP. Q-switched ruby laser treatment for postsclerotherapy hyperpigmentation. *Dermatol Surg.* 2000;26:653-656.
52. Goldman MP. How to utilize compression after sclerotherapy. *Dermatol Surg.* 2002;28:860-862.
53. Craft N. Keloids: current concepts in pathogenesis and treatment. *Cosmet Dermatol.* 2002;15:35-39.
54. Nouri K, Elsaie ML, Vejjabhinanta V, et al. Comparison of the effects of short-and-long-pulse durations when using a 585-nm pulsed dye laser in the treatment of new surgical scars. *Lasers Med Sci.* 2010;25:121-126.
55. Bailey JK, Burkes SA, Visscher MO, et al. Multimodal quantitative analysis of early pulsed-dye-laser treatment of scars at a pediatric burn hospital. *Dermatol Surg.* 2012;38:1490-1496.
56. Asilian A, Darougheh A, Shariati F. New combination of triamcinolone, 5-fluorouracil, and pulsed-dye laser for treatment of keloid and hypertrophic scars. *Dermatol Surg.* 2006;32:907-915.
57. Goldman MP, Fitzpatrick RE. Laser treatment of scars. *Dermatol Surg.* 1995; 21:685-687.
58. Koo J. Population-based epidemiologic study of psoriasis with emphasis on quality of life assessment. *Dermatol Clin.* 1996;14:485-496.
59. Hacker SM, Rasmussen JE. The effect of flash lamp-pulsed dye laser on psoriasis. *Arch Dermatol.* 1992;128:853-855.
60. De Leeuw J, Tank B, Bjerring P, et al. Concomitant treatment of psoriasis of the hands and feet with the pulsed dye laser and topical calcipotriol, salicylic acid, or both; a prospective open study in 41 patients. *J Am Acad Dermatol.* 2006;54:266-271.
61. Oram Y, Karincoaoglu Y, Koyuncu E, et al. Pulsed dye laser in the treatment of nail psoriasis. *Dermatol Surg.* 2010;36:377-381.
62. Treewittayapoom C, Singvahanont P, Chanprapaph K, et al. The effect of different pulse durations in the treatment of nail psoriasis with the 595-nm pulsed dye laser: a randomized, double blind, intrapatient left-to-right study. *J Am Acad Dermatol.* 2012;66:807-812.

63. Huang YC, Chou CL, Chiang YY. Efficacy of pulsed dye laser plus topical tazarotene versus topical tazarotene alone in psoriatic nail disease: a single-blind, intrapatient left-to-right controlled study. *Lasers Surg Med.* 2013;45:102-107.
64. Bónis B, Kemény L, Dobozy A, et al. 308-nm excimer laser for psoriasis. *Lancet.* 1997;350:1522.
65. Kopera D. Verrucae vulgaris: flashlamp-pumped pulsed dye laser treatment of 120 patients. *Int J Dermatol.* 2003;42:904-908.
66. Lui A, Moy R, Ross EV, et al. Pulsed dye laser and pulsed dye laser-mediated photodynamic therapy in the treatment of dermatologic disorders. *Dermatol Surg.* 2012;38:351-366.
67. Kawada A, Shiraishi H, Mutsuyo A, et al. Clinical improvement of solar lentigines and ephelides with an intense pulsed light source. *Dermatol Surg.* 2002;28:504-508.
68. Wang CC, Sue YM, Yang CH, et al. A comparison of Q switched alexandrite laser and intense pulsed light for the treatment of freckles and lentigines in Asian persons: a randomized, physician-blinded, split face comparison trial. *J Am Acad Dermatol.* 2006;54:804-810.
69. Watanabe S, Takahashi H. Treatment of nevus of Ota with the Q-switched ruby laser. *N Engl J Med.* 1994;331:1745-1750.
70. Chan HH, Ying SY, Ho WS, et al. An in vivo trial comparing the clinical efficacy and complications of Q-switched 755-nm alexandrite and Q-switched 1064-nm (Nd-YAG) lasers in the treatment of nevus of Ota. *Dermatol Surg.* 2000;26:919-922.
71. Kim EH, Kim YC, Lee E-S, et al. The vascular characteristics of melasma. *J Derm Sci.* 2007;46:111-116.
72. Ortonne JP, Arellano I, Berneburg M, et al. A global survey of the role of ultraviolet radiation and hormonal influences in the development of melasma. *J Eur Acad Dermatol Vernereol.* 2009;23:1254-1262.
73. Arora P, Sarkar R, Garg WK, et al. Lasers for treatment of melasma and post-inflammatory hyperpigmentation. *J Cutan Aesthet Surg.* 2012;5:93-103.
74. Wattanakrai P, Mornchan R, Eimpunth S. Low-fluence Q-switched neodymium-doped yttrium aluminum garnet (1,064 nm) laser for the treatment of facial melasma in Asians. *Dermatol Surg.* 2010;36:76-87.
75. Arora P, Sarkar R, Garg VK, et al. Lasers for treatment of melasma and post-inflammatory hyperpigmentation. *J Cutan Aesthet Surg.* 2012;5:93-103.
76. Sheth VM, Panndya AG. Melasma: a comprehensive update: part II. *J Am Acad Dermatol.* 2011;65:699-714.
77. Li TH, Chen JZ, Wei HC, et al. Efficacy and safety of intense pulsed light in treatment of melasma in Chinese patients. *Dermatol Surg.* 2008;34:693-700.
78. Negishi K, Kushikata N, Tezuka Y, et al. Study of the incidence and nature of "very subtle epidermal melasma" in relation to intense pulsed light treatment. *Dermatol Surg.* 2004;30:881-886.
79. Goldberg DJ, Berlin AL, Phleps R. Histologic and ultrastructural analysis of melasma after fractional resurfacing. *Lasers Surg Med.* 2008;40:134-138.
80. Lee HS, Won CH, Lee DH, et al. Treatment of melasma in Asian skin using a fractional 1,550 nm: an open clinical study. *Dermatol Surg.* 2009;35: 1499-1504.
81. Zelickson BD, Kilmer SL, Bernstein E. Pulsed dye laser therapy for sun damage skin. *Lasers Surg Med.* 1999;25:229-236.
82. Hsu TS, Zelickson B, Dover JS, et al. Multicenter study of the safety and efficacy of a 585 nm pulsed-dye laser for the nonablative treatment of facial rhytides. *Dermatol Surg.* 2005;31:1-9.
83. Moody BR, McCarthy JE, Hruza GJ. Collagen remodeling after 585-nm pulsed dye laser irradiation: an ultrasonographic analysis. *Dermatol Surg.* 2003;29:997-999.
84. Negishi K, Tezuka Y, Kudshikata N, et al. Photorejuvenation for Asian skin by intense pulsed light. *Dermatol Surg.* 2001;27:627-632.
85. Chan HH, Chan E, Kono T, et al. The use of variable pulse width frequency doubled Nd:YAG 532 nm laser in the treatment of port-wine stain in Chinese patients. *Dermatol Surg.* 2000:26:657-661.
86. Hernandez-Perez E, Ibiett E. Gross and microscopic findings in patients submitted to nonablative full face resurfacing using intense pulsed light: a preliminary study. *Dermatol Surg.* 2001;27:627-632.
87. Braverman S. One in five U.S. adults now has a tattoo: yet over two in five without a tattoo say adult tattoos are less attractive. http://www.Harrisinterative.com/vault/harris%20poll%2022%20-tatoos_2.23.12.pdf. Accessed February 23, 2012.
88. Kilmer S. Laser treatment of tattoos. *Dermatol Clin.* 1997;15:409-417.
89. Anderson R, Geronemus R, Kilmer S, et al. Cosmetic tattoo ink darkening. A complication of Q-switched and pulsed-laser treatment. *Arch Dermatol.* 1993;129:1010-1014.
90. Bernstein L, Geronemus R. Keloid formation with the 585-nm pulsed dye laser during isotretinoin treatment. *Arch Dermatol.* 1997;133:111-112.
91. Alissa A. Concomitant use of laser and isotretinoin, how safe. Grapevine, TX: American Society for Laser Medicine and Surgery; 2011.
92. Taylor C. Laser ignition of traumatically embedded firework debris. *Lasers Surg Med.* 1998;22:157-158.
93. Almoallium H, Klinkhoff A, Arthur A, et al. Laser induced chrysiasis: disfiguring hyperpigmentation following Q-switched laser therapy in a woman previously treated with gold. *J Rheumatol.* 2006;33:620-621.
94. Bencini PL, Cazzaniga S, Tourlaki A, et al. Removal of tattoos by Q-switched laser. *Arch Dermatol.* 2012;148:1364-1369.
95. Ross V, Naseef G, Lin G, et al. Comparison of responses to tattoos to picosecond and nanosecond Q-switched neodymium: YAG lasers. *Arch Dermatol.* 1998:134:167-171.
96. Nazanin S, Metelista A, Petrell K, et al. Treatment of tattoos with a picosecond alexandrite laser. A prospective trial. *Arch Dermatol.* 2012;148:1360-1363.
97. Izikson L, Farinelli W, Sakamoto F, et al. Safety and effectiveness of black tattoo clearance in a pig model after a single treatment with a novel 758 nm 500 picosecond laser: a pilot study. *Lasers Surg Med.* 2010;42:640-646.
98. Kaufmann R, Hibst R. Pulsed erbium: YAGla-ser ablation in cutaneous surgery. *Lasers Surg Med.* 1996;19:324-330.
99. Burgess CM, et al. Laser skin resurfacing. In: Alster TS, ed. *Cosmetic Dermatology.* Springer, Berlin; 2005:118-126.
100. Alster TS. Clinical and histologic evaluation of six erbium: YAG lasers for cutaneous resurfacing. *Lasers Surg Med.* 1999;24:87-92.
101. Goldberg DJ, Cutler K. The use of the erbium: YAG laser for the treatment of class III rhytides. *Dermatol Surg.* 1999;24: 619-621.
102. Weiss RA, Harrington AC, Pfau RC, et al. Per-orbital skin resurfacing using high-energy erbium:YAG laser: results in 50 patients. *Lasers Surg Med.* 1999;24:81-86.
103. Kye YC. Resurfacing of pitted facial scars with a pulsed Er: YAG laser. *Dermatol Surg.* 1997;23:880-883.
104. Polnikorn N, Goldberg DJ, Suwanchinda A, et al. Erbium: YAG laser resurfacing in Asians. *Dermatol Surg.* 1998;24:1303-1307.
105. Chathra N, Mysore V. Resurfacing of facial acne scars with a new variable-pulsed Er:YAG laser in Fitzpatrick skin types IV and V. *J Cutan Aesthet Surg.* 2018;11(1):20-25.
106. Burgess C. Aerolase light pod neo elite clinical insights. www.aerolase.com.
107. Roberts WE, Henry M, Burgess C, Saedi N, Chilukuri S, Campbell-Chambers DA. Laser treatment of skin of color for medical and aesthetic uses with a new 650-microsecond nd:YAG 1064nm laser. *J Drugs Dermatol.* 2019;18(4): s135-s137.
108. Lipper GM, Perez M. Nonablative acne scar reduction after a series of treatments with a short-pulsed 1,064-nm neodymium: YAG laser. *Dermatol Surg.* 2006;32(8):998-1006.
109. Badawi A, Tome MA, Atteya A, Sami N, Morsy IA. Retrospective analysis of non-ablative scar treatment in dark skin types using the sub-millisecond nd:YAG 1,064 nm laser. *Lasers Surg Med.* 2011;43(2):130-136.
110. Greywal T, Ortiz A. Treating melasma with the 1064 nm nd: YAG laser with a 650-microsecond pulse duration: a clinical evaluation. *J Cosmet Dermatol.* 2021;20(12):3889-3892.
111. Campbell-Chambers A. Combination therapy for PIH in skin of colour. *PMFA J.* 2022;10(1).
112. Alexis AF. Lasers and light-based therapies in ethnic skin: treatment options and recommendations for Fitzpatrick skin types V and VI. *Br J Dermatol.* 2013;169 suppl 3:91-97.
113. Chan HH, Manstein D, Yu CS, Shek S, Kono T, Wei WI. The prevalence and risk factors of post-inflammatory hyperpigmentation after fractional resurfacing in Asians. *Lasers Surg Med.* 2007;39(5):381-385.
114. Tierney EP, Hanke CW. Review of the literature: treatment of dyspigmentation with fractionated resurfacing. *Dermatol Surg.* 2010;36(10): 1499-1508.
115. Kaushik SB, Alexis AF. Nonablative fractional laser resurfacing in skin of color: evidence-based review. *J Clin Aesthet Dermatol.* 2017;10(6):51-67.
116. Graber EM, Tanzi EL, Alster TS. Side effects and complications of fractional laser photothermolysis: Experience with 961 treatments. *Dermatol Surg.* 2008;34(3):301-307.
117. Brauer JA, McDaniel DH, Bloom BS, Reddy KK, Bernstein LJ, Geronemus RG. Nonablative 1927 nm fractional resurfacing for the treatment of facial photopigmentation. *J Drugs Dermatol.* 2014;13(11):1317-1322.
118. Alharbi MA. 1927 nm thulium laser successfully treats postinflammatory hyperpigmentation in skin of color. *Dermatol Res Pract.* 2021;2021:5560386.
119. Brody HJ, Monheit GD, Resnik SS, Alt TH. A history of chemical peeling. *Dermatol Surg.* 2000;26:405-409.
120. Brody H. History and classification of chemical peels. In: Patterson AN, ed. *Chemical Peeling.* St. Louis, MO: Mosby; 1992:7-22.

121. Resnik SS, Lewis LA, Cohen BH. TCA peeling. *Cutis*. 1976;17:127-129.
122. Alt TH. Occluded Baker-Gordon chemical peel: review and update. *J Dermatol Surg Oncol*. 1989;15:980-993.
123. Van Scott EJ, Yu RJ. Hyperkeratinization, corneocyte cohesion, and alpha hydroxyl acids. *J Am Acad Dermatol*. 1984;11:867-879
124. Tung RC, Bergfeld WF, Vidimos AT, Remzi BK. Alfa-Hydroxy acid-based cosmetic procedures: guidelines for patient management. *Am J Clin Dermatol*. 2000;1:1-88.
125. Roberts WE. Chemical peeling in ethnic/-dark skin. *Dermatol Ther*. 2004;17(2):196-205.
126. Kakita LS. The use of chemical peels in Asian skin. In: Moy R, Luftman D, Kakita LS, eds. *Glycolic Acid Peels*. New York, NY: Marcel Dekker; 2002:141-153.
127. Grimes PE. Glycolic acid peels in blacks. In: Moy R, Luftman D, Kakita LS, eds. *Glycolic Acid Peels*. New York, NY: Marcel Dekker; 2002:179-186.
128. Rendon M, Berson DS, Cohen JL, et al. Evidence and considerations in the application of chemical peels in skin disorders and aesthetic resurfacing. *J Clin Aesthet Dermatol*. 2010;3:32-43.
129. Corcuff P, Fiat F, Minodo AM, et al. A comparative ultrastructural study of hydroxyacids induced desquamation. *Eur J Dermatol*. 2002;12:XXXIX-XLIII.
130. Sarkar R, Bansal S, Garg VK. Chemical peels for melasma in dark-skinned patients. *J Cutan Aesthet Surg*. 2012;5:247-253.
131. Kadhim KA, Al-Waiz M. Treatment of periorbital wrinkles by repeated medium-depth chemical peels in dark-skinned individuals. *J Cosmet Dermatol*. 2005;4:18-22.
132. Burgess CM, ed. *Cosmetic Dermatology*. Berlin: Springer; 2005.
133. Resnik SS, Resnik BI. Complications of chemical peeling: cosmetic dermatology. *Dermatol Clin*. 1995;13:309-331.
134. Brody HJ. Skin resurfacing: chemical peels. In: Freedberg IM, Eisen AZ, Wolf K, eds. *Fitzpatrick's Dermatology in General Medicine*. 6th ed. New York, NY: McGraw-Hill; 2003:2530-2535.
135. Roberts WE. Chemical peeling in ethnic/-dark skin. *Dermatol Ther*. 2004;17(2):196-205.
136. Newman N, Newman A, Moy LS, et al. Clinical improvement of photoaged skin with 50% glycolic acid: a double-blinded vehicle-controlled study. *Dermatol Surg*. 1996;22:455-460.
137. Khunger N, Sarkar R, Jain RK. Tretinoin peels versus glycolic acid peels in the treatment of melasma in dark-skinned patients. *Dermatol Surg*. 2004;30:756-760.
138. Burns RL, Prevot-Blank PL, Lawry MA, et al. Glycolic acid peels for postinflammatory hyperpigmentation in black patients: a comparative study. *Dermatol Surg*. 1997;23:171-175.
139. Marrero GM, Katz BE. The new fluor-hydroxy pulse peel: a combination of s-fluorouracil and glycolic acid. *Dermatol Surg*. 1998;24:973-978.
140. Moy LS, Howe K, Moy RL. Glycolic acid modulation of collagen production in human skin fistulation of collagen production. *Dermatol Surg*. 1996;22:439-441.
141. Grimes PE. The safety and efficacy of salicylic acid chemical peels in darker racial-ethnic groups. *Dermatol Surg*. 1999;25:18-22.
142. Kligman D, Kligman AM. Salicylic acid peels for the treatment of photoaging. *Dermatol Surg*. 1988;24:325-328.
143. Monheit GD. The Jessner's and TCA peel: a medium depth chemical peel. *J Dermatol Surg Oncol*. 1989;15:945-950.
144. Stagnone JI. Superficial peeling. *J Dermatol Surg Oncol*. 1989;15:924-930.
145. Roenigk RK, Brodland DG. A primer of facial chemical peel. *Dermatol Clin*. 1993;11:349-359.
146. Gersetich I, Brazzini B, Peris K, et al. Pyruvic acid peels for the treatment of photoaging. *Dermatol Surg*. 2004;30:32-36.
147. Brody HJ. *Chemical Peeling and Resurfacing*. St Louis, MO: Mosby; 1997.
148. Monheit GD, Chastain, MA. Chemical peels. *Facial Plast Surg Clin of North Am*. 2001;9(2):239-255.
149. Mendelsohn JE. update on chemical peels. *Otolaryngol Clin North Am*. 2002;35(1).
150. Gersetich I, Brazzini B, Peris K, et al. Pyruvic acid peels for the treatment of photoaging. *Dermatol Surg*. 2004;30:32-36.
151. Marrero GM, Katz BE. The new fluor-hydroxy pulse peel: a combination of s-fluorouracil and glycolic acid. *Dermatol Surg*. 1998;24:973-978.
152. Monheit GD. Medium-depth chemical peels. *Dermtol Clin*. 2001;19(3): 413-425.
153. Chun E, Lee B, Lee KH. Focal trichloroacetic acid peel method for benign pigmented lesions in dark-skinned patients. *Dermatol Surg*. 2004;30:512-516.
154. Monheit GD, Chastain, MA. Chemical peels. *Facial Plast Surg Clin North Am*. 2001;9(2): 239-255.
155. Obagi S, Obagi Z, Bridenstine JB. Isotretinoin use during chemical skin resurfacing: a review of complications. *Am J Cosmet Surg*. 2002;19:9-13.
156. Tse Y, Ostad A, Lee HS, et al. A clinical and histologic evaluation of two medium depth peels. glycolic acid versus Jessner's, trichloroacetic acid. *Dermatol Surg*. 1996;22:781-786.
157. Monheit GD, Chastian MA. Chemical and mechanical skin resurfacing. In: Bolognia JL, Jorizzo JL, Rapini RP, eds. *Dermatology*. Philadelphia, PA: Mosby; 2003:2379-2398.
158. Manaloto RMP, Alster TS. Periorbital rejuvenation: a review of dermatologic treatments. *Dermatol Surg*. 1999;25(1):1-9.
159. Pandya AG, Guevara IL. Disorders of hyperpigmentation. *Dermatol Clin*. 2000;18:91-98.
160. Glogau RG, Matarasso SL. Chemical peels: trichloroacetic acid and phenol. *Dermatol Clin*. 1995;13(2):263-276.
161. Kindred C, Okereke UR, Callender VD. Skin lightening agents: an overview of prescription, office-dispensed and OTC products. *Cosmet Dermatol*. 2012;5:18-26.
162. Grimes PE. Skin of color: disease and cosmetic issues of major concern. *Cosmet Dermatol*. 2003;16:1-4.
163. Koch RJ, Hanasono M. Microdermabrasion. *Facial Plast Surg Clin of North Am*. 2001;9(3):377-382.
164. Tan MH, Spencer JM, Pires LM, Ajmeri L, Skover G. The evaluation of aluminum oxide crystal microdermabrasion for photodamage. *Dermatol Surg*. 2001;27:943-949.
165. Rubin MG, Greenbaum SS. Histologic effects of aluminum oxide microdermabrasion on facial skin. *J Aesth Derm Cosmetic Surg*. 2000;1:237.
166. Bernard R, Beran SI, et al. Microdermabrasion in clinical practice. *Clin Plast Surg*. 2000;27(4):571-577.
167. Hernandez-Perez E, Ibiett EV. Gross and microscopic findings in patients undergoing micro dermabrasion for facial rejuvenation. *Dermatol Surg*. 2001;27:637-640.
168. Freeman MS. Microdermabrasion. *Facial Plast Surg Clin North Am*. 2001;9(2):257-266.
169. Tsai RY, Wang CN, Chan HL. Aluminum oxide crystal microdermabrasion: a new technique for treating facial scarring. *Dermatol Surg*. 1995;21:539-542.
170. McCollough EG, Langdon PR. chemical peeling with phenol. In: Roenigk H, Roenigk R, eds. *Dermatologic Surgery: Principles and Practice*. New York, NY: Marcel Dekker; 1989:997-1016.
171. Warmuth IP, Bader R, Scarborough DA, et al. Herpes simplex infection after microdermabrasion. *Cosmet Dermatol*. 1999;12:13.
172. Lim JT. Microdermabrasion. In: Grimes PE, ed. *Aesthetic and Cosmetic Surgery for Darker Skin Types*. Philadelphia, PA: Lippincott Williams & Wilkins; 2008:147-153.
173. Lloyd J. The use of micordermabrasion for acne: a pilot study. *Dermatol Surg*. 2001;27:329-331.
174. Shim EK, Barnette D, Hughes K, et al. Microdermabrasion: a clinical and histopathologic study. *Dermatol Surg*. 2001;27:524-530.
175. Tsai RY, Wang CN, Chan HL. Aluminum oxide crystal microdermabrasion: a new technique for treating facial scarring. *Dermatol Surg*. 1995;21: 539-542.
176. Farajzadeh S, Daraei Z, Esfandiarpour I, et al. The efficacy of pimecrolimus 1% cream combined with microdermabrasion in the treatment of nonsegmental childhood vitiligo: a randomized placebo-controlled study. *Pediatr Dermatol*. 2009;26:286-291.
177. Sethi S, Mahajan BB, Guptta RR, et al. Comparative evaluation of the therapeutic efficacy of dermabrasion, dermabrasion combined with topical 5% 5-fluorouracil cream, and dermabrasion combined with topical placentrex gel in localized stable vitiligo. *Int J Dermatol*. 2007;46:875-879.
178. Alam M, Omura N, Dover JS, Arndt KA. Glycolic acid peels compared to microdermabrasion: a right-left controlled trial of efficacy and patient satisfaction. *Dermatol Surg*. 2002;28:475-479.
179. Juhasz MLW, Cohen JL. microneedling for the treatment of scars: an update for clinicians. *Clin Cosmet Investig Dermatol*. 2020;13:997-1003.
180. Cohen BE, Elbuluk N. microneedling in skin of color: a review of uses and efficacy. *J Am Acad Dermatol*. 2016;74(2):348-355.
181. Moftah NH, El Khayyat MAM, Ragai MH, Alaa H. carboxytherapy versus skin microneedling in treatment of atrophic postacne scars: a comparative clinical, histopathological, and histometrical study. *Dermatol Surg*. 2018;44(10):1332-1341.
182. Bhargava S, Kumar U, Varma K. Subcision and microneedling as an inexpensive and safe combination to treat atrophic acne scars in dark skin: a prospective study of 45 patients at a tertiary care center. *J Clin Aesthet Dermatol*. 2019;12(8):18-22.

183. Fertig RM, Gamret AC, Cervantes J, Tosti A. Microneedling for the treatment of hair loss? *J Eur Acad Dermatol Venereol.* 2018;32(4):564-569.
184. Desai M, Gill J, Luke J. Cosmetic procedures in patients with skin of color: clinical pearls and pitfalls. *J Clin Aesthet Dermatol.* 2023;16(3):37-40.
185. Yadav S, Dogra S. Cutaneous A. reaction to microneedling for post-acne scarring caused by nickel hypersensitivity. *Aesthet Surg J.* 2016;36: NP168-NP170.

CHAPTER 95

Laser Treatments

Mandy W. M. Chan
Henry Hin-Lee Chan

KEY POINTS

- The term "skin of color" refers to individuals with Fitzpatrick skin type III to VI. Variations in skin complexion is determined by the amount and distribution of melanin produced by melanocytes. The use of lasers in individuals with skin of color requires an understanding of laser physics and laser tissue interaction to allow for successful clinical outcome.
- Within the electromagnetic spectrum, melanin has a broad absorption spectrum. Higher epidermal melanin content in ethnic skin acts as a competing chromophore, which absorbs laser energy intended for other targets, but can also cause nonselective thermal injury to the epidermis.
- In individuals with skin of color, it is important to choose appropriate laser parameters including skin cooling, longer laser pulse width to protect the epidermis, longer laser wavelength to reduce absorption by competing epidermal melanin, and conservative fluence to achieve desired clinical outcome.
- In this chapter, we will discuss the use of lasers in pigmented lesions, skin rejuvenation, noninvasive body contouring, and common skin disorders.

INTRODUCTION

The U.S. Census Bureau projects that racial minorities will make up more than 50% of the population by 2044,[1] as a result, dermatologists must also welcome this growth by increasing their understanding in treating patients with skin of color, understand the clinical implications in variations in skin structure and function, and appreciate different cultural perceptions of beauty to deliver quality dermatological treatment to patients of all skin types.

LASER-TISSUE INTERACTION IN SKIN OF COLOR

The possibility of stimulated emission of radiation was first conceived by Einstein in 1917,[2] and Maiman operated the first laser using ruby as the active medium.[3] Laser, an acronym for light amplification by the stimulated emission of radiation, is made up of a pumping system, the lasing medium, and optical cavity. The instrument is a device that produces orderly beams of light. Laser radiation is coherent, monochromatic, temporally coherent, and of high energy, allowing for selective optical absorption and selective tissue heating.[4] Once the laser light hits the skin, it can be transmitted, scattered, reflected, or absorbed, depending on the type of tissue and wavelength of the light. For a laser to have an effect, the radiation needs to be absorbed and converted to heat, therefore it requires a "target" chromophore. There are three main endogenous chromophores within the skin: melanin, hemoglobin, and water. Each chromophore in the skin absorbs light of different wavelengths—they each have a specific peak absorption in the electromagnetic spectrum. Through Anderson and Parish theory of *selective photothermolysis*, the use of lasers has revolutionized in the field of dermatology and other subspecialties.[5] The three elements needed to achieve selective photothermolysis are: (1) emitted laser wavelength should be highly absorbed by target structures; (2) sufficient fluence provided to radiant energy into heat to induce thermal damage to target; and (3) duration of tissue exposure to laser should be short enough to inflict damage to target without heat transmission to surrounding tissues. The laser pulse duration must be less or equal to the thermal relaxation time of the target.

LASER TREATMENT IN SKIN OF COLOR

Skin of color is characterized by an increased number of larger and dispersed melanosomes, and increased tyrosinase activity yielding higher melanin content. It also has larger and more fibroblast content with increased activity, therefore a higher prevalence of hypertrophic scarring and keloid formation may result after injury. The use of lasers and light sources in skin of color is more challenging due to a higher epidermal melanin content, leading to increased risks of unwanted side effects. Melanin has a wide absorption wavelength of 250 to 1200 nm,[6] and is the target of all visible and near-infrared dermatologic lasers. Epidermal melanin not only decreases the effect of the laser treatment, but it may also cause nonselective thermal injury to the epidermis, acting as a competing chromophore that absorbs laser energy intended for other targets such as hemoglobin in blood vessels and pigment in hair follicles. Unwanted side effects such as blistering, crust, pigmentary discoloration, scarring can be a result of laser treatment in skin of color, therefore special considerations much be given to the appropriate use of the laser parameters. To counter these risks, special considerations must be considered when using lasers in skin of color including longer laser wavelength to reduce absorption by melanin-rich epidermis; longer pulse width duration to protect the epidermis; efficient skin cooling; and conservative fluences to prevent too much heat within the epidermis and surrounding tissues. A test spot can be performed on patients prior to treatment on a large area.

Prior to laser treatment, a thorough medical history including history of recurrent herpes simplex, keloid or hypertrophic scarring, and vitiligo should be elicited. History of oral retinoid use in the last 6 months and photosensitivity including consumption of photosensitizing agents should be detailed. Patient counseling on expectations, frequency of treatment, potential cost, and complications should also be discussed. Realistic expectations from treatments are also pivotal to successful clinical outcome. Informed consent should also be obtained from the patient, and pre- and posttreatment photos should be documented. Post-laser wound care is also important, and advice on sun avoidance and sunblock is pertinent. In this chapter, we will discuss the use of lasers in pigmented lesions, skin rejuvenation, noninvasive body contouring, and common skin disorders.

LASERS AND LIGHTS IN PIGMENTED LESIONS IN SKIN OF COLOR

In patients with skin of color, the incidence of both congenital and acquired pigmentary disorders is increased, including epidermal pigmented lesions such as lentigines, ephelides, melasma, and dermal pigmented lesions such as Hori nevus, seborrheic keratosis, and nevus of Ota. It is imperative that a pigmented lesion is assessed whether it is benign or malignant, and that a melanoma is excluded prior to laser treatment.

SOLAR LENTIGINES AND EPHELIDES [FIGURE 95-1]

The earliest signs of photoaging in ethnic skin is the appearance of solar lentigines and ephelides.[7] They respond well to laser treatment and usually clear within one to three treatments, but recurrence is common.

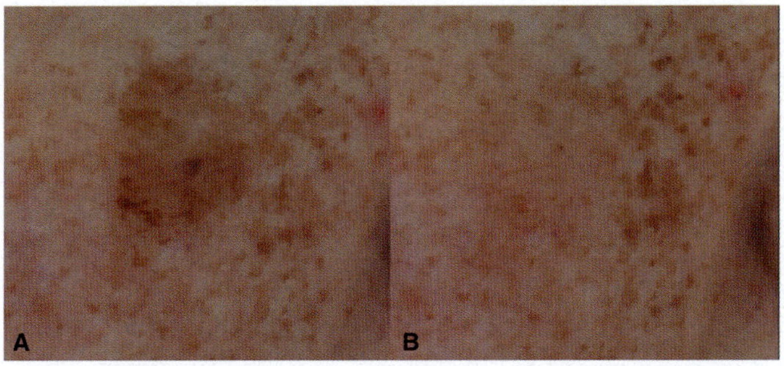

FIGURE 95-1. Solar lentigines **(A)** and **(B)** 3 months after 2 treatments of picosecond 532 nm (0.4 J/cm^2, 2 Hz, 4 mm).

Various lasers [**Table 95-1**] can be used for the treatment of lentigines and ephelides including frequency-doubled Q-switched (QS) lasers such as QS 532-nm neodymium-doped yttrium-aluminum-garnet (Nd:YAG) laser, QS ruby laser (694nm), QS alexandrite laser (755nm), intense pulsed light (IPL) source, long-pulsed 532nm Nd:YAG laser, and long-pulse pulsed dye laser (LPDL) (595 nm).

Nano and picosecond lasers are effective in treating lentigines and ephelides but are associated with a higher risk of postinflammatory hyperpigmentation (PIH) as compared to long pulsed laser or IPL.[8] The Nano and picosecond lasers destroy melanin through both photomechanical and photothermal effects when short bursts of wavelength specific energy is delivered to the skin, and the photomechanical effect inflicts damage to adjacent oxyhemoglobin causing inflammation to superficial blood vessels and change in melanocyte activity causing PIH. Wang et al also found similar findings of higher rate of PIH when comparing QS alexandrite laser compared with IPL for the treatment of lentigines and freckles in Asian patients, especially in treating patients with lentigines (47%) than in those with freckles (7%).[9] Kono et al demonstrated PIH was more frequently found after nanosecond laser treatment (22%), compared to long-pulsed laser treatment (6%).[10] In our previous study, the rate of PIH was 10.2% with 532 nm picosecond laser in treating lentigines.[11]

LPDL 595 nm targets both hemoglobin and melanin. Kono et al demonstrated the use of diascopy with compression of the skin with a flat glass window on the handpiece, leading to emptying of blood vessels, reducing the risk of bruising and PIH.[12] The longer pulse duration with LPDL is better suited to target the basal layer; however due to theoretical risk of dermal injury and scar formation due to thermal diffusion injury from the epidermis to the dermis, the pulse duration should be shorter or equal to the thermal relaxation time of the epidermal basal layer.

The IPL system emits broadband of visible light (400-1200 nm) from noncoherent filtered flashlamp and destroys pigment through photothermal effects. The lack of photomechanical effects gives IPL an advantage in the treatment of lentigines and freckles in Asians.[9] However, the large spot size between lesional and nonlesional skin may be a limitation, and excessive outcome affecting normal skin may lead to "footprint" injury. IPL is not suitable for patients with skin phototypes V or VI.

With multiple treatment options, it is imperative for the ultimate choice of laser treatment to be decided on after discussion with the patient and willingness to accept possible complications such as PIH, with PIH risk being around 5% to 10%[13] using QS nano- or picosecond laser requiring one to two sessions and downtime for 1 week, or a more conservative approach and lower risk of PIH with long-pulsed lasers, requiring more sessions, typically three to four treatments.

TABLE 95-1 Treatment options and suggested parameters for lentigines and ephelides in skin of color

	Laser	Spot size	Fluence (J/cm^2)
Lentigines and ephelides	Long-pulsed 532 KTP	3 mm (with cooling 10°C)	8.8-9.6, 2 ms
	Long-pulsed 595 nm	7 mm	11-13, 1.5 ms
	Q-switched 532 nm	2 mm	0.6
	Picosecond 532 nm	4 mm	0.3-0.4

KTP, potassium titanyl phosphate.

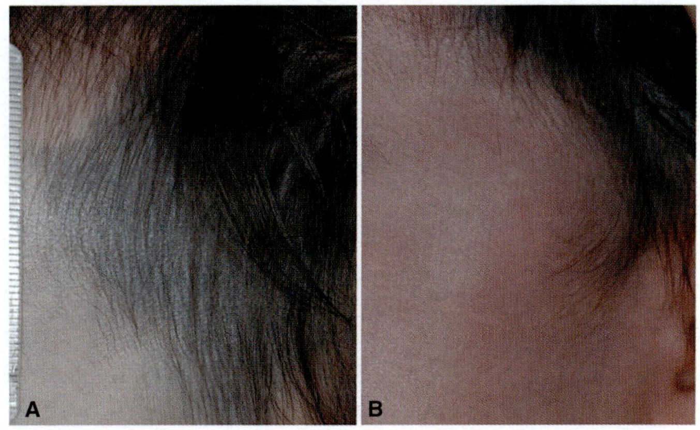

FIGURE 95-2. Nevus of Ota **(A)** and **(B)** 6 months post 11th laser treatment.

DERMATOSIS PAPULOSE NIGRA

Dermatosis papulosa nigra is a benign pigmented skin lesion associated with darker skin phenotypes. A comparison of 532 nm potassium-titanyl-phosphate (KTP) laser treatment with electrodesiccation found the laser to be safe, well tolerated, and even less painful for patients.[14] The smallest spot size (ie, 1-2 mm) should be used to treat individual lesions and avoiding injury to normal skin.

NEVUS OF OTA AND NEVUS OF ITO [FIGURE 95-2]

Nevus of Ota is a dermal melanocytic hamartoma that appears as a bluish grey hyperpigmentation along the first of second branches of the trigeminal nerve, and can sometimes affect the sclera. They are apparent at birth or early childhood and are commonly found in female Asians and Blacks. Nevus of Ito is a bluish-gray patch usually found on the shoulder where the posterior supraclavicular and lateral brachial cutaneous nerves innervate. Due to the anatomical position of these lesions, social stigmatization and disfigurement can be significant. Treatment with various lasers such as QSRL,[15] QS alexandrite 755 nm,[16] and QS ND: YAG 1064 nm,[17] and PS alexandrite 755 nm laser treatments have demonstrated excellent clinical results.[18,19]

QS alexandrite appeared to be better tolerated by patients in terms of postoperative discomfort when compared with QS ND:YAG 1064,[20] but in terms of clinical efficacy, QS ND:YAG 1064 nm laser appears to be superior after three or more laser treatment sessions.[21] PS alexandrite lasers (parameters: 1.75-4.80 J/cm^2, 2.5-5 Hz, 2.3-3.8 mm spot size) has shown to be effective with minimal adverse effects, where a total of 4 to 8 treatments are typically required. Possible side effects include PIH, hypopigmentation, and recurrence of pigmentation.[18] Picosecond laser poses an advantage as the number of sessions are found to be fewer without increase in complication. This is particularly advantageous as patients often present in the pediatric age group, and sedation for treatment is often required. Early treatment is advised as it not only prevents psychosocial impact of the lesion but treatment at younger age tend to require less treatment sessions and less complication rate.[22]

HORI NEVUS/ACQUIRED BILATERAL NEVUS OF OTA-LIKE MACULES [FIGURE 95-3]

Acquired bilateral nevus of Ota-like macules (ABNOM) or Hori nevus are bluish-gray or slate brown speckles found bilaterally over the malar region of the face. Unlike nevus of Ota, they develop at around 20 years of age. QSRL, QS alexandrite, and QS Nd:YAG lasers have all be reported to be effective.[23] Picosecond alexandrite laser is the authors' current clinical practice (parameters: 1.76-3.03 J/cm^2, 1.0-2.5 Hz, and 2.9-3.8 mm spot size).[24] Patients are counselled on risks of PIH, and hypopigmentation that are usually temporary.

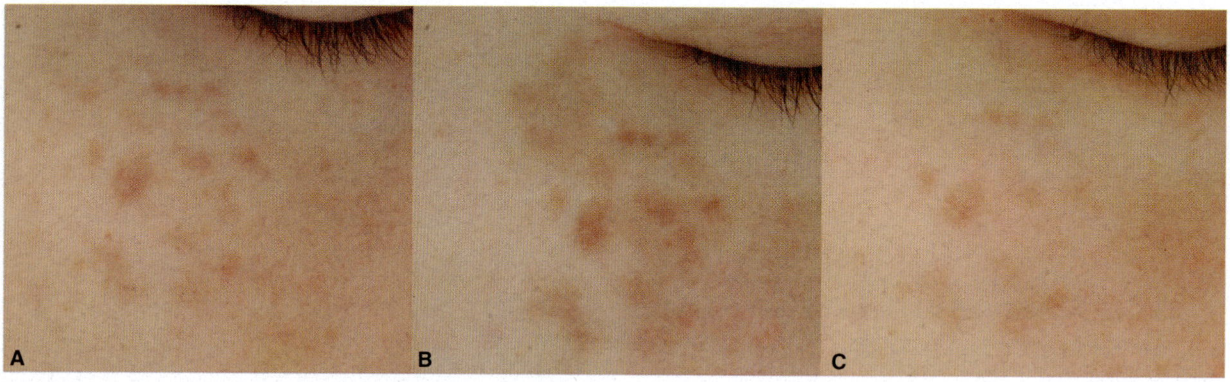

FIGURE 95-3. Hori macules **(A)** and **(B)** postinflammatory hyperpigmentation (PIH) after one laser treatment, **(C)** PIH resolved.

MELASMA [FIGURE 95-4]

Melasma is an acquired common pigmentary disorder characterized by brown hypermelanosis on sun-exposed areas of the face with histological findings of increased basal layer melanin. Increased dermal vascularity and expression of angiogenic factors play a role in melasma.[25] It is associated with multiple factors including pregnancy, hormonal dysfunction, hereditary predisposition, and sun exposure.

Recommended treatment options include sun protection and topical depigmenting agents that inhibit tyrosinase activity, remove melanin, and cause destruction of melanin granules.[26] Current treatment includes hydroquinone, azelaic acid, tretinoin, topical corticosteroids, vitamin C, α- and β-hydroxyacids in monotherapy or in combination therapy.[27]

Melasma is difficult to treat due to its resistance to treatment and relapsing nature. Triple combination cream consisting of hydroquinone, tretinoin, and fluocinolone is recommended by the Latin American Pigmentary Disorders Academy as the first line of treatment for mild, moderate, and severe melasma.[28] Arellano et al[26] found that after initial phase of daily application of triple combination cream for 8 weeks, followed by a maintenance phase of twice weekly application showed better effectiveness in postponing relapse in severe melasma cases than compared to a tapering regimen, with 53% patients relapse free after 6 months of maintenance therapy. A review by Rivas et al[29] also found topical depigmenting agents to be most effective in treating moderate-to-severe melasma with combination therapies such as triple combination therapy yielding the best results.

Tranexamic acid (TA) is a synthetic derivative of lysine and has been used as an off-label drug for the treatment of melasma in recent years. TA is found to inhibit plasminogen-keratinocyte interaction decreasing the tyrosinase activity causing decreased melanin synthesis from melanocytes.[30] Na et al[31] reported that both topical and oral TA reduces melasma-associated epidermal pigmentation and reverses melasma-related changes in the dermis. It has been demonstrated to be effective in treatment of melasma in combination with topical depigmentation cream, alone, and in combination with lasers.[32] Caution is to be noted to exclude a history of pro-thrombotic disease prior to prescribing oral TA.[33]

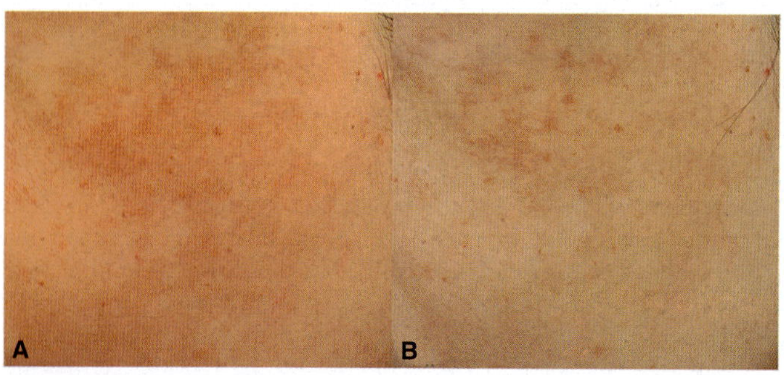

FIGURE 95-4. Melasma **(A)** and **(B)** 3 months post 9th picosecond laser treatment (1064 nm, 0.54-1.22 J/cm^2, 3 Hz, 6 mm).

The authors stress that lasers and IPL should be reserved for those who are resistant to topical therapy and should be avoided in skin types V and VI. A review done by Halachmi et al[34] found that the response of melasma to lasers was not consistent, and that adverse event of PIH was reported in several studies. The durability of melasma improvement was also limited in all cases where laser was used as monotherapy. The analysis suggested that the use of lasers for the treatment of melasma could not be recommended due to the unpredictable safety and efficacy, time-limited clinical improvement, and no clear benefit over conventional treatment. Shankar et al[35] also concluded that the recommendation for the treatment of melasma remains as triple combination cream as first line, addition of selective peels if required in second line, and lasers as a last resort.

Fractional 1550 nm laser[36] and 1927 nm thulium fiber laser,[37] QSRL,[38] QS Nd:YAG (1064 nm),[39] QSAL (755 nm),[40] CO_2 (10,600 nm),[41] Er: YAG (2940 nm),[42] and vascular[43] lasers have been studied; however, sustained response in the treatment of melasma has not been demonstrated. Complications include hypopigmentation,[44] recurrence and rebound hyperpigmentation. Hypopigmentation is postulated to be due to possible excess fluence, skin uneven pigmentation, additive of sub-threshold effects, and possibly phototoxic effect similar to PUVA-induced leukoderma.[45]

The authors use lasers (picosecond alexandrite 755 nm, and fractionated picosecond Nd:YAG 1064 nm)[46,47] in the treatment of melasma, only in resistant cases or patients who request a rapid means of induction. The laser parameters used for fractionated 1064 nm picosecond laser were 1.3 to 1.9 mJ/μbeam, 10 Hz, 6 mm, 4 passes. Recurrence, PIH, potential hypopigmentation, and rebound are explained to the patient. The reduction of frequency and lowering energy is likely to reduce complication risks. Combination therapy with topicals as mentioned above, IPL,[48] and oral TA[49] have demonstrated better response than laser alone.

LASERS AND LIGHT BASED COSMETIC TREATMENTS IN SKIN OF COLOR

SKIN REJUVENATION

In the past ablative lasers with CO_2 or Erbium:YAG were used to remove the epidermis and part of the dermis, thereby removing signs of photoaging and scarring, leading to neocollagenesis and skin rejuvenation. However, long downtime, potential complications including infection and even scarring has made ablative lasers less appealing. In particular, patients with skin of color are more prone to developing PIH.[50] The development of fractional photothermolysis has revolutionized skin rejuvenation by trying to achieve the clinical results to that of ablative lasers but with a safety profile comparable to that of nonablative technologies.[51] The main objective of fractional resurfacing is to cause microvolumes of full thickness thermal injury, from epidermis to reticular dermis while the stratum corneum remains intact. These microthermal wound zones heal as necrotic debris and melanin are eliminated by keratinocyte migration and rapid expulsion leading to resurfacing and remodeling effects. Skin barrier function remains intact due to the low water content of stratum corneum. Fractional photothermolysis has shown to be effective in photoaging, dyschromia, scarring, poikiloderma, and rhytides.[52] For patients with skin of color, PIH is of particular concern and studies have shown that treatment density rather than energy is the strongest determining factor.[53] In skin of color, the principle of reducing posttreatment erythema to minimize the risk of PIH is important. Therefore, the authors emphasize that a reduction in energy and density as well as increasing the number of treatments can help with reduction of risk of PIH and can still yield efficacious clinical results.

Nonablative skin rejuvenation with laser and light source has become popular in skin of color with less downtime and limited risks of complications. Nonablative rejuvenation involves lasers or light source with the use of a cooling device to protect the epidermis reducing the risk of erythema and oedema that may lead to PIH. This targets and improves signs of photoaging including lentigines, telangiectasia, pore size, wrinkles, skin texture, and skin laxity. A combination of lasers are usually deployed including PDL, Nd:YAG, 1450 nm diode, 1540 nm erbium:glass, and radiofrequency.[54,55] To avoid cumulative heat generation, lower fluency is used. Monthly treatments are required for good effect.

Intradermal high energy focal point technology involves the use of intradermal 1550 nm laser focusing that allows much higher energy (FDA approved 150 mJ) to be delivered to the dermis with relative sparring of the epidermis. In doing so, it can be particularly applicable to skin rejuvenation among skin of color.

TATTOO REMOVAL [FIGURE 95-5]

The estimated overall prevalence of tattooing is around 10% to 20% in the United States, Europe, or Australia.[56] Laser-assisted removal is considered the gold-standard treatment for tattoo removal. Tattoos are amenable to laser removal but factors such as tattoo color, tattoo composition (such as containing heavy metals), professional or amateur tattooist affect the number of sessions required for removal. Complications such as PIH, partial removal, and sometimes even scarring can occur.

A particular laser wavelength can be chosen depending on the absorption spectrum of the ink. In skin of color, black tattoo ink is treated with 1064 nm laser (picosecond 1064 nm laser, spot size 4-8 mm, fluence 0.8-3.5 J/cm^2). Picosecond laser also has advantages of over nanosecond lasers due to greater degree of photomechanical effect, allowing for more effective destruction without greater risk of complication.[57] In addition to PS laser, fractional laser can be deployed to reduce the risk of blister formation that can be associated with PS laser (PS 755 nm alexandrite laser, spot size 3.5-3.8 mm, fluence 1.76-2.08 J/cm^2, nonablative fractional laser 1550 nm, 50-65 mJ).[58]

Red inks are best treated with 532 nm laser (picosecond 532 nm, spot size 4-8mm, fluence 0.4-0.6 J/cm^2), and green tattoos are best treated with 755 nm lasers (picosecond 755 nm alexandrite, spot size 3.6 mm, fluence 1.96 J/cm^2).

In cases where an allergic reaction develops at the site of tattoo, surgical removal of tattoo, or ablative laser is recommended. Skin colored or white ink tattoos may contain ferric oxide and can undergo immediate darkening reduction to ferrous oxide by Q-switched lasers.[59] Therefore, a test spot should be deployed prior to treating the whole tattoo. Caution should be taken in patients who are keloid prone and those who have taking oral isotretinoin in the last 6 months. Tattoo ink using combustible ingredients such as gunpowder or fireworks can also ignite when treated with Q-switched lasers.[60]

NONINVASIVE BODY CONTOURING

Noninvasive body contouring is gaining popularity over traditional liposuction in body contouring due to high safety profile and limited recovery time, although multiple sessions are generally required. Four major categories exist for noninvasive body contouring devices that decrease adipose tissue and they include high-intensity focused ultrasound (HIFU), radiofrequency, cryolipolysis, and laser.

HIGH-INTENSITY FOCUSED ULTRASOUND

HIFU uses the nonionizing ultrasonic waves to heat up and destroy adipose tissue while sparing superficial and surrounding structure. At high frequencies (2 MHz), the ultrasound energy targets tissue at a specific depth focusing injury to a focal point, causing thermal effects and mechanical coagulative necrosis of adipocyte, which are then engulfed and removed by macrophages. Apart from adipocyte apoptosis, HIFU can induce gradual skin tightening through collagen contraction and remodeling.[61] HIFU has been reported to be associated with erythema, edema, induration, bruising that is temporary, and pain during treatment.[62] In rare cases, fibrosis has been reported.[63]

Pulsed (nonthermal) focused ultrasound transmits bursts of pulsed ultrasonic energy allowing for precise control over temperature elevation ($<0.5°C$) and allow for mechanical fat destruction in the selective subcutaneous fat layer. The selective damage to adipocyte leaves surrounding tissues unharmed and maybe more favorable as it lacks the typical adverse effects associated with thermal-based treatment modalities as discussed above.[64]

RADIOFREQUENCY

The use of radiofrequency (RF) is based on oscillating electrical current forcing collisions between charged molecules and ions that are then converted to heat.[65] It is independent of skin type and chromophore and not dependent on selective photothermolysis. RF devices causes skin tightening via collagen remodeling, and volumetric heating of fat leading to adipocyte death, sparing the overlying epidermal and dermal tissue with effecting cooling of the epidermis. RF can be delivered using monopolar, bipolar, and unipolar devices. In monopolar devices, the patient is grounded with RF delivered through the skin into the body and ending with grounding electrode. This is why patients who have indwelling metal devices such as pacemakers, or hip and knee replacement, are not candidates for RF devices. In clinical practice, the authors find that using unipolar RF device with multiple passes with lower energy resulted in less pain and more tolerable for patients.[65]

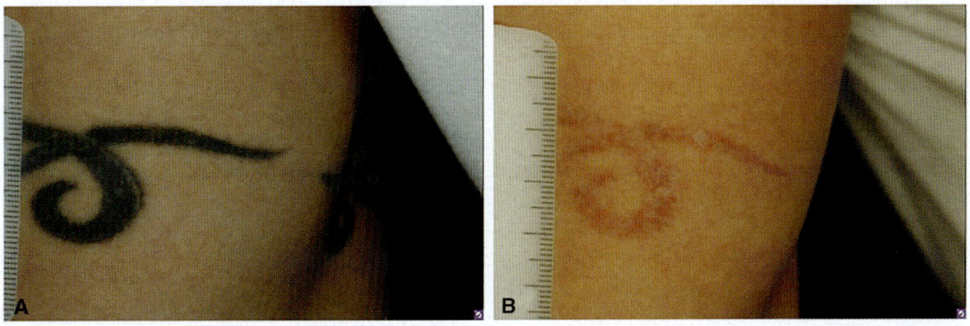

FIGURE 95-5. Tattoo **(A)** and **(B)** 4 months post 7th laser treatment.

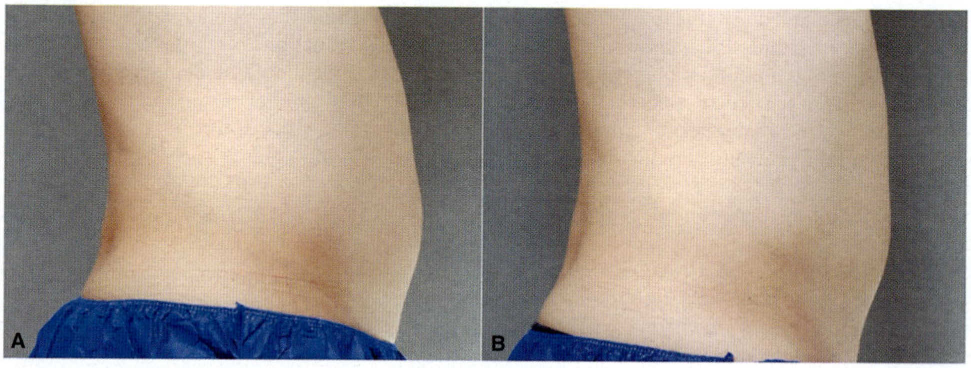

FIGURE 95-6. Cryolipolysis on body contouring. **(A)** Abdomen at baseline and **(B)** 3 months after two treatments.

CRYOLIPOLYSIS [FIGURE 95-6]

Cryolipolysis involves the controlled cooling of adipose cells to temperature below normal, but above freezing, to induce adiposity apoptosis without compromising the epidermis or dermis. The inflammatory response occurs 72 hours after treatment, and fat reduction gradually occurs between 30 and 90 days after treatment.[66] Localization of undesirable fat is first identified, and an applicator is applied to the area and sucks the bulge into a vacuum after applying coupling gel, and selected cooling then targets the adipose tissue. Side effects are usually temporary and include bruising, erythema, pain, and numbness.

LASER

The 1060-nm high-energy diode laser with cooling delivery delivers laser energy to adipose cells and induces injury at 42 to 47°C. The subsequent laser delivery and cooling protects the outer layer of the skin. The maximum number of applicators applied is 4, and the authors use one 25-minute treatment cycle to the abdominal area. Side effects include discomfort during treatment, redness, temporary nodules, and even burns and prolonged tenderness.[67]

COMMON SKIN DISORDERS

ACNE VULGARIS

In skin of color, acne hyperpigmentation can persist for months or even longer. Ice-pick scarring and hypertrophic, keloidal scarring can affect a patient's self-esteem and have significant psychosocial impact.[68] In terms of lasers and light therapy in acne vulgaris, ablative lasers have been shown to be effective in treating atrophic scars, but in skin of color, hyperpigmentation and significant downtime can be a problem. Blue light activates endogenous porphyrins in Propionibacterium acne and kills the bacteria, but in skin of color increased pigmentation can occur after prolonged blue light exposure.[52,54] Photodynamic therapy using short contact aminolaevulinic acid (10-hour occlusion) followed by activation using an IPL source has been demonstrated to be effective in Asians, but erythema can be a complication.[54] Fractional photothermolysis as discussed earlier can also be a treatment option for treatment of acne scarring and skin rejuvenation, with emphasis on high energy, and low-density treatment being preferred, and adjunctive cooling.

Novel therapy with 1726-nm laser with epidermal contact cooling has recently been demonstrated to induce selective photothermolysis of sebaceous glands in the treatment of mild to moderate acne vulgaris.[69] Goldberg et al demonstrated that the high-power 1726-nm laser reduced the total number of inflammatory lesions by more than 52% within 1 month of treatment and 56% by third-month post final laser treatment.[70]

HYPERTROPHIC SCARRING AND KELOID SCARRING

Skin of color tends to have larger and more numerous fibroblasts with increased activity, resulting in higher occurrence of hypertrophic and keloidal scarring. Silicone gel and sheets are used with some success. Intralesional corticosteroids have been established in treating hypertrophic and keloidal scars every 4 to 6 weeks, but clinicians must be aware for potential side effects including skin atrophy, telangiectasia, and pigmentary changes. As vascular proliferation plays a key role in scar formation, the 595 nm PDL is used to improve scar color, texture, and pruritus. This can be used in combination with intralesional corticosteroid or combined with 5-fluorouracil. Longer pulse duration, with conservative fluences to achieve subpurpuric result is recommended.

PSORIASIS

Psoriasis is more common in Caucasians than in Asians and Africans. Treatment ranges from conventional topical therapies including corticosteroid, tar, calcipotriene, to light therapy (ultraviolet-B light and psoralen plus UVA [PUVA]), oral immunosuppressants, and biologics.

VASCULAR DISORDERS

Vascular lesions including salmon patch, port wine stain (PWS), vascular malformation, and hemangiomas are difficult to treat in skin of color as melanin acts as a competing chromophore for hemoglobin. As a result, PIH, hypopigmentation, and atrophic scarring may present as side effect post PDL.[71] The use of epidermal cooling, extended pulse duration in PDL, and fractional resurfacing has led to improved clinical outcome and reduction in side effects.

Different laser devices can be used for vascular lesions including 532 nm Nd:YAG, 585/595 nm PDL, LP 755 nm Alex laser, LP 1964 nm ND:YAG laser, IPL, and fractional resurfacing. The choice of wavelength, fluence, pulse duration, spot size, and skin cooling techniques depends on the type of vascular lesion and skin type. It is crucial that test spots are performed on patients prior to treatment of the whole lesion—this allows for determination of fluence for the best clinical outcome. Stacked of double pulsing is not recommended, and patients should return 1 month to review outcome of test spot. The aim of subpurpuric tissue response is optimal, and a transient violaceous discoloration post PDL laser is normal. Patients should be counselled on limitation to sun exposure, heat, and exercise to prevent recanalization of blood vessels after laser treatment.

PORT WINE STAIN [FIGURE 95-7]

Wavelength Longer wavelengths penetrate into deeper tissue. In skin of color, 532 nm Nd:YAG or long-pulsed nm PDL is used to treat more superficial telangiectasia, while shorter wavelength treatments should be avoided in the treatment of PWS and hemangiomas.

595 nm PDL equipped with cooling is the ideal laser for treating PWS in skin of color as it allows for deeper penetration into the dermis targeting ectatic vasculature of PWS.[72] LP 755 nm Alex laser together with LP 595 nm PDL has been demonstrated to be effective in PWS cases that are resistant to PDL.[73] 1064 nm Nd:YAG laser has demonstrated to be effected in the treatment for hypertrophic PWS on the lips to minimize discoloration caused by PDL.[74]

Pulse Duration Based on the principle of selective thermolysis, pulse duration should be equal or less than the thermal relaxation time of the

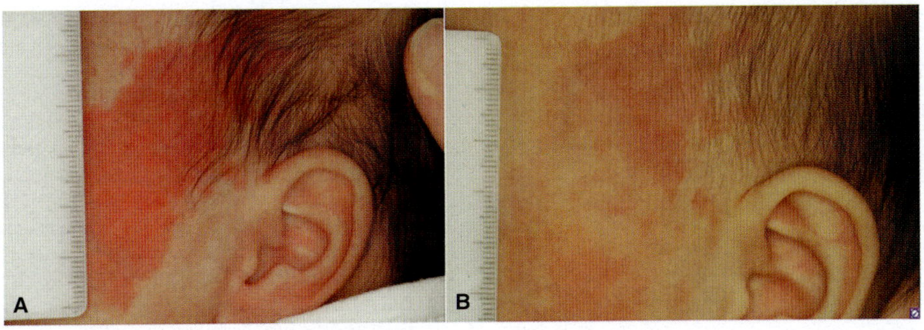

FIGURE 95-7. Port wine stain **(A)** and **(B)** one month post 5th laser treatment.

blood vessels being treated. For smaller vessels (≤20 μm), a pulse duration of 450 μs is adequate, while larger vessels (30-150 μm) should have a pulse duration of approximately 1 to 10 ms.[75] In the treatment of PWS, purpura is the target endpoint.

Spot Size Larger spot size of laser allows for greater depth of thermal injury using the same fluence, and lesser degree of scattering. In general, when using PDL, IPL, 532 nm Nd:YAG lasers, larger spot size (>10 cm) can be used, whereas smaller spot size should be used when using alexandrite and 1064 nm Nd:YAG lasers to reduce the risk of bulk tissue heating that can lead to scarring.

Epidermal Cooling Epidermal cooling is defined as the use of cooling substance to lower the skin surface temperature before, during, and after laser therapy. It has been shown to reduce thermal injury to epidermis and improve the clinical efficacy of vascular lasers. The development of dynamic cooling with Cryogen Spray Cooling (CSC), where a cryogen spurt is applied to the skin surface, reduces the skin surface temperature from 30°C to 0 to −5°C for epidermal cooling, leaving the temperature of deeper PWS vessels unchanged. Chang et al demonstrated that epidermal cooling enhanced clinical efficacy and higher fluence was achieved without increase in side effects.[76]

PWS Redarkening Unfortunately, despite clinical response of treatment with PWS, redarkening of PWS can occur. Redarkening of PWS has been hypothesized to several reasons; natural darkening with age from progressive ectasia of remaining vessels; neovascularization resulting from posttreatment thrombus formation; and angiogenesis from deeper parts of PWS that were unreachable from PDL.[77]

Combing PDL with antiangiogenic agents has been tried including imiquimod,[78] and topical and oral rapamycin has yielded some success.[79,80]

Hemangiomas Hemangiomas are benign vascular tumors characterized by a rapid intermittent growth phase usually within first year of life, reaching its maximum size by 9 months of age, followed by spontaneous involution and resolution in majority of cases. During the proliferation phase, complications may arise including bleeding, ulceration, infection, or even obstruction to organs.[81] Treatment includes topical β-blocker, topical and oral glucocorticoids, intralesional steroid injections, lasers, and surgical excision.

In general, β-blockers are the first choice for treatment of hemangiomas. If lasers are considered during the weaning of β-blocker to counteract potential rebound growth of the hemangioma, 595 nm PDL can be considered, and this is patient variable. The number of laser treatments depends on the lesion response and the target is subpurpuric changes in the skin as with PWS lesions.

CONCLUSION

We have discussed how skin structures and function vary in patients with skin of color and how this poses a challenge when using lasers and light therapy in treatment of different dermatological conditions. An understanding of laser and light treatment in skin of color including test spots, skin cooling, lower fluence, and postoperative advice on skin care and sun avoidance is imperative in achieving good clinical outcomes and preventing unwanted side effects.

REFERENCES

1. Brown X, Rucker JM, Richeson JA. Political ideology moderates White Americans' reactions to racial demographic change. *Group Process Intergroup Relat*. 2022;25(3):642-660.
2. Houk LD, Humphreys T. Masers to magic bullets: an updated history of lasers in dermatology. *Clin Dermatol*. 2007;25(5):434-442.
3. Geiges ML. History of lasers in dermatology. *Curr Probl Dermatol*. 2011;42:1-6.
4. Arndt KA, Noe JM. Lasers in dermatology. *Arch Dermatol*. 1982;118(5):293-295.
5. Anderson RR, Parrish JA. Selective photothermolysis: precise microsurgery by selective absorption of pulsed radiation. *Science*. 1983;220(4596):524-527.
6. Anderson RR, Parrish JA. The optics of human skin. *J Invest Dermatol*. 1981;77(1):13-19.
7. Chung JH. Photoaging in Asians. *Photodermatol Photoimmunol Photomed*. 2003;19(3):109-121.
8. Chan HH, Fung WK, Ying SY, Kono T. An in vivo trial comparing the use of different types of 532 nm Nd:YAG lasers in the treatment of facial lentigines in Oriental patients. *Dermatol Surg*. 2000;26(8):743-749.
9. Wang CC, Sue YM, Yang CH, Chen CK. A comparison of Q-switched alexandrite laser and intense pulsed light for the treatment of freckles and lentigines in Asian persons: a randomized, physician-blinded, split-face comparative trial. *J Am Acad Dermatol*. 2006;54(5):804-810.
10. Kono T, Shek SY, Chan HH, Groff WF, Imagawa K, Akamatsu T. Theoretical review of the treatment of pigmented lesions in Asian skin. *Laser Ther*. 2016;25(3):179-184.
11. Chan MWM, Shek SY, Yeung CK, Chan HH. A prospective study in the treatment of lentigines in Asian skin using 532 nm picosecond Nd:YAG laser. *Lasers Surg Med*. 2019;51(9):767-773.
12. Kono T, Chan HH, Groff WF, et al. Long-pulse pulsed dye laser delivered with compression for treatment of facial lentigines. *Dermatol Surg*. 2007;33(8):945-950.
13. Shek SY, Negishi K, Tanaka S, Yeung CK, Chan HHL. A prospective multicenter study of a dual-wavelength laser picosecond for the treatment of melasma and lentigines in Asian skin. *Lasers Surg Med*. 2016;48(4):421.
14. Kundu RV, Joshi SS, Suh KY, et al. Comparison of electrodesiccation and potassium-titanyl-phosphate laser for treatment of dermatosis papulosa nigra. *Dermatol Surg*. 2009;35(7):1079-1083.
15. Geronemus RG. Q-switched ruby laser therapy of nevus of Ota. *Arch Dermatol*. 1992;128(12):1618-1622.
16. Chan HH, Leung RS, Ying SY, et al. A retrospective analysis of complications in the treatment of nevus of Ota with the Q-switched alexandrite and Q-switched Nd:YAG lasers. *Dermatol Surg*. 2000;26(11):1000-1006.
17. Aurangabadkar S. QYAG5 Q-switched Nd:YAG laser treatment of Nevus of Ota: an Indian study of 50 patients. *J Cutan Aesthet Surg*. 2008;1(2):80-84.
18. Hu S, Yang CS, Chang SL, Huang YL, Lin YF, Lee MC. Efficacy and safety of the picosecond 755-nm alexandrite laser for treatment of dermal pigmentation in Asians-a retrospective study. *Lasers Med Sci*. 2020;35(6):1377-1383.
19. Sakio R, Ohshiro T, Sasaki K, Ohshiro T. Usefulness of picosecond pulse alexandrite laser treatment for nevus of Ota. *Laser Ther*. 2018;27(4):251-255.
20. Chan HH, King WW, Chan ES, et al. In vivo trial comparing patients' tolerance of Q-switched Alexandrite (QS Alex) and Q-switched neodymium:yttrium-aluminum-garnet (QS Nd:YAG) lasers in the treatment of nevus of Ota. *Lasers Surg Med*. 1999;24(1):24-28.
21. Chan HH, Ying SY, Ho WS, Kono T, King WW. An in vivo trial comparing the clinical efficacy and complications of Q-switched 755 nm alexandrite and Q-switched 1064 nm Nd:YAG lasers in the treatment of nevus of Ota. *Dermatol Surg*. 2000;26(10):919-922.

22. Kono T, Chan HH, Ercocen AR, et al. Use of Q-switched ruby laser in the treatment of nevus of ota in different age groups. *Lasers Surg Med.* 2003;32(5):391-395.
23. Kaur H, Sarma P, Kaur S, et al. Therapeutic options for management of Hori's nevus: a systematic review. *Dermatol Ther.* 2020;33(1):e13167.
24. Chan JC, Shek SY, Kono T, Yeung CK, Chan HH. A retrospective analysis on the management of pigmented lesions using a picosecond 755-nm alexandrite laser in Asians. *Lasers Surg Med.* 2016;48(1):23-29.
25. Kim EH, Kim YC, Lee ES, Kang HY. The vascular characteristics of melasma. *J Dermatol Sci.* 2007;46(2):111-116.
26. Arellano I, Cestari T, Ocampo-Candiani J, et al. Preventing melasma recurrence: prescribing a maintenance regimen with an effective triple combination cream based on long-standing clinical severity. *J Eur Acad Dermatol Venereol.* 2012;26(5):611-618.
27. Bandyopadhyay D. Topical treatment of melasma. *Indian J Dermatol.* 2009;54(4):303-309.
28. Cestari T, Arellano I, Hexsel D, Ortonne JP, Latin American Pigmentary Disorders A. Melasma in Latin America: options for therapy and treatment algorithm. *J Eur Acad Dermatol Venereol.* 2009;23(7):760-772.
29. Rivas S, Pandya AG. Treatment of melasma with topical agents, peels and lasers: an evidence-based review. *Am J Clin Dermatol.* 2013;14(5):359-376.
30. Maeda K, Tomita Y. Mechanism of the inhibitory effect of tranexamic acid on melanogenesis in cultured human melanocytes in the presence of keratinocyte-conditioned medium. *J Health Sci.* 2007;53(4):389-396.
31. Na JI, Choi SY, Yang SH, Choi HR, Kang HY, Park KC. Effect of tranexamic acid on melasma: a clinical trial with histological evaluation. *J Eur Acad Dermatol Venereol.* 2013;27(8):1035-1039.
32. Tse TW, Hui E. Tranexamic acid: an important adjuvant in the treatment of melasma. *J Cosmet Dermatol.* 2013;12(1):57-66.
33. Lee HC, Thng TG, Goh CL. Oral tranexamic acid (TA) in the treatment of melasma: a retrospective analysis. *J Am Acad Dermatol.* 2016;75(2):385-392.
34. Halachmi S, Haedersdal M, Lapidoth M. Melasma and laser treatment: an evidenced-based analysis. *Lasers Med Sci.* 2014;29(2):589-598.
35. Shankar K, Godse K, Aurangabadkar S, et al. Evidence-based treatment for melasma: expert opinion and a review. *Dermatol Ther (Heidelb).* 2014;4(2):165-186.
36. Lee HS, Won CH, Lee DH, et al. Treatment of melasma in Asian skin using a fractional 1,550-nm laser: an open clinical study. *Dermatol Surg.* 2009;35(10):1499-1504.
37. Ho SG, Yeung CK, Chan NP, Shek SY, Chan HH. A retrospective study of the management of Chinese melasma patients using a 1927 nm fractional thulium fiber laser. *J Cosmet Laser Ther.* 2013;15(4):200-206.
38. Yoshimura K, Sato K, Aiba-Kojima E, et al. Repeated treatment protocols for melasma and acquired dermal melanocytosis. *Dermatol Surg.* 2006;32(3): 365-371.
39. Cho SB, Kim JS, Kim MJ. Melasma treatment in Korean women using a 1064-nm Q-switched Nd:YAG laser with low pulse energy. *Clin Exp Dermatol.* 2009;34(8):e847-850.
40. Angsuwarangsee S, Polnikorn N. Combined ultrapulse CO2 laser and Q-switched alexandrite laser compared with Q-switched alexandrite laser alone for refractory melasma: split-face design. *Dermatol Surg.* 2003;29(1):59-64.
41. Nouri K, Bowes L, Chartier T, Romagosa R, Spencer J. Combination treatment of melasma with pulsed CO2 laser followed by Q-switched alexandrite laser: a pilot study. *Dermatol Surg.* 1999;25(6):494-497.
42. Manaloto RM, Alster T. Erbium:YAG laser resurfacing for refractory melasma. *Dermatol Surg.* 1999;25(2):121-123.
43. Lee HI, Lim YY, Kim BJ, et al. Clinicopathologic efficacy of copper bromide plus/yellow laser (578 nm with 511 nm) for treatment of melasma in Asian patients. *Dermatol Surg.* 2010;36(6):885-893.
44. Chan NP, Ho SG, Shek SY, Yeung CK, Chan HH. A case series of facial depigmentation associated with low fluence Q-switched 1,064 nm Nd:YAG laser for skin rejuvenation and melasma. *Lasers Surg Med.* 2010;42(8):712-719.
45. Kim MJ, Kim JS, Cho SB. Punctate leucoderma after melasma treatment using 1064-nm Q-switched Nd:YAG laser with low pulse energy. *J Eur Acad Dermatol Venereol.* 2009;23(8):960-962.
46. Lee YJ, Shin HJ, Noh TK, Choi KH, Chang SE. Treatment of melasma and post-inflammatory hyperpigmentation by a Picosecond 755-nm Alexandrite laser in Asian patients. *Ann Dermatol.* 2017;29(6):779-781.
47. Wong CSM, Chan MWM, Shek SYN, Yeung CK, Chan HHL. Fractional 1064 nm picosecond laser in treatment of melasma and skin rejuvenation in Asians, a prospective study. *Lasers Surg Med.* 2021;53(8):1032-1042.
48. Na SY, Cho S, Lee JH. Intense pulsed light and low-fluence Q-switched Nd:YAG laser treatment in melasma patients. *Ann Dermatol.* 2012;24(3):267-273.
49. Cho HH, Choi M, Cho S, Lee JH. Role of oral tranexamic acid in melasma patients treated with IPL and low fluence QS Nd:YAG laser. *J Dermatolog Treat.* 2013;24(4):292-296.
50. Nanni CA, Alster TS. Complications of carbon dioxide laser resurfacing. An evaluation of 500 patients. *Dermatol Surg.* 1998;24(3):315-320.
51. Manstein D, Herron GS, Sink RK, Tanner H, Anderson RR. Fractional photothermolysis: a new concept for cutaneous remodeling using microscopic patterns of thermal injury. *Lasers Surg Med.* 2004;34(5):426-438.
52. Tierney EP, Kouba DJ, Hanke CW. Review of fractional photothermolysis: treatment indications and efficacy. *Dermatol Surg.* 2009;35(10):1445-1461.
53. Kono T, Chan HH, Groff WF, et al. Prospective direct comparison study of fractional resurfacing using different fluences and densities for skin rejuvenation in Asians. *Lasers Surg Med.* 2007;39(4):311-314.
54. Chan HH. Effective and safe use of lasers, light sources, and radiofrequency devices in the clinical management of Asian patients with selected dermatoses. *Lasers Surg Med.* 2005;37(3):179-185.
55. Alam M, Hsu TS, Dover JS, Wrone DA, Arndt KA. Nonablative laser and light treatments: histology and tissue effects–a review. *Lasers Surg Med.* 2003;33(1):30-39.
56. Kluger N. Epidemiology of tattoos in industrialized countries. *Curr Probl Dermatol.* 2015;48:6-20.
57. Ross V, Naseef G, Lin G, et al. Comparison of responses of tattoos to picosecond and nanosecond Q-switched neodymium: YAG lasers. *Arch Dermatol.* 1998;134(2):167-171.
58. Au S, Liolios AM, Goldman MP. Analysis of incidence of bulla formation after tattoo treatment using the combination of the picosecond Alexandrite laser and fractionated CO2 ablation. *Dermatol Surg.* 2015;41(2):242-245.
59. Anderson RR, Geronemus R, Kilmer SL, Farinelli W, Fitzpatrick RE. Cosmetic tattoo ink darkening. A complication of Q-switched and pulsed-laser treatment. *Arch Dermatol.* 1993;129(8):1010-1014.
60. Taylor CR. Laser ignition of traumatically embedded firework debris. *Lasers Surg Med.* 1998;22(3):157-158.
61. Minkis K, Alam M. Ultrasound skin tightening. *Dermatol Clin.* 2014;32(1):71-77.
62. Shek SY, Yeung CK, Chan JC, Chan HH. Efficacy of high-intensity focused ultrasonography for noninvasive body sculpting in Chinese patients. *Lasers Surg Med.* 2014;46(4):263-269.
63. Greenhaw BN, Cook J. Painful subcutaneous fibrosis: a complication after high-intensity focused ultrasound for lipolysis. *Dermatol Surg.* 2015;41(6):744-746.
64. Weinstein Velez M, Ibrahim O, Petrell K, Dover JS. Nonthermal pulsed ultrasound treatment for the reduction in abdominal fat: a pilot study. *J Clin Aesthet Dermatol.* 2018;11(9):32-36.
65. Weiss RA. Noninvasive radio frequency for skin tightening and body contouring. *Semin Cutan Med Surg.* 2013;32(1):9-17.
66. Jewell ML, Solish NJ, Desilets CS. Noninvasive body sculpting technologies with an emphasis on high-intensity focused ultrasound. *Aesthetic Plast Surg.* 2011;35(5):901-912.
67. Bass LS, Doherty ST. Safety and efficacy of a non-invasive 1060 nm diode laser for fat reduction of the abdomen. *J Drugs Dermatol.* 2018;17(1):106-112.
68. Taylor SC, Cook-Bolden F, Rahman Z, Strachan D. Acne vulgaris in skin of color. *J Am Acad Dermatol.* 2002;46(2 Suppl Understanding):S98-106.
69. Scopelliti MG, Kothare A, Karavitis M. A novel 1726-nm laser system for safe and effective treatment of acne vulgaris. *Lasers Med Sci.* 2022;37(9):3639-3647.
70. Goldberg D, Kothare A, Doucette M, et al. Selective photothermolysis with a novel 1726 nm laser beam: a safe and effective solution for acne vulgaris. *J Cosmet Dermatol.* 2023;22(2):486-496.
71. Sommer S, Sheehan-Dare RA. Pulsed dye laser treatment of port-wine stains in pigmented skin. *J Am Acad Dermatol.* 2000;42(4):667-671.
72. Brightman LA, Geronemus RG, Reddy KK. Laser treatment of port-wine stains. *Clin Cosmet Investig Dermatol.* 2015;8:27-33.
73. Izikson L, Nelson JS, Anderson RR. Treatment of hypertrophic and resistant port wine stains with a 755 nm laser: a case series of 20 patients. *Lasers Surg Med.* 2009;41(6):427-432.
74. Kono T, Frederick Groff W, Chan HH, Sakurai H, Yamaki T. Long-pulsed neodymium:yttrium-aluminum-garnet laser treatment for hypertrophic port-wine stains on the lips. *J Cosmet Laser Ther.* 2009;11(1):11-13.
75. Kenneth A. Arndt, Jeffrey S. Dover, Suzanne M. Olbricht. Lasers in cutaneous and aesthetic surgery. Philadelphia, Pa.; Lippincott-Raven Publishers, *New York*, 1997:36-41.
76. Chang CJ, Nelson JS. Cryogen spray cooling and higher fluence pulsed dye laser treatment improve port-wine stain clearance while minimizing epidermal damage. *Dermatol Surg.* 1999;25(10):767-772.
77. Huikeshoven M, Koster PH, de Borgie CA, Beek JF, van Gemert MJ, van der Horst CM. Redarkening of port-wine stains 10 years after pulsed-dye-laser treatment. *N Engl J Med.* 2007;356(12):1235-1240.
78. Chang CJ, Hsiao YC, Mihm MC Jr, Nelson JS. Pilot study examining the combined use of pulsed dye laser and topical Imiquimod versus laser alone for treatment of port wine stain birthmarks. *Lasers Surg Med.* 2008;40(9):605-610.

79. Griffin TD Jr, Foshee JP, Finney R, Saedi N. Port wine stain treated with a combination of pulsed dye laser and topical rapamycin ointment. *Lasers Surg Med*. 2016;48(2):193-196.
80. Nelson JS, Jia W, Phung TL, Mihm MC Jr. Observations on enhanced port wine stain blanching induced by combined pulsed dye laser and rapamycin administration. *Lasers Surg Med*. 2011;43(10):939-942.
81. Drolet BA, Esterly NB, Frieden IJ. Hemangiomas in children. *N Engl J Med*. 1999;341(3):173-181.

CHAPTER 96

Soft Tissue Augmentation and Neuromodulators

Janeth R. Campbell
Alicia Edwards
Valerie Callender
Cheryl Burgess

KEY POINTS

- Individuals of racial minorities underwent 34% of the cosmetic procedures performed in the United States 2020.
- Hispanics account for 13%, Blacks 11%, Asians 8%, and other non-White 2% of all cosmetic procedures.
- Although photodamage is less of a concern in skin of color, all races experience brow furrows, frown lines, and crow feet from repeated facial muscle contractions that are amenable to relaxation with botulinum toxin treatment.
- Soft tissue augmentation with dermal fillers is used in the treatment and correction of fine lines, nasolabial fold creases, marionette lines, tear trough depressions, lip augmentation, volume loss, and acne scars in the skin of color population.

INTRODUCTION

By 2044, the U.S. Census Bureau predicts that the United States will be more racially and ethnically pluralistic.[1] This demographic trend, in addition to increased awareness and availability of cosmetic treatments, has in turn led to an increase in the number of people of color (POC) receiving aesthetic services. According to the 2019 Aesthetic Plastic Surgery National Databank Statistics report, 32% of procedures were performed on racial minorities, a 2% increase from 2018 report.[2,3] Given that clinicians are performing more cosmetic procedures on POC, acquiring a comprehensive understanding of aesthetics used within ethnic populations is imperative. Of the non-surgical cosmetic procedures, soft-tissue fillers and neuromodulators are of growing popularity in the aesthetic industry. In 2017, botulinum toxin and soft tissue augmentation were, respectively, the first and second most sought after minimally invasive procedures.[4] This chapter seeks to provide an overview of the evidence, skin characteristics, anatomical variations, aesthetic preferences, and augmentation strategies regarding soft-tissue fillers and neuromodulators in POC. Importantly, this chapter defines POC as individuals with darker skin tones, in the range of Fitzpatrick IV to VI phototypes. This includes but is not limited to those of Asian, African, Hispanic/Latino, Middle Eastern, and mixed racial (bi- and multiracial) backgrounds. The descriptions herein will be comparisons to the European White population.

EVIDENCE FOR SOFT TISSUE FILLER USE IN POC

Informed use of soft tissue fillers and neuromodulators in POC begins with clinicians reviewing the literature on these procedures to practice evidence-based medicine. Soft tissue fillers, also known as dermal fillers, are used to augment facial volume, contour, and definition. They are ideal to address midface aging-associated changes and temporal fossa hollowing. The U.S. Food and Drug Administration (FDA) has approved 13 brands of soft tissue fillers for the treatment of nasolabial folds, cheeks, chin, lips, and/or dorsal hands.[5] According to the FDA, fillers may contain absorbable or nonabsorbable material. Common absorbable, nonpermanent material includes hyaluronic acid (HA), calcium hydroxyapatite (CAHA), and poly-l-lactic acid (PLLA). Polymethylmethacrylate beads (PMMA) is a nonabsorbable or permanent filler. Of these, HA is the most injected type of filler.[5] CAHA and PLLA increase collagen and elastin formation through fibroplasia, ultimately leading to dermal remodeling.[6] Five clinical studies have demonstrated that soft tissue augmentation with certain types of filler can be quite successful in POC.

Through a randomized, evaluator-blinded, split-face trial, Taylor et al examined nonanimal stabilized HA filler to correct moderate to severe nasolabial folds in Fitzpatrick skin phototypes (FST) IV to VI. This study enrolled 150 patients at 10 sites. Clinicians used a fan, linear threading approach or droplet with serial puncture technique for injections. Large-particle gel HA filler was injected into the deep dermis to the superficial subcutaneous tissue, while small-particle gel HA filler was injected into the mid to deep dermis. Efficacy was maintained at 24 weeks, and only mild pigmentation changes occurred in 6% of the large-particle gel group, and 9% of the small-particle gel group. Pigmentation changes were associated with multiple or serial puncture sites. Notably, slowing of injection time reduced pigmentation changes. All but three patients had resolution of pigmentation changes in 12 weeks.[7]

To evaluate the use of CAHA filler for the correction of facial wrinkles and folds in FST IV to VI, Marmur et al conducted an open-label, nonrandomized prospective trial. Specifically, 100 patients were included to undergo treatment for the nasolabial folds with 0.6 to 2.8 mL CAHA injected subdermally with a 24- to 27- gauge needle. No keloid formation, hypertrophic scarring, hypo- or hyperpigmentation, or any other adverse events were reported at 3- and 6-month evaluations. Deeper injections used for CAHA could have contributed to the lack of pigmentation side effects.[8]

Downie et al enrolled a total of 93 subjects into an open-label, multicenter trial to assess the safety of a cohesive, polydensified HA filler for nasolabial fold treatment in FST IV to VI. The left nasolabial fold was injected with 1.46 mL, while the right was injected with 1.47 mL. Seventy-two percent of patients required touch up at week 2. Improvement in the Wrinkle Severity Rating Sale and the Global Aesthetic Improvement scale was observed. While one patient developed mild hypopigmentation, and two developed mile hyperpigmentation, there was no association found between cohesive polydensified HA filler and pigment changes or scarring.[9]

More recently, two clinical trials examined the safety and effectiveness of HA fillers for lip and perioral augmentation.[10,11] While these trials looked at all FST, Taylor et al pooled the data for phototypes IV to VI for a meta-analysis. The subjects were injected with 1.58 mL of filler, with 55.8% requiring a touch up. Data from 72 participants showed similar effectiveness of HA fillers for lip and perioral augmentation when compared to all phototypes from the original studies. Numerically, at 3 months the mean Lip Fullness Scale improved by 1.1, which was sustained at 6 months. It was also found that FST IV to VI experienced fewer side effects than participants of lower phototypes.[12]

While these five clinical trials detail the safe and effective use of some dermal fillers in POC, there are currently no controlled studies regarding the use of PLLA fillers in this population.

EVIDENCE FOR NEUROMODULATORS USE IN POC

Neuromodulators are commonly used to treat lines of facial expression in POC. Movements of underlying facial muscles, such as the corrugator superciliaris and/or procerus muscles lead to the creation of glabellar lines that are a sign of aging.[13] The U.S. FDA has approved Botulinum

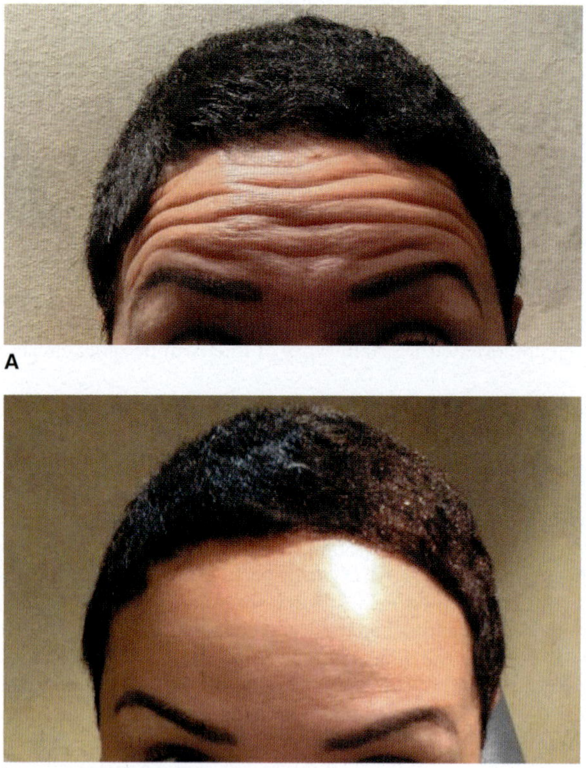

A

B

FIGURE 96-1. (A and B) Botulinum toxin A to relax the glabellar complex and forehead muscles. (Used with permission from Cheryl Burgess, MD, FAAD.)

toxin type A (BoNTA) for the treatment of frown lines and crow feet. BoNTA inhibits the release of acetylcholine into the synaptic cleft that paralyzes muscles temporarily. BoNTA containing neurotoxins, onabotulinumtoxinA, abobotulinumtoxinA, prabotulinumtoxinA, incobotulinumtoxinA, and daxibotulinumtoxinA, have also been approved by the FDA to treat glabellar lines. OnabulinumtoxinA (BoNTA-ABO) is the only FDA-approved treatment of lateral canthal lines (LCL) and forehead frontalis lines. The corrugator, crow feet, forehead, platysmal neckbands, and the marionette lines are frequent sites of neuromodulator injection[14] [**Figure 96-1**]. There is limited U.S. clinical data available on the use of neuromodulators in POC.

Grimes et al conducted a randomized control trial of 31 African American women (FST IV and V) to evaluate the degree and duration of efficacy of 20 and 30 U of BoNTA for the treatment of glabellar lines. Wrinkle severity was graded by both the investigator and patient using a four-point facial wrinkle scale. BoNTA was injected into the procerus muscle, each corrugator muscle, and a site above the midpupillary line on each side. After 120 days, it was concluded that 20 and 30 U of BoNTA demonstrated efficacy and safety in African American women with skin types V and VI. Adverse events were mild and transient and did not differ between the groups.[15]

In a meta-analysis of six clinical trials, Taylor et al aimed to compare the effectiveness and tolerability of BoNTA-ABO for glabellar lines in POC. Three groups were examined: a safety population of 472 POC, an efficacy population of 50U BoNTA-ABO of 117 POC, and an efficacy population adjusted to muscle mass containing 160 POC. Efficacy, tolerability, and adverse event rates were similar in White patients and POC.[16]

In 2021, Taylor et al conducted a post hoc analysis of 492 patients treated with 20U prabotulinumtoxinA for the treatment of glabellar lines. The subjects were separated into POC (FST IV-VI) and non-POC (FST I-III). The proportion of responders with a one or more-point improvement from baseline at maximum frown was graded using the four-point glabellar line scale. It was found that a single dose of 20U prabotulinumtoxinA resulted in similar effectiveness across both groups with good tolerability.[17]

Recently in 2023, Solish et al enrolled 2785 patients in a randomized open-label trial to evaluate DaxibotulinumtoxinA for injection (DAXI) in the treatment of glabellar lines. Efficacy and safety were analyzed by age and race (Asian, Black and African American, and White). Over 96% of patients in all age and race subgroups achieved none or mild glabellar line severity at maximum frown (IGA-FWS) after DAXI treatment at week 4. Glabellar line severity of none or mild by composite IGA-FWS rating was maintained for a median of 27.0 weeks in Asian, 25.3 weeks in Black, and 24.0 weeks in White subgroups. Across all subgroups, treatment emergent adverse events were similar.[18]

While these studies demonstrate the safe and effective use of neuromodulators in POC, more studies are needed as an increasing number of POC seek neuromodulator treatment.

IDENTIFICATION OF RACE AND ETHNICITY

The discussion and identification of race and ethnicity within POC who seek augmentation using soft tissue fillers and/or neuromodulators should occur at the first visit. Bi- or multiracial patients should be asked with which race they physically identify. It is best practice to ask, rather than assume based on skin color, about a patient's racial or ethnic background. Once correct identification of race and ethnicity is completed, the clinician may better understand the associated skin property differences, pattern of aging, and anatomical variations among POC that influence soft tissue filler and neuromodulator use in this group.

SKIN DIFFERENCES AND AGING

Understanding skin properties and patterns of aging in POC gives clinicians foundational knowledge needed for the correct selection and administration of fillers and/or neuromodulators. From a histological standpoint, there are functional differences in skin properties of POC compared to their White counterparts. Melanosomes, for example, are larger and more heavily concentrated throughout the epidermal layer in individuals with POC.[19] Increased melanin production by melanosomes within the melanocytes coincides with darker skin tones. Melanin offers a photoprotective role by acting as a neutral density filter, reducing all wavelengths of light equally. It was found that ultraviolet light (UVB and UVA) reaches the upper dermis of White skin five times as much than that of POC.[20] Subsequently, POC have delayed and decreased photoaging due to photoprotection by increased melanin. Although increased melanin protects against photodamage, it also makes POC more vulnerable to dyspigmentation. Hypo- and hyperpigmentation is a sign of photoaging in POC.[21] There are other components in POC that lead to differences in aging. Asian and Black skin have a thicker, more compact dermis. Rhytides are believed to be caused by progressive dermal atrophy leading to folds and wrinkles. A thicker dermis in Asian and Black skin may contribute to the lower incidence of facial rhytids in these patients compared to lighter skin types.[21-23] Delayed signs of aging in POC is also due to the characteristics of fibroblasts in this skin type. The fibroblasts are increased and larger, containing smaller more compact collagen bundles that are surrounded by proteoglycans.[24] While increased fibroblasts delay aging, it also increases the likelihood of the development of hypertrophic or keloidal scars. Overall, all these biological factors contribute to POC experiencing age-related changes 10 to 20 years after their White counterparts.[25,26]

Signs of aging vary among POC and non-POC. For White patients, some features of skin aging include forehead, glabellar, and perioral rhytids, brow ptosis, crow feet, reduced lip volume, displacement of the orbital fat pad, and descent of the melolabial fat pad [**Figure 96-2**].[27] In contrast, African American patients experience malar fat pad sagging, tear-trough deformity, deepening of the nasolabial folds, and jowl formation.[25,28,29] With respect to lip aging, patients of African descent mainly develop rhytids in the body of the lip below the vermilion border. Loss of volume in the upper lip leads to this phenomenon, while the lower lip usually maintains its same appearance. Given this aging

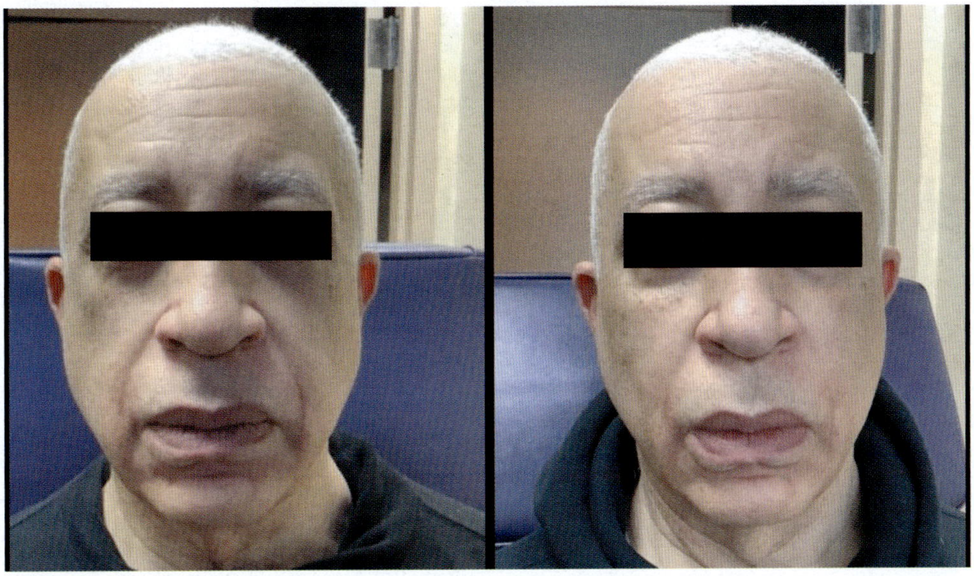

FIGURE 96-2. (A and B) Mid-face enhancement with hyaluronic acid filler. (Used with permission from Cheryl Burgess, MD, FAAD.)

pattern, collagen enhancement of the vermilion border is rarely performed in African American women, as opposed to their White counterparts. Black patients mostly seek lip augmentation to restore their lip size to that of their youth, unlike White patients who obtain lip filler primarily to increase their natural lip size.[30]

Hispanic patients experience eyebrow and eyelid drooping, infraorbital hollowing, and thickening of nasolabial folds as they age.[22,28,31] Aging in East Asian patients consists of soft-tissue laxity of the midface in addition to tear trough formation likely due to thicker skin and a weaker skeletal framework.[21,28] For aging in South Asian patients, they experience more facial fullness and descent of the mid-face tissue.[32] The aging pattern in Middle Eastern patients is more commonly mid-face sagging and jowl formation.[33]

ANATOMIC VARIATIONS

There are many anatomical differences among POC. Clinicians should understand morphological patterns in POC as these variations may influence cultural standards of beauty. Importantly, clinicians must recognize that there is a high degree of intraracial anatomical variation for each group described below.

White patients facial structure includes a narrow nasal base, large tip projections, and thin lips. This groups face is narrow with a greater vertical height than other ethnic groups.[21,34]

The term Black or African American describes people of African or Afro-Caribbean descent. Black patients tend to have a depressed nasal root, short nasal spine, squared chin, rounded supraorbital margins, and temporal lines. Increased midface soft tissue, prominent fuller lips, and increased facial convexity is also characteristic of Black patients.[21,34]

Hispanic refers to individuals from Mexico, Central and South America, and those of Spanish-Caribbean descent. Distinctive facial features of Latinx patients include increased bizygomatic distance, bimaxillary protrusion, broader nose, round face, and receded chin.[21,34,35] Intraracial variations exist in the Hispanic population. The term Mestizos describes a sub-racial group with Native American and White backgrounds. Mestizos typically have a flat, more vertical forehead, broad face with prominent malar eminences, broad nose with widened alar base, and slightly retrusive chins.[36] Hispanics of Caribbean origin have similar features to African Americans, while those of Central and South American origin have features more like Whites.[21,37–40]

The term East Asian refers to those of Chinese, Japanese, Korean, and Taiwanese backgrounds. For East Asians, anatomical variations consist of a flat nasal region, round/square anterior nasal aperture, short nasal spine, and a single frontal boss. Notably, East Asians also have hooding of the upper eyelid/lateral brow, prominent mandibular angle, more protuberant lips, and are flat or concave in the medial maxilla and midface.[21,34,41] Within this group, Chinese patients have slim faces with narrow noses and long jaws, while Korean patients have shorter faces with prominent cheeks.[42,43]

South Asian refers to those from Bangladesh, Pakistan, India, and Sri Lanka. Southeast Asian patients typically have a low nasal bridge with voluminous thick skin, low dorsum, wide and hanging ala, bulbous tip, and retracted premaxilla. This group also has large eyes, and a greater nasal projection than East Asians.[21,34,41,44]

Patients of Middle Eastern descent describes those from the Arabian Gulf (Bahrain, Kuwait, Saudi Arabia, United Arab Emirates), Egypt, Iran, and Lebanon. A convex profile with a longer forehead, longer midface, and shorter lower face is typical of Middle Eastern patients.[45] Additionally, Middle Eastern patients have wider nasal widths, increased upper lip protrusion, and a decreased lower lip height-depth ratio.[46] Intraracially, Persian patients have noses that are less prominent than that of Arabian patients.[45]

SCALES FOR CATEGORIZATION OF SKIN TYPE

Beyond the scope of ethnicity and race, which often correlates to skin characteristics, patterns of aging, and anatomical variations, POC can be further categorized by skin type. The most used classification system in dermatologic practice is the Fitzpatrick skin type (FST), developed to assess the propensity of the skin to burn during phototherapy. Over time, clinicians have used the FST to categorize skin color and identify subjects in clinical trials. While clinician reported FSTs have correlated with race, race does not consistently correlate with objective measures of pigmentation or self-reported FSTs.[47,48] Other limitations of this scale include poor correlation with constitutive skin color and minimal erythema dose values.[47,49] Finally, FST does not consider anatomic difference or age-related changes.[48] For example, Latino and Middle Eastern patients can both be Fitzpatrick phototypes IV and yet have very different facial anatomy. Specific description terms should thus be identified in conjunction with the patient. Another system for classifying skin type is the Robert Skin Type (RST) Classification System. This system allows clinicians to predict the skin response to injury from cosmetic procedures by recording a patients phototype, hyperpigmentation, photoaging, and scarring capability.[50] Other classifications of skin type include the Goldman World Classification of Skin Type and the Taylor Hyperpigmentation Scale.[51,52] While these scales offer clinicians some benefit in classification, no scale captures the nuances of underlying facial morphology variation.[50,53] Thus, a more comprehensive and encompassing classification system is required for POC.

COSMETIC PREFERENCES AND TECHNIQUES

Aesthetic trends for POC are influenced by the factors discussed above, such as race, ethnicity, patterns of aging, and anatomical variations, in addition to cultural preferences. POC come from diverse backgrounds and beauty standards from across the world. Given this notion, one can predict that beauty standards for POC will differ from that of western standards. Clinicians must practice cultural competency and awareness to understand and meet aesthetic goals in POC. Importantly, some patients may deviate from standards of beauty inherent to their race, and thus, it is imperative that patients be consulted on their individual goals. Chapter 89 provides a detailed discussion of cultural beauty standards around the world.

An example of a cosmetic trend in an ethnic group is lip enhancement with fillers in African American patients. While there is a common misconception that this group does not seek lip filler treatment due to the presence of full lips, this is not the case. African American patients tend to restore the 50:50 lip proportion from their youth, while White patients aim to increase the size of their lips.[54] Age associated volume loss in patients of African descent occur below the vermillion border of the upper mucosal lip, with the preservation of the lower lip volume.[21,24,34,55] Additionally, this group of patients present at a more advanced age than White patients for lip enhancement with soft tissue filler.[53]

With East Asians, hyaluronic acid fillers are often sought to address mid-face structural retrusion. However, clinicians must also consider the increased bizygomatic width of East Asians. As a result, soft tissue fillers should be placed in the central face to provide anterior projection while avoiding widening of the face.[56]

Specific filler types should be considered for POC as they have compact and increased collagen bundles, which provide a scaffold for volumization. Stimulatory soft tissue fillers, including calcium hydroxyapatite and poly-L-lactic acid, thus may be preferred.[29] Overall, POC achieve the desired outcome after fewer treatments; this results in a longer interval between treatments to avoid overcorrection.[57,58]

There are important pearls to note regarding PLLA fillers. Unlike most traditional fillers, PLLA is not intended for the treatment of specific wrinkles. Instead, it is used almost exclusively for volume restoration in areas of "sinking and sagging" skin that require contouring and sculpting. PLLA is injected into deeper regions for creating supportive structure and foundation [**Figure 96-3**]. It can be used to build up the maxillary fat pads, and it cannot be injected into the lips.[59] Also, unlike traditional fillers, PLAA exploits a unique mechanism of action in soft tissue augmentation. Upon injection into the deep dermis or dermal subcutaneous plane, PLLA results in immediate physical improvement. However, this improvement is temporary and diminishes over the first week as water is absorbed. Over the next 3 to 6 months, PLLA microparticles induce collagen formation and ultimate dermal thickening.[30] Given that PLLA does not result in immediate correction, as in the case of most traditional fillers, PLLA use requires a markedly different approach and treatment plan. Both clinicians and patients must have great patience through the span of treatment sessions. Clinicians should treat, wait, assess, and then decide how to proceed forward with PLLA treatment. Sufficient training is most critical to successful PLAA injection. Techniques include aiming treatment toward volume restoration, rather than specific lines, and injection into the dermal-subcutaneous plane, unlike collagen or hyaluronic acids. Additionally, PLLA injections should be accompanied by a massage of the treatment area and continued by the patient posttreatment.[59,60] The effects of volume restoration with PLLA are not permanent but can persist anywhere from 18 to 24 months.[59,61] PLLA is approved by the FDA for the treatment of HIV-associated lipoatrophy,

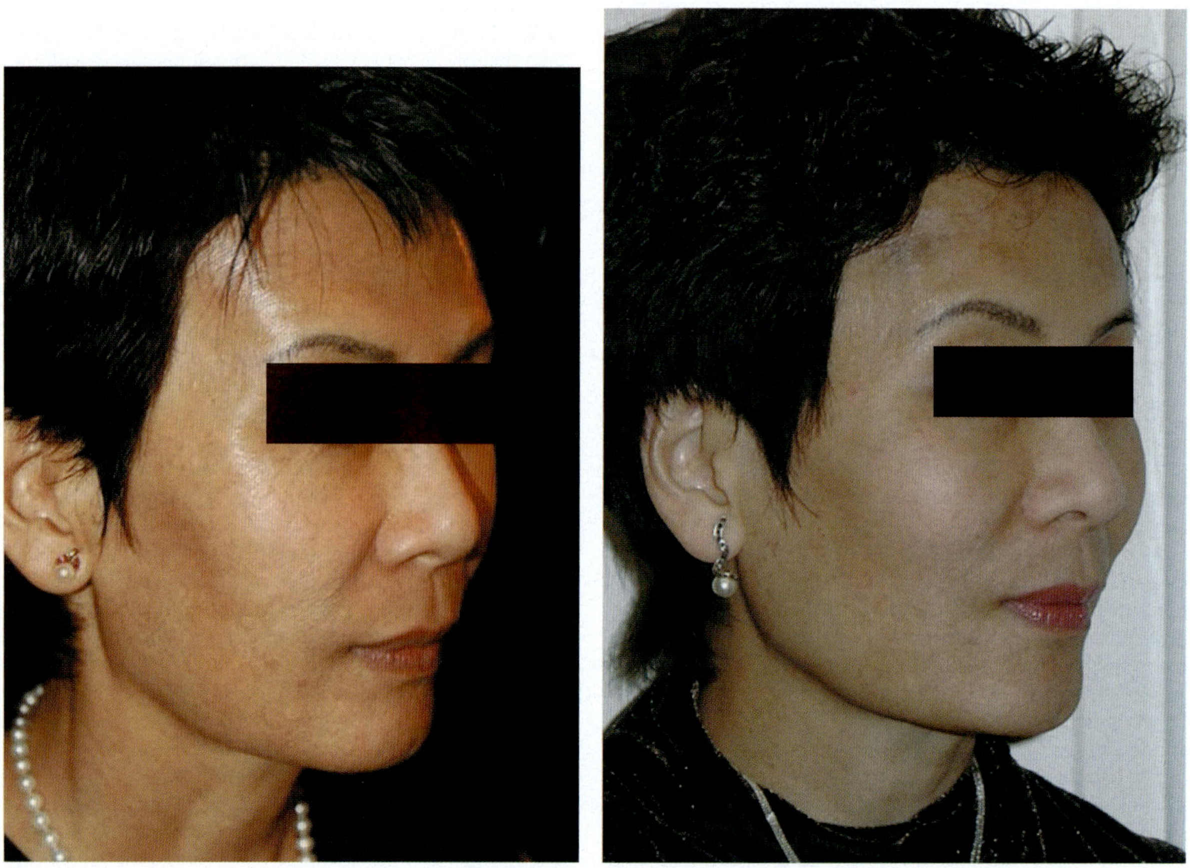

A B

FIGURE 96-3. (**A** and **B**) Facial volumization and enhancement with Poly-L-lactic acid. (Used with permission from Cheryl Burgess, MD, FAAD.)

correction of shallow to deep nasolabial folds, contour deficiencies, and other facial rhytids.[30]

Regarding neuromodulators, both anatomical differences and cultural standards of beauty in specific ethnic groups may require dosage adjustments for botulinum toxin cosmetic injection. For example, in East Asians, corrugator muscles were identified to be smaller in mass and shorter, narrower, and less hyperdynamic than White patients. Thus, it is recommended that a dosage lower than the typical 20U of BoNTA be injected into the glabellar complex in East Asian populations.[34,62,63] In contrast, Asians tend to have more prominent masseter muscles than Whites. Consequently, bilateral BoNTA injection for the cosmetic modification of prominent masseters, commonly referred to as jaw contouring, is frequently performed in Asian patients to create a more tapered appearance of the lower face. This application of BoNTA off-label in the United States. It is suggested to inject three to five injection points per masseter and four to six U per injection point, for a total of 20 to 30U per side.[34,62]

Of note, differences in BoNTA efficacy between POC and White patients have been demonstrated. In one study, 30 day response rates for 50U abobotulinumtoxinA was higher in POC than in White subjects.[64] In contrast, responder rates of improvement in maximum glabellar frown in POC (IV-VI) were lower with prabotulinumtoxinA than for non-POC by 5.9%.[17]

SAFETY AND ADVERSE EVENTS

The current literature details that POC can safely undergo both filler and neuromodulator treatments. Regarding fillers, patients of all skin tones may develop mild and transient bruising, edema, tenderness, and erythema. In a case review of 60 patients, it was found that there was no difference in complication rates for HA filler injections between POC and non-POC.[65] No studies report an increased risk of permanent discoloration, such as hyperpigmentation, or scarring, such as keloids, for POC with soft tissue filler treatments. To reduce these risks, clinicians should minimize the total number of punctures to the skin. Slower injection times reduce pigmentation changes.[8] Additionally, placing fillers in the mid-dermis to avoid direct disruption of the epidermal dermal junction may also reduce the risk of discoloration and scarring.[8,9] An adverse event of filler treatments is the Tyndall effect, which describes blue discoloration due to light scattering. This can occur if fillers are placed too superficially.[66] Often this occurs in an area with thin skin, such as the periorbital area. Due to thicker skin properties and increased degree of pigmentation, the risk of the Tyndall effect may be minimized in POC.[67] Regardless, superficial placement of hyaluronic acid fillers in the periorbital area should be avoided. The most dangerous complications result from inadvertent intra-arterial injections of filler. This can lead to tissue necrosis or embolism that can cause stroke or blindness. The most commonly injection locations that lead to blindness in a review of the literature were reported as the nose (55%), glabella (35%), and forehead (11%).[68] Importantly, a higher incidence of blindness as a complication of filler injections has been reported in East Asian Countries, such as Korea (40%) and China (19%).[68,69] Asians tend to have a flat central facial profile, and nonsurgical rhinoplasties and other techniques utilize fillers to increase three-dimensionality of the central face.[56] The uptake of these techniques likely contributes to the higher incidence. Additionally, anatomic differences may also play a role in this increased incidence among Asians. As the dorsal nasal artery directly feeds into the ophthalmic artery, inadvertent injection of the dorsal nasal artery can cause blindness. Sixty percent of East Asian cadavers had a single oblique vessel for the dorsal nasal artery, in contrast to bilateral vessels in an anatomic study.[70] Consequently, direct injections to higher risk areas such as the glabella and nasal tip should be avoided, and filler placement should be at the periosteal layer.[71] Ultimately, only highly experienced physician injectors should complete such an advanced technique given the complexity of anatomical considerations and the associated risks. Notably, PLLA use in older or aging patients results in a greater likelihood of bruising due to diminished thickness of the dermis plane. In these patients, clinicians should allow 8 weeks between treatment sessions, as opposed to the regular 4 to 6 week waiting period.[59,72]

With respect to neuromodulators, adverse effects include minor bruising with injection, headache, and injection-site reactions.[73] Less commonly, temporary blepharoptosis and eyebrow ptosis may occur.[74] Administration of NSAIDs prior to and after treatment may prevent headache. Proper training and technique should be practiced such to prevent the occurrence of blepharoptosis and eyebrow ptosis. One study reports that the rate of adverse events associated with neuromodulator use in POC are similar to that of White patients.[64] Interestingly, a significantly greater incidence of eyelid sensory disorder (tightness, pressure, heaviness, and feeling of droopiness), eyelid ptosis, and eyelid edema was found in Asian patients compared to White patients. In this meta-analysis of nine studies, the authors identified differences in Asian and Caucasian eyelid anatomy. This group advised that Asian patients should be informed of possible eyelid sensory disorder and eyelid edema before treatment.[75]

Notably, clinicians must understand forehead anatomy when administering neuromodulators to avoid eyebrow ptosis in all skin types. This may be done through identification of the line of convergence (C-line). The C-line is where the lower forehead moves cranially and meets the upper overhead moving caudally. It is located at the second horizontal forehead line, when counting from superior to inferior in all subjects. Injections above the C-line are believed to mitigate the risk of neuromodulator-induced brow ptosis.[76]

CONCLUSION

There is an ongoing need for education and research on the safety and efficacy of neuromodulator and soft tissue filler use in POC. Premarket trials must incorporate POC in larger numbers to further demonstrate safety and efficacy among this group. Increased education regarding cosmetic treatments in POC among clinicians is needed. While the Fitzpatrick scale is a tool used to identify subjects in clinical trials, new classifications are needed that consider skin pigmentation, skin characteristics, and anatomical variations. Overall, understanding of racial and ethnic similarities in combination with clinician training and education is key to the successful and safe administration of cosmetics procedures for POC.

REFERENCES

1. Bureau, US Census. "2014 National Population Projections Datasets." *Census.gov*, 8 Oct. 2021, https://www.census.gov/data/datasets/2014/demo/popproj/2014-popproj.html.
2. Surgery. ASfAP. Aesthetics Plastic Surgery National Databank Statistics 2019.
3. The American Society for Aesthetic Plastic Surgery's Cosmetic Surgery National Data Bank: Statistics 2018. *Aesthet Surg J*. 2019;39(Suppl_4):1-27.
4. The American Society for Aesthetic Plastic Surgery. Procedural statistics. https://www.surgery.org/sites/default/files/ASAPS-Stats2017.pdf. Assessed January 19, 2023.
5. Center for Devices and Radiological Health. (n.d.). *FDA-approved dermal fillers*. U.S. Food and Drug Administration. https://www.fda.gov/medical-devices/aesthetic-cosmetic-devices/fda-approved-dermal-fillers.
6. Berlin A, Cohen JL, Goldberg DJ. Calcium hydroxylapatite for facial rejuvenation. *Semin Cutan Med Surg*. 2006;25(3):132-137.
7. Taylor SC, Burgess CM, Callender VD. Safety of nonanimal stabilized hyaluronic acid dermal fillers in patients with skin of color: a randomized, evaluator-blinded comparative trial. *Dermatol Surg*. 2009;35(Suppl 2):1653-1660.
8. Marmur ES, Taylor SC, Grimes PE, Boyd CM, Porter JP, Yoo JY. Six-month safety results of calcium hydroxylapatite for treatment of nasolabial folds in Fitzpatrick skin types IV to VI. *Dermatol Surg*. 2009;35(Suppl 2):1641-1645.
9. Downie JB, Grimes PE, Callender VD. A multicenter study of the safety and effectiveness of hyaluronic acid with a cohesive polydensified matrix for treatment of nasolabial folds in subjects with Fitzpatrick skin types IV, V, and VI. *Plast Reconstr Surg*. 2013;132(4 Suppl 2):41S-47S.
10. Dayan S, Bruce S, Kilmer S, et al. Safety and effectiveness of the hyaluronic acid filler, HYC-24L, for lip and perioral augmentation. *Dermatol Surg*. 2015;41(Suppl 1):S293-301.

11. Geronemus RG, Bank DE, Hardas B, Shamban A, Weichman BM, Murphy DK. Safety and effectiveness of VYC-15L, a hyaluronic acid filler for lip and perioral enhancement: one-year results from a randomized, controlled study. *Dermatol Surg.* 2017;43(3):396-404.
12. Taylor SC, Downie JB, Shamban A, et al. Lip and perioral enhancement with hyaluronic acid dermal fillers in individuals with skin of color. *Dermatol Surg.* 2019;45(7):959-967.
13. Frampton JE, Easthope SE. Botulinum toxin A (botox cosmetic): a review of its use in the treatment of glabellar frown lines. *Am J Clin Dermatol.* 2003;4(10):709-725.
14. Dessy LA, Fallico N, Mazzocchi M, Scuderi N. Botulinum toxin for glabellar lines: A review of the efficacy and safety of currently available products. *Am J Clin Dermatol.* 2012;12(6):377-388.
15. Grimes PE, Shabazz D. A four-month randomized, double-blind evaluation of the efficacy of botulinum toxin type A for the treatment of glabellar lines in women with skin types V and VI. *Dermatol Surg.* 2009;35(3):429-436.
16. Taylor SC, Callender VD, Albright CD, Coleman J, Axford-Gatley RA, Lin X. AbobotulinumtoxinA for reduction of glabellar lines in patients with skin of color: post hoc analysis of pooled clinical trial data. *Dermatol Surg.* 2012;38(11):1804-1811.
17. Taylor SC, Grimes PE, Joseph JH, Jonker A, Avelar RL. PrabotulinumtoxinA for the treatment of moderate-to-severe glabellar lines in adult patients with skin of color: post hoc analyses of the US phase III clinical study data. *Dermatol Surg.* 2021;47(4):516-521.
18. Solish N, Burgess CM, Weinkle SH, et al. Efficacy and safety of DaxibotulinumtoxinA for injection in the treatment of glabellar lines by age and race: subgroup analysis of the SAKURA clinical trials. *Aesthet Surg J.* 2023;43(2):205-214.
19. Montagna W, Carlisle K. The architecture of black and white facial skin. *J Am Acad Dermatol.* 1991;24(6 Pt 1):929-937.
20. Kaidbey KH, Agin PP, Sayre RM, Kligman AM. Photoprotection by melanin–a comparison of black and Caucasian skin. *J Am Acad Dermatol.* 1979;1(3):249-260.
21. Vashi NA, de Castro Maymone MB, Kundu RV. Aging differences in ethnic skin. *J Clin Aesthet Dermatol.* 2016;9(1):31-38.
22. Lapière CM. The ageing dermis: the main cause for the appearance of 'old' skin. *Br J Dermatol.* 1990;122 Suppl 35:5-11.
23. Montagna W, Prota G, Kenney J. The structure of black skin. In: Montagna W, Prota G, Kenney J, eds. *Black Skin Structure and Function.* Houston, TX: Gulf Professional Publishing; 1993.
24. Brissett AE, Naylor MC. The aging African-American face. *Facial Plast Surg.* 2010;26(2):154-163.
25. Alexis A, Boyd C, Callender V, Downie J, Sangha S. Understanding the female African American facial aesthetic patient. *J Drugs Dermatol.* 2019;18(9):858-866.
26. Nouveau-Richard S, Yang Z, Mac-Mary S, et al. Skin ageing: a comparison between Chinese and European populations. A pilot study. *J Dermatol Sci.* 2005;40(3):187-193.
27. Venkatesh S, Maymone MBC, Vashi NA. Aging in skin of color. *Clin Dermatol.* 2019;37(4):351-357.
28. Talakoub L, Wesley NO. Differences in perceptions of beauty and cosmetic procedures performed in ethnic patients. *Semin Cutan Med Surg.* 2009;28(2): 115-129.
29. Burgess C, Awosika O. Ethnic and gender considerations in the use of facial injectables: African-American patients. *Plast Reconstr Surg.* 2015;136(5 Suppl):28S-31S.
30. Burgess C, Awosika O. Ethnic and gender considerations in the use of facial injectables: African-American patients. *Plast Reconstr Surg.* 2015;136(5 Suppl): 28S-31S.
31. Grimes PE. Beauty: an historical and societal perspective. In: Grimes PE, Soriano T, Hexsel DM, Kim J, eds. *Aesthetics and Cosmetic Surgery for Darker Skin Types.* Philadelphia, PA: Lippincott Williams & Wilkins; 2008:15-36.
32. Shetty R. Outer circle versus inner circle: special considerations while rejuvenating an Indian face using fillers. *J Cutan Aesthet Surg.* 2015;8(3): 169-172.
33. Kashmar M, Alsufyani MA, Ghalamkarpour F, et al. Consensus opinions on facial beauty and implications for aesthetic treatment in Middle Eastern women. *Plast Reconstr Surg Glob Open.* 2019;7(4):e2220.
34. Quiñonez RL, Agbai ON, Burgess CM, Taylor SC. An update on cosmetic procedures in people of color. Part 2: neuromodulators, soft tissue augmentation, chemexfoliating agents, and laser hair reduction. *J Am Acad Dermatol.* 2022;86(4):729-739.
35. Sanchez AE. Rhinoplasty in the "Chata" nose of the Caribbean. *Aesthetic Plast Surg.* 1980;4(1):169-177.
36. Aguilera SB, Hall M, Carvajal DCS, Gaviria A. Frontoplasty technique for the Mestizo patient. *J Clin Aesthet Dermatol.* 2021;14(3):14-16.
37. Porter JP, Olson KL. Anthropometric facial analysis of the African American woman. *Arch Facial Plast Surg.* 2001;3(3):191-197.
38. Sugiyama-Nakagiri Y, Sugata K, Hachiya A, Osanai O, Ohuchi A, Kitahara T. Ethnic differences in the structural properties of facial skin. *J Dermatol Sci.* 2009;53(2):135-139.
39. Alexis AF. New and emerging treatments for hyperpigmentation. *J Drugs Dermatol.* 2014;13(4):382-385.
40. Milgrim LM, Lawson W, Cohen AF. Anthropometric analysis of the female Latino nose. Revised aesthetic concepts and their surgical implications. *Arch Otolaryngol Head Neck Surg.* 1996;122(10):1079-1086.
41. Liew S, Wu WT, Chan HH, et al. Consensus on changing trends, attitudes, and concepts of Asian beauty. *Aesthetic Plast Surg.* 2016;40(2):193-201.
42. Lee JS, Kim HK, Kim YW. Anthropometric analysis of the attractive and normal faces in Korean female. *J Korean Soc Plast Reconstr Surg.* 7 2004;31(4):526-531.
43. Zhao Q, Zhou R, Zhang X, et al. Morphological quantitative criteria and aesthetic evaluation of eight female Han face types. *Aesthetic Plast Surg.* 2013;37(2):445-453.
44. Yap EC. Rhinoplasty for South East Asian nose. *Facial Plast Surg Clin North Am.* 2018;26(3):389-402.
45. Kashmar M, Alsufyani MA, Ghalamkarpour F, et al. Consensus opinions on facial beauty and implications for aesthetic treatment in Middle Eastern women. *Plast Reconstr Surg Glob Open.* 2019;7(4):e2220.
46. Al-Sebaei MO. The validity of three neo-classical facial canons in young adults originating from the Arabian Peninsula. *Head Face Med.* 2015;11:4.
47. Ware OR, Dawson JE, Shinohara MM, Taylor SC. Racial limitations of Fitzpatrick skin type. *Cutis.* 2020;105(2):77-80.
48. He SY, McCulloch CE, Boscardin WJ, Chren MM, Linos E, Arron ST. Self-reported pigmentary phenotypes and race are significant but incomplete predictors of Fitzpatrick skin phototype in an ethnically diverse population. *J Am Acad Dermatol.* 2014;71(4):731-737.
49. Leenutaphong V. Relationship between skin color and cutaneous response to ultraviolet radiation in Thai. *Photodermatol Photoimmunol Photomed.* 1995;11(5-6):198-203.
50. Roberts WE. Skin type classification systems old and new. *Dermatol Clin.* 2009;27(4):529-viii.
51. Goldman MP. Universal classification of skin type. In: Shiffman MA, Mirrafati SJ, Lam SM, Cueteaux CG, eds. *Simplified Facial Rejuvenation.* Berlin: Springer; 2008:47-50.
52. Taylor S, Westerhof W, Im S, Lim J. Noninvasive techniques for the evaluation of skin color. *J Am Acad Dermatol.* 2006;54(5 Suppl 2):S282-S290.
53. CM. B. Dermal fillers in ethnic skin. In: Alexis AF BV, eds. *Skin of Color: A Practical Guide to Dermatologic Diagnosis and Treatment* New York, NY: Springer; 2013:247-262.
54. Burgess C, Awosika O. Ethnic and gender considerations in the use of facial injectables: African-American patients. *Plast Reconstr Surg.* 2015;136(5 Suppl):28S-31S.
55. Henry M, Sadick N. Aesthetic considerations in female skin of color: what you need to know. *Semin Cutan Med Surg.* 2018;37(4):210-216.
56. Liew S. Ethnic and gender considerations in the use of facial injectables: Asian patients. *Plast Reconstr Surg.* 2015;136(5 Suppl):22S-27S.
57. Burgess CM. Special considerations in African American skin. In: Alam M, Bhatia AC, Kundu RV, Yoo SS, Chan H, eds. *Cosmetic Dermatology for Skin of Color.* New York, NY: McGraw-Hill Companies; 2008:163-167.
58. Hamilton TK, Burgess CM. Considerations for the use of injectable poly-L-lactic acid in people of color. *J Drugs Dermatol.* 2010;9(5):451-456.
59. Burgess CM. Principles of soft tissue augmentation for the aging face. *Clin Interv Aging.* 2006;1(4):349-355.
60. Werschler P. Advances in recognizing and treating facial lipoatrophy. *Cosmet Dermatol.* 2005;18:3-8.
61. Mest D. 2005. Experience with injectable poly-L-lactic acid in clinical practice. *Cosmet Dermatol.* 2005;18(2 S2):5-8.
62. Sundaram H, Huang PH, Hsu NJ, et al. Aesthetic applications of botulinum toxin A in Asians: an international, multidisciplinary, Pan-Asian consensus. *Plast Reconstr Surg Glob Open.* 2016;4(12):e872.
63. Jiang H, Zhou J, Chen S. Different glabellar contraction patterns in Chinese and efficacy of botulinum toxin type A for treating glabellar lines: a pilot study. *Dermatol Surg.* 2017;43(5):692-697.
64. Taylor SC, Callender VD, Albright CD, Coleman J, Axford-Gatley RA, Lin X. AbobotulinumtoxinA for reduction of glabellar lines in patients with skin of color: post hoc analysis of pooled clinical trial data. *Dermatol Surg.* 2012;38(11):1804-1811.
65. Odunze M, Cohn A, Few JW. Restylane and people of color. *Plast Reconstr Surg.* 2007;120(7):2011-2016.
66. King M. Management of Tyndall effect. *J Clin Aesthet Dermatol.* 2016; 9(11):E6-E8.

67. Choi HS, Whipple KM, Oh SR, et al. Modifying the upper eyelid crease in Asian patients with hyaluronic acid fillers. *Plast Reconstr Surg.* 2011;127(2):844-849.
68. Sorensen EP, Council ML. Update in soft-tissue filler-associated blindness. *Dermatol Surg.* 2020;46(5):671-677.
69. Beleznay K, Carruthers JDA, Humphrey S, Carruthers A, Jones D. Update on avoiding and treating blindness from fillers: a recent review of the world literature. *Aesthet Surg J.* 2019;39(6):662-674.
70. Tansatit T, Apinuntrum P, Phetudom T. Facing the worst risk: confronting the dorsal nasal artery, implication for non-surgical procedures of nasal augmentation. *Aesthetic Plast Surg.* 2017;41(1):191-198.
71. Liew S, Scamp T, de Maio M, et al. Efficacy and safety of a hyaluronic acid filler to correct aesthetically detracting or deficient features of the Asian nose: a prospective, open-label, long-term study. *Aesthet Surg J.* 2016;36(7):760-772.
72. Burgess C, Lowe N. 2006. NewFill for skin augmentation: a filler or a failure. Letter to the editor. *Dermatol Surg.* 32:1530-1532.
73. Dessy LA, Fallico N, Mazzocchi M, Scuderi N. Botulinum toxin for glabellar lines: a review of the efficacy and safety of currently available products. *Am J Clin Dermatol.* 2011;12(6):377-388.
74. Small R, M.D. Botulinum toxin injection for facial wrinkles. *Am Fam Physician.* 2014;90(3):168-175.
75. Brin MF, Boodhoo TI, Pogoda JM, et al. Safety and tolerability of onabotulinumtoxinA in the treatment of facial lines: a meta-analysis of individual patient data from global clinical registration studies in 1678 participants. *J Am Acad Dermatol.* 2009;61(6):961-70.e711.
76. Cotofana S, Freytag DL, Frank K, et al. The bidirectional movement of the frontalis muscle: introducing the line of convergence and its potential clinical relevance. *Plast Reconstr Surg.* 2020;145(5):1155-1162.

CHAPTER 97

Liposuction

Kimberly Huerth
Shanae N. Henry
Ugonna Nwannunu
DiAnne S. Davis

KEY POINTS

- Liposuction is a surgical body sculpting technique that aims to reduce cosmetically unappealing, localized areas of adipose tissue to engender more aesthetically pleasing proportions and contours.
- Patient selection should be informed by current health status, skin quality, and the location, volume, and character of the adipose tissue being targeted. Those with more melanin-rich skin and a history of postinflammatory pigment alteration and/or hypertrophic scar/keloid formation should be extensively counseled on the risk of these complications with tumescent liposuction.
- Racial differences in body habitus and beauty standards must be considered and openly discussed so that the goals of the patient can be reconciled with the vision of the physician, and the limitations of the procedure.
- Suctioning technique, port placement, fat and skin quality, supplemental technology use, and duration of postoperative compression will vary by anatomic region. The physician must familiarize themselves with these varying considerations to optimize patient outcomes.

INTRODUCTION

Liposuction is a body sculpting technique that aims to reduce cosmetically unappealing, localized areas of adipose tissue, to achieve more pleasing proportions and contours. In a postpandemic world, liposuction has, according to some data, become the most popular aesthetic surgical procedure performed in the United States.[1] According to the American Society of Plastic Surgeons Cosmetic Surgery 2022 Insights and Trends Report, liposuction is particularly popular among those aged 31 to 45 who are seeking to address changes in appearance born of pandemic stress, optimize their appearance as the world returns to in-person interaction, undergo elective surgery that may not have been feasible during lockdown, address undesirable features that became discernible for the first time or amplified during video calls, and generally improve confidence and self-esteem.[1] Anatomic areas where liposuction is commonly performed for aesthetic improvement include the neck, breasts/chest, upper arms, abdomen, flanks, trochanteric region, lumbar region, medial/lateral thighs, and gluteal region. Liposuction may also be utilized to address fibrofatty changes resulting from various medical conditions [**Table 97-1**],[2-5] though an in-depth discussion of these indications is unfortunately beyond the scope of this chapter.

TABLE 97-1 Noncosmetic indications for liposuction

Lipomas and angiolipomas
Lipedema in the lower extremities where subcutaneous fat deposits may inhibit daily activities
Lymphedema (refractory to traditional conservative treatments)
Lipodystrophy syndromes (congenital or acquired)
Cervicodorsal lipodystrophy
Reduction of excess fat deposits at surgical sites in obese patients who are undergoing tracheostomy, colostomy, or urostomy procedures

Source: Adapted from Wu S, Coombs D, Gurunian R. Liposuction: Concepts, safety, and techniques in body-contouring surgery. *Cleve Clin J Med.* 2020;87(6):367-375.

EVOLUTION OF MODERN LIPOSUCTION

Since 1921,[6,7] we have sought ways to contour the body by removing aesthetically undesirable adipose tissue [**Table 97-2**].[6-23] In the years following, physicians from many different countries and many different specialties have innovated, refined techniques, and experienced complications so that those who perform liposuction today can provide patients maximal aesthetic outcomes with minimal risk of adverse events. We have evolved from tissue resection surgery to the use of sharp curettes to remove fat manually to a wide array of modern-day suction-assisted cannulae. Early "wet" infiltration techniques[12] have been supplanted by the use of tumescent anesthesia.[14] Regarding tumescent anesthesia, this too has been widely modified from Klein's original recipe of 1L normal saline, 100 mg lidocaine, 1.0 mg epinephrine, 12.5 mL of 8.4% sodium bicarbonate, ± 10 mg of triamcinolone,[14] to suit the needs and expertise of the physicians using it.[24] Energy-based devices have been developed to help promote efficiency, fat liquefaction, and overlying skin contraction, thereby improving aesthetic outcomes while decreasing procedural fatigue for the physician. Guidelines have been established that provide valuable direction on patient selection and preoperative evaluation, choice and dosing of anesthesia, anxiolytics, and sedatives, intraoperative technique, fat removal volume, as well as post-operative care, all in the name of optimizing patient safety and outcomes.[15,25]

PREOPERATIVE CONSIDERATIONS

PATIENT SELECTION

A healthy adult who is no more than 20% to 30% over their ideal body weight that seeks to address isolated areas of fat that are unresponsive to diet and exercise is an appropriate candidate for tumescent liposuction, in the absence of other chronic medical conditions that may be disqualifying [**Table 97-3**].[26] Full-thickness "pinch-tests" of the skin from proposed sites bilaterally can allow the surgeon to assess underlying muscle integrity, estimate fat removal volumes, evaluate symmetry, and test skin quality and elasticity.[27] The presence of markedly excess skin, stretch marks, and/or delayed rebound with manual manipulation may

TABLE 97-2 Timeline of techniques for removing aesthetically undesirable adipose tissue

Year	Event
1921	French surgeon Dujarrier attempts to remove localized fat on a dancer legs. The postoperative course is complicated by tissue necrosis necessitating amputation.[6,7]
1964	German surgeon Schrudde utilizes a uterine curette in an attempt to contour fat on the legs. The postoperative course is complicated by hematoma and seroma formation.[8]
1969	Brazilian surgeon Pitanguy performs en bloc resections of skin and fat for thigh contouring, but the consequent scars are deemed aesthetically unacceptable.[9]
1975-1977	Italian surgeons Arpard and Fischer, and Swiss surgeons Kesserling and Meyer, work to develop their own respective iterations of modified curettes attached to suction devices. These techniques, however, required broad undermining before fat could be removed via suction unit, with associated complications stemming from large-scale tissue disruption.[10,11]
Late 1970s	France surgeon, Illouz, pioneers the "wet technique" in which infiltrated saline and hyaluronidase facilitate deeper and easier suction, while preserving neurovascular bundles.[12] Fournier subsequently develops the "dry technique," initially believing fluid infiltration to compromise precision, though he did eventually embrace the "wet technique" for its hemostatic advantages.[13]
1982	American ENT Newman coins the term "liposuction," teaches the first liposuction course in the United States, and founded the American Society of Liposuction Surgery.[7]
1987	American dermatologist Klein describes liposuction using tumescent anesthesia.[14]
1991	The American Academy of Dermatology becomes the first society to publish liposuction guidelines.[15]
1992	Italian surgeon Zocchi describes ultrasonic-assisted liposculpturing utilizing 20 to 30 MHz of cannula-delivered ultrasonic energy to facilitate fat liquefaction prior to suction.[16] American surgeon Apfelberg describes the use of a 600-μm 40-W YAG laser fiber to minimize edema, ecchymosis, and pain during liposuction.[17]
1998	U.S. Food and Drug Administration (FDA) approves MicroAire power-assisted liposuction (PAL) device (MicroAire Surgical Instruments, LLC, Charlottesville, VA).[18]
2002	Brazilian surgeon Goldman and Argentinian surgeons Schavelzon and Blugerman describe the use of a 300-μm 6-W 1064-nm Nd:YAG laser fiber to promote fat liquefaction, hemostasis, and dermal injury.[19]
2006	U.S. FDA approves SmartLipo (Cynosure, Inc., Westford, MA), the first laser-assisted lipolysis system.[20]
2008	U.S. FDA approves Body-Jet water-assisted liposuction device (Human Med AG c/o TUV SUD America, Inc, New Brighton, Minnesota).[21]
2011	U.S. FDA approves Vaser 2.1 Lipo System (Sound Surgical Technologies, LLC, Louisville, CO).[22] The use of BodyTite radiofrequency-assisted liposuction (InMode MD, LTD, Yoqneam Illit, Israel) is described.[23]

indicate poor elasticity, and patients should be counseled accordingly on how this will bear upon their anticipated outcome. Striae, hyperpigmentation, and cellulite should be brought to the attention of the patient and meticulously documented with photographs during the preoperative evaluation. Patients with more heavily melanated skin or a history of known pigmentary changes induced by trauma and/or inflammation should be counseled on the risk of postinflammatory pigmentary alteration with liposuction. Prior hypertrophic scar or keloid formation also warrants additional preoperative patient counseling and anticipatory postoperative intervention.

A detailed past medical and past surgical history should be obtained to inform both a general assessment of the patient's current state of health, as well as procedural planning. For example, past major abdominal or orthopedic surgeries and their resultant scarring can have present day consequences for where suction-cannula ports are placed. Laboratory

TABLE 97-3 Contraindications to liposuction

Bleeding diatheses	Poor wound healing
Body dysmorphic disorder	**Pregnancy***
Chronic lymphedema	Psychiatric illness
Concomitant infection	**Severe cardiovascular disease***
Diabetes mellitus	**Severe coagulopathy***
Liver disease	Thromboembolic disease
Morbid obesity	

*Conditions in bold represent absolute contraindications to liposuction.

Source: Adapted from Coleman K, Coleman III K, Flynn TC. Body contouring: liposuction and noninvasive modalities. In: Bologna J, Schaffer J, Cerroni L, eds. *Dermatology*. 4th ed. Amsterdam: Elsevier; 2018:2627-2636.

investigations including a comprehensive metabolic panel, complete blood counts, coagulation profiles, hepatitis panel, human immunodeficiency virus (HIV) testing, and pregnancy test (if applicable) should be obtained. Some advocate obtaining a preoperative chest x-ray and electrocardiogram for patients over the age of 40.[27] Women undergoing breast liposuction should have a baseline mammogram, while correctable causes of male gynecomastia and pseudogynecomastia should be excluded by history and physical examination.[28-30] Irregularities in any of the aforementioned will warrant clearance and/or intervention by relevant physicians involved in the patient's care.

A list of current medications should be obtained from the patient. Lidocaine is metabolized by cytochrome P_{450} 3A4,[31] and drugs that inhibit this enzyme [see **Table 97-4**][28,31] place a patient at heightened risk of lidocaine toxicity. The same holds true for medications or disease states that result in impaired liver function or reduced hepatic blood flow. Drugs that inhibit cytochrome P_{450} 3A4 should be discontinued 2 weeks prior to surgery if possible. If this is not possible, then the maximum dose of lidocaine delivered via tumescent solution should not exceed 35 mg/kg.[32] Over-the-counter medications and supplements that increase the risk of bleeding should also be discontinued 1 to 2 weeks before tumescent liposuction.

EQUIPMENT

The fundamental components needed to perform tumescent liposuction include a variety of blunt-tipped cannulae, an aspirator and

TABLE 97-4 Drugs that inhibit cytochrome P_{450} isozyme 3A[28,31]

Antibiotics	erythromycin, clarithromycin, ciprofloxacin, fluconazole, isoniazid, itraconazole, ketoconazole, metronidazole, miconazole, tetracycline,
Analgesics	alfentanil, fentanyl, methadone
Antiarrhythmics	Amiodarone
Anticonvulsants	carbamazepine, valproic acid
Antihistamines	Terfenadine
Antihypertensives	amlodipine, calcium channel blockers, dihydralazine, diltiazem, losartan, nifedipine, propranolol, verapamil,
Antidepressants	amitriptyline, fluoxetine, nefazodone, sertraline
Benzodiazepines	alprazolam, diazepam, flurazepam, triazolam, midazolam
Histamine 2 Receptor Antihistamines	Cimetidine
Hypnotic	Propofol
Immunosuppressants	Cyclosporine
Phosphodiesterase Inhibitors	Sildenafil
Proton Pump Inhibitors	Omeprazole
Statins	atorvastatin, lovastatin, pravastatin, simvastatin

Source: Adapted from Klein JA. *Tumescent Technique: Tumescent Anesthesia and Microcannular Liposuction*. St. Louis, MO: Mosby, Inc.; 2000.

TABLE 97-5 Types of liposuction technique

Type of technique	Description	Devices (with year)
Laser-assisted Liposuction (LAL)	An optical laser fiber within an introducer cannula inserts through a small incision in direct contact with adipose tissue to induce lysis of the adipose fat with thermal damage that also tightens the surrounding soft tissue[33]	• Smartlipo™ (2006)[20] • Cellulaze™ (2013)[34] • SculpSure™ (2015)[35]
Ultrasound-assisted liposuction (UAL)	Ultrasonic energy is used to selectively emulsify excess fat prior to its removal[16]	• LySonix™ (1998)[36] • Vaser Lipo (2011)[22] • UltraShape® (2017)[37]
Power-assisted liposuction (PAL)	Incorporates the use of an electric vacuum pump to reduce operator fatigue, while aiding in the removal of large volumes of fat in densely fibrous areas (flanks, back, and chest)[38]	• MicroAire Power-Assisted Liposuction (PAL) System (????)
Water jet-assisted liposuction (WAL)	Utilizes a pressurized stream of tumescent solution to anesthetize and dislodge fat lobules while simultaneously suctioning the fatty tissue and instilled fluid[39]	• BodyJet® (2008)[21] • HydraSolve® Lipoplasty System (2013)[40]
Radiofrequency-assisted liposuction (RFAL)	Delivers radiofrequency energy to the tissue through electrodes that leads to concurrent liquefaction of fat, coagulation of blood vessels, and modified skin tightening[41,42]	• BodyTite® (2016)[43] • FaceTite® (2016)[44] • AccuTite (2018)[45]

canisters, and an infiltration pump. Ancillary equipment for patient safety includes the ability to monitor vital signs and respond accordingly with supplemental oxygen and a "crash cart" in the event that any are compromised. There are also a number of supplementary technologies that have come to market during the past two decades that aim to make tumescent liposuction less labor intensive for the physician while also aiming to decrease scarring and increase skin contraction [**Table 97-5**].

OPERATIVE PLANNING AND TECHNIQUE

There is a robust body of dermatology and plastic surgery literature that describes how to prep and mark the patient for tumescent liposuction. Likewise, much had been published on tumescent anesthesia formulation,[24] infiltration, and suctioning technique. For example, Chapter 83 in this textbook's second edition offers helpful guidance on these topics.[27] However, reading a textbook chapter or published guidelines on how to perform liposuction is no substitute for experiential learning in the form of residency training, procedural fellowship, peer-to-peer training, or a dedicated training course. Individual facility and technique is further honed through a feedback loop of performing cases, observing outcomes and complications, and continued education. For these reasons, an in-depth discussion of operative planning and technique will not be included in this chapter.

PRACTICAL AND AESTHETIC CONSIDERATIONS INFORMED BY RACE AND ETHNICITY

According to the American Society of Plastic Surgeons Plastic Surgery Statistics Report, non-Caucasians represented 39% of patients seeking liposuction in 2020, specifically comprising 15% African Americans, 5% Asian and Pacific Islanders, 18% Hispanics, and 1% other non-Caucasians.[1] Given this degree of patient diversity, it may be helpful to anticipate how character and distribution of fat varies by racial group to inform operative planning (eg, using power-assisted or other energy based devices or selecting cannulae).

There is some research-based evidence to suggest that African Americans, Hispanics, and Asians possess more subcutaneous fat than age-matched Caucasians.[33-37] Furthermore, some authors have anecdotally observed that African Americans and Latinos tend to accumulate fat in the upper and lower abdomen, while Asians and East Indians do so in the lower abdomen.[27] It has also been claimed (though not to our knowledge substantiated by histologic studies of this anatomic region) that the truncal fat of African American men feels more dense and fibrous during liposuction than that of other groups.[27] Histologic studies have shown that fibroblasts in the facial skin of individuals of African descent are larger, multinucleated, more numerous, and contain more biosynthetically active organelles.[38] It is possible that these cellular characteristics are also demonstrated in the fibrous septa of adipose tissue in this population, potentially accounting for the aforementioned tactile observation.

It may be possible to anticipate some differences in body habitus based on race, but making race-based assumptions about a patient's aesthetic goals is somewhat problematic. While some have described trends in waist, gluteal, and thigh proportions sought by African American, Hispanic, and Asian female liposuction patients,[27,39] it must be remembered that these are anecdotal observations limited to specific practice settings during a set interval of time. In contrast, the influence of race and ethnicity on body image and perceptions of attractiveness has been widely examined in the psychology literature, resulting in numerous studies that have reached variable conclusions, many of them opposing.[40,41] It is also of importance to note that a significant number of published studies on these topics have used convenience samples of college students (in which men rate the attractiveness of women's bodies, or women rate other women according to how attractive they are likely to be perceived by men), and have failed to account for the impact of confounding variables including age, body weight, and socioeconomic status.[40,41] It is therefore overly simplistic to endorse broad generalizations about how beauty standards vary by racial and ethnic group. In fact, it may be possible that articulating an incorrect assumption about how a patient is seeking to contour their body could cause offense, thereby compromising the physician/patient relationship.

Old adages, though often trite, do not needlessly endure. We believe that beauty is in the eye of the beholder—namely, the individual who beholds their own form in the mirror. The surgeon performing liposuction should therefore eschew assumptions, and instead take time in consultation to understand what the patient is seeking.

UNIQUE CONSIDERATIONS INFORMED BY ANATOMIC REGION

SUBMANDIBULAR, SUBMENTAL, JOWL, AND NECK REGIONS

The principal target for liposuction in this region is the fat that is superficial to the platysma and medial to the sternocleidomastoid muscles. To access this area, the patient should be recumbent with the neck moderately extended so that an entry point in the submental crease can facilitate access to an area laterally bounded by the angles of the mandible and inferiorly bounded by the cricoid cartilage. Subauricular incisions permit access to the submental fat. Internal cannula diameter should not exceed 3 mm when treating this area. Removal of only 35 to 100 mL of adipose tissue can result in immediate improvement in the patient's profile [**Fig. 97.1 A & B**], while gently abrading the underside of the dermis with the cannula is particularly effective at promoting skin contraction. The marginal branch of the mandibular nerve can be avoided by lifting the skin away from the mandible and orienting the cannula medially and inferiorly.[28] Refer to **Table 97-6** for complications unique to this area. Postoperative compression garments are worn for 3 to 7 days.

BREASTS/CHEST

Tumescent liposuction can remove 30% to 50% of a woman's breast volume but may not be suitable for those who require a greater than 50% reduction, or for those whose breasts are pendulous or largely devoid

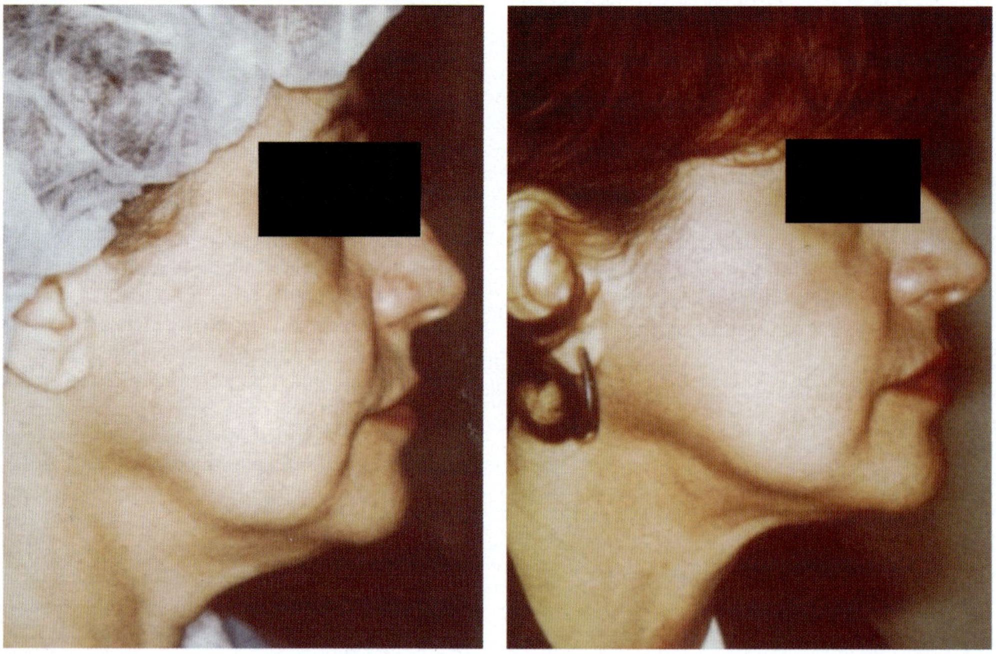

FIGURE 97-1. Hispanic woman before **(A)** and after **(B)** of liposuction of the neck and submandibular region.

of fat.[28] In male patients, the endpoint of suctioning is when the skin lies completely flat against the chest wall. The entry point is placed in the anterior axillary line at the level of the serratus anterior muscle. The use of aggressive grater and loop cannulas should be avoided beneath the areolar complex. Compression is worn for at least 3 weeks to promote maximum skin contraction. Refer to Table 97-6 for complications unique to this area.

UPPER ARMS

Deep fat targeted by liposuction is situated around 75% of the arm's circumference, excepting the volar aspect. One entry point over the olecranon fossa is often sufficient for both infiltration and suction. The use of nonaggressive technique and cannulae that are no more than 3-mm in diameter are recommended, as the skin of the upper arms is particularly susceptible to postoperative surface irregularities. Care should be taken when approaching the axilla to avoid brachial plexus injury. In females, a thin layer of fat should be spared to preserve a softened appearance, unless the patient's desires run explicitly counter to this aesthetic. Some may elect to simultaneously treat fat overlying the lateral portions of the latissimus dorsi, teres major, and teres minor muscles.[28] Compression garments should be worn for 2 weeks.

TABLE 97-6 Complications from liposuction[27]

Cardiac arrythmias	Keloids
Contour deformity	Lidocaine toxicity
Deep vein thrombosis	Lymphedema
Ecchymosis	Paresthesias
Edema	Postinflammatory pigmentary alteration
Fat embolism	Pulmonary embolism
Hematoma	Seroma
Hemorrhage	Skin necrosis and ulceration
Hospitalization	Soft tissue damage
Hypertrophic scarring	Volume overload
Hypotension	Wound infection
Intrathoracic or intraperitoneal perforations	Death
Complications unique to the submandibular, submental, Jowl, and neck regions	
Laryngeal edema (secondary to hemorrhage into the thyroid gland or trauma to and obstruction of the venous and lymphatic vessels)	
Hemorrhage into the neck, deep to the investing fascia of the larynx (that may put external pressure on the trachea causing airway obstruction)	
Complications unique to the breast/chest region	
Galactorrhea	
Postoperative calcifications that may hinder the mammographic detection of breast cancers (hence mammograms should be performed 3-6 months postprocedure)	

ABDOMEN

The abdomen, waist, and upper flanks should in most cases be treated simultaneously to optimize aesthetic outcome. To access the lower abdomen, entry points can be placed (and hidden) in the umbilicus and midway between the femoral canal and the anterosuperior iliac spine. Access to the upper abdomen requires additional entry points. Suctioning is preferentially performed in the deep fat planes. Because the upper abdomen is more fibrous, prone to post-treatment surface irregularities, and sensitive to pain, microcannulae tend to make the procedure more comfortable while yielding even and predictable results.[28] Patients should be informed of possible scrotal or vulvar swelling that may persist for up to a week before resolving without sequelae. Compression garments should be worn for 2 to 4 weeks.

FLANKS

Because of their fibrous nature, the flanks can be challenging to treat in certain individuals, particularly men. For small to medium flanks, one entry point overlying the tubercle of the iliac crest will usually suffice for infiltration and suctioning, while larger flanks (>350 mL) will likely require a second entry point overlying the tenth rib in the midaxillary line. The lower back and waistline may also be accessed from these sites. The use of more aggressive cannulae and technique, or power-assisted cannulae, may be helpful when treating the flanks.[28] Despite the need for these aggressive measures, the skin of the flanks tends to contract nicely. Compression garments should be worn for around 2 weeks.

HIP/LATERAL THIGH/BUTTOCKS

The adipose tissue of the hip and lateral thigh is similar in quality, and less aggressive suctioning techniques are often able to achieve

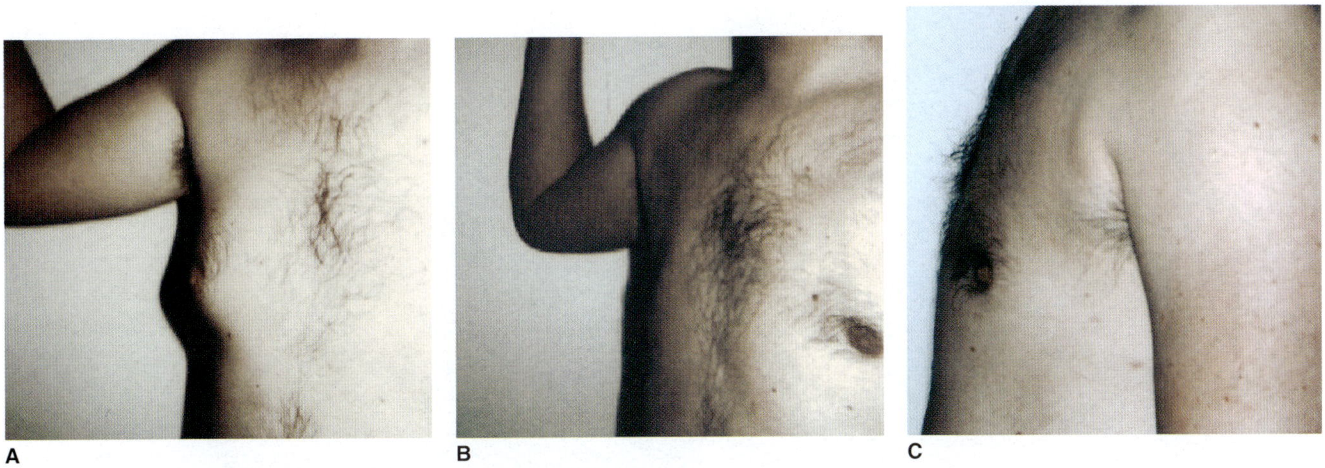

FIGURE 97-2. Before (A) and after (B and C) photos of liposuction to the breast region of a Hispanic man.

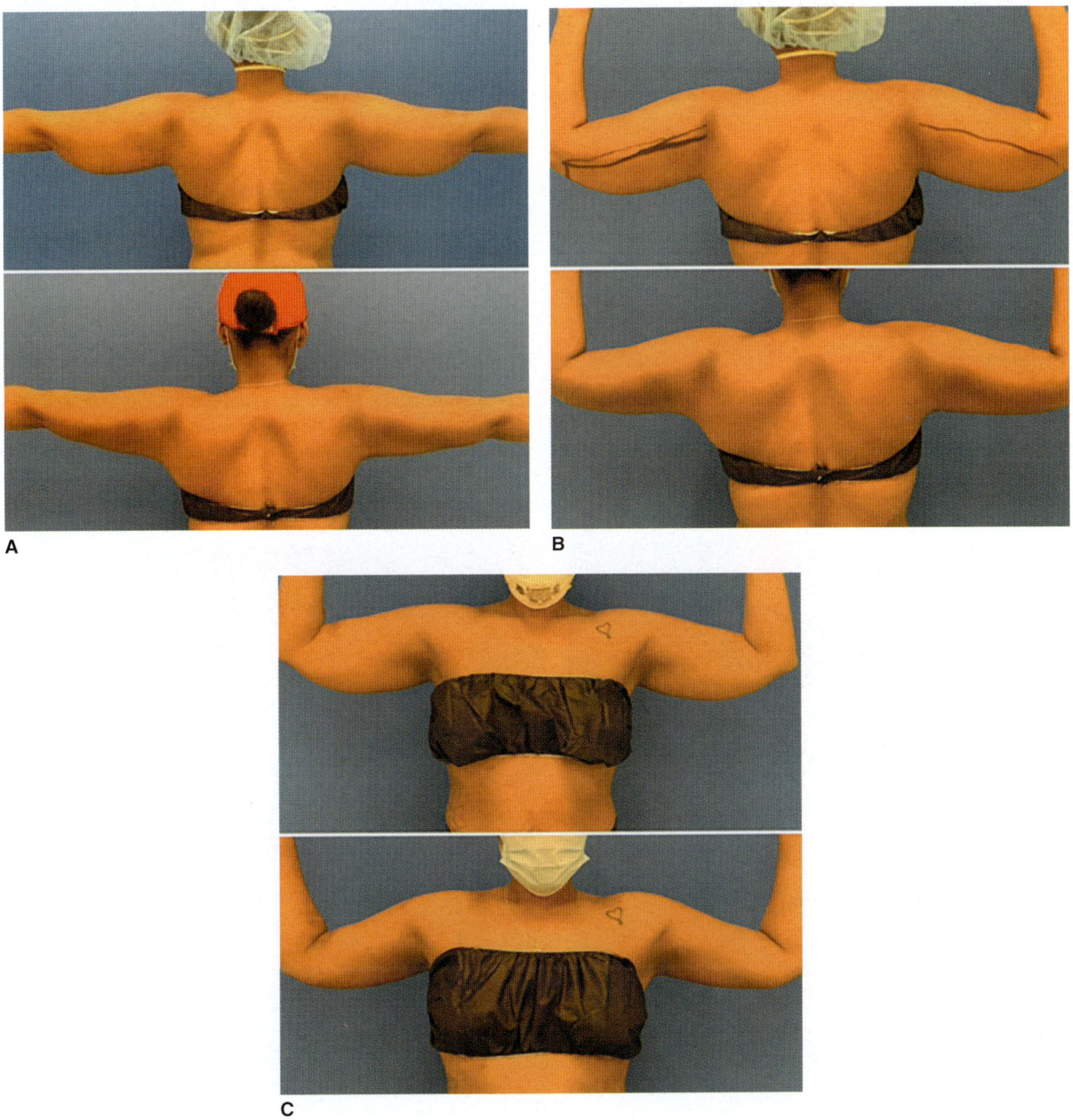

FIGURE 97-3. (A-C) Before and 3 month after photos of liposuction to the upper arms. (Courtesy of DiAnne Davis, MD, FAAD; Dallas, TX.)

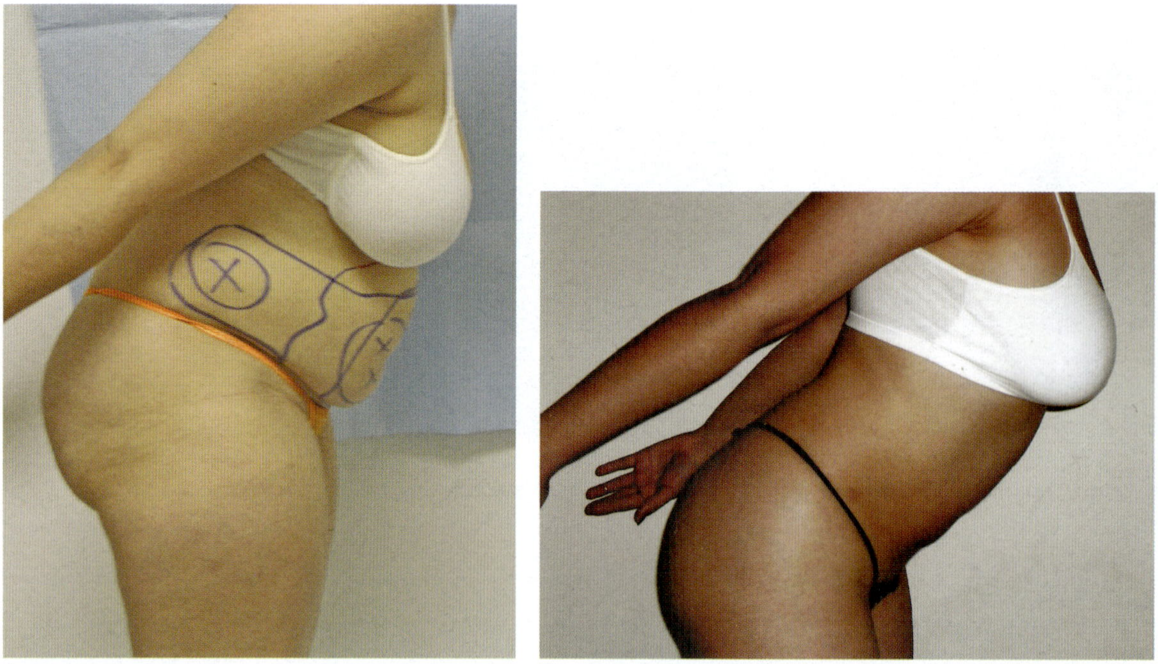

A B

FIGURE 97-4. Before (**A**, with topographic markings) and after (**B**) photos of SmartLipo of the abdomen in an African American woman.

the soft downward slope from waistline to hip, and gentle curve of the lateral thigh, that many female patients seek. An entry point is made in the anterior gluteal region to access the hip, while the infragluteal crease can hide the lateral thigh entry point. Having the patient stand intraoperatively may allow for better assessment of symmetry and silhouette.[28] Compression garments should be worn for around 10 days.

MEDIAL THIGH

The skin of the medial thigh extending from the labia majora to the inner knee resembles that of the upper arm in its tendency to display surface irregularities postoperatively. Less aggressive suctioning of only the deeper fat, with microcannulas inserted in multiple entry points and crisscrossed in diagonal and longitudinal directions, can help avoid the "doll" medial thigh appearance. The appearance of medial thigh skin that is excessively crepey or rugose may be worsened by performing liposuction—in these patients a medial thigh lift should be discussed.[28] Compression garments should be worn for at least 3 weeks.

OUTCOMES FOR SKIN OF COLOR PATIENTS

Postinflammatory hyper- or hypopigmentation, as well as hypertrophic scarring or keloid formation, where the dermis has been breached at cannula entry points, may be observed in skin of color patients following tumescent liposuction. Those who have experienced these alterations with

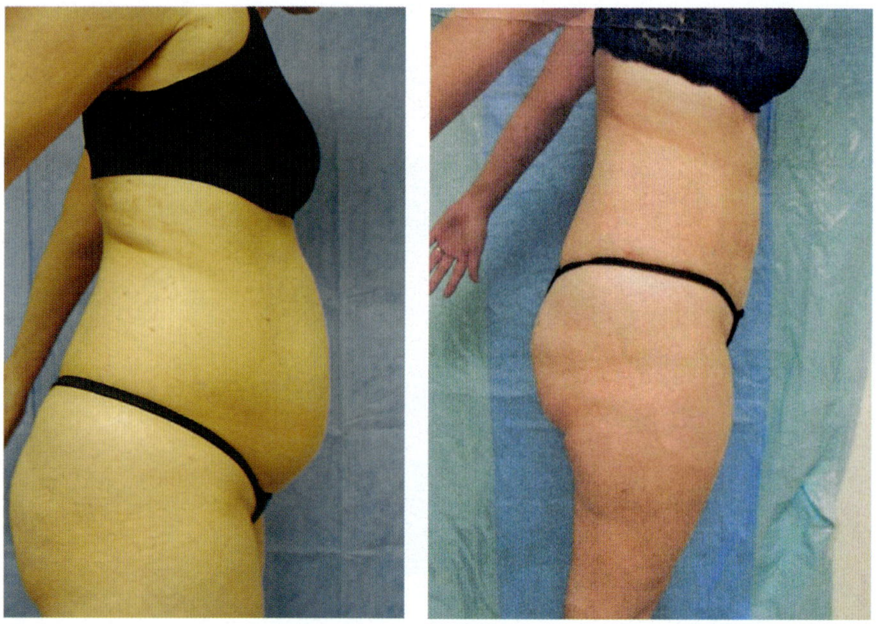

A B

FIGURE 97-5. Before (**A**) and after (**B**) photos of SmartLipo of the abdomen and flanks in an African American woman.

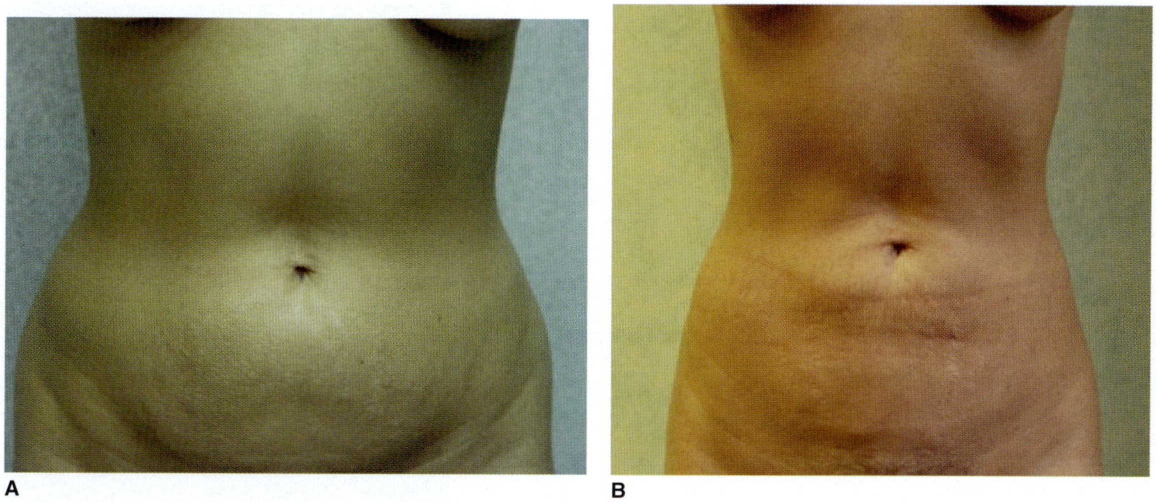

FIGURE 97-6. Before **(A)** and after **(B)** photos of liposuction to the abdomen and flanks in a Hispanic woman.

previous cutaneous injury are likely at relatively higher risk. Fortunately, these changes are not permanent and usually respond reasonably well to therapy that is both appropriately selected and initiated in a timely manner. To our knowledge, there have been no reported differences in serious healing complications or other adverse outcomes resulting from tumescent liposuction in skin of color patients compared with Caucasians.

Early intervention of persistent erythema or hyperpigmentation with hydroquinone 4% cream applied twice daily to intact skin should be initiated. Patients may concurrently apply a low- to mid-potency topical corticosteroid if inflammation is also present.[27] The physician may elect to treat focal areas of persistent inflammation with low concentration intralesional corticosteroid, before pigmentary alteration has the opportunity to manifest. There are also a number of topical cosmeceutical skin lightening agents that patients may use to supplement the medical management of their hyperpigmentation, but an in-depth discussion of these agents is unfortunately beyond the scope of this chapter. Finally, picosecond or Q-switched 755-nm alexandrite and 1064-nm Nd:YAG lasers may also be effective in managing hyperpigmentation in skin of color.

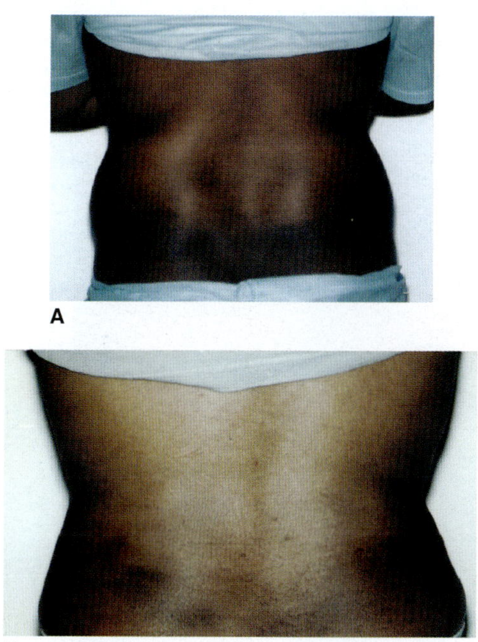

FIGURE 97-7. Before **(A)** and after **(B)** photos of liposuction to the flanks and lower back in an East Indian man.

Hypertrophic scar or keloid formation can be managed with a combination of intralesional corticosteroids and fractional nonablative and ablative lasers that can assist with collagen remodeling, drug-delivery, and improving concurrent hyperpigmentation.

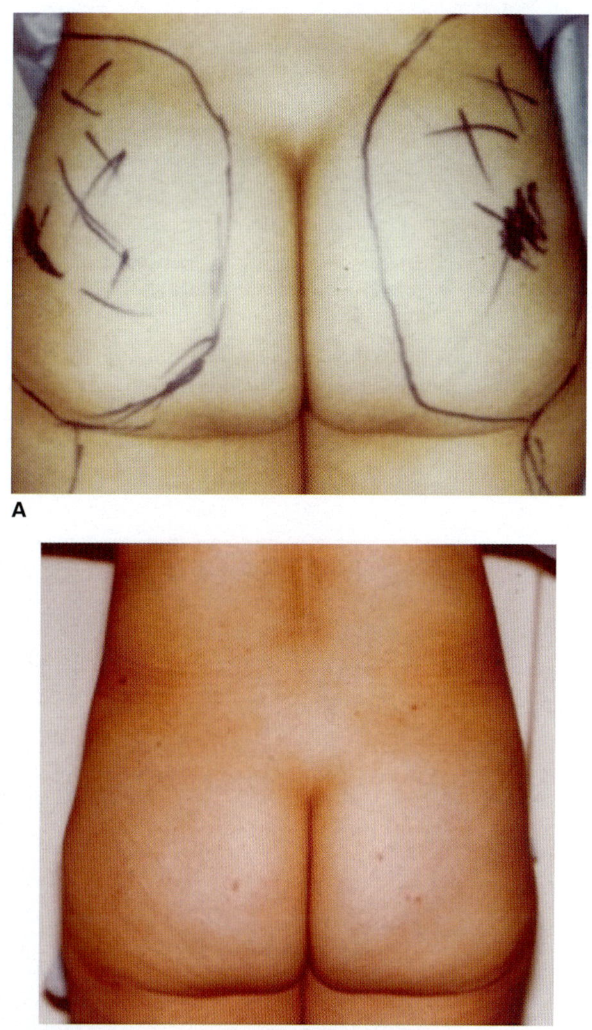

FIGURE 97-8. Before **(A)** and after **(B)** photos of liposuction to the hips, thighs, and buttocks in a Hispanic woman.

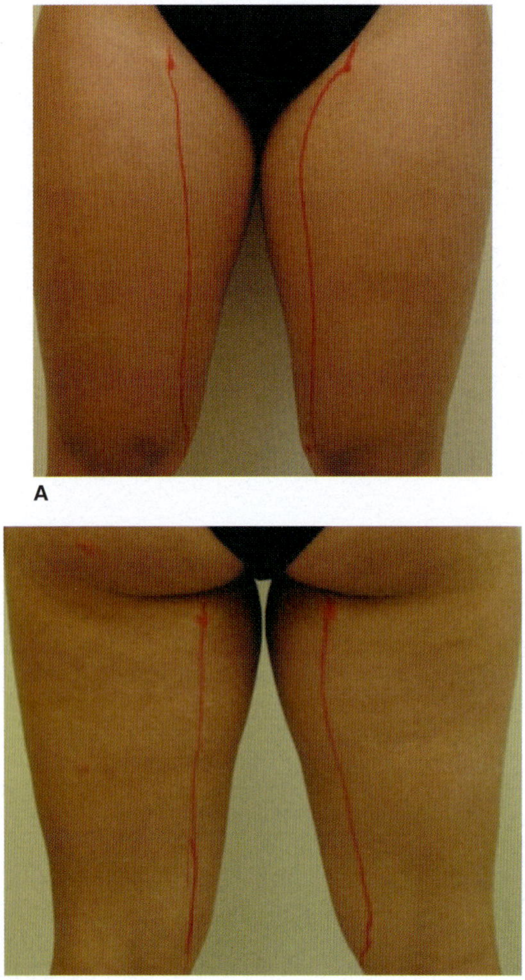

A

B

FIGURE 97-9. **(A** and **B)** Topographic markings for liposuction to the medial thighs prior to liposuction (after photos are shown in Figure 97-10A and B).

For patients with a known history of hypertrophic/keloid scar formation following cutaneous injury, the physician may also consider intralesional corticosteroid or neuromodulator[42] at incision sites at the conclusion of the procedure as an early and ideally preventive intervention.

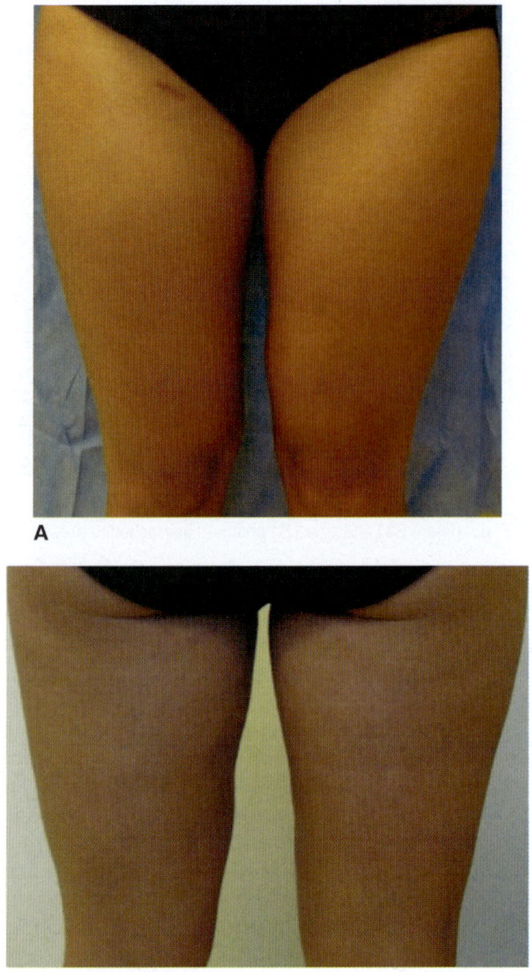

A

B

FIGURE 97-10. Anterior **(A)** and posterior **(B)** views after liposuction to the medial thighs in a Hispanic woman (before photos are shown in Figure 97-9A and B).

COMPLICATIONS

Dermatologists, who perform approximately one-third of liposuction procedures in the United States,[43] have demonstrated outpatient tumescent liposuction to be extraordinarily safe, with a serious adverse event

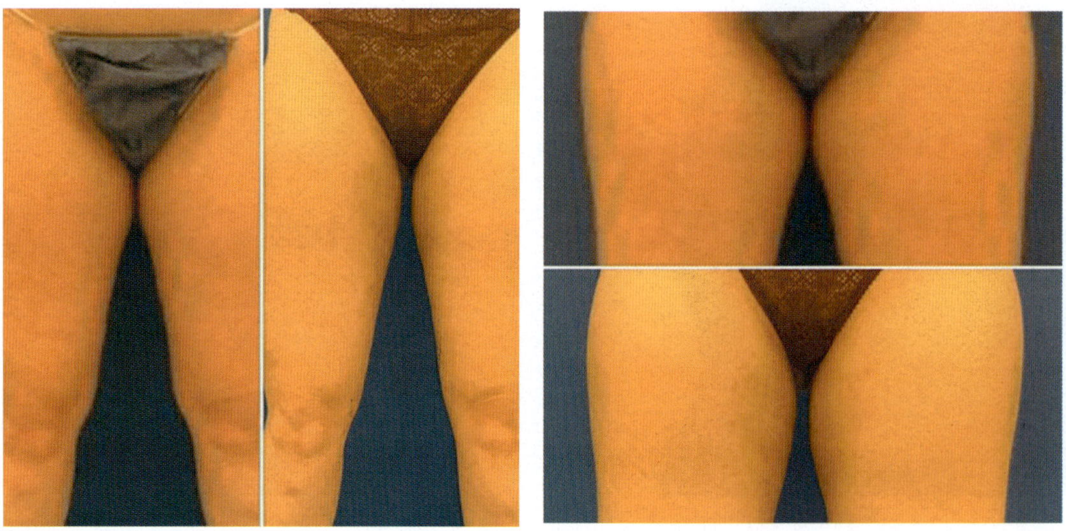

A B

FIGURE 97-11. **(A** and **B)** Before and after photos of liposuction to the medial thighs. (Courtesy of Dr. DiAnne Davis, MD, FAAD; Dallas, TX.)

rate of 0.68 per 1000 cases and no deaths reported. By comparison, hospital-based liposuction has been shown to result in up to 3.5 times as many malpractice claims.[44,45] Despite the likelihood of an uneventful recovery, complications [Table 97-6] do occur and therefore must be discussed with patients in consultation and when obtaining informed consent. Furthermore, additional counseling may be required when a normal part of the postoperative course is regarded by the patient as a complication. This may include weeks to months of position and activity dependent migratory swelling, transient nodule formation, and a delay of up to 6 months before full skin contraction is observed. The risk of complications can be mitigated by ensuring adequate physician training, appropriate patient selection, proper technique, careful formulation and administration of anesthesia, and meticulous pre-, intra-, and postoperative assessment and care.[27]

FUTURE PERSPECTIVES

If the past decades are to be used as an indicator, we can anticipate that many new supplemental, energy-based technologies will come to market over the next several years that will improve liposuction efficiency and deliver additional improvements in skin quality for enhanced patient outcomes. While patients have historically been counseled that weight gain and redistribution of fat is possible following tumescent liposuction, and that maintaining healthy diet, lifestyle, and exercise habits are important preventative measures against this, it remains to be seen how the advent of GLP-1 receptor agonists as weight loss agents will alter the liposuction landscape. Will some patients elect to use these drugs in the postoperative period to help maintain their results? Will certain anatomic areas emerge as more common targets for liposuction? Will liposuction shift to targeting much smaller but more recalcitrant areas of localized fat? Will there be a trend toward more high-definition liposuction, thereby making modalities such as power-assisted liposuction less necessary? Perhaps we will have enough data to address these issues in a future edition of this textbook.

REFERENCES

1. Inaugural American Society of Plastic Surgeons Insights and Trends Report: Cosmetic Surgery 2022. https://www.plasticsurgery.org/documents/News/Trends/2022/trends-report-cosmetic-surgery-2022.pdf. Accessed June 26, 2023.
2. Wu S, Coombs D, Gurunian R. Liposuction: concepts, safety, and techniques in body-contouring surgery. *Cleve Clin J Med.* 2020;87(6):367-375.
3. Field L. Liposuction surgery (suction-assisted lipectomy) for symmetric lipomatosis. *J Am Acad Dermatol.* 1988;18:1370.
4. Pinski K, Roenigk Jr. H. Liposuction of lipomas. *Dermatol Clin.* 1990;8:483-492.
5. Brorson H, Svensson H. Complete reduction of lymphedema of the arm by liposuction after breast cancer. *Scand J Plast Reconstr Surg Hand Surg.* 1997;31:137-143.
6. Sterodimas A, Boriani F, Magarakis E, Nicaretta B, Pereira LH, Illouz YG. Thirtyfour years of liposuction: past, present, and future. *Eur Rev Med Pharmacol Sci.* 2012;16:393-406.
7. Flynn TC, Coleman WP, Field LM, Klein JA, Hanke CW. History of Liposuction. *Dermatol Surg.* 2000;26:515-520.
8. Shrudde J. Lipexheresis (liposuction) for body contouring. *Clin Plast Surg.* 1982;11:455-456.
9. Pitanguy I. Trochanteric lipodystrophy. *Plast Reconstr Surg.* 1964;34:280-286.
10. Kesselring U. Regional fat aspiration for body contouring. *Plast Reconstr Surg.* 1983;72:610-619.
11. Fischer A, Fischer G. First surgical treatment for molding body's cellulite with three 5mm incisions. *Bull Int Acad Cosmet Surg.* 1976;3:35.
12. Illouz YG. Body contouring by lipolysis: a 5-year exeperience with over 3000 cases. *Plast Reconstr Surg.* 1983;72:591-597.
13. Fournier P, Otteni F. Lipodissection in body sculpturing: the dry procedure. *Plast Reconstr Surg.* 1983;72:598-609.
14. Klein JA. The tumescent technique for liposuction surgery. *Am J Cosmetic Surg.* 1987;4:263-267.
15. Drake L, Ceilley R, Cornelison R, et al. Guidelines of care for liposuction. Commiitee on Guidelines of Care. *J Am Acad Dermatol.* 1991;24:489-494.
16. Zocchi M. Ultrasonic liposculpturing. *Aesthetic Plast Surg.* 1992;16(4):287-298.
17. Apfelberg D. Laser-assisted lipousction may benefit surgeons and subjects. *Clin Laser Mon.* 1992;10(12):193-194.
18. U.S. Food and Drug Administration. *Device Approval Package: MicroAire Power-Assisted Liposuction (PAL) Infiltration System.* 1998. https://www.accessdata.fda.gov/cdrh_docs/pdf22/K220318.pdf. Accessed June 26, 2023.
19. Goldman A, Schavelzon D, Blugerman G. Laser lipolysis: liposuction using Nd-YAG laser. *Rev Soc Bras Cir Plast.* 2002;17:17-26.
20. U.S. Food and Drug Administration. *Device Approval Package: Smart Lipo.* https://www.accessdata.fda.gov/cdrh_docs/pdf6/K062321.pdf. Accessed June 26, 2023.
21. U.S. Food and Drug Administration. *Device Approval Package: Body-Jet.* 2008. https://www.accessdata.fda.gov/cdrh_docs/pdf8/k082025.pdf. Accessed June 26, 2023.
22. U.S. Food and Drug Administration. *Device Approval Package: Vaser 2.1 Lipo System*; 2011. https://www.accessdata.fda.gov/cdrh_docs/pdf11/K110306.pdf. Accessed June 26, 2023.
23. U.S. Food and Drug Administration. *Device Approval Package*; 2011. Accessed June 26, 2023.
24. Hanke CW, Dent M. Tumescent anesthesia: a brief history regarding the evolution of tumescent solution. *J Drugs Dermatol.* 2021;20(12):1283-1287.
25. Svedman K, Coldiron B, Coleman WP, et al. ASDS guidelines of care for tumescent liposuction. *Dermatol Surg.* 2006;32(5):709-716.
26. Coleman K, Coleman III K, Flynn TC. Body contouring: liposuction and non-invasive modalities. In: Bologna J, Schaffer J, Cerroni L, eds. *Dermatology.* 4th ed. Amsterdam: Elsevier; 2018:2627-2636.
27. Nijhawan R, Perez M, Ara-Honore C. Liposuction. In: Taylor S, Kelly A, Lim H, Serrano A, eds. *Dermatology for Skin of Color.* 2nd ed. New York, NY: McGraw Hill Professional; 2016:581-590.
28. Klein JA. *Tumescent Technique: Tumescent Anesthesia and Microcannular Liposuction.* St. Louis, MO: Mosby, Inc.; 2000.
29. GD B, HA G. Gynecomastia. *Curr Ther Endocrinol Meds.* 1997;6:401-404.
30. Thompson D, Carter J. Drug-induced gynecomastia. *Pharmacotherapy.* 1993;13:37-45.
31. Taro D. Cytochrome P450 enzyme drug interactions. *Drug Newsletter.* 1995;14:59-61.
32. Lozinski A, Huq N. Tumescent liposuction. *Plastic Surg.* 2013;40(4):593-613.
33. Deurenberg P, Bhaskaran K, Lian P. Singaporean Chinese adolescents have more subcutaneous adipose tissue than Dutch Caucasians of the same age and body mass index. *Asia Pac J Clin Nutr.* 2003;12:261-265.
34. Huang T, Johnson M, Figueroa-Colon R, Dwyer J, Goran M. Growth of visceral fat, subcutaneous abdominal fat, and total body fat in children. *Obes Res.* 2001;9:283-289.
35. Okosun I, Liao Y, Rotimi C, Dever G, Cooper R. Impact of birth weight on ethnic variations in subcutaneous and central adiposity in American children aged 5-11 years. A study from the Third National Health and Nutrition Examination Survey. *Int J Obes Relat Metab Disord.* 2000;24:479-484.
36. Lovejoy J, Smith S, Rood J. Comparison of regional fat distribution and health risk factors in middle-aged white and African American women: the Healthy Transitions Study. *Obes Res.* 2001;9:10-16.
37. Lovejoy J, de la Bretonne J, Klemperer M, Tulley R. Abdominal fat distribution and metabolic risk factors: effects of race. *Metabolism.* 1996;45:1119-1124.
38. Montagna W, Carlisle K. The architecture of black and white facial skin. *J Am Acad Dermatol.* 1991;24(6)(Pt 1):929-937.
39. Lee E, Roberts T, Bruner T. Ethnic considerations in buttock aesthetics *Semin Plast Surg.* 2009;23:232-243.
40. Cachelin F, Rebeck R, Chung G, Pelayo E. Does ethnicity influence body-size preference? A comparison of body image and body size. *Obes Res.* 2002;10(3):158-166.
41. Swami V, Jones J, Einon D, Furnham A. Men's preferences for women's profile waist-to-hip ratio, breast size, and ethnic group in Britain and South Africa. *Br J Psychol.* 2009;(100)(Pt 2):313-325.
42. Xiao Z, Zhang M, Liu Y, Ren L. Botulinum toxin type a inhibits connective tissue growth factor expression in fibroblasts derived from hypertrophic scar. *Aesthetic Plast Surg.* 2011;35(5):802-807.
43. Yu T, Perez M. Dermatologic liposuction: safety record and techniques. *Cosmet Dermatol.* 2004;17:209-212.
44. Coleman WP, Hanke CW, Glogau R. Does the specialty of the physician affect fatality rates in liposuction? A comparison of specialty specific data. *Dermatol Surg.* 2000;26:611-615.
45. Housman T, Lawrence N, Mellen B, et al. The safety of liposuction: results of a national survey. *Dermatol Surg.* 2002;28:971-978.

CHAPTER 98

Tissue Tightening Treatments

Mansee Desai
Sabrina Guillen Fabi

KEY POINTS

- Genetic and environmental factors impact the development, extent, and unique patterns of skin laxity in aging.
- The facelift is a longstanding surgical treatment for reducing skin laxity; however, patients now opt for less invasive tissue laxity treatments including utilization of lasers and light sources, radiofrequency energy, focused ultrasound, laser-assisted lipolysis, or a combination of approaches.
- Most patients require a combination of treatments and modalities to achieve desired results.
- Larger, controlled trials are necessary to achieve an objective comparison of various tissue-tightening treatments, especially with regard to the use of these modalities in people with skin of color.

INTRODUCTION

Tissue laxity is one of the most recognizable signs of aging. Both genetic and environmental factors contribute to the morphologic appearance of aged skin. Extrinsic aging, caused by external factors, results from a cumulative exposure to ultraviolet light and is manifested by signs of photodamage such as dyspigmentation, roughness, and keratosis.[1,2] Intrinsic aging, which is tied to internal factors, is linked with an individual's unique biological makeup and is largely genetically predetermined.

Although the presence or lack of epidermal melanin is central to the differential phenotype of aged skin, recent research has begun to uncover heretofore unrecognized histologic, molecular, and genetic factors that contribute to the pathogenesis of tissue laxity, both via their interplay with melanin and in its absence.[3] Fantasia et al[4] studied the levels of elastin fibers and transforming growth factor-β (TGF-β) were compared between skin biopsies of African Americans and Caucasians. TGF-β is critical to the resilience of human skin through its ability to upregulate the expression of elastin and other extracellular matrix proteins.[4] Chronologic aging compromises the structural integrity of dermal connective tissue, and there is a loss of elasticity, which manifests as skin thinning, wrinkling, and sagging. Interestingly, both TGF-β and TGF-β receptor expression were found to be higher in African American skin compared with Caucasian skin that points to the notion that Caucasians often display earlier signs of wrinkling and tissue laxity than those with darker skin of color.[5]

Although facelift remains the gold standard and results in the most significant improvement in skin laxity, it is associated with a substantial recovery time, expense, and risk.[1,6] Thus, many of today's discerning cosmetic patients are demanding less invasive approaches and are willing to settle for, and at times prefer, a less dramatic outcome. Today's options include both invasive and noninvasive modalities including the utilization of lasers and light sources, radiofrequency (RF) energy, focused ultrasound (US), laser-assisted lipolysis, and combination approaches.[6]

In addition, there is a paradigm shift toward lower energy settings, multiple treatments and emphasis on optimizing patient comfort to ultimately deliver a more palatable and safe patient experience.[6] Patient selection plays a key role in treatment success as clinical studies consistently have shown that areas of sagging skin with attached muscular fibers tend to respond best to tissue-tightening procedures.[6] In addition, patients must be appropriately counseled that the benefits of tissue tightening extend well beyond the immediate treatment phase; patients can expect to see continued improvement up to 6 months.[7]

Much of the latest cutting-edge research evaluating novel tissue-tightening devices in skin of color has been generated from studies investigating these techniques in Asian patients, classically Fitzpatrick skin types II to V. Unfortunately, there remains a relative paucity of data about these modalities being used in heavily pigmented skin, such as phototype VI. This chapter will discuss current tissue-tightening techniques and review the available data on their safety and efficacy in skin of color.

LASERS

This following section will review the current research and techniques particular to lasers and their use in skin tightening. For a discussion of the general principles and uses of lasers in skin of color, please refer to Chapter 94.

Lasers used in tissue tightening can be divided into two main categories: nonablative and ablative. Unlike ablative devices, nonablative lasers leave the epidermis intact while generating a large amount of heat in the dermis. The use of nonablative lasers for tissue tightening has become increasingly more widespread due to their relative safety in pigmented skin and the minimal associated down time. While fractional nonablative lasers have great utility in treatment of photoaging and scars, there is inconsistent data on its efficacy in tissue tightening.[8] A fundamental impediment to the laser's efficacy is the result of the light scatter that occurs during the transmission of the laser energy through the tissue. This property makes it difficult to achieve significant depths of penetration without the use of sufficiently higher energy, which could damage the epidermis and result in postinflammatory hyperpigmentation (PIH) or scarring in those with darker skin of color.[9] One way to increase the amount of deliverable energy has been the adjunctive use of superficial cooling devices during treatment.[10] In this way, the epidermis is protected, and somewhat deeper penetration and heat can be generated while minimizing the pain and adverse effects. A well-studied and commonly used nonablative laser is the long-pulse 1064-nm neodymium-doped yttrium-aluminum-garnet (Nd:YAG) laser.[11] This laser has a long proven history of efficacy and safety in epilation in darker skin of color, including Fitzpatrick skin types IV through VI.[12] The advantage of using this laser in skin of color is a longer wavelength, allowing for penetration that bypasses the epidermal melanin.[11] A noteworthy obstacle to the use of the Nd:YAG laser, especially in sensitive areas, is the discomfort associated with this treatment.[11] At times, the pain can be so severe that it necessitates aborting the procedure. Kono et al[13] addressed this issue by comparing two different mechanisms to reduce the pain during treatment sessions: cryogen spray cooling (CSC) versus pneumatic skin flattening (PSF). In this split-face trial, Asian patients with skin phototypes III and IV who had facial skin laxity were subjected to Nd:YAG laser and CSC on one side of the face, while the other side was treated with Nd:YAG laser and PSF. The authors reported that the use of PSF with the Nd:YAG laser was associated with less pain than the use of CSC with the Nd:YAG laser. Neither of the adjunctive measures affected the efficacy of the procedure.[13]

Recently, Lee et al[14] reported that a single session of 1444-nm pulsed Nd:YAG laser therapy resulted in a mild to moderate improvement in both the cheek laxity and the nasolabial fold depth in a small study of 10 Korean patients. A histologic analysis of posttreatment biopsy specimens from five volunteers showed increases in skin thickness, collagen fibers, and the expression of Ki-67, a marker of cell proliferation.[15] Additionally, real-time reverse transcriptase polymerase chain reaction revealed a substantial increase in levels of TGF-β from the baseline, which persisted at the 3-month follow-up.[15] The 1444-nm pulsed Nd:YAG laser was initially introduced for use in laser-assisted lipolysis, as it has a greater affinity for water and a prior study showed that it is more lipolytic than the 1064-nm Nd:YAG laser.[15]

Ablative lasers, such as the high-energy pulsed CO_2 and erbium-doped yttrium-aluminum-garnet (Er:YAG) lasers, function by vaporizing the intact epidermis while simultaneously generating a large amount of thermal energy in the dermis. Although it has been demonstrated that this technique is extremely effective for tissue tightening and facial rejuvenation, it is also associated with a lengthy recovery period and an increased potential for infection. These adverse effects mean this treatment is often

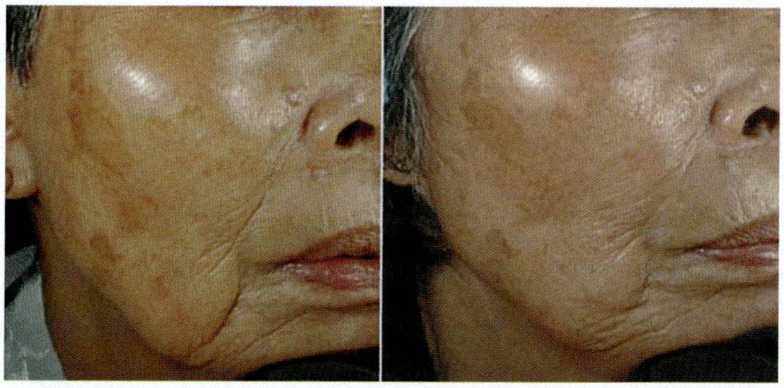

FIGURE 98-1. Before **(A)** and 7 months after **(B)** a single fractional CO_2 ablative laser treatment. (Used with permission from Dr. Henry Hin Lee Chan.)

unappealing for today's patients. Importantly, the use of these lasers in much darker skin of color is relatively contraindicated, due to the significant risk of postinflammatory dyspigmentation and scarring. An alternative to the classic ablative laser is fractional laser resurfacing. In this technique, microscopic thermal zones are created with intervening areas of intact epidermis. This allows for a more rapid repair of the damaged tissue and a decreased propensity for infection.[12] This approach has nearly revolutionized the use of lasers in facial rejuvenation because it can cause a significant clinical improvement in photodamage while minimizing both risks and down time.[16]

Another device that has been shown to induce tissue tightening is fractional delivery of the ablative 10,600-nm CO_2 laser [**Figure 98-1**]. Although fractional ablative CO_2 laser has demonstrated an average improvement of 57% in superficial skin tightening of the neck at 2 months, it too comes at the risk of dyspigmentation and scarring in highly pigmented skin.[17]

INFRARED LIGHT

Broadband infrared light has also gained popularity in the armamentarium of nonablative tissue-tightening modalities ranging from 800 to 1800 nm with water as the target chromophore.[18] This technique delivers thermal energy to the tissues that promotes a wound-healing response with collagen contraction and dermal remodeling over time. An infrared light source has the ability to operate at fluences significantly lower than that of other nonablative RF devices. This potentially provides a less painful alternative for the treatment of facial sagging.[18] Chua et al[19] investigated the use of infrared light with epidermal cooling for facial skin laxity in Asian patients with Fitzpatrick skin types IV and V. In this study, patients were exposed to infrared light in three treatment sessions at 4-week intervals. Both physicians and patients performed a final analysis of the outcome at a 6-month follow-up. It was noted that in all subjects, there were varying degrees of mild to moderate improvement in their skin laxity after treatment.[19] Additionally, there was a high rate of patient satisfaction, with only minimal discomfort reported during the procedure. The most common side effect was blistering, which was transient and resolved without sequelae. A more recent split face study by Tanaka et al studied the effects of a water filtered near infrared device (1000-1800 nm) with contact cooling on facial tightening in 20 Japanese patients.[20] The treated cheek was objectively evaluated by three-dimensional (3-D) color imaging and volumetric measurements that showed a mean volume reduction of 2.554 mL at 3 months posttreatment. There were no reports of epidermal burns or resultant scars.[20] Thus, a nonablative infrared device with contact cooling appears to be a viable option for mild to moderate tissue tightening in skin of color.

RADIOFREQUENCY

One of the earliest modalities developed to specifically target tissue laxity in a noninvasive manner was RF energy.[21] The electromagnetic spectrum of RF energy ranges from 300 MHz to 3 kHz.[21] This results in an immediate tissue contraction and damage to the dermal collagen, with a subsequent wound-healing response that occurs over months. However, unlike lasers, RF energy creates an electric field that is transduced through the skin, independent of a chromophore presence. The number of devices using RF energy has increased dramatically since the introduction of the first monopolar RF device in 2003.[21] Additionally, the modifications to existing devices, and the development of new protocols for their use, have further expanded the available options for the delivery of RF energy. RF devices are categorized as monopolar, bipolar, or tripolar, based on the arrangement of electrodes used in the treatment.[21]

Monopolar RF devices contain a single electrode that transmits current through to a grounding plate. When compared with a bipolar system, the delivery of electromagnetic energy via a monopolar device allows for an increased penetration depth but a less controlled current distribution.[21] Kushikata et al[22] used a monopolar RF device to evaluate skin tightening in Japanese females with skin phototypes III and IV who had lower facial laxity and wrinkles. At the 3- and 6-month assessment points, 30.5% and 25.6% of the patients reported a substantial improvement in their jowls, respectively.[22] A smaller number of patients admitted to a similarly positive outcome in the severity of their nasolabial folds and marionette lines over the same time frame. A physician assessment, largely based on before and after photography, revealed a slightly greater percentage of improvement after treatment. The patients experienced only minor complications such as edema, mild blistering, and PIH, all of which were transient.[22]

Although monopolar RF is a well-studied modality for facial laxity treatment, numerous small-scale studies with varying treatment parameters and grading systems have failed to show a significant and consistent degree of improvement.[23] A large-scale study by Dover et al[23] attempted to remedy this discrepancy and, in the process, develop a reproducible and effective protocol for this device. The authors compared a high-energy, single-pass treatment technique with a low-energy, multiple-pass technique using monopolar RF in 5700 patients.[23] The results revealed that the multiple-pass protocol was associated with less pain and a significantly better outcome in terms of immediate and long-term (6 months) tissue tightening. Importantly, the patient feedback on heat sensation was found to be crucial in determining the optimum energy parameters to be used during treatments.[23]

More recently, Tanaka et al demonstrated full face use of noninsulated microneedle radiofrequency (NIMNRF) on 20 Japanese patients with marked skin tightening of the lower two-thirds of the face. Specifically, patients achieved a 12.1-mL volumetric reduction as evidenced by superimposed 3-D volumetric assessments 6 months postprocedure. Patient experienced transitory erythema and slight burning that resolved within 5 hours posttreatment.[24]

In addition, Dayan et al did a prospective analysis of 247 patients who underwent combination RF microneedling with bipolar RF (FaceTite, InMode Aesthetic Solutions) for neck laxity and jowling with a post treatment improvement of 1.4 points on the Baker Face Neck Classification.[25] Notable postoperative side effects included edema lasting greater than 6 weeks, induration of treated area for 12 weeks or more and neuropraxia, all of which self-resolved.[25] While clinical studies show a consistent qualitative improvement in subdermal tissue tightening, many newer study results are predicated on subjective scales. Efforts on the development of objective scales for better surface area measurements are ongoing.[25]

FOCUSED ULTRASOUND

Ultrasonography has been a mainstay of diagnostic clinical medicine for many years. Micro-focused ultrasound (MFU) uses transducers to localize acoustic energy to a specific target in the dermal region at relatively higher energy and lower frequency than traditional diagnostic ultrasound.[26] The recipient tissue is heated to up to 65°C, thereby denaturing proteins, creating a controlled wound that causes immediate contraction of existing collagen fibrils and ultimately stimulating neocollagenesis that results in improved skin laxity[26] [**Figure 98-2**]. MFU is

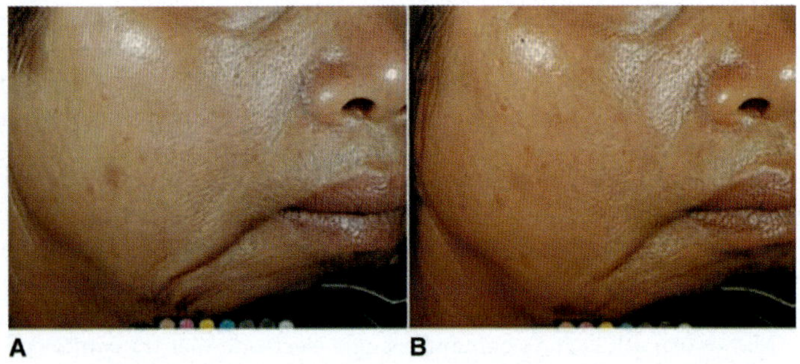

FIGURE 98-2. Baseline (A) and 5 months after (B) a single treatment with a focused ultrasound. (Used with permission from Dr. Henry Hin Lee Chan.)

FDA cleared for lifting lax skin of the submental area as well as providing a nonsurgical brow lift. MFU for tissue-tightening purposes delivers millisecond pulses of 0.5 to 10 J/cm^2 of energy, as opposed to the approximately 100 J/cm^2 used in HIFU. A significant advantage of MFU is its depth of penetration. It can deliver up to 65°C of heat to 4.5 mm, as opposed to the 1- to 3-mm depth achieved by other deep tissue heating devices such as RF, laser, and infrared light sources.[26-28] Precise visualization of tissue layers becomes paramount due to individual variability in depth and thickness of key anatomic structures. For instance, Asian subjects tend to have thinner skin with higher lipid concentration of the stratum corneum coupled with a more dense Superficial Muscular Aponeurotic System (SMAS).[29] The adjunct of real time visualization in the form of microfocused ultrasound with visualization (MFU-V) delivers low energy to three different depths (1.5, 3.0, and 4.5) with targeted treatment of the reticular dermis down to the SMAS without adversely heating the overlying superficial layers. The result is a 1-mm inverted cylinder lesion known as a thermal coagulation point (TCP). Subsequent wound healing around the TCP induces de novo collagen growth.[30] This technology is FDA cleared for the noninvasive lifting of the brow, submental neck skin, and reductions of décolleté wrinkles.[30] Studies have shown that dual depth treatments in one setting provides greater improvement in lax skin of the face, neck, abdomen, extremities and buttocks, compared to single depth.[30]

A consensus paper on optimal microfocused ultrasound with visualization in Asian patients summarized MFU lines and transducers in a set of flagship studies. Lee at al utilized 4-MHz/4.5-mm and 7-MHz/3.0-mm transducers to deliver on average of 238 lines at the dermal and fibrous layers of the lower face and neck with a decreased skin laxity in 90% of the subjects at 90 days posttreatment.[31] Jung et al utilized a 4-MHz/4.5-mm transducer to deliver 100 to 120 lines for facial skin laxity with a comparable outcome.[32]

In a study by Suh et al,[33] 22 Korean patients with Fitzpatrick skin types III to VI were exposed to one session of an MFU-V treatment for the treatment of facial skin laxity. All of the patients were noted to have some degree of objective (physician-graded) improvement, while more than 70% of the patients reported subjective improvement in the severity of their nasolabial folds and jaw line laxity 2 months after their treatment. A histologic analysis of the biopsy samples from a subset of patients revealed a more parallel arrangement of their elastic fibers and increased collagen in their dermis.[33]

Another report specifically investigated the safety and adverse effect profile of MFU-V treatment in Chinese patients with skin phototypes III and IV.[26] In this study, volunteers underwent between one and three treatments at 4-week intervals with transcutaneous focused U.S. technology. As per the protocol, a lower frequency transducer was used to deliver energy to regions of the face with an increased concentration of subcutaneous fat, such as the cheek and preauricular region. A higher frequency hand piece was used to treat thin-skinned areas such as the forehead and temple. Immediately after the treatment, erythema and edema were noted in 77.9% and 60.3% of the patients, respectively. However, this was transient and largely resolved within 1 week.[34] Focal bruising was experienced in 25% of cases but was no longer noticeable 1 month after the procedure.[26] Two patients developed minor, localized PIH on the forehead when the 4.5-mm depth transducer was used, and heat bounced off the bone. The PIH did slowly improved. Importantly, upon changing the transducer to a more superficial one, the 3.0 mm/7mHz, to avoid heat bouncing off the bone, no further cases of PIH occurred. Although no anesthetic agents were used in this study, it is suggested that more adequate pain control measures be pursued because severe pain was reported in more than half of the participants.[26] This study illustrates that although the MFU-V device is currently considered as the most effective nonablative modality for tissue tightening, even small modifications in treatment parameters and using proper visualization to avoid treating the bone in areas with overlying thin skin, can have a significant impact on potential adverse effects. While the absorption of ultrasonic energy is not affected by melanin, the thermal injury produced can still pose a risk of PIH in patients with darker skin of color, especially at high energies in areas of thin skin.[26]

LASER LIPOLYSIS

Laser lipolysis entails controlled injury of adipocyte deposits leading to noninvasive fat reduction with resultant skin tightening.[35] A purported advantage of this procedure over conventional liposuction is the potential for reduced scarring and shorter recovery times. Hyperthermia induces adipocyte apoptosis resulting in an inflammatory response with downstream removal of cellular debris by macrophage phagocytosis.[36] The heat generated leads to vessel coagulation and dermal remodeling. In 2017, the FDA cleared the use of 1060 nm diode laser for noninvasive lipolysis of adipose deposits of the abdomen, back, and thighs, among other sites. The 1060-nm laser energy has low affinity for pigment, making it theoretically safe for use in skin of color.[36] Doherty et al conducted a two-center study with single laser treatment to one flank among 49 patients ranging from Fitzpatrick skin Type I to VI. Ultrasound images and high-resolution photos taken preprocedure and at 12 weeks were reviewed by independent evaluators and yielded a statistically significant fat reduction of 2.6mm ± 1.1 mm.[37] In addition, Wan et al demonstrated statistically significant reduction of medial knee fat among 19 Asian female patients treated with a single session of 1060 nm wavelength at powers ranging from 1.0 to 1.4 W/cm^2.[36] Ultrasound-guided knee circumference measurements were taken in the axial and sagittal dimensions at 1, 3, and 6 months.[36]

COMBINATION APPROACHES

Treatment of the aging face, regardless of genetic makeup, often requires multiple modalities to achieve the desired cosmetic outcome. Same day multi-modal treatment is feasible for tissue tightening. Ultrasound therapies engender minimal edema or erythema enabling efficacious adjunctive treatment of neck laxity with laser-based therapies. For instance, patients first treated with microfocused ultrasound with visualization at maximal energy settings who were subsequently treated with ablative fractional laser demonstrated greater improvement in neck laxity compared to either therapy alone.[34,38,39] A retrospective analysis by Gao et al also demonstrated the safety of radiofrequency technology with fractional ablative laser of the periocular region in a Chinese cohort of 15 patients that significant differences in the following indices compared to baseline: skin elasticity, wrinkles, and textural irregularity. Patients reported variable degrees of erythema, hyperpigmentation, and edema that resolved within 10 days of treatment.[40] Park et al examined the efficacy of combination treatment for periocular rejuvenation in a study with 20 Korean patients and demonstrated that MFU-V followed by filler and botulinum toxin showed an average eyebrow height increase of 3.5 mm at 12 weeks.[41] Given the majority studies on multimodal treatment for skin tightening are pilot studies, randomized control trials with larger patient populations are needed for the reproducibility of results and to establish standardized treatment parameters.

CONCLUSION

Over the years, there has been substantial progress in the development of new devices and methodologies seeking to achieve tissue tightening. However, further research and testing are still required to establish a more complete body of knowledge in this area. Most laser and light sources have only been successful in improving skin laxity in small studies with stringent parameters in a select subset of patients. Head-to-head controlled trials are necessary to objectively compare the efficacy of the tissue-tightening techniques reviewed in this chapter. Nonablative lasers are often a more readily available and attractive option. However, they have yet to rival long-proven devices such as RF and newer modalities such as focused U.S. devices in the improvement of wrinkles and skin laxity. Similarly, patients need to be cautioned that while the technology of noninvasive tissue tightening is advancing at a rapid pace, there is nothing that can deliver results comparable to those obtained by interventional approaches such as the face lift or ablative CO_2 resurfacing. As such, physicians must carefully tailor an appropriate treatment regimen for each individual's unique presentation and concerns. Finally, a thorough discussion of risks, benefits, and limitations of each procedure is of the utmost importance in managing patient expectations and ensuring a satisfactory outcome.

REFERENCES

1. Alexiades-Armenakas M, Rosenberg D, et al. Blinded, randomized, quantitative grading comparison of minimally invasive, fractional radiofrequency and surgical face-lift to treat skin laxity. *Arch Dermatol.* 2010;146:396-405.
2. Rabe JH, Mamelak AJ, McElgunn PJ, et al. Photoaging: mechanisms and repair. *J Am Acad Dermatol.* 2006;55:1-19.
3. Rawlings AV. Ethnic skin types: are there differences in skin structure and function? *Int J Cosmetic Sci.* 2006;28:79-93.
4. Fantasia J, Lin CB, Wiwi C, et al. Differential levels of elastin fibers and TGF-beta signaling in the skin of Caucasians and African Americans. *J Dermatol Sci.* 2013;70:159-165.
5. Kahari VM, Olsen DR, Rhudy RW, et al. Transforming growth factor-beta up-regulates elastin gene expression in human skin fibroblasts. Evidence for post-transcriptional modulation. *Lab Invest.* 1992;66:580-588.
6. Bogle MA, Dover JS. Tissue tightening technologies. *Dermatol Clin.* 2009;27:491-499, vii.
7. Chan HH, Yu CS, Shek S, et al. A prospective, split face, single-blinded study looking at the use of an infrared device with contact cooling in the treatment of skin laxity in Asians. *Laser Surg Med.* 2008;40:146-152.
8. Kauvar AN. Fractional nonablative laser resurfacing: is there a skin tightening effect? *Dermatol Surg.* 2014;40 Suppl 12:S157-S163.
9. Chan HH, Lam LK, Wong DS, et al. Role of skin cooling in improving patient tolerability of Q-switched Alexandrite (QS Alex) laser in nevus of Ota treatment. *Laser Surg Med.* 2003;32:148-151.
10. Yeung CK, Shek SY, Chan HH. Hair removal with neodymium-doped yttrium aluminum garnet laser and pneumatic skin flattening in Asians. *Dermatol Surg.* 2010;36:1664-1670.
11. Alster TS, Bryan H, Williams CM. Long-pulsed Nd:YAG laser-assisted hair removal in pigmented skin: a clinical and histological evaluation. *Arch Dermatol.* 2001;137:885-889.
12. Manstein D, Herron GS, Sink RK, et al. Fractional photothermolysis: a new concept for cutaneous remodeling using microscopic patterns of thermal injury. *Laser Surg Med.* 2004;34:426-438.
13. Kono T, Kikuchi Y, Groff WF, et al. Split-face comparison study of cryogen spray cooling versus pneumatic skin flattening in skin tightening treatments using a long-pulsed Nd:YAG laser. *J Cosmet Laser Ther.* 2010;12:87-91.
14. Lee SH, Roh MR, Jung JY, et al. Effect of subdermal 1,444-nm pulsed neodymium-doped yttrium aluminum garnet laser on the nasolabial folds and cheek laxity. *Dermatol Surg.* 2013;39:1067-1078.
15. Tark KC, Jung JE, Song SY. Superior lipolytic effect of the 1,444 nm Nd:YAG laser: comparison with the 1,064 nm Nd:YAG laser. *Laser Surg Med.* 2009;41:721-727.
16. Jih MH, Kimyai-Asadi A. Fractional photothermolysis: a review and update. *Semin Cutan Med Surg.* 2008;27:63-71.
17. Tierney EP, Hanke CW. Ablative fractionated CO2, laser resurfacing for the neck: prospective study and review of the literature. *J Drugs Dermatol.* 2009;8(8):723-731.
18. Ruiz-Esparza J. Near [corrected] painless, nonablative, immediate skin contraction induced by low-fluence irradiation with new infrared device: a report of 25 patients. *Dermatol Surg.* 2006;32:601-610.
19. Chua SH, Ang P, Khoo LS, et al. Nonablative infrared skin tightening in type IV to V Asian skin: a prospective clinical study. *Dermatol Surg.* 2007;33:146-151.
20. Tanaka Y, Tsunemi Y, Kawashima M, Tatewaki N, Nishida H. Objective assessment of skin tightening in Asians using a water-filtered near-infrared (1,000-1,800 nm) device with contact-cooling and freezer-stored gel. *Clin Cosmet Investig Dermatol.* 2013;6:167-176.
21. Krueger N, Sadick NS. New-generation radiofrequency technology. *Cutis.* 2013;91:39-46.
22. Kushikata N, Negishi K, Tezuka Y, et al. Non-ablative skin tightening with radiofrequency in Asian skin. *Lase Surg Med.* 2005;36:92-97.
23. Dover JS, Zelickson B, 14-Physician Multispecialty Consensus Panel. Results of a survey of 5,700 patient monopolar radiofrequency facial skin tightening treatments: assessment of a low-energy multiple-pass technique leading to a clinical end point algorithm. *Dermatol Surg.* 2007;33:900-907.
24. Tanaka Y. Long-term three-dimensional volumetric assessment of skin tightening using a sharply tapered non-insulated microneedle radiofrequency applicator with novel fractionated pulse mode in asians. *Lasers Surg Med.* 2015;47(8):626-633.
25. Dayan E, Chia C, Burns AJ, et al. Adjustable depth fractional radiofrequency combined with bipolar radiofrequency: a minimally invasive combination treatment for skin laxity. *Aesthet Surg J* 2019;39:(suppl_3)S112-S119.
26. Chan NP, Shek SY, Yu CS, et al. Safety study of transcutaneous focused ultrasound for non-invasive skin tightening in Asians. *Laser Surg Med.* 2011;43:366-375.
27. Gliklich RE, White WM, Slayton MH, et al. Clinical pilot study of intense ultrasound therapy to deep dermal facial skin and subcutaneous tissues. *Arch Facial Plast Surg.* 2007;9:88-95.
28. White WM, Makin IR, Barthe PG, et al. Selective creation of thermal injury zones in the superficial musculoaponeurotic system using intense ultrasound therapy: a new target for noninvasive facial rejuvenation. *Arch Facial Plast Surg.* 2007;9:22-29.
29. Park JY, Lin F, Suwanchinda A, et al. Customized treatment using microfocused ultrasound with visualization for optimized patient outcomes: a review of skin-tightening energy technologies and a Pan-Asian adaptation of the expert panel's gold standard consensus. *J Clin Aesthet Dermatol.* 2021;14(5):E70-E79.
30. Fabi SG, Joseph J, Sevi J, Green JB, Peterson JD. Optimizing patient outcomes by customizing treatment with microfocused ultrasound with visualization: gold standard consensus guidelines from an expert panel. *J Drugs Dermatol.* 2019;18(5):426-432.
31. Lee HS, Jang WS, Cha YJ et al. Multiple pass ultrasound tightening of skin laxity of the lower face and neck. *Dermatol Surg.* 2012;38(1):20-27.
32. Jung HJ, Min J, Seo HM, Kim WS. Comparison of effect between high intense focused ultrasound devices for facial tightening: Evaluator-blinded, split-face study. *J Cosmet Laser Ther.* 2016;18(5):252-256.
33. Suh DH, Oh YJ, Lee SJ, et al. An intense-focused ultrasound tightening for the treatment of infraorbital laxity. *J Cosmet Laser Ther.* 2012;14:290-292.
34. Guss L, Bolton JG, Fabi SG. Combination therapy in skin of color including injectables, laser, and light devices. *Semin Cutan Med Surg.* 2016;35(4):211-217.
35. Wolfenson M, Hochman B, Ferreira LM. Laser lipolysis: skin tightening in lipoplasty using a diode laser. *Plast Reconstr Surg.* 2015;135(5):1369-1377.
36. Yan C, Wanitphakdeedecha R, Evangelista KER, et al. Efficacy of noninvasive 1060-nm diode laser for medial knee fat reduction. *Dermatol Ther (Heidelb).* 2022;12(5):1253-1261.
37. Katz B, Doherty ST. Safety and efficacy of a noninvasive 1060 nm diode laser for fat reduction of the flanks. *Dermatol Surg.* 2018;44:388-396.
38. Vanaman M, Fabi SG, Cox SE. Neck rejuvenation using a combination approach: our experience and a review of the literature. *Dermatol Surg.* 2016;42 Suppl 2:S94-S100.
39. Woodward JA, Fabi SG, Alster T, Colon-Acevedo B. Safety and efficacy of combining microfocused ultrasound with fractional CO2 laser resurfacing for lifting and tightening the face and neck. *Dermatol Surg.* 2014;40 Suppl 12:S190-S193.
40. Gao L, Kang H, Li Y, et al. Clinical efficacy and safety of 3DEEP multisource radiofrequency therapy combined with fractional skin resurfacing for periocular skin aging. *J Clin Aesthet Dermatol.* 2020;13(3):41-44.
41. Park JY, Byun EJ, Kim HS. Rejuvenation of periocular region in Koreans: a multimodal approach combining botulinum toxin, fillers, and microfocused ultrasound with visualization for optimal results. *Dermatol Ther.* 2020;33(1):e13159.

CHAPTER 99

Body Contouring

DiAnne S. Davis

KEY POINTS

- The desire and increased demand for noninvasive cosmetic procedures that focus on body contouring and/or fat reduction has prompted the rise and innovation of options pioneered by dermatologists.
- Advanced methods, including cryolipolysis, radiofrequency, high-intensity focused ultrasound, lasers, electromagnetic stimulation, and injectable agents all leverage different properties of adipose cells and the surrounding connective tissue, with a common goal of achieving a desired aesthetic outcome.
- Cryolipolysis selectively targets and reduces fat cells through controlled cooling that not only reduces the thickness of fat layers but also results in simultaneous tightening of the skin in the areas of fat reduction.
- High-intensity focused ultrasound utilizes negative acoustic wave pressure and heat to induce adipocyte cell death.
- Radiofrequency devices employ controlled heat energy to target fat, improve body contour, and enhance skin quality, all while demonstrating a favorable safety profile.
- In vitro studies have demonstrated the effectiveness of selective photothermolysis in targeting adipose tissue by utilizing the infrared vibrational absorption bands of lipids.
- High-intensity focused electromagnetic muscle stimulation simultaneously increases fat metabolism while strengthening muscles in the target area by delivering pulses in a frequency that produces a vast amount of muscle contractions not achievable voluntarily.
- In the wake of the COVID-19 pandemic, the "zoom effect" phenomenon sparked a renewed interest in aesthetic enhancements as people sought to address concerns about their face, jaw line, and neck regions, with deoxycholic acid becoming an attractive solution, based on its efficacy, convenience, and minimal downtime.
- Collagenase clostridium histolyticum-aaes incorporates two purified forms of the bacteria to induce an enzymatic reaction that disrupts the organization of collagen fibrils and targets the fibrous septae in cellulite to improve the overlying topography of the skin surface.
- Minimally invasive and noninvasive modalities have gained significant traction, and the array of different treatment modalities for targeting focal fat deposits is only destined to grow with simplistic use, tolerability, and negligible downtime.

INTRODUCTION

The desire for cosmetic procedures that focus on body contouring and/or fat reduction have continued to increase in popularity over the last decade.[1] This desire has prompted a specific focus within cosmetic dermatology known as noninvasive body sculpting, shaping, or contouring.[2] Over the past 7 years, there has been a fourfold rise in popularity, attributed to factors such as sedentary lifestyles, unbalanced diets,[3] and the pervasive influence of beauty standards projected by mass media. Additional factors include the growing receptiveness of individuals to seek cosmetic treatments to address their overall body dissatisfaction and achieve desired aesthetic goals. Moreover, the advent of innovative and less invasive procedures for targeted fat reduction, coupled with minimal downtime and a low risk of complications, has contributed to the rise of body contouring.[1,4] Coinciding with consumer demand, an increasing number of minimally invasive options, pioneered by dermatologists, have emerged to specifically target localized fat deposits, some with the added benefit of tissue tightening or muscle toning. These advanced methods, including cryolipolysis, radiofrequency, high-intensity focused ultrasound, lasers, electromagnetic stimulation, and injectable agents all leverage different properties of adipose cells and the surrounding connective tissue, with a common goal of achieving a desired aesthetic outcome.

PATIENT CONSIDERATIONS

When considering body contouring procedures, several factors should be taken into consideration. First and foremost, it's important that patients have realistic expectations and understand the limitations of the procedure. Body contouring can enhance and improve the body's appearance, but it cannot achieve drastic or overnight transformations. Patients should have a clear understanding of the potential outcomes and discuss their goals and expectations with a board-certified dermatologist. Another crucial consideration is the overall health and suitability of the patient for the procedure. It's essential to disclose and review any preexisting medical conditions, allergies, or medications that may impact treatment. The dermatologist should also perform a physical examination to determine if they are a suitable candidate for the recommended procedure. An accurate calculation of the Body Mass Index (BMI) is instrumental in assessing obesity and its associated factors such as visceral fat and widespread subcutaneous adiposity, in particular when considering body procedures focused on the abdomen. In cases where obesity is present, it is highly recommended to prioritize weight loss and achieve a BMI below 30 kg/m^2 before considering aesthetic fat reduction treatments. This approach ensures that adequate weight loss has occurred and sets a foundation for more effective outcomes in subsequent procedures.[1] In cases where there is a substantial amount of abdominal adipose tissue, noninvasive modalities would necessitate an impractical number of sessions, resulting in exorbitant costs and ultimately yielding insignificant or unappreciable results. Open communication, adherence to pre- and postprocedure instructions, and realistic expectations are key for any successful body contouring experience.

TREATMENT OPTIONS

Currently, there exists a wide range of therapeutic options for body contouring on different areas. These available methods employ various approaches, including ablation techniques such as cooling, heating, disrupting or dissolving adipocytes, nonablative effects that stimulate adipocyte lipolysis or the modification of their structure,[1] targeting muscle groups via motor neuron stimulation to provoke repetitive contractions while simultaneously enhancing fat metabolism,[4] acoustic waves, and injectable agents. The optimal choice for your patient will vary based on their unique clinical presentation, treatment objectives, and their personal preference.

CRYOLIPOLYSIS

Cryolipolysis was first described as "popsicle panniculitis" in 1970, by Epstein and Oren, who reported a case where an infant was sucking on a popsicle that resulted in the development of a nodule on the cheek that prompted temporary tissue death. These observations brought about the realization that tissues rich in lipids were more vulnerable to cold injury compared to surrounding tissues with higher water content.[5] Manstein and colleagues were able to demonstrate that prolonged controlled cooling of local skin regions induced selective damage and subsequent fat cell death without damaging the overlying skin,[5,6] followed by additional studies showing a 30% reduction in the thickness of fat layers.[7]

The mechanism of action involves programmed apoptotic fat cell death secondary to the application of cold temperatures, which are then engulfed and digested by macrophages. This stimulates an inflammatory process leading to the digestion of lipid cells and overall reduction in

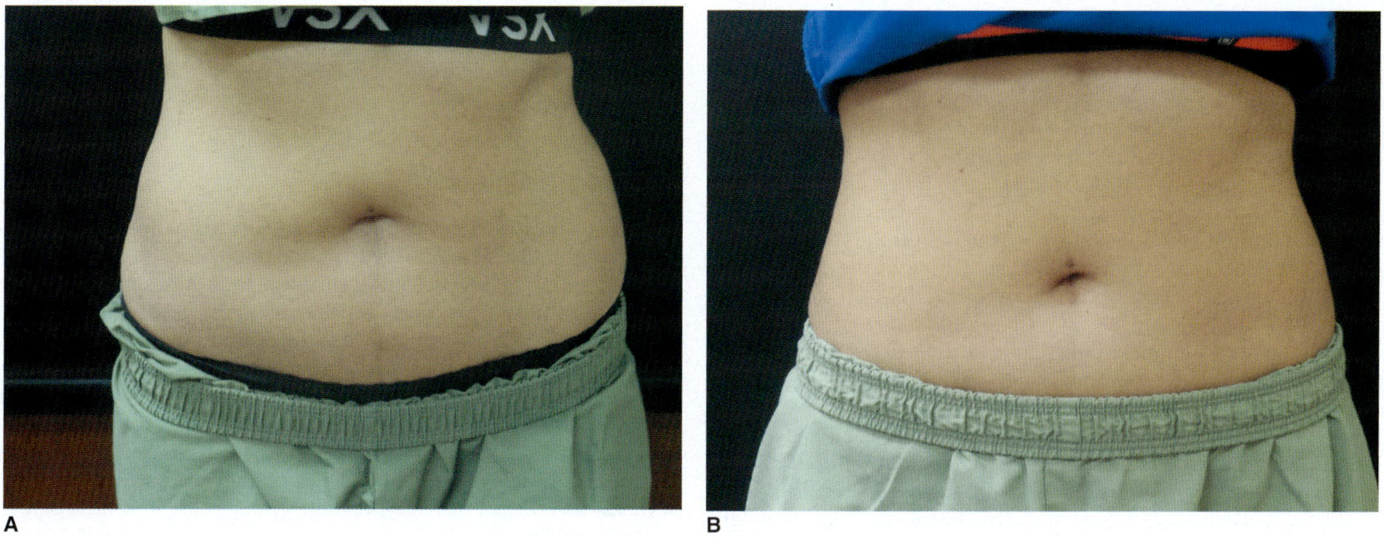

FIGURE 99-1. Before (A) and after (B) of CoolSculpting on the abdomen. (Courtesy of Peterson Pierre, MD, FAAD; Thousand Oaks, CA.)

adipocyte volume. With time, the interlobular septa thicken and account for the majority of tissue volume in the treated area.[8,9] Initial clinical studies involving human subjects indicated that cryolipolysis was successful in reducing fat on the flanks and back areas.[10] In 2010, the first U.S. Federal Drug Administration (FDA)-cleared cryolipolytic device (CoolSculpting®; ZELTIQ Aesthetics, Inc., Pleasanton, CA) was approved for the reduction of fat on the flanks and abdomen [**Figure 99-1A** and **B**], with the approval for treatment on the thighs in 2014.[11] Since then, the arms, knees, and submental region [**Figure 99-2**] have received expanded FDA clearance with the development of customized applicators unique for different treatment areas. The technology currently utilizes a vacuum to draw in and compress a specific fold of tissue between two opposing cooling plates, which compress cutaneous blood flow and apply noninvasive cooling for a predetermined duration based on the area being treated (35-75 minutes). Thermoelectric elements determine the appropriate temperature and it is regulated by sensors that monitor the heat

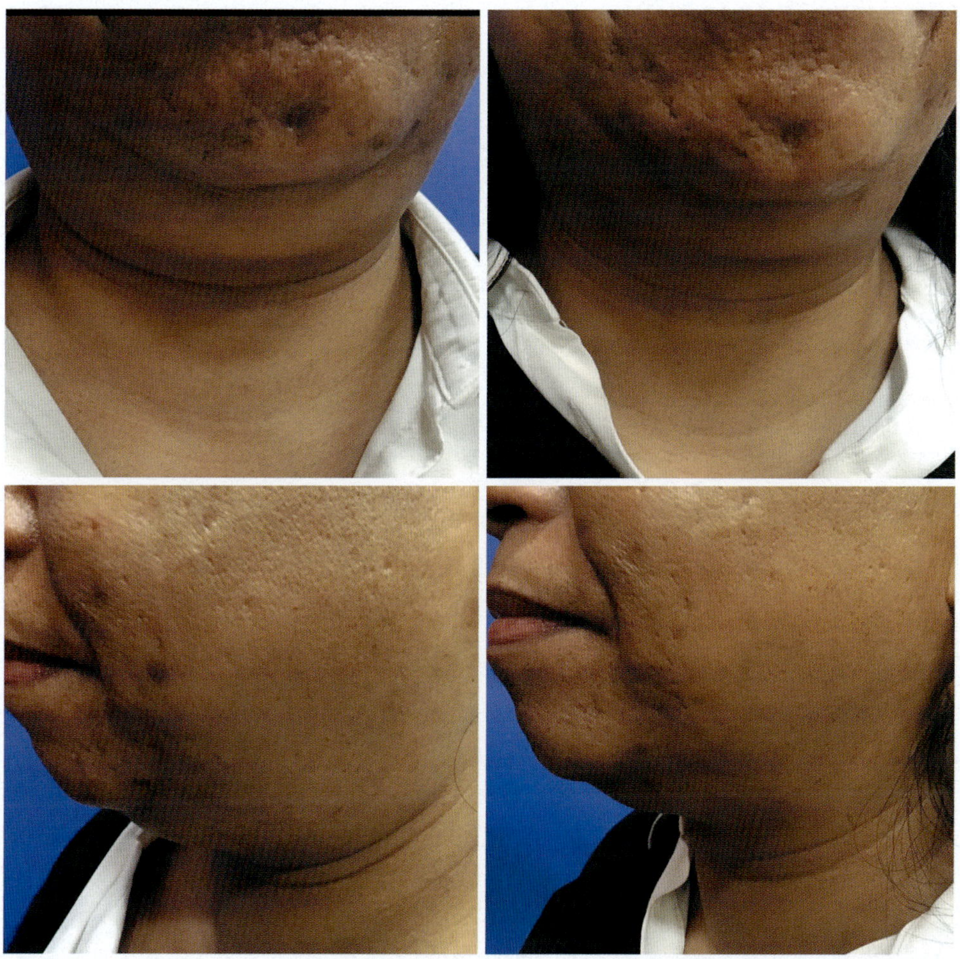

FIGURE 99-2. Before and after of CoolSculpting to the submental region on an African American woman. (Courtesy of Mara Weinstein Velez, MD, FAAD; Rochester, NY.)

flow emanating from the tissue.[12] Immediately after, the skin exhibits a cool firm texture, often in the shape of the treatment applicator. Vigorous massaging for 2 minutes instantaneously after treatment helps to break up crystallized adipocytes[13] and has demonstrated greater reductions in fat thickness by 44% and overall improved outcomes.[14] In addition to fat reduction, skin tightening was also anecdotally reported as a sequalae of cryolipolysis by Carruthers et al, based on independent assessments by patients and investigators.[5] The researchers postulated that the application of vacuum suction, which pulls the tissue into the treatment applicator and induces mild stretching of the skin, stimulates neocollagenesis, leading to improvements in both skin texture and laxity.

Both human and animal studies have demonstrated the safety of this procedure with no significant changes in lipid levels, liver function tests, or long-term peripheral nerve function.[15,16] Common but transient side effects include edema, erythema, bruising, and numbness, with most resolving weeks after treatment.[1,5,17] While no significant adverse events have been reported, increasing reports have documented well-demarcated, bulky, tender masses at the treatment site, consistent with paradoxical adipose hyperplasia (PAH) as a rare (1 in 20,000) and challenging complication.[17,18] PAH usually presents 2 to 3 months postprocedure and results from the unintended stimulation of tissue growth (either as a result of the recruitment of circulating stem cells and/or preadipocytes or hypoxic injury supported by increased vascularity and septal thickening).[17,18] Should PAH present itself, liposuction or abdominoplasty have been employed to correct the adverse event. Since its introduction to the market, the CoolSculpting® device has undergone continuous evolution, incorporating various applicators designed for specific body areas, including the elite handpieces that allow for more tissue contact, suction, cooling, and faster treatment times.[13]

HIGH-INTENSITY FOCUSED ULTRASOUND

High-intensity focused ultrasound (HIFU) is a noninvasive alternative to ablate adipose tissue by utilizing ultrasound waves to generate precise and controlled thermal energy to specific treatment areas. The technology combines the mechanical (cavitational) effects that disrupts cell membranes via negative acoustic pressure while utilizing heat to raise the local temperature of tissue (above 58°C), resulting in instantaneous adipocyte cell death via coagulative necrosis. All the while, sparing the surrounding tissue and overlying skin.[19,20] Following treatment, the induced adipocyte cell death triggers a wound healing response attracting macrophages that engulf and carry away lipids and cellular debris. The wound healing cascade activates fibroblasts and the production of new collagen, accompanied by tightening of the septal fibers and skin. After approximately 18 weeks, 95% of the destroyed adipocytes are resorbed, resulting in a significant reduction in the volume of localized fat. This process contributes to an overall improvement in the appearance and contour of the treated area.[21]

Several studies have demonstrated the safety and efficacy of HIFU contouring of the abdomen and flanks.[19,20,22] Jewell et al conducted research on 180 subjects using the FDA-approved Liposonix device (Solta Medical, Bausch, Bothell, WA), and demonstrated a statistically significant reduction in waist circumference.[22] A significant advantage of HIFU compared to other thermal ablative techniques is the absence of the need to transcutaneously insert probes into the target tissue. Adverse events that are short-lived include paresthesias, erythema, edema, ecchymosis, and transient discomfort or pain.[1,20] Operators are encouraged to exercise caution when applying these therapeutic devices over bony areas to avoid wave reflection and the potential for cutaneous injury.[23]

In contrast to HIFU, low intensity/low frequency nonthermal focused ultrasound technology ablates adipocytes through mechanical disruption.[1] The Ultrashape System (Syneron Candela, Marlborough, MA) was approved in 2014 for the treatment of excess adipose tissue. Several trials demonstrated remarkable enhancements in abdominal fat reduction and waist circumference improvement, some within the initial 14 days postprocedure.[24-26] Following the treatment, all studies documented minor and localized adverse events confined to the treatment sites, including temporary pain, erythema, purpura, and blistering.

RADIOFREQUENCY

Radiofrequency (RF) devices harness the power of RF energy to selectively target and heat adipose tissue beneath the skin's surface. By utilizing the capacity of an oscillating electrical field to generate alternating currents (AC), controlled heat is delivered to the desired areas through the movement and interaction of water molecules (which create friction in the tissue). Because of its high electrical impedance and relatively low heat transfer coefficient, adipose tissue is easily heated to the optimal temperature with the heat confined to the adipocytes, therefore sparing more superficial tissues.[13] This phenomenon stimulates the lipase-mediated enzymatic breakdown and elimination of stubborn fat deposits, along with partial collagen denaturation followed by collagen contraction and thickening.[1,27,28]

Currently RF energy can be delivered via monopolar, unipolar, bipolar, and multipolar options. [See **Table 99-1**.] RF devices have been extensively studied in clinical trials to evaluate their safety and efficacy for body contouring. Numerous studies have demonstrated positive

TABLE 99-1 Different radiofrequency (RF) delivery mechanisms[1,28]

RF delivery mechanism	Description
Monopolar RF	• Utilizes a single electrode that contacts the skin to deliver RF energy by producing an electrical current (requires a grounding path to complete the circuit to ensure the energy is focused on the treatment area • The RF energy penetrates the skin and reaches the underlying adipose tissue inducing controlled volumetric heating • Effectively targets deeper layers of fat, promoting fat reduction and skin tightening • Often used for larger body areas
Unipolar RF	• Employs an active electrode (typically a handpiece) and a large grounding pad to heat tissue through high-frequency electromagnetic radiation • Known for its ability to deeply penetrate the skin (up to 15-20 mm), stimulating collagen production, and promoting fat reduction • Commonly used for body contouring on larger areas such as the abdomen, thighs, and buttocks and for irregularities of the fibrous septa seen in cellulite
Bipolar RF	• Involves two adjacent electrodes that delivers the current between the two for controlled RF energy delivery • Depth of penetration is equal to half the distance between the two electrodes • Known for its precision and ability to deliver consistent heating to the desired depth, making it suitable for smaller treatment areas (neck, arms) or delicate skin (face) • May be combined with other modalities for synergistic treatment enhancements
Multipolar RF	• Utilizes multiple (three or more) electrodes to simultaneously heat dermal and subcutaneous tissues • Electrodes are strategically placed creating a more uniform and controlled heat distribution • The multipolar configuration allows for better targeting of specific body areas while minimizing the risk of discomfort or overheating • Ideal for both superficial and deep fat layers, promoting fat reduction, skin tightening, and even cellulite improvement

Please note this table provides a general overview and there may be specific brands or models that offer additional features or variations.

outcomes, highlighting the effectiveness of RF devices in reducing fat and improving one's contour without invasive modalities.[29] RF treatments have consistently demonstrated reductions in fat thickness and circumference measurements on various body locations,[30] with synergistic results when combined with other treatment modalities on skin laxity, firmness, texture, and tightening.[13,22,31-35]

In terms of safety, clinical trials consistently report minimal adverse events associated with RF treatments. Commonly observed side effects include temporary redness (erythema), mild swelling, and transient discomfort during or immediately after the procedure. These adverse events are typically mild, localized, and temporary, with no long-term complications reported in the literature. Although relatively uncommon, certain adverse events, including postinflammatory hyperpigmentation superficial burns, blisters, and subcutaneous erythematous papules and nodules have been reported.[28] For certain devices, primary monopolar RF, contraindications include implantable medical devices such as pacemakers and defibrillators, and caution should be displayed in patients with radiated skin or those prone to viral outbreaks.[28]

While the specific protocols and treatment parameters may vary among studies, the overall consensus from clinical trials supports the safety and efficacy of RF devices for body contouring. However, it's worth noting that individual results may vary, and a personalized treatment plan should be determined in consultation with a board-certified dermatologist.

INFRARED AND LOW-LEVEL LASER THERAPY

In the pursuit of body contouring, numerous light sources and lasers have been integrated into liposuction procedures. While the inclusion of light-based technologies into liposuction aims to enhance the precision and efficacy, the fundamental nature of the procedure remains invasive. In vitro studies have demonstrated the effectiveness of selective photothermolysis in targeting adipose tissue by utilizing the infrared vibrational absorption bands of lipids.[36] This innovative approach harnesses the unique properties of lipids to absorb specific wavelengths of light, allowing for precise and targeted thermal energy delivery to adipose cells. By exploiting this phenomenon, researchers have successfully shown the potential of using infrared light to selectively heat and disrupt adipose tissue, leading to fat reduction and body contouring effects. These findings provide valuable insights into the development of noninvasive treatments that specifically target adipose tissue through the application of wavelengths in the near-infrared regions, as well as other light-based sources.

Low-level laser therapy (LLLT) has garnered attention as a potential noninvasive method for body contouring and fat reduction. Numerous studies have explored the efficacy of LLLT in the context of body contouring, although the evidence remains somewhat mixed.[37-39] Some clinical trials have reported positive outcomes, demonstrating a reduction in abdominal circumference measurements following LLLT treatments; however, they are not without limitations.[40-42] The effectiveness of LLLT for body contouring varies among individuals, and the results may be modest compared to surgical interventions. While LLLT shows promise as a noninvasive option for fat reduction in body contouring, more robust evidence is needed to fully assess its clinical efficacy, establish optimal treatment protocols, including the number of sessions and treatment duration, and long-term sustainability of the effects.

FOCUSED ELECTROMAGNETIC STIMULATION

While many of the aforementioned modalities have focused on adipose cells for body contouring, there are some consumers who despite undergoing abdominal fat removal procedures remain dissatisfied. This often stems from the presence of a bulging mid-section that can be attributed to weak abdominal muscles and/or a condition called diastasis recti (separation of the abdominal muscles). Furthermore, those patients with a lower BMI may not have an excessive amount of adipose tissue that would respond to certain body contouring procedures.[43,44] These factors have led to a focus on muscle strengthening and toning to achieve a desired physique. Electrical muscle stimulation[45,46] (EMS) and electromagnetic (EM) stimulation[47-49] have emerged as techniques for muscle toning and body contouring. The latter, EM, penetrates deeper into the tissue without the risk of pain or burns associated with easily available electrical devices. This noninvasive approach utilizes electromagnetic energy to induce strong muscle contractions, simulating an intense workout without physical exertion. The repetitive muscle contractions lead to muscle strengthening and toning.[47-49] Additionally, intensive muscle training has been shown to induce lipolysis.[50,51] The combination of the two principles led to the development of high-intensity focused electromagnetic (HIFEM) field technology targeting both musculature and adipose tissue for optimal and refined aesthetic results.[52]

HIFEM, first introduced in 2018 with the EMSCULPT (BTL Medical Technologies, Boston, MA) device, was FDA approved to enhance and sculpt the abdomen, buttocks, arms, and calves [**Figure 99-3**].[53] By generating an oscillating magnetic field at a low frequency (3-5 Hz), HIFEM targets motor neurons for muscular contractions, given their size and lower threshold for depolarization, compared to sensory neurons.[54] This is beneficial as it prevents the dispersion of thermal energy to the surrounding tissues resulting in enhanced patient comfort.[55] The literature has demonstrated the efficacy in HIMEM building muscles for enhanced

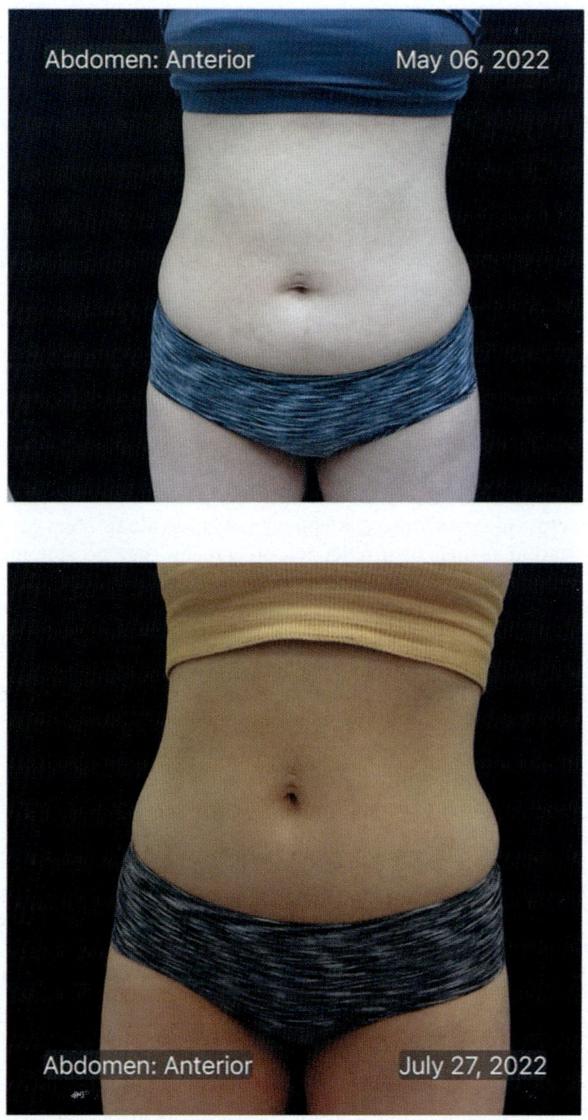

FIGURE 99-3. Before and after high-intensity focused electromagnetic (HIFEM) (EMSCULPT) to the abdomen on an Asian woman. (Courtesy of Sophia Reid, MD, FAAD; Closter, NJ.)

tone with the elimination of fat cells.[56-58] Jacob and colleagues observed an average 4.37 cm reduction in waist circumference in 19 subjects attributed to augmented muscle tone and a decrease in adipose tissue.[44] Katz et al studied 33 subjects who underwent four treatment sessions and reported a reduction in subcutaneous fat thickness across the abdomen by 19% and 23%, at 1- and 3-month follow-up, respectively.[43]

Synergistic effects have been demonstrated when HIFEM was used in conjunction with other treatment modalities. Jacob and colleagues demonstrated combined HIFEM and RF technologies in the EMSCULPT NEO (BTL Industries Inc., Boston, MA), harnessed effects to induce adipose tissue reduction, abdominal muscle hypertrophy, and overall waist circumference reduction.[59] An advisory board unanimously agreed that the combination of HIFEM + RF for muscle stimulation and lipolysis was superior to HIFEM alone.[57] The combination of HIFEM and cryolipolysis was investigated by Kilmer et al in 50 subjects. There was a 15-mm reduction in abdominal circumference when HIFEM + cyrolipolysis were used together, compared to subjects that were only treated with cryolipolysis or HIFEM alone (which only showed 10-mm and 4-mm reductions, respectively).[60] There continues to be an rise in investigative studies regarding combined treatment regimens using HIFEM with other noninvasive body contouring modalities yielding superior results.[61,62]

HIFEM is well tolerated with minimal to no discomfort and transient muscle fatigue and soreness, usually observed for 1 to 2 days post treatment.[43,44,52] There was one occurrence of chest discomfort/soreness and five instances of menstrual cycle irregularities, all of which resolved spontaneously during the course of one study.[63] High patient satisfaction has been demonstrated in a number of studies[43,44,59] with patients having increased motivation to maintain the results with exercise months after their treatments.[63] This is partially attributed to motivation patients have after seeing their results and the sustained elevation in basal metabolism as a result of muscle thickening, enhanced lipolysis, and prolonged programmed cell death of fat tissue that persists.[64-66] In summary, there is a burgeoning collection of evidence that supports the use of HIFEM for body contouring, given it is painless and noninvasive with favorable outcomes and patient satisfaction.

INJECTION ADIPOLYSIS WITH DEOXYCHOLIC ACID

While most of this chapter has focused on body contouring for the abdomen and other areas, the demand for contouring procedures for the face and neck has been on the rise. In the wake of the pandemic, there was a notable surge in the demand for aesthetic procedures, fueled in part by the widespread use of video conferencing. As individuals spent countless hours staring at their own reflection on screens, they became increasingly aware of perceived imperfections and newfound self-consciousness about their appearance. This phenomenon, often referred to as the "zoom effect," sparked a renewed interest in aesthetic enhancements as people sought to address concerns about their face, jaw line, and neck regions. The shape and contour of the chin and neck are integral to personal aesthetics, playing key roles in facial harmony and overall appearance. Unfortunately, the accumulation of fat in this area can distort its natural shape and definition, impacting the overall balance of the face. Excess fat deposits can disrupt the smooth contours of the chin and submental region, leading to a less defined and less desirable appearance,[67,68] sometimes referred to as a "double chin."

Deoxycholic acid (DCA) (deoxycholic acid 10 mg/mL injection; Kybella, Kythera Biopharmaceuticals, Inc., Parsippany, NJ), is an injectable agent FDA approved for moderate to severe convexity of submental fat (SMF).[69] DCA is a naturally occurring bile acid, found in the human body, with remarkable ability to break down and absorb dietary fat. It selectively targets and destroys fat cells in the submental region, offering a tailored approach to contouring and improving the profile of the chin and neck [**Figure 99-4A** and **B**].[67] Following the injection, adipocyte cell membranes are destabilized, causing the leakage of cytoplasmic content, after which a neutrophilic inflammatory response with macrophages clears cellular debris and lipids by day 7.[70] Because of its protein-poor properties, DCA has a higher affinity for adipose tissue, compared to skin, muscle, and blood vessels that are all protein-rich.[71] By the 28th day, atrophic fat lobules with surrounding fibroblastic septal thickening are identified supporting an overall reduction of fat. Given the time it takes for resolution of the inflammatory process, 1 month intervals are recommended between each treatment session.[70] The efficacy and safety of DCA treatments in reducing SMF, improving satisfaction with facial/chin appearance, and alleviating the psychological impact of fullness of the submental region were demonstrated in several randomized, placebo-controlled phase 3 trials.[72-75] Farina and colleagues summarized all of the clinical trials that tested the efficacy and safety of DCA.[68] The literature also supports 77% of men who were treated with DCA achieved a clinically significant decrease in SMF.[76] Chestnut et al conducted MRI studies that demonstrated a 23.8% reduction in preplatysmal SMF following DCA injections.[77]

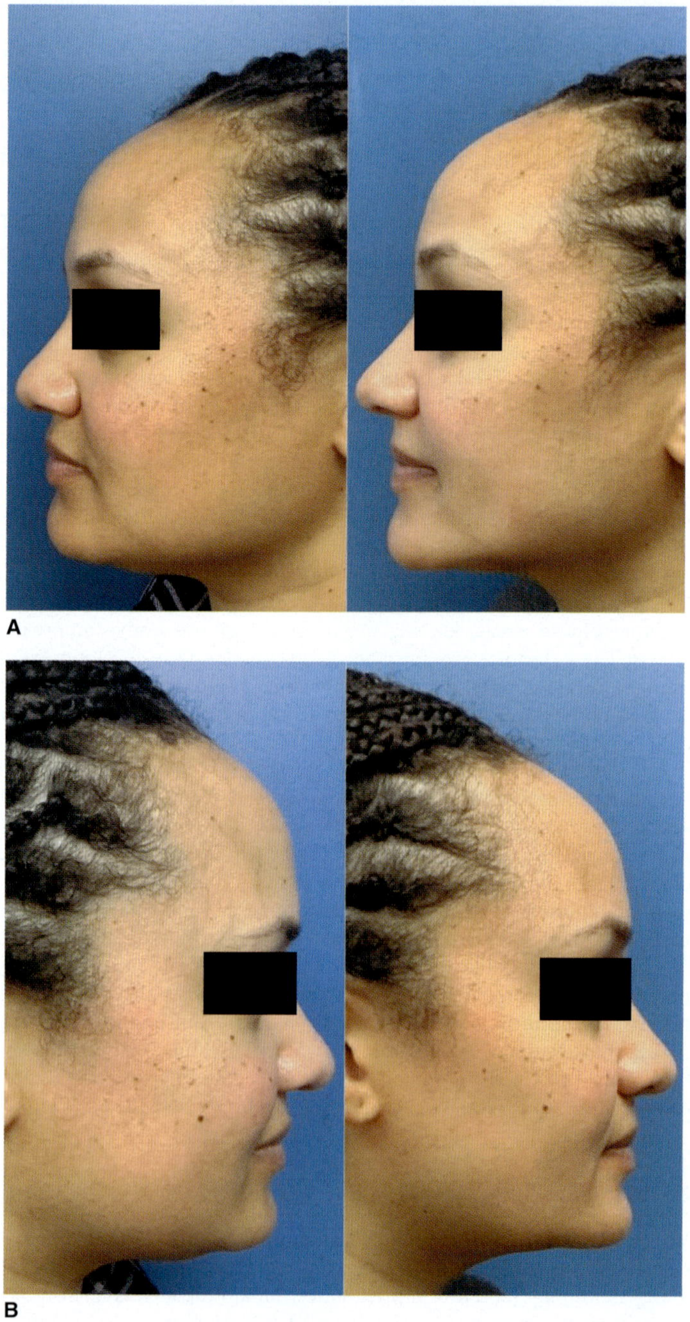

A

B

FIGURES 99-4 A AND B. Before **(A)** and after **(B)** photos of Kybella injections to the submental region on an African American woman. (Courtesy of Corey Hartman, MD, FAAD; Birmingham, AL.)

Furthermore, many of the trials provided valuable insights into the safety profile of DCA. The treatment is generally well tolerated, with most reported adverse events mild to moderate in nature. The adverse advents comprise transient injection site discomfort, swelling, numbness, bruising, erythema, and local induration, which all correlate to the inflammatory process that takes place histologically.[1] DCA is rapidly absorbed by the human body with plasma concentrations returning to baseline 12 to 24 hours after administration. There have been reports of marginal mandibular nerve damage leading to paresthesia and an asymmetrical smile due to muscle paralysis. This is attributed to temporary demyelination of the nerve and inflammation, not intra-neural injury, and is transient in nature.[74] The occurrence of alopecia after DCA injections in male patients is gaining recognition. Initial reports by Souyoul et al highlighted alopecia affecting the beard area in the submental region.[78] The precise mechanism remains unclear, as this adverse reaction exhibits variable characteristics, ranging from transient to permanent in different cases. Direct injury to the bulb of the hair follicle is one hypothesis, while too superficial injections has also been proposed.[79] Additional investigations are needed to fully understand the underlying factors. As such, this is an important consideration to discuss with patients prior to treatment. In the literature, cases of inadvertent intra-arterial injection of DCA resulting in skin necrosis have been documented, without a clear mechanism of damage.[80-82] However, it is known that DCA possesses vasoconstrictive properties and can disrupt the cell membrane, leading to cell lysis, cell death, and tissue inflammation.[81] To prevent intravascular injection, it is crucial to perform reflux before the injection procedure. This precautionary step helps ensure the avoidance of unintended intravascular administration.[68]

With its proven efficacy, convenience, and minimal downtime, DCA has become an attractive solution for individuals looking to enhance their facial aesthetics without undergoing surgery, with the added benefit of presenting their best self in virtual meetings and online interactions.

COLLAGENASE

Cellulite, a common cosmetic concern affecting individuals of various ages and body types, has long been a subject of interest in the field of body contouring. This unique form of adipose tissue dimpling, predominantly found on the thighs, buttocks, and abdomen, has proven challenging to address effectively. With its distinct appearance caused by structural changes in the underlying connective tissue, including excess fat herniation through perpendicularly oriented collagen fibrous septae, overlying skin laxity, and areas of volume loss, cellulite poses a significant hurdle in achieving desired body contours and a smooth skin texture.[83] Collagenase clostridium histolyticum-aaes (CCH-aaes) (Qwo®; Endo Aesthetics LLC, Malvern, PA) was approved by the FDA in 2020 for the treatment of moderate-to-severe cellulite in the buttocks of adult women [**Figure 99-5**].[84] The mechanism of action includes two purified bacterial collagenases that induce the enzymatic reaction to disrupt the triple helical configuration of collagen and targeting the fibrous collagen septae in cellulite, to release the depressions and improve the overlying topography of the skin surface. Studies have shown neocollagenesis and the reorganization of adipose tissue following CCH-aaes injections.[85] The significant improvement in the appearance of cellulite compared to placebo was demonstrated by Sadick et al.[86] The efficacy, safety, and tolerability profile of CCH-aaes was demonstrated in both phase 2 and phase 3 clinical trials.[86-88] However, the same phase 2 and phase 3 clinical trials also reported the common injection site adverse events associated with CCH-aaes, which were bruising, as did the Randomized Evaluation of Cellulite Reduction by Collagenase Clostridium Histolyticum (RELEASE) phase 3 trials. RELEASE-1 and RELEASE-2 placebo-controlled trials reported bruising in 84.4% of 424 female subjects who received up to three CCH-aaes treatment sessions. An interim analysis on the effectiveness of CCH-aaes on thigh cellulite evaluated 22 subjects and demonstrated a high percentage of responders at day 90 for either one or both thighs at 86.4% and 72.7%, respectively.[84]

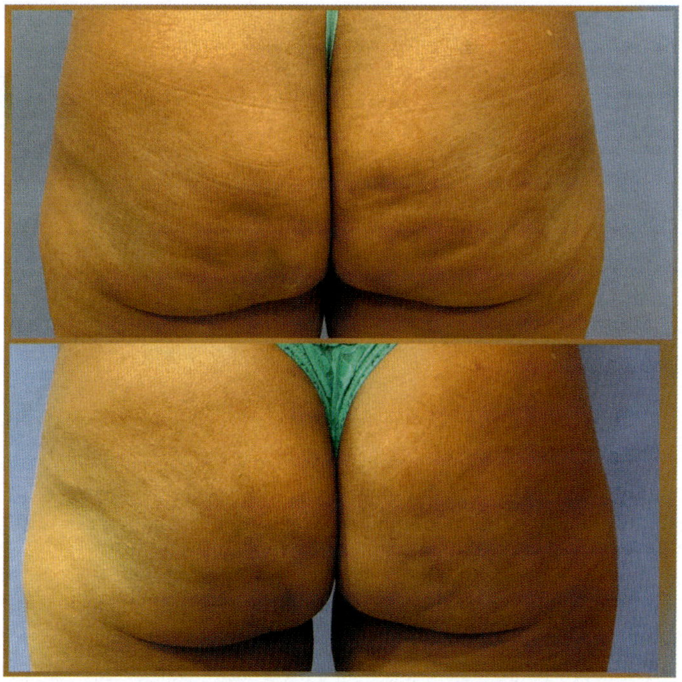

FIGURE 99-5. Before and after photo of Collagenase clostridium histolyticum-aaes (CCH-aaes) (QWO) injections to the buttocks on a Hispanic woman. (Courtesy of Mara Weinstein Velez, MD, FAAD; Rochester, NY.)

The abrupt cease in the manufacturing and distribution of the product was announced in December 2022 by the manufacturer, hypothesized to be due to excessive and unpredictable bruising as well as prolonged skin discoloration.

Understanding the multifactorial nature of the pathophysiology of cellulite is essential in formulating comprehensive approaches for its evaluation and potential treatment interventions. Given the extensive literature and sources that review and discuss cellulite, **Table 99-2** lists the different modalities that have been used to target cellulite for body contouring. As research strives to gain a deeper understanding of cellulite with the development of innovative techniques and therapeutic approaches, the field of body contouring can provide improved solutions to individuals seeking to enhance their overall physique and confidence.

CONCLUSION

Body contouring, a rapidly growing field in cosmetic surgery, offers individuals a solution to achieve the desired shape and proportion for their body. A variety of body contouring technologies are available, including low-energy devices that utilize low-frequency ultrasound, radiofrequency, light energy, or a combination of these, often accompanied by mechanical manipulation, to enhance and improve body appearance. Whether it's stubborn fat that refuses to budge despite diet and exercise

TABLE 99-2 Devices and modalities available for the treatment of cellulite[89-93]

Device name	Manufacturer	Treatment method	FDA clearance year
Velashape	Syneron Medical Ltd	Radiofrequency	FDA cleared—2007
Thermage	Solta Medical, Inc.	Radiofrequency	FDA cleared—2013
Cellfina	Merz Aesthetics (previously Ulthera, Inc).	Subcision	FDA Cleared—2014
Sofwave	Sofwave Medical Ltd	Synchronous Ultrasound Parallel Beam Technology	FDA Cleared—2022
Aveli	Revelle Aesthetics, Inc.	Targeted Verifiable Subcision	FDA Cleared—TBD

or loose skin following significant weight loss, body contouring procedures provide a transformative solution. With advancements in noninvasive technology, more and more people are turning to body contouring to sculpt their bodies and regain their confidence with their achieved aesthetic goals.

REFERENCES

1. Friedmann D. A review of the aesthetic treatment of abdominal subcutaneous adipose tissue: background, implications, and therapeutic options. *Dermatol Surg*. 2015;41:18-34.
2. Orringer J, Dover J, Alam M. *Procedures in Cosmetic Dermatology*. Amsterdam: Elsevier; 2016.
3. Survey on dermatologic procedures: report of 2018 procedures. https://www.asds.net/portals/0/PDF/procedures-survey-results-presentation-2018.pdf. Accessed June 30, 2023.
4. Wang J, Murgia R, Albornoz C. Millennial perspectives on body-contouring procedures: a national survey. *Dermatol Surg*. 2021;47(6):866-867.
5. Carruthers J, Stevens W, Carruthers A, Humphrey S. Cryolipolysis and skin tightening. *Dermatol Surg*. 2014;40: S184-S189.
6. Manstein D, Laubach H, Watanabe K, Farinelli W, Zurakowski D, Anderson R. Selective cryolysis: a novel method of non-invasive fat removal. *Lasers Surg Med*. 2008;40:595-604.
7. Zelickson B, Egbert B, Preciado J, et al. Cryolipolysis for noninvasive fat cell destruction: initial results from a pig model. *Dermatol Surg*. 2009;35: 1462-1470.
8. Nelson A, Wasserman D, Avram M. Cryolipolysis for reduction of excess adipose tissue. *Semin Cutan Med Surg*. 2009;28(4):244-249.
9. Avram M, Harry R. Cryolipolysis for subcutaneous fat layer reduction. *Lasers Surg Med*. 2009;41(10):703-708.
10. Dover J, Burns J, Coleman S, et al. A prospective clinical study of noninvasive cryolipolysis for subcutaneous fat layer reduction—interim report of available subject data. 2009.
11. U.S. Food and Drug Administration. Device approval package: ZELTIQ CoolSculpting System 2014. http://www.accessdata.fda.gov/cdrh_docs/pdf13/K133212.pdf. Accessed June 30, 2023.
12. Krueger N, Mai S, Luebberding S, Sadick N. Cryolipolysis for noninvasive body contouring: clinical efficacy and patient satisfaction. *Clin Cosmet Investig Dermatol*. 2014;7:201-205.
13. Bonati L, Ibrahim O. Nonsurgical Body Contouring of Fat. In: Dover J, Alam M, eds. *Procedures in Cosmetic Dermatology: Lasers, Lights, and Energy Devices*. 5th ed. Amsterdam: Elsevier, Inc.; 2023:152-166.
14. Boey G, Wasilenchuk J. Enhanced clinical outcome with manual massage following cryolipolysis treatment: a 4-month study of safety and efficacy. *Lasers Surg Med*. 2014;46:20-26.
15. Klein K, Zelickson B, Riopelle J, et al. Non-invasive cryolipolysis for subcutaneous fat reduction does not affect serum lipid levels or liver function tests. *Lasers Surg Med*. 2009;41:785-790.
16. Coleman S, Sachdeva K, Egbert B, Preciado J, Allison J. Clinical efficacy of noninvasive cryolipolysis and its effects on peripheral nerves. *Aesthetic Plast Surg*. 2009;33:482-488.
17. Karcher C, Katz B, Sadick N. Paradoxical hyperplasia post cryolipolysis and management. *Dermatol Surg*. 2017;43(3):467-470.
18. Jalian H, Avram M, Garibyan L, Mihm M, Anderson R. Paradoxical adipose hyperplasia after cryolipolysis. *JAMA Dermatol*. 2014;150(3):317-319.
19. Fatemi A, Kane M. High-intensity focused ultrasound effectively reduces waist circumference by ablating adipose tissue from the abdomen and flanks: a retrospective case series. *Aesthetic Plast Surg*. 2010;34:577-582.
20. Fatemi A. High-intensity focused ultrasound effectively reduces adipose tissue. *Semin Cutan Med Surg*. 2009;28:257-262.
21. Fodor P, Smoller B, Stecco K, Desilets C. Biochemical changes in adipocytes and lipid metabolism secondary to the use of high-intensity focused ultrasound for non-invasive body sculpting. Presented at the Annual Meeting of the American Society of Aesthetic Plastic Surgery, April, 2006, Orlando, FL.
22. Jewell M, Baxter R, Cox S, et al. Randomized sham-controlled trial to evaluate the safety and effectiveness of a high-intensity focused ultrasound device for noninvasive body sculpting. *Plast Reconstr Surg*. 2011;128:253-262.
23. Haar G, Coussios C. High intensity focused ultrasound: physical principles and devices. *Int J Hyperthermia*. 2007;23:89-104.
24. Teitelbaum S, Burns J, Kubota J, et al. Noninvasive body conttouring by focused ultrasound: safety and efficacy of the Contour I device in a multicenter, controlled, clinical study. *Plast Reconstr Surg*. 2007;120(3):779-789.
25. Moreno-Moraga J, Valero-Altes T, Riquelme A, Isarria-Marcosy M, de la Torre J. Body contouring by non-invasive transdermal focused ultrasound. *Lasers Surg Med*. 2007;39:315-323.
26. Ascher B. Safety and efficacy of UltraShape Contour I treatments to improve the appearance of body contours: multiple treatments in shorter intervals. *Aesthet Surg J*. 2010;30:217-224.
27. Weiss R. Noninvasive radio frequency for skin tightening and body contouring. *Semin Cutan Med Surg*. 2013;32:9-17.
28. Lolis M, Goldberg D. Radiofrequency in cosmetic dermatology: a review. *Dermatol Surg*. 2012;38:1765-1776.
29. Boisnic S, Divaris M, Nelson A, Gharavi N, Lask G. A clinical and biological evaluation of a novel, noninvasive radiofrequency device for the long-term reduction of adipose tissue. *Lasers Surg Med*. 2014;46:94-103.
30. Goldberg D, Fazeli A, Berlin A. Clinical, laboratory, and MRI analysis of cellulite treatment with a unipolar radiofrequency device. *Dermatol Surg*. 2007;34:204-209.
31. Chang S, Huang Y, Lee M, et al. Combination therapy of focused ultrasound and radiofrequency for noninvasive body contouring in Asians with MRI photographic documentation. *Lasers Surg Med*. 2014;29:165-172.
32. Brightman L, Weiss E, Chapas A, Karen J. Improvement in arm and postpartum abdominal and flank subcutaneous fat deposits and skin laxity using a bipolar radiofrequency, infrared, vacuum and mechanical massage device. *Lasers Surg Med*. 2009;41:791-798.
33. Winter M. Post-pregnancy body contouring using a combined radiofrequency, infrared light and tissue manipulation device. *J Cosmet Laser Ther*. 2009;11:229-235.
34. Wanitphakdeedecha R, Manuskiatti W. Treatment of cellulite with a bipolar radiofrequency, infrared heat, and pulsatile suction device: a pilot study. *J Cosmet Dermatol*. 2006;5:284-288.
35. Adatto M, Adatto-Neilson R, Moren G. Reduction in adipose tissue volume using a new high-power radiofrequency technology combined with infrared light and mechanical manipulation for body contouring. *Lasers Surg Med*. 2014;29:1627-1631.
36. Anderson R, Farinelli W, Laubach H, et al. Selective photothermolysis of lipid-rich tissues: a free electron laser study. *Lasers Surg Med*. 2006;38(10): 913-919.
37. Medrado A, Trindade E, Reis S, Andrade Z. Action of low-level laser therapy on living fatty tissue of rats. *Lasers Surg Med*. 2006;21(1):19-23.
38. Brown S, Rohrich R, Kenkel J, Young V, Hoopman J, Coimbra M. Effect of low-level laser therapy on abdominal adipocytes before lipoplasty procedures. *Plast Reconstr Surg*. 2004;113(6):1796-1804.
39. Caruso-Davis M, Guillot T, Podichetty V, et al. Efficacy of low-level laser therapy for body contouring and spot fat reduction. *Obes Surg*. 2011;21(6): 722-729.
40. Jackson R, Stern F, Neira R, Ortiz-Neira C, Maloney J. Application of low-level laser therapy for noninvasive body contouring. *Lasers Surg Med*. 2012;44(3):211-217.
41. Jackson R, Dedo D, Roche G, Turok D, Maloney R. Low-level laser therapy as a non-invasive approach for body contouring: a randomized, controlled study. *Lasers Surg Med*. 2009;41(10):799-809.
42. McRae E, Boris J. Independent evaluation of low-level laser therapy at 635 nm for non-invasive body contouring of the waist, hips, and thighs. *Lasers Surg Med*. 2013;45(1):1-7.
43. Katz B, Bard R, Goldfarb R, Shiloh A, Kenolova D. Ultrasound assessment of subcutaneous abdominal fat thickness after treatments with a high-intensity focused electromagnetic field device: a multicenter study. *Dermatol Surg*. 2019;45:1542-1548.
44. Jacob C, Paskova K. Safety and efficacy of a novel high-intensity focused electromagnetic technology device for noninvasive abdominal body shaping. *J Cosmet Dermatol*. 2018;17(5):643-944.
45. Langeard A, Bigot L, Chastan N, Gauthier A. Does neuromuscular electrical stimulation training of the lower limb have functional effects on the elderly? A systematic review. *Exp Gerontol*. 2017;91(C):88-98.
46. Matsuse H, Hashida R, Takano Y, et al. Walking exercise simultaneously combined with neuromuscular electrical stimulation of antagonists resistance improved muscle strength, physical function, and knee pain in symptomatic knee osteoarthritis: a single-arm study. *J Strength Cond Res*. 2017;31(1):171-180.
47. Han T, Shin H, Kim I. Magnetic stimulation of the quadriceps femoris muscle: comparison of pain with electrical stimulation. *AM J Phys Med Rehabil*. 2006;85:593-599.
48. Abulhasan J, Rumble Y, Morgan E, Slatter W, Grey M. Peripheral electrical and magnetic stimulation to augment resistance training. *J Funct Morphol Kinesiol*. 2016;1:328-342.

49. Galloway N, El-Galley R, Sand P, Appell R, Russell H, Carlan S. Extracorporeal magnetic innervation therapy for stress urinary incontinence. *Urology*. 1999;53(6):1108-1111.
50. Chatzinikolaou A, Fatouros I, Petridou A, et al. Adipose tissue lipoly- sis is upregulated in lean and obese men during acute resistance exercise. *Diabetes Care*. 2008;31(7):1397-1399.
51. Ormsbee M, Thyfault J, Johnson E, Kraus R, Choi M, Hickner R. Fat metabolism and acute resistance exercise in trained men. *J Appl Physiol*. 2007;102(5):1767-1772.
52. Rambhia P, Turner L, Ugonabo N, Chapas A. Muscle stimulation for aesthetic body shaping: a comprehensive and critical review. *Dermatol Surg*. 2022;48(10):1076-1082.
53. U.S. Food and Drug Administration. Device approval package: EMSCULPT. https://www.accessdata.fda.gov/cdrh_docs/pdf16/K160992.pdf. Accessed July 3, 2023.
54. Weiss R, Bernardy J. Induction of fat apoptosis by a non-thermal device: mechanism of action of non-invasive high-intensity electro- magnetic technology in a porcine model. *Lasers Surg Med*. 2019;51(1):47-53.
55. KatZ B. MRI assessment of arm and calf muscle toning with high-intensity focused electromagnetic technology: case study. *J Drugs Dermatol*. 2020;19(5):556-558.
56. Alexiades M. High intensity focused electromagnetic field (HIFEM) devices in dermatology. *J Drugs Dermatol*. 2019;18(11):1088.
57. Goldberg D, Enright K, Goldfarb R, Katz B, Gold M. The role and clinical benefits of high-intensity focused electromagnetic devices for non-invasive lipolysis and beyond: a narrative review and position paper. *J Cosmet Dermatol*. 2021;20(7):2096-2101.
58. Dunacan D, Dinev I. Duncan D, Dinev I. Noninvasive induction of muscle fiber hypertrophy and hyperplasia: effects of high-intensity focused electromagnetic field evaluated in an in-vivo porcine model: a pilot study. *Aesthet Surg J*. 2020;40(5):568-574.
59. Jacob C, Kent D, Ibrahim O. Efficacy and safety of simultaneous application of HIFEM and synchronized radiofrequency for abdominal fat reduction and muscle toning: a multicenter magnetic resonance imaging evaluation study. *Dermatol Surg*. 2021;47(7):969-973.
60. Kilmer S, Cox S, Zelickson B, et al. Feasibility study of electromagnetic muscle stimulation and cryolipolysis for abdominal contouring. *Dermatol Surg*. 2020;46(1)(1):S14-S21.
61. Samuels J, Weiss R, Katz B. Radiofrequency heating and HIFEM delivered simultaneously – the first sham-controlled randomized trial. *Plast Reconstr Surg*. 2022;149(5):893e-900e.
62. Goldberg D. Deletion of adipocytes induced by a novel device simultaneously delivering synchronized radiofrequency and HIFEM: human histological study. *J Cosmet Dermatol*. 2021;20(4):1104-1109.
63. Fabi S, Dover J, Tanzi E, Bowes L, Fu F, Odusan A. A 12-week, prospective, non-comparative, non-randomized study of magnetic muscle stimu- lation for improvement of body satisfaction with the abdomen and buttocks. *Lasers Surg Med*. 2021;53(1):79-88.
64. Kinney B, Lozanova P. High intensity focused electromagnetic therapy evaluated by magnetic resonance imaging: safety and efficacy study of a dual tissue effect based non-invasive abdominal body shaping. *Lasers Surg Med*. 2019;51(1):40-46.
65. Jacob C, Rank B. Abdominal remodeling in postpartum women by using a high-intensity focused electromagnetic (HIFEM) procedure: an investigational magnetic resonance imaging (MRI) pilot study. *J Clin Aesthet Dermatol*. 2020;13(9)(1):S16-S20.
66. Kinney B, Kent D. MRI and CT assessment of abdominal tissue composition in patients after high-intensity focused electromagnetic therapy treatments: one-year follow-up. *Aesthet Surg J*. 2020;40(12):NP686-NP693.
67. Shridharani S, Behr K. ATX-101 (deoxycholic acid injection) treatment in men: insights from our clinical experience. *Dermatol Surg*. 2017;43(2):S225 -S230.
68. Farina G, Cherubini K, Zancanaro de Figueiredo M, Salum F. Deoxycholic acid in the submental fat reduction: a review of properties, adverse effects, and complications. *J Cosmet Dermatol*. 2020;19:2497-2504.
69. U.S. Food and Drug Administration. Device approval package: Kybella. https://www.accessdata.fda.gov/drugsatfda_docs/nda/2015/206333Orig1s000Approv.pdf. Accessed July 10, 2023.
70. Walker P, Lee D, Toth B, Bowen B. Histological analysis of the effect of ATX-101 (deoxycholic acid injection) on subcutaneous fat: results from a phase 1 open-label study. *Dermatol Surg*. 2020;46:70-77.
71. Dayan S, Humphrey S, Jones D, et al. Overview of ATX-101 (deoxycholic acid Injection): a nonsurgical approach for reduction of submental fat. *Dermatol Surg*. 2016;42:S263-S270.
72. Ascher B, Hoffman K, Walker P, Lippert S, Wollina U, Havlickova B. Efficacy, patient-reported outcomes and safety profile of ATX-101 (deoxycholic acid), an injectable drug for the reduction of unwanted submental fat: results from a phase III, randomized, placebo-controlled study. *J Eur Acad Dermatol Venereol*. 2014;28(12):1707-1715.
73. Humphrey S, Sykes S, Kantor J, et al. ATX-101 for reduction of submental fat: a phase III randomized controlled trial. *J Am Acad Dermatol*. 2016;75:788-797.
74. Jones D, Carruthers J, Joseph J, et al. REFINE-1, a multicenter, randomized, double-blind, placebo-controlled, phase 3 trial with ATX-101, an injectable drug for submental fat reduction. *Dermatol Surg*. 2016;42(1):38-49.
75. Rzany B, Griffiths T, Walker P, Lippert S, McDiarmid J, Havlickova B. Reduction of unwanted submental fat with ATX-101 (deoxycholic acid), an adipocytolytic injectable treatment: results from a phase III, randomized, placebo-controlled study. *Br J Dermatol*. 2014;170(2):445-453.
76. Bertucci V, Carruthers J, Schlessinger J, Gross T, Beddingfield F III. Deoxycholic acid injection (ATX-101) is safe and effective in men: results of a pooled analysis from the REFINE trials 2015.
77. Chestnut C, Branting N, Joseph J, Gross T, Lizzul P, Beddingfield III F. Deoxycholic acid injection (ATX-101) treatment markedly reduces platysmal fat. *J Am Acad Dermatol*. 2016;74(5):AB15-AB15.
78. Souyoul S, Gioe O, Emerson A, Hooper D. Alopecia after injection of ATX-101 for reduction of submental fat. *JAAD Case Reports*. 2017;3(3):250-252.
79. Grady B, Porphirio F, Rokhsar C. Submental alopecia at deoxycholic acid injection site. *Dermatol Surg*. 2017;43(8):1105-1108.
80. McKay C, Price C, Pruett L. Vascular injury after deoxycholic acid injection. *Dermatol Surg*. 2019;45(2):306-309.
81. Lindgren A, Welsh K. Inadvertent intra-arterial injection of deoxycholic acid: a case report and proposed protocol for treatment. *J Cosmet Dermatol*. 2020;19(7):1614-1618.
82. Sachdev D, Mohammadi T, Fabi S. Deoxycholic acid–induced skin necrosis: prevention and management deoxycholic. *Dermatol Surg*. 2018;44(7): 1037-1039.
83. Davis D, Boen M, Fabi S. Cellulite: Patient selection and combination treatments for optimal results-a review and our experience. *Dermatol Surg*. 2019;45(9):1171-1184.
84. Joseph J, Dayan S, Bhatia A, et al. Real-world effectiveness and safety of collagenase clostridium histolyticum-aaes injections for the treatment of thigh cellulite in women. *J Cosmet Dermatol*. 2023;22:177-185.
85. Shridharani S, Vijayan S, Napekoski K, Dalton S, Bhatia A. Characterization of tissue histology for the injectable cellulite treatment collagenase clostridium histolyticum-aaes: results in swine. *Aesthet Surg J Open Forum*. 2023;5:ojad034.
86. Sadick N, Goldman M, Liu G, et al. Collagenase clostridium histolyticum for the treatment of edematous fibrosclerotic panniculopathy (cellulite): a randomized trial. *Dermatol Surg*. 2019;45(8):1047-1056.
87. Kaufman-Janette J, Bass L, Xiang Q, McLane M, Kirby M, Vijayan S. Efficacy, safety, and durability of response of collagenase clostridium histolyticum-aaes for treating cellulite. *Plast Reconstr Surg Glob Open*. 2020;8(12):e3316.
88. Kaufman-Janette J, Joseph J, Kaminer M, et al. Collagenase clostridium histolyticum-aaes for the treatment of cellulite in women: results from two phase 3 randomized, placebo-controlled trials. *Dermatol Surg*. 2021;47(5):649-656.
89. U.S. Food and Drug Administration. Device approval package: Velashape. https://www.accessdata.fda.gov/cdrh_docs/pdf7/K071872.pdf. Accessed August 28, 2023.
90. U.S. Food and Drug Administration. Device approval package: Thermage. https://www.accessdata.fda.gov/cdrh_docs/pdf13/k132431.pdf. Accessed August 28, 2023.
91. U.S. Food and Drug Administration. Device approval package: Sofwave. https://www.accessdata.fda.gov/cdrh_docs/pdf22/K223237.pdf. Accessed August 28, 2023.
92. U.S. Food and Drug Administration. Device approval package: Aveli. https://www.accessdata.fda.gov/cdrh_docs/pdf21/K212399.pdf. Accessed August 28, 2023.
93. U.S. Food and Drug Administration. Device approval package: Celfina. https://www.accessdata.fda.gov/cdrh_docs/pdf16/k161885.pdf. Accessed August 28, 2023.

CHAPTER 100

Platelet-Rich Plasma and Hair Transplantation as Novel Therapeutic Agents in the Treatment of Alopecia: Applications and Considerations for Skin of Color

Kaelynn Workman
Mikayla Woodard
Ugonna Nwannunu
Meena Singh
Chesahna Kindred

KEY POINTS

- Platelet-rich plasma is a novel therapeutic agent with minimal reported side effects. This therapy has been shown to have clinical success in hair regrowth in nonscarring alopecias like androgenetic alopecia and alopecia areata. More studies are needed to assess the impact of PRP with scarring alopecias like CCCA.
- Platelet-rich plasma is defined as plasma with a minimum platelet concentration of 1,000,000/uL or an approximate fivefold increase in platelets from baseline.
- PRP is thought to be effective in hair regrowth due to the abundance of platelet growth factors and anti-inflammatory molecules present in solution.
- While PRP offers promising results in alopecia patients, steps to standardize point of care devices, centrifugation speed and time, anticoagulant use, and treatment schedule must be taken.
- Follicular unit transplantation (FUT) and follicular unit extraction (FUE) may be successfully performed in patients of African descent.
- When performing FUT or FUE in patients with curly or textured hair, care must be taken to avoid transection of the hair follicle due to the elliptical shape.
- When treating scarring and inflammatory alopecias with FUT or FUE, it is important that such inflammatory alopecias are currently and have historically been inactive before the start of treatment.
- Access to PRP remains limited due to the high cost of treatment and lack of coverage by health insurance companies. This decreases equitable access to PRP among skin of color populations.

INTRODUCTION

BRIEF OVERVIEW OF PLATELET-RICH PLASMA (PRP)

PRP, also known as platelet-rich growth factors or platelet-concentrated plasma, is a human by-product that contains a highly concentrated solution of platelets with small amounts of residually filtrated leukocytes and erythrocytes, suspended in low volume plasma.[1] While the clinical utilization of PRP first began in the field of hematology in the 1970s, its medical uses has since been expanded and it is currently at the forefront of innovative therapies in many medical specialties, including but not limited to dermatology, orthopedic surgery, ophthalmology, and plastic surgery.[1] The term PRP was first coined by Kingsley et al and was used to refer to the platelet concentrate that was used for transfusion.[2,3] PRP was initially used for the treatment of thrombocytopenia for bleeding prevention. Later, PRP would make its introduction into the world of surgical repair and procedures when used as a sealant to promote clotting and expedite wound healing.[4] Today, PRP has seen promising results in the world of cosmetics with facial rejuvenation, wound healing, and tissue repair in orthopedic surgery and hair follicle stimulation and regrowth in patients experiencing alopecia in the field of dermatology.

IMPORTANCE OF CONSIDERING SKIN OF COLOR IN PRP TREATMENTS

Alopecia or hair loss is one of the primary reasons for people of African descent to seek a dermatologist.[5,6] This is in stark contrast to patient populations that do not fall under the category of skin of color, where the primary reason for dermatologic care is usually cutaneous precancer and cancer screening and treatment.[6] Traction alopecia (TA) and central centrifugal cicatricial alopecia (CCCA) are two common forms of alopecia in the African American community resulting from continuous and prolonged internal or external damaging and inflammatory processes to the hair follicle.[7] Both forms of alopecia are limited in therapeutic tools to promote hair growth/regrowth in the affected area(s). As such, PRP may offer a significant therapeutic benefit for these patients via stimulation of the hair follicle through growth factors and cytokines, and modulation of tissue repair and inflammatory processes. Alopecia areata (AA) is a nonscarring auto-immune form of hair loss with a disease burden that disproportionately affects skin of color populations. Reported prevalence ratios of AA among Asian, Black, and Hispanic/Latinx relative to Caucasian patients from a large cross-sectional study were 2.47 (95% CI, 2.17-2.81), 1.35 (95% CI, 1.26-1.44), and 1.26 (95% CI, 1.03-1.55), respectively.[8] Alopecia areata has recently seen advances in therapies in the field of small molecule immunomodulating drugs like Janus kinase (JAK) inhibitors. While these medications have been studied with significant proven success in hair regrowth among patients with extensive hair loss, PRP may offer an efficacious alternative with lessened systemic side effects seen with JAK inhibitors. Androgenetic alopecia is another common form of hair loss and although equivalent in prevalence among communities of color and noncommunities of color, PRP may be of significant benefit to these patients if hair loss is extensive and first-line agents like minoxidil have been adequately tried without success.

CHAPTER PURPOSE AND SCOPE

PRP in the field of dermatology is a recent therapeutic advent, and as such, extensive literature on how it is used, the indications for its use, and the science behind its efficacy has not been well developed. Further, the medical benefit and positive impact of this therapy with regard to conditions seen among patient populations of color has not been thoroughly described. PRP has undergone extensive research in numerous medical fields and has seen promising results in the world of tissue repair, regeneration, and rejuvenation.[9] This chapter will largely focus on the dermatological utility of PRP with regards to alopecia and hair regrowth, with specific interest paid to alopecias highly prevalent in skin of color populations. Additionally, this chapter will expound upon the scientific theory behind PRP as a medical therapy, methods of preparation, limitations of therapy, future directions, and future potential of PRP in the field of dermatology.

BASICS OF PLATELET RICH PLASMA

DEFINITION AND COMPOSITION OF PRP

Human blood is roughly composed of 55% plasma (the majority of which is water with a minority of dissolved sugars, gases, and proteins), 44% red blood cells, and 1% platelets and white blood cells, known as the buffy coat.[10] In contrast, platelet-rich plasma is a centrifugated product that contains platelets in a concentration that is two to nine times greater than the physiologic concentration. In addition, depending on the centrifugation process, PRP can contain leukocytes and red blood cells referred to as leukocyte and platelet-rich plasma (L-PRP) or can contain little to no leukocytes or RBCs, referred to as leukocyte-poor or pure PRP (P-PRP).[11] While the composition of PRP is highly variable due to the lack of standardization in centrifugation and processing techniques, on average PRP is composed of 4% erythrocytes, 95% platelets, and 1% leukocytes.[12] Platelets remain a rich source of stimulating growth factors and cytokines when activated. These growth factors play an integral role in tissue repair and regeneration and have also been studied to have positive effects on hair growth, hair cycling, and follicle stimulation [**Table 100-1**]. While any plasma volume with a platelet concentration above that of normal blood is considered platelet-rich plasma, the working definition is shifting to a minimum platelet concentration of 1,000,000/uL—an approximate fivefold increase from baseline.[13]

MECHANISM OF ACTION

To properly understand the role of PRP and the effect on the structure of the hair follicle and its cycle, it is important to understand hair follicle anatomy and the phases of the hair cycle. Anatomically, the hair follicle can be divided into three main sections—the inferior follicle, the isthmus, and the infundibulum.[14] The inferior follicle consists of the bulb, which is the most inferior part of the hair follicle, and the suprabulbar region.[14] Inside the bulb is the dermal papilla and hair matrix keratinocytes that undergo proliferation to form the hair shaft. In the suprabulbar region, there are three concentric layers—those being the inner root sheath, outer root sheath, and the connective tissue layer sheath from inside to out, respectively.[14] The inner root sheath is responsible for providing the structure to shape the cells of the hair matrix as they proliferate and form the hair shaft. The cells of the outer root sheath are responsible for the provision and storage of glycogen to meet the metabolic needs of the hair follicle and also the generation of growth factors like IGF-1 and TGF-β that play significant roles in hair follicle cycling.[14]

Every hair follicle progresses through the hair cycle over the course of its lifetime. The three main components of the hair cycle are the anagen phase (growing phase), the catagen phase (resting phase), and the telogen phase (shedding phase).[14] The maintenance and subsequent transition of the hair follicle into each of these cycles is governed by locally released growth factors generated by the outer root sheath keratinocytes, among other internal and external signals.[14] Due to many hair disorders being caused by premature disruption of the hair cycle, PRP offers a therapeutic benefit through provision of growth factors and cytokines that are known to have positive modulatory effects on hair growth. When platelets are activated, growth factors like PDGF, IGF-1, etc, are released into the area provisioned with PRP.[4] The multitude of growth factors released by platelets are known to work by stimulating angiogenesis, stimulating activation of the dermal papilla cells, or promoting induction and/or extension of the anagen phase of the hair cycle.[4]

PRP is also known to have anti-inflammatory mechanisms due to the presence of TGF-β. TGF-β inhibits the function of natural killer cells and CD8+ T cells and suppresses MCP-1.[15,16] MCP-1 is a chemotactic cytokine that aids in recruitment of T lymphocytes and is thought to play a role in the pathogenesis of AA by recruiting T lymphocytes to the hair bulb.[16] The suppression of CD8+ T cells and MCP-1 may hold an important key in the treatment of AA, as AA is a cytotoxic T lymphocyte mediated autoimmune form of alopecia. It is hypothesized that TGF-β acts in part in creating the immune privilege experienced by the hair follicle in its nonpathological state.[17]

PREPARATION TECHNIQUES FOR PRP

PRP can be produced through laboratory techniques or through commercially available point of care devices. As PRP is an autologous blood product, the first step in production is obtaining blood from the patient through venipuncture. A 30 cc venous blood draw will approximately yield 3 to 5 cc of PRP but is variable depending on the baseline platelet level of the patient.[18] When drawing the blood, it is necessary to add an anticoagulant, usually in the form of acid citrate dextrose (ACD-A) or sodium citrate.[11] The dextrose in ACD-A serves as an energy reservoir for the platelets, the citrate chelates calcium ions to prevent activation of the clotting cascade prior to injection, and sodium citrate maintains platelet viability.[11] The goal of PRP preparation is near-complete to complete separation of solid blood components from liquid blood components through application of an acceleration force so that cellular constituents separate according to their specific gravity.[4] This can be achieved via a process known as differential centrifugation. Gravity filtration is another

TABLE 100-1 Summary of platelet growth factors, their systemic effects, and their actions on the hair follicle

Platelet-released growth factors and their systemic and follicular functions		
Growth factor	**Biochemical function**	**Hair growth function**
PDGF	• Chemotactic and mitogen for fibroblasts, glial cells, and smooth muscle cells. • Regulates collagen synthesis and collagenase secretion.	• Increases hair growth through increased vascularization via stimulation of angiogenesis.
TGF-β	• Mitogen for endothelial cells, fibroblasts, and osteoblasts. • Regulates collagen synthesis and collagenase secretion. • Regulates mitogenic effects of other growth factors. • Stimulates angiogenesis. • Inhibits the function of natural killer cells and CD8+ T-cells.	• Inhibits hair growth in vitro and in vivo via androgen-mediated induction when secreted by the dermal papilla cells. • Induces the catagen phase.
VEGF	• Mitogen for endothelial cells. • Increases angiogenesis.	• Highly expressed in the dermal papilla cells in the anagen phase and increases perifollicular angiogenesis and perifollicular vessel size.
EGF	• Mitogenic for endothelial cells. • Promotes proliferation of keratinocytes and fibroblasts.	• Promotion of the proliferation and migration of outer root sheath cells and modulation of the expression of follicle-regulatory genes via Wnt/β-catenin signaling.
HGF	• Regulates cell growth in epithelial cells and supports vascularization during wound healing.	• Acts on follicular epithelial cells to promote follicular growth.
FGF	• Mitogenic for mesenchymal cells, chondrocytes, and osteoblasts.	• Induces the anagen phase of hair follicles. • Increases the size of the hair shaft.
IGF-1	• Major mediator of prenatal and postnatal growth. • Fibroblast chemotactic. • Stimulates protein synthesis. • Increases bone formation via proliferation of osteoblasts.	• One of the most potent anagen prolonging growth factors in hair follicles. • Prevents entrance of the hair follicle into a catagen-like state. • IGF-1 receptors are expressed on the hair matrix and outer root sheath keratinocytes of hair follicles, where their signaling with IGF-1 promotes maintenance of the anagen phase and hair follicle proliferation.

Abbreviations: EGF, epidermal growth factor; FGF, fibroblast growth factor; HGF, hepatocyte growth factor; IGF-1, insulin-like growth factor-1; PDGF, platelet-derived growth factors; TGF-β, transforming growth factor-β; VEGF, vascular endothelial growth factor.

Source: Modified from Alves R, Grimalt R [4] and Everts et al [9].

TABLE 100-2 List of point of care PRP kits and their respective mean platelet concentrations delivered in their production of PRP

Point of care PRP kits with PRP platelet concentrations above 1000 × 10³/uL	
Point of care PRP devices	**Platelet concentration of PRP (Platelet × 10³/uL)**
Biomet GPS II (Biomet Biologics Drucker centrifuge)	1546.5
Biomet GPS III (Biomet Biologics Drucker centrifuge)	1519.03
Biomet GPS III Mini	1135.20 ± 422.15
Emcyte GenesisCS	1643 ± 421
Emcyte PurePRP	1128 ± 319
Friadent-Schutze Protocol	1440.5 ± 501.7
Harvest Smart PreP	1228 ± 312
KYOCERA	1312
DePuy PEAK	1242.4
Arteriocyte MagellanPRP	1520
Biomet 3i PCCS	939 ± 284

Source: Modified by Fadadu et al [19].

process that can also be used for component separation. Size and density of the individual constituents are the two key factors in determining the separation of blood components when utilizing centrifugation.[11] In contrast, pore size/diameter of the filter is the key factor when separating blood components using gravity filtration. With regard to density and size, erythrocytes are the largest and heaviest solid component of blood, with leukocytes being the second largest and platelets being the smallest.[11] As such, when blood is put through a centrifuge for the first time, erythrocytes will be the first to settle, then leukocytes and platelets last. The first spin is referred to as a soft spin. Soft spin centrifugation systems will create three separate layers: the top layer, which is the supernatant acellular plasma, the buffy coat, which is the layer rich in platelets, and white blood cells and the erythrocyte layer.[18] After transfer of the top layer and the buffy coat, a second spin, known as the hard spin, would be required to remove the remaining leukocytes and platelets, as platelets are much smaller and less dense.[18] The centrifuged platelets are homogenized by mixing them with the lower third volume of plasma. Most preparations require the addition of platelet activators such as thrombin or calcium. Release of growth factors begin within 10 minutes of activation, with 95% of growth factors being released within an hour of activation.[12] Platelet growth factor synthesis can continue for 7 days.[12]

There are a number of commercially available devices used for PRP preparation, each with their own systems and settings for blood collection and centrifugation. A study was performed by Fadadu et al that assessed platelet concentration yields in commercially available PRP kits. Out of 33 different commercially available PRP systems studied, only 11 were found to deliver PRP with a platelet concentration that met the definition of PRP set by Marx—1,000,000/uL.[19] A summary of commercially available point of care devices that provide PRP with a platelet concentration greater or equal to 1,000,000/uL is provided in **Table 100-2**. When utilizing commercially available point of care devices for PRP preparation, a closed technique is employed. A closed technique refers to a collection system in which the patient's autologous sample is not in contact with the environment.[4] This is the most recommended method, as opposed to an open technique whereby the sample comes into contact with laboratory devices such as pipettes and tubes, as seen with gravity filtration.

DERMATOLOGIC APPLICATIONS OF PRP

HAIR LOSS

Overview of Common Hair Disorders in Individuals with Skin of Color

Traction Alopecia Traction alopecia is a common form of hair loss in Black women, arising from the long-term use of hair prosthetics including braids, ponytails, and hair weaves, along with styling techniques that apply significant tension on the hair follicle. Primary management and progression prevention in traction alopecia is comprehensive patient counseling and education on the etiology of this type of hair loss and methods to mitigate excessive follicular tension and resulting alopecia.[14] To encourage hair regrowth in alopecic areas, therapies such as minoxidil have been and are currently still recommended.[14] PRP is a therapy that has been explored among many clinical practices with numerous patients seeing significant positive results in hair regrowth. However, no studies or case reports have been documented in the literature. Still, it is important to recognize this form of hair loss and present PRP as a treatment option that is being used in many practices with good success, while recognizing an opportunity for future studies for PRP in the treatment of traction alopecia.

Central Centrifugal Cicatricial Alopecia (CCCA) Central centrifugal cicatricial alopecia (CCCA) is another common form of alopecia seen in patients of African descent that is characterized by permanent hair loss and loss of follicular ostia.[14] CCCA develops in a roughly circular patch on the crown or vertex region of the scalp, with the area of inflammation and scarring increasing in circumference as the condition progresses. The scalp is often smooth and the hair remaining in the scarred zone is short and brittle. While therapies for this form of hair loss are limited and potential novel therapies are under current investigation, PRP shines a light into a future therapy for the treatment of CCCA, with promising results reported in clinical practice and preliminary studies [**Figure 100-1**]. The studies are discussed in the section on Central Centrifugal Cicatricial Alopecia in Chapter 42.

Alopecia Areata Alopecia areata is a nonscarring, painless form of alopecia, that is autoimmune in origin and driven by loss of immune privilege within the hair follicle.[14] While treatment of AA is often directed at modulating the immune response in the hair follicle to prevent subsequent hair loss, PRP has been reported to have success among a handful of randomized controlled trials, pilot studies, and case reports. The results are discussed in section Alopecia Areata.

Androgenetic Alopecia (AGA) Androgenetic alopecia is a common alopecic disorder seen across all racial and ethnic groups that more commonly affects men than women. Androgenetic alopecia is thought to be due to the interaction of androgens, like DHT, within the scalp hair follicle, promoting miniaturization and regression of the hair follicle.[14] As such, therapies targeted toward blocking DHT and reducing DHT levels on the scalp have seen significant success among some patients with androgenetic alopecia.[14] While antiandrogen and anagen phase promoting medications like finasteride and minoxidil are the current mainstay of treatment for patterned hair loss, many experts see PRP as a useful adjuvant therapy when a patient has maximized their results on

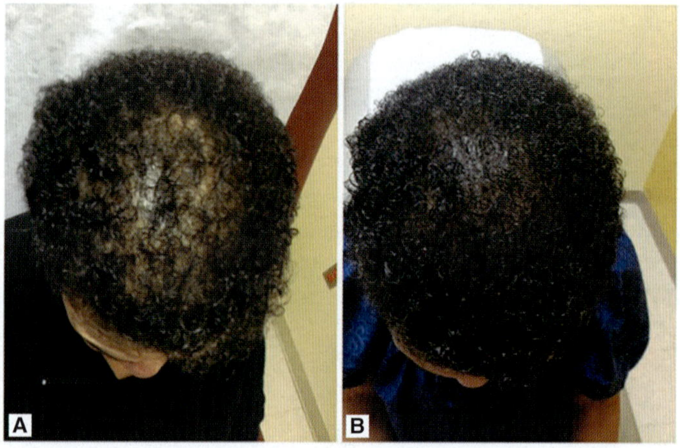

FIGURE 100-1. (A) A 73-year-old Black woman with biopsy-proven CCCA after achieving good control via medical management (topical corticosteroids and intralesional triamcinolone). **(B)** The same patient 3 months after receipt of three courses of platelet rich fibrin matrix (PRFM). (Courtesy of Dr. Chesahna Kindred, Kindred Hair & Skin Center.)

those therapies. Numerous studies have reported success using PRP as a treatment option for AGA; however, administration protocols, therapy schedules, and preparation methods are not standardized, making it difficult to comparatively assess results among published studies. The results of some of these studies are discussed in section Androgenetic Alopecia.

Patient Selection and Assessment

Beneficial Candidates For PRP Patients that have experienced extensive hair loss over a prolonged amount of time will take longer to regrow their hair due to the dormancy of the hair follicles. In some cases, like in late-stage AGA, regrowth of hair is not likely.[20] In these cases, PRP may see limited value. Patients that respond best to PRP are patients with AGA who still have some hair but may notice that it is thinning. Additionally, patients that are good candidates for PRP should have a platelet count within normal limits. Patients who have active disease may not experience significant benefit from PRP initially and would likely see the most utility after adequately medically controlling the underlying process.

Pretreatment Counseling and Informed Consent Due to the large amount of variation in PRP composition between patients, but also in the same patient over time, it is important to engage in patient education and counseling on the variability of hair regrowth. Appropriately setting expectations on the amount of potential hair regrowth based on the extent of current hair loss will allow for the patient to weigh all options, assess cost versus potential benefit, and make an informed decision. As with any medical procedure, informed consent and thoroughly explaining to the patient all parts of the procedure along with side effects is required.

Efficacy and Safety of PRP in Treating Hair Loss in Diverse Populations

Central Centrifugal Cicatricial Alopecia A case report by Dina and Aguh described the implementation of PRP in a 53-year-old African American woman with biopsy-proven CCCA with concomitant mild AGA.[21] Whole blood (9 cc's) was obtained from the patient with sodium citrate used as the anti-coagulant. A single spin at 1100 *g* for 6 minutes was performed to yield 4 to 5 cc of plasma. Calcium was then added to activate the platelets for subsequent growth factor release. The patient received 4 to 4.2 cc's of PRP along the vertex and temporal hairline for three consecutive treatments, each separated by 1 month. The authors concluded at the end of the three treatments, there was greater than 50% improvement in hair density along the portion of the scalp that was biopsied for CCCA.

In another case study, Larrondo et al discussed the usage of PRP in two African American female patients with stable, clinically diagnosed CCCA in the first patient and biopsy-proven CCCA in the second patient.[22]

The first case described a 50-year-old female with a 4-year history of alopecia who was stabilized with topical and intralesional corticosteroids. Injections were scheduled monthly for 3 months, followed by a fourth injection that was spaced 6 months from the third monthly session.

The second case described a woman in her 50s with a 6-year history of alopecia and biopsy-proven CCCA. The patient was stabilized following a routine of topical and intralesional corticosteroids along with spironolactone 50 mg/day. The injection schedule followed the same timeline as the first patient in the study described above.

In both scenarios, researchers found that the patients experienced an increase in follicular density during the monthly treatments × 3 months but saw a subsequent reduction in follicular density at the last treatment session, 6 months after the last monthly treatment.

Alopecia Areata Few studies assessing the impact of PRP in the treatment of alopecia areata have been reported. Recent studies are discussed in detail and summarized in **Table 100-3**. This table has been modified from Paichitrojjana and Paichitrojjana, and Alves and Grimalt.[23,24]

One of the first studies to trial PRP for this type of hair loss was published in 2013 by Trink et al.[25] Forty-five patients with chronic, recurring alopecia areata of at least 2 years in duration were randomized in this half-head, parallel group study to receive either PRP injections, triamcinolone acetonide injections, or a placebo to half of the scalp, with three injections separated by 1 month. The researchers found that PRP increased hair regrowth, decreased hair dystrophy, decreased symptoms of burning and itching, and increased cell proliferation through measurement of Ki-67 activity. Ki-67 is a proliferation marker highly expressed by dermal papilla cells during the anagen phase.

El Taieb et al studied the impact of PRP on 90 patients diagnosed with patchy alopecia areata, alopecia totalis, alopecia universalis, and ophiasis pattern alopecia areata in a randomized control trial.[26] Patients were randomized to receive topical minoxidil 5% twice daily ($N = 30$), PRP injections every 4 weeks ($N = 30$) and topical panthenol cream twice daily ($N = 30$). Patients receiving PRP received three treatments 1 month apart. Researchers found that both PRP and minoxidil showed a significant increase in hair growth. Patients treated with PRP showed a significant decrease in short vellus hairs, dystrophic hairs, and yellow dots unlike patients treated with minoxidil. PRP was most effective in treating patchy alopecia than alopecia universalis. PRP was not effective in treating alopecia totalis.

A case report published by Tordova and Abadjeva described a 46-year-old woman experiencing extensive patchy AA for 17 months who saw significant success with PRP treatment.[27] She received three treatments separated by 1 month. The researchers found after the third session she had a 13% reduction in severity of alopecia tool (SALT) score, a 50% reduction in the Dermatology Quality of Life Index (DQLI) and an increase in the number of pigmented, thick, regrowing hairs.

The ophiasis pattern of alopecia areata is a subtype of AA associated with being refractory to many of the current medical treatments available for treatment along with poor prognosis. A case report published by Jeff Donovan in 2015 described a case of a 41-year-old woman who had poor response to intralesional triamcinolone injections but saw significant improvement in growth following treatment with PRP.[28] PRP was prepared using the Arthrex Angel System, creating PRP with a final platelet concentration 3.5 times above the baseline. Nine milliliter total was injected. After 3 months, the researchers noted significant hair regrowth.

In a case series analyzing the effect of PRP on 25 patients with chronic (>2 year) and severe (SALT > 50) AA, d'Ovidio and Roberto reported positive results from three consecutive PRP treatments separated by 45 to 60 days.[29] Researchers closely followed the protocol developed by Trink et al in designing this study. Patient follow-up was at the 8-month and 1-year mark. Only nine patients completed all three PRP treatments, eight patients completed two PRP treatments, and eight patients completed one PRP treatment session. Of the nine patients that completed the treatment, six patients saw regrowth of terminal pigmented hair and three saw growth of nonpigmented vellus hairs at 8 months. None of the patients maintained regrown hair from PRP treatments at the 1-year mark. Researchers concluded PRP may have utility in some cases of AA, with greater results more likely to be seen with increasing treatment sessions. The authors hypothesize TGF-β may be one of the growth factors responsible for the positive clinical response seen in AA patients, as it is a potent immunosuppressive cytokine and found in high concentrations in PRP preparations.

Khademi et al studied the effect of PRP on 10 patients (five males and five females) who had been clinically diagnosed with alopecia totalis for 3 years and had not received treatment within 3 months prior to the start of the study.[30] Each patient received four treatments, separated by 1 month. In eight patients, no hair regrowth was seen after 4 months and in two patients, less than 10% of hair regrowth was seen.

Androgenetic Alopecia Numerous studies have been conducted assessing PRP in the treatment of AGA, including randomized controlled trials, prospective studies, retrospective studies and case studies. While multiple studies are published, for the sake of brevity, only the most recent randomized controlled trials will be discussed in detail in this section and a summary of the remaining studies are available in **Table 100-4** for reference.

TABLE 100-3 Summary of studies assessing the efficacy of PRP in hair regrowth in alopecia areata

Summary of clinical studies assessing the impact of PRP on patients with alopecia areata						
Author, year, and type of study	**Number of participants**	**Participants demographic**	**Endpoints**	**PRP preparation**	**Number of treatments**	**Results**
Randomized controlled trials						
Trink et al, 2013[25] Randomized double-blind half-head, parallel group study.	45	20 men and 25 women with mean age of 28.	Hair regrowth, hair dystrophy (dermoscopy), burning/itching, cell proliferation (Ki-67 levels).	36 mL of blood was obtained and centrifuged for 8 minutes at 70 *g*. Calcium gluconate was added to preparation.	Three treatments separated by 1 month.	PRP resulted in a significant increase in hair regrowth, decreased hair dystrophy, decreased burning and itching symptoms, and increased cell proliferation.
El Taieb et al, 2017[26] Randomized, placebo-controlled trial	90	39 men and 51 women between the ages of 10 and 40 years old with patchy AA, alopecia totalis, alopecia universalis and ophiasis pattern.	Clinical evaluation and trichoscopic findings (percentage of hair growth, short vellus hairs and yellow dots.	10 mL of blood was obtained and centrifuged rpm for 10 minutes. Calcium gluconate was added to the preparation.	Three treatments separated by 1 month.	PRP resulted in significant decrease in vellus hairs, yellow dots and dystrophic hair by end of 3 months.
Case reports/series and pilot studies						
Todorova and Abadjivea, 2023[27] Case report	1	46 year-old-female with patchy AA.	Clinical photography, scalp hair loss assessment (SALT), digital trichoscopy and dermatology quality of life index (DLQI).	8-10 mL of blood drawn and centrifuged for 10 minutes a 3500 rpm. 5-6 mL of PRP remained and was intradermally injected.	Three treatments separated by 1 month.	Beginning of treatment: SALT = 18%; trichoscopy = predominantly yellow dots and shot vellus hairs; DLQI = 20. End of treatment: SALT = 5%; trichoscopy = upright regrowing hairs and longer, thicker, pigmented hairs; DLQI = 10.
Donovan, 2015[28] Case report	1	41-year-old woman with alopecia ophiasis.	Clinical assessment.	120 mL of blood was obtained using Arthrex Angel System at a platelet concentration of 3.5 times above the baseline.	1 treatment.	Robust regrowth of hairs measuring 2.8 cm was noted 3 months after treatment.
d'Ovidio and Roberto, 2014[29] Case series	25 (nine completed all three treatment sessions, eight completed one treatment session, and eight completed two treatment sessions).	Chronic (>2 years), severe AA (>50% of scalp involved).	Clinical assessment.	PRP preparation performed with Technica Centric 90® and centrifuged at 1200 rpm for 8 minutes.	Three treatments every 45-60 days.	Of the 9 patients, 6 patients obtained regrowth of terminal pigmented hair at 8 months. At 1 year, none of the patients maintained the hair grown with PRP.
Khademi et al, 2019[30] Pilot Study	10	Alopecia totalis patients; five male, five females; 28.9 ± 6.28 years.	Clinical photography and assessment using SALT.	8 mL of blood collected and centrifuged for 5 min at 3500 rpm and 20°C. Collection tube contained calcium gluconate and 95% ethanol.	Four treatments separated by 1 month.	In 8 patients, no hair regrowth was seen after 4 months. In 2 patients, >10% hair regrowth was observed.

Source: Modified from Paichitrojjana and Paichitrojjana [23], and Alves and Grimalt [24].

Male Androgenetic Alopecia RCTs Pakhomova and Smirnova performed a comparative analysis of the clinical efficacy of PRP versus topical 5% minoxidil among 69 male patients aged 18 to 53 years with AGA stages I to IV on the Norwood-Hamilton scale.[31] Patients were randomized into three groups: (1) PRP injections only, (2) PRP w/topical 5% minoxidil, and (3) topical 5% minoxidil only. Injections were performed monthly for 4 months. Clinical efficacy was assessed using hair density, average hair diameter, proportion of vellus hairs, and proportion of telogen hairs. Researchers found in patients receiving PRP therapy compared to topical 5% minoxidil solution, there was not a significant difference in improvement of hair density between the groups. In all other factors like hair diameter, vellus hair proportion, and telogen hair proportion, PRP demonstrated statistically significant higher efficacy. In the PRP group versus minoxidil group, the average hair diameter was 6.3 times higher, vellus hair proportion decreased by 11.8 times, and telogen hair proportion decreased by 3.1 times. When comparing combination therapy with minoxidil only therapy, hair density increased by 1.74 times, hair shaft thickness increased by 14.3 times, proportion of vellus hairs decreased 19.1 times, and proportion of telogen hairs decreased 9.3 times, all statistically significant. When comparing after treatment results to baseline in patients receiving PRP therapy, hair density and hair diameter increased by 12% and proportion of vellus hairs and telogen hairs decreased by 17% and 16%, respectively.

Female Androgenetic Alopecia RCTs Dubin DP et al conducted a randomized placebo-controlled patient blinded trial to study the efficacy of monthly PRP injections for women with AGA stages I to III on the Ludwig scale.[38] Thirty women were recruited to participate in the study and randomized to either the treatment group or placebo group (normal saline) at week 0, 4, and 8. Patients were evaluated at week 24. Four milliliters of PRP was injected subdermally with each injection delivering 0.2 mL of PRP and spaced 1 to 2 cm apart. Injections were performed in a ring around the scalp and along the midline. The same protocol was performed for patients in the control group with normal saline. Twenty-eight patients completed all components of the study. Researchers found at week 8 compared to baseline, mean hair density improved significantly in the PRP treated group, whereas in the placebo group it did not (+71.1 vs −26.7 hairs/cm^2). Improvement of mean hair density was sustained at week 24 for the PRP treated group (+105.9 vs −52.4 hairs/cm^2). In terms of hair diameter, researchers also found at week 8 compared to baseline there was significant improvement in the PRP-treated group, whereas there was not an improvement in the control group (+0.0043 mm vs

TABLE 100-4 Summary of studies assessing the efficacy of PRP on hair regrowth in androgenetic alopecia

Summary of clinical studies assessing the impact of PRP on patients with androgenetic alopecia

Author, year, and type of study	Number of participants	Participant demographics	Endpoints	PRP preparation	Number of treatments	Results
Randomized controlled trials for male androgenetic alopecia						
Pakhomova and Smirnova[31] Randomized controlled trial	69	Men aged 18-53 years with grades I-IV AGA on the Norwood-Hamilton scale. Average AGA duration was 3.3 ± 0.61 years.	Trichoscopy and phototrichogram.	18 mL of blood was obtained and added to a tube containing sodium citrate as the anti-coagulant. The sample underwent double centrifuge (first spin at 570 g for 5 min; second spin at 1200 g at 10 minutes). 2 mL of supernatant was added to calcium chloride for activation.	Four treatments separated by 1 month.	In patients who received PRP, hair density, and hair diameter increased by 12%, proportion of vellus and telogen hairs decreased by 17% and 16%, respectively, from baseline.
Dicle et al., 2020[32] Randomized controlled trial	30 (25 completed the study).	Male patients with average age of 32.2 ± 7.4 years and grades III-V on the Norwood-Hamilton scale.	Number of terminal and vellus hairs.	28 cc of blood was drawn and prepared according to Genesis PRP/centrifuge system. 2 cc of citrate dextrose was used as the anti-coagulant.	Six injection sessions (three PRP sessions, three saline sessions) separated by 1 month with PRP first (Group 1) (10) vs saline first (Group 2) (15). Participants injected at months 0, 1, 2, 6, 7, and 8. Groups crossed over at month 4.	Mean total hair count was increased in groups 1 and 2. The increase was statistically significant for group 2. Researchers detected no statistically significant difference between hair densities on the primary endpoints (M0 and M4) after PRP injections vs placebo injections.
Singh et al, 2020[33] Randomized controlled trial	80	Male patients with AGA grades II-V on the Norwood-Hamilton scale between the ages of 18 and 60 years.	Improvement in hair density and a patient self-assessment score.	18 mL of blood was collected and mixed with 2 mL of 3.8% sodium citrate and centrifuged at 2200 rpm for 12 minutes on first spin. The second spin was done at 3000 rpm for 6 minutes.	Three sessions separated by 1 month.	Patient satisfaction and maximum improvement in hair density was highest in the group that received PRP injections with topical 5% minoxidil.
Rodrigues et al, 2020[34] Randomized controlled trial	26	Male patients diagnosed with AGA-III-vertex on the Norwood-Hamilton scale and between the ages of 18 and 50 years.	Hair growth, hair density and percentage of anagen hairs.	Blood was collected in eight 8.5 mL tubes (six containing acid citrate dextrose, one containing ethylenediaminetetraacetic acid and one without anticoagulant). The sample was centrifuged at 1258 g for 15 minutes.	Four sessions separated by 15 days.	Significant increase in hair count, hair density and percentage of anagen hairs in the PRP group vs control.
Jha et al, 2019[35] Pilot study	93	Male patients with clinically diagnosed AGA grades 1-5 on the Norwood-Hamilton scale.	Hair pull test, hair growth and patient self-satisfaction score.	20 mL of whole blood was collected with sodium citrate used as the anticoagulant. The samples were centrifuged first at 160 g for 10 minutes. The top layer was aspirated and centrifuged again at 400 g for 10 minutes.	Four sessions separated by 3-week intervals.	At the end of treatment, hair pull test was negative in patients receiving topical 5% minoxidil twice daily + PRP + microneedling and in patients receiving topical 5% minoxidil twice daily + PRP. Increased hair growth and higher patient satisfaction was reported among patients receiving all three therapies adjuvantly.
Gentile et al, 2017[36] Randomized controlled trial	18	Male patients between the ages of 19 and 63 years of age with diagnosed AGA stages II-IV on the Norwood-Hamilton scale.	Hair count and hair density.	55 mL of blood was collected with sodium citrate used as the anticoagulant. The sample was centrifuged at 1200 rpm for 10 minutes.	Three sessions separated by 1 month.	Both hair count and hair density in PRP-treated scalp area showed statistically significant improvement over placebo-treated scalp area.
Cervelli et al, 2014[37] Retrospective	10	Male patients aged 22-60 years old with clinically diagnosed AGA on the Norwood-Hamilton scale.	Hair count, hair density, terminal hair density and vellus hair density.	18 cc of whole blood was collected. Sodium citrate was used as the anticoagulant. The sample was centrifuged at 1100 g for 10 minutes. Calcium was added to activate the PRP after.	Three treatments separated by 1 month.	In PRP the treated area of the scalp, there was a statistically significant increase in mean hair count, total hair density, and terminal hair density compared to controlled areas of the scalp at the end of the treatment cycles.

(*Continued*)

TABLE 100-4 Summary of studies assessing the efficacy of PRP on hair regrowth in androgenetic alopecia (*Continued*)

Summary of clinical studies assessing the impact of PRP on patients with androgenetic alopecia

Author, year, and type of study	Number of participants	Participant demographics	Endpoints	PRP preparation	Number of treatments	Results
Randomized controlled trials for female androgenetic alopecia						
Dubin DP et al, 2020[38] Randomized controlled trial	30 (28 participants completed the study).	Female patients diagnosed with AGA stages I-III on the Ludwig scale.	Mean hair density and hair shaft diameter.	22 mL of whole blood was drawn and prepared using Eclipse PRP System (Eclipse Aesthetics LLC, Dallas, TX). The sample was centrifuged at 3500 rpm for 10 minutes.	Three sessions separated by 1 month.	Significant improvement in mean hair density in PRP group vs placebo group at week 8. At week 24, there was sustained improvement of mean hair density in the PRP group vs placebo group.
Bruce et al, 2019[39] Randomized controlled trial	20	Female patients aged 18 years or older diagnosed with grade I or II AGA using the Ludwig scale.	Hair count, vellus hair density, terminal hair density, and cumulative thickness.	60 mL of blood was obtained from the patient. Citrate dextrose solution A was used as the anticoagulant. Blood was centrifuged twice - the first at 1500 rpm for 10 minutes and the second at 3500 rpm for 10 minutes.	Patients were randomized into group A or B. Group A received three treatments of PRP separated by 1 month, had an 8-week washout period followed by topical application of 5% minoxidil for 12 weeks. Patients in group B received the same treatment in reverse order.	For PRP, there were significant increases in hair count and vellus hair density from baseline to week 12. For minoxidil, there were significant increases in hair density, hair count, vellus hair density, terminal hair density and cumulative thickness from baseline to week 12. Comparatively, there was a greater degree of improvement with minoxidil over PRP for hair density, hair count, terminal hair density, and cumulative thickness from baseline to week 12.
Tawfik and Osman, 2018[40] Randomized controlled trial	30	Female patients between the ages of 20 and 45 years old with clinically diagnosed female androgenetic alopecia using the Ludwig scale.	Hair growth, hair density, hair diameter and hair volume.	10 mL of fresh blood was obtained from the patient and drawn into 1.5 mL tubes containing sodium citrate. The sample was centrifuged at 1200 g for 15 minutes. The buffy coat with platelet poor plasma was collected and centrifuged at 2000 g for 10 minutes. Calcium gluconate was added for platelet activation.	Four treatments were given to each patient with each session separated by 1 week. Patients were followed up at 6 months.	At 6 months, areas treated with PRP resulted in a statistically significant increase in hair density and hair thickness compared with baseline. Areas injected with normal saline did not statistically significantly improve compared with baseline.
Lee et al, 2015[41] Randomized controlled trial	40	Korean female patients with the mean age of 33.9 with clinically diagnosed female pattern hair loss.	Hair count and hair fiber diameter.	60 mL of whole blood was obtained from the patient and transferred to 8 mL tubes containing sodium citrate. Blood was centrifuged with the SmartPReP2 system.	One PRP injection 1 week prior to the start of 12 sessions of polydeoxyribonucleotide injections (PDRN) separated by 1-week intervals.	In both the PRP + (polydeoxyribonucleotide) PDRN and PDRN treatment groups, improvements in mean hair counts and mean hair diameter improved 1 week after the final treatment session. Comparative analysis between the groups showed PRP+PDRN therapy resulted in greater improvement in hair diameter but not in hair count, than PDRN alone.

Combined studies for male and female androgenetic alopecia						
Shah et al, 2023[42] Randomized controlled trial	72	Male ($N = 36$) and female ($N = 36$) patients between the ages of 20 and 60 years old diagnosed with AGA via the Norwood-Hamilton scale and Ludwig scale respectively.	Hair count, hair pull tests and AGA grade.	N/A	Three treatments separated by 1 month.	Before treatment: positive hair pull test for all patients. After treatment: 91.7% of patients receiving PRP had a negative hair pull test vs 69.4% for the 5% topical minoxidil group.
Qu et al, 2021[43] Randomized controlled trial	52	32 male patients with grades II-V AGA on Norwood-Hamilton scale and 20 female patients grades I-III AGA on Ludwig scale.	Mean hair count, density, diameter anagen hair ratio.	40 mL of blood was collected in the Tricell kit. Two-step centrifugation was performed (310 g for 4 minutes on first spin and 300 g for 3 minutes on second spin) to produce 4 mL of PRP.	Three treatments separated by 1 month.	Mean hair count, density and diameter showed statistically significant improvement at 3 and 6 months. Anagen hair ratio showed statistically significant improvement at 6 months.
Shapiro et al, 2020[44] Randomized controlled trial	35	17 females and 18 males aged 18-58 years with AGA grades III-V on the Norwood-Hamilton scale and I-II on the Ludwig scale.	Hair density and mean hair shaft diameter.	10 mL of blood was collected and centrifuged at 1500 g for 5 minutes using the Regen Blood Cell Therapy kit (Regan Lab, Le Mont-sur-Lausanne, Switzerland).	Three treatment sessions separated by 1 month.	Hair density in the PRP treated region saw a statistically significant increase of ~20 hairs/cm^2 from before to after treatment. No significant difference was found between PRP-treated areas and placebo areas.
Alves and Grimalt, 2016[45] Randomized controlled trial	25 (13 women, 12 men). Twenty-two patients completed the entire study (11 men and 11 women).	12 men and 13 women aged 18-65 with AGA grades II to V and I to III on the Norwood-Hamilton scale and Ludwig scale, respectively.	Half head studies assessing hair count, hair density, terminal hair density, anagen %, telogen % and anagen/telogen ratio.	20 mL of blood was centrifuged at 460 g for 8 minutes.	Three sessions of PRP separated by 3 months.	PRP-treated scalp areas was found to have a significant increase in mean total hair density when compared to placebo treated scalp areas at 3 and 6 months. No significant differences were found for total hair count and vellus hair density.

Source: Modified from Paichitrojjana and Paichitrojjana [23], and Alves and Grimalt [24].

−0.0034 mm). The increase in hair diameter was sustained at week 24 in the PRP-treated group (+0.0053 mm vs −0.0060 mm).

Combined Male and Female Androgenetic Alopecia RCTs Shah et al compared the efficacy of PRP to 5% topical minoxidil among male and female patients with androgenetic alopecia in a randomized control trial.[42] In this study, 72 patients (60 male, 12 female) with all stages of AGA with ages ranging from 20 to 60 years were included in the trial and randomized for treatment. PRP treatments were performed monthly on the PRP treatment group, while patients in the minoxidil group were instructed to apply 1 mL of 5% minoxidil twice daily. Patients were followed over the course of 3 months. Details on the preparation of PRP were not provided in the study. At the beginning of the study, all patients were noted to have a positive pull test. At the end of treatment, 91.7% of PRP patients were found to have negative hair pull tests and 69.4% of minoxidil patients were found to have negative hair pull tests. The difference between the groups was statistically significant. However, when stratified by age, no significant difference was found between the PRP and minoxidil groups for age stratas 20 to 30 and 31 to 40. When accounting for sex, female patients had no significant differences among the PRP group and minoxidil group in hair pull test results.

Qu et al conducted a randomized placebo-controlled double-blind half-head study to delineate the efficacy of PRP.[43] Fifty-two male and female Chinese patients with AGA were recruited for the study. Patients were excluded if finasteride, dutasteride, or minoxidil was used within 1 year of starting the study. Patients were also excluded if they were immunosuppressed or had hematological or autoimmune disorders. PRP was prepared using the Tricell kit and underwent two-step centrifugation. Four milliliters of PRP was administered to half the head using a 30-gauge needle. PRP was injected according to a machine-generated allocation sequence. Saline was injected to the opposite half of the scalp as a control. Treatment sessions were scheduled monthly for 3 months with follow-up at 3 and 6 months. The authors found that mean hair count, hair density, and hair diameter were both significantly increased at the 3- and 6-month follow-up after treatment. Anagen hair ratios were found to be statistically significantly increased in the half of the scalp treated with PRP at the 6-month mark.

HAIR TRANSPLANTATION IN TREATMENT OF ALOPECIA IN SKIN OF COLOR POPULATIONS: OVERVIEW OF TECHNIQUE, INDICATIONS, COMPLICATIONS, AND THE POTENTIAL FOR PRP AS ADJUVANT THERAPY

Platelet-Rich Fibrin (PRF) and Platelet-Rich Plasma in Hair Transplantation Platelet-rich fibrin (PRF) is based on similar mechanistic principles as PRP in the treatment of alopecia. The difference lies in PRF having a higher concentration of platelets and as such, can produce a higher cumulative release of growth factors.[46] PRF comparably uses the process of differential centrifugation for preparation, with minor noted differences in technique. The centrifugation process is short and rapid to allow for slight separation of blood components. An anticoagulant is not used to allow for clotting. A fibrin rich matrix is then formed in the platelet-rich layer, trapping the platelets and prolonging the release of growth factors over time. PRF has also been found to contain greater concentrations of collagen 1 and TGF-β.[46] The beneficial properties of TGF-β in relation to hair growth has been described in detail in section Mechanism of Action. While the authors of this chapter want to note the enhanced results seen with PRF utilization over PRP in hair transplantation in their individual practices, studies utilizing PRF in hair transplantation have not yet been reported. However, a few studies examining the impact and utility of PRP have been reported. A prospective study examining the efficacy of intra-operative PRP injections during hair transplantation was described by Garg Suruchi. Further, a study examining the effect of hair follicle viability during follicular unit transplantation has also recently been reported by Thuangtong et al. Both of these studies are detailed below in section Assessing the role of PRP in hair restoration surgery.

Before delving into the use of PRP in hair transplantation, this section will start off by discussing hair transplantation, candidate selection, contraindications, and techniques involved in transplantation. The section will then move into describing the role and utility of PRP in hair transplantation and highlight current studies that have examined the impact of intraoperative PRP and extension of follicular graft viability when adding PRP to the culture medium.

Hair Transplantation Background Hair transplantation techniques have evolved and improved tremendously over the years. The two main techniques utilized in hair transplantation are follicular unit transplantation (FUT) and follicular unit extraction (FUE). FUT was developed to provide a more natural appearing cosmetic result in men with straight hair who were diagnosed with androgenetic alopecia.[47] Since then, hair transplantation has become more popular and has expanded to include women diagnosed with scarring and nonscarring forms of alopecia, along with patients of ethnic groups where curly hair is predominant. According to the International Society of Hair Restoration Surgery Practice Census, there were approximately 703,183 hair transplant procedures performed worldwide in 2021, and of these, 149,254 were performed in the United States.[48] Although the exact number of hair transplant procedures performed in persons of color is unknown, it is clear that as the awareness of alopecia grows, the number of hair transplantations in minority and female patient populations will increase. Thus, there are several racial differences in hair morphology, surgical instrumentation, and surgical technique in hair transplant surgery that are important to understand in order to appropriately provide this service to diverse populations. These considerations are discussed below.

FUT involves removing follicular groups or follicular units (FU) from the permanently hair-bearing rim hair (donor area) and inserting them into small incisions produced in the area of hair loss (recipient area). FUE involves widespread extraction of follicular units across the donor area and transplanting those units into the recipient area. Racial variation in hair follicle morphology is by far the most important difference when performing hair transplant surgery in diverse populations. Patients of African descent have extremely curly hair and an elliptical hair follicle [**Figure 100-2**]. This is in contrast to the extremely straight hair and circular hair follicle seen in White and Asian patients. Larger grafts are typically used in patients of color because of the distinct follicular morphology within the dermis. The larger grafts allow for avoidance of hair follicle transection—a major concern that exists during donor harvesting and graft preparation that is known to affect graft survival.

Racial differences in hair density also exist. Patients of African descent exhibit decreased densities when compared with other races, resulting in fewer number of donor grafts needed for hair transplantation.[47,49] In addition, the curliness and dark coloration of the hair provides enhanced scalp coverage and decreased contrast between the hair and scalp. Therefore, surgeons should be less deterred in Blacks with lower donor supply.

Candidate Selection The most common indication for hair transplantation is for the management of androgenetic alopecia. Medical therapy with oral or topical minoxidil 5% or finasteride is recommended

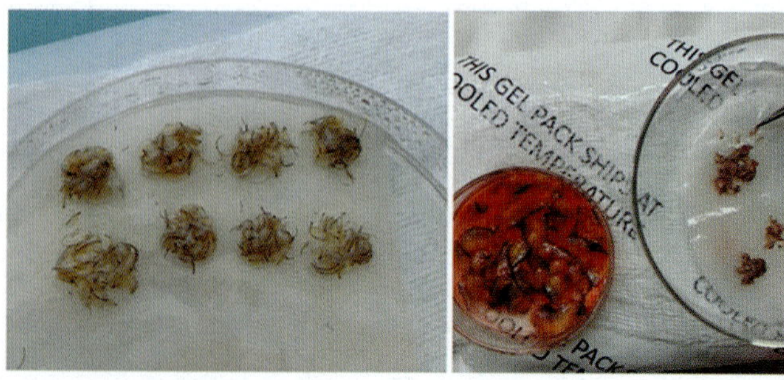

FIGURE 100-2. Visual demonstration of typical "C"-shaped curly hair grafts. (Courtesy of Dr. Meena Singh, KMC Hair Center.)

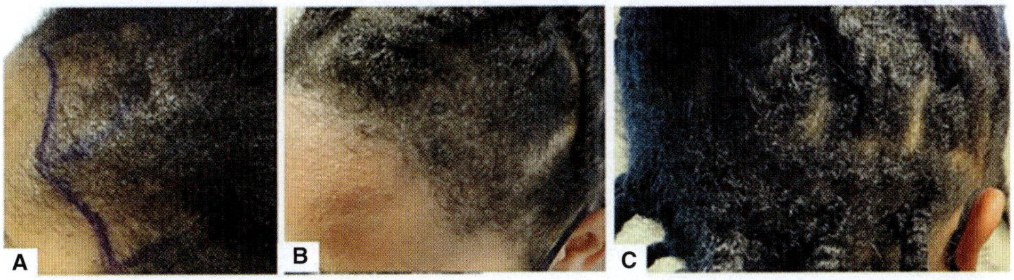

FIGURE 100-3. Follicular unit transplantation in a woman with traction alopecia. **(A)** Preoperative hair line design for TA treatment. **(B)** Regrowth after 6 months. **(C)** Well-healed strip excision scar 6 months status post follicular unit transplantation. (Courtesy of Dr. Meena Singh, KMC Hair Center.)

as first-line treatment in younger patients to slow the progression of AGA before considering a hair transplantation procedure. The medical and surgical treatment of AGA in men of African descent is similar to that in other racial groups; however, Black men who wear their hair closely shaved in a "fade haircut" will have difficulty camouflaging the resulting donor scar produced by the strip technique of follicular unit transplantation.[50,51]

Androgenetic alopecia in women or female pattern hair loss (FPHL) is characterized by a diffuse thinning of the hair over the crown and frontal scalp with preservation of the anterior hairline. In all ethnicities, topical or oral minoxidil is the mainstay of medical therapy for FPHL. However, an increasingly popular option for women with FPHL is hair transplantation.

Hair transplantation surgery is an effective treatment for traction alopecia (TA), or traumatic alopecia marginalis [**Figure 100-3**].[49,52] The distribution of hair loss in TA is often seen along the frontotemporal scalp but not limited to that distribution. While traction alopecia is considered a form of nonscarring alopecia and is generally reversible in its early stages, end-stage traction alopecia is characterized by permanent scarring and the inability for hair to regrow in the affected area(s). Hair transplantation is an excellent treatment for end-stage traction alopecia, as end-stage traction is often stable so long as the inciting traumatic hairstyles have been discontinued. In addition, the curliness common in Afro-textured hair provides increased scalp coverage compared to straight hair. Therefore, even with severe loss of the frontotemporal hairline, an excellent cosmetic outcome can still be achieved.

CCCA is another form of alopecia commonly seen in women of African descent that is cicatricial in nature and may see improvement with hair transplantation [**Figure 100-4**]. Prior to hair transplantation, it is important to ensure the recipient site is not actively inflamed. Proper medical treatment for a minimum of 9 to 12 months to suppress ongoing inflammation is required prior to hair transplantation in order to achieve the best results. Medical treatments are tailored to controlling the inflammatory process with topical and intralesional corticosteroids, immunosuppressants, and anti-inflammatory agents like doxycycline. Surgical correction for biopsy-proven end stage CCCA is an option to help cover the scarred areas. However, special technical considerations are important with hair transplantation in scarring alopecia.

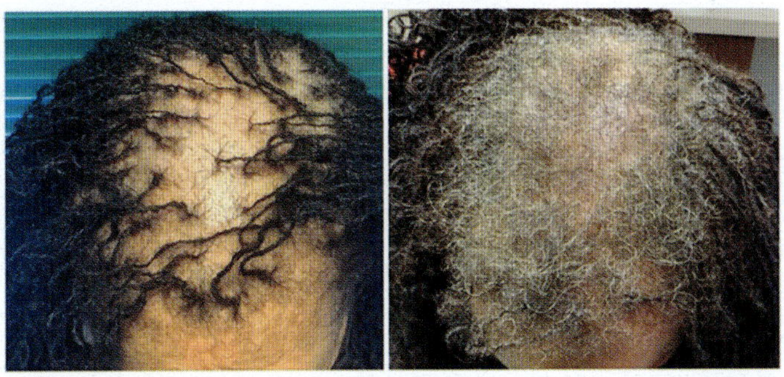

FIGURE 100-4. Left photograph—preoperative photo of a woman with CCCA. Right photograph—6 months status post follicular unit transplantation. (Courtesy of Dr. Meena Singh, KMC Hair Center.)

When transplanting scarring alopecias, the same general principles apply. The main differences tend to be with candidate selection, donor harvesting, recipient site creation, the total number of surgeries performed, and management of patients' expectations. To determine if an individual with CCCA is a proper candidate, a detailed history and scalp examination should be performed. The donor supply, density, and caliber of the hair should be assessed. Recipient areas with scarring alopecia often have decreased blood supply and thickened fibrotic tissue, which can lead to decreased graft survival. Therefore, preoperatively, scalp thickness and available blood supply should be determined as best can be achieved. Hair transplantation should only be considered if the involved areas have been inactive for 1 to 2 years. The CCCA should be quiescent with no anticipation of further disease activity. This decreases the risk of targeted inflammation of the transplanted hairs and likelihood of disease flare. A postoperative biopsy may be warranted to evaluate for disease reactivation, if graft survival is less than expected or with any signs of inflammation.

Contraindications The contraindications for hair transplantation are similar in all racial groups, but patients of color have a higher incidence of keloid and hypertrophic scarring.[53] Keloids are a relative contraindication, as those patients have the option of undergoing a hair transplantation with FUE in lieu of follicular unit transplantation. A careful and detailed history of keloid formation along with a physical examination to check for other scars should be performed. Very few incidences of scalp keloid after hair transplantation have been documented.

Surgical Technique Performing hair transplantation in patients with curly hair can be challenging and steps to avoid transection of the hair follicle within the grafts demand special attention and skill. Anesthesia is obtained by utilizing local infiltration and regional blocks for the donor and recipient areas. In addition, normal saline is injected into the donor area prior to excision of the donor strip to provide maximum skin turgor and to straighten the hair and hair follicles, thus decreasing the rate of follicular transection while harvesting the donor strip. There are four steps in performing a hair transplantation procedure that will be discussed: donor harvesting, graft preparation, recipient-site creation, and graft placement.

Donor Harvesting

Follicular Unit Transplantation (FUT) The initial step in FUT involves excision of a single strip of donor tissue from the occipital scalp [**Figure 100-5**]. Care is taken to ensure that transection of hair follicles is limited and the resulting scar is undetectable. Strip excision is favorable in patients with longer hair lengths, which tends to hide the linear scar. This procedure is generally carried out by a single 10 or 15 blade scalpel. The length and width of the harvested tissue is determined by the hair density of the individual and the number of grafts needed to cover the area of hair loss. Trichophytic closure is a technique currently used to minimize the scar by trimming the epidermis of one edge of the wound before suturing the wound margins together.[54] Undermining the wound margins and limiting the width to less than 1 cm results in less tension along the scar and aids in minimizing the size of the donor scar.

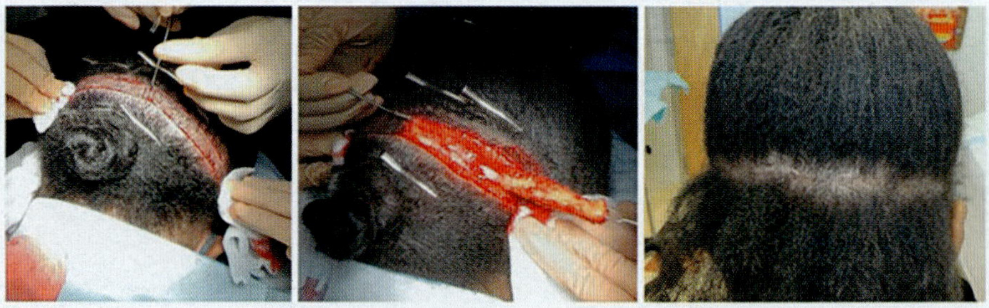

FIGURE 100-5. Depiction of follicular unit transplantation. Left and middle photographs—the epidermis is scored with a scalpel and the strip of skin is dissected away from surrounding structures utilizing blunt dissection techniques. Right photograph—depiction of a typical well-healed scar 6 months status post FUT. (Courtesy of Dr. Meena Singh, KMC Hair Center.)

Follicular unit extraction (FUE) FUE poses advantages over FUT. One advantage is that FUE avoids linear scar formation and disturbance of the natural growth alignment of the donor site. It is a minimally invasive procedure resulting in microscopic scars, which is beneficial in patient populations prone to keloids. Additional advantages of this method of hair transplantation include a relatively fast healing time and avoidance of stitches.

In Black males who wear shorter hairstyles, FUE is the preferred method of hair transplant surgery. FUT is less favorable due to scar visibility with low-cropped hair. Major drawbacks with FUE in comparison to FUT include increased follicular transection and increased donor harvesting time. Using punch excisions greater than 1 mm has been proven to decrease transection of the hair follicles in Black patients, however, larger-diameter punches increase the risk of hypopigmented macular scars. With tightly curled hair, angling the punch instrument parallel to the angle of hair exit may improve donor harvesting.

The first step in performing a follicular unit extraction involves prepping the surgical site by trimming the hairs in the donor safe area. This area is then injected with local anesthetic, so that the physician may begin extracting the grafts from this region using a micropunch tool. The tool may be manual, motorized, or robotic. The scalp is scored and the micropunch tool twists into the scalp for removal of the follicular unit [**Figure 100-6**]. The hair grafts are then extracted from the scalp and held in a solution until they are transplanted into the recipient area.

In FUE of curly hair grafts, a larger punch graft (1-1.2 mm) is encouraged due to an observed smaller number of follicular units per square centimeter (lower density) and higher number of hairs per follicular unit in populations of African descent. Larger punch grafts also allow for better survival of transplanted follicles, especially in areas of scar tissue. Incisions of slightly wider girth are made for curly graft transplantation.

Graft Preparation When utilizing FUT, the donor strip is converted into individual grafts of different sizes. Caution must be taken with curly hair to avoid transection of the hair follicle, so a curved blade may be used to match the curvature of the hair. The grafts that are created contain one to four hair follicular units and are placed in a holding solution until they are ready to be inserted into the recipient sites. When utilizing FUE, the grafts may be trimmed and counted prior to transplantation into the recipient area.

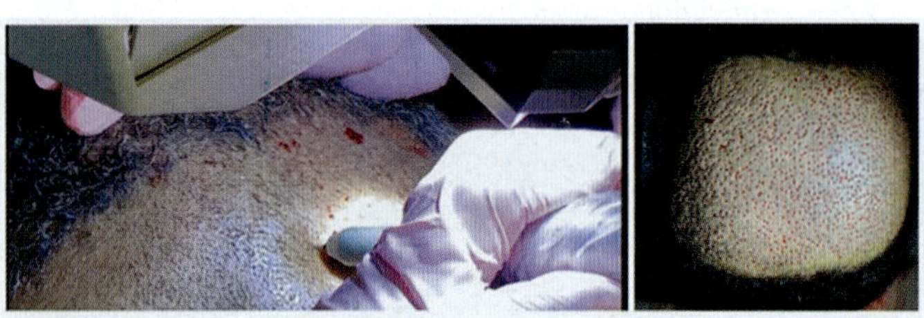

FIGURE 100-6. Depiction of follicular unit extraction with a punch device. Left photograph—before FUT. Right photograph—immediately after FUT. (Courtesy of Dr. Meena Singh, KMC Hair Center.)

Recipient Site Creation and Graft Placement A number of surgical instruments can be used to create recipient sites in areas of hair loss. Instrumentation is based on the degree of curl of the hair—the greater the curl, the larger the recipient site. Typically, the recipient site ranges from 1.2 to 2.0 mm in size in patients with a significant curl pattern. The grafts are then placed using microvascular forceps or implanters [**Figure 100-7**].

Hairline Design The hairline can contribute to a youthful facial shape and appearance. Patients with hairline recession often hope to regain the appearance they had prior to their hair loss. Thus, the perceived success of the hair transplant may rest on the hair line design. It is important to create a natural appearance with an appropriate hair density. The same general principles of hairline design apply to Black males. Smaller follicular unit grafts should be used. A straight, flat hairline is more desirable and can look natural in Black men [**Figure 100-8**]. When creating a frontal hairline in Black men, the patient should be counseled that the hairline will appear more natural over time. The patient should also be informed of the possibility of continued hairline recession and thinning.

Complications Most patients have excellent cosmetic results from hair transplantation surgery and experience a low risk of keloidal scarring. However, at least one case of a large keloidal scar following hair transplantation has been reported. This was reported in a 60-year-old African American male with androgenetic alopecia and no previous history of keloidal scarring.[55] The scar developed over a large portion of the patient's scalp. This represents a significant potential complication, particularly in Black and Asian patients with a history of scarring. To avoid this complication, test grafting is recommended in some patients before a hair transplantation procedure. If normal healing occurs in the donor area and recipient site after 3 months, the patient is a good candidate for a full transplantation procedure.

Assessing the Role of PRP in Hair Restoration Surgery Intraoperative PRP has been used by the authors in clinical settings, with delivery of positive results in hair regrowth [**Figure 100-9**]. The use of intraoperative PRP in FUE has also been explored in a prospective, randomized study of 40 patients.[56] Forty male FUE hair transplant patients with stages III to VII AGA on the Norwood-Hamilton scale between 20 and 55 years of age were randomized to either receive or not receive PRP. PRP collection was uniform throughout the study and done using the YCELL BIO kit. PRP preparation utilized a double spin centrifugation with the first spin at 3200 rpm for 4 minutes and the second spin at 3200 rpm for 1 minute. A total of 3 mL of PRP was collected from 20 mL of blood. PRP was prepared while slits were being made. PRP was injected into the dermis and subcutis 1-cm apart in the slits of the recipient area. Patients randomized to receive PRP received 0.2 to 0.3 mL of PRP and patients randomized for control received 0.2 to 0.3 mL of normal saline. Only scalp hairs were harvested for PRP and only grafts with intact roots were implanted. The density of implantation was maintained at 40 to 45 grafts/cm^2. Patients were evaluated for improvement at the end of 2 weeks, 4 weeks, 8 weeks, 3 months and 6 months on measures of hair density, hair shaft length, hair thickness, and measures of scalp post-surgical recovery. In the PRP group, all patients achieved greater than 75% hair regrowth at 6 months, whereas in the control group only four patients had achieved greater than 75% hair regrowth at 6 months.

Further, activity in dormant follicles was seen in all 20 PRP randomized patients at 3 months and greater, as noted by the appearance of fine hair

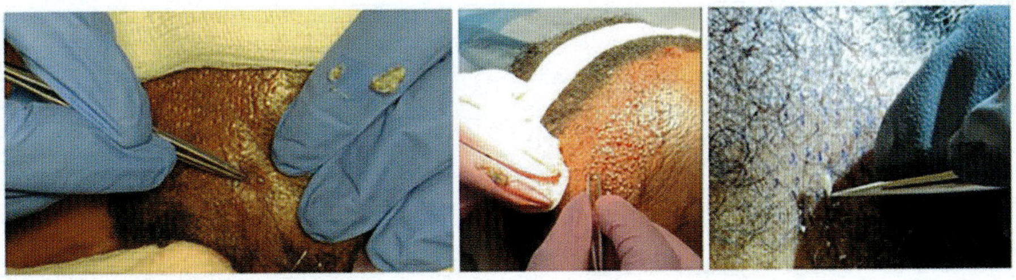

FIGURE 100-7. Follicular unit grafts being placed in patients with traction alopecia. (Courtesy of Dr. Meena Singh, KMC Hair Center.)

in addition to the thick transplanted hair. This is in contrast to the control group, where fine vellus hairs were noted in 13 patients at 4 months and greater.

Patients receiving PRP were also noted to have longer hairs. After 6 months of hair transplant, 13/20 patients had 10 mm or longer hairs while only 2/20 patients in the non-PRP group had 10 mm or longer hairs. Finally, scalp redness was significantly decreased in the PRP treated group. After 3 months of hair transplant, 5% of patients in the PRP group experienced scalp redness. This is in contrast to the placebo treated group, where 30% of patients had scalp redness.

A randomized controlled trial performed by Thuangtong et al described the impact of PRP on hair graft preservation in follicular unit transplantation (FUT).[57] The researchers recruited 10 androgenetic alopecia patients who received follicular unit transplantation. After FUT, human hair follicles were collected from each patient. The study consisted of a 2 ×2 × 2 design, allowing for eight different culture conditions: (1) William medium or Ringer Lactate Solution, (2). 4°C or 37°C, and (3) with PRP supplementation or without PRP supplementation. Forty follicles were randomized to the eight culture conditions, with each culture condition containing five hair follicles.

PRP underwent single spin centrifugation for 5 minutes at 200 g at room temperature. The first half of the PRP sample was added to the culture medium on day 0 and the second half was added on day 4. Hair follicles were examined and photographed on days 0, 4, and 7. The authors found that the growth of hair follicle grafts cultured with 10% PRP was not statistically different from the growth of hair follicle grafts cultured without PRP. However, researchers also found that hair follicle grafts with PRP supplementation had a higher expression of CK15, which is a marker of the outer root sheath cells in the hair follicle. This potentially suggests the addition of PRP may maintain hair follicle viability during storage.

SAFETY AND CONSIDERATIONS

REVIEW OF POTENTIAL SIDE EFFECTS AND COMPLICATIONS

PRP is considered a very safe therapeutic option with minimal to no reported negative side effects. Due to the blood product being autologous, the patient does not have to worry about reactions to the injected product. Among the minor side effects reported from PRP are bruising and pain at the injection site. Lightheadedness and dizziness have been reported from the partial removal of blood from the patient in order to prepare PRP. As with any procedure that involves making breaks in the skin, infection is always a risk but again remains minimal. Absolute and relative contraindications to PRP were reported by Garg and Manchanda. Absolute contraindications include critical thrombocytopenia, hemodynamic instability, local infection at injection site, or a platelet dysfunction syndrome. Relative contraindications to PRP include consistent use of NSAIDs within 48 hours of procedure, corticosteroid injection at treatment site within 1 month, systemic use of corticosteroids within 2 weeks, use of tobacco, recent fever/illness, cancer—especially hematopoietic or bone, hemoglobin < 10 g/dL, platelet count < $10^5/\mu L$.[58]

VARIABILITY IN PROCESSING AND PRODUCT COMPOSITION

The greatest concern surrounding the field of PRP as a medical therapy today is the current lack of standardization in processing and preparation methods and the high variability in the final composition of the injected product. While many methods have been proposed for the classification of PRP for medical usage, none have been universally adopted. The first classification system to be suggested was by Dohan Ehrenfest et al in 2009, where he suggested the classification system should be based on three variables—those being platelets, fibrin, and leukocytes.[59] Subsequently, a new classification system called PAW, standing for platelets, activation, and white blood cells, called for the classification system to be based upon platelets, platelet-activating substances, and the presence or absence of leukocytes.[9] Continuous changes have been made over the years in the parameters of PRP classification, with the most recent classification suggestion being the system of the International Society on Thrombosis and Hemostasis. This was proposed by the Scientific Standardization Committee in 2018.[9]

The failure to standardize has led to high variability in patient results and can lead to patient disappointment if inappropriately counseled on

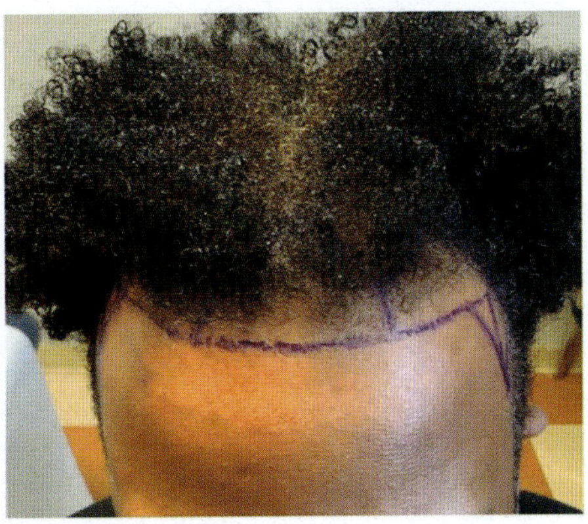

FIGURE 100-8. Depiction of a flat hairline design in an African American male patient. (Courtesy of Dr. Meena Singh, KMC Hair Center.)

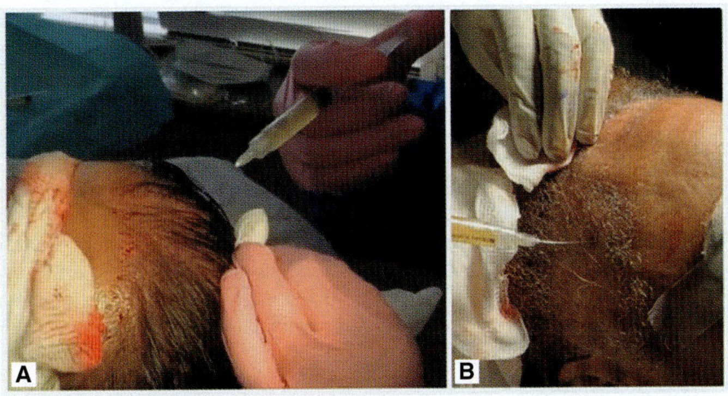

FIGURE 100-9. Visual depiction of intraoperative PRP injections during hair restoration surgery in two different patients. **(A)** Left photograph—patient with straight hair undergoing hair transplantation and PRP injections. **(B)** Right photograph—patient with afro-textured hair undergoing hair transplantation and PRP injections. (Courtesy of Dr. Meena Singh, KMC Hair Center.)

the high level of outcome variability. In addition, while standardization of methods can help to reduce variability in patient outcomes, a baseline level will always persist as the composition of the final product and available growth factors is dependent on the health and vitality of the patient and their blood at the time of the procedure. The lack of a standardized therapy and high variability in patient outcomes also creates a gap in accessibility and affordability. This is because many insurance companies recognize PRP as an experimental form of treatment and therefore will not cover the cost, as opposed to conventional and proven therapies that are often covered.

EXPENSE

One session of PRP can range from US$500 to 1200 with a series of three sessions needed for visual improvement. The schedule of PRP may vary depending on the type of hair loss and extent of hair loss present. However, in general many PRP therapies require three treatments 4 to 6 weeks apart as induction therapy and maintenance treatment every 4 to 6 months. Currently, PRP for hair loss is not covered with medical insurance, requiring patients to bear the financial cost. This creates a gap in accessibility to care among skin of color patient populations, who often lack the resources to take on the extra financial burden.

FUTURE DIRECTIONS AND EMERGING RESEARCH

ONGOING STUDIES AND RESEARCH ON PRP IN SKIN OF COLOR

Due to the novelty of PRP, there is much room for advancement of practice in PRP application technique, standardization of preparation, and discovery of effectiveness among numerous dermatologic pathologies. While PRP has been used in the treatment of AGA, AA, and CCCA, it is recently starting to be explored among FFA and LPP. In addition to hair loss, PRP therapy is also being studied in wound healing and vitiligo, which could potentially have profound impacts on skin of color populations. As PRP continues to be studied and advances toward standardization in preparation and application are made, new implementations for a variety of dermatological conditions and skin of color pathologies can be studied.

CONCLUSION

PRP is a safe, effective treatment for hair loss but also a simple procedure. Dermatologists are indeed the hair loss experts of the medical field and should add PRP to their toolbox for alopecia. Compared to common dermatologic procedures, dermatologists should find incorporating PRP into their practice to be straightforward.

REFERENCES

1. Justicz N, Derakhshan A, Chen JX, Lee LN. Platelet-rich plasma for hair restoration. *Facial Plast Surg Clin N Am.* 2020;28(2):181-187.
2. Gonçalves NJN, Frantz N, de Oliveira RM. Platelet-rich plasma (PRP) therapy: an approach in reproductive medicine based on successful animal models. *Anim Reprod.* 16(1):93-98.
3. Kingsley CS. Blood Coagulation: evidence of an antagonist to factor VI in platelet-rich human plasma. *Nature.* 1954;173(4407):723-724.
4. Alves R, Grimalt R. A review of platelet-rich plasma: history, biology, mechanism of action, and classification. *Skin Appendage Disord.* 2017;4(1):18-24.
5. Halder RM, Grimes PE, McLaurin CI, Kress MA, Kenney JA. Incidence of common dermatoses in a predominantly black dermatologic practice. *Cutis.* 1983;32(4):388, 390.
6. Alexis AF, Sergay AB, Taylor SC. Common dermatologic disorders in skin of color: a comparative practice survey. *Cutis.* 2007;80(5):387-394.
7. Semble A, McMichael A. Hair loss in patients with skin of color. *Semin Cutan Med Surg.* 2015;34(2):81-88.
8. Sy N, Mastacouris N, Strunk A, Garg A. Overall and racial and ethnic subgroup prevalences of alopecia areata, alopecia totalis, and alopecia universalis. *JAMA Dermatol.* 2023;159(4):419-423.
9. Everts P, Onishi K, Jayaram P, Lana JF, Mautner K. Platelet-rich plasma: new performance understandings and therapeutic considerations in 2020. *Int J Mol Sci.* 2020;21(20):7794.
10. Dean L. Blood and the cells it contains. In: *Blood Groups and Red Cell Antigens [Internet].* National Center for Biotechnology Information (US); 2005. https://www.ncbi.nlm.nih.gov/books/NBK2263/. Accessed December 2, 2023.
11. Schnabel LV, Boone L, Peroni JF. Chapter 8—Regenerative medicine. In: Auer JA, Stick JA, Kümmerle JM, Prange T, eds. *Equine Surgery.* 5th ed. Philadelphia, PA: W.B. Saunders; 2019:104-122.
12. Liebig BE, Kisiday JD, Bahney CS, Ehrhart NP, Goodrich LR. The platelet-rich plasma and mesenchymal stem cell milieu: a review of therapeutic effects on bone healing. *J Orthop Res Off Publ Orthop Res Soc.* 2020;38(12):2539-2550.
13. Marx RE. Platelet-rich plasma (PRP): what is PRP and what is not PRP? *Implant Dent.* 2001;10(4):225-228.
14. Miteva M. *Alopecia.* Amsterdam: Elsevier; 2018.
15. Yang L, Pang Y, Moses HL. TGF-β and immune cells: an important regulatory axis in the tumor microenvironment and progression. *Trends Immunol.* 2010;31(6):220-227.
16. Almohanna HM, Ahmed AA, Griggs JW, Tosti A. Platelet-rich plasma in the treatment of alopecia areata: a review. *J Investig Dermatol Symp Proc.* 2020;20(1):S45-S49.
17. Paus R, Ito N, Takigawa M, Ito T. The hair follicle and immune privilege. *J Investig Dermatol Symp Proc.* 2003;8(2):188-194.
18. Dhurat R, Sukesh M. Principles and methods of preparation of platelet-rich plasma: a review and author's perspective. *J Cutan Aesthetic Surg.* 2014;7(4):189-197.
19. Fadadu PP, Mazzola AJ, Hunter CW, Davis TT. Review of concentration yields in commercially available platelet-rich plasma (PRP) systems: a call for PRP standardization. *Reg Anesth Pain Med.* 2019;44(6):652-659.
20. Workman K, Piliang M. Approach to the patient with hair loss. *J Am Acad Dermatol.* 2023;89(2, Supplement):S3-S8.
21. Dina Y, Aguh C. Use of Platelet-rich plasma in cicatricial alopecia. *Dermatol Surg Off Publ Am Soc Dermatol Surg Al.* 2019;45(7):979-981.
22. Larrondo J, Petela J, McMichael AJ. Transitory hair growth using platelet-rich plasma therapy in stabilized central centrifugal cicatricial alopecia. *Dermatol Ther.* 2022;35(11):e15798.
23. Paichitrojjana A, Paichitrojjana A. Platelet rich plasma and its use in hair regrowth: a review. *Drug Des Devel Ther.* 2022;16:635-645.
24. Alves R, Grimalt R. Platelet-rich plasma and its use for cicatricial and non-cicatricial alopecias: a narrative review. *Dermatol Ther.* 2020;10(4):623-633.
25. Trink A, Sorbellini E, Bezzola P, et al. A randomized, double-blind, placebo- and active-controlled, half-head study to evaluate the effects of platelet-rich plasma on alopecia areata. *Br J Dermatol.* 2013;169(3):690-694.
26. El Taieb MA, Ibrahim H, Nada EA, Seif Al-Din M. Platelets rich plasma versus minoxidil 5% in treatment of alopecia areata: a trichoscopic evaluation. *Dermatol Ther.* 2017;30(1).
27. Todorova LN, Abadjieva TI. Platelet-rich plasma in alopecia areata: a case report with a mini review of literature. *Cureus.* 15(5):e38751.
28. Donovan J. Successful treatment of corticosteroid-resistant ophiasis-type alopecia areata (AA) with platelet-rich plasma (PRP). *JAAD Case Rep.* 2015;1(5):305-307.
29. Roberto M. Limited Effectiveness of platelet-rich-plasma treatment on chronic severe alopecia areata. *Hair Ther Transplant.* 2014;04(01).
30. Khademi F, Tehranchinia Z, Abdollahimajd F, Younespour S, Kazemi-Bajestani SMR, Taheri K. The effect of platelet rich plasma on hair regrowth in patients with alopecia areata totalis: A clinical pilot study. *Dermatol Ther.* 2019;32(4):e12989.
31. Pakhomova EE, Smirnova IO. Comparative evaluation of the clinical efficacy of prp-therapy, minoxidil, and their combination with immunohistochemical study of the dynamics of cell proliferation in the treatment of men with androgenetic alopecia. *Int J Mol Sci.* 2020;21(18):6516.
32. Dicle Ö, Bilgic Temel A, Gülkesen KH. Platelet-rich plasma injections in the treatment of male androgenetic alopecia: a randomized placebo-controlled crossover study. *J Cosmet Dermatol.* 2020;19(5):1071-1077.
33. Singh SK, Kumar V, Rai T. Comparison of efficacy of platelet-rich plasma therapy with or without topical 5% minoxidil in male-type baldness: a randomized, double-blind placebo control trial. *Indian J Dermatol Venereol Leprol.* 2020;86(2):150-157.
34. Rodrigues BL, Montalvão SAL, Cancela RBB, et al. Treatment of male pattern alopecia with platelet-rich plasma: a double-blind controlled study with analysis of platelet number and growth factor levels. *J Am Acad Dermatol.* 2019;80(3):694-700.

35. Jha AK, Vinay K, Zeeshan M, Roy PK, Chaudhary RKP, Priya A. Platelet-rich plasma and microneedling improves hair growth in patients of androgenetic alopecia when used as an adjuvant to minoxidil. *J Cosmet Dermatol.* 2019;18(5):1330-1335.
36. Gentile P, Cole JP, Cole MA, et al. Evaluation of not-activated and activated PRP in hair loss treatment: role of growth factor and cytokine concentrations obtained by different collection systems. *Int J Mol Sci.* 2017;18(2):408.
37. Cervelli V, Garcovich S, Bielli A, et al. The effect of autologous activated platelet rich plasma (AA-PRP) injection on pattern hair loss: clinical and histomorphometric evaluation. *BioMed Res Int.* 2014;2014:760709.
38. Dubin DP, Lin MJ, Leight HM, et al. The effect of platelet-rich plasma on female androgenetic alopecia: a randomized controlled trial. *J Am Acad Dermatol.* 2020;83(5):1294-1297.
39. Bruce AJ, Pincelli TP, Heckman MG, et al. A randomized, controlled pilot trial comparing platelet-rich plasma to topical minoxidil foam for treatment of androgenic alopecia in women. *Dermatol Surg Off Publ Am Soc Dermatol Surg Al.* 2020;46(6):826-832.
40. Tawfik AA, Osman MAR. The effect of autologous activated platelet-rich plasma injection on female pattern hair loss: A randomized placebo-controlled study. *J Cosmet Dermatol.* 2018;17(1):47-53.
41. Lee SH, Zheng Z, Kang JS, Kim DY, Oh SH, Cho SB. Therapeutic efficacy of autologous platelet-rich plasma and polydeoxyribonucleotide on female pattern hair loss. *Wound Repair Regen Off Publ Wound Heal Soc Eur Tissue Repair Soc.* 2015;23(1):30-36.
42. A randomized control trial comparing the efficacy of platelet-rich plasma and 5% topical minoxidil for the treatment of androgenetic alopecia. *J Drugs Dermatol.* https://jddonline.com/articles/a-randomized-control-trial-comparing-the-efficacy-of-platelet-rich-plasma-and-5-topical-minoxidil-for-the-treatment-of-androgenetic-alopecia-s1545961623p0905x/. Accessed December 3, 2023.
43. Qu Q, Zhou Y, Shi P, et al. Platelet-rich plasma for androgenic alopecia: a randomized, placebo-controlled, double-blind study and combined mice model experiment. *J Cosmet Dermatol.* 2021;20(10):3227-3235.
44. Shapiro J, Ho A, Sukhdeo K, Yin L, Lo Sicco K. Evaluation of platelet-rich plasma as a treatment for androgenetic alopecia: a randomized controlled trial. *J Am Acad Dermatol.* 2020;83(5):1298-1303.
45. Alves R, Grimalt R. Randomized placebo-controlled, double-blind, half-head study to assess the efficacy of platelet-rich plasma on the treatment of androgenetic alopecia. *Dermatol Surg Off Publ Am Soc Dermatol Surg Al.* 2016;42(4):491-497.
46. Diab NAF, Ibrahim A shimaa M, Abdallah AM. Fluid platelet-rich fibrin (PRF) versus platelet-rich plasma (PRP) in the treatment of atrophic acne scars: a comparative study. *Arch Dermatol Res.* 2023;315(5):1249-1255.
47. Bernstein RM, Rassman WR. The aesthetics of follicular transplantation. *Dermatol Surg Off Publ Am Soc Dermatol Surg Al.* 1997;23(9):785-799.
48. 2022 ISHRS Practice Census Results. Published online 2022.
49. Sperling LC. Hair density in African Americans. *Arch Dermatol.* 1999;135(6):656-658.
50. Pierce HE. The uniqueness of hair transplantation in black patients. *J Dermatol Surg Oncol.* 1977;3(5):533-535.
51. Rm E. Hair transplantation, scalp reduction, and flap rotation in black men. *J Dermatol Surg Oncol.* 1986;12(1).
52. Callender VD, McMichael AJ, Cohen GF. Medical and surgical therapies for alopecias in black women. *Dermatol Ther.* 2004;17(2):164-176.
53. Shaffer JJ, Taylor SC, Cook-Bolden F. Keloidal scars: a review with a critical look at therapeutic options. *J Am Acad Dermatol.* 2002;46(2 Suppl Understanding):S63-97.
54. Marzola M. Trichophytic closure of the donor area. *Hair Transpl Forum Int.* 2005;15(4):113-116.
55. Brown MD, Johnson T, Swanson NA. Extensive keloids following hair transplantation. *J Dermatol Surg Oncol.* 1990;16(9):867-869.
56. Garg S. Outcome of intra-operative injected platelet-rich plasma therapy during follicular unit extraction hair transplant: a prospective randomised study in forty patients. *J Cutan Aesthetic Surg.* 2016;9(3):157-164.
57. Thuangtong R, Chaweekulrat P, Thanomkitti K, Triwongwaranat D, Rujitharanawong C. Effect of platelet-rich plasma and other key factors on hair follicle preservation. *Int J Trichology.* 2023;15(2):50.
58. Garg S, Manchanda S. Platelet-rich plasma—an 'Elixir' for treatment of alopecia: personal experience on 117 patients with review of literature. *Stem Cell Investig.* 2017;4:64.
59. Dohan Ehrenfest DM, Rasmusson L, Albrektsson T. Classification of platelet concentrates: from pure platelet-rich plasma (P-PRP) to leucocyte- and platelet-rich fibrin (L-PRF). *Trends Biotechnol.* 2009;27(3):158-167.

SECTION 14

Populations with Unique Considerations

CHAPTER 101 Considerations in Sexual and Gender Diverse Dermatology

Nicholas Tan
Iain Noel Encarnacion
Erica Dommasch
Klint Peebles

KEY POINTS

- Sexual and gender diverse (SGD) individuals are a unique, understudied, and growing population with more than 7% of individuals in the United States currently identifying as SGD. These populations experience disproportionate rates of marginalization and stigma compared to their non-SGD peers, impacting healthcare access and outcomes.
- Inclusive terminology, language, and communication are critical when interacting with SGD individuals across the lifespan. Terminology can be fluid and evolves over time.
- SGD individuals are not a monolithic community. There is substantial diversity and intersectionality inherent within these populations that must be recognized and affirmed in order to provide culturally humble care that reflects a trauma-informed approach while acknowledging structural barriers to equitable care.
- A standardized approach to routine demographic data collection inclusive of sexual orientation and gender identity is of paramount importance when identifying and mitigating the health disparities SGD individuals face.
- Dermatologists have important roles in gender-affirming care, including management of side effects or complications of hormone therapy, preparation for gender-affirming surgical procedures, and provision of minimally invasive dermatologic procedures that facilitate congruence of gender expression with gender identity.
- Individuals with differences of sex development or variations of sex characteristics have unique health needs that are understudied and often inappropriately conflated with those of the broader SGD population.

INTRODUCTION

Sexual and gender diverse (SGD) individuals represent a diverse and growing population subject to historic and ongoing marginalization and stigma with consequential impacts on their healthcare needs, access, and outcomes. National surveys show that the number of individuals identifying as LGBTQ (lesbian, gay, bisexual, transgender, queer) continues to increase, currently at 7.1% of the population, with 0.6%, or 1.6 million adults, identifying as transgender.[1] While these numbers are stable in older generations, numbers are increasing particularly in younger generations. The transgender population is also more racially and ethnically diverse than the general population. In general, SGD individuals remain poorly studied within dermatology, particularly from an intersectional lens. Moreover, while health disparities are well-described in SGD people, standardized curricular integration of these topics and routine clinical exposure during training are lacking.

This chapter aims to equip dermatologists with an awareness of the unique health needs of SGD persons, dermatologic considerations, and a broader approach to inclusive, compassionate care for this population within the framework of cultural humility. Given the complexity of the topic, this section is not intended to be comprehensive.

LANGUAGE AND CORE TERMINOLOGY

Language and terminology are essential components of competent care for SGD persons and are the foundation upon which a therapeutic, trusting patient-physician alliance is built. First, it is critical to distinguish among the concepts of identity, body, and behavior. Identity refers to the innumerable ways in which an individual may personally identify. From an SGD lens, this can refer to gender identity and sexual orientation. Body refers to one's biology, anatomy, sexual development, and reproductive capacity, just to name several. Behavior refers, in a manner of speaking, to how one engages with their body both alone and with others, which would include the spectrum of sexual behaviors, or the lack thereof. In order to have a holistic understanding of an individual, one must understand all three of these components: the ways in which the individual self-identifies, the body and organs the individual possesses, and the behaviors in which the individual engages.

"Sexual diverse" refers to those individuals whose sexual identity, sexual orientation, or sexual behaviors differ from the presumed majority of the population. "Gender diverse" refers to those whose gender identity (eg, man, woman, nonbinary, or other) or gender expression (masculine, feminine, nonconforming, or other) differs from their sex assigned at birth. Sex assigned at birth is typically determined by observation of one's anatomy at birth (eg, male, female, intersex, or other). Transgender is an umbrella term referring to an individual for whom gender identity does not align with sex assigned at birth. There are numerous terms under the transgender umbrella that can be used to describe gender-diverse identities. It is essential to recognize that sexual orientation, attraction, sexual behavior, gender identity, and gender expression are all distinct concepts that do not define each other and cannot be assumed based upon each other. Common terminology is summarized in **Table 101-1**.

Of note, terminology used by SGD people is fluid and will continue to evolve. As there is no universal consensus regarding terminology among individuals, not every term will resonate with each person. In some cases, terms that one individual may wholly embrace may be deemed offensive by another. Clinicians must continuously elicit a patient's identifiers and normalize routine questions regarding gender identity, sexual orientation, sexual behaviors, and pronouns, among others, while recognizing that these identifiers can change over time.

The concept of intersectionality, first introduced by Professor Kimberle Crenshaw, draws upon the lens of critical legal theory within the experience of Black feminism. The term describes the numerous social forces and ideological paradigms by which power and privilege are exerted and how oppressive systems overlap to create distinct lived experiences for individuals belonging to multiple minority identity categories.[2] Dermatologists should be aware of how intersectionality impacts SGD patients of color. By doing so, providers may better recognize and address the social determinants of health as well as the resulting disparities experienced by marginalized groups with multiple social identities in both clinical care and research.

TABLE 101-1 Summary of sexual and gender diverse terminology

Term	Definition
Gender identity	An individual's sense of their internal self and their gender (eg masculine, feminine, both, or neither). Gender identity may differ from one's sex assigned at birth.
Gender expression	A person's external expression of their gender identity (eg, through clothing, grooming, behavior, speech, etc)
Gender affirmation	Refers to processes and steps by which one's internal gender identity is affirmed. In some cases known as 'transitioning,' gender affirmation encompasses a variety of domains, including psychological or self-affirmation, social, legal affirmation, and medical affirmation, the latter of which includes interventions such as hormonal therapy and a host of surgical procedures. Not all gender diverse people will desire all or any of these domains of affirmation.
Gender dysphoria	Clinically significant distress arising from conflict between a person's gender identity and their sex assigned at birth.
Sexual and Gender minority	Encompasses both sexually and gender diverse (SGD) individuals and is used as to inclusively encompass the entirety of the LGBTQIA+ spectrum.
Cisgender	An individual whose current gender identity aligns with their sex assigned at birth.
Gender diverse	An individual whose gender identity and expression differ from their sex assigned at birth.
Transgender	Umbrella term referring to an individual for whom gender identity does not align with sex assigned at birth, identifies individuals whose gender identity or expression differs from their sex assigned at birth based on genital anatomy.
Transgender woman/MTF Transgender person/Trans woman	An individual who was assigned male at birth but currently identifies as female.
Transgender man/FTM Transgender person/Trans man	An individual who was assigned female at birth but currently identifies as male.
Transmasculine and Transfeminine	Broader terms to encompass individuals who express or identify as predominantly masculine or feminine, respectively.
Genderqueer	An umbrella term for gender identities that exist outside binary definitions of male or female. This Includes people who view themselves as a blend of both male and female, neither male nor female, different gender at different times, or no specific gender at all.
Gender nonconforming	A person whose gender does not conform to the predominant cultural and social gender norms, roles, or expectations of their perceived gender.
Nonbinary	Gender identities that exist outside of traditional binary identities of male and female.
Genderfluid	An individual whose gender is not identified to be static across time or contexts.
Agender	An individual who does not identify with having a gender.
Intersex	Relating to congenital sex characteristics outside of the typical binary of male and female. This may include gonads and chromosomes. Also termed "variations of sex characteristics" and "differences of sex development."
Sexual orientation	An individual's pattern of emotional, romantic, and/or sexual attraction (or lack of attraction) to other gender identities, independent of their own gender identity. Self-identified sexual orientation may not always reflect one's sexual practices, level of sexual activity, or the gender and sexual orientation of one's sexual and romantic partners.
Heterosexual/Straight	Relating to sexual or emotional attraction to persons of the opposite sex or gender.
Sexual diverse	Refers to those individuals whose sexual identity, sexual orientation, or sexual behaviors differ from the presumed majority of the population.
Gay	Relating to sexual or emotional attraction to persons of the same sex or gender.
Men who have sex with men (MSM)/ women who have sex with women (WSW)	Useful in research to classify persons that engage in any same-sex sexual behaviors irrespective of sexual orientation.
Lesbian	A woman who is emotionally or sexually attracted to women. Note: some women may also identify as being gay.
Bisexual	Relating to sexual or emotional attraction to both men and women.
Pansexual	An individual who is emotionally or sexually attracted to any sex or gender.
Asexual	An individual who does not experience sexual attraction toward any individual, regardless of sex or gender identity. However, they may or may not still be emotionally or romantically attracted to others.

Source: Gao, J. L., Kamal, K., & Peebles, K. (2023). Equity for sexual and gender diverse persons in medicine and dermatology. *Dermatologic Clinics, 41*(2), 299-308. https://www.derm.theclinics.com/article/S0733-8635(22)00094-8/abstract

OVERVIEW OF HEALTH DISPARITIES AND INEQUITY

Compared to non-LGBT populations, SGD people experience numerous health disparities with greater risk of mood disorders, depression, and anxiety as well as eating disorders, alcohol and substance abuse, tobacco use, and suicidality, with 41% of transgender individuals having attempted suicide.[3] SGD people also experience higher rates of chronic illnesses and earlier onset of disabilities.[4] Men who have sex with men (MSM) continue to face higher risks of HIV infection and STDs, especially among communities of color. Lesbians are less likely to receive preventative services for cancer. Moreover, transgender individuals are less likely to have health insurance than their heterosexual or LGB counterparts.[5]

Compounding these burdens, SGD individuals face significant barriers in accessing healthcare due to discrimination, mistreatment, refusal of care, and scarcity of competent providers. Twenty-five percent of transgender individuals report denial of health insurance coverage for these services, with 55% of transition-related surgeries and 25% of hormone therapy authorizations denied.[6] Fear of mistreatment and discrimination remains a significant barrier to access for transgender populations, particularly for those of color and those living with disabilities. A startling 33% of transgender individuals report at least one negative healthcare experience related to being transgender whether due to refusal of treatment, verbal harassment, physical and sexual assault, or the burden of having to educate providers to receive culturally humble care. As a result, transgender patients may hesitate to seek care when needed. Further, social determinants such as housing instability, lower educational attainment, and lack of family support especially impact transgender health outcomes.[6]

Healthcare access and outcomes are shaped by innumerable variables with clear sociopolitical intersections. While progress has been made in recent years, particularly in the Supreme Court decisions of Obergefell v Hodges (2015) and Bostock v Clayton County (2020), which legalized marriage equality nationwide and banned employment discrimination on the basis of sexual orientation and gender identity, respectively, structural inequality remains a major barrier. Numerous state-based efforts have been undertaken to dismantle LGBTQ protections with 2022 seeing record legislation introduced across the states, aimed to place limitations on the lives of transgender Americans. These restrictions exist across a variety of domains, including transgender participation in athletics, limitations on discussion of LGBTQ issues and people in school curricula, and prohibitions on the ability of healthcare workers to provide various aspects of gender-affirming care.

DERMATOLOGICAL CARE: SEXUAL DIVERSE POPULATIONS

STIs are covered in detail in Chapters 62 and 63 and will not be specifically discussed in this section with the exception of specific considerations related to HPV.

HPV AND ANAL DYSPLASIA

HPV is the leading cause of anal dysplasia and anal squamous cell carcinoma, which disproportionately affects the SGD community, particularly those who are living with HIV infection. The incidence of anal cancer is increasing and is markedly higher among MSM living with HIV infection compared to HIV seronegative MSM and U.S. men overall.[7] Additionally, MSM have a higher prevalence of anal, penile, and oral HPV infection compared to heterosexual men. Evidence-based screening protocols have yet to be established despite the increasing incidence of anal cancer and clear risk factors for the disease. Reported anal cancer risk factors include a high number of lifetime sexual partners, receptive anal intercourse, other concurrent sexually transmitted infections, cigarette smoking, immunosuppression, and previous history of lower genital tract dysplasia or carcinoma.

Anal cytology and high-resolution anoscopy are the most common screening modalities; until more robust recommendations emerge for anal cancer screening, dermatologists should consider referral for screening based on each patient's unique risk factors, clinical presentation (including perianal warts), and resource availability within their respective institutions. Dermatologists should also encourage HPV vaccination as well as risk mitigation measures based on sexual behaviors.

SKIN CANCER

Sexual diverse men may be at higher risk for skin cancer, likely driven by behavioral risk factors related to variable population-based sun-protection behaviors, including higher rates of indoor tanning, which is estimated to be up to six times more common in gay and bisexual men compared to heterosexual men. Reasons for this disproportionate indoor tanning frequency are unclear though may be influenced by body dissatisfaction and social pressures. Previous national and state-based surveys demonstrate that MSM are up to twice as likely to report a history of nonmelanoma skin cancer compared to heterosexual men.[8]

"POPPERS" DERMATITIS

Volatile alkyl nitrates, or "poppers," serve as recreational inhalants that induce a brief rush of euphoria and sexual arousal. They are used within social contexts as well as sexual intercourse due to their properties of vasodilation and smooth muscle relaxation. The amyl nitrites and fragrances within these substances can cause irritant or allergic contact dermatitis, known as "poppers" dermatitis, which often presents as an eczematous eruption around the nares, perioral region, cheeks, or upper chest.[9] Careful history taking and high clinical suspicion may warrant examination for dermatitis in areas corresponding to pockets or socks where vials of poppers may be carried or on genitals where the chemical may make inadvertent contact.[9] Chronic use may eventually cause perinasal chemical leukoderma, acrocyanosis, and methemoglobinemia.[10]

DERMATOLOGIC CARE: GENDER DIVERSE POPULATIONS

INCLUSIVE PRACTICES

The creation of a safe, inclusive, validating clinic environment is of paramount importance when serving the gender-diverse population. Tenets of such spaces include gender neutrality (eg, gender-neutral language and restroom facilities); inclusive paperwork and forms; inclusive signage and advertisements; and cultural humility training for physicians and staff. Electronic medical records should allow for routine and standardized collection of patient information such as sex assigned at birth, gender identity, pronouns, anatomic inventory, and sexual partners and behaviors. Whether provided verbally or in nonverbal form, patients should be able to opt out of providing any information they are not comfortable disclosing and should also be able to provide free-response answers to these questions in the event that they do not identify with common categories or terms. Furthermore, it is important to recognize that identity information can be fluid and may evolve over time, highlighting the need to periodically confirm this information and to update records accordingly. An approach to gender-inclusive history-taking and language is summarized in **Figure 101-1**.

TRANSMASCULINE DERMATOLOGY

For simplicity and clarity, note that this section will utilize the terminology of "transmasculine" and "transfeminine," recognizing that the binary framework is not ideal when discussing gender-diverse populations.

Many of the medical dermatologic complications seen in transmasculine men are related to complications or side effects of masculinizing hormone therapy (MHT). MHT consists of testosterone preparations, which are most commonly administered via the intramuscular route in the United States. Testosterone therapy produces desired male secondary sex characteristics such as increased facial and body hair growth, subcutaneous fat redistribution, vocal virilization, amenorrhea, breast reduction, and clitoral enlargement.[11] The dermatologic effects of hormonal therapies are summarized in **Table 101-2**.

Acne Vulgaris Cutaneous complications of testosterone therapy include an increased risk of acne vulgaris, which impacts the majority of transgender men; some studies indicate that as many as 9 out of 10 transmasculine patients will develop acne within 4 to 6 months of MHT initiation.[13] Current research suggests that risk factors for acne in the setting of MHT include higher BMI, high serum testosterone levels, smoking, younger age, and a history of acne prior to MHT initiation.[14] Given a heightened risk of mental health disorders, substance use, depression, and suicide among transgender people, these populations may be especially vulnerable to the psychosocial effects of acne such as decreased self-esteem and overall quality of life, poor body image, and social withdrawal.[14] While older dogma surrounding acne in this population suggested that acne severity would peak within a few years of starting MHT and later decrease, some studies and growing anecdotal experience indicate that acne burden may be more persistent.[15] Acne therapy in the setting of MHT often mirrors the approach in cisgender patients with some important considerations. First, spironolactone should be avoided in transmasculine persons on MHT given its interference with testosterone and its intended masculinizing effects. Second, isotretinoin is an effective therapeutic option for acne during MHT, though with several important nuances.

Because of the teratogenicity of isotretinoin, it is important to consider the patient's potential for pregnancy based on individual anatomy and sexual behaviors. All of these dimensions must be evaluated in order to deliver quality, nonstigmatizing, and empowering care. Important to note, testosterone does not provide reliable contraception; pregnancy has indeed occurred in transmasculine individuals on MHT.

In the United States, the Food and Drug Administration (FDA) requires registration of any patient initiating isotretinoin in the Risk Evaluation and Mitigation Strategies program known as iPLEDGE. Recent modifications to iPLEDGE have resulted in welcome changes, namely that the patient categorization model is now based on pregnancy potential alone without the problematic conflation of pregnancy potential with gender. Individuals with anatomy capable of producing a pregnancy must be registered as "patient who can become pregnant." If a patient who can become pregnant engages in sexual behaviors with an individual in a manner that could result in pregnancy, then two forms of acceptable contraception are required. It should be noted that MHT is not a contraindication to any form of hormonal or nonhormonal contraception. Contraception choice should always be determined through shared decision-making with the patient and their gender providers.

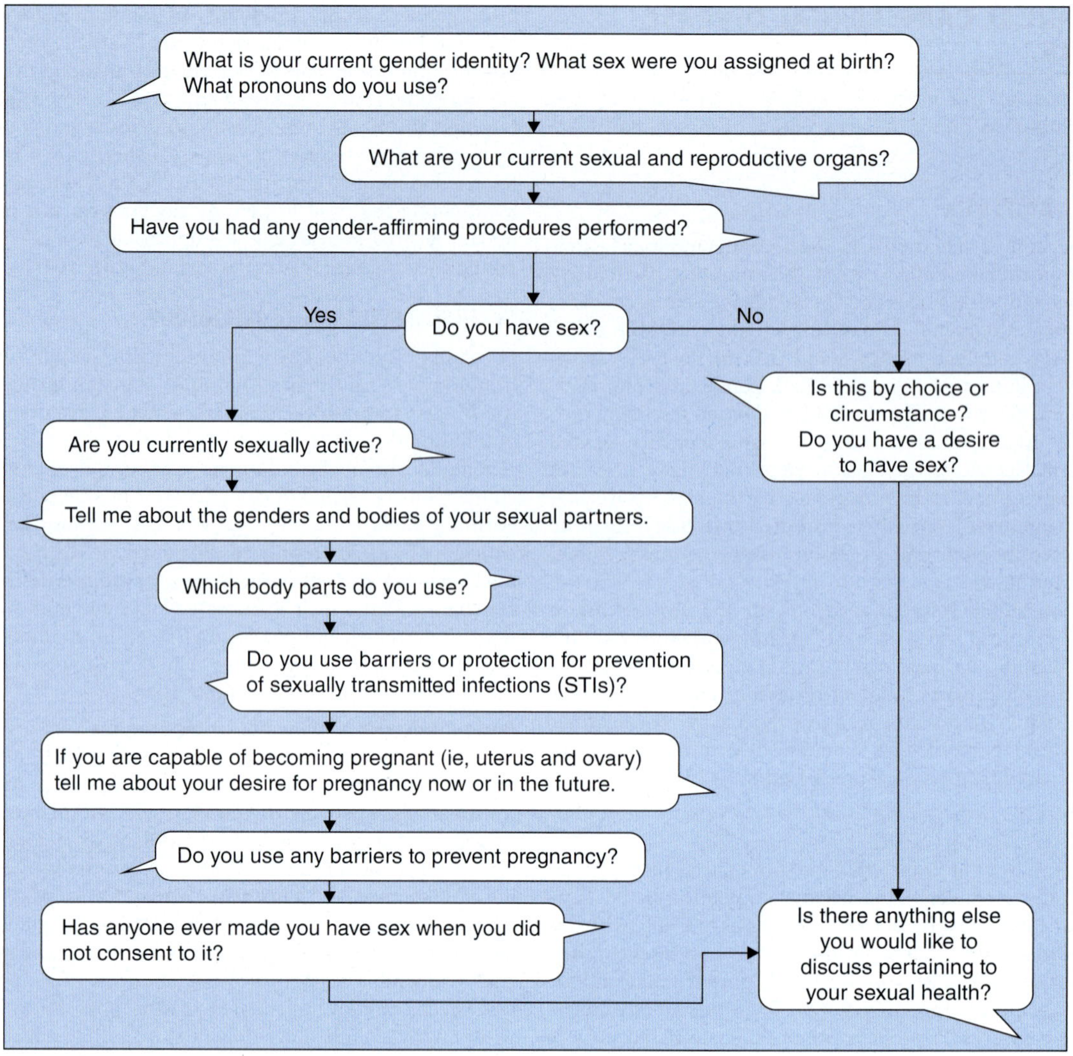

FIGURE 101-1. Sample approach for an inclusive gender and sexual history.

Unfortunately, rigorous evidence-based guidelines for isotretinoin dosing and duration in transmasculine individuals on MHT are lacking. Anecdotal and general consensus among SGD dermatology experts as of this writing support cumulative weight-based dosing for patients undergoing MHT, similar to the approach with cisgender patients. However, low-dose maintenance therapy may be needed in some cases to ensure adequate acne control and durability. Laboratory monitoring in MHT patients does not differ from the standard protocol for cisgender patients. When necessary, pregnancy testing should be offered as a serologic test as an alternative to urine given that some transmasculine patients may experience dysphoria while providing a urine sample.

TABLE 101-2 Dermatologic effects of masculinizing and feminizing hormone therapies[12]

Testosterone therapy
Increased facial and body hair
Increased sebum production of skin
Redistribution of body fat mass
Thinning of hair on the crown and receding hairline
Estrogen and antiandrogen therapy
Decreased facial and body hair
Decreased sebum production of skin
Redistribution of body fat mass
Increased pigmentation due to melanocyte stimulation
Sweat and odor changes

Source: From Hembree WC, Cohen-Kettenis PT, Gooren L, et al. Endocrine treatment of gender-dysphoric/gender-incongruent persons: an Endocrine Society clinical practice guideline. *J Clin Endocrinol Metab.* 2017;102(11):3869-3903.

Androgenetic Alopecia Androgenetic alopecia (AGA) can impact both transmasculine and transfeminine people, requiring an individualized approach to therapy. The prevalence of AGA in transgender populations remains unknown, though research suggests as much as an eightfold frequency of hair loss in the setting of testosterone therapy. Onset of AGA may occur years following testosterone initiation and appears to correlate with the treatment duration, though more research is needed.[16]

While rigorous evidence is lacking and off-label medication use is common, AGA therapy generally mirrors that of cisgender people, though with nuances. Based on the limited literature regarding AGA treatment, first-line approaches include minoxidil 5% foam or solution, as well as finasteride 1 mg oral daily. For transfeminine individuals, spironolactone may be used. Importantly, 5-α-reductase inhibitors (eg, finasteride) do not appear to interfere with serum testosterone levels. However, they may impact secondary sex characteristics depending on the timing of therapy in the context of gender affirmation. Second-line options include oral minoxidil, finasteride solution, oral dutasteride, and a range of procedures such as hairline advancement and hairline transplantation.[16]

Binding Through breast tissue compression, chest binding is a common practice of many transmasculine individuals who desire a flatter chest. As many as 90% of transmasculine individuals chest bind; unfortunately, the majority experience complications. Dermatologic complications that arise include acne, miliaria, dermatitis, scarring, swelling, pruritus, and infection.[17] Potential nondermatologic complications include rib fractures and pneumothorax. Dermatologists should be keen to emphasize the importance of professional and appropriately sized binding garments; removal of garments while sleeping; and limitation of binding to no more than 8 to 12 hours per day. Nonprofessional binding garments, such as elastic bandages, duct tape, and plastic wrap, should be avoided.

TRANSFEMININE DERMATOLOGY

Feminizing hormone therapy (FHT) most commonly consists of an estrogen preparation along with an antiandrogen, such as spironolactone. These interventions help to achieve affirmation through breast development; reduction of body and facial hair; redistribution of subcutaneous fat; and femininizing facial changes.[12] The dermatologic effects of hormonal therapies are summarized in Table 101-2.

Hirsutism and Hair Removal While FHT will often reduce male-pattern hair growth to some degree, it does not result in complete cessation, thus incompletely addressing dysphoria for some transfeminine individuals. As such, hair removal treatments are not only sought after for gender affirmation but also often medically necessary as part of preoperative preparation for procedures such as vaginoplasty to prevent postoperative hair complications. Such complications include trapping of moisture and secretions, infections, pruritus, and dyspareunia. Thorough preoperative treatment is imperative given the challenging nature of postoperative hair removal from the neovaginal cavity or neourethra as these areas are largely inaccessible to laser and electrolysis.

Therapies for undesired facial hair growth include plucking, threading, waxing, or topical eflornithine.[18] Insurance coverage and access to options such as laser hair removal or electrolysis are slowly improving though coverage remains a challenge for the majority of patients. A consequence of frequent shaving and plucking in transfeminine patients, however, is pseudofolliculitis barbae, a chronic inflammatory disorder frequently referred to as "razor bumps." This primarily affects individuals with curled hair, especially transgender women of color, and favors the beard area though also seen at the axillae, pubic area, and legs. Particularly of concern in individuals of color are complications such as postinflammatory hyperpigmentation or keloid scarring, highlighting the importance of early referral to dermatology. A detailed review of this condition can be found in Chapters 45 and 47.

Subcutaneous Injections and "Fillers" Soft tissue augmentation is an increasingly sought-after intervention for many transfeminine patients, favored in part because of its minimally invasive nature. These fillers are subcutaneous injections used for feminization and broader gender affirmation. As previously discussed, access to this care in the medical setting is limited by numerous structural barriers, including availability, lack of competent and knowledgeable providers, cost, inadequate insurance coverage, and fear of discrimination. Consequently, unmet needs prompt many transgender women to seek care outside the medical system through social networks and shadow economies. Such practices are most common among the socioeconomically marginalized, and some studies show disproportionate engagement in sex work among trans women who have used fillers. Despite the safety issues of illicit fillers, many trans women seek these interventions to achieve affirmation that is otherwise unattainable and, more importantly, to "pass" in a manner that conceals their transgender identity. Aligning gender identity with gender expression is amenable to safer social navigation and can also be protective against victimization and violence.

These unregulated fillers are often referred to as "silicone" though they can take many forms, including industrial-grade silicone, paraffin, petroleum jelly, lanolin, beeswax, tire sealant, cement glue, automobile transmission fluid, mineral oil, cooking oil, and saline. These understandably contrast to safer FDA-approved materials such as collagen, hyaluronic acid, calcium hydroxylapatite, poly-L-lactic acid, and polymethylmethacrylate.[19] In fact, the U.S. FDA has warned against large-scale use of injectable silicone for the purposes of aesthetics and body contouring. Though likely underestimated, survey studies show that as many as 10% of trans women have used fillers,[20] with even higher rates in larger urban settings.[21]

Numerous complications can arise from filler injections that can be immediate or significantly delayed. Such complications include pain, erythema, hematoma, lymphedema, anatomic distortion, hypersensitivity reactions, scarring, ulceration, numbness, and foreign-body granulomas. Infectious complications may also occur, including bacterial cellulitis and atypical mycobacterial infection.[22] Rarer complications include sepsis, pneumonitis, silicone emboli, pulmonary embolism, hypercalcemia, and death.[21]

Infectious complications from illicit fillers should be treated with antimicrobials as appropriate. For complications such as granulomas and nodules, surgical excision is considered definitive, which in some cases may be challenging or precluded by the size of the affected area. Medical options mirror those in the broader granuloma therapeutic armamentarium, including intralesional corticosteroids, hydroxychloroquine, minocycline, methotrexate, and biologics (eg, anti-TNF-α).[22] With a gradual reduction in stigma and discrimination toward the transgender community, improved access to affordable affirming care, and heightened awareness of the potential harms of unlicensed filler use, complications of these injections are anticipated to hopefully decrease in frequency. However, as the prevalence of filler use in transgender women remains disproportionately high, clinicians should be familiar with these practices as well as their complications and management in order to provide necessary, empathic, and validating care.

Lichen Sclerosus Lichen sclerosus has been reported in transfeminine patients. Without careful examination and a low threshold for consideration, this diagnosis is easily missed in the context of postoperative anatomy. Lichen sclerosus can augment dysphoria and undermine otherwise welcome results of gender-affirming surgery if symptoms develop and functionality is impaired. Timely management is critical to avoid scarring and development of malignancy. More information can be found in Chapter 37, under inflammatory diseases.

GENDER-AFFIRMING PROCEDURES AND SURGERIES

An overview of gender-affirming surgeries and procedures can be found in **Tables 101-3** and **101-4**.

Preoperative laser hair removal at the donor skin site is usually required to optimize surgical outcomes. Additionally, referral for internal examination may be warranted, especially in patients with histories of external genital warts, as condyloma acuminata[26] and carcinomas[27] of the neovagina have been reported.

Potential complications of gender-affirming surgeries include infection; keloid scarring; squamous cell carcinoma within the neovagina or neo-urethra; and Koebnerization of preexisting dermatologic conditions, such as psoriasis and lichen planus.[28]

Scars Like any surgery, gender-affirmation procedures risk the development of hypertrophic scars and keloids, consequences of fibrous proliferation following dermal injury.[29] Such scarring may be accompanied by pain or pruritus and may undermine a patient's satisfaction with their gender-affirming procedures.[30] These postsurgical scars tend to develop over weeks or months and are often recalcitrant or recurrent, emphasizing the importance of dermatology referral for scar prevention and management as well as continued monitoring months following the procedure. Particularly at risk for keloid development are patients of color, those with a family or personal history of keloids, and those undergoing procedures in high-tension skin areas, especially the chest.[31] Typical treatments for postsurgical keloids apply, including intralesional corticosteroids, radiofrequency devices, and laser therapy.[32] Repeated triamcinolone injections have moderate efficacy in scar reduction; however, a 50% recurrence rate should be noted with this regimen.[33] Treatment-resistant keloids may be addressed with surgical excision, which unfortunately carries a similarly high recurrence rate.[30]

TABLE 101-3 Overview of gender-affirming procedures[23,24]

	Transmasculine	Transfeminine
"Top surgery"/ reconstruction of the chest wall	• Mastectomy • Pectoral implants	• Mammoplasty
"Bottom surgery"/ genital surgery	• Hysterectomy and oophorectomy • Vaginectomy • Metoidioplasty (procedure that utilizes hormonally enlarged clitoral tissue to create a neophallus) • Phalloplasty[a] (procedure to create a neophallus utilizing a skin flap, typically from the forearm • Scrotoplasty	• Labiaplasty • Clitoroplasty • Vaginoplasty • Orchiectomy
Other Procedures	• Minimally invasive procedures[b] (eg, botulinum toxins and soft tissue augmentation) • Facial masculinization surgery	• Minimally invasive procedures[b] (eg, botulinum toxins and soft tissue augmentation) • Facial feminization surgery • Laser hair removal • Body contouring • Thyroid chondroplasty • Speech therapy or vocal cord surgery

[a]Note that tattoo placement on the forearm may complicate tissue flap selection in patients undergoing phalloplasty. Clinicians may consider discussing these concerns with patients who are considering tattoos prior to gender-affirming surgery.

[b]See Table 101-4 for an overview of conventional masculine and feminine facial features.

Sources: From Pan S, Honig SC. Gender-affirming surgery: current concepts. *Curr Urol Rep*. 2018;19(8):62; Benson TA, Boskey ER, Ganor O. The effect of forearm tattoos on flap choice in transmasculine phalloplasty patients. *MDM Policy Pract*. 2020;5(1):2381468320938740.

DIFFERENCES OF SEX DEVELOPMENT AND VARIATION OF SEX CHARACTERISTICS

Differences of sex development (DSD), also known as intersex or variation of sex characteristics, refer to gonads, chromosomes, and genitals that are not typical of binary notions of male and female sex characteristics. Although individuals with DSD have unique health needs, there is a general lack of research and understanding related to their overall health and well-being. Reasons for this have their origins in historic medical pathologization and consequent overmedicalization of individuals with DSD in an effort to "correct" perceived ambiguities without recognizing them as uncommon variations otherwise within the normal spectrum of human anatomy.[34] Recent work has shown significant health disparities, including a higher prevalence of mental health concerns, in the DSD population as well as a paucity of longitudinal research across the lifespan. Additionally, intersectional-focused research is lacking with underrepresentation of individuals of color.[34]

Within the scant available literature, a study characterizing skin concerns in Turner syndrome (TS), reported that the presence of lymphedema, commonly seen in TS, may be associated with underlying cardiac disease and its progression. Further, despite increased numbers of nevi in this population, the incidence of melanoma appears to be markedly reduced, potentially suggesting the presence of a protective factor yet to be described.[35]

TABLE 101-4 Overview of conventional masculine versus feminine facial features[25]

Masculine Features	Feminine Features
• Facial hair or coarse lower facial skin	• Heart-shaped/smaller lower face proportions relative to upper face
• Wider and longer chin/lower face	• Fuller lips
• Wider mouth with thinner lips	• Wider nasolabial angle
• Shorter nasolabial angle	• Prominent cheek structures
• Flat eyebrows with prominent brow structure above the eyes	• Arching eyebrows with smoother forehead
• Wider forehead with higher hairline	• Smaller forehead with lower hairline

Source: From MacGregor JL, Chang YC. Minimally invasive procedures for gender affirmation. *Dermatol Clin*. 2020;38(2):249-260.

CONCLUSION

This chapter intends to provide a brief overview of SGD healthcare with an emphasis on dermatologic concerns for these diverse populations. While it is important to understand that SGD individuals have unique needs, it is similarly critical to recognize that they are not a homogeneous population. SGD patient care should be approached within the framework of cultural humility and empathy with a commitment to shared decision-making and patient autonomy. Social determinants of health continue to shape the lives and outcomes of SGD people—the intersections of race and ethnicity with sexual orientation and gender identity play a crucial role, meriting further research. We hope the information presented in this chapter will inspire further exploration of these topics and greater confidence when providing care for patients of all identities.

REFERENCES

1. Herman J, Flores A, O'Neill K. *How Many Adults and Youth Identify as Transgender in the United States?* Los Angeles, CA: The Williams Institute, UCLA; 2022. https://williamsinstitute.law.ucla.edu/wp-content/uploads/Trans-Pop-Update-Jun-2022.pdf.
2. de Vries KM. Transgender people of color at the center: conceptualizing a new intersectional model. *Ethnicities*. 2015;15(1):3-27.
3. Haas A, Rodgers P, Herman J. *Suicide Attempts among Transgender and Gender Non-Conforming Adults*. American Foundation for Suicide Prevention; The Williams Institute, UCLA; 2014. https://queeramnesty.ch/docs/AFSP-Williams-Suicide-Report-Final.pdf.
4. Lick DJ, Durso LE, Johnson KL. Minority stress and physical health among sexual minorities. *Perspect Psychol Sci*. 2013;8(5):521-548.
5. Lesbian, Gay, Bisexual, and Transgender Health | Healthy People 2020. https://www.healthypeople.gov/2020/topics-objectives/topic/lesbian-gay-bisexual-and-transgender-health. Accessed August 28, 2022.
6. James S, Herman J, Rankin S, Keisling M, Mottet L, Anafi M. The Report of the 2015 U.S. Transgender Survey. Published online 2016. https://transequality.org/sites/default/files/docs/usts/USTS-Full-Report-Dec17.pdf. Accessed July 14, 2022.
7. Goldstone S, Palefsky JM, Giuliano AR, et al. Prevalence of and risk factors for human papillomavirus (HPV) infection among HIV-seronegative men who have sex with men. *J Infect Dis*. 2011;203(1):66-74.
8. Mansh M, Katz KA, Linos E, Chren MM, Arron S. Association of skin cancer and indoor tanning in sexual minority men and women. *JAMA Dermatol*. 2015;151(12):1308-1316.
9. Schauber J, Herzinger T. "Poppers" dermatitis. *Clin Exp Dermatol*. 2012;37(5):587-588.
10. Hunter L, Gordge L, Dargan PI, Wood DM. Methaemoglobinaemia associated with the use of cocaine and volatile nitrites as recreational drugs: a review. *Br J Clin Pharmacol*. 2011;72(1):18-26.
11. Hembree WC, Cohen-Kettenis PT, Gooren L, et al. Endocrine treatment of gender-dysphoric/gender-incongruent persons: an Endocrine Society clinical practice guideline. *J Clin Endocrinol Metab*. 2017;102(11):3869-3903.
12. Hembree WC, Cohen-Kettenis PT, Gooren L, et al. Endocrine Treatment of gender-dysphoric/gender-incongruent persons: an Endocrine Society clinical practice guideline. *J Clin Endocrinol Metab*. 2017;102(11):3869-3903.
13. Motosko CC, Zakhem GA, Pomeranz MK, Hazen A. Acne: a side-effect of masculinizing hormonal therapy in transgender patients. *Br J Dermatol*. 2019;180(1):26-30.
14. Thoreson N, Park JA, Grasso C, et al. Incidence and factors associated with acne among transgender patients receiving masculinizing hormone therapy. *JAMA Dermatology*. 2021;157(3):290-295.

15. Wierckx K, Van de Peer F, Verhaeghe E, et al. Short- and long-term clinical skin effects of testosterone treatment in trans men. *J Sex Med.* 2014;11(1):222-229.
16. Gao JL, Streed CG, Thompson J, Dommasch ED, Peebles JK. Androgenetic alopecia in transgender and gender diverse populations: a review of therapeutics. *J Am Acad Dermatol.* 2023;89(4):774-783.
17. Peitzmeier S, Gardner I, Weinand J, Corbet A, Acevedo K. Health impact of chest binding among transgender adults: a community-engaged, cross-sectional study. *Cult Health Sex.* 2017;19(1):64-75.
18. Xia Y, Cho S, Howard RS, Maggio KL. Topical eflornithine hydrochloride improves the effectiveness of standard laser hair removal for treating pseudofolliculitis barbae: a randomized, double-blinded, placebo-controlled trial. *J Am Acad Dermatology.* 2012;67(4):694-699.
19. Health C for D and R. FDA-approved dermal fillers. FDA. https://www.fda.gov/medical-devices/aesthetic-cosmetic-devices/fda-approved-dermal-fillers. Accessed January 18, 2023.
20. Sergi FD, Wilson EC. Filler use among trans women: correlates of feminizing subcutaneous injections and their health consequences. *Transgender Health.* 2021;6(2):82-90.
21. Wilson E, Rapues J, Jin H, Raymond HF. The use and correlates of illicit silicone or "fillers" in a population-based sample of transwomen, San Francisco, 2013. *J Sex Med.* 2014;11(7):1717-1724.
22. Paul S, Goyal A, Duncan LM, Smith GP. Granulomatous reaction to liquid injectable silicone for gluteal enhancement: review of management options and success of doxycycline. *Dermatol Ther.* 2015;28(2):98-101.
23. Pan S, Honig SC. Gender-affirming surgery: current concepts. *Curr Urol Rep.* 2018;19(8):62.
24. Benson TA, Boskey ER, Ganor O. The effect of forearm tattoos on flap choice in transmasculine phalloplasty patients. *MDM Policy Pract.* 2020;5(1):2381468320938740.
25. MacGregor JL, Chang YC. Minimally invasive procedures for gender affirmation. *Dermatol Clin.* 2020;38(2):249-260.
26. Liguori G, Trombetta C, Bucci S, et al. Condylomata acuminata of the neovagina in a HIV-seropositive male-to-female transsexual. *Urol Int.* 2004;73(1):87-88.
27. Fernandes HM, Manolitsas TP, Jobling TW. Carcinoma of the neovagina after male-to-female reassignment. *J Low Genit Tract Dis.* 2014;18(2):E43-45.
28. Coulton A, Devkota M. P44: dermatological issues in the transgender population: a review of the literature. *Brit J Dermatol.* 2021;185(S1):45-46.
29. Ogawa R. Keloid and hypertrophic scars are the result of chronic inflammation in the reticular dermis. *Int J Mol Sci.* 2017;18(3):606.
30. Chike-Obi CJ, Cole PD, Brissett AE. Keloids: pathogenesis, clinical features, and management. *Semin Plast Surg.* 2009;23(3):178-184.
31. Hage JJ, van Kesteren PJ. Chest-wall contouring in female-to-male transsexuals: basic considerations and review of the literature. *Plast Reconstr Surg.* 1995;96(2):386-391.
32. Ginsberg BA. Dermatologic care of the transgender patient. *Int J Womens Dermatol.* 2016;3(1):65-67.
33. Trisliana Perdanasari A, Torresetti M, Grassetti L, et al. Intralesional injection treatment of hypertrophic scars and keloids: a systematic review regarding outcomes. *Burns Trauma.* 2015;3:14.
34. Rosenwohl-Mack A, Tamar-Mattis S, Baratz AB, et al. A national study on the physical and mental health of intersex adults in the U.S. *PLoS One.* 2020;15(10):e0240088.
35. Lowenstein EJ, Kim KH, Glick SA. Turner's syndrome in dermatology. *J Am Acad Dermatol.* 2004;50(5):767-776.

CHAPTER 102 Pregnancy

Marita Yaghi
Daniel Butler
Divya Sharma
Kelly KyungHwa Park
Jenny E. Murase

KEY POINTS

- Striae gravidarum, keloids, melasma, and intrahepatic cholestasis of pregnancy have a predilection for pregnant women of color.
- Seventy percent of the world's patients with human immunodeficiency virus/acquired immunodeficiency virus live in sub-Saharan Africa and African women of childbearing age have a heightened susceptibility for acquiring HIV.
- Mycosis fungoides (MF), sarcoidosis, scleroderma, and lupus erythematosus (SLE) are more aggressive and confer a poorer prognosis when it comes to pregnancy outcomes in pregnant women of color.
- It is important that patients understand that the risks associated with MF, sarcoidosis, scleroderma, or SLE during pregnancy are largely due to poorly controlled disease.
- It is important to stress contraception to patients whose MF, sarcoidosis, scleroderma, or SLE is currently active or has been in remission for less than 6 months. Planning a pregnancy 6 months after disease control can help ensure the safety of the mother and child.

INTRODUCTION

Pregnant women of color constitute a unique population. Maternal morbidity and mortality disproportionately affect women of color as compared to other racial groups, a phenomenon that has been linked to systemic racism.[1,2] It is important to note that there are dermatologic conditions that are seen exclusively in this group. These conditions could be primary cutaneous conditions or skin manifestations of conditions that are more prevalent in populations with skin of color. Awareness of these conditions are essential to render proper diagnosis and institute proper therapeutic plans. Furthermore, there are special considerations when selecting and starting therapies for pregnant women of color who have common dermatologic conditions.

DERMATOLOGIC CONDITIONS IN PREGNANCY: A FOCUS ON WOMEN OF COLOR

CONNECTIVE TISSUE CHANGES

Striae Gravidarum

Epidemiology, Presentation, and Diagnosis Striae gravidarum (SG) are striae distensae (SD), or stretch marks, that occur during pregnancy. SG are the most common connective tissue change observed during gestation with an overall incidence between 50% and 88%.[3-7] A risk factor for SG is race/ethnicity, specifically individuals of African American, Hispanic, East Asian, and South Asian descent.[8] The specific incidence of SG in different ethnic groups has been found to be 55% in Afro-Caribbean women, 69% in Chinese women, and 85% in Malay and Indian women.[9,10] Family history of striae, younger maternal age, maternal weight gain, higher pre-pregnancy body mass index, premature birth, and newborn size are also risk factors.[11-13]

SG can appear in primigravidas or alternately develop for the first time in subsequent pregnancies in any trimester, although they most commonly appear in the second and third trimesters. SG occurs most often on the abdomen and breasts. Initially, they appear as striae rubra and become longer, wider, and raised over time. They then become striae alba, or mature striae, which are wrinkled, white, and atrophic [**Figure 102-1**]. SG can be associated with pruritis, burning, and discomfort. SD in darker skin types are often referred to as striae nigrae.[14] A mechanobiologic process is likely to activate or inhibit melanogenesis in this population, but there is no evidence of any topical preparation that would prevent SG.[15] Topical vitamin A therapy with tretinoin (retinoic acid) 0.1% improves SG, but no study has been done exclusively in skin of color.[16] Combined therapies may improve striae alba in skin types I to V.[17]

Treatment The treatment of SG is generally performed following delivery and has significantly improved in recent years with advances made through many techniques including lasers and microneedling.[13] Fractional photothermolysis using the erbium-doped 1550-nm fractional laser is one such laser, but it comes with the risk of pigmentary changes.[18] As melanin does not absorb the 1550-nm wavelength, the use of this laser in skin of color has significantly less risk of postinflammatory

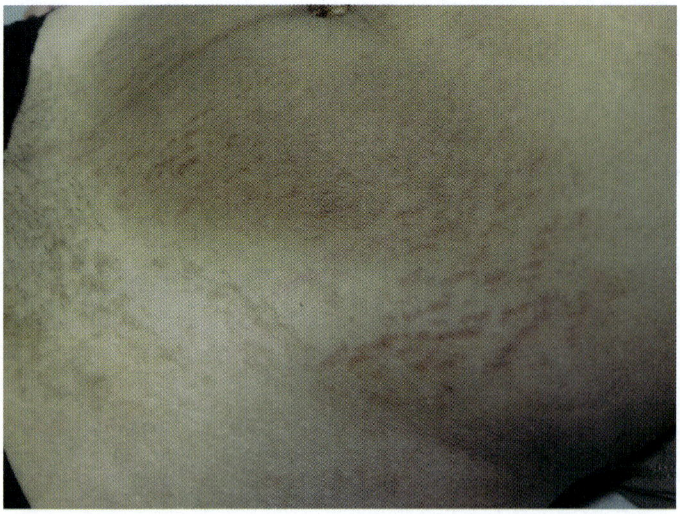

FIGURE 102-1. Stretch marks on an East Indian woman postpartum after her first pregnancy. In this patient, both striae rubra and evolving striae alba are present.

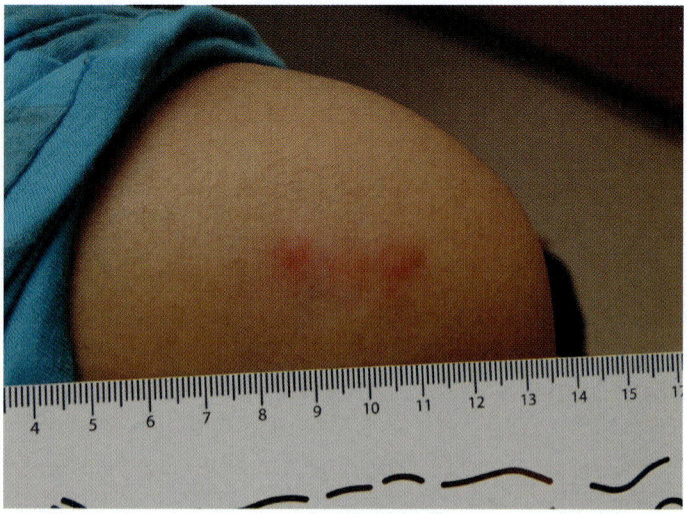

FIGURE 102-2. Keloid on the shoulder of an East Indian female that became inflamed during pregnancy, requiring intralesional triamcinolone injections.

pigmentation than other lasers.[18] The laser has been used in striae (both immature and mature) with graded improvement and better results in white rather than red striae.[19] An overview of various lasers studied for the treatment of SG and their indication in SOC can be found in **Table 102-1**. For skin types IV to VI, the use of preoperative treatment such as hydroquinone may help in preventing or ameliorating pigmentary side effects.[19-21]

Microneedling has been shown to be effective in treating SD in darker skin types.[22] A disk microneedle therapy system was found to improve SD in Koreans with type III and IV skin with both striae rubra and stria alba.[23] Microneedling was also found to be as effective as both fractional CO_2 laser therapy and fractional nonablative laser therapy on striae alba.[24-26]

TABLE 102-1 An overview of lasers for striae gravidarum in skin of color

Laser type	Indication	Notes
2940-nm Er:YAG	Striae alba (III-IV)	
1540-nm fractional nonablative erbium:glass	Striae rubra and alba (ST II-IV)	Postinflammatory hyperpigmentation
1550-nm erbium-doped nonablative fractional	Striae distensae (ST VI-VI)	Self-limited side effects
1064-nm Nd:YAG long-pulsed	Striae distensae (ST II-IV)	
1064-nm fractional picosecond	Stria alba (ST IV-V)	
585-nm ablative CO_2 fractional (short-pulsed) laser	Striae distensae	Lack of improvement (ST IV) Hyperpigmentation (ST VI) Not recommended for use unless with great caution
313, 360, and 420 nm nbUVB and UVA1	Striae alba (ST II-IV)	For short-term repigmentation
308-nm excimer	Striae alba	Pigment splaying noted Less maintenance required for ST III-IV
Broadband visible light pulsed light flashlamp	Striae distensae (Hispanic with ST III-IV)	
TriPollar radiofrequency	Striae distensae (ST VI-V)	
Intradermal radiofrequency combined with autologous PRP	Striae distensae (Asian with ST IV)	

Abbreviations: Er:YAG, erbium-yttrium-aluminum-garnet; nbUVB, narrowband ultraviolet B; Nd:YAG: neodymium-doped yttrium-aluminum-garnet; PRP, platelet-rich plasma; ST, skin type; UVA1, ultraviolet A1.

Additionally, microneedling was found to be more effective than microdermabrasion with sonophoresis (combination of ultrasound and topical therapy) when treating SD in female patients with skin types III and IV.[27]

Hypertrophic Scars and Keloids Hypertrophic scars and keloids (for a more in-depth discussion of keloids, see Chapter 33) are the result of abnormal wound healing and are common in African Americans, Hispanics, and Asians, along with those with a family history.[28] Formation occurs in areas of high melanocyte concentration, including the chest, shoulder [**Figure 102-2**], upper back, neck, and earlobes.[29] Keloid formation is a concern in surgical sites, particularly in cesarean sections. In a prospective study of 429 cesarean sections, keloids occurred in 1.6% of Hispanics, 5.2% of Asians, and 7.1% of African Americans, and those with keloid formation were found to have a higher risk of intraabdominal adhesions.[30]

There is no way to prevent hypertrophic scars or keloids; however, there are ways to reduce risk of occurrence. In pregnancy-related surgery, surgical technique should be atraumatic and precise with hemostasis and skin edge eversion closure. Proper wound care and debridement and infection prevention should be practiced. Cesarean sections using absorbable subcuticular stitch closure have better cosmetic results with reduced pain than surgical staples.[31] Bilayered closures with running polyglactin 910 sutures left in place have better appearance and less erythema.

Intralesional corticosteroids are often first-line therapy. Simple excision and primary closure when caused by complicated wounds or delayed closure for hypertrophic scars is an option. However, complete surgical resection for keloids as monotherapy is associated with a high recurrence rate. Additionally, pulsed dye laser therapy along with intralesional triamcinolone injection can help improve the appearance of cesarean-section scars following surgical removal.[32] Bleomycin has also shown to be effective in the treatment of hypertrophic scars and keloids; however, it was found to be teratogenic in rats and should be avoided when pregnant.[33,34] There is limited data regarding the safety of intralesional bleomycin when breastfeeding. Thus, it is recommended to be avoided if possible when nursing.[34] For treatment of keloids, refer to Chapter 33.

PIGMENTARY CHANGES

Hyperpigmentation, which is common in pregnancy, is seen in up to 90% of women and may be related to pregnancy hormones.[35] Commonly, it presents as a mild generalized hyperpigmentation with darkening of normally pigmented areas, such as the areola, genital skin, nipples, axillae, and inner thighs, and at time, nevi, freckles, and scars. Linea alba can darken to become linea nigra [**Figure 102-3**].[36]

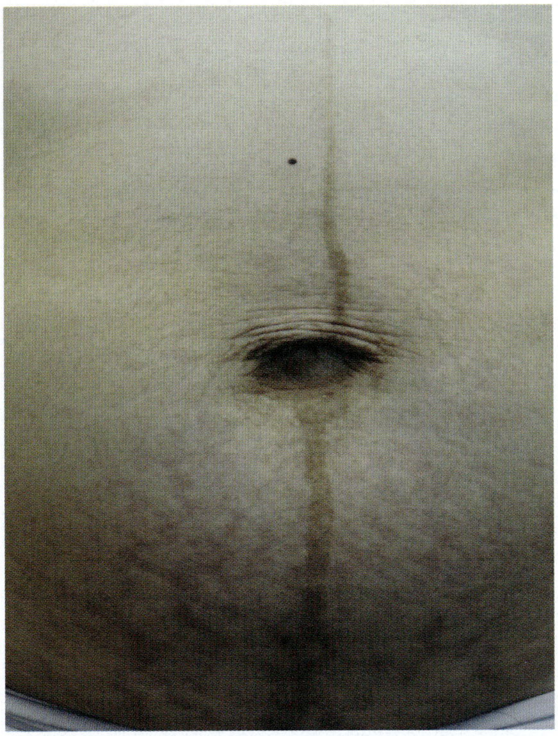

FIGURE 102-3. Linea nigra in a Chinese female that began to develop in the second trimester. Linea nigra appears in three quarters of pregnancies and is due to the increased melanocyte-stimulating hormone made by the placenta, which also results in melasma and darkening of the nipples.

Melasma (chloasma), an acquired hyperpigmentation of the face, is commonly seen in women with skin of color, particularly those of African American, Hispanic, and Asian ancestry. The gestational type may resolve in the postpartum period but is worsened by both visible and ultraviolet light. It may recur with another pregnancy or the use of the use of oral contraceptives. Epidermal melasma, as opposed to dermal melasma, is treatable.

Treatment options include counseling regarding sun protection and the use of broad-spectrum sunscreens. (For treatment of melasma, see Chapter 56.)

Persistent melasma may be treated after delivery with topical agents such as hydroquinone, tretinoin, or azelaic acid. Topical use of hydroquinone has shown high levels of systemic absorption and thus should be avoided in pregnancy due to unknown risks to the fetus.[37-40] Glycolic acid peels are safe in patients with darker skin types because they are generally classified as superficial chemical peels. The use of glycolic acid peels in pregnancy is also generally considered safe due to negligible dermal penetration.[41] Intense pulsed light treatment combined with hydroquinone was studied in skin types III and IV with noticeable improvement; however, due to a lack of safety data, intense pulsed light treatment is not indicated for cosmetic procedures during pregnancy.[42] A fractional 1064-nm picosecond laser has been shown to improve the severity of melasma in patients with skin types III and IV.[43] Fractional thermolysis has been used in patients with skin types III to V with improvement and limited postinflammatory hyperpigmentation. However, those with type V skin did not respond to therapy. With any treatment, the risk in darker skin types of postinflammatory hyperpigmentation is high; therefore, patients should be adequately counseled. Oral tranexamic acid has also been shown to be efficacious in treating melasma in Asian skin, although its safety profile in pregnancy has not been thoroughly studied.[44] Additionally, due to the increased risk of thromboembolism while pregnant, pregnancy should be considered an exclusion criterion for the use of tranexamic acid when treating melasma.[44] The use of tranexamic acid while breastfeeding has not been found to result in adverse outcomes to infants; however, it has been detected in breast milk and thus is recommended to be avoided.[45-47]

DERMATOSES OF PREGNANCY

Certain skin diseases appear only in pregnant women and thus are known as the dermatoses of pregnancy. The specific dermatoses of pregnancy have been classified into four entities: polymorphic eruption of pregnancy (PEP, previously known as pruritic urticarial papules and plaques of pregnancy [PUPPP]), atopic eruption of pregnancy (AEP), pemphigoid gestationis formally known as herpes gestationis (PG), and intrahepatic cholestasis of pregnancy (ICP). Pustular psoriasis of pregnancy (PPP) is a fifth possible dermatosis of pregnancy. ICP is more common in women of color, with greater incidences found in Asian Indian and Pakistani populations (1.2-1.5%) as well as Hispanic populations (5.6%).[48,49] While PEP is found less commonly in women of color, PG [**Figure 102-4**] and AEP do not have a specific predilection for women with skin of color.[50] It is important for the clinician to counsel patients on the safety of therapy when treating these conditions in pregnancy.

POLYMORPHIC ERUPTION OF PREGNANCY

PEP is unique to pregnancy and typically appears in the third trimester of primigravid women [**Figure 102-5**]. When examining the prevalence of dermatoses of pregnancy in East Indian populations, PEP was the most common, representing close to 65% of cases.[51] Its incidence has been estimated to be 1 in 200 pregnancies (0.5%) but largely varies depending on the population.[52] A large Israeli study found a rate of 0.03% while a similar study in India found a higher rate of PEP of 2.3%.[51,53] While the condition is more frequently seen in non-Hispanic White females, it is also seen in other populations including those of Asian descent as well

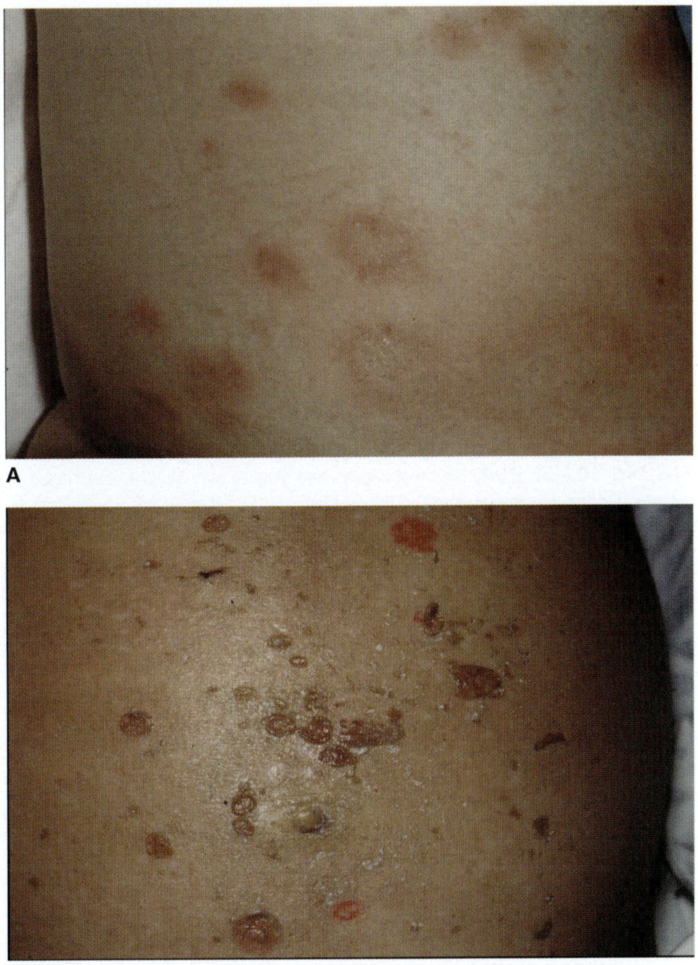

A

B

FIGURE 102-4. **(A)** Pemphigoid gestationis (PG) in pregnant African American female. **(B)** PG was originally called "herpes gestationis" because of the blistering appearance shown here, although it is not associated with the herpes virus.

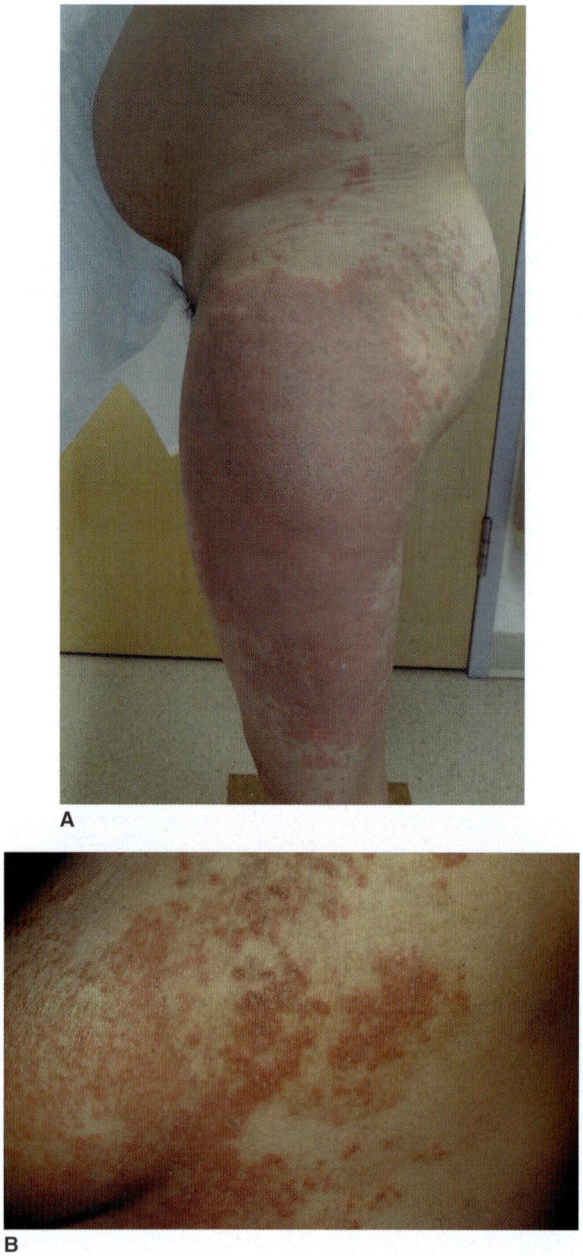

FIGURE 102-5. Pruritic urticarial papules and plaques of pregnancy, also known as polymorphic eruption of pregnancy, on the **(A)** legs and **(B)** chest in a Taiwanese female. This often begins on the abdomen and subsequently can spread to the thighs, legs, feet, arms, chest, and neck.

as African and Afro-Caribbean descent.[54] Studies show that the condition is rarely associated with fetal or maternal complications and usually regresses 1 week postpartum.[55,56]

PEP is characterized by an acute eruption of pruritic papules coalescing into plaques usually over the distended gravid abdomen, classically sparing the palms, soles, face, mucosae, and the umbilicus allowing the differential diagnosis with pemphigoid gestationis. PEP is additionally associated with striae gravidarum.[57] Treatment is mainly symptomatic. The use of emollients and low-potency topical corticosteroids are usually enough to cause remission. For more severe cases, antihistamines and higher potency topical steroids may be needed. (Refer to section "Medication management in pregnancy.") PEP usually resolves shortly postpartum.

ATOPIC ERUPTION OF PREGNANCY

AEP is defined as either an exacerbation *or* the first occurrence of eczematous manifestations during pregnancy in atopic individuals. Eighty percent of patients fall in the latter category. AEP is the most common dermatoses of pregnancy and manifests before the third trimester in 75% of patients.[58,59] AEP does not appear to have a racial or ethnic predilection.

Classic "eczematous" lesions, mainly scattered small erythematous papules, on the face, neck, and flexural extremities constitute the most common presentation alongside other signs of atopy.[60] The exclusion of other dermatosis of pregnancy, through the lack of association with striae and normal bile levels, precedes diagnosis. It is also important to rule out other general pruritic dermatoses, such as drug eruptions.

There are no associated fetal risks and AEP usually resolves after delivery. Treatment is mainly symptomatic with the use of emollients and topical steroids.

PEMPHIGOID GESTATIONIS

PG is a rare autoimmune pregnancy-associated bullous disease. Its incidence has been estimated between 1 in 70,000 and 1 in 50,000 pregnancies and is associated with the development of Graves disease.[61-63] No association with race or ethnicity has been described. PG may develop during any trimester and usually recurs earlier in every subsequent pregnancy. Pruritic, painful, disfiguring, polymorphous papulovesicular, or larger bullous eruptions on the gravid abdomen, mostly confined to the umbilicus, chest, back, and on the distal extremities, including the palms and soles, are pathognomonic of PG.[64] The face and mucosal surfaces are usually spared, but involvement has been described.[65] Nikolsky sign I and II may be positive.[64]

Treatment is highly challenging. Oral corticosteroids are the therapeutic mainstay during pregnancy and IVIG has proven efficacious in refractory cases. Options for the postpartum period include methotrexate, cyclosporine, and azathioprine among others.[64] PG self-resolves after delivery, with rare residual hyperpigmentation and without scarring, but affects up to 5% of neonates born to affected mothers.[65]

Importantly, PG has been rarely associated with trophoblastic tumors (ie, hydatidiform mole, choriocarcinoma) and its manifestation outside the pregnancy and immediate postpartum period warrants additional investigation.[63,66,67]

INTRAHEPATIC CHOLESTASIS OF PREGNANCY

This condition has been referred to by a variety of names including prurigo gravidarum, jaundice of pregnancy, and obstetric cholestasis. It is caused by genetic and hormonal effects on the gallbladder, which results in spillage of bile from the liver into the bloodstream. Patients present with significant pruritus and evidence of whole-body excoriation.

While this condition is seen across all population groups, an increased incidence has been appreciated in women with skin of color from several locales. Initially, the Indigenous people of South America were identified to have an increased incidence of the condition during pregnancy, but subsequent studies have extended that demographic to both North and South American populations.[68,69] There appears to be a genetic predisposition for these populations.[69] There is also increased prevalence in other populations including women of Indian and Pakistani descent.[70]

Pruritus during the third trimester is the most common presenting symptom, with resultant subtle skin excoriations or even frank prurigo nodularis. Symptoms usually worsen as the pregnancy progresses. Clinical jaundice is rare, affecting approximately 10% to 15% of pregnant women with ICP.[71] Assessment of jaundice can be difficult in skin of color patients. Ideal locations to assess color changes associated with jaundice are the buccal mucosa and the sclera of the eyes. Additionally, patients should be screened with questions regarding recent urine color changes or feelings of depression, both of which can indicate elevated bilirubin levels in the blood. The optimal screening test is serum bile acids.

Systemic dexamethasone and ursodeoxycholic acid are first-line treatment for ICP. (Refer to section "Medication management in pregnancy.")

PUSTULAR PSORIASIS OF PREGNANCY

PPP is a rare autoimmune inflammatory dermatosis that usually manifests as of the second trimester of pregnancy. Its incidence remains uncharacterized as the entity has only been described in a number of case reports.[72]

PPP classically manifests with sterile pustules over annular erythematous patches, beginning in the intertriginous areas and spreading radially, sparing the face, palms, and soles.[73-75] Fever, chills, malaise, and gastrointestinal symptoms may occur, and laboratory findings include leukocytosis with marked neutrophilia, increased erythrocyte sedimentation rate, and electrolyte derangements.[73,75-77] PPP can be life-threatening with a reported case of maternal severe hypocalcemia leading to tetany, delirium, and convulsions and another of maternal death.[78,79] PPP also jeopardized fetal health and the association is incremental with disease severity.[80]

Early induction of labor remains first-line treatment.[80] Alternatives include systemic corticosteroids. A treatment algorithm has been suggested by Robinson et al for a similar disease, generalized pustular psoriasis, and included cyclosporine, infliximab, topical corticosteroids, and topical calcipotriene as the first-line treatment options, in addition to systemic prednisone.[81] However, apart from corticosteroids, most of these medications are not safe for use during pregnancy.[82] PPP usually dramatically resolves after delivery but may recur in subsequent pregnancies.[80]

CONNECTIVE TISSUE DISEASE AND SARCOIDOSIS: SPECIAL CONSIDERATIONS IN WOMEN WITH SKIN OF COLOR

SYSTEMIC LUPUS ERYTHEMATOSUS

Systemic lupus erythematosus is a disease that typically presents in female patients during their fourth decade of life. It more commonly occurs in African Americans, African Caribbeans, and Asians, than in non-Hispanic Whites and tends to present earlier in these populations.[83,84] As disease onset occurs during the childbearing years, lupus affects regularly in pregnant females. Approximately 45,000 women with lupus become pregnant each year in the United States alone.[85]

The literature supports a two- to threefold increase in disease flares when patients are pregnant. The most common manifestation, which occurs in 25% to 90% of patients, is dermatologic, followed by lupus nephritis in up to 75% of patients.[86,87] The recognition of a lupus flare during pregnancy may be difficult because the signs and symptoms may mimic those of normal pregnancy.[88] Skin of color patients affected by the discoid lupus erythematosus subtype are more likely to experience postinflammatory hyperpigmentation than their non-Hispanic White counterparts.[89] Additionally, healthcare providers report significantly less confidence in diagnosing cutaneous manifestations of lupus in skin of color compared to lighter skin.[90] Special attention on pigmentation changes, a sign of erythema in darker pigmented skin, may aid in the identification of cutaneous lupus exacerbations.

While skin manifestations can be initial indicators of active disease, it is underlying kidney disease that carries significant comorbid consequence and requires prompt response. It is essential that nephritis be identified and properly evaluated. Differentiating preeclampsia from lupus nephritis can be difficult due to the overlap of hypertension, proteinuria, and hematuria in both disorders. This differentiation is paramount due to differences in treatment: eclampsia required delivery, and lupus exacerbation can be managed pharmacologically.[85] Similarly to nonpregnant populations, racial differences in pregnancy revealed a higher prevalence of adverse outcomes in African American and Hispanic women with lupus, including hypertensive disorders, intrauterine growth retardation, or cesarean deliveries.[87,91] Both biological factors and low household income play a role in the observed outcome differences, which highlight the impact of inequity in access to healthcare.[91] As kidney disease is frequently responsible for fetal and maternal complications in lupus pregnancies, it is recommended that all clinicians carefully monitor for these serious complications. In addition, maternal anti-SSA/Ro antibodies are associated with congenital heart block and hydroxychloroquine can reduce the risk of fetal cardiac disease.[92,93]

SCLERODERMA

Scleroderma is a rare multisystem connective tissue disease characterized by skin fibrosis and vasculopathy with a predilection for females.[94] In addition, the scleroderma literature suggests a significant difference between Black and White patients in regard to increased incidence and severity of disease. A 20-year study revealed that African American females from the ages of 15 to 24 have the greatest incidence.[95] Additionally, it was found that women of color are more likely to develop multiorgan disease, be diagnosed at a younger age, have a higher incidence of inflammatory features, and have worse age-adjusted prognosis.[96] In fact, the survival rate of African American patients with scleroderma is half that of non-African American patients. The differences in survival are attenuated following adjustment for socioeconomic covariates, highlighting once again the detrimental impact of health inequities.[97]

Knowledge about differential disease presentations across various populations is essential for timely diagnosis and management. Data suggest that African American patients are more likely to present with diffuse skin involvement as compared to their White or Asian counterparts.[98] Conversely, both African American and Asian patients are more likely to suffer from underlying pulmonary and vascular involvement,[98] putting in focus the higher need for monitoring noncutaneous involvement in these populations, given the higher risk on both the mother and the fetus associated with systemic disease.[99] Interestingly, data have shown a high prevalence of Scl-70 antibody positivity in South Asian population with pulmonary involvement, suggesting the highly efficient use of this biomarker in disease classification in this specific group.[100]

Although active, multiorgan disease can be harmful during pregnancy due to placental vascular abnormalities, poor outcomes can be prevented with adequate disease control.[101] The first step is screening the patient during early pregnancy. It is proposed that clinicians, particularly dermatologists, ask general screening questions regarding common rheumatologic disease manifestations including sun sensitivity, Raynaud phenomenon, and localized skin changes.[102] One study revealed that clinicians are 30% more likely to find undiagnosed rheumatic diseases if these simple screening questions are performed during the first trimester.[103]

Data on disease activity in pregnancy are encouraging, as pregnancy has not been associated with exacerbation, as seen with other autoimmune spectrum conditions.[104] However, good disease control still needs to be prioritized in these women prior to conception, to avoid harmful mother or fetal effects.

SJÖGREN SYNDROME

Sjögren syndrome (SS) is a systemic autoimmune disease that most commonly affects middle-aged women.[105] SS presents with oral and/or ocular dryness, either as primary SS or in association with an underlying connective tissue disease, most frequently systemic lupus erythematosus or rheumatoid arthritis.[106,107]

The majority of SS patients are women, with an increased female-to-male ratio in South American populations.[108] The latter also demonstrates a higher rate of positivity of antinuclear antibodies and rheumatoid factor.[108] On the other hand, African American patients suffer from the highest degree of disease severity as compared to White, Asian, or Hispanic patients.[109]

SS is likely to worsen during pregnancy, and mutually affect pregnancy outcomes. Several studies have reported an increased rate of spontaneous abortion and fetal loss associated with SS, as well as adverse fetal outcomes, such as preterm deliveries, lower neonatal birth weight, or fetal growth restriction.[110] Most importantly, infant congenital heart block is one of the most dreaded complications of SS in pregnant women with anti-SS-A positive disease.[111,112] Hence, early diagnosis and treatment are of utmost importance.[113] Oral steroids are the mainstay of therapy (refer to section "Medication management in pregnancy").

DERMATOMYOSITIS

Dermatomyositis (DM) is an acquired systemic inflammatory disease that presents with cutaneous manifestations and proximal muscle myopathy. It typically manifests in White females and may be associated with concomitant malignancy.[114,115]

Disease presentation varies across races. Cutaneous calcinosis is more prevalent in African American patients and some data suggest that DM manifests at an earlier age in this population.[114,116] While DM is associated with a wide range of malignancy in Caucasians, nasopharyngeal carcinoma is the most common associated cancer in Asians.[115]

Pregnancy does not appear to be a trigger for DM, but data remain controversial. A single center prospective study in Spain described improved clinical disease during pregnancy with postpartum symptom relapse.[117] However, a case series described disease onsetting in the postpartum period in three patients.[118] On the other hand, the literature describes the complications during pregnancy in patients with active DM, such as neonatal prematurity, low birth weight, congenital anomalies, or morality as well as higher rates of spontaneous abortions and obstetric complications.[119] Overall, these findings emphasize the critical role of good control of disease for optimum pregnancy outcomes. Systemic steroids and intravenous immunoglobulin (IVIG) are the mainstay of treatment for DM. (Refer to section "Medication management in pregnancy.")

ALOPECIA AREATA

Alopecia areata (AA) has a lifetime prevalence of 1.7% and equally affects both sexes.[120] AA is most common in patients with African American descent and least common in those of Asian descent.[121] Most patients affected with AA are adults under the age of 40.[120,122,123] Data suggest that females are more likely to be affected by extensive disease and have comorbid nail involvement and concomitant autoimmune disease, particularly thyroid disease.[124,125] (Refer to Chapter 41 for clinical findings and classification.)

A large national database analysis in Korea reported higher rates of pregnancy loss, pelvic inflammatory disease, and ectopic pregnancy in patients with AA as compared to healthy controls, suggesting that AA is both a cutaneous and systemic disorder that can affect pregnancy outcomes.[126] Another similar study revealed a lower pregnancy rate in women with AA, especially in patients with long-standing disease, as compared to controls.[127] This impact was larger in older fertile women as compared to younger women.[127] Hence, disease control in the preconception and pregnancy period is of utmost importance.

Minoxidil is considered part of the first-line therapy regimens for AA. Its topical use during pregnancy has been associated with fetal malformations and should therefore be avoided.[128] The use of topical corticosteroids is favored (refer to section "Medication Management in Pregnancy").

SARCOIDOSIS

Sarcoidosis is another disease that occurs commonly in skin of color populations [**Figure 102-6**]. African Americans have a threefold higher age-adjusted annual incidence than Whites. African American females between the ages of 30 and 39 are at the highest risk of developing the disease.[129] Although lung disease is the most common presentation of sarcoidosis, there are a variety of dermatologic presentations as well, including erythema nodosum, lupus pernio, and macular, plaque, and subcutaneous nodular sarcoidosis.

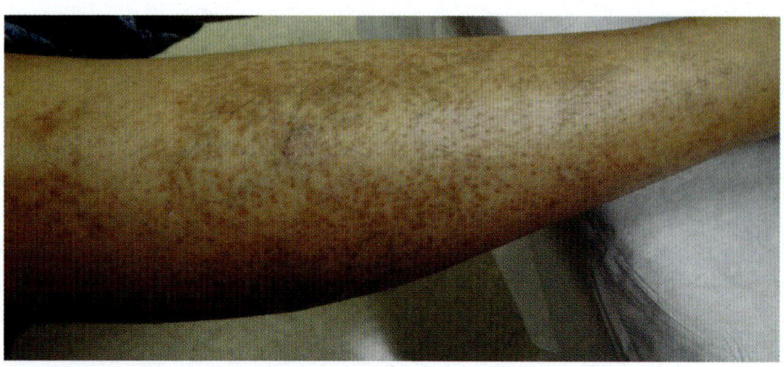

FIGURE 102-6. Cutaneous sarcoidosis in a Hispanic female. Note the numerous dermal papules with minimal epidermis surface change.

Sarcoidosis has recently been shown to be associated with a higher risk of adverse pregnancy outcomes such as preeclampsia, eclampsia, and preterm birth.[130,131] Significant uncontrolled disease including hypercalcemia, respiratory failure, or heart failure secondary to restrictive disease can threaten pregnancy.[132,133] To avoid fetal compromise, pregnancy should be discouraged for patients with active disease. Pregnancy can be revisited once the disease is under appropriate medical control.

TREATMENT

The management of connective tissue disease and sarcoidosis can be challenging. It is important that patients understand that the risks associated with these diseases during pregnancy are largely due to poorly controlled disease. Planning a pregnancy 6 months after the disease has been controlled can help ensure the safety of the mother and child.[134] Toward this end, it is important to stress contraception to patients whose disease is currently active or has been in remission for less than 6 months. Patients may be reassured that they are likely to have more successful than unsuccessful pregnancies with these disorders, and with appropriate management and close follow-up, they can have a healthy pregnancy and favorable outcome.

MEDICATION MANAGEMENT IN PREGNANCY

Dermatologists are frequently faced with questions about the safety of commonly prescribed topical and systemic medications during pregnancy and lactation from women of childbearing age who are pregnant, considering pregnancy, or breastfeeding. Safety data, particularly regarding medications that are unique to dermatology, can be increasingly found in emerging literature focusing on these topics.[82,135] The safety of dermatologic procedures has also been reported.[136] In this section, we herein focus on the medications most relevant to conditions discussed in the sections above.

Since some of the dermatoses of pregnancy rarely result in complications and often remit postpartum, the goal of treatment is the management of symptoms. The overriding complaint is pruritus, which is effectively treated with first-line topical agents and oral medications when needed.

TREATING SPECIFIC DERMATOSES OF PREGNANCY

Topical Steroids Previously, the U.S. Food and Drug Administration (FDA) categorized corticosteroids as a "class C" medication for use during pregnancy. The Pregnancy and Lactation Labeling Rule removed these pregnancy letter categories in 2015 in order to facilitate greater emphasis on risk versus benefit assessment.[137] In general, there is inadequate human data available to prove safety, particularly with long-term usage, location of usage, strength of topical steroid, and body surface area covered; there is evidence to warrant their safe use. Although there is a risk of fetal harm, including intrauterine growth restriction, studies have shown no increase in congenital malformations or abnormalities including cleft palates for infants exposed in utero and no increase in preterm delivery. Conversely, there is evidence to support retarded fetal growth for those exposed to potent or super potent topical corticosteroids. Studies have further classified the use of different strengths of topical corticosteroids. They found minimal growth retardation with high-strength steroids used in the first trimester, but there was a significant association of lower birth weight infants, smaller placental size, and lower plasma cortisol levels when the strongest topical steroids were used in the third trimester.[138,139] Additionally, a stratified analysis based on topical corticosteroid potency of 14 studies conducted over a 26-year span found no association between maternal use of corticosteroids with birth defects, fetal death, or preterm delivery.[140] From these data, recommendations were made regarding the use of topical corticosteroids during pregnancy. Potent and very potent corticosteroids should be avoided, whereas mild to moderate strength corticosteroids should be preferentially used. If potent or very potent strengths are needed, they should be used for minimal time periods and patients should be warned about potential fetal growth restriction.

Antihistamines First- and second-generation antihistamines can be used safely during pregnancy in low doses. Used in high doses in the third trimester, antihistamines have two potential toxicities: oxytocin-like effects, causing early uterine contractions and resulting in fetal hypoxia, and postpartum withdrawal in infants, which can result in seizure-like activity. Clinicians should make patients aware of the risk of retrolental fibroplasia, or retinopathy of prematurity, when using antihistamines within 2 weeks of delivery, specifically with preterm infants.[141]

When selecting an antihistamine, first-generation medications such as chlorpheniramine or diphenhydramine should be first line.[142] If the first-line agents cannot be tolerated, cetirizine and loratadine can be used after the first trimester.[143] It is important to absolutely avoid use of doxepin because of significant anticholinergic withdrawal effects including agitation, impaired cardiorespiratory function, and poor fetal continence.

Ursodeoxycholic Acid Used specifically for cholestatic disease of pregnancy, ursodeoxycholic acid proved to be both safe and effective in pregnancy. When pruritus is uncontrolled or liver enzymes are elevated, ursodeoxycholic acid can improve liver function tests and diminish pruritus. In an older study of over 500 pregnant women, maternal side effects were reported to be minimal, and fetal outcome was improved with respect to reducing fetal distress and premature births.[144] However, a few recent studies have questioned the effectiveness of ursodeoxycholic acid in reducing adverse perinatal outcomes.[145,146]

TREATING NEOPLASTIC CONDITIONS

There are certain neoplastic conditions that appear more commonly in young females of color. Early-onset mycosis fungoides, defined as before age 40, is most common in African American and Hispanic women. Moreover, African American women diagnosed with early-onset disease have worse prognoses.[147]

Another rare but concerning cancer in skin of color patients is melanoma. While less prevalent in skin of color populations, melanoma is more likely to metastasize, resulting in worse survival rates. Among Asian, Pacific Islander, and Latin American populations, the incidence of melanoma has steadily risen since 1996. Additionally, Black patients are more likely to experience a longer delay from diagnosis of melanoma to the time of definitive surgery when compared to White patients.[148] Research continues to elucidate risks factors for skin of color populations, with the hope of establishing standard preventative and detection measures.[149]

TREATING INFLAMMATORY CONDITIONS

Systemic Corticosteroids Similar to topical corticosteroids, oral corticosteroids can be safe and effective to use during pregnancy, but due to greater bioavailability, there are increased risks to consider when using this medication. The literature shows evidence of intrauterine growth retardation, premature rupture of membranes, and preterm delivery in exposed infants and increases in cleft palates with exposure up to 12 weeks after conception. However, these results are challenged by much larger population studies that fail to show significant increases in cleft palates or other congenital malformations. There is also uncertainty as to whether the underlying disease, which is often associated with similar fetal outcomes, is the cause for these outcomes or if it is indeed a complication of the medication.[150]

Placental metabolism plays a role in which oral corticosteroid should be selected for treatment. Nonfluorinated corticosteroids, such as prednisone, are largely inactivated by placental enzymes and thus are minimally passed to the child. Fluorinated steroids such as betamethasone and dexamethasone pass freely through the placenta, which make them ideal for when fetal effects, such as promotion of lung maturity, are the desired outcome. In the case of a desired maternal effect, prednisone is the recommended medication. While there are challenges in using the oral corticosteroids, they remain an important option during pregnancy. However, they must be accompanied by a thorough assessment and discussion of the risk-benefit ratio with the patient.

Antimalarial and Disease Modifying Agents The antimalarial drugs, hydroxychloroquine and chloroquine, are used to treat cutaneous lesions of systemic and discoid lupus erythematosus because of their immune-modulating properties. Several studies support the safe use of hydroxychloroquine not only for malaria prophylaxis but also cutaneous disease in pregnancy. While animal models have shown some auditory and retinal effects of antimalarials, a 2009 meta-analysis found no increase in congenital defects, spontaneous abortions, fetal death, or even prematurity.[151] In addition to hydroxychloroquine's strong safety profile, it allows for decreased dosage of systemic steroids and diminishes the degree of lupus activity for patients during pregnancy.

Other antimalarials, such as chloroquine, were also proven safe, but hydroxychloroquine has the lowest placental concentration, which makes it the preferred choice. Its beneficial effects go beyond the skin by decreasing the risk of neonatal lupus and heart block in the mother. However, due to the development of chloroquine-resistant malarial infections, the use of newer, less-studied antimalarials may be necessary. The World Health Organization (WHO) states the use of quinine and clindamycin is the safest treatment regimen for women in the first trimester; however, they are less utilized in the second and third trimester due to an increased risk of hypoglycemia in late pregnancy.[152] Additionally, the WHO states artemisinin-based combination therapy should be used to treat uncomplicated falciparum malaria in the second and third trimesters.[152]

SPECIAL CONSIDERATIONS IN TREATING PREGNANT WOMEN WITH INFLAMMATORY OR AUTOIMMUNE SKIN CONDITIONS

Vitiligo Although no direct factors have been attributed to precipitating or exacerbating vitiligo (except the Koebner phenomenon), patients do report pregnancy as a cause [**Figure 102-7**]. Traditionally, it has

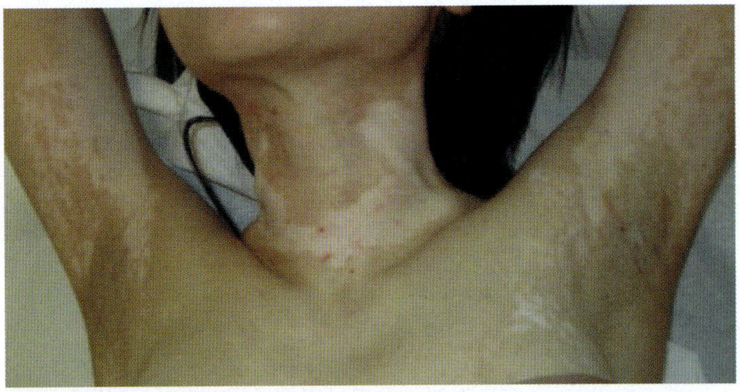

A

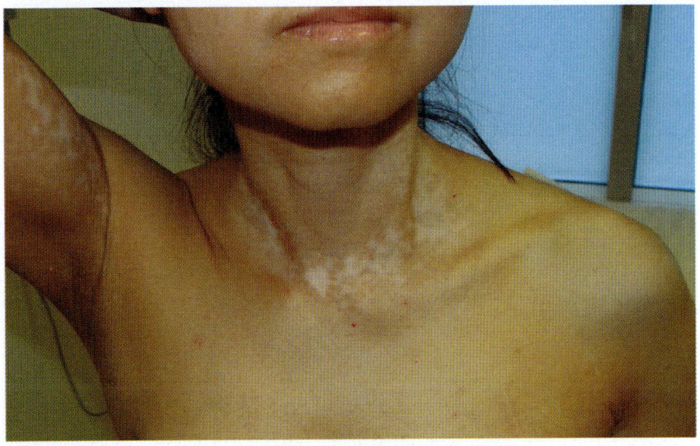

B

FIGURE 102-7. (A) Vitiligo initial presentation in a Japanese female. **(B)** The same patient following two to three times weekly narrowband ultraviolet B (UVB) therapy between 700 and 800 mJ after 72 weeks of therapy. Narrowband UVB therapy is a safe option for pregnant women who take adequate folic acid supplementation.

been thought that pregnancy in patients with vitiligo was not found to be associated with adverse pregnancy outcomes, including labor issues, and birth outcomes. However, pregnancy in Korean and Taiwanese patients with vitiligo was found to be associated with an increased risk of spontaneous abortion, with one study finding a decreased risk of abortion among patients on oral treatment including steroids and methotrexate.[153,154] There are no guidelines for the treatment of vitiligo in pregnancy. The safest option may be simply camouflage using cosmetics and makeup. Low- to moderate-potency corticosteroids, narrowband UVB [Figure 102-7], and broadband UVB are also options. With UVB phototherapy, regardless of the condition being treated, folate supplementation should be provided to prevent folate deficiency, which would increase risk of neural tube defects in the first trimester.[155] Only one case has been reported in the literature of a neural tube defect potentially related to folate deficiency from phototherapy.[82,156]

Psoriasis Psoriasis is a chronic inflammatory disorder that has characteristic erythematous plaques with scale. It is the sixth most common diagnosis of African American patient visits to the dermatologist, the fourth most common in Asian or Pacific Islander patient visits, and the third most common in Hispanic or Latino patient visits.[157] There are approximately 65,000 to 107,000 births to women with psoriasis annually.[158] Of pregnant women with psoriasis, 55% have reported improvement, 21% no change, and 23% worsening, whereas the majority have flaring in the postpartum period.[159,160] Notably, pregnant women with psoriasis have been found to have an increased risk for ectopic pregnancy.[161] The Medical Board of the National Psoriasis Foundation released treatment options for pregnant and lactating women with psoriasis.[162] First-line treatments for pregnant women with mild psoriasis are emollients and low- to moderate-potency topical steroids. Second-line treatment is usually narrowband UVB phototherapy or broadband UVB phototherapy. UVB phototherapy can precipitate melasma, so patients should be counseled. Third-line therapies include tumor necrosis factor-α inhibitors (eg, adalimumab, etanercept, infliximab) and cyclosporine. More recent data have shown certolizumab and etanercept as preferred agents due to their minimal transplacental transfer when compared to infliximab and adalimumab.[163] Systemic steroids for pustular psoriasis, which may occur in the later stages of pregnancy, can be used with caution in the second and third trimesters. The use of methotrexate and acitretin is absolutely contraindicated in pregnancy due to their teratogenicity.[164]

For lactating women, first-line treatment includes moisturizers and topical steroids. UVB phototherapy in lactating women is also safe. If unavoidable, systemic steroids should be ingested 4 hours prior to breastfeeding to minimized amounts found in breast milk. It is recommended to avoid the use of cyclosporine during lactation as well.[165]

Atopic Dermatitis Atopic dermatitis (AD) is the most common dermatosis during pregnancy, accounting for 36% to 49.7% of disorders.[59,166] It has been reported that up to 52% of pregnant patients with preexisting AD experienced worsening of disease [**Figure 102-8**].[167] It is reported that only 20% to 40% of patients have preexisting eczema.[59,166] Up to 2% of lactating mothers will develop areola and/or nipple eczema.[168] The basis of treatment should focus on emollient usage and avoidance of irritants and allergens.[169]

First-line therapy includes judicious use of low- to mid-potency topical corticosteroids and oral second-generation antihistamines. UVB phototherapy is considered the safest second-line treatment in pregnancy. For very severe AD, oral corticosteroids may be used short term in the second and third trimester in low doses. Topical immunomodulators (ie, pimecrolimus, tacrolimus) in small areas are also likely safe. Third-line therapy includes topical Janus kinase (JAK) inhibitors or humanized monoclonal IgG4 antibody dupilumab injections for severe AD. There is a scarcity of data on the safety of Janus kinase (JAK) inhibitors in pregnancy; however, animal studies have shown fetal abnormalities with exposure to baricitinib 10 and 39 times that of therapeutic human exposure.[170] Additionally, human doses of upadacitinib led to increased skeletal and cardiovascular malformations in animal studies. Thus, the use of baricitinib, upadacitinib, and abrocitinib is contraindicated in pregnancy.[170] Dupilumab is the only biologic approved for the treatment of AD. No pregnancy, puerperium, and perinatal adverse drug reactions were found to be associated with the use of dupilumab following the analysis of outcomes from a large global pharmacovigilance database.[171] However, no randomized clinical trials exist investigating its safety in the pregnancy, and its use should balance the clinical need with the possible related adverse effects that could affect the fetus. For bacterial superinfection, penicillin and cephalosporins are first-line, and for herpetic superinfections, acyclovir is safe in pregnancy.

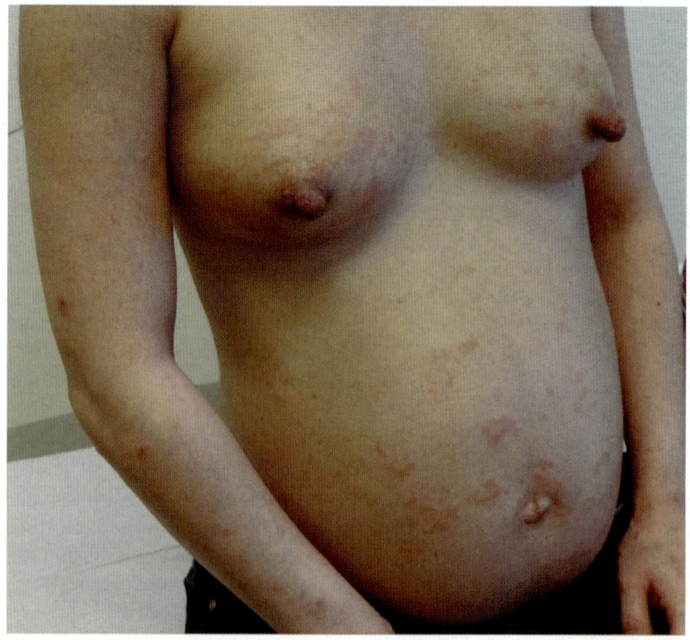

FIGURE 102-8. Atopic eruption of pregnancy in a Japanese female during the second trimester of pregnancy. This patient had longstanding atopic dermatitis and experienced a significant worsening of her condition during the latter half of her pregnancy.

SPECIAL CONSIDERATIONS: DISEASES MORE COMMON IN SKIN OF COLOR POPULATIONS AND PREGNANCY

HUMAN IMMUNODEFICIENCY VIRUS

Seventy percent of the world's human immunodeficiency virus (HIV)/acquired immunodeficiency (AIDS) patients live in sub-Saharan Africa, and this is the only region in the world where more females than males are infected. African women of childbearing age have a heightened susceptibility for acquiring this infection.[172] The infection is responsible for a unique group of skin manifestations that necessitate knowledge and skill for accurate diagnosis and management.

Infectious

Coccidioidomycosis Pregnancy is known as a risk factor for a severe, diffuse form of coccidioidomycosis, a fungal infection that has a special predilection for immunosuppressed patients as well as African Americans. This puts HIV-positive females with skin of color at significantly heightened risk of this life-threatening disease for mother and child.[173,174] While the immunologic reason for the predilection is unknown, there is significant literature that shows that being of African descent is a risk factor for disseminated disease. Additionally, individuals of Filipino and Mexican descent are 175 and 3 times more likely, respectively, to have disseminated coccidioidomycosis.[175,176] While coccidioidomycosis has a variety of disease presentations, the most common presentations to a dermatologist include erythema nodosum or erythema multiforme.

Miscellaneous Infections Studies show that across HIV-positive populations, 90% of patients will have skin disease.[177,178] While not unique to pregnant patients, common infections include methicillin-resistant

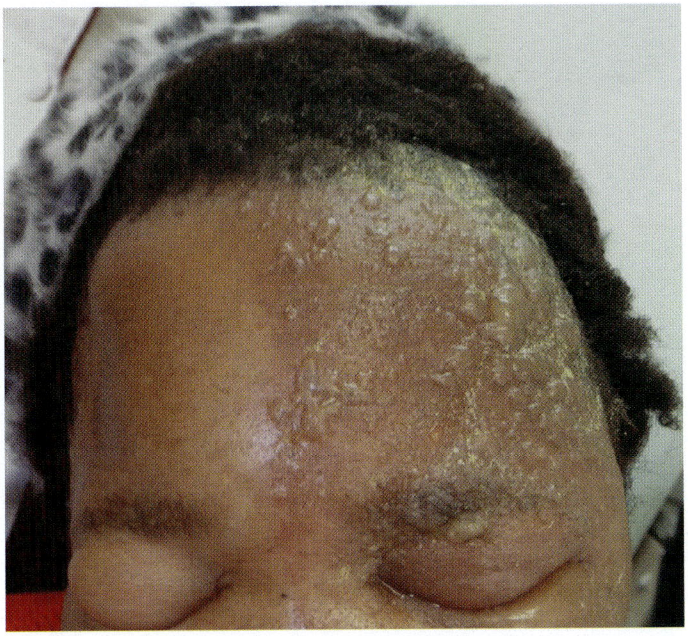

FIGURE 102-9. Human immunodeficiency virus (HIV)-positive African female with herpes zoster infection in a V_1 distribution. Unlike zoster in individuals without HIV infection, the dermatomal eruption may be particularly bullous, hemorrhagic, necrotic, and painful in HIV-infected persons. (Used with permission from Dr. Deepti Gupta.)

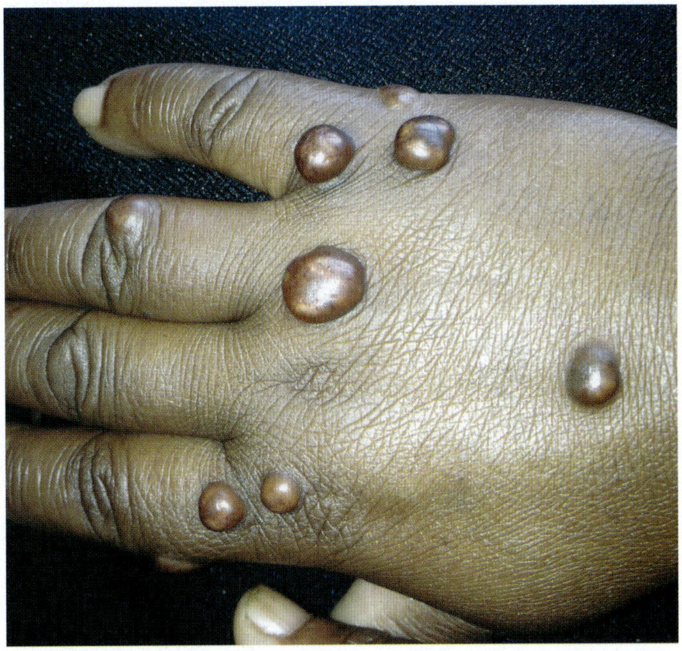

FIGURE 102-11. Molluscum contagiosum infection in a human immunodeficiency virus (HIV)-positive African female. Once CD4 count falls below 200/μL, the lesions tend to proliferate, and extensive molluscum contagiosum is a cutaneous marker of advanced HIV disease. (Used with permission from Dr. Deepti Gupta.)

Staphylococcus aureus, human papilloma virus, herpes simplex virus, varicella zoster virus [**Figure 102-9**], scabies [**Figure 102-10**], molluscum contagiosum [**Figure 102-11**], and primary and secondary [**Figure 102-12**] syphilis.[179]

Pruritus and Inflammatory Skin Conditions

Pruritus Close to 30% of HIV-positive individuals will experience some degree of itching. Studies have shown a relationship between increased pruritus and HIV in pregnant females, but it is unclear if the pruritus is a product of the pregnancy itself or of HIV progression.[180,181] Chronic pruritus often leads to prurigo nodularis particularly when the itch-scratch cycle has continued for weeks to months. The goal of management is to identify the cause of the pruritus with the ultimate goal of breaking the itch-scratch cycle.[182]

Papular Pruritic Eruption Papular pruritic eruption is found more commonly in African and other tropical environments. This disease likely represents an exaggerated immune response to arthropod antigens in a subset of susceptible HIV-infected patients. Patients will often complain of pruritic lesions that last longer than a typical insect bite.

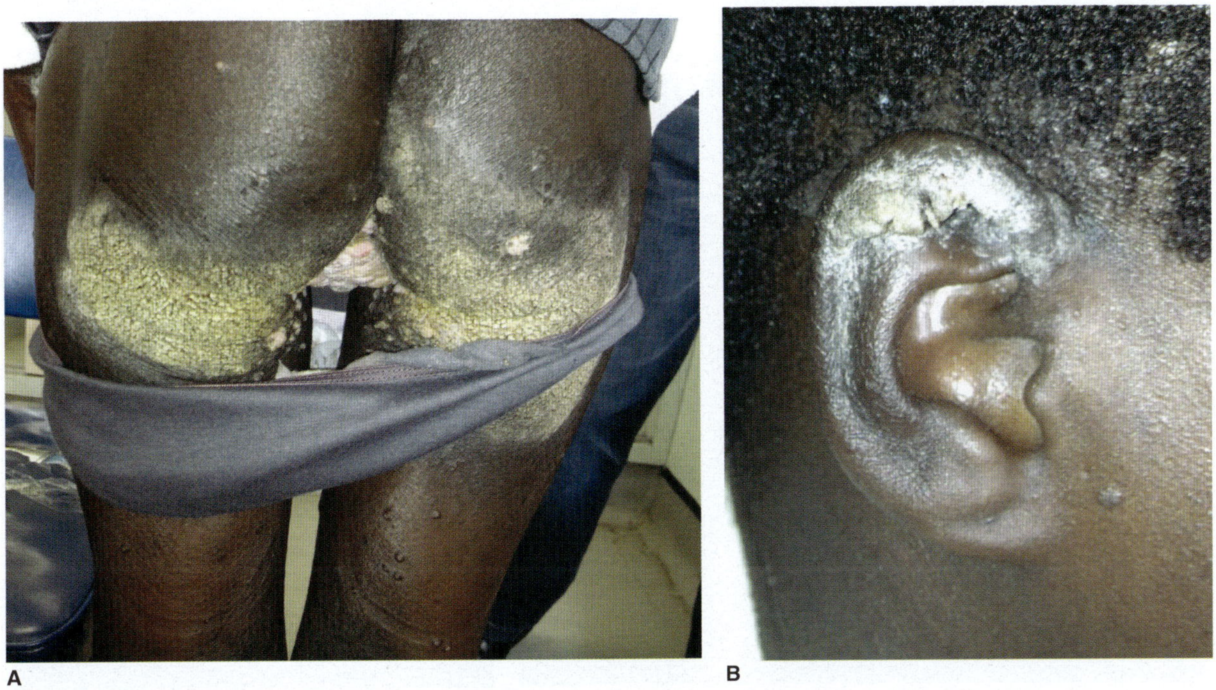

FIGURE 102-10. Scabies infection in human immunodeficiency virus (HIV)-positive African female. **(A)** HIV patients have higher likelihood of developing Norwegian crusted scabies. **(B)** Patients are also more likely to present with lesions on the head and neck, which is less common in immunocompetent individuals. Scabies can be treated safely with permethrin 5% cream, benzoyl benzoate in Europe, and topical sulfur 5% or 10% ointment in pregnancy. (Used with permission from Dr. Deepti Gupta.)

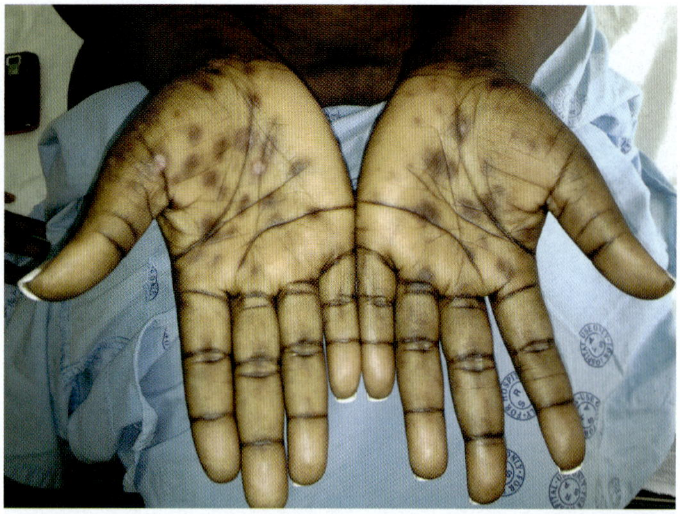

FIGURE 102-12. Secondary syphilis in a human immunodeficiency virus (HIV)-positive African female. The copper-colored maculopapular rash on the palms harbors bacteria and is contagious. (Used with permission from Dr. Deepti Gupta.)

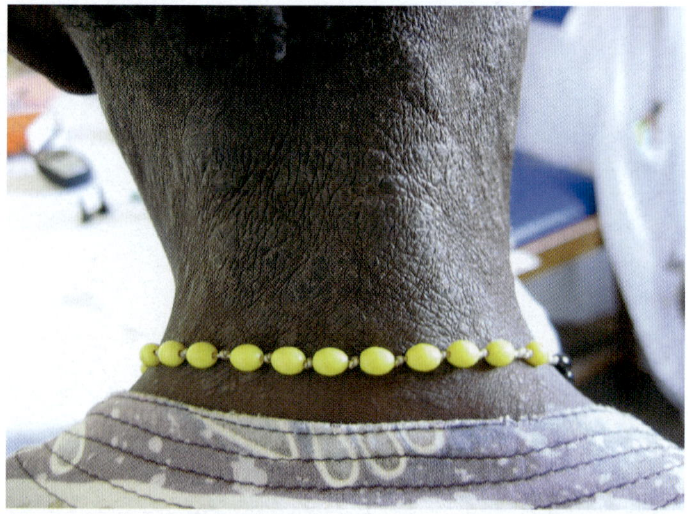

FIGURE 102-14. Atopic dermatitis flare in a human immunodeficiency virus (HIV)-positive female. HIV-infected adults with a previous history of atopic disease may note recurrence of atopy in advanced HIV disease as well as in pregnancy.

The typical primary lesions is a firm, discrete, erythematous, urticarial papule.[183] In HIV patients, the condition can recur episodically and is often resistant to oral antihistamines and topical steroids. Most patients scratch the lesions because of the severe pruritus, leading to excoriated papules, marked postinflammatory hyperpigmentation, and, eventually, scarred nodules [**Figure 102-13**].[184]

Photodermatitis There can be several etiologic causes of photodermatologic reactions in pregnant patients with HIV. Not only can HIV itself have a photosensitizing effect, but several medications including azithromycin, tetracyclines, quinolones, and several anti-parasitics taken for the infection can cause a similar reaction.[182]

Eczematous Dermatitis and Psoriasis These inflammatory skin disorders are common in African HIV-positive patients [**Figure 102-14**]. They can present with greater severity in HIV patients, such as new-onset erythroderma. Patients may or may not have a history of disease prior to HIV diagnosis.[182]

Cutaneous Drug Reactions in HIV

Sulfonamides Sulfonamides are uniquely noted to cause drug eruptions, particularly trimethoprim-sulfamethoxazole, which is often used in HIV patients to treat pneumocystis pneumonia. Drug eruptions to sulfa-containing antibiotics can present in a variety of ways, with Stevens-Johnson syndrome and toxic epidermal necrolysis as the most severe presentations. The literature reveals that almost two-thirds of HIV-positive patients experience adverse reactions requiring discontinuation of the medication [**Figure 102-15**], and the rates of adverse reaction are particularly high in East Africa.[182,185] The medication can also contribute to hyperbilirubinemia and kernicterus in an unborn fetus; for that reason, sulfa antibiotics should be avoided 6 weeks prior to birth.

Nevirapine While the side effect profile of this antiretroviral spans all HIV-infected individuals, it has a particular proclivity for causing reactions in pregnant HIV-positive females. It is associated with several adverse reactions, the most common being an erythematous drug rash

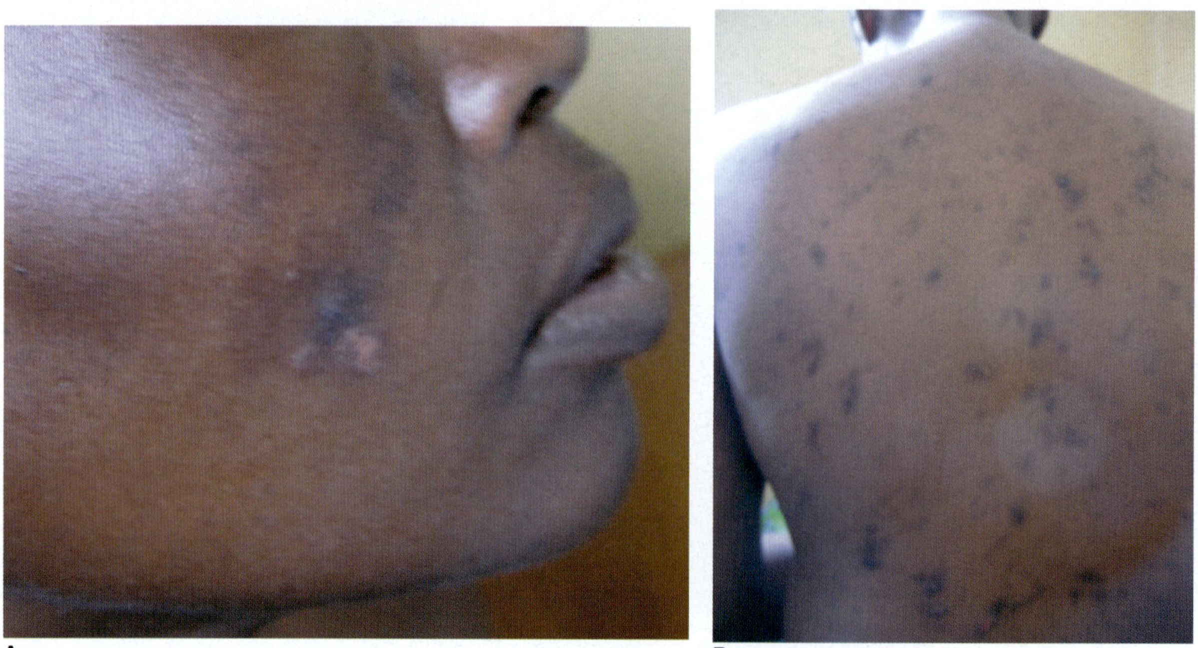

A B

FIGURE 102-13. Pruritic papular eruption is thought to reflect an altered and exaggerated immune response to arthropod antigens in human immunodeficiency virus (HIV)-infected patients. The concentration of the lesions is highest on the extremities, but the face **(A)** and the trunk **(B)** are also involved in half of patients.

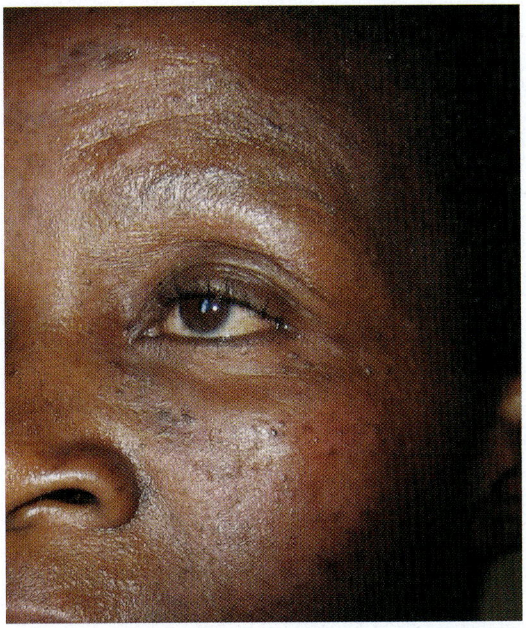

FIGURE 102-15. Photosensitivity secondary to sulfonamides in an African human immunodeficiency virus (HIV)-positive female. This patient was being treated for pneumocystis pneumonia.

that can precede liver toxicity. Two risk factors identified for a potentially life-threatening drug reaction include initiation of the drug late in pregnancy and those with a CD4 count greater than 250/μL upon initiation.[186] It is suggested to start the medication early in the pregnancy and only when HIV has progressed significantly.

Antiretroviral Therapy (ART) The World Health Organization recommends an initial antiretroviral regimen consisting of zidovudine, lamivudine, and nevirapine. This three-drug ART regimen is remarkably effective at preventing vertical transmission.[187] If patients cannot tolerate zidovudine, stavudine, which has also proven safe in pregnancy, may be substituted. As previously mentioned, nevirapine has a significant adverse effect profile, but the key is the initiation of the medication early in pregnancy.[188] Efavirenz is commonly used in antiretroviral regimens, but it should be avoided given possible neural tube defects if administered in the first trimester. While the evidence is not overly compelling, it should be avoided in favor of the aforementioned therapies.[189,190]

Current trials are investigating the safety and efficacy of bictegravir and doravirine, two recently marketed ARTs.[191] Additionally, davipirine-containing vaginal rings, currently used for pre-exposure prophylaxis, are expected to be used in lactating women in countries with a high incidence of HIV.[191]

SICKLE CELL DISEASE

Treatment of sickle cell disease (SCD) with hydroxyurea has been reported to result in utero death or spontaneous abortion.[192] The National Toxicology Program expert does not recommend the use of hydroxyurea in pregnancy.[193] Chronic narcotic treatment for SCD patients is not uncommon, and it has been reported that pain control required for pregnant women with SCD has not been associated with congenital defects. Chronic narcotic treatment is associated with a risk of neonatal abstinence syndrome, but the risk was not found to be dependent on dose.[194]

In pregnancy, there is an increased risk of the development of ulcers due to increased blood volume. Sickle cell ulceration is often recalcitrant to treatment and often recurs.[195] There have been two case reports of spontaneous healing of sickle cell ulcers during pregnancy, which was hypothesized to be due to fetal stem cell circulation. However, relapse occurred in both women 3 to 4 months after delivery.[196,197]

There is some research that suggest both micro- and macronutrient deficiencies are associated with SCD.[198] For SCD-related leg ulceration, zinc deficiency may play a role in pathogenesis.[198] In pregnant women with SCD, iron deficiency is common.[198] There are currently no specific recommended guidelines for zinc and iron supplementation for pregnant women with SCD, and clinicians must make decisions for patients on an individual basis.

CONCLUSION

SG, melasma, and ICP are disorders that occur not uncommonly in pregnant women of color. Additionally, serious systemic diseases including MF, sarcoidosis, scleroderma, and lupus appear to be more aggressive and confer a worse prognosis in pregnant women of color. The approach to these patients must include aggressive control of the underlying disease.

REFERENCES

1. Fink DA, Kilday D, Cao Z, et al. Trends in maternal mortality and severe maternal morbidity during delivery-related hospitalizations in the United States, 2008 to 2021. *JAMA Network Open*. 2023;6(6):e2317641.
2. Njoroge WF, White LK, Waller R, et al. Association of COVID-19 and endemic systemic racism with postpartum anxiety and depression among black birthing individuals. *JAMA Psychiatry*. 2022;79(6):600-609.
3. Ghasemi A, Gorouhi F, Rashighi-Firoozabadi M, Jafarian S, Firooz A. Striae gravidarum: associated factors. *J Eur Acad Dermatol Venereol*. 2007;21(6):743-746.
4. Hoefel IDR, Weber MB, Manzoni APD, Lovato BH, Bonamigo RR. Striae gravidarum, acne, facial spots, and hair disorders: risk factors in a study with 1284 puerperal patients. *J Pregnancy*. 2020;2020:8036109.
5. Picard D, Sellier S, Houivet E, et al. Incidence and risk factors for striae gravidarum. *J Am Acad Dermatol*. 2015;73(4):699-700.
6. J-Orh R, Titapant V, Chuenwattana P, Tontisirin P. Prevalence and associate factors for striae gravidarum. *J Med Assoc Thai*. 2008;91(4):445-451.
7. Kasielska-Trojan A, Sobczak M, Antoszewski B. Risk factors of striae gravidarum. *Int J Cosmet Sci*. 2015;37(2):236-240.
8. Chang AL, Agredano YZ, Kimball AB. Risk factors associated with striae gravidarum. *J Am Acad Dermatol*. 2004;51(6):881-885.
9. Buchanan K, Fletcher HM, Reid M. Prevention of striae gravidarum with cocoa butter cream. *Int J Gynaecol Obstet*. 2010;108(1):65-68.
10. Tang-Lin L, Liew HM, Koh MJ, Allen JC, Tan TC. Prevalence of striae gravidarum in a multi-ethnic Asian population and the associated risk factors. *Australas J Dermatol*. 2017;58(3):e154-e155.
11. Osman H, Rubeiz N, Tamim H, Nassar AH. Risk factors for the development of striae gravidarum. *Am J Obstet Gynecol*. 2007;196(1):62.e1-e5.
12. Yamaguchi K, Suganuma N, Ohashi K. Quality of life evaluation in Japanese pregnant women with striae gravidarum: a cross-sectional study. *BMC Res Notes*. 2012;5:450.
13. Farahnik B, Park K, Kroumpouzos G, Murase J. Striae gravidarum: risk factors, prevention, and management. *Int J Womens Dermatol*. 2017;3(2):77-85.
14. Piérard-Franchimont C, Hermanns JF, Hermanns-Lê T, Piérard GE. Striae distensae in darker skin types: the influence of melanocyte mechanobiology. *J Cosmet Dermatol*. 2005;4(3):174-178.
15. Brennan M, Young G, Devane D. Topical preparations for preventing stretch marks in pregnancy. *Cochrane Database Syst Rev*. 2012;11:Cd000066.
16. Rangel O, Arias I, García E, Lopez-Padilla S. Topical tretinoin 0.1% for pregnancy-related abdominal striae: an open-label, multicenter, prospective study. *Adv Ther*. 2001;18(4):181-186.
17. Ash K, Lord J, Zukowski M, McDaniel DH. Comparison of topical therapy for striae alba (20% glycolic acid/0.05% tretinoin versus 20% glycolic acid/10% L-ascorbic acid). *Dermatol Surg*. 1998;24(8):849-856.
18. Sherling M, Friedman PM, Adrian R, et al. Consensus recommendations on the use of an erbium-doped 1,550-nm fractionated laser and its applications in dermatologic laser surgery. *Dermatol Surg*. 2010;36(4):461-469.
19. Bak H, Kim BJ, Lee WJ, et al. Treatment of striae distensae with fractional photothermolysis. *Dermatol Surg*. 2009;35(8):1215-1220.
20. Vaiyavatjamai P, Wattanakrai P. Side effects and complications of fractional 1550-nm erbium fiber laser treatment among Asians. *J Cosmet Dermatol*. 2011;10(4):313-316.
21. Cohen SR, Goodacre A, Lim S, et al. Clinical outcomes and complications associated with fractional lasers: a review of 730 patients. *Aesthetic Plast Surg*. 2017;41(1):171-178.

22. Alster TS, Li MK. Microneedling treatment of striae distensae in light and dark skin with long-term follow-up. *Dermatol Surg*. 2020;46(4):459-464.
23. Park KY, Kim HK, Kim SE, Kim BJ, Kim MN. Treatment of striae distensae using needling therapy: a pilot study. *Dermatol Surg*. 2012;38(11):1823-1828.
24. Saki N, Rahimi F, Pezeshkian FS, Parvar SY. Comparison of the efficacy of microneedling versus CO_2 fractional laser to treat striae alba: a randomized clinical trial. *Dermatol Ther*. 2022;35(1):e15212.
25. Khater MH, Khattab FM, Abdelhaleem MR. Treatment of striae distensae with needling therapy versus CO_2 fractional laser. *J Cosmet Laser Ther*. 2016; 18(2):75-79.
26. Naspolini AP, Boza JC, da Silva VD, Cestari TF. Efficacy of microneedling versus fractional non-ablative laser to treat striae alba: a randomized study. *Am J Clin Dermatol*. 2019;20(2):277-287.
27. Nassar A, Ghomey S, El Gohary Y, El-Desoky F. Treatment of striae distensae with needling therapy versus microdermabrasion with sonophoresis. *J Cosmet Laser Ther*. 2016;18(6):330-334.
28. Shridharani SM, Magarakis M, Manson PN, Singh NK, Basdag B, Rosson GD. The emerging role of antineoplastic agents in the treatment of keloids and hypertrophic scars: a review. *Ann Plast Surg*. 2010;64(3):355-361.
29. Bayat A, Arscott G, Ollier WE, Ferguson MW, Mc Grouther DA. Description of site-specific morphology of keloid phenotypes in an Afrocaribbean population. *Br J Plast Surg*. 2004;57(2):122-133.
30. Tulandi T, Al-Sannan B, Akbar G, Ziegler C, Miner L. Prospective study of intraabdominal adhesions among women of different races with or without keloids. *Am J Obstet Gynecol*. 2011;204(2):132.e1-e4.
31. Alderdice F, McKenna D, Dornan J. Techniques and materials for skin closure in caesarean section. *Cochrane Database Syst Rev*. 2003;(2):Cd003577.
32. Kim JW, Huh CH, Na JI, Hong JS, Yoon Park J, Shin JW. Evaluating outcomes of pulsed dye laser therapy combined with intralesional triamcinolone injection after surgical removal of hypertrophic cesarean section scars. *J Cosmet Dermatol*. 2022;21(4):1471-1476.
33. Payapvipapong K, Niumpradit N, Piriyanand C, Buranaphalin S, Nakakes A. The treatment of keloids and hypertrophic scars with intralesional bleomycin in skin of color. *J Cosmet Dermatol*. 2015;14(1):83-90.
34. Saitta P, Krishnamurthy K, Brown LH. Bleomycin in dermatology: a review of intralesional applications. *Dermatol Surg*. 2008;34(10):1299-1313.
35. Kroumpouzos G, Cohen LM. Dermatoses of pregnancy. *J Am Acad Dermatol*. 2001;45(1):1-19.
36. Cummings K. Dermatoses associated with pregnancy. *Cutis*. 1967;3:120-126.
37. Briggs G, Freeman R, Yaffe S. Drugs in pregnancy and lactation 8th edition: a reference guide to fetal and neonatal risk. *Obstet Med*. 2009;2(2):89.
38. Wester RC, Melendres J, Hui X, et al. Human in vivo and in vitro hydroquinone topical bioavailability, metabolism, and disposition. *J Toxicol Environ Health A*. 1998;54(4):301-317.
39. Krasavage WJ, Blacker AM, English JC, Murphy SJ. Hydroquinone: a developmental toxicity study in rats. *Fundam Appl Toxicol*. 1992;18(3):370-375.
40. Mahé A, Perret JL, Ly F, Fall F, Rault JP, Dumont A. The cosmetic use of skin-lightening products during pregnancy in Dakar, Senegal: a common and potentially hazardous practice. *Trans R Soc Trop Med Hyg*. 2007;101(2): 183-187.
41. Andersen F. Final report on the safety assessment of glycolic acid, ammonium, calcium, potassium, and sodium glycolates, methyl, ethyl, propyl, and butyl glycolates, and lactic acid, ammonium, calcium, potassium, sodium, and TEA-lactates, methyl, ethyl, isopropyl, and butyl lactates, and lauryl, myristyl, and cetyl lactates. *Int J Toxicol*. 1998;17(1_suppl):1-241.
42. Trivedi M, Inouye T, Murase J. Safety of cosmetic procedures during pregnancy and lactation: a review [24E]. *Obstet Gynecol*. 2017;129(5):58S.
43. Wong CSM, Chan MWM, Shek SYN, Yeung CK, Chan HHL. Fractional 1064 nm picosecond laser in treatment of melasma and skin rejuvenation in asians, a prospective study. *Lasers Surg Med*. 2021;53(8):1032-1042.
44. Bala HR, Lee S, Wong C, Pandya AG, Rodrigues M. Oral tranexamic acid for the treatment of melasma: a review. *Dermatol Surg*. 2018;44(6):814-825.
45. Gilad O, Merlob P, Stahl B, Klinger G. Outcome following tranexamic acid exposure during breastfeeding. *Breastfeed Med*. 2014;9(8):407-410.
46. Tranexamic Acid. In: Drugs and Lactation Database (LactMed®) [Internet]. Bethesda (MD): National Institute of Child Health and Human Development; 2006. Available from: https://www.ncbi.nlm.nih.gov/books/NBK501734/ Accessed March 7, 2023.
47. Caballero T, Farkas H, Bouillet L, et al. International consensus and practical guidelines on the gynecologic and obstetric management of female patients with hereditary angioedema caused by C1 inhibitor deficiency. *J Allergy Clin Immunol*. 2012;129(2):308-320.
48. Lee RH, Goodwin TM, Greenspoon J, Incerpi M. The prevalence of intrahepatic cholestasis of pregnancy in a primarily Latina Los Angeles population. *J Perinatol*. 2006;26(9):527-532.
49. Abedin P, Weaver JB, Egginton E. Intrahepatic cholestasis of pregnancy: prevalence and ethnic distribution. *Ethn Health*. 1999;4(1-2):35-37.
50. Taylor D, Pappo E, Aronson IK. Polymorphic eruption of pregnancy. *Clin Dermatol*. 2016;34(3):383-391.
51. Kumari R, Jaisankar T, Thappa DM. A clinical study of skin changes in pregnancy. *Indian J Dermatol Venereol Leprol*. 2007;73(2):141.
52. Taylor D, Pappo E, Aronson IK. Polymorphic eruption of pregnancy. *Clin Dermatol*. 2016;34(3):383-391.
53. Ohel I, Levy A, Silberstein T, Holcberg G, Sheiner E. Pregnancy outcome of patients with pruritic urticarial papules and plaques of pregnancy. *J Matern Fetal Neonatal Med*. 2006;19(5):305-308.
54. Rudolph C, Al-Fares S, Vaughan-Jones SA, Müllegger RR, Kerl H, Black MM. Polymorphic eruption of pregnancy: clinicopathology and potential trigger factors in 181 patients. *Br J Dermatol*. 2006;154(1):54-60.
55. Yancey KB, Hall RP, Lawley TJ. Pruritic urticarial papules and plaques of pregnancy: clinical experience in twenty-five patients. *J Am Acad Dermatol*. 1984;10(3):473-480.
56. Alcalay J, Ingber A, Kafri B, et al. Hormonal evaluation and autoimmune background in pruritic urticarial papules and plaques of pregnancy. *Am J Obstet Gynecol*. 1988;158(2):417-420.
57. Brandão P, Sousa-Faria B, Marinho C, Vieira-Enes P, Melo A, Mota L. Polymorphic eruption of pregnancy: review of literature. *J Obstet Gynaecol*. 2017; 37(2):137-140.
58. Ambros-Rudolph CM. Dermatoses of pregnancy-clues to diagnosis, fetal risk and therapy. *Ann Dermatol*. 2011;23(3):265-275.
59. Ambros-Rudolph CM, Müllegger RR, Vaughan-Jones SA, Kerl H, Black MM. The specific dermatoses of pregnancy revisited and reclassified: results of a retrospective two-center study on 505 pregnant patients. *J Am Acad Dermatol*. 2006;54(3):395-404.
60. Sävervall C, Sand FL, Thomsen SF. Dermatological diseases associated with pregnancy: pemphigoid gestationis, polymorphic eruption of pregnancy, intrahepatic cholestasis of pregnancy, and atopic eruption of pregnancy. *Dermatol Res Pract*. 2015;2015:979635.
61. Kolodny RC. Herpes gestationis: a new assessment of incidence, diagnosis, and fetal prognosis. *Am J Obstet Gynecol*. 1969;104(1):39-45.
62. Roger D, Vaillant L, Fignon A, et al. Specific pruritic diseases of pregnancy: a prospective study of 3192 pregnant women. *Arch Dermatol*. 1994;130(6): 734-739.
63. Shornick JK, Black MM. Secondary autoimmune diseases in herpes gestationis (pemphigoid gestationis). *J Am Acad Dermatol*. 1992;26(4): 563-566.
64. Lipozenčić J, Ljubojevic S, Bukvić-Mokos Z. Pemphigoid gestationis. *Clin Dermatol*. 2012;30(1):51-55.
65. Braun-Falco O, Plewig G, Wolff HH, Burgdorf WHC. Blistering diseases. In: *Dermatology*. Springer Berlin, Heidelberg; 2000:649-695.
66. Djahansouzi S, Nestle-Kraemling C, Dall P, Bender HG, Hanstein B. Herpes gestationis may present itself as a paraneoplastic syndrome of choriocarcinoma—a case report. *Gynecol Oncol*. 2003;89(2):334-337.
67. Jenkins J, Hern H, Black B. Clinical features and management of 87 patients with pemphigoid gestationis. *Clin Exp Dermatol*. 1999;24(4):255-259.
68. Reyes H, Gonzalez MC, Ribalta J, et al. Prevalence of intrahepatic cholestasis of pregnancy in Chile. *Ann Intern Med*. 1978;88(4):487-493.
69. Reyes H, Wegmann ME, Segovia N, et al. HLA in Chileans with intrahepatic cholestasis of pregnancy. *Hepatology*. 1982;2(4):463S-466S.
70. Abedin P, Weaver JB, Egginton E. Intrahepatic cholestasis of pregnancy: prevalence and ethnic distribution. *Ethn Health*. 1999;4(1–2):35-37.
71. Geenes V, Williamson C. Intrahepatic cholestasis of pregnancy. *World J Gastroenterol*. 2009;15(17):2049.
72. Roth M-M. Pregnancy dermatoses: diagnosis, management, and controversies. *Am J Clin Dermatol*. 2011;12:25-41.
73. Kondo RN, Araújo FM, Pereira AM, Lopes VC, Martins LM. Pustular psoriasis of pregnancy (Impetigo herpetiformis)-Case report. *An Bras Dermatol*. 2013;88:186-189.
74. Green M, Bragg J, Rosenman KS, Pomeranz MK. Pustular psoriasis of pregnancy in a patient whose dermatosis showed features of acute generalized exanthematous pustulosis. *Int J Dermatol*. 2009;48(3):299-303.
75. Bangale-Daflapurkar S, Danve A. Pustular psoriasis of pregnancy successfully treated with cyclosporine. *Am J Ther*. 2016;23(5):e1250-e1252.
76. Breier-Maly J, Ortel B, Breier F, Schmidt JB, Hönigsmann H. Generalized pustular psoriasis of pregnancy (impetigo herpetiformis). *Dermatology*. 1999;198(1):61-64.
77. Oosterling RJ, Nobrega RE, Du Boeuff JA, Van Der Meer JB. Impetigo herpetiformis or generalized pustular psoriasis? *Arch Dermatol*. 1978; 114(10): 1527-1529.

78. Kroumpouzos G, Cohen LM. Dermatoses of pregnancy. *J Am Acad Dermatol.* 2001;45(1):1-22.
79. Hebra F. Über einzelne während der Schwangerschaft, dem Wochenbett und bei Uterinalerkrankungen zu beobachtende Hautkrankheiten. *Wien. med. Wschr.* 1872;22(48):737-740.
80. Benjegerdes KE, Hyde K, Kivelevitch D, Mansouri B. Pustular psoriasis: pathophysiology and current treatment perspectives. *Psoriasis.* 2016;6: 131-144.
81. Robinson A, Van Voorhees AS, Hsu S, et al. Treatment of pustular psoriasis: from the Medical Board of the National Psoriasis Foundation. *J Am Acad Dermatol.* 2012;67(2):279-288.
82. Murase JE, Heller MM, Butler DC. Safety of dermatologic medications in pregnancy and lactation: Part I. Pregnancy. *J Am Acad Dermatol.* 2014;70(3): 401.e1-401.e14.
83. Barrouq DM, Jibril NI. Systemic lupus erythematosus: a narrative review of disease. *East African Scholars J Med Sci.* 2022;5(9):259-267.
84. Petri M. Epidemiology of systemic lupus erythematosus. *Best Pract Res Clin Rheumatol.* 2002;16(5):847-858.
85. Clowse ME, Jamison M, Myers E, James AH. A national study of the complications of lupus in pregnancy. *Am J Obstet Gynecol.* 2008;199(2):127.e1-127.e6.
86. Clowse ME. Lupus activity in pregnancy. *Rheum Dis Clin North Am.* 2007; 33(2):237-252.
87. Chakravarty EF, Nelson L, Krishnan E. Obstetric hospitalizations in the United States for women with systemic lupus erythematosus and rheumatoid arthritis. *Arthritis Rheum.* 2006;54(3):899-907.
88. Baer AN, Witter FR, Petri M. Lupus and pregnancy. *Obstet Gynecol Surv.* 2011;66(10):639-653.
89. Jeon C, Agbai O, Butler D, Murase J. Dermatologic conditions in patients of color who are pregnant. *Int J Womens Dermatol.* 2017;3(1):30-36.
90. Kannuthurai V, Murray J, Chen L, Baker EA, Zickuhr L. Health care practitioners' confidence assessing lupus-related rashes in patients of color. *Lupus.* 2021;30(12):1998-2002.
91. Contreras G, Lenz O, Pardo V, et al. Outcomes in African Americans and Hispanics with lupus nephritis. *Kidney Int.* 2006;69(10):1846-1851.
92. Dalal DS, Patel KA, Patel MA. Systemic lupus erythematosus and pregnancy: a brief review. *J Obstet Gynecol India.* 2019;69:104-109.
93. Izmirly P, Kim M, Friedman DM, et al. Hydroxychloroquine to prevent recurrent congenital heart block in fetuses of anti-SSA/Ro-positive mothers. *J Am Coll Cardiol.* 2020;76(3):292-302.
94. Calderon LM, Pope JE. Scleroderma epidemiology update. *Curr Opin Rheumatol.* 2021;33(2):122-127.
95. Steen VD, Oddis CV, Conte CG, Janoski J, Casterline GZ, Medsger TA Jr. Incidence OF systemic sclerosis in allegheny county, Pennsylvania. A twenty-year study of hospital-diagnosed cases, 1963–1982. *Arthritis Rheum.* 1997;40(3):441-445.
96. Laing TJ, Gillespie BW, Toth MB, et al. Racial differences in scleroderma among women in Michigan. *Arthritis Rheum.* 1997;40(4):734-742.
97. Moore DF, Kramer E, Eltaraboulsi R, Steen VD. Increased morbidity and mortality of scleroderma in African Americans compared to non–African Americans. *Arthritis Care Res.* 2019;71(9):1154-1163.
98. Jaeger VK, Tikly M, Xu D, et al. Racial differences in systemic sclerosis disease presentation: a European Scleroderma Trials and Research group study. *Rheumatology.* 2020;59(7):1684-1694.
99. Clark KE, Etomi O, Ong VH. Systemic sclerosis in pregnancy. *Obstet Med.* 2020;13(3):105-111.
100. Janardana R, Nair AM, Surin AK, Prakash JAJ, Gowri M, Danda D. Unique clinical and autoantibody profile of a large Asian Indian cohort of scleroderma—do South Asians have a more aggressive disease? *Clin Rheum.* 2019;38:3179-3187.
101. Rabhi M, Tiev KP, Genereau T, Cabane J. Scleroderma and pregnancy. *Ann Med Interne (Paris).* 2002;153(3):193-200.
102. Spinillo A, Beneventi F, Ramoni V, et al. Prevalence and significance of previously undiagnosed rheumatic diseases in pregnancy. *Ann Rheum Dis.* 2012;71(6):918-923.
103. Spinillo A, Beneventi F, Epis OM, et al. Prevalence of undiagnosed autoimmune rheumatic diseases in the first trimester of pregnancy. Results of a two-steps strategy using a self-administered questionnaire and autoantibody testing. *BJOG.* 2008;115(1):51-57.
104. Deshauer S, Junek M, Baron M, Beattie KA, Larché MJ. Effect of pregnancy on scleroderma progression. *J Scleroderma Relat Disord.* 2023;8(1):27-30.
105. Brito-Zerón P, Baldini C, Bootsma H, et al. Sjögren syndrome. *Nat Rev Dis Primers.* 2016;2(1):1-20.
106. Ramos-Casals M, Brito-Zerón P, Sisó-Almirall A, Bosch X. Primary Sjögren syndrome. *BMJ.* 2012;344:e3821.
107. Tincani A, Andreoli L, Cavazzana I, et al. Novel aspects of Sjögren's syndrome in 2012. *BMC Med.* 2013;11:1-18.
108. Restrepo-Jiménez P, Molano-González N, Anaya J-M. Geoepidemiology of Sjögren's syndrome in Latin America. *Joint Bone Spine.* 2019;86(5): 620-626.
109. Brito-Zerón P, Acar-Denizli N, Ng WF, et al. Epidemiological profile and north–south gradient driving baseline systemic involvement of primary Sjögren's syndrome. *Rheumatology.* 2020;59(9):2350-2359.
110. Gupta S, Gupta N. Sjögren syndrome and pregnancy: a literature review. *Perm J.* 2017;21:16-47.
111. Brucato A, Frassi M, Franceschini F, et al. Risk of congenital complete heart block in newborns of mothers with anti-Ro/SSA antibodies detected by counterimmunoelectrophoresis: a prospective study of 100 women. *Arthritis Rheum.* 2001;44(8):1832-1835.
112. Brucato A, Cimaz R, Caporali R, Ramoni V, Buyon J. Pregnancy outcomes in patients with autoimmune diseases and anti-Ro/SSA antibodies. *Clin Rev Allergy Immunol.* 2011;40:27-41.
113. Rosenthal D, Druzin M, Chin C, Dubin A. A new therapeutic approach to the fetus with congenital complete heart block: preemptive, targeted therapy with dexamethasone. *Obstet Gynecol.* 1998;92(4):689-691.
114. Phillippi K, Hoeltzel M, Byun Robinson A, Kim S, Childhood Arthritis and Rheumatology Research Alliance (CARRA) Legacy Registry Investigators. Race, income, and disease outcomes in juvenile dermatomyositis. *J Pediatr.* 2017;184:38-44.e1.
115. Liu WC, Ho M, Koh WP, et al. An 11-year review of dermatomyositis in Asian patients. *Ann Acad Med Singap.* 2010;39(11):843.
116. Chinniah KJ, Mody GM. The spectrum of idiopathic inflammatory myopathies in South Africa. *Clin Rheumatol.* 2021;40:1437-1446.
117. Pinal-Fernandez I, Selva-O'Callaghan A, Fernandez-Codina A, et al. "Pregnancy in adult-onset idiopathic inflammatory myopathy": Report from a cohort of myositis patients from a single center. *Semin Arthritis Rheum.* 2014;44(2):234-240.
118. Yassaee M, Kovarik CL, Werth VP. Pregnancy-associated dermatomyositis. *Arch Dermatol.* 2009;145(8):952-953.
119. Munira S, Christopher-Stine L. Pregnancy in myositis and scleroderma. *Best Pract Res Clin Obstet Gynaecol.* 2020;64:59-67.
120. Safavi KH, Muller SA, Suman VJ, Moshell AN, Melton LJ 3rd. Incidence of alopecia areata in Olmsted County, Minnesota, 1975 through 1989. *Mayo Clin Proc.* 1995;70(7):628-633.
121. Lee H, Jung SJ, Patel AB, Thompson JM, Qureshi A, Cho E. Racial characteristics of alopecia areata in the United States. *J Am Acad Dermatol.* 2020;83(4): 1064-1070.
122. Darwin E, Hirt PA, Fertig R, Doliner B, Delcanto G, Jimenez JJ. Alopecia areata: review of epidemiology, clinical features, pathogenesis, and new treatment options. *Int J Trichology.* 2018;10(2):51.
123. Villasante Fricke AC, Miteva M. Epidemiology and burden of alopecia areata: a systematic review. *Clin Cosmet Investig Dermatol.* 2015;8:397-403.
124. Tan E, Tay YK, Giam YC. A clinical study of childhood alopecia areata in Singapore. *Pediatric Dermatol.* 2002;19(4):298-301.
125. Lundin M, Chawa S, Sachdev A, Bhanusali D, Seiffert-Sinha K, Sinha AA. Gender differences in alopecia areata. *J Drugs Dermatol.* 2014;13(4): 409-413.
126. Cho SI, Yu DA, Kim SI, Lee SM, Kwon O. Pregnancy outcomes in female patients with alopecia areata: a nationwide population-based study. *J Invest Dermatol.* 2021;141:1844-1847.
127. Kim JC, Choi JW. Impact of alopecia areata on subsequent pregnancy rate: a retrospective cohort study. *Australas J dermatol.* 2021;62(1):e121-e123.
128. Smorlesi C, Caldarella A, Caramelli L, Di Lollo S, Moroni F. Topically applied minoxidil may cause fetal malformation: a case report. *Birth Defects Res Part A Clin Mol Teratol.* 2003;67(12):997-1001.
129. Rybicki BA, Major M, Popovich J Jr, Maliarik MJ, Iannuzzi MC. Racial differences in sarcoidosis incidence: a 5-year study in a health maintenance organization. *American J Epidemiol.* 1997;145(3):234-241.
130. Köcher L, Rossides M, Remaeus, K et al. Maternal and infant outcomes in sarcoidosis pregnancy: a Swedish population-based cohort study of first births. *Respir Res.* 2020;21(1):225.
131. Hadid V, Patenaude V, Oddy L, Abenhaim HA. Sarcoidosis and pregnancy: obstetrical and neonatal outcomes in a population-based cohort of 7 million births. *J Perinat Med.* 2015;43(2):201-7.
132. Subramanian P, Chinthalapalli H, Krishnan M, et al. Pregnancy and sarcoidosis: an insight into the pathogenesis of hypercalciuria. *Chest.* 2004;126(3): 995-998.
133. Ellafi M, Valeyre D, Sarcoidosis and pregnancy. *Revue de Pneumologie Clinique.* 1999;55(5):335-337.
134. Lateef A, Petri M. Management of pregnancy in systemic lupus erythematosus. *Nat Rev Rheumatol.* 2012;8(12):710-718.
135. Butler DC, Heller MM, Murase JE, Safety of dermatologic medications in pregnancy and lactation: Part II. Lactation. *J Am Acad Dermatol.* 2014;70(3):417.e1-417.e10.

136. Garg AM, Mysore V. Dermatologic and cosmetic procedures in pregnancy. *J Cutan Aesthet Surg*. 2022;15(2):108.
137. U.S. Food and Drug Administration, Pregnancy and Lactation Labeling (Drugs) Final Rule. 2021.
138. Mygind H, Thulstrup AM, Pedersen L, Larsen H. Risk of intrauterine growth retardation, malformations and other birth outcomes in children after topical use of corticosteroid in pregnancy. *Acta Obstet Gynecol Scand*. 2002;81(3):234-239.
139. Mahé A, Perret JL, Ly F, Fall F, Rault JP, Dumont A. The cosmetic use of skin-lightening products during pregnancy in Dakar, Senegal: a common and potentially hazardous practice. *Trans R Soc Trop Med Hyg*. 2007;101(2): 183-187.
140. Chi CC, Wang SH, Wojnarowska F, Kirtschig G, Davies E, Bennett C. Safety of topical corticosteroids in pregnancy. *Cochrane Database Syst Rev*. 2015;2015(10):CD007346.
141. Zierler S, Purohit D. Prenatal antihistamine exposure and retrolental fibroplasia. *Am J Epidemiol*. 1986;123(1):192-196.
142. Kar S, Krishnan A, Mohankar A. A review of antihistamines used during pregnancy. *J Pharmacol Pharmacother*. 2012;3(2):105-108.
143. The use of newer asthma and allergy medications during pregnancy. *Ann Allergy Asthma Immunol*. 2000;84(5):475-480.
144. Bacq Y, Sentilhes L, Reyes HB, et al. Efficacy of ursodeoxycholic acid in treating intrahepatic cholestasis of pregnancy: a meta-analysis. *Gastroenterology*. 2012;143(6):1492-1501.
145. Chappell LC, Bell JL, Smith A, et al. Ursodeoxycholic acid versus placebo in women with intrahepatic cholestasis of pregnancy (PITCHES): a randomised controlled trial. *Lancet*. 2019;394(10201):849-860.
146. Walker KF, Chappell LC, Hague WM, Middleton P, Thornton JG. Pharmacological interventions for treating intrahepatic cholestasis of pregnancy. *Cochrane Database Syst Rev*. 2020;7(7):CD000493.
147. Sun G, Berthelot C, Li Y, et al. Poor prognosis in non-Caucasian patients with early-onset mycosis fungoides. *J Am Acad Dermatol*. 2009;60(2):231-235.
148. Tripathi R, Archibald LK, Mazmudar RS, et al. Racial differences in time to treatment for melanoma. *J Am Acad Dermatol*. 2020;83(3):854-859.
149. Shoo BA, Kashani-Sabet M. Melanoma arising in African-, Asian-, Latino- and native-American populations. *Semin Cutan Med Surg*. 2009;28(2):96-102.
150. Fitzsimons R, Greenberger PA, Patterson R. Outcome of pregnancy in women requiring corticosteroids for severe asthma. *J Allergy Clin Immunol*. 1986;78(2):349-353.
151. Sperber K, Hom C, Chao CP, Shapiro D, Ash J. Systematic review of hydroxychloroquine use in pregnant patients with autoimmune diseases. *Pediatr Rheumatol*. 2009;7:1-9.
152. World Health Organization. WHO guidelines for malaria. 2022.
153. Park KY, Kwon HJ, Wie JH, et al. Pregnancy outcomes in patients with vitiligo: a nationwide population-based cohort study from Korea. *J Am Acad Dermatol*. 2018;79(5):836-842.
154. Hung CT, Huang HH, Wang CK, et al. Pregnancy outcomes in women with vitiligo: a Taiwanese nationwide cohort study. *PLoS One*. 2021;16(3):e0248651.
155. Park KK, Murase JE. Narrowband UV-B phototherapy during pregnancy and folic acid depletion. *Arch Dermatol*. 2012;148(1):132-133.
156. Kebria AS, Hosseini M, Khafri S. The effect of narrowband ultraviolet B phototherapy on serum folate level. *Caspian J Intern Med*. 2021;12(2):180.
157. Davis SA, Narahari S, Feldman SR, Huang W, Pichardo-Geisinger RO, McMichael AJ. Top dermatologic conditions in patients of color: an analysis of nationally representative data. *J Drugs Dermatol*. 2012;11(4):466-473.
158. Horn EJ, Chambers CD, Menter A, Kimball AB, International Psoriasis Council. Pregnancy outcomes in psoriasis: why do we know so little? *J Am Acad Dermatol*. 2009;61(2):e5-e8.
159. Murase JE, Chan KK, Garite TJ, Cooper DM, Weinstein GD. Hormonal effect on psoriasis in pregnancy and post partum. *Arch Dermatol*. 2005;141(5): 601-606.
160. Boyd AS, Morris LF, Phillips CM, Menter MA. Psoriasis and pregnancy: hormone and immune system interaction. *Int J Dermatol*. 1996;35(3):169-172.
161. Johansen CB, Egeberg A, Jimenez-Solem E, Skov L, Thomsen SF. Psoriasis and adverse pregnancy outcomes: a nationwide case-control study in 491,274 women in Denmark. *JAAD Int*. 2022;7:146-155.
162. Bae Y-SC, Van Voorhees AS, Hsu S, et al. Review of treatment options for psoriasis in pregnant or lactating women: from the Medical Board of the National Psoriasis Foundation. *J Am Acad Dermatol*. 2012;67(3):459-477.
163. Kaushik SB, Lebwohl MG. Psoriasis: which therapy for which patient: focus on special populations and chronic infections. *J Am Acad Dermatol*. 2019;80(1):43-53.
164. Murase JE, Heller MM, Butler DC. Safety of dermatologic medications in pregnancy and lactation: Part I. Pregnancy. *J Am Acad Dermatol*. 2014;70(3):401.e1-14.
165. Butler DC, Heller MM, Murase JE. Safety of dermatologic medications in pregnancy and lactation: Part II. Lactation. *J Am Acad Dermatol*. 2014;70(3):417.e1-10.
166. Vaughan Jones S, Hern S, Nelson-Piercy C, Seed PT, Black MM. A prospective study of 200 women with dermatoses of pregnancy correlating clinical findings with hormonal and immunopathological profiles. *Br J Dermatol*. 1999;141(1):71-81.
167. Kemmett D, Tidman M. The influence of the menstrual cycle and pregnancy on atopic dermatitis. *Br J Dermatol*. 1991;125(1):59-61.
168. Weatherhead S, Robson SC, Reynolds NJ. Eczema in pregnancy. *BMJ*. 2007;335(7611):152-154.
169. Koutroulis I, Papoutsis J, Kroumpouzos G. Atopic dermatitis in pregnancy: current status and challenges. *Obstet Gynecol Surv*. 2011;66(10):654-663.
170. Balakirski G, Novak N. Atopic dermatitis and pregnancy. *J Allergy Clin Immunol*. 2022;149(4):1185-1194.
171. Khamisy-Farah R, Damiani G, Kong JD, Wu JH, Bragazzi NL. Safety profile of Dupilumab during pregnancy: A data mining and disproportionality analysis of over 37,000 reports from the WHO individual case safety reporting database (VigiBase™). *Eur Rev Med Pharmacol Sci*. 2021;25(17):5448-5451.
172. Glynn JR, Caraël M, Auvert B, et al. Why do young women have a much higher prevalence of HIV than young men? A study in Kisumu, Kenya and Ndola, Zambia. *AIDS*. 2001;15:S51-S60.
173. Woods CW, McRill C, Plikaytis BD, et al. Coccidioidomycosis in human immunodeficiency virus-infected persons in Arizona, 1994–1997: incidence, risk factors, and prevention. *J Infect Dis*. 2000;181(4):1428-1434.
174. Vaughan J, Ramirez H. Coccidioidomycosis as a complication of pregnancy. *Calif Med*. 1951;74(2):121.
175. Smith CE, Beard RR. Varieties of coccidioidal infection in relation to the epidemiology and control of the diseases. *Am J Public Health Nations Health*. 1946;36(12):1394-1402.
176. Ruddy BE, Mayer AP, Ko MG, et al. Coccidioidomycosis in African Americans. *Mayo Clinic Proc*. 2011;86:63–69.
177. Gibbs S. Skin disease and socioeconomic conditions in rural Africa: Tanzania. *Int J Dermatol*. 1996;35(9):633-639.
178. Mosam A, Irusen EM, Kagoro H, Aboobaker J, Dlova N. The impact of human immunodeficiency virus/acquired immunodeficiency syndrome (HIV/AIDS) on skin disease in KwaZulu-Natal, South Africa. *International J Dermatol*. 2004;43(10):782-783.
179. Rodgers S, K.S. Leslie KS. Skin infections in HIV-infected individuals in the era of HAART. *Curr Opin Infect Dis*. 2011;24(2):124-129.
180. Alonso N, Lugo-Somolinos A, Torres-Paoli D, Sánchez JL. Prevalence of skin disease in HIV-positive pregnant women. *Int J Dermatol*. 2003;42(7): 521-523.
181. Coopman SA, Johnson RA, Platt R, Stern RS. Cutaneous disease and drug reactions in HIV infection. *N Engl J Med*. 1993;328(23):1670-1674.
182. Amerson EH, Maurer TA. Dermatologic manifestations of HIV in Africa. *Top HIV Med*. 2010;18(1):16-22.
183. Resneck JS Jr, Van Beek M, Furmanski L, et al. Etiology of pruritic papular eruption with HIV infection in Uganda. *JAMA*. 2004;292(21):2614-2621.
184. Hevia O, Jimenez-Acosta F, Ceballos PI, Gould EW, Penneys NS. Pruritic papular eruption of the acquired immunodeficiency syndrome: a clinicopathologic study. *J Am Acad Dermatol*. 1991;24(2):231-235.
185. Gordin FM, Simon GL, Wofsy CB, Mills J. Adverse reactions to trimethoprim-sulfamethoxazole in patients with the acquired immunodeficiency syndrome. *Ann Intern Med*. 1984;100(4):495-499.
186. Kondo W, Carraro EA, Prandel E, et al. Nevirapine-induced side effects in pregnant women: experience of a Brazilian university hospital. *Braz J Infect Dis*. 2007;11:544-548.
187. Eke AC, Mirochnick M, Lockman S. Antiretroviral therapy and adverse pregnancy outcomes in people living with HIV. *N Engl J Med*. 2023;388(4): 344-356.
188. de Ruiter A, Taylor GP, Clayden P, et al. British HIV Association guidelines for the management of HIV infection in pregnant women 2012 (2014 interim review). *HIV Med*. 2014;15(Suppl 4):1-77.
189. Ford N, Mofenson L, Kranzer K, et al. Safety of efavirenz in first-trimester of pregnancy: a systematic review and meta-analysis of outcomes from observational cohorts. *AIDS*. 2010;24(10):1461-1470.
190. Ford N, Calmy A, Mofenson L. Safety of efavirenz in the first trimester of pregnancy: an updated systematic review and meta-analysis. *AIDS*. 2011;25(18):2301-2304.
191. Eke AC, Olagunju A, Momper J, et al. Optimizing pharmacology studies in pregnant and lactating women using lessons from HIV: a consensus statement. *Clin Pharmacol Ther*. 2021;110(1):36-48.
192. Thauvin-Robinet C, Maingueneau C, Robert E, et al. Exposure to hydroxyurea during pregnancy: a case series. *Leukemia*. 2001;15(8):1309-1311.

193. Lanzkron S, Strouse JJ, Wilson R, et al. Systematic review: hydroxyurea for the treatment of adults with sickle cell disease. *Ann Intern Med*. 2008;148(12): 939-955.
194. Cleary BJ, Donnelly J, Strawbridge J, et al. Methadone dose and neonatal abstinence syndrome—systematic review and meta-analysis. *Addiction*. 2010;105(12):2071-2084.
195. Cackovic M, Chung C, Bolton LL, Kerstein MD. Leg ulceration in the sickle cell patient. *J Am Coll Surg*. 1998;187(3):307-309.
196. Droitcourt C, Khosrotehrani K, Girot R, Aractingi S. Healing of sickle cell ulcers during pregnancy: a favourable effect of foetal cell transfer? *J Eur Acad Dermatol Venereol*. 2008;22(10):1256-1257.
197. Bleet T, Spontaneous healing of sickle cell anemia ulcer in pregnancy. *JAMA*. 1952;148(12):1025-1026.
198. Reed JD, Redding-Lallinger R, Orringer EP. Nutrition and sickle cell disease. *Am J Hematol*. 1987;24(4):441-455.

CHAPTER 103

Pediatrics

Domenica Del Pozo
Nanette Silverberg
Joni Mazza-McCrann
Candrice R. Heath

KEY POINTS

- The population of children with skin of color in the United States is growing rapidly.
- There are clinical findings and treatment caveats in children with skin of color due to biologic properties of the hair, skin, and nails.
- Cultural practices and, for many, the impact of social determinants of health influence disease presentation, severity, and treatment.

INTRODUCTION

Children of color are often underserved in their needs as the majority of dermatology textbooks have been written about Caucasian children and most prescription drugs have been tested primarily in Caucasian children.[1] Ten percent of visits to pediatricians are for skin issues, and 30% of all dermatology appointments are made for children.[2] By the year 2050, almost half of the U.S. population will be non-Caucasian.[3] Thus, dermatologic education for those caring for children with skin of color is a priority.

Children of color have specific reactions to injury. They are more susceptible to keloid and hypertrophic scar development.[2] Most children with darker skin tones will develop a pigmentary alteration in response to inflammatory skin conditions, including, but not limited to, atopic dermatitis, pityriasis rosea, and acne.[3] Pigmentation, both hyperpigmentation and hypopigmentation, may be more noticeable and consequently more disturbing to children, particularly adolescents of color and their parents. Furthermore, lichenoid dermatologic responses are more common in children of color, resulting in cases of lichenoid atopic dermatitis, hypertrophic lichen planus, and lichenoid contact dermatitis.

Immunologic and metabolic reaction patterns in children of color are different as well. Higher rates of diabetes, poor vitamin D levels due to melanin-related sun protection, and alterations in enzymes such as low levels of glucose-6-phosphate dehydrogenase (G6PD) may all serve to contribute to skin disease development and ability to tolerate standard dermatologic therapeutics (eg, dapsone).

African American children are more susceptible to dry scalp, traction related hair loss, and tinea capitis. Other concerns include elliptical hair follicles and reduced flow of sebum on the hair shaft,[4] leaving the African American child more susceptible to dry hair and traction-related hair loss.

This chapter is meant to provide an overview of skin conditions seen in children of color and includes 10 sections: newborn skin conditions, dermatitis, papulosquamous disorders, acneiform skin conditions, autoimmune and collagen vascular diseases, vascular birthmarks, pigmentary diseases, traumatic, hair disorders, and infections. The sections will be limited to conditions not covered elsewhere in the text or will provide added information pertinent to pediatric patients supplemental to other chapters. Due to the complexity of the topic, only a limited number of conditions are covered in depth.

SECTION I: NEWBORN SKIN CONDITIONS

NORMAL VARIATION

From birth to adulthood, skin pigmentation changes gradually. In children with skin of color, pigmentation at birth is concentrated in the hair and other regions of the body. A cross-sectional study of 1000 newborns in India, examined in the first 4 years of life, found that there were areas of pigmentation change on the skin due to melanin including linea nigra (44.5%), outer ear (49.6%), knuckles (57.6%), genital (20.2%), axillary pigmentation (25.6%), and dermal melanocytosis (84.7%).[5] Infants with skin of color have thin, straighter hair in the first months of life and begins to undulate or thicken with age. Newborns are often covered with soft, fine lanugo hair. As newborns mature, the lanugo hair is reduced and replaced with body site-dependent vellus and terminal hairs.

Other normal variants of infancy and childhood include pigmentary mosaicism and greater tendency toward postinflammatory hypopigmentation.

CONGENITAL DERMAL MELANOCYTOSIS

Congenital dermal melanocytosis (CDM), previously known as Mongolian spots, are benign lesions typically seen over the lumbar and sacral-gluteal regions of infants and children. These areas of hyperpigmentation are due to the incomplete migration of melanocytes from the dermis to the epidermis. Gray, green to blue pigmentation of lesions is dependent on the depth of melanocytes in the dermis and the quantity of melanin carried in melanocytes. CDM is predominantly seen among infants and children with skin of color. A study found that 96% of African American children presented with CDM lesions in comparison to 10% of Caucasian children.[6]

CDM are either present at birth or develop within the first few weeks of life and tend to fade by first year of life and may persist past 6 years of life. Commonly, CDM presents in well-appearing infants and children as asymptomatic hyperpigmented 2- to 8-cm macules and patches. Rare associations with congenital anomalies, such as lysosomal storage disorders and other inborn errors of metabolism, have been documented in literature.

Other blue gray hyperpigmented lesions like blue nevi, nevus of Ota, nevus of Ito, and dermal melanocyte hamartoma are in the differential diagnosis of CDM. Also, extensive spots in atypical locations can make it difficult to distinguish CDM from child abuse. Children with extensive CDM lesions are at a higher risk of being mistakenly categorized as victims of child abuse, especially if there is poor documentation of lesions in infancy.[7] If there is uncertainty with the diagnosis, lesions should be documented and reevaluated within a couple days. Ecchymoses will tend to change colors while evolving into later stages and CDM lesions go unchanged. Physicians with limited exposure to CDM characteristics and localization can contribute to inaccuracy of diagnosis. Congenital dermal melanocytosis spontaneously improves or resolves with age, so treatment is focused on observation. Persistent CDM lesion can be covered up with medical makeup or removed with laser therapy if desired.

TRANSIENT NEONATAL PUSTULAR MELANOSIS

Transient neonatal pustular melanosis (TNPM) is a benign, asymptomatic, and self-limiting vesicopustular disease of the newborn.[8] TNPM is a neonatal pustular rash mainly affecting Black infants. Nonerythematous cutaneous lesions present as vesicles or pustules that can rupture within the first hours of life and heal to become hyperpigmented macules with collarette scaling.[9] Subsequent macules fade within 4 weeks but may persist for several months. This rash is often seen on the forehead, chin, retroauricular area, torso, palms, and soles of infants and has no associated systemic symptoms.[9] TNPM have no associated mortality and morbidity. The different stages of TNPM may be associated with gestational age as vesicular lesions are usually present on term infants, while hyperpigmented macules are often seen on postterm infants upon birth.

The etiology of this neonatal condition is not fully understood. Biopsy of lesions can be done but not advised. On Tzanck smear, pustules will predominately contain neutrophils with some cellular debris. On histopathology, collections of subcorneal and intracorneal neutrophils with few eosinophils can be visualized.[10] Furthermore, vesicopustular lesions are not exclusive to TNPM and may also be seen in infectious illnesses like neonatal impetigo, herpes simplex, varicella zoster, candidiasis, syphilis, and scabies.[11] Misdiagnosing TNPM can lead to inappropriate antibiotic use. Further still, other neonatal cutaneous disorders should be considered in the differential diagnosis like sterile neonatal pustulosis and erythema toxicum neonatorum.

TNPM is a benign condition that does not require pharmaceutical management. Nature and progression of rash should be adequately explained to parents. TNPM does not have long-term effects and should not impede infants from meeting childhood milestones.

CLEAR CELL PAPULOSIS

Clear cell papulosis (CCP) is a rare skin condition that presents before 6 years of age as eruptions of flat-topped papules and hypopigmented macules. These macules can vary in coloration as they can appear flesh-colored or completely depigmented. Abdominal distribution of these lesions is common, but they can also be seen in the pubic and axillary regions. CCP has an Asian predominance as there have only been six documented cases in non-Asian children and zero in African individuals.[12-15] Researchers hypothesize that the inheritance of CCP may be autosomal recessive and may have a female predominance.[15]

Biopsy of lesions demonstrates epidermal acanthosis with normal melanocytes, yet minimal epidermal pigmentation. On histopathology, clear cells have a centrally located nuclei with ample, pale cytoplasm.[12] These cells are significantly larger than normal appearing keratinocytes and are usually scattered in the basal cell layer of epidermis. Clear cells consistently stain negative for S-100 and CD1a but can stain positive for mucin, CEA, epithelial membrane antigen, Cytokeratin AE1 and/or AE3, and many others.[12,15] Due to decreased melanin staining, it appears as if CCP may have a defect in melanogenesis.

Similar to TNPM, etiology is unknown. CCP is a clinical diagnosis but can be confirmed via biopsy, histopathology, and immunohistochemical studies. Differential diagnosis such as verruca plana, tinea versicolor-like epidermodysplasia verruciformis, lichen sclerosus, pityriasis lichenoides chronica, guttate morphea, and guttate vitiligo. CCP lesions will completely or partially self-resolve in early to late childhood with 11.5 years being the median age. There is no treatment for CCP, but patients should be monitored for resolution or exacerbation of lesions. A 2010 report by Tseng et al followed 19 patients with biopsy-proven CCP. Some patients had complete resolution, some had decreased lesion counts, and others had the same the same number of lesions, but the lesions lightened over time. No cases developed malignant transformation, with the longest observation period being 21 years.[16] Malignant transformation seems low based on the reported cases highlighting the natural history of CCP but may still occur. More information is needed on the pathogenesis of this rare condition.[17]

SECTION II: DERMATITIS

SEBORRHEIC DERMATITIS

Seborrheic dermatitis is a chronic inflammatory skin condition characterized by erythema, greasy scaling, and pruritus. This condition is often seen on the nasolabial folds of the face, scalp, anterior chest, and upper back, which are areas highly dense with sebaceous glands.[18] In infants, the two most common presentations are cradle cap and diaper distribution. Seborrheic dermatitis affecting the scalp may be accompanied by hair loss. The degree of severity in seborrheic dermatitis can range from a simple dermatitis to psoriasiform plaques. In patients with skin of color, this condition may present with postinflammatory hypopigmentation and petaloid patches and plaques.[19] Individuals with a darker complexion tend to have limited erythema when compared to those with lighter complexion. Seborrheic dermatitis affects all ages and has a peak between 2 and 12 months of age and another peak after 18 years of age.

The underlying mechanism of seborrheic dermatitis is multifactorial, as it is associated with changes in microbiology, immunology, and genetics. There are different phases in the pathogenesis. It is theorized that sebaceous glands secrete lipids and *Malassezia* fungus (*M. restricta and M. globosa)* colonize the skin surface lipid.[20] These colonies release lipase, which breaks down lipids to free fatty acids and lipid peroxides activating an inflammatory reaction. Different cytokines and leukotrienes stimulate keratinocyte proliferation. This process disrupts skin barrier function and contributes to the clinical presentation of seborrheic dermatitis. The genetic component of seborrheic dermatitis is unclear, but researchers have noted that there are certain HLA alleles that are more prevalent among individuals with seborrheic dermatitis.

The differential diagnosis for this cutaneous skin condition varies with age. In infants and children, Langerhans cell histiocytosis and tinea capitis must be considered. Tinea capitis can be ruled out via a fungal culture. Other differential diagnoses include psoriasis, atopic dermatitis, pityriasis versicolor, and nutritional efficiency.[20] Infantile seborrheic dermatitis is self-limiting as it tends to resolve within 6 to 12 months of age. Emollient can be used for the softening and removal of the white/yellow scales.[20] Ketoconazole 1% to 2% cream can be used twice daily for 2 weeks if needed. Low to mid potency corticosteroid cream can be used to reduce inflammation.[20,21] In patients with skin of color, haircare management should be discussed in detail as some antidandruff shampoos may be drying. [22]

ATOPIC DERMATITIS

Atopic dermatitis is a chronic inflammatory disease primarily seen in children. This disorder presents within the first 5 years of life and is associated with the development of additional atopic comorbidities. Further still, the atopic march is a notion that claims that children who develop atopic dermatitis will subsequently develop allergic rhinitis, food allergies, and asthma. Some literature has reported an increased risk of allergic rhinitis in White children and an increased risk of asthma in Black children after atopic dermatitis onset.[23] Recently, the traditional atopic march hypothesis has been challenged as some argue that the atopic march does not have a racial predilection.[24,25] In the United States, 18% of children are affected by atopic dermatitis.[26] While often a disorder of childhood, patients may have symptoms persisting into adulthood. The pathogenesis of atopic dermatitis is multifactorial in that immune dysregulation, skin barrier defect, genetics, and environmental factors may play a role in the onset and severity of disease. In a cohort of 741 children with atopic dermatitis, researchers found that the filaggrin loss of function variants were higher among White children in comparison to African American children.[27]

The prevalence, severity, and management of AD among different populations may be influenced by social, environmental, and economic factors. A recent prospective cohort study found that children who were female, Black, or multiracial living in urban communities had a higher prevalence of persistent AD.[28] Moreover, the financial commitment to appropriately manage AD has been found to be heavier among Black individuals as they are often under- or uninsured.[29] While unclear what role social determinates of health have on the pathophysiology of atopic dermatitis, it plays a role in overall AD management.

Atopic dermatitis is characterized by eczematous and pruritic plaques. Children with darker complexions commonly present with papulation, lichenification,[30] follicular prominence, nummular plaques, lichenoid papules, and dyspigmentation.[22] Black patients tend to have hyperlinearity of the palms, darkened periorbital circles, Dennie-Morgan lines, and prurigo nodularis. The distribution of atopic dermatitis lesions varies with age. Among Asian patients, psoriasiform features are common.[31] In infants, eczematous lesions are on the face or extensor surfaces. In school-aged children, common locations of lesions are flexural areas.

Atopic dermatitis is a clinical diagnosis. The American academy of dermatology has diagnostic criterion for atopic dermatitis that describes the presence of essential, important, and associated features.[32] Patients with suspected atopic dermatitis must have essential features like pruritis, eczema, typical morphology, and chronic or relapse history. Patients with atopic dermatitis are increased risk of acquiring *Staphylococcus aureus*, *Beta-hemolytic Streptococcus,* and at times herpes simplex infection. Management of lesions includes topical corticosteroids, calcineurin inhibitors, JAK inhibitors, Il-4 and IL-13 inhibitors, as well as immunosuppressants. Dupilumab, a monoclonal antibody that inhibits Il-4 and Il-3 activity, was approved to treat moderate-to-severe AD in children and is first-choice treatment among providers. JAK inhibitors usage is increasing as it has shown rapid improvement within a week of atopic dermatitis symptoms. Among children with severe AD, methotrexate can be used as a first-line treatment option. Further still, acute AD flares are often managed with short-term topical steroids.[33]

ALLERGIC CONTACT DERMATITIS

Allergic contact dermatitis is a type IV hypersensitivity reaction to inorganic and/or organic antigens. Allergens that cause allergic contact dermatitis varies among races and are often detected via patch testing. Positive patch tests are easier to ascertain on lighter complexions and more difficult on darker complexions.[34] Detection of nuance skin changes for patch tests requires training in assessing skin of color patients. Additionally, allergic contact dermatitis tends to present differently among darker complexions with lichenification and hyperpigmentation being more common than erythematous vesicles.[34] Scalp contact dermatitis can be erroneously diagnosed as seborrheic dermatitis due to its atypical presentation in minority populations.[34] Being unfamiliar with how contact dermatitis presents in skin of color patients can delay diagnosis and negatively affect disease management. Children of color tend to be exposed to antigens at an earlier age via cultural practices. For example, children from some cultural backgrounds, including those from some Spanish-speaking nations are accustomed to getting their ears pierced within the first months of life. While the quality of the earrings varies, nickel-laden earrings may precipitate an allergic contact dermatitis reaction in children. Prevention of allergic contact dermatitis is avoidance of exacerbating antigens and management is via avoidance and topical anti-inflammatory agents. Patch testing, which is typically used to elucidate new allergens in patients with allergic contact dermatitis, is completed less often for children with darker complexions. This disparity is multifactorial as socioeconomic factors may limit patients with skin of color from adequately receiving patch testing.[35]

SECTION III: PAPULOSQUAMOUS DISORDERS

PSORIASIS

Psoriasis is a noncommunicable, immune-mediated inflammatory disease. This cutaneous disorder is seen in children, adolescents, and adults. In children, psoriasis may be more subtle and thus difficult to diagnose. Psoriasis is a common skin condition across different racial groups. Among Black and Hispanic individuals, psoriasis may be underdiagnosed when compared to their White counterparts. In the United States, the combined prevalence of psoriasis in Hispanic and Black adults is 3.6% and in Black children is 0.06%.[36] Studies done in Asia estimate psoriasis prevalence in adults at 0.05% to 0.47% and studies done in Mexico and South America have found a 1.3% to 4.2% prevalence of psoriasis among Latinx populations.[36] The development of Psoriasis is multifactorial as genetics and environmental factors may play a role in its development.

Clinical presentation and distribution of psoriasis lesions varies within age categories. In infants, lesions are erythematous plaques without scaling in the genital region, specifically in the inguinal folds. Infants may present on the scalp with thick scaly plaques. In toddlers, plaques are thin with a white scale often localized to the face, scalp, and flexures. Older children can present with psoriasis lesions in the ear canal, the medial upper eyelids, as well as, pitting of the nail plate. Children can also present with guttate psoriasis, which is transient and presents as scaly papules after a streptococcal or viral infection. Typical psoriasis lesions differ between patients with skin of color and those who are White. In African American patients, cutaneous lesions can be hyperpigmented or violaceous, plaques are thicker, and erythema is minimal.[36,37] In White individuals, lesions are red or pink with silver scaling. Additionally, patients with skin of color typically have postinflammatory hyperpigmentation.

Psoriasis in children is a clinical diagnosis. A consensus-agreed diagnostic criteria was recently developed to accurately diagnose psoriasis in children. A UK multicenter case-control study looked at the diagnostic accuracy of 16 diagnostic criteria. Criteria includes scale and erythema involving the hairline, persistent well-demarcated facial rash, nail pitting, and many more.[38,39] Researchers found that if at least two of the seven best predictive diagnostic criteria were met, psoriasis would be identified in greater than 70% of children.[38] Biologic medications have been approved for management of moderate to severe psoriasis in pediatric populations. There are biologic medications approved for psoriasis for pediatric patients including adalimumab, etanercept, ustekinumab,[40] and ixekizumab. Additionally, changes in hair products can help reduce exacerbation of scalp lesions. Psoriasis is a relapsing skin disorder that will require consideration of polytherapy to reduce flares.[41]

PITYRIASIS ROSEA

Pityriasis Rosea was first discovered in 1860 and was described as pink, fine branny scales. This exanthematous cutaneous disease is closely associated with human herpes virus 6 and 7.[42] This disease starts as two distinct stages: single erythematous Herald plaque on the trunk or face followed by a second eruption on torso cleavage lines (Langer lines). Atypical manifestations of pityriasis rosea includes atypical herald patch location, PR gigantic of Darier, limb-girdle distribution, and atypical papular and papulovesicular morphology.[43] The Christmas tree presentation is the most common Pityriasis rosea variant. Pityriasis Rosea affects healthy children and presents with the classic oval and scaly herald patch lesion. It takes up to 21 days for the secondary lesions to form.

In a study done to assess the prevalence of pityriasis rosea in the United States, researchers found that out of 327,624 patients about 0.21% had a diagnosis of pityriasis rosea.[44] When looking at the prevalence of pityriasis rosea in specific racial groups, Black, Asian, Hispanic, and White patients had similar prevalence.[44] While the prevalence may be similar across racial groups, presentation of disease is different. In White children, salmon-colored plaques are limited to the central body and inner arms. In patients with darker complexions, pityriasis rosea presents as pruritic violaceous plaques and often has an inverse pattern. A descriptive study of 50 Black children with pityriasis rosea found that 80% of those patients had scalp lesions.[45] There is literature suggesting that face and scalp involvement is common among children with darker complexions. Postinflammatory hyperpigmented or hypopigmented plaques were also common among African patients as the papulosquamous plaques flattened and cleared.

Pityriasis rosea is a clinical diagnosis. Diagnostic criteria includes the presence of discrete oval or circular scaly macules or plaques and peripheral collarette scales on at least two lesions. Skin biopsy can be done to exclude other cutaneous disorders as histology will typically show focal parakeratosis, spongiosis, and acanthosis in the epidermis as well as red blood cells and white blood cells in the dermis.[43] Differential diagnosis includes lichen planus, nummular eczema, pityriasis rosea-like medication-induced eruption, guttate psoriasis, and tinea corporis. Cutaneous disorders listed above can be distinguished clinically with a thorough history and physical exam as well as a skin biopsy of lesions. Pityriasis rosea is a self-limiting disorder that resolves within 3 to 6 weeks. Disease relapse is uncommon with an occurrence of 2% to 3%.[43,46] In children with skin of color, postinflammatory lesions will resolve with months or years from onset. Patients with pityriasis rosea are managed symptomatically. Topical corticosteroids may be used for pruritic symptoms, if present.[47]

LICHEN PLANUS

Lichen Planus is an inflammatory disorder that affects skin, oral mucosa, scalp, and nails. Its classic clinical presentation are flat-topped, violaceous polygonal papules or plaques associated with pruritis and erythema. A white lacy lesion, known as Wickham striae, can also be seen in oral mucosa. This cutaneous disease is more commonly seen in adults and rarely in children. Of all documented cases of lichen planus, children and infants make up less than 4%.[48] In a systemic review looking at pediatric lichen planus, investigators found that among their study group 51% of pediatric patients presented with classic lichen planus features with 22% of patients also having mucosal involvement.[48] The classic pattern of lichen planus has been noted as the most occurring pattern in pediatric populations. In sub-Saharan Africa, pigmented form of lichen planus can sometimes be seen, but literature has found it to be most common among Afro-American, Afro-Caribbean, Hispanics, and Asians.[49,50] While oral lichen planus is extremely rare in children, a recent Italian case series of 13 children documented the presence of oral lesions of varying patterns (reticular, plaque-like, papular, and erythematous).[51] Oral lichen planus has been documented in literature to be most prevalent in Asian patients. As mentioned prior, lichen planus in children is not well looked into due to sparsity of data. In adults and children, lichen planus does not have a racial preference, but it must be noted that a lot of the case reports in literature look at a predominately Indian patient population. A retrospective study done in the United States found a predominance of classic lichen planus in African American children and more atypical patterns in Caucasian patients.[49] Postinflammatory hyperpigmentation may last for months to years.[52]

Moreover, differential diagnosis of lichen planus may include discoid lupus erythematosus, linear psoriasis, and inflammatory linear verrucous epidermal nevus. Biopsy of lichen planus lesions shows degeneration of basal layer of epidermis with lymphocytic infiltrates along the dermo-epidermal junction. Destruction of the basal layer can result in a "saw-tooth" pattern at the dermo-epidermal junction alongside of epidermal hyperplasia and orthokeratosis.

Treatment guidelines for pediatric lichen planus have not been established. In a systemic review looking at lichen planus in a pediatric population, medium to high potency topical corticosteroids were the most common medications used and systemic corticosteroids were second-most common.[48] Children with limited disease or lighter skin complexion should be initiated on topical steroids. Children with generalized disease or darker complexions should be initiated on systemic corticosteroids as they may prevent post inflammatory hyperpigmentation.[48] Phototherapy is rarely used for children with lichen planus. Symptoms such as pruritis can be managed with antihistamines.[48] Pediatric lichen planus has a good prognosis and rate of recurrence is minimal.

MYCOSIS FUNGOIDES

Mycosis Fungoides (MF) is a cutaneous T-cell lymphoma seen primarily in adults and in less than 1% of children. The cases that have been reported in children are characterized as atypical variants of Mycosis Fungoides. Because these atypical variants are rare, little is known about prognosis. A systemic review found that in a cohort of 567 children, 54.5% presented with the hypopigmented variant of mycosis fungoides.[53] Hypopigmented mycosis fungoides is a variant commonly seen in children and more so in children with darker complexions (Fitzpatrick skin type IV-VI). While in adults, CD4+ T-cells predominate, in children, studies have found a CD8+ T-cell predominance.[53,54] Loss of CD7 is a specific finding associated with mycoides fungoides.[54] Knowing that childhood-onset mycosis fungoides has a CD8+ T-cell predominance will assist in diagnosing mycosis fungoides at a young age. Delayed diagnosis of MF is common due to its phenotypic similarities to other childhood cutaneous conditions.

Hypopigmented mycosis fungoides clinically presents as scaly erythema on a hypopigmented patch. Erythema may be absent. These patches can present alongside telangiectasia and poikilodermatous lesions. These patches can be biopsied, and histopathology will show atypical lymphocytes with hyperchromatic, cerebriform nuclei in the epidermis and dermis. Differential diagnosis of hypopigmented MF include atopic dermatitis, vitiligo, tinea versicolor, PLEVA, and PLC. Management of hypopigmented MF includes phototherapy (NBUVB, ultraviolet A, and psoralen), topical corticosteroids, and nitrogen mustard. More specifically, among the pediatric population, NBUVB, UVA therapies have been found to be the most effective at managing folliculotropic and nonfolliculotropic MF variants in children under 18 years of age.[55] In a study of nine children with hypopigmented MF, researchers found that four patients achieved partial resolution of MF with NBUVB, while one patient achieved complete resolution.[54] Early diagnosis and treatment of childhood MF is ideal to achieve good prognosis.

PITYRIASIS LICHENOIDES ET VARIOLIFORMIS ACUTA AND PITYRIASIS LICHENOIDES CHROMONICUM (PLEVA AND PLC)

Pityriasis lichenoides has three documented variants: PLEVA, PLC, and febrile ulceronecrotic Mucha-Habermann disease.[56] PLEVA is a rare inflammatory rash present in patients of different races and primarily among children and young adults. PLEVA has been noted to occur after administration of childhood vaccines, such as influenza, MMR, and human papillomavirus. PLEVA presents with erythematous macules and transition into inflammatory papules with scaling. These lesions are self-limiting and resolve between 1 and 3 years but can ulcerate into red-brown crusts or transform into chronic PLC lesions. The characteristic red, scaly macules of PLC can persist for several years. PLEVA and PLC lesions are localized to the chest and back. Diagnosis of PLEVA and PLC is clinical, but biopsy of lesions should be done to rule out other diagnosis. Differential diagnosis such as pityriasis rosea, guttate psoriasis, and hypopigmented mycosis fungoides should be considered. Phototherapy, oral antibiotics, and topical corticosteroids have been trialed for management of pityriasis lichenoides.[57] Erythromycin is given to children to reduce inflammation and is usually given until lesion resolution.[57] If lesions persist, ultraviolet B light phototherapy can be used in children. Overall, pityriasis lichenoides has a great prognosis, except for febrile ulceronecrotic Mucha-Habermann disease, which may be lethal.

SECTION IV: ACNEIFORM SKIN CONDITIONS

ACROPUSTULOSIS OF INFANCY

Acropustulosis of infancy is a pruritic rash affecting palms and soles. These lesions may transition from vesicles to pustules and, subsequently, postinflammatory hyperpigmentation. The onset of infantile acropustulosis is within the first year of life and is frequently seen among Black children.[58,59] Acropustulosis of infancy is cyclic with relapses frequently until complete resolution, which occurs by 2 to 3 years of age.[60] Management of disease is symptomatic. Potent topical corticosteroids are primarily used to relieve itching. Dapsone has been used in severe infantile acropustulosis cases but requires careful hematologic monitoring.[61,62] Differential diagnosis for infantile acropustulosis includes scabies, erythema toxicum neonatorum, bacterial skin infection, and coxsackievirus infection. Scabies can be ruled out using scabies prep, as it may co-occur with or happen before acropustulosis ensues. Some have hypothesized that acropustulosis of infancy may be a hypersensitivity response to scabies.[63]

ACNE

Acne is an inflammatory skin disease characterized by open and closed comedones, papules, and pustules commonly seen in adolescents and adults. Acne among children can be categorized based on age as neonatal (less than 6 weeks old), infantile (6 weeks to 12 months), and mid-childhood (1-7 years).[64] Neonatal and infantile acne have been associated with increased androgen production by adrenal glands, which subsequently stimulates sebum production inducing inflammatory lesions. Mid-childhood acne is extremely uncommon since healthy children between the ages of 1 and 7 are not producing androgen via adrenal glands.[64] While exogenous production of androgens should be ruled out in all childhood acne categories, mid-childhood acne should be worked-up thoroughly for underlying systemic pathology. Endocrine work-up should include assessment of bone age, DHEA, testosterone, FSH, prolactin, and 17-hydroxy-progesterone levels.

Pomade acne is a subtype of comedonal and papular acne localized to the forehead and temples. Pomades are hair products used to manage hair texture, hair strength, and overall scalp health and are commonly used by skin of color individuals.[65] Skin of color patients are more likely to use comedogenic hair products and thus are more likely to present with forehead acne. While most of these associations have been primarily studied in adults, children of parents with similar hair textures and routines may present with similar acne distributions. Pomade acne in children of color begins on the forehead with open and closed comedones and small papules, progressing at times to papules and pustules.

Acne should be managed conservatively as to avoid scarring or depigmentation. In children, acne management should be kept simple and targeted. Neonatal and infantile acne are self-limiting and require no pharmacological treatment as it resolves within a couple months or by 5 years of age, respectively.[64] Acne regimen will vary based on severity of disease and age of patient as certain medications are contraindicated in children. Topical retinoid and benzoyl peroxide are recommended for targeting comedones or papules. Oral antibiotics are used for moderate disease and isotretinoin for severe or scarring acne. A recent study assessing shared decision-making (SDM) on acne care found that skin of color patients were 1.8 times more likely to engage in SDM than White individuals.[66] This participation in SDM may be due to patient advocacy for culturally competent care and increased physician knowledge on skin of color disorders. There are still barriers to care, such as language and accessibility, that need to be optimized to improve dermatological care satisfaction among skin of color patients.

PERIORIFICIAL DERMATITIS

Periorificial dermatitis is a benign acneiform eruption of the face. Erythematous monomorphic papules are localized to perioral, perinasal, and periocular regions. Among children, periorificial dermatitis can be seen as early as 3 months of age and has a female preference. The two variants seen in pediatric populations are childhood granulomatous periorificial dermatitis (CGPD) and lupus miliaris. CGPD is a benign red-brown papular rash that affects children with darker complexions.[67] Pediatric periorificial dermatitis is associated with atopic comorbidities like asthma and atopic dermatitis, family history of atopies, and steroid exposure.

Periorificial dermatitis is a clinical diagnosis as additional laboratory exams and biopsy are typically unrevealing and will not change management of disease. The standard treatment is topical metronidazole twice daily and/or oral erythromycin. Average resolution with pharmaceutical management is 1 to 2 months. Similarly, CGPD can be managed with a topical and oral antibiotic but has a slightly longer time of resolution of up to 6 months.[67]

SECTION V: AUTOIMMUNE AND COLLAGEN VASCULAR DISORDERS

SARCOIDOSIS

As a systemic granulomatous disease, sarcoidosis affects multiple organs and is primarily seen in young adults during the third or fourth decades of life. Sarcoidosis in children is rare but when seen under the age of 4, it presents as rashes, arthritis, and uveitis, and in older children, it primarily manifest as uveitis and pulmonary dysfunction.[68] Sarcoidosis is strongly associated with race in adults as prevalence and incidence are significantly higher in African American individuals compared to Caucasian patients. This racial predilection has also been noted in children as most pediatric cases have been documented in Black children. In African American patients, sarcoidosis is more severe and occurs at a younger age than White patients.[69] Sarcoidosis being a multisystem disease will have varying and at times nonspecific clinical presentations. Cutaneous lesions can be red or brown flat-topped papules localized to the face or larger plaque-like lesions on trunk and extremities. In young children, systemic-onset juvenile rheumatoid arthritis should be ruled out as it presents with a similar triad as sarcoidosis. Diagnosis of sarcoidosis in children may be done using imaging, blood work, and biopsy. Symptomatic children are managed with topical, oral, or inhaled corticosteroids.

LUPUS

Lupus erythematous is a chronic autoimmune disorder that is typified by the production of antinuclear antibodies and immune complexes for multi-organ damage. Lupus affects both adults and children, with children presenting more acutely and across several organ systems.[70] Systemic lupus erythematous (SLE) is the most common variant, while cutaneous lupus erythematosus (CLE) variants like discoid lupus, acute cutaneous lupus, and subacute cutaneous lupus are less prevalent. Childhood SLE occurs prior to 18 years old and is more severe than adult SLE. There is an SLE predominance in minority children with Native American, Black, Asian, and Hispanic children being predominately affected.[71] There are racial disparities associated with childhood SLE. Black children with SLE were at higher risk of adverse renal outcomes and non-White children with SLE were at higher risk of developing depression.[71] Contributors to racial disparities in childhood SLE are not fully understood, but socioeconomic factors may play a role.

Neonatal lupus is acquired in utero via the transplacental passage of maternal autoantibodies to fetus.[72] A recent retrospective cohort study found that patients with skin of color were significantly more likely to have cutaneous neonatal lupus at birth, as well as a maternal history of SLE.[73] Neonatal lupus skin findings are characterized as annular erythematous plaques with co-occurring periorbital erythema, or atrophic, scaly, telangiectatic discoid lesions that can be present at birth or after sun exposure. Lesions are typically apparent in sun-exposed areas such as face, neck, and upper extremities. In general, children with cutaneous neonatal lupus are at increased risk of developing cardiac complications, this is especially true among children with skin of color.[71] Other organs may be involved in neonatal lupus, although less common. Cutaneous lesions resolve within a few months, but hypopigmentation may remain for at least a year. Interestingly, there is a correlation between absence of maternal autoantibodies in infant blood and resolution of skin findings.[74] Multi-disciplinary management should be expected for infants with neonatal lupus for monitoring of extracutaneous manifestations of disease, especially heart blocks.

SECTION VI: VASCULAR BIRTHMARKS

INFANTILE HEMANGIOMAS

Infantile hemangiomas are the most common pediatric vascular tumors, which affects about 5% to 10% of infants.[75] Risk factors for infantile hemangiomas includes female sex, Caucasian race, prematurity, and family history of infantile hemangiomas. Caucasian children had increased risk of infantile hemangiomas than African American, Asian, and Native American children.[76] While children with infantile hemangiomas is typically managed outpatient, some require hospitalization. In a recent study, researchers have documented racial discrepancies among infants hospitalized for infantile hemangiomas. Among those with infantile hemangiomas, Black infants were older upon hospitalization than White infants and had a higher prevalence of hematological disorders, umbilical hernias, and retinal disorders.[76] It is hypothesized that the later age of hospitalization seen among Black infants is likely due to healthcare disparities. This suggests that Black infants had limited access to care and so often had more severe presentation of disease. Misdiagnosis of infantile hemangiomas in Black infants can occur due to lack of medical provider education on how infantile hemangiomas present in darker skin tones. A retrospective cohort study of 804 children seen at a large academic center found that children with lower socioeconomic status (SES) had a higher odds of presenting for care later; however, those enrolled in their institution-facilitated managed care program did not present any later than peers within the institution-facilitated managed care program from higher SES.[77] The authors highlighted that the patients having pediatricians in the same institution allowed ease of communication, and a scheduling protocol that facilitated timely hemangioma evaluations likely contributed to these findings.[77]

Clinical presentation of infantile hemangiomas varies as it can be located between the superficial dermis all the way down to the subcutaneous tissue. Those that are within the superficial dermis will present as red plaques, while infantile hemangiomas that are deeper in the dermis will present as skin-color or blue subcutaneous mass.[75] Furthermore, infantile hemangiomas vary in pattern of involvement as they can be focal covering a single localized area or segmental as they cover larger, expansive areas. Infantile hemangiomas can go beyond cutaneous presentation with its association with PHACE and LUMBAR syndrome.[75] Hispanic infants had stronger associations with PHACE syndrome and had higher rates of complications. The infantile hemangioma severity scale is one of many scales that can be used to guide management of disease. While infantile hemangiomas can resolve with time, some require systemic treatment. Propranolol is the first-line agent for infantile hemangioma management.[78] Other systemic treatments like atenolol, nadolol, corticosteroids, and sirolimus could be considered in specific cases. Topical therapy with timolol could be considered for superficial infantile hemangiomas.[78] Ulceration is the most common complication of infantile hemangiomas and should be managed with appropriate wound care.

SECTION VII: PIGMENTARY DISEASES

VITILIGO

Vitiligo is an autoimmune condition that has multifactorial etiology including genetic tendency and environmental triggers including trauma, sun exposure, and infections, which results in loss of melanocyte function and/or destruction of melanocytes at the site of inflammation. Vitiligo has been loosely subtyped into nonsegmental vitiligo, which encompasses all generalized forms including periorificial localizations, folds, flexures, and acrofacial. Segmental vitiligo affects one-third of children and is localized to a broad stripe corresponding to the lines of Blaschko. A recent study looked at proxy reported vitiligo prevalence yielding 1.52% in children and 2.16% in adolescents.[79,80] Clinician-adjudicated prevalence is 0.84% and 1.19%, respectively. Two-thirds are nonsegmental. Around the world pockets of increased prevalence exist including on the Indian subcontinent, which can be associated with stigma.[81]

Vitiligo pathogenesis is felt to occur when an injury or trauma causes the melanocytes antigens to be exposed to autoimmune attack. Contribution of loss of tolerance, polymorphisms of the melanocytic genes, and a complex of genetic alterations to innate immunity, T- and B-cell activation occurs. The currently recognized pathogenesis involves activated CD8+ T-cells attacking the skin producing interferon gamma that in turn binds to the receptor through a JAK/STAT dependent pathway, releasing substances that promote keratinocyte release of CXCL9/10 that home more T-cells to the region, in a self-promoting feedback loop. Finally, IL 15 + T-cells of the SALT system home to the area and set up long-term residence in the disease regions.[82-86]

The differential diagnosis includes all conditions that are Woods lamp positive, which can range from benign magic marker marks to milk moustaches, to illnesses such as mycosis fungoides, which requires biopsy to distinguish. It is important to note that overlap or mimic can occur between vitiligo and lichen sclerosis et atrophicus in the groin [87] and genetic disorders of pigmentation such as piebaldism.[88,89]

Treatment is a four-pronged approach of screening for secondary autoimmunity, such as thyroid disease, whether through careful history and examination or via laboratory examinations including thyroid function testing, antibodies to thyroid that can identify subclinical thyroid disease, complete blood counts that can identify early signs of pernicious anemia, and Vitamin D levels that can reflect increased autoimmune tendency. Prong two is a good topical skin care regimen that will include the usage of agents shown to have efficacy including topical corticosteroids, topical calcineurin inhibitors for segmental facial and genital regions, and topical ruxolitinib 1.5% cream that has been FDA approved in the United States for nonsegmental vitiligo in children ages 12 years and over.[90] Excimer/308-nm laser can enhance repigmentation especially in facial and segmental disease.[91] Narrow-band UVB can stabilize and repigment in generalized disease, with 2 to 3 sessions a week for a year being required for best outcomes.[92] Systemic medications can be used in severe cases and JAK inhibitors are being tested for long-term usage in vitiligo at this time. The long-term prognosis is that segmental vitiligo repigmentation is fastest in the first 6 months and thereafter may be resistant to therapy, while nonsegmental vitiligo may take a slow, progressive course over time if left untreated.

ACROPIGMENTATION OF DOHI

Acropigmentation of Dohi, also known as dyschromatosis symmetrica hereditaria and symmetrical dyschromatosis, is a rare genetic disorder with autosomal dominant inheritance[93,94] with high penetrance.[95] There have also been reports of recessive inheritance.[95-97] The gene identified in acropigmentation of Dohi is adenosine deaminase acting on RHA 1 (*ADAR1*).[96] Most cases of acropigmentation of Dohi in the literature detail patients from Japan, but patients from other places, like India, have also been reported.[93,94]

Characteristically, the depigmentation is mottled, patchy, and reticulated. The dyspigmentation is most commonly limited to the dorsal hands and dorsal feet. However, it may also appear on the arms and legs. The pigmentation begins before the age of 6 years. The pigmentation spreads to the extremities only in 50% of those affected. The other 50% also have involvement of the face. By adolescence, the total amount of skin involvement is solidified, remains stable, and is permanent.[95,96] The differential diagnosis includes Dowling-Degos disease, reticulate pigmentation of Kitamura, dyschromatosis universalis hereditaria, and xeroderma pigmentosa. Dermatoscopy may be useful in diagnosis as it depicts honeycomb pattern reticulate pigment networks on a pink to brown background. This condition is genetic and not preventable. The skin involvement remains stable after adolescence, but there are reports of patients developing dystonia and mental deterioration.[95]

COLE SYNDROME

Cole syndrome, also known as dyskeratosis congenita of Zinsser-Cole-Engman, Zinsser-Cole-Engman syndrome, dyskeratosis congenita, Hoyeraal-Hreidarsson syndrome, or Revesz syndrome, results from defects in *DKC1* (X-linked), which codes for dyskerin, *TERC* (autosomal dominant), which codes for mRNA for telomeres, *TERT* (autosomal dominant), which codes for telomerase enzyme, and *NOP10* (autosomal recessive). These four genes only account for 40% of the people with Cole syndrome.[98] *NHP2, TIN2, C16orf57*, and *TCAB1* genes may also cause Cole syndrome. Patients with Cole syndrome have short telomeres and difficulty properly maintaining the telomeres.[99]

Patients with Cole syndrome have dystrophic nails, oral leukoplakia, and reticulated hyperpigmentation of the face, neck, and shoulders. Other organ systems affected include the gastrointestinal, dental, genitourinary, neurologic, pulmonary, ophthalmic, and skeletal systems. The presenting findings are most commonly reticulated hyperpigmentation and nail dystrophy. The most life-threatening feature of this syndrome is bone marrow failure, which usually appears in early adulthood. Half of Cole syndrome patients develop aplastic anemia by the time they are 20 years old, and most patients will have bone marrow failure by age 30 years. Specific early childhood variants exist; these are called Hoyeraal-Hreidarsson syndrome and Revesz syndrome. Those with

Hoyeraal-Hreidarsson syndrome demonstrate low T- and B-cells during childhood.[100]

The diagnosis can be made when the classic clinical findings are present, despite the patient having no hematologic abnormality. However, in a patient with hematologic abnormalities without the classic clinical findings, flow cytometry with fluorescence in situ hybridization can be used to evaluate the length of the telomeres in leukocytes. Unlike other acquired forms of aplastic anemia, the telomeres are short in all subsets of leukocytes in patients with Cole syndrome.[100]

The differential diagnosis includes graft-versus-host disease and Rothmund-Thomson syndrome. The treatment of choice is stem cell transplantation from a matched sibling. Alternative treatments for those with hematopoietic dysfunction that have shown varied success include androgens with or without granulocyte colony-stimulating factor.[98]

The prognosis is grim. While those with autosomal dominant inheritance have milder disease, those with X-linked inherited disease have a severe course. Neuropsychiatry problems are more common in patients with dyskeratosis congenital.[100] Patients usually succumb to aplastic anemia, failed bone marrow transplant, or malignancies. There is a risk of head, neck, oropharyngeal, and gastrointestinal system cancers and squamous cell carcinomas.[98]

ERYTHEMA DYSCHROMICUM PERSTANS

Erythema dyschromicum perstans (EDP), also known as ashy dermatosis, or los cientos is uncommon.[101] EDP, a pigmentation disorder, most commonly affects the young adult population in patients of color.[101,102] However, pediatric cases have been reported. EDP was initially described in South Americans and most commonly affects Hispanics. It has also been reported in people of other racial groups including those of African descent, Caucasians, Asians, and East Indians[102] Prepubertal cases are more common in Caucasians compared with Hispanics.[102,103] No sex predilection has been found in children, but in adults, the disease is more common in females.[102,104]

Some cases of EDP have followed exposure to pharmaceutical drugs, infections, ammonium nitrate, intestinal parasites, oral contrast media, cobalt, and chlorothalonil, among others, but the exact cause of EDP is unknown.[102,104] Genetic susceptibility also likely plays a role. In EDP, the clinical hue of the 0.5- to 3-cm macules and patches is slate gray to blue. The slate gray oval macules, patches, and plaques begin on the trunk and spread centrifugally, also affecting the extremities.[102] The lesions may also be polycyclic or irregularly shaped.[104] When the lesions first appear, they are often surrounded by erythema, but the erythema resolves as lesions expand. Not only may the border of the lesion be erythematous, but it may also be elevated. Although the histologic pattern of EDP itself is nonspecific, skin biopsy can help distinguish EDP from other pigment disorders. The differential diagnosis includes extensive fixed drug eruption, lichen planus, lichen planus pigmentosus, lichen planus-like drug eruption, incontinentia pigmenti, pinta, Addison disease, contact dermatitis, hemochromatosis, and leprosy.[102-104]

EDP is difficult to treat and often lasts for many years in adults, whereas it often resolves after 2 to 3 years in children.[102,103] Treatments that have been tried for EDP include clofazimine, dapsone, antibiotics, corticosteroids, chemical peels, vitamins, tetracyclines, antihistamines, griseofulvin, isoniazid, chloroquine, and psychotherapy.[101] A recent case series found that when used at the earliest inflammatory disease state of EDP, prednisone can be used to improve dyspigmentation within 3 weeks of steroid use. Further still, researchers noted that isotretinoin can be used in addition to prednisone to clear any remaining hyperpigmentation and promote a remission state of disease.[105] Photoprotection is essential in preventing further darkening of the lesions. The exact etiology of EDP is unknown. EDP may pose a significant cosmetic problem for those affected. However, EDP does not lead to any systemic abnormalities.

LONGITUDINAL MELANONYCHIA

Longitudinal melanonychia is more common in those with darker skin tones. When longitudinal melanonychia is present, the initial worry is often if the patient has melanoma, which is rare in pediatric patients. However, the most common cause of longitudinal melanonychia in the pediatric population is a nevus of the nail matrix. The signs that may suggest melanoma in adults include Hutchinson sign, new onset of pigmentation, multiple irregular bands of color, hazy band borders and onychodystrophy. However, in pediatric patients, these signs do not consistently predict those with melanoma.[106,107] Lee et al studied 381 Asian children with 703 longitudinal melanonychia and 17 had biopsies performed; none were melanoma,[108] but biopsy should still be considered if there is high concern.[107] Some lesions may regress after several years, but more studies are needed.[107,108] Watchful waiting with reexamination and progress photos is recommended as part of conservative management.

MUCOSAL PIGMENTATION

Mucosal pigmentation (also known as black gums),[109] particularly of the gingiva, is a prominent feature found in patients with skin of color (see Chapter 56).[110] The gingival and oral mucosal pigmentation often correlates with the cutaneous pigmentation.[111] In a study of 600 people of African descent, those with darkly pigmented skin were more likely to have darkly pigmented gingiva. However, many of the patients with darkly pigmented skin did not have darkly pigmented gingiva.[112,113] Patients with this disease have confluent brown gingiva or brown patches present on gingiva. The pigmentation may even have a gray-blue hue.

The differential diagnosis includes benign pigmentation, Addison disease, Albright syndrome, blue nevi, melanocytic macule, oral melanoacanthoma, oral nevi, Peutz-Jeghers syndrome, smoker's melanosis, melanoma, and amalgam tattoo.[114] Once underlying systemic conditions causing oral mucosal pigmentation have been excluded (eg, Addison disease), treatment options or reassurance can be discussed. Gingival hyperpigmentation in itself is not dangerous; therefore, medically, it requires no treatment.

However, adolescents or parents of children may be concerned about the cosmetic appearance. Various cosmetic techniques have been used to lighten the pigmentation of the gingiva including electrosurgery, scalpel surgical excision, surgical abrasion,[115] liquid nitrogen application,[116] and acellular dermal matrix with partial-thickness flap.[117] Prevention is not possible if a child's mucosal pigment is due solely to the level of genetically predetermined cutaneous pigmentation. However, acquired gingival pigmentation has been seen in the children who have at least one parent who smokes.[118] In this case, limiting a child's exposure to secondhand smoke and discouraging teens from smoking may prevent not only acquired gingival pigmentation but also exacerbation of other diseases, like asthma.

SECTION VIII: TRAUMATIC

CUPPING AND COINING (CAO GIO)

Cupping and cao gio is a therapeutic practice common in Southeast Asian cultures for cleansing and healing. This practice can be divided into two phases: (1) a smooth stone, coin, or spoon is used to create linear bruises along a participant's back and (2) a heated cup is placed on the skin creating a suction effect that promotes edematous and ecchymosed lesions. These annular and linear purpuric lesions can be mistaken for early signs of physical child abuse. Physicians who are unaware of such cultural practice are at a higher risk of misdiagnosis and escalating benign findings to child protective services.[119] To minimize diagnosing errors, culturally competent pediatric dermatologists or child abuse teams should be consulted for confirmation.

KELOIDS [FIGURE 103-1]

Keloids are reviewed elsewhere in this textbook; however, some specific clinical points in childhood bear review. Keloids are more common in individuals of color.[120] For children of color with a family history of keloids, careful evaluation regarding elective procedures is needed. Although younger children are less likely to form keloids, keloids can occur at any age.[120] In the pediatric population, a complete history

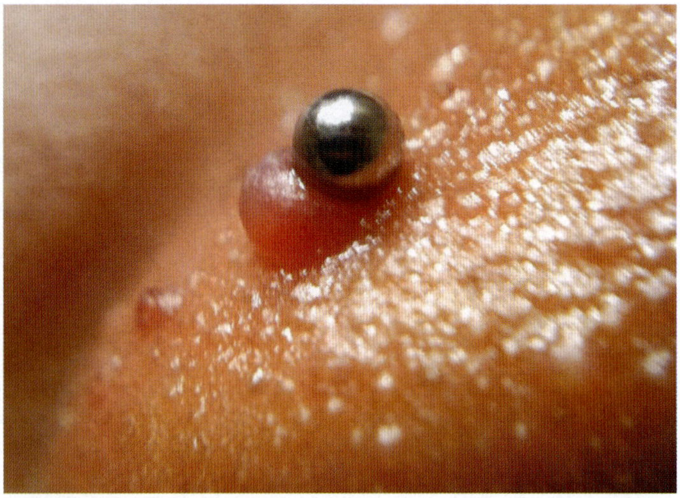

FIGURE 103-1. This 15-year-old African American girl developed a keloid adjacent to her nose piercing.

should be obtained. Keloids most commonly follow skin trauma; however, spontaneous keloid development may occur as a feature of a genetic syndrome like Rubstein-Taybi syndrome,[121] Dubowitz syndrome,[122] or nodular or keloidal scleroderma.[123]

Often parents with keloids or a family history of keloids inquire about the risks of piercing their child's ears. One study found that children who pierced their ears early in life (before age 11 years) were less likely to develop keloids.[124] However, Tirgan et al[125] reported bilateral earlobe keloids in a 9-month-old child following ear piercing at age 3 months. The child had a family history of keloid development. Although early ear piercing is recommended if desired by parents, there is still no guarantee that keloids will not develop.

If keloids occur, treatments such as intralesional triamcinolone are appropriate, but special comfort measures should be taken in the pediatric population.[126] Topical numbing medication and/or distractors such as cellphone games or videos may reduce the child's anxiety about the procedure. In children who undergo surgical keloid repair, care must be taken to evaluate whether the child will be able to tolerate postoperative measures (intralesional triamcinolone, pressure earrings, silicone dressings, or pressure dressings). If general anesthesia is used, the risks and benefits should be weighed.[127]

SECTION IX: HAIR DISORDERS

TRICHORRHEXIS NODOSA

Trichorrhexis nodosa is a hair shaft anomaly in which broomstick deformity occurs in the hair shaft causing brittle hair and breakage at the site of the deformity. While trichorrhexis nodosa can be seen in several genodermatoses, the condition can also be acquired. Acquired proximal trichorrhexis nodosa has been described in skin of color patients as fragile, easily breakable hair that clinically resembles hair that has been cut very close to the scalp, without evidence of alopecia or hair loss. Large areas of the scalp can be involved, often the occiput or frontal scalp but not the entire scalp. This condition is likely related to chemical, thermal, or mechanical hair treatments and can occur even after years of hair processing with no adverse effects. The hair breakage can also persist for years after the discontinuation of traumatic hair processing. An underlying genetic susceptibility has been suggested.[128] Diagnosis can be made via clipped hair mounts or through trichoscopy of hair in vivo for lighter-skinned patients or via dermoscopy of clipped hairs against a white background.[129]

BUBBLE HAIRS

Bubble hair occurs in people of all races. In children of African descent, various techniques are used to help with hair manageability. Due to tightly coiled hair shafts, braids, chemical relaxers, and heat are often used to straighten the hair shafts for ease of hair styling in children and adults. Bubble hair, with air-filled spaces in the hair shaft, is caused by the application of thermal heat to the hair shaft. The bubbles in the hair shaft are filled with a gas. The heat may be delivered by an overheating blow dryer, curling iron, or flat iron. Blow dryers operating at ≥175°C may cause bubble hair.[130]

Clinical examination may reveal dry, wiry, coarse, lusterless hair or areas of alopecia due to hair breakage.[130,131] Trichorrhexis nodosa and trichoptilosis may also be present. Bubbles are visible on light microscopy, while electron microscopy demonstrates loss of cortical and medulla cells at the affected sites along the hair shaft.[132] The differential diagnosis includes trichorrhexis nodosa, trichoptilosis, and monilethrix.

Cutting off the damaged hair may be a quick fix. However, without proper prevention practices like limiting the amount or temperature of heat applied to the hair shaft, bubble hair may recur. Patients should be advised to avoid prolonged exposure to hot dryers and curling irons.[131] Detwiler et al[130] suggest that hair trapped in the coils of hair dryers contributes to overheating of the hair dryer. Hair dryer coils should be free of hair and free of any obstruction. Bubble hair is an acquired hair shaft abnormality. New hair, unexposed to the heat necessary to form bubble hair, inherently will not have the bubble hair abnormality.

HYPERTRICHOSIS

A child's genetic predisposition drives the amount of normal hair that is present. Some ethnic groups like Hispanics and those of Indian descent commonly have a higher density of body hair. A study performed on 422 Caucasian girls and 434 African American girls revealed that 8.9% and 48.8%, respectively, were observed to have upper lip hair. The limitation highlighted in the study concerned whether the authors found more hair on the upper lips of African American girls because it was just easier to see.[133] Hypertrichosis, unlike nonidiopathic hirsutism, is not driven by androgens. In addition to genetic predisposition, hypertrichosis may be caused by medications.[134]

After establishing an underlying diagnosis, some patients or parents may seek cosmetic improvement. On a patient-by-patient basis, hair removal methods may be explored. Lasers, including the long-pulse alexandrite (755 nm) with cooling, long-pulse Nd:YAG (1064 nm) with cooling, and long-pulse ruby (694 nm), have been used successfully in treating children.[135] Children are at risk for the well-known potential side effects of lasers including burns, discomfort, postinflammatory pigment alteration, and damage to the eyes. The child's Fitzpatrick skin type should determine the specific laser chosen and settings. To increase pediatric patient comfort, topical anesthetics are often used. However, care must be taken to abide by dosage guidelines to avoid systemic side effects.[136]

Depilatories are commonly used among adults but have also been used in children with hypertrichosis. Irritation is a potential side effect, and therefore, a test spot should be performed. Increasing the time between depilatory applications will also decrease irritation. Topical hydrocortisone may be applied following the depilatory treatment to reduce irritation.[137]

TRACTION ALOPECIA

Traction alopecia typically presents as thinning at the temporal and frontal regions of the scalp and represents years of prolonged tension on the hair, typically from tight hairstyles such as braiding. In early stages, the traction can also cause an associated folliculitis. This preventable condition, if recognized early, can be corrected by discontinuing the tight hairstyles and removing the tension and pull on the hair follicle. Full regrowth can be demonstrated within months. However, if these practices continue into adulthood, the perifollicular inflammation can lead to permanent scar formation. In these cases, treatment with intralesional steroid injections may be helpful to prevent further scarring.[128] Despite early intervention with hair care practice modifications being key to prevent permanent scarring from traction alopecia, discussing traction alopecia with parents may be challenging but is necessary.[22]

Alopecia areata, particularly the ophiasis pattern, is the main differential diagnosis of traction alopecia. These conditions can occasionally be distinguished by the presence of terminal hairs still present in the affected areas of patients with traction alopecia.[138]

CENTRAL CENTRIFUGAL CICATRICIAL ALOPECIA

Central centrifugal cicatricial alopecia (CCCA) is often diagnosed in adult Black women; however, it may present during childhood and adolescence. CCCA is covered in another section of this textbook, but there are some caveats in children and adolescents.

Barriers to early diagnosis may include low clinical suspicion, decreased awareness of CCCA occurring in this age group, and inadequate scalp examination due to clinician discomfort with examining tightly coiled hair.[139]

Treatments are like those in adults with potent topical steroids, oral antibiotics (ie, doxycycline in those 8 years and above), and intralesional corticosteroids as tolerated. Tetracyclines, like doxycycline, can cause teeth staining in those under 8 years old.

SECTION X: INFECTIONS

TINEA CAPITIS

Tinea capitis (TC, commonly known as ringworm) is a dermatophyte infection of the hair and scalp. Although tinea capitis can affect any age group, children between the ages of 3 and 11 years are most likely to develop disease. In the United States, tinea capitis disproportionately affects African American children, followed by Hispanic children.[140] While the cause of this is unknown, genetic susceptibilities and socioeconomic factors have been postulated.[140] Prior to the 1970s, most tinea capitis was caused by highly inflammatory zoonotic dermatophytes that fluoresced under Wood lamp. From 1974 to 1994, a rise in the number of *Trichophyton tonsurans* cases in San Francisco, CA, was reported.[141] *T. tonsurans*, which causes an endothrix, does not fluoresce and is found only in humans. *T. tonsurans* remains the most common dermatophyte to cause tinea capitis (>95%).[140]

Tinea capitis is generally a clinical diagnosis in the setting of alopecia, hyperkeratosis (scale) and often occipital lymphadenopathy, though this latter finding is nonspecific.[142,143] A case series of TC pediatric patients in NYC found that the presence of scalp hyperkeratosis and alopecia was associated with mycologically confirmed TC in 82.1% of patients.[144] Visualization of "black dots" occurs in TC caused by endothrix and remains a helpful diagnostic finding. Trichoscopy can also aid in this diagnosis with comma hairs and corkscrew hairs common in both curly and straight-haired patients.[145] In more inflammatory presentations of TC, V-shaped hairs, scale, follicular hyperkeratosis, crusts, pustules, and erythema can also be seen.[145,146]

A scalp fungal culture may be performed for suspected tinea capitis by rubbing a cotton-tipped applicator over the scalp.[147] If there is a suppurative inflammatory reaction present, as in the setting of kerion, it is appropriate to perform a bacterial culture to rule out a bacterial superinfection.

Wood lamps were frequently used to examine the scalp of a person with suspected tinea capitis because zoonotic fluorescing *Microsporum* species (*Microsporum canis* and *Microsporum audouinii*) were the leading cause of infection in the United States in the 1950s. However, *T. tonsurans*, the most common cause of tinea capitis in the United States, does not fluoresce.[148] Kerions and inflammatory tinea capitis may still be caused by *Microsporum* species, and fluorescing the scalp with a Wood lamp may be helpful in that setting. *M. canis* fluoresces white and *M. audouinii* fluoresces blue-green.[149]

It is important to note that *T. tonsurans* causes minimal to no inflammation in the early stages of disease. Additionally, the seborrheic dermatitis-like presentation may be initially "treated" by parents with scalp oils, pomades, and grease camouflaging the TC even further and leading to delayed presentation for treatment or more difficulty for clinicians in making the diagnosis. These subtle finding significantly increase the rate of silent transmission among family members through the shared use of combs, brushes, hats, etc.

To ensure treatment of all the keratinized hair extending into the follicles, systemic treatment is necessary to eradicate tinea capitis. *T. tonsurans* is the most common dermatophyte causing tinea capitis in the United States. The most common treatment options include terbinafine and griseofulvin. Griseofulvin suspension was originally prescribed at 5 to 10 mg/kg/day, but higher, off-label dosages of 20 to 25 mg/kg/day are more commonly used. The higher dosing of griseofulvin can be estimated by adding a zero to the weight in pounds. For example, a 25-pound child would receive 250 mg daily.[150] In a recent systematic review of the literature, terbinafine (dosing per FDA-approved weight-based dosing) and itraconazole (5 mg/kg/day) had the highest mycological cure rate for *T. tonsurans* infection, while griseofulvin and terbinafine had the highest clinical cure rates,[151] and treat non-*Tonsurans* spp. *Trichophyton* TC.[152] For *Microsporum* species, griseofulvin remains the treatment of choice.

Prevention begins with avoidance of shared household items (hairstyling tools, clothing, pillowcases) and the washing or replacing of such items weekly during active infection. Although children are the most commonly affected by tinea capitis, consider undiagnosed adults in the home who many have tinea capitis in families with multiple episodes of tinea capitis.

Children diagnosed with tinea capitis may return to school after instituting systemic treatment. However, those engaged in contact sports with a lot of skin-to-skin contact, like wrestling or judo, require special "return to play" instructions.

Tinea capitis is a benign condition. The alopecia associated with tinea capitis is usually temporary and typically nonscarring. However, permanent alopecia may occur following extensive cases of kerion. Recurrence and reinfection are not uncommon, and vigilance in monitoring for signs of disease (especially hyperkeratosis and alopecia) is required even after successful therapy.

TINEA VERSICOLOR

Tinea versicolor is an overgrowth of *Malassezia* species in the seborrheic distribution, usually over the chest, back, and shoulders. Tinea versicolor is rarely seen in infants, with most cases occurring in adolescence through young adulthood, particularly seasonally in warm weather. Significant pigment changes can be seen in adolescents of color. In contrast to lighter-skinned patients where lesions can present as pink, or hypo or hyperpigmented, TV lesions in darker-skinned patients are often hypopigmented, as well as more likely to be present on the head and neck.[152] Treatment involves topical agents such as selenium sulfide or topical azole antifungals and, in more extensive cases, brief courses of oral antifungals. Continued use of weekly lotion or shampoo applications can be helpful at preventing recurrence in warmer months. Excessive sun exposure while infected is ill advised due to aggravation of color disparity.

WHITE PIEDRA

White piedra (trichosporosis) is a superficial fungal/saprophytic yeast infection caused by *Trichosporon* species.[153,154] *Trichosporon* are found in soil, water, air, animal feces, and sewage.[155] Most cases of white piedra occur in tropical regions, but it can occur in any country, regardless of climate. Transmission to humans occurs, but the exact mechanism is unknown.[153-155]

Increased incidence of white piedra has been noted in patients who frequently use head coverings. Shivaprakash et al [155] suggest that the absence of hair's exposure to "germicidal properties" of sunlight and humid temperature under head coverings may be contributory factors. Kiken et al [153] reported eight children with white piedra, two of whom were siblings and seven of whom had long hair. Most of the children were from Latin America or the Middle East. Close contact and long hair may also be factors in developing white piedra.[153]

Upon examination of the hair shaft, white to tan/brown nodules are present. The white-tan nodules are irregularly shaped and feel gritty.

Unlike pediculosis capitis and black piedra, white piedra can easily be removed from the hair shaft. White piedra may affect any hair-bearing area including the scalp, face (beard, mustache, eyebrows, eyelashes), axillae, and pubic area.[153]

Direct microscopy of the hair shaft with 10% potassium hydroxide mount helps to distinguish white piedra from pediculosis.[153,156] Hyphae and arthroconidia are visualized in white piedra.[154] White piedra does not fluoresce under Wood lamp examination, in contrast to trichomycosis axillaris, which fluoresces coral pink. Fungal and bacterial cultures will distinguish white piedra from trichomycosis axillaris.[154] The differential diagnosis includes pediculosis capitis, trichomycosis axillaris, monilethrix, and peripilar keratin cast.

Cutting off all of the hair is one treatment option. However, Kiken et al [153] report achieving clearance of white piedra with a combination of oral antifungals and antifungal shampoo, without cutting the hair. Therapeutic regimens that can be used include oral ketoconazole or oral fluconazole for a 1-month period accompanied by frequent use of topical ketoconazole 2% shampoo to eliminate the reservoir of fungus on the scalp. Shampoos should be continued until a month after fungal concretions have been eliminated.[153] *Trichosporon* is ubiquitous in South America and the Middle East and is therefore difficult to avoid. Avoidance of sharing hats, combs, brushes, and pillowcases is the best prevention; however, the actual mode of transmission of the disease is unknown, so prevention is difficult. The prognosis is excellent. Most cases can be cleared with therapy similar to that of tinea capitis.

REFERENCES

1. Silverberg NB. *Atlas of Pediatric Cutaneous Biodiversity*. New York, NY: Springer, 2012.
2. Schachner LA, Hansen RG. Preface. In: Schachner LA, Hansen RC, eds. *Pediatric Dermatology*. 2nd ed. New York, NY: Churchill-Livingstone; 1995.
3. U.S. Census estimates. http://www.census.gov/compendia/statab/cats/population/estimates_and_projections_by_age_sex_raceethnicity.html. Accessed August 26, 2013.
4. Trowers A. Chapter 78: pediatric dermatology. In: Taylor S, Kelley P, eds. *Dermatology for Skin of Color*. New York, NY: McGraw Hill; 2009.
5. Haveri FT, Inamadar AC. A cross-sectional prospective study of cutaneous lesions in newborn. *ISRN Dermatol*. 2014;2014:360590.
6. Cordova A. The Mongolian spot: a study of ethnic differences and a literature review. *Clin Pediatr (Phila)*. 1981;20(11):714-719.
7. Kolbe V, Boy D, Büttner A. Mongolian Spots–a challenging clinical sign. *Forensic Sci Int*. 2021;327:110964.
8. Reginatto FP, Muller FM, Peruzzo J, Cestari TF. Epidemiology and predisposing factors for erythema toxicum neonatorum and transient neonatal pustular: a multicenter study. *Pediatr Dermatol*. 2017;34(4):422-426.
9. Van Praag MC, Van Rooij RW, Folkers E, Spritzer R, Menke HE, Oranje AP. Diagnosis, and treatment of pustular disorders in the neonate. *Pediatr Dermatol*. 1997;14(2):131-143.
10. Wyre HW Jr, Murphy MO. Transient neonatal pustular melanosis. *Arch Dermatol*. 1979;115(4):458.
11. Fölster-Holst R. Vesikeln, Pusteln und Vesikulopusteln im frühen Kindesalter [Vesicles, pustules and vesiculopustules in early childhood]. *Hautarzt*. 2020;71(10):809-826. [German].
12. Leerunyakul K, Kanokrungsee S, Rutnin S. Clear cell papulosis: dermatoscopic findings and literature review. *Pediatr Dermatol*. 2019;36(5):655-657.
13. Wang D, Ho MS, Koh MJ, Giam YC. A case report of clear cell papulosis and a review of the literature. *Ann Acad Med Singapore*. 2017;46 (4):160-166.
14. Seykora CM, Dalton SR, Brown P. Clear cell papulosis: report and review. *Dermatol Online J*. 2018;24(1):15.
15. Tan KWJ, Chong JH, Koh JAM. Clear cell papulosis: a rare pediatric dermatosis. *Case Rep Pediatr*. 2018;2018:3908505.
16. Tseng FW, Kuo TT, Lu PH, et al. Long-term follow-up study of clear cell papulosis. *J Am Acad Dermatol*. 2010;63(2):266-273.
17. Seykora CM, Dalton SR, Brown PJ. Clear cell papulosis: report and review. *Dermatol Online J*. 2018;24(1).
18. McColl M, Boozalis E, Aguh C, Eseonu AC, Okoye GA, Kwatra SG. Pruritus in black skin: unique molecular characteristics and clinical features. *J Natl Med Assoc*. 2021;113(1):30-38.
19. Williams KA, Wondimu B, Ajayi AM, Sokumbi O. Skin of color in dermatopathology: does color matter? *Hum Pathol*. 2023;140:240-266.
20. Clark GW, Pope SM, Jaboori KA. Diagnosis and treatment of seborrheic dermatitis. *Am Fam Physician*. 2015;91(3):185-190.
21. Mangion SE, Mackenzie L, Roberts MS, Holmes AM. Seborrheic dermatitis: topical therapeutics and formulation design. *Eur J Pharm Biopharm*. 2023;185:148-164.
22. Grayson C, Heath CR. Counseling about traction alopecia: a "Compliment, Discuss, and Suggest" method. *Cutis*. 2021;108(1):20-22.
23. Cunningham J, Dockery DW, Speizer FE. Race, asthma, and persistent wheeze in Philadelphia schoolchildren. *Am J Public Health*. 1996;86(10):1406-1409.
24. Del Pozo DV, Zhu Y, Mitra N, Hoffstad OJ, Margolis DJ. The risk of atopic comorbidities and atopic march progression among Black and White children with mild-to-moderate atopic dermatitis: a cross-sectional study. *J Am Acad Dermatol*. 2022;87(5):1145-1147.
25. Takeshita J, Gupta J, Zhu Y, Berna R, Chiesa Fuxench ZC, Margolis DJ. Atopic dermatitis and the atopic march: Considering racial and ethnic diversity in atopic disease progression. *J Allergy Clin Immunol*. 2022;149(5):1590-1591.
26. Huang E, Ong PY. Severe atopic dermatitis in children. *Curr Allergy Asthma Rep*. 2018;18:35.
27. Margolis DJ, Mitra N, Wubbenhorst B, et al. Association of filaggrin loss-of-function variants with race in children with atopic dermatitis. *JAMA Dermatol*. 2019;155(11):1269-1276.
28. McKenzie C, Silverberg JI. The prevalence and persistence of atopic dermatitis in urban United States children. *Ann Allergy Asthma Immunol*. 2019;123(2):173-178.e1.
29. Chovatiya R, Begolka WS, Thibau IJ, Silverberg JI. Financial burden and impact of atopic dermatitis out-of-pocket healthcare expenses among black individuals in the United States. *Arch Dermatol Res*. 2022;314(8):739-747.
30. Sangha AM. Dermatological conditions in skin of color: managing atopic dermatitis. *J Clin Aesthet Dermatol*. 2021;14(3 Suppl 1):S20-S22.
31. Lopez Carrera YI, Al Hammadi A, Huang YH, et al. Epidemiology, diagnosis, and treatment of atopic dermatitis in the developing countries of Asia, Africa, Latin America, and the Middle East: a review. *Dermatol Ther (Heidelb)*. 2019;9:685-705.
32. Chong JH. Atopic dermatitis in children: when topical steroid treatment "does not work". *BMJ*. 2021;372:n297.
33. Dodein R, Abdul-Wahab A, Banerjee P. Systemic treatments for atopic dermatitis in children and adolescents: review of current practice and new treatments. *Apollo Med*. 2023;20(1):61-70.
34. Scott I, Atwater AR, Reeder M. Update on contact dermatitis and patch testing in patients with skin of color. *Cutis*. 2021;108(1):10-12.
35. Young K, Collis RW, Sheinbein D, et al. Retrospective review of pediatric patch testing results in skin of color. *J Am Acad Dermatol*. 2023;88(4):953-954.
36. Kaufman BP, Alexis AF. Psoriasis in skin of color: insights into the epidemiology, clinical presentation, genetics, quality-of-life impact, and treatment of psoriasis in non-white racial/ethnic groups. *Am J Clin Dermatol*. 2018;19(3):405-423.
37. Cardwell LA, Kesty C, Feldman SR, McMichael AJ. Psoriasis in skin of color. In: Orfanos C, Zouboulis, C, Assaf C, eds. *Pigmented Ethnic Skin and Imported Dermatoses*. Cham: Springer; 2018.
38. Burden-Teh E, Murphy R, Gran S, et al. Identifying the best predictive diagnostic criteria for psoriasis in children (< 18 years): a UK multicentre case-control diagnostic accuracy study (DIPSOC study). *Br J Dermatol*. 2022;186(2):341-351.
39. Pinson R, Sotoodian B, Fiorillo L. Psoriasis in children. *Psoriasis (Auckl)*. 2016:6:121-129.
40. Diotallevi F, Simonetti O, Rizzetto G, Molinelli E, Radi G, Offidani A. Biological treatments for pediatric psoriasis: state of the art and future perspectives. *Int J Mol Sci*. 2022;23(19):11128.
41. Pietrzak A, Grywalska E, Walankiewicz M, et al. Psoriasis and metabolic syndrome in children: current data. *Clin Exp Dermatol*. 2017;42(2):131-136.
42. Drago F, Ciccarese G, Rebora A, Broccolo F, Parodi A. Pityriasis rosea: a comprehensive classification. *Dermatology*. 2016;232(4):431-437.
43. Zawar V, Jerajani H. Current trends in pityriasis rosea. *Expert Rev Dermatol*. 2010;5(3):325-333.
44. Joshi TP, Calderara GA, Lipoff JB. Prevalence of pityriasis rosea in the United States: a cross-sectional study using the *All of Us* database. *JAAD Int*. 2022;8:45-46.
45. Amer A, Fischer H, Li X. The natural history of pityriasis rosea in black American children: how correct is the "classic" description? *Arch Pediatr Adolesc Med*. 2007;161(5):503-506.
46. González LM, Allen R, Janniger CK, Schwartz RA. Pityriasis rosea: an important papulosquamous disorder. *Int J Dermatol*. 2005;44(9):757-764.

47. Mayfield J, Solomon M, Plamoottil CI, Ganti L. Childhood pityriasis rosea with multiple herald patches. *Cureus*. 2020;12(8):e9876.
48. Merhy R, Sarkis AS, Assaf J, et al. Pediatric lichen planus: a systematic review of 985 published cases. *Int J Dermatol*. 2022;61(4):416-421.
49. Diop A, Ly F, Ndiaye MT, et al. Epidemiology, clinical features, and associated factors in 78 cases of lichen planus on black skin. *Int J Dermatol*. 2020;59(2):137-142.
50. Walton KE, Bowers EV, Drolet BA, Holland KE. Childhood lichen planus: demographics of a U.S. population. *Pediatr Dermatol*. 2010;27(1):34-38.
51. Spirito F, Caponio VCA, Lo Muzio E, et al. Oral lichen planus in children: an Italian case series. *Pediatr Dermatol*. 2023;40(3):489-493.
52. Pandhi D, Singal A, Bhattacharya SN. Lichen planus in childhood: a series of 316 patients. *Pediatr Dermatol*. 2014;31(1):59-67.
53. Jung JM, Lim DJ, Won CH, Chang SE, Lee MW, Lee WJ. Mycosis fungoides in children and adolescents: a systematic review. *JAMA Dermatol*. 2021;157(4):431-438.
54. Chen Y, Xu J, Qiu L, et al. Hypopigmented mycosis fungoides: a clinical and histopathology analysis in 9 children. *Am J Dermatopathol*. 2021;43(4):259-265.
55. Reiter O, Amitay-Laish I, Oren-Shabtai M, Feinmesser M, Ben-Amitai D, Hodak E. Paediatric mycosis fungoides - characteristics, management and outcomes with particular focus on the folliculotropic variant. *J Eur Acad Dermatol Venereol*. 2022;36(5):671-679. Erratum in: J Eur Acad Dermatol Venereol. 2022;36(7):1143.
56. Ankad BS, Beergouder SL. Pityriasis lichenoides et varioliformis acuta in skin of color: new observations by dermoscopy. *Dermatol Pract Concept*. 2017;7(1):27-34.
57. Jung F, Sibbald C, Bohdanowicz M, Ingram JR, Piguet V. Systematic review of the efficacies and adverse effects of treatments for pityriasis lichenoides. *Br J Dermatol*. 2020;183(6):1026-1032.
58. McLaurin CI. Pediatric dermatology in black patients. *Dermatol Clin*. 1988;6(3):457-473.
59. Paloni G, Berti I, Cutrone M. Acropustulosis of infancy. *Arch Dis Child Fetal Neonatal Ed*. 2013;98(4):F340.
60. Jennings JL, Burrows WM. Infantile acropustulosis. *J Am Acad Dermatol*. 1983;9(5):733-738.
61. Boccara O, Blanche S, de Prost Y, Brousse N, Bodemer C, Fraitag S. Cutaneous hematologic disorders in children. *Pediatr Blood Cancer*. 2012;58:226-232.
62. Truong AL, Esterly NB. Atypical acropustulosis in infancy. *Int J Dermatol*. 1997;36(9):688-691.
63. Mancini AJ, Frieden IJ, Paller AS. Infantile acropustulosis revisited: history of scabies and response to topical corticosteroids. *Pediatr Dermatol*. 1998;15(5):337-341.
64. Solman L, Layton AM. Acne in childhood. *Pediatrics and Child Health*. 2019;29:85-89.
65. Taylor SC, Cook-Bolden F, Rahman Z, Strachan D. Acne vulgaris in skin of color. *J Am Acad Dermatol*. 2002;46(2 Suppl Understanding):S98-106.
66. Kingston P, Yee D, Huang MY, et al. Shared decision-making and satisfaction with care: a population-based study in acne patients with skin of color in the United States. *Clin Exp Dermatol*. 2023;48(9):1032-1035.
67. Kellen R, Silverberg NB. Pediatric periorificial dermatitis. *Cutis*. 2017; 100(6):385-388.
68. Shetty AK, Gedalia A. Sarcoidosis: a pediatric perspective. *Clin Pediatr (Phila)*. 1998;37(12):707-717.
69. Haimovic A, Sanchez M, Judson MA, Prystowsky S. Sarcoidosis: a comprehensive review and update for the dermatologist: part I. Cutaneous disease. *J Am Acad Dermatol*. 2012;66(5):699.e1-18.
70. Charras A, Smith E, Hedrich CM. Systemic lupus erythematosus in children and young people. *Curr Rheumatol Rep*. 2021;23(3):20.
71. Rubinstein TB, Knight AM. Disparities in childhood-onset lupus. *Rheum Dis Clin North Am*. 2020;46(4):661-672.
72. Vanoni F, Lava SAG, Fossali EF, et al. Neonatal systemic lupus erythematosus syndrome: a comprehensive review. *Clin Rev Allergy Immunol*. 2017;53(3):469-476.
73. Kleitsch J, Mazori DR, Masson M, et al. Cutaneous neonatal lupus in patients with skin of color: A retrospective cohort study from a national registry. *J Am Acad Dermatol*. 2023;89:364-366.
74. Levy R, Briggs L, Silverman E, Pope E, Lara-Corrales I. Cutaneous sequelae in neonatal lupus: a retrospective cohort study. *J Am Acad Dermatol*. 2020;83(2):440-446.
75. Jung HL. Update on infantile hemangioma. *Clin Exp Pediatr*. 2021;64(11): 559-572.
76. Kumar KD, Desai AD, Shah VP, Lipner SR. Racial discrepancies in presentation of hospitalized infantile hemangioma cases using the Kids' Inpatient Database. *Health Sci Rep*. 2023;6(2):e1092.
77. Lie E, Psoter KJ, Püttgen KB. Lower socioeconomic status is associated with delayed access to care for infantile hemangioma: a cohort study. *J Am Acad Dermatol*. 2023;88(5):e221-e230.
78. Sebaratnam DF, Rodríguez Bandera AL, Wong LF, Wargon O. Infantile hemangioma. Part 2: management. *J Am Acad Dermatol*. 2021;85(6):1395-1404.
79. Jin Y, Andersen G, Yorgov D, et al. Genome-wide association studies of autoimmune vitiligo identify 23 new risk loci and highlight key pathways and regulatory variants. *Nat Genet*. 2016;48(11):1418-1424.
80. Van Driessche F, Silverberg N. Current management of pediatric vitiligo. *Paediatr Drugs*. 2015;17(4):303-313.
81. Silverberg NB. The epidemiology of vitiligo. *Curr Derm Rep*. 2015;4:36-43.
82. Jin Y, Birlea SA, Fain PR, et al. Variant of TYR and autoimmunity susceptibility loci in generalized vitiligo. *N Engl J Med*. 2010;362(18):1686-1697.
83. Iannella G, Greco A, Didona D, et al. Vitiligo: pathogenesis, clinical variants and treatment approaches. *Autoimmun Rev*. 2016;15(4):335-343.
84. Sandoval-Cruz M, García-Carrasco M, Sánchez-Porras R, et al. Immunopathogenesis of vitiligo. *Autoimmun Rev*. 2011;10(12):762-765.
85. Regazzetti C, Joly F, Marty C, et al. Transcriptional analysis of vitiligo skin reveals the alteration of WNT pathway: a promising target for repigmenting vitiligo patients. *J Invest Dermatol*. 2015;135(12):3105-3114.
86. Mosenson JA, Zloza A, Nieland JD, et al. Mutant HSP70 reverses autoimmune depigmentation in vitiligo. *Sci Transl Med*. 2013;5(174):174ra28.
87. Dennin MH, Stein SL, Rosenblatt AE. Vitiligoid variant of lichen sclerosus in young girls with darker skin types. *Pediatr Dermatol*. 2018;35(2):198-201.
88. Silverberg JI, Silverberg NB. False "highlighting" with Wood's lamp. *Pediatr Dermatol*. 2014;31(1):109-110.
89. Richards KA, Fukai K, Oiso N, Paller AS. A novel KIT mutation results in piebaldism with progressive depigmentation. *J Am Acad Dermatol*. 2001;44(2):288-292.
90. Renert-Yuval Y, Ezzedine K, Grimes P, et al. Vitiligo evidence-based expert consensus recommendations for paediatric and adolescent patients: part I—topical therapeutics. *Br J Dermatol*. 2023;188(Supplement_1). doi:10.1093/bjd/ljac106.007.
91. Sethi S, Silverberg N. Short and long-term outcomes of 308-nm laser for pediatric vitiligo. *J Drugs Dermatol*. 2022;21(7):773-775.
92. Njoo MD, Bos JD, Westerhof W. Treatment of generalized vitiligo in children with narrow-band (TL-01) UVB radiation therapy. *J Am Acad Dermatol*. 2000;42(2 Pt 1):245-253.
93. Mohana D, Verma U, Amar AJ, Choudhary RKP. Reticulate acropigmentation of Dohi: a case report with insight into genodermatoses with mottled pigmentation. *Indian J Dermatol*. 2012;57:42-44.
94. Dhar S, Kanwar AJ, Jebraili R, Dawn G, Das A. Spectrum of reticular flexural and acral pigmentary disorder in Northern India. *J Dermatol*. 1994;21:598-603.
95. Hayashi M, Suzuki T. Dyschromatosis symmetrica hereditaria. *J Dermatol*. 2013;40:336-340.
96. Xing QH, Wang MT, Chen XD, et al. A gene locus responsible for dyschromatosis symmetrica hereditaria (DSH) maps to chromosome 6q24.2-q25.2. *Am J Hum Genet*. 2003;73:377-382.
97. Taki T, Kozuka S, Izawa Y, et al. Surgical treatment of speckled skin caused by dyschromatosis symmetrica hereditaria: case report. *J Dermatol*. 1986;13:471-473.
98. Gupta V, Kumar A. Dyskeratosis congenita. *Adv Exp Med Biol*. 2010;685: 215-219.
99. Dokal I. Dyskeratosis congenita. *Hematology Am Soc Hematol Educ Program*. 2011;2011:480-486.
100. Rackley S, Pao M, Seratti GF, et al. Neuropsychiatric conditions among patients with dyskeratosis congenita: a link with telomere biology? *Psychosomatics*. 2012;5:230-235.
101. Keisham C, Sarkar R, Garg VK, Chugh S. Ashy dermatosis in an 8-year-old Indian child. *Indian Dermatol Online J*. 2013;4:30-32.
102. Silverberg NB, Herz J, Wagner A, Paller AS. Erythema dyschromicum perstans in prepubertal children. *Pediatr Dermatol*. 2003;20:398-403.
103. Torrelo A, Zaballos P, Colmenero I, Mediero IG, de Prada I, Zambrano A. Erythema dyschromicum perstans in children: a report of 14 cases. *J Eur Acad Dermatol Venereol*. 2005;19:422-426.
104. Schwartz RA, Centurian SA. Erythema dyschromicum perstans. *Medscape*, May 22, 2012. http://emedicine.medscape.com/article/1122807-overview. Accessed March 22, 2013.
105. Diaz A, Gillihan R, Motaparthi K, Rees A. Combination therapy with prednisone and isotretinoin in early erythema dyschromicum perstans: a retrospective series. *JAAD Case Rep*. 2020;6(3):207-213.
106. Smith RJ, Rubin AI. Pediatric nail disorders: a review. *Curr Opin Pediatr*. 2020;32(4):506-515.

107. Heymann WR. Pediatric longitudinal melanonychia: delaying the bottom line. *J Am Acad Dermatol.* 2022;87(2):296-297.
108. Lee JS, Kim S, Kim DH, Lee JW, Mun JH, Lee SH. Clinical features and natural course of pediatric longitudinal melanonychia: a retrospective cohort study in Korea. *J Am Acad Dermatol.* 2022;87(2):366-372.
109. Talebi M, Farmanbar N, Abolfazli S, Shirazi, AS. Management of physiological hyperpigmentation of oral mucosa by cryosurgical treatment: a case report. *J Dent Res Dent Clin Dent Prospects.* 2012;6:148-151.
110. Laude TA. Approach to dermatologic disorders in black children. *Sem Dermatol.* 1995;14:15-20.
111. Bhanusali D, Coley M, Silverberg JI, Alexis A, Silverberg NB. Treatment outcomes for tinea capitis in a skin of color population. *J Drugs Dermatol.* 2012;11(7):852-856.
112. Dummett CO. Colour changes in the oral mucosa. *J Can Dent Assoc.* 1967;33:206-212.
113. Dummett CO. Overview of normal oral pigmentations. *J Indiana Dent Assoc.* 1980;59:13-18.
114. Najjar T. Disorders of oral pigmentation. *Medscape.* http://emedicine.medscape.com/article/1078143-overview. Accessed March 16, 2013.
115. Kasagani SK, Nutalapati R, Muttthineni RB. Esthetic depigmentation of anterior gingiva. A case series. *N Y State Dent J.* 2012;78:26-31.
116. Mitchell KN, Tay YK, Heath CR, Trachtman R, Silverberg NB. Review article: Emerging issues in pediatric skin of color, part 1. *Pediatr Dermatol.* 2021;38(Suppl 2):20-29.
117. Pontes AEF, Pontes CC, Souza SLS, Novales AB, Grisi MFM, Taba M. Evaluation of the efficacy of the acellular dermal matrix allograft with partial thickness flap in the elimination of gingival melanin pigmentation. A comparative clinical study with 12 months of follow-up. *J Esthet Restor Dent.* 2006;18:135-143.
118. Hanioka T, Tanaka K, Ojima M, Yuuki K. Association of melanin pigmentation in the gingiva of children with parents who smoke. *Pediatrics.* 2005;116:e186.
119. Manan MR, Rahman S, Komer L, Manan H, Iftikhar S. A multispecialty approach to the identification and diagnosis of nonaccidental trauma in children. *Cureus.* 2022;14(7):e27276.
120. Kelly AP. Update on the management of keloids. *Semin Cutan Med Surg.* 2009;28:71-76.
121. Goodfellow A, Emmerson RW, Calvert HT. Rubstein-Taybi syndrome and spontaneous keloids. *Clin Exp Dermatol.* 1980;5:369-371.
122. Halder R, Grimes P, McLaurin C, Kress M, Kenney J. Incidence of common dermatoses in a predominantly black dermatologic practice. *Cutis.* 1983;32;388-390.
123. Wriston CC, Rubin AI, Elenitsas R, Crawford GH. Nodular scleroderma: a report of 2 cases. *Am J Dermatopathol.* 2008;30:385-388.
124. Lane JE, Waller JL, Davis LS. Relationship between age of ear piercing and keloid formation. *Pediatrics.* 2005;115:1312-1314.
125. Tirgan MH, Shutty CM, Park TH. Nine-month-old patient with bilateral earlobe keloids. *Pediatrics.* 2013;131:e313-e317.
126. Hamrick M, Boswell W, Carney D. Successful treatment of earlobe keloids in the pediatric population. *J Pediatr Surg.* 2009;44:286-288.
127. Mellon RD, Simone AF, Rappaport BA. Use of anesthetic agents in neonates and young children. *Anesth Analg.* 2007;104:509-520.
128. Fu JM, Price VH. Approach to hair loss in women of color. *Semin Cutan Med Surg.* 2009;28:109-114.
129. Silverberg NB, Silverberg JI, Wong ML. Trichoscopy using a handheld dermoscope: an in-office technique to diagnose genetic disease of the hair. *Arch Dermatol.* 2009;145:600-601.
130. Detwiler SP, Carson JL, Woosley JT, Gambling TM, Briggaman RA. Bubble hair. Case caused by an overheating hair dryer and reproducibility in normal hair with heat. *J Am Acad Dermatol.* 1994;30:54-60.
131. Savitha AS, Sacchidanand S, Revathy TN. Bubble hair and other acquired hair shaft anomalies due to hot ironing on wet hair. *Int J Trichol.* 2011;3:118-120.
132. Elston DM, Bergfeld WF, Whiting DA, et al. Bubble hair. *J Cutan Pathol.* 1992;19:439-444.
133. Lucky AW, Biro FM, Daniels SR, Cedars MI, Khoury PR, Morrison JA. The prevalence of upper lip hair in black and white girls during puberty: a new standard. *J Pediatr.* 2001;138:134-136.
134. Paller AS, Mancini A. *Hurwitz Clinical Pediatric Dermatology.* 3rd ed. New York, NY: Elsevier-Saunders; 2006.
135. Cordisco MR. An update on lasers in children. *Curr Opin Pediatr.* 2009;21:499-504.
136. Cantatore JL, Kriegel DA. Laser surgery: an approach to the pediatric patient. *J Am Acad Dermatol.* 2004;50:165-184.
137. Wendelin DS, Mallory GB, Mallory SB. Depilation in a 6-month-old with hypertrichosis: a case report. *Pediatric Dermatol.* 1999;16:311-313.
138. Heath CR, Taylor SC. Alopecia in an ophiasis pattern: traction alopecia versus alopecia areata. *Cutis.* 2012;89:213-216.
139. Grayson C, Heath C. An approach to examining tightly coiled hair among patients with hair loss in race-discordant patient-physician interactions. *JAMA Dermatol.* 2021;157(5):505-506.
140. Mirmirani P, Tucker LY. Epidemiologic trends in pediatric tinea capitis: a population-based study from Kaiser Permanente Northern California. *J Am Acad Dermatol.* 2013;69(6):916-921.
141. Wilmington M, Aly R, Frieden IJ. *Trichophyton tonsurans* tinea capitis in the San Francisco Bay area: increased infection demonstrated in a 20-year survey of fungal infections from 1974 to 1994. *J Med Vet Mycol.* 1996;34:285-287.
142. Silverberg NB. Scalp hyperkeratosis in children with skin of color: diagnostic and therapeutic considerations. *Cutis.* 2015;95(4):199-204, 207.
143. Williams JV, Eichenfield LF, Burke BL, Barnes-Eley M, Friedlander SF. Prevalence of scalp scaling in prepubertal children. *Pediatrics.* 2005;115(1):e1-e6.
144. Coley MK, Bhanusali DG, Silverberg JI, Alexis AF, Silverberg NB. Scalp hyperkeratosis and alopecia in children of color. *J Drugs Dermatol.* 2011; 10(5):511-516.
145. Nguyen J, Chapman LW, Smith J. Trichoscopic features of tinea capitis in a straight-haired Hispanic woman. *Dermatol Online J.* 2018;24(11):13030/qt8cw0s639.
146. Aqil N, BayBay H, Moustaide K, Douhi Z, Elloudi S, Mernissi FZ. A prospective study of tinea capitis in children: making the diagnosis easier with a dermoscope. *J Med Case Rep.* 2018;12(1):383.
147. Friedlander SF, Pickering B, Cunningham BB, Gibbs NF, Eichenfield LF. Use of the cotton swab method in diagnosing tinea capitis. *Pediatrics.* 1999;104:276-279.
148. Laude TA, Shah BR, Lynfield Y. Tinea capitis in Brooklyn. *Am J Dis Child.* 1982;136:1047-1050.
149. Andrews MD, Burns M. Common tinea infections in children. *Am Fam Physician.* 2008;77:1415-1420.
150. Silverberg NB. Easy griseofulvin dosing. *Pediatr Dermatol.* 2008;25(5):577.
151. Grigoryan KV, Tollefson MM, Olson MA, Newman CC. Pediatric tinea capitis caused by trichophyton violaceum and trichophyton soudanense in Rochester, Minnesota, United States. *Int J Dermatol.* 2019;58(8):912-915.
152. Gupta AK, Mays RR, Versteeg SG, et al. Tinea capitis in children: a systematic review of management. *J Eur Acad Dermatol Venereol.* 2018;32(12): 2264-2274.
153. Kiken DA, Sekaran A, Antaya RJ, Davis A, Imaeda S, Silverberg NB. White piedra in children. *J Am Acad Dermatol.* 2006;55:956-961.
154. de Almeida Júnior HL, Rivitti EA, Jaeger RG. White piedra: ultrastructure and a new microecological aspect. *Mycoses.* 1990;33:491-497.
155. Shivaprakash MR, Singh G, Gupta P, Dhaliwal M, Kanwar AJ, Chakrabarti A. Extensive white piedra of the scalp caused by *Trichosporon* inkin: a case report and review of literature. *Mycopathologia.* 2011;172:481-486.
156. Figueras MJ, Guarro J. Ultrastructural aspect of the keratinolytic activity of piedra. *Rev Iberoam Micol.* 2000;17:136-141.

CHAPTER 104 Adolescence

Patricia Treadwell
Candrice R. Heath

KEY POINTS

- Dyspigmentation is often a major concern for adolescents with skin of color
- Epidermal nevus is the primary differential diagnosis for lichen striatus
- The erythema in atopic dermatitis is often underestimated in skin of color resulting in poor characterization of severity of the disorder
- Nevus sebaceous, although present from birth, may become more prominent at puberty
- Phytophotodermatitis can be misdiagnosed as ecchymoses from abuse
- Prevention of permanent hair loss from traction alopecia and central centrifugal cicatricial alopecia begins with early recognition, counseling, and treatment.

ACNE

Acne is one of the most common dermatologic disorders in adolescence. It is estimated that approximately 85% of adolescents have acne lesions.[1,2] The incidence of acne in adolescents with skin of color is similar to that in adolescents of European ancestry; however, special attention is necessary for treatment choices and anticipated pigmentary changes.[3,4]

Acne is an inflammatory dermatosis that is primarily located in areas with increased sebaceous gland concentration. Those areas include face, upper chest, and back. Factors driving the development of acne include: (1) abnormal keratinization leading to follicular plugging; (2) androgenic stimulation of the sebaceous glands; (3) the effect of *Cutibacterium acnes* (formerly *Propionibacterium acnes*); and (4) inflammation.

Characteristic acne lesions include open comedones (blackheads), closed comedones (whiteheads) inflammatory papules, pustules, nodules, and cysts.

Differential diagnoses include perioral dermatitis, folliculitis, rosacea, adenoma sebaceum, and drug-induced acneiform eruptions.

Treatment regimens are addressed in review articles[1-5] and Chapters 47 and 48 in this textbook. Of note, topical retinoids, which are considered the foundation for treatment of acne, should be prescribed cautiously in adolescents with skin of color. It is important to avoid irritation, retinoid dermatitis, and subsequent dyspigmentation. Noncomedogenic facial moisturizers with sunscreen are recommended for use daily in addition to other acne therapies to specifically avoid further darkening of the hyperpigmented areas.

ACNE KELOIDALIS NUCHAE

Individuals who develop acne keloidalis nuchae (AKN) may be noted to have their initial lesions around puberty.[6] This condition is more common in individuals who identify as males, however, may also be seen in females. This specific topic is covered extensively in Chapter 33. The inciting agents are noted to be androgens, inflammation, infection, trauma, genetics, and ingrowing hairs. Specifically, close shaving and friction from clothing are contributing factors.

Initially folliculitis with follicular-based papules and pustules is noted. This may progress to form firm papules of the posterior neck and occipital scalp [**Figure 104-1**]. In severe cases, keloidal plaques develop and, in some cases, scarring alopecia may occur. Other patients may have crusting and purulent drainage. The lesions are noted following shaving and later the dermis is exposed to the hair that then acts as a foreign body. Histopathology often demonstrates a granulomatous foreign body reaction.

Medical treatments include benzoyl peroxide, retinoids, and topical and intralesional corticosteroids. Antibiotics (topical and systemic) may result in some improvement. Oral isotretinoin and ultraviolet therapy have been reported as effective.[6,7] Comprehensive review of surgical treatments is presented in Chapter 33.

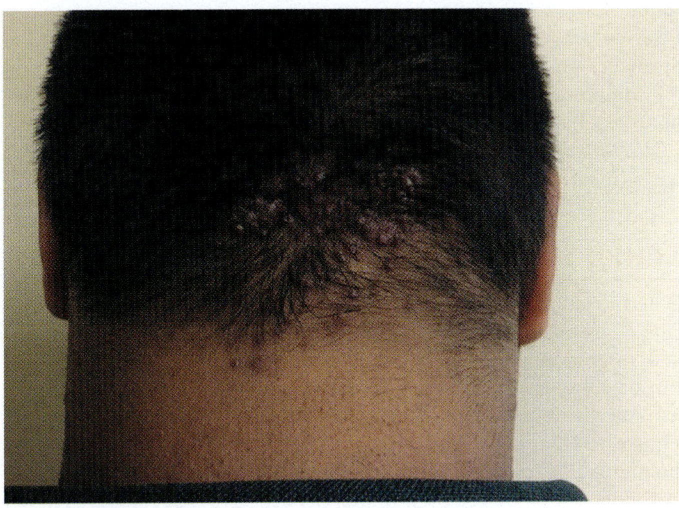

FIGURE 104-1. Firm papules of the occipital scalp in AKN.

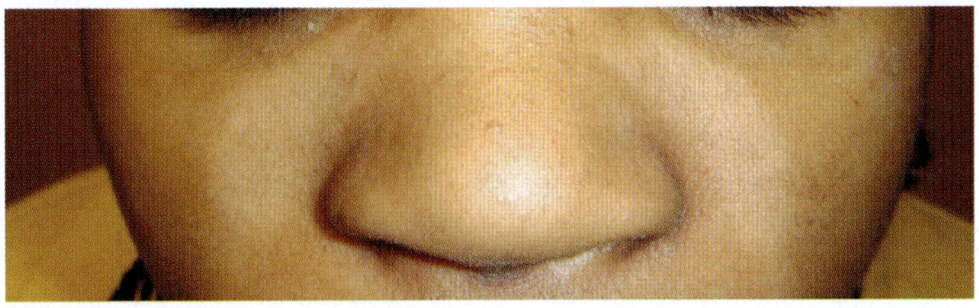

FIGURE 104-2. Hypopigmentation associated with seborrheic dermatitis.

SEBORRHEIC DERMATITIS

Seborrheic dermatitis (SD) occurs in 3% to 10% of the population.[8] The incidence of SD has been described as occurring both more frequently and less frequently in patients with skin of color.[8,9] Further studies may be necessary to clarify this point. This condition is characterized by two different subtypes: (1) infantile seborrheic dermatitis and (2) adolescent and adult type. In adolescents and adults, this disorder is noted to have diffuse scale in the scalp and eyebrows along with erythematous papules with "greasy" scale of the paranasal area. In individuals with skin of color, the facial lesions may present as "petaloid seborrheic dermatitis" (polycyclic coalescing rings)[8] and/or with some associated dyspigmentation [**Figure 104-2**].[8]

The inflammatory process in SD is mediated by free fatty acids in susceptible individuals. Localized lipase activity has also been implicated in the pathogenesis of SD. There are documented differences in adolescents and adults demonstrating colonization of Malassezia species in SD skin versus healthy skin. There is an increased incidence of SD in immunodeficiency, diabetes, malabsorption, and neurologic disorders.[9]

Differential diagnoses for the scalp involvement include psoriasis, tinea capitis, and eczema. Differential diagnoses for the facial involvement include perioral dermatitis, psoriasis, secondary syphilis (especially when annular lesions are noted), tinea faciei, tinea versicolor, and psoriasis.

An extensive review of treatments is available.[10] Topical antifungals and shampoos have been beneficial in the treatment of SD.[10] In patients with tightly coiled hair, often more prone to dryness and breakage, some medicated shampoos can be very drying for the hair.[11] Applying the medicated shampoo only to the scalp is helpful; in addition, following up with a moisturizing shampoo and conditioner may help to lessen dryness.[11]

Topical anti-inflammatory agents (eg, corticosteroids and topical calcineurin inhibitors) have also been shown to be useful.[10] Other topical treatments include metronidazole, keratolytic agents, and sodium sulfacetamide. Asking the patient which medication vehicle they prefer is important. The patient's preference may depend on hairstyling and cultural practices.[11] Systemic agents with reported efficacy include itraconazole, terbinafine, fluconazole, ketoconazole, and isotretinoin.[10]

PITYRIASIS ROSEA

Pityriasis rosea (PR) is a self-limited papulosquamous condition. Seventy-five percent of patients are between the ages of 10 and 35 years. Thus, adolescents constitute an important portion of those affected. Considering the seasonal variations and evident clustering, a viral etiology is probable. The condition can be proceeded by symptoms of a viral illness. Association of PR and COVID-19 virus and vaccine has been reported.[12,13]

Typically, the initial lesion noted is a herald patch. The lesion is generally 2 to 5 cm in diameter and can be located anywhere on the body, especially on the proximal legs or arms, trunk, or neck. The herald patch is often circular, erythematous, and has fine white scales. Within a few days, multiple smaller oval lesions with a similar morphology are noted.

These lesions tend to be oriented parallel to the lines of skin cleavage. On the back, this results in a "fir tree" pattern. On the flank, a "school of minnows" pattern is evident. In inverse PR, the lesions are located in flexural areas and on the face. In patients with skin of color, the lesions may be more papular and/or follicular centered, crusted, and may sometimes have dyspigmentation.[14] There have been reports of increased facial and scalp involvement in children with skin of color.[14]

The eruption may persist for 6 to 8 weeks following the onset of the herald patch. Generally, the lesions are asymptomatic but on occasion may be pruritic. Additional information is available on pityriasis rosea in Chapter 27.

Some of the differential diagnoses are tinea corporis (especially the herald patch), guttate psoriasis, nummular eczema, secondary syphilis, and pityriasis lichenoides chronica among others.

Treatment can be considered if the lesions are symptomatic. Topical corticosteroids and antipruritics have some efficacy. Other possible treatment recommendations include macrolides, antivirals, and ultraviolet light therapy.[14]

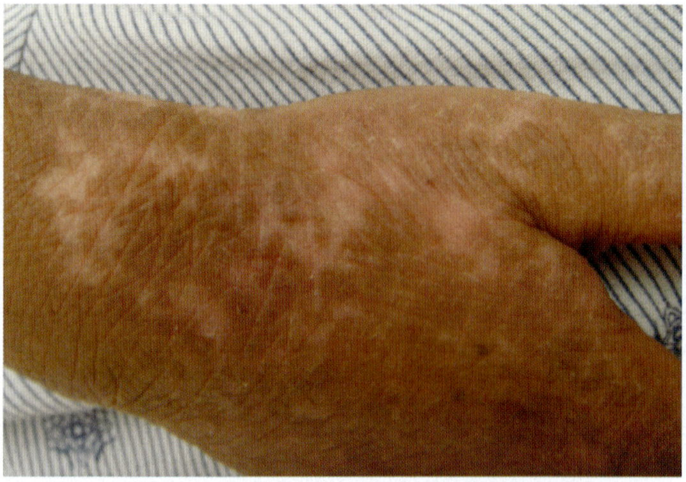

FIGURE 104-4. Lichenification, hypopigmentation, and hyperpigmentation in a patient with atopic dermatitis.

ATOPIC DERMATITIS

Atopic dermatitis in the adolescent age group has a similar appearance to that in younger children. It does tend to be more difficult to treat and often has widespread dyspigmentation and lichenification due to the chronic nature of dermatitis. Often thought of as a childhood condition, atopic dermatitis is more persistent in Black patients, with severe cases even persisting into adolescent years and beyond. Socioeconomic factors and racism have been implicated in disease severity.[15]

In patients with skin of color, erythema may not be as evident when the skin is darkly pigmented. The severity of the atopic dermatitis may not be recognized because of the underappreciation of the erythema using the standard scoring instruments: Eczema Area and Severity Index (EASI) and Scoring Atopic Dermatitis (SCORAD).[16] Since the erythema is less evident in richly pigmented skin, the lower scores may not accurately reflect disease severity.

The distribution of lesions tends to vary with age, adolescents and adults will tend to have lesions on the eyelids, genital area, and fold areas. Pruritus is a frequent symptom. Of note, the papular variant (consisting of discrete eczematous papules) of atopic dermatitis (also known as papular eczema) is more common in patients with skin of color [**Figure 104-3**].[5] In addition, pityriasis alba (irregular hypopigmented macules and patches with fine scale) is more common in patients with skin of color. In patients with skin of color, dyspigmentation can also be a significant issue occurring following inflammation or noted with scarring [**Figure 104-4**].[5]

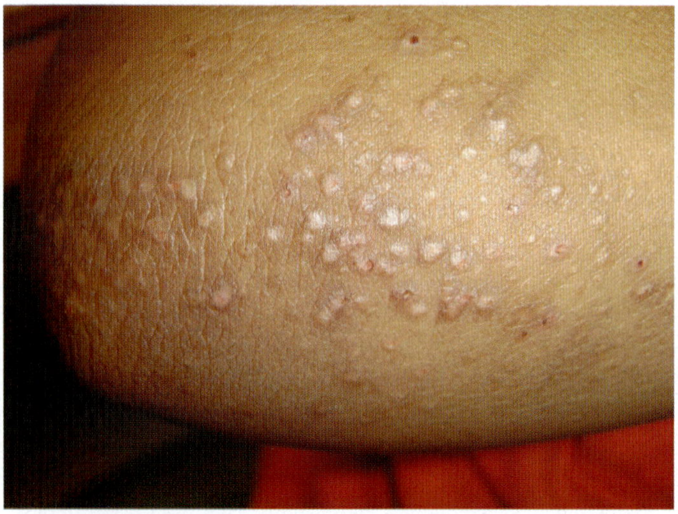

FIGURE 104-3. Papular eruption in a patient with atopic dermatitis.

Filaggrin mutations have been identified in a subset of patients with atopic dermatitis and are associated with epidermal barrier dysfunction. Patients in both African and European ancestry have been noted to have loss-of-function filaggrin mutations; however, the mutation seems to play less of a role in pathogenesis in patients with African ancestry. The mutation is much less common in African Americans when compared to individuals of European and Asian ancestry.

Patch testing should be considered since the disrupted epidermal barrier can allow allergens to penetrate.[16]

An extra rinse of the laundry and avoidance of dryer fabric softeners can minimize the effects of irritants in clothing. Trimming the fingernails can result in fewer linear erosions. Dilute bleach baths can be useful to decrease the colonization of *Staphylococcus aureus* (*S. aureus*) that can frequently be present in patients with atopic dermatitis. Treatment of atopic dermatitis in adolescents includes repairing the epidermal barrier with daily short soaks/showers and liberal use of topical emollients. Emollients are more effective if applied while the skin is damp. Topical corticosteroids are prescribed for the most affected areas.[4] Topical calcineurin inhibitors and phosphodiaesterase-4 inhibitors can be prescribed especially for facial and Intertriginous involvement and in particular areas where topical corticosteroids are contraindicated.[5]

Patients with secondary bacterial infections should continue daily treatments (including emollients and topical corticosteroids) to improve the epidermal barrier. Topical antibiotics can be used to decrease colonization of the *S. aureus* applied to lesions, under fingernails, and intranasally.

Antihistamine use has been questioned recently; however, they can be useful for sleep disturbances.[16]

Severe and chronic cases of atopic dermatitis can be treated with ultraviolet therapy, systemic immunosuppressives, biologics, and/or JAK inhibitors. A comprehensive discussion of treatment options can be found in Chapter 29.

The differential diagnoses for atopic dermatitis include irritant dermatitis, psoriasis (especially guttate), and contact dermatitis.

LICHEN STRIATUS

Lichen striatus is a cutaneous disorder that is characterized by grouped papules arranged in a linear pattern. The groupings follow along embryonal migration patterns and/or Blaschko lines. In adolescents with skin of color, the papules often appear hypopigmented in contrast to being erythematous or hyperpigmented in less pigmented individuals [**Figure 104-5**].[17] The disorder typically lasts for a few years and then spontaneously resolves. There have been reports of lichen striatus following vaccination (hepatitis B and COVID-19).[18] Occurrences in siblings and unrelated individuals residing in the same household may

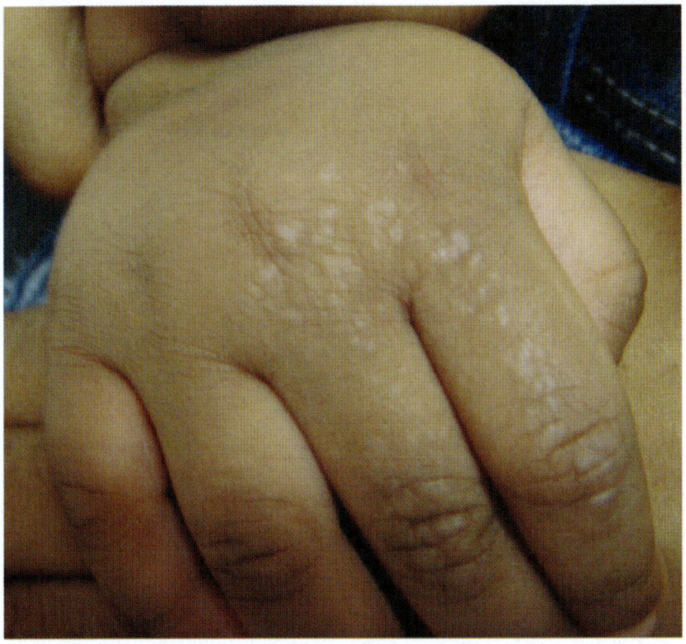

FIGURE 104-5. Hypopigmented papules of lichen striatus.

suggest a possible inflammatory response following exposure to the same environmental trigger.[17]

If the fingers are involved, the nail bed may be affected, and nail dystrophy can be seen.[19]

Differential diagnoses include epidermal nevus (which would be present from birth), lichen planus, papular eczema, and incontinentia pigmenti.

This disorder can be managed with reassurance and expectant monitoring. If symptoms are present, topical corticosteroids and/or antipruritics can be used.

TINEA VERSICOLOR

Tinea versicolor (TV) is a fungal infection of the skin caused by *Malassezia species* (formerly known as *Pityrosporum ovale* and *Pityrosporum orbiculare*) that are part of the normal flora of the skin. The organisms are nourished by the sebum and convert from the yeast form to the mycelial form that causes this disorder. TV often is noted in adolescence. Additionally, the incidence is increased in diabetes, pregnancy, immunosuppression, and with hot, humid weather.[20,21]

The patches with fine powdery scale are typically seen on the upper back, chest, and proximal arms. These are also the areas of the highest concentrations of sebum. TV occurs with a similar incidence for all races; however, adolescents with skin of color often have a different clinical presentation. The lesions are more often hypopigmented and/or follicular centered in patients with skin of color [**Figure 104-6**].[5,20]

Diagnosis can be made based on the clinical findings or with a Wood lamp examination. Short hyphae and spores (spaghetti and meatballs) will be seen on a potassium hydroxide plus India ink preparation [**Figure 104-7**]. Culture of the *Malassezia species* is not feasible because the specific conditions needed to grow the organism are not easily achieved.

Differential diagnoses include vitiligo, pityriasis rosea, pityriasis rubra pilaris, and confluent and reticulated papillomatosis of Gougerot and Carteaud.

A variety of treatment regimens have been proposed in the literature. If the TV is limited, a topical antifungal such as ketoconazole cream can be efficacious. Topical selenium sulfide lotion or ketoconazole shampoo can be applied to larger areas of involvement. The liquid preparations are left on for 5 to 10 minutes and then rinsed off. They can be applied nightly for a few weeks, and subsequently used intermittently as needed.

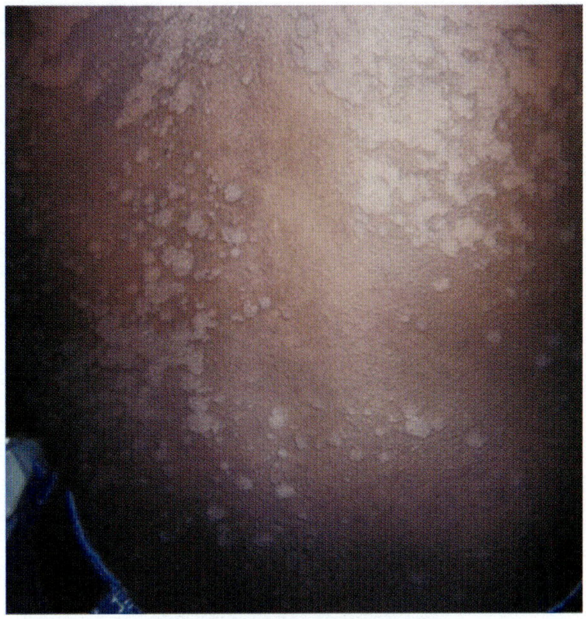

FIGURE 104-6. Tinea versicolor on the back.

Oral medications such as ketoconazole, itraconazole, and fluconazole have been used in a variety of treatment regimens.[5,20]

PHYTOPHOTODERMATITIS

Phytophotodermatitis may have a more prominent clinical appearance in adolescents with skin of color. Phytophotodermatitis is a phototoxic cutaneous reaction that results from the exposure of the skin to furocoumarin derivatives and subsequent sun exposure. Furocoumarins can be found in lemons and limes, other citrus fruits, species of Umbelliferae (celery, cow parsley, giant hogwood, cowbane, carrot, parsnips, dill, fennel, and anise) rue, meadow grass, figs, and some perfumes.[22] Bullae can develop with significant furocoumarin derivatives exposure.[23] Dermatitis may be painful and ruptured bullae can be susceptible to secondary to bacterial infection. Less intense concentration of furocoumarin derivatives may result in pigment changes without bullae formation [**Figure 104-8**]. Unusual patterns can be seen. Phytophotodermatitis may on occasion be misdiagnosed as child abuse especially if there are fingerprints or streaks.

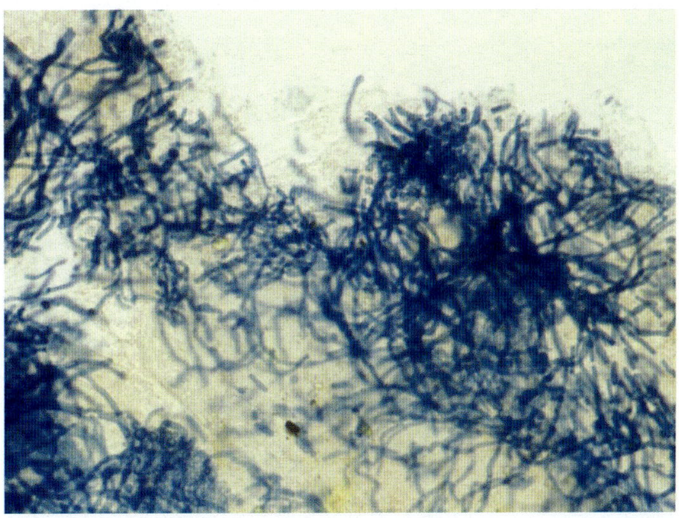

FIGURE 104-7. Potassium hydroxide and India ink preparation in tinea versicolor showing "spaghetti and meatballs."

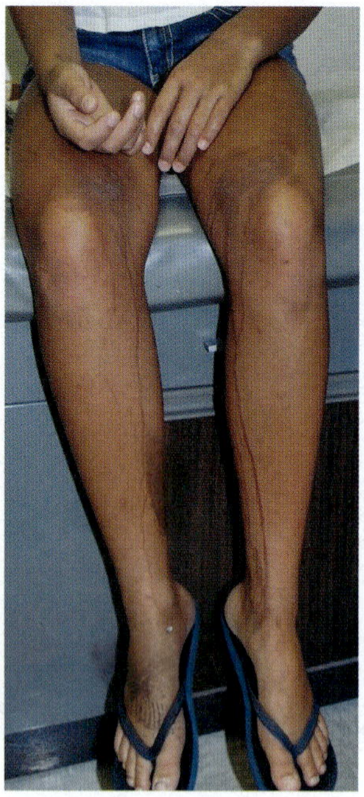

FIGURE 104-8. "Drip" pattern of hyperpigmentation in phytophotodermatitis.

Differential diagnoses include allergic contact dermatitis, sunburn, cellulitis, or other photosensitive eruptions.

Treatment (if needed) consists of topical corticosteroids, topical or systemic antibiotics, and sun protection.[22,23]

Washing the derivatives from the skin and/or protection from the sun following exposure can be preventative.[23]

BECKER NEVUS

Becker nevus (BN), a benign cutaneous hamartoma, typically develops in the peripubertal period. Although the incidence in not increased in individuals with skin of color, the clinical appearance may be different. Clinically, the hamartoma is typically unilateral and hyperpigmented. In addition, the lesion has an irregular outline and surface. The nevus is most often located on the shoulders, anterior chest, and upper back near the scapula [**Figure 104-9**].[24] The nevus is more frequent in males and in many cases will have increased overlying hair and/or acne within the lesion. In adolescents with more richly pigmented skin, the hyperpigmentation may be significant. The nevi tend to be asymptomatic; however, Becker nevus syndrome (BNS) has been described.[25,26] The syndrome is characterized by associated abnormalities including hypoplasia, limb asymmetry, scoliosis, and supernumerary nipples (among other abnormalities).

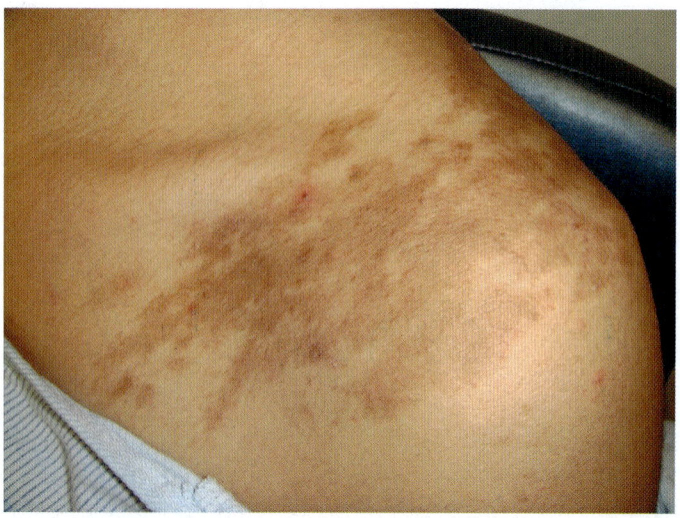

FIGURE 104-9. Becker nevus.

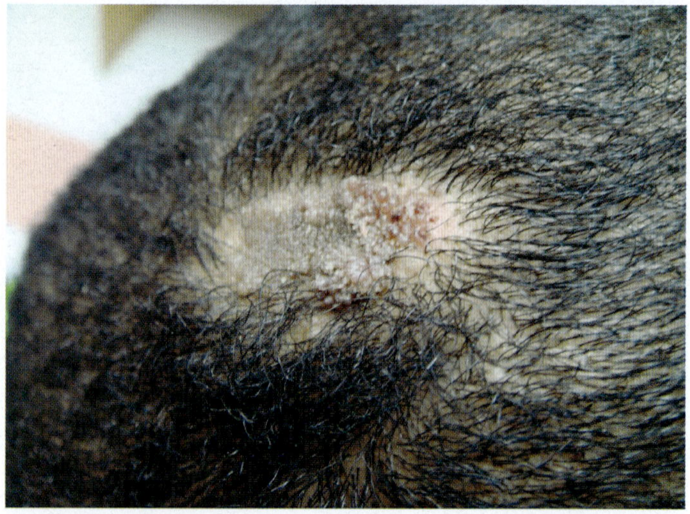

FIGURE 104-10. Nevus sebaceous of Jadassohn on the scalp.

The histopathologic findings are acanthosis, papillomatosis, and increased pigmentation of the basal layer.[24,25]

It has been reported that BN and BNS are caused by postzygotic lethal mutations of the *ACTB* gene that codes for Beta-actin.[26]

Differential diagnoses include congenital melanocytic nevus, café-au-lait macule, and hamartoma.

There have been isolated reports of the use of spironolactone for treatment of BNS.[25]

NEVUS SEBACEOUS

Nevus sebaceous of Jadassohn is a hamartomatous lesion that is present from birth but often becomes more raised and prominent in adolescence. The occurrence rate is 0.3% of newborns. The lesion is generally considered sporadic, but autosomal dominant cases have been reported. The literature describes the lesions as yellow, yellow-brown, and orange. In patients with skin of color, the lesions tend to be more darkly pigmented. Clinically, the nevus sebaceous is a hairless plaque with an irregular surface. The most common location is on the scalp [**Figure 104-10**].

Malignancy may occur within the nevus at a rate of approximately 1%.[27,28] Basal cell carcinoma is the most common malignancy that may develop within the lesion.[28] Other tumors, such as trichoblastoma, syringocystadenoma papilliferum, apocrine cystadenoma, squamous cell carcinoma, sebaceous epithelioma, and sebaceous carcinoma have been reported.

Histopathology shows increased sebaceous glands, papillomatosis, and hyperkeratosis.

Differential diagnoses are aplasia cutis congenita (at birth), epidermal nevus (in adolescence), and mastocytoma.[27]

Sebaceous nevus syndrome is a subset of epidermal nevus syndrome. These syndromes are characterized by neurologic, ocular, and skeletal abnormalities in addition to the nevus.[29]

Excision can be considered for tumors or because of cosmetic concerns.

TRACTION ALOPECIA

Traction alopecia is a common type of hair loss occurring due to tension on the hair. In those with more tightly coiled hair, the tension often begins at an early age with hair styling practices.

The process of caring for the hair of a child or teen with tightly coiled hair can be time intensive with care being taken to detangle and style the hair.[30] Hairstyles are not only created for convenience but are a reflection of creativity.[30] In the pediatric and early adolescent population, hair may also be perceived as a reflection of parenting ability.[30] This contributes to the emphasis on meticulous hairstyling, including high-tension hairstyles, which ultimately may lead to an increased risk of traction alopecia.[30]

Traction alopecia is a biphasic hair disorder. Early on traction alopecia is reversible, but with continued hair tension, the affected areas become permanently scarred. The clinical findings, time course, differential diagnoses, and treatment are covered in Chapter 39.

Counseling about high tension hairstyles with cultural humility is crucial in preventing permanent scarring.[31]

CENTRAL CENTRIFUGAL CICATRICIAL ALOPECIA (CCCA)

Central centrifugal cicatricial alopecia (CCCA) is often thought of as a scarring alopecia occurring in Black women. However, the age of onset may occur in the pediatric and adolescent population. Early suspicion and treatment is critical.[32]

The clinical findings, time course, differential diagnoses, and treatment are covered in Chapter 42.

REFERENCES

1. Conforti C, Chello C, Giuffrida R, di Meo N, Zalaudek I, Dianzani C. An overview of treatment options for mild-to-moderate acne based on American Academy of Dermatology, European Academy of Dermatology and Venereology, and Italian Society of Dermatology and Venereology guidelines. *Dermatol Ther.* 2020;33:e13548.
2. Mwanthi M, Zaenglein A. Update in the management of acne in adolescence. *Curr Opin Pediatr.* 2018;30:492-498.
3. Alexis AF, Woolery-Lloyd H, Williams K, et al. Racial/Ethnic variations in acne: implications for treatment and skin care recommendations for acne patients with skin of color. *J Drugs Dermatol.* 2021;20:716-725.
4. Mitchell KN, Tay YK, Heath CR, Silverberg N. Review article: emerging issues in pediatric skin of color, part 2. *Pediatr Dermatol.* 2021;38(Suppl 2):30-36.
5. Maymone MBC, Watchmaker JD, Dubiel M, Wirya SA, Shen LY, Vashi NA. Common skin disorders in pediatric skin of color. *J Pediatr Health Care.* 2019; 33:727-737.
6. Ogunbiyi A. Acne keloidalis nuchae: prevalence, impact, and management challenges. *Clin Cosmet Investig Dermatol.* 2016;9:483-489.
7. Brahe C, Peters K, Meunier N. Acne keloidalis nuchae in the armed forces. *Cutis.* 2020;105:223-226.
8. Elgash M, Dlova N, Ogunleye T, Taylor S. Seborrheic dermatitis in skin of color: clinical considerations. *J Drugs Dermatol.* 2019;18:24-27.
9. Saunte DML, Gaitanis G, Hay RJ. Malassezia-associated skin diseases, the use of diagnostics and treatment. *Front Cell Infect Microbiol.* 2020;10:112.
10. Borda LJ, Perper M, Keri JE. Treatment of seborrheic dermatitis: a comprehensive review. *J Dermatolog Treat.* 2019;30:158-169.
11. Grayson C, Heath CR. Tips for addressing common conditions affecting pediatric and adolescent patients with skin of color. *Pediatr Dermatol.* 2021;38 (Suppl 2):155-157.
12. Vazquez AM, Morgado B. Pityriasis rosea-like eruption after Pfizer-BioNTech COVID-19 vaccination. *Br J Dermatol.* 2021;185:e34.
13. Veraldi S, Spigariolo CB. Pityriasis rosea and COVID-19. *J Med Virol.* 2021; 93:4068.
14. Villalon-Gomez JM. Pityriasis rosea: diagnosis and treatment. *Am Fam Physician.* 2018;97:38-44.
15. Tackett KJ, Jenkins F, Morrell DS, McShane DB, Burkhart CN. Structural racism and its influence on the severity of atopic dermatitis in African American children. *Pediatr Dermatol.* 2020;37:142-146.
16. Stander S. Atopic dermatitis. *N Engl J Med.* 2021;389:1136-1143.
17. Tripathy T, Singh BSTP, Kar BR. Co-occurrence of lichen striatus in twins. *Indian J Dermatol Venereol Leprol.* 2019;85:632-634.
18. Belina ME, Sarver MM, Al-Rohil R, Fresco A. Lichen striatus post-COVID-19 vaccination. *JAAD Case Rep.* 2021:16;16-18.
19. Leung AKC, Leong KF, Barankin B. Lichen striatus with nail involvement in a 6-year-old boy. *Case Rep Pediatr.* 2020;1494760.
20. Saleem MD, Oussedik E, Picardo M, Schoch JJ. Acquired disorders with hypopigmentation: a clinical approach to diagnosis and treatment. *J Am Acad Dermatol.* 2019;80:1233-1250.
21. Alam HS, Ward JM, Davis LS. Generalized tinea versicolor following initiation of ixekizumab therapy. *JAAD Case Rep.* 2021;18:54-56.
22. Abugroun A, Gaznabi S, Natarajan A, Daoud H. Lime-induced phytophotodermatitis. *Oxf Med Case Reports.* 2019;11:470-472.
23. Maniam G, Light KM, Wilson J. Margarita burn: recognition and treatment of phytophotodermatitis. *J Am Board Fam Med.* 2021;34:398-401.
24. Baalann KP, Krishman M. Becker's nevus. *Pan Afr Med J.* 2022;41:142.
25. Chikani UN, Ohuche IN, Bisi-Onyemaechi AI. Becker's nevus syndrome: a case report. *J Med Case Reports.* 2021:15:395.
26. Tochia D. Becker nevus syndrome: a 2020 update. *J Am Acad Dermatol.* 2021;85:e101-e103.
27. Lopaez AS, Lam J. Nevus sebaceus. *CMAJ.* 2019;191:E765.
28. Goel P, Wolfswinkel EM, Fahradyan A, et al. Sebaceous nevus of the scalp. *J Craniofac Surg.* 2020;31:257-260.
29. El Ezzi O, de Buys Roessingh AS, Bigorra M, Captier Gl. Syndromic sebaceous nevus: current findings. *Int J Dermatol.* 2018;57:509-604.
30. Jones NL, Heath CR. Hair at the intersection of dermatology and anthropology: a conversation on race and relationships. *Pediatr Dermatol.* 2021;38(Suppl 2):155-157.
31. Grayson C, Heath CR. Counseling about traction alopecia: a "compliment, discuss, and suggest" method. *Cutis.* 2021;108:20-22.
32. Eginli AN, Dlova NC, McMichael A. Central centrifugal cicatricial alopecia in children: a case series and review of the literature. *Pediatr Dermatol.* 2017;34:133-137.

CHAPTER 105 Geriatrics

Natalie M. Villa
Shanice McKenzie
Jennifer L. Hsiao

KEY POINTS

- Aging changes in individuals with skin of color typically occurs 10 to 20 years later than those of age-matched White counterparts.
- Common clinical signs of photoaging in darker-skinned individuals include lentigines, rhytids, telangiectasia, and loss of elasticity.
- Cleansers with lubricating products that contain emollients should also be employed and appropriate photoprotection should be practiced.
- Maturational dyschromia (uneven skin tone) was a chief complaint in more than one-third of women with skin of color.

BASIC SCIENCE OF SKIN AGING

DEFINITION OF AGING

Skin aging refers to the changes that skin undergoes over time, both clinically and microscopically. Clinically, aging skin demonstrates rhytids, dyspigmentation, and laxity, although the extent to which these occur vary based on intrinsic factors such as race and external factors such as sun exposure or tobacco smoking.[1]

TYPES OF SKIN AGING: INTRINSIC AGING VERSUS PHOTOAGING

Intrinsic aging in photoprotected areas is subtle, while photoaging results in effacement of the dermal-epidermal junction (DEJ) and atrophy of both the epidermis and dermis. Over time, the architecture of fibrillin-rich microfibrils (FRM) becomes distorted and elastin deposits accumulate in a process called solar elastosis. Decreased collagen production by dermal fibroblasts results in dermal thinning.[2] Overall, these processes lead to loss of skin elasticity, manifesting as laxity and wrinkles.[3]

In a study specifically evaluating aging in skin of color, both photoaged and intrinsically aged skin had decreased elasticity, disruption of elastic fiber architecture, loss of structural proteins including FRMs, collagens, and fibulin-5, and reduced epidermal thickness. Photoaged skin also exhibited decreased elasticity, significant effacement of rete ridges, and flattening of the DEJ.[3]

FUNCTIONAL CONSEQUENCES OF AGING

Epidermal atrophy results in decreased skin barrier function, leading to xerosis [**Figure 105-1**] and increased risk of infection.[2] Xerosis may also lead to pruritus and excoriations, which also increases risk of secondary infection.

RACIAL DIFFERENCES IN SKIN AGING

Photoaging in skin of color has a delayed onset, clinically by around 10 to 20 years and molecularly by up to 40 to 50 years. The difference in onset of intrinsic aging is less marked, with a difference of a decade or less.[1,3] Skin of color has several structural differences that may contribute to this phenomenon: there is (1) increased thickness of the stratum corneum, (2) increased number of fibroblasts, resulting in more abundant and more well-organized collagen, and (3) increased melanin dispersion and content, which provides higher protection from UV radiation.[1,4] As a result, there is delayed onset of wrinkles and decreased solar elastosis in skin of color compared to lightly pigmented skin.[3,4] Higher amounts of pigment content is associated with higher susceptibility to dyspigmentation due to slower melanin degradation and labile melanocytes.[1] Pigmentary disorders including melasma and postinflammatory hyperpigmentation have been reported more commonly in, and are more bothersome to, patients with skin of color compared to patients with lower skin phototypes.[5,6] Patients with skin of color have been demonstrated to develop pigmented lesions, such as seborrheic keratoses [**Figure 105-2**], dermatosis papulosa nigra, and solar lentigines [**Figure 105-3**] earlier and in greater numbers than patients with lightly pigmented skin.[1]

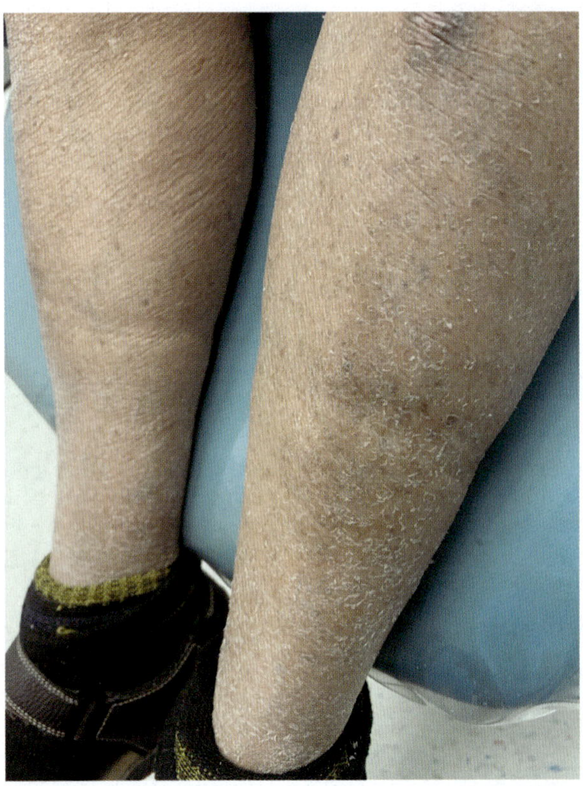

FIGURE 105-1. Xerosis. Diffuse xerosis on the lower legs. Photo credit: Shanice McKenzie, MD.

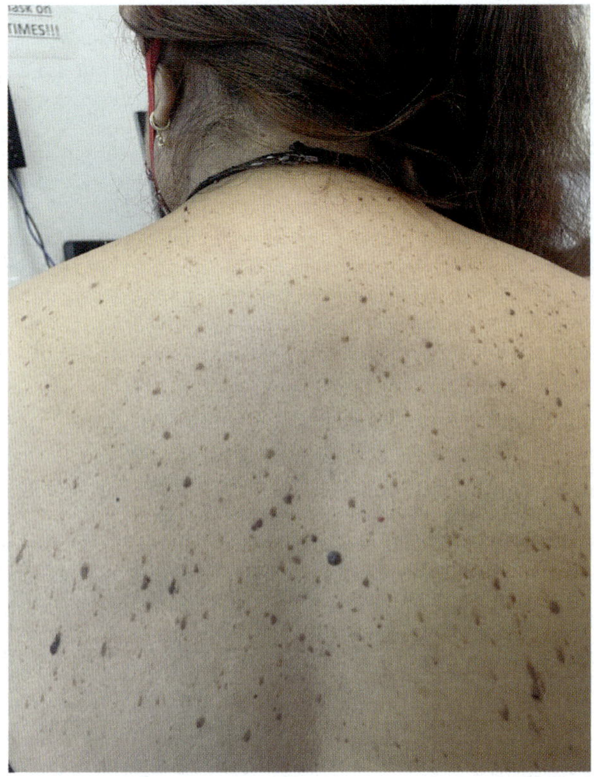

FIGURE 105-2. Seborrheic keratoses. Scattered waxy stuck-on papules on the back. Photo credit: Shanice McKenzie, MD.

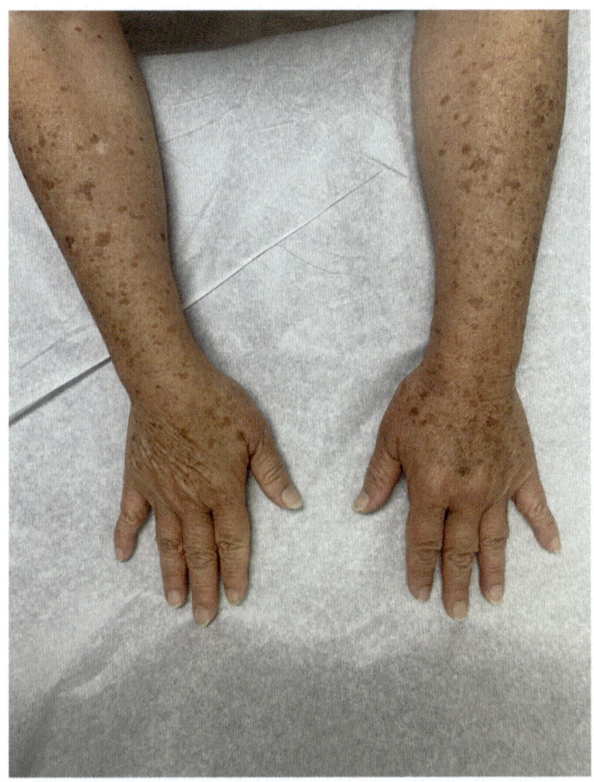

FIGURE 105-3. Lentigines. Light brown macules and patches with scalloped borders in a photodistributed pattern on the dorsal forearms and hands. Photo credit: Shanice McKenzie, MD.

SPECIAL CONSIDERATIONS IN THE ELDERLY POPULATION

MEDICAL ETHICS

Principles of medical ethics should be adhered to during all patient interactions, but especially when dealing with a vulnerable population such as the elderly.[7] Sometimes clinicians will face complex ethical dilemmas when treating geriatric patients. For example, patients should be empowered to make their own medical decisions (principle of autonomy); however, this may not be so straightforward in a patient with cognitive deficits. Elderly patients should be considered for all appropriate treatment modalities for their skin conditions (principle of justice). However, the potential negative impact of an aggressive treatment option on one patient's quality of life may outweigh that patient's perceived benefit from prolonging life (principles of beneficence, nonmaleficence).

For example, when considering a superficial basal cell carcinoma (BCC) on the forearm, patients may often opt for a surgical excision to achieve the highest cure rate. However, an elderly patient who already has mobility restrictions may be hesitant to have sutures placed, which would require wound care. The patient might prefer a topical treatment such as 5-fluorouracil or imiquimod if mobility is the most important factor. The patient may also prefer to avoid pain associated with the procedure. Conversely, the inconvenience associated with a topical treatment modality stretching across several weeks may not be tolerable to the patient who may prefer a procedure such as electrodessication and curettage to condense treatment and healing times. Finally, an elderly patient may not feel the need or desire to treat the superficial BCC at all. In cases like this one, a patient's priorities must be elicited.

POLYPHARMACY AND MEDICATION SIDE EFFECTS

During the aging process, the body undergoes several physiologic changes that affect pharmacology: (1) renal clearance decreases leading to increases in drug concentration and half-life for a given dose; (2) gastric acid secretion decreases, which also decreases absorption for some medications; (3) muscle mass decreases and the proportion of adipose tissue increases that alters drug distribution; and (4) metabolism decreases leading to altered half-life of medications.[8] These factors can alter the impact of medications in elderly patients that may not be seen in other populations. It is important to avoid medications on the Beers Criteria list of potentially inappropriate medications for the elderly. For example, when recommending antihistamines for itching or hives, avoid anticholinergic antihistamines such as hydroxyzine or diphenhydramine that may result in sedation or confusion.[8,9] When selecting a nonsteroidal anti-inflammatory drug, avoid indomethacin that may also have undesirable central nervous system side effects.[8]

Polypharmacy is an issue for many older patients. As number of comorbidities increases, patients may be placed on additional medications, which increases risk of adverse effects and medication interactions. Attempts to manage adverse effects may then further lead to additional medications.[8]

Medications used to treat common conditions in the elderly, such as infection, pain, hypertension, and diabetes, may cause rash or cutaneous symptoms including[8]: lichenoid eruptions (β-blockers, angiotensin-converting enzyme (ACE) inhibitors, thiazides), morbilliform/exanthematous eruptions (penicillin, cephalosporins, sulfonamides, ACE inhibitors), bullous pemphigoid (gliptins), photosensitivity (sulfonamides, tetracyclines, non-steroidal anti-inflammatory drugs [NSAIDs]), and pruritus (ACE inhibitors, salicylates, calcium channel blockers).[10]

DECREASED MOBILITY AND FUNCTION

The elderly patient may experience decreased mobility and function, which is reflected in cutaneous conditions such as pressure ulcers, incontinence dermatitis, or dermatitis neglecta. Pressure ulcers occur when physical pressure on local blood vessels prevents blood flow, resulting in skin breakdown and ulceration.[11] They commonly occur on dependent areas such as the sacrum, buttocks, hips, and heels. Prevention of pressure ulcers is key, with frequent position changes and use of donut pillows.[12] In patients with skin of color, the early erythema that may herald an early stage pressure ulcer may be more difficult to detect, which can lead to delays in diagnosis, treatment, and prevention of further injury. A 2021 observational study of 142 nursing home residents noted that more Black individuals than patients of other races had stage 4 pressure ulcers, and Black and Hispanic individuals had deeper tissue injuries.[13]

Incontinence dermatitis is skin irritation and/or damage that arises due to contact with physical and chemical irritants found in feces and urine.[14] Contact that results in a dermatitis may be as short as 10 to 15 minutes. Cutaneous findings include erythema, edema, and erosion. Incontinence dermatitis can be painful and become secondarily infected, prolonging hospital or long-term care facility stays.[14] The prevalence of any type of incontinence in the elderly has been reported to be as high as 46%, and incontinence dermatitis may be present in up to 25% of patients upon admission to a facility.[14] Cleansing agents with a pH between 4 and 6.8, nutritional support, and optimized body positioning may all help prevent incontinence dermatitis.[14]

Dermatitis neglecta presents as a hyperkeratotic plaque on the skin in an area where the patient does not perform adequate cleansing, either consciously or unconsciously. It is typically asymptomatic but may be cosmetically bothersome to the patient, and can be easily removed by cleansing with soap and water, revealing normal skin underneath.[15] This condition may be exacerbated by functional decline in elderly patients.

It is also important for dermatologists to be able to recognize signs of elder abuse. A 2021 study of 628 participants living in New York State found an overall prevalence of 11.4% of any form of elder mistreatment.[16] Elder abuse has been reported to be more prevalent in skin of color patients, with reported odds of experiencing any form of elder mistreatment ranging from 2.6 to 4.0 times more likely in non-Hispanic Black or non-White patients compared to non-Hispanic White patients.[16,17] Skin tears and bruising can occur during activities of daily living, especially given the weakened skin barrier in the elderly as discussed above. However, special attention should be paid to any signs of traumatized skin in an abnormal location, such as the face, thighs, or back; or in an abnormal pattern: linear/rectangular (such as from a belt or belt buckle), fingertip distribution, or any marks that could be consistent with blunt trauma.[12] Other injuries that are usually nonaccidental include immersion burns or when a patient presents with multiple similar lesions in different stages of healing. Neglect may also be a sign of elder abuse, and may manifest as severe decubitus ulcers, dehydration, malnutrition, or lack of cleanliness.

HEALTHCARE BARRIERS IN THE ELDERLY POPULATION

PHYSICAL FACTORS

Declining physical function may impact an elderly patient's ability to treat their skin conditions. In a survey study of 200 participants, 41.5% reported they had difficulty reading or opening their medication bottles, while almost 10% reported difficulty hearing directions about the medication.[18] Elderly patients may have difficulty applying topical medications or performing wound care that can negatively impact their treatment. Dermatologists should try to simplify regimens whenever possible, and consider providing instructions with large fonts for improved readability. Medication adherence issues are compounded by the reduced health literacy that has been found among skin of color populations, particularly among elderly skin of color patients compared to elderly White patients.[19,20]

COGNITIVE FACTORS

A quarter to a third of adults over age 65 have some form of cognitive impairment.[9] Older patients with cognitive impairment may not be fully able to participate in medical decision-making regarding their care, and thus family or designated caregivers may need to be consulted. Patients with cognitive decline may become confused and combative during administration of local anesthesia or may not understand the purpose of wound care dressings. They may have difficulties with adherence to medication regimens due to forgetfulness.[8] In a survey of 96 patients with diagnosed mild cognitive impairment, 55% reported memory issues as a barrier to medication adherence.[18]

SOCIAL FACTORS

Elderly patients may rely on caregivers for healthcare-related activities such as attending appointments, applying topical treatments, obtaining medications, or performing wound care. Older patients who do not have caregivers may have practical difficulty obtaining medications if they do not drive and must use a home delivery pharmacy. This may have additional downstream consequences for the patient. For example, a patient who relies on a mail order pharmacy may experience a delay in treatment initiation, and their condition may worsen during this delay. Delays in obtaining refills also interfere with treatment adherence.

Elderly patients may also experience financial difficulty obtaining medications. Among Medicare beneficiaries who reported having trouble getting needed healthcare, almost a third cited financial reasons, and 26% of 200 patients aged 65 or greater in a 2016 survey study reported that cost was a barrier to medication adherence.[18,21] Black and Hispanic Medicare beneficiaries also have more limited financial resources compared to White beneficiaries.[22]

SELECT CUTANEOUS CONDITIONS IN THE ELDERLY

PRURITUS

A systematic review including over 28,000 patients found that pruritus without primary skin findings was a common dermatologic concern among the elderly with a prevalence of 21%, (range 5.6-66.9%).[10] Pruritus is over twice as common in men (18.65%) than in women (8.26%).[10]

There are numerous mechanisms that are purported to cause itching, including xerosis due to changes in the function of the skin barrier with aging, immunosenescence, and neuropathic changes.[23] With aging, xerosis develops through increased skin barrier transepidermal water loss, decreased ceramides, decreased activity of sebaceous and sweat glands, and, in women, decreased production of estrogen.[23] Immunosenesence, or age-related changes in the immune system, results in increased autoreactivity, with diseases such as bullous pemphigoid.[23] Neuropathic itch may be due to postherpetic neuritis, diabetes mellitus, or radiculopathy such as brachioradial pruritus or notalgia paresthetica.[23] Senile pruritus without primary skin lesions is associated with a nonvaried diet (odds ratio (OR) 1.22), smoking (OR 1.26), and excessive alcohol use (OR 25.03), and may also be seen as a medication side effect.[10] Common dermatologic and systemic conditions may also cause itching, such as xerosis, kidney disease, and liver failure.

DERMATOSIS PAPULOSA NIGRA (DPN)

Dermatosis papulosa nigra (DPN) consists of pigmented stuck-on papules on the face, neck, and other sun-exposed areas, usually one to several millimeters in size. This condition is considered a variant of seborrheic keratosis. Lesions are usually asymptomatic but may impact quality of life.[24] DPN occurs in up to 70% of Black individuals, twice as frequently in women as in men.[24] Onset is in adulthood and usually patients have a strong family history; 84% of 50 patients in one survey study had an affected first-degree relative.[24]

SOLAR PURPURA

Solar purpura [**Figure 105-4**] presents as violaceous to erythematous ecchymotic patches that are distributed on sun-exposed areas on the extensor forearms. They arise after even minimal trauma, which may be so minor that patients do not recall it occurring. Patients may be more prone to developing solar purpura when they are taking anti-coagulants or systemic prednisone. They should be counseled to take care to avoid pressure on the forearms and may consider protective clothing. In the absence of any concern for nonaccidental trauma or a nutritional deficiency, patients may be counseled that these are benign and will slowly self-resolve.

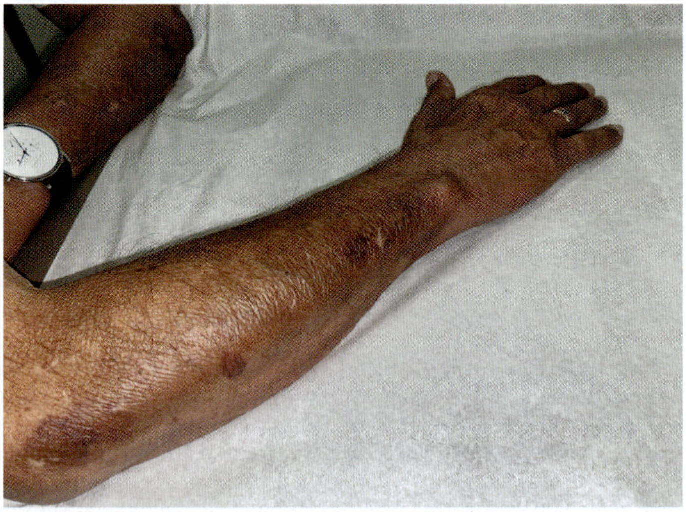

FIGURE 105-4. Solar purpura. Violaceous patches on the extensor surface of the forearm. Photo credit: Shanice McKenzie, MD.

NUTRITIONAL DEFICIENCIES

Nutritional deficiencies, such as pellagra and scurvy, are more common in the elderly. Pellagra results from vitamin B3 (niacin) deficiency. Niacin is a required cofactor for several components of cellular metabolism. Patients with restricted diets (including diets low in protein or high in corn), excess alcohol consumption, intake of isoniazid or 6-mercaptopurine for extended periods, or with chronic malabsorptive diseases may develop niacin deficiency.[25] Patients initially experience fatigue, weight loss, glossitis, and weakness, before developing the classic triad of diarrhea, dementia, and a sharply demarcated bilateral, photo-exposed dermatitis on the neck, face, dorsal hands, and back.[25] The rash starts with the eruption of erythematous papules, vesicles and bullae, and progresses to lichenified scaly plaques. Niacin must be supplemented for treatment.

Scurvy [**Figure 105-5**] is caused by vitamin C (ascorbic acid) deficiency. Humans are required to obtain vitamin C through the diet, as it cannot be synthesized endogenously. Patients with extremely limited diets are at risk. Vitamin C is essential for the cross-linking of collagen, and therefore for the proper structure and function of skin and blood vessels.[25] Scurvy presents on the skin with perifollicular hemorrhage, easy bruising/bleeding including from the gums, impaired wound healing, splinter hemorrhages on the nails, and corkscrew hair.[25] Patients may also feel general fatigue. Treatment is with daily vitamin C supplementation.

TREATMENT OF ACTINIC KERATOSES AND SKIN CANCERS IN THE ELDERLY

INTRODUCTION

Precancerous and malignant cutaneous neoplasms are more common in the elderly, with a higher prevalence in lightly pigmented individuals compared to patients with skin of color.[26] Despite this, squamous cell carcinoma (SCC)-specific mortality in Black and Hispanic men is increased compared to White men, and a similar disparity exists between the incidence of melanoma and disease severity in non-White patients.[26] Presentation of skin cancers is different in patients with skin of color, which may lead to delayed diagnosis. For example, basal cell carcinoma (BCC) is more likely to be pigmented [**Figure 105-6**] in skin of

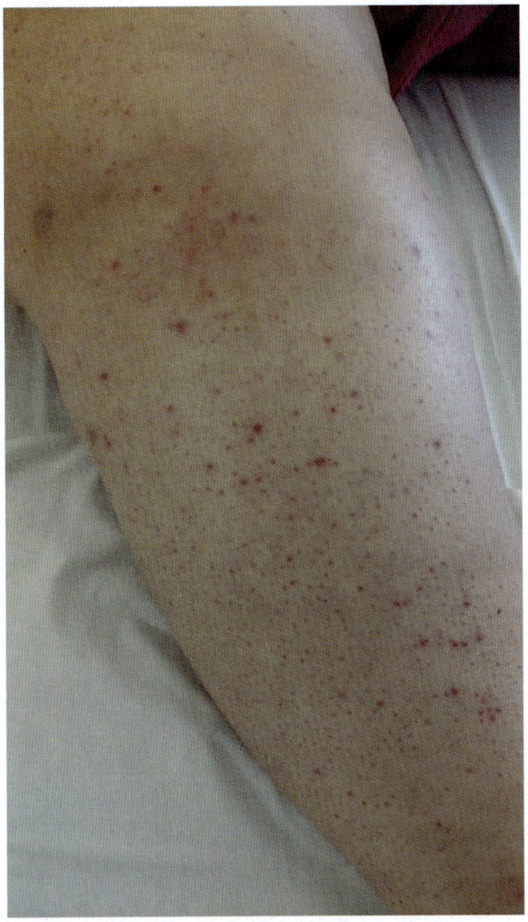

FIGURE 105-5. Scurvy. Perifollicular hemorrhages on the leg.

color patients, and SCC is more likely to occur in scars, chronic ulcers, or photo-protected areas, as compared to White patients.[26] Increased education and awareness regarding the presentation of skin cancers in patients with skin of color is needed in order to facilitate early diagnosis, which in turn can help minimize treatment invasiveness.

TREATMENT OF ACTINIC KERATOSIS (AK)

Management options for AKs include cryosurgery, topical modalities, and surveillance in patients who are not bothered by them and have a low likelihood of future benefit from treatment.[9,27] Efficacy of cryosurgery depends on freeze duration, which may be limited by patient's ability to tolerate the procedure.[27] Topical treatments include 5-fluorouracil, with or without calcipotriene; imiquimod; and diclofenac applied across several days to weeks. Side effects include skin irritation and photosensitivity. Photodynamic therapy (PDT) may also be used to treat AKs, requiring in-office incubation of 5-aminolevulanic acid (ALA) on the area(s) to be treated, followed by exposure to red or blue light or daylight for varying amounts of time to activate the ALA. Patient pain and discomfort may again limit treatment. Factors to consider when selecting a treatment modality, especially in an elderly population, include occupational status, desire to participate in any outdoor work or hobbies, importance of cosmetic outcome to patient, and ability to tolerate pain/discomfort.[7,9]

TREATMENT OF BASAL CELL CARCINOMA (BCC) AND SQUAMOUS CELL CARCINOMA (SCC)

Topical therapies, cryosurgery, and PDT all may be utilized for the treatment of some BCCs and SCCs in select patients, especially those who decline surgery or are not surgical candidates. Electrodessication and curettage (ED&C) is a surgical procedure with a lower cure rate and poorer cosmetic outcome compared to other surgical modalities such as Mohs surgery or elliptical excision; however, its use may be warranted in patients who cannot tolerate a long procedure or the wound care required for a sutured wound. Patients who prioritize a high cure rate should be offered either elliptical excision or Mohs surgery, if appropriate depending on specific subtype of the skin cancer and its location.

CONSIDERATIONS RELATED TO AK AND SKIN CANCER TREATMENT

Elderly skin of color patients face several barriers to care that result in more advanced tumors at presentation. There may be an element of neglect in some cases, either by the patient or a caregiver. Other factors associated with advanced age such as decreased access to healthcare, attribution of their symptoms to skin aging, physical inability to monitor hard-to-reach areas such as the back, and social isolation also may contribute to geriatric patients presenting with more advanced tumors.[28,29] Diagnosis of skin cancer is more likely to be delayed in patients with skin of color as well.[26] Importantly, these factors are compounded by racial disparities in access to care, which may further exacerbate delays in presentation and treatment for elderly skin of color patients.[26]

Age does not necessarily determine life expectancy as other factors such as an individual's comorbidities and lifestyle choices play an important role. Both age and life expectancy should be considered when making treatment decisions with elderly patients.[9] A 2016 systematic review found that patient age and life expectancy are not always taken into account when considering skin cancer treatment.[30] However, patients with limited life expectancy have a higher incidence of complications

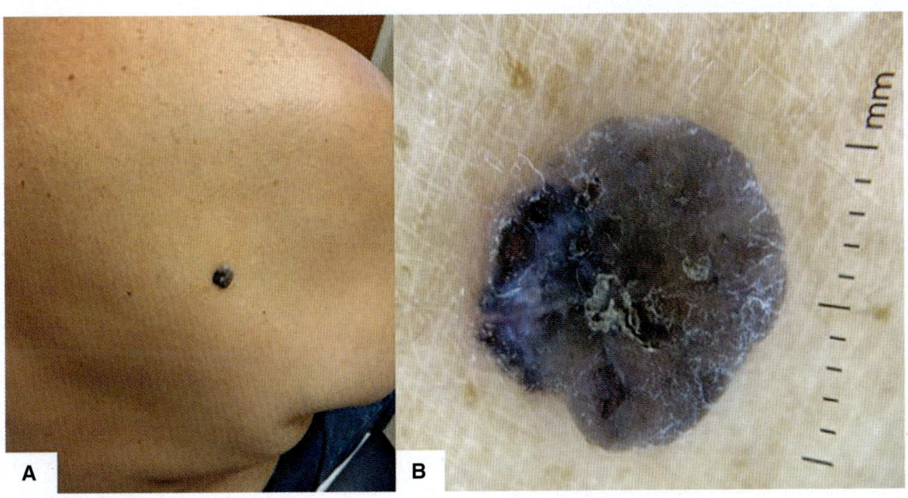

FIGURE 105-6. Pigmented basal cell carcinoma. **(A)** Solitary heavily pigmented plaque on the upper back. **(B)** Dermoscopy image of pigmented basal cell carcinoma showing areas of ulceration. Photo credit: Natalie M. Villa, MD.

after surgery.[30,31] The risk of an AK transforming into an SCC is low and cumulates over time, thus elderly patients may feel that the pain and inconvenience of AK treatments are not worth minimizing that risk. It is important to consider each individual patient's situation holistically when discussing and recommending treatment options. In addition, specific considerations when discussing procedural treatments in skin of color patients include increased risk of dyspigmentation and keloid scars after procedures.[24,32]

HAIR CONDITIONS IN THE ELDERLY

ANDROGENETIC ALOPECIA

Androgenetic alopecia [**Figure 105-7**] comprises specific patterns of hair loss due to hair follicular miniaturization. The "male" pattern involves loss at the temples bilaterally and the vertex, while the "female" pattern produces a Christmas-tree pattern of loss in the central part, although these patterns can be observed in either sex. Dermoscopy will not reveal a loss of follicular openings, which can distinguish androgenetic alopecia from central centrifugal cicatricial alopecia, another form of alopecia that can present with central hair loss and is more commonly seen in Black patients.[32] Treatment of androgenetic alopecia includes topical or oral minoxidil, oral spironolactone, or oral finasteride. Procedures such as platelet-rich plasma (PRP) injections or hair transplantation are at times utilized.

HAIR GRAYING

Onset of hair graying [**Figure 105-8**] varies with ethnicity, and is typically 5 to 10 years later for skin of color populations compared to populations with lightly pigmented skin.[33] Over time, melanocyte stem cells become senescent.[2] Gray hair follicles have fewer active, properly functioning melanocytes, with disrupted melanosomes and melanin transfer to the hair follicle.[34] Eventually all pigment is lost, although some amelanotic melanocytes may still persist in the follicle.[34] Part of this is due to genetics, which is incompletely understood. In addition, oxidative stress, due to internal reactive oxygen species (ROS) generation during melanin production and external stimuli such as smoking and ultraviolet (UV) radiation, causes damage to the hair follicle pigmentary unit (HFPU) and likely plays a role in aging.[33,34]

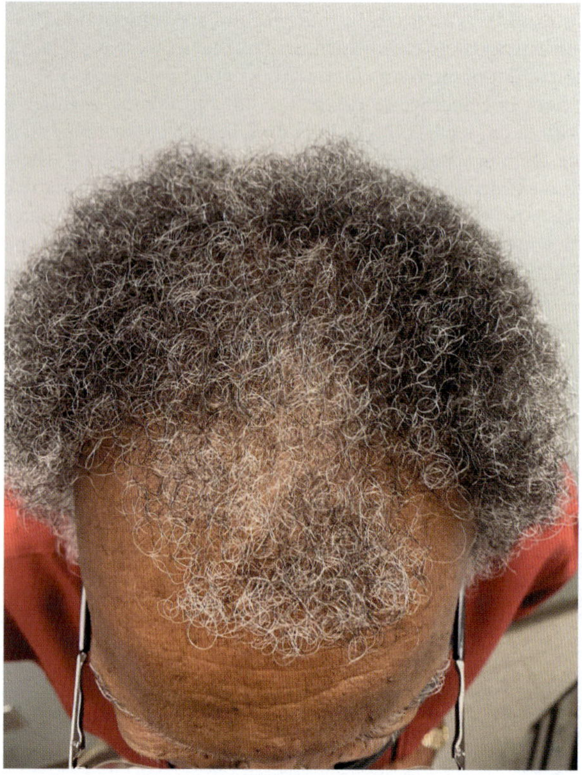

FIGURE 105-7. Androgenetic alopecia. Recession of frontal hairline at the bilateral temples. Photo credit: Shanice McKenzie, MD.

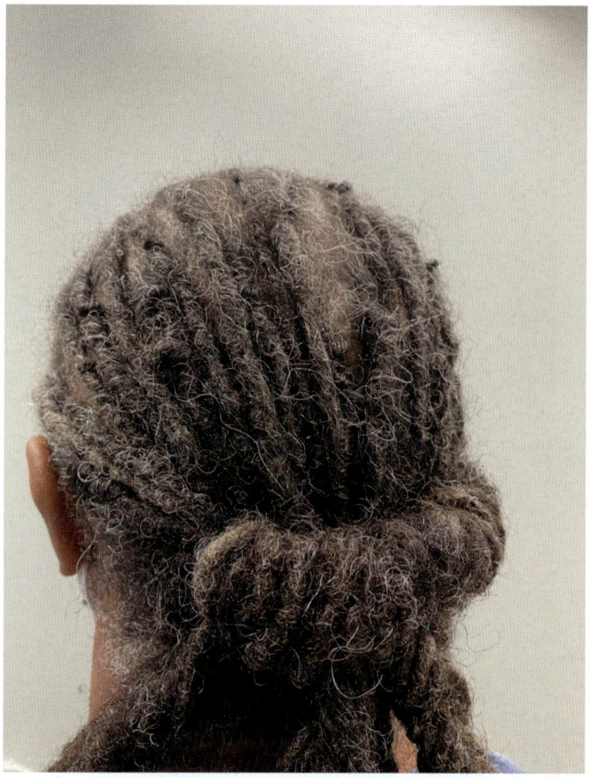

FIGURE 105-8. Hair graying. Gray hairs admixed among darker hairs on the scalp. Photo credit: Shanice McKenzie, MD.

PALLIATIVE SKIN CARE

Geriatric dermatology also includes skin care for patients receiving palliative and hospice care, though unfortunately, skin of color patients are less likely to have access to palliative care.[35] In one study, over one-third of 65 patients admitted to a palliative care unit had a dermatologic condition, including 7.7% of patients presenting with decubitus ulcers on admission to the unit and 10.8% of patients with decubitus ulcers that developed after admission.[36] Patients in all hospital or long-term acute care facilities, and especially those in palliative care settings, should be monitored regularly for pressure sores and their caregivers should perform regular turning and repositioning. Painful pressure ulcers can be treated with moist dressings such as gel or colloid dressings and appropriate analgesia.[11] Trauma caused by medication delivery such as intravenous (IV) line insertions[36] may also be upsetting or painful to patients, therefore any unnecessary medications are usually discontinued or given via other modalities when possible. Patients with xerosis should be moisturized with thick emollients such as petroleum jelly, and any residual pruritus can be treated with topical corticosteroids.[11]

CONCLUSION

It is important for dermatologists to be aware of special considerations for elderly patients with skin of color, who face additional healthcare barriers compared to White patients. Patients with skin of color experience delayed onset of photoaging skin changes and hair graying by up to 10 to 20 years compared to patients with lower skin phototypes.

Conversely, patients with skin of color may develop pigmented lesions earlier in life and are more susceptible to dyspigmentation. Elderly patients have higher risks of experiencing medication side effects and polypharmacy may compound these effects. Treatment of skin cancers and precancerous lesions should include consideration of a patient's age, functional status, and goals of care. As elderly patients come to represent an increasingly larger portion of the population, dermatologists will commonly encounter the topics covered in this chapter.

REFERENCES

1. Vashi NA, De Castro Maymone MB, Kundu R V. Aging differences in ethnic skin. *J Clin Aesthet Dermatol.* 2016;9(1):31-38.
2. Lowry WE. Its written all over your face: the molecular and physiological consequences of aging skin. *Mech Ageing Dev.* 2020;190:111315.
3. Langton AK, Alessi S, Hann M, et al. Aging in skin of color: disruption to elastic fiber organization is detrimental to skin's biomechanical function. *J Invest Dermatol.* 2019;139(4):779-788.
4. Alexis AF, Obioha JO. Ethnicity and aging skin. *J Drugs Dermatol.* 2017;16(6): s77-s80.
5. Davis EC, Callender VD. Postinflammatory hyperpigmentation: a review of the epidemiology, clinical features, and treatment options in skin of color. *J Clin Aesthet Dermatol.* 2010;3(7):20./pmc/articles/PMC2921758/. Accessed September 24, 2023.
6. Callender VD, Baldwin H, Cook-Bolden FE, Alexis AF, Stein Gold L, Guenin E. Effects of topical retinoids on acne and post-inflammatory hyperpigmentation in patients with skin of color: a clinical review and implications for practice. *Am J Clin Dermatol.* 2022;23(1):69.
7. Fontanella D, Grant-Kels JM, Patel T, Norman R. Ethical issues in geriatric dermatology. *Clin Dermatol.* 2012;30(5):511-515.
8. Carneiro SC da S, Azevedo-e-Silva MC, Ramos-e-Silva M. Drug eruptions in the elderly. *Clin Dermatol.* 2011;29(1):43-48.
9. Linos E, Chren MM, Covinsky K. Geriatric dermatology—a framework for caring for older patients with skin disease. *JAMA Dermatology.* 2018;154(7): 757-758.
10. Chen S, Zhou F, Xiong Y. Prevalence and risk factors of senile pruritus: a systematic review and meta-analysis. *BMJ Open.* 2022;12(2):e051694.
11. Regnard C, Allport S, Stephenson L. ABC of palliative care: mouth care, skin care, and lymphoedema. *BMJ.* 1997;315(7114):1002-1005.
12. Clarysse K, Kivlahan C, Beyer I, Gutermuth J. Signs of physical abuse and neglect in the mature patient. *Clin Dermatol.* 2018;36(2):264-270.
13. Bates-Jensen BM, Anber K, Chen MM, et al. Natural history of pressure injury among ethnically/racially diverse nursing home residents: the pressure ulcer detection study. *J Gerontol Nurs.* 2021;47(3):37-46.
14. Banharak S, Panpanit L, Subindee S, et al. Prevention and care for incontinence-associated dermatitis among older adults: a systematic review. *J Multidiscip Healthc.* 2021;14:2983-3004.
15. Pérez-Rodríguez IM, Muñoz-Garza FZ, Ocampo-Candiani J. An unusually severe case of dermatosis neglecta: a diagnostic challenge. *Case Rep Dermatol.* 2014;6(2):194.
16. Burnes D, Hancock DW, Eckenrode J, Lachs MS, Pillemer K. Estimated incidence and factors associated with risk of elder mistreatment in New York State. *JAMA Netw Open.* 2021;4(8).
17. Lachs MS, Williams C, O'Brien S, Hurst L, Horwitz R. Risk factors for reported elder abuse and neglect: a nine-year observational cohort study. *Gerontologist.* 1997;37(4):469-474.
18. Campbell NL, Zhan J, Tu W, et al. Self-reported medication adherence barriers among ambulatory older adults with mild cognitive impairment. *Pharmacotherapy.* 2016;36(2):196-202.
19. Chesser AK, Woods NK, Smothers K, Rogers N. Health literacy and older adults: a systematic review. *Gerontol Geriatr Med.* 2016;2:233372141663049.
20. Gerber BS, Cho YI, Arozullah AM, Lee SYD. Racial differences in medication adherence: a cross-sectional study of medicare enrollees. *Am J Geriatr Pharmacother.* 2010;8(2):136-145.
21. McClintock HF, Kurichi JE, Kwong PL, et al. Disability stages and trouble getting needed health care among medicare beneficiaries. *Am J Phys Med Rehabil.* 2017;96(6):408.
22. Fields C, Cubanski J, Boccuti C, Neuman T. *Profile of Medicare Beneficiaries by Race and Ethnicity: A Chartpack*; 2016. http://files.kff.org/attachment/chartpack-profile-of-medicare-beneficiaries-by-race-and-ethnicity-a-chartpack. Accessed September 1, 2022.
23. Valdes-Rodriguez R, Stull C, Yosipovitch G. Chronic pruritus in the elderly: pathophysiology, diagnosis and management. *Drugs Aging.* 2015;32(3): 201-215.
24. Uwakwe LN, De Souza B, Subash J, McMichael AJ. Dermatosis papulosa nigra: a quality of life survey study. *J Clin Aesthet Dermatol.* 2020;13(2):17-19.
25. Schneider JB, Norman RA. Cutaneous manifestations of endocrine-metabolic disease and nutritional deficiency in the elderly. *Dermatol Clin.* 2004;22(1): 23-31.
26. Shao K, Feng H. Racial and Ethnic healthcare disparities in skin cancer in the united states: a review of existing inequities, contributing factors, and potential solutions. *J Clin Aesthet Dermatol.* 2022;15(7):16-22.
27. Eisen DB, Asgari MM, Bennett DD, et al. Guidelines of care for the management of actinic keratosis. *J Am Acad Dermatol.* 2021;85(4):e209-e233.
28. Legrand A, Quintard B, Garrouteigt C, Beylot-Barry M, Broc G. From neglect to earlier diagnosis: a qualitative meta-synthesis of psycho-social factors associated with consultation delay in advanced basal cell carcinoma. *Psychol Heal Med.* 2022;27(8):1793-1804.
29. Manjunath J, Friedman A. Assessing dermatology provider perceptions and attitudes about the unique needs of older adult patients. *J Drugs Dermatol.* 2022;21(3):331-332.
30. Linos E, Chren MM, Stijacic Cenzer I, Covinsky KE. Skin cancer in U.S. elderly adults: does life expectancy play a role in treatment decisions? *J Am Geriatr Soc.* 2016;64(8):1610-1615.
31. Haisma MS, Bras L, Aghdam MA, et al. Effect of patient characteristics on treatment decisions regarding keratinocyte carcinoma in elderly patients: a review of the current literature. *Acta Derm Venereol.* 2020;100(13):1-7.
32. Lawson CN, Hollinger J, Sethi S, et al. Updates in the understanding and treatments of skin & hair disorders in women of color. *Int J Women Dermatology.* 2017;3(1 Suppl):S21.
33. Maymone MBC, Laughter M, Pollock S, et al. Hair aging in different races and ethnicities. *J Clin Aesthet Dermatol.* 2021;14(1):38-44.
34. O'Sullivan JDB, Nicu C, Picard M, et al. The biology of human hair greying. *Biol Rev Camb Philos Soc.* 2021;96(1):107-128.
35. Estrada L V., Harrison JM, Dick AW, Luchsinger JA, Dhingra L, Stone PW. Examining regional differences in nursing home palliative care for Black and Hispanic residents. *J Palliat Med.* 2022;25(8):1228-1235.
36. Barnabé C, Daeninck P. "Beauty is only skin deep": prevalence of dermatologic disease on a palliative care unit. *J Pain Symptom Manage.* 2005;29(4).

Index

Note: Page numbers followed by f and t indicate figures and tables respectively.

M

N

T